Contributors and consultants

At the time of publication, the contributors and consultants held the following positions.

Tricia M. Berry, PharmD, BCPS
Director of Experiential Programs and
    Professor of Pharmacy Practice
St. Louis College of Pharmacy

Lawrence Carey, PharmD
Associate Director and Academic
    Coordinator
Philadelphia University

Jason C. Cooper, PharmD
Clinical Specialist, Drug Information
Medical University of South Carolina
Charleston

Melissa M. Devlin, PharmD
Clinical Pharmacist
Excellerx, Inc.
Philadelphia

Tatyana Gurvich, PharmD
Clinical Pharmacologist
USC School of Pharmacy
UCI Senior Health Center
Orange, Calif.

Toshal Hallowell, BS Pharm
Clinical Pharmacist
Great Brook Valley Health Center
Worcester, Mass.

Collette Bishop Hendler, RN, MS
Infection Control Nurse
Abington (Pa.) Memorial Hospital

**Samantha P. Jellinek, PharmD, BCPS,
CGP**
Clinical Pharmacy Manager for
    Medication Reconciliation and Safety
Maimonides Medical Center
Brooklyn, N.Y.

Mary Kate Kelly, PharmD
Clinical Pharmacist
Buckley Pharmacy
King of Prussia, Pa.

Patrick J. Kiel, PharmD, BCPS
Clinical Pharmacy Specialist,
    Hematology/Bone Marrow Transplant
Indiana University Hospital
Indianapolis

Judith L. Kristeller, PharmD, BCPS
Associate Professor
Wilkes University
Wilkes-Barre, Pa.

William Lai, RPh, PharmD
Senior Manager, Medical Affairs
Endo Pharmaceuticals
Collegeville, Pa.

Kristy H. Lucas, PharmD
Associate Professor, Clinical Pharmacy
    and Internal Medicine
West Virginia University
Schools of Pharmacy and Medicine
Charleston

Zoe Ngo, PharmD
Investigational Drug Pharmacist and
    Assistant Clinical Professor
Department of Clinical Pharmacy
University of California
San Francisco

**Robert Lee Page II, PharmD, FCCP,
FAHA, BCPS, CGP**
Associate Professor of Clinical Pharmacy
    and Physical Medicine
University of Colorado Schools of
    Pharmacy & Medicine
Aurora

Priti N. Patel, PharmD, BCPS
Assistant Clinical Professor
St. John's University
Queens, N.Y.

Dawn Pollitt, PharmD
Medical Information Manager
AstraZeneca Pharmaceuticals
Wilmington

Leigh Ann Trujillo, RN, BSN
Nurse Educator
St. James Hospital
Olympia Fields, Ill.

Joanne Whitney, PhD, PharmD, RPh
Associate Clinical Professor
University of California
San Francisco

How to use *Nursing2010 Drug Handbook*

Nursing2010 Drug Handbook, created by pharmacists and nurses, focuses on drug information that nurses need to know. *Nursing2010 Drug Handbook* emphasizes nursing aspects of drugs without trying to replace detailed pharmacology texts. The unique book design makes the content readily accessible and applicable in any clinical setting. this edition also emphasizes safety to help you avoid medication errors.

Features in this edition
The 30th edition offers features that enhance nursing knowledge and skills and promote drug safety:
- New monographs for 14 new, FDA-approved drugs
- New "Black Box Warning" logo indicating FDA-issued black box warnings.
- New appendices on recommended pediatric and adult immunizations.
- Pronunciation key for generic drug names
- Administration section that gives step-by-step guidance on safely preparing, giving, and storing drugs by all routes
- "Safety Alert!" label for drugs that present an avoidable danger for you or your patient and the sidesteps for you to take
- A symbol in the drug monographs (✔) indicating that the drug is illustrated in the color photoguide
- A symbol that shows off-label uses at a glance (♦)
- "Adjust-a-dose" logos to highlight dosage adjustments that may be needed in certain patient populations
- Pharmacologic class for each drug entry
- "Incompatibilities" section to highlight I.V. drugs that shouldn't be given together
- Tables that show the route, onset, peak, and duration of each drug
- Half-life listed for each drug entry
- An "Alert" logo that signals cautionary tips to help you avoid common medication errors, with a special "look alike–sound alike" logo for drug names easily confused with a similar name
- An "Effects on lab test results" section in every monograph

- In the "Interactions" section, drugs that cause a rapid- and delayed-onset interaction highlighted
- A guide to common abbreviations approved by The Joint Commission as safe to use throughout the book, with an appendix on which abbreviations to avoid
- An appendix on drugs affected by cytochrome P-450 enzymes
- Appendices on drugs that affect the QTc interval, vitamins and minerals, pregnancy risk categories, controlled substance schedules, dialyzable drugs, therapeutic drug monitoring guidelines, indications and dosages of vaccines and toxoids, and combination drugs.
- A Web Toolkit on NDHnow.com, the *Nursing2010 Drug Handbook* Web site, provides new drug updates, news, warnings, and patient teaching aids; herbal information; 200 most common drugs along with their patient-teaching sheets; dosage calculator; drug safety and administration videos; pharmacology animations; English-Spanish audio medical phrases; NCLEX-style questions; and continuing education tests.

Introductory chapters
Chapter 1 explains generally how drugs work. It includes drug actions, interactions, and reactions. Chapter 2 gives general guidelines about drug use in pregnancy and the presence of drugs in breast milk. It also covers the unique problems of giving drugs to children and elderly patients and offers suggestions to minimize problems in these areas. Chapter 3 discusses techniques and provides guidelines for safe drug administration. Chapter 4 provides an overview of more than 60 drug classes including a list of drugs in that class; indications; actions; and contra-indications and cautions.

Therapeutic class chapters
Chapters 5 to 98 classify all drugs according to their approved therapeutic uses. Drugs with more than one therapeutic use are classified according to their most common use; they're also listed (with a cross-reference to the major drug entry) in drug

groups that share their secondary applications. For example, nadolol, a beta-blocker, is described in the chapter that covers antianginals because its major therapeutic application is the management of angina pectoris. Less commonly, nadolol is used to treat hypertension, so it's also listed among the generic drugs grouped as antihypertensives, with a cross-reference to Chapter 21, Antianginals.

Such classification by therapeutic use offers several advantages. It helps you identify an unknown drug by its clinical application alone. It also identifies all other drugs that share the same use and provides easy comparison of their dosages and effects. In this way, it quickly lets you refer to similar drugs for patients who can't tolerate or don't respond to a particular drug.

Each chapter, representing a major therapeutic use, begins with an alphabetical list of the generic drugs described in the chapter. Specific information on each drug is arranged under the following headings: *Pronunciation, Pharmacologic class, Pregnancy risk category, Controlled substance schedule, Available forms, Indications & dosages, Administration (with I. V. incompatibilities), Action* (with quick-reference table), *Adverse reactions, Interactions, Effects on lab test results, Contraindications & cautions, Nursing considerations,* and *Patient teaching.*

In each drug entry, drugs may have received a "Safety Alert!" label. This label is reserved for drugs, designated by the Institute for Safe Medication Practices, that are dangerous to you or your patient, either because they're powerful and hazardous or prone to accidental error.

Further into the entry, the generic name and pronunciation are followed by an alphabetized list of one or more brand names. A brand name followed by an open diamond (◊) indicates an OTC drug. Canadian brands are designated with a dagger (†). Brand names that appear in the Photoguide to Tablets and Capsules are highlighted with a capsule symbol (✔). A brand name with no symbol is available in the United States, and possibly Canada. The mention of a brand name in no way implies endorsement of that product or guarantees its legality.

Available forms
This section lists the preparations available for each drug (for example, tablets, capsules, solutions for injection) and specifies available dosage forms and strengths. Dosage strengths specifically available in Canada are designated with a dagger (†). Preparations that don't require a prescription are marked with an open diamond (◊).

Indications & dosages
This section lists general dosage information for adults, children, and elderly patients. Dosage instructions reflect current trends in therapeutics and can't be considered absolute or universal. For individual patients, dosage instructions must be considered in light of the patient's condition.

Indications for dosages that aren't approved by the FDA are followed by a closed diamond (♦). The logo for "Adjust-a-dose" indicates dosage adjustments for certain patients, such as those with renal impairment.

Administration
This section provides guidelines for safely administering drugs by all applicable routes. For instance, an I.V. section would describe reconstituting and mixing I.V. drugs, giving them safely, and storing them properly.

I.V. incompatibilities
This section lists drugs incompatible with the I.V. solution being discussed, detailing all of the known information.

Action
This section succinctly describes the mechanism of action—that is, how the drug provides its therapeutic effect. For example, although all antihypertensives lower blood pressure, they don't all do so by the same process.

Also included, in table form, are the onset, peak (described in terms of effect or peak blood level), and duration of drug action for each route of administration, if data are available or applicable. Values listed are for patients with normal renal function, unless specified otherwise.

Adverse reactions
This section lists adverse reactions to each drug by body system. The most common adverse reactions (those experienced by at least 10% of people taking the drug in clinical trials) appear in *italic* type; less common reactions are in roman type; life-threatening reactions are in ***bold italic*** type; and reactions that are common *and* life-threatening are in BOLD CAPITAL LETTERS.

Interactions
This section lists each drug's confirmed, clinically significant interactions with other drugs (additive effects, potentiated effects, and antagonistic effects); herbs; foods; beverages; and lifestyle behaviors. Rapid-onset interactions are highlighted in color in this section.

Drug interactions are listed under the drug that's adversely affected. For example, because magnesium trisilicate, an antacid ingredient, interacts with tetracycline to decrease tetracycline absorption, this interaction is listed under tetracycline. To check on the possible effects of using two or more drugs simultaneously, refer to the interaction entry for each drug in question.

Effects on lab test results
This section lists increased and decreased levels, counts, and other values in laboratory test results, which may be caused by the drug's systemic effects. It also indicates false-positive, false-negative, and otherwise altered results of laboratory tests a drug may cause.

Contraindications & cautions
This section lists any conditions, especially diseases, in which the use of the drug is undesirable, as well as those for which the drug should be given with caution.

Nursing considerations
This section provides information useful to nurses, such as monitoring techniques and suggestions for prevention and treatment of adverse reactions. Also included are suggestions for ensuring patient comfort and for preparing, giving, and storing the drug.

An "Alert" logo gives important advice about life-threatening effects of the drug and its administration.

A special "Look alike–sound alike" alert provides information to avoid medication errors that may occur when drug names that sound or look alike are confused.

Patient teaching
This section gives the nurse guidelines on teaching the patient about each drug. It includes instructions for explaining the drug's purpose, promoting compliance, ensuring proper use and storage of the drug, and preventing or minimizing adverse reactions.

Photoguide to tablets and capsules
To make drug identification easier and to enhance patient safety, *Nursing2010 Drug Handbook* offers a 32-page full-color photoguide to the most commonly prescribed tablets and capsules. Shown in actual size, the drugs are arranged alphabetically for quick reference, along with their most common dosage strengths. Below the name of each drug, you'll find a cross-reference to information on the drug. Brand names of drugs that appear in the photoguide are shown in the text with a special capsule symbol (✐). Page references to the drug photos appear in boldface type in the index (for example, **C12**).

Guide to abbreviations

ACE	angiotensin-converting enzyme	GABA	gamma-aminobutyric acid
ADH	antidiuretic hormone	GFR	glomerular filtration rate
AIDS	acquired immunodeficiency syndrome	GGT	gamma-glutamyltransferase
		GI	gastrointestinal
ALT	alanine transaminase	gtt	drops
ANA	antinuclear antibody	GU	genitourinary
AST	aspartate transaminase	G6PD	glucose-6-phosphate dehydrogenase
AV	atrioventricular		
b.i.d.	twice daily	H_1	histamine$_1$
BPH	benign prostatic hypertrophy	H_2	histamine$_2$
		HDL	high-density lipoprotein
BSA	body surface area	HIV	human immunodeficiency virus
BUN	blood urea nitrogen		
cAMP	cyclic 3′, 5′ adenosine monophosphate	HMG-CoA	3-hydroxy-3-methylglutaryl coenzyme A
CBC	complete blood count	I.D.	intradermal
CK	creatine kinase	I.M.	intramuscular
CMV	cytomegalovirus	INR	International Normalized Ratio
CNS	central nervous system		
COPD	chronic obstructive pulmonary disease	IPPB	intermittent positive-pressure breathing
CSF	cerebrospinal fluid	I.V.	intravenous
CV	cardiovascular	kg	kilogram
D_5W	dextrose 5% in water	L	liter
DEHP	di(2-ethylhexyl)phthalate	lb	pound
DIC	disseminated intravascular coagulation	LDH	lactate dehydrogenase
		LDL	low-density lipoprotein
dl	deciliter	M	molar
DNA	deoxyribonucleic acid	m^2	square meter
ECG	electrocardiogram	MAO	monoamine oxidase
EEG	electroencephalogram		
EENT	eyes, ears, nose, throat	mcg	microgram
FDA	Food and Drug Administration	mEq	milliequivalent
		mg	milligram
g	gram	MI	myocardial infarction
G	gauge	min	minute

ml	milliliter	t.i.d.	three times daily
mm³	cubic millimeter	tsp	teaspoon
mo	month	USP	United States Pharmacopeia
msec	millisecond	UTI	urinary tract infection
NNRI	non-nucleoside reverse transcriptase inhibitor	WBC	white blood cell
NSAID	nonsteroidal anti-inflammatory drug	wk	week
OTC	over-the-counter		
oz	ounce		
PABA	para-aminobenzoic acid		
PCA	patient-controlled analgesia		
P.O.	by mouth		
P.R.	by rectum		
p.r.n.	as needed		
PT	prothrombin time		
PTT	partial thromboplastin time		
PVC	premature ventricular contraction		
q.i.d.	four times daily		
RBC	red blood cell		
RDA	recommended daily allowance		
REM	rapid eye movement		
RNA	ribonucleic acid		
RSV	respiratory syncytial virus		
SA	sinoatrial		
Subcut.	subcutaneous		
sec	second		
SIADH	syndrome of inappropriate antidiuretic hormone		
S.L.	sublingual		
SSNRI	selective serotonin and norepinephrine reuptake inhibitor		
SSRI	selective serotonin reuptake inhibitor		
T_3	triiodothyronine		
T_4	thyroxine		

1

Drug actions, interactions, and reactions

Any drug a patient takes causes a series of physical and chemical events in his body. The first event, when a drug combines with cellular drug receptors, is the drug action. What happens next is the drug effect. Depending on the type of cellular drug receptors affected by a given drug, an effect can be local, systemic, or both. A systemic drug effect can follow a local effect. For example, when you apply a drug to the skin, it causes a local effect. But transdermal absorption of that drug can then produce a systemic effect. A local effect can also follow systemic absorption. For example, the peptic ulcer drug cimetidine produces a local effect after it's swallowed by blocking histamine receptors in the stomach's parietal cells. Diphenhydramine, on the other hand, causes a systemic effect by blocking histamine receptors throughout the body.

Drug properties

Drug absorption, distribution, metabolism, and excretion make up a drug's pharmacokinetics. These parts also describe a drug's onset of action, peak level, duration of action, and bioavailability.

Absorption

Before a drug can act in the body, it must be absorbed into the bloodstream—usually after oral administration, the most common route. Before an oral drug can be absorbed, it must disintegrate into particles small enough to dissolve in gastric juices. Only after dissolving can the drug be absorbed. Most absorption of orally given drugs occurs in the small intestine because the mucosal villi provide extensive surface area. Once absorbed and circulated in the bloodstream, the drug is bioavailable, or ready to produce a drug effect. The speed of absorption and whether absorption is complete or partial depend on the drug's effects, dosage form, administration route, interactions with other substances in the GI tract, and various patient characteristics. Oral solutions and elixirs bypass the need for disintegration and dissolution and

are usually absorbed faster. Some tablets have enteric coatings to prevent disintegration in the acidic environment of the stomach; others have coatings of varying thickness that simply delay release of the drug.

Drugs given I.M. must first be absorbed through the muscle into the bloodstream. Rectal suppositories must dissolve to be absorbed through the rectal mucosa. Drugs given I.V. are injected directly into the bloodstream and are bioavailable completely and immediately.

Distribution

After absorption, a drug moves from the bloodstream into the fluids and tissues in the body, a movement known as distribution. All of the area to which a drug is distributed is known as volume of distribution. Individual patient variations can change the amount of drug distributed throughout the body. For example, in an edematous patient, a given dose must be distributed to a larger volume than in a nonedematous patient. Occasionally, a dose is increased to account for this difference. In this case, the dose should be decreased after the edema is corrected. Conversely, a dose given to a dehydrated patient must be decreased to allow for its distribution to a much smaller volume. Patients who are very obese may present another problem when considering drug distribution. Some drugs—such as digoxin, gentamicin, and tobramycin—aren't well-distributed to fatty tissue. Sometimes, doses based on actual body weight may lead to overdose and serious toxicity. In these cases, doses must be based on lean body weight, or adjusted body weight, which may be estimated from actuarial tables that give average weight range for height.

Metabolism

Most drugs are metabolized in the liver. Hepatic diseases may affect the liver's metabolic functions and may increase or decrease a drug's usual metabolism. Closely monitor all patients with hepatic disease for drug effect and toxicity.

The rate at which a drug is metabolized varies from person to person. Some patients metabolize drugs so quickly that the drug levels in their blood and tissues prove therapeutically inadequate. In other patients, the rate of metabolism is so slow that ordinary doses can produce toxicity.

Excretion

The body eliminates drugs by metabolism (usually hepatic) and excretion (usually renal). Drug excretion is the movement of a drug or its metabolites from the tissues back into circulation and from the circulation into the organs of excretion, where they're removed from the body. Most drugs are excreted by the kidneys, but some can be eliminated through the lungs, exocrine glands (sweat, salivary, or mammary), liver, skin, and intestinal tract. Drugs also may be removed artificially by direct mechanical intervention, such as peritoneal dialysis or hemodialysis.

Other modifying factors

One important factor influencing a drug's action and effect is its tendency to bind to plasma proteins, especially albumin, and other tissue components. Because only a free, unbound drug can act in the body, protein binding greatly influences the amount and duration of effect. Malnutrition, renal failure, and the presence of other protein-bound drugs can influence protein binding. When protein binding changes, the drug dose may need to be changed also.

The patient's age is another important factor. Elderly patients usually have decreased hepatic function, less muscle mass, diminished renal function, and lower albumin levels. These patients need lower doses and sometimes longer dosage intervals to avoid toxicity. Neonates have underdeveloped metabolic enzyme systems and inadequate renal function, so they need highly individualized dosages and careful monitoring.

Underlying disease also may affect drug action and effect. For example, acidosis may cause insulin resistance. Genetic diseases, such as G6PD deficiency and hepatic porphyria, may turn drugs into toxins, with serious consequences. Patients with G6PD deficiency may develop hemolytic anemia when given certain drugs, such as sulfonamides. A genetically susceptible patient can develop acute porphyria if given a barbiturate. A patient with a highly active hepatic enzyme system, such as a rapid acetylator, can develop hepatitis when treated with isoniazid because of the quick intrahepatic buildup of a toxic metabolite.

Drug administration issues

How a drug is given can also influence a drug's action in the body. The dosage form of a drug is important. Some tablets and capsules are too large to be easily swallowed by sick patients. An oral solution may be substituted, but it will produce higher drug levels than a tablet because the liquid is more easily and completely absorbed. When a potentially toxic drug (such as digoxin) is given, its increased absorption can cause toxicity. Sometimes a change in dosage form also requires a change in dosage.

Routes of administration aren't interchangeable. For example, diazepam is readily absorbed P.O. but is slowly and erratically absorbed I.M. On the other hand, gentamicin must be given parenterally because oral administration results in drug levels too low for systemic infections.

Improper storage can alter a drug's potency. Store most drugs in tight containers protected from direct sunlight and extremes in temperature and humidity that can cause them to deteriorate. Some drugs require special storage conditions, such as refrigeration. Caution patients not to store drugs in a bathroom because of the constantly changing environment.

The timing of drug administration can be important. Sometimes, giving an oral drug during or shortly after a meal decreases the amount of drug absorbed. In most drugs, this isn't significant and may even be desirable with irritating drugs such as aspirin. But penicillins and tetracyclines shouldn't be taken at mealtimes because certain foods can inactivate them. If in doubt about the effect of food on a certain drug, check with a pharmacist.

Consider the patient's age, height, and weight. The prescriber will need this information when calculating the dosage for many drugs. Record all information accu-

rately on the patient's chart. The chart should also include all current laboratory data, especially renal and liver function studies, so the prescriber can adjust the dosage as needed.

Watch for metabolic changes and physiologic changes (depressed respiratory function, acidosis, or alkalosis) that might alter drug effect.

Know the patient's medical history. Whenever possible, obtain a comprehensive family history from the patient or his family. Ask about past reactions to drugs, possible genetic traits that might affect drug response, and the current use of other prescription, OTC, and illicit drugs, herbal remedies, and vitamin supplements. Multiple drug therapies can cause serious and fatal drug interactions and dramatically change many drugs' effects.

Drug interactions
A drug interaction occurs when a drug given with or shortly after another drug alters the effect of either or both drugs. Usually the effect of one drug is increased or decreased. For instance, one drug may inhibit or stimulate the metabolism or excretion of the other or free it for further action by releasing the drug from protein-binding sites.

Combination therapy is based on drug interaction. One drug may be given to complement the effects of another. Probenecid, which blocks the excretion of penicillin, is sometimes given with penicillin to maintain an adequate level of penicillin for a longer time. In many cases, two drugs with similar actions are given together precisely because of the additive effect. For instance, aspirin and codeine are commonly given in combination because together they provide greater pain relief than if either is given alone.

Drug interactions are sometimes used to prevent or antagonize certain adverse reactions. The diuretics hydrochlorothiazide and spironolactone are often given together because the former is potassium-depleting and the latter potassium-sparing.

Not all drug interactions are beneficial: many drugs interact and decrease efficacy or increase toxicity. An example of decreased efficacy occurs when a tetracycline is given with drugs or foods that

contain calcium or magnesium (such as antacids or milk). These bind with tetracycline in the GI tract and cause inadequate drug absorption. An example of increased toxicity can be seen in a patient taking a diuretic and lithium. The diuretic may increase the lithium level, causing lithium toxicity. This drug effect is known as *antagonism*. Avoid drug combinations that produce these effects, if possible.

Adverse reactions
Drugs cause adverse *effects*; patients have adverse *reactions*. An adverse reaction may be tolerated to obtain a therapeutic effect, or it may be hazardous and unacceptable. Some adverse reactions subside with continued use. For example, the drowsiness caused by paroxetine and the orthostatic hypotension caused by prazosin usually subside after several days when the patient develops tolerance. But many adverse reactions are dosage related and lessen or disappear only if the dosage is reduced. Most adverse reactions aren't therapeutically desirable, but a few can be put to clinical use. An outstanding example of this is the drowsiness caused by diphenhydramine, which makes it useful as a mild sedative.

Drug hypersensitivity, or drug allergy, is the result of an antigen–antibody immune reaction that occurs in the body when a drug is given to a susceptible patient. One of the most dangerous of all drug hypersensitivities is penicillin allergy. In its most severe form, penicillin anaphylaxis can rapidly become fatal.

Rarely, idiosyncratic reactions occur. These reactions are highly unpredictable and unusual. One of the best-known idiosyncratic adverse reactions is aplastic anemia caused by the antibiotic chloramphenicol. This reaction may appear in only 1 of 24,000 patients, but when it does occur, it can be fatal. A more common idiosyncratic reaction is extreme sensitivity to very low doses of a drug or insensitivity to higher-than-normal doses.

To deal with adverse reactions correctly, you need to be alert to even minor changes in the patient's clinical status. Such minor changes may be an early warning of pending toxicity. Listen to the patient's complaints about his reactions to a drug, and

consider each objectively. You may be able to reduce adverse reactions in several ways. Obviously, dosage reduction can help. But, in many cases, so does a simple rescheduling of the dose. For example, pseudoephedrine may produce stimulation that will be no problem if it's given early in the day. Similarly, drowsiness from antihistamines or tranquilizers can be harmless if these drugs are given at bedtime. Most important, your patient needs to be told which adverse reactions to expect so that he won't become worried or even stop taking the drug on his own. Always advise the patient to report adverse reactions to the prescriber immediately.

Your ability to recognize signs and symptoms of drug allergies or serious idiosyncratic reactions may save your patient's life. Ask each patient about the drugs he's taking currently or has taken in the past and whether he experienced any unusual reactions from taking them. If a patient claims to be allergic to a drug, ask him to tell you exactly what happens when he takes it. He may be calling a harmless adverse reaction, such as upset stomach, an allergic reaction, or he may have a true tendency toward anaphylaxis. In either case, you and the prescriber need to know this. Of course, you must record and report clinical changes throughout the patient's course of treatment. If you suspect a severe adverse reaction, withhold the drug until you can check with the pharmacist and the prescriber.

Toxic reactions
Chronic drug toxicities are usually caused by the cumulative effect and resulting buildup of the drug in the body. These effects may be extensions of the desired therapeutic effect. For example, normal doses of glyburide normalize the glucose level, but higher doses can produce hypoglycemia.

Drug toxicities occur when a drug level rises as a result of impaired metabolism or excretion. For example, hepatic dysfunction impairs the metabolism of theophylline, raising its levels. Similarly, renal dysfunction may cause digoxin toxicity because this drug is eliminated from the body by the kidneys. Of course, excessive dosage can cause toxic levels also. For instance, tinnitus is usually a sign that the safe dose of aspirin has been exceeded.

Most drug toxicities are predictable, dosage-related, and reversible upon dosage adjustment. So, monitor patients carefully for physiologic changes that might alter drug effect. Watch especially for hepatic and renal impairment. Warn the patient about signs of pending toxicity, and tell him what to do if a toxic reaction occurs. Also, make sure to emphasize the importance of taking a drug exactly as prescribed. Warn the patient that serious problems could arise if he changes the dose or schedule or stops taking the drug without his prescriber's knowledge.

2

Drug therapy across the lifespan

Drug therapy is a fact of life for millions of people of all ages, and certain aspects of a patient's life, such as age, growth, and development, can affect drug therapy.

Drugs and pregnancy

Drug administration during pregnancy has been a source of serious medical concern and controversy since the thalidomide tragedy of the late 1950s, when thousands of malformed infants were born after their mothers were given this mild sedative–hypnotic while pregnant. To identify drugs that may cause such teratogenic effects, preclinical drug studies always include tests on pregnant laboratory animals. These studies may reveal gross teratogenicity but don't establish absolute safety. This is because different animal species react to drugs in different ways. Consequently, animal studies can't reveal all possible teratogenic effects in humans. For example, the preliminary studies on thalidomide gave no warning of teratogenic effects, and it was subsequently released for general use in Europe.

What about the placental barrier? Once thought to protect the fetus from drug effects, the placenta isn't much of a barrier at all. Almost every drug a pregnant woman takes crosses the placenta and enters the fetal circulation, except for drugs with exceptionally large molecular structure, such as heparin, the injectable anticoagulant. By this standard, heparin could be used in a pregnant woman without fear of harming the fetus, but even heparin carries a warning for cautious use during pregnancy. Conversely, just because a drug crosses the placenta doesn't necessarily mean it's harmful to the fetus. The relative risk to the fetus is expressed by the drug's pregnancy risk category.

Actually, only one factor—stage of fetal development—seems clearly related to greater risk during pregnancy. During the first and third trimesters of pregnancy, the fetus is especially vulnerable to damage from maternal use of drugs. During these times, give *all* drugs with extreme caution.

Organogenesis—when fetal organs differentiate—occurs in the first trimester. This is the most sensitive period for drug-induced fetal malformation. Withhold all drugs except those in category A or B during this time, unless this would jeopardize the mother's health. Strongly advise your patient to avoid *all* self-prescribed drugs during early pregnancy.

Fetal sensitivity to drugs is also of special concern during the last trimester. At birth, when separated from his mother, the neonate must rely on his own metabolism to eliminate any remaining drug. Because his detoxifying systems aren't fully developed, any residual drug may take a long time to be metabolized, and thus may induce prolonged toxic reactions. For this reason, discourage pregnant patients from taking drugs except when absolutely necessary and advised by their prescriber during the last 3 months of pregnancy.

Of course, in many circumstances, pregnant women must continue to take certain drugs. For example, a woman with a seizure disorder that is well-controlled with an anticonvulsant should keep taking the drug during pregnancy. Similarly, a pregnant woman with a bacterial infection must receive antibiotics. In such cases, the potential risk to the fetus is outweighed by the mother's medical needs.

Complying with these general guidelines can prevent indiscriminate and harmful use of drugs in pregnancy:
● Before a drug is prescribed for a woman of childbearing age, ask the date of her last menstrual period and whether she may be pregnant. If a drug is a known teratogen (for example, isotretinoin), some manufacturers may recommend special precautions to ensure that the drug isn't given to a woman of childbearing age until pregnancy is ruled out and that contraceptives are used throughout the course of therapy.
● Caution a pregnant woman to avoid all drugs except those essential to maintain her pregnancy or health—especially during the first and third trimesters.

• Topical drugs are subject to the same warning against use during pregnancy. Many topically applied drugs can be absorbed in large enough amounts to be harmful to the fetus.
• When a pregnant woman needs a drug, use the safest drug in the lowest possible dose to minimize harm to the fetus.
• Instruct a pregnant woman to check with her prescriber before taking any drug.

Drugs and breast-feeding
Most drugs a breast-feeding mother takes appear in breast milk. Drug levels in breast milk tend to be high when drug levels in maternal blood are high, especially right after each dose. Advise the mother to breast-feed *before* taking each drug dose, not *after.*

A mother who wants to breast-feed usually may continue to do so with her prescriber's advice. However, breast-feeding should be temporarily interrupted and replaced with bottle-feeding when the mother must take tetracycline, chloramphenicol, a sulfonamide (during the first 2 weeks postpartum), an oral anticoagulant, a drug that contains iodine, or an antineoplastic.

Caution the breast-feeding patient to protect her infant by not taking drugs indiscriminately. Instruct the mother to first check with her prescriber to be sure she's taking the safest drug at the lowest dose. Also instruct her to give her prescriber a list of all drugs and herbs she's currently taking.

Drug therapy in children
Providing drug therapy to infants, children, and adolescents is challenging. Physiologic differences between children and adults, including those in vital organ maturity and body composition, significantly influence a drug's effectiveness.

Physiologic changes affecting drug action
A child's absorption, distribution (including drug binding to plasma proteins), metabolism, and excretion processes undergo profound changes that affect drug dosage. To ensure optimal drug effect and minimal toxicity, consider these factors when giving drugs to a child.

Absorption
Drug absorption in children depends on the form of the drug, its physical properties, simultaneous ingestion of other drugs or food, physiologic changes, and concurrent disease.

The pH of neonatal gastric fluid is neutral or slightly acidic; it becomes more acidic as the infant matures, which affects drug absorption. For example, nafcillin and penicillin G are better absorbed in an infant than in an adult because of low gastric acidity.

Various infant formulas or milk products may increase gastric pH and impede absorption of acidic drugs. If possible, give a child oral drugs on an empty stomach.

Gastric emptying time and transit time through the small intestine—which takes longer in children than in adults—can affect absorption. Also, intestinal hypermotility (as occurs in patients with diarrhea) can diminish the drug's absorption.

A child's comparatively thin epidermis allows increased absorption of topical drugs.

Distribution
As with absorption, changes in body weight and physiology during childhood can significantly influence a drug's distribution and effects. In a premature infant, body fluid makes up about 85% of total body weight; in a full-term infant, it makes up 55% to 70%; in an adult, 50% to 55%. Extracellular fluid (mostly blood) constitutes 40% of a neonate's body weight, compared with 20% in an adult. Intracellular fluid remains fairly constant throughout life and has little effect on drug dosage.

Extracellular fluid volume influences a water-soluble drug's concentration and effect because most drugs travel through extracellular fluid to reach their receptors. Compared with adults, distribution area in children is proportionately greater because their fluid-to-solid body weight proportion is larger.

Because the proportion of fat to lean body mass increases with age, the distribution of fat-soluble drugs is more limited in children than in adults. As a result, a drug's fat or water solubility affects the dosage for a child.

Plasma protein binding

A decrease in albumin level or intermolecular attraction between drug and plasma protein causes many drugs to be less bound to plasma proteins in infants than in adults.

Strongly protein-bound drugs may displace endogenous compounds, such as bilirubin or free fatty acids. Displacement of bound bilirubin can increase unbound bilirubin, which can lead to increased risk of kernicterus at normal bilirubin levels. Conversely, an endogenous compound may displace a weakly bound drug.

Because only an unbound (free) drug has a pharmacologic effect, a change in ratio of a protein-bound to an unbound active drug can greatly influence its effect.

Several diseases and disorders, such as nephrotic syndrome and malnutrition, can decrease plasma protein and increase the level of an unbound drug, which can either intensify the drug's effect or produce toxicity.

Metabolism

A neonate's ability to metabolize a drug depends on the integrity of the hepatic enzyme system, intrauterine exposure to the drug, and the nature of the drug itself.

Certain metabolic mechanisms are underdeveloped in neonates. Glucuronidation is a metabolic process that renders most drugs more water soluble, facilitating renal excretion. This process isn't developed enough to permit full pediatric doses until the infant is age 1 month. The use of chloramphenicol in a neonate may cause gray baby syndrome because the infant's immature liver can't metabolize the drug and toxic levels accumulate in the blood. Reduce dosage in a neonate and periodically monitor his levels.

Conversely, intrauterine exposure to drugs may induce precocious development of hepatic enzyme mechanisms, increasing the infant's capacity to metabolize potentially harmful substances.

Older children can metabolize some drugs (theophylline, for example) more rapidly than adults. This ability may come from their increased hepatic metabolic activity. Doses larger than those recommended for adults may be required.

Also, more than one drug given to a child simultaneously may change the hepatic metabolism and initiate production of hepatic enzymes. Phenobarbital, for example, accelerates the metabolism of drugs taken with it and causes hepatic enzyme production.

Excretion

Renal excretion of a drug is the net result of glomerular filtration, active tubular secretion, and passive tubular reabsorption. Many drugs are excreted in the urine. The degree of renal development or presence of renal disease can greatly affect a child's dosage requirements because if a child can't excrete a drug renally, the drug may accumulate to toxic levels.

Physiologically, an infant's kidneys differ from an adult's because infants have a high resistance to blood flow and their kidneys receive a smaller proportion of cardiac output. Infants have incomplete glomerular and tubular development and short, incomplete loops of Henle. (A child's GFR reaches an adult value between ages 2½ and 5 months; his tubular secretion rate may reach an adult value between ages 7 and 12 months.) Infants also are less able to concentrate urine or reabsorb certain filtered compounds. The proximal tubules in infants also are less able to secrete organic acids.

Children and adults have diurnal variations in urine pH that correlate with sleep patterns.

Special administration considerations

Biochemically, a drug displays the same mechanisms of action in all people. But the response to a drug can be affected by a child's age and size, as well as by the maturity of the target organ. To ensure optimal drug effect and minimal toxicity, consider the following factors when giving drugs to children.

Adjusting dosages for children

When calculating children's dosages, don't use formulas that just modify adult dosages. Base pediatric dosages on either body weight (mg/kg) or body surface area (mg/m^2). A child isn't a scaled-down version of an adult.

Reevaluate dosages at regular intervals to ensure needed adjustments as the child

develops. Although body surface area provides a useful standard for adults and older children, use the body weight method instead in premature or full-term infants. Don't exceed the maximum adult dosage when calculating amounts per kilogram of body weight (except with certain drugs such as theophylline, if indicated).

Obtain an accurate maternal drug history, including prescription and nonprescription drugs, vitamins, herbs, or other health foods taken during pregnancy. Drugs passed into breast milk can have adverse effects on the breast-feeding infant. Before giving a drug to a breast-feeding mother, investigate its potential effects on the infant.

For example, a sulfonamide given to a breast-feeding mother for a UTI appears in breast milk and may cause kernicterus in an infant with low levels of unconjugated bilirubin. Also, high levels of isoniazid appear in the breast milk of a mother taking this drug. Because this drug is metabolized by the liver, the infant's immature hepatic enzyme mechanisms can't metabolize the drug, and he may develop CNS toxicity.

Giving oral drugs

Remember the following when giving oral drugs to a child:

If the patient is an infant, give drugs in liquid form, if possible. For accuracy, measure and give the preparation by oral syringe. It's very important to remove the syringe cap to keep the infant from aspirating it. Be sure to instruct parents to do the same. Never use a vial or cup. Lift the patient's head to prevent aspiration of the drug, and press down on his chin to prevent choking. You may also place the drug in a nipple and allow the infant to suck the contents.

If the patient is a toddler, explain how you're going to give him the drug. If possible, have the parents enlist the child's cooperation. Don't mix the drug with food or call it "candy," even if it has a pleasant taste. Let the child drink a liquid drug from a calibrated medication cup rather than a spoon. It's easier and more accurate. If the preparation is available only in tablet form, crush and mix it with an appropriate buffer, such as jelly or apple-

sauce. (First, verify with the pharmacist that the tablet can be crushed without compromising its effectiveness.)

If the patient is an older child who can swallow a tablet or capsule by himself, have him place the drug on the back of his tongue and swallow it with water or nonacidic fruit juice, because milk and milk products may interfere with drug absorption.

Giving I.V. infusions

For I.V. infusions, in infants, use a peripheral vein or a scalp vein in the temporal region. The scalp vein is safe because the needle isn't likely to dislodge. However, the head must be shaved around the site, and the needle and infiltrated fluids may cause temporary disfigurement. For these reasons, scalp veins aren't used as commonly today as they were in the past.

The arms and legs are the most accessible insertion sites, but because patients tend to move about, take these precautions:
● Protect the insertion site to keep the catheter or needle from being dislodged.
● Use a padded arm board to reduce the risk of dislodgment. Remove the arm board during range-of-motion exercises.
● Place the clamp out of the child's reach. If extension tubing is used to allow the child greater mobility, securely tape the connection.
● Explain in simple terms to the child why he must be restrained while asleep, to alleviate anxiety and maintain trust.

During an infusion, monitor flow rates and check the child's condition and insertion site at least every hour. Titrate the flow rate only while the patient is composed; crying and emotional upset can constrict blood vessels. Flow rate may vary if a pump isn't used. Flow should be adequate because some drugs (calcium, for example) can be irritating at low flow rates. Infants, small children, and children with compromised cardiopulmonary status are especially vulnerable to fluid overload with I.V. drug administration. To prevent this problem and help ensure that a limited amount of fluid is infused in a controlled manner, use a volume-control device in the I.V. tubing and an infusion pump or a syringe. Don't place more than

2 hours of I.V. fluid in the volume-control set at a time.

Giving I.M. injections

I.M. injections are preferred when a drug can't be given by other parenteral routes and rapid absorption is needed.

The vastus lateralis muscle is the preferred injection site in children younger than age 2. The ventrogluteal area or gluteus medius muscle can be used in older children. To select the correct needle size, consider the patient's age, muscle mass, nutritional status, and drug viscosity.

Record and rotate injection sites. Explain to the patient that the injection will hurt but that the drug will help him. Restrain him during the injection, if needed, and comfort him afterward.

Giving topical drugs and inhalants

When you give a child a topical drug or inhalant, consider the following:

Use eardrops warmed to room temperature. Cold drops can cause pain and vertigo. To give drops, turn the patient on his side, with the affected ear up. If he's younger than age 3, pull the pinna down and back; if age 3 or older, pull the pinna up and back.

Avoid using inhalants in young children because it's difficult to get them to cooperate. Before you try to give a drug to an older child through a metered-dose nebulizer, explain the inhaler to him. Then have him hold the nebulizer upside down and close his lips around the mouthpiece. Have him exhale and pinch his nostrils shut. When he starts to inhale, release one dose of the drug into his mouth. Tell the patient to continue inhaling until his lungs feel full; then he can breathe normally and unpinch his nostrils. Most inhaled drugs aren't useful if the drug remains in the mouth or throat—if you doubt the patient's ability to use the inhalant correctly, don't use it. Such devices as spacers or assist devices may help. Check with a pharmacist, the prescriber, or a respiratory therapist.

Use topical corticosteroids cautiously because prolonged use in children may delay growth. When you apply topical corticosteroids to the diaper area of infants, don't cover the area with plastic or rubber pants, which act as an occlusive dressing and may enhance systemic absorption.

Giving parenteral nutrition

Give I.V. nutrition to patients who can't or won't take adequate food orally and to patients with hypermetabolic conditions who need supplementation. The latter group includes premature infants and children with burns or other major trauma, intractable diarrhea, malabsorption syndromes, GI abnormalities, emotional disorders (such as anorexia nervosa), and congenital abnormalities.

Before giving fat emulsions to infants and children, weigh the potential benefits against any possible risks. Fats—supplied as 10% or 20% emulsions—are given both peripherally and centrally. Their use is limited by the child's ability to metabolize them. For example, an infant or child with a diseased liver can't efficiently metabolize fats.

Some fats, however, must be supplied both to prevent essential fatty acid deficiency and to permit normal growth and development. A minimum of calories (2% to 4%) must be supplied as linoleic acid—an essential fatty acid found in lipids. In infants, fats are essential for normal neurologic development.

Nevertheless, fat solutions may decrease oxygen perfusion and may adversely affect children with pulmonary disease. This risk can be minimized by supplying only the minimum fat needed for essential fatty acid requirements and not the usual intake of 40% to 50% of the child's total calories.

Fatty acids can also displace bilirubin bound to albumin, causing a rise in free, unconjugated bilirubin and an increased risk of kernicterus. But fat solutions may interfere with some bilirubin assays and cause falsely elevated levels. To avoid this complication, draw a blood sample 4 hours after infusion of the lipid emulsion; or if the emulsion is introduced over 24 hours, be sure the laboratory is aware so they can centrifuge the blood sample before the assay is performed.

Drug therapy in elderly patients

If you're giving drugs to elderly patients, you'll need to understand the physiologic

and pharmacokinetic changes that may affect drug dosage, cause common adverse reactions, or create compliance problems.

Physiologic changes affecting drug action

As a person ages, gradual physiologic changes occur. Some of these age-related changes may alter the therapeutic and toxic effects of drugs.

Body composition

Proportions of fat, lean tissue, and water in the body change with age. Total body mass and lean body mass tend to decrease, but the proportion of body fat tends to increase.

Body composition varies from person to person, and these changes in body composition affect the relationship between a drug's concentration and distribution in the body.

For example, a water-soluble drug such as gentamicin isn't distributed to fat. Because there's relatively less lean tissue in an elderly person, more drug remains in the blood.

Gastrointestinal function

In elderly patients, decreases in gastric acid secretion and GI motility slow the emptying of stomach contents and movement through the entire intestinal tract. Also, research suggests that elderly patients may have more difficulty absorbing drugs than younger patients. This is an especially significant problem with drugs that have a narrow therapeutic range, such as digoxin, in which any change in absorption can be crucial.

Hepatic function

The liver's ability to metabolize certain drugs decreases with age. This decrease is caused by diminished blood flow to the liver, which results from an age-related decrease in cardiac output, and from the lessened activity of certain liver enzymes. When an elderly patient takes a sleep medication such as flurazepam, for example, the liver's reduced ability to metabolize the drug can produce a hangover effect the next morning.

Decreased hepatic function may result in more intense drug effects caused by higher levels, longer-lasting drug effects because of prolonged levels, and a greater risk of drug toxicity.

Renal function

An elderly person's renal function is usually sufficient to eliminate excess body fluid and waste, but the ability to eliminate some drugs may be reduced by 50% or more.

Many drugs commonly used by elderly patients, such as digoxin, are excreted primarily through the kidneys. If the kidneys' ability to excrete the drug is decreased, high blood levels may result. Digoxin toxicity can be relatively common in elderly patients who don't receive a reduced digoxin dosage to accommodate decreased renal function.

Drug dosages can be modified to compensate for age-related decreases in renal function. Aided by results of laboratory tests, such as BUN and creatinine levels, adjust drug dosages so the patient receives therapeutic benefits without the risk of toxicity. Also, observe the patient for signs and symptoms of toxicity. A patient taking digoxin, for example, may experience anorexia, nausea, vomiting, or confusion.

Special administration considerations

Aging is usually accompanied by a decline in organ function that can affect drug distribution and clearance. This physiologic decline is likely to be worsened by a disease or a chronic disorder. Together, these factors can significantly increase the risk of adverse reactions and drug toxicity, as well as noncompliance.

Adverse reactions

Compared with younger people, elderly patients experience twice as many adverse drug reactions, mostly from greater drug use, poor compliance, and physiologic changes.

Signs and symptoms of adverse drug reactions—confusion, weakness, agitation, and lethargy—are often mistakenly attributed to senility or disease. If the adverse reaction isn't identified, the patient may continue to receive the drug. He may receive other, unnecessary drugs to treat complications caused by the original drug. This regi-

men can sometimes result in a pattern of inappropriate and excessive drug use.

Any drug can cause adverse reactions, but most of the serious reactions in the elderly are caused by relatively few drugs. Be particularly alert for toxicities resulting from diuretics, antihypertensives, digoxin, corticosteroids, anticoagulants, sleeping aids, and OTC drugs.

Diuretic toxicity

Because total body water content decreases with age, a normal dosage of a potassium-wasting diuretic, such as hydrochlorothiazide or furosemide, may result in fluid loss and even dehydration in an elderly patient.

These diuretics may deplete a patient's potassium level, making him feel weak, and they may raise blood uric acid and glucose levels, complicating gout and diabetes mellitus.

Antihypertensive toxicity

Many elderly patients experience light-headedness or fainting when taking antihypertensives, partly in response to atherosclerosis and decreased elasticity of the blood vessels. Antihypertensives can lower blood pressure too rapidly, resulting in insufficient blood flow to the brain, which can cause dizziness, fainting, or even a stroke.

Consequently, dosages of antihypertensives must be carefully individualized. In elderly patients, aggressive treatment of high blood pressure may be harmful. Treatment goals should be reasonable. Blood pressure needs to be reduced more slowly in elderly patients.

Digoxin toxicity

As the body's renal function and rate of excretion decline, the digoxin level in the blood of an elderly patient may increase to the point of causing nausea, vomiting, diarrhea, and, most seriously, cardiac arrhythmias. Monitor the patient's digoxin level and observe him for early signs and symptoms of inotropic toxicity, such as appetite loss, confusion, or depression.

Corticosteroid toxicity

Elderly patients taking a corticosteroid may experience short-term effects, including fluid retention and psychological effects ranging from mild euphoria to acute psychotic reactions. Long-term toxic effects, such as osteoporosis, can be especially severe in elderly patients who have been taking prednisone or related steroidal compounds for months or even years. To prevent serious toxicity, carefully monitor patients on long-term regimens. Observe them for subtle changes in appearance, mood, and mobility; for impaired healing; and for fluid and electrolyte disturbances.

Anticoagulant effects

Elderly patients taking an anticoagulant have an increased risk of bleeding, especially when they take NSAIDs at the same time, which is common. They're also at increased risk of bleeding and bruising because they are more likely to fall. Observe the patient's INR carefully, and monitor him for bruising and other signs of bleeding.

Sleeping aid toxicity

Sedatives and sleeping aids such as flurazepam may cause excessive sedation or drowsiness. Keep in mind that consuming alcohol may increase depressant effects, even if the sleeping aid was taken the previous evening. Use these drugs sparingly in elderly patients.

Over-the-counter drug toxicity

Toxicity is minimal when aspirin, aspirin-containing analgesics, and other OTC NSAIDs (such as ibuprofen, ketoprofen, and naproxen) are used in moderation. But prolonged ingestion may cause GI irritation—even ulcers—and gradual blood loss resulting in severe anemia. Prescription NSAIDs may cause similar problems. Anemia from prolonged aspirin consumption can affect all age groups, but elderly patients may be less able to compensate because of their already reduced iron stores.

Laxatives may cause diarrhea in elderly patients, who are extremely sensitive to drugs such as bisacodyl. Long-term oral use of mineral oil as a lubricating laxative may result in lipid pneumonia from aspiration of small residual oil droplets in the patient's mouth.

Noncompliance

Poor compliance can be a problem with patients of any age. Many hospitalizations result from noncompliance with a medical regimen. In elderly patients, factors linked to aging, such as diminished visual acuity, hearing loss, forgetfulness, the need for multiple drug therapy, and socioeconomic factors, can combine to make compliance a special problem. About one-third of elderly patients fail to comply with their prescribed drug therapy. They may fail to take prescribed doses or to follow the correct schedule. They may take drugs prescribed for previous disorders, stop drugs prematurely, or indiscriminately use drugs that are to be taken as needed. Elderly patients may also have multiple prescriptions for the same drug and inadvertently take an overdose.

Review the patient's drug regimen with him. Make sure he understands the dose amount, the time and frequency of doses, and why he's taking the drug. Also, explain in detail if a drug is to be taken with food, with water, or separate from other drugs.

Help the patient avoid drug therapy problems by suggesting that he use drug calendars, pill sorters, or other aids to help him comply. Refer him to the prescriber, a pharmacist, or social services if he needs further information or assistance with his drug therapy.

Safe drug administration

In the state where you practice nursing, a number of different health care professionals, including doctors, nurse practitioners, dentists, podiatrists, and optometrists, may be legally permitted to prescribe, dispense, and give drugs. Most often, however, doctors prescribe drugs, pharmacists dispense them, and nurses give them.

That means you're almost always on the front line when it comes to patients and their drugs. It also means you bear a major share of the responsibility for avoiding drug errors. Besides following your institution's administration policies, you can help prevent drug mistakes by reviewing the common errors outlined below and ways to prevent them.

Also included in this chapter is a section on important points to teach your patients so they may take their drugs safely at home.

Drug orders
Prescribing and filling drug orders must be done carefully to avoid potential problems.

Pharmacy computer systems
Error: The Institute for Safe Medication Practices (ISMP) performed a field test on 307 pharmacy computer systems; only four detected all of the unsafe orders. Many didn't detect potentially lethal orders, including doses that exceeded safe limits, drug ingredient duplications, and orders to give oral solutions I.V.
Best practice or prevention: Don't rely on the pharmacy computer system to detect all unsafe orders. Before you give a drug, understand the correct dosage, indications, and adverse effects. If necessary, check a current drug reference guide.

Confusing drug names
Error: According to the USP, insulin was the drug most often involved in medication errors in 2003. One type of error stems from name confusion. For instance, Humulin may easily be confused with

Humalog insulin. This mix-up could happen with either a verbal or a written order.
Best practice or prevention: Be aware of the drugs your patient takes regularly, and question any deviations from his regular routine. As with any drug, take your time and read the label carefully.

Abbreviations
Error: Abbreviating drug names is risky. A cancer patient with anemia may receive epoetin alfa, commonly abbreviated EPO, to stimulate RBC production. In one case, when a cancer patient was admitted to a hospital, the doctor wrote, "May take own supply of EPO." But the patient wasn't anemic. Sensing that something was wrong, the pharmacist interviewed the patient, who confirmed that he was taking "EPO"—evening primrose oil—to lower his cholesterol level.
Best practice or prevention: Ask all prescribers to spell out drug names.

Unclear orders
Error: A patient was supposed to receive one dose of the antineoplastic lomustine to treat brain cancer. (Lomustine is typically given as a single oral dose once every 6 weeks.) The doctor's order read "Administer h.s." Because this was misinterpreted to mean every night, the patient received nine daily doses, developed severe thrombocytopenia and leukopenia, and died.
Best practice or prevention: If you're unfamiliar with a drug, check a drug reference before giving it. If a prescriber uses "h.s." but doesn't specify the frequency of administration, clarify the order. When documenting orders, note "h.s. nightly" or "h.s.—one dose today."

Misreading orders
Error: Two reports concerned incorrect use of the tricyclic antidepressant nortriptyline (Pamelor or Aventyl) when ordered for neuropathic pain syndromes. The cases involved 10-mg and 20-mg orders that were misread as 100 mg and 200 mg, respectively. One patient who

received an incorrect dose required hospitalization; the other developed sedation and orthostatic hypotension after two doses, which led to recognition of the error.

Best practice or prevention: Nortriptyline and other tricyclic antidepressants aren't prescribed as frequently as they once were. To make sure you're familiar with recommended dosages, refer to a drug handbook and then ask a pharmacist, if necessary.

Misinterpretation of orders

Error: The ISMP reports that insulin orders may be especially prone to misinterpretation. In one case, an order was written as "add 10U of regular insulin to each TPN bag," and the pharmacist preparing the solution misinterpreted the dose as 100 units. In another case, a pharmacy technician entering orders misinterpreted a sliding scale when the insulin order used "u" for units, an error that could have caused a 10-fold overdose if a nurse hadn't caught it. Yet another report involved a nurse who received a verbal order to resume an insulin drip but wrote "resume heparin drip." Fortunately, the pharmacist caught the error.

Best practice or prevention: Before you give a drug ordered in units, such as insulin or heparin, always check the prescriber's written order against the provided dose. Never abbreviate "units." If you must accept a verbal order, have another nurse listen in; then transcribe that order directly onto an order form and repeat it to make sure that you've transcribed it correctly.

Inadvertent overdose

Error: The inadvertent prescribing of harmful acetaminophen doses has become a disturbing trend. To relieve pain, prescribers may write orders for combined acetaminophen and opioid analgesic tablets (Lortab, Tylox, Darvocet-N) without realizing that the total acetaminophen dose could be toxic.

Consider this order: "Tylox, 1 to 2 tablets every 4 hours, as needed, for pain." By taking the higher dose, the patient would receive 1,000 mg of acetaminophen every 4 hours, exceeding the maximum recommended dose of 4 g/day.

Best practice or prevention: To prevent an acetaminophen overdose from combined analgesics, note the amount of acetamino-

phen in each drug. Beware of substitutions by the pharmacy because the amount of acetaminophen may vary.

Lipid-based drugs

Error: Serious drug errors, some fatal, have occurred because of confusion between certain lipid-based (liposomal) drugs and their conventional counterparts. The drugs involved include:

• lipid-based amphotericin B (Abelcet, Amphotec, AmBisome) and conventional amphotericin B for injection (available as Fungizone as well as generically)

• the pegylated liposomal form of doxorubicin (Doxil) and its conventional form, doxorubicin hydrochloride

• a liposomal form of daunorubicin (DaunoXome, daunorubicin citrate liposomal) and conventional daunorubicin hydrochloride (Cerubidine).

Best practice or prevention: Lipid-based products have different dosages than their conventional counterparts. Check the original order and labels carefully to avoid confusion.

Drug preparation

When preparing to give a drug, be alert for potential problems.

Syringe tip caps and children

Error: A syringe tip cap poses a potential choking hazard to a small child: If you forget to remove the cap from an oral syringe before you give a drug, the cap could blow off into the child's mouth when you press the plunger. If a cap from an oral or a hypodermic syringe gets lost in the linens, the child may find it later and swallow or aspirate it.

Best practice or prevention: Remove and discard the cap in a secure sharps container before you give the drug; don't place it in a trash can where the child may find it later.

Teach parents about the potential danger of syringe tip caps. Tell them to store a capped syringe where children can't reach it and to remove the cap before giving the drug.

Inattentiveness

Error: When a hospital pharmacy received an order for Fludara (fludarabine), a phar-

macy technician asked the pharmacist if Navelbine (vinorelbine) was the same as Fludara (both are antineoplastics). The preoccupied pharmacist said "yes." The technician prepared the Navelbine, but labeled it as Fludara. The pharmacist checked the preparation but didn't notice the error, and the patient received the wrong drug.

Best practice or prevention: To prevent errors of this type, the hospital posted tables of antineoplastics and their dosing guidelines in the pharmacy. As an added safeguard, the pharmacy now sends the empty drug vial or box top with the prepared solution for the nurse to double-check before infusing the drug.

Solution color changes

Error: In two cases, alert nurses noticed that antineoplastics prepared in the pharmacy didn't look the way they should.

In the first error, a 6-year-old child was to receive 12 mg of methotrexate intrathecally. In the pharmacy, a 1-g vial was mistakenly selected instead of a 20-mg vial, and the drug was reconstituted with 10 ml of normal saline solution. The vial containing 100 mg/ml was incorrectly labeled as containing 2 mg/ml, and 6 ml of the solution was drawn into a syringe. Although the syringe label indicated 12 mg of drug, the syringe actually contained 600 mg of drug.

When the nurse received the syringe and noted that the drug's color didn't appear right, she returned it to the pharmacy for verification. The pharmacist retrieved the vial used to prepare the dose and drew the remaining solution into another syringe. The solutions in both syringes matched, and no one noticed the vial's 1-g label. The pharmacist concluded that a manufacturing change caused the color difference.

The child received the 600-mg dose and experienced seizures 45 minutes later. A pharmacist responding to the emergency detected the error. The child received an antidote and recovered.

In the second error, a 20-year-old patient with leukemia received mitomycin instead of mitoxantrone. The nurse had questioned the drug's unusual bluish tint, but the pharmacist had assured her that the color difference was the result of a

change in manufacturer. Fortunately, the patient didn't suffer any harm.

Best practice or prevention: If a familiar drug has an unfamiliar appearance, find out why. If the pharmacist cites a manufacturing change, ask him to double-check whether he has received verification from the manufacturer. Document the appearance discrepancy, your actions, and the pharmacist's response in the patient record.

Dropper confusion

Error: Ordering drugs such as liquid ferrous sulfate by the dropperful is a dangerous practice. One person might correctly consider the dropper full when the liquid meets the upper calibration mark; another might incorrectly fill the entire length of the dropper. Also, parents giving the drug at home may use a different dropper, which could significantly change the dose given.

Best practice or prevention: Dosing directions for liquid drugs should always be expressed as weight per volume, such as 15 mg/0.6 ml. Verify the correct dose and teach parents to use only the dropper provided. Show them the mark on the dropper that indicates a full dose and ask them to demonstrate the proper technique.

Incorrect allergy history

Error: After a patient was admitted to the hospital, a nurse faxed a list of the patient's allergies to the pharmacy. The pharmacist couldn't read it, so he accessed the files from the patient's previous admission. However, these records didn't reflect an allergy to the anti-infective cefazolin that the patient had recently developed.

A consulting doctor ordered cefazolin, and the pharmacy processed the order. The medication administration record (MAR) generated by the pharmacy's database didn't indicate the allergy, and the nurse didn't know about it either.

The patient received cefazolin and became hypotensive and unresponsive. The nurse immediately notified the doctor and gave the antihistamine diphenhydramine. The patient recovered and was discharged the next day.

Best practice or prevention: Obtain a new allergy history with each admission. If the patient's history must be faxed, name the

drugs, note how many are included, and follow the facility's faxing safeguards. If the pharmacy also adheres to strict guidelines, the computer-generated MAR should be accurate.

Drug administration

According to the USP, the number of medication errors caused by administration problems declined almost 10% between 1999 and 2003. However, administration errors are still the most common type of medication error. When you give a drug, be careful to avoid the following potential problems.

Misidentifying patients

Error: Two common errors are inadvertently failing to check the patient's identification and confusing patients with similar names. Using a tactic that helps prevent wrong-site surgery—involving the patient in the identification process—can also help prevent these drug errors.

Best practice or prevention: Urge the patient to clearly state his full name, even without being asked, at admission and before accepting drugs, procedures, or treatments. Teach him to offer his identification bracelet for inspection when anyone arrives with drugs and to insist on having it replaced if it's removed.

Herbal remedies

Error: Surveys suggest that about one-third of Americans use herbs as medicine. Some people take them with conventional drugs; others use them as replacements. Herbs are available without a prescription. Because government quality assurance standards don't apply to herbs' manufacturing and labeling, their ingredients may be misrepresented or contaminated.

Research on the effects of herbs is limited. Because these products may contain a mixture of chemicals, their use carries risks.

Best practice or prevention: Ask the patient about his use of alternative therapies, including herbs, and record your findings in his medical record. Monitor the patient carefully and report unusual events. Ask the patient to keep a diary of all therapies he uses and to take the diary for review each time he visits a health care professional.

Calculation errors

Error: A physician assistant wrote the following order for a woman being admitted to the hospital for neck surgery: "methyl-prednisolone 10.6 g (30 mg/kg) over 1 hour IVPB before surgery" to minimize inflammation. The patient weighed 154 lb (70 kg), so the dose should have been 2.1 g, and not 10.6 g. Because neither the pharmacist nor the nurse independently checked the calculation, the patient received an overdose. She developed significant hyperglycemia and hypokalemia but recovered without injury.

Best practice or prevention: Writing the mg/kg or mg/m^2 dose and the calculated dose provides a safeguard against calculation errors. Whenever a prescriber provides the calculation, double-check it and document that the dose was verified.

Eyedrops for two or more

Error: Using one bottle of eyedrops to treat several patients may seem like a good way to prevent waste, control cost, and save time. Some facilities, for example, give shared eyedrops to multiple patients undergoing outpatient cataract surgery. But this practice has risks.

Eyedrops contain preservatives to prevent bacterial growth, but contaminants may remain on the bottle top's inner surfaces or outer grooves. The dropper can also become contaminated if it accidentally touches an infected eye. (Cross-infections have been reported.)

Giving the wrong drug or wrong concentration is more likely when containers are shared because patient names don't appear on the containers. A patient may receive the wrong drops because the nurse can't check the bottle label against the patient's identification.

Best practice or prevention: Just as sharing any drug is poor practice, eyedrops shouldn't be used for more than one patient. If unit doses aren't available for surgical patients, each patient should fill his prescriptions before admission and bring his drugs with him.

Trouble with liquids

Error: Liquid drugs may be more error-prone than solid drugs because of the calculations and dosage measurements

needed. Here are a few examples: A 5-year-old boy who was receiving imipramine to treat his enuresis was given a fivefold overdose because of an incorrectly compounded suspension. A prescription of Augmentin was dispensed with the instruction to take 2½ tsp instead of 2½ ml. In another case, a mother who misunderstood the written directions gave her child 7 ml instead of 0.7 ml of a liquid drug.

Best practice or prevention: Don't assume that liquid drugs are less likely to cause harm than parenteral ones. Pediatric and geriatric patients often receive liquid drugs and may be especially sensitive to the effects of an inaccurate dose. If a unit-dose form isn't available, calculate carefully, and double-check your math and the drug label.

Labels and toxicity

Error: A container of 5% acetic acid, used to clean tracheostomy tubing, was left near nebulization equipment in the room of a 10-month-old infant. A respiratory therapist mistook the liquid for normal saline solution and used it to dilute albuterol for the child's nebulizer treatment. During treatment, the child experienced bronchospasm, hypercapnic dyspnea, tachypnea, and tachycardia.

Best practice or prevention: Leaving potentially dangerous chemicals near patients is extremely risky, especially when the container labels don't indicate toxicity. To prevent such problems, read the label on every drug you prepare and never give anything that isn't labeled.

Dosage equations

Error: A 13-month study at Albany (N.Y.) Medical Center examined 200 prescribing errors arising from the use of dosage equations. Almost 70% involved children, for whom dosage equations are commonly used. Mistakes in decimal point placement, mathematical calculation, or expression of the regimen accounted for more than 50% of the errors. Examples include prescribing the entire day's drug as a single dose instead of at intervals and giving an entire day's dose at each interval. Use of dosage equations invites drug errors.

Best practice or prevention: Alternatives to dosage equations include using

preestablished ranges or tables, incorporating a calculator into a computer order entry system, and requiring both the calculated dose and dosage equation on orders to facilitate independent checks.

After you calculate a drug dosage, always have another nurse calculate it independently to double-check your results. If doubts or questions remain or if the calculations don't match, ask a pharmacist to calculate the dose before you give the drug.

Air bubbles in pump tubing

Error: After starting an I.V. drip to give insulin, 2 units/hour, to a 9-year-old patient, a nurse noted air bubbles in the tubing and pump chamber. To remove them and promote proper flow, she disconnected the tubing and increased the pump rate to 200 ml/hour. When the bubbles were cleared, she reconnected the tubing and restarted the infusion without resetting the rate. The child received about 50 units of insulin before the error was detected. Fortunately, the child wasn't harmed.

Best practice or prevention: To clear bubbles from I.V. tubing, never increase the pump's flow rate to flush the line. Instead, remove the tubing from the pump, disconnect it from the patient, and use the flow-control clamp to establish gravity flow. When the bubbles have been removed, return the tubing to the pump, restart the infusion, and recheck the flow rate.

Misplacing decimals

Error: A patient in the intensive care unit was to receive the opioid fentanyl, 12.5 to 25 mcg I.V. every 4 to 6 hours, p.r.n., for pain. Unit stock consisted of 5-ml ampules of fentanyl 0.05 mg/ml, so each ampule contained 0.25 mg (250 mcg). A nurse preparing a dose confused the volume needed when she converted from milligrams to micrograms and gave 5 ml, thinking it contained 25 mcg. The patient suffered respiratory arrest but was resuscitated.

Best practice or prevention: Numerous serious fentanyl errors have been reported, and a misplaced decimal point caused many of them. A safer alternative for intermittent dosing is I.V. morphine. Fentanyl doses are best prepared in the pharmacy

rather than in the unit. If a fentanyl dose must be prepared, refer to dosing charts, follow the facility's protocols, and ask another nurse to check your calculations.

Incorrect administration route

Error: A nurse was caring for a patient who had a jejunostomy tube for oral drugs and a central I.V. line for hyperalimentation and I.V. drugs. At the bedside was a stock bottle of digoxin elixir. After checking the concentration, the nurse used a syringe to withdraw 2.5 ml of elixir for a 0.125-mg dose. She then mistakenly gave the elixir through the central line rather than the jejunostomy tube.

Using an incorrect route put the patient at risk for overdose and secondary infection from unsterile I.V. administration. Fortunately, he was receiving antibiotics for a preexisting infection and suffered no adverse reactions.

Best practice or prevention: This case emphasizes the need to ensure that the right route is being used to give any drug. When the patient has multiple lines, label the distal end of each line. Using a parenteral syringe to prepare oral liquid drugs increases the chance for error because the syringe tip fits easily into I.V. ports. To safely give an oral drug through a feeding tube, use a dose prepared by the pharmacy and a syringe with the appropriate tip.

Stress

Error: A nurse-anesthetist gave the sedative midazolam to the wrong patient. When she discovered the error, she grabbed what she thought was a vial of the antidote flumazenil (Romazicon), withdrew 2.5 ml, and gave it. When the patient didn't respond, she realized she'd grabbed a vial of ondansetron (Zofran), an antiemetic, instead. Another practitioner assisted with proper I.V. administration of flumazenil, and the patient recovered without harm.

Best practice or prevention: Committing a serious error can cause enormous stress and cloud your judgment. If you're involved in a drug error, ask another professional to give the antidote.

Patient teaching

Patients being discharged from an acute care setting may be at a greater risk for adverse drug reactions arising from drug-drug interactions. Changes are frequently made to a patient's regular drug regimen before discharge, either by altering the dose or adding one or more new drugs. Adverse effects may go unnoticed by the practitioner or unreported when the patient is at home. Carefully review the patient's drugs upon discharge, inform him of any potential adverse drug effects to be aware of, and tell him to call the prescriber if adverse effects become bothersome.

The following general guidelines will help to ensure that the patient receives the maximum therapeutic benefit and avoids adverse reactions, accidental overdose, and harmful changes in effectiveness.

● Instruct the patient to learn the brand and generic names of all drugs he's taking and to inform his regular prescriber about their use. Before you give a patient a drug, ask him to report unusual reactions experienced in the past, allergies to foods and other substances, special medical problems, and drugs taken over the last few weeks, including OTC drugs or herbs.

● Advise the patient to always read the label before taking a drug, to take it exactly as prescribed, and never to share prescription drugs.

● Warn the patient not to change brands of a drug without consulting his prescriber, to avoid harmful changes in effectiveness. Certain generic preparations aren't equivalent in effect to brand-name preparations of the same drug.

● Tell the patient to check the expiration date before taking a drug.

● Instruct the patient to safely discard drugs that are outdated or no longer needed and to keep discarded drugs out of the reach of children and pets.

● Tell the patient to store each drug in its original container, at room temperature (unless directed otherwise), and in places that aren't accessible to children or exposed to sunlight. Discourage storage in the bathroom medicine cabinet, in the kitchen close to heat, or in the glove compartment or trunk of an automobile, where extremes of temperature and humidity will cause deterioration.

● Caution the patient about mixing different drugs in a single container, removing a drug from its original container, or remov-

ing the label. Relying on memory to identify a drug and specific directions for its use is dangerous.

● If the patient must remove pills from their original container to use a daily or weekly "medication planner" as a reminder, tell him to keep an index card with the planner that includes the drug's name, strength, dosage instructions, and physical description written on the card. This is particularly important when he's taking more than one prescription.

● Stress how important it is for the patient to tell the prescriber about adverse reactions he experiences during drug therapy.

● Advise the patient to have all prescriptions filled at the same pharmacy so that the pharmacist can identify and warn against potentially harmful drug interactions. Also, tell the patient to inform the pharmacist and prescriber about any OTC drugs or herbs he takes.

● Instruct the patient to call the prescriber, poison control center, or pharmacist immediately if he or someone else has taken an overdose. The National Poison Control Center phone number is 1-800-222-1222. Tell the patient to keep this and other emergency telephone numbers handy at all times.

● Advise the patient to inform medical personnel about use of drugs before undergoing surgery (including dental surgery).

● Tell the patient to have a sufficient supply of drugs when traveling. He should carry them with him in their original containers and not pack them in his luggage. Also, recommend that a patient who travels abroad should carry a letter from his prescriber authorizing the use of the drug, especially if the drug is a controlled substance.

4

Drug classifications

Alkylating drugs

busulfan
carboplatin
carmustine
chlorambucil
cisplatin
cyclophosphamide
dacarbazine
ifosfamide
lomustine
mechlorethamine hydrochloride
melphalan
oxaliplatin
thiotepa

INDICATIONS
➤ **Various tumors, especially those with large volume and slow cell-turnover rate**

ACTION
Alkylating drugs appear to act independently of a specific cell-cycle phase. They're polyfunctional compounds that can be divided chemically into five groups: nitrogen mustards, ethylene imines, alkyl sulfonates, triazines, and nitrosoureas. These drugs are highly reactive; they primarily target nucleic acids and form links with the nuclei of different molecules. This allows the drugs to cross-link double-stranded DNA and to prevent strands from separating for replication, which may contribute to these drugs' ability to destroy cells.

ADVERSE REACTIONS
The most common adverse reactions are bone marrow depression, chills, diarrhea, fever, flank pain, hair loss, leukopenia, nausea, redness or pain at the injection site, sore throat, swelling of the feet or lower legs, thrombocytopenia, secondary leukemia, infertility, and vomiting.

CONTRAINDICATIONS & CAUTIONS
● Contraindicated in patients hypersensitive to these drugs.

● Use cautiously in patients receiving other cell-destroying drugs or radiation therapy.
● In pregnant women, use only when potential benefits to the mother outweigh known risks to the fetus. Breast-feeding women should stop breast-feeding during therapy because drugs are found in breast milk. In children, safety and effectiveness of many alkylating drugs haven't been established. Elderly patients have an increased risk of adverse reactions; monitor these patients closely.

Alpha blockers (peripherally acting)

doxazosin mesylate
phentolamine mesylate
prazosin hydrochloride
terazosin hydrochloride

INDICATIONS
➤ **Hypertension, or mild to moderate urinary obstruction in men with BPH**

ACTION
Selective alpha blockers decrease vascular resistance and increase vein capacity, thereby lowering blood pressure and causing nasal and scleroconjunctival congestion, ptosis, orthostatic and exercise hypotension, mild to moderate miosis, interference with ejaculation, and pink, warm skin. They also relax nonvascular smooth muscle, especially in the prostate capsule, which reduces urinary problems in men with BPH. Because alpha$_1$ blockers don't block alpha$_2$ receptors, they don't cause transmitter overflow.

Nonselective alpha blockers antagonize both alpha$_1$ and alpha$_2$ receptors. Generally, alpha blockade results in tachycardia, palpitations, and increased renin secretion because of abnormally large amounts of norepinephrine (from transmitter overflow) released from adrenergic nerve endings as a result of the

blockade of alpha$_1$ and alpha$_2$ receptors. Norepinephrine's effects are counterproductive to the major uses of nonselective alpha blockers.

ADVERSE REACTIONS
Alpha blockers may cause severe orthostatic hypotension and syncope, especially with the first few doses, an effect commonly called the "first-dose effect." The most common adverse effects of alpha$_1$ blockade are dizziness, headache, drowsiness, somnolence, and malaise. These drugs also may cause tachycardia, palpitations, fluid retention (from excess renin secretion), nasal and ocular congestion, and aggravation of respiratory tract infection.

CONTRAINDICATIONS & CAUTIONS
• Contraindicated in patients with MI, coronary insufficiency, or angina or with hypersensitivity to these drugs or any of their components. Also contraindicated in combination therapy with phosphodiesterase type 5 inhibitors (sildenafil, tadalafil, vardenafil), although tadalafil may be taken with tamsulosin 0.4 mg daily.
• In pregnant or breast-feeding women, use cautiously. In children, the safety and effectiveness of many alpha blockers haven't been established; use cautiously. In elderly patients, hypotensive effects may be more pronounced.

Alzheimer disease drugs

donepezil hydrochloride
galantamine hydrobromide
memantine hydrochloride
rivastigmine tartrate
tacrine hydrochloride

INDICATIONS
➤ **Treatment of mild to moderate dementia of the Alzheimer type**

ACTION
Current theories attribute signs and symptoms of Alzheimer disease to a deficiency of cholinergic neurotransmission. It's suggested that these drugs improve cholinergic function by increasing acetylcholine through reversible inhibition of its hydro-

lysis by cholinesterase. Memantine is an N-methyl-D-aspartate (NMDA) receptor antagonist. Persistent activation of the NMDA receptors is thought to contribute to symptoms of Alzheimer disease. There is no evidence that any of the drugs alter the course of the underlying disease process.

ADVERSE REACTIONS
Weight loss, diarrhea, anorexia, nausea, vomiting, dizziness, headache, bradyarrhythmias, elevated liver function test results (tacrine); hypertension and constipation (memantine).

CONTRAINDICATIONS & CAUTIONS
• Contraindicated in patients hypersensitive to any of the drug components.
• May exaggerate neuromuscular blocking effects of succinylcholine-type and similar neuromuscular blocking agents used during anesthesia.
• Use cautiously with concomitant drugs that slow heart rate. There is an increased risk for heart block.
• Use cautiously with NSAIDs because the drug increases gastric acid secretion. There is increased risk of developing ulcers and active or occult GI bleeding.
• Use cautiously in patients with moderate hepatic or renal impairment. The drugs are not recommended in severe hepatic impairment or severe renal impairment (creatinine clearance less than 9 ml/minute).
• Use cautiously in patients with a history of asthma or COPD.

Aminoglycosides

amikacin sulfate
gentamicin sulfate
neomycin sulfate
streptomycin sulfate
tobramycin sulfate

INDICATIONS
➤ **Septicemia; postoperative, pulmonary, intra-abdominal, and urinary tract infections; skin, soft tissue, bone, and joint infections; aerobic gram-negative bacillary meningitis not susceptible to other antibiotics; serious staphylococcal, *Pseudomonas***

aeruginosa, and *Klebsiella* infections; enterococcal infections; nosocomial pneumonia; anaerobic infections involving *Bacteroides fragilis;* tuberculosis; initial empiric therapy in febrile, leukopenic patients

ACTION
Aminoglycosides are bactericidal. They bind directly and irreversibly to 30S ribosomal subunits, inhibiting bacterial protein synthesis. They're active against many aerobic gram-negative and some aerobic gram-positive organisms and can be used in combination with other antibiotics for short courses of therapy.

ADVERSE REACTIONS
Ototoxicity and nephrotoxicity are the most serious complications. Neuromuscular blockade also may occur. Oral forms most commonly cause diarrhea, nausea, and vomiting. Parenteral drugs may cause vein irritation, phlebitis, and sterile abscess.

CONTRAINDICATIONS & CAUTIONS
● Contraindicated in patients hypersensitive to these drugs.
● Use cautiously in patients with a neuromuscular disorder and in those taking neuromuscular blockades.
● Use at lower dosages in patients with renal impairment.
● In pregnant women, use cautiously. In breast-feeding women, safety hasn't been established. In neonates and premature infants, the half-life of aminoglycosides is prolonged because of immature renal systems. In infants and children, dosage adjustment may be needed. Elderly patients have an increased risk of nephrotoxicity and commonly need a lower dose and longer intervals; they're also susceptible to ototoxicity and superinfection.

Angiotensin-converting enzyme inhibitors

benazepril hydrochloride
captopril
enalaprilat
enalapril maleate
fosinopril sodium
lisinopril
perindopril erbumine
quinapril hydrochloride
ramipril
trandolapril

INDICATIONS
➤ Hypertension, heart failure, left ventricular dysfunction (LVD), MI (with ramipril and lisinopril), and diabetic nephropathy (with captopril)

ACTION
ACE inhibitors prevent conversion of angiotensin I to angiotensin II, a potent vasoconstrictor. Besides decreasing vasoconstriction and thus reducing peripheral arterial resistance, inhibiting angiotensin II decreases adrenocortical secretion of aldosterone. This reduces sodium and water retention and extracellular fluid volume. ACE inhibition also causes increased levels of bradykinin, which results in vasodilation. This decreases heart rate and systemic vascular resistance.

ADVERSE REACTIONS
The most common adverse effects of therapeutic doses are angioedema of the face and limbs, dry cough, dysgeusia, fatigue, headache, hyperkalemia, hypotension, proteinuria, rash, and tachycardia. Severe hypotension may occur at toxic drug levels.

CONTRAINDICATIONS & CAUTIONS
● Contraindicated in patients hypersensitive to these drugs.
● Use cautiously in patients with impaired renal function or serious autoimmune disease and in those taking other drugs known to decrease WBC count or immune response.
● Women of childbearing potential taking ACE inhibitors should report suspected pregnancy immediately to prescriber. High

risks of fetal morbidity and mortality are linked to ACE inhibitors, especially in the second and third trimesters. Some ACE inhibitors appear in breast milk. To avoid adverse effects in infants, instruct patient to stop breast-feeding during therapy. In children, safety and effectiveness haven't been established; give drug only if potential benefits outweigh risks. Elderly patients may need lower doses because of impaired drug clearance.

Antacids

aluminum hydroxide
calcium carbonate
magnesium oxide
sodium bicarbonate

INDICATIONS
➤ **Hyperacidity; hyperphosphatemia (aluminum hydroxide); hypomagnesemia (magnesium oxide); postmenopausal hypocalcemia (calcium carbonate)**

ACTION
Antacids reduce the total acid load in the GI tract and elevate gastric pH to reduce pepsin activity. They also strengthen the gastric mucosal barrier and increase esophageal sphincter tone.

ADVERSE REACTIONS
Antacids containing aluminum may cause aluminum intoxication, constipation, hypophosphatemia, intestinal obstruction, and osteomalacia. Antacids containing magnesium may cause diarrhea or hypermagnesemia (in renal failure). Calcium carbonate, magaldrate, magnesium oxide, and sodium bicarbonate may cause constipation, milk-alkali syndrome, or rebound hyperacidity.

CONTRAINDICATIONS & CAUTIONS
• Calcium carbonate and magnesium oxide are contraindicated in patients with severe renal disease. Sodium bicarbonate is contraindicated in patients with hypertension, renal disease, or edema; patients who are vomiting; patients receiving diuretics or continuous GI suction; and patients on sodium-restricted diets.

• In patients with mild renal impairment, give magnesium oxide cautiously.
• Give aluminum preparations and calcium carbonate cautiously in elderly patients; in those receiving antidiarrheals, antispasmodics, or anticholinergics; and in those with dehydration, fluid restriction, chronic renal disease, or suspected intestinal absorption problems.
• Pregnant women should consult their prescriber before using antacids. Breast-feeding women may take antacids. In infants, serious adverse effects are more likely from changes in fluid and electrolyte balance; monitor them closely. Elderly patients have an increased risk of adverse reactions; monitor them closely; also, give these patients aluminum preparations, calcium carbonate, and magnesium oxide cautiously.

Antianginals

Beta blockers
atenolol
esmolol hydrochloride
metoprolol
nadolol
propranolol hydrochloride

Calcium channel blockers
amlodipine besylate
diltiazem hydrochloride
nicardipine hydrochloride
nifedipine
verapamil hydrochloride

Nitrates
isosorbide dinitrate
isosorbide mononitrate
nitroglycerin

INDICATIONS
➤ **Moderate to severe angina (beta blockers); classic, effort-induced angina and Prinzmetal angina (calcium channel blockers); recurrent angina (long-acting nitrates and topical, transdermal, transmucosal, and oral extended-release nitroglycerin); acute angina (S.L. nitroglycerin and S.L. or chewable isosorbide dinitrate); unstable angina (I.V. nitroglycerin)**

ACTION

Beta blockers decrease catecholamine-induced increases in heart rate, blood pressure, and myocardial contraction. Calcium channel blockers inhibit the flow of calcium through muscle cells, which dilates coronary arteries and decreases systemic vascular resistance, known as afterload. Nitrates decrease afterload and left ventricular end-diastolic pressure, or preload, and increase blood flow through collateral coronary vessels.

ADVERSE REACTIONS

Beta blockers may cause bradycardia, cough, diarrhea, disturbing dreams, dizziness, dyspnea, fatigue, fever, heart failure, hypotension, lethargy, nausea, peripheral edema, and wheezing. Calcium channel blockers may cause bradycardia, confusion, constipation, depression, diarrhea, dizziness, dyspepsia, edema, elevated liver enzyme levels (transient), fatigue, flushing, headache, hypotension, insomnia, nervousness, and rash. Nitrates may cause flushing, headache, orthostatic hypotension, reflex tachycardia, rash, syncope, and vomiting.

CONTRAINDICATIONS & CAUTIONS

● Beta blockers are contraindicated in patients hypersensitive to them and in patients with cardiogenic shock, sinus bradycardia, heart block greater than first degree, or bronchial asthma. Calcium channel blockers are contraindicated in patients with severe hypotension or heart block greater than first degree (except with functioning pacemaker). Nitrates are contraindicated in patients with severe anemia, cerebral hemorrhage, head trauma, glaucoma, or hyperthyroidism or in patients using phosphodiesterase type 5 inhibitors (sildenafil, tadalafil, vardenafil).
● Use beta blockers cautiously in patients with nonallergic bronchospastic disorders, diabetes mellitus, or impaired hepatic or renal function. Use calcium channel blockers cautiously in patients with hepatic or renal impairment, bradycardia, heart failure, or cardiogenic shock. Use nitrates cautiously in patients with hypotension or recent MI.
● In pregnant women, use beta blockers cautiously. Recommendations for breast-feeding vary by drug; use beta blockers and calcium channel blockers cautiously. In children, safety and effectiveness haven't been established. Check with prescriber before giving these drugs to children. Elderly patients have an increased risk of adverse reactions; use cautiously.

Antiarrhythmics

adenosine

Class IA
disopyramide
procainamide hydrochloride
quinidine bisulfate
quinidine gluconate
quinidine sulfate

Class IB
lidocaine hydrochloride
mexiletine hydrochloride
phenytoin sodium

Class IC
flecainide acetate
propafenone hydrochloride

Class II (beta blockers)
amiodarone hydrochloride
dofetilide
ibutilide fumarate
sotalol hydrochloride

Class IV (calcium channel blocker)
verapamil hydrochloride

INDICATIONS
➤ **Atrial and ventricular arrhythmias**

ACTION
Class I drugs reduce the inward current carried by sodium ions, which stabilizes neuronal cardiac membranes. Class IA drugs depress phase 0, prolong the action potential, and stabilize cardiac membranes. Class IB drugs depress phase 0, shorten the action potential, and stabilize cardiac membranes. Class IC drugs block the transport of sodium ions, which

decreases conduction velocity but not re-polarization rate. Class II drugs decrease the heart rate, myocardial contractility, blood pressure, and AV node conduction. Class III drugs prolong the action potential and refractory period. Class IV drugs decrease myocardial contractility and oxygen demand by inhibiting calcium ion influx; they also dilate coronary arteries and arterioles.

ADVERSE REACTIONS
Most antiarrhythmics can aggravate existing arrhythmias or cause new ones. They also may produce CNS disturbances, such as dizziness or fatigue, GI problems, such as nausea, vomiting, or altered bowel elimination; hypersensitivity reactions; and hypotension. Some antiarrhythmics may worsen heart failure. Class II drugs may cause bronchoconstriction.

CONTRAINDICATIONS & CAUTIONS
• Contraindicated in patients hypersensitive to these drugs.
• Many antiarrhythmics are contraindicated or require cautious use in patients with cardiogenic shock, digitalis toxicity, and second- or third-degree heart block (unless patient has a pacemaker or implantable cardioverter defibrillator).
• In pregnant women, use only if potential benefits to the mother outweigh risks to the fetus. In breast-feeding women, use cautiously; many antiarrhythmics appear in breast milk. In children, monitor closely because they have an increased risk of adverse reactions. In elderly patients, use these drugs cautiously because these patients may exhibit physiologic alterations in CV system.

Antibiotic antineoplastics

bleomycin sulfate
daunorubicin hydrochloride
doxorubicin hydrochloride
epirubicin hydrochloride
idarubicin hydrochloride
mitomycin

INDICATIONS
➤ Various tumors

ACTION
Although classified as antibiotics, these drugs destroy cells, thus ruling out their use as antimicrobials alone. They interfere with proliferation of malignant cells in several ways. Their action may be specific to cell-cycle phase, not specific to cell-cycle phase, or both. Some of these drugs act like alkylating drugs or antimetabolites. By binding to or creating complexes with DNA, antibiotic antineoplastics directly or indirectly inhibit DNA, RNA, and protein synthesis.

ADVERSE REACTIONS
The most common adverse reactions include anxiety, bone marrow depression, chills, confusion, diarrhea, fever, flank or joint pain, hair loss, nausea, redness or pain at the injection site, sore throat, swelling of the feet or lower legs, vomiting, and cardiomyopathy.

CONTRAINDICATIONS & CAUTIONS
• Contraindicated in patients hypersensitive to these drugs.
• In pregnant women, avoid antineoplastics. Breast-feeding during therapy isn't recommended. In children, safety and effectiveness of some drugs haven't been established; use cautiously. In elderly patients, use cautiously because of their increased risk of adverse reactions.

Anticholinergics

atropine sulfate
benztropine mesylate
dicyclomine hydrochloride
scopolamine

INDICATIONS
➤ **Prevention of motion sickness, preoperative reduction of secretions and blockage of cardiac reflexes, adjunct treatment of peptic ulcers and other GI disorders, blockage of cholinomimetic effects of cholinesterase inhibitors or other drugs, and (for benztropine) various spastic conditions, including acute dystonic reactions, muscle rigidity, parkinsonism, and extrapyramidal disorders**

ACTION

Anticholinergics competitively antagonize the actions of acetylcholine and other cholinergic agonists at muscarinic receptors.

ADVERSE REACTIONS

Therapeutic doses commonly cause blurred vision, constipation, cycloplegia, decreased sweating or anhidrosis, dry mouth, headache, mydriasis, palpitations, tachycardia, and urinary hesitancy and retention. These reactions usually disappear when therapy stops. Toxicity can cause signs and symptoms resembling psychosis (disorientation, confusion, hallucinations, delusions, anxiety, agitation, and restlessness); dilated, nonreactive pupils; blurred vision; hot, dry, flushed skin; dry mucous membranes; dysphagia; decreased or absent bowel sounds; urine retention; hyperthermia; tachycardia; hypertension; and increased respirations.

CONTRAINDICATIONS & CAUTIONS

● Contraindicated in patients hypersensitive to these drugs and in those with angle-closure glaucoma, renal or GI obstructive disease, reflux esophagitis, or myasthenia gravis.
● Use cautiously in patients with heart disease, GI infection, open-angle glaucoma, prostatic hypertrophy, hypertension, hyperthyroidism, ulcerative colitis, autonomic neuropathy, or hiatal hernia with reflux esophagitis.
● In pregnant women, safe use hasn't been established. In breast-feeding women, avoid anticholinergics because they may decrease milk production; some may appear in breast milk and cause infant toxicity. In children, safety and effectiveness haven't been established. Patients older than age 40 may be more sensitive to these drugs. In elderly patients, use cautiously and give a reduced dosage, as indicated.

Anticoagulants

Coumarin derivative
warfarin sodium

Heparin derivative
heparin sodium

Low-molecular-weight heparins
dalteparin sodium
enoxaparin sodium
tinzaparin sodium

Selective factor Xa inhibitor
fondaparinux sodium

Thrombin inhibitors
argatroban
bivalirudin
desirudin

INDICATIONS

➤ Pulmonary emboli, deep vein thrombosis, thrombus, blood clotting, DIC, unstable angina, MI, atrial fibrillation

ACTION

Heparin derivatives accelerate formation of an antithrombin III-thrombin complex. It inactivates thrombin and prevents conversion of fibrinogen to fibrin. The coumarin derivative warfarin inhibits vitamin K–dependent activation of clotting factors II, VII, IX, and X, which are formed in the liver. Thrombin inhibitors directly bind to thrombin and inhibit its action. Selective factor Xa inhibitors bind to antithrombin III, which in turn initiates the neutralization of factor Xa.

ADVERSE REACTIONS

Anticoagulants commonly cause bleeding and may cause hypersensitivity reactions. Warfarin may cause agranulocytosis, alopecia (long-term use), anorexia, dermatitis, fever, nausea, tissue necrosis or gangrene, urticaria, and vomiting. Heparin derivatives may cause thrombocytopenia and may increase liver enzyme levels. Nonhemorrhagic adverse reactions associated with thrombin inhibitors may include back pain, bradycardia, and hypotension.

CONTRAINDICATIONS & CAUTIONS
● Contraindicated in patients hypersensitive to these drugs or any of their components; in patients with aneurysm, active bleeding, CV hemorrhage, hemorrhagic blood dyscrasias, hemophilia, severe hypertension, pericardial effusions, or pericarditis; and in patients undergoing major surgery, neurosurgery, or ophthalmic surgery.
● Use cautiously in patients with severe diabetes, renal impairment, severe trauma, ulcerations, or vasculitis.
● Most anticoagulants (except warfarin) may be used in pregnancy only if clearly necessary. In pregnant women and those who have just had a threatened or complete spontaneous abortion, warfarin is contraindicated. Women should avoid breast-feeding during therapy. Infants, especially neonates, may be more susceptible to anticoagulants because of vitamin K deficiency. Elderly patients are at greater risk for hemorrhage because of altered hemostatic mechanisms or age-related deterioration of hepatic and renal functions.

Anticonvulsants

carbamazepine
clonazepam
diazepam
fosphenytoin sodium
gabapentin
lamotrigine
levetiracetam
magnesium sulfate
oxcarbazepine
phenobarbital
phenobarbital sodium
phenytoin sodium
phenytoin sodium (extended)
primidone
tiagabine hydrochloride
topiramate
valproate sodium
valproic acid
zonisamide

INDICATIONS
➤ Seizure disorders; acute, isolated seizures not caused by seizure disorders; status epilepticus; prevention of seizures after trauma or craniotomy; neuropathic pain

ACTION
Anticonvulsants include six classes of drugs: selected hydantoin derivatives, barbiturates, benzodiazepines, succinimides, iminostilbene derivatives (carbamazepine), and carboxylic acid derivatives. Magnesium sulfate is a miscellaneous anticonvulsant. Some hydantoin derivatives and carbamazepine inhibit the spread of seizure activity in the motor cortex. Some barbiturates and succinimides limit seizure activity by increasing the threshold for motor cortex stimuli. Selected benzodiazepines and carboxylic acid derivatives may increase inhibition of GABA in brain neurons. Magnesium sulfate interferes with the release of acetylcholine at the myoneural junction.

ADVERSE REACTIONS
Anticonvulsants can cause adverse CNS effects, such as ataxia, confusion, somnolence, and tremor. Many anticonvulsants also cause CV disorders, such as arrhythmias and hypotension; GI effects, such as vomiting; and hematologic disorders, such as agranulocytosis, bone marrow depression, leukopenia, and thrombocytopenia. Stevens-Johnson syndrome, other severe rashes, and abnormal liver function test results may occur with certain anticonvulsants.

CONTRAINDICATIONS & CAUTIONS
● Contraindicated in patients hypersensitive to these drugs.
● Carbamazepine is contraindicated within 14 days of MAO inhibitor use.
● Use cautiously in patients with blood dyscrasias. Also, use barbiturates cautiously in patients with suicidal ideation.
● In pregnant women, therapy usually continues despite the fetal risks caused by some anticonvulsants (barbiturates, phenytoin). In breast-feeding women, the safety of many anticonvulsants hasn't been established. Children, especially young ones, are sensitive to the CNS depression of some anticonvulsants; use cautiously. Elderly patients are sensitive to CNS effects and may require lower doses. Also, some anticonvulsants may

take longer to be eliminated because of decreased renal function, and parenteral use is more likely to cause apnea, hypotension, bradycardia, and cardiac arrest.

Antidepressants, tricyclic

amitriptyline hydrochloride
clomipramine hydrochloride
desipramine hydrochloride
doxepin hydrochloride
imipramine hydrochloride
imipramine pamoate
nortriptyline hydrochloride

INDICATIONS
➤ **Depression, anxiety (doxepin hydrochloride), obsessive-compulsive disorder (clomipramine), enuresis in children older than age 6 (imipramine), neuropathic pain**

ACTION
Tricyclic antidepressants may inhibit reuptake of norepinephrine and serotonin in CNS nerve terminals (presynaptic neurons), thus enhancing the concentration and activity of neurotransmitters in the synaptic cleft. Tricyclic antidepressants also exert antihistaminic, sedative, anticholinergic, vasodilatory, and quinidine-like effects.

ADVERSE REACTIONS
Adverse reactions include anticholinergic effects, orthostatic hypotension, and sedation. The tertiary amines (amitriptyline, doxepin, and imipramine) exert the strongest sedative effects; tolerance usually develops in a few weeks. Amoxapine is most likely to cause seizures, especially with overdose. Tricyclic antidepressants may cause CV effects such as T-wave abnormalities, conduction disturbances, and arrhythmias.

CONTRAINDICATIONS & CAUTIONS
● Contraindicated in patients hypersensitive to these drugs and in patients with urine retention or angle-closure glaucoma.
● Tricyclic antidepressants are contraindicated within 2 weeks of MAO inhibitor therapy.

● Use cautiously in patients with suicidal tendencies, schizophrenia, paranoia, seizure disorders, CV disease, or impaired hepatic function.
● In pregnant and breast-feeding women, safety hasn't been established; use cautiously. In children younger than age 12, tricyclic antidepressants aren't recommended. Elderly patients are more sensitive to therapeutic and adverse effects; they need lower dosages.

Antidiabetics

acarbose
chlorpropamide
glimepiride
glipizide
glyburide
metformin hydrochloride
miglitol
nateglinide
pioglitazone hydrochloride
pramlintide acetate
repaglinide
rosiglitazone maleate
sitagliptin phosphate

INDICATIONS
➤ **Mild to moderately severe, stable, nonketotic, type 2 diabetes mellitus that can't be controlled by diet alone**

ACTION
Oral antidiabetics come in several types. Sulfonylureas are sulfonamide derivatives that aren't antibacterial. They lower glucose levels by stimulating insulin release from the pancreas. These drugs work only in the presence of functioning beta cells in the islet tissue of the pancreas. After prolonged administration, they produce hypoglycemia by acting outside of the pancreas, including reduced glucose production by the liver and enhanced peripheral sensitivity to insulin. The latter may result from an increased number of insulin receptors or from changes after insulin binding. Sulfonylureas are divided into first-generation drugs, such as chlorpropamide, and second-generation drugs, such as glyburide, glimepiride, and glipizide. Although their mechanisms of action are

similar, the second-generation drugs carry a more lipophilic side chain, are more potent, and cause fewer adverse reactions. Their most important difference is their duration of action.

Meglitinides, such as nateglinide and repaglinide, are nonsulfonylurea antidiabetics that stimulate the release of insulin from the pancreas.

Metformin decreases hepatic glucose production, reduces intestinal glucose absorption, and improves insulin sensitivity by increasing peripheral glucose uptake and utilization. With metformin therapy, insulin secretion remains unchanged, and fasting insulin levels and all-day insulin response may decrease.

Alpha-glucosidase inhibitors, such as acarbose and miglitol, delay digestion of carbohydrates, resulting in a smaller rise in glucose levels. Pramlintide, a human amylin analogue, slows the rate at which food leaves the stomach, decreasing postprandial increase in glucose level, and reduces appetite.

Rosiglitazone and pioglitazone are thiazolidinediones, which lower glucose levels by improving insulin sensitivity. These drugs are potent and highly selective agonists for receptors found in insulin-sensitive tissues, such as adipose, skeletal muscle, and liver.

Sitagliptin increases insulin release by inhibiting the enzyme DPP-4.

ADVERSE REACTIONS

Sulfonylureas cause dose-related reactions that usually respond to decreased dosage: anorexia, headache, heartburn, nausea, paresthesia, vomiting, and weakness. Hypoglycemia may follow excessive dosage, increased exercise, decreased food intake, or alcohol use.

The most serious adverse reaction linked to metformin is lactic acidosis. It's a rare effect and most likely to occur in patients with renal dysfunction. Other reactions to metformin include dermatitis, GI upset, megaloblastic anemia, rash, and unpleasant or metallic taste.

Thiazolidinediones may cause fluid retention leading to or exacerbating heart failure. Alpha-glucosidase inhibitors can cause abdominal pain, diarrhea, and flatulence.

CONTRAINDICATIONS & CAUTIONS

● Contraindicated in patients hypersensitive to these drugs and in patients with diabetic ketoacidosis with or without coma. Metformin is also contraindicated in patients with renal disease or metabolic acidosis and generally should be avoided in patients with hepatic disease.

● Use sulfonylureas cautiously in patients with renal or hepatic disease. Use metformin cautiously in patients with adrenal or pituitary insufficiency and in debilitated and malnourished patients. Alpha-glucosidase inhibitors should be used cautiously in patients with mild to moderate renal insufficiency. Thiazolidinediones aren't recommended in patients with edema, heart failure, or liver disease.

● In pregnant or breast-feeding women, use is contraindicated. Oral antidiabetics appear in small amounts in breast milk and may cause hypoglycemia in the infant. In children, oral antidiabetics aren't effective in type 1 diabetes mellitus. Elderly patients may be more sensitive to these drugs, usually need lower dosages, and are more likely to develop neurologic symptoms of hypoglycemia; monitor these patients closely. In elderly patients, avoid chlorpropamide use because of its long duration of action.

Antidiarrheals

bismuth subsalicylate
calcium polycarbophil
diphenoxylate hydrochloride and atropine sulfate
kaolin and pectin mixtures
loperamide hydrochloride
octreotide acetate

INDICATIONS

➤ **Mild, acute, or chronic diarrhea. Octreotide acetate is indicated for certain cancers that cause diarrhea**

ACTION

Bismuth preparations may have a mild water-binding capacity, may absorb toxins, and provide a protective coating for the intestinal mucosa. Kaolin and pectin mixtures decrease fluid in the stool by absorbing bacteria and toxins that cause diarrhea.

ADVERSE REACTIONS

Bismuth preparations may cause salicylism (with high doses) or temporary darkening of tongue and stools. Kaolin and pectin mixtures may cause constipation and fecal impaction or ulceration.

CONTRAINDICATIONS & CAUTIONS

• Contraindicated in patients hypersensitive to these drugs.

• Some antidiarrheals may appear in breast milk; check individual drugs for specific recommendations. For infants younger than age 2, don't give kaolin and pectin mixtures. For children or teenagers recovering from flu or chickenpox, consult prescriber before giving bismuth subsalicylate. For elderly patients, use caution when giving antidiarrheal drugs.

Antiemetics

aprepitant
dimenhydrinate
dronabinol
franisetron hydrochloride
meclizine hydrochloride
metoclopramide hydrochloride
nabilone
ondansetron hydrochloride
palonosetron hydrochloride
prochlorperazine
scopolamine
scopolamine hydrobromide
trimethobenzamide hydrochloride

INDICATIONS

➤ **Nausea, vomiting, motion sickness, and vertigo**

ACTION

For antihistamines (dimenhydrinate, meclizine hydrochloride, trimethobenzamide) the mechanism of action is unclear. Phenothiazines (prochlorperazine) work by blocking the dopaminergic receptors in the chemoreceptor trigger zone of the brain. Serotonin-receptor antagonists (dolasetron, granisetron, ondansetron) block serotonin stimulation centrally in the chemoreceptor trigger zone and peripherally in vagal nerve terminals. Nabilone works on the cannabinoid receptor system, and should be used only in those who have failed other antiemetics.

ADVERSE REACTIONS

Antiemetics may cause asthenia, fatigue, dizziness, headache, insomnia, abdominal pain, anorexia, constipation, diarrhea, epigastric discomfort, gastritis, heartburn, nausea, vomiting, neutropenia, hiccups, tinnitus, dehydration, and fever.

CONTRAINDICATIONS & CAUTIONS

• Contraindicated in patients hypersensitive to any of the drug components.

• Contraindicated in severe vomiting until etiology of vomiting is established.

• Use cautiously in patients with tartrazine and sulfite sensitivities. Antiemetics may cause allergic type reactions including hives, itching, wheezing, asthma, and anaphylaxis.

Antifungals

amphotericin B cholesteryl sulfate
amphotericin B desoxycholate
amphotericin B lipid complex
amphotericin B liposomal
anidulafungin
caspofungin acetate
fluconazole
flucytosine
griseofulvin
itraconazole
ketoconazole
micafungin sodium
nystatin
posaconazole
terbinafine hydrochloride
voriconazole

INDICATIONS

➤ **Use to treat a variety of fungal infections**

ACTION

The amphotericin products bind to sterols in the fungal cell membrane, altering permeability and allowing intracellular components to leak out. These drugs usually inhibit fungal growth and multiplication, but if the level is high enough, the drugs can destroy fungi. The azole class of drugs includes fluconazole, itraconazole, keto-

conazole, and voriconazole. Fluconazole inhibits fungal cytochrome P450, which weakens fungal cell walls. Itraconazole and voriconazole interfere with fungal wall synthesis by inhibiting ergosterol formation and increasing cell wall permeability and osmotic instability. Ketoconazole interferes with sterol synthesis in fungal cells, damaging cell membranes and increasing permeability. Caspofungin inhibits the synthesis of an integral component of fungal cell walls. Flucytosine penetrates the fungal cell wall and alters protein synthesis. Nystatin binds to sterols in fungal cell membranes and alters membrane permeability. Terbinafine inhibits fungal cell growth by inhibiting an enzyme responsible for the manufacture of ergosterol.

ADVERSE REACTIONS

Fluconazole may cause transient elevations of liver enzymes, alkaline phosphatase and bilirubin levels, dizziness, nausea, vomiting, abdominal pain, diarrhea, rash, headache, hypokalemia, elevated BUN and creatinine levels. Itraconazole adverse reactions include headache and nausea. The most common adverse reactions to ketoconazole are nausea and vomiting. Adverse reactions to voriconazole are uncommon. However, the drug may alter renal function and cause vision changes. Common adverse reactions to caspofungin include paresthesia, tachycardia, anorexia, anemia, pain, myalgia, tachypnea, chills, and sweating. Flucytosine may cause bone marrow suppression leading to leukopenia, thrombocytopenia, anemia, pancytopenia, or granulocytopenia. Reactions to nystatin seldom occur, but may include diarrhea, nausea, vomiting, and abdominal pain. Terbinafine may cause abdominal pain, jaundice, diarrhea, flatulence, nausea, anaphylaxis, headache, rash, and vision disturbances.

CONTRAINDICATIONS & CAUTIONS

• Contraindicated in patients hypersensitive to any of the drug components.
• Administer I.V. amphotericin under close clinical observation. Acute infusion reactions can occur including fever, shaking chills, hypotension, anorexia, nausea, vomiting, and tachypnea.

• Caspofungin is contraindicated with concomitant use of cyclosporine because of the possibility of elevated liver enzymes.
• The amphotericin drugs aren't interchangeable and are each prescribed differently.

Antihistamines

azelastine hydrochloride
brompheniramine maleate
cyproheptadine hydrochloride
desloratadine
diphenhydramine hydrochloride
fexofenadine hydrochloride
hydroxyzine embonate
hydroxyzine hydrochloride
hydroxyzine pamoate
loratadine
meclizine hydrochloride
promethazine hydrochloride

INDICATIONS
➤ **Allergic rhinitis, urticaria, pruritus, vertigo, motion sickness, nausea and vomiting, sedation, dyskinesia, parkinsonism**

ACTION
Antihistamines are structurally related chemicals that compete with histamine for histamine H_1-receptor sites on smooth muscle of bronchi, GI tract, and large blood vessels, binding to cellular receptors and preventing access to and subsequent activity of histamine. They don't directly alter histamine or prevent its release.

ADVERSE REACTIONS
Most antihistamines cause drowsiness and impaired motor function early in therapy. They also can cause blurred vision, constipation, and dry mouth and throat. Some antihistamines, such as promethazine, may cause cholestatic jaundice, which may be a hypersensitivity reaction, and may predispose patients to photosensitivity. Promethazine may also cause extrapyramidal reactions with high doses.

CONTRAINDICATIONS & CAUTIONS
• Contraindicated in patients hypersensitive to these drugs and in those with angle-closure glaucoma, stenosing peptic

ulcer, pyloroduodenal obstruction, or bladder neck obstruction. Also contraindicated in those taking MAO inhibitors.

• In pregnant women, safe use hasn't been established. During breast-feeding, antihistamines shouldn't be used because many of these drugs appear in breast milk and may cause unusual excitability in the infant. Neonates, especially premature infants, may experience seizures. Children, especially those younger than age 6, may experience paradoxical hyperexcitability with restlessness, insomnia, nervousness, euphoria, tremors, and seizures; give cautiously. Elderly patients usually are more sensitive to the adverse effects of antihistamines, especially dizziness, sedation, hypotension, and urine retention; use cautiously and monitor these patients closely.

Antihypertensives

Angiotensin-converting enzyme inhibitors
benazepril hydrochloride
captopril
enalaprilat
enalapril maleate
fosinopril sodium
lisinopril
perindopril erbumine
quinapril hydrochloride
ramipril
trandolapril

Angiotensin II receptor blockers
candesartan cilexetil
eprosartan mesylate
irbesartan
losartan potassium
olmesartan medoxomil
telmisartan
valsartan

Beta blockers
atenolol
carvedilol
labetalol hydrochloride
metoprolol tartrate
nadolol
pindolol
propranolol hydrochloride
timolol maleate

Calcium channel blockers
amlodipine besylate
diltiazem hydrochloride
felodipine
nicardipine hydrochloride
nifedipine
nisoldipine
verapamil hydrochloride

Centrally acting alpha blockers (sympatholytics)
clonidine hydrochloride
guanfacine hydrochloride
methyldopa

Peripherally acting alpha blockers
doxazosin mesylate
prazosin hydrochloride
terazosin hydrochloride

Vasodilators
hydralazine hydrochloride
nitroglycerine
nitroprusside sodium

INDICATIONS
➤ Essential and secondary hypertension

ACTION
For information on the action of ACE inhibitors, alpha blockers, angiotensin II receptor blockers, beta blockers, calcium channel blockers, and diuretics, see their individual drug class entries. Centrally acting sympatholytics stimulate central alpha-adrenergic receptors, reducing cerebral sympathetic outflow, thereby decreasing peripheral vascular resistance and blood pressure. Rauwolfia alkaloids bind to and gradually destroy the norepinephrine-containing storage vesicles in central and peripheral adrenergic neurons. Vasodilators act directly on smooth muscle to reduce blood pressure.

ADVERSE REACTIONS
Antihypertensives commonly cause orthostatic changes in heart rate, headache, hypotension, nausea, and vomiting. Other reactions vary greatly among different drug types. Centrally acting sympatholytics may cause constipation, depression, dizziness, drowsiness, dry mouth, head-

ache, palpitations, severe rebound hypertension, and sexual dysfunction; methyldopa also may cause aplastic anemia and thrombocytopenia. Rauwolfia alkaloids may cause anxiety, depression, drowsiness, dry mouth, hyperacidity, impotence, nasal stuffiness, and weight gain. Vasodilators may cause ECG changes, diarrhea, dizziness, heart failure, palpitations, pruritus, and rash.

CONTRAINDICATIONS & CAUTIONS
● Contraindicated in patients hypersensitive to these drugs and in those with hypotension.
● Use cautiously in patients with hepatic or renal dysfunction.
● In pregnant women, use cautiously when potential benefits to the mother outweigh risks to the fetus. Check each drug because some are safe only in the first trimester. In breast-feeding women, use cautiously; some antihypertensives appear in breast milk. In children, safety and effectiveness of many antihypertensives haven't been established; give these drugs cautiously and monitor children closely. Elderly patients are more susceptible to adverse reactions and may need lower maintenance doses; monitor these patients closely.

Antilipemics

atorvastatin calcium
cholestyramine
colesevelam hydrochloride
ezetimibe
fenofibrate
fluvastatin sodium
gemfibrozil
lovastatin
pravastatin sodium
rosuvastatin calcium
simvastatin

INDICATIONS
➤ **Hyperlipidemia, hypercholesterolemia**

ACTION
Antilipemics lower elevated lipid levels. Bile-sequestering drugs (cholestyramine and colesevelam) lower LDL level by forming insoluble complexes with bile salts, thus triggering cholesterol to leave the bloodstream and other storage areas to make new bile acids. Fibric acid derivatives (gemfibrozil) reduce cholesterol formation, increase sterol excretion, and decrease lipoprotein and triglyceride synthesis. HMG-CoA reductase inhibitors (atorvastatin, fluvastatin, lovastatin, pravastatin, rosuvastatin, simvastatin) interfere with the activity of enzymes that generate cholesterol in the liver. Selective cholesterol absorption inhibitors (ezetimibe) inhibit cholesterol absorption by the small intestine, reducing hepatic cholesterol stores and increasing cholesterol clearance from the blood.

ADVERSE REACTIONS
Antilipemics commonly cause GI upset. Bile-sequestering drugs may cause bloating, cholelithiasis, constipation, and steatorrhea. Fibric acid derivatives may cause cholelithiasis and have other GI or CNS effects. Use of gemfibrozil with lovastatin may cause myopathy. HMG-CoA reductase inhibitors may affect liver function or cause rash, pruritus, increased CK levels, rhabdomyolysis, and myopathy.

CONTRAINDICATIONS & CAUTIONS
● Contraindicated in patients hypersensitive to these drugs. Also, bile-sequestering drugs are contraindicated in patients with complete biliary obstruction. Fibric acid derivatives are contraindicated in patients with primary biliary cirrhosis or significant hepatic or renal dysfunction. HMG-CoA reductase inhibitors and cholesterol absorption inhibitors are contraindicated in patients with active liver disease or persistently elevated transaminase levels.
● Use bile-sequestering drugs cautiously in constipated patients. Use fibric acid derivatives cautiously in patients with peptic ulcer. Use HMG-CoA inhibitors cautiously in patients who consume large amounts of alcohol or who have a history of liver or renal disease.
● In pregnant women, use bile-sequestering drugs and fibric acid derivatives cautiously and avoid using HMG-CoA inhibitors. In breast-feeding women, avoid using fibric acid derivatives and HMG-CoA inhibitors; give bile-sequestering drugs cautiously. In

children ages 10 to 17, certain antilipemics have been approved to treat heterozygous familial hypercholesterolemia. Elderly patients have an increased risk of severe constipation; use bile-sequestering drugs cautiously and monitor patients closely.

Antimetabolite antineoplastics

capecitabine
cytarabine
fludarabine phosphate
fluorouracil
hydroxyurea
mercaptopurine
methotrexate
premetrexed

INDICATIONS
➤ **Various tumors and hematologic conditions**

ACTION
Antimetabolites are structurally similar to naturally occurring metabolites and can be divided into three subcategories: purine, pyrimidine, and folinic acid analogues. Most of these drugs interrupt cell reproduction at a specific phase of the cell cycle. Purine analogues are incorporated into DNA and RNA, interfering with nucleic acid synthesis (by miscoding) and replication. They also may inhibit synthesis of purine bases through pseudofeedback mechanisms. Pyrimidine analogues inhibit enzymes in metabolic pathways that interfere with biosynthesis of uridine and thymine. Folic acid antagonists prevent conversion of folic acid to tetrahydrofolate by inhibiting the enzyme dihydrofolic acid reductase.

ADVERSE REACTIONS
The most common adverse effects include anxiety, bone marrow depression (anemia, leukopenia, thrombocytopenia), chills, diarrhea, fever, flank or joint pain, hair loss, nausea, redness or pain at injection site, stomatitis, swelling of the feet or lower legs, and vomiting.

CONTRAINDICATIONS & CAUTIONS
● Contraindicated in patients hypersensitive to these drugs.

● Pregnant women should be informed of the risks to the fetus. Breast-feeding isn't recommended for women taking these drugs. In children, safety and effectiveness of some drugs haven't been established; use cautiously. Elderly patients have an increased risk of adverse reactions; monitor them closely.

Antimigraine drugs

almotriptan
eletriptan hydrobromide
frovatriptan succinate
naratriptan hydrochloride
rizatriptan benzoate
sumatriptan succinate
zolmitriptan

INDICATIONS
➤ **Treatment of migraines with or without aura**

ACTION
The antimigraine drugs are serotonin 5HT-1 agonists. These drugs constrict cranial vessels, inhibit neuropeptide release and reduce transmission in the trigeminal nerve pathway.

ADVERSE REACTIONS
These drugs have a wide range of adverse reactions. These include tingling, warmth or hot sensations, flushing, nasal discomfort, visual disturbances, parasthesias, dizziness, fatigue, somnolence, chest pain, neck, throat or jaw pain, weakness, dry mouth, dyspepsia, nausea, sweating, and injection site reactions. Intranasal sumatriptan can cause nasal or throat discomfort and taste disturbances.

CONTRAINDICATIONS & CAUTIONS
● Contraindicated in patients hypersensitive to any of the drug components.
● Contraindicated in patients with ischemic heart disease, angina, previous MI, uncontrolled hypertension or other significant underlying CV conditions, cerebrovascular disease, peripheral vascular disease, and ischemic bowel disease.

Antiparkinsonians

amantadine hydrochloride
apomorphine hydrochloride
benztropine mesylate
bromocriptine mesylate
diphenhydramine hydrochloride
entacapone
levodopa
levodopa and carbidopa
levodopa, carbidopa, and
   entacapone
pramipexole dihydrochloride
rasagiline mesylate
ropinirole hydrochloride
selegiline hydrochloride
tolcapone

INDICATIONS
➤ **Signs and symptoms of Parkinson disease and drug-induced extrapyramidal reactions**

ACTION
Antiparkinsonians include synthetic anticholinergics, dopaminergics, and the antiviral amantadine. Anticholinergics probably prolong the action of dopamine by blocking its reuptake into presynaptic neurons and by suppressing central cholinergic activity. Dopaminergics act in the brain by increasing dopamine availability, thus improving motor function. Entacapone is a reversible inhibitor of peripheral catechol-O-methyltransferase (commonly known as COMT), which is responsible for elimination of various catecholamines, including dopamine. Blocking this pathway when giving levodopa and carbidopa should result in higher levels of levodopa, thereby allowing greater dopaminergic stimulation in the CNS and leading to a greater effect in treating parkinsonian symptoms. Amantadine is thought to increase dopamine release in the substantia nigra.

ADVERSE REACTIONS
Anticholinergics may cause blurred vision, cycloplegia, constipation, decreased sweating or anhidrosis, dry mouth, headache, mydriasis, palpitations, tachycardia, and urinary hesitancy and urine retention. Dopaminergics may cause arrhythmias, confusion, disturbing dreams, dystonias,

hallucinations, headache, muscle cramps, nausea, orthostatic hypotension, and vomiting. Amantadine also causes irritability, insomnia, and livedo reticularis (with prolonged use).

CONTRAINDICATIONS & CAUTIONS
● Contraindicated in patients hypersensitive to these drugs.
● Use cautiously in patients with prostatic hyperplasia or tardive dyskinesia and in debilitated patients.
● Neuroleptic malignant-like syndrome involving muscle rigidity, increased body temperature, and mental status changes may occur with abrupt withdrawal of antiparkinsonians.
● In pregnant women, safe use hasn't been established. Antiparkinsonians may appear in breast milk; a decision should be made to stop the drug or stop breast-feeding, taking into account the importance of the drug to the mother. In children, safety and effectiveness haven't been established. Elderly patients have an increased risk for adverse reactions; monitor them closely.

Antiplatelet drugs

abciximab
cilostazol
clopidogrel bisulfate
dipyridamole
eptifibatide
oprelvekin
ticlopidine hydrochloride
tirofiban hydrochloride

INDICATIONS
➤ **Reduction of thrombolytic events by reducing platelet aggregation; adjunct to percutaneous catheter intervention, prevention of cardiac ischemic complications, or unstable angina not responding to conventional therapy when percutaneous catheter intervention is planned within 24 hours (abciximab); acute coronary syndrome and percutaneous catheter interventions (eptifibatide); acute coronary syndrome (tirofiban); non-ST-segment elevation acute coronary syndrome and ST-segment elevation MI, recent MI,**

recent stroke or peripheral vascular disease (clopidogrel and ticlopidine)

ACTION
The I.V. drugs abciximab, eptifibatide, and tirofiban antagonize the GPIIb/IIIa receptors located on platelets, which are involved in platelet aggregation. Clopidogrel is an inhibitor of platelet aggregation by inhibiting the binding of adenosine diphosphate (ADP) to its platelet receptor and the subsequent ADP mediated activation of the glycoprotein (GP)IIb/IIIa complex. Ticlopidine inhibits the binding of fibrinogen to platelets.

ADVERSE REACTIONS
The I.V. drugs can cause serious bleeding, thrombocytopenia, and anaphylaxis. The most common adverse reactions to the oral agents include anaphylaxis, rash, stomach pain, nausea, and headache. Ticlopidine may cause neutropenia and elevated alkaline phosphatase and serum transaminase levels.

CONTRAINDICATIONS & CAUTIONS
● Contraindicated in patients hypersensitive to any of the drug components.
● Contraindicated in active bleeding, bleeding disorders, intracranial neoplasm, AV malformation or aneurysm, cerebrovascular accident (within 2 years), recent major surgery or trauma, severe uncontrolled hypertension, or thrombocytopenia.

Antirheumatics

abatacept
adalimumab
auranofin
aurothioglucose
entacapone
gold sodium thiomalate
leflunomide

INDICATIONS
➤ **Rheumatoid arthritis, ankylosing spondylitis, Crohn disease, psoriatic arthritis**

ACTION
Inhibits T-cell activation by binding to CD80 and CD86, thereby blocking inter-

action with CD28. Activated T lymphocytes are found in the synovium of patients with rheumatoid arthritis. Some drugs bind to tumor necrosis factor (TNF) so it can't bind to a receptor and exert an effect. TNF plays an important role in pathologic inflammation and joint destruction.

ADVERSE REACTIONS
The most serious adverse reactions include serious infections and malignancies in patients treated with abatacept and adalimumab. The most common adverse reactions include rash, pruritus, hair loss, urticaria, nausea, vomiting, anorexia, flatulence, dyspepsia, anemia, leukopenia, thrombocytopenia, elevated liver enzymes, stomatitis, hypertension, headache, and hematuria. Serious adverse reactions from gold therapy include anaphylactic shock, bradycardia, and angioneurotic edema. The most common adverse reactions from gold therapy include dermatitis, pruritus, and stomatitis.

CONTRAINDICATIONS & CAUTIONS
● Contraindicated in patients hypersensitive to any of the drug components.
● Use cautiously in patients receiving two antirheumatics with similar mechanisms of action.
● Use with caution in patients with a history of recurrent infections, COPD, CNS disorders, demyelinating disorders, heart failure, and immunosuppression.

Antituberculotics

cycloserine
ethambutol
isoniazid
rifabutin
rifampin
rifapentine

INDICATIONS
➤ **Acute pulmonary and extrapulmonary tuberculosis, acute UTIs**

ACTION
Inhibits cell wall synthesis in susceptible strains of gram-positive and gram-negative bacteria and if *Mycobacterium tuberculosis* is identified.

ADVERSE REACTIONS

Adverse reactions primarily affect the GI tract, peripheral nervous system and hepatic system. Isoniazid may precipitate seizures in patients with a seizure disorder and produce optic or peripheral neuritis, as well as elevated liver enzymes. Optic neuritis is the only significant reaction to ethambutol. The most common adverse reactions to rifampin include epigastric pain, nausea, vomiting, flatulence, abdominal cramps, anorexia and diarrhea. Cycloserine can cause seizures, confusion, dizziness, headache, and somnolence.

CONTRAINDICATIONS & CAUTIONS

● Contraindicated in patients hypersensitive to any of the drug components.
● Drugs should be discontinued or dosage reduced if patients develop signs of CNS toxicity including convulsions, psychosis, somnolence, depression, confusion, hyperreflexia, headache, tremor, vertigo, paresis, or dysarthria.

Barbiturates

pentobarbital sodium
phenobarbital
phenobarbital sodium
secobarbital sodium

INDICATIONS

➤ Sedation, preanesthetic, short-term treatment of insomnia, seizure disorders

ACTION

Barbiturates act throughout the CNS, especially in the mesencephalic reticular activating system, which controls the CNS arousal mechanism. The main anticonvulsant actions are reduced nerve transmission and decreased excitability of the nerve cell. Barbiturates decrease presynaptic and postsynaptic membrane excitability by promoting the actions of GABA. They also depress respiration and GI motility and raise the seizure threshold.

ADVERSE REACTIONS

CNS depression, drowsiness, headache, lethargy, and vertigo are common with barbiturates. After hypnotic doses, a hangover effect, subtle distortion of mood, and impaired judgment and motor skills may continue for many hours. After dosage reduction or discontinuation, rebound insomnia or increased dreaming or nightmares may occur. Barbiturates cause hyperalgesia in subhypnotic doses. They can also cause paradoxical excitement at low doses, confusion in elderly patients, and hyperactivity in children. High fever, severe headache, stomatitis, conjunctivitis, or rhinitis may precede potentially fatal skin eruptions. Withdrawal symptoms may occur after as little as 2 weeks of uninterrupted therapy.

CONTRAINDICATIONS & CAUTIONS

● Contraindicated in patients hypersensitive to these drugs and in those with bronchopneumonia, other severe pulmonary insufficiency, or liver dysfunction.
● Use cautiously in patients with blood pressure alterations, pulmonary disease, and CV dysfunction. Use cautiously, if at all, in patients who are depressed or have suicidal tendencies.
● Barbiturates can cause fetal abnormalities; avoid use in pregnant women. Barbiturates appear in breast milk and may result in infant CNS depression; use cautiously. Premature infants are more susceptible to depressant effects of barbiturates because of their immature hepatic metabolism. Children may experience hyperactivity, excitement, or hyperalgesia; use cautiously and monitor closely. Elderly patients may experience hyperactivity, excitement, or hyperalgesia; use cautiously.

Benzodiazepines

alprazolam
chlordiazepoxide hydrochloride
clonazepam
diazepam
estazolam
flurazepam hydrochloride
lorazepam
midazolam hydrochloride
oxazepam
temazepam
triazolam

INDICATIONS

➤ **Seizure disorders (clonazepam, diazepam, midazolam, parenteral lorazepam); anxiety, tension, and insomnia (chlordiazepoxide, diazepam, estazolam, flurazepam, lorazepam, oxazepam, quazepam, temazepam, triazolam); conscious sedation or amnesia in surgery (diazepam, lorazepam, midazolam); skeletal muscle spasm and tremor (oral forms of chlordiazepoxide and diazepam); delirium**

ACTION

Benzodiazepines act selectively on polysynaptic neuronal pathways throughout the CNS. Precise sites and mechanisms of action aren't fully known. However, benzodiazepines enhance or facilitate the action of GABA, an inhibitory neurotransmitter in the CNS. These drugs appear to act at the limbic, thalamic, and hypothalamic levels of the CNS to produce anxiolytic, sedative, hypnotic, skeletal muscle relaxant, and anticonvulsant effects.

ADVERSE REACTIONS

Therapeutic dose may cause drowsiness, impaired motor function, constipation, diarrhea, vomiting, altered appetite, urinary changes, visual disturbances, and CV irregularities. Toxic dose may cause continuing problems with short-term memory, confusion, severe depression, shakiness, vertigo, slurred speech, staggering, bradycardia, shortness of breath, difficulty breathing, or severe weakness. Prolonged or frequent use of benzodiazepines can cause physical dependency and withdrawal syndrome when drug is stopped.

CONTRAINDICATIONS & CAUTIONS

● Contraindicated in patients hypersensitive to these drugs, in those with acute angle-closure glaucoma, and in those with depressive neuroses or psychotic reactions in which anxiety isn't prominent.
● Avoid use in patients with suicidal tendencies and patients with a history of drug abuse.
● Use cautiously in patients with chronic pulmonary insufficiency or sleep apnea and in those with hepatic or renal insufficiency.
● In pregnant patients, benzodiazepines increase the risk of congenital malformation if taken in the first trimester. Use during labor may cause neonatal flaccidity. A neonate whose mother took a benzodiazepine during pregnancy may have withdrawal symptoms. In breast-feeding women, benzodiazepines may cause sedation, feeding difficulties, and weight loss in the infant. In children, use caution; they're especially sensitive to CNS depressant effects. In elderly patients, benzodiazepine elimination may be prolonged; consider a lower dosage.

Beta blockers

Beta₁ blockers
atenolol
esmolol hydrochloride
metoprolol tartrate

Beta₁ and beta₂ blockers
carvedilol
labetalol hydrochloride
nadolol
propranolol hydrochloride
sotalol hydrochloride
timolol maleate

INDICATIONS

➤ **Hypertension (most drugs), angina pectoris (atenolol, metoprolol, nadolol, and propranolol), arrhythmias (esmolol, propranolol, and sotalol), glaucoma (betaxolol and timolol), prevention of MI (atenolol, metoprolol, propranolol, and timo-**

lol), prevention of recurrent migraine and other vascular headaches (propranolol and timolol), pheochromocytomas or essential tremors (selected drugs), heart failure (atenolol, carvedilol, metoprolol)

ACTION
Beta blockers compete with beta agonists for available beta receptors; individual drugs differ in their ability to affect beta receptors. Some drugs are nonselective: they block $beta_1$ receptors in cardiac muscle and $beta_2$ receptors in bronchial and vascular smooth muscle. Several drugs arc cardioselective and, in lower doses, inhibit mainly $beta_1$ receptors. Some beta blockers have intrinsic sympathomimetic activity and stimulate and block beta receptors, and thereby have less affect on slowing heart rate. Others stabilize cardiac membranes, which affects cardiac action potential.

ADVERSE REACTIONS
Therapeutic dose may cause bradycardia, dizziness, and fatigue; some may cause other CNS disturbances, such as depression, hallucinations, memory loss, and nightmares. Toxic dose can produce severe hypotension, bradycardia, heart failure, or bronchospasm.

CONTRAINDICATIONS & CAUTIONS
● Contraindicated in patients hypersensitive to these drugs and in patients with cardiogenic shock, sinus bradycardia, heart block greater than first degree, and bronchial asthma.
● Use cautiously in patients with nonallergic bronchospastic disorders, diabetes mellitus, impaired hepatic or renal function, and congestive heart failure.
● Use caution in discontinuing drug; dose should be tapered. Suddenly stopping can worsen angina or precipitate MI.
● In pregnant women, use cautiously. Drugs appear in breast milk. In children, safety and effectiveness haven't been established; use only if the benefits outweigh the risks. In elderly patients, use cautiously; these patients may need reduced maintenance doses because of increased bioavailability, delayed metabolism, and increased adverse effects.

Calcium channel blockers

amlodipine besylate
diltiazem hydrochloride
felodipine
nicardipine hydrochloride
nifedipine
nisoldipine
verapamil hydrochloride

INDICATIONS
➤ Prinzmetal variant angina, chronic stable angina, unstable angina, mild-to-moderate hypertension, arrhythmias

ACTION
The main physiologic action of calcium channel blockers is to inhibit calcium influx across the slow channels of myocardial and vascular smooth muscle cells. By inhibiting calcium flow into these cells, calcium channel blockers reduce intracellular calcium levels. This, in turn, dilates coronary arteries, peripheral arteries, and arterioles and slows cardiac conduction.
  When used to treat Prinzmetal variant angina, calcium channel blockers inhibit coronary spasm, which then increases oxygen delivery to the heart. Peripheral artery dilation reduces afterload, which decreases myocardial oxygen use. Inhibiting calcium flow into specialized cardiac conduction cells in the SA and AV nodes slows conduction through the heart. Verapamil and diltiazem have the greatest effect on the AV node, which slows the ventricular rate in atrial fibrillation or flutter and converts supraventricular tachycardia to a normal sinus rhythm.

ADVERSE REACTIONS
Verapamil may cause bradycardia, hypotension, various degrees of heart block, and worsening of heart failure after rapid I.V. delivery. Prolonged oral verapamil therapy may cause constipation. Nifedipine may cause flushing, headache, heartburn, hypotension, lightheadedness, and peripheral edema. The most common adverse reactions with diltiazem are anorexia and nausea; it also may induce bradycardia, heart failure, peripheral edema, and various degrees of heart block.

CONTRAINDICATIONS & CAUTIONS

• Contraindicated in patients hypersensitive to these drugs and in those with second- or third-degree heart block (except those with a pacemaker) and cardiogenic shock. Use diltiazem and verapamil cautiously in patients with heart failure.

• In pregnant women, use cautiously. Calcium channel blockers may appear in breast milk; instruct patient to stop breast-feeding during therapy. In neonates and infants, adverse hemodynamic effects of parenteral verapamil are possible, but safety and effectiveness of other calcium channel blockers haven't been established; avoid use, if possible. In elderly patients, the half-life of calcium channel blockers may be increased as a result of decreased clearance; use cautiously.

Cephalosporins

First generation
cefadroxil monohydrate
cefazolin sodium
cephalexin monohydrate

Second generation
cefaclor
cefoxitin sodium
cefprozil
cefuroxime axetil
cefuroxime sodium

Third generation
cefdinir
cefotaxime sodium
cefpodoxime proxetil
ceftazidime
ceftizoxime sodium
ceftriaxone sodium

INDICATIONS
➤ **Infections of the lungs, skin, soft tissue, bones, joints, urinary and respiratory tracts, blood, abdomen, and heart; CNS infections caused by susceptible strains of *Neisseria meningitidis, Haemophilus influenzae,* and *Streptococcus pneumoniae;* meningitis caused by *Escherichia coli* or *Klebsiella;* infections that develop after surgical procedures classified as contaminated or potentially contaminated; penicillinase-producing *N. gonorrhoeae;* otitis media and ampicillin-resistant middle ear infection caused by *H. influenzae***

ACTION
Cephalosporins are chemically and pharmacologically similar to penicillin; they act by inhibiting bacterial cell wall synthesis, causing rapid cell destruction. Their sites of action are enzymes known as penicillin-binding proteins. The affinity of certain cephalosporins for these proteins in various microorganisms helps explain the differing actions of these drugs. They are bactericidal: they act against many aerobic gram-positive and gram-negative bacteria and some anaerobic bacteria but don't kill fungi or viruses.

First-generation cephalosporins act against many gram-positive cocci, including penicillinase-producing *Staphylococcus aureus* and *S. epidermidis, S. pneumoniae,* group B streptococci, and group A beta-hemolytic streptococci. Susceptible gram-negative organisms include *Klebsiella pneumoniae, E. coli, Proteus mirabilis,* and *Shigella.*

Second-generation cephalosporins are effective against all organisms attacked by first-generation drugs and have additional activity against *Moraxella catarrhalis, H. influenzae, Enterobacter, Citrobacter, Providencia, Acinetobacter, Serratia,* and *Neisseria. Bacteroides fragilis* are susceptible to cefoxitin.

Third-generation cephalosporins are less active than first- and second-generation drugs against gram-positive bacteria but are more active against gram-negative organisms, including those resistant to first- and second-generation drugs. They have the greatest stability against beta-lactamases produced by gram-negative bacteria. Susceptible gram-negative organisms include *E. coli, Klebsiella, Enterobacter, Providencia, Acinetobacter, Serratia, Proteus, Morganella,* and *Neisseria.* Some third-generation drugs are active against *B. fragilis* and *Pseudomonas.*

ADVERSE REACTIONS
Many cephalosporins have similar adverse effects. Hypersensitivity reactions range from mild rashes, fever, and eosino-

philia to fatal anaphylaxis and are more common in patients with penicillin allergy. Adverse GI reactions include abdominal pain, diarrhea, dyspepsia, glossitis, nausea, tenesmus, and vomiting. Hematologic reactions include positive direct and indirect antiglobulin in Coombs' test, thrombocytopenia or thrombocythemia, transient neutropenia, and reversible leukopenia. Minimal elevation of liver function test results occurs occasionally. Adverse renal effects may occur with any cephalosporin; they are most common in older patients, those with decreased renal function, and those taking other nephrotoxic drugs.

Local venous pain and irritation are common after I.M. injection; these reactions occur more often with higher doses and long-term therapy. Bacterial and fungal superinfections may result from suppression of normal flora.

CONTRAINDICATIONS & CAUTIONS
● Contraindicated in patients hypersensitive to these drugs.
● Use cautiously in patients with renal or hepatic impairment, history of GI disease, or allergy to penicillins.
● In pregnant women, use cautiously; safety hasn't been definitively established. In breast-feeding women, use cautiously because drugs appear in breast milk. In neonates and infants, half-life is prolonged; use cautiously. Elderly patients are susceptible to superinfection and coagulopathies, commonly have renal impairment, and may need a lower dosage; use cautiously.

CNS stimulants

doxapram hydrochloride
modafinil
phentermine hydrochloride
sibutramine hydrochloride

INDICATIONS
➤ To stimulate respiration in patients with drug-induced postanesthesia respiratory depression or CNS depression caused by overdose and as temporary measure in acute respiratory insufficiency (doxapram and modafinil); obesity (phentermine and sibutramine)

ACTION
Doxapram and modafinil produce respiratory stimulation through the peripheral carotid chemoreceptors. Phentermine is a sympathomimetic amine. The exact mechanism of action in treating obesity isn't established. Sibutramine blocks the reuptake of serotonin and norepinephrine.

ADVERSE REACTIONS
Phentermine's adverse reactions are related to its stimulatory effect including hypertension, palpitations, tachyarrhythmias, urticaria, constipation, diarrhea, dizziness, excitement, insomnia, tremor, and restlessness. Sibutramine can cause headache, insomnia, constipation, and rash.

CONTRAINDICATIONS & CAUTIONS
● Contraindicated in patients hypersensitive to any of the drug components.
● Doxapram and modafinil are contraindicated in epilepsy, seizure disorders, mechanical disorders of ventilation such as muscle paresis, flail chest, pneumothorax, asthma, pulmonary fibrosis, head injury, stroke, cerebral edema, uncompensated congestive heart failure, severe coronary disease, and severe hypertension.
● Delay administration of doxapram and modafinil in patients who have received general anesthesia utilizing a volatile agent until the volatile agent has been excreted. This will lessen the chance for arrhythmias including ventricular tachycardia or ventricular fibrillation.
● Administer doxapram and modafinil cautiously in patients taking MAO inhibitors or sympathomimetics because an added pressor effect may occur.
● Administer doxapram and modafinil cautiously in patients taking aminophylline or theophylline because agitation and hyperactivity may occur.
● Phentermine is contraindicated in agitated states, CV disease, history of drug abuse, severe hypertension, hyperthyroidism, glaucoma, and during or within 14 days following use of MAO inhibitors.
● Sibutramine is contraindicated with concomitant MAO inhibitor use.

Corticosteroids

betamethasone
dexamethasone
dexamethasone acetate
dexamethasone sodium
    phosphate
fludrocortisone acetate
hydrocortisone
hydrocortisone acetate
hydrocortisone cypionate
hydrocortisone sodium phosphate
hydrocortisone sodium succinate
methylprednisolone
methylprednisolone acetate
methylprednisolone sodium
    succinate
prednisolone
prednisolone acetate
prednisolone sodium phosphate
prednisolone tebutate
prednisone
triamcinolone

INDICATIONS
➤ **Hypersensitivity; inflammation, particularly of eye, nose, and respiratory tract; to initiate immunosuppression; replacement therapy in adrenocortical insufficiency, dermatologic diseases, respiratory disorders, rheumatic disorders**

ACTION
Corticosteroids suppress cell-mediated and humoral immunity by reducing levels of leukocytes, monocytes, and eosinophils; by decreasing immunoglobulin binding to cell-surface receptors; and by inhibiting interleukin synthesis. They reduce inflammation by preventing hydrolytic enzyme release into the cells, preventing plasma exudation, suppressing polymorphonuclear leukocyte migration, and disrupting other inflammatory processes.

ADVERSE REACTIONS
Systemic corticosteroid therapy may suppress the hypothalamic-pituitary-adrenal (HPA) axis. Excessive use may cause cushingoid symptoms and various systemic disorders, such as diabetes and osteoporosis. Other effects may include dermatologic disorders, edema, euphoria, fluid and electrolyte imbalances, gastritis or GI irritation, hypertension, immunosuppression, increased appetite, insomnia, psychosis, and weight gain.

CONTRAINDICATIONS & CAUTIONS
● Contraindicated in patients hypersensitive to these drugs or any of their components and in those with systemic fungal infection.
● Use cautiously in patients with GI ulceration, renal disease, hypertension, osteoporosis, varicella, vaccinia, exanthema, diabetes mellitus, hypothyroidism, thromboembolic disorder, seizures, myasthenia gravis, heart failure, tuberculosis, ocular herpes simplex, hypoalbuminemia, emotional instability, or psychosis.
● In pregnant women, avoid use, if possible, because of risk to the fetus. Women should stop breast-feeding because these drugs appear in breast milk and could cause serious adverse effects in infants. In children, long-term use should be avoided whenever possible because stunted growth may result. Elderly patients may have an increased risk of adverse reactions; monitor them closely.

Diuretics, loop

bumetanide
ethacrynate sodium
ethacrynic acid
furosemide
torsemide

INDICATIONS
➤ **Edema from heart failure, hepatic cirrhosis, or nephrotic syndrome; mild-to-moderate hypertension; adjunct treatment in acute pulmonary edema or hypertensive crisis**

ACTION
Loop diuretics inhibit sodium and chloride reabsorption in the ascending loop of Henle, thus increasing excretion of sodium, chloride, and water. Like thiazide diuretics, loop diuretics increase excretion of potassium. Loop diuretics produce more diuresis and electrolyte loss than thiazide diuretics.

ADVERSE REACTIONS

Therapeutic dose commonly causes metabolic and electrolyte disturbances, particularly potassium depletion. It also may cause hyperglycemia, hyperuricemia, hypochloremic alkalosis, and hypomagnesemia. Rapid parenteral administration may cause hearing loss (including deafness) and tinnitus. High doses can produce profound diuresis, leading to hypovolemia and CV collapse. Photosensitivity also may occur.

CONTRAINDICATIONS & CAUTIONS

● Contraindicated in patients hypersensitive to these drugs and in patients with anuria, hepatic coma, or severe electrolyte depletion.

● Use cautiously in patients with severe renal disease. Also use cautiously in patients with severe hypersensitivity to sulfonamides because allergic reaction may occur.

● In pregnant women, use cautiously. In breast-feeding women, don't use. In neonates, use cautiously; the usual pediatric dose can be used, but dosage intervals should be extended. In elderly patients, use a lower dose, if needed, and monitor patient closely; these patients are more susceptible to drug-induced diuresis.

Diuretics, potassium-sparing

spironolactone
triamterene

INDICATIONS

➤ **Edema from hepatic cirrhosis, nephrotic syndrome, and heart failure; mild or moderate hypertension; diagnosis of primary hyperaldosteronism; metabolic alkalosis produced by thiazide and other kaliuretic diuretics; recurrent calcium nephrolithiasis; lithium-induced polyuria secondary to lithium-induced nephrogenic diabetes insipidus; aid in the treatment of hyperkalemia; prophylaxis of hypokalemia in patients taking cardiac glycosides; precocious puberty and female hirsutism; adjunct to treatment of myasthenia gravis and familial periodic paralysis**

ACTION

Triamterene acts directly on the distal renal tubules, inhibiting sodium reabsorption and potassium excretion, thereby reducing potassium loss. Spironolactone competitively inhibits aldosterone at the distal renal tubules, also promoting sodium excretion and potassium retention.

ADVERSE REACTIONS

Hyperkalemia is the most serious adverse reaction; it may occur with all drugs in this class and could lead to arrhythmias. Other adverse reactions include nausea, vomiting, headache, weakness, fatigue, bowel disturbances, cough, and dyspnea.

CONTRAINDICATIONS & CAUTIONS

● Contraindicated in patients hypersensitive to these drugs, those with a potassium level above 5.5 mEq/L, those taking other potassium-sparing diuretics or potassium supplements, and those with anuria, acute or chronic renal insufficiency, or diabetic nephropathy.

● Use cautiously in patients with severe hepatic insufficiency, because electrolyte imbalance may lead to hepatic encephalopathy, and in patients with diabetes, who are at increased risk for hyperkalemia.

● In pregnant women, no controlled studies exist. Women who wish to breast-feed should consult prescriber because drug may appear in breast milk. In children, use cautiously; they're more susceptible to hyperkalemia. In elderly and debilitated patients, observe closely and reduce dosage, if needed; they're more susceptible to drug-induced diuresis and hyperkalemia.

Diuretics, thiazide and thiazide-like

Thiazide
hydrochlorothiazide

Thiazide-like
indapamide
metolazone

INDICATIONS

➤ **Edema from right-sided heart failure, mild-to-moderate left-sided heart failure, or nephrotic syndrome;**

edema and ascites caused by hepatic cirrhosis; hypertension; diabetes insipidus, particularly nephrogenic diabetes insipidus

ACTION
Thiazide and thiazide-like diuretics interfere with sodium transport across the tubules of the cortical diluting segment in the nephron, thereby increasing renal excretion of sodium, chloride, water, potassium, and calcium.

Thiazide diuretics also exert an antihypertensive effect. Although the exact mechanism is unknown, direct arteriolar dilation may be partially responsible. In diabetes insipidus, thiazides cause a paradoxical decrease in urine volume and an increase in renal concentration of urine, possibly because of sodium depletion and decreased plasma volume. This increases water and sodium reabsorption in the kidneys.

ADVERSE REACTIONS
Therapeutic doses cause electrolyte and metabolic disturbances, most commonly potassium depletion. Other abnormalities include elevated cholesterol levels, hypercalcemia, hyperglycemia, hyperuricemia, hypochloremic alkalosis, hypomagnesemia, and hyponatremia. Photosensitivity also may occur.

CONTRAINDICATIONS & CAUTIONS
● Contraindicated in patients hypersensitive to these drugs and in those with anuria.
● Use cautiously in patients with severe renal disease, impaired hepatic function, or progressive liver disease.
● In pregnant women, use cautiously. In breast-feeding women, thiazides are contraindicated because they appear in breast milk. In children, safety and effectiveness haven't been established. In elderly patients, reduce dosage, if needed, and monitor patient closely; these patients are more susceptible to drug-induced diuresis.

Estrogens

esterified estrogens
estradiol
estradiol cypionate
estradiol hemihydrate
estradiol valerate
estrogenic substances, conjugated
estropipate

INDICATIONS
➤ **Prevention of moderate to severe vasomotor symptoms linked to menopause, such as hot flushes and dizziness; stimulation of vaginal tissue development, cornification, and secretory activity; inhibition of hormone-sensitive cancer growth; female hypogonadism; female castration; primary ovulation failure; ovulation control; prevention of conception**

ACTION
Estrogens promote the development and maintenance of the female reproductive system and secondary sexual characteristics. They inhibit the release of pituitary gonadotropins and have various metabolic effects, including retention of fluid and electrolytes, retention and deposition in bone of calcium and phosphorus, and mild anabolic activity. Of the six naturally occurring estrogens in humans, estradiol, estrone, and estriol are present in significant quantities.

Estrogens and estrogenic substances given as drugs have effects related to endogenous estrogen's mechanism of action. They can mimic the action of endogenous estrogen when used as replacement therapy and can inhibit ovulation or the growth of certain hormone-sensitive cancers. Conjugated estrogens and estrogenic substances are normally obtained from the urine of pregnant mares. Other estrogens are manufactured synthetically.

ADVERSE REACTIONS
Acute adverse reactions include abdominal cramps; bloating caused by fluid and electrolyte retention; breast swelling and tenderness; changes in menstrual bleeding patterns, such as spotting and prolongation or

absence of bleeding; headache; loss of appetite; loss of libido; nausea; photosensitivity; swollen feet or ankles; and weight gain.

Long-term effects include benign hepatomas, cholestatic jaundice, elevated blood pressure (sometimes into the hypertensive range), endometrial carcinoma (rare), and thromboembolic disease (risk increases greatly with cigarette smoking, especially in women older than age 35).

CONTRAINDICATIONS & CAUTIONS
• Contraindicated in women with thrombophlebitis or thromboembolic disorders, unexplained abnormal genital bleeding, or estrogen-dependent neoplasia.
• Use cautiously in patients with hypertension; metabolic bone disease; migraines; seizures; asthma; cardiac, renal, or hepatic impairment; blood dyscrasia; diabetes; family history of breast cancer; or fibrocystic disease.
• In pregnant or breast-feeding women, use is contraindicated. In adolescents whose bone growth isn't complete, use cautiously because of effects on epiphyseal closure. Postmenopausal women with a history of long-term estrogen use have an increased risk of endometrial cancer and stroke. Postmenopausal women also have increased risk for breast cancer, MI, stroke, and blood clots with long-term use of estrogen plus progestin.

Fluoroquinolones

ciprofloxacin
gemifloxacin
levofloxacin
moxifloxacin
norfloxacin
ofloxacin

INDICATIONS
➤ Bone and joint infection, bacterial bronchitis, endocervical and urethral chlamydial infection, bacterial gastroenteritis, endocervical and urethral gonorrhea, intra-abdominal infection, empiric therapy for febrile neutropenia, pelvic inflammatory disease, bacterial pneumonia, bacterial prostatitis, acute sinusitis, skin and soft tissue infection, typhoid fever, bacterial UTI (prevention and treatment), chancroid, meningococcal carriers, and bacterial septicemia caused by susceptible organisms

ACTION
Fluoroquinolones produce a bactericidal effect by inhibiting intracellular DNA topoisomerase II (DNA gyrase), which prevents DNA replication. These enzymes are essential catalysts in the duplication, transcription, and repair of bacterial DNA.

Fluoroquinolones are broad-spectrum, systemic antibacterial drugs active against a wide range of aerobic gram-positive and gram-negative organisms. Gram-positive aerobic bacteria include *Staphylococcus aureus, S. epidermis, S. hemolyticus, S. saprophyticus;* penicillinase- and non–penicillinase-producing staphylococci and some methicillin-resistant strains; *Streptococcus pneumoniae;* group A (beta) hemolytic streptococci *(S. pyogenes);* group B streptococci *(S. agalactiae);* viridans streptococci; groups C, F, and G streptococci and nonenterococcal group D streptococci; *Enterococcus faecalis.* These drugs are active against gram-positive aerobic bacilli including *Corynebacterium* species, *Listeria monocytogenes,* and *Nocardia asteroides.*

Fluoroquinolones are also effective against gram-negative aerobic bacteria including, but not limited to, *Neisseria meningitidis* and most strains of penicillinase- and non–penicillinase-producing *Haemophilus ducreyi, H. influenzae, H. parainfluenzae, Moraxella catarrhalis, N. gonorrhoeae,* and most clinically important *Enterobacteriaceae,* and *Vibrio parahaemolyticus.* Certain fluoroquinolones are active against *Chlamydia trachomatis, Legionella pneumophila, Mycobacterium avium-intracellulare, Mycoplasma hominis, M. pneumoniae,* and *Pseudomonas aeruginosa.*

ADVERSE REACTIONS
Adverse reactions that are rare but need medical attention include CNS stimulation (acute psychosis, agitation, hallucinations, tremors), hepatotoxicity, hypersensitivity reactions, interstitial nephritis, phlebitis, pseudomembranous colitis, and tendinitis or tendon rupture. Adverse reactions that

need no medical attention unless they persist or become intolerable include CNS effects (dizziness, headache, nervousness, drowsiness, insomnia), GI reactions, and photosensitivity.

CONTRAINDICATIONS & CAUTIONS
• Contraindicated in patients hypersensitive to fluoroquinolones because serious, possibly fatal, reactions can occur.
• Use cautiously in patients with known or suspected CNS disorders that predispose them to seizures or lower seizure threshold, cerebral ischemia, severe hepatic dysfunction, or renal insufficiency.
• In pregnant women, these drugs cross the placenta and may cause arthropathies. Breast-feeding isn't recommended because these drugs may cause arthropathies in newborns and infants, although it isn't known if all fluoroquinolones appear in breast milk. In children, fluoroquinolones aren't recommended because they can cause joint problems. In elderly patients, reduce dosage, if needed, because these patients are more likely to have reduced renal function.

Hematopoietic agents

colony-stimulating factors
darbepoetin alfa
epoetin alfa

INDICATIONS
➤ **To reduce the incidence of infection in myelosuppressive chemotherapy; to reduce time for neutrophil recovery and fever in patients with acute myelogenous leukemia and other cancers in patients undergoing chemotherapy (colony-stimulating factors)**
➤ **Anemia associated with chronic renal failure, zidovudine therapy in patients with HIV and cancer patients on chemotherapy; to reduce the need for allogeneic blood transfusions in surgical patients (epoetin alpha and related products)**

ACTION
Epoetin and darbopoetin stimulate RBC production in the bone marrow, while the CSF products help increase production of neutrophils and other white blood cell components.

ADVERSE REACTIONS
Hematopoietic agents may cause fatigue, headache, weakness, chest pain, hypertension, tachycardia, nausea, vomiting diarrhea, constipation, mucositis, stomatitis, anorexia, myalgias, neutropenic fever, dyspnea, cough, sore throat, alopecia, rash, urticaria, and stinging at the injection site.

CONTRAINDICATIONS & CAUTIONS
• Contraindicated in patients hypersensitive to any of the drug components or human albumin.
• Contraindicated in uncontrolled hypertension.
• Use cautiously in patients with cardiac disease, seizures, and porphyria.

Histamine₂-receptor antagonists

cimetidine
famotidine
ranitidine hydrochloride

INDICATIONS
➤ **Acute duodenal or gastric ulcer, Zollinger-Ellison syndrome, gastroesophageal reflux**

ACTION
All H_2-receptor antagonists inhibit the action of H_2-receptors in gastric parietal cells, reducing gastric acid output and concentration, regardless of stimulants, such as histamine, food, insulin, and caffeine, or basal conditions.

ADVERSE REACTIONS
H_2-receptor antagonists rarely cause adverse reactions. Cardiac arrhythmias, dizziness, fatigue, gynecomastia, headache, mild and transient diarrhea, and thrombocytopenia are possible.

CONTRAINDICATIONS & CAUTIONS
• Contraindicated in patients hypersensitive to these drugs.
• Use cautiously in patients with impaired renal or hepatic function.

• In pregnant women, use cautiously. In breast-feeding women, H$_2$-receptor antagonists are contraindicated because they may appear in breast milk. In children, safety and effectiveness haven't been established. Elderly patients have increased risk of adverse reactions, particularly those affecting the CNS; use cautiously.

Immunosuppressants

alefacept
anakinra
azathioprine
basiliximab
cyclosporine
daclizumab
efalizumab
etanercept
glatiramer acetate
infliximab
lymphocyte immune globulin
muromonab-CD3
mycophenolate mofetil
sirolimus

INDICATIONS
➤ **For prevention of rejection in organ transplants and in the management of severe rheumatoid arthritis**

ACTION
The exact mechanism of action is not fully known. They act by suppressing cell-mediated hypersensitivity reactions and produce various alterations in antibody production, blocking the activity of interleukin, inhibiting helper T cells and suppressor T cells and antagonizing the metabolism of purine, therefore inhibiting ribonucleic acid and deoxyribonucleic acid structure and synthesis.

ADVERSE REACTIONS
Immunosuppressants may cause albuminuria, hematuria, proteinuria, renal failure, hepatotoxicity, oral *Candida* infections, gingival hyperplasia, tremors, and headache. The most serious reactions include leukopenia, thrombocytopenia, and risk of secondary infection.

CONTRAINDICATIONS & CAUTIONS
• Contraindicated in patients hypersensitive to any of the drug components.
• Use cautiously in patients with severe renal disease, severe hepatic disease, or pregnancy.

Inotropics

digoxin
inamrinone
milrinone

INDICATIONS
➤ **Heart failure and supraventricular arrhythmias including supraventricular tachycardia, atrial fibrillation, and atrial flutter (digoxin); short-term heart failure and patients awaiting heart transplantation (inamrinone, milrinone)**

ACTION
The drugs help move calcium into the cells which increases cardiac output by strengthening contractility. Digoxin also acts on the central nervous system to slow heart rate. Inamrinone and milrinone relax vascular smooth muscle, decreasing peripheral vascular resistance (afterload) and the amount of blood returning to the heart (preload).

ADVERSE REACTIONS
Inotropics may cause arrhythmias, nausea, vomiting, diarrhea, headache, fever, mental disturbances, visual changes, and chest pain. Inamrinone and milrinone may cause thrombocytopenia, hypotension, hypokalemia, and elevated liver enzymes.

CONTRAINDICATIONS & CAUTIONS
• Contraindicated in patients hypersensitive to any of the drug components.
• Inamrinone is contraindicated in patients with a sulfite allergy and severe aortic or pulmonic valve disease. Use cautiously in patients with hypertrophic subaortic stenosis and acute MI.
• Digoxin is contraindicated in ventricular fibrillation.
• Use digoxin cautiously in patients with renal insufficiency because of the potential

for digoxin toxicity. Use digoxin cautiously in patients with sinus node disease or AV block because of the potential for advanced heart block.

Laxatives

Bulk-forming
calcium polycarbophil

Emollient
docusate calcium
docusate sodium

Hyperosmolar
glycerin
lactulose
lubiprostone
magnesium citrate
magnesium hydroxide
magnesium sulfate
sodium phosphates

Stimulant
bisacodyl

INDICATIONS
➤ **Constipation, irritable bowel syndrome, diverticulosis**

ACTION
Laxatives promote movement of intestinal contents through the colon and rectum in several ways: bulk-forming, emollient, hyperosmolar, and stimulant.

ADVERSE REACTIONS
All laxatives may cause flatulence, diarrhea, abdominal discomfort, weakness, and dependence. Bulk-forming laxatives may cause intestinal obstruction, impaction, or (rarely) esophageal obstruction. Emollient laxatives may cause a bitter taste or throat irritation. Hyperosmolar laxatives may cause fluid and electrolyte imbalances. Stimulant laxatives may cause urine discoloration, malabsorption, and weight loss.

CONTRAINDICATIONS & CAUTIONS
• Contraindicated in patients with GI obstruction or perforation, toxic colitis, megacolon, nausea and vomiting, or acute surgical abdomen.

• Use cautiously in patients with rectal or anal conditions such as rectal bleeding or large hemorrhoids.
• For pregnant women and breast-feeding women, recommendations vary for individual drugs. Infants and children have an increased risk of fluid and electrolyte disturbances; use cautiously. In elderly patients, dependence is more likely to develop because of age-related changes in GI function. Monitor these patients closely.

Macrolide anti-infectives

azithromycin
clarithromycin
erythromycin estolate
erythromycin ethylsuccinate
erythromycin lactobionate
erythromycin stearate

INDICATIONS
➤ **Various common infections**

ACTION
Inhibit RNA-dependent protein synthesis by acting on a small portion of the 50S ribosomal unit.

ADVERSE REACTIONS
These drugs may cause nausea, vomiting, diarrhea, abdominal pain, palpitations, chest pain, vaginal candidiasis, nephritis, dizziness, headache, vertigo, somnolence, rash, and photosensitivity.

CONTRAINDICATIONS & CAUTIONS
• Contraindicated in patients hypersensitive to any of the drug components.
• Contraindicated in patients with concomitant use of terfenadine, astemizole, or cisapride due to the potential for cardiac arrhythmias. These drugs also have the potential to cause many other drug interactions when given with other drugs; screen carefully.

Neuromuscular blockers

atracurium besylate
cisatracurium besylate
pancuronium bromide
rocuronium bromide
succinylcholine chloride
vecuronium bromide

INDICATIONS
➤ **Relax skeletal muscle during surgery to reduce the intensity of muscle spasms in drug- or electrically induced seizures and to manage patients who are fighting mechanical ventilation**

ACTION
Nondepolarizing blockers (atracurium, cisatracurium, pancuronium, rocuronium, vecuronium) compete with acetylcholine at cholinergic receptor sites on the skeletal muscle membrane. This action blocks acetylcholine's neurotransmitter actions, preventing muscle contraction. Succinylcholine is a depolarizing blocker. This drug isn't inactivated by cholinesterase, thereby preventing repolarization of the motor endplate and causing muscle paralysis.

ADVERSE REACTIONS
Neuromuscular blockers may cause apnea, hypotension, hypertension, arrhythmias, tachycardia, bronchospasm, excessive bronchial or salivary secretions, and skin reactions.

CONTRAINDICATIONS & CAUTIONS
● Contraindicated in patients hypersensitive to any of the drug components.
● The drugs should be used only by personnel skilled in airway management and respiratory support.

Nonsteroidal anti-inflammatory drugs

aspirin
celecoxib
diclofenac potassium
diclofenac sodium
diflunisal
etodolac
ibuprofen
indomethacin
indomethacin sodium trihydrate
ketoprofen
ketorolac tromethamine
meloxicam
nabumetone
naproxen
naproxen sodium
piroxicam
sulindac

INDICATIONS
➤ **Mild to moderate pain, inflammation, stiffness, swelling, or tenderness caused by headache, arthralgia, myalgia, neuralgia, dysmenorrhea, rheumatoid arthritis, juvenile arthritis, osteoarthritis, or dental or surgical procedures**

ACTION
The analgesic effect of NSAIDs may result from interference with the prostaglandins involved in pain. Prostaglandins appear to sensitize pain receptors to mechanical stimulation or to other chemical mediators. NSAIDs inhibit synthesis of prostaglandins peripherally and possibly centrally.

Like salicylates, NSAIDs exert an anti-inflammatory effect that may result in part from inhibition of prostaglandin synthesis and release during inflammation. The exact mechanism isn't clear.

ADVERSE REACTIONS
Adverse reactions chiefly involve the GI tract, particularly erosion of the gastric mucosa. The most common symptoms are abdominal pain, dyspepsia, epigastric distress, heartburn, and nausea. CNS and skin reactions also may occur. Flank pain with other evidence of nephrotoxicity occurs occasionally. Fluid retention may aggravate hypertension or heart failure.

CONTRAINDICATIONS & CAUTIONS

• Contraindicated in patients with GI lesions or GI bleeding and in patients hypersensitive to these drugs.

• Use cautiously in patients with heart failure, hypertension, risk of MI, fluid retention, renal insufficiency, or coagulation defects.

• In pregnant women, use cautiously in the first and second trimesters; don't use in the third trimester. For breast-feeding women, NSAIDs aren't recommended. In children younger than age 14, safety of long-term therapy hasn't been established. Patients older than age 60 may be more susceptible to toxic effects of NSAIDs because of decreased renal function.

Nucleoside reverse transcriptase inhibitors

abacavir sulfate
didanosine
emtricitabine
lamivudine
stavudine
tenofovir disoproxil fumarate
zidovudine

INDICATIONS

➤ **HIV infection, AIDS, prevention of maternal-fetal HIV transmission, prevention of HIV infection after occupational exposure (as by needle stick) or nonoccupational exposure to blood, genital secretions, or other potentially infectious body fluids of an HIV-infected person when there's substantial risk of transmission**

ACTION

Nucleoside reverse transcriptase inhibitors (NRTIs) suppress HIV replication by inhibiting HIV DNA polymerase. Competitive inhibition of nucleoside reverse transcriptase inhibits DNA viral replication by chain termination, competitive inhibition of reverse transcriptase, or both.

ADVERSE REACTIONS

Because of the complexity of HIV infection, it's often difficult to distinguish between disease-related symptoms and adverse drug reactions. The most frequently reported adverse effects of NRTIs are anemia, leukopenia, and neutropenia. Thrombocytopenia is less common. Rare adverse effects of NRTIs are hepatotoxicity, myopathy, and neurotoxicity. Any of these adverse effects requires prompt medical attention.

Adverse effects that don't need medical attention unless they persist or are bothersome include headache, severe insomnia, myalgias, nausea, or hyperpigmentation of nails.

CONTRAINDICATIONS & CAUTIONS

• Contraindicated in patients hypersensitive to these drugs and patients with moderate to severe hepatic impairment (abacavir) or pancreatitis (didanosine).

• Use cautiously in patients with mild hepatic impairment or risk factors for liver impairment, risk for pancreatitis (didanosine), or compromised bone marrow function (zidovudine).

• In pregnant women, use drug only if benefits outweigh risks. HIV-infected mothers shouldn't breast-feed to reduce the risk of transmitting the virus. It isn't known if NRTIs appear in breast milk. The pharmacokinetic and safety profile of NRTIs is similar in children and adults. NRTIs may be used in children age 3 months and older, but the half-life may be prolonged in neonates. In elderly patients, elimination half-life may be prolonged.

Opioids

codeine phosphate
codeine sulfate
diphenoxylate hydrochloride
fentanyl citrate
hydrocodone bitartrate
hydromorphone hydrochloride
meperidine hydrochloride
methadone hydrochloride
morphine sulfate
nalbuphine hydrochloride
oxycodone hydrochloride
oxymorphone hydrochloride
pentazocine hydrochloride
propoxyphene hydrochloride
propoxyphene napsylate

INDICATIONS
➤ **Moderate to severe pain from acute and some chronic disorders; diarrhea; dry, nonproductive cough; management of opioid dependence; anesthesia support; sedation**

ACTION
Opioids act as agonists at specific opioid-receptor binding sites in the CNS and other tissues, altering the patient's perception of pain.

ADVERSE REACTIONS
Respiratory and circulatory depression (including orthostatic hypotension) are the major hazards of opioids. Other adverse CNS effects include agitation, coma, depression, dizziness, dysphoria, euphoria, faintness, mental clouding, nervousness, restlessness, sedation, seizures, visual disturbances, and weakness. Adverse GI effects include biliary colic, constipation, nausea, and vomiting. Urine retention or hypersensitivity also may occur. Tolerance to the drug and psychological or physical dependence may follow prolonged therapy.

CONTRAINDICATIONS & CAUTIONS
● Contraindicated in patients hypersensitive to these drugs and in those who have recently taken an MAO inhibitor. Also contraindicated in those with acute or severe bronchial asthma or respiratory depression.

● Use cautiously in patients with head injury, increased intracranial or intraocular pressure, hepatic or renal dysfunction, mental illness, emotional disturbances, or drug-seeking behaviors.
● In pregnant or breast-feeding women, use cautiously; codeine, meperidine, methadone, morphine, and propoxyphene appear in breast milk. Breast-feeding infants of women taking methadone may develop physical dependence. In children, safety and effectiveness of some opioids haven't been established; use cautiously. Elderly patients may be more sensitive to opioids, and lower doses are usually given.

Penicillins

Natural penicillins
penicillin G benzathine
penicillin G potassium
penicillin G procaine
penicillin G sodium
penicillin V potassium

Aminopenicillins
amoxicillin and clavulanate
    potassium
amoxicillin trihydrate
ampicillin
ampicillin sodium and sulbactam
    sodium
ampicillin trihydrate

Extended-spectrum penicillins
piperacillin sodium and
    tazobactam sodium
ticarcillin disodium and clavulanate
    potassium

Penicillinase-resistant penicillins
nafcillin sodium

INDICATIONS
➤ **Streptococcal pneumonia; enterococcal and nonenterococcal group D endocarditis; diphtheria; anthrax; meningitis; tetanus; botulism; actinomycosis; syphilis; relapsing fever; Lyme disease; pneumococcal infections; rheumatic fever; bacterial endocarditis; neonatal group B streptococcal disease; septicemia;**

gynecologic infections; infections of
urinary, respiratory, and GI tracts;
infections of skin, soft tissue, bones,
and joints

ACTION

Penicillins are generally bactericidal. They
inhibit synthesis of the bacterial cell wall,
causing rapid cell destruction. They're
most effective against fast-growing susceptible bacteria. Their sites of action are
enzymes known as penicillin-binding proteins (PBPs). The affinity of certain penicillins for PBPs in various microorganisms helps explain the different activities
of these drugs.

Susceptible aerobic gram-positive cocci
include *Staphylococcus aureus;* nonenterococcal group D streptococci; groups A, B,
D, G, H, K, L, and M streptococci; *Streptococcus viridans;* and *Enterococcus* (usually with an aminoglycoside). Susceptible
aerobic gram-negative cocci include *Neisseria meningitidis* and non–penicillinase-
producing *N. gonorrhoeae.*

Susceptible aerobic gram-positive
bacilli include *Corynebacterium, Listeria,*
and *Bacillus anthracis.* Susceptible anaer-
obes include *Peptococcus, Peptostreptococcus, Actinomyces, Clostridium, Fusobacterium, Veillonella,* and non–beta-
lactamase–producing strains of *Streptococcus pneumoniae.* Susceptible spirochetes
include *Treponema pallidum, T. pertenue,
Leptospira, Borrelia recurrentis,* and, possibly, *B. burgdorferi.*

Aminopenicillins have uses against
more organisms, including many gram-
negative organisms. Like natural penicillins, aminopenicillins are vulnerable to
inactivation by penicillinase. Susceptible
organisms include *Escherichia coli, Proteus mirabilis, Shigella, Salmonella,
S. pneumoniae, N. gonorrhoeae, Haemophilus influenzae, S. aureus, S. epidermidis*
(non–penicillinase-producing *Staphylococcus*), and *Listeria monocytogenes.*

Penicillinase-resistant penicillins are
semisynthetic penicillins designed to remain stable against hydrolysis by most
staphylococcal penicillinases and thus are
the drugs of choice against susceptible
penicillinase-producing staphylococci.
They also act against most organisms susceptible to natural penicillins.

Extended-spectrum penicillins offer a
wider range of bactericidal action than the
other three classes and usually are given in
combination with aminoglycosides. Susceptible strains include *Enterobacter,
Klebsiella, Citrobacter, Serratia, Bacteroides fragilis, Pseudomonas aeruginosa,
Proteus vulgaris, Providencia rettgeri,* and
Morganella morganii. These penicillins
are also vulnerable to beta-lactamase and
penicillinases.

ADVERSE REACTIONS

With all penicillins, hypersensitivity reactions range from mild rash, fever, and
eosinophilia to fatal anaphylaxis. Hematologic reactions include hemolytic anemia, leukopenia, thrombocytopenia, and
transient neutropenia. Certain adverse
reactions are more common with specific
classes. For example, bleeding episodes
are usually seen with high doses of
extended-spectrum penicillins, whereas
GI adverse effects are most common with
ampicillin. In patients with renal disease,
high doses, especially of penicillin G,
irritate the CNS, causing confusion,
twitching, lethargy, dysphagia, seizures,
and coma. Hepatotoxicity may occur
with penicillinase-resistant penicillins,
and hyperkalemia and hypernatremia
have been reported with extended-
spectrum penicillins. Local irritation
from parenteral therapy may be severe
enough to warrant administration by subclavian or centrally placed catheter or
stopping therapy.

CONTRAINDICATIONS & CAUTIONS

● Contraindicated in patients hypersensitive to these drugs.

● Use cautiously in patients with history
of asthma or drug allergy, mononucleosis, renal impairment, CV diseases,
hemorrhagic condition, or electrolyte
imbalance.

● In pregnant women, use cautiously. For
breast-feeding patients, recommendations
vary depending on the drug. For children,
dosage recommendations have been established for most penicillins. Elderly patients are susceptible to superinfection and
renal impairment, which decreases excretion of penicillins; use cautiously and at a
lower dosage.

Phenothiazines

chlorpromazine hydrochloride
fluphenazine
perphenazine
prochlorperazine maleate
promethazine hydrochloride
thioridazine hydrochloride
thiothixene
trifluoperazine hydrochloride

INDICATIONS
➤ Agitated psychotic states, hallucinations, manic-depressive illness, excessive motor and autonomic activity, nausea and vomiting, moderate anxiety, behavioral problems caused by chronic organic mental syndrome, tetanus, acute intermittent porphyria, intractable hiccups, itching, symptomatic rhinitis

ACTION
Phenothiazines are believed to function as dopamine antagonists by blocking postsynaptic dopamine receptors in various parts of the CNS. Their antiemetic effects result from blockage of the chemoreceptor trigger zone. They also produce varying degrees of anticholinergic effects and alpha-adrenergic–receptor blocking.

ADVERSE REACTIONS
Phenothiazines may produce extrapyramidal symptoms, such as dystonic movements, torticollis, oculogyric crises, and parkinsonian symptoms ranging from akathisia during early treatment to tardive dyskinesia after long-term use. A neuroleptic malignant syndrome resembling severe parkinsonism may occur, most often in young men taking fluphenazine.

Other adverse reactions include abdominal pain, agitation, anorexia, arrhythmias, confusion, constipation, dizziness, dry mouth, endocrine effects, fainting, hallucinations, hematologic disorders, local gastric irritation, nausea, orthostatic hypotension with reflex tachycardia, photosensitivity, seizures, skin eruptions, urine retention, visual disturbances, and vomiting.

CONTRAINDICATIONS & CAUTIONS
• Contraindicated in patients with CNS depression, bone marrow suppression, heart failure, circulatory collapse, coronary artery or cerebrovascular disorders, subcortical damage, or coma. Also contraindicated in patients receiving spinal and epidural anesthetics and adrenergic blockers.
• Use cautiously in debilitated patients and in those with hepatic, renal, or CV disease; respiratory disorders; hypocalcemia; seizure disorders; suspected brain tumor or intestinal obstruction; glaucoma; and prostatic hyperplasia.
• In pregnant women, use only if clearly necessary; safety hasn't been established. Women shouldn't breast-feed during therapy because most phenothiazines appear in breast milk and directly affect prolactin levels. For children younger than age 12, phenothiazines aren't recommended unless otherwise specified; use cautiously for nausea and vomiting. Acutely ill children, such as those with chickenpox, measles, CNS infections, or dehydration have a greatly increased risk of dystonic reactions. Elderly patients are more sensitive to therapeutic and adverse effects, especially cardiac toxicity, tardive dyskinesia, and other extrapyramidal effects; use cautiously and give reduced doses, adjusting dosage to patient response.

Protease inhibitors

amprenavir
atazanavir sulfate
fosamprenavir calcium
indinavir sulfate
lopinavir
nelfinavir mesylate
ritonavir
saquinavir
tipranavir

INDICATIONS
➤ HIV infection and AIDS

ACTION
Protease inhibitors bind to the protease active site and inhibit HIV protease activity. This enzyme is required for the proteolysis of viral polyprotein precursors into

individual functional proteins found in infectious HIV. The net effect is formation of noninfectious, immature viral particles.

ADVERSE REACTIONS
The most common adverse effects, which require immediate medical attention, include kidney stones, pancreatitis, diabetes or hyperglycemia, ketoacidosis, and paresthesia.

Common adverse effects that don't need medical attention unless they persist or are bothersome include generalized weakness, GI disturbances, headache, insomnia, and taste disturbance. Less common adverse effects include dizziness and somnolence.

CONTRAINDICATIONS & CAUTIONS
● Contraindicated in patients hypersensitive to these drugs or their components, patients taking a drug highly dependent on CYP3A4 for metabolism, and patients with renal failure (amprenavir oral solution).
● Use cautiously in patients with impaired hepatic or renal function and those with diabetes mellitus or hemophilia.
● In pregnant women, use drug only if benefits outweigh risks. Contact the pregnancy registry at 1-800-258-4263 or www.apregistry.com to report pregnant women on therapy. HIV-infected mothers shouldn't breast-feed to reduce the risk of transmitting HIV to the infant.

Proton pump inhibitors

esomeprazole
lansoprazole
omeprazole
pantoprazole
rabeprazole

INDICATIONS
➤ **Duodenal ulcers, gastric ulcers, erosive esophagitis, and GERD (all proton pump inhibitors); hypersecretory conditions (Zollinger-Ellison syndrome) (lansoprazole, omeprazole, pantoprazole, rabeprazole)**

ACTION
The drugs reduce stomach acid production by combining with hydrogen, potassium and adenosine triphosphate in parietal cells of the stomach to block the last step in gastric acid secretion.

ADVERSE REACTIONS
Proton pump inhibitors may cause abdominal pain, diarrhea, constipation, flatulence, nausea, dry mouth, headache, asthenia, cough, abnormal liver function test results, and hyperglycemia.

CONTRAINDICATIONS & CAUTIONS
● Contraindicated in patients hypersensitive to the drug components.

Selective serotonin reuptake inhibitors

citalopram hydrobromide
escitalopram oxalate
fluoxetine hydrochloride
fluvoxamine maleate
paroxetine hydrochloride
sertraline hydrochloride

INDICATIONS
➤ **Major depression, obsessive-compulsive disorder, bulimia nervosa, premenstrual dysphoric disorders, panic disorders, post-traumatic stress disorder (sertraline)**

ACTION
SSRIs selectively inhibit the reuptake of serotonin with little or no effects on other neurotransmitters such as norepinephrine or dopamine, in the CNS.

ADVERSE REACTIONS
Common adverse effects include headache, tremor, dizziness, sleep disturbances, GI disturbances, and sexual dysfunction. Less common adverse effects include bleeding (ecchymoses, epistaxis), akathisia, breast tenderness or enlargement, extrapyramidal effects, dystonia, fever, hyponatremia, mania or hypomania, palpitations, serotonin syndrome, weight gain or loss, rash, urticaria, or pruritus.

CONTRAINDICATIONS & CAUTIONS
● Contraindicated in patients hypersensitive to these drugs or their components.
● Use cautiously in patients with hepatic, renal, or cardiac insufficiency.

• In pregnant women, use drug only if benefits outweigh risks; use of certain SSRIs in the first trimester may cause birth defects. Neonates born to women who took an SSRI during the third trimester may develop complications that warrant prolonged hospitalization, respiratory support, and tube feeding. In breast-feeding women, use isn't recommended. SSRIs appear in breast milk and may cause diarrhea and sleep disturbance in neonates. However, risks and benefits to both the woman and infant must be considered. Children and adolescents may be more susceptible to increased suicidal tendencies when taking SSRIs or other antidepressants. Elderly patients may be more sensitive to the insomniac effects of SSRIs.

Skeletal muscle relaxants

baclofen
carisoprodol
cyclobenzaprine hydrochloride
dantrolene sodium
tizanidine hydrochloride

INDICATIONS
➤ **Painful musculoskeletal disorders, spasticity caused by multiple sclerosis**

ACTION
Skeletal muscle relaxant baclofen may reduce impulse transmission from the spinal cord to skeletal muscle. Carisoprodol, cyclobenzaprine, and tizanidine's mechanism of action is unclear. Dantrolene acts directly on skeletal muscle to decrease excitation and reduce muscle strength by interfering with intracellular calcium movement.

ADVERSE REACTIONS
Skeletal muscle relaxants may cause ataxia, confusion, depressed mood, dizziness, drowsiness, dry mouth, hallucinations, headache, hypotension, nervousness, tachycardia, tremor, and vertigo. Baclofen also may cause seizures.

CONTRAINDICATIONS & CAUTIONS
• Contraindicated in patients hypersensitive to these drugs.

• Use cautiously in patients with impaired renal or hepatic function.
• In pregnant women and breast-feeding women, use only when potential benefits to the patient outweigh risks to the fetus or infant. In children, recommendations vary. Elderly patients have an increased risk of adverse reactions; monitor them carefully.

Sulfonamides

co-trimoxazole (trimethoprim and sulfamethoxazole)
sulfasalazine

INDICATIONS
➤ **Bacterial infections, nocardiosis, toxoplasmosis, chloroquine-resistant *Plasmodium falciparum* malaria**

ACTION
Sulfonamides are bacteriostatic. They inhibit biosynthesis of tetrahydrofolic acid, which is needed for bacterial cell growth. They're active against some strains of staphylococci, streptococci, *Nocardia asteroides* and *brasiliensis, Clostridium tetani* and *perfringens, Bacillus anthracis, Escherichia coli,* and *Neisseria gonorrhoeae* and *meningitidis.* Sulfonamides are also active against organisms that cause UTIs, such as *E. coli, Proteus mirabilis* and *vulgaris, Klebsiella, Enterobacter,* and *Staphylococcus aureus,* and genital lesions caused by *Haemophilus ducreyi* (chancroid).

ADVERSE REACTIONS
Many adverse reactions stem from hypersensitivity, including bronchospasm, conjunctivitis, erythema multiforme, erythema nodosum, exfoliative dermatitis, fever, joint pain, pruritus, leukopenia, Lyell syndrome, photosensitivity, rash, Stevens-Johnson syndrome, and toxic epidermal necrolysis. GI reactions include anorexia, diarrhea, folic acid malabsorption, nausea, pancreatitis, stomatitis, and vomiting. Hematologic reactions include agranulocytosis, granulocytopenia, hypoprothrombinemia, thrombocytopenia, and, in G6PD deficiency, hemolytic anemia. Renal effects usually result from crystalluria caused by precipitation of sulfonamide in renal system.

CONTRAINDICATIONS & CAUTIONS
● Contraindicated in patients hypersensitive to these drugs.
● Use cautiously in patients with renal or hepatic impairment, bronchial asthma, severe allergy, or G6PD deficiency.
● In pregnant women at term and in breast-feeding women, use is contraindicated; sulfonamides appear in breast milk. In infants younger than age 2 months, sulfonamides are contraindicated unless there's no therapeutic alternative. In children with fragile X chromosome and mental retardation, use cautiously. Elderly patients are susceptible to bacterial and fungal superinfection and have an increased risk of folate deficiency anemia and adverse renal and hematologic effects.

Tetracyclines

doxycycline
doxycycline hyclate
doxycycline hydrochloride
doxycycline monohydrate
minocycline hydrochloride
oxytetracycline hydrochloride
tetracycline hydrochloride

INDICATIONS
➤ **Bacterial, protozoal, rickettsial, and fungal infections**

ACTION
Tetracyclines are bacteriostatic but may be bactericidal against certain organisms. They bind reversibly to 30S and 50S ribosomal subunits, which inhibits bacterial protein synthesis.

Susceptible gram-positive organisms include *Bacillus anthracis, Actinomyces israelii, Clostridium perfringens* and *tetani, Listeria monocytogenes,* and *Nocardia.*

Susceptible gram-negative organisms include *Neisseria meningitidis, Pasteurella multocida, Legionella pneumophila, Brucella, Vibrio cholerae, Yersinia enterocolitica, Yersinia pestis, Bordetella pertussis, Haemophilus influenzae, H. ducreyi, Campylobacter fetus, Shigella,* and many other common pathogens.

Other susceptible organisms include *Rickettsia akari, typhi, prowazekii,* and *tsutsugamushi; Coxiella burnetii; Chlamydia trachomatis* and *psittaci; Mycoplasma pneumoniae* and *hominis; Leptospira; Treponema pallidum* and *pertenue;* and *Borrelia recurrentis.*

ADVERSE REACTIONS
The most common adverse effects involve the GI tract and are dose related; they include abdominal discomfort; anorexia; bulky, loose stools; epigastric burning; flatulence; nausea; and vomiting. Superinfections also are common.

Photosensitivity reactions may be severe. Renal failure may be caused by Fanconi syndrome after use of outdated tetracycline. Permanent discoloration of teeth occurs if drug is given during tooth formation in children younger than age 8.

CONTRAINDICATIONS & CAUTIONS
● Contraindicated in patients hypersensitive to these drugs.
● Use cautiously in patients with renal or hepatic impairment.
● In pregnant or breast-feeding women, use is contraindicated; tetracyclines appear in breast milk. Children younger than age 8 shouldn't take tetracyclines; these drugs can cause permanent tooth discoloration, enamel hypoplasia, and a reversible decrease in bone calcification. Elderly patients may have decreased esophageal motility; use these drugs cautiously, and monitor patients for local irritation from slow passage of oral forms. Elderly patients also are more susceptible to superinfection.

Thrombolytics

alteplase
drotrecogin alfa
reteplase
streptokinase
tenecteplase
urokinase

INDICATIONS
➤ **To dissolve a preexisting clot or thrombus, often in acute or emergency situations**
➤ **Acute MI, acute ischemic stroke, pulmonary embolism and peripheral**

vascular occlusion; to restore patency to clotted grafts and I.V. access devices (alteplase); acute MI (reteplase and tenecteplase); acute MI, pulmonary embolism, and DVT (streptokinase); pulmonary embolism, coronary artery thrombosis, and catheter clearance (urokinase)

ACTION
Thrombolytics convert plasminogen to plasma, which lyse thrombi, fibrinogen and other plasma proteins.

ADVERSE REACTIONS
The most common with streptokinase are bleeding, allergic responses, reperfusion arrhythmias, hemorrhage infarct at the site of myocardial necrosis, and temperature elevation. Other adverse reactions common to all are bleeding, allergic reactions, flushing, headache, musculoskeletal pain, nausea, and hypotension.

CONTRAINDICATIONS & CAUTIONS
• Contraindicated in patients hypersensitive to any of the drug components.
• Contraindicated in active bleeding, history of stroke, recent intracranial or intraspinal surgery or trauma, intracranial neoplasm, arteriovenous malformation or aneurysm, bleeding diathesis, or severe uncontrolled hypertension.

Vasopressors

dobutamine hydrochloride
dopamine hydrochloride
ephedrine sulfate
norepinephrine bitartrate
phenylephrine hydrochloride

INDICATIONS
➤ Correction of hemodynamic imbalances present in cardiogenic shock due to MI, trauma, septicemia, cardiac surgical procedures, spinal anesthesia, drug reactions, renal failure, and heart failure
➤ As vasoconstrictor in regional analgesia and to overcome paroxysmal supraventricular tachycardia (phenylephrine hydrochloride)

➤ Stokes-Adams syndrome with complete heart block, narcolepsy, and myasthenia gravis (ephedrine sulfate)

ACTION
Dobutamine is a direct-acting inotropic whose primary activity results from stimulation of the beta receptors of the heart while producing mild chronotropic, hypertensive, arrhythmogenic, and vasodilatory effects. Dobutamine increases cardiac output by decreasing peripheral vascular resistance, reducing ventricular filling pressure, and increasing AV node conduction. Dopamine is a natural catecholamine, a precursor to norepinephrine in noradrenergic nerves, and a neurotransmitter in certain areas of the central nervous system. It produces positive chronotropic and inotropic effects on the myocardium, resulting in increased heart rate and cardiac contractility. This is accomplished by directly exerting an agonist action on beta-adrenoreceptors.

ADVERSE REACTIONS
Adverse reactions to vasopressors may include ventricular arrhythmias, tachycardia, angina, palpitations, cardiac conduction abnormalities, widened QRS complex, bradycardia, hypotension, hypertension, vasoconstriction, headache, anxiety, azotemia, dyspnea, phlebitis, peripheral cyanosis, and gangrene of extremities. Difficult or painful urination can be seen with ephedrine. Less common are hypotension, thrombocytopenia, hypokalemia, nausea, and shortness of breath.

CONTRAINDICATIONS & CAUTIONS
• Contraindicated in patients hypersensitive to any of the drug components.
• Contraindicated in patients with pheochromocytoma, uncorrected tachyarrhythmias, or ventricular fibrillation.
• Dobutamine is contraindicated in idiopathic hypertropic subaortic stenosis.
• Before treatment, hypovolemia should be corrected.
• Some vasopressors must be used cautiously in patients with a sulfite allergy, particularly asthmatic patients. Allergic type reactions, including anaphylactic symptoms and severe asthmatic episodes can occur.

• Infusion should be given into a large vein to prevent extravasation into surrounding tissue because this can cause tissue necrosis.

• Patients taking MAO inhibitors or who have been treated with MAO inhibitors 2 to 3 weeks before infusion will require substantially reduced dosage of dopamine.

• Norephinephrine bitartrate shouldn't be used during cyclopropane and halothane anesthesia because of the risk of ventricular tachycardia or fibrillation.

• Use cautiously in elderly patients and in patients with hyperthyroidism, bradycardia, partial heart block, myocardial disease, or severe arteriosclerosis.

• Safety and effectiveness in pediatric patients haven't been established. Phenylephrine can be used to treat hypotension during spinal anesthesia in children.

• Drugs should be given to pregnant woman only if clearly indicated.

• Caution should be used when these drugs are administered to breast-feeding women.

Xanthine derivatives

aminophylline
theophylline

INDICATIONS
➤ **Asthma and bronchospasm from emphysema and chronic bronchitis**

ACTION
Xanthine derivatives are structurally related; they directly relax smooth muscle, stimulate the CNS, induce diuresis, increase gastric acid secretion, inhibit uterine contractions, and exert weak inotropic and chronotropic effects on the heart. Of these drugs, theophylline exerts the greatest effect on smooth muscle.

The action of xanthine derivatives isn't completely caused by inhibition of phosphodiesterase. Current data suggest that inhibition of adenosine receptors or unidentified mechanisms may be responsible for therapeutic effects. By relaxing smooth muscle of the respiratory tract, they increase airflow and vital capacity. They also slow onset of diaphragmatic fatigue and stimulate the respiratory center in the CNS.

ADVERSE REACTIONS
Adverse effects, except for hypersensitivity, are dose related and can be controlled by dosage adjustment. Common reactions include arrhythmias, headache, hypotension, irritability, nausea, palpitations, restlessness, urine retention, and vomiting.

CONTRAINDICATIONS & CAUTIONS
• Contraindicated in patients hypersensitive to these drugs.

• Use cautiously in patients with arrhythmias, cardiac or circulatory impairment, cor pulmonale, hepatic or renal disease, active peptic ulcers, hyperthyroidism, or diabetes mellitus.

• In pregnant women, use cautiously. In breast-feeding women, avoid these drugs because they appear in breast milk, and infants may have serious adverse reactions. Small children may have excessive CNS stimulation; monitor them closely. In elderly patients, use cautiously.

atovaquone
chloroquine phosphate
(See Chapter 8, ANTIMALARIALS.)
mebendazole
metronidazole
metronidazole hydrochloride
nitazoxanide
pentamidine isethionate
tinidazole

atovaquone
a-TOE-va-kwon

Mepron

Pharmacologic class: ubiquinone
analogue
Pregnancy risk category C

AVAILABLE FORMS
Suspension: 750 mg/5 ml

INDICATIONS & DOSAGES
➤ **Acute, mild to moderate** *Pneumo-*
cystis jiroveci (carinii) **pneumonia**
in patients who can't tolerate
co-trimoxazole
Adults and adolescents ages 13 to 16:
Give 750 mg P.O. b.i.d. with food for
21 days.
➤ **To prevent** *P. jiroveci (carinii)*
pneumonia in patients who are un-
able to tolerate co-trimoxazole
Adults and adolescents ages 13 to 16:
Give 1,500 mg (10 ml) P.O. daily with
food.

ADMINISTRATION
P.O.
• Give drug with meals to enhance
absorption.

ACTION
May interfere with electron transport in
protozoal mitochondria, inhibiting enzymes needed to synthesize nucleic acids
and adenosine triphosphate.

Route	Onset	Peak	Duration
P.O.	Unknown	Unknown	Unknown

Half-life: 2 to 3 days.

ADVERSE REACTIONS
CNS: *headache, insomnia, fever, pain,*
asthenia, anxiety, dizziness.
CV: hypotension.
EENT: sinusitis, rhinitis.
GI: *abdominal pain, nausea, diarrhea,*
oral candidiasis, vomiting, constipation,
anorexia, dyspepsia, taste perversion.
Hematologic: *neutropenia,* anemia.
Metabolic: *hypoglycemia,* hyponatremia.
Respiratory: *cough.*
Skin: *rash, diaphoresis,* pruritus.

INTERACTIONS
Drug-drug. *Rifabutin, rifampin:* May
decrease atovaquone's steady-state level.
Avoid using together.

EFFECTS ON LAB TEST RESULTS
• May increase alkaline phosphatase, ALT,
and AST levels. May decrease glucose,
hemoglobin, and sodium levels.
• May decrease neutrophil count.

CONTRAINDICATIONS & CAUTIONS
• Contraindicated in patients hypersensitive to drug.
• Use cautiously in breast-feeding patients; it's unknown if drug appears in
breast milk.
• Use cautiously with other highly protein-
bound drugs; if used together, assess patient for toxicity.

NURSING CONSIDERATIONS
• *Alert:* Monitor patient closely during
therapy because of risk of pulmonary
infection.

PATIENT TEACHING
• Instruct patient to take drug with meals
because food significantly enhances
absorption.

mebendazole
me-BEN-da-zole

Pharmacologic class: benzimidazole
Pregnancy risk category C

AVAILABLE FORMS
Tablets (chewable): 100 mg

INDICATIONS & DOSAGES
➤ **Pinworm**
Adults and children older than age 2:
Give 100 mg P.O. as a single dose; repeat
if infestation persists 3 weeks later.
➤ **Roundworm, whipworm, and
hookworm**
Adults and children older than age 2:
Give 100 mg P.O. b.i.d. for 3 days; repeat
if infestation persists 3 weeks later.
➤ **Trichinosis ♦**
Adults: 200 to 400 mg P.O. t.i.d. for 3 days;
then 400 to 500 mg t.i.d. for 10 days.
➤ **Capillariasis ♦**
Adults and children: 200 mg P.O. b.i.d. for
20 days.
➤ **Dracunculiasis ♦**
Adults: 400 to 800 mg P.O. daily for 6 days.

ADMINISTRATION
P.O.
● Tablets may be chewed, swallowed
whole, or crushed and mixed with food.

ACTION
Selectively and irreversibly inhibits uptake
of glucose and other nutrients by susceptible helminths.

Route	Onset	Peak	Duration
P.O.	Unknown	2–4 hr	Variable

Half-life: 3 to 9 hours.

ADVERSE REACTIONS
CNS: *seizures,* fever.
GI: transient abdominal pain and diarrhea
in massive infestation and during expul-
sion of worms.
Skin: urticaria.

INTERACTIONS
Drug-drug. *Carbamazepine, hydantoin:*
May decrease mebendazole level, which
may decrease drug's effect. Monitor
patient for drug effectiveness.
Cimetidine: May increase mebendazole
level. Monitor patient for increased
adverse effects.

EFFECTS ON LAB TEST RESULTS
None reported.

CONTRAINDICATIONS & CAUTIONS
● Contraindicated in patients hypersensitive to drug.
● Safe use in children younger than age 2
hasn't been established.

NURSING CONSIDERATIONS
● Give drug to all family members to decrease risk of spreading the infestation.
● No dietary restrictions, laxatives, or ene-
mas are needed.

PATIENT TEACHING
● Teach patient about personal hygiene,
especially good hand-washing technique.
Advise him to refrain from preparing food
for others.
● To avoid reinfestation, teach patient to
wash perianal area daily, change under-
garments and bedclothes daily, and wash
hands and clean fingernails before meals
and after bowel movements.

metronidazole
me-troe-NI-da-zole

Flagyl, Flagyl 375, Flagyl ER,
Florazole ER†, Novo-Nidazol†

metronidazole hydrochloride
Flagyl IV RTU

Pharmacologic class: nitroimidazole
Pregnancy risk category B

AVAILABLE FORMS
Capsules: 375 mg
Injection: 500 mg/100 ml in vials or
ready-to-use minibags
Powder for injection: 500-mg single-dose
vials
Tablets: 250 mg, 500 mg
Tablets (extended-release): 750 mg

INDICATIONS & DOSAGES

■ **Black Box Warning** Use metronidazole only for the conditions for which it's indicated. ■

➤ **Amebic liver abscess**
Adults: 500 to 750 mg P.O. t.i.d. for 5 to 10 days; or 2.4 g P.O. once daily for 1 to 2 days. Or, 500 mg I.V. every 6 hours for 10 days if patient can't tolerate P.O. route.
Children: 35 to 50 mg/kg daily in three divided doses for 10 days. Maximum, 750 mg/dose.

➤ **Intestinal amebiasis**
Adults: 750 mg P.O. t.i.d. for 5 to 10 days; then treat with a luminal amebicide, such as iodoquinol or paromomycin.
Children: 35 to 50 mg/kg daily in three divided doses for 10 days; then treat with a luminal amebicide, such as iodoquinol or paromomycin.

➤ **Trichomoniasis**
Adults: 500 mg P.O. b.i.d. for 7 days, or 2 g P.O. in single dose (may give the 2-g dose in two 1-g doses, both on the same day); wait 4 to 6 weeks before repeating course.
Children: 5 mg/kg P.O. t.i.d. for 7 days.

➤ **Refractory trichomoniasis**
Adults: 500 mg P.O. b.i.d. for 7 days.

➤ **Bacterial infections caused by anaerobic microorganisms**
Adults: Loading dose is 15 mg/kg I.V. infused over 1 hour. Maintenance dose is 7.5 mg/kg I.V. or P.O. every 6 hours. Give first maintenance dose 6 hours after loading dose. Maximum dose shouldn't exceed 4 g daily.

➤ **To prevent postoperative infection in contaminated or potentially contaminated colorectal surgery**
Adults: Infuse 15 mg/kg I.V. over 30 to 60 minutes and complete about 1 hour before surgery. Then, infuse 7.5 mg/kg I.V. over 30 to 60 minutes at 6 and 12 hours after first dose.

➤ **Bacterial vaginosis**
Adults: 750 mg Flagyl ER P.O. daily for 7 days.

➤ *Clostridium difficile*–**associated diarrhea and colitis** ◆
Adults: Usually 250 mg P.O. q.i.d. or 500 mg P.O. t.i.d. for 10 days. Or, 500 mg to 750 mg I.V. every 6 to 8 hours when P.O. route isn't practical.

Children: 30 to 50 mg/kg/day P.O. given in three to four equally divided doses for 7 to 10 days. Don't exceed adult dose.

➤ **Pelvic inflammatory disease (PID)** ◆
Adults: 500 mg I.V. every 8 hours with ofloxacin or with I.V. levofloxacin. For ambulatory patients, 500 mg P.O. b.i.d. with ofloxacin for 14 days.

➤ **Bacterial vaginosis** ◆
Nonpregnant women: 500 mg P.O. b.i.d. for 7 days. Or, 2 g P.O. as a single dose.
Pregnant women: 250 mg P.O. t.i.d. or 500 mg P.O. b.i.d. for 7 days.

ADMINISTRATION

P.O.
● Give drug with food.

I.V.
● Flagyl IV ready-to-use (RTU) minibags need no preparation.
● Don't use aluminum needles or hubs to reconstitute the drug or to transfer reconstituted drug. Equipment that contains aluminum will turn the solution orange; the potency isn't affected.
● To reconstitute lyophilized vials, add 4.4 ml of sterile water for injection, bacteriostatic water for injection, sterile normal saline solution for injection, or bacteriostatic normal saline solution for injection. Reconstituted drug contains 100 mg/ml. Add contents of vial to 100 ml of D_5W, lactated Ringer's injection, or normal saline solution to yield 5 mg/ml. Neutralize this highly acidic solution by carefully adding 5 mEq sodium bicarbonate to each 500 mg; the carbon dioxide gas that forms may need to be vented.
● Infuse drug over at least 1 hour. Don't give by I.V. push.
● Don't refrigerate the neutralized diluted solution; precipitation may occur. Refrigerated Flagyl IV RTU may form crystals, which disappear after the solution warms to room temperature.
● **Incompatibilities:** Aluminum, amino acid 10%, amoxicillin sodium and clavulanate potassium, amphotericin B, aztreonam, ceftriaxone, dopamine, filgrastim, meropenem, other I.V. drugs, warfarin.

ACTION

Direct-acting trichomonacide and amebicide that works inside and outside the

intestines. It's thought to enter the cells of microorganisms that contain nitroreductase, forming unstable compounds that bind to DNA and inhibit synthesis, causing cell death.

Route	Onset	Peak	Duration
P.O.	Unknown	2 hr	Unknown
I.V.	Immediate	1 hr	Unknown

Half-life: 6 to 8 hours.

ADVERSE REACTIONS
CNS: *headache, seizures,* fever, vertigo, ataxia, dizziness, syncope, incoordination, confusion, irritability, depression, weakness, insomnia, peripheral neuropathy.
CV: flattened T wave, edema, flushing, thrombophlebitis after I.V. infusion.
EENT: rhinitis, sinusitis, pharyngitis.
GI: *nausea,* abdominal cramping or pain, stomatitis, epigastric distress, vomiting, anorexia, diarrhea, constipation, proctitis, dry mouth, metallic taste.
GU: *vaginitis,* darkened urine, polyuria, dysuria, cystitis, dyspareunia, dryness of vagina and vulva, vaginal candidiasis, genital pruritus.
Hematologic: *transient leukopenia, neutropenia.*
Musculoskeletal: transient joint pains.
Respiratory: upper respiratory tract infection.
Skin: rash.
Other: decreased libido, overgrowth of nonsusceptible organisms, especially *Candida.*

INTERACTIONS
Drug-drug. Busulfan: May increase busulfan toxicity. Avoid using together.
Cimetidine: May increase risk of metronidazole toxicity because of inhibited hepatic metabolism. Monitor patient for toxicity.
Disulfiram: May cause acute psychosis and confusion. Avoid giving metronidazole within 2 weeks of disulfiram.
Lithium: May increase lithium level, which may cause toxicity. Monitor lithium level.
Phenobarbital, phenytoin: May decrease metronidazole effectiveness; may reduce total phenytoin clearance. Monitor patient.

Warfarin: May increase anticoagulant effects and risk of bleeding. Reduce warfarin as needed.
Drug-lifestyle. *Alcohol use:* May cause disulfiram-like reaction, including nausea, vomiting, headache, cramps, and flushing. Warn patient to avoid alcohol during and for 3 days after completing drug therapy.

EFFECTS ON LAB TEST RESULTS
● May decrease WBC and neutrophil counts.
● May falsely decrease triglyceride and aminotransferase levels.

CONTRAINDICATIONS & CAUTIONS
● Contraindicated in patients hypersensitive to drug or other nitroimidazole derivatives and in patients in first trimester of pregnancy.
● **Alert:** If drug must be given to a pregnant woman for trichomoniasis, use the 7-day regimen, not the 2-g single-dose regimen. The 2-g dose produces a high level that's more likely to reach fetal circulation.
● Use cautiously in patients with history of blood dyscrasia, CNS disorder, or retinal or visual field changes.
● Use cautiously in patients who take hepatotoxic drugs or have hepatic disease or alcoholism.

NURSING CONSIDERATIONS
● Monitor liver function test results carefully in elderly patients.
● Observe patient for edema, especially if he's receiving corticosteroids; Flagyl IV RTU may cause sodium retention.
● Record number and character of stools when drug is used to treat amebiasis. Give drug only after *Trichomonas vaginalis* infection is confirmed by wet smear or culture or *Entameba histolytica* is identified.
● Sexual partners of patients being treated for *T. vaginalis* infection, even if asymptomatic, must also be treated to avoid reinfection.

PATIENT TEACHING
● Instruct patient to take extended-release tablets at least 1 hour before or 2 hours after meals but to take all other oral forms with food to minimize GI upset.

Reactions may be *common,* uncommon, *life-threatening,* or COMMON AND LIFE-THREATENING.
Interaction may have a *rapid* onset or *delayed onset.*

• Inform patient of need for sexual partners to be treated simultaneously to avoid reinfection.
• Instruct patient in proper hygiene.
• Tell patient to avoid alcohol and alcohol-containing drugs during and for at least 3 days after treatment course.
• Tell patient he may experience a metallic taste and have dark or red-brown urine.
• Tell patient to report to prescriber symptoms of candidal overgrowth.
• Tell patient to report to prescriber immediately any neurologic symptoms (seizures, peripheral neuropathy).

nitazoxanide
nye-te-ZOCKS-a-nide

Alinia

Pharmacologic class: antiprotozoal
Pregnancy risk category B

AVAILABLE FORMS
Oral suspension: 100 mg/5 ml
Tablets: 500 mg

INDICATIONS & DOSAGES
➤ **Diarrhea caused by *Cryptosporidium parvum* or *Giardia lamblia***
Adults and children age 12 and older: 500 mg P.O. with food every 12 hours for 3 days.
Children ages 4 to 11: Give 10 ml (200 mg) P.O. with food every 12 hours for 3 days.
Children ages 1 to 3: Give 5 ml (100 mg) P.O. with food every 12 hours for 3 days.

ADMINISTRATION
P.O.
• Give drug with food.
• Discard unused suspension after 7 days.

ACTION
May interfere with an enzyme-dependent electron transfer reaction, essential for anaerobic energy metabolism.

Route	Onset	Peak	Duration
P.O.	Rapid	1–4 hr	Unknown

Half-life: Unknown.

ADVERSE REACTIONS
CNS: headache.
GI: abdominal pain, diarrhea, nausea, vomiting.

INTERACTIONS
Drug-drug. *Drugs that are highly protein-bound:* May compete for binding sites. Use together cautiously.

EFFECTS ON LAB TEST RESULTS
• May increase creatinine and glutamate pyruvate transaminase levels.

CONTRAINDICATIONS & CAUTIONS
• Contraindicated in patients hypersensitive to nitazoxanide.
• Use cautiously in patients with renal or hepatic dysfunction. Safety and effectiveness haven't been established in HIV-positive patients, other immunodeficient patients, or infants younger than age 1.

NURSING CONSIDERATIONS
• *Alert:* A single tablet contains more of the drug than is recommended for pediatric doses and shouldn't be given to children age 11 or younger.
• Monitor glucose level in patients with diabetes who are taking the suspension.

PATIENT TEACHING
• Tell caregiver or patient to give drug with food.
• Instruct caregiver or patient to keep container tightly closed and to shake it well before each use.
• Advise caregiver or patient that drug may be stored at room temperature.
• Advise caregiver or patient to discard suspension after 7 days.
• Inform diabetic patient or his caregiver that suspension contains 1.48 g of sucrose per 5 ml.

pentamidine isethionate
pen-TA-ma-deen

NebuPent, Pentam 300

Pharmacologic class: diamidine
derivative
Pregnancy risk category C

AVAILABLE FORMS
Aerosol, injection, powder for injection:
300-mg vial

INDICATIONS & DOSAGES
➤ *Pneumocystis jiroveci (carinii)*
pneumonia
*Adults and children age 4 months and
older:* 3 to 4 mg/kg I.V. or I.M. once daily
for 14 to 21 days.
➤ **To prevent** *P. jiroveci (carinii)*
pneumonia in high-risk patients
*Adults and children capable of using a
nebulizer effectively:* 300 mg by inhalation
using a Respirgard II nebulizer once every
4 weeks.
➤ **Visceral leishmaniasis caused by**
Leishmania donovani ◆
Adults and children: 2 to 4 mg/kg I.V. or
I.M. once daily or once every other day
for up to 15 doses.
➤ **Cutaneous leishmaniasis** ◆
Adults and children: 2 mg/kg I.M. every
other day for seven doses or 3 mg/kg I.M.
every other day for four doses.

ADMINISTRATION
I.V.
● Reconstitute drug with 3 ml sterile water
for injection.
● Dilute reconstituted drug in 50 to 250 ml
D₅W.
● Infuse over at least 60 minutes.
● To minimize risk of hypotension, infuse
drug slowly with patient lying down.
Closely monitor blood pressure.
● **Incompatibilities:** Aldesleukin, cephalo-
sporins, fluconazole, foscarnet, linezolid.
I.M.
● Reconstitute drug with 3 ml sterile water
for a solution containing 100 mg/ml.
● Give deep into muscle.
● Patient may have pain and induration at
injection site.
● Rotate injection sites.

Inhalational
● Give aerosol form only by Respirgard II
nebulizer. Dosage recommendations are
based on particle size and delivery rate of
this device. To give aerosol, mix contents
of one vial in 6 ml sterile water for injection. Don't use normal saline solution.
Don't mix with other drugs.
● Don't use low-pressure (less than
20 pounds per square inch [psi]) com-
pressors. The flow rate should be 5 to
7 L/minute from 40- to 50-psi air or
oxygen source.

ACTION
May interfere with biosynthesis of DNA,
RNA, phospholipids, and proteins in sus-
ceptible organisms.

Route	Onset	Peak	Duration
I.V.	Unknown	1 hr	Unknown
I.M., inhalation	Unknown	30 min	Unknown

Half-life: 9 to 13 hours for I.M., about
6½ hours for I.V. Unknown for inhalation.

ADVERSE REACTIONS
CNS: *dizziness, fatigue,* confusion, hallu-
cinations, headache.
CV: *chest pain,* **severe hypotension, ven-
tricular tachycardia,** edema.
EENT: *pharyngitis,* burning in throat
(with inhaled form).
GI: *nausea, metallic taste, decreased ap-
petite, vomiting,* **pancreatitis,** diarrhea,
abdominal pain, anorexia.
GU: *acute renal failure.*
Hematologic: *leukopenia, thrombocy-
topenia,* anemia.
Metabolic: *hypoglycemia,* hyperglyce-
mia, hypocalcemia.
Musculoskeletal: myalgia.
Respiratory: *congestion, cough, short-
ness of breath,* **bronchospasm,** pneumothorax.
Skin: **Stevens-Johnson syndrome,** rash.
Other: *night sweats, chills, sterile ab-
scess, pain, induration at injection site.*

INTERACTIONS
Drug-drug. *Aminoglycosides, amphotericin B, capreomycin, cisplatin,
methoxyflurane, polymyxin B, vancomycin:* May increase risk of nephrotoxi-

---

Reactions may be *common*, uncommon, *life-threatening*, or COMMON AND LIFE-THREATENING.
Interaction may have a *rapid onset* or *delayed onset*.

city. Monitor renal function test results closely.

Antineoplastics: May cause additive bone marrow suppression. Use together cautiously; monitor hematologic study results.

Drugs that prolong the QT interval (antipsychotics; antiarrhythmics, such as amiodarone, disopyramide, procainamide, quinidine, and sotalol; fluoroquinolones; macrolides; tricyclic antidepressants): May cause additive effect. Use together cautiously; monitor patient for adverse cardiac effects.

EFFECTS ON LAB TEST RESULTS
• May increase BUN, creatinine, and potassium levels. May decrease hemoglobin level and hematocrit. May increase or decrease glucose level.
• May decrease WBC and platelet counts.

CONTRAINDICATIONS & CAUTIONS
• Contraindicated in patients with history of anaphylactic reaction to drug.
• Use cautiously in patients with hypertension, hypotension, hypoglycemia, hypocalcemia, leukopenia, thrombocytopenia, anemia, diabetes, pancreatitis, Stevens-Johnson syndrome, or hepatic or renal dysfunction.
• Use cautiously in breast-feeding women; it's unknown if drug appears in breast milk.

NURSING CONSIDERATIONS
• *Alert:* Monitor glucose, calcium, creatinine, and BUN levels daily. After parenteral administration, glucose level may decrease initially; hypoglycemia may be severe in 5% to 10% of patients. After several months of therapy, this may be followed by hyperglycemia and type 1 diabetes mellitus, which may be permanent because of pancreatic cell damage.
• In patients with AIDS, drug may produce less severe adverse reactions than co-trimoxazole.

PATIENT TEACHING
• Instruct patient to use the aerosol device until the chamber is empty, which may take up to 45 minutes.
• Warn patient that I.M. injection is painful.

• Instruct patient to complete the full course, even if he's feeling better.

tinidazole
teh-NID-ah-zol

Tindamax

Pharmacologic class: antiprotozoal
Pregnancy risk category C

AVAILABLE FORMS
Tablets: 250 mg, 500 mg

INDICATIONS & DOSAGES
■ **Black Box Warning** Use tinidazole only for the conditions for which it's indicated. ■

➤ **Bacterial vaginosis in nonpregnant adult women**
Adults: 2 g once daily for 2 days with food, or 1 g once daily for 5 days with food.

➤ **Trichomoniasis caused by *Trichomonas vaginalis***
Adults: 2 g P.O. as a single dose taken with food. Sexual partners should be treated at the same time with the same dose.

➤ **Giardiasis caused by *Giardia lamblia (G. duodenalis)***
Adults: 2 g P.O. as a single dose taken with food.
Children older than age 3: Give 50 mg/kg (up to 2 g) as a single dose taken with food.

➤ **Intestinal amebiasis caused by *Entamoeba histolytica***
Adults: 2 g P.O. daily for 3 days, taken with food.
Children older than age 3: Give 50 mg/kg (up to 2 g) P.O. daily for 3 days, taken with food.

➤ **Amebic liver abscess (amebiasis)**
Adults: 2 g P.O. daily for 3 to 5 days, taken with food.
Children older than age 3: Give 50 mg/kg (up to 2 g) P.O. daily for 3 to 5 days, taken with food.

Adjust-a-dose: For patients receiving hemodialysis, give an additional dose equal to one-half the recommended dose after the hemodialysis session.

ADMINISTRATION
P.O.
● Give drug with food to minimize adverse GI effects.
● For children who can't swallow pills, crush tablet into fine powder and mix with artificial cherry syrup.

ACTION
For *Trichomonas,* drug reduces the compound's nitro group into a free nitro radical that may be responsible for the antiprotozoal activity. Mechanism of action against *Giardia* and *Entamoeba* is unknown.

Route	Onset	Peak	Duration
P.O.	Unknown	1½ hr	Unknown

Half-life: 12 to 14 hours.

ADVERSE REACTIONS
CNS: *seizures,* dizziness, fatigue, headache, malaise, peripheral neuropathy, weakness.
GI: anorexia, constipation, cramps, dyspepsia, metallic taste, nausea, vomiting.

INTERACTIONS
Drug-drug. *Cyclosporine, tacrolimus:* May increase cyclosporine or tacrolimus level. Monitor patient closely for toxicity, including headache, nausea, vomiting, nephrotoxicity, and electrolyte abnormalities.
Disulfiram: May increase abdominal cramping, nausea, vomiting, headaches, and flushing. Separate doses by 2 weeks.
Drugs that induce CYP-450, such as fosphenytoin, phenobarbital, phenytoin, and rifampin: May increase tinidazole elimination. Monitor patient.
Drugs that inhibit CYP-450, such as cimetidine and ketoconazole: May prolong tinidazole half-life and decrease clearance. Monitor patient.
Fluorouracil: May decrease fluorouracil clearance, increasing adverse effects without added benefit. Monitor patient for rash, nausea, vomiting, stomatitis, and leukopenia.
Fosphenytoin, phenytoin: May prolong phenytoin half-life and decrease clearance of I.V. drug. Monitor patient for toxicity.

Lithium: May increase lithium level. Monitor patient; monitor lithium and creatinine levels.
Oxytetracycline: May counteract tinidazole. Assess patient for lack of effect.
Warfarin and other oral anticoagulants: May increase anticoagulant effect. Anticoagulant dosage may need adjustment during and for up to 8 days after tinidazole therapy.
Drug-herb. *St. John's wort:* May increase or decrease drug level. Discourage use together.
Drug-lifestyle. *Use of alcohol and alcohol-containing products:* May increase abdominal cramping, nausea, vomiting, headaches, and flushing. Discourage use together and for 3 days after stopping drug.

EFFECTS ON LAB TEST RESULTS
● May increase AST, ALT, glucose, LDH, and triglyceride levels.
● May decrease WBC count.

CONTRAINDICATIONS & CAUTIONS
● Contraindicated in patients hypersensitive to drug, its component, or other nitroimidazole derivatives.
● Contraindicated in pregnant women during first trimester.
● Use cautiously in patients with CNS disorders and in those with blood dyscrasias or hepatic dysfunction.

NURSING CONSIDERATIONS
● If therapy exceeds 3 days, monitor children closely.
● Patient should take drug with food to minimize adverse GI effects.
● **Alert:** If abnormal neurologic signs, such as seizures or numbness of the arms or legs, occur, stop drug immediately.
● If candidiasis develops during therapy, the patient may need an antifungal.
● Women shouldn't breast-feed during therapy and for 3 days after the last dose.
● An elderly patient may have decreased liver or kidney function or other medical conditions and may be taking other drugs that may affect dosage.

PATIENT TEACHING
● Tell patient to take drug with food.
● **Alert:** Tell patient to report to prescriber seizures and numbness in arms or legs.

Reactions may be *common,* uncommon, *life-threatening,* or COMMON AND LIFE-THREATENING.
Interaction may have a *rapid onset* or *delayed onset.*

- Warn patient not to drink alcohol or use alcohol-containing products while taking drug and for 3 days afterward.
- Advise woman to immediately notify her prescriber if she becomes pregnant.
- Tell woman to stop breast-feeding during therapy and for 3 days after the last dose.
- If patient is being treated for a sexually transmitted infection, explain that his sexual partners should be treated at the same time.

6

Aminoglycosides

amikacin sulfate
gentamicin sulfate
neomycin sulfate
streptomycin sulfate
tobramycin sulfate

---

amikacin sulfate
am-i-KAY-sin

Amikin

Pharmacologic class:
aminoglycoside
Pregnancy risk category D

AVAILABLE FORMS
Injection: 50 mg/ml (pediatric) vial,
250 mg/ml vial, 250 mg/ml disposable
syringe

INDICATIONS & DOSAGES
➤ **Serious infections caused by sensitive strains of *Pseudomonas aeruginosa, Escherichia coli, Proteus, Klebsiella,* or *Staphylococcus***
Adults and children: 15 mg/kg/day I.M. or
I.V. infusion, in divided doses every 8 to
12 hours for 7 to 10 days.
Neonates: Initially, loading dose of
10 mg/kg I.V.; then 7.5 mg/kg every
12 hours for 7 to 10 days.
➤ **Uncomplicated UTI caused by organisms not susceptible to less toxic drugs**
Adults: 250 mg I.M. or I.V. b.i.d.
➤ **Active tuberculosis, with other antituberculotics** ◆
Adults and children age 15 and older:
15 mg/kg (up to 1 g) I.M. or I.V. once
daily five to seven times per week for 2 to
4 months or until culture conversion. Then
reduce dose to 15 mg/kg daily given two
or three times weekly depending on other
drugs in regimen. Patients older than
age 59 may receive a reduced dose of
10 mg/kg (up to 750 mg) daily.
Children younger than age 15: Give 15 to
30 mg/kg (up to 1 g) I.M. or I.V. once
daily or twice weekly.

➤ *Mycobacterium avium* **complex
(MAC) infection** ◆
Adults: 15 mg/kg/day I.V. in divided doses
every 8 to 12 hours as part of a multiple-
drug regimen.
Adjust-a-dose: For adults with impaired
renal function, initially, 7.5 mg/kg I.M. or
I.V. Subsequent doses and frequency determined by amikacin levels and renal
function studies. For adults receiving hemodialysis, give supplemental doses of
50% to 75% of initial loading dose at end
of each dialysis session. Monitor drug
levels and adjust dosage accordingly.

ADMINISTRATION
I.V.
● Obtain specimen for culture and sensitivity tests before giving first dose. Begin
therapy while awaiting results.
● For adults, dilute I.V. drug in 100 to
200 ml of D_5W or normal saline solution.
For children, the amount of fluid will
depend on the ordered dose.
● In adults and children, infuse over 30 to
60 minutes. In infants, infuse over 1 to
2 hours.
● After infusion, flush line with normal
saline solution or D_5W.
● **Incompatibilities:** Allopurinol, aminophylline, amphotericin B, ampicillin,
azithromycin, bacitracin, cefazolin, ceftazidime, chlorothiazide sodium, cisplatin,
heparin sodium, hetastarch in 0.9% sodium
chloride, oxacillin, phenytoin, propofol,
thiopental, vancomycin, vitamin B complex with C.
I.M.
● Obtain specimen for culture and sensitivity tests before giving first dose. Begin
therapy while awaiting results.
● Obtain blood for peak level 1 hour after
I.M. injection and 30 minutes to 1 hour
after I.V. infusion ends; for trough levels,
draw blood just before next dose. Don't
collect blood in a heparinized tube; heparin is incompatible with aminoglycosides.

Reactions may be *common,* uncommon, *life-threatening,* or COMMON AND LIFE-THREATENING.
Interaction may have a *rapid onset* or *delayed onset.*

ACTION
Inhibits protein synthesis by binding directly to the 30S ribosomal subunit; bactericidal.

Route	Onset	Peak	Duration
I.V.	Immediate	30 min	8–12 hr
I.M.	Unknown	1 hr	8–12 hr

Half-life: Adults, 2 to 3 hours. Patients with severe renal damage, 30 to 86 hours.

ADVERSE REACTIONS
CNS: *neuromuscular blockade.*
EENT: *ototoxicity.*
GU: *azotemia,* **nephrotoxicity,** increase in urinary excretion of casts.
Musculoskeletal: arthralgia.
Respiratory: *apnea.*

INTERACTIONS
Drug-drug. ■ **Black Box Warning** *Acyclovir, amphotericin B, bacitracin, cephalosporins, cidofovir, cisplatin, methoxyflurane, vancomycin, other aminoglycosides:* May increase nephrotoxicity. Use together cautiously, and monitor renal function test results. ■
Atracurium, pancuronium, rocuronium, vecuronium: May increase effects of nondepolarizing muscle relaxants, including prolonged respiratory depression. Use together only when necessary, and expect to reduce dosage of nondepolarizing muscle relaxant.
Dimenhydrinate: May mask ototoxicity symptoms. Monitor patient's hearing.
General anesthetics: May increase neuromuscular blockade. Monitor patient for increased effects.
Indomethacin: May increase trough and peak amikacin levels. Monitor amikacin level.
■ **Black Box Warning** *I.V. loop diuretics such as furosemide:* May increase ototoxicity. Use together cautiously, and monitor patient's hearing. ■
Parenteral penicillins: May inactivate amikacin in vitro. Don't mix.

EFFECTS ON LAB TEST RESULTS
● May increase BUN, creatinine, nonprotein nitrogen, and urine urea levels.

CONTRAINDICATIONS & CAUTIONS
● Contraindicated in patients hypersensitive to drug or other aminoglycosides.
● Use cautiously in patients with impaired renal function or neuromuscular disorders, in neonates and infants, and in elderly patients.

NURSING CONSIDERATIONS
■ **Black Box Warning** Due to increased risk of ototoxicity, evaluate patient's hearing before and during therapy if he'll be receiving the drug for longer than 2 weeks. Notify prescriber if patient has tinnitus, vertigo, or hearing loss. ■
● Weigh patient and review renal function studies before therapy begins.
● Correct dehydration before therapy because of increased risk of toxicity.
● Peak drug levels more than 35 mcg/ml and trough levels more than 10 mcg/ml may be linked to a higher risk of toxicity.
■ **Black Box Warning** Due to increased risk of nephrotoxicity, monitor renal function: urine output, specific gravity, urinalysis, BUN and creatinine levels, and creatinine clearance. Report to prescriber evidence of declining renal function. ■
● Watch for signs and symptoms of superinfection (especially of upper respiratory tract), such as continued fever, chills, and increased pulse rate.
■ **Black Box Warning** Neuromuscular blockage and respiratory paralysis have been reported after aminoglycoside administration. Monitor patient closely. ■
● Therapy usually continues for 7 to 10 days. If no response occurs after 3 to 5 days, stop therapy and obtain new specimens for culture and sensitivity testing.
● *Look alike-sound alike:* Don't confuse Amikin with Amicar. Don't confuse amikacin with anakinra.

PATIENT TEACHING
● Instruct patient to promptly report adverse reactions to prescriber.
● Encourage patient to maintain adequate fluid intake.

gentamicin sulfate
jen-ta-MYE-sin

Pharmacologic class:
aminoglycoside
Pregnancy risk category D

AVAILABLE FORMS
Injection: 40 mg/ml (adults), 10 mg/ml (children)
I.V. infusion (premixed): 40 mg, 60 mg, 70 mg, 80 mg, 100 mg, 120 mg, in normal saline solution

INDICATIONS & DOSAGES
➤ **Serious infections caused by sensitive strains of *Pseudomonas aeruginosa, Escherichia coli, Proteus, Klebsiella, Serratia,* or *Staphylococcus***
Adults: 3 mg/kg daily in three divided doses I.M. or I.V. infusion every 8 hours. For life-threatening infections, may give up to 5 mg/kg daily in three or four divided doses; reduce dosage to 3 mg/kg daily as soon as patient improves.
Children: 2 to 2.5 mg/kg every 8 hours I.M. or I.V. infusion.
Neonates older than 1 week and infants: 2.5 mg/kg every 8 hours I.M. or by I.V. infusion.
Neonates younger than 1 week and preterm infants: 2.5 mg/kg every 12 hours I.M. or by I.V. infusion.
➤ **To prevent endocarditis before GI or GU procedure or surgery**
Adults: 1.5 mg/kg I.M. or I.V. 30 minutes before procedure or surgery. Maximum dose is 80 mg. Give with ampicillin (vancomycin in penicillin-allergic patients).
Children: 2 mg/kg I.M. or I.V. 30 minutes before procedure or surgery. Maximum dose is 80 mg. Give with ampicillin (vancomycin in penicillin-allergic patients).
Adjust-a-dose: For adults with impaired renal function, doses and frequency are determined by drug level and renal function. To maintain therapeutic levels, adults should receive 1 to 1.7 mg/kg I.M. or by I.V. infusion after each dialysis session, and children should receive 2 to 2.5 mg/kg I.M. or by I.V. infusion after each dialysis session.

ADMINISTRATION
I.V.
• Obtain specimen for culture and sensitivity tests before giving. Begin therapy while awaiting results.
• For intermittent infusion, dilute with 50 to 200 ml of D_5W or normal saline solution for injection.
• Infuse over 30 minutes to 2 hours.
• After completing infusion, flush the line with normal saline solution or D_5W.
• **Incompatibilities:** Allopurinol, amphotericin B, ampicillin, azithromycin, cefazolin, cefepime, cefotaxime, ceftazidime, ceftriaxone sodium, cefuroxime, certain parenteral nutrition formulations, cytarabine, dopamine, fat emulsions, furosemide, heparin, hetastarch, idarubicin, indomethacin sodium trihydrate, nafcillin, propofol, ticarcillin, warfarin.

I.M.
• Obtain specimen for culture and sensitivity tests before giving. Begin therapy while awaiting results.
• Obtain blood for peak level 1 hour after I.M. injection or 30 minutes after I.V. infusion finishes; for trough levels, draw blood just before next dose. Don't collect blood in a heparinized tube; heparin is incompatible with aminoglycosides.

ACTION
Inhibits protein synthesis by binding directly to the 30S ribosomal subunit; bactericidal.

Route	Onset	Peak	Duration
I.V.	Immediate	30–90 min	Unknown
I.M.	Unknown	30–90 min	Unknown

Half-life: 2 to 3 hours.

ADVERSE REACTIONS
CNS: *encephalopathy, seizures,* fever, headache, lethargy, confusion, dizziness, numbness, peripheral neuropathy, vertigo, ataxia, tingling.
CV: hypotension.
EENT: *ototoxicity,* blurred vision, tinnitus.
GI: vomiting, nausea.
GU: *nephrotoxicity,* possible increase in urinary excretion of casts.
Hematologic: *agranulocytosis, leukopenia, thrombocytopenia,* anemia, eosinophilia.

Reactions may be *common,* uncommon, *life-threatening,* or COMMON AND LIFE-THREATENING.
Interaction may have a *rapid onset* or *delayed onset.*

Musculoskeletal: muscle twitching, myasthenia gravis–like syndrome.
Respiratory: *apnea.*
Skin: rash, urticaria, pruritus, injection site pain.
Other: *anaphylaxis.*

INTERACTIONS
Drug-drug. ■ **Black Box Warning** *Acyclovir, amphotericin B, cephalosporins, cidofovir, cisplatin, methoxyflurane, vancomycin, other aminoglycosides:* May increase ototoxicity and nephrotoxicity. Monitor hearing and renal function test results. ■
Atracurium, pancuronium, rocuronium, vecuronium: May increase effects of nondepolarizing muscle relaxants, including prolonged respiratory depression. Use together only when necessary, and expect to reduce dosage of nondepolarizing muscle relaxant.
Dimenhydrinate: May mask ototoxicity symptoms. Monitor patient's hearing.
General anesthetics: May increase neuromuscular blockade. Monitor patient closely.
Indomethacin: May increase peak and trough levels of gentamicin. Monitor gentamicin level.
■ **Black Box Warning** *I.V. loop diuretics (such as furosemide):* May increase risk of ototoxicity. Monitor patient's hearing. ■
Parenteral penicillins (such as ampicillin and ticarcillin): May inactivate gentamicin in vitro. Don't mix together.

EFFECTS ON LAB TEST RESULTS
● May increase ALT, AST, bilirubin, BUN, creatinine, LDH, and nonprotein nitrogen levels. May decrease hemoglobin level.
● May increase eosinophil count. May decrease granulocyte, platelet, and WBC counts.

CONTRAINDICATIONS & CAUTIONS
● Contraindicated in patients hypersensitive to drug or other aminoglycosides.
● Use cautiously in neonates, infants, elderly patients, and patients with impaired renal function or neuromuscular disorders.

NURSING CONSIDERATIONS
■ **Black Box Warning** Evaluate patient's hearing before and during therapy. Notify prescriber if patient complains of tinnitus, vertigo, or hearing loss. ■
● Weigh patient and review renal function studies before therapy begins.
● **Alert:** Use preservative-free form when intrathecal route is used adjunctively for serious CNS infections, such as meningitis and ventriculitis.
● Maintain peak levels at 4 to 12 mcg/ml and trough levels at 1 to 2 mcg/ml. The maximum peak level is usually 8 mcg/ml, except in patients with cystic fibrosis, who need increased lung penetration. Prolonged peak levels of 10 to 12 mcg/ml or prolonged trough levels greater than 2 mcg/ml may increase risk of toxicity.
■ **Black Box Warning** Monitor renal function: urine output, specific gravity, urinalysis, BUN and creatinine levels, and creatinine clearance. Report to prescriber evidence of declining renal function. ■
● Hemodialysis for 8 hours may remove up to 50% of drug from blood.
● Watch for signs and symptoms of superinfection (especially of upper respiratory tract), such as continued fever, chills, and increased pulse rate.
● Therapy usually continues for 7 to 10 days. If no response occurs in 3 to 5 days, stop therapy and obtain new specimens for culture and sensitivity testing.

PATIENT TEACHING
● Instruct patient to promptly report adverse reactions, such as dizziness, vertigo, unsteady gait, ringing in the ears, hearing loss, numbness, tingling, or muscle twitching.
● Encourage patient to drink plenty of fluids.
● Warn patient to avoid hazardous activities if adverse CNS reactions occur.

neomycin sulfate
nee-o-MYE-sin

Neo-fradin

Pharmacologic class: aminoglycoside
Pregnancy risk category D

AVAILABLE FORMS
Oral solution: 125 mg/5 ml
Tablets: 500 mg

INDICATIONS & DOSAGES
➤ **Infectious diarrhea caused by enteropathogenic** *Escherichia coli*
Adults: 50 mg/kg daily P.O. in four divided doses for 2 to 3 days; maximum of 3 g/day.
Children: 50 to 100 mg/kg daily P.O. in divided doses every 4 to 6 hours for 2 to 3 days.

➤ **To suppress intestinal bacteria before surgery**
Adults: After saline cathartic, 1 g neomycin with 1 g erythromycin base P.O. at 1 p.m., 2 p.m., and 11 p.m. on day before 8 a.m. surgery; or 2 g neomycin with 2 g metronidazole P.O. at 7 p.m. and 11 p.m. on day preceding surgery.
Children: After saline cathartic, 40 to 100 mg/kg daily P.O. in divided doses every 4 to 6 hours. Or, 88 mg/kg in equally divided doses every 4 hours.

➤ **Adjunctive treatment for hepatic coma**
Adults: 1 to 3 g P.O. q.i.d. for 5 to 6 days; or 200 ml of 1% solution. For patients with chronic hepatic insufficiency, 4 g/day indefinitely may be needed.
Children: 100 mg/kg/day P.O. in 4 divided doses for maximum of 7 days.

ADMINISTRATION
P.O.
• For preoperative disinfection, provide a low-residue diet and a cathartic immediately before therapy.

ACTION
Inhibits protein synthesis by binding directly to the 30S ribosomal subunit; bactericidal.

Route	Onset	Peak	Duration
P.O.	Unknown	1–4 hr	8 hr

Half-life: 2 to 3 hours.

ADVERSE REACTIONS
EENT: *ototoxicity.*
GI: nausea, vomiting, diarrhea, malabsorption syndrome, *Clostridium difficile*–related colitis.
GU: *nephrotoxicity,* possible increase in urinary excretion of casts.

INTERACTIONS
Drug-drug. ■ **Black Box Warning** *Acyclovir, amphotericin B, cephalosporins,* *cidofovir, cisplatin, methoxyflurane, vancomycin, other aminoglycosides:* May increase nephrotoxicity. Monitor renal function test results. ■

■ **Black Box Warning** *Atracurium, pancuronium, rocuronium, vecuronium:* May increase effects of nondepolarizing muscle relaxants, including prolonged respiratory depression. Use together only when necessary, and expect to reduce dosage of nondepolarizing muscle relaxants. ■

Digoxin: May decrease digoxin absorption. Monitor digoxin level.

■ **Black Box Warning** *I.V. loop diuretics (such as furosemide):* May increase ototoxicity. Monitor patient's hearing. ■

Oral anticoagulants: May inhibit vitamin K–producing bacteria; may increase anticoagulant effect. Monitor PT and INR.

EFFECTS ON LAB TEST RESULTS
• May increase BUN, creatinine, and nonprotein nitrogen levels.

CONTRAINDICATIONS & CAUTIONS
• Contraindicated in patients hypersensitive to other aminoglycosides and in those with intestinal obstruction.
• Use cautiously in elderly patients and in those with impaired renal function, neuromuscular disorders, or ulcerative bowel lesions.

NURSING CONSIDERATIONS
■ **Black Box Warning** Due to increased risk of nephrotoxicity, monitor renal function: urine output, specific gravity, urinalysis, BUN and creatinine levels, and creatinine clearance. Report to prescriber evidence of declining renal function. ■

■ **Black Box Warning** Due to increased risk of ototoxicity, evaluate patient's hearing before and during prolonged therapy. Notify prescriber if patient has tinnitus, vertigo, or hearing loss. Deafness may start several weeks after drug is stopped. ■

• Watch for signs and symptoms of superinfection, such as fever, chills, and increased pulse rate.

■ **Black Box Warning** Neuromuscular blockage and respiratory paralysis have been reported after administration of aminoglycosides. Monitor patient closely. ■

Reactions may be *common,* uncommon, **life-threatening,** or COMMON AND LIFE-THREATENING.
Interaction may have a *rapid onset* or **delayed onset.**

• For adjunctive treatment for hepatic coma, decrease patient's dietary protein and assess neurologic status frequently during therapy.
• The ototoxic and nephrotoxic properties of drug limit its usefulness.

PATIENT TEACHING
• Instruct patient to report adverse reactions promptly.
• Encourage patient to maintain adequate fluid intake.

streptomycin sulfate
strep-toe-MYE-sin

Pharmacologic class:
aminoglycoside
Pregnancy risk category D

AVAILABLE FORMS
Injection: 1-g/2.5-ml ampules

INDICATIONS & DOSAGES
➤ **Streptococcal endocarditis**
Adults: 1 g every 12 hours I.M. for 1 week; then 500 mg I.M. every 12 hours for 1 week, given with penicillin.
Adjust-a-dose: In patients older than age 60, give 500 mg I.M. every 12 hours for entire 2 weeks, with penicillin.
➤ **Second-line treatment of tuberculosis (TB), given with other antituberculotics**
Adults: 15 mg/kg (maximum of 1 g) I.M. daily, continued long enough to prevent relapse. For intermittent use, 25 to 30 mg/kg (maximum of 1.5 g) two to three times weekly.
Children: 20 to 40 mg/kg (maximum of 1 g) I.M. daily. Give with other antituberculotics, except capreomycin; continue until sputum test result becomes negative. For intermittent use, 25 to 30 mg/kg (maximum of 1.5 g) two to three times weekly.
Adults older than 59: Give 10 mg/kg I.M. daily.
➤ **Enterococcal endocarditis**
Adults: 1 g I.M. every 12 hours for 2 weeks; then 500 mg I.M. every 12 hours for 4 weeks, given with penicillin.
➤ **Tularemia**
Adults: 1 to 2 g I.M. daily in divided doses injected deep into upper outer quadrant of buttocks; continued for 7 to 14 days or until patient is afebrile for 5 to 7 days.

ADMINISTRATION
I.M.
• Obtain specimen for culture and sensitivity tests before giving, except when treating TB. Begin therapy while awaiting results.
• Obtain blood for peak level 1 to 2 hours after I.M. injection; obtain blood for trough level just before next dose. Don't use a heparinized tube; heparin is incompatible with aminoglycosides.
• To avoid irritation, protect hands when preparing drug.
• Inject deep into upper outer quadrant of buttocks or midlateral thigh. Rotate injection sites.
• In children, give injection in midlateral thigh, if possible, to minimize possibility of damaging sciatic nerve.

ACTION
Inhibits protein synthesis by binding directly to the 30S ribosomal subunit; bactericidal.

Route	Onset	Peak	Duration
I.M.	Unknown	1–2 hr	Unknown

Half-life: 2 to 3 hours.

ADVERSE REACTIONS
CNS: *neuromuscular blockade,* vertigo, facial paresthesia.
EENT: *ototoxicity.*
GI: vomiting, nausea.
GU: *nephrotoxicity,* increase in urinary excretion of casts.
Hematologic: *leukopenia, thrombocytopenia, hemolytic anemia,* eosinophilia.
Respiratory: *apnea.*
Skin: exfoliative dermatitis.
Other: *anaphylaxis,* hypersensitivity reactions.

INTERACTIONS
Drug-drug. ■ **Black Box Warning** *Acyclovir, amphotericin B, cephalosporins, cidofovir, cisplatin, methoxyflurane, vancomycin, other aminoglycosides:* May increase nephrotoxicity. Monitor renal function test results. ■

■ **Black Box Warning** *Atracurium, pancuronium, rocuronium, vecuronium:* May increase effects of nondepolarizing muscle relaxants, including prolonged respiratory depression. Use together only when necessary, and expect to reduce dosage of nondepolarizing muscle relaxant. ■
General anesthetics: May increase neuromuscular blockade. Monitor patient closely.
I.V. loop diuretics such as furosemide: May increase ototoxicity. Monitor patient's hearing.
Penicillins: May inactivate streptomycin, decreasing the therapeutic effects. Don't mix together.

EFFECTS ON LAB TEST RESULTS
● May increase BUN, creatinine, and non-protein nitrogen levels. May decrease hemoglobin level.
● May increase eosinophil count. May decrease WBC and platelet counts.
● May cause false-positive reaction in copper sulfate tests for urine glucose, such as Benedict's reagent and Diastix.

CONTRAINDICATIONS & CAUTIONS
● Contraindicated in patients hypersensitive to drug or other aminoglycosides.
● Use cautiously in elderly patients and in patients with impaired renal function or neuromuscular disorders.

NURSING CONSIDERATIONS
■ **Black Box Warning** Evaluate patient's hearing before therapy and for 6 months afterward. Notify prescriber if patient has hearing loss, feels fullness in ears, or hears roaring noises. ■
● Drug has been given off-label as I.V. infusion over 30 to 60 minutes without unusual adverse effects in patients who can't tolerate I.M. injections.
● Watch for signs and symptoms of superinfection, such as continued fever, chills, and increased pulse rate.
■ **Black Box Warning** Due to increased risk of nephrotoxicity, monitor renal function: urine output, specific gravity, urinalysis, BUN and creatinine levels, and creatinine clearance. Report to prescriber evidence of declining renal function. Nephrotoxicity occurs less frequently with streptomycin than with other aminoglycosides. ■

● When drug is used as primary treatment of TB, stop therapy when sputum test result becomes negative.
● Total dose for TB shouldn't exceed 120 g over the course of therapy unless there are no other treatment options.

PATIENT TEACHING
● Instruct patient to report adverse reactions promptly.
● Encourage patient to maintain adequate fluid intake.
● Emphasize need for blood tests to monitor levels and determine effectiveness of therapy.

tobramycin sulfate
toe-bra-MYE-sin

TOBI

Pharmacologic class:
aminoglycoside
Pregnancy risk category D

AVAILABLE FORMS
Multidose vials (pediatric): 10 mg/ml, 40 mg/ml
Nebulizer solution (for inhalation): 300 mg/5 ml
Prefilled syringe (pediatric): 40 mg/ml
Premixed parenteral injection for infusion: 60 mg or 80 mg in normal saline solution

INDICATIONS & DOSAGES
➤ **Serious infection by sensitive strains of** *Escherichia coli, Proteus, Klebsiella, Enterobacter, Serratia, Morganella morganii, Staphylococcus aureus, Citrobacter, Pseudomonas,* **or** *Providencia*
Adults: 3 mg/kg/day I.M. or I.V. in divided doses. For life-threatening infections, give up to 5 mg/kg/day in divided doses every 6 to 8 hours; reduce to 3 mg/kg daily as soon as clinically indicated.
Children: 6 to 7.5 mg/kg/day I.M. or I.V., divided t.i.d. or q.i.d.
Neonates younger than age 1 week or premature infants: Up to 4 mg/kg/day I.V. or I.M. in two equal doses every 12 hours.
Adjust-a-dose: For patients with renal impairment, give loading dose of 1 mg/kg; then give decreased doses at 8-hour inter-

vals or same dose at prolonged intervals. For patients with severe cystic fibrosis, initial dose is 10 mg/kg/day I.V. or I.M., divided q.i.d.

➤ **To manage cystic fibrosis patients with *Pseudomonas aeruginosa***
Adults and children age 6 and older:
300 mg via nebulizer every 12 hours for 28 days. Continue cycle of 28 days on drug and 28 days off.

ADMINISTRATION
I.V.
• Obtain specimen for culture and sensitivity tests before giving. Begin therapy while awaiting results.
• For adults, dilute in 50 to 100 ml of normal saline solution or D_5W; use a smaller volume for children.
• Infuse over 20 to 60 minutes.
• After infusion, flush line with normal saline solution or D_5W.
• Obtain blood for peak level 30 minutes after infusion stops; draw blood for trough level just before next dose. Don't collect blood in a heparinized tube because of incompatibility.
• **Incompatibilities:** Allopurinol; amphotericin B; azithromycin; beta lactam antibiotics; cefepime; clindamycin; dextrose 5% in Isolyte E, M, or P; heparin sodium; hetastarch; indomethacin; propofol; sargramostim; solutions containing alcohol.
I.M.
• Obtain specimen for culture and sensitivity tests before giving. Begin therapy while awaiting results.
• Obtain blood for peak level 1 hour after I.M. injection; draw blood for trough level just before next dose. Don't collect blood in a heparinized tube because of incompatibility.
Inhalational
• Obtain specimen for culture and sensitivity tests before giving. Begin therapy while awaiting results.
• Give nebulizer solution over 10 to 15 minutes using handheld Pari LC Plus reusable nebulizer with DeVilbiss Pulmo-Aide compressor.

ACTION
Generally bactericidal. Inhibits protein synthesis by binding directly to the 30S ribosomal subunit.

Route	Onset	Peak	Duration
I.V.	Immediate	30 min	8 hr
I.M.	Unknown	30–60 min	8 hr
Inhalation	Unknown	Unknown	Unknown

Half-life: 2 to 3 hours.

ADVERSE REACTIONS
CNS: *seizures,* headache, lethargy, confusion, disorientation, fever.
EENT: *ototoxicity, hoarseness, pharyngitis.*
GI: vomiting, nausea, diarrhea.
GU: *nephrotoxicity,* possible increase in urinary excretion of casts.
Hematologic: anemia, eosinophilia, *leukopenia, thrombocytopenia, agranulocytosis.*
Metabolic: electrolyte imbalances.
Musculoskeletal: muscle twitching.
Respiratory: *bronchospasm.*
Skin: rash, urticaria, pruritus.

INTERACTIONS
Drug-drug. ■ Black Box Warning *Acyclovir, amphotericin B, cephalosporins, cidofovir, cisplatin, methoxyflurane, vancomycin, other aminoglycosides:* May increase nephrotoxicity. Monitor renal function test results. ■
Atracurium, pancuronium, rocuronium, vecuronium: May increase effects of nondepolarizing muscle relaxants, including prolonged respiratory depression. Use together only when necessary, and expect to reduce dosage of nondepolarizing muscle relaxant.
Dimenhydrinate: May mask symptoms of ototoxicity. Monitor patient's hearing.
General anesthetics: May increase neuromuscular blockade. Monitor patient for increased clinical effects.
■ Black Box Warning *I.V. loop diuretics such as furosemide:* May increase ototoxicity. Monitor patient's hearing. ■
Parenteral penicillins: May inactivate tobramycin in vitro. Don't mix together.

EFFECTS ON LAB TEST RESULTS
• May increase BUN, creatinine, nonprotein nitrogen, and urine urea levels. May decrease calcium, magnesium, and potassium levels.
• May increase eosinophil count. May decrease WBC, platelet, and granulocyte counts.

CONTRAINDICATIONS & CAUTIONS
• Contraindicated in patients hypersensitive to drug or other aminoglycosides.
• Use cautiously in patients with impaired renal function or neuromuscular disorders and in elderly patients.

NURSING CONSIDERATIONS
• Weigh patient and review renal function studies before therapy.
• *Alert:* Evaluate patient's hearing before and during therapy. If patient complains of tinnitus, vertigo, or hearing loss, notify prescriber.
• Don't dilute or mix with dornase alpha in a nebulizer.
• Unrefrigerated drug, which is normally slightly yellow, may darken with age. This change doesn't indicate a change in product quality.
• Avoid exposing ampules to intense light.
■ **Black Box Warning** Peak levels over 12 mcg/ml and trough levels over 2 mcg/ml may increase the risk of toxicity. Reserve higher peak levels for cystic fibrosis patients, who need a greater lung penetration. ■
■ **Black Box Warning** Due to increased risk of nephrotoxicity, monitor renal function: urine output, specific gravity, urinalysis, creatinine clearance, and BUN and creatinine levels. Notify prescriber about signs and symptoms of decreasing renal function. ■
• Watch for signs and symptoms of superinfection, such as continued fever, chills, and increased pulse rate.
• If no response occurs in 3 to 5 days, therapy may be stopped and new specimens obtained for culture and sensitivity testing.
• *Look alike–sound alike:* Don't confuse tobramycin with Trobicin.

PATIENT TEACHING
• Instruct patient to report adverse reactions promptly.
• Caution patient not to perform hazardous activities if adverse CNS reactions occur.
• Encourage patient to maintain adequate fluid intake.
• Teach patient how to use and maintain nebulizer.
• Tell patient using several inhaled therapies to use this drug last.
• Instruct patient not to use if the inhalation solution is cloudy or contains particles or if it has been stored at room temperature for longer than 28 days.

Reactions may be *common*, uncommon, *life-threatening*, or COMMON AND LIFE-THREATENING.
Interaction may have a *rapid onset* or *delayed onset*.

7

Antifungals

amphotericin B cholesteryl
   sulfate complex
amphotericin B desoxycholate
amphotericin B lipid complex
amphotericin B liposomal
anidulafungin
caspofungin acetate
fluconazole
flucytosine
griseofulvin microsize
griseofulvin ultramicrosize
itraconazole
ketoconazole
micafungin sodium
nystatin
posaconazole
terbinafine hydrochloride
voriconazole

SAFETY ALERT!

amphotericin B cholesteryl sulfate complex
am-foe-TER-i-sin

Amphotec

Pharmacologic class: polyene
antibiotic
Pregnancy risk category B

AVAILABLE FORMS
Injection: 50 mg/20 ml, 100 mg/50 ml

INDICATIONS & DOSAGES
➤ **Invasive aspergillosis in patients
whose renal impairment or unacceptable toxicity precludes use of
effective doses of amphotericin B
deoxycholate or whose previous
amphotericin B deoxycholate therapy has failed**
■ **Black Box Warning** Don't use to treat
noninvasive forms of fungal disease in patients with normal neutrophil counts. ■
Adults and children: 3 to 4 mg/kg/day I.V.
Dilute in D_5W and give by continuous infusion at 1 mg/kg/hour. Give a test dose
before beginning new course of treatment;
infuse 10 ml of final preparation containing 1.6 to 8.3 mg of drug over 15 to
30 minutes and monitor patient for next
30 minutes. May shorten infusion time to
2 hours or lengthen infusion time based on
patient's tolerance.
➤ *Candida* or *Cryptococcus* infections in patients who can't tolerate
or who failed to respond to conventional amphotericin B ♦
Adults: 3 to 6 mg/kg/day I.V. Dosages up
to 7.5 mg/kg/day I.V. have been used for
invasive fungal infections in bone marrow
transplant patients.

ADMINISTRATION
I.V.
● Don't give undiluted drug.
● Reconstitute 50-mg vial by rapidly
adding 10 ml sterile water for injection;
reconstitute 100-mg vial by rapidly adding
20 ml sterile water for injection. Shake
vial gently.
● Don't use any diluent except sterile
water for injection. Don't reconstitute
lyophilized powder with saline or dextrose
solution or mix reconstituted liquid with
saline solution or electrolytes. A bacteriostatic product in the solution may cause
drug to precipitate.
● Reconstituted drug should be clear or
opalescent.
● Add reconstituted drug to D_5W to yield
about 0.6 mg/ml.
● Don't use a filter (including an in-line
filter), and don't freeze.
● If given through an existing I.V. line,
flush line with D_5W before infusion.
● Infuse drug over at least 2 hours.
● Store unopened vials at room temperature; store reconstituted drug in refrigerator, where it's stable for 24 hours.
● Discard partially used vials.
● **Incompatibilities:** Bacteriostatic agents,
electrolyte solutions, saline solutions.
Don't mix with other drugs.

ACTION
Binds to sterols of fungal cell membranes,
altering cell permeability and causing cell
death.

---

†Canada   ◇ OTC   ♦ Off-label use   ✐Photoguide   *Liquid contains alcohol.

Route	Onset	Peak	Duration
I.V.	Unknown	3 hr	Unknown

Half-life: Biphasic, with initial half-life of 24 hours and a second phase of about 15 days.

ADVERSE REACTIONS

CNS: *fever, seizures,* abnormal thinking, anxiety, agitation, confusion, depression, dizziness, hallucinations, headache, hypertonia, neuropathy, nervousness, paresthesia, psychosis, somnolence, speech disorder, stupor, asthenia, syncope.

CV: *tachycardia, arrhythmias, bradycardia, cardiac arrest, heart failure, hemorrhage, shock, supraventricular tachycardia,* atrial fibrillation, hypertension, hypotension, phlebitis, chest pain, orthostatic hypotension, vasodilation, edema.

EENT: amblyopia, deafness, epistaxis, eye hemorrhage, pharyngitis, tinnitus, rhinitis, sinusitis.

GI: *nausea, vomiting, GI hemorrhage,* abdominal pain, anorexia, diarrhea, dry mouth, gingivitis, glossitis, hematemesis, melena, mouth ulceration, oral candidiasis, stomatitis.

GU: *renal failure,* albuminuria, dysuria, glycosuria, hematuria, oliguria, urinary incontinence or urine retention.

Hematologic: *leukopenia, thrombocytopenia,* anemia, coagulation disorders, ecchymosis, hypochromic anemia, leukocytosis, petechiae.

Hepatic: *hyperbilirubinemia, hepatic failure,* jaundice.

Metabolic: *hypokalemia, hypoglycemia, hyperkalemia,* weight changes, acidosis, dehydration, hypocalcemia, hypoproteinemia, hyperglycemia, hypervolemia, hypophosphatemia, hyponatremia, hyperlipemia, hypernatremia, *hypomagnesemia.*

Musculoskeletal: arthralgia, myalgia, neck or back pain.

Respiratory: *apnea,* asthma, dyspnea, hemoptysis, hyperventilation, *hypoxia,* increased cough, lung or respiratory tract disorders, pleural effusion, *pulmonary edema.*

Skin: acne, alopecia, pruritus, rash, sweating, skin discoloration, nodules, ulcers, urticaria, pain or reaction at injection site.

Other: *chills, anaphylaxis, sepsis,* allergic reaction, peripheral or facial edema, infection, mucous membrane disorder.

INTERACTIONS

Drug-drug. *Antineoplastics:* May enhance renal toxicity, bronchospasm, and hypotension. Use together cautiously.

Cardiac glycosides: May enhance potassium excretion and increase digitalis toxicity. Monitor potassium level closely.

Corticosteroids: May enhance potassium depletion, which may increase risk of cardiac dysfunction. Monitor electrolyte levels.

Cyclosporine, tacrolimus: May increase creatinine level. Monitor renal function.

Flucytosine: May increase toxicity by amphotericin. Use together cautiously.

Imidazoles (clotrimazole, fluconazole, ketoconazole, miconazole): May antagonize effects of amphotericin by inducing fungal resistance. Monitor patient closely.

Leukocyte transfusions: May increase risk of pulmonary reactions, such as acute dyspnea, tachypnea, hypoxemia, hemoptysis, and interstitial infiltrates. Use together cautiously; separate doses as much as possible, and monitor pulmonary function.

Nephrotoxic drugs (such as aminoglycosides, pentamidine): May enhance renal toxicity. Monitor renal function closely.

Skeletal muscle relaxants: May enhance muscle relaxant effects because of amphotericin. Monitor potassium level closely.

EFFECTS ON LAB TEST RESULTS

• May increase alkaline phosphatase, ALT, AST, bilirubin, BUN, creatinine, GGT, and LDH levels. May decrease calcium, magnesium, phosphate, protein, and hemoglobin levels. May increase or decrease glucose, sodium, and potassium levels.

• May decrease platelet count and INR. May increase or decrease WBC count and PT.

CONTRAINDICATIONS & CAUTIONS

• Contraindicated in patients hypersensitive to drug or its components, unless the benefits outweigh the risks.

• It's unknown if drug appears in breast milk; if it does, breast-fed infants are at risk for serious adverse reactions. Patient should either stop breast-feeding or stop drug.

Reactions may be *common,* uncommon, *life-threatening,* or **COMMON AND LIFE-THREATENING.**
Interaction may have a *rapid onset* or **delayed onset.**

NURSING CONSIDERATIONS

• **Alert:** Dosages of different amphotericin B preparations will vary because the preparations aren't interchangeable. Confusing the preparations may cause permanent damage or death.

• **Alert:** Monitor vital signs every 30 minutes during initial therapy. Acute infusion-related reactions, including fever, chills, hypotension, nausea, and tachycardia, usually occur 1 to 3 hours after the I.V. infusion starts and are usually most severe after first dose, usually diminishing with each dose. If severe respiratory distress occurs, stop infusion immediately and don't restart.

• Reduce acute infusion-related reactions by pretreating with antihistamines, antipyretics, and corticosteroids; reducing infusion rate; and maintaining sodium balance.

• Hydrate patient before infusion to reduce risk of nephrotoxicity.

• Monitor intake and output; report changes in urine appearance or volume.

• Monitor renal and hepatic function test results, electrolyte levels (especially potassium, magnesium, and calcium), CBC, and PT.

PATIENT TEACHING

• Instruct patient to immediately report symptoms of hypersensitivity.

• Warn patient of possible discomfort at I.V. site.

• Advise patient of potential adverse reactions, such as fever, chills, nausea, and vomiting. Tell patient that these can be severe with first dose but usually subside with repeated doses.

SAFETY ALERT!

---

amphotericin B desoxycholate
am-foe-TER-i-sin

Amphocin, Fungizone

Pharmacologic class: polyene antibiotic
Pregnancy risk category B

AVAILABLE FORMS
Powder for injection: 50 mg

INDICATIONS & DOSAGES

➤ **Systemic fungal infection (histoplasmosis, coccidioidomycosis, blastomycosis, cryptococcosis, disseminated candidiasis, aspergillosis, phycomycosis, zygomycosis) or meningitis**

■ **Black Box Warning** Don't use to treat noninvasive forms of fungal disease in patients with normal neutrophil counts. Use caution to prevent inadvertent overdose with amphotericin B. Verify product name and dosage if dose exceeds 1.5 mg/kg. ■

Adults: Initially, test dose of 1 mg in 20 ml of D_5W infused I.V. over 20 to 30 minutes. If that dosage is tolerated, start daily dose at 0.25 to 0.3 mg/kg by slow I.V. infusion (0.1 mg/ml) over 2 to 6 hours. Daily dose is gradually increased to maximum of 1.5 mg/kg in patients with potentially fatal infections. If drug is stopped for 1 week or longer, resume at 0.25 mg/kg I.V. and increase gradually.

➤ **To prevent fungal infection in bone marrow transplant patients** ♦
Adults: 0.1 mg/kg/day as I.V. infusion.

ADMINISTRATION
I.V.

• Reconstitute drug with 10 ml of sterile water.

• If solution contains precipitate or foreign matter, don't use.

• Drug seems to be compatible with limited amounts of heparin sodium, hydrocortisone sodium succinate, and methylprednisolone sodium succinate.

• Choose I.V. sites in distal veins. If veins become thrombosed, alternate administration sites.

• Use an infusion pump and in-line filter with mean pore diameter larger than 1 micron.

• After giving test dose, monitor patient's pulse, respiratory rate, temperature, and blood pressure for at least 4 hours.

• Rapid infusion may cause CV collapse.

• Monitor vital signs every 30 minutes; fever, shaking chills, and hypotension may appear 1 to 2 hours after start of infusion and should subside within 4 hours after stopping drug.

• Store the dry form at 36° to 46° F (2° to 8° C). Protect from light.

• Reconstituted solution is stable 1 week refrigerated or 24 hours at room temperature. It's stable 8 hours in room light.

• **Incompatibilities:** Amikacin, calcium chloride, chlorpromazine, cimetidine, diphenhydramine, edetate calcium disodium, gentamicin, kanamycin, lactated Ringer's injection, melphalan, methyldopate, normal saline solution, paclitaxel, penicillin G potassium, penicillin G sodium, polymyxin B, potassium chloride, prochlorperazine mesylate, streptomycin, verapamil. To avoid precipitation, don't mix with solutions containing sodium chloride, other electrolytes, or bacteriostatic products such as benzyl alcohol. Give antibiotics separately; don't mix or piggyback them with amphotericin B.

ACTION

Binds to sterols of fungal cell membranes, altering cell permeability and causing cell death.

Route	Onset	Peak	Duration
I.V.	Immediate	Unknown	Unknown

Half-life: Adults and children older than age 9, 24 hours; children age 9 and younger, 18 hours.

ADVERSE REACTIONS

CNS: *headache, fever, malaise,* **seizures,** peripheral neuropathy, transient vertigo.
CV: **arrhythmias, asystole,** hypertension, hypotension, tachycardia, flushing, *phlebitis, thrombophlebitis.*
EENT: hearing loss, tinnitus, blurred vision, diplopia.
GI: *anorexia, nausea, vomiting, dyspepsia, diarrhea, epigastric pain, cramping,* **hemorrhagic gastroenteritis,** melena, steatorrhea.
GU: *abnormal renal function with azotemia, hyposthenuria, renal tubular acidosis, nephrocalcinosis,* **permanent renal impairment, anuria,** oliguria.
Hematologic: *normochromic anemia, normocytic anemia,* **thrombocytopenia, leukopenia, agranulocytosis,** eosinophilia, leukocytosis.
Hepatic: *acute liver failure, hepatitis,* jaundice.
Metabolic: *weight loss, hypokalemia,* **hypoglycemia,** hyperglycemia, hyperuricemia, hypomagnesemia.

Musculoskeletal: arthralgia, myalgia.
Respiratory: *bronchospasm,* dyspnea, tachypnea, wheezing.
Skin: *maculopapular rash, pain at injection site,* pruritus, tissue damage with extravasation.
Other: *chills, generalized pain,* **anaphylactoid reaction.**

INTERACTIONS

Drug-drug. *Antineoplastics (such as mechlorethamine):* May cause renal toxicity, bronchospasm, and hypotension. Use together cautiously.
Cardiac glycosides: May increase risk of digitalis toxicity in potassium-depleted patients. Monitor digoxin level closely.
Corticosteroids: May increase potassium depletion. Monitor potassium level.
Flucytosine: May have synergistic effect; may cause increased toxicity of flucytosine. Monitor patient closely for toxicity.
Leukocyte transfusions: May increase risk of pulmonary reactions, such as acute dyspnea, tachypnea, hypoxemia, hemoptysis, and interstitial infiltrates. Use together cautiously; separate doses as much as possible and monitor pulmonary function if drugs are used together.
Nephrotoxic drugs such as antibiotics, pentamidine: May cause additive renal toxicity. Use together cautiously and monitor renal function studies.
Thiazides: May intensify depletion of electrolytes, especially potassium. Monitor patient for hypokalemia.
Drug-herb. *Gossypol:* May increase risk of renal toxicity. Discourage use together.

EFFECTS ON LAB TEST RESULTS

• May increase alkaline phosphatase, ALT, AST, bilirubin, BUN, creatinine, GGT, LDH, urine urea, and uric acid levels. May decrease hemoglobin, magnesium, and potassium levels. May increase or decrease glucose level.

• May decrease granulocyte and platelet counts. May increase or decrease eosinophil and WBC counts.

CONTRAINDICATIONS & CAUTIONS

• Contraindicated in patients hypersensitive to drug.

• Use cautiously in patients with impaired renal function.

Reactions may be *common,* uncommon, *life-threatening,* or **COMMON AND LIFE-THREATENING.**
Interaction may have a *rapid onset* or *delayed onset.*

NURSING CONSIDERATIONS

• Because of drug's dangerous adverse effects, it's used primarily to treat patients with progressive and potentially fatal fungal infections.

• Infusion-related reactions, including fever, shaking chills, hypotension, anorexia, nausea, vomiting, headache, dyspnea, and tachypnea, may occur 1 to 3 hours after starting infusion.

• *Alert:* Different amphotericin B preparations aren't interchangeable, so dosages will vary. Confusing the preparations may cause permanent damage or death.

• *Alert:* To reduce severe adverse effects, premedicate with antipyretics, antihistamines, antiemetics, or small doses of corticosteroids on an alternate-day schedule. For severe reactions, stop drug and notify prescriber.

• Infusion-related reactions occur most frequently with initial doses and usually lessen with subsequent doses.

• Monitor fluid intake and output; report change in urine appearance or volume. Monitor BUN and creatinine levels or creatinine clearance two or three times weekly. If BUN level exceeds 40 mg/100 ml or if creatinine level exceeds 3 mg/100 ml, prescriber may reduce or stop drug until renal function improves. Kidney damage may be reversible if drug is stopped at first sign of renal dysfunction.

• Hydrate patient before infusion to reduce risk of nephrotoxicity.

• Obtain liver function studies once or twice weekly. Drug may be stopped if alkaline phosphatase or bilirubin level increases. Monitor CBC weekly.

• Monitor potassium level closely and report signs of hypokalemia. Hypokalemia occurs commonly and can be life-threatening. Potassium supplementation may be needed.

• Check calcium and magnesium levels twice weekly.

• Drug may be ototoxic. Report evidence of hearing loss, tinnitus, vertigo, or unsteady gait.

PATIENT TEACHING

• Warn patient of possible discomfort at I.V. site and other potential adverse reactions. Instruct patient to report signs and symptoms of hypersensitivity immediately.

• Inform patient that therapy may take several months. Stress importance of compliance and follow-up.

SAFETY ALERT!

amphotericin B lipid complex
am-foe-TER-i-sin

Abelcet

Pharmacologic class: polyene antibiotic
Pregnancy risk category B

AVAILABLE FORMS

Suspension for injection: 100 mg/20-ml vial

INDICATIONS & DOSAGES

➤ **Invasive fungal infections, including *Aspergillus* and *Candida* species, in patients refractory to or intolerant of conventional amphotericin B therapy**

■ **Black Box Warning** Don't use to treat noninvasive forms of fungal disease in patients with normal neutrophil counts. ■

Adults and children: 5 mg/kg daily I.V. as a single infusion given at rate of 2.5 mg/kg/hour.

ADMINISTRATION

I.V.

• To prepare, shake vial gently until there's no yellow sediment. Using aseptic technique, withdraw calculated dose into one or more 20-ml syringes using an 18G needle. More than one vial will be needed.

• Attach a 5-micron filter needle to syringe and inject dose into I.V. bag of D_5W. Volume of D_5W should be sufficient to yield 1 mg/ml. One filter needle can be used for up to four vials of amphotericin B lipid complex.

• For children and patients with CV disease, dilute to 2 mg/ml.

• Don't use an in-line filter.

• If infusing through an existing I.V. line, flush first with D_5W.

• Use an infusion pump, and give by continuous infusion at 2.5 mg/kg/hour.

• If infusion time exceeds 2 hours, mix contents by shaking infusion bag every 2 hours.

• Monitor vital signs closely. Fever, shaking chills, and hypotension may appear within 2 hours of starting infusion. Slowing infusion rate may decrease risk of infusion-related reactions.

• If severe respiratory distress occurs, stop infusion, provide supportive therapy for anaphylaxis, and notify prescriber. Don't restart drug.

• Reconstituted drug is stable up to 48 hours if refrigerated (36° to 46° F [2° to 8° C]) and up to 6 hours at room temperature.

• Discard any unused drug because it contains no preservative.

• **Incompatibilities:** Electrolytes, other I.V. drugs, saline solutions.

ACTION
Binds to sterols of fungal cell membranes, altering cell permeability and causing cell death.

Route	Onset	Peak	Duration
I.V.	Unknown	Unknown	Unknown

Half-life: About 1 week.

ADVERSE REACTIONS
CNS: *fever,* headache, pain.
CV: *cardiac arrest,* chest pain, hypertension, hypotension.
GI: *GI hemorrhage,* abdominal pain, diarrhea, nausea, vomiting.
GU: *renal failure.*
Hematologic: *leukopenia, thrombocytopenia,* anemia.
Hepatic: bilirubinemia.
Metabolic: hypokalemia.
Respiratory: *respiratory failure,* dyspnea, respiratory disorder.
Skin: rash.
Other: MULTIPLE ORGAN FAILURE, *chills, sepsis,* infection.

INTERACTIONS
Drug-drug. *Antineoplastics:* May increase risk of renal toxicity, bronchospasm, and hypotension. Use together cautiously.
Cardiac glycosides: May increase risk of digitalis toxicity from amphotericin B–induced hypokalemia. Monitor potassium level closely.

Clotrimazole, fluconazole, itraconazole, ketoconazole, miconazole: May counteract effects of amphotericin B by inducing fungal resistance. Monitor patient closely.
Corticosteroids, corticotropin: May enhance hypokalemia, which could lead to cardiac toxicity. Monitor electrolyte levels and cardiac function.
Cyclosporine: May increase renal toxicity. Monitor renal function test results closely.
Flucytosine: May increase risk of flucytosine toxicity from increased cellular uptake or impaired renal excretion. Use together cautiously.
Leukocyte transfusions: May increase risk of pulmonary reactions, such as acute dyspnea, tachypnea, hypoxemia, hemoptysis, and interstitial infiltrates. Use together with caution; separate doses as much as possible, and monitor pulmonary function.
Nephrotoxic drugs (such as aminoglycosides, pentamidine): May increase risk of renal toxicity. Use together cautiously and monitor renal function closely.
Skeletal muscle relaxants: May enhance skeletal muscle relaxant effects of amphotericin B–induced hypokalemia. Monitor potassium level closely.
Zidovudine: May increase myelotoxicity and nephrotoxicity. Monitor renal and hematologic function.

EFFECTS ON LAB TEST RESULTS
• May increase alkaline phosphatase, ALT, AST, bilirubin, BUN, creatinine, GGT, and LDH levels. May decrease hemoglobin and potassium levels.
• May decrease platelet and WBC counts.

CONTRAINDICATIONS & CAUTIONS
• Contraindicated in patients hypersensitive to amphotericin B or its components.
• Use cautiously in patients with renal impairment. Adjust dosage based on patient's overall condition. Renal toxicity is more common at higher dosages.
• It's unknown if drug appears in breast milk. Encourage the patient to stop either breast-feeding or treatment.

NURSING CONSIDERATIONS
• *Alert:* Different amphotericin B preparations aren't interchangeable, so dosages will vary. Confusing the preparations may cause permanent damage or death.

Reactions may be *common,* uncommon, *life-threatening,* or COMMON AND LIFE-THREATENING.
Interaction may have a *rapid onset* or *delayed onset.*

• Premedicate patient with acetaminophen, antihistamines, or corticosteroids to prevent or lessen severity of infusion-related reactions, such as fever, chills, nausea, and vomiting, which occur 1 to 2 hours after start of infusion.
• Hydrate before infusion to reduce risk of nephrotoxicity.
• Monitor creatinine and electrolyte levels (especially magnesium and potassium), liver function, and CBC during therapy.

PATIENT TEACHING
• Inform patient that he may develop fever, chills, nausea, and vomiting during infusion, but that these symptoms usually subside with subsequent doses.
• Instruct patient to report any redness or pain at infusion site.
• Teach patient to recognize and report to prescriber signs and symptoms of acute hypersensitivity, such as respiratory distress.
• Warn patient that therapy may take several months.
• Tell patient to expect frequent laboratory testing to monitor kidney and liver function.

SAFETY ALERT!

amphotericin B liposomal
am-foe-TER-i-sin

AmBisome

Pharmacologic class: polyene antibiotic
Pregnancy risk category B

AVAILABLE FORMS
Powder for injection: 50-mg vial

INDICATIONS & DOSAGES
➤ **Empirical therapy for presumed fungal infection in febrile, neutropenic patients**
Adults and children: 3 mg/kg I.V. infusion over 2 hours daily.
➤ **Systemic fungal infections caused by *Aspergillus* species, *Candida* species, or *Cryptococcus* species refractory to amphotericin B deoxycholate or in patients for whom renal impairment or unacceptable toxicity precludes use of amphotericin B deoxycholate**
Adults and children: 3 to 5 mg/kg I.V. infusion over 2 hours daily.
➤ **Visceral leishmaniasis in immunocompetent patients**
Adults and children: 3 mg/kg I.V. infusion over 2 hours daily on days 1 to 5, day 14, and day 21. A repeat course of therapy may be beneficial if initial treatment fails to clear parasites.
➤ **Visceral leishmaniasis in immunocompromised patients**
Adults and children: 4 mg/kg I.V. infusion over 2 hours daily on days 1 to 5, day 10, day 17, day 24, day 31, and day 38.
➤ **Cryptococcal meningitis in patients with HIV infection**
Adults and children: 6 mg/kg/day I.V. infusion over 2 hours. Reduce infusion time to 1 hour if treatment is well tolerated, and increase infusion time if discomfort occurs.
■ **Black Box Warning** Don't use to treat noninvasive forms of fungal disease in patients with normal neutrophil counts. ■

ADMINISTRATION
I.V.
• Don't reconstitute with bacteriostatic water for injection, and don't allow bacteriostatic product in solution.
• Don't reconstitute with saline solution, add saline solution to reconstituted concentration, or mix with other drugs.
• Reconstitute each 50-mg vial with 12 ml of sterile water for injection to yield 4 mg/ml.
• After reconstitution, shake vial vigorously for 30 seconds or until particulate matter disperses.
• Dilute to 1 to 2 mg/ml by withdrawing calculated amount of reconstituted solution into a sterile syringe and injecting it through a 5-micron filter into D₅W. Use only 1 filter needle per vial. Concentrations of 0.2 to 0.5 mg/ml may provide sufficient volume of infusion for children.
• Flush existing I.V. line with D₅W before infusing drug. If this isn't possible, give drug through a separate line.
• Use a controlled infusion device and an in-line filter with a mean pore diameter of 1 micron or larger.

- Initially, infuse drug over at least 2 hours. If drug is tolerated well, reduce infusion time to 1 hour. If discomfort occurs, increase infusion time.
- Store unopened vial at 36° to 46° F (2° to 8° C). Store reconstituted drug for up to 24 hours at 36° to 46° F. Use within 6 hours of dilution with D₅W. Don't freeze.
- **Incompatibilities:** Other I.V. drugs, saline solutions.

ACTION

Binds to sterols of fungal cell membranes, altering cell permeability and causing cell death.

Route	Onset	Peak	Duration
I.V.	Unknown	Unknown	Unknown

Half-life: About 4 to 6 days.

ADVERSE REACTIONS

CNS: *fever, anxiety, confusion, headache, insomnia, asthenia, pain.*
CV: *chest pain, hypotension, tachycardia, hypertension, edema, flushing.*
EENT: *epistaxis, rhinitis.*
GI: *nausea, vomiting, abdominal pain, diarrhea,* **GI hemorrhage.**
GU: *hematuria,* **renal failure.**
Hepatic: *bilirubinemia,* **hepatotoxicity.**
Metabolic: *hyperglycemia, hypernatremia, hypocalcemia, hypokalemia,* **hypomagnesemia.**
Musculoskeletal: *back pain.*
Respiratory: *increased cough, dyspnea, hypoxia, pleural effusion, lung disorder, hyperventilation.*
Skin: *pruritus, rash, sweating.*
Other: *chills, infection,* **anaphylaxis, sepsis,** *blood product infusion reaction.*

INTERACTIONS

Drug-drug. *Antineoplastics:* May enhance potential for renal toxicity, bronchospasm, and hypotension. Use together cautiously.
Cardiac glycosides: May increase risk of digitalis toxicity caused by amphotericin B–induced hypokalemia. Monitor potassium level closely.
Clotrimazole, fluconazole, ketoconazole, miconazole: May induce fungal resistance to amphotericin B. Use together cautiously.
Corticosteroids, corticotropin: May increase potassium depletion, which could cause cardiac dysfunction. Monitor electrolyte levels and cardiac function.
Flucytosine: May increase flucytosine toxicity by increasing cellular reuptake or impairing renal excretion of flucytosine. Use together cautiously.
Leukocyte transfusions: May increase risk of pulmonary reactions, such as acute dyspnea, tachypnea, hypoxemia, hemoptysis, and interstitial infiltrates. Use together cautiously; separate doses as much as possible, and monitor pulmonary function.
Other nephrotoxic drugs, such as antibiotics and antineoplastics: May cause additive nephrotoxicity. Use together cautiously; monitor renal function closely.
Skeletal muscle relaxants: May enhance effects of skeletal muscle relaxants resulting from amphotericin B–induced hypokalemia. Monitor potassium level.

EFFECTS ON LAB TEST RESULTS

- May increase alkaline phosphatase, ALT, AST, bilirubin, BUN, creatinine, GGT, glucose, LDH, and sodium levels. May decrease calcium, magnesium, and potassium levels.

CONTRAINDICATIONS & CAUTIONS

- Contraindicated in patients hypersensitive to drug or its components.
- Use cautiously in patients with impaired renal function, in elderly patients, and in pregnant women.
- It's unknown if drug appears in breast milk. Because of risk of serious adverse reactions in breast-fed infants, encourage patient to stop either breast-feeding or therapy, taking into account importance of drug.

NURSING CONSIDERATIONS

- Patients also receiving chemotherapy or bone marrow transplantation are at greater risk for additional adverse reactions, including seizures, arrhythmias, and thrombocytopenia.

Reactions may be *common,* uncommon, **life-threatening,** or **COMMON AND LIFE-THREATENING.**
Interaction may have a *rapid onset* or **delayed onset.**

• *Alert:* Different amphotericin B preparations aren't interchangeable, so dosages will vary. Confusing the preparations may cause permanent damage or death.
• Premedicate patient with antipyretics, antihistamines, antiemetics, or corticosteroids.
• Hydrate before infusion to reduce the risk of nephrotoxicity.
• Monitor BUN and creatinine and electrolyte levels (particularly magnesium and potassium), liver function, and CBC.
• Watch for signs and symptoms of hypokalemia (ECG changes, muscle weakness, cramping, drowsiness).
• Patients treated with this drug have a lower risk of chills, elevated BUN level, hypokalemia, hypertension, and vomiting than patients treated with conventional amphotericin B.
• Therapy may take several weeks or months.
• Observe patient closely for adverse reactions during infusion. If anaphylaxis occurs, stop infusion immediately, provide supportive therapy, and notify prescriber.

PATIENT TEACHING
• Teach patient signs and symptoms of hypersensitivity, and stress importance of reporting them immediately.
• Warn patient that therapy may take several months; teach personal hygiene and other measures to prevent spread and recurrence of lesions.
• Instruct patient to report any adverse reactions that occur while receiving drug.
• Tell patient to watch for and report signs and symptoms of low levels of potassium in the blood (muscle weakness, cramping, drowsiness).
• Advise patient that frequent laboratory testing will be needed.

anidulafungin
an-ah-DOO-lah-fun-gin

Eraxis

Pharmacologic class: echinocandin
Pregnancy risk category C

AVAILABLE FORMS
Powder for injection: 50 mg/vial with companion diluent

INDICATIONS & DOSAGES
➤ **Candidemia and other** *Candida* **infections (intra-abdominal abscess, peritonitis)**
Adults: A single 200-mg loading dose given by I.V. infusion at no more than 1.1 mg/minute on day 1; then 100 mg daily for at least 14 days after last positive culture result.
➤ **Esophageal candidiasis**
Adults: A single 100-mg loading dose given by I.V. infusion at no more than 1.1 mg/minute on day 1; then 50 mg daily for at least 14 days and for at least 7 more days after symptoms resolve.

ADMINISTRATION
I.V.
• Obtain specimens for culture and sensitivity tests and baseline laboratory tests before starting therapy.
• Reconstitute each vial with 15 ml of supplied diluent.
• Further dilute with D_5W or normal saline solution to a final concentration of 0.5 mg/ml.
• For 50-mg dose, add to 85 ml for final infusion volume of 100 ml. For 100-mg dose, add to 170 ml for final infusion volume of 200 ml. For 200-mg dose, add to 340 ml for final infusion volume of 400 ml.
• Don't infuse at more than 1.1 mg/minute.
• Store at room temperature; don't freeze. Use reconstituted solution within 24 hours of preparation.
• **Incompatibilities:** Unknown. Only use supplied diluent to reconstitute and D_5W or normal saline solution to further dilute.

ACTION
Inhibits glucan synthase, which in turn inhibits formation of 1,3-β-D-glucan, an essential component of fungal cell walls.

Route	Onset	Peak	Duration
I.V.	< 24 hr	Unknown	Unknown

Half-life: 40 to 50 hours.

ADVERSE REACTIONS
CNS: headache.
CV: *deep vein thrombosis,* hypotension.

GI: abdominal pain, dyspepsia, nausea, vomiting.
Hematologic: *leukopenia, neutropenia.*
Metabolic: hypokalemia.
Skin: flushing, pruritus, rash, urticaria.

INTERACTIONS
None reported.

EFFECTS ON LAB TEST RESULTS
• May increase AST, ALT, alkaline phosphatase, GGT, hepatic enzymes, amylase, lipase, bilirubin, CK, creatinine, urea, calcium, glucose, potassium, and sodium levels. May decrease potassium and magnesium levels.
• May increase PT. May decrease neutrophil and WBC counts. May increase or decrease platelet count.

CONTRAINDICATIONS & CAUTIONS
• Contraindicated in patients hypersensitive to drug, other echinocandins, or any component of the drug.
• Use cautiously in patients with liver impairment and in pregnant or breast-feeding women.

NURSING CONSIDERATIONS
• Use only the supplied diluent to reconstitute powder.
• To avoid histamine-mediated symptoms, such as rash, urticaria, flushing, itching, dyspnea, and hypotension, don't infuse faster than 1.1 mg/minute.
• Monitor patient closely for changes in liver function and blood cell counts during therapy.
• Notify prescriber about signs or symptoms of liver toxicity, such as dark urine, jaundice, abdominal pain, and fatigue.
• Patients with esophageal candidiasis who are HIV positive may need suppressive antifungal therapy after drug to prevent relapse.
• Safety and effectiveness in children haven't been established.

PATIENT TEACHING
• Tell patient to call the nurse if he develops a rash, itching, trouble breathing, or other adverse effects during infusion.
• Explain that blood tests will be needed to monitor the drug's effects.

caspofungin acetate
KAS-po-fun-gin

Cancidas

Pharmacologic class: echinocandin
Pregnancy risk category C

AVAILABLE FORMS
Lyophilized powder for injection: 50-mg, 70-mg single-use vials

INDICATIONS & DOSAGES
➤ **Invasive aspergillosis in patients who are refractory to or intolerant of other therapies (amphotericin B, lipid forms of amphotericin B, or itraconazole); candidemia and *Candida*-caused intra-abdominal abscesses, peritonitis, and pleural space infections**
Adults: Single 70-mg I.V. loading dose on day 1, followed by 50 mg/day I.V. over about 1 hour. Base treatment duration on severity of patient's underlying disease, recovery from immunosuppression, and clinical response.
➤ **Empirical treatment of presumed fungal infections in febrile, neutropenic patients**
Adults: Single 70-mg I.V. loading dose on day 1, followed by 50 mg/day I.V. over 1 hour thereafter. Continue empirical therapy until neutropenia resolves. If fungal infection is confirmed, treat for a minimum of 14 days and continue therapy for at least 7 days after neutropenia and symptoms resolve. May increase daily dose to 70 mg if the 50-mg dose is well tolerated but clinical response is suboptimal.
➤ **Esophageal candidiasis**
Adults: 50 mg I.V. daily over 1 hour. After treatment, patients with HIV may require oral suppressive therapy to reduce risk of relapse.
Adjust-a-dose: For patients with Child-Pugh score 7 to 9, after initial 70-mg loading dose (when indicated), give 35 mg/day. Dosage adjustment in patients with Child-Pugh score of more than 9 is unknown.

Reactions may be *common*, uncommon, *life-threatening*, or COMMON AND LIFE-THREATENING.
Interaction may have a *rapid onset* or **delayed onset**.

ADMINISTRATION
I.V.
- Let refrigerated vial warm to room temperature.
- For patients on fluid restriction, dilute the 35-mg and 50-mg doses in 100 ml normal saline solution. For other patients, dilute 35-mg, 50-mg, and 70-mg doses in 250 ml normal saline solution.
- Give drug by slow infusion over about 1 hour.
- Monitor site carefully for phlebitis.
- Use reconstituted vials within 1 hour or discard.
- The final product for infusion (solution in I.V. bag or bottle) can be stored at room temperature for 24 hours.
- **Incompatibilities:** Don't mix or infuse with other drugs or dextrose solutions.

ACTION
Inhibits synthesis of 1,3-β-D-glucan, an essential component of the cell wall, in susceptible *Aspergillus* and *Candida* species. Drug is extensively distributed and has a prolonged half-life.

Route	Onset	Peak	Duration
I.V.	Unknown	Unknown	Unknown

Half-life: 9 to 11 hours.

ADVERSE REACTIONS
CNS: *paresthesia,* fever, headache.
CV: *tachycardia,* phlebitis, infused vein complications.
GI: *anorexia,* nausea, vomiting, diarrhea, abdominal pain.
GU: proteinuria, hematuria.
Hematologic: *anemia,* eosinophilia.
Metabolic: hypokalemia.
Musculoskeletal: *pain, myalgia.*
Respiratory: *tachypnea.*
Skin: histamine-mediated symptoms, including rash, facial swelling, pruritus, sensation of warmth.
Other: *chills, sweating.*

INTERACTIONS
Drug-drug. *Cyclosporine:* May increase caspofungin level. May increase risk of elevated ALT level; avoid using together unless benefit outweighs risk.
Inducers of drug clearance or mixed inducer-inhibitors (carbamazepine, dexamethasone, efavirenz, nelfinavir, nevirap-ine, phenytoin, rifampin): May reduce caspofungin level. May need to adjust dosage upwards to 70 mg in patients who are clinically unresponsive.
Tacrolimus: May reduce tacrolimus level. Monitor tacrolimus level; expect to adjust dosage.

EFFECTS ON LAB TEST RESULTS
- May increase alkaline phosphatase and liver enzyme levels. May decrease albumin, calcium, hemoglobin, potassium, and protein levels.
- May increase eosinophil count.

CONTRAINDICATIONS & CAUTIONS
- Contraindicated in patients hypersensitive to drug or its components.
- Safety and efficacy in children younger than age 18 aren't known.
- It's unknown if drug appears in breast milk. Use cautiously in breast-feeding women.

NURSING CONSIDERATIONS
- Safety information is limited, but drug is well tolerated for therapy lasting longer than 2 weeks.
- Observe patients for histamine-mediated reactions, including rash, facial swelling, pruritus, and a sensation of warmth.

PATIENT TEACHING
- Instruct patient to report signs and symptoms of phlebitis.
- Instruct patient to immediately report any signs of a hypersensitivity reaction.

---

fluconazole
floo-KON-a-zole

Diflucan🖉

Pharmacologic class: bis-triazole derivative
Pregnancy risk category C

AVAILABLE FORMS
Injection: 200 mg/100 ml, 400 mg/200 ml
Powder for oral suspension: 10 mg/ml, 40 mg/ml
Tablets: 50 mg, 100 mg, 150 mg, 200 mg

INDICATIONS & DOSAGES
➤ **Oropharyngeal candidiasis**
Adults: 200 mg P.O. or I.V. on first day, then 100 mg once daily for at least 2 weeks.
Children: 6 mg/kg P.O. or I.V. on first day, then 3 mg/kg daily for 2 weeks.
➤ **Esophageal candidiasis**
Adults: 200 mg P.O. or I.V. on first day, then 100 mg once daily. Up to 400 mg daily has been used, depending on patient's condition and tolerance of treatment. Patients should receive drug for at least 3 weeks and for 2 weeks after symptoms resolve.
Children: 6 mg/kg P.O. or I.V. on first day, then 3 mg/kg daily for at least 3 weeks and for at least 2 weeks after symptoms resolve. Maximum daily dose 12 mg/kg.
➤ **Vulvovaginal candidiasis**
Adults: 150 mg P.O. for one dose only.
➤ **Systemic candidiasis**
Adults: 400 mg P.O. or I.V. on first day, then 200 mg once daily for at least 4 weeks and for 2 weeks after symptoms resolve. Doses up to 400 mg/day may be used.
Children: 6 to 12 mg/kg/day P.O. or I.V.
➤ **Cryptococcal meningitis**
Adults: 400 mg P.O. or I.V. on first day, then 200 mg once daily for 10 to 12 weeks after CSF culture result is negative. Doses up to 400 mg/day may be used.
Children: 12 mg/kg/day P.O. or I.V. on first day, then 6 mg/kg/day for 10 to 12 weeks after CSF culture result is negative.
➤ **To prevent candidiasis in bone marrow transplant**
Adults: 400 mg P.O. or I.V. once daily. Start treatment several days before anticipated agranulocytosis, and continue for 7 days after neutrophil count exceeds 1,000/mm³.
➤ **To suppress relapse of cryptococcal meningitis in patients with AIDS**
Adults: 200 mg P.O. or I.V. daily.
Children: 6 mg/kg/day P.O. or I.V.
Adjust-a-dose: If creatinine clearance is less than 50 ml/minute and patient isn't receiving dialysis, reduce dosage by 50%. Patients receiving regular hemodialysis treatment should receive usual dose after each dialysis session.

ADMINISTRATION
P.O.
● Give drug without regard for food.
● Shake oral suspension well before giving.
I.V.
● To ensure product sterility, don't remove protective wrap from I.V. bag until just before use.
● The plastic container may show some opacity from moisture absorbed during sterilization. This doesn't affect drug and diminishes over time.
● To prevent air embolism, don't connect in series with other infusions.
● Use an infusion pump.
● Give by continuous infusion at no more than 200 mg/hour.
● **Incompatibilities:** Amphotericin B, amphotericin B cholesteryl sulfate complex, ampicillin sodium, calcium gluconate, cefotaxime sodium, ceftazidime, ceftriaxone, cefuroxime sodium, chloramphenicol sodium succinate, clindamycin phosphate, co-trimoxazole, diazepam, digoxin, erythromycin lactobionate, furosemide, haloperidol lactate, hydroxyzine hydrochloride, imipenem and cilastatin sodium, pentamidine, piperacillin sodium, ticarcillin disodium, trimethoprim-sulfamethoxazole. Don't add other drugs to I.V. bag.

ACTION
Inhibits fungal cytochrome P-450 (responsible for fungal sterol synthesis); weakens fungal cell walls.

Route	Onset	Peak	Duration
P.O.	Unknown	1–2 hr	30 hr
I.V.	Immediate	Immediate	Unknown

Half-life: 20 to 50 hours.

ADVERSE REACTIONS
CNS: *headache,* dizziness.
GI: nausea, vomiting, abdominal pain, diarrhea, dyspepsia, taste perversion.
Hematologic: *leukopenia, thrombocytopenia.*
Skin: rash.
Other: *anaphylaxis.*

INTERACTIONS
Drug-drug. *Alprazolam, chlordiazepoxide, clonazepam, clorazepate, diazepam,*

estazolam, flurazepam, midazolam, quazepam, triazolam: May increase and prolong levels of these drugs, CNS depression, and psychomotor impairment. Avoid using together.

Cimetidine: May decrease fluconazole level. Monitor patient's response to fluconazole.

Cyclosporine, phenytoin, theophylline: May increase levels of these drugs. Monitor cyclosporine, phenytoin, and theophylline levels.

HMG-CoA reductase inhibitors (atorvastatin, fluvastatin, lovastatin, pravastatin, simvastatin): May increase levels and adverse effects of these drugs. Avoid using together or reduce dosage of HMG-CoA reductase inhibitor.

Isoniazid, oral sulfonylureas, phenytoin, rifampin, valproic acid: May increase hepatic transaminase level. Monitor liver function test results closely.

Oral sulfonylureas (such as glipizide, glyburide, tolbutamide): May increase levels of these drugs. Monitor patient for enhanced hypoglycemic effect.

Proton pump inhibitors: May decrease fluconazole effect. Give fluconazole 2 hours or more before proton pump inhibitors.

Rifampin: May enhance fluconazole metabolism. Monitor patient for lack of response to fluconazole.

Tacrolimus: May increase tacrolimus level and nephrotoxicity. Monitor patient carefully.

Warfarin: May increase risk of bleeding. Monitor PT and INR.

Zidovudine: May increase zidovudine activity. Monitor patient closely.

EFFECTS ON LAB TEST RESULTS
● May increase alkaline phosphatase, ALT, AST, bilirubin, and GGT levels.
● May decrease platelet and WBC counts.

CONTRAINDICATIONS & CAUTIONS
● Contraindicated in patients hypersensitive to drug and breast-feeding patients.
● Use cautiously in patients hypersensitive to other antifungal azole compounds.

NURSING CONSIDERATIONS
● Serious hepatotoxicity has occurred in patients with underlying medical conditions.

● If patient develops mild rash, monitor him closely. Stop drug if lesions progress.
● Likelihood of adverse reactions may be greater in HIV-infected patients.

PATIENT TEACHING
● Tell patient to take drug as directed, even after he feels better.
● Instruct patient to report adverse reactions promptly.

---

flucytosine
(5-FC, 5-fluorocytosine)
floo-SYE-toe-seen

Ancobon

Pharmacologic class: fluorinated pyrimidine
Pregnancy risk category C

AVAILABLE FORMS
Capsules: 250 mg, 500 mg

INDICATIONS & DOSAGES
➤ **Severe fungal infections from susceptible strains of *Candida* (including septicemia, endocarditis, and urinary tract or pulmonary infection), and of *Cryptococcus* (including meningitis and urinary tract or pulmonary infection)**
Adults: 50 to 150 mg/kg daily P.O. in four equally divided doses every 6 hours.

ADMINISTRATION
P.O.
● Give patient a few capsules at a time over 15 minutes to reduce adverse GI reactions.

ACTION
Appears to penetrate fungal cells and cause defective protein synthesis.

Route	Onset	Peak	Duration
P.O.	Unknown	1–2 hr	Unknown

Half-life: 2½ to 6 hours.

ADVERSE REACTIONS
CNS: headache, vertigo, sedation, fatigue, weakness, confusion, hallucinations,

psychosis, ataxia, hearing loss, paresthesia, parkinsonism, peripheral neuropathy.
CV: *cardiac arrest,* chest pain.
GI: *hemorrhage,* nausea, vomiting, diarrhea, abdominal pain, dry mouth, duodenal ulcer, ulcerative colitis, anorexia.
GU: *renal failure,* azotemia, crystalluria.
Hematologic: *agranulocytosis, aplastic anemia, leukopenia, bone marrow suppression, thrombocytopenia,* anemia, eosinophilia.
Hepatic: jaundice.
Metabolic: *hypoglycemia,* hypokalemia.
Respiratory: *respiratory arrest,* dyspnea.
Skin: rash, pruritus, urticaria, photosensitivity.

INTERACTIONS
Drug-drug. *Amphotericin B:* May cause synergistic effects, increasing risk of toxicity. Monitor patient for increased adverse reactions and toxicity.

EFFECTS ON LAB TEST RESULTS
● May increase alkaline phosphatase, ALT, AST, bilirubin, BUN, creatinine, and urine urea levels. May decrease glucose, hemoglobin, and potassium levels.
● May increase eosinophil count. May decrease granulocyte, platelet, and WBC counts.

CONTRAINDICATIONS & CAUTIONS
● Contraindicated in patients hypersensitive to drug.
■ **Black Box Warning** Use with extreme caution in patients with impaired hepatic or renal function or bone marrow suppression. ■

NURSING CONSIDERATIONS
■ **Black Box Warning** Due to increased risk of bone marrow, hepatic, and renal toxicities, monitor blood, liver, and renal function studies frequently during therapy; obtain susceptibility tests weekly to monitor drug resistance. ■
● Regularly perform drug level assays to maintain therapeutic level of 40 to 60 mcg/ml. Levels above 100 mcg/ml may be toxic.
● Monitor fluid intake and output; report marked changes.

PATIENT TEACHING
● Instruct patient to take a few capsules at a time over 15 minutes to reduce adverse GI reactions.
● Tell patient that drug may cause photosensitivity and to avoid prolonged exposure to sun or ultraviolet light, such as tanning beds, to use sunscreen, and to wear protective clothing.
● Tell patient that therapeutic response may take weeks or months.
● Advise patient to report adverse reactions promptly.

---

griseofulvin microsize
gris-ee-oh-FUHL-vin

Grifulvin V

griseofulvin ultramicrosize
Gris-PEG

Pharmacologic class: penicillium antibiotic
Pregnancy risk category C

AVAILABLE FORMS
microsize
Oral suspension: 125 mg/5 ml
Tablets: 500 mg
ultramicrosize
Tablets (film-coated): 125 mg, 250 mg

INDICATIONS & DOSAGES
➤ **Tinea corporis, tinea capitis, tinea barbae, tinea cruris, tinea pedis, or tinea unguium infections**
Microsize
Adults: 500 mg P.O. daily. For more difficult fungal infections, such as tinea pedis or unguium, give 1 g P.O. daily.
Children: About 5 mg/lb of body weight daily. For children who weigh 14 to 23 kg (30 to 50 lb), acceptable range is 125 to 250 mg daily; children who weigh more than 23 kg, acceptable range is 250 to 500 mg daily.
Ultramicrosize
Adults: 375 mg P.O. daily. For more difficult fungal infections, such as tinea pedis or unguium, give 750 mg P.O. daily in divided doses.
Children older than age 2: About 3.3 mg/lb of body weight daily. For chil-

dren who weigh 16 to 27 kg (35 to 60 lb), acceptable range is 125 to 187.5 mg daily; children who weigh more than 27 kg, acceptable range is 187.5 mg to 375 mg daily.

ADMINISTRATION
P.O.
● Confirm identity of organism before starting treatment.
● Give with or after meals, preferably high-fat meals if allowed, to minimize GI distress.

ACTION
Active against *Trichophyton, Microsporum,* and *Epidermophyton* species. Drug disrupts fungal cells' mitotic spindle, interfering with cell division; also may inhibit DNA replication. Drug enters keratin precursor cells, slowing fungal growth.

Route	Onset	Peak	Duration
P.O.	Unknown	4–8 hr	Unknown

Half-life: 9 to 24 hours.

ADVERSE REACTIONS
CNS: dizziness, fatigue, headache, impaired performance, insomnia, mental confusion, paresthesia of the hands and feet, psychotic symptoms.
EENT: oral thrush, transient decrease in hearing.
GI: *bleeding,* diarrhea, epigastric distress, flatulence, nausea, vomiting.
GU: menstrual irregularities, proteinuria.
Hematologic: *granulocytopenia, leukopenia,* porphyria.
Hepatic: *hepatotoxicity.*
Skin: erythema multiforme–like reaction, photosensitivity, *rash, urticaria.*
Other: *angioedema,* hypersensitivity reactions, systemic lupus erythematosus.

INTERACTIONS
Drug-drug. *Barbiturates:* May impair griseofulvin absorption. Increase dosage as needed.
Cyclosporine, salicylates: May decrease levels of these drugs. Monitor patient for decreased drug effects.
Hormonal contraceptives: May decrease contraceptive efficacy. Suggest alternative method of contraception.

Warfarin: May decrease PT and INR. Adjust dosage if needed.
Drug-food. *High-fat meals:* May increase absorption. Give together if permissible.
Drug-lifestyle. *Alcohol use:* May increase alcohol effect, producing tachycardia, diaphoresis, and flushing. Discourage alcohol use.

EFFECTS ON LAB TEST RESULTS
● May decrease WBC and granulocyte counts.

CONTRAINDICATIONS & CAUTIONS
● Contraindicated in patients hypersensitive to drug, women who intend to become pregnant during therapy, and patients with porphyria or hepatocellular failure.
● Use cautiously in penicillin-sensitive patients.

NURSING CONSIDERATIONS
● Ask patient if he's allergic to penicillin; cross-sensitivity may exist.
● Treatment duration depends on location of infection: for tinea capitis, 4 to 6 weeks; for tinea corporis, 2 to 4 weeks; for tinea pedis, 4 to 8 weeks. Treatment duration for tinea unguium depends on growth rate of nails—fingernails, at least 4 months; toenails, at least 6 months.
● Tinea pedis may need combined oral and topical therapy.
● *Alert:* Because griseofulvin ultramicrosize is dispersed in polyethylene glycol, it's absorbed more rapidly and completely than microsize and is effective at half to two-thirds the usual griseofulvin dose. Don't interchange preparations.
● Check CBC regularly for adverse effects; monitor renal and liver function studies periodically.

PATIENT TEACHING
● Tell patient to take drug with or after meals, preferably high-fat meals if allowed, to minimize GI distress.
● Encourage patient to maintain adequate nutritional intake.
● Stress importance of completing prescribed regimen, even if symptoms subside quickly, to prevent relapse.
● Tell patient to report adverse reactions immediately.

---

†Canada ◇ OTC ♦ Off-label use ✐Photoguide *Liquid contains alcohol.

• Advise patient to avoid exposure to intense indoor light and sunlight to reduce the risk of photosensitivity reactions.
• Explain that drug may increase the effects of alcohol, and advise patient to avoid alcohol during therapy.

---

itraconazole
eye-tra-KON-a-zole

Sporanox

Pharmacologic class: synthetic triazole
Pregnancy risk category C

AVAILABLE FORMS
Capsules: 100 mg
Oral solution: 10 mg/ml

INDICATIONS & DOSAGES
➤ **Pulmonary and extrapulmonary blastomycosis, nonmeningeal histoplasmosis**
Adults: 200 mg P.O. daily; increase as needed and tolerated by 100 mg to maximum of 400 mg daily. Give dosages exceeding 200 mg P.O. daily in two divided doses. Continue treatment for at least 3 months. In life-threatening illness, give a loading dose of 200 mg P.O. t.i.d. for 3 days.
➤ **Aspergillosis**
Adults: 200 to 400 mg P.O. daily.
➤ **Onychomycosis of the toenail (with or without fingernail involvement)**
Adults: 200 mg P.O. once daily for 12 consecutive weeks.
➤ **Onychomycosis of the fingernail**
Adults: 200 mg P.O. b.i.d. for 1 week, followed by 3 weeks drug free. Repeat dosage.
➤ **Oropharyngeal candidiasis**
Adults: 200 mg oral solution swished in mouth vigorously and swallowed daily, for 1 to 2 weeks.
➤ **Oropharyngeal candidiasis in patients unresponsive to fluconazole tablets**
Adults: 100 mg oral solution swished in mouth vigorously and swallowed b.i.d., for 2 to 4 weeks.

➤ **Esophageal candidiasis**
Adults: 100 to 200 mg oral solution swished in mouth vigorously and swallowed daily, for at least 3 weeks. Treatment should continue for 2 weeks after symptoms resolve.

ADMINISTRATION
P.O.
• Before starting therapy, confirm diagnosis of onychomycosis by sending nail specimens for testing.
• Don't interchange capsules and oral solution.

ACTION
Interferes with fungal cell-wall synthesis by inhibiting ergosterol formation and increasing cell-wall permeability, leading to osmotic instability.

Route	Onset	Peak	Duration
P.O.	Unknown	3–4 hr	Unknown

Half-life: 1 to 8¼ hours.

ADVERSE REACTIONS
CNS: *headache,* fever, dizziness, somnolence, fatigue, malaise, asthenia, pain, tremor, abnormal dreams, anxiety, depression.
CV: *heart failure,* hypertension, edema, orthostatic hypotension.
EENT: rhinitis, sinusitis, pharyngitis.
GI: *nausea,* vomiting, diarrhea, abdominal pain, anorexia, dyspepsia, flatulence, increased appetite, constipation, gastritis, gastroenteritis, ulcerative stomatitis, gingivitis.
GU: albuminuria, impotence, cystitis, UTI.
Hematologic: *neutropenia.*
Hepatic: *hepatotoxicity, liver failure,* impaired hepatic function.
Metabolic: hypokalemia, hypertriglyceridemia.
Musculoskeletal: myalgia.
Respiratory: *pulmonary edema,* upper respiratory tract infection.
Skin: rash, pruritus.
Other: decreased libido, injury, herpes zoster, *hypersensitivity reactions (urticaria, angioedema, Stevens-Johnson syndrome).*

Reactions may be *common,* uncommon, *life-threatening,* or COMMON AND LIFE-THREATENING.
Interaction may have a *rapid onset* or *delayed onset.*

INTERACTIONS

Drug-drug. *Alprazolam, midazolam, triazolam:* May increase and prolong drug levels, CNS depression, and psychomotor impairment. Avoid using together.

Antacids, carbamazepine, H₂-receptor antagonists, isoniazid, phenobarbital, **phenytoin,** *rifabutin, rifampin:* May decrease itraconazole level. Avoid using together.

Chlordiazepoxide, clonazepam, clorazepate, diazepam, estazolam, flurazepam, quazepam: May increase and prolong drug levels, CNS depression, and psychomotor impairment. Avoid using together.

Clarithromycin, erythromycin: May increase itraconazole levels. Monitor patient for signs of itraconazole toxicity.

Cyclosporine, **digoxin,** *tacrolimus:* May increase levels of these drugs. Monitor drug levels.

■ **Black Box Warning** *Dofetilide, pimozide, quinidine:* May increase levels of these drugs by cytochrome P-450 metabolism, causing serious CV events, including torsades de pointes, QT interval prolongation, ventricular tachycardia, cardiac arrest, and sudden death. Avoid using together. ■

HMG-CoA reductase inhibitors (atorvastatin, fluvastatin, lovastatin, pravastatin, simvastatin): May increase levels and adverse effects of these drugs. Avoid using together, or reduce dose of HMG-CoA reductase inhibitor. Don't use itraconazole with lovastatin or simvastatin.

Indinavir, ritonavir, saquinavir: May increase levels of these drugs; indinavir and ritonavir may increase itraconazole levels. Monitor patient for toxicity.

Oral anticoagulants: May enhance anticoagulant effect. Monitor PT and INR.

Oral antidiabetics: May cause hypoglycemia, similar to effect of other antifungals. Monitor glucose level. Avoid using together.

Drug-food. *Grapefruit and orange juice:* May decrease drug level and therapeutic effect. Discourage use together.

EFFECTS ON LAB TEST RESULTS

● May increase alkaline phosphatase, ALT, AST, bilirubin, triglyceride, and GGT levels. May decrease potassium level.

CONTRAINDICATIONS & CAUTIONS

■ **Black Box Warning** Contraindicated in patients hypersensitive to drug or those receiving alprazolam, dofetilide, lovastatin, midazolam, pimozide, quinidine, simvastatin, or triazolam; in those with ventricular dysfunction or a history of heart failure; and in those who are breast-feeding. If signs and symptoms of heart failure occur, stop itraconazole. ■

● Use cautiously in patients with hypochlorhydria; they may not absorb drug readily.

● Use cautiously in HIV-infected patients because hypochlorhydria can accompany HIV infection.

● Use cautiously in patients receiving other highly bound drugs.

NURSING CONSIDERATIONS

● *Alert:* Capsules and oral solution aren't interchangeable.

● Perform baseline liver function tests and monitor results periodically. In patients with baseline hepatic impairment, give drug only if patient's condition is life threatening. If liver dysfunction occurs during therapy, notify prescriber immediately.

PATIENT TEACHING

● Teach patient to recognize and report signs and symptoms of liver disease (anorexia, dark urine, pale stools, unusual fatigue, and jaundice).

● Instruct patient not to use oral solution interchangeably with capsules.

● For the oral solution, tell patient to take 10 ml at a time.

● Advise patient to take solution without food and to take capsules with a full meal.

● Urge patient to list the other drugs he's taking for prescriber, to avoid drug interactions.

● Advise women of childbearing age that an effective form of contraception must be used during therapy and for two menstrual cycles after stopping therapy with capsules.

ketoconazole
kee-toe-KOE-na-zole

Nizoral

Pharmacologic class: imidazole derivative
Pregnancy risk category C

AVAILABLE FORMS
Tablets: 200 mg

INDICATIONS & DOSAGES
➤ **Systemic candidiasis, chronic mucocutaneous candidiasis, oral candidiasis, candiduria, coccidioidomycosis, blastomycosis, histoplasmosis, chromomycosis, and paracoccidioidomycosis; severe cutaneous dermatophyte infections that are resistant to therapy with topical or oral griseofulvin**
Adults and children who weigh more than 40 kg (88 lb): Initially, 200 mg P.O. daily in a single dose. Dosage may be increased to 400 mg once daily in patients who don't respond.
Children age 2 and older: 3.3 to 6.6 mg/kg P.O. daily in a single dose.
➤ **Onychomycosis (caused by *Trichophyton* and *Candida* species); tinea versicolor; tinea pedis, tinea corporis, and tinea cruris ♦**
Adults: 200 to 400 mg P.O. daily.
➤ **Tinea capitis ♦**
Adults: 3.3 to 6.6 mg/kg P.O. daily.

ADMINISTRATION
P.O.
● For patient with achlorhydria, dissolve each tablet in 4 ml aqueous solution of 0.2 N hydrochloric acid and have patient sip solution through a glass or plastic straw. Then have patient drink a glass of water because drug needs gastric acidity for dissolution and absorption.
● Patient should wait at least 2 hours after dose before taking antacids.

ACTION
Interferes with fungal cell-wall synthesis by inhibiting formation of ergosterol and increasing cell-wall permeability that makes the fungus susceptible to osmotic instability.

Route	Onset	Peak	Duration
P.O.	Unknown	1–2 hr	Unknown

Half-life: 8 hours.

ADVERSE REACTIONS
CNS: *suicidal tendencies,* fever, headache, nervousness, dizziness, somnolence, severe depression.
EENT: photophobia.
GI: *nausea, vomiting,* abdominal pain, diarrhea.
GU: impotence.
Hematologic: *leukopenia, thrombocytopenia,* hemolytic anemia.
Hepatic: *fatal hepatotoxicity.*
Metabolic: hyperlipidemia.
Skin: pruritus.
Other: gynecomastia with tenderness, chills.

INTERACTIONS
Drug-drug. *Antacids, anticholinergics, H₂-receptor antagonists:* May decrease absorption of ketoconazole. Wait at least 2 hours after ketoconazole dose before giving these drugs.
Chlordiazepoxide, clonazepam, clorazepate, diazepam, estazolam, flurazepam, midazolam, quazepam: May increase and prolong levels of these drugs. May cause CNS depression and psychomotor impairment. Avoid using together.
Cyclosporine, methylprednisolone, tacrolimus: May increase drug levels. Monitor drug levels, if appropriate.
Digoxin: May increase digoxin level. Monitor digoxin level.
Isoniazid, rifampin: May increase ketoconazole metabolism. Monitor patient for decreased antifungal effect.
HMG-CoA reductase inhibitors (atorvastatin, fluvastatin, lovastatin, pravastatin, simvastatin): May increase levels and adverse effects of these drugs. Avoid using together, or reduce dose of HMG-CoA reductase inhibitor.
Midazolam, triazolam: May increase and prolong levels of these drugs. May cause CNS depression and psychomotor impairment. Avoid using together.

Reactions may be *common,* uncommon, *life-threatening,* or **COMMON AND LIFE-THREATENING.**
Interaction may have a *rapid onset* or **delayed onset.**

Oral antidiabetics: May cause hypoglycemia. Monitor glucose level.

Paclitaxel: May inhibit metabolism. Use together cautiously.

Phenytoin: May alter the metabolism of one or both drugs. Monitor patient for adverse effects.

Rifampin, isoniazid: May decrease ketoconazole level. Avoid using together.

Theophylline: May decrease theophylline level. Monitor theophylline level.

Warfarin: May enhance effects of anticoagulant. Monitor PT and INR and adjust dosage, as needed.

Drug-herb. *Yew:* May inhibit drug metabolism. Discourage use together.

EFFECTS ON LAB TEST RESULTS
● May increase lipid, alkaline phosphatase, ALT, and AST levels. May decrease hemoglobin level.
● May decrease platelet and WBC counts.

CONTRAINDICATIONS & CAUTIONS
■ **Black Box Warning** Contraindicated in patients hypersensitive to drug and in those taking midazolam or oral triazolam. ■
■ **Black Box Warning** Due to increased risk of hepatotoxicity, use cautiously in patients with hepatic disease and in those taking other hepatotoxic drugs. ■

NURSING CONSIDERATIONS
● *Alert:* Because of risk of hepatotoxicity, drug shouldn't be used for less serious conditions, such as fungal infections of skin or nails.
■ **Black Box Warning** Due to increased risk of hepatotoxicity, monitor patient for signs and symptoms of hepatotoxicity, including elevated liver enzyme levels, nausea that doesn't subside, and unusual fatigue, jaundice, dark urine, or pale stool. ■
● Doses up to 800 mg/day can be used to treat fungal meningitis and intracerebral fungal lesions.
● *Alert:* Drug is a potent inhibitor of the cytochrome P-450 enzyme system. Giving this drug with drugs metabolized by the cytochrome P-450 3A4 enzyme system may lead to increased drug levels, which could increase or prolong therapeutic and adverse effects.

PATIENT TEACHING
● Instruct patient with achlorhydria to dissolve each tablet in 4 ml aqueous solution of 0.2 N hydrochloric acid, sip mixture through a glass or plastic straw, and then drink a glass of water because drug needs gastric acidity for dissolution and absorption.
● Instruct patient to wait at least 2 hours after dose before taking antacids.
● Make sure patient understands that treatment should continue until all tests indicate that active fungal infection has subsided. If drug is stopped too soon, infection will recur. Minimum treatment for candidiasis is 7 to 14 days; for other systemic fungal infections, 6 months; for resistant dermatophyte infections, at least 4 weeks.
● Reassure patient that nausea is common early in therapy but will subside. To minimize nausea, instruct patient to divide daily amount into two doses or take drug with meals.
● Review signs and symptoms of hepatotoxicity with patient; instruct him to stop drug and notify prescriber if they occur.
● Advise patient to discuss any new drugs or herbal supplements with prescriber.

---

micafungin sodium
mick-a-FUN-gin

Mycamine

Pharmacologic class: echinocandin
Pregnancy risk category C

AVAILABLE FORMS
Lyophilized powder for injection: 50 mg, 100-mg single-use vial

INDICATIONS & DOSAGES
✷*NEW INDICATION:* **Candidemia, acute disseminated candidiasis, and** *Candida* **peritonitis and abscesses**
Adults: 100 mg I.V. daily for 10 to 47 days (mean duration 15 days).
➤ **Esophageal candidiasis**
Adults: 150 mg I.V. daily for 10 to 30 days.
➤ **To prevent candidal infection in hematopoietic stem cell transplant recipients**
Adults: 50 mg I.V. daily for 6 to 51 days.

ADMINISTRATION
I.V.
- Use aseptic technique when preparing drug.
- Reconstitute each 50-mg or 100-mg vial with 5 ml of normal saline solution or D_5W for injection. To minimize foaming, dissolve powder by swirling the vial; don't shake it.
- Dilute dose in 100 ml of normal saline solution or D_5W for injection.
- Flush line with normal saline solution for injection before infusing drug.
- Infuse drug over 1 hour.
- Reconstituted product and diluted infusion may be stored for up to 24 hours at room temperature.
- Protect diluted solution from light.
- **Incompatibilities:** Drug may precipitate when mixed with commonly used drugs.

ACTION
Inhibits synthesis of an essential component of fungal cell walls. Drug is active against *Candida albicans, C. glabrata, C. krusei, C. parapsilosis,* and *C. tropicalis.*

Route	Onset	Peak	Duration
I.V.	Unknown	Unknown	Unknown

Half-life: Unknown.

ADVERSE REACTIONS
CNS: headache.
GI: abdominal pain, diarrhea, nausea, vomiting.
Hematologic: *leukopenia, neutropenia, thrombocytopenia,* anemia.
Metabolic: hypocalcemia, hypokalemia, *hypomagnesemia,* hypophosphatemia.
Skin: infusion site inflammation, phlebitis, pruritus, rash.
Other: pyrexia, rigors.

INTERACTIONS
Drug-drug. *Nifedipine:* May increase nifedipine level. Monitor blood pressure, and decrease nifedipine dose if needed.
Sirolimus: May increase sirolimus level. Monitor patient for evidence of toxicity, and decrease sirolimus dose if needed.

EFFECTS ON LAB TEST RESULTS
- May increase alkaline phosphatase, ALT, AST, bilirubin, BUN, creatinine, and LDH levels. May decrease calcium, magnesium, phosphorus, potassium, and hemoglobin levels and hematocrit.
- May decrease neutrophil and platelet counts.

CONTRAINDICATIONS & CAUTIONS
- Contraindicated in patients hypersensitive to drug.
- Use cautiously in patients with severe hepatic disease.

NURSING CONSIDERATIONS
- Injection site reactions occur more often in patients receiving drug by peripheral I.V.
- To reduce the risk of histamine-mediated reactions, infuse drug over at least 1 hour.
- **Alert:** If patient develops signs of serious hypersensitivity reaction, including shock, stop infusion and notify prescriber.
- Monitor hepatic and renal function during therapy.
- Monitor patient for hemolysis and hemolytic anemia.
- Use drug in pregnant women only if clearly needed.
- It's unknown whether drug appears in breast milk. Use cautiously in breast-feeding women.

PATIENT TEACHING
- Advise patient to report pain or redness at infusion site.
- Tell patient he'll likely need laboratory tests to monitor his hematologic, renal, and hepatic function.

---

nystatin
nye-STAT-in

Mycostatin, Nilstat

Pharmacologic class: polyene macrolide
Pregnancy risk category C

AVAILABLE FORMS
Lozenges: 200,000 units
Oral suspension: 100,000 units/ml
Powder (bulk): 50, 150, or 500 million units; 1, 2, or 5 billion units
Tablets: 500,000 units
Vaginal tablets: 100,000 units

Reactions may be *common,* uncommon, *life-threatening,* or COMMON AND LIFE-THREATENING.
Interaction may have a *rapid onset* or *delayed onset.*

INDICATIONS & DOSAGES
➤ **Intestinal candidiasis**
Adults: 500,000 to 1 million units P.O. as tablets t.i.d.
➤ **Oral candidiasis (thrush)**
Adults and children: 400,000 to 600,000 units P.O. as oral suspension q.i.d. or 200,000 to 400,000 units P.O. as lozenges four to five times daily for up to 14 days.
Infants: 200,000 units P.O. as oral suspension q.i.d.
Neonates and premature infants: 100,000 units P.O. oral suspension q.i.d.
➤ **Vaginal candidiasis**
Adults: 100,000 units, as vaginal tablets, inserted high into vagina, daily at bedtime or b.i.d. for 14 days.

ADMINISTRATION
P.O.
● To treat oral candidiasis, after the patient's mouth is clean of food debris, have him hold suspension in mouth for several minutes before swallowing. When treating infants, swab medication on oral mucosa.
● Suspension made with bulk powder contains no preservatives. Use immediately; don't store.
● Patient shouldn't chew or swallow lozenge but should allow it to dissolve slowly in mouth.
● Prescriber may instruct immunosuppressed patients to suck on vaginal tablets (100,000 units) because this provides prolonged contact with oral mucosa.
Vaginal
● Vaginal tablets can be used by pregnant patients up to 6 weeks before term to treat maternal infection that may cause oral candidiasis in neonates.

ACTION
Probably binds to sterols in fungal cell membrane, altering cell permeability and allowing leakage of intracellular components.

Route	Onset	Peak	Duration
P.O., vaginal	Unknown	Unknown	Unknown

Half-life: Unknown.

ADVERSE REACTIONS
GI: transient nausea, vomiting, diarrhea.

GU: irritation, sensitization, vulvovaginal burning (vaginal form).
Skin: rash.

INTERACTIONS
None significant.

EFFECTS ON LAB TEST RESULTS
None reported.

CONTRAINDICATIONS & CAUTIONS
● Contraindicated in patients hypersensitive to drug.

NURSING CONSIDERATIONS
● Drug isn't effective against systemic infections.

PATIENT TEACHING
● Instruct patient not to chew or swallow lozenge but to allow it to dissolve slowly in mouth.
● Advise patient to continue taking drug for at least 2 days after signs and symptoms disappear. Consult prescriber for exact length of therapy.
● Instruct patient to continue therapy during menstruation.
● Explain that factors predisposing women to vaginal infection include use of antibiotics, hormonal contraceptives, and corticosteroids; diabetes; reinfection by sexual partner; and tight-fitting pantyhose. Encourage woman to wear cotton underwear.
● Instruct woman in careful hygiene for affected areas, including cleaning perineal area from front to back.
● Advise patient to report redness, swelling, or irritation.
● Tell patient, especially an older patient, that overusing mouthwash or wearing poorly fitting dentures may promote infection.

posaconazole
pahs-ah-KON-ah-zall

Noxafil

Pharmacologic class: triazole antifungal
Pregnancy risk category C

AVAILABLE FORMS
Oral suspension: 40 mg/ml

INDICATIONS & DOSAGES
➤ **Prevention of invasive *Aspergillus* and *Candida* infections in high-risk immunocompromised patients**
Adults and children age 13 and older:
200 mg (5 ml) P.O. t.i.d. with a full meal or a liquid nutritional supplement; duration of therapy is based on recovery from neutropenia or immunosuppression.
➤ **Oropharyngeal candidiasis**
Adults and children age 13 and older:
100 mg (2.5 ml) P.O. b.i.d. on first day, then 100 mg (2.5 ml) once daily for 13 days with a full meal or a liquid nutritional supplement.
➤ **Oropharyngeal candidiasis resistant to itraconazole or fluconazole treatment**
Adults and children age 13 and older:
400 mg (10 ml) P.O. b.i.d. with a full meal or a liquid nutritional supplement; duration of treatment is based on severity of underlying disease and patient response.

ADMINISTRATION
P.O.
● Give drug with a full meal or a liquid nutritional supplement.
● Shake the suspension well before giving it.
● Measure doses using calibrated spoon provided with the drug, which has two markings, one for 2.5 ml and one 5 ml. After patient takes dose, fill spoon with water and have him drink it to ensure a full dose.
● Store oral suspension at room temperature.

ACTION
Blocks the synthesis of ergosterol, a vital component of the fungal cell membrane.

Route	Onset	Peak	Duration
P.O.	Unknown	3–5 hr	Unknown

Half-life: 35 hours.

ADVERSE REACTIONS
CNS: *anxiety, dizziness, fatigue, fever, headache, insomnia, weakness.*
CV: *edema, hypertension, hypotension, tachycardia.*
EENT: *epistaxis, pharyngitis,* altered taste, blurred vision.

GI: *abdominal pain, constipation, diarrhea, dyspepsia, mucositis, nausea, vomiting.*
GU: VAGINAL HEMORRHAGE.
Hematologic: *anemia, petechiae,* FEBRILE NEUTROPENIA, NEUTROPENIA, THROMBOCYTOPENIA.
Hepatic: *bilirubinemia.*
Metabolic: *anorexia, hyperglycemia, hypokalemia,* **hypomagnesemia,** hypocalcemia.
Musculoskeletal: *arthralgia, back pain, pain.*
Respiratory: *cough, dyspnea,* upper respiratory tract infection.
Other: *bacteremia, CMV infection, herpes simplex, rigors.*

INTERACTIONS
Drug-drug. *Cimetidine,phenytoin:* May decrease level and effectiveness of posaconazole. Avoid using together.
Calcium channel blockers, cyclosporine, HMG-CoA reductase inhibitors, midazolam, phenytoin, sirolimus, tacrolimus, vinca alkaloids: May increase levels of these drugs. Reduce dosages, increase monitoring of levels, and observe patient for adverse effects.
Rifabutin: May decrease level and efficacy of posaconazole while increasing rifabutin level and risk of toxicity. Avoid using together. If unavoidable, monitor patient for uveitis, leukopenia, and other adverse effects.
Drug-food. *Food, liquid nutritional supplements:* May greatly enhance absorption of drug. Always give drug with liquid supplement or food.

EFFECTS ON LAB TEST RESULTS
● May increase AST, ALT, bilirubin, creatinine, alkaline phosphatase, and glucose levels. May decrease potassium, magnesium, and calcium levels.
● May decrease WBC, RBC, and platelet counts.

CONTRAINDICATIONS & CAUTIONS
● Contraindicated in patients hypersensitive to drug or its components and in patients taking ergot derivatives, pimozide, or quinidine.
● Use cautiously in patients hypersensitive to other azole antifungals, patients

---

Reactions may be *common,* uncommon, *life-threatening,* or COMMON AND LIFE-THREATENING.
Interaction may have a *rapid onset* or *delayed onset.*

with potentially proarrhythmic conditions, and patients with hepatic or renal insufficiency.

NURSING CONSIDERATIONS
• Correct electrolyte imbalances, especially potassium, magnesium, and calcium imbalances, before therapy.
• Monitor patient for signs and symptoms of electrolyte imbalance including a slow, weak, or irregular pulse; ECG change; nausea; neuromuscular irritability; and tetany.
• Obtain baseline liver function tests, including bilirubin level, before therapy and periodically during treatment. Notify prescriber if patient develops signs or symptoms of hepatic dysfunction.
• Monitor patient who has severe vomiting or diarrhea for breakthrough fungal infection.

PATIENT TEACHING
• If patient can't take a liquid supplement or eat a full meal, instruct him to notify prescriber. A different anti-infective may be needed, or monitoring may need to be increased.
• Tell patient to notify prescriber about an irregular heartbeat, fainting, or severe diarrhea or vomiting.
• Explain the signs and symptoms of liver dysfunction, including abdominal pain, yellowing skin or eyes, pale stools, and dark urine.
• Urge patient to contact the prescriber or pharmacist before taking other prescription or OTC drugs, and herbal or dietary supplements.
• Tell patient to shake the suspension well before taking it.
• Instruct patient to measure doses using the spoon provided with the drug. Household spoons vary in size and may yield an incorrect dose.
• Point out that the calibrated spoon has two markings: one for 2.5 ml and one for 5 ml. Make sure patient understands which mark to use for his prescribed dose.
• After patient takes dose, tell him to fill the spoon with water and drink it, to ensure a full dose. Tell him to clean the spoon with water before putting it away.

terbinafine hydrochloride
ter-BIN-ah-fin

Lamisil

Pharmacologic class: synthetic allylamine derivative
Pregnancy risk category B

AVAILABLE FORMS
Oral granules (packets): 125 mg, 187.5 mg
Tablets: 250 mg

INDICATIONS & DOSAGES
➤ **Fingernail onychomycosis caused by dermatophytes (tinea unguium)**
Adults: 250 mg P.O. once daily for 6 weeks.
➤ **Tinea capitus**
Children age 4 and older: One dose of granules daily for 6 weeks based on body weight. For < 25 kg, give 125 mg; 25 to 35 kg, 187.5 mg; > 35 kg, 250 mg.
➤ **Toenail onychomycosis caused by dermatophytes (tinea unguium)**
Adults: 250 mg P.O. once daily for 12 weeks.

ADMINISTRATION
P.O.
• Obtain pretreatment transaminase levels for all patients taking drug. Tablets aren't recommended for patients with acute or chronic liver disease.
• Give tablets without regard for food.
• Sprinkle entire contents of granule packet on a spoonful of nonacidic food, such as pudding or mashed potatoes. Have patient swallow spoonful without chewing.

ACTION
Prevents biosynthesis of ergosterol, causing a deficiency of this essential component of fungal cell membranes.

Route	Onset	Peak	Duration
P.O.	Unknown	2 hr	Unknown

Half-life: Unknown.

ADVERSE REACTIONS
CNS: *headache.*
EENT: vision disturbances.

GI: taste disturbances, diarrhea, dyspepsia, abdominal pain, nausea, flatulence.
Hematologic: *neutropenia.*
Hepatic: hepatobiliary dysfunction, including cholestatic jaundice.
Skin: *Stevens-Johnson syndrome, toxic epidermal necrolysis,* rash, pruritus, urticaria.
Other: *anaphylaxis,* hypersensitivity reactions.

INTERACTIONS
Drug-drug. *Caffeine:* May decrease I.V. caffeine clearance. Use cautiously together.
Cimetidine: May decrease clearance of terbinafine by one-third. Avoid using together.
Cyclosporine: May increase cyclosporine clearance. Monitor cyclosporine level.

EFFECTS ON LAB TEST RESULTS
● May increase AST and ALT levels.
● May decrease neutrophil and lymphocyte counts.

CONTRAINDICATIONS & CAUTIONS
● Contraindicated in patients hypersensitive to drug, pregnant or breast-feeding women, those with liver disease, and those with creatinine clearance less than 50 ml/ minute.

NURSING CONSIDERATIONS
● *Alert:* Rarely, patients with or without liver disease may suffer life-threatening liver failure.
● Monitor CBC and hepatic enzyme levels in patients receiving drug for longer than 6 weeks. Stop drug if hepatobiliary dysfunction or cholestatic hepatitis develops.
● *Look alike–sound alike:* Don't confuse terbinafine with terbutaline or Lamisil with Lamictal.

PATIENT TEACHING
● Inform patient that successful treatment may take 10 weeks for toenail infections and 4 weeks for fingernail infections.
● Tell patient to report vision disturbances immediately; changes in the ocular lens and retina may occur. Patient should also immediately report persistent nausea, anorexia, fatigue, vomiting, right upper quadrant pain, jaundice, dark urine, or pale stools.

● Teach patient or caregiver to sprinkle entire contents of granule packet on spoonful of nonacidic food, such as pudding or mashed potatoes, and to swallow spoonful without chewing.

---

voriconazole
vor-ah-KON-ah-zole

Vfend

Pharmacologic class: synthetic triazole
Pregnancy risk category D

AVAILABLE FORMS
Oral suspension: 40 mg/ml (after reconstitution)
Powder for injection: 200 mg
Tablets: 50 mg, 200 mg

INDICATIONS & DOSAGES
➤ **Esophageal candidiasis**
Adults who weigh 40 kg (88 lb) or more: 200 mg P.O. every 12 hours. Treat for a minimum of 14 days and for at least 7 days after symptoms resolve.
Adults who weigh less than 40 kg: 100 mg P.O. every 12 hours. Treat for a minimum of 14 days and for at least 7 days after symptoms resolve.
➤ **Invasive aspergillosis; serious infections caused by *Fusarium* species and *Scedosporium apiospermum* in patients intolerant of or refractory to other therapy**
Adults: Initially, 6 mg/kg I.V. every 12 hours for two doses; then maintenance dose of 4 mg/kg I.V. every 12 hours. If patient can't tolerate 4-mg dose, decrease to 3 mg/kg. Switch to P.O. form as tolerated, using the maintenance dosages shown here.
Adults who weigh more than 40 kg: 200 mg P.O. every 12 hours. May increase to 300 mg P.O. every 12 hours, if needed. If unable to tolerate the 300-mg dose, reduce dose in 50-mg decrements to a minimum of 200 mg every 12 hours.
Adults who weigh less than 40 kg: 100 mg P.O. every 12 hours. May increase to 150 mg P.O. every 12 hours, if needed. If unable to tolerate the 150-mg dose, reduce dose to 100 mg every 12 hours.

Reactions may be *common*, uncommon, *life-threatening*, or COMMON AND LIFE-THREATENING.
Interaction may have a *rapid onset* or *delayed onset.*

➤ **Candidemia in nonneutropenic patients;** *Candida* **infections of the kidney, abdomen, bladder wall, or wounds and disseminated skin infections**

Adults: Initially, 6 mg/kg I.V. every 12 hours for two doses, then 3 to 4 mg/kg I.V. every 12 hours for maintenance, depending on severity of the infection. If patient can't tolerate 4-mg dose, decrease to 3 mg/kg. Switch to P.O. form as tolerated. For adults who weigh 40 kg or more, give 200 mg P.O. every 12 hours. May increase to 300 mg P.O. every 12 hours, if needed. If unable to tolerate the 300-mg dose, reduce dose in 50-mg decrements to a minimum of 200 mg every 12 hours. For adults who weigh less than 40 kg, give 100 mg P.O. every 12 hours. May increase to 150 mg P.O. every 12 hours, if needed. If unable to tolerate the 150-mg dose, reduce dose to 100 mg every 12 hours. Treat patients with candidemia for at least 14 days after symptoms resolve or after the last positive culture result, whichever is longer.

Adjust-a-dose: For patients in Child-Pugh classes A or B, decrease the maintenance dosage by 50%. In patients with a creatinine clearance of less than 50 ml/minute, use oral form instead of I.V. form to prevent accumulation of a component of the I.V. mixture. In patients also receiving phenytoin, increase maintenance dose of voriconazole to 5 mg/kg I.V. every 12 hours, or increase P.O. dose from 100 mg to 200 mg (in patients weighing 40 kg or less) or from 200 mg to 400 mg (in patients weighing more than 40 kg).

ADMINISTRATION

P.O.
● Give drug at least 1 hour before or 1 hour after a meal.
● For the oral suspension, use only the dispenser provided in the medication package.
● Don't mix oral suspension with other drugs or beverages.
● Discard unused portion of suspension after 14 days.

I.V.
● In patients with creatinine clearance less than 50 ml/minute, use cautiously.

● Reconstitute the powder with 19 ml of water for injection to obtain a volume of 20 ml of clear concentrate containing 10 mg/ml of drug. Discard the vial if a vacuum doesn't pull the diluent into the vial. Shake the vial until all the powder is dissolved. Use the reconstituted solution immediately.
● Further dilute the 10-mg/ml solution to 5 mg/ml or less. Follow the manufacturer's instructions for diluting.
● Infuse over 1 to 2 hours at 5 mg/ml or less and a maximum hourly rate of 3 mg/kg/hour.
● **Incompatibilities:** Blood products, electrolyte supplements, 4.2% sodium bicarbonate infusion.

ACTION

Inhibits the cytochrome P-450–dependent synthesis of ergosterol, a vital component of fungal cell membranes.

Route	Onset	Peak	Duration
P.O., I.V.	Immediate	1–2 hr	12 hr

Half-life: Depends on dose.

ADVERSE REACTIONS

CNS: fever, headache, hallucinations, dizziness.
CV: tachycardia, hypertension, hypotension, vasodilatation.
EENT: *abnormal vision,* photophobia, chromatopsia, dry mouth.
GI: abdominal pain, nausea, vomiting, diarrhea.
Hepatic: cholestatic jaundice.
Metabolic: hypokalemia, hypomagnesemia.
Skin: rash, pruritus.
Other: chills, peripheral edema.

INTERACTIONS

Drug-drug. *Benzodiazepines, calcium channel blockers, methadone, omeprazole, sulfonylureas, vinca alkaloids:* May increase levels of these drugs. Adjust dosages of these drugs; monitor patient for adverse reactions.
Carbamazepine, long-acting barbiturates, rifabutin, rifampin, ritonavir (high-dose therapy): May decrease voriconazole level. Use together is contraindicated.

Cyclosporine, tacrolimus: May increase levels of these drugs. Adjust dosages; monitor levels.

Efavirenz: May significantly decrease voriconazole levels while significantly increasing efavirenz levels. Use together is contraindicated.

Ergot alkaloids (such as ergotamine), sirolimus: May increase levels of these drugs. Use together is contraindicated.

HIV protease inhibitors (amprenavir, nelfinavir, ritonavir, saquinavir), nonnucleoside reverse transcriptase inhibitors (delavirdine): May increase levels of both drugs. Monitor patient for adverse reactions and toxicity.

HMG-CoA reductase inhibitors (atorvastatin, fluvastatin, lovastatin, pravastatin, rosuvastatin, simvastatin): May increase levels and adverse effects, including rhabdomyolysis, of these drugs. Monitor patient closely and reduce dose of HMG-CoA reductase inhibitor as needed.

Oral contraceptives containing ethinyl estradiol and norethindrone: May increase levels and adverse effects of these drugs. Monitor patient closely.

Phenytoin: May decrease voriconazole level and increase phenytoin level. Increase voriconazole maintenance dose; monitor phenytoin level.

Pimozide, quinidine: May increase levels of these drugs, leading to torsades de pointes and prolonged QT interval. Use together is contraindicated.

Warfarin: May significantly increase PT. Monitor PT and other anticoagulant test results.

Drug-herb. *St. John's wort:* May increase drug level. Discourage use together.

Drug-lifestyle. *Sun exposure:* May cause photosensitivity. Advise patient to avoid excessive sunlight exposure.

EFFECTS ON LAB TEST RESULTS
● May increase alkaline phosphatase, AST, ALT, bilirubin, and creatinine levels. May decrease potassium and hemoglobin levels and hematocrit.
● May decrease platelet, WBC, and RBC counts.

CONTRAINDICATIONS & CAUTIONS
● Contraindicated in patients hypersensitive to drug or its components; in those

with rare, hereditary galactose intolerance, Lapp lactase deficiency, or glucose-galactose malabsorption; and in those taking carbamazepine, efavirenz, ergot alkaloid, a long-acting barbiturate, pimozide, quinidine, rifabutin, rifampin, ritonavir, or sirolimus.
● Use cautiously in patients hypersensitive to other azoles.

NURSING CONSIDERATIONS
● Infusion reactions, including flushing, fever, sweating, tachycardia, chest tightness, dyspnea, faintness, nausea, pruritus, and rash, may occur as soon as infusion starts. If reaction occurs, notify prescriber; infusion may need to be stopped.
● Monitor liver function test results at start of and during therapy. Monitor patients who develop abnormal liver function test results for more severe hepatic injury. If patient develops signs and symptoms of liver disease, drug may need to be stopped.
● Monitor renal function during treatment. For patients with creatinine clearance less than 50 ml/minute, give the oral form.
● If treatment lasts longer than 28 days, vision changes may occur.

PATIENT TEACHING
● Tell patient to take oral form at least 1 hour before or 1 hour after a meal.
● Tell patient taking the oral suspension to only use the dispenser provided with the medication pack.
● Advise patient not to mix oral suspension with other drugs or beverages.
● Tell patient to discard any unused portion of suspension after 14 days.
● Advise patient to avoid driving or operating machinery while taking drug, especially at night, because vision changes, including blurring and photophobia, may occur.
● Tell patient to avoid strong, direct sunlight during therapy.
● Advise patient to avoid becoming pregnant during therapy because of the risk of fetal harm.

8
Antimalarials

atovaquone and proguanil hydrochloride
chloroquine phosphate
doxycycline
(See Chapter 19, TETRACYCLINES.)
hydroxychloroquine sulfate
mefloquine hydrochloride
quinidine gluconate
(See Chapter 22, ANTIARRHYTHMICS.)
primaquine phosphate
pyrimethamine
pyrimethamine with sulfadoxine
tetracycline hydrochloride
(See Chapter 19, TETRACYCLINES.)

---

atovaquone and proguanil hydrochloride
a-TOE-va-kwon

Malarone, Malarone Pediatric

Pharmacologic class:
hydroxynaphthoquinone and
biguanide derivative
Pregnancy risk category C

AVAILABLE FORMS
Tablets (adult-strength): 250 mg atovaquone and 100 mg proguanil hydrochloride
Tablets (pediatric-strength): 62.5 mg
atovaquone and 25 mg proguanil hydrochloride

INDICATIONS & DOSAGES
➤ **To prevent *Plasmodium falciparum* malaria, including in areas
where chloroquine resistance has
been reported**
*Adults and children who weigh more than
40 kg (88 lb):* 1 adult-strength tablet P.O.
once daily with food or milk, beginning
1 or 2 days before entering a malaria-
endemic area. Continue prophylactic
treatment during stay and for 7 days after
return.
*Children who weigh 31 to 40 kg (68 to
88 lb):* 3 pediatric-strength tablets P.O.
once daily with food or milk, beginning

1 or 2 days before entering endemic area.
Continue prophylactic treatment during
stay and for 7 days after return.
*Children who weigh 21 to 30 kg (46 to
66 lb):* 2 pediatric-strength tablets P.O.
once daily with food or milk, beginning
1 or 2 days before entering endemic area.
Continue prophylactic treatment during
stay and for 7 days after return.
*Children who weigh 11 to 20 kg (24 to
44 lb):* 1 pediatric-strength tablet P.O.
daily with food or milk, beginning
1 or 2 days before entering endemic
area. Continue prophylactic treatment
during stay and for 7 days after
return.
➤ **Acute, uncomplicated *P. falciparum* malaria**
*Adults and children who weigh more than
40 kg (88 lb):* 4 adult-strength tablets P.O.
once daily, with food or milk, for 3 consecutive days.
*Children who weigh 31 to 40 kg (68 to
88 lb):* 3 adult-strength tablets P.O. once
daily, with food or milk, for 3 consecutive
days.
*Children who weigh 21 to 30 kg (46 to
66 lb):* 2 adult-strength tablets P.O. once
daily, with food or milk, for 3 consecutive
days.
*Children who weigh 11 to 20 kg (24 to
44 lb):* 1 adult-strength tablet P.O. once
daily, with food or milk, for 3 consecutive
days.
*Children who weigh 9 to 10 kg (20 to
22 lb):* 3 pediatric-strength tablets P.O.
once daily, with food or milk, for
3 consecutive days.
*Children who weigh 5 to 8 kg (11 to
18 lb):* 2 pediatric-strength tablets P.O.
once daily, with food or milk, for
3 consecutive days.

ADMINISTRATION
P.O.
● Give dose at same time each day, with
food or milk.
● If child has difficulty swallowing tablets,
parents may crush tablet and mix it in
condensed milk.

● Store tablets at controlled room temperature of 59° to 86° F (15° to 30° C).

ACTION

Thought to interfere with nucleic acid replication in the malarial parasite. Atovaquone selectively inhibits mitochondrial electron transport in the parasite. Cycloguanil, an active metabolite of proguanil hydrochloride, inhibits dihydrofolate reductase. Atovaquone and cycloguanil, an active metabolite of proguanil hydrochloride, are active against the erythrocytic and exoerythrocytic stages of *Plasmodium* species.

Route	Onset	Peak	Duration
P.O.	Unknown	Unknown	Unknown

Half-life: atovaquone: 2 to 3 days in adults; proguanil: 12 to 21 hours in adults and children.

ADVERSE REACTIONS

CNS: *headache,* fever, asthenia, dizziness, dreams, insomnia.
GI: *abdominal pain, nausea, vomiting,* diarrhea, anorexia, dyspepsia, gastritis, oral ulcers.
Respiratory: cough.
Skin: pruritus.

INTERACTIONS

Drug-drug. *Metoclopramide:* May decrease atovaquone bioavailability. Use another antiemetic.
Rifampin, rifabutin: May decrease atovaquone level by about 50%. Avoid using together.
Tetracycline: May decrease atovaquone level by about 40%. Monitor patient with parasitemia closely.

EFFECTS ON LAB TEST RESULTS

● May increase alkaline phosphatase, ALT, and AST levels. May decrease hemoglobin level and hematocrit.
● May decrease WBC count.

CONTRAINDICATIONS & CAUTIONS

● Contraindicated in patients hypersensitive to atovaquone, proguanil hydrochloride, or any component of the drug.
● Use cautiously in patients with severe renal impairment and in those who are vomiting.

● Use cautiously in elderly patients because they have a greater frequency of decreased renal, hepatic, and cardiac function.
● It isn't known if atovaquone appears in breast milk, but proguanil does in small amounts. Use cautiously in breast-feeding women.
● Safety and effectiveness haven't been established for prevention in children who weigh less than 11 kg or for treatment in children who weigh less than 5 kg.

NURSING CONSIDERATIONS

● Persistent diarrhea or vomiting may decrease drug absorption. Patients with these symptoms may need a different antimalarial.

PATIENT TEACHING

● Tell patient to take dose at the same time each day with food or milk.
● Tell parents that if child has difficulty swallowing tablets, to crush and mix in condensed milk.
● Tell patient to repeat dose if he vomits within 1 hour.
● Advise patient to notify prescriber if he can't complete the course of therapy as prescribed.
● Instruct patient to supplement preventive malarial with use of protective clothing, bed nets, and insect repellents.

chloroquine phosphate
KLO-ro-kwin

Aralen Phosphate

Pharmacologic class:
aminoquinoline
Pregnancy risk category C

AVAILABLE FORMS

Tablets: 250 mg (equivalent to 150 mg base), 500 mg (equivalent to 300 mg base)

INDICATIONS & DOSAGES

■ **Black Box Warning** Prescribers should be completely familiar with this drug before prescribing. ■

➤ **Acute malarial attacks caused by**
Plasmodium vivax, P. malariae,
P. ovale, **and susceptible strains of**
P. falciparum
Adults: Initially, 600 mg base P.O.; then
300 mg base at 6, 24, and 48 hours.
Children: Initially, 10 mg/kg base P.O.;
then 5 mg/kg base at 6, 24, and 48 hours.
Don't exceed adult dose.

➤ **To prevent malaria**
Adults: 300 mg base P.O. once weekly
on the same day each week, for 1 to
2 weeks before entering a malaria-
endemic area and continued for 4 weeks
after leaving the area. If treatment begins after exposure, give 600 mg base
P.O. initially, in two divided doses
6 hours apart, followed by the usual
dosing regimen.
Children: 5 mg/kg base P.O. once weekly
on the same day each week, for 1 to
2 weeks before entering a malaria-
endemic area and continued for 4 weeks
after leaving the area. Don't exceed
300 mg. If treatment begins after exposure, give 10 mg/kg base P.O. initially,
in two divided doses 6 hours apart,
followed by the usual dosing regimen.

➤ **Extraintestinal amebiasis**
Adults: 600 mg base P.O. once daily for
2 days; then 300 mg base daily for 2 to
3 weeks. Treatment is usually combined
with an intestinal amebicide.
Children: 10 mg/kg base P.O. once daily
for 2 to 3 weeks. Maximum dose is
300 mg base daily.

ADMINISTRATION
P.O.
● *Alert:* Drug dosage may be discussed
in "mg" or "mg base"; be aware of the
difference.
● To improve compliance when drug is
used for prevention, advise patient to take
drug immediately before or after a meal
on the same day each week.

ACTION
May bind to and alter the properties of
DNA in susceptible parasites.

Route	Onset	Peak	Duration
P.O.	Unknown	1–3 hr	Unknown

Half-life: 1 to 2 months.

ADVERSE REACTIONS
CNS: *seizures,* mild and transient headache, psychic stimulation, dizziness,
neuropathy.
CV: hypotension, ECG changes.
EENT: blurred vision, difficulty in focusing, reversible corneal changes, typically
irreversible, sometimes progressive or delayed retinal changes such as narrowing of
arterioles, macular lesions, pallor of optic
disk, optic atrophy, patchy retinal pigmentation, typically leading to blindness, ototoxicity, nerve deafness, vertigo, tinnitus.
GI: anorexia, abdominal cramps, diarrhea, nausea, vomiting, stomatitis.
Hematologic: *agranulocytosis, aplastic*
anemia, thrombocytopenia, hemolytic
anemia.
Skin: pruritus, lichen planus eruptions,
skin and mucosal pigmentary changes,
pleomorphic skin eruptions.

INTERACTIONS
Drug-drug. *Aluminum salts (kaolin),*
magnesium: May decrease GI absorption.
Separate dose times.
Cimetidine: May decrease hepatic metabolism of chloroquine. Monitor patient for
toxicity.
Drug-lifestyle. *Sun exposure:* May worsen
drug-induced dermatoses. Advise patient
to avoid excessive sun exposure.

EFFECTS ON LAB TEST RESULTS
● May decrease hemoglobin level.
● May decrease granulocyte and platelet
counts.

CONTRAINDICATIONS & CAUTIONS
● Contraindicated in patients hypersensitive to drug and in those with retinal or
visual field changes or porphyria.
● Use cautiously in patients with severe
GI, neurologic, or blood disorders; hepatic
disease or alcoholism; or G6PD deficiency
or psoriasis.

NURSING CONSIDERATIONS
● Ensure that baseline and periodic ophthalmic examinations are performed.
Check periodically for ocular muscle
weakness after long-term use.
● Make sure patient is tested with an audiometer before, during, and after therapy,
especially if therapy is long-term.

• Monitor CBC and liver function studies periodically during long-term therapy. If a severe blood disorder—not caused by the disease—develops, drug may need to be stopped.

• *Alert:* Monitor patient for overdose, which can quickly lead to toxic symptoms: headache, drowsiness, visual disturbances, CV collapse, seizures, and then cardiopulmonary arrest. Children are extremely susceptible to toxicity; avoid long-term treatment.

PATIENT TEACHING

• To improve compliance when using drug for prevention, advise patient to take drug immediately before or after a meal on the same day each week.

• Instruct patient to avoid excessive sun exposure to prevent worsening of drug-induced dermatoses.

• Tell patient to report adverse reactions promptly, especially blurred vision, increased sensitivity to light, tinnitus, hearing loss, or muscle weakness.

• Instruct patient to keep drug out of reach of children. Overdose may be fatal.

---

hydroxychloroquine sulfate
hye-drox-ee-KLOR-oh-kwin

Plaquenil

Pharmacologic class:
aminoquinoline
Pregnancy risk category C

AVAILABLE FORMS
Tablets: 200 mg (equivalent to 155 mg base)

INDICATIONS & DOSAGES
■ **Black Box Warning** Prescribers should be completely familiar with this drug before prescribing. ■

➤ **Suppressive prevention of malaria attacks caused by *Plasmodium vivax, P. malariae, P. ovale,* and susceptible strains of *P. falciparum***
Adults: 310 mg base P.O. weekly on the same day each week, beginning 1 to 2 weeks before entering malaria-endemic area and continuing for 4 weeks after leaving area. If not started before exposure,

double first dose to 620 mg base in two divided doses 6 hours apart.
Children: 5 mg/kg base P.O. weekly on the same day each week, beginning 1 to 2 weeks before entering malaria-endemic area and continuing for 4 weeks after leaving area. Don't exceed adult dose. If not started before exposure, double first dose to 10 mg/kg base in two divided doses, 6 hours apart.

➤ **Acute malarial attacks**
Adults: Initially, 620 mg base P.O., followed by 310 mg base 6 to 8 hours after first dose; then 310 mg base daily for 2 days.
Children: Initially, 10 mg/kg base P.O.; then 5 mg/kg base at 6 hours, 24 hours, and 48 hours after the first dose.

➤ **Lupus erythematosus**
Adults: 310 mg base P.O. daily or b.i.d., continued for several weeks or months, depending on response. For prolonged maintenance dose, 155 to 310 mg base daily.

➤ **Rheumatoid arthritis**
Adults: Initially, 310 to 465 mg base P.O. daily. When good response occurs, usually in 4 to 12 weeks, cut dosage in half.

ADMINISTRATION
P.O.
• *Alert:* Drug dosage may be discussed in "mg" or "mg base"; be aware of the difference.
• To improve compliance when drug is used for prevention, advise patient to take drug immediately before or after a meal on the same day each week.

ACTION
May bind to and alter the properties of DNA in susceptible organisms.

Route	Onset	Peak	Duration
P.O.	Unknown	2–4½ hr	Unknown

Half-life: 32 to 50 days.

ADVERSE REACTIONS
CNS: *seizures,* irritability, nightmares, ataxia, psychosis, vertigo, dizziness, hypoactive deep tendon reflexes, lassitude, headache.
CV: T-wave inversion or depression, widening of QRS complex.

Reactions may be *common,* uncommon, *life-threatening,* or COMMON AND LIFE-THREATENING.
Interaction may have a *rapid onset* or **delayed onset.**

EENT: blurred vision, difficulty in focusing, reversible corneal changes, typically irreversible nystagmus, sometimes progressive or delayed retinal changes such as narrowing of arterioles, macular lesions, pallor of optic disk, optic atrophy.

GI: anorexia, abdominal cramps, diarrhea, nausea, vomiting.

Hematologic: *agranulocytosis, leukopenia, thrombocytopenia, hemolysis in patients with G6PD deficiency, aplastic anemia.*

Metabolic: weight loss.

Musculoskeletal: skeletal muscle weakness.

Skin: pruritus, lichen planus eruptions, skin and mucosal pigmentary changes, pleomorphic skin eruptions, worsened psoriasis, alopecia, bleaching of hair.

INTERACTIONS
Drug-drug. *Aluminum salts (kaolin), magnesium:* May decrease GI absorption. Separate dose times.
Cimetidine: May decrease hepatic metabolism of hydroxychloroquine. Monitor patient for toxicity.
Digoxin: May increase digoxin level. Monitor drug levels; monitor patient for toxicity.

EFFECTS ON LAB TEST RESULTS
• May decrease hemoglobin level.
• May decrease granulocyte, WBC, and platelet counts.

CONTRAINDICATIONS & CAUTIONS
• Contraindicated in patients hypersensitive to drug and in those with retinal or visual field changes or porphyria.
• Contraindicated for long-term therapy for children.
• Use with caution in patients with severe GI, neurologic, or blood disorders.
• Use with caution in patients with hepatic disease or alcoholism because drug concentrates in liver.
• Use with caution in those with G6PD deficiency or psoriasis because drug may worsen these conditions.

NURSING CONSIDERATIONS
• Ensure that baseline and periodic ophthalmic examinations are performed.

Check periodically for ocular muscle weakness after long-term use.
• Make sure patient is examined with an audiometer before, during, and after therapy, especially if therapy is long-term.
• Monitor CBC and liver function studies periodically during long-term therapy; if severe blood disorder—not caused by disease—develops, drug may need to be stopped.
• *Alert:* Monitor patient for possible overdose, which can quickly lead to toxic signs or symptoms: headache, drowsiness, visual disturbances, CV collapse, seizures, then cardiopulmonary arrest. Children are extremely susceptible to toxicity.

PATIENT TEACHING
• Advise patient taking drug for prevention to take drug immediately before or after a meal on the same day each week, to improve compliance.
• Instruct patient to report adverse reactions promptly.

---

mefloquine hydrochloride
MEH-flow-kwin

Lariam

Pharmacologic class: quinine derivative
Pregnancy risk category C

AVAILABLE FORMS
Tablets: 250 mg

INDICATIONS & DOSAGES
➤ **Acute malaria infections caused by mefloquine-sensitive strains of Plasmodium falciparum or P. vivax**
Adults: 1,250 mg (5 tablets) P.O. as a single dose with food and at least 8 ounces of water. Patients with *P. vivax* infections should receive further therapy with primaquine or other 8-aminoquinolines to avoid relapse after treatment of the initial infection.
Children: 20 to 25 mg/kg P.O. as a single dose with food and at least 8 ounces of water. Maximum dose 1,250 mg. Dosage may be divided into two doses given 6 to 8 hours apart to reduce the incidence and severity of adverse effects. Patients with

---

P. vivax infections should receive further therapy with primaquine or other 8-aminoquinolines to avoid relapse after treatment of the initial infection.

➤ **To prevent malaria**
Adults and children weighing more than 45 kg (99 lb): 250 mg P.O. once weekly. Prevention therapy should start 1 week before entering endemic area and continue for 4 weeks after returning. If patient returns to an area without malaria after a prolonged stay in an endemic area, prevention therapy should end after three doses.
Children who weigh 31 to 45 kg (68 to 99 lb): 187.5 mg (¾ of a 250-mg tablet) P.O. once weekly.
Children who weigh 20 to 30 kg (44 to 66 lb): 125 mg (½ of a 250-mg tablet) P.O. once weekly.
Children who weigh 15 to 19 kg (33 to 42 lb): 62.5 mg (¼ of a 250-mg tablet) P.O. once weekly.
Children who weigh less than 15 kg (33 lb): 3 to 5 mg/kg P.O. once weekly.

ADMINISTRATION
P.O.
● Because giving quinine and mefloquine together poses a health risk, give mefloquine no sooner than 12 hours after the last dose of quinine or quinidine.
● Patient should avoid taking drug on empty stomach and should always take it with at least 8 ounces of water.

ACTION
May be caused by drug's ability to form complexes with hemin and to raise intravesicular pH in parasite acid vesicles.

Route	Onset	Peak	Duration
P.O.	Unknown	7–24 hr	Unknown

Half-life: About 21 days.

ADVERSE REACTIONS
CNS: *seizures, suicidal behavior,* fever, dizziness, syncope, headache, psychotic changes, hallucinations, confusion, anxiety, fatigue, vertigo, depression, tremor, ataxia, mood changes, panic attacks.
CV: chest pain, edema.
EENT: tinnitus, visual disturbances.
GI: anorexia, vomiting, *nausea,* loose stools, diarrhea, abdominal discomfort or pain, dyspepsia.

Hematologic: *leukopenia, thrombocytopenia.*
Musculoskeletal: myalgia.
Skin: rash.
Other: chills.

INTERACTIONS
Drug-drug. *Beta blockers, quinidine, quinine:* May cause ECG abnormalities and cardiac arrest. Avoid using together.
Carbamazepine, phenobarbital, phenytoin, valproic acid: May decrease drug levels and loss of seizure control at start of mefloquine therapy. Monitor anticonvulsant level.
Chloroquine, quinine: May increase risk of seizures and ECG abnormalities. Give mefloquine at least 12 hours after last dose.
Valproic acid: May decrease valproic acid level and loss of seizure control at start of mefloquine therapy. Monitor anticonvulsant level.

EFFECTS ON LAB TEST RESULTS
● May increase transaminase level. May decrease hematocrit.
● May decrease WBC and platelet counts.

CONTRAINDICATIONS & CAUTIONS
● Contraindicated in patients hypersensitive to mefloquine or related compounds.
● Contraindicated for prevention of malaria in patients with a history of seizures or an active or recent history of depression, generalized anxiety disorder, psychosis, schizophrenia, or other major psychiatric disorders.
● Use cautiously when treating patients with cardiac disease or seizure disorders.

NURSING CONSIDERATIONS
● Patients with *P. vivax* infections are at high risk for relapse because drug doesn't eliminate the hepatic-phase exoerythrocytic parasites. Give follow-up therapy with primaquine.
● Monitor liver function test results periodically.
● If overdose is suspected, induce vomiting or perform gastric lavage because of risk of cardiotoxicity. Mefloquine has produced cardiac reactions similar to quinidine and quinine.

• *Alert:* When drug is used preventively, psychiatric symptoms (acute anxiety, depression, restlessness, confusion) that occur may precede onset of a more serious event. Replace drug with other therapy.

PATIENT TEACHING
• Advise patient taking drug for prevention to take dose immediately before or after a meal on the same day each week, to improve compliance beginning 1 week before arrival at endemic area.
• Tell patient not to take drug on an empty stomach and always to take it with at least 8 ounces of water.
• Advise patient to use caution when performing activities that require alertness and coordination because dizziness, disturbed sense of balance, and neuropsychiatric reactions may occur.
• Instruct patient taking drug for prevention to stop drug and notify prescriber if signs or symptoms of impending toxicity, such as anxiety, depression, confusion, or restlessness, occur.
• Advise patient undergoing long-term therapy to have periodic ophthalmic exams because drug may cause ocular lesions.
• Advise women of childbearing age to use reliable contraception during treatment.

primaquine phosphate
PRIM-uh-kween

Pharmacologic class: aminoquinoline
Pregnancy risk category NR

AVAILABLE FORMS
Tablets: 26.3 mg (equivalent to 15-mg base)

INDICATIONS & DOSAGES
■ **Black Box Warning** Prescribers should be completely familiar with this drug before prescribing. ■
➤ **Relapsing *Plasmodium vivax* malaria, eliminating symptoms and infection completely; to prevent relapse**
Adults: 15 mg base P.O. daily for 14 days. Begin therapy during the last 2 weeks of,

or after, a course of suppression with chloroquine or comparable drug.
Children: 0.3 mg/kg/day base P.O. for 14 days. Maximum 15 mg base/dose. Begin therapy during the last 2 weeks of, or after, a course of suppression with chloroquine or comparable drug.

ADMINISTRATION
P.O.
• *Alert:* Drug dosage may be discussed in "mg" or "mg base"; be aware of the difference.
• Give drug with meals.

ACTION
May bind to and alter the properties of DNA in susceptible parasites.

Route	Onset	Peak	Duration
P.O.	Unknown	1–3 hr	Unknown

Half-life: 4 to 10 hours.

ADVERSE REACTIONS
GI: nausea, vomiting, epigastric distress, abdominal cramps.
Hematologic: *hemolytic anemia, leukopenia, methemoglobinemia.*

INTERACTIONS
Drug-drug. *Aluminum salts, magnesium:* Decreases GI absorption. Separate dose times.

EFFECTS ON LAB TEST RESULTS
• May decrease hemoglobin level.
• May decrease RBC count. May increase or decrease WBC count.

CONTRAINDICATIONS & CAUTIONS
• Contraindicated in patients with systemic diseases in which agranulocytosis may develop, such as lupus erythematosus or rheumatoid arthritis, and in those taking a bone marrow suppressant, quinacrine, or hemolytic drugs.
• Use cautiously in patients with previous idiosyncratic reaction involving hemolytic anemia, methemoglobinemia, or leukopenia; in those with a family or personal history of favism; and in those with erythrocytic G6PD or nicotinamide-adenine-dinucleotide (NADH) methemoglobin reductase deficiency.

NURSING CONSIDERATIONS
● Use drug with a fast-acting antimalarial such as chloroquine to reduce possibility of drug-resistant strains.
● Obtain frequent blood studies and urinalysis in light-skinned patients taking more than 30 mg base daily, dark-skinned patients taking more than 15 mg base daily, and patients with severe anemia or suspected sensitivity.
● Monitor patient for markedly darkened urine and for suddenly reduced hemoglobin level or erythrocyte or leukocyte count, which suggest impending hemolytic reactions. Stop drug immediately and notify prescriber.
● Safe use during pregnancy hasn't been established.

PATIENT TEACHING
● Instruct patient to take drug with meals to minimize stomach upset. If nausea, vomiting, or stomach pain persists, tell patient to notify prescriber.
● Tell patient to report to prescriber chills, fever, chest pain, and bluish skin discoloration; these signs and symptoms may suggest a hemolytic reaction.
● Tell patient to stop drug and notify prescriber immediately if urine darkens markedly.
● Stress importance of completing full course of therapy.

---

pyrimethamine
pihr-ih-METH-ah-meen

Daraprim

pyrimethamine with sulfadoxine
Fansidar

Pharmacologic class: folic acid antagonist
Pregnancy risk category C

AVAILABLE FORMS
pyrimethamine
Tablets: 25 mg
pyrimethamine with sulfadoxine
Tablets: 25 mg pyrimethamine and 500 mg sulfadoxine

INDICATIONS & DOSAGES
➤ **To prevent and control transmission of malaria**
pyrimethamine
Adults and children age 10 and older: 25 mg P.O. weekly for 6 to 10 weeks or longer after leaving malaria-endemic areas.
Children ages 4 to 10: Give 12.5 mg P.O. weekly continued for 6 to 10 weeks or longer after leaving malaria-endemic areas.
Children younger than age 4: Give 6.25 mg P.O. weekly continued for 6 to 10 weeks or longer after leaving malaria-endemic areas.
pyrimethamine with sulfadoxine
Adults and children age 14 and older: 1 tablet weekly or 2 tablets every 2 weeks during exposure and for 4 to 6 weeks after exposure.
Children ages 9 to 14: Give ¾ tablet weekly, or 1½ tablets every 2 weeks during exposure and for 4 to 6 weeks after exposure.
Children ages 4 to 8: Give ½ tablet weekly or 1 tablet every 2 weeks during exposure and for 4 to 6 weeks after exposure.
Children younger than age 4: Give ¼ tablet weekly, or ½ tablet every 2 weeks during exposure and for 4 to 6 weeks after exposure.
➤ **Acute attacks of malaria**
pyrimethamine
Adults: 50 mg P.O. daily for 2 days; then 25 mg once weekly for at least 10 weeks.
Children ages 4 to 10: Give 25 mg P.O. once daily for 2 days; then 12.5 mg once weekly for at least 10 weeks.
pyrimethamine with sulfadoxine
Adults and children age 14 and older: 2 to 3 tablets as a single dose, given on the last day of quinine therapy.
Children ages 9 to 14: Give 2 tablets as a single dose, given on the last day of quinine therapy.
Children ages 4 to 8: Give 1 tablet as a single dose, given on the last day of quinine therapy.
Children ages 1 to 3: Give ½ tablet as a single dose, given on the last day of quinine therapy.
Children ages 2 to 11 months: Give ¼ tablet as a single dose, given on the last day of quinine therapy.

Reactions may be *common*, uncommon, *life-threatening*, or COMMON AND LIFE-THREATENING.
Interaction may have a *rapid onset* or **delayed onset**.

➤ **Toxoplasmosis**
pyrimethamine
Adults: Initially, 50 to 75 mg P.O. with
1 to 4 g sulfadiazine; continue for 1 to
3 weeks. After 3 weeks, reduce dosage by
half and continue for 4 to 5 weeks.
Children: Initially, 1 mg/kg/day P.O. in
two equally divided doses for 2 to 4 days;
then 0.5 mg/kg daily for 4 weeks, along
with 100 mg sulfadiazine/kg P.O. daily,
divided every 6 hours. Don't exceed
100 mg.

➤ **Primary prevention of toxoplasmosis in patients with HIV
infection ◆**
Adults and adolescents: 50 mg P.O., once
weekly, with leucovorin 25 mg P.O. once
weekly and dapsone 50 mg P.O. daily; or
75 mg pyrimethamine with leucovorin
25 mg and dapsone 200 mg P.O., all once
weekly.

➤ **Secondary prevention of toxoplasmosis in patients with HIV
infection ◆**
Adults and adolescents: 25 to 50 mg P.O.,
once daily, with leucovorin 10 to 25 mg
P.O. once daily and either sulfadiazine
0.5 to 1 g P.O. q.i.d. or clindamycin 300 to
450 mg every 6 to 8 hours.

ADMINISTRATION
P.O.
● Patient should take first preventive dose
1 to 2 days before traveling.
● Give drug with meals.

ACTION
Blocks creation of folic acid, which is required for the reproduction of the infecting organism. Sulfadoxine competitively
inhibits use of PABA.

Route	Onset	Peak	Duration
P.O.	Unknown	1½–8 hr	2 wk

Half-life: 4 days.

ADVERSE REACTIONS
CNS: *seizures,* headache, peripheral neuritis, mental depression, ataxia, hallucinations, fatigue.
CV: *arrhythmias,* allergic myocarditis.
EENT: scleral irritation, periorbital
edema.
GI: anorexia, vomiting, atrophic glossitis.

Hematologic: *agranulocytosis, aplastic
anemia, leukopenia, thrombocytopenia,
pancytopenia,* megaloblastic anemia.
Skin: *Stevens-Johnson syndrome,* generalized skin eruptions, urticaria, pruritus,
photosensitivity.

INTERACTIONS
Drug-drug. *Co-trimoxazole, methotrexate, sulfonamides:* May increase risk of
bone marrow suppression. Avoid using
together.
Lorazepam: May increase risk of hepatotoxicity. Avoid using together.
PABA: May decrease action against toxoplasmosis. May need to adjust dosage.

EFFECTS ON LAB TEST RESULTS
● May decrease hemoglobin level.
● May decrease granulocyte, WBC,
platelet, and RBC counts.

CONTRAINDICATIONS & CAUTIONS
● Pyrimethamine is contraindicated in patients hypersensitive to drug and in those
with megaloblastic anemia from folic acid
deficiency. Pyrimethamine with sulfadoxine is contraindicated in patients with
porphyria.
● Repeated use of pyrimethamine with
sulfadoxine is contraindicated in patients
with severe renal insufficiency, marked
parenchymal damage to the liver, blood
dyscrasias, hypersensitivity to pyrimethamine or sulfonamides, or documented
megaloblastic anemia from folic-acid
deficiency.
● Contraindicated in infants younger than
age 2 months and in pregnant (at term)
and breast-feeding women.
● Use cautiously after treatment with
chloroquine and in patients with impaired
hepatic or renal function, severe allergy or
bronchial asthma, G6PD deficiency, or
seizure disorders (smaller doses may be
needed).

NURSING CONSIDERATIONS
● Pyrimethamine alone isn't recommended for malaria. Use drug with faster-acting antimalarials, such as chloroquine,
for 2 days to start transmission control and
suppressive cure.
● For toxoplasmosis, obtain twice-weekly
blood counts, including platelets, because

usual dosages approach toxic levels. If signs of folic- or folinic-acid deficiency develop, reduce dosage or stop drug and give parenteral folinic acid (leucovorin) until blood counts return to normal.

● Adverse drug reactions related to sulfadiazine are similar to those related to sulfonamides.

● When used for toxoplasmosis in patients with AIDS, therapy may be lifelong.

● Use pyrimethamine with sulfadoxine only in areas where chloroquine-resistant malaria is prevalent and only if the traveler plans to stay longer than 3 weeks.

PATIENT TEACHING

● Instruct patient to take drug with meals.

● Inform patient with toxoplasmosis of importance of frequent laboratory studies and compliance with therapy. Tell patient he may need long-term therapy.

● Warn patient taking pyrimethamine with sulfadoxine to stop drug and notify prescriber at first sign of rash, sore throat, or glossitis.

● Tell patient to take first preventive dose 1 to 2 days before traveling.

9

Antiretrovirals

abacavir sulfate
atazanavir sulfate
darunavir ethanolate
delavirdine mesylate
didanosine
efavirenz
emtricitabine
enfuvirtide
etravirine
fosamprenavir calcium
indinavir sulfate
lamivudine
lopinavir and ritonavir
maraviroc
nelfinavir mesylate
nevirapine
raltegravir
ritonavir
saquinavir mesylate
stavudine
tenofovir disoproxil fumarate
tipranavir
zidovudine

---

abacavir sulfate
ah-BAK-ah-veer

Ziagen

Pharmacologic class: nucleoside
reverse transcriptase inhibitor
Pregnancy risk category C

AVAILABLE FORMS
Oral solution: 20 mg/ml
Tablets: 300 mg

INDICATIONS & DOSAGES
➤ **HIV-1 infection**
Adults: 300 mg P.O. b.i.d. or 600 mg P.O.
daily with other antiretrovirals.
Children ages 3 months to 16 years: Give
8 mg/kg P.O. b.i.d., up to maximum of
300 mg P.O. b.i.d., with other antiretrovirals.
Adjust-a-dose: In patients with mild hepatic impairment (Child-Pugh score 5 to
6), give 200 mg (oral solution) P.O. b.i.d.
Don't use in patients with moderate to
severe hepatic impairment.

ADMINISTRATION
P.O.
● Always give drug with other antiretro-
virals, never alone.
● Patient may take drug with or without
food.

ACTION
Converted intracellularly to the active
metabolite carbovir triphosphate, which
inhibits activity of HIV-1 reverse transcriptase, terminating viral DNA growth.

Route	Onset	Peak	Duration
P.O.	Unknown	Unknown	Unknown

Half-life: 1 to 2 hours.

ADVERSE REACTIONS
CNS: fever, headache, insomnia and sleep
disorders.
GI: *anorexia, diarrhea, nausea, vomiting.*
Skin: rash.
Other: *hypersensitivity reaction.*

INTERACTIONS
Drug-lifestyle. *Alcohol use:* May decrease elimination of drug, increasing
overall exposure. Monitor alcohol consumption. Discourage use together.

EFFECTS ON LAB TEST RESULTS
● May increase GGT, glucose, and triglyceride levels.

CONTRAINDICATIONS & CAUTIONS
■ **Black Box Warning** Patients who carry
the HLA-B*5701 allele are at high risk for
hypersensitivity reactions; patients should
be screened prior to beginning therapy. ■
● Contraindicated in patients hypersensitive to drug or its components.
● Contraindicated in patients with moderate to severe hepatic impairment.
■ **Black Box Warning** Due to increased
risk of hepatotoxicity, use cautiously when
giving drug to patients at risk for liver
disease. Lactic acidosis and severe hepatomegaly with steatosis, including fatal
cases, have been reported with the use
of nucleoside analogues alone or in

---

combination, including abacavir and other antiretrovirals. Stop treatment with drug if events occur. ■

● Use cautiously in pregnant women because the effects are unknown. Use during pregnancy only if the potential benefits outweigh the risk. Register pregnant women with the Antiretroviral Pregnancy Registry at 1-800-258-4263.

NURSING CONSIDERATIONS

● Women are more likely than men to experience lactic acidosis and severe hepatomegaly with steatosis. Obesity and prolonged nucleoside exposure may be risk factors.

■ **Black Box Warning** Drug can cause fatal hypersensitivity reactions; if patient develops signs or symptoms of hypersensitivity (such as fever, rash, fatigue, nausea, vomiting, diarrhea, or abdominal pain), stop drug and notify prescriber immediately. ■

■ **Black Box Warning** Don't restart drug after a hypersensitivity reaction because severe signs and symptoms will recur within hours and may include life-threatening hypotension and death. To facilitate reporting of hypersensitivity reactions, register patients with the Abacavir Hypersensitivity Reaction Registry at 1-800-270-0425. ■

● Because of a high rate of early virologic resistance, triple antiretroviral therapy with abacavir, lamivudine, and tenofovir shouldn't be used as new treatment regimen for naïve or pretreated patients. Monitor patients currently controlled with this combination and those who use this combination in addition to other antiretrovirals, and consider modification of therapy.

● Drug may mildly elevate glucose level.

● **Look alike–sound alike:** Don't confuse abacavir with amprenavir.

PATIENT TEACHING

● Inform patient that drug can cause a life-threatening hypersensitivity reaction. Warn patient who develops signs or symptoms of hypersensitivity (such as fever, rash, severe tiredness, achiness, a generally ill feeling, nausea, vomiting, diarrhea, or stomach pain) to stop taking drug and notify prescriber immediately.

● Include information leaflet about drug with each new prescription and refill. Patient also should receive, and be instructed to carry, a warning card summarizing signs and symptoms of hypersensitivity reaction.

● Inform patient that this drug doesn't cure HIV infection. Tell patient that drug doesn't reduce the risk of transmission of HIV to others through sexual contact or blood contamination and that its long-term effects are unknown.

● Tell patient to take drug exactly as prescribed.

● Inform patient that drug can be taken with or without food.

---

atazanavir sulfate
ah-TAZ-ah-nah-veer

Reyataz❦

Pharmacologic class: protease inhibitor
Pregnancy risk category B

AVAILABLE FORMS
Capsules: 100 mg, 150 mg, 200 mg, 300 mg

INDICATIONS & DOSAGES
➤ **HIV-1 infection, with other anti-retrovirals**
Adults: Give antiretroviral-experienced patients 300 mg (as one 300-mg capsule or two 150-mg capsules) once daily, plus 100 mg ritonavir once daily with food. Give antiretroviral-naive patients 400 mg (as two 200-mg capsules) once daily with food. When drug is given with efavirenz in antiretroviral-naive patients, give atazanavir 300 mg, ritonavir 100 mg, and efavirenz 600 mg as a single daily dose with food. Dosage recommendations for efavirenz and atazanavir in treatment-experienced patients haven't been established.
Adolescents at least age 13 and weighing at least 39 kg (86 lb) who are treatment-naive and unable to tolerate ritonavir: 400 mg P.O. once daily with food.
Children and adolescents ages 6 to 18 who are treatment-naive: Weighing 15 to less than 25 kg (33 to less than

---

55 lb), give 150 mg P.O. once daily with 80 mg ritonavir; 25 to less than 32 kg (55 to less than 70 lb), give 200 mg P.O. once daily with 100 mg ritonavir; 32 to less than 39 kg (70 to less than 86 lb), give 250 mg P.O. once daily with 100 mg ritonavir; at least 39 kg (86 lb), give 300 mg once daily with 100 mg ritonavir.

Children and adolescents ages 6 to 18 who are treatment-experienced: Weighing 25 to less than 32 kg, give 200 mg P.O. once daily with 100 mg ritonavir; 32 to less than 39 kg, give 250 mg P.O. once daily with 100 mg ritonavir; at least 39 kg, give 300 mg P.O. once daily with 100 mg ritonavir.

Adjust-a-dose: In patients with Child-Pugh class B hepatic insufficiency who haven't experienced prior virologic failure, reduce dosage to 300 mg P.O. once daily.

ADMINISTRATION
P.O.
• Give drug with food.
• Give drug to pregnant woman only if potential benefit justifies fetal risk.

ACTION
Inhibits viral maturation in HIV-1–infected cells, resulting in the formation of immature noninfectious viral particles.

Route	Onset	Peak	Duration
P.O.	Unknown	2½ hr	Unknown

Half-life: About 7 hours.

ADVERSE REACTIONS
CNS: *headache,* depression, dizziness, fatigue, fever, insomnia, pain, peripheral neurologic symptoms.
CV: prolonged PR interval.
EENT: scleral yellowing.
GI: *abdominal pain, diarrhea, nausea,* vomiting.
Hepatic: hyperbilirubinemia, jaundice.
Metabolic: lipodystrophy.
Musculoskeletal: arthralgia, back pain.
Respiratory: increased cough.
Skin: *rash.*

INTERACTIONS
Drug-drug. *Amiodarone, lidocaine (systemic), quinidine, tricyclic antidepres-*

sants: May increase levels of these drugs. Monitor drug levels.
Antacids, buffered drugs, didanosine: May decrease atazanavir level. Give atazanavir 2 hours before or 1 hour after these drugs.
Atorvastatin: May increase atorvastatin levels, increasing the risk of myopathy and rhabdomyolysis. Use together cautiously.
Clarithromycin: May increase clarithromycin level and prolong QTc interval while reducing active metabolite. Avoid using together, except to treat *Mycobacterium avium* complex infection. Decrease clarithromycin by 50% when using together.
Cyclosporine, sirolimus, tacrolimus: May increase immunosuppressant level. Monitor immunosuppressant level.
Diltiazem, felodipine, nicardipine, nifedipine, verapamil: May increase calcium channel blocker level. Use together cautiously, with close ECG monitoring. Adjust calcium channel blocker dosage as needed. Decrease diltiazem dose by 50%.
Efavirenz: May alter atazanavir level. Reduce atazanavir dosage.
Ergot derivatives, pimozide: May cause serious or life-threatening reactions. Avoid using together.
Ethinyl estradiol and norethindrone: May increase ethinyl estradiol and norethindrone levels. Use cautiously together; give the lowest effective dose of hormonal contraceptive.
H₂-receptor antagonists: May decrease atazanavir level, reducing therapeutic effect. Separate doses by at least 12 hours.
Indinavir: May increase risk of indirect (unconjugated) hyperbilirubinemia. Avoid using together.
Irinotecan: May interfere with irinotecan metabolism and increase irinotecan toxicity. Avoid using together.
Lovastatin, simvastatin: May cause myopathy and rhabdomyolysis. Avoid using together.
Midazolam, triazolam: May cause prolonged or increased sedation or respiratory depression. Avoid using together.
Proton-pump inhibitors, *rifampin:* May significantly reduce atazanavir level. Avoid using together.
Rifabutin: May increase rifabutin level. Reduce rifabutin dose up to 75%.

Ritonavir: May increase atazanavir level. Decrease atazanavir dose to 300 mg.

Saquinavir (soft-gelatin capsules): May increase saquinavir level. Avoid using together.

Sildenafil, tadalafil, vardenafil: May increase levels of these drugs, causing hypotension, visual changes, and priapism. Use together cautiously and reduce sildenafil dose to 25 mg every 48 hours, tadalafil dose to 10 mg every 72 hours, and vardenafil dose to 2.5 mg every 72 hours.

Tenofovir: May decrease atazanavir level, causing resistance. Give both drugs with ritonavir.

Warfarin: May increase warfarin level, which may cause life-threatening bleeding. Monitor INR.

Drug-herb. *St. John's wort:* May decrease drug level, reducing therapeutic effect and causing drug resistance. Discourage use together.

Drug-food. *Any food:* May increase bioavailability of drug. Tell patient to take drug with food.

EFFECTS ON LAB TEST RESULTS
• May increase ALT, amylase, AST, bilirubin, and lipase levels. May decrease hemoglobin level.
• May decrease neutrophil count.

CONTRAINDICATIONS & CAUTIONS
• Contraindicated in patients hypersensitive to drug or its ingredients.
• Contraindicated in patients taking drugs cleared mainly by CYP3A4 or drugs that can cause serious or life-threatening reactions at high levels (dihydroergotamine, ergonovine, ergotamine, midazolam, methylergonovine, pimozide, triazolam).
• Don't use in patients with Child-Pugh class C hepatic insufficiency.
• Use cautiously in patients with conduction system disease or hepatic impairment.
• Use cautiously in elderly patients because of the increased likelihood of other disease, additional drug therapy, and decreased hepatic, renal, or cardiac function.

NURSING CONSIDERATIONS
• *Alert:* Drug may prolong the PR interval.
• Monitor the patient for hyperglycemia and new-onset diabetes or worsened diabetes. Insulin and oral hypoglycemic dosages may need adjustment.
• Monitor a patient with hepatitis B or C for elevated liver enzymes or hepatic decompensation.
• Watch for life-threatening lactic acidosis syndrome and symptomatic hyperlactatemia, especially in women and obese patients.
• If the patient has hemophilia, watch for bleeding.
• Monitor patient for renal colic; drug may cause nephrolithiasis.
• Most patients have an asymptomatic increase in indirect bilirubin, possibly with yellowed skin or sclerae. This hyperbilirubinemia will resolve when therapy stops.
• Although cross resistance occurs among protease inhibitors, resistance to drug doesn't preclude use of other protease inhibitors.
• Register pregnant women for monitoring of maternal-fetal outcomes by calling the Antiretroviral Pregnancy Registry at 1-800-258-4263.

PATIENT TEACHING
• Urge patient to take drug with food every day and to take other antiretrovirals as prescribed.
• Explain that drug doesn't cure HIV infection and that the patient may develop opportunistic infections and other complications of HIV disease.
• Caution the patient that drug doesn't reduce the risk of transmitting the HIV virus to others.
• Tell patient that drug may cause altered or increased body fat, central obesity, buffalo hump, peripheral wasting, facial wasting, breast enlargement, and a cushingoid appearance.
• Tell patient to report yellowed skin or eyes, dizziness, or light-headedness.
• Caution patient not to take other prescriptions or OTC or herbal medicines without first consulting his prescriber.

Reactions may be *common*, uncommon, *life-threatening*, or COMMON AND LIFE-THREATENING.
Interaction may have a *rapid onset* or *delayed onset*.

darunavir ethanolate
duh-ROO-nah-veer

Prezista

Pharmacologic class: protease inhibitor
Pregnancy risk category B

AVAILABLE FORMS
Tablets: 300 mg, 600 mg

INDICATIONS & DOSAGES
➤ **With ritonavir and other antiretrovirals, for IIIV infection in antiretroviral treatment-experienced patients**
Adults: 600 mg P.O. b.i.d., given with 100 mg ritonavir P.O. b.i.d. and food.

ADMINISTRATION
P.O.
● Always give with ritonavir and food.

ACTION
Binds to the protease-active site and inhibits enzyme activity. This inhibition prevents cleavage of viral polyproteins, resulting in the formation of immature, noninfectious viral particles.

Route	Onset	Peak	Duration
P.O.	Unknown	2½–4 hr	Unknown

Half-life: About 15 hours when combined with ritonavir.

ADVERSE REACTIONS
CNS: *headache,* altered mood, anxiety, asthenia, confusion, disorientation, fatigue, hypoesthesia, irritability, memory impairment, nightmares, paresthesia, peripheral neuropathy, somnolence, transient ischemic attack, vertigo.
CV: *MI,* hypertension, tachycardia.
EENT: nasopharyngitis.
GI: *diarrhea, nausea,* abdominal distension, abdominal pain, anorexia, constipation, dry mouth, dyspepsia, flatulence, polydipsia, vomiting.
GU: *acute renal failure,* renal insufficiency, nephrolithiasis, polyuria.
Hematologic: LEUKOPENIA, *neutropenia, thrombocytopenia.*
Hepatic: *hepatotoxicity.*

Metabolic: decreased appetite, diabetes mellitus, hypercholesterolemia, hyperlipidemia, hypernatremia, hyperuricemia, hyponatremia, obesity.
Musculoskeletal: arthralgia, myalgia, osteopenia, osteoporosis, pain in extremity.
Respiratory: cough, dyspnea, hiccups.
Skin: *erythema multiforme, Stevens-Johnson syndrome,* allergic dermatitis, alopecia, dermatitis medicamentosa, eczema, folliculitis, increased sweating, inflammation, lipoatrophy, maculopapular rash, night sweats, toxic skin eruption.
Other: fat redistribution, gynecomastia, hyperthermia, peripheral edema, pyrexia, rigors.

INTERACTIONS
Drug-drug. *Amiodarone, bepridil, cyclosporine, felodipine, fluticasone, lidocaine, nicardipine, nifedipine, quinidine, rifabutin, sildenafil, sirolimus, tacrolimus, tadalafil, trazodone, vardenafil:* May increase levels of these drugs, increasing the risk of adverse reactions. Use caution, and monitor patient carefully.
Ergot derivatives, midazolam, pimozide, terfenadine, triazolam: May cause life-threatening reactions. Use together is contraindicated.
Atorvastatin, pravastatin: May increase levels of these drugs. Start at the lowest possible dose, and monitor patient carefully.
Clarithromycin: May increase clarithromycin level. Reduce clarithromycin dose in patients with renal impairment.
CYP3A inducers (carbamazepine, dexamethasone, phenobarbital, phenytoin, rifabutin, rifampin), efavirenz, lopinavir, saquinavir: May increase darunavir clearance and decrease darunavir level. Avoid using together.
Ethinyl estradiol, norethindrone: May decrease estrogen level. Recommend alternative or additional contraception.
Itraconazole, ketoconazole: May increase levels of these drugs and darunavir. Don't exceed 200 mg of itraconazole or ketoconazole daily.
Lovastatin, simvastatin (HMG-CoA reductase inhibitors): May increase risk of myopathy, including rhabdomyolysis. Use extreme caution.

Methadone: May decrease methadone level. Monitor patient for opioid abstinence syndrome, and consider increasing methadone dosage.

Rifabutin: May decrease darunavir level. If used together, give rifabutin as 150 mg every other day.

SSRIs (paroxetine, sertraline): May decrease levels of these drugs. Adjust dosage carefully based on antidepressant response.

Trazodone: May increase trazodone level and risk of toxicity. Decrease trazodone dosage.

Warfarin: May decrease warfarin level. Monitor patient carefully.

Drug-herb. *St. John's wort:* May decrease drug level significantly. Discourage use together.

Drug-food. *Food:* Increases drug absorption, which is needed for adequate therapeutic effect. Advise patient to take with food.

EFFECTS ON LAB TEST RESULTS

• May increase AST, ALT, GGT, alkaline phosphatase, bilirubin, pancreatic amylase, pancreatic lipase, cholesterol, triglyceride, and uric acid levels. May decrease albumin, bicarbonate, and calcium levels. May increase or decrease sodium and glucose levels.

• May decrease WBC, neutrophil, lymphocyte, and platelet counts.

CONTRAINDICATIONS & CAUTIONS

• Contraindicated in patients hypersensitive to any component of drug and patient taking drugs metabolized by CYP3A (dihydroergotamine, ergonovine, ergotamine, methylergonovine, midazolam, pimozide, triazolam).

• Use cautiously in patients with liver or renal impairment, diabetes mellitus, hemophilia, known sulfonamide allergy, or a history of opportunistic infections.

• Safety and effectiveness in children haven't been established

NURSING CONSIDERATIONS

• **Alert:** Because of an increased risk of hepatotoxicity, especially in patients with prior hepatic dysfunction, check liver function tests before beginning treatment

and periodically thereafter. Discontinue treatment in patients with elevated liver enzyme levels and signs and symptoms of liver dysfunction.

• Make sure patient isn't taking any drugs that are incompatible with darunavir.

• If patient has diabetes, monitor glucose level.

• Risks and benefits of drug in treatment-naïve patients aren't known.

PATIENT TEACHING

• Explain that many drugs interact with darunavir; advise patient to report all drugs he takes, including OTC products.

• **Alert:** Instruct patient to take darunavir and ritonavir at the same time every day, with food.

• Tell patient that drug doesn't cure HIV infection or AIDS and doesn't reduce the risk of passing HIV to others.

• Explain that opportunistic infections and other complications of HIV infection may still develop.

• If patient misses a dose by more than 6 hours, tell him to wait and take the next dose at the regularly scheduled time. If he remembers within 6 hours, tell him to take the missed dose immediately.

---

delavirdine mesylate
dell-ah-VUR-den

Rescriptor

Pharmacologic class:
nonnucleoside reverse
transcriptase inhibitor
Pregnancy risk category C

AVAILABLE FORMS
Tablets: 100 mg, 200 mg

INDICATIONS & DOSAGES
➤ **HIV-1 infection**
Adults: 400 mg P.O. t.i.d. with other appropriate antiretrovirals.
■ **Black Box Warning** Resistant virus emerges rapidly when delavirdine is administered as monotherapy. Always administer with appropriate antiretroviral therapy. ■

ADMINISTRATION

P.O.

- Patient may take drug with or without food.
- For patient who doesn't have gastric hydrochloric acid, drug should be taken with an acidic beverage, such as orange juice or cranberry juice.
- Patient should separate doses of delavirdine and antacid by at least 1 hour.
- Drug may be dispersed in water before ingestion. Add four 100-mg tablets to at least 3 ounces (90 ml) of water, allow to stand for a few minutes, and stir until a uniform dispersion occurs. Tell patient to drink dispersion promptly, rinse glass, and swallow the rinse to ensure that entire dose is consumed. Don't try to disperse 200-mg tablets because they don't disperse well; take 200-mg tablets intact.

ACTION

A nonnucleoside reverse transcriptase inhibitor of HIV-1 that binds directly to reverse transcriptase and blocks RNA- and DNA-dependent DNA polymerase activities.

Route	Onset	Peak	Duration
P.O.	Unknown	1 hr	Unknown

Half-life: 5¼ hours.

ADVERSE REACTIONS

CNS: *asthenia, fatigue, headache,* depression, fever, insomnia, pain.
EENT: pharyngitis, sinusitis.
GI: *nausea,* abdominal cramps, diarrhea, distention or pain, vomiting.
GU: epididymitis, hematuria, hemospermia, impotence, metrorrhagia, nocturia, polyuria, proteinuria, renal calculi, renal pain, vaginal candidiasis.
Respiratory: bronchitis, cough, upper respiratory tract infection.
Skin: *rash.*
Other: flulike syndrome.

INTERACTIONS

Drug-drug. *Amphetamines, nonsedating antihistamines, benzodiazepines, calcium channel blockers, clarithromycin, dapsone, ergot alkaloid preparations, indinavir, quinidine, rifabutin, sedative-hypnotics, warfarin:* May increase or prolong therapeutic and adverse effects of these drugs. Avoid using together or, if use together is unavoidable, reduce doses of indinavir and clarithromycin.
Antacids: May reduce absorption of delavirdine. Separate doses by at least 1 hour.
Carbamazepine, phenobarbital, phenytoin: May decrease delavirdine level. Use together cautiously.
Clarithromycin, fluoxetine, ketoconazole: May cause a 50% increase in delavirdine bioavailability. Monitor patient and reduce dose of clarithromycin.
Didanosine: May decrease absorption of both drugs by 20%. Separate doses by at least 1 hour.
H₂-receptor antagonists: May increase gastric pH and reduce absorption of delavirdine. Long-term use together isn't recommended.
HMG-CoA reductase inhibitors, such as atorvastatin, lovastatin, simvastatin: May increase levels of these drugs, which increases risk of myopathy, including rhabdomyolysis. Avoid using together.
Rifabutin, rifampin: May decrease delavirdine level. May increase rifabutin level by 100%. Avoid using together.
Saquinavir: May increase bioavailability of saquinavir fivefold. Monitor AST and ALT levels frequently when used together.
Sildenafil: May increase sildenafil level and may increase sildenafil adverse events, including hypotension, visual changes, and priapism. Tell patient not to exceed 25 mg of sildenafil in 48 hours.
Drug-herb. *St. John's wort:* May decrease drug level. Discourage use together.

EFFECTS ON LAB TEST RESULTS

- May increase alkaline phosphatase, ALT, amylase, AST, CK, creatinine, GGT, and lipase levels. May decrease glucose and hemoglobin levels and hematocrit.
- May increase eosinophil count, PT, and PTT. May decrease granulocyte, neutrophil, platelet, RBC, and WBC counts.

CONTRAINDICATIONS & CAUTIONS

- Contraindicated in patients hypersensitive to drug or its components.
- Use cautiously in patients with impaired hepatic function.

NURSING CONSIDERATIONS
- Because drug's effects in patients with hepatic or renal impairment haven't been studied, monitor renal and liver function test results carefully.
- Drug-induced diffuse, maculopapular, erythematous, pruritic rash occurs most commonly on upper body and arms of patients with lower CD4 cell counts, usually within first 3 weeks of treatment. Dosage adjustment doesn't seem to affect rash. Treat symptoms with diphenhydramine, hydroxyzine, or topical corticosteroids.
- Drug doesn't reduce risk of transmission of HIV-1.
- Monitor patient's fluid balance and weight.

PATIENT TEACHING
- Tell patient to stop drug and call prescriber if severe rash or such symptoms as fever, fatigue, headache, nausea, abdominal pain, or cough occur.
- Inform patient that drug doesn't cure HIV-1 infection and that he may continue to acquire illnesses including opportunistic infections related to HIV-1 infection. Therapy hasn't been shown to reduce the risk or frequency of such illnesses. Drug hasn't been shown to reduce transmission of HIV.
- Advise patient to remain under medical supervision when taking drug because the long-term effects aren't known.
- Tell patient to take drug as prescribed and not to alter doses without prescriber's approval. If a dose is missed, tell patient to take the next dose as soon as possible; he shouldn't double the next dose.
- Inform patient that drug may be dispersed in water before ingestion. Add four 100-mg tablets to at least 3 ounces (90 ml) of water, allow to stand for a few minutes, and stir until a uniform dispersion occurs. Tell patient to drink dispersion promptly, rinse glass, and swallow the rinse to ensure that entire dose is consumed.
- Instruct patient to take 200-mg tablets whole; 200-mg tablets don't disperse well in water.
- Tell patient that drug may be taken with or without food.
- Tell patient without hydrochloric acid in the stomach to take drug with an acidic

beverage, such as orange or cranberry juice.
- Instruct patient to take drug and antacids at least 1 hour apart.
- Advise patient to report use of other prescription or nonprescription drugs, including herbal remedies.
- Advise patient taking sildenafil about an increased risk of sildenafil-related adverse events, including low blood pressure, visual changes, and painful penile erection. Tell him to promptly report any symptoms to his prescriber. Tell patient not to exceed 25 mg of sildenafil in 48 hours.

didanosine (ddl, dideoxyinosine)
dye-DAN-oh-seen

Videx, Videx EC

Pharmacologic class: nucleoside reverse transcriptase inhibitor
Pregnancy risk category B

AVAILABLE FORMS
Delayed-release capsules: 125 mg, 200 mg, 250 mg, 400 mg
Powder for oral solution (pediatric): 2 g/4-ounce glass bottle, 4 g/8-ounce glass bottle

INDICATIONS & DOSAGES
➤ **HIV infection**
Adults who weigh 60 kg (132 lb) or more: 400-mg capsule P.O. daily. Or, 200 mg b.i.d. (preferred dosing) or 400 mg P.O. once daily of the pediatric powder for oral solution.
Adults who weigh less than 60 kg: 250 mg capsule P.O. daily. Or, 125 mg b.i.d. (preferred dosing) or 250 mg P.O. once daily of the pediatric powder for oral solution.
Children older than 8 months: 120 mg/m² P.O. b.i.d. of the pediatric powder for oral solution; Videx EC hasn't been studied in children.
Children 2 weeks to 8 months: 100 mg/m² P.O. b.i.d. of the pediatric powder for oral solution.
Adjust-a-dose: For dialysis patients who weigh 60 kg (132 lb) or more, 100 mg once daily of the pediatric powder for oral solution. For dialysis patients who weigh

less than 60 kg, give 75 mg once daily of the pediatric powder for oral solution. For dialysis patients who weigh 60 kg or more, give 125 mg of Videx EC once daily. Don't use in dialysis patients who weigh less than 60 kg. If creatinine clearance is less than 10 ml/minute, don't give a supplemental dose after hemodialysis for either drug.

In adults who weigh 60 kg or more with creatinine clearance of 30 to 59 ml/minute, give 200-mg capsule once daily; or, 200 mg once daily or 100 mg b.i.d. of the pediatric powder for oral solution. If clearance is 10 to 29 ml/minute, give 125-mg capsule, or 150 mg of the pediatric powder for oral solution once daily. If clearance is less than 10 ml/minute, give 125-mg capsule, or 100 mg of the pediatric powder for oral solution once daily.

In adults who weigh less than 60 kg and have a clearance of 30 to 59 ml/minute, give 125-mg capsule once daily; or, 150 mg once daily or 75 mg b.i.d. of the pediatric powder for oral solution. If clearance is 10 to 29 ml/minute, give 125-mg capsule, or 100 mg of the pediatric powder for oral solution once daily. For clearance less than 10 ml/minute, give 75 mg of the pediatric powder for oral solution once daily; capsule not indicated for these patients.

For adult patients taking tenofovir who weigh 60 kg or more with a creatinine clearance greater than or equal to 60 ml/minute, reduce Videx dose to 250 mg once daily. Avoid concomitant therapy in patients with a creatinine clearance less than 60 ml/minute. For adult patients taking tenofovir who weigh less than 60 kg with a creatinine clearance greater than or equal to 60 ml/minute, reduce Videx dose to 200 mg once daily. Avoid concomitant therapy in patients with a creatinine clearance less than 60 ml/minute.

ADMINISTRATION
P.O.
● Give drug on an empty stomach, at least 30 minutes before or 2 hours after eating; giving drug with meals can decrease absorption by 50%.
● *Alert:* The pediatric powder for oral solution must be prepared by a pharmacist be-

fore dispensing. It must be constituted with purified USP water and then diluted with an antacid (Mylanta Double Strength Liquid, Extra Strength Maalox Plus Suspension, or Maalox TC Suspension) to a final concentration of 10 mg/ml. The admixture is stable for 30 days at 36° to 46° F (2° to 8° C). Shake the solution well before measuring dose.

ACTION
Inhibits the enzyme HIV-RNA–dependent DNA polymerase (reverse transcriptase) and terminates DNA chain growth.

Route	Onset	Peak	Duration
P.O.	Unknown	15–90 min	Unknown
P.O., E.C.	Unknown	2 hr	Unknown

Half-life: 48 minutes.

ADVERSE REACTIONS
CNS: *dizziness, fever, headache, peripheral neuropathy, seizures,* abnormal thinking, anxiety, asthenia, confusion, depression, insomnia, nervousness, pain, twitching.
CV: *heart failure,* hypertension, edema.
EENT: optic neuritis, retinal changes.
GI: *abdominal pain, diarrhea, nausea, vomiting, pancreatitis,* anorexia, dry mouth.
Hematologic: *leukopenia, thrombocytopenia,* anemia, granulocytosis.
Hepatic: *hepatic failure.*
Metabolic: hyperuricemia.
Musculoskeletal: myopathy.
Respiratory: dyspnea, pneumonia.
Skin: alopecia, pruritus, rash.
Other: *chills, sarcoma,* allergic reactions, infection.

INTERACTIONS
Drug-drug. *Amprenavir, delavirdine, indinavir, nelfinavir, ritonavir, saquinavir:* May alter pharmacokinetics of didanosine or these drugs. Separate dosage times.
Antacids containing magnesium or aluminum hydroxides: May enhance adverse effects of the antacid component (including diarrhea or constipation) when given with didanosine tablets or pediatric suspension. Avoid using together.
Co-trimoxazole, pentamidine, other drugs linked to pancreatitis: May increase risk of pancreatic toxicity. Use together

cautiously; consider temporarily stopping didanosine during administration of these drugs.

Dapsone, drugs that require gastric acid for adequate absorption, ketoconazole: May decrease absorption from buffering action. Give these drugs 2 hours before didanosine.

Fluoroquinolones, tetracyclines: May decrease absorption from buffering products in didanosine tablets or antacids in pediatric suspension. Separate dosage times by at least 2 hours.

Itraconazole: May decrease itraconazole level. Avoid using together.

■ **Black Box Warning** *Stavudine, other antiretrovirals:* Fatal lactic acidosis has been reported in pregnant women. Use only if potential benefits clearly outweigh potential risks. ■

Tenofovir: May increase didanosine levels and risk of life-threatening adverse effects including lactic acidosis and pancreatitis. Adjust didanosine dosage.

Drug-herb. *St. John's wort:* May decrease drug level, decreasing therapeutic effects. Discourage use together.

Drug-food. *Any food:* May decrease rate of absorption. Advise patient to take drug on an empty stomach at least 30 minutes before a meal.

EFFECTS ON LAB TEST RESULTS

● May increase alkaline phosphatase, ALT, AST, bilirubin, and uric acid levels. May decrease hemoglobin level.

● May decrease granulocyte, platelet, and WBC counts.

CONTRAINDICATIONS & CAUTIONS

● Contraindicated in patients hypersensitive to drug or its components.

■ **Black Box Warning** Contraindicated in patients with confirmed pancreatitis. ■

■ **Black Box Warning** Use cautiously in patients with history of pancreatitis; deaths have occurred. ■

■ **Black Box Warning** Lactic acidosis and severe hepatomegaly with steatosis, including fatal cases, have been reported. ■

● Use cautiously in patients with peripheral neuropathy, renal or hepatic impairment, or hyperuricemia. Monitor liver and renal function tests.

NURSING CONSIDERATIONS

● Patients with advanced HIV disease or history of peripheral neuropathy may develop numbness, tingling, or pain in the hands and feet resulting in dosage reduction or stopping drug.

● Patients may tolerate a reduced dose of Videx after symptoms of peripheral neuropathy resolve; if symptoms recur, consider permanently stopping drug.

● Because of a high rate of early virologic failure and emergence of resistance, using tenofovir with didanosine and lamivudine isn't recommended as a new treatment regimen for therapy-naïve or -experienced patients with HIV infection. Patients on this regimen should be considered for treatment modification.

● *Look alike–sound alike:* Don't confuse drug with other antiretrovirals that use abbreviations for identification.

PATIENT TEACHING

● Instruct patient to take drug on an empty stomach, 30 minutes before or 2 hours after eating.

● Inform patient that drug doesn't cure HIV infection, that opportunistic infections and other complications of HIV infection may continue to occur, and that transmission of HIV to others through sexual contact or blood contamination is still possible.

● Tell patient to report symptoms of inflammation of the pancreas, such as abdominal pain, nausea, vomiting, diarrhea, or symptoms of peripheral neuropathy.

---

efavirenz
eff-ah-VYE-renz

Sustiva

Pharmacologic class:
nonnucleoside reverse
transcriptase inhibitor
Pregnancy risk category D

AVAILABLE FORMS
Capsules: 50 mg, 100 mg, 200 mg
Tablets: 600 mg

Reactions may be *common*, uncommon, *life-threatening*, or COMMON AND LIFE-THREATENING.
Interaction may have a *rapid onset* or **delayed onset**.

INDICATIONS & DOSAGES
➤ **HIV-1 infection, with a protease inhibitor or nucleoside analogue reverse transcriptase inhibitors**
Adults and children age 3 and older who weigh 40 kg (88 lb) or more: 600 mg (three 200-mg capsules or one 600-mg tablet) P.O. once daily on an empty stomach, preferably at bedtime.
Children age 3 and older who weigh 33 to less than 40 kg (72 to less than 88 lb): 400 mg P.O. once daily on an empty stomach, preferably at bedtime.
Children age 3 and older who weigh 25 to less than 33 kg (55 to less than 72 lb): 350 mg P.O. once daily on an empty stomach, preferably at bedtime.
Children age 3 and older who weigh 20 to less than 25 kg (44 to less than 55 lb): 300 mg P.O. once daily on an empty stomach, preferably at bedtime.
Children age 3 and older who weigh 15 to less than 20 kg (33 to less than 44 lb): 250 mg P.O. once daily on an empty stomach, preferably at bedtime.
Children age 3 and older who weigh 10 to less than 15 kg (22 to less than 33 lb): 200 mg P.O. once daily on an empty stomach, preferably at bedtime.
Adjust-a-dose: For adults also taking voriconazole, increase voriconazole maintenance dose to 400 mg every 12 hours and decrease efavirenz capsules to 300 mg once daily.

ADMINISTRATION
P.O.
● Give drug at bedtime to decrease CNS adverse effects.

ACTION
Inhibits the transcription of HIV-1 RNA to DNA, a critical step in the viral replication process, suppressing viral replication.

Route	Onset	Peak	Duration
P.O.	Unknown	3–5 hr	Unknown

Half-life: 40 to 76 hours.

ADVERSE REACTIONS
CNS: *dizziness,* abnormal dreams or thinking, agitation, amnesia, confusion, depersonalization, depression, euphoria, fever, fatigue, hallucinations, headache, hypoesthesia, impaired concentration, insomnia, nervousness, somnolence.
GI: *diarrhea, nausea,* abdominal pain, anorexia, dyspepsia, flatulence, vomiting.
GU: hematuria, renal calculi.
Skin: *rash, erythema multiforme, Stevens-Johnson syndrome, toxic epidermal necrolysis,* increased sweating, pruritus.

INTERACTIONS
Drug-drug. *Amprenavir, clarithromycin, indinavir, lopinavir:* May decrease levels of these drugs. Consider alternative therapy or dosage adjustment.
Atorvastatin, calcium channel blockers, itraconozole, pravastatin, rifampin, simvastatin: May decrease levels of these drugs. Dosage adjustments may be necessary.
Bepridil, ergot derivatives, midazolam, pimozide, triazolam: May inhibit metabolism of these drugs and cause serious or life-threatening adverse events (such as arrhythmias, prolonged sedation, or respiratory depression). Avoid using together.
Drugs that induce the cytochrome P-450 enzyme system (such as phenobarbital phenytoin, rifampin): May result in lower drug levels of efavirenz. Avoid using together.
Estrogens, ritonavir: May increase drug levels. Monitor patient.
Hormonal contraceptives: May increase ethinyl estradiol level. Advise use of a reliable method of barrier contraception in addition to use of hormonal contraceptives.
Psychoactive drugs: May cause additive CNS effects. Avoid using together.
Rifabutin: May decrease rifabutin level. Increase daily rifabutin dosage by 50%. Consider doubling rifabutin dosage when rifabutin is given two or three times per week.
Ritonavir: May increase levels of both drugs. Monitor patient and liver function closely.
Saquinavir: May decrease saquinavir level and efavirenz exposure to the body. Don't use with saquinavir as sole protease inhibitor.
Voriconazole (in standard doses): Decreases voriconazole levels significantly, while efavirenz levels significantly

increase. Avoid using together unless doses of each are adjusted.

Warfarin: May increase or decrease level and effects of warfarin. Monitor INR.

Drug-herb. *St. John's wort:* May decrease drug level. Discourage use together.

Drug-food. *High-fat meals:* May increase absorption of drug. Instruct patient to maintain a proper low-fat diet.

Drug-lifestyle. *Alcohol use:* May enhance CNS effects. Discourage use together.

EFFECTS ON LAB TEST RESULTS
• May increase ALT, AST, and cholesterol levels.
• May cause false-positive urine cannabinoid test results.

CONTRAINDICATIONS & CAUTIONS
• Contraindicated in patients hypersensitive to drug or its components and in those taking astemizole, bepridil, cisapride, midazolam, pimozide, triazolam, or ergot derivatives.
• Use cautiously in patients with hepatic impairment and in those receiving hepatotoxic drugs. Monitor liver function test results in patients with history of hepatitis B or C and in those taking ritonavir.

NURSING CONSIDERATIONS
• Monitor cholesterol level.
• *Alert:* Drug shouldn't be used as monotherapy or added on as a single drug to a regimen failing because of viral resistance.
• Using drug with ritonavir may increase liver enzyme levels and adverse effects (such as dizziness, nausea, paresthesia).
• Pregnancy must be ruled out before starting therapy in women of childbearing age.
• Children may be more prone to adverse reactions, especially diarrhea, nausea, vomiting, and rash.

PATIENT TEACHING
• Instruct patient to take drug with water, preferably at bedtime and on an empty stomach.
• Inform patient about need for scheduled blood tests to monitor liver function and cholesterol level.
• Tell patient to use a barrier contraceptive with a hormonal contraceptive and to

notify prescriber immediately if pregnancy is suspected; drug is a known risk to the fetus.
• Inform patient that drug doesn't cure HIV infection, that opportunistic infections and other complications of HIV infection may continue to occur, and that transmission of HIV to others through sexual contact or blood contamination is still possible.
• Instruct patient to take drug at the same time daily and always with other antiretrovirals.
• Tell patient to take drug exactly as prescribed and not to stop it without medical approval. Also instruct patient to report adverse reactions.
• Inform patient that rash is the most common adverse effect. Tell patient to report rash immediately because it may be serious in rare cases.
• Advise patient to report use of other drugs.
• Advise patient that dizziness, difficulty sleeping or concentrating, drowsiness, or unusual dreams may occur during the first few days of therapy. Reassure him that these symptoms typically resolve after 2 to 4 weeks and may be less problematic if drug is taken at bedtime.
• Tell patient to avoid alcohol, driving, or operating machinery until the drug's effects are known.

---

emtricitabine
em-tra-SYE-tah-ben

Emtriva

Pharmacologic class: nucleoside reverse transcriptase inhibitor
Pregnancy risk category B

AVAILABLE FORMS
Capsules: 200 mg
Oral solution: 10 mg/ml

INDICATIONS & DOSAGES
➤ **HIV-1 infection, with other antiretrovirals**
Adults: One 200-mg capsule or 240 mg (24 ml) oral solution P.O. once daily.
Children ages 3 months to 18 years: For children who weigh more than 33 kg

---

(73 lb) and can swallow intact capsules, give one 200-mg capsule P.O. once daily. Otherwise, give 6 mg/kg, up to a maximum dose of 240 mg (24 ml) oral solution once daily.

Children younger than age 3 months:
3 mg/kg oral solution P.O. once daily.

Adjust-a-dose: In adults with creatinine clearance of 30 to 49 ml/minute, give one 200-mg capsule every 48 hours or 120 mg oral solution every 24 hours; if clearance is 15 to 29 ml/minute, give one 200-mg capsule every 72 hours or 80 mg oral solution every 24 hours; if clearance is less than 15 ml/minute or patient is receiving dialysis, give one 200-mg capsule every 96 hours or 60 mg oral solution every 24 hours. Give dose after dialysis session. In children with renal insufficiency, consider a dose reduction and increased dosing interval.

■ **Black Box Warning** Emtricitabine isn't indicated for the treatment of chronic hepatitis B virus (HBV) infection; safety and efficacy of drug haven't been established in patients coinfected with HBV and HIV. ■

ADMINISTRATION
P.O.
● Give drug with or without food.
● Refrigerate oral solution; if stored at room temperature, use within 3 months.

ACTION
Inhibits replication of HIV by blocking viral DNA synthesis and inhibits reverse transcriptase by acting as an alternative for the enzyme's substrate, deoxycytidine triphosphate.

Route	Onset	Peak	Duration
P.O.	Unknown	1–2 hr	Unknown

Half-life: About 10 hours.

ADVERSE REACTIONS
CNS: *abnormal dreams, asthenia, dizziness, headache, insomnia,* depressive disorders, neuritis, paresthesia, peripheral neuropathy.
EENT: *rhinitis.*
GI: *abdominal pain, diarrhea, nausea,* dyspepsia, vomiting.
Hepatic: *hepatotoxicity.*
Musculoskeletal: arthralgia, myalgia.

Respiratory: *increased cough.*
Skin: *allergic skin reaction, discoloration, maculopapular rash, pruritus, urticarial and purpuric lesions, vesiculobullous rash.*

INTERACTIONS
None reported.

EFFECTS ON LAB TEST RESULTS
● May increase ALT, amylase, AST, bilirubin, CK, lipase, glucose, and triglyceride levels.
● May decrease neutrophil count.

CONTRAINDICATIONS & CAUTIONS
● Contraindicated in patients hypersensitive to drug or its ingredients.
● In elderly patients, use cautiously because of the potential for other diseases and drug therapies and for decreased hepatic, renal, or cardiac function.
● Use cautiously in patients with impaired renal function.
■ **Black Box Warning** Lactic acidosis and severe hepatomegaly, including fatal cases, have been reported. ■

NURSING CONSIDERATIONS
● Test all patients for HBV before starting drug.
■ **Black Box Warning** Hepatitis B may worsen after emtricitabine therapy stops. Patients with both HIV and HBV need close clinical and laboratory follow-up for several months or longer after stopping drug. ■
● Like other antiretrovirals, emtricitabine may cause changes or increases in body fat, including central obesity, buffalo hump, peripheral wasting, facial wasting, breast enlargement, and a cushingoid appearance.
● Use drug only if clearly needed in pregnant women.

PATIENT TEACHING
● Remind patient that anti-HIV medicine must be taken for life.
● Inform patient that drug doesn't cure HIV infection, that opportunistic infections and other complications of HIV infection may continue to occur, and that transmission of HIV to others through sexual contact or blood contamination is still possible.

• Explain possible adverse reactions, including lactic acidosis, hepatotoxicity, and changes or increases in body fat.
• Tell woman to notify prescriber immediately if she is or could be pregnant.
• Inform patient the drug may be taken with or without food.
• Tell patient to refrigerate oral solution but if stored at room temperature, to use within 3 months.

---

enfuvirtide
en-foo-VEER-tide

Fuzeon

Pharmacologic class: fusion inhibitor
Pregnancy risk category B

AVAILABLE FORMS
Powder for injection: 108-mg single-use vials (90 mg/ml after reconstitution)

INDICATIONS & DOSAGES
➤ **To help control HIV-1 infection, with other antiretrovirals, in patients who have continued HIV-1 replication despite antiretroviral therapy**
Adults: 90 mg subcutaneously b.i.d., injected into the upper arm, anterior thigh, or abdomen.
Children ages 6 to 16: Give 2 mg/kg subcutaneously b.i.d.; maximum 90 mg per dose.

ADMINISTRATION
Subcutaneous
• Reconstitute vial with 1.1 ml sterile water for injection. Tap vial for 10 seconds and then gently roll to prevent foaming. Let drug stand for up to 45 minutes to ensure reconstitution. Or, gently roll vial between hands until product is completely dissolved. Then draw up correct dose and inject drug.
• If you won't be using drug immediately after reconstitution, refrigerate in original vial and use within 24 hours. Don't inject drug until it's at room temperature.
• Vial is for single use; discard unused portion.

• Rotate injection sites. Don't inject into the same site for two consecutive doses, and don't inject into moles, scar tissue, bruises, or the navel.
• Store unreconstituted vials at room temperature.

ACTION
Interferes with entry of HIV-1 into cells by inhibiting fusion of HIV-1 to cell membranes.

Route	Onset	Peak	Duration
Subcut.	Unknown	4–8 hr	Unknown

Half-life: 4 hours.

ADVERSE REACTIONS
CNS: *fatigue, insomnia,* anxiety, asthenia, depression, peripheral neuropathy.
EENT: conjunctivitis, sinusitis, taste disturbance.
GI: *diarrhea, nausea, **pancreatitis,*** abdominal pain, constipation.
Metabolic: anorexia, weight decrease.
Musculoskeletal: myalgia.
Respiratory: *bacterial pneumonia,* cough.
Skin: *injection site reactions,* pruritus, skin papilloma.
Other: herpes simplex, influenza, influenza-like illness, lymphadenopathy.

INTERACTIONS
None reported.

EFFECTS ON LAB TEST RESULTS
• May increase ALT, amylase, AST, CK, GGT, lipase, and triglyceride, levels. May decrease hemoglobin level.
• May decrease eosinophil count.

CONTRAINDICATIONS & CAUTIONS
• Contraindicated in patients hypersensitive to drug and in those not infected with HIV.
• Use in pregnant women only if clearly needed. Pregnant women can be registered in the Antiretroviral Pregnancy Registry by calling 1-800-258-4263.
• Safety and effectiveness haven't been established in children younger than age 6.

NURSING CONSIDERATIONS
• Injection site reactions (pain, discomfort, induration, erythema, pruritus, nodules,

---

Reactions may be *common,* uncommon, *life-threatening,* or COMMON AND LIFE-THREATENING.
Interaction may have a *rapid onset* or *delayed onset.*

cysts, ecchymosis) are common and may require analgesics or rest.
- **Alert:** Monitor patient closely for evidence of bacterial pneumonia. Patients at high risk include those with a low initial CD4 count or high initial viral load, those who use I.V. drugs or smoke, and those with history of lung disease.
- Hypersensitivity may occur with the first dose or later doses. If symptoms occur, stop drug.

PATIENT TEACHING
- Teach patient how to prepare and give drug and how to safely dispose of used needlcs and syringes.
- Tell patient to rotate injection sites and to watch for cellulitis or local infection.
- Urge patient to immediately report evidence of pneumonia, such as cough with fever, rapid breathing, or shortness of breath.
- Tell patient to stop taking drug and seek medical attention if evidence of hypersensitivity develops, such as rash, fever, nausea, vomiting, chills, rigors, and hypotension.
- Teach patient that drug doesn't cure HIV infection and that it must be taken with other antiretrovirals.
- Tell patient to inform prescriber if she's pregnant, plans to become pregnant, or is breast-feeding while taking this drug. Because HIV could be transmitted to the infant, HIV-infected mothers shouldn't breast-feed.
- Tell patient that drug may affect his ability to drive or operate machinery.

✳ NEW DRUG

etravirine
eh-trah-VIGH-reen

Intelence

Pharmacologic class: antiviral
Pregnancy risk category B

AVAILABLE FORMS
Tablets: 100 mg

INDICATIONS & DOSAGES
➤ **HIV-1 in patients who have had previous treatment and have replication of HIV-1 strains resis-**

tant to an NNRTI and other antiretrovirals.
Adults: 200 mg P.O. b.i.d. after meals. Given with other antiretrovirals.

ACTION
Binds to reverse transcriptase, an enzyme that replicates HIV.
Absorption: Unknown.
Distribution: Protein-bound.
Metabolism: By CYP3A4, CYP2C9, CYP2C19 enzymes in the liver.
Excretion: In feces.

Route	Onset	Peak	Duration
P.O.	Unknown	2.5–4 hours	Unknown

Half-life: About 41 hours.

ADVERSE REACTIONS
CNS: abnormal dreams, amnesia, anxiety, confusion, disorientation, fatigue, headache, hypoesthesia, insomnia, paresthesia, peripheral neuropathy, *seizures,* sluggishness, syncope, tremors.
CV: angina, *atrial fibrillation,* hypertension, *MI.*
EENT: blurred vision, vertigo.
GI: abdominal distension, abdominal pain, anorexia, constipation, diarrhea, dry mouth, flatulence, gastritis, gastroesophageal reflux disease, hematemesis, *nausea,* pancreatitis, retching, stomatitis, vomiting.
GU: *renal failure.*
Hepatic: *hepatitis,* hepatomegaly, increased liver enzyme levels.
Hematologic: anemia, hemolytic anemia.
Metabolic: *diabetes,* dyslipidemia.
Respiratory: *bronchospasm,* dyspnea.
Skin: *rash.*
Other: facial wasting, fat redistribution or accumulation, gynecomastia, hypersensitivity, immune reconstitution syndrome.

INTERACTIONS
Drug-drug. *Amiodarone, bepridil, disopyramide, flecainide, lidocaine, mexiletine, propafenone, quinidine:* May decrease levels of these drugs. Use caution, and monitor patient closely.
Amprenavir and ritonavir: May increase amprenavir level. Avoid use together.
Atazanavir and ritonavir: May decrease atazanavir level and increase etravirine level. Avoid use together.

Atorvastatin, lovastatin, simvastatin: May decrease levels of these drugs. Adjust dosage, if needed.

Clarithromycin: May decrease clarithromycin level and increase etravirine level. Consider using azithromycin for treating *Mycobacterium avium* complex.

CYP3A4 inhibitors (such as itraconazole, ketoconazole): May decrease levels of these drugs. Adjust dosage, if needed.

CYP450 inducers (such as carbamazepine, phenobarbital, phenytoin): May decrease etravirine level. Avoid use together.

Delavirdine: May increase etravirine level. Avoid use together.

Dexamethasone: May decrease etravirine level. Avoid use together.

Diazepam: May increase diazepam level. Reduce diazepam dose, as needed.

Efavirenz, nevirapine: May decrease etravirine level. Avoid use together.

Fluconazole, posaconazole: May increase etravirine level. Use together cautiously.

Fluvastatin: May increase fluvastatin level. Adjust dosage, if needed.

Immunosuppressants (such as cyclosporine, sirolimus, tacrolimus): May decrease levels of these drugs. Use together cautiously, and monitor patient closely.

Lopinavir and ritonavir: May increase etravirine level. Use together cautiously.

Methadone: May cause withdrawal symptoms. Monitor patient, and consider increasing methadone dosage.

Phosphodiesterase-5 inhibitors (sildenafil, tadalafil, vardenafil): May decrease effectiveness of these drugs. Adjust dosage, as needed.

Protease inhibitors (such as atazanavir, fosamprenavir, indinavir, nelfinavir): May alter protease inhibitor level if given without ritonavir. Avoid use together unless given with low-dose ritonavir.

Rifabutin: May decrease etravirine and rifabutin levels. If etravirine isn't given with a protease inhibitor and ritonavir, give rifabutin 300 mg daily. If etravirine is given with darunavir and ritonavir or with raquinavir and ritonavir, avoid rifabutin.

Rifampin, rifapentine: May decrease etravirine level. Avoid use together.

Ritonavir: May decrease etravirine level. Avoid use together.

Ritonavir and tipranavir: May decrease etravirine level. Avoid use together.

Warfarin: May increase warfarin level. Monitor INR closely, and adjust warfarin dosage if needed.

Drug-herb. *St. John's wort:* May decrease etravirine level. Avoid use together.

EFFECTS ON LAB TEST RESULTS
● May increase amylase, lipase, creatinine, total cholesterol, LDL, triglyceride, AST, ALT, and glucose levels. May decrease hemoglobin level.
● May decrease RBC, neutrophil, and platelet count.

CONTRAINDICATIONS & CAUTIONS
● Contraindicated in patients hypersensitive to etravirine or its components.
● Use cautiously in elderly patients and patients with hepatic impairment or hepatitis B or C.

NURSING CONSIDERATIONS
● *Alert:* Etravirine may interact with many drugs. Review patient's complete drug regimen.
● If patient can't swallow the tablet whole, dissolve it in water and have patient drink it immediately. To make sure patient receives entire dose, refill the glass several times and have patient drink.
● Monitor patient closely for skin reactions. If severe rash develops, stop therapy.
● Monitor patient for signs of fat redistribution, including central obesity, buffalo hump, peripheral wasting, breast enlargement, and cushingoid appearance.
● Notify prescriber if signs, symptoms, or laboratory abnormalities suggest pancreatitis. Monitor amylase and lipase levels.
● Monitor patient's CBC, platelet count, and renal and liver function studies. Report abnormalities.

Pregnant patients
● Pregnant women should take etravirine only if potential benefits to mother outweigh risks to fetus.
● Pregnant women who take etravirine should be enrolled in the Antiretroviral Pregnancy Registry, which monitors maternal-fetal outcomes, by calling 1-800-258-4263.

Reactions may be *common,* uncommon, *life-threatening,* or COMMON AND LIFE-THREATENING.
Interaction may have a *rapid onset* or *delayed onset.*

Breast-feeding patients
• HIV-infected women shouldn't breast-feed because of the risk of transmitting HIV to the infant.

Pediatric patients
• Safety and efficacy haven't been established.

Geriatric patients
• Use cautiously in elderly patients.

PATIENT TEACHING
• Advise patient to take etravirine after a meal.
• Warn patient to tell prescriber about any other prescription drugs, over-the-counter drugs, and herbal supplements he takes.
• Advise patient to report adverse effects to prescriber.
• Inform patient that drug doesn't cure HIV infection, that opportunistic infections and other complications of HIV infection may still occur, and that HIV may still be transmitted to others through sexual contact or blood contamination.
• Advise patient to take drug as prescribed and not to alter dose or stop drug without medical approval.
• If patient misses a dose, tell him to take it as soon as possible and then return to his normal schedule. Advise patient not to double the dose.
• Tell patient that routine blood tests will be needed to assess how he is tolerating drug therapy.

---

fosamprenavir calcium
foss-am-PREN-ah-ver

Lexiva

Pharmacologic class: protease inhibitor
Pregnancy risk category C

AVAILABLE FORMS
Oral suspension: 50 mg/ml
Tablets: 700 mg

INDICATIONS & DOSAGES
➤ **HIV infection, with other anti-retrovirals**
Adults: In patients not previously treated, 1,400 mg P.O. b.i.d. (without ritonavir). Or, 1,400 mg P.O. once daily and ritonavir 200 mg P.O. once daily. Or, 1,400 mg P.O. once daily and ritonavir 100 mg P.O. once daily. Or, 700 mg P.O. b.i.d. and ritonavir 100 mg P.O. b.i.d. In patients previously treated with a protease inhibitor, 700 mg P.O. b.i.d. plus ritonavir 100 mg P.O. b.i.d.
Children ages 6 and older: In patients not previously treated, 30 mg/kg oral suspension b.i.d., not to exceed adult dosage of 1,400 mg b.i.d., or 18 mg/kg oral suspension plus ritonavir 3 mg/kg b.i.d., not to exceed adult dosage of fosamprenavir 700 mg plus ritonavir 100 mg b.i.d. In therapy-experienced children, 18 mg/kg oral suspension plus ritonavir 3 mg/kg b.i.d., not to exceed adult dosage of fosamprenavir 700 mg plus ritonavir 100 mg b.i.d. When administered without ritonavir, adult regimen of fosamprenavir 1,400 mg tablets b.i.d. may be used for children weighing at least 47 kg (104 lb). When administered with ritonavir, fosamprenavir tablets may be used for children weighing at least 39 kg (86 lb); ritonavir capsules may be used for children weighing at least 33 kg (73 lb).
Children ages 2 to 5: In patients not previously treated, 30 mg/kg oral suspension b.i.d., not to exceed adult dosage of 1,400 mg b.i.d. Don't use in therapy-experienced children in this age-group.
Adjust-a-dose: If the patient receives efavirenz, fosamprenavir, and ritonavir once daily, give an additional 100 mg/day of ritonavir (300 mg total). If the patient has mild hepatic impairment (Child-Pugh score of 5 to 6), reduce dosage to 700 mg P.O. b.i.d. without ritonavir (in therapy-naive patients) or 700 mg b.i.d. plus ritonavir 100 mg once daily (in therapy-naive or protease inhibitor–experienced patients). If the patient has moderate hepatic impairment (Child-Pugh score of 7 to 9), reduce dosage to 700 mg b.i.d. (in therapy-naive patients) without ritonavir or 450 mg b.i.d. plus ritonavir 100 mg once daily (in therapy-naive or protease inhibitor–experienced patients). If the patient has severe hepatic impairment

(Child-Pugh score of 10 to 12), reduce dosage to 350 mg b.i.d. without ritonavir (in therapy-naive patients). Don't use in combination with ritonavir.

ADMINISTRATION
P.O.
- Give drug with other antiretrovirals.
- Tablets may be taken with or without food.
- Adults should take oral suspension without food. Children should take oral suspension with food. If patient vomits within 30 minutes after taking medication, dose should be repeated.
- Shake oral suspension before using.

ACTION
Converts rapidly to amprenavir, which binds to the active site of HIV-1 protease and forms immature noninfectious viral particles.

Route	Onset	Peak	Duration
P.O.	Unknown	1½–4 hr	Unknown

Half-life: 7¼ hours.

ADVERSE REACTIONS
CNS: *depression, fatigue, headache, oral paresthesia.*
GI: *abdominal pain, diarrhea, nausea, vomiting.*
Metabolic: *hyperglycemia.*
Skin: *rash,* pruritus.

INTERACTIONS
Drug-drug. *Amitriptyline, cyclosporine, imipramine, rapamycin, tacrolimus:* May increase levels of these drugs. Monitor drug levels.
Antiarrhythmics (amiodarone, systemic lidocaine, quinidine): May increase antiarrhythmic level. Use together cautiously and monitor antiarrhythmic levels.
Atorvastatin: May increase atorvastatin level. Give 20 mg/day or less of atorvastatin and monitor patient carefully. Or, consider other HMG-CoA reductase inhibitors, such as fluvastatin, pravastatin, or rosuvastatin.
Benzodiazepines (alprazolam, clorazepate, diazepam, flurazepam): May increase benzodiazepine level. Decrease benzodiazepine dosage as needed.

Bepridil: May increase bepridil level, possibly leading to arrhythmias. Use together cautiously.
Calcium channel blockers (amlodipine, diltiazem, felodipine, isradipine, nifedipine, nicardipine, nimodipine, nisoldipine, verapamil): May increase calcium channel blocker level. Use together cautiously.
Carbamazepine, dexamethasone, H₂-receptor antagonists, phenobarbital, phenytoin, proton-pump inhibitors: May decrease amprenavir level. Use together cautiously.
Delavirdine: May cause loss of virologic response and resistance to delavirdine. Avoid using together.
Dihydroergotamine, ergonovine, ergotamine, flecainide, methylergonovine, midazolam, pimozide, propafenone, triazolam: May cause serious adverse reactions. Avoid using together.
Efavirenz, nevirapine, saquinavir: May decrease amprenavir level. Appropriate combination doses haven't been established.
Efavirenz with ritonavir: May decrease amprenavir level. Increase ritonavir by 100 mg/day (300 mg total) when giving efavirenz, fosamprenavir, and ritonavir once daily. No change needed in ritonavir when giving efavirenz, fosamprenavir, and ritonavir twice daily.
Ethinyl estradiol and norethindrone: May increase ethinyl estradiol and norethindrone levels. Recommend nonhormonal contraception.
Indinavir, nelfinavir: May increase amprenavir level. Appropriate combination doses haven't been established.
Ketoconazole, itraconazole: May increase ketoconazole and itraconazole levels. Reduce ketoconazole or itraconazole dosage as needed if patient receives more than 400 mg/day. (More than 200 mg/day isn't recommended.)
Lopinavir with ritonavir: May decrease amprenavir and lopinavir levels. Appropriate combination doses haven't been established.
Lovastatin, simvastatin: May increase risk of myopathy, including rhabdomyolysis. Avoid using together.
Methadone: May decrease methadone level. Increase methadone dosage as needed.

Reactions may be *common,* uncommon, **life-threatening,** or **COMMON AND LIFE-THREATENING.**
Interaction may have a *rapid onset* or **delayed onset.**

Rifabutin: May increase rifabutin level. Obtain CBC weekly to watch for neutropenia, and decrease rifabutin dosage by at least half. If patient receives ritonavir, decrease dosage by at least 75% from the usual 300 mg/day. (Maximum, 150 mg every other day or three times weekly.)

Rifampin: May decrease amprenavir level and drug effect. Avoid using together.

Sildenafil, vardenafil: May increase sildenafil and vardenafil levels. Recommend cautious use of sildenafil at 25 mg every 48 hours or vardenafil at no more than 2.5 mg every 24 hours. If patient receives ritonavir, advise no more than 2.5 mg vardenafil every 72 hours, and tell patient to report adverse events.

Warfarin: May alter warfarin level. Monitor INR.

Drug-herb. *St. John's wort:* May cause loss of virologic response and resistance to drug or its class of protease inhibitors. Discourage use together.

EFFECTS ON LAB TEST RESULTS
● May increase ALT, AST, glucose, lipase, and triglyceride levels.
● May decrease neutrophil count.

CONTRAINDICATIONS & CAUTIONS
● Contraindicated in patients hypersensitive to drug or its components.
● Contraindicated with dihydroergotamine, ergonovine, ergotamine, flecainide, methylergonovine, midazolam, pimozide, propafenone, and triazolam.
● Use cautiously in patients allergic to sulfonamides and those with mild to moderate hepatic impairment.
● Use in pregnant woman only when benefit to mother justifies risk to fetus.
● Tell woman not to breast-feed during therapy.

NURSING CONSIDERATIONS
● Patients with hepatitis B or C or marked increase in transaminases before treatment may have increased risk of transaminase elevation. Monitor patient closely during treatment.
● Monitor triglyceride, lipase, ALT, AST, and glucose levels before starting therapy and periodically throughout treatment.
● Ask patient if he's allergic to sulfa drugs.

● Monitor patient with hemophilia for spontaneous bleeding.
● During first treatment, monitor patient for opportunistic infections, such as mycobacterium avium complex, CMV, *Pneumocystis jiroveci (carinii)* pneumonia, and tuberculosis.
● Assess patient for redistribution or accumulation of body fat, as in central obesity, dorsocervical fat enlargement (buffalo hump), peripheral wasting, facial wasting, breast enlargement, and a cushingoid appearance.

PATIENT TEACHING
● Tell patient that drug doesn't reduce the risk of transmitting HIV to others.
● Inform patient that the drug may reduce the risk of progression to AIDS.
● Explain that fosamprenavir must be used with other antiretrovirals.
● Tell patient not to alter the dose or stop taking drug without consulting prescriber.
● Drug interacts with many other drugs; urge patient to tell prescriber about any prescription, OTC, or herbal medicines he's taking (especially St. John's wort).
● Explain that body fat may redistribute or accumulate.

indinavir sulfate
in-DIN-ah-ver

Crixivan♦

Pharmacologic class: protease inhibitor
Pregnancy risk category C

AVAILABLE FORMS
Capsules: 100 mg, 200 mg, 333 mg, 400 mg

INDICATIONS & DOSAGES
➤ **HIV infection, with other antiretrovirals, when antiretrovirals are warranted**
Adults: 800 mg P.O. every 8 hours.
Adjust-a-dose: For patients with mild to moderate hepatic insufficiency from cirrhosis, reduce dosage to 600 mg P.O. every 8 hours.

ADMINISTRATION
P.O.
• Give drug on an empty stomach with water 1 hour before or 2 hours after a meal. Or, give it with other liquids (such as skim milk, juice, coffee, or tea) or a light meal. A meal high in fat, calories, and protein reduces drug absorption.
• Store capsules in the original container and keep desiccant in the bottle; capsules are sensitive to moisture.

ACTION
Inhibits HIV protease by binding to the protease-active site and inhibiting activity of the enzyme, preventing cleavage of the viral polyproteins and forming immature noninfectious viral particles.

Route	Onset	Peak	Duration
P.O.	Unknown	< 1 hr	Unknown

Half-life: 2 hours.

ADVERSE REACTIONS
CNS: asthenia, dizziness, fatigue, headache, insomnia, malaise, somnolence.
CV: chest pain, palpitations.
EENT: blurred vision, eye pain or swelling.
GI: *nausea,* abdominal pain, acid regurgitation, anorexia, diarrhea, dry mouth, taste perversion, vomiting.
GU: hematuria, nephrolithiasis.
Hematologic: *neutropenia, thrombocytopenia,* anemia.
Metabolic: *hyperbilirubinemia,* hyperglycemia.
Musculoskeletal: back pain.
Other: flank pain.

INTERACTIONS
Drug-drug. *Amprenavir, saquinavir:* May increase levels of these drugs. Dosage adjustments not needed.
Carbamazepine: May decrease indinavir exposure to the body. Consider an alternative drug.
Clarithromycin: May alter clarithromycin level. Dosage adjustments not needed.
Delavirdine, itraconazole, ketoconazole: May increase indinavir level. Consider reducing indinavir to 600 mg every 8 hours.
Didanosine: May alter absorption of indinavir. Separate doses by 1 hour and give on an empty stomach.

Efavirenz, nevirapine: May decrease indinavir level. Increase indinavir to 1,000 mg every 8 hours.
HMG-CoA reductase inhibitors: May increase levels of these drugs and increase risk of myopathy and rhabdomyolysis. Avoid using together.
Lopinavir and ritonavir combination: May increase indinavir level. Adjust indinavir dosage to 600 mg b.i.d.
Midazolam, triazolam: May inhibit metabolism of these drugs, which may cause serious or life-threatening events, such as arrhythmias or prolonged sedation. Avoid using together.
Nelfinavir: May increase indinavir level by 50% and nelfinavir by 80%. May need to adjust dosage to indinavir 1,200 mg b.i.d. and nelfinavir 1,250 mg b.i.d. Monitor patient closely.
Proton-pump inhibitors (lansoprazole, omeprazole, pantoprazole, rabeprazole): May reduce the antiviral activity of indinavir. Avoid using together.
Rifabutin: May increase rifabutin level and decrease indinavir level. Give indinavir 1,000 mg every 8 hours and decrease the rifabutin dose to either 150 mg daily or 300 mg two to three times a week.
Rifampin: May decrease indinavir level. Avoid using together.
Rifapentine: May decrease indinavir level. Use with extreme caution, if at all.
Ritonavir: May increase indinavir level twofold to fivefold. Adjust dosage to indinavir 400 mg b.i.d. and ritonavir 400 mg b.i.d., or indinavir 800 mg b.i.d. and ritonavir 100 to 200 mg b.i.d.
Sildenafil, tadalafil, vardenafil: May increase levels of these drugs and increase adverse effects (hypotension, visual changes, and priapism). Tell patient not to exceed prescribed dosage.
Drug-herb. *St. John's wort:* May reduce drug level by more than half. Discourage use together.
Drug-food. *Grapefruit and grapefruit juice:* May decrease drug level and therapeutic effect. Discourage use together.

EFFECTS ON LAB TEST RESULTS
• May increase ALT, AST, bilirubin, amylase, hemoglobin, and glucose levels.
• May decrease neutrophil and platelet counts.

Reactions may be *common,* uncommon, *life-threatening,* or COMMON AND LIFE-THREATENING.
Interaction may have a *rapid onset* or *delayed onset.*

CONTRAINDICATIONS & CAUTIONS
• Contraindicated in patients hypersensitive to drug or its components.
• Use cautiously in patients with hepatic insufficiency from cirrhosis.
• Safety and effectiveness in children haven't been established.

NURSING CONSIDERATIONS
• Drug must be taken at 8-hour intervals.
• Drug may cause nephrolithiasis. If signs and symptoms of nephrolithiasis occur, prescriber may stop drug for 1 to 3 days during acute phases.
• To prevent nephrolithiasis, patient should maintain adequate hydration (at least 48 ounces or 1.5 L of fluids every 24 hours while taking indinavir).

PATIENT TEACHING
• Tell patient that drug doesn't cure HIV infection and that he may continue to develop opportunistic infections and other complications of HIV infection. Drug hasn't been shown to reduce the risk of HIV transmission.
• Advise patient to use barrier protection during sexual intercourse.
• Caution patient not to adjust dosage or stop therapy without first consulting prescriber.
• Advise patient that if a dose is missed, he should take the next dose at the regularly scheduled time and shouldn't double the dose.
• Instruct patient to take drug on an empty stomach with water 1 hour before or 2 hours after a meal. Or, he may take it with other liquids (such as skim milk, juice, coffee, or tea) or a light meal. Inform patient that a meal high in fat, calories, and protein reduces absorption of drug.
• Instruct patient to store capsules in the original container and to keep desiccant in the bottle; capsules are sensitive to moisture.
• Tell patient to drink at least 48 ounces (1.5 L) of fluid daily.
• Advise woman to avoid breast-feeding because drug may appear in breast milk. Also, to prevent transmitting virus to infant, advise an HIV-positive woman not to breast-feed.

lamivudine (3TC)
lam-ah-VEW-den

Epivir, Epivir-HBV, Heptovir†

Pharmacologic class: nucleoside reverse transcriptase inhibitor
Pregnancy risk category C

AVAILABLE FORMS
Epivir
Oral solution: 10 mg/ml
Tablets: 150 mg, 300 mg
Epivir-HBV
Oral solution: 5 mg/ml
Tablets: 100 mg

INDICATIONS & DOSAGES
■ **Black Box Warning** Epivir tablets and oral solution (used to treat HIV infection) contain a higher dose of the active ingredient than Epivir-HBV tablets and oral solution (used to treat chronic hepatitis B infection). Patient with HIV infection should receive only dosing forms appropriate for HIV treatment. ■
➤ **HIV infection, with other antiretrovirals**
Adults and children older than age 16: Give 300 mg Epivir P.O. once daily or 150 mg P.O. b.i.d.
Children ages 3 months to 16 years: 4 mg/kg Epivir solution P.O. b.i.d. Maximum dose is 150 mg b.i.d.
Children 14 kg (31 lb) or more who can reliably swallow tablets: Weighing 14 to 21 kg (46 lb), give ½ tablet (75 mg) P.O. b.i.d.; 21 to less than 30 kg (66 lb), give ½ tablet (75 mg) P.O. in morning and 1 tablet (150 mg) P.O. in evening; 30 kg or more, give 150 mg P.O. b.i.d.
Neonates age 30 days and younger♦ : 2 mg/kg Epivir P.O. b.i.d.
Adjust-a-dose: For patients with creatinine clearance of 30 to 49 ml/minute, give 150 mg Epivir P.O. daily. If clearance is 15 to 29 ml/minute, give 150 mg P.O. on day 1 and then 100 mg daily; if it's 5 to 14 ml/minute, give 150 mg on day 1 and then 50 mg daily; if it's less than 5 ml/minute, give 50 mg on day 1 and then 25 mg daily.

➤ **Chronic hepatitis B with evidence of hepatitis B virus (HBV) replication and active liver inflammation**
Adults: 100 mg Epivir-HBV P.O. once daily.
Children ages 2 to 17 years: 3 mg/kg Epivir-HBV P.O. once daily, up to a maximum dose of 100 mg daily. Optimum duration of treatment isn't known; safety and effectiveness of treatment beyond 1 year haven't been established.
Adjust-a-dose: For adult patients with creatinine clearance of 30 to 49 ml/minute, give first dose of 100 mg Epivir-HBV; then give 50 mg P.O. once daily. If clearance is 15 to 29 ml/minute, give first dose of 100 mg; then give 25 mg P.O. once daily. If clearance is 5 to 14 ml/minute, give first dose of 35 mg; then give 15 mg P.O. once daily. If clearance is less than 5 ml/minute, give first dose of 35 mg; then give 10 mg P.O. once daily.

ADMINISTRATION
P.O.
● Give without regard for food.

ACTION
A synthetic nucleoside analogue that inhibits HIV and HBV reverse transcription via viral DNA chain termination. RNA- and DNA-dependent DNA polymerase activities.

Route	Onset	Peak	Duration
P.O.	Unknown	1–3 hr	Unknown

Half-life: 5 to 7 hours.

ADVERSE REACTIONS
Adverse reactions pertain to the combination therapy of lamivudine and zidovudine.
CNS: *dizziness, fatigue, fever, headache, insomnia and other sleep disorders, malaise, neuropathy, depressive disorders.*
EENT: *nasal symptoms.*
GI: *anorexia, diarrhea, nausea, vomiting, pancreatitis,* abdominal cramps, abdominal pain, dyspepsia.
Hematologic: *neutropenia, thrombocytopenia,* anemia.
Hepatic: *hepatotoxicity.*
Metabolic: *lactic acidosis.*
Musculoskeletal: *musculoskeletal pain,* arthralgia, myalgia.

Respiratory: *cough.*
Skin: rash.
Other: *chills.*

INTERACTIONS
Drug-drug. *Trimethoprim and sulfamethoxazole:* May increase lamivudine level because of decreased clearance of drug. Monitor patient for toxicity.
Zalcitabine: May inhibit activation of both drugs. Avoid using together.
Zidovudine: May increase zidovudine level. Monitor patient closely for adverse reactions.

EFFECTS ON LAB TEST RESULTS
● May increase ALT and bilirubin levels. May decrease hemoglobin level.
● May decrease neutrophil and platelet counts.

CONTRAINDICATIONS & CAUTIONS
■ **Black Box Warning** Lactic acidosis and severe hepatomegaly with steatosis, including fatal cases, have been reported. ■
● Contraindicated in patients hypersensitive to drug.
● Use cautiously in patients with renal impairment.
● *Alert:* Use drug cautiously, if at all, in children with history of pancreatitis or other significant risk factors for development of pancreatitis.
● The Antiretroviral Pregnancy Registry monitors maternal-fetal outcomes of pregnant women exposed to lamivudine. To register a pregnant woman, call the Antiretroviral Pregnancy Registry at 1-800-258-4263.

NURSING CONSIDERATIONS
● *Alert:* Stop treatment immediately and notify prescriber if signs, symptoms, or laboratory abnormalities suggest pancreatitis. Monitor amylase level.
● *Alert:* Lactic acidosis and hepatotoxicity have been reported. Notify prescriber if signs of lactic acidosis or hepatotoxicity occurs.
■ **Black Box Warning** Hepatitis may recur in some patients with chronic HBV when they stop taking drug. ■
■ **Black Box Warning** Safety and effectiveness of Epivir-HBV for longer than 1 year haven't been established; optimum

Reactions may be *common,* uncommon, *life-threatening,* or COMMON AND LIFE-THREATENING.
Interaction may have a *rapid onset* or *delayed onset.*

duration of treatment isn't known. Test patients for HIV before starting treatment and during therapy because form and dosage of lamivudine in Epivir-HBV aren't appropriate for those infected with both HBV and HIV. If lamivudine is given to patients with HBV and HIV, use the higher dosage indicated for HIV therapy as part of an appropriate combination regimen. ■

• Because of a high rate of early virologic resistance, don't use triple antiretroviral therapy with abacavir or didanosine, lamivudine, and tenofovir as new treatment for never-treated or pretreated patients. Monitor patients currently taking this therapy and those who take it with other antiretrovirals, and consider a different therapy.

• Monitor patient's CBC, platelet count, and renal and liver function studies. Report abnormalities.

PATIENT TEACHING
• Inform patient that long-term effects of drug aren't known.
• Stress importance of taking drug exactly as prescribed.
• Inform patient that drug doesn't cure HIV infection, that opportunistic infections and other complications of HIV infection may still occur, and that transmission of HIV to others through sexual contact or blood contamination is still possible.
• Teach parents or guardians the signs and symptoms of pancreatitis. Advise them to report signs and symptoms immediately.

lopinavir and ritonavir
low-PIN-ah-ver

Kaletra*✔

Pharmacologic class: protease inhibitor
Pregnancy risk category C

AVAILABLE FORMS
Tablets: lopinavir 100 mg and ritonavir 25 mg; lopinavir 200 mg and ritonavir 50 mg
Solution: lopinavir 400 mg and ritonavir 100 mg/5 ml (80 mg and 20 mg/ml)*

INDICATIONS & DOSAGES
➤ **HIV infection, with other antiretrovirals in treatment-naive adults**
Adults: 800 mg lopinavir and 200 mg ritonavir (4 tablets of 200 mg lopinavir and 50 mg ritonavir strength or 10 ml) P.O. once daily or divided evenly b.i.d.
➤ **HIV infection, with other antiretrovirals in treatment-experienced patients**
Adults and children older than age 12 years: 400 mg lopinavir and 100 mg ritonavir (2 tablets of 200 mg lopinavir and 50 mg ritonavir strength or 5 ml) P.O. b.i.d.
Children ages 6 months to 12 years, who weigh 15 to 40 kg (33 to 88 lb): 10 mg/kg (lopinavir content) P.O. b.i.d. with food up to a maximum of 400 mg lopinavir and 100 mg ritonavir.
Children ages 6 months to 12 years, who weigh 7 to 15 kg (15 to 33 lb): 12 mg/kg (lopinavir content) P.O. b.i.d. with food.
Children ages 14 days to 6 months: Kaletra oral solution lopinavir 16 mg/kg with ritonavir 4 mg/kg b.i.d. Don't use in combination with efavirenz, nevirapine fosamprenavir, or nelfinavir.
Adjust-a-dose: In treatment-experienced patients older than age 12 also taking efavirenz, nevirapine, fosamprenavir without ritonavir, or nelfinavir, consider dosage of 600 mg lopinavir and 150 mg ritonavir (3 tablets) P.O. b.i.d. For patients using oral solution and also taking efavirenz, nevirapine, amprenavir, or nelfinavir, 533 mg lopinavir and 133 mg ritonavir (6.5 ml) b.i.d. with food is recommended.

In treatment-experienced children age 6 months to 12 years who also take amprenavir, efavirenz, or nevirapine and who weigh 7 to 15 kg, give 13 mg/kg (lopinavir content) P.O. b.i.d. with food. For those who weigh 15 to 45 kg, give 11 mg/kg (lopinavir content) P.O. b.i.d. with food up to a maximum dose of 533 mg lopinavir, and 133 mg ritonavir b.i.d. in children who weigh more than 45 kg.

ADMINISTRATION
P.O.
• *Alert:* Many drug interactions are possible. Review all drugs patient is taking.
• Give oral solution with food. Give tablets without regard for food.

- Tablets must be swallowed whole; don't crush or divide, and tell patient not to chew.
- Refrigerated drug remains stable until expiration date on package. If stored at room temperature, use drug within 2 months.

ACTION

Lopinavir is an HIV protease inhibitor, which produces immature, noninfectious viral particles. Ritonavir, also an HIV protease inhibitor, slows lopinavir metabolism, thereby increasing lopinavir level.

Route	Onset	Peak	Duration
P.O.	Unknown	4 hr	5–6 hr

Half-life: About 6 hours.

ADVERSE REACTIONS

CNS: *encephalopathy,* abnormal dreams, abnormal thinking, agitation, amnesia, anxiety, asthenia, ataxia, confusion, depression, dizziness, dyskinesia, emotional lability, fever, headache, hypertonia, insomnia, malaise, nervousness, neuropathy, pain, paresthesia, peripheral neuritis, somnolence, tremors.
CV: chest pain, *deep vein thrombosis,* edema, hypertension, palpitations, thrombophlebitis, vasculitis.
EENT: abnormal vision, eye disorder, otitis media, sinusitis, tinnitus.
GI: *hemorrhagic colitis, pancreatitis, diarrhea, nausea,* abdominal pain, abnormal stools, anorexia, cholecystitis, constipation, dry mouth, dyspepsia, dysphagia, enterocolitis, eructation, esophagitis, fecal incontinence, flatulence, gastritis, gastroenteritis, GI disorder, increased appetite, inflammation of the salivary glands, stomatitis, taste perversion, ulcerative stomatitis, vomiting.
GU: abnormal ejaculation, hypogonadism, renal calculus, urine abnormality.
Hematologic: *leukopenia, neutropenia, thrombocytopenia in children,* anemia.
Hepatic: hyperbilirubinemia in children.
Metabolic: Cushing's syndrome, dehydration, decreased glucose tolerance, hyperglycemia, hyperuricemia, hyponatremia in children, hypothyroidism, *lactic acidosis,* weight loss.
Musculoskeletal: arthralgia, arthrosis, back pain, myalgia.

Respiratory: bronchitis, dyspnea, lung edema.
Skin: acne, alopecia, benign skin neoplasm, dry skin, exfoliative dermatitis, furunculosis, nail disorder, pruritus, rash, skin discoloration, sweating.
Other: chills, decreased libido, facial edema, flu syndrome, gynecomastia, lymphadenopathy, viral infection.

INTERACTIONS

Drug-drug. *Amiodarone, bepridil, lidocaine, quinidine:* May increase antiarrhythmic level. Use together cautiously. Monitor levels of these drugs, if possible.
Amprenavir, efavirenz, nelfinavir, nevirapine: May decrease lopinavir level. Consider increasing lopinavir-ritonavir combination dose. Don't use a once-daily regimen of lopinavir-ritonavir combination with these drugs.
Antiarrhythmics (flecainide, propafenone), pimozide: May increase risk of cardiac arrhythmias. Avoid using together.
Atorvastatin: May increase level of this drug. Use lowest possible dose and monitor patient carefully.
Atovaquone, methadone: May decrease levels of these drugs. Consider increasing doses of these drugs.
Carbamazepine, dexamethasone, phenobarbital, phenytoin: May decrease lopinavir level. Use together cautiously.
Clarithromycin: May increase clarithromycin level in patients with renal impairment. Adjust clarithromycin dosage.
Cyclosporine, rapamycin, tacrolimus: May increase levels of these drugs. Monitor therapeutic levels.
Delavirdine: May increase lopinavir level. Avoid using together.
Didanosine: May decrease absorption of didanosine because lopinavir-ritonavir combination is taken with food. Give didanosine 1 hour before or 2 hours after lopinavir-ritonavir combination.
Disulfiram, metronidazole: May cause disulfiram-like reaction. Avoid using together.
Ergot derivatives (dihydroergotamine, ergonovine, ergotamine, methylergonovine): May increase risk of ergot toxicity characterized by peripheral vasospasm and ischemia. Avoid using together.

Reactions may be *common,* uncommon, *life-threatening,* or COMMON AND LIFE-THREATENING.
Interaction may have a *rapid onset* or **delayed onset.**

Felodipine, nicardipine, nifedipine: May increase levels of these drugs. Use together cautiously.

Hormonal contraceptives (ethinyl estradiol): May decrease effectiveness of contraceptives. Recommend nonhormonal contraceptives.

Indinavir, saquinavir: May increase levels of these drugs. Avoid using together.

Itraconazole, ketoconazole: May increase levels of these drugs. Don't give more than 200 mg/day of these drugs.

Lovastatin, simvastatin: May increase risk of adverse reactions, such as myopathy, rhabdomyolysis. Avoid using together.

Midazolam (parenteral), triazolam: May cause prolonged or increased sedation or respiratory depression. Avoid using together. Don't give with oral midazolam.

Rifabutin: May increase rifabutin level. Decrease rifabutin dose by 75%. Monitor patient for adverse effects.

Rifampin: May decrease effectiveness of Kaletra. Avoid using together.

Sildenafil, tadalafil, vardenafil: May increase level of these drugs and adverse effects, such as hypotension and prolonged erection. Warn patient not to take more than 25 mg of sildenafil in 48 hours, more than 10 mg of tadalafil in 72 hours, or more than 2.5 mg vardenafil in 72 hours.

Warfarin: May affect warfarin level. Monitor PT and INR.

Drug-herb. *St. John's wort:* Loss of virologic response and possible resistance to drug. Discourage use together.

Drug-food. *Any food:* May increase absorption of oral solution. Tell patient to take with food.

EFFECTS ON LAB TEST RESULTS

● May increase amylase, cholesterol, and triglyceride levels. May decrease hemoglobin level and hematocrit.
● May decrease RBC, WBC, neutrophil, and platelet counts.

CONTRAINDICATIONS & CAUTIONS

● Contraindicated in patients hypersensitive to drug or any of its components.
● Use cautiously in patients with a history of pancreatitis or with hepatic impairment, hepatitis B or C, marked elevations in liver enzyme levels, or hemophilia.

● Use cautiously in elderly patients.
● The Antiretroviral Pregnancy Registry monitors maternal-fetal outcomes of pregnant women taking Kaletra. Health care providers are encouraged to enroll women by calling 1-800-258-4263.

NURSING CONSIDERATIONS

● Monitor patient for signs of fat redistribution, including central obesity, buffalo hump, peripheral wasting, breast enlargement, and cushingoid appearance.
● Monitor total cholesterol and triglycerides before starting therapy and periodically thereafter.
● Monitor patient for signs and symptoms of pancreatitis (nausea, vomiting, abdominal pain, or increased lipase and amylase values).
● Monitor patient for signs and symptoms of bleeding (hypotension, rapid heart rate).
● *Look alike–sound alike:* Don't confuse Kaletra with Keppra.

PATIENT TEACHING

● Tell patient to take oral solution with food. Tablets may be taken without regard to food.
● *Alert:* Tablets must be swallowed whole; don't crush or divide, and tell patient not to chew.
● Tell patient also taking didanosine to take it 1 hour before or 2 hours after lopinavir-ritonavir combination.
● Advise patient to report side effects to prescriber.
● Tell patient to immediately report severe nausea, vomiting, or abdominal pain.
● Inform patient that drug doesn't cure HIV infection, that opportunistic infections and other complications of HIV infection may still occur, and that transmission of HIV to others through sexual contact or blood contamination remains possible.
● Advise patient taking an erectile dysfunction drug of an increased risk of adverse effects, including low blood pressure, visual changes, and painful erections, and to promptly report any symptoms to his prescriber. Tell him not to take more often than directed.
● Warn patient to tell prescriber about any other prescription or nonprescription

medicine that he's taking, including herbal supplements.

maraviroc
mahr-AY-vih-rok

Selzentry

Pharmacologic class: CCR5 co-receptor antagonist
Pregnancy risk category B

AVAILABLE FORMS
Tablets: 150 mg, 300 mg

INDICATIONS & DOSAGES
➤ **Combined with CYP3A4 inhibitors including protease inhibitors to treat CCR5-tropic HIV-1 infection with evidence of viral replication or HIV-1 strains resistant to multiple antiretrovirals**
Adults: 150 mg P.O. b.i.d.
➤ **Combined with nucleoside reverse transcriptase inhibitors, tipranavir/ritonavir, nevirapine, or other drugs that aren't strong CYP3A inhibitors or CYP3A inducers, to treat CCR5-tropic HIV-1 infection with evidence of viral replication or HIV-1 strains resistant to multiple antiretrovirals**
Adults: 300 mg P.O. b.i.d.
➤ **Combined with CYP3A inducers, to treat CCR5-tropic HIV-1 infection with evidence of viral replication or HIV-1 strains resistant to multiple antiretrovirals**
Adults: 600 mg P.O. b.i.d.

ADMINISTRATION
P.O.
● Give drug without regard for food.

ACTION
Blocks viral entry into cells by binding to chemokine receptor 5 co-receptor and preventing the initiation of HIV replication cycle.

Route	Onset	Peak	Duration
P.O.	Unknown	½–4 hr	Unknown

Half-life: 14–18 hours

ADVERSE REACTIONS
CNS: dizziness, paresthesias, sensory abnormalities, peripheral neuropathy, sleep disturbances, depressive disorders, *pyrexia,* pain, disturbances in consciousness, **stroke.**
CV: unstable angina, ***acute cardiac failure,*** coronary artery disease, ***MI,*** myocardial ischemia, vascular hypertensive disorders.
GI: abdominal pain, constipation, dyspepsia, stomatitis, appetite disorders.
GU: urinary tract signs and symptoms.
Hepatic: ***cirrhosis, hepatic failure,*** cholestatic jaundice.
Musculoskeletal: muscle pains, joint pain, myositis, osteonecrosis, ***rhabdomyolysis.***
Respiratory: *upper respiratory tract infection,* bronchitis, sinusitis, *cough,* pneumonia.
Skin: rash, pruritus, dermatitis, eczema, folliculitis, condyloma acuminatum.
Other: herpes infection, influenza.

INTERACTIONS
Drug-drug. *CYP3A inhibitors (protease inhibitors except tipranavir/ritonavir), delavirdine, ketoconazole, itraconazole, clarithromycin, nefazodone, telithromycin:* May increase levels of maraviroc. Decrease dose of maraviroc.
CYP3A inducers including efavirenz: May decrease levels of maraviroc. Increase dose of maraviroc.
Drug-herb. *St. John's wort:* May decrease levels of maraviroc. Discourage use together.

EFFECTS ON LAB TEST RESULTS
● May increase AST, ALT, bilirubin, amylase, lipase, and CK levels.
● May decrease absolute neutrophil count.

CONTRAINDICATIONS & CAUTIONS
● Contraindicated in patients hypersensitive to drug or its components.
● Use cautiously in patients with preexisting liver dysfunction or patients who are infected with viral hepatitis B or C.
● Use cautiously in patients at risk for CV events, with a history of postural hypotension, or taking another medication known to lower blood pressure.

Reactions may be *common,* uncommon, ***life-threatening***, or COMMON AND LIFE-THREATENING.
Interaction may have a *rapid onset* or ***delayed onset.***

- Safety and efficacy haven't been established in treatment-naive or pediatric patients.
- Patient shouldn't breast-feed while taking drug because of the potential for HIV transmission and serious drug side effects in infants.
- Pregnant women exposed to drug should be registered in the Antiretroviral Pregnancy Registry 1-800-258-4263.

NURSING CONSIDERATIONS
- Effectiveness hasn't been established in patients with dual, mixed, or CXCR4–tropic HIV-1 infection.
- Monitor patient closely for signs and symptoms of infection.
- **Black Box Warning** Due to increased risk of hepatotoxicity, monitor patient closely. Systemic allergic reaction with pruritic rash, eosinophilia, or elevated IgE may precede hepatotoxicity. Patients with signs or symptoms of hepatitis or allergic reaction should be evaluated immediately. ■

PATIENT TEACHING
- Instruct patient to promptly report signs or symptoms of hepatitis or allergic reaction (rash, yellow eyes or skins, dark urine, vomiting, and abdominal pain).
- Caution patients that drug doesn't cure HIV infection and that they may still develop HIV-related illness, including opportunistic infections.
- Caution patient that drug doesn't reduce risk of transmission of HIV to others.
- If patient feels dizzy while taking drug, advise him to avoid driving or operating machinery.
- Instruct woman to tell her prescriber if she's pregnant or planning to become pregnant while taking drug.
- Advise patient to take drug every day as prescribed with other antiretrovirals. Tell patient not to change the dose or dosing schedule or stop any antiretroviral without consulting prescriber.

nelfinavir mesylate
nell-FIN-ah-veer

Viracept

Pharmacologic class: protease inhibitor
Pregnancy risk category B

AVAILABLE FORMS
Powder: 50 mg/g powder in 144-g bottle
Tablets: 250 mg, 625 mg

INDICATIONS & DOSAGES
➤ **HIV infection**
Adults: 1,250 mg b.i.d. or 750 mg P.O. t.i.d. with meals or light snack.
Children ages 2 to 13: 45 to 55 mg/kg P.O. b.i.d. or 25 to 35 mg/kg P.O. t.i.d. with meals or light snack; don't exceed 750 mg t.i.d.
➤ **To prevent infection after occupational exposure to HIV ◆**
Adults: 750 mg P.O. t.i.d. with two other antiretrovirals (zidovudine and lamivudine, lamivudine and stavudine, or didanosine and stavudine) for 4 weeks.

ADMINISTRATION
P.O.
- Give oral powder to children unable to take tablets. May mix oral powder with small amount of water, milk, formula, soy formula, soy milk, or dietary supplements. Patient should consume entire amount.
- Don't reconstitute with water in the original container.
- Use reconstituted powder within 6 hours.
- Mixing with acidic foods or juice isn't recommended because of bitter taste.

ACTION
An HIV-1 protease inhibitor, which prevents cleavage of the viral polyprotein, resulting in the production of immature, noninfectious virus.

Route	Onset	Peak	Duration
P.O.	Unknown	2–4 hr	Unknown

Half-life: 3½ to 5 hours.

ADVERSE REACTIONS
CNS: *seizures, suicidal ideation.*
GI: *diarrhea, pancreatitis,* flatulence, nausea.
Hematologic: *leukopenia, thrombocytopenia.*
Hepatic: *hepatitis.*
Metabolic: *hypoglycemia,* dehydration, diabetes mellitus, hyperlipidemia, hyperuricemia.
Skin: rash.
Other: redistribution or accumulation of body fat.

INTERACTIONS
Drug-drug. *Amiodarone, ergot derivatives, lovastatin, midazolam, pimozide, quinidine, simvastatin, triazolam:* May increase levels of these drugs, causing increased risk of life-threatening adverse events. Avoid using together.
Atorvastatin: May increase atorvastatin level. Use lowest possible dose or consider using pravastatin or fluvastatin instead.
Azithromycin: May increase azithromycin level. Monitor patient for liver impairment.
Carbamazepine, phenobarbital: May reduce the effectiveness of nelfinavir. Use together cautiously.
Cyclosporine, sirolimus, tacrolimus: May increase levels of these immunosuppressants. Use cautiously together.
Delavirdine, HIV protease inhibitors (indinavir, saquinavir): May increase levels of protease inhibitors. Use together cautiously.
Didanosine: May decrease didanosine absorption. Take nelfinavir with food at least 2 hours before or 1 hour after didanosine.
Ethinyl estradiol: May decrease contraceptive level and effectiveness. Advise patient to use alternative contraceptive measures during therapy.
Methadone, phenytoin: May decrease levels of these drugs. Adjust dosage of these drugs accordingly.
Rifabutin: May increase rifabutin level and decrease nelfinavir level. Reduce dosage of rifabutin to half the usual dose and increase nelfinavir to 1,250 mg b.i.d.
Sildenafil: May increase adverse effects of sildenafil. Caution patient not to exceed 25 mg of sildenafil in a 48-hour period.
Drug-herb. *St. John's wort:* May decrease drug level. Discourage use together.

EFFECTS ON LAB TEST RESULTS
● May increase ALT, AST, alkaline phosphatase, bilirubin, GGT, amylase, CK, and lipid levels. May decrease hemoglobin level. May increase or decrease glucose level.
● May decrease WBC and platelet counts.

CONTRAINDICATIONS & CAUTIONS
● Contraindicated in patients hypersensitive to drug or its components and in patients receiving amiodarone, ergot derivatives, lovastatin, midazolam, pimozide, quinidine, simvastatin, or triazolam.
● Contraindicated in pregnant women unless no other treatment option exists because of the presence of the carcinogen ethyl methanesulfonate (EMS) in Viracept. Children currently receiving Viracept may continue, but children shouldn't be started on this drug.
● Use cautiously in patients with hepatic dysfunction or hemophilia types A or B. Monitor liver function test results.
● It's not known if drug appears in breast milk. Because safety hasn't been established, advise HIV-infected women not to breast-feed, to avoid transmitting virus to the infant.

NURSING CONSIDERATIONS
● Drug dosage is the same whether drug is used alone or with other antiretrovirals.
● *Look alike–sound alike:* Don't confuse nelfinavir with nevirapine.

PATIENT TEACHING
● Advise patient to take drug with food.
● Inform patient that drug doesn't cure HIV infection.
● Tell patient that long-term effects of drug are unknown and that there are no data stating that nelfinavir reduces risk of HIV transmission.
● Advise patient to take drug daily as prescribed and not to alter dose or stop drug without medical approval.
● If patient misses a dose, tell him to take it as soon as possible and then return to his normal schedule. Advise patient not to double the dose.
● Tell patient that diarrhea is the most common adverse effect and that it can be controlled with loperamide, if needed.

Reactions may be *common,* uncommon, *life-threatening,* or COMMON AND LIFE-THREATENING.
Interaction may have a *rapid onset* or **delayed onset.**

• Instruct patient taking hormonal contraceptives to use alternative or additional contraceptive measures while taking nelfinavir.

• Advise patient taking sildenafil about an increased risk of sildenafil-related adverse events, including low blood pressure, visual changes, and painful erections. Tell him to promptly report any symptoms. Tell him not to exceed 25 mg of sildenafil in a 48-hour period.

• Warn patient with phenylketonuria that powder contains 11.2 mg phenylalanine per gram.

• Advise patient to report use of other prescribed or OTC drugs because of possible drug interactions.

---

nevirapine
neh-VEER-ah-pine

Viramune

Pharmacologic class:
nonnucleoside reverse
transcriptase inhibitor
Pregnancy risk category C

AVAILABLE FORMS
Oral suspension: 50 mg/5 ml
Tablets: 200 mg

INDICATIONS & DOSAGES
➤ **Adjunct treatment in HIV-infected adults who have experienced clinical or immunologic deterioration; used with other antiretrovirals**
■ **Black Box Warning** Adhere strictly to 14-day lead-in period with nevirapine 200-mg-daily dosing. ■
Adults: 200 mg P.O. daily for the first 14 days; then 200 mg P.O. b.i.d.
Adjust-a-dose: For patients on dialysis, give an additional 200-mg dose after each dialysis treatment. Patients with a creatinine clearance equal to or greater than 20 ml/minute don't require dosage adjustment.
➤ **Adjunct treatment in HIV-infected children**
Children age 8 and older: 4 mg/kg P.O. once daily for first 14 days; then 4 mg/kg P.O. b.i.d. thereafter. Maximum daily dose is 400 mg.

Children ages 2 months to 8 years:
4 mg/kg P.O. once daily for first 14 days; then 7 mg/kg P.O. b.i.d. thereafter. Maximum daily dose is 400 mg.

ADMINISTRATION
P.O.
• Use drug with at least one other antiretroviral.

ACTION
Binds directly to reverse transcriptase and blocks RNA-dependent and DNA-dependent DNA polymerase activities by disrupting the enzyme's catalytic site.

Route	Onset	Peak	Duration
P.O.	Unknown	4 hr	Unknown

Half-life: 25 to 30 hours.

ADVERSE REACTIONS
CNS: *fever,* headache, paresthesia.
GI: *nausea,* abdominal pain, diarrhea, ulcerative stomatitis.
Hematologic: *neutropenia.*
Hepatic: *hepatitis.*
Musculoskeletal: myalgia.
Skin: *blistering, rash, Stevens-Johnson syndrome.*

INTERACTIONS
Drug-drug. *Drugs extensively metabolized by cytochrome P-450:* May lower levels of these drugs. Dosage adjustment of these drugs may be needed.
Ketoconazole: May decrease ketoconazole level. Avoid using together.
Protease inhibitors or hormonal contraceptives: May decrease levels of these drugs. Use together cautiously.
Rifabutin, rifampin: Dosage adjustment may be needed. Monitor patient closely.
Drug-herb. *St. John's wort:* May decrease drug level. Discourage use together.

EFFECTS ON LAB TEST RESULTS
• May increase ALT, AST, GGT, and bilirubin levels. May decrease hemoglobin level.
• May decrease neutrophil count.

CONTRAINDICATIONS & CAUTIONS
• Contraindicated in patients hypersensitive to drug.

• For patients with severe hepatic impairment from drug accumulation, don't give.
• In patients with mild to moderate hepatic function, use cautiously; pharmacokinetics haven't been evaluated in these patients.
• Drug appears in breast milk. Don't use drug in breast-feeding women.

NURSING CONSIDERATIONS
• Perform laboratory tests, including renal function tests, before therapy and regularly throughout.
• Increased AST or ALT levels or coinfection with hepatitis B or C at the start of therapy suggest a greater risk of hepatic adverse events.
■**Black Box Warning** Severe and, in some cases, fatal hepatotoxicity, particularly in the first 18 weeks of treatment, has been reported and may occur in all patients, including those receiving the drug for postexposure prophylaxis, an approved use. Hepatotoxicity is often linked with rash and fever. Women and patients with higher CD4+ cell counts are at increased risk. Women with CD4+ cell counts greater than 250/mm³, including pregnant women receiving long-term treatment for HIV infection, are at considerably higher risk for hepatotoxicity. ■
• Monitor patient for signs and symptoms of hepatitis including rash. Closely monitor liver function tests at baseline and during the first 18 weeks of treatment; then monitor frequently thereafter.
• Perform liver function tests immediately if hepatitis or hypersensitivity reactions are suspected.
■ **Black Box Warning** Severe, life-threatening skin reactions, including fatalities, have occurred. The greatest risk of reaction is within the first 6 weeks of therapy. Monitor patient for blistering, oral lesions, conjunctivitis, muscle or joint aches, or general malaise. Especially look for a severe rash or rash accompanied by fever. Report these signs and symptoms to prescriber. Patients who experience a rash or hypersensitivity reactions must discontinue nevirapine and seek medical evaluation immediately. ■
• *Alert:* If hepatitis occurs, permanently stop drug and don't restart after recovery.

In some cases, hepatic injury progresses anyway.
• Patients who have stopped therapy for more than 7 days should restart therapy as if receiving drug for the first time.
• Antiretroviral therapy may be changed if disease progresses while patient is receiving this drug.
• *Look alike–sound alike:* Don't confuse nevirapine with nelfinavir.

PATIENT TEACHING
• Inform patient that drug doesn't cure HIV and that illnesses from advanced HIV infection still may occur. Explain that drug doesn't reduce risk of HIV transmission.
• Instruct patient to report rash immediately and to stop drug until told to resume.
• Tell patient with signs or symptoms of hepatitis (such as fatigue, malaise, anorexia, nausea, jaundice, liver tenderness or hepatomegaly, with or without initially abnormal transaminase levels) to stop drug and seek medical evaluation immediately.
• Stress importance of taking drug exactly as prescribed. If a dose is missed, tell patient to take the next dose as soon as possible and not to double next dose.
• Tell patient not to use other drugs unless approved by prescriber.
• Advise woman of childbearing age that hormonal contraceptives and other hormonal methods of birth control shouldn't be used with this drug.

---

raltegravir
rahl-TEH-gra-vear

Isentress

Pharmacologic class: HIV integrase strand transfer inhibitor
Pregnancy risk category C

AVAILABLE FORMS
Tablets: 400 mg

INDICATIONS & DOSAGES
➤ **HIV-1 infection, with other anti-retrovirals, in treatment-experienced patients who have continued HIV-1**

---

replication despite antiretroviral therapy
Adults: 400 mg P.O. b.i.d.

ADMINISTRATION
P.O.
● Give drug without regard for meals.

ACTION
Inhibits HIV-1 integrase, an enzyme required for HIV-1 replication.

Route	Onset	Peak	Duration
P.O.	Rapid	3 hr	Unknown

Half-life: About 9 hours.

ADVERSE REACTIONS
CNS: *headache,* fever, fatigue, dizziness.
GI: *diarrhea, nausea,* abdominal pain, vomiting.
Hematologic: anemia, *neutropenia, thrombocytopenia.*
Metabolic: hyperglycemia.
Musculoskeletal: asthenia, myopathy, *rhabdomyolysis.*
Skin: lipodystrophy.

INTERACTIONS
Drug-drug. *UGT1A1 inhibitors, such as rifampin:* May decrease raltegravir level. Use together cautiously.
Atazanavir: May increase raltegravir level. Use together cautiously.

EFFECTS ON LAB TEST RESULTS
● May increase bilirubin, AST, ALT, alkaline phosphatase, amylase, lipase, glucose, and CK levels. May decrease hemoglobin level.
● May decrease neutrophil and platelet counts.

CONTRAINDICATIONS & CAUTIONS
● Contraindicated in patients hypersensitive to drug or its components.
● Use cautiously in patients taking drugs known to cause myopathy or rhabdomyolysis such as statins.
● Use cautiously in elderly patients, especially those with hepatic, renal, and cardiac insufficiency.

NURSING CONSIDERATIONS
● Perform laboratory tests, including CBC, platelet count, and liver function studies, before therapy and regularly throughout.
● Use drug with at lease one other antiretroviral.
● Drug should be reserved for patients who demonstrate resistance to other regimens.
● Watch for signs of myopathy.
● Give drug to a pregnant woman only if the potential benefit justifies the risk to the fetus.
● Register pregnant women for monitoring of maternal-fetal outcomes by calling the Antiretroviral Pregnancy Registry at 1-800-258-4263.
● Safety and efficacy haven't been establish in children younger than age 16.
● Breast-feeding isn't recommended during therapy.

PATIENT TEACHING
● Inform patient that drug doesn't cure HIV infection. He may continue to develop opportunistic infections and other complications of HIV infection, and transmission of HIV to others through sexual contact or blood contamination is still possible.
● Advise patient to use barrier protection during sexual intercourse.
● Tell women that breast-feeding isn't recommended during therapy.
● Advise patient to immediately report worsening symptoms or unexplained muscle pain, tenderness, or weakness while taking the drug.
● Instruct patient to avoid missing any doses to decrease the risk of developing HIV resistance.
● Tell patient if a dose is missed to take the next dose as soon as possible and not to double the next dose.
● Advise patient to report use of other drugs, including OTC drugs; this drug interacts with other drugs.
● Tell patient that drug may be taken without regard for meals.

ritonavir
ri-TON-ah-veer

Norvir*

Pharmacologic class: protease inhibitor
Pregnancy risk category B

AVAILABLE FORMS
Capsules: 100 mg
Oral solution: 80 mg/ml*

INDICATIONS & DOSAGES
➤ **HIV infection, with other anti-retrovirals**
Adults: 600 mg P.O. b.i.d. with meals. To reduce adverse GI effects, begin with 300 mg P.O. b.i.d. and increase by 100 mg b.i.d. at 2- to 3-day intervals.
Children older than age 1 month: 350 to 400 mg/m² P.O. b.i.d.; don't exceed 600 mg P.O. b.i.d. Initially, start with 250 mg/m² b.i.d. and increase by 50 mg/m² P.O. every 12 hours at 2- to 3-day intervals. If children can't reach b.i.d. doses of 400 mg/m² because of adverse effects, consider alternate therapy.

ADMINISTRATION
P.O.
• When giving oral solution to children, use a calibrated dosing syringe, if possible.

ACTION
An HIV-1 and HIV-2 protease inhibitor. Drug binds to the protease-active site and inhibits activity of the enzyme, preventing cleavage of the viral polyproteins and causing formation of immature, noninfectious viral particles.

Route	Onset	Peak	Duration
P.O.	Unknown	2–4 hr	Unknown

Half-life: Unknown.

ADVERSE REACTIONS
CNS: *asthenia,* **generalized tonic-clonic seizure,** anxiety, circumoral paresthesia, confusion, depression, dizziness, fever, headache, insomnia, malaise, pain, paresthesia, peripheral paresthesia, somnolence, thinking abnormality.

CV: syncope, vasodilation.
EENT: pharyngitis.
GI: *diarrhea, nausea, taste perversion, vomiting,* **pancreatitis, pseudomembranous colitis,** abdominal pain, anorexia, constipation, dyspepsia, flatulence.
Hematologic: *leukopenia,* **thrombocytopenia.**
Hepatic: *hepatitis.*
Metabolic: *diabetes mellitus,* weight loss.
Musculoskeletal: arthralgia, myalgia.
Skin: rash, sweating.
Other: hypersensitivity reactions, fat redistribution or accumulation.

INTERACTIONS
Drug-drug. ■ **Black Box Warning** *Alfuzosin, amiodarone, bepridil, ergot derivatives, flecainide, midazolam, pimozide, propafenone, quinidine, triazolam, voriconazole:* May cause life-threatening adverse reactions. Use together is contraindicated. ■
Atovaquone, divalproex, lamotrigine, phenytoin, warfarin: May decrease levels of these drugs. Use together cautiously and monitor drug levels closely.
Beta blockers, disopyramide, fluoxetine, mexiletine, nefazodone: May increase levels of these drugs, causing cardiac and neurologic events. Use together cautiously.
Bupropion, buspirone, calcium channel blockers, carbamazepine, clonazepam, clorazepate, cyclosporine, desipramine, dexamethasone, diazepam, **digoxin,** *dronabinol, estazolam, ethosuximide, flurazepam, lidocaine, methamphetamine, metoprolol, perphenazine, prednisone, propoxyphene, quinine, risperidone, sirolimus, SSRIs, tacrolimus, tricyclic antidepressants, thioridazine, timolol, tramadol, zolpidem:* May increase levels of these drugs. Use cautiously together and consider decreasing the dosage of these drugs by almost 50%. Monitor therapeutic levels.
Clarithromycin: May increase clarithromycin level. If creatinine clearance is 30 to 60 ml/minute, reduce clarithromycin dose by 50%. If creatinine clearance is less than 30 ml/minute, reduce clarithromycin dose by 75%.
Clozapine, piroxicam: May increase levels and toxicity of these drugs. Avoid using together.

Reactions may be *common*, uncommon, *life-threatening*, or COMMON AND LIFE-THREATENING.
Interaction may have a *rapid onset* or **delayed onset.**

Delavirdine: May increase ritonavir level. Adjusted dose recommendations aren't established. Use together cautiously.

Didanosine: May decrease didanosine absorption. Separate doses by 2½ hours.

Disulfiram, metronidazole: May increase risk of disulfiram-like reactions because ritonavir formulations contain alcohol. Monitor patient.

Ethinyl estradiol: May decrease ethinyl estradiol level. Use an alternative or additional method of birth control.

Fluticasone: May significantly increase fluticasone exposure, significantly decreasing cortisol concentrations and causing systemic corticosteroid effects (including Cushing's syndrome). Don't use together, if possible.

HMG-CoA reductase inhibitors: May cause large increase in statin levels, resulting in myopathy. Avoid using with lovastatin and simvastatin. Use cautiously with atorvastatin. Consider using fluvastatin or pravastatin.

Indinavir: May increase indinavir levels. Use together cautiously.

Ketoconazole, itraconazole: May increase levels of these drugs. Don't exceed 200 mg/day of these drugs.

Meperidine: May decrease levels of meperidine and its metabolite. Dosage increases and long-term use together aren't recommended because of CNS effects. Use cautiously together.

Methadone: May decrease methadone levels. Consider increasing methadone dosage.

PDE5 inhibitors (sildenafil, tadalafil, vardenafil): May increase levels of PDE5 inhibitor, causing hypotension, syncope, visual changes, or prolonged erection. Use together cautiously and increase monitoring for adverse reactions. Tell patient not to exceed 25 mg of sildenafil in a 48-hour period, 10 mg of tadalafil in a 72-hour period, or 2.5 mg of vardenafil in a 72-hour period.

Rifabutin: May increase rifabutin levels. Monitor patient and reduce rifabutin daily dosage by at least 75% of usual dose.

Rifampin, rifapentine: May decrease ritonavir levels. Consider using rifabutin.

Saquinavir: May increase saquinavir plasma levels. Adjust dose by taking saquinavir 400 mg b.i.d. and ritonavir 400 mg b.i.d.

Theophylline: May decrease theophylline levels. Increase dose based on blood levels.

Trazodone: May increase trazodone level causing nausea, dizziness, hypotension and syncope. Avoid using together. If unavoidable, use cautiously and lower trazodone dose.

Drug-herb. St. John's wort: May substantially reduce drug levels. Discourage use together.

Drug-food. *Any food:* May increase absorption. Advise patient to take drug with food.

Drug-lifestyle. *Smoking:* May decrease drug levels. Discourage smoking.

EFFECTS ON LAB TEST RESULTS

● May increase ALT, AST, GGT, glucose, triglyceride, lipid, CK, and uric acid levels. May decrease hemoglobin level and hematocrit.

● May decrease WBC, RBC, platelet, and neutrophil counts.

CONTRAINDICATIONS & CAUTIONS

● Contraindicated in patients hypersensitive to drug or its components.

● Use cautiously in patients with hepatic insufficiency.

● Safety and effectiveness in children younger than 1 month haven't been established.

● It's unknown if ritonavir appears in breast milk. Use cautiously in breast-feeding women.

NURSING CONSIDERATIONS

● Patients beginning regimens with ritonavir and nucleosides may improve GI tolerance by starting ritonavir alone and then adding nucleosides before completing 2 weeks of ritonavir.

● ***Look alike–sound alike:*** Don't confuse Norvir with Norvasc.

PATIENT TEACHING

● Inform patient that drug doesn't cure HIV infection. He may continue to develop opportunistic infections and other complications of HIV infection. Drug hasn't been shown to reduce the risk of transmitting HIV to

others through sexual contact or blood contamination.

• Caution patient to take drug as prescribed and not to adjust dosage or stop therapy without first consulting prescriber.

• Tell patient that taste of oral solution may be improved by mixing it with chocolate milk, Ensure, or Advera within 1 hour of the scheduled dose.

• Instruct patient to take drug with a meal to improve absorption.

• Tell patient that if a dose is missed, he should take the next dose as soon as possible. If a dose is skipped, he shouldn't double the next dose.

• Advise patients taking a PDE5 inhibitor for erectile dysfunction to promptly report hypotension, dizziness, visual changes, and prolonged erection to their prescriber. Caution against exceeding the recommended reduced dosage.

• Advise patient to report use of other drugs, including OTC drugs; this drug interacts with many drugs.

saquinavir mesylate
sa-KWEN-ah-veer

Invirase

Pharmacologic class: protease inhibitor
Pregnancy risk category B

AVAILABLE FORMS
Capsules (hard gelatin): 200 mg
Tablets (film-coated): 500 mg

INDICATIONS & DOSAGES
■ **Black Box Warning** Saquinavir mesylate capsules and tablets and saquinavir soft gelatin capsules aren't bioequivalent and can't be used interchangeably. Saquinavir mesylate should be used only if it's combined with ritonavir, which significantly inhibits saquinavir's metabolism to provide plasma saquinavir levels at least equal to those achieved with saquinavir soft gelatin capsules. When saquinavir is used as the sole protease inhibitor in an antiviral regimen, saquinavir soft gelatin capsules are the recommended formulation. ■

➤ **Adjunct treatment of advanced HIV infection in selected patients**
Adults and adolescents age 16 and older: 1,000 mg P.O. b.i.d. given at the same time with 100 mg ritonavir P.O. b.i.d.

ADMINISTRATION
P.O.
• Give drug with food or within 2 hours of a full meal to increase drug absorption.

ACTION
Inhibits the activity of HIV protease and prevents the cleavage of HIV polyproteins, which are essential for HIV maturation.

Route	Onset	Peak	Duration
P.O.	Unknown	Unknown	Unknown

Half-life: 1 to 2 hours.

ADVERSE REACTIONS
CNS: anxiety, asthenia, depression, dizziness, headache, insomnia, numbness, paresthesia.
CV: chest pain.
GI: *diarrhea, nausea, pancreatitis,* altered taste, abdominal pain, constipation, dyspepsia, flatulence, ulcerated buccal mucosa, vomiting.
Hematologic: *pancytopenia, thrombocytopenia.*
Musculoskeletal: musculoskeletal pain.
Respiratory: bronchitis, cough.
Skin: rash.

INTERACTIONS
Drug-drug. *Amprenavir:* May decrease amprenavir level. Use together cautiously.
Carbamazepine, phenobarbital, phenytoin: May decrease saquinavir level. Avoid using together.
Delavirdine: May increase saquinavir level. Use cautiously and monitor hepatic enzymes. Decrease dose when used together.
Dexamethasone: May decrease saquinavir level. Avoid using together.
Efavirenz: May decrease levels of both drugs. Avoid using together.
HMG-CoA reductase inhibitors: May increase levels of these drugs, which increases risk of myopathy, including rhabdomyolysis. Avoid using together.
Indinavir, lopinavir and ritonavir combination, nelfinavir, ritonavir: May increase saquinavir level. Use together cautiously.

Reactions may be *common,* uncommon, *life-threatening,* or COMMON AND LIFE-THREATENING.
Interaction may have a *rapid onset* or **delayed onset.**

Macrolide antibiotics, such as clarithromycin: May increase levels of both drugs. Use together cautiously.

Nevirapine: May decrease saquinavir level. Monitor patient.

PDE5 inhibitors (sildenafil, tadalafil, vardenafil): May increase levels of these drugs. Reduce dose and frequency of PDE5 inhibitor and monitor patient closely for adverse reactions.

Rifabutin, rifampin: May decrease saquinavir level. Use with rifabutin cautiously. Don't use with rifampin.

Drug-herb. *Garlic supplements,* **St. John's wort:** May substantially reduce drug level, causing loss of therapeutic effects. Discourage use together.

Drug-food. *Any food:* May increase drug absorption. Advise patient to take drug with food.

Grapefruit juice: May increase drug level. Tell patient to take with liquid other than grapefruit juice.

EFFECTS ON LAB TEST RESULTS
• May decrease WBC, RBC, and platelet counts.

CONTRAINDICATIONS & CAUTIONS
• Contraindicated in patients hypersensitive to drug or its components.
• Safety of drug hasn't been established in pregnant or breast-feeding women or in children younger than age 16.

NURSING CONSIDERATIONS
• Evaluate CBC, platelets, electrolytes, uric acid, liver enzymes, and bilirubin before therapy begins and at appropriate intervals throughout therapy.
• If serious toxicity occurs during treatment, stop drug until cause is identified or toxicity resolves. Drug may be resumed without dosage modifications.
• Monitor patient's hydration if adverse GI reactions occur.

PATIENT TEACHING
• Advise patient to take drug with food or within 2 hours of a full meal to increase drug absorption.
• Instruct patient to avoid missing any doses, to decrease the risk of developing HIV resistance.

• Inform patient that drug doesn't cure HIV infection, that opportunistic infections and other complications of HIV infection may continue to occur, and that transmission of HIV to others through sexual contact or blood contamination is still possible.
• Advise patient to keep an updated list of the drugs he's taking and to contact his prescriber before using any prescription or OTC drug because of the many interactions.

---

stavudine (2' 3'-didehydro-3-deoxythymidine, d4T)
stay-VYOO-deen

Zerit

Pharmacologic class: nucleoside reverse transcriptase inhibitor
Pregnancy risk category C

AVAILABLE FORMS
Capsules: 15 mg, 20 mg, 30 mg, 40 mg
Oral solution: 1 mg/ml

INDICATIONS & DOSAGES
➤ **HIV-infection, with other anti-retrovirals**
Adults who weigh 60 kg (132 lb) or more: 40 mg P.O. regular-release every 12 hours.
Adults who weigh 30 kg (66 lb) to 60 kg: 30 mg P.O. regular-release every 12 hours.
Children who weigh 60 kg or more: 40 mg P.O. regular-release every 12 hours.
Children who weigh 30 kg to 60 kg: 30 mg P.O. regular-release every 12 hours.
Neonates 14 days and older and children who weigh less than 30 kg: 1 mg/kg P.O. regular-release every 12 hours.
Neonates age 13 days and younger: 0.5 mg/kg P.O. regular-release every 12 hours.
Adjust-a-dose: For patients experiencing peripheral neuropathy, stop temporarily; then resume therapy at 50% recommended dose. Consider stopping therapy if neuropathy recurs. For patients with creatinine clearance 26 to 50 ml/minute, adjust dosage to 20 mg (if weight exceeds 60 kg) or 15 mg (if weight is less than 60 kg) P.O. every 12 hours; if clearance is 10 to

25 ml/minute, 20 mg (if weight exceeds 60 kg) or 15 mg (if weight is less than 60 kg) P.O. every 24 hours.

ADMINISTRATION
P.O.
• Give drug without regard for meals.
• For patient who has difficulty swallowing, extended-release capsules can be opened and contents mixed with 2 tablespoons of yogurt or applesauce. Patient shouldn't chew or crush the beads while swallowing.

ACTION
A thymidine nucleoside analogue that prevents replication of retroviruses, including HIV, by inhibiting the enzyme reverse transcriptase and causing termination of DNA chain growth.

Route	Onset	Peak	Duration
P.O.	Unknown	1 hr	Unknown

Half-life: 1 to 2 hours.

ADVERSE REACTIONS
CNS: asthenia, *fever,* anxiety, depression, dizziness, headache, insomnia, malaise, motor weakness, nervousness, peripheral neuropathy.
CV: chest pain.
EENT: conjunctivitis.
GI: *abdominal pain, anorexia, diarrhea, nausea, vomiting, **pancreatitis,*** constipation, dyspepsia.
Hematologic: *neutropenia, thrombocytopenia,* anemia.
Hepatic: *hepatotoxicity,* severe hepatomegaly with steatosis.
Metabolic: *lactic acidosis,* weight loss.
Musculoskeletal: *arthralgia, back pain, myalgia.*
Respiratory: *dyspnea.*
Skin: *diaphoresis, pruritus, rash,* maculopapular rash.
Other: *chills,* **pancreatitis.**

INTERACTIONS
Drug-drug. *Didanosine, hydroxyurea:* Coadministration may increase risk for lactic acidosis, hepatotoxicity, pancreatitis, or peripheral neuropathy. Monitor closely for adverse effects.
Methadone: May decrease stavudine absorption and level. Separate dosage times

and monitor patient for clinical effect if drugs must be used together.
Zidovudine: May inhibit phosphorylation of stavudine. Avoid using together.

EFFECTS ON LAB TEST RESULTS
• May increase ALT and AST levels. May decrease hemoglobin level.
• May decrease neutrophil and platelet count.

CONTRAINDICATIONS & CAUTIONS
• Contraindicated in patients hypersensitive to drug.
■ **Black Box Warning** Lactic acidosis and severe hepatomegaly with steatosis, including fatal cases, have been reported. ■
• Use cautiously in patients with renal impairment or history of peripheral neuropathy. Adjust dosage for creatinine clearance of less than 50 ml/minute; adjust dosage or stop drug in patients with peripheral neuropathy.
■ **Black Box Warning** Use cautiously in pregnant women; fatal lactic acidosis may occur in pregnant women who receive stavudine and didanosine with other antiretrovirals. ■

NURSING CONSIDERATIONS
■ **Black Box Warning** Due to increased risk of pancreatic toxicity, monitor patient for signs and symptoms of pancreatitis, especially if he takes stavudine with didanosine or hydroxyurea. If patient has pancreatitis, reinstate drug cautiously. ■
• Monitor liver function test results.
■ **Black Box Warning** Motor weakness mimicking the signs and symptoms of Guillain-Barré syndrome (including respiratory failure) in HIV patients taking stavudine with other antiretrovirals may occur, especially in patients with lactic acidosis. Monitor patient for characteristics of lactic acidosis, including generalized fatigue, GI problems, tachypnea, and dyspnea. Patients with these symptoms should promptly interrupt antiretroviral therapy and rapidly receive a full medical workup. Consider permanently stopping drug. Symptoms may continue or worsen when drug is stopped. ■

Reactions may be *common,* uncommon, *life-threatening,* or COMMON AND LIFE-THREATENING.
Interaction may have a *rapid onset* or **delayed onset.**

- **Alert:** Peripheral neuropathy may be the major dose-limiting adverse effect; it may or may not resolve after drug is stopped.
- Monitor CBC results and creatinine.

PATIENT TEACHING

- Tell patient that drug may be taken without regard to meals.
- Warn patient not to take other drugs for HIV or AIDS unless prescriber has approved them.
- Inform patient that drug doesn't cure HIV infection, that opportunistic infections and other complications of HIV infection may still occur, and that transmission of HIV to others through sexual contact or blood contamination is still possible.
- Teach patient signs and symptoms of peripheral neuropathy (pain, burning, aching, weakness, or pins and needles in the limbs) and tell him to report these immediately.
- Tell patient to report symptoms of lactic acidosis, including fatigue, GI problems, dyspnea, or tachypnea.
- Tell patient to report symptoms of pancreatitis, including abdominal pain, nausea, vomiting, weight loss, or fatty stools.
- Tell patient to monitor weight patterns and report weight loss or gain.
- Explain to patient who has difficulty swallowing that extended-release capsules can be opened and contents mixed with 2 tablespoons of yogurt or applesauce. Caution patient not to chew or crush the beads while swallowing.

---

tenofovir disoproxil fumarate
te-NOE-fo-veer

Viread♪

Pharmacologic class: nucleotide reverse transcriptase inhibitor
Pregnancy risk category B

AVAILABLE FORMS

Tablets: 300 mg as the fumarate salt (equivalent to 245 mg of tenofovir disoproxil)

INDICATIONS & DOSAGES
➤ **HIV-1 infection, with other anti-retrovirals**
Adults: 300 mg P.O. once daily.
Adjust-a-dose: For patients with creatinine clearance of 30 to 49 ml/minute, 300 mg P.O. every 48 hours. For a clearance of 10 to 29 ml/minute, 300 mg P.O. twice weekly. For patients receiving hemodialysis, 300 mg P.O. every 7 days or after a total of about 12 hours of hemodialysis. Give dose after session. There are no recommendations for patients with a creatinine clearance of less than 10 ml/minute not receiving hemodialysis.

ADMINISTRATION
P.O.
- Give drug with a meal to enhance bioavailability.
- For patients receiving tenofovir and didanosine (buffered or enteric-coated form), give tenofovir 2 hours before or 1 hour after didanosine.

ACTION
Hydrolyzed to produce tenofovir, a nucleoside analogue of adenosine monophosphate that yields tenofovir diphosphate. Tenofovir diphosphate inhibits HIV replication.

Route	Onset	Peak	Duration
P.O.	Unknown	1–2 hr	Unknown

Half-life: Unknown.

ADVERSE REACTIONS
CNS: asthenia, headache.
GI: *nausea,* abdominal pain, anorexia, diarrhea, flatulence, vomiting.
GU: glycosuria.
Hematologic: *neutropenia.*
Hepatic: hepatomegaly.
Metabolic: hyperglycemia, *lactic acidosis.*

INTERACTIONS
Drug-drug. *Atazanavir:* May decrease atazanavir levels, causing resistance. Give both drugs with ritonavir.
Didanosine (buffered or enteric-coated form): May increase didanosine bioavailability. Monitor patient for didanosine-related adverse effects, such as bone marrow suppression, GI distress, and

---

peripheral neuropathy. Give tenofovir 2 hours before or 1 hour after didanosine. *Drugs that reduce renal function or compete for renal tubular secretion (acyclovir, cidofovir, ganciclovir, valacyclovir, valganciclovir):* May increase levels of tenofovir or other renally eliminated drugs. Monitor patient for adverse effects.

EFFECTS ON LAB TEST RESULTS
- May increase amylase, AST, ALT, CK, serum and urine glucose, creatinine, phosphate, and triglyceride levels.
- May decrease neutrophil count.

CONTRAINDICATIONS & CAUTIONS
- Contraindicated in patients hypersensitive to any component of the drug.
- Use very cautiously in patients with risk factors for liver disease or with hepatic impairment.
- Don't use triple antiretroviral therapy with abacavir, lamivudine, and tenofovir as new regimen for naive or pretreated patient with HIV infection because of high rate of early virologic resistance.

NURSING CONSIDERATIONS
- **Black Box Warning** Drug may cause lactic acidosis and hepatomegaly with steatosis, even fatal cases. These effects may occur without elevated transaminase levels. Risk factors include long-term antiretroviral use, obesity, and being female. Monitor all patients closely. ∎
- Drug may cause body fat to accumulate and be redistributed, resulting in central obesity, peripheral wasting, and buffalo hump. Monitor patient for changes in body fat.
- Drug may be linked to osteomalacia and decreased bone mineral density and increased creatinine and phosphaturia levels. Monitor patient carefully during long-term treatment.
- Drug may lead to decreased HIV RNA level and CD4+ cell counts.
- In elderly patients, use drug cautiously because these patients may be taking other drugs and may be at higher risk for decreased renal function.
- Because of a high rate of early virologic resistance, triple antiretroviral therapy with abacavir, lamivudine, and tenofovir shouldn't be used as new regimen for

naive or pretreated patient with HIV infection. Monitor patients currently controlled with this regimen and those who use this regimen with other antiretrovirals, and consider a different therapy.
- Because the effects of drug on pregnant women aren't known, use during pregnancy only if benefits clearly outweigh risks.

PATIENT TEACHING
- Instruct patient to take drug with a meal to enhance bioavailability.
- Inform patient that drug doesn't cure HIV infection, that opportunistic infections and other complications of HIV infection may still occur, and that transmission of HIV to others through sexual contact or blood contamination is still possible.
- If patient takes tenofovir and didanosine (buffered or enteric-coated form), instruct him to take tenofovir 2 hours before or 1 hour after didanosine.
- Tell patient to report adverse effects, including nausea, vomiting, diarrhea, flatulence, and headache.

tipranavir
tih-PRAN-uh-veer

Aptivus

Pharmacologic class: protease inhibitor
Pregnancy risk category C

AVAILABLE FORMS
Capsules: 250 mg
Oral solution: 100 mg/ml

INDICATIONS & DOSAGES
➤ **HIV-1 in patients with viral replication who are highly treatment experienced or have HIV-1 strains resistant to multiple protease inhibitors**
Adults: 500 mg P.O. twice daily with 200 mg of ritonavir twice daily. Give with or without food.
Children ages 2 to 18: Tipranavir 14 mg/kg with ritonavir 6 mg/kg (or tipranavir 375 mg/m^2 with ritonavir 150 mg/m^2) b.i.d., not to exceed dosage of tipranavir 500 mg with ritonavir 200 mg

b.i.d. For children who develop intolerance or toxicity, prescribers may consider decreasing dosage to tipranavir 12 mg/kg with ritonavir 5 mg/kg b.i.d. provided the virus isn't resistant to multiple protease inhibitors.

ADMINISTRATION
P.O.
- Give with 200 mg ritonavir and other antiretrovirals.
- Give drug with or without food.
- Do not freeze or refrigerate oral solution.

ACTION
Inhibits virus-specific processing of polyproteins in HIV-1 infected cells, preventing formation of mature virions.

Route	Onset	Peak	Duration
P.O.	Unknown	3 hr	Unknown

Half-life: 5 to 6 hours.

ADVERSE REACTIONS
CNS: asthenia, depression, dizziness, fatigue, headache, insomnia, malaise, peripheral neuropathy, pyrexia, sleep disorder, somnolence.
GI: *diarrhea, pancreatitis,* abdominal distention, abdominal pain, dyspepsia, flatulence, GERD, nausea, vomiting.
GU: renal insufficiency.
Hematologic: *neutropenia, thrombocytopenia,* anemia.
Hepatic: *hepatic failure,* hepatitis.
Metabolic: anorexia, decreased appetite, dehydration, diabetes mellitus, facial wasting, hyperglycemia, weight loss.
Musculoskeletal: muscle cramps, myalgia.
Respiratory: bronchitis, cough, dyspnea.
Skin: *rash,* acquired lipodystrophy, exanthem, lipoatrophy, lipohypertrophy, pruritus.
Other: flulike illness, hypersensitivity, reactivation of herpes simplex and varicella zoster.

INTERACTIONS
Drug-drug. *Amiodarone, bepridil, flecainide, propafenone, quinidine:* May increase levels of these drugs and risk of life-threatening arrhythmias. Avoid using together.

Atorvastatin: May increase levels of both drugs. Start with lowest dose of atorvastatin, and monitor patient closely or consider other drugs.
Clarithromycin: May increase levels of both drugs. If patient's creatinine clearance is 30 to 60 ml/minute, decrease clarithromycin dose by 50%. If patient's creatinine clearance is less than 30 ml/minute, decrease clarithromycin dose by 75%.
Cyclosporine, sirolimus, tacrolimus: May cause unpredictable interaction. Monitor drug levels closely until they've stabilized.
Desipramine: May increase desipramine level. Decrease dose and monitor desipramine level.
Diltiazem, felodipine, nicardipine, nisoldipine, verapamil: May cause unpredictable interaction. Use together cautiously, and monitor patient closely.
Disulfiram, metronidazole: May cause disulfiram-like reaction. Use together cautiously.
Ergot derivatives (dihydroergotamine, ergonovine, ergotamine, methylergonovine): May cause acute ergot toxicity, including peripheral vasospasm and ischemia of extremities. Avoid using together.
Estrogen-based hormone therapy: May decrease estrogen level, and rash may occur. Monitor patient carefully. Advise using nonhormonal contraception.
Fluoxetine, paroxetine, sertraline: May increase levels of these drugs. Adjust dosages as needed.
Glimepiride, glipizide, glyburide, pioglitazone, repaglinide, tolbutamide: May affect glucose levels. Monitor glucose level carefully.
Lovastatin, simvastatin: May increase risk of myopathy and rhabdomyolysis. Avoid using together.
Meperidine: May increase normeperidine metabolite. Avoid using together.
Methadone: May decrease methadone level by 50%. Consider increased methadone dose.
Midazolam, triazolam: May cause prolonged or increased sedation or respiratory depression. Don't use together.
Pimozide: May cause life-threatening arrhythmias. Avoid using together.
Rifampin: May lead to loss of virologic response and resistance to tipranavir and

other protease inhibitors. Avoid using together.

Rifabutin: May increase rifabutin level. Decrease rifabutin dose by 75%.

Sildenafil, tadalafil, vardenafil: May increase levels of these drugs. Use together cautiously. Tell patient not to exceed 25 mg sildenafil in 48 hours, 10 mg tadalafil every 72 hours, or 2.5 mg vardenafil every 72 hours.

Warfarin: May cause unpredictable reaction. Check INR often.

Drug-herb. *St. John's wort:* May lead to loss of virologic response and resistance to this drug and other antiretrovirals. Warn patient to avoid using together.

EFFECTS ON LAB TEST RESULTS

• May increase total cholesterol, triglyceride, blood glucose, amylase, lipase, ALT, and AST levels.
• May decrease WBC count.

CONTRAINDICATIONS & CAUTIONS

■ **Black Box Warning** Administration of tipranavir with ritonavir 200 mg has been associated with fatal and nonfatal intracranial hemorrhage, clinical hepatitis, and hepatic decompensation. ■
• Contraindicated in patients hypersensitive to any ingredients of the product, patients with moderate (Child-Pugh class B) and severe (Child-Pugh class C) hepatic insufficiency, and patients taking drugs that depend on CYP3A for clearance, such as amiodarone, astemizole, bepridil, cisapride, ergot derivatives (dihydroergotamine, ergonovine, ergotamine, methylergonovine), flecainide, midazolam, pimozide, propafenone, quinidine, terfenadine, and triazolam.
• Use cautiously in patients with sulfonamide allergy, diabetes, liver disease, hepatitis B or C, or hemophilia A or B.

NURSING CONSIDERATIONS

• *Alert:* Don't give drug to treatment-naive patients.
• To be effective, drug must be given with 200 mg ritonavir and with other antiretrovirals.
• Monitor patient for signs and symptoms of intracranial hemorrhage, including headache, nausea and vomiting, change in mental status, speech or balance difficulties, and seizures.
• *Alert:* Obtain thorough patient drug history. Many drugs may interact with tipranavir.
• Monitor liver function tests at start of treatment and often during treatment.
• Assess for evidence of hepatitis, such as fatigue, malaise, anorexia, nausea, jaundice, bilirubinemia, acholic stools, liver tenderness, and hepatomegaly.
• If patient develops signs or symptoms of hepatitis, notify prescriber.
• *Alert:* Patients with chronic hepatitis B or C are at increased risk of hepatotoxicity.
• In diabetic patients, monitor glucose level closely; hyperglycemia may occur.
• Obtain baseline cholesterol and triglyceride levels at start of and periodically during therapy.
• Monitor patient for cushingoid symptoms, such as central obesity, buffalo hump, peripheral wasting, facial wasting, and breast enlargement.
• Use cautiously in elderly patients because they are more likely to have decreased organ function, multidrug therapy, and other illnesses.

PATIENT TEACHING

• Explain that drug doesn't cure HIV infection and doesn't reduce the risk of transmitting the virus to others.
• *Alert:* Many drugs may interfere with this drug. Urge patient to tell prescriber about all prescription drugs, OTC drugs, and herbal products he takes.
• Tell patient that drug is effective only when taken with ritonavir and other antiretrovirals.
• Instruct patient to take drug with food.
• Urge patient to stop drug and contact prescriber if he has evidence of hepatitis, such as fatigue, malaise, anorexia, nausea, jaundice, bilirubinemia, acholic stools, or liver tenderness.
• If woman uses hormonal contraceptives, advise use of barrier contraception.
• Tell patient that redistribution or accumulation of body fat may occur.
• Advise woman that breast-feeding isn't recommended during therapy.

zidovudine (azidothymidine, AZT, Compound S)
zid-oh-VEW-den

Novo-AZT†, Retrovir*⚬*

Pharmacologic class: nucleoside reverse transcriptase inhibitor
Pregnancy risk category C

AVAILABLE FORMS
Capsules: 100 mg
Injection: 10 mg/ml
Syrup: 50 mg/5 ml
Tablets: 300 mg

INDICATIONS & DOSAGES
➤ **HIV infection, with other anti-retrovirals**
Adults: 600 mg daily P.O. in divided doses, with other antiretrovirals. If patient is unable to tolerate oral drug, give 1 mg/kg I.V. over 1 hour five to six times daily.
Children ages 6 weeks to 12 years: 160 mg/m² every 8 hours (480 mg/m²/day up to a maximum of 200 mg every 8 hours) with other antiretrovirals. Some prescribers recommend 120 mg/m² I.V. every 6 hours, or 20 mg/m²/hour continuous I.V. infusion.
➤ **To prevent maternal-fetal transmission of HIV**
Pregnant women at more than 14 weeks' gestation: 100 mg P.O. five times daily until the start of labor. Then, 2 mg/kg I.V. over 1 hour followed by a continuous I.V. infusion of 1 mg/kg/hour until the umbilical cord is clamped.
Neonates: 2 mg/kg P.O. every 6 hours starting within 12 hours after birth and continuing until 6 weeks old. Or, give 1.5 mg/kg via I.V. infusion over 30 minutes every 6 hours.
Adjust-a-dose: In patients with significant anemia (hemoglobin level less than 7.5 g/dl or more than 25% below baseline) or significant neutropenia (granulocyte count less than 750 cells/mm³ or more than 50% below baseline), interrupt therapy until evidence proves marrow has recovered. In patients receiving hemodialysis or peritoneal dialysis, give 100 mg P.O. or 1 mg/kg I.V. every 6 to 8 hours. For patients with mild to moderate hepatic dysfunction or liver cirrhosis, daily dose may need to be reduced.

ADMINISTRATION
P.O.
● Drug should be taken on an empty stomach. To avoid esophageal irritation, patient should take drug with adequate fluids, while sitting upright.
● Capsules shouldn't be kept in the kitchen, bathroom, or other places that may be damp or hot. Heat and moisture may cause the drug to break down and affect the intended results.
I.V.
● Give by this route only until oral drug can be tolerated.
● Remove the calculated dose from the vial; add to D_5W to achieve a concentration no greater than 4 mg/ml.
● Infuse drug over 1 hour at a constant rate. Avoid rapid infusion or bolus injection.
● Protect undiluted vials from light.
● Give diluted solution within 8 hours if stored at room temperature or 24 hours if refrigerated.
● **Incompatibilities:** Biological or colloidal solutions, such as blood products or protein-containing solutions; meropenem.

ACTION
Nucleoside reverse transcriptase inhibitor that inhibits replication of HIV by blocking DNA synthesis.

Route	Onset	Peak	Duration
P.O., I.V.	Unknown	30–90 min	Unknown

Half-life: 1 hour.

ADVERSE REACTIONS
CNS: *asthenia, dizziness, fever, headache, malaise, **seizures,** insomnia, paresthesia, somnolence.*
GI: *anorexia, nausea, vomiting, **pancreatitis,** abdominal pain, constipation, diarrhea, dyspepsia, taste perversion.*
Hematologic: *agranulocytosis, severe bone marrow suppression, thrombocytopenia, anemia.*
Hepatic: *hepatomegaly.*
Metabolic: *lactic acidosis.*
Musculoskeletal: *myalgia.*
Respiratory: *cough, wheezing.*
Skin: *rash, diaphoresis.*

INTERACTIONS

Drug-drug. *Acetaminophen:* May decrease bioavailability of zidovudine. Adjust zidovudine dosage, as needed.

Atovaquone, fluconazole, methadone, probenecid, trimethoprim, valproic acid: May increase bioavailability of zidovudine. May need to adjust dosage.

Doxorubicin, ribavirin, stavudine: May have antagonistic effects. Avoid using together.

Ganciclovir, interferon alfa, other bone marrow suppressive or cytotoxic drugs: May increase hematologic toxicity of zidovudine. Use together cautiously.

Phenytoin: May alter phenytoin level and decrease zidovudine clearance by 30%. Monitor patient closely.

EFFECTS ON LAB TEST RESULTS

• May increase ALT, AST, alkaline phosphatase, and LDH levels. May decrease hemoglobin level.

• May decrease granulocyte and platelet counts.

CONTRAINDICATIONS & CAUTIONS

• Contraindicated in patients hypersensitive to drug.

■ **Black Box Warning** Use cautiously and with close monitoring in patients with advanced symptomatic HIV infection and in those with severe bone marrow depression. ■

• Use cautiously in patients with hepatomegaly, hepatitis, or other risk factors for liver disease and in those with renal insufficiency. Monitor renal and liver function tests.

■ **Black Box Warning** Prolonged use has been associated with myopathy. ■

NURSING CONSIDERATIONS

■ **Black Box Warning** Although rare, lactic acidosis without hypoxemia and severe hepatomegaly with steatosis may occur. Notify prescriber if patient develops unexplained tachypnea, dyspnea, or a decrease in bicarbonate level. Therapy may need to be suspended until lactic acidosis is ruled out. ■

• Monitor blood studies every 2 weeks to detect anemia or agranulocytosis. Patients may need reduced dosage or temporary stop to therapy.

• Drug may temporarily decrease morbidity and mortality in certain patients with AIDS.

• ***Look alike–sound alike:*** Don't confuse Retrovir with ritonavir.

PATIENT TEACHING

• Instruct patient to take drug on an empty stomach. To avoid esophageal irritation, tell patient to take drug while sitting upright and with adequate fluids.

• Tell patient to take drug exactly as directed and not to share it with others.

• Remind patient to comply with the dosage schedule. Suggest ways to avoid missing doses, perhaps by using an alarm clock.

• Tell patient that dosages vary among patients and not to change his dosing instructions unless directed to do so by his prescriber.

• Warn patient not to take other drugs for AIDS unless prescriber has approved them.

• Advise patient that monotherapy isn't recommended and to discuss any questions with prescriber.

• Advise patient that blood transfusions may be needed during therapy because of drug-related anemia.

• Tell patient that his gums may bleed. Recommend good mouth care with a soft toothbrush.

• Advise pregnant, HIV-infected patient that drug therapy only reduces the risk of HIV transmission to her newborn. Long-term risks to infants are unknown.

• Tell patient not to keep capsules in the kitchen, bathroom, or other places that may be damp or hot. Heat and moisture may cause the drug to break down and affect the intended results.

• Advise health care worker considering prophylactic use after occupational exposure (such as needlestick injury) that drug's safety and effectiveness haven't been established.

Reactions may be *common,* uncommon, *life-threatening,* or COMMON AND LIFE-THREATENING.
Interaction may have a *rapid onset* or ***delayed onset.***

10

Antituberculotics

cycloserine
ethambutol hydrochloride
isoniazid
rifabutin
rifampin
rifapentine
streptomycin sulfate
(See Chapter 6, AMINOGLYCOSIDES.)

---

cycloserine
sye-kloe-SER-een

Seromycin

Pharmacologic class: isoxazolidine
derivative, d-alanine analogue
Pregnancy risk category C

AVAILABLE FORMS
Capsules: 250 mg

INDICATIONS & DOSAGES
➤ **Adjunctive treatment for
pulmonary or extrapulmonary
tuberculosis (TB)**
Adults: Initially, 250 mg P.O. every
12 hours for 2 weeks; then, if levels are
below 25 to 30 mcg/ml and no toxicity has
developed, increase dosage to 250 mg
every 8 hours for 2 weeks. If optimum
levels still aren't achieved and no toxicity
has developed, then increase dosage to
250 mg every 6 hours. Maximum dosage
is 1 g daily. If CNS toxicity occurs, stop
drug for 1 week, then resume at 250 mg
daily for 2 weeks. If no serious toxic effects occur, increase dosage by 250-mg increments every 10 days until level of 25 to
30 mcg/ml is obtained.
Children ♦: 10 to 20 mg/kg/day P.O. in
two divided doses. Maximum dosage is
1 g daily.
➤ **Acute UTIs**
Adults: 250 mg P.O. every 12 hours for
2 weeks.

ADMINISTRATION
P.O.
● Drug is considered a second-line drug in
TB treatment and should always be given
with other antituberculotics to prevent the
development of resistant organisms.

ACTION
Inhibits cell-wall biosynthesis by interfering with the bacterial use of amino acids;
may be bacteriostatic or bactericidal, depending on the drug level attained at the
site of infection and the organism's
susceptibility.

Route	Onset	Peak	Duration
P.O.	Unknown	4–8 hr	Unknown

Half-life: 10 hours.

ADVERSE REACTIONS
CNS: *coma, seizures, suicidal behavior,*
drowsiness, somnolence, headache,
tremor, dysarthria, vertigo, confusion, loss
of memory, psychosis, hyperirritability,
paresthesia, paresis, hyperreflexia.
CV: *sudden heart failure.*
Other: hypersensitivity reactions (rash,
photosensitivity).

INTERACTIONS
Drug-drug. *Ethionamide:* May increase
neurotoxic adverse reactions. Monitor
patient closely.
Isoniazid: May increase risk of CNS toxi-
city, causing dizziness or drowsiness.
Monitor patient closely.
Drug-lifestyle. *Alcohol use:* May increase
risk of CNS toxicity, causing seizures.
Discourage use together.

EFFECTS ON LAB TEST RESULTS
● May increase transaminase levels.

CONTRAINDICATIONS & CAUTIONS
● Contraindicated in patients hypersensitive to drug, in those who use
alcohol excessively, and in those with
seizure disorders, depression, severe
anxiety, psychosis, or severe renal
insufficiency.

---

†Canada ◇OTC ♦Off-label use ✐Photoguide *Liquid contains alcohol.

• Use cautiously in patients with impaired renal function; reduce dosage in these patients.

NURSING CONSIDERATIONS

• Obtain specimen for culture and sensitivity tests before therapy begins and then periodically to detect possible resistance.
• Use to treat UTIs only when better alternatives are contraindicated and susceptibility to cycloserine is confirmed.
• Monitor level periodically, especially in patients receiving high dosages (more than 500 mg daily), because toxic reactions may occur with levels above 30 mcg/ml.
• Watch patient receiving dosages of more than 500 mg daily for signs and symptoms of CNS toxicity, such as seizures, anxiety, and tremor. Giving 200 to 300 mg pyridoxine daily may help prevent neurotoxic effects.
• Monitor results of hematologic tests and renal and liver function tests.
• Observe patient for psychotic symptoms, hallucinations, and suicidal behavior.
• Monitor patient for hypersensitivity reactions, such as allergic dermatitis.
• Give anticonvulsant, tranquilizer, or sedative to relieve adverse reactions.

PATIENT TEACHING

• Warn patient to avoid alcohol, which may cause serious neurologic reactions.
• Advise patient not to perform hazardous activities if drowsiness occurs.
• Tell patient to report adverse reactions promptly; dosage may need to be adjusted or other drugs prescribed to relieve adverse reactions.

---

ethambutol hydrochloride
e-THAM-byoo-tole

Etibi†, Myambutol

Pharmacologic class: synthetic antituberculotic
Pregnancy risk category B

AVAILABLE FORMS
Tablets: 100 mg, 400 mg

INDICATIONS & DOSAGES
➤ **Adjunctive treatment for pulmonary tuberculosis**
Adults and children older than age 13: In patients who haven't received prior antitubercular therapy, 15 mg/kg P.O. daily as a single dose, combined with other antituberculotics. For retreatment, 25 mg/kg P.O. daily as a single dose for 60 days (or until bacteriologic smears and cultures become negative) with at least one other antituberculotic; then decrease to 15 mg/kg/day as a single dose.

ADMINISTRATION
P.O.
• Always give drug with other antituberculotics to prevent development of resistant organisms.
• Giving drug with food doesn't significantly alter absorption.
• Administer on a once-every-24-hour basis only.

ACTION
May inhibit synthesis of one or more metabolites of susceptible bacteria, changing cell metabolism during cell division; bacteriostatic.

Route	Onset	Peak	Duration
P.O.	Unknown	2–4 hr	Unknown

Half-life: About 3½ hours.

ADVERSE REACTIONS
CNS: dizziness, fever, hallucinations, headache, malaise, mental confusion, peripheral neuritis.
EENT: optic neuritis.
GI: abdominal pain, anorexia, GI upset, nausea, vomiting.
Hematologic: *thrombocytopenia.*
Metabolic: hyperuricemia.
Musculoskeletal: joint pain.
Respiratory: bloody sputum.
Skin: *toxic epidermal necrolysis,* dermatitis, pruritus.
Other: *anaphylactoid reactions,* precipitation of acute gout.

INTERACTIONS
Drug-drug. *Aluminum salts:* May delay and reduce absorption of ethambutol. Separate doses by several hours.

Reactions may be *common,* uncommon, *life-threatening,* or COMMON AND LIFE-THREATENING.
Interaction may have a *rapid onset* or *delayed onset.*

EFFECTS ON LAB TEST RESULTS
• May increase ALT, AST, bilirubin, and uric acid levels. May decrease glucose level.
• May decrease platelet count.

CONTRAINDICATIONS & CAUTIONS
• Contraindicated in children younger than age 13, patients hypersensitive to drug, and patients with optic neuritis.
• Use cautiously in patients with impaired renal function, cataracts, recurrent eye inflammation, gout, or diabetic retinopathy.

NURSING CONSIDERATIONS
• Perform visual acuity and color discrimination tests before and during therapy.
• Ensure that any changes in vision don't result from an underlying condition.
• Obtain AST and ALT levels before therapy, and monitor these levels every 3 to 4 weeks.
• In patients with impaired renal function, base dosage on drug level.
• Monitor uric acid level; observe patient for signs and symptoms of gout.

PATIENT TEACHING
• Reassure patient that visual disturbances usually disappear several weeks to months after drug is stopped. Inflammation of the optic nerve is related to dosage and duration of treatment.
• Inform patient that drug is given with other antituberculotics.
• Stress importance of compliance with drug therapy.
• Advise patient to report adverse reactions to prescriber.

isoniazid (INH, isonicotinic acid hydrazide)
Isotamine†, Nydrazid

Pharmacologic class: isonicotinic acid hydrazine
Pregnancy risk category C

AVAILABLE FORMS
Injection: 100 mg/ml
Oral solution: 50 mg/5 ml
Tablets: 100 mg, 300 mg

INDICATIONS & DOSAGES
➤ **Actively growing tubercle bacilli**
Adults and children age 15 and older:
5 mg/kg daily P.O. or I.M. in a single dose, up to 300 mg/day, with other drugs, continued for 6 months to 2 years. For intermittent multiple-drug regimen, 15 mg/kg (up to 900 mg) P.O. or I.M. up to three times a week.
Infants and children: 10 to 15 mg/kg daily P.O. or I.M. in a single dose, up to 300 mg/day, continued long enough to prevent relapse. Give with at least one other antituberculotic. For intermittent multidrug regimen, 20 to 40 mg/kg (up to 900 mg) P.O. or I.M. two or three times weekly.
➤ **To prevent tubercle bacilli in those exposed to tuberculosis (TB) or those with positive skin test results whose chest X-rays and bacteriologic study results indicate non-progressive TB**
Adults: 300 mg daily P.O. in a single dose, continued for 6 months to 1 year.
Infants and children: 10 mg/kg daily P.O. in a single dose, up to 300 mg/day, continued for up to 1 year.

ADMINISTRATION
P.O.
• Always give drug with other antituberculotics to prevent development of resistant organisms.
• Give drug 1 hour before or 2 hours after meals.
I.M.
• Solution may crystallize at a low temperature. Warm vial to room temperature before use to redissolve crystals.

ACTION
May inhibit cell-wall biosynthesis by interfering with lipid and DNA synthesis; bactericidal.

Route	Onset	Peak	Duration
P.O., I.M.	Unknown	1–2 hr	Unknown

Half-life: 1 to 4 hours.

ADVERSE REACTIONS
CNS: *peripheral neuropathy, seizures, toxic encephalopathy,* memory impairment, toxic psychosis.
EENT: optic neuritis and atrophy.
GI: epigastric distress, nausea, vomiting.

Hematologic: *agranulocytosis, aplastic anemia, thrombocytopenia,* eosinophilia, hemolytic anemia, sideroblastic anemia.
Hepatic: *hepatitis,* bilirubinemia, jaundice.
Metabolic: hyperglycemia, hypocalcemia, hypophosphatemia, *metabolic acidosis.*
Skin: irritation at injection site.
Other: gynecomastia, hypersensitivity reactions, pyridoxine deficiency, rheumatic and lupuslike syndromes.

INTERACTIONS
Drug-drug. *Antacids and laxatives containing aluminum:* May decrease isoniazid absorption. Give isoniazid at least 1 hour before antacid or laxative.
Benzodiazepines, such as diazepam, triazolam: May inhibit metabolic clearance of benzodiazepines that undergo oxidative metabolism, possibly increasing benzodiazepine activity. Monitor patient for adverse reactions.
Carbamazepine, phenytoin: May increase levels of these drugs. Monitor drug levels closely.
Cycloserine: May increase CNS adverse reactions. Use safety precautions.
Disulfiram: May cause neurologic symptoms, including changes in behavior and coordination. Avoid using together.
Enflurane: In rapid acetylators of isoniazid, may cause high-output renal failure because of nephrotoxic inorganic fluoride level. Monitor renal function.
Ketoconazole: May decrease ketoconazole level. Monitor patient for lack of efficacy.
Meperidine: May increase CNS adverse reactions and hypotension. Use safety precautions.
Oral anticoagulants: May enhance anticoagulant activity. Monitor PT and INR.
Phenytoin: May inhibit phenytoin metabolism and increase phenytoin level. Monitor patient for phenytoin toxicity.
Rifampin: May increase the risk of hepatotoxicity. Monitor liver function tests closely.
Drug-food. *Foods containing tyramine (such as aged cheese, beer, and chocolate):* May cause hypertensive crisis. Tell patient to avoid such foods or eat in small quantities.

Drug-lifestyle. *Alcohol use:* May increase risk of drug-related hepatitis. Discourage use of alcohol.

EFFECTS ON LAB TEST RESULTS
● May increase transaminase, glucose, and bilirubin levels. May decrease calcium, phosphate, and hemoglobin levels.
● May increase eosinophil count. May decrease granulocyte and platelet counts.
● May alter result of urine glucose tests that use cupric sulfate method, such as Benedict's reagent and Diastix.

CONTRAINDICATIONS & CAUTIONS
■ **Black Box Warning** Contraindicated in patients with acute hepatic disease or isoniazid-related liver damage. Severe and sometimes fatal hepatitis associated with isoniazid therapy may occur even after months of treatment. If signs or symptoms suggest hepatic damage, discontinue isoniazid because a more severe form of liver damage can occur. ■
● Use cautiously in elderly patients, in those with chronic non–isoniazid-related liver disease or chronic alcoholism, in those with seizure disorders (especially if taking phenytoin), and in those with severe renal impairment.

NURSING CONSIDERATIONS
■ **Black Box Warning** Drug's pharmacokinetics vary among patients because drug is metabolized in the liver by genetically controlled acetylation. Fast acetylators metabolize drug up to five times faster than slow acetylators. About 50% of blacks and whites are fast acetylators; more than 80% of Chinese, Japanese, and Inuits are fast acetylators. A report suggests the risk of fatal hepatitis increases in black and hispanic women and in the postpartum period. ■
● Peripheral neuropathy is more common in patients who are slow acetylators, malnourished, alcoholic, or diabetic.
● Monitor hepatic function closely for changes. Monitor patients older than age 35 monthly and measure hepatic enzyme levels before starting treatment. Elevated liver function study results occur in about 15% of patients; most abnormalities are mild and transient, but some may persist throughout treatment.

Reactions may be *common,* uncommon, *life-threatening,* or COMMON AND LIFE-THREATENING.
Interaction may have a *rapid onset* or *delayed onset.*

• Give pyridoxine to prevent peripheral neuropathy, especially in malnourished patients.

PATIENT TEACHING
• Instruct patient to take drug exactly as prescribed; warn against stopping drug without prescriber's consent.
• Advise patient to take drug 1 hour before or 2 hours after meals.
■ **Black Box Warning** Tell patient to notify prescriber immediately if signs and symptoms of liver impairment occur, such as appetite loss, fatigue, malaise, yellow skin or eye discoloration, and dark urine. ■
• Advise patient to avoid alcoholic beverages while taking drug. Also tell him to avoid certain foods: fish, such as skipjack and tuna, and products containing tyramine, such as aged cheese, beer, and chocolate, because drug has some MAO inhibitor activity.
• Encourage patient to comply fully with treatment, which may take months or years.

rifabutin
rif-ah-BYOO-tin

Mycobutin

Pharmacologic class: semisynthetic ansamycin
Pregnancy risk category B

AVAILABLE FORMS
Capsules: 150 mg

INDICATIONS & DOSAGES
➤ **To prevent disseminated *Mycobacterium avium* complex in patients with advanced HIV infection**
Adults: 300 mg P.O. daily as a single dose or divided b.i.d.

ADMINISTRATION
P.O.
• For patient who has difficulty swallowing, mix drug with soft foods such as applesauce.
• Patient experiencing GI adverse effects, such as nausea or vomiting, may divide total daily dose into two doses and take with food.

ACTION
Inhibits DNA-dependent RNA polymerase in susceptible bacteria, blocking bacterial protein synthesis.

Route	Onset	Peak	Duration
P.O.	Unknown	2–4 hr	Unknown

Half-life: About 2 days.

ADVERSE REACTIONS
CNS: headache, fever.
EENT: eye inflammation.
GI: dyspepsia, eructation, flatulence, diarrhea, nausea, vomiting, abdominal pain, anorexia, taste perversion.
GU: discolored urine.
Hematologic: *neutropenia, leukopenia, thrombocytopenia,* eosinophilia.
Musculoskeletal: myalgia.
Skin: *rash.*

INTERACTIONS
Drug-drug. *Benzodiazepines, beta blockers, buspirone,* **corticosteroids, cyclosporine,** *delavirdine, doxycycline, fluconazole, hydantoins, indinavir, itraconazole, ketoconazole, losartan, macrolides, methadone, morphine, nelfinavir, quinidine, quinine,* **tacrolimus,** *theophylline, tricyclic antidepressants, zolpidem:* May decrease effectiveness of these drugs. Monitor patient for drug effects.
Hormonal contraceptives: May decrease contraceptive effectiveness. Tell patient to use another form of birth control.
Indinavir: May increase rifabutin level. Decrease rifabutin dosage by 50%.
Ritonavir: May increase the risk of rifabutin hematologic toxicity. Use together is contraindicated.
Voriconazole: May decrease therapeutic effects of voriconazole while increasing the risk of rifabutin adverse effects. Use together is contraindicated.
Warfarin: May decrease effectiveness of warfarin. May require higher dosages of anticoagulants. Monitor PT and INR.
Drug-food. *High-fat foods:* May reduce rate but not extent of absorption. Discourage use together.

EFFECTS ON LAB TEST RESULTS
• May increase aminotransferase level.
• May decrease neutrophil, WBC, and platelet counts.

CONTRAINDICATIONS & CAUTIONS

● Contraindicated in patients hypersensitive to drug or other rifamycin derivatives, such as rifampin, and in patients with active tuberculosis because single-drug therapy with rifabutin increases risk of inducing bacterial resistance to both rifabutin and rifampin.

● Use cautiously in patients with neutropenia and thrombocytopenia.

NURSING CONSIDERATIONS

● In patients with neutropenia or thrombocytopenia, obtain baseline hematologic studies and repeat periodically.

● *Look alike–sound alike:* Don't confuse rifabutin with rifampin or rifapentine.

PATIENT TEACHING

● Instruct patient to take drug for as long as prescribed, exactly as directed, even after feeling better.

● Tell patient experiencing GI adverse effects, such as nausea or vomiting, to divide total daily dose into 2 doses and to take with food.

● Tell patient that drug may cause brownish orange staining of urine, feces, sputum, saliva, tears, and skin. Tell him to avoid wearing soft contact lenses because they may be permanently stained.

● Instruct patient to report sensitivity to light, excessive tears, or eye pain immediately.

● Advise patient to report tingling and joint stiffness, swelling, or tenderness.

---

rifampin (rifampicin)
RIF-am-pin

Rifadin, Rimactane, Rofact†

Pharmacologic class: semisynthetic rifamycin
Pregnancy risk category C

AVAILABLE FORMS

Capsules: 150 mg, 300 mg
Powder for injection: 600 mg

INDICATIONS & DOSAGES

➤ **Pulmonary tuberculosis, with other antituberculotics**
Adults: 10 mg/kg P.O. or I.V. daily in single dose. Give oral doses 1 hour before or 2 hours after meals with a full glass of water. Maximum daily dose is 600 mg.
Children age 5 and older: 10 to 20 mg/kg P.O. or I.V. daily in single dose. Give oral doses 1 hour before or 2 hours after meals with a full glass of water. Maximum daily dose is 600 mg. Give with other antituberculotics.

➤ **Meningococcal carriers**
Adults: 600 mg P.O. or I.V. every 12 hours for 2 days; or 600 mg P.O. or I.V. once daily for 4 days.
Children ages 1 month to 12 years: 10 mg/kg P.O. or I.V. every 12 hours for 2 days, not to exceed 600 mg/day; or 20 mg/kg once daily for 4 days.
Neonates: 5 mg/kg P.O. or I.V. every 12 hours for 2 days.

➤ ***Mycobacterium avium* complex ◆**
Adults: 600 mg P.O. or I.V. daily as part of a multiple-drug regimen.

ADMINISTRATION

P.O.
● Give drug with at least one other antituberculotic.
● For best absorption, give capsules 1 hour before or 2 hours after meals.
● For the patient who can't tolerate capsules on an empty stomach, give drug with meals and a full glass of water.
I.V.
● Reconstitute drug with 10 ml of sterile water for injection to yield 60 mg/ml.
● Add to 100 ml of D_5W and infuse over 30 minutes, or add to 500 ml of D_5W and infuse over 3 hours.
● When dextrose is contraindicated, dilute with normal saline solution for injection.
● Once prepared, dilutions in D_5W are stable for up to 4 hours and dilutions in normal saline solution are stable for up to 24 hours at room temperature.
● **Incompatibilities:** Diltiazem, minocycline, other IV solutions.

ACTION

Inhibits DNA-dependent RNA polymerase, which impairs RNA synthesis; bactericidal.

Reactions may be *common,* uncommon, *life-threatening,* or COMMON AND LIFE-THREATENING.
Interaction may have a *rapid onset* or **delayed onset.**

Route	Onset	Peak	Duration
P.O.	Unknown	2–4 hr	Unknown
I.V.	Unknown	Unknown	Unknown

Half-life: 1¼ to 5 hours.

ADVERSE REACTIONS

CNS: headache, fatigue, drowsiness, behavioral changes, dizziness, mental confusion, generalized numbness, ataxia.
CV: *shock.*
EENT: visual disturbances, exudative conjunctivitis.
GI: *pancreatitis, pseudomembranous colitis,* epigastric distress, anorexia, nausea, vomiting, abdominal pain, diarrhea, flatulence, sore mouth and tongue.
GU: *acute renal failure,* hemoglobinuria, hematuria, menstrual disturbances.
Hematologic: *thrombocytopenia, transient leukopenia,* eosinophilia, hemolytic anemia.
Hepatic: *hepatotoxicity.*
Metabolic: hyperuricemia.
Musculoskeletal: osteomalacia.
Respiratory: shortness of breath, wheezing.
Skin: pruritus, urticaria, rash.
Other: flulike syndrome, discoloration of body fluids, porphyria exacerbation.

INTERACTIONS

Drug-drug. *Acetaminophen, amiodarone, analgesics, anticonvulsants, barbiturates, beta blockers, cardiac glycosides, chloramphenicol, clofibrate,* **corticosteroids, cyclosporine,** *dapsone, delavirdine, diazepam, digoxin, disopyramide, doxycycline, enalapril, fluoroquinolones, hormonal contraceptives, hydantoins, losartan, methadone, mexiletine, midazolam, nifedipine, ondansetron, opioids, progestins, propafenone, quinidine,* **ritonavir,** *sulfonylureas,* **tacrolimus,** *theophylline, tocainide, triazolam, tricyclic antidepressants, verapamil, zidovudine, zolpidem:* May decrease effectiveness of these drugs. Monitor effectiveness.
Anticoagulants: May increase requirements for anticoagulant. Monitor PT and INR closely and adjust dosage of anticoagulants.
Halothane: May increase risk of hepatotoxicity. Monitor liver function test results.

Isoniazid: May increase risk of hepatotoxicity. Monitor liver function test results.
Ketoconazole, para-aminosalicylate sodium: May interfere with absorption of rifampin. Separate doses by 8 to 12 hours.
Macrolide antibiotics, protease inhibitors: May inhibit rifampin metabolism but increase metabolism of other drug. Monitor patient for clinical and adverse effects.
Probenecid: May increase rifampin levels. Use together cautiously.
Voriconazole: May decrease voriconazole's therapeutic effects while increasing the risk of rifampin adverse effects. Use together is contraindicated.
Drug-lifestyle. *Alcohol use:* May increase risk of hepatotoxicity. Discourage use together.

EFFECTS ON LAB TEST RESULTS

- May increase ALT, AST, alkaline phosphatase, bilirubin, and uric acid levels. May decrease hemoglobin level.
- May increase eosinophil counts. May decrease platelet and WBC counts.
- May alter standard folate and vitamin B_{12} assay results.

CONTRAINDICATIONS & CAUTIONS

- Contraindicated in patients hypersensitive to rifampin or related drugs.
- Use cautiously in patients with liver disease.
- Use in pregnant women only if potential benefit justifies potential risk to fetus.

NURSING CONSIDERATIONS

- Monitor hepatic function, hematopoietic studies, and uric acid levels. Drug's systemic effects may asymptomatically raise liver function test results and uric acid level.
- Watch for and report to prescriber signs and symptoms of hepatic impairment.
- Drug may cause hemorrhage in neonates and mother when drug is given during last few weeks of pregnancy. Monitor clotting parameters closely, and treat with vitamin K as needed.
- *Look alike–sound alike:* Don't confuse rifampin with rifabutin or rifapentine.

---

†Canada   ◊ OTC   ♦ Off-label use   ✐Photoguide   *Liquid contains alcohol.

PATIENT TEACHING
● Instruct patient who can't tolerate capsules on an empty stomach to take drug with meals and a full glass of water.
● Advise patient who is unable to swallow capsules whole that an oral suspension can be prepared by the pharmacist.
● Warn patient that he may feel drowsy and that drug can turn body fluids red-orange and permanently stain contact lenses.
● Advise a woman using hormonal contraceptive to consider another form of birth control.
● Advise patient to contact prescriber if he experiences fever, loss of appetite, malaise, nausea, vomiting, dark urine, or yellow discoloration of the eyes or skin.
● Advise patient to avoid alcohol during drug therapy.

rifapentine
rif-ah-PIN-ten

Priftin

Pharmacologic class: synthetic rifamycin
Pregnancy risk category C

AVAILABLE FORMS
Tablets (film-coated): 150 mg

INDICATIONS & DOSAGES
➤ **Pulmonary tuberculosis (TB), with at least one other antituberculotic to which the isolate is susceptible**
Adults: During intensive phase of short-course therapy, 600 mg P.O. twice weekly for 2 months, with an interval between doses of at least 3 days (72 hours). During continuation phase of short-course therapy, 600 mg P.O. once weekly for 4 months, combined with isoniazid or another drug to which the isolate is susceptible.

ADMINISTRATION
P.O.
● Give drug with pyridoxine (vitamin B_6) in malnourished patients; in those predisposed to neuropathy, such as alcoholics and diabetics; and in adolescents.
● *Alert:* Give drug with appropriate daily companion drugs. Compliance with all

drug regimens, especially with daily companion drugs on the days when rifapentine isn't given, is crucial for early sputum conversion and protection from relapse of TB.

ACTION
Inhibits DNA-dependent RNA polymerase in susceptible strains of *Mycobacterium tuberculosis.* Demonstrates bactericidal activity against the organism both intracellularly and extracellularly.

Route	Onset	Peak	Duration
P.O.	Unknown	5–6 hr	Unknown

Half-life: 13 hours.

ADVERSE REACTIONS
CNS: headache, dizziness, pain.
CV: hypertension.
GI: anorexia, nausea, vomiting, dyspepsia, diarrhea.
GU: pyuria, proteinuria, hematuria, urinary casts.
Hematologic: *leukopenia, neutropenia,* anemia, *thrombocytosis.*
Metabolic: *hyperuricemia.*
Musculoskeletal: arthralgia.
Respiratory: hemoptysis.
Skin: rash, pruritus, acne, maculopapular rash.

INTERACTIONS
Drug-drug. *Antiarrhythmics (disopyramide, mexiletine, quinidine, tocainide), antibiotics (chloramphenicol, clarithromycin, dapsone, doxycycline, fluoroquinolones), anticonvulsants (phenytoin), antifungals (fluconazole, itraconazole, ketoconazole), barbiturates, benzodiazepines (diazepam), beta blockers, calcium channel blockers (diltiazem, nifedipine, verapamil), cardiac glycosides, clofibrate,* **corticosteroids,** *haloperidol, HIV protease inhibitors (indinavir, nelfinavir, ritonavir, saquinavir), hormonal contraceptives,* **immunosuppressants (cyclosporine, tacrolimus),** *levothyroxine, opioid analgesics (methadone), oral anticoagulants (warfarin), oral hypoglycemics (sulfonylureas), progestins, quinine, reverse transcriptase inhibitors (delavirdine, zidovudine), sildenafil, theophylline, tricyclic antidepressants (amitriptyline, nortriptyline):* May decrease activity of these

drugs because of cytochrome P-450 enzyme metabolism. May need to adjust dosage.

Ritonavir: May decrease ritonavir levels. Carefully monitor patient's response.

EFFECTS ON LAB TEST RESULTS
• May increase uric acid, ALT, and AST levels. May decrease hemoglobin level.
• May increase platelet count. May decrease neutrophil and WBC counts.
• May alter folate and vitamin B_{12} assay results.

CONTRAINDICATIONS & CAUTIONS
• Contraindicated in patients hypersensitive to rifamycins (rifapentine, rifampin, or rifabutin).
• Use drug cautiously and with frequent monitoring in patients with liver disease.

NURSING CONSIDERATIONS
• Rifamycin antibiotics may cause hepatotoxicity. Obtain baseline liver function test results before therapy.
• If used during the last 2 weeks of pregnancy, drug may lead to postnatal hemorrhage in mother or infant. Monitor clotting parameters closely if drug is used at that time.
• *Look alike–sound alike:* Don't confuse rifapentine with rifabutin or rifampin.

PATIENT TEACHING
• Stress importance of strict compliance with this drug regimen and that of daily companion drugs, as well as needed follow-up visits and laboratory tests.
• Advise woman to use nonhormonal birth control methods.
• Tell patient to take drug with food if nausea, vomiting, or GI upset occurs.
• Instruct patient to report to prescriber fever, appetite loss, malaise, nausea, vomiting, darkened urine, yellowish skin and eyes, joint pain or swelling, or excessive loose stools or diarrhea.
• Instruct patient to protect pills from excessive heat.
• Tell patient that drug may turn body fluids red-orange and permanently stain contact lenses.

11

Antivirals

acyclovir
acyclovir sodium
adefovir dipivoxil
amantadine hydrochloride
   (See Chapter 40, ANTIPARKINSONIANS.)
cidofovir
entecavir
famciclovir
foscarnet sodium
ganciclovir
oseltamivir phosphate
ribavirin
telbivudine
valacyclovir hydrochloride
valganciclovir
zanamivir

---

acyclovir
ay-SYE-kloe-ver

Zovirax

acyclovir sodium
Zovirax

Pharmacologic class: synthetic
purine nucleoside
Pregnancy risk category B

AVAILABLE FORMS
Capsules: 200 mg
Injection: 500 mg/vial, 1 g/vial
Suspension: 200 mg/5 ml
Tablets: 400 mg, 800 mg

INDICATIONS & DOSAGES
➤ **First and recurrent episodes of
mucocutaneous herpes simplex
virus (HSV-1 and HSV-2) infections
in immunocompromised patients;
severe first episodes of genital herpes in patients who aren't immunocompromised**
Adults and children age 12 and older:
5 mg/kg given I.V. over 1 hour every
8 hours for 7 days. Give for 5 to
7 days for severe first episode of
genital herpes.

Children younger than age 12: Give
10 mg/kg I.V. over 1 hour every 8 hours
for 7 days.
➤ **First genital herpes episode**
Adults: 200 mg P.O. every 4 hours
while awake, five times daily; or
400 mg P.O. every 8 hours. Continue for
10 days.
➤ **Intermittent therapy for recurrent genital herpes**
Adults: 200 mg P.O. every 4 hours while
awake, five times daily. Continue for
5 days. Begin therapy at first sign of
recurrence.
➤ **Long-term suppressive therapy
for recurrent genital herpes**
Adults: 400 mg P.O. b.i.d. for up to
12 months. Or, 200 mg P.O. three to five
times daily for up to 12 months.
➤ **Varicella (chickenpox) infections
in immunocompromised patients**
Adults and children age 12 and older:
10 mg/kg I.V. over 1 hour every 8 hours
for 7 days. Dosage for obese patients is
10 mg/kg based on ideal body weight
every 8 hours for 7 days. Don't exceed
maximum dosage equivalent of 20 mg/kg
every 8 hours.
Children younger than age 12: Give
20 mg/kg I.V. over 1 hour every 8 hours
for 7 days.
➤ **Varicella infection in immunocompetent patients**
*Adults and children who weigh more than
40 kg (88 lb):* 800 mg P.O. q.i.d. for
5 days.
*Children age 2 and older, who weigh
less than 40 kg:* 20 mg/kg (maximum
800 mg/dose) P.O. q.i.d. for 5 days. Start
therapy as soon as symptoms appear.
➤ **Acute herpes zoster infection in
immunocompetent patients**
Adults and children age 12 and older:
800 mg P.O. every 4 hours five times daily
for 7 to 10 days.
➤ **Herpes simplex encephalitis**
Adults and children age 12 and older:
10 mg/kg I.V. over 1 hour every 8 hours
for 10 days.

Reactions may be *common*, uncommon, *life-threatening*, or COMMON AND LIFE-THREATENING.
Interaction may have a *rapid onset* or *delayed onset*.

Children ages 3 months to 12 years:
20 mg/kg I.V. over 1 hour every 8 hours
for 10 days.

➤ **Neonatal herpes simplex virus
infection**
Neonates to 3 months old: 10 mg/kg I.V.
over 1 hour every 8 hours for 10 days.

Adjust-a-dose: For patients receiving the
I.V. form, if creatinine clearance is 25 to
50 ml/minute, give 100% of dose every
12 hours; if clearance is 10 to 24 ml/
minute, give 100% of dose every 24 hours;
if clearance is less than 10 ml/minute, give
50% of dose every 24 hours.

For patients receiving the P.O. form, if
normal dose is 200 mg every 4 hours five
times daily and creatinine clearance is less
than 10 ml/minute, give 200 mg P.O. every
12 hours. If normal dose is 400 mg every
12 hours and clearance is less than 10 ml/
minute, give 200 mg every 12 hours. If
normal dose is 800 mg every 4 hours
five times daily and clearance is 10 to
25 ml/minute, give 800 mg every 8 hours;
if clearance is less than 10 ml/minute, give
800 mg every 12 hours.

ADMINISTRATION
P.O.
• Give drug without regard for meals, but
give with food if stomach irritation occurs.
• Patient should take drug as prescribed,
even after he feels better.
I.V.
• Solutions concentrated at 7 mg/ml or
more may cause a higher risk of
phlebitis.
• Encourage fluid intake because patient
must be adequately hydrated during infusion.
• Bolus injection, dehydration (decreased
urine output), renal disease, and use with
other nephrotoxic drugs increase the risk
of renal toxicity. Don't give by bolus
injection.
• Give I.V. infusion over at least 1 hour to
prevent renal tubular damage.
• Monitor intake and output, especially
during the first 2 hours after administration.
• *Alert:* Don't give I.M. or subcutaneously.
• **Incompatibilities:** Amifostine, aztreonam, biological or colloidal solutions, cefepime, cisatracurium besylate, diltiazem
hydrochloride, dobutamine hydrochloride,

dopamine hydrochloride, fludarabine
phosphate, foscarnet sodium, gemcitabine
hydrochloride, idarubicin hydrochloride,
levofloxacin, meperidine hydrochloride,
meropenem, morphine sulfate, ondansetron
hydrochloride, parabens, piperacillin sodium and tazobactam sodium, sargramostim,
tacrolimus, vinorelbine tartrate.

ACTION
Interferes with DNA synthesis and inhibits viral multiplication.

Route	Onset	Peak	Duration
P.O.	Unknown	2½ hr	Unknown
I.V.	Immediate	Immediate	Unknown

Half-life: 2 to 3½ hours with normal renal
function; up to 19 hours with renal
impairment.

ADVERSE REACTIONS
CNS: *headache, malaise, encephalopathic
changes (including lethargy, obtunda-
tion, tremor, confusion, hallucinations,
agitation, seizures, coma).*
GI: *nausea, vomiting,* diarrhea.
GU: *acute renal failure,* hematuria.
Hematologic: *leukopenia, thrombocytopenia,* thrombocytosis.
Skin: *inflammation or phlebitis at injection site,* itching, rash, urticaria.

INTERACTIONS
Drug-drug. *Interferon:* May have syner-
gistic effect. Monitor patient closely.
Probenecid: May increase acyclovir level.
Monitor patient for possible toxicity.
Zidovudine: May cause drowsiness or
lethargy. Use together cautiously.

EFFECTS ON LAB TEST RESULTS
• May increase BUN and creatinine levels.
• May decrease WBC count. May increase
or decrease platelet count.

CONTRAINDICATIONS & CAUTIONS
■ **Black Box Warning** Lactic acidosis and
severe hepatomegaly with steatosis, including fatal cases, have been reported. ■
■ **Black Box Warning** HIV resistance
may occur in chronic hepatitis B patients
with unrecognized or untreated HIV
infection treated with anti-hepatitis B
therapies. ■

■ **Black Box Warning** Patients who discontinue therapy for hepatitis B may experience severe, acute exacerbations of hepatitis. Monitor hepatic function closely. ■
• Contraindicated in patients hypersensitive to drug.
• Use cautiously in patients with neurologic problems, renal disease, or dehydration, and in those receiving other nephrotoxic drugs.
• Adequate studies haven't been done in pregnant women; use only if potential benefits outweigh risks to fetus.

NURSING CONSIDERATIONS
■ **Black Box Warning** Long-term acyclovir use may result in nephrotoxicity. In patients with renal disease or dehydration and in those taking other nephrotoxic drugs, monitor renal function. ■
• Encephalopathic changes are more likely to occur in patients with neurologic disorders and in those who have had neurologic reactions to cytotoxic drugs.
• *Look alike–sound alike:* Don't confuse acyclovir sodium (Zovirax) with acetazolamide sodium (Diamox) vials, which may look alike.
• *Look alike–sound alike:* Don't confuse Zovirax with Zyvox.

PATIENT TEACHING
• Tell patient to take drug as prescribed, even after he feels better.
• Tell patient drug is effective in managing herpes infection but doesn't eliminate or cure it. Warn patient that drug won't prevent spread of infection to others.
• Tell patient to avoid sexual contact while visible lesions are present.
• Teach patient about early signs and symptoms of herpes infection (such as tingling, itching, or pain). Tell him to notify prescriber and get a prescription for drug before the infection fully develops. Early treatment is most effective.

adefovir dipivoxil
ah-DEF-oh-veer

Hepsera

Pharmacologic class: acyclic nucleotide analogue
Pregnancy risk category C

AVAILABLE FORMS
Tablets: 10 mg

INDICATIONS & DOSAGES
➤ **Chronic hepatitis B infection**
Adults: 10 mg P.O. once daily.
Adjust-a-dose: In patients with creatinine clearance of 20 to 49 ml/minute, give 10 mg P.O. every 48 hours. In patients with clearance of 10 to 19 ml/minute, give 10 mg P.O. every 72 hours. In patients receiving hemodialysis, give 10 mg P.O. every 7 days, after dialysis session.

ADMINISTRATION
P.O.
• Give drug without regard for meals.

ACTION
An acyclic nucleotide analogue that inhibits hepatitis B virus reverse transcription via viral DNA chain termination.

Route	Onset	Peak	Duration
P.O.	Unknown	1–4 hr	Unknown

Half-life: Unknown.

ADVERSE REACTIONS
CNS: *asthenia,* fever, headache.
EENT: pharyngitis, sinusitis.
GI: abdominal pain, diarrhea, dyspepsia, flatulence, nausea, vomiting.
GU: *renal failure, renal insufficiency, hematuria,* glycosuria.
Hepatic: *hepatic failure,* hepatomegaly with steatosis.
Metabolic: *lactic acidosis.*
Respiratory: cough.
Skin: pruritus, rash.

INTERACTIONS
Drug-drug. *Ibuprofen:* May increase adefovir bioavailability. Monitor patient for adverse effects.

Reactions may be *common,* uncommon, *life-threatening,* or COMMON AND LIFE-THREATENING.
Interaction may have a *rapid onset* or **delayed onset.**

Nephrotoxic drugs (aminoglycosides, cyclosporine, NSAIDs, tacrolimus, vancomycin): May increase risk of nephrotoxicity. Use together cautiously.

EFFECTS ON LAB TEST RESULTS
• May increase ALT, amylase, AST, CK, creatinine, and lactate levels.

CONTRAINDICATIONS & CAUTIONS
• Contraindicated in patients hypersensitive to any component of the drug.
• Use cautiously in patients with renal dysfunction, in those receiving nephrotoxic drugs, and in those with known risk factors for hepatic disease.
• In elderly patients, use cautiously because they're more likely to have decreased renal and cardiac function.
• Safety and effectiveness in children haven't been established.

NURSING CONSIDERATIONS
■ **Black Box Warning** Due to increased risk of nephrotoxicity, monitor renal function, especially in patients with renal dysfunction or those taking nephrotoxic drugs. ■
■ **Black Box Warning** Patients may develop lactic acidosis and severe hepatomegaly with steatosis during treatment. Women, obese patients, and those taking antiretrovirals are at higher risk. ■
■ **Black Box Warning** Due to increased risk of hepatotoxicity, monitor hepatic function. Notify prescriber if patient develops signs or symptoms of lactic acidosis and severe hepatomegaly with steatosis. Stop drug, if needed. ■
■ **Black Box Warning** Stopping adefovir may cause severe worsening of hepatitis. Monitor hepatic function closely in patients who stop antihepatitis B therapy. ■
• The ideal length of treatment hasn't been established.
■ **Black Box Warning** Offer patients HIV antibody testing; drug may promote resistance to antiretrovirals in patients with unrecognized or untreated HIV infection. ■
• For pregnant women, call the Antiretroviral Pregnancy Registry at 1-800-258-4263 to monitor fetal outcome.

PATIENT TEACHING
• Inform the patient that drug may be taken without regard to meals.

• Tell patient to immediately report weakness, muscle pain, trouble breathing, stomach pain with nausea and vomiting, dizziness, light-headedness, fast or irregular heartbeat, and feeling cold, especially in arms and legs.
• Warn patient not to stop taking this drug unless directed because it could cause hepatitis to become worse.
• Instruct woman to tell her prescriber if she becomes pregnant or is breast-feeding. It's unknown if drug appears in breast milk. Use cautiously in breast-feeding women.

---

cidofovir
sye-DOE-fo-veer

Vistide

Pharmacologic class: nucleotide analogue
Pregnancy risk category C

AVAILABLE FORMS
Injection: 75 mg/ml in 5-ml vial

INDICATIONS & DOSAGES
➤ **CMV retinitis in patients with AIDS**
Adults: Initially, 5 mg/kg I.V. infused over 1 hour once weekly for 2 consecutive weeks; then maintenance dose of 5 mg/kg I.V. infused over 1 hour once every 2 weeks. Give probenecid and prehydration with normal saline solution I.V. simultaneously to reduce risk of nephrotoxicity.
Adjust-a-dose: For patients with creatinine level of 0.3 to 0.4 mg/dl above baseline, reduce dosage to 3 mg/kg at same rate and frequency. If creatinine level reaches 0.5 mg/dl or more above baseline, or patient develops 3+ or higher proteinuria, stop drug.

ADMINISTRATION
I.V.
■ **Black Box Warning** Drug has mutagenic effects; prepare it in a class II laminar flow biological safety cabinet and wear surgical gloves and a closed-front surgical gown with knit cuffs. ■
• If drug contacts skin, wash and flush thoroughly with water.

- Place excess drug and all materials used to prepare and give it in a leak-proof, puncture-proof container.
- Let drug reach room temperature before use.
- Using a syringe, withdraw prescribed dose and add to an I.V. bag containing 100 ml of normal saline solution.
- Infuse over 1 hour using an infusion pump.
- Because of the risk of nephrotoxicity, don't exceed recommended dosages or frequency or rate of infusion.
- Discard any partially used vials.
- Give within 24 hours of preparing. Admixture may be refrigerated at 36° to 46° F (2° to 8° C) for up to 24 hours.
- ■ **Black Box Warning** Due to increased risk of nephrotoxicity, give 1 L normal saline solution I.V. over 1- to 2-hour period, immediately before giving drug. ■
- **Alert:** Give probenecid with cidofovir.
- Compatibility of admixture with Ringer's, lactated Ringer's, and bacteriostatic solutions hasn't been evaluated.
- **Incompatibilities:** Other drugs or supplements.

ACTION
Suppresses CMV replication by selective inhibition of viral DNA synthesis.

Route	Onset	Peak	Duration
I.V.	Unknown	Unknown	Unknown

Half-life: Unknown.

ADVERSE REACTIONS
CNS: *asthenia, fever, headache,* **seizures,** abnormal gait, amnesia, anxiety, confusion, depression, dizziness, hallucinations, insomnia, neuropathy, paresthesia, somnolence, malaise.
CV: hypotension, orthostatic hypotension, pallor, syncope, tachycardia, vasodilation.
EENT: *ocular hypotony,* abnormal vision, amblyopia, conjunctivitis, eye disorders, iritis, pharyngitis, retinal detachment, rhinitis, sinusitis, uveitis.
GI: *abdominal pain, anorexia, diarrhea, nausea, vomiting,* aphthous stomatitis, colitis, constipation, dry mouth, dyspepsia, dysphagia, flatulence, gastritis, melena, mouth ulcers, oral candidiasis, rectal disorders, stomatitis, taste perversion, tongue discoloration.

GU: *proteinuria,* **nephrotoxicity,** glycosuria, hematuria, urinary incontinence, UTI.
Hematologic: *anemia,* **neutropenia, thrombocytopenia.**
Hepatic: hepatomegaly.
Metabolic: fluid imbalance, hyperglycemia, hyperlipemia, hypocalcemia, hypokalemia, weight loss.
Musculoskeletal: arthralgia, myalgia, myasthenia, pain in back, chest, or neck.
Respiratory: *dyspnea,* asthma, bronchitis, coughing, hiccups, increased sputum, lung disorders, pneumonia.
Skin: *alopecia, rash,* acne, dry skin, pruritus, skin discoloration, sweating, urticaria.
Other: *chills, infections,* **sarcoma, sepsis,** allergic reactions, facial edema, herpes simplex.

INTERACTIONS
Drug-drug. *Nephrotoxic drugs (such as aminoglycosides, amphotericin B, foscarnet, I.V. pentamidine):* May increase nephrotoxicity. Avoid using together.

EFFECTS ON LAB TEST RESULTS
- May increase alkaline phosphatase, ALT, AST, BUN, creatinine, LDH, and urine protein levels. May decrease bicarbonate and hemoglobin levels.
- May decrease neutrophil and platelet counts.

CONTRAINDICATIONS & CAUTIONS
- Contraindicated in patients hypersensitive to drug, probenecid, and other sulfa drugs.
- ■ **Black Box Warning** Renal failure has occurred with as few as one or two doses of cidofovir. Contraindicated in patients receiving other drugs with nephrotoxic potential (stop such drugs at least 7 days before starting cidofovir therapy) and in those with creatinine level exceeding 1.5 mg/dl, creatinine clearance of 55 ml/minute or less, or urine protein level of 100 mg/dl or more (equivalent to 2+ proteinuria or more). ■
- Use within 1 month of placement of a ganciclovir ocular implant may cause profound hypotony.
- Safety and effectiveness in children haven't been established.

Reactions may be *common,* uncommon, *life-threatening,* or COMMON AND LIFE-THREATENING.
Interaction may have a *rapid onset* or **delayed onset.**

• Use cautiously in patients with renal impairment. Monitor renal function tests and patient's fluid balance.

NURSING CONSIDERATIONS
■ **Black Box Warning** Safety and effectiveness of drug haven't been established for treating other CMV infections, congenital or neonatal CMV disease, or CMV disease in patients not infected with HIV. ■

■ **Black Box Warning** Due to increased risk of nephrotoxicity and bone marrow suppression, monitor creatinine and urine protein levels and WBC counts with differential before each dose. ■

• Drug may cause Fanconi syndrome and decreased bicarbonate level with renal tubular damage. Monitor patient closely.

• Drug may cause granulocytopenia.

• Stop zidovudine therapy or reduce dosage by 50% on the days when cidofovir is given; probenecid reduces metabolic clearance of zidovudine.

PATIENT TEACHING
• Inform patient that drug doesn't cure CMV retinitis and that regular ophthalmologic examinations are needed.

• Alert patient taking zidovudine that he'll need to obtain dosage guidelines on days cidofovir is given.

• Tell patient that close monitoring of kidney function will be needed and that abnormalities may require a change in therapy.

• Stress importance of completing a full course of probenecid with each cidofovir dose. Tell patient to take probenecid after a meal to decrease nausea.

• Patients with AIDS should use effective contraception, especially during and for 1 month after treatment.

• Advise men to practice barrier contraception during and for 3 months after treatment.

entecavir
en-TEK-ah-veer

Baraclude

Pharmacologic class: guanosine nucleoside analogue
Pregnancy risk category C

AVAILABLE FORMS
Oral solution: 0.05 mg/ml
Tablets: 0.5 mg, 1 mg

INDICATIONS & DOSAGES
➤ **Chronic hepatitis B virus (HBV) infection in patients with active viral replication and either persistently increased aminotransferase levels or histologically active disease**
Adults and adolescents age 16 and older who have had no previous nucleoside treatment: 0.5 mg P.O. once daily at least 2 hours before or after a meal.
Adjust-a-dose: If creatinine clearance is 30 to 49 ml/minute, give 0.25 mg P.O. once daily. If clearance is 10 to 30 ml/minute, give 0.15 mg P.O. once daily. If clearance is less than 10 ml/minute or patient is undergoing hemodialysis or continuous ambulatory peritoneal dialysis, give 0.05 mg P.O. once daily.
Adults and adolescents age 16 and older who have a history of viremia and are taking lamivudine or have resistance mutations: 1 mg P.O. once daily at least 2 hours before or after a meal.
   If creatinine clearance is 30 to 49 ml/minute, give 0.5 mg P.O. once daily. If clearance is 10 to 30 ml/minute, give 0.3 mg P.O. once daily. If clearance is less than 10 ml/minute or patient is undergoing hemodialysis or continuous ambulatory peritoneal dialysis, give 0.1 mg P.O. once daily.

ADMINISTRATION
P.O.
• Drug should be taken on an empty stomach at least 2 hours before or after a meal to increase absorption.

ACTION
Inhibits HBV polymerase and reduces viral DNA levels.

Route	Onset	Peak	Duration
P.O.	Unknown	½ –1½ hr	Unknown

Half-life: About 5 or 6 days.

ADVERSE REACTIONS
CNS: dizziness, fatigue, headache.
GI: diarrhea, dyspepsia, nausea.
GU: glycosuria, hematuria.
Hepatic: hepatomegaly.
Metabolic: *lactic acidosis.*

INTERACTIONS
Drug-drug. *Cyclosporine, tacrolimus:* May further decrease renal function. Monitor renal function carefully.
Drugs that reduce renal function or compete for active tubular secretion: May increase level of either drug. Monitor renal function, and watch for adverse effects.
Drug-food. *All foods:* Delays absorption and decreases drug level. Give drug at least 2 hours before or after a meal.

EFFECTS ON LAB TEST RESULTS
• May increase ALT, amylase, AST, blood glucose, creatinine, lipase, and total bilirubin levels.
• May decrease platelet count.

CONTRAINDICATIONS & CAUTIONS
• Contraindicated in patients hypersensitive to drug or its components.
• Use cautiously in patients with renal impairment and in patients who have had a liver transplant.
• Use in patients coinfected with HIV/ HBV who aren't receiving effective anti-HIV treatment. Use caution with these patients.

NURSING CONSIDERATIONS
■ **Black Box Warning** Drug may cause life-threatening lactic acidosis and severe hepatomegaly with steatosis. ■
■ **Black Box Warning** HBV infection may worsen severely after therapy stops. ■
• Monitor hepatic function for several months in patients who stop therapy. If appropriate, start therapy for HBV infection.
• Use cautiously in pregnant women only if maternal benefit outweighs fetal risk. For monitoring of fetal outcome

data, call the pregnancy registry at 1-800-258-4263.
• It's unknown if drug appears in breast milk. Avoid use in breast-feeding women.
• In elderly patients, adjust dosage for age-related decrease in renal function.

PATIENT TEACHING
• Tell patient to take drug on an empty stomach at least 2 hours before or after a meal.
• Caution against mixing or diluting oral solution with any other substance. Teach proper use of dosing spoon.
• Tell patient to report to prescriber any new adverse effects from this drug and any new drugs he's taking.
• Explain that drug doesn't reduce the risk of HBV transmission to others.
• Teach patient the signs and symptoms of lactic acidosis, such as muscle pain, weakness, dyspnea, GI distress, cold hands and feet, dizziness, or fast or irregular heartbeat.
• Teach patient the signs and symptoms of hepatotoxicity, such as jaundice, dark urine, light-colored stool, loss of appetite, nausea, and stomach pain.
• Warn patient not to stop drug abruptly.

---

famciclovir
fam-SYE-kloe-vir

Famvir

Pharmacologic class: synthetic acyclic guanine derivative
Pregnancy risk category B

AVAILABLE FORMS
Tablets: 125 mg, 250 mg, 500 mg

INDICATIONS & DOSAGES
➤ **Acute herpes zoster infection (shingles)**
Adults: 500 mg P.O. every 8 hours for 7 days.
Adjust-a-dose: For patients with creatinine clearance of 40 to 59 ml/minute, give 500 mg P.O. every 12 hours; if clearance is 20 to 39 ml/minute, give 500 mg P.O. every 24 hours; if clearance is less than 20 ml/minute, give 250 mg P.O. every 24 hours.

For hemodialysis patients, give 250 mg P.O. after each hemodialysis session.

➤ **Recurrent genital herpes**
Adults: 1,000 mg P.O. b.i.d. for a single day. Begin therapy at the first sign or symptom.
Adjust-a-dose: For patients with creatinine clearance of 40 to 59 ml/minute, give 500 mg every 12 hours for 1 day; for clearance of 20 to 39 ml/minute, give 500 mg P.O. as a single dose; if clearance is less than 20 ml/minute, give 250 mg as a single dose. For hemodialysis patient, give 250 mg single dose following dialysis session.

➤ **Suppression of recurrent genital herpes**
Adults: 250 mg P.O. b.i.d. for up to 1 year.
Adjust-a-dose: For patients with creatinine clearance of 20 to 39 ml/minute, give 125 mg P.O. every 12 hours; if clearance is less than 20 ml/minute, give 125 mg P.O. every 24 hours. For hemodialysis patients, give 125 mg P.O. after each hemodialysis session.

➤ **Recurrent mucocutaneous herpes simplex infections in HIV-infected patients**
Adults: 500 mg P.O. b.i.d. for 7 days.
Adjust-a-dose: For patients with creatinine clearance of 20 to 39 ml/minute, give 500 mg P.O. every 24 hours; if clearance is less than 20 ml/minute, give 250 mg P.O. every 24 hours. For hemodialysis patients, give 250 mg P.O. after each hemodialysis session.

➤ **Recurrent herpes labialis (cold sores)**
Adults: 1,500 mg P.O. for one dose. Give at the first sign or symptom of cold sore.
Adjust-a-dose: For patients with creatinine clearance of 40 to 59 ml/minute, give 750 mg as a single dose; for clearance of 20 to 39 ml/minute, give 500 mg P.O. as a single dose; if clearance is less than 20 ml/minute, give 250 mg as a single dose. For hemodialysis patient, give 250 mg single dose following dialysis session.

ADMINISTRATION
P.O.
• Give drug without regard for meals.

ACTION
A guanosine nucleoside that is converted to penciclovir, which enters viral cells and inhibits DNA polymerase and viral DNA synthesis.

Route	Onset	Peak	Duration
P.O.	Unknown	1 hr	Unknown

Half-life: 2 to 3 hours.

ADVERSE REACTIONS
CNS: *headache,* fatigue, fever, dizziness, paresthesia, somnolence.
EENT: pharyngitis, sinusitis.
GI: *nausea,* abdominal pain, anorexia, constipation, diarrhea, vomiting.
Musculoskeletal: arthralgia, back pain.
Skin: pruritus.
Other: zoster-related signs, symptoms, and complications.

INTERACTIONS
Drug-drug. *Probenecid:* May increase level of penciclovir, the active metabolite of famciclovir. Monitor patient for increased adverse reactions.

EFFECTS ON LAB TEST RESULTS
None reported.

CONTRAINDICATIONS & CAUTIONS
• Contraindicated in patients hypersensitive to drug.
• Use cautiously in patients with renal or hepatic impairment.

NURSING CONSIDERATIONS
• In patients with renal or hepatic impairment, adjust dosage as needed.
• Monitor renal and liver function tests in these patients.

PATIENT TEACHING
• Inform patient that drug doesn't cure genital herpes but can decrease the length and severity of symptoms.
• Teach patient how to avoid spreading infection to others.
• Urge patient to recognize the early signs and symptoms of herpes infection, such as tingling, itching, and pain, and to report them. Therapy is more effective if started within 48 hours of rash onset.

foscarnet sodium
(PFA, phosphonoformic acid)
foss-CAR-net

Foscavir

Pharmacologic class:
pyrophosphate analogue
Pregnancy risk category C

AVAILABLE FORMS
Injection: 24 mg/ml in 250- and 500-ml
bottles

INDICATIONS & DOSAGES
■ **Black Box Warning** Drug is only indicated for use in immunocompromised
patients with cytomegalovirus (CMV)
retinitis and mucocutaneous acyclovir-
resistant herpes simplex virus (HSV)
infections. ■
➤ **CMV retinitis in patients with
AIDS**
Adults: Initially, for induction, 60 mg/kg
I.V. over a minimum of 1 hour every
8 hours or 90 mg/kg I.V. over 1½ to
2 hours every 12 hours for 2 to 3 weeks,
depending on patient response. Follow
with a maintenance infusion of 90 to
120 mg/kg over 2 hours daily.
➤ **Acyclovir-resistant HSV
infections**
Adults: 40 mg/kg I.V. over 1 hour every
8 to 12 hours for 2 to 3 weeks or until
healed.
Adjust-a-dose: Adjust dosage when
creatinine clearance is less than
1.4 ml/minute/kg. If clearance falls below
0.4 ml/minute/kg, stop drug. Consult manufacturer's package insert for specific
dosage adjustments.

ADMINISTRATION
I.V.
■ **Black Box Warning** To minimize
renal toxicity, make sure patient is
adequately hydrated before and during
infusion. ■
● Don't exceed the recommended dosage,
rate, or frequency of infusion. Doses must
be individualized according to patient's
renal function.
● Drug may be infused via a central or peripheral vein with enough blood flow for
rapid distribution and dilution. If infusing
into a central vein, don't dilute the commercially available form (24 mg/ml). If
infusing into a peripheral vein, dilute to
12 mg/ml with D_5W or normal saline
solution to decrease risk of local irritation.
Use an infusion pump.
● Give induction treatment over 1 to
2 hours, depending on the dose, and maintenance infusions over 2 hours.
● **Incompatibilities:** Acyclovir, amphotericin B, co-trimoxazole, dextrose 30%,
diazepam, digoxin, diphenhydramine,
dobutamine, droperidol, ganciclovir,
haloperidol, lactated Ringer's solution,
leucovorin, lorazepam, midazolam, pentamidine, phenytoin, prochlorperazine,
promethazine, solutions containing
calcium (such as total parenteral nutrition), trimetrexate, vancomycin.

ACTION
Inhibits herpes virus replication in vitro
by blocking the pyrophosphate-binding
site on DNA polymerases and reverse
transcriptases.

Route	Onset	Peak	Duration
I.V.	Unknown	Immediate	Unknown

Half-life: 3 hours.

ADVERSE REACTIONS
CNS: *asthenia, dizziness, fatigue, fever,
headache, hypoesthesia, malaise, neuropathy, paresthesia,* **seizures,** abnormal
coordination, agitation, aggression,
amnesia, anxiety, aphasia, ataxia, cerebrovascular disorder, confusion, dementia, depression, EEG abnormalities,
generalized spasms, hallucinations, insomnia, meningitis, nervousness, pain,
sensory disturbances, somnolence,
stupor, tremor.
CV: *ECG abnormalities, first-degree AV
block, flushing, hypertension, hypotension,
palpitations, sinus tachycardia,* chest pain,
edema.
EENT: conjunctivitis, eye pain,
pharyngitis, rhinitis, sinusitis, visual
disturbances.
GI: *abdominal pain, anorexia, diarrhea,
nausea, vomiting,* **pancreatitis,** constipation, dysphagia, dry mouth, dyspepsia,
flatulence, melena, rectal hemorrhage,
taste perversion, ulcerative stomatitis.

Reactions may be *common*, uncommon, *life-threatening*, or COMMON AND LIFE-THREATENING.
Interaction may have a *rapid onset* or **delayed onset**.

GU: *acute renal failure, abnormal renal function,* albuminuria, candidiasis, dysuria, polyuria, urethral disorder, urinary retention, UTI.
Hematologic: *anemia, bone marrow suppression, granulocytopenia, leukopenia, thrombocytopenia,* thrombocytosis.
Hepatic: abnormal hepatic function.
Metabolic: *hyperphosphatemia, hypocalcemia, hypokalemia,* HYPOMAGNE-SEMIA, *hypophosphatemia, hyponatremia.*
Musculoskeletal: arthralgia, back pain, leg cramps, myalgia.
Respiratory: *bronchospasm, cough, dyspnea,* hemoptysis, pneumonitis, *pneumothorax,* pulmonary infiltration, *respiratory insufficiency,* stridor.
Skin: *diaphoresis, rash,* erythematous rash, facial edema, pruritus, seborrhea, skin discoloration, skin ulceration.
Other: *sarcoma, sepsis,* abscess, bacterial or fungal infections, flulike symptoms, inflammation and pain at infusion site, lymphadenopathy, lymphoma-like disorder, rigors.

INTERACTIONS
Drug-drug. *Nephrotoxic drugs (such as aminoglycosides, amphotericin B):* May increase risk of nephrotoxicity. Avoid using together.
Pentamidine: May increase risk of nephrotoxicity; severe hypocalcemia also has been reported. Monitor renal function tests and electrolytes.
Zidovudine: May increase risk or severity of anemia. Monitor blood counts.

EFFECTS ON LAB TEST RESULTS
• May increase alkaline phosphatase, ALT, AST, bilirubin, creatinine, and phosphate levels. May decrease calcium, hemoglobin, magnesium, phosphate, potassium, and sodium levels.
• May increase platelet count. May decrease granulocyte, platelet, and WBC counts.

CONTRAINDICATIONS & CAUTIONS
• Contraindicated in patients hypersensitive to drug.
■ **Black Box Warning** In patients with abnormal renal function, use cautiously and reduce dosage. Drug is nephrotoxic

and can worsen renal impairment. Some degree of nephrotoxicity occurs in most patients. ■

NURSING CONSIDERATIONS
• *Alert:* Because drug is highly toxic, which is probably dose-related, always use the lowest effective maintenance dose.
• Monitor creatinine clearance frequently during therapy because of drug's adverse effects on renal function. Obtain a baseline 24-hour creatinine clearance. Monitor level two to three times weekly during induction and at least once every 1 to 2 weeks during maintenance.
■ **Black Box Warning** Drug can alter electrolyte levels; monitor levels using a schedule similar to that established for creatinine clearance. Assess patient for tetany and seizures caused by abnormal electrolyte levels. ■
• Monitor patient's hemoglobin level and hematocrit. Anemia occurs in about a third of patients and may be severe enough to require transfusions.
• Drug may cause a dose-related transient decrease in ionized calcium, which may not always show up in patient's laboratory values.

PATIENT TEACHING
• Explain the importance of adequate hydration throughout therapy.
• Advise patient to report tingling around the mouth, numbness in the arms and legs, and pins-and-needles sensations.
• Tell patient to alert nurse about discomfort at I.V. insertion site.

ganciclovir (DHPG)
gan-SYE-kloe-vir

Cytovene

Pharmacologic class: synthetic purine nucleoside analogue of guanine
Pregnancy risk category C

AVAILABLE FORMS
Capsules: 250 mg, 500 mg
Injection: 500 mg/vial

INDICATIONS & DOSAGES
➤ **CMV retinitis in immunocompromised patients, including those with AIDS and normal renal function**
Adults and children older than age 3 months: Induction treatment is 5 mg/kg I.V. every 12 hours for 14 to 21 days. Don't use capsules for induction. Maintenance treatment is 5 mg/kg I.V. daily 7 days per week or 6 mg/kg I.V. daily five times weekly. Or, for maintenance therapy, give 1,000 mg P.O. t.i.d. with food or 500 mg P.O. every 3 hours while awake (six times daily).

➤ **To prevent CMV disease in patients with advanced HIV infection and normal renal function**
Adults: 1,000 mg P.O. t.i.d. with food.

➤ **To prevent CMV disease in transplant recipients with normal renal function**
Adults: 5 mg/kg I.V. (given at a constant rate over 1 hour) every 12 hours for 7 to 14 days; then 5 mg/kg daily 7 days per week or 6 mg/kg daily five times weekly. Duration of therapy depends on degree of immunosuppression.

Adjust-a-dose: Adjust dosage in patients with renal impairment according to the table. If patient is receiving hemodialysis, give dose shortly after session is complete.

Initial I.V. therapy

Creatinine clearance (ml/min)	Dose (mg/kg)	Interval
50–69	2.5	12 hr
25–49	2.5	24 hr
10–24	1.25	24 hr
< 10	1.25	3 times weekly after hemodialysis

Maintenance I.V. therapy

Creatinine clearance (ml/min)	Dose (mg/kg)	Interval
50–69	2.5	24 hr
25–49	1.25	24 hr
10–24	0.625	24 hr
< 10	0.625	3 times weekly after hemodialysis

P.O. therapy

Creatinine clearance (ml/min)	Dose (mg)	Interval
50–69	1,500	24 hr
	500	8 hr
25–49	1,000	24 hr
	500	12 hr
10–24	500	24 hr
< 10	500	3 times weekly after hemodialysis

ADMINISTRATION
P.O.
- Give drug with a meal.
- Don't crush or open capsule.

I.V.
- To reconstitute, add 10 ml sterile water for injection to 500-mg vial. Shake vial well to dissolve drug.
- Further dilute in 50 to 250 ml (usually 100 ml) of compatible I.V. solution.
- If fluids are being restricted, dilute to no more than 10 mg/ml.
- Don't give as bolus.
- Use an infusion pump.
- Infuse over at least 1 hour.
- Infusing drug too rapidly has toxic effects.
- Use caution when preparing solution, which is alkaline.
- *Alert:* Don't give subcutaneously or I.M.
- **Incompatibilities:** Aldesleukin, amifostine, aztreonam, cefepime, cytarabine, doxorubicin hydrochloride, fludarabine, foscarnet, ondansetron, other I.V. drugs, paraben (bacteriostatic agent), piperacillin sodium with tazobactam, sargramostim, vinorelbine.

ACTION
Inhibits binding of deoxyguanosine triphosphate to DNA polymerase, resulting in inhibition of DNA synthesis.

Route	Onset	Peak	Duration
P.O.	Unknown	2–3 hr	Unknown
I.V.	Unknown	Immediate	Unknown

Half-life: About 3 hours.

ADVERSE REACTIONS

CNS: *fever, coma, seizures,* abnormal thinking, agitation, altered dreams, amnesia, anxiety, asthenia, ataxia, confusion, dizziness, headache, somnolence, tremor, neuropathy, paresthesia.
EENT: retinal detachment in CMV retinitis patients.
GI: *abdominal pain, anorexia, diarrhea, nausea, vomiting,* dry mouth, dyspepsia, flatulence.
Hematologic: *anemia, agranulocytosis, leukopenia, thrombocytopenia.*
Respiratory: pneumonia.
Skin: *rash, sweating,* inflammation, pruritus, pain and phlebitis at injection site.
Other: *sepsis,* chills, infection.

INTERACTIONS

Drug-drug. *Amphotericin B, cyclosporine, other nephrotoxic drugs:* May increase risk of nephrotoxicity. Monitor renal function.
Imipenem and cilastatin: May increase seizure activity. Use together only if potential benefits outweigh risks.
Cytotoxic drugs: May increase toxic effects, especially hematologic effects and stomatitis. Monitor patient closely.
Immunosuppressants (such as azathioprine, corticosteroids, cyclosporine): May enhance immune and bone marrow suppression. Use together cautiously.
Probenecid: May increase ganciclovir level. Monitor patient closely.
Zidovudine: May increase risk of agranulocytosis. Use together cautiously; monitor hematologic function closely.

EFFECTS ON LAB TEST RESULTS

● May increase alkaline phosphatase, ALT, AST, creatinine, and GGT levels. May decrease hemoglobin level.
● May decrease granulocyte, neutrophil, platelet, and WBC counts.

CONTRAINDICATIONS & CAUTIONS

■ **Black Box Warning** Contraindicated in patients hypersensitive to drug or acyclovir and in those with an absolute neutrophil count below 500/mm³ or a platelet count below 25,000/mm³. ■
● Use cautiously and reduce dosage in patients with renal dysfunction. Monitor renal function tests.

■ **Black Box Warning** Ganciclovir caused aspermatogenesis and was carcinogenic and teratogenic in animal studies. ■

NURSING CONSIDERATIONS

■ **Black Box Warning** Because of the frequency of agranulocytosis and thrombocytopenia, obtain neutrophil and platelet counts every 2 days during twice-daily doses and at least weekly thereafter. ■
■ **Black Box Warning** Ganciclovir capsules are associated with a risk of more rapid rate of CMV retinitis progression. Use capsules as maintenance treatment only in patients for whom this risk is balanced by benefit associated with avoiding daily I.V. infusions. ■

PATIENT TEACHING

● Explain importance of drinking plenty of fluids during therapy.
● Instruct patient to report adverse reactions promptly.
● Tell patient to report discomfort at I.V. insertion site.
● Advise patient that drug causes birth defects. Instruct women to use effective birth control; men should use barrier contraception during and for at least 90 days after therapy.
● Tell patient to take capsule with food and to swallow whole. Tell patient not to crush, open, or chew capsule.

oseltamivir phosphate
oz-el-TAM-ah-ver

Tamiflu

Pharmacologic class: selective neuraminidase inhibitor
Pregnancy risk category C

AVAILABLE FORMS

Capsules: 30 mg, 45 mg, 75 mg
Oral suspension: 12 mg/ml after reconstitution

INDICATIONS & DOSAGES

➤ **Uncomplicated, acute illness caused by influenza infection in**

patients who have had symptoms for 2 days or less
Adults and adolescents age 13 and older: 75 mg P.O. b.i.d. for 5 days.
Children age 1 and older who weigh more than 40 kg (88 lb): 75 mg oral suspension P.O. b.i.d. for 5 days.
Children age 1 and older who weigh 23 to 40 kg (51 to 88 lb): 60 mg oral suspension P.O. b.i.d. for 5 days.
Children age 1 and older who weigh 15 to 23 kg (33 to 51 lb): 45 mg oral suspension P.O. b.i.d. for 5 days.
Children age 1 and older who weigh 15 kg (33 lb) or less: 30 mg oral suspension P.O. b.i.d. for 5 days.
Adjust-a-dose: For adults and adolescents with creatinine clearance of 10 to 30 ml/minute, reduce dosage to 75 mg P.O. once daily for 5 days.
➤ **To prevent influenza after close contact with infected person within 2 days of exposure**
Adults and adolescents age 13 and older: 75 mg P.O. once daily for at least 10 days.
Children age 1 and older who weigh more than 40 kg (88 lb): 75 mg P.O. once daily for 10 days.
Children age 1 and older who weigh 23 to 40 kg (51 to 88 lb): 60 mg P.O. once daily for 10 days.
Children age 1 and older who weigh 15 to 23 kg (33 to 51 lb): 45 mg P.O. once daily for 10 days.
Children age 1 and older who weigh 15 kg (33 lb) or less: 30 mg oral suspension P.O. once daily for 10 days.
Adjust-a-dose: For adults and adolescents with creatinine clearance of 10 to 30 ml/minute, reduce dosage to 75 mg P.O. every other day or 30 mg once daily.
➤ **To prevent influenza during a community outbreak**
Adults and adolescents age 13 and older: 75 mg P.O. once daily for up to 6 weeks.

ADMINISTRATION
P.O.
● Give drug with meals to decrease GI adverse effects.
● Store at controlled room temperature (59° to 86° F [15° to 30° C]).
● Capsules may be opened and mixed with sweetened liquids such as chocolate syrup.

ACTION
Inhibits influenza A and B virus enzyme neuraminidase, which is thought to play a role in viral particle aggregation and release from the host cell and appears to interfere with viral replication.

Route	Onset	Peak	Duration
P.O.	Unknown	Unknown	Unknown

Half-life: 1 to 10 hours.

ADVERSE REACTIONS
CNS: dizziness, fatigue, headache, insomnia, vertigo.
GI: abdominal pain, diarrhea, nausea, vomiting.
Respiratory: bronchitis, cough.

INTERACTIONS
None significant.

EFFECTS ON LAB TEST RESULTS
None reported.

CONTRAINDICATIONS & CAUTIONS
● Contraindicated in patients hypersensitive to drug or its components.
● Use cautiously in patients with chronic cardiac or respiratory diseases, or any medical condition that may require imminent hospitalization. Also use cautiously in patients with renal failure.
● It's unknown if drug or its metabolite appears in breast milk. Use only if benefits to patient outweigh risks to infant.

NURSING CONSIDERATIONS
● Drug must be given within 2 days of onset of symptoms.
● Safety and effectiveness of repeated treatment courses haven't been established.
● *Alert:* Closely monitor patients with influenza for neuropsychiatric symptoms, such as hallucinations, delirium, and abnormal behavior. Risks and benefits of continuing drug should be evaluated.

PATIENT TEACHING
● Instruct patient to begin treatment as soon as possible after appearance of flu symptoms.
● Inform patient that drug may be taken with or without meals. If nausea or vomiting occurs, he can take drug with food or milk.

Reactions may be *common*, uncommon, *life-threatening*, or COMMON AND LIFE-THREATENING.
Interaction may have a *rapid onset* or *delayed onset*.

• Tell patient that, if a dose is missed, he should take it as soon as possible. However, if next dose is due within 2 hours, tell him to skip the missed dose and take the next dose on schedule.

• Advise patient to complete the full course of treatment, even if symptoms resolve.

• Alert patient that drug isn't a replacement for the annual influenza vaccination. Patients for whom vaccine is indicated should continue to receive the vaccine each fall.

ribavirin
rye-ba-VYE-rin

Copegus, Rebetol, Ribaspheres, Virazole

Pharmacologic class: synthetic nucleoside
Pregnancy risk category X

AVAILABLE FORMS
Capsules: 200 mg
Oral solution: 40 mg/ml
Powder to be reconstituted for inhalation: 6 g in 100-ml glass vial
Tablets: 200 mg, 400 mg, 600 mg

INDICATIONS & DOSAGES
➤ **Hospitalized infants and young children infected by respiratory syncytial virus (RSV)**
Infants and young children: Solution in concentration of 20 mg/ml delivered via the Viratek Small Particle Aerosol Generator (SPAG-2) and mechanical ventilator or oxygen hood, face mask, or oxygen tent at a rate of about 12.5 L of mist/minute. Treatment is given for 12 to 18 hours/day for at least 3 days, and no longer than 7 days.
➤ **Chronic hepatitis C**
■ **Black Box Warning** Ribavirin alone isn't effective for treatment of chronic hepatitis C. ■
Adults who weigh more than 75 kg (165 lb): 1,200 mg Rebetol P.O. divided b.i.d. (600 in morning, 600 mg in evening) with interferon alfa-2b, 3 million units subcutaneously three times weekly. Or, 1,200 mg

Copegus with 180 mcg of peginterferon alfa-2a.
Adults who weigh 75 kg or less: 1,000 mg Rebetol P.O. daily in divided dose (400 mg in morning, 600 mg in evening) with interferon alfa-2b, 3 million units subcutaneously three times weekly. Or, 1,000 mg Copegus with 180 mcg of peginterferon alfa-2a.
Children age 3 and older who weigh 50 to 61 kg (110 to 134 lb): 400 mg P.O. (Rebetol) every morning and 400 mg P.O. every evening with interferon alfa-2b, 3 million units/m² subcutaneously three times weekly.
Children age 3 and older who weigh 37 to 49 kg (81 to 108 lb): 200 mg P.O. (Rebetol) every morning and 400 mg P.O. every evening with interferon alfa-2b, 3 million units/m² subcutaneously three times weekly.
Children age 3 and older who weigh 25 to 36 kg (55 to 79 lb): 200 mg P.O. (Rebetol) every morning and 200 mg P.O. every evening with interferon alfa-2b, 3 million units/m² subcutaneously three times weekly.
➤ **Chronic hepatitis C (regardless of genotype) in HIV-infected patients who haven't previously been treated with interferon**
Adults: 800 mg Copegus P.O. daily given in two divided doses with peginterferon alfa-2a, 180 mcg subcutaneously weekly for 48 weeks.
Adjust-a-dose: In patient with no cardiac history and hemoglobin level less than 10 g/dl, reduce dosage to 600 mg daily (200 mg in a.m., 400 mg in p.m.) for adults and 7.5 mg/kg daily for children. If hemoglobin level is less than 8.5 g/dl, stop drug. In patient with cardiac history and whose hemoglobin level falls 2 g/dl or more during any 4-week period, reduce dosage to 600 mg daily (200 mg in a.m., 400 mg in p.m.) for adults and 7.5 mg/kg daily for children. If hemoglobin level is less than 12 g/dl after 4 weeks of reduced dosage, stop drug.

ADMINISTRATION
Inhalational
• Give by the Viratek SPAG-2 only. Don't use any other aerosol-generating device.

• Use sterile USP water for injection, not bacteriostatic water. Water used to reconstitute this drug must not contain any antimicrobial product.
• Discard solutions placed in the SPAG-2 unit at least every 24 hours before adding newly reconstituted solution.
• Store reconstituted solutions at room temperature for 24 hours.

P.O.
• Give drug without regard for meals at the same time every day.

ACTION
Inhibits viral activity by an unknown mechanism, possibly by inhibiting RNA and DNA synthesis by depleting intracellular nucleotide pools.

Route	Onset	Peak	Duration
Inhalation	Unknown	Unknown	Unknown
P.O.	Unknown	2 hr	Unknown

Half-life: First phase, 9¼ hours; second phase, 40 hours.

ADVERSE REACTIONS
CV: *bradycardia, cardiac arrest,* hypotension.
EENT: conjunctivitis, rash or erythema of eyelids.
Hematologic: anemia, reticulocytosis.
Respiratory: *apnea, bronchospasm,* bacterial pneumonia, *pneumothorax, pulmonary edema,* worsening respiratory state.

INTERACTIONS
Drug-drug. *Acetaminophen, antacids that contain magnesium, aluminum, or simethicone, aspirin, cimetidine:* May affect drug level. Monitor patient.
Didanosine: May increase toxicity. Avoid using together.
Stavudine, zidovudine: May decrease antiretroviral activity. Use together cautiously.

EFFECTS ON LAB TEST RESULTS
• May increase ALT, AST, and bilirubin levels. May decrease hemoglobin level.
• May increase reticulocyte count.

CONTRAINDICATIONS & CAUTIONS
■ **Black Box Warning** Aerosol form contraindicated in patients hypersensitive to drug, and isn't indicated for use in adults. ■
■ **Black Box Warning** Ribavirin may cause hemolytic anemia and worsen cardiac disease, leading to potentially fatal MI. ■
■ **Black Box Warning** Oral form is contraindicated in patients hypersensitive to drug, pregnant women, men whose partners are pregnant or may become pregnant within 6 months, patients with thalassemia major or sickle cell anemia, patients with a history of significant or unstable cardiac disease, and patients whose creatinine clearance is less than 50 ml/minute. ■
■ **Black Box Warning** In infants, aerosolized ribavirin has been associated with sudden deterioration of respiratory function. Monitor respiratory function carefully and stop treatment if sudden respiratory deterioration occurs. ■
• Use cautiously in elderly patients and patients with hepatic or renal insufficiency.

NURSING CONSIDERATIONS
Aerosol form
• *Alert:* The long-term and cumulative effects to health care personnel exposed to this form aren't known. Eye irritation and headache may occur. Advise pregnant women to avoid unnecessary exposure.
■ **Black Box Warning** Monitor ventilator function frequently. Drug may precipitate in ventilator, causing equipment to malfunction with serious consequences. ■
• This form is indicated only for severe lower respiratory tract infection caused by RSV. Although you should begin treatment while awaiting test results, an RSV infection must be documented eventually.
• Most infants and children with RSV infection don't require treatment with antivirals because the disease is commonly mild and self-limiting. Premature infants or those with cardiopulmonary disease experience RSV in its severest form and benefit most from treatment with ribavirin aerosol.
Oral form
• Don't start therapy until a negative pregnancy test is confirmed in patient or partner of patient; they should take a

---

Reactions may be *common,* uncommon, *life-threatening,* or **COMMON AND LIFE-THREATENING.**
Interaction may have a *rapid onset* or *delayed onset.*

pregnancy test every month during therapy and for 6 months afterward.
• Women or female partner of patient should use two reliable forms of contraception before and during treatment and for 6 months afterward.
• Report pregnancies that occur during treatment by calling 800-727-7064 for capsules and 800-593-2214 for tablets.
• Monitor hematologic status, liver function, and thyroid-stimulating hormone level at baseline and throughout therapy.
• *Alert:* Monitor patient for suicidal ideation, severe depression, hemolytic anemia, bone marrow suppression, autoimmune and infective disorders, pulmonary dysfunction, pancreatitis, and diabetes.
• Stop drug if pulmonary infiltrates or severe pulmonary impairment occur.

PATIENT TEACHING
• Inform parents of need for drug, and answer any questions.
• Encourage parents to immediately report any subtle change in child.
• Inform patient that oral form may be taken without regard to meals but should be taken in a consistent manner.

---

telbivudine
tell-BIV-you-deen

Tyzeka, Sebivo†

Pharmacologic class: synthetic thymidine nucleoside analogue
Pregnancy risk category B

AVAILABLE FORMS
Tablets: 600 mg

INDICATIONS & DOSAGES
➤ **Chronic hepatitis**
Adults and children age 16 or older: 600 mg P.O. daily.
Adjust-a-dose: If creatinine clearance is 30 to 49 ml/minute, give 600 mg every 48 hours; if creatinine clearance is less than 30 ml/minute and patient doesn't require dialysis, give 600 mg every 72 hours; for patients with end-stage renal disease, give 600 mg every 96 hours after dialysis.

ADMINISTRATION
P.O.
• Give drug without regard for meals.

ACTION
Inhibits HBV replication by interrupting DNA polymerase activity.

Route	Onset	Peak	Duration
P.O.	Immediate	1–4 hr	Unknown

Half-life: 40 to 49 hours.

ADVERSE REACTIONS
CNS: fatigue, headache, malaise, pyrexia.
Hematologic: NEUTROPENIA.
Musculoskeletal: muscle-related symptoms, *myopathy.*
Respiratory: nasopharyngitis, *upper respiratory tract infection.*
Other: influenza and influenza-like symptoms.

INTERACTIONS
Drug-drug. *Other drugs that alter renal function (aminoglycosides, cyclosporine, NSAIDs, tacrolimus, vancomycin):* May increase risk of nephrotoxicity and cause decreased telbivudine elimination. Monitor renal function closely and adjust drug dose if necessary.

EFFECTS ON LAB TEST RESULTS
• May increase CK, ALT, AST, lipase, creatinine, and lactate levels.
• May increase neutrophil count.

CONTRAINDICATIONS & CAUTIONS
• Contraindicated in patients hypersensitive to drug or its components.
• Use cautiously in those with renal impairment.
• Use cautiously in those with lamivudine-resistant hepatitis B infection.
• Give drug to pregnant woman only if potential benefit outweighs fetal risk. Register patient in the Antiretroviral Pregnancy Registry by calling 1-800-258-4263 to monitor fetal outcomes.
• Drug may appear in breast milk. Don't use drug in breast-feeding women.
• Safety and efficacy in children haven't been established.

NURSING CONSIDERATIONS

• Monitor hepatic and renal function test results for liver transplant patients.

■ **Black Box Warning** The patient may develop lactic acidosis and severe hepatomegaly with steatosis during treatment. Risk factors include female gender, obesity, and concurrent antiretroviral therapy. ■

• Monitor patient for symptoms of myopathy.

■ **Black Box Warning** Stopping telbivudine may cause worsening of hepatitis B. Monitor hepatic function closely during therapy and for several months after stopping the drug. Therapy may need to be restarted. ■

PATIENT TEACHING

• Teach patient to report immediately signs and symptoms of lactic acidosis, such as weakness, muscle pain, difficulty breathing, nausea and vomiting, coldness in arms and legs, dizziness, lightheadedness, and fast or irregular heartbeat.

• Advise patient not to change the dose or stop the drug because symptoms may worsen.

• Teach patient to report signs and symptoms of worsening liver disease, such as jaundice, dark urine, light-colored stool, decreased appetite, nausea, and stomach pain.

• Remind the patient that telbivudine won't cure HBV and doesn't stop the spread of HBV to others.

---

valacyclovir hydrochloride
val-ah-SYE-kloe-ver

Valtrex

Pharmacologic class: synthetic purine nucleoside
Pregnancy risk category B

AVAILABLE FORMS
Tablets: 500 mg, 1,000 mg

INDICATIONS & DOSAGES
➤ **Herpes zoster infection (shingles)**
Adults: 1 g P.O. t.i.d. for 7 days.
Adjust-a-dose: For patients with creatinine clearance of 30 to 49 ml/minute, give 1 g P.O. every 12 hours; if clearance is 10 to 29 ml/minute, give 1 g P.O. every 24 hours; if clearance is less than 10 ml/minute, give 500 mg P.O. every 24 hours.

➤ **First episode of genital herpes**
Adults: 1 g P.O. b.i.d. for 10 days.
Adjust-a-dose: For patients with creatinine clearance of 10 to 29 ml/minute, give 1 g P.O. every 24 hours; if clearance is less than 10 ml/minute, give 500 mg P.O. every 24 hours.

➤ **Recurrent genital herpes in immunocompetent patients**
Adults: 500 mg P.O. b.i.d. for 3 days, given at the first sign or symptom of an episode.
Adjust-a-dose: For patients with creatinine clearance of 29 ml/minute or less, give 500 mg P.O. every 24 hours.

➤ **Long-term suppression of recurrent genital herpes**
Adults: 1 g P.O. once daily. In patients with a history of nine or fewer recurrences per year, use alternative dose of 500 mg once daily.
Adjust-a-dose: For patients with creatinine clearance of 29 ml/minute or less, 500 mg P.O. every 24 hours (every 48 hours if patient has nine or fewer occurrences per year).

➤ **Cold sores (herpes labialis)**
Adults: 2 g P.O. every 12 hours for two doses.
Adjust-a-dose: For patients with creatinine clearance of 30 to 49 ml/minute, give 1 g every 12 hours for two doses; if clearance is 10 to 29 ml/minute, give 500 mg every 12 hours for two doses; if clearance is less than 10 ml/minute, give 500 mg as a single dose.

➤ **Long-term suppression of recurrent genital herpes in HIV-infected patients with CD4 cell count of 100 cells/mm³ or more**
Adults: 500 mg P.O. b.i.d.
Adjust-a-dose: For patients with creatinine clearance of 29 ml/minute or less, give 500 mg P.O. every 24 hours.

➤ **To reduce transmission of genital herpes in patients with history of nine or fewer occurrences per year**
Adults: 500 mg P.O. daily for source partner.

Reactions may be *common*, uncommon, *life-threatening*, or COMMON AND LIFE-THREATENING.
Interaction may have a *rapid onset* or **delayed onset**.

ADMINISTRATION
P.O.
● Give drug without regard for meals.

ACTION
Rapidly converts to acyclovir, which in turn becomes incorporated into viral DNA, thereby terminating growth of the DNA chain; inhibits viral DNA polymerase, causing inhibition of viral replication.

Route	Onset	Peak	Duration
P.O.	30 min	Unknown	Unknown

Half-life: 2½ to 3¼ hours.

ADVERSE REACTIONS
CNS: *headache,* depression, dizziness.
GI: *nausea,* abdominal pain, diarrhea, vomiting.
GU: dysmenorrhea.
Musculoskeletal: arthralgia.

INTERACTIONS
Drug-drug. *Cimetidine, probenecid:* May reduce rate but not extent of conversion of valacyclovir to acyclovir and may decrease renal clearance of acyclovir, thus increasing acyclovir level. Monitor patient for acyclovir toxicity.

EFFECTS ON LAB TEST RESULTS
● May increase alkaline phosphatase, ALT, AST, and creatinine levels. May decrease hemoglobin level.
● May decrease platelet and WBC counts.

CONTRAINDICATIONS & CAUTIONS
● Contraindicated in patients hypersensitive to or intolerant of valacyclovir, acyclovir, or components of the formulation.
● **Alert:** Drug isn't recommended for use in patients with HIV infection or in bone marrow or renal transplant recipients because thrombotic thrombocytopenic purpura and hemolytic uremic syndrome may occur in these patients at doses of 8 g/day.
● Use cautiously in elderly patients, those with renal impairment, and those receiving other nephrotoxic drugs. Monitor renal function test results.
● Give drug to pregnant woman only if potential benefits outweigh fetal risk.
● If patient is breast-feeding, drug may need to be stopped.

● Safety and effectiveness in prepubertal children haven't been established.

NURSING CONSIDERATIONS
● Safety and effectiveness of therapy beyond 6 months haven't been established.
● Start treatment for herpes zoster infection at earliest signs or symptoms. It's most effective when started within 48 hours of onset of rash.
● Although there are no reports of overdose, precipitation of acyclovir in renal tubules may occur when solubility (2.5 mg/ml) is exceeded in the intratubular fluid. With acute renal failure and anuria, the patient may benefit from hemodialysis until renal function is restored.
● **Look alike–sound alike:** Don't confuse valacyclovir (Valtrex) with valganciclovir (Valcyte).

PATIENT TEACHING
● Inform patient that drug may be taken without regard for meals.
● Teach patient the signs and symptoms of herpes infection (rash, tingling, itching, and pain), and advise him to notify prescriber immediately if they occur. Treatment should begin as soon as possible after symptoms appear, preferably within 48 hours of the onset of zoster rash.
● Tell patient that drug isn't a cure for herpes but may decrease the length and severity of symptoms.

valganciclovir
val-gan-SYE-kloe-veer

Valcyte

Pharmacologic class: synthetic nucleoside
Pregnancy risk category C

AVAILABLE FORMS
Tablets: 450 mg

INDICATIONS & DOSAGES
➤ **To prevent CMV disease in heart, kidney, and kidney-pancreas transplantation in patients at high risk**

(donor CMV seropositive or recipient CMV seronegative)
Adults: 900 mg P.O. once daily with food starting within 10 days of transplantation until 100 days after transplantation.
➤ **Active CMV retinitis in patients with AIDS**
Adults: 900 mg P.O. b.i.d. with food for 21 days; maintenance dose is 900 mg P.O. daily with food.
➤ **Inactive CMV retinitis**
Adults: 900 mg P.O. daily with food.
Adjust-a-dose: For patients with creatinine clearance of 40 to 59 ml/minute, induction dosage is 450 mg b.i.d.; maintenance dosage is 450 mg daily. If clearance is 25 to 39 ml/minute, induction dosage is 450 mg daily; maintenance dosage is 450 mg every 2 days. If clearance is 10 to 24 ml/minute, induction dosage is 450 mg every 2 days; maintenance dosage is 450 mg twice weekly.

ADMINISTRATION
P.O.
● Give drug with food.

ACTION
Converted to the active drug ganciclovir, which inhibits replication of CMV.

Route	Onset	Peak	Duration
P.O.	Unknown	1–3 hr	Unknown

Half-life: 4 hours.

ADVERSE REACTIONS
CNS: *headache, insomnia, pyrexia, **seizures,** agitation, confusion, hallucinations, paresthesia, peripheral neuropathy, psychosis.*
EENT: *retinal detachment.*
GI: *abdominal pain, diarrhea, nausea, vomiting.*
Hematologic: NEUTROPENIA, *anemia, **aplastic anemia, bone marrow depression, pancytopenia, thrombocytopenia.***
Other: *sepsis,* catheter-related infection, hypersensitivity reactions, local or systemic infections.

INTERACTIONS
Drug-drug. *Didanosine:* May increase absorption of didanosine. Monitor patient closely for didanosine toxicity.

Immunosuppressants, zidovudine: May enhance neutropenia, anemia, thrombocytopenia, and bone marrow depression. Monitor CBC results.
Mycophenolate mofetil: May increase levels of both drugs in renally impaired patients. Use together cautiously.
Probenecid: May decrease renal clearance of ganciclovir. Monitor patient for ganciclovir toxicity.
Drug-food. *Any food:* May increase drug absorption. Give drug with food.

EFFECTS ON LAB TEST RESULTS
● May decrease hemoglobin level and hematocrit.
● May decrease neutrophil, platelet, RBC, and WBC counts.

CONTRAINDICATIONS & CAUTIONS
● Contraindicated in patients hypersensitive to valganciclovir or ganciclovir. Don't use in patients receiving hemodialysis.
● Drug isn't indicated for use in liver transplant patients.
● The safety and effectiveness of drug for the prevention of CMV disease in other solid organ transplant patients, such as lung transplant patients, haven't been established.
● Use cautiously in patients with cytopenias and in those who have received immunosuppressants or radiation.

NURSING CONSIDERATIONS
● Adhere to dosing guidelines for valganciclovir because ganciclovir and valganciclovir aren't interchangeable and overdose may occur.
■ **Black Box Warning** Toxicities include severe leukopenia, neutropenia, anemia, pancytopenia, bone marrow depression, aplastic anemia, and thrombocytopenia. Don't use if patient's absolute neutrophil count is less than 500/mm³, platelet count is less than 25,000/mm³, or hemoglobin level is less than 8 g/dl. ■
● Monitor CBC, platelet counts, and creatinine level or creatinine clearance values frequently during treatment.
● Cytopenia may occur at any time during treatment and increase with continued use. Counts usually recover 3 to 7 days after stopping drug.

Reactions may be *common*, uncommon, *life-threatening*, or COMMON AND LIFE-THREATENING.
Interaction may have a *rapid onset* or *delayed onset*.

• No drug interaction studies have been conducted but, because drug is converted to ganciclovir, assume that drug interactions will be similar.

■ **Black Box Warning** Drug may cause temporary or permanent inhibition of spermatogenesis. ■

• *Look alike–sound alike:* Don't confuse valganciclovir hydrochloride (Valcyte) with valacyclovir (Valtrex).

PATIENT TEACHING
• Tell patient to take drug with food.
• Tell patient to follow dosage instructions precisely. Ganciclovir capsules and valganciclovir tablets aren't interchangeable.
• Advise patient that blood tests are needed during treatment. Doses may need to be adjusted based on blood counts.
• Tell woman of childbearing potential to use contraception during treatment. Tell man to use barrier contraception during and for 90 days after treatment.
• Advise patient that ganciclovir is a carcinogen.
• Tell patient that CNS effects (seizures, ataxia, dizziness) can occur and to use care in driving or operating machinery.
• Advise patient that this drug isn't a cure for CMV retinitis and that the condition may recur. Tell patient to see an ophthalmologist at least every 4 to 6 weeks during treatment.

---

zanamivir
zan-AM-ah-ver

Relenza

Pharmacologic class: selective neuraminidase inhibitor
Pregnancy risk category C

AVAILABLE FORMS
Powder for inhalation: 5 mg/blister

INDICATIONS & DOSAGES
➤ **Uncomplicated acute illness caused by influenza virus A and B in patients who have had symptoms for no longer than 2 days**
Adults and children age 7 and older:
2 oral inhalations (one 5-mg blister per inhalation for total dose of 10 mg) b.i.d.

using the dry-powder inhalation device for 5 days. Give two doses on first day of treatment, allowing at least 2 hours to elapse between doses. Give subsequent doses about 12 hours apart (in the morning and evening) at about the same time each day.
➤ **Prevention of influenza in a household setting**
Adults and children age 5 and older:
2 oral inhalations (one 5-mg blister per inhalation for total dose of 10 mg) once daily for 10 days.
➤ **Prevention of influenza in a community setting**
Adults and adolescents: 2 oral inhalations (one 5-mg blister per inhalation for total dose of 10 mg) once daily for 28 days.

ADMINISTRATION
Inhalational
• Dry-powder inhaler should be kept level when patient loads and inhales drug. Patient should check inside the mouthpiece of the inhaler before each use to make sure it's free of foreign objects.
• Patient should exhale fully before putting the mouthpiece in his mouth; then, keeping the dry-powder inhaler level, he should close his lips around the mouthpiece and inhale steadily and deeply. Patient should hold his breath for a few seconds after inhaling to keep drug in lungs.

ACTION
Inhibits neuraminidase on the surface of the influenza virus, altering virus particle aggregation and release.

Route	Onset	Peak	Duration
Inhalation	Unknown	1–2 hr	Unknown

Half-life: 2½ to 5¼ hours.

ADVERSE REACTIONS
CNS: dizziness, headache.
EENT: ear, nose, and throat infections, nasal signs and symptoms, sinusitis.
GI: diarrhea, nausea, vomiting.
Respiratory: *bronchospasm,* bronchitis, cough.
Skin: serious rash.
Other: *anaphylaxis.*

INTERACTIONS
None significant.

EFFECTS ON LAB TEST RESULTS
• May increase CK and liver enzyme levels.
• May decrease lymphocyte and neutrophil counts.

CONTRAINDICATIONS & CAUTIONS
• Contraindicated in patients hypersensitive to drug or its components.
• Not recommended for patients with severe or decompensated COPD, asthma, or other underlying respiratory disease.

NURSING CONSIDERATIONS
• For a patient with underlying respiratory disease, have a fast-acting bronchodilator readily available and carefully monitor respiratory status. Patients using an inhaled bronchodilator for asthma simultaneously with this drug should use the bronchodilator first.
• Start drug within 48 hours of symptoms or as prevention after household contact, within 36 hours, or community outbreak, within 5 days.
• Drug doesn't replace annual influenza vaccine.
• Monitor patient for bronchospasm and decline in lung function. Stop drug in such situations.
• Closely monitor patients with influenza for signs and symptoms of abnormal behavior. If neuropsychiatric symptoms occur, risks and benefits of continuing treatment should be evaluated.

PATIENT TEACHING
• Tell patient to carefully read the instructions for the dry-powder inhalation device.
• Teach parents how to give the drug to a child and to properly supervise use.
• Advise patient to keep the dry-powder inhaler level when loading and inhaling drug. Tell him to always check inside the mouthpiece of the dry-powder inhaler before each use to make sure it's free of foreign objects.
• Tell patient to exhale fully before putting the mouthpiece in his mouth; then, keeping the dry-powder inhaler level, to close his lips around the mouthpiece and inhale steadily and deeply. Advise patient to hold his breath for a few seconds after inhaling to help drug stay in the lungs.
• Instruct patient simultaneously using a bronchodilator with this drug, to use the bronchodilator first. Tell patient to have a fast-acting bronchodilator readily available in case of wheezing.
• *Alert:* Advise all patients to immediately report worsening of respiratory symptoms, wheezing, shortness of breath, and bronchospasm.
• Advise patient that it's important to finish the entire treatment course.
• Tell patient that drug doesn't reduce the risk of transmitting the influenza virus to others.

12

Cephalosporins

cefaclor
cefadroxil
cefazolin sodium
cefdinir
cefepime hydrochloride
cefotaxime sodium
cefoxitin sodium
cefpodoxime proxetil
cefprozil
ceftazidime
ceftizoxime sodium
ceftriaxone sodium
cefuroxime axetil
cefuroxime sodium
cephalexin

---

cefaclor
SEF-ah-klor

Ceclor, Raniclor

Pharmacologic class: second-
generation cephalosporin
Pregnancy risk category B

AVAILABLE FORMS
Capsules: 250 mg, 500 mg
Oral suspension: 125 mg/5 ml,
187 mg/5 ml, 250 mg/5 ml, 375 mg/5 ml
Tablets (chewable): 125 mg, 187 mg,
250 mg, 375 mg
Tablets (extended-release): 375 mg,
500 mg

INDICATIONS & DOSAGES
➤ **Respiratory tract infections,
UTIs, skin and soft-tissue infections,
and otitis media caused by *Haemophilus influenzae, Streptococcus
pneumoniae, S. pyogenes, Escherichia
coli, Proteus mirabilis, Klebsiella*
species, and staphylococci**
Adults: 250 to 500 mg P.O. every 8 hours.
For pharyngitis or otitis media, daily dose
may be given in two equally divided doses
every 12 hours. For extended-release
forms in bronchitis, 500 mg P.O. every
12 hours for 7 days; for extended-release
forms in pharyngitis or skin and skin-

structure infections, 375 mg P.O. every
12 hours for 10 days and 7 to 10 days,
respectively.
Children: 20 mg/kg daily P.O. in divided
doses every 8 hours. For pharyngitis or
otitis media, daily dose may be given in
two equally divided doses every 12 hours.
In more serious infections, 40 mg/kg daily
is recommended, not to exceed 1 g daily.

ADMINISTRATION
P.O.
● Before giving, ask patient if he's allergic
to penicillins or cephalosporins.
● Obtain specimen for culture and sensitivity tests before giving. Begin therapy
while awaiting results.
● Give drug with meals.
● Extended-release tablets shouldn't be
crushed, cut, or chewed and should be
taken with meals.
● Store reconstituted suspension in refrigerator. Suspension is stable for 14 days if
refrigerated. Shake well before use.

ACTION
Inhibits cell-wall synthesis, promoting
osmotic instability; usually bactericidal.

Route	Onset	Peak	Duration
P.O.	Unknown	30–60 min	Unknown
P.O. (extended)	Unknown	1½–2½ hr	Unknown

Half-life: ½ to 1 hour.

ADVERSE REACTIONS
CNS: fever, dizziness, headache, somnolence, malaise.
GI: *diarrhea, nausea, pseudomembranous colitis,* vomiting, anorexia, dyspepsia, abdominal cramps, oral candidiasis.
GU: vaginal candidiasis, vaginitis.
Hematologic: *thrombocytopenia, transient leukopenia,* anemia, eosinophilia,
lymphocytosis.
Skin: *maculopapular rash,* dermatitis,
pruritus.
Other: *anaphylaxis,* hypersensitivity reactions, serum sickness.

INTERACTIONS
Drug-drug. *Aminoglycosides:* May increase risk of nephrotoxicity. Avoid using together.
Antacids: May decrease absorption of extended-release cefaclor if taken within 1 hour. Separate doses by 1 hour.
Anticoagulants: May increase anticoagulant effects. Monitor PT and INR.
Chloramphenicol: May cause antagonistic effect. Avoid using together.
Probenecid: May inhibit excretion and increase cefaclor level. Monitor patient for increased adverse reactions.

EFFECTS ON LAB TEST RESULTS
• May increase alkaline phosphatase, ALT, AST, bilirubin, GGT, and LDH levels. May decrease hemoglobin level.
• May increase eosinophil count. May decrease platelet and WBC counts.
• May falsely increase serum or urine creatinine level in tests using Jaffe reaction. May cause false-positive results of Coombs' test and urine glucose tests that use cupric sulfate, such as Benedict's reagent and Clinitest.

CONTRAINDICATIONS & CAUTIONS
• Contraindicated in patients hypersensitive to drug or other cephalosporins.
• Use cautiously in patients hypersensitive to penicillin because of the possibility of cross-sensitivity with other beta-lactam antibiotics.
• Use cautiously in breast-feeding women and in patients with a history of colitis or renal insufficiency.

NURSING CONSIDERATIONS
• If large doses are given, therapy is prolonged, or patient is at high risk, monitor patient for signs and symptoms of superinfection.
• *Look alike–sound alike:* Don't confuse drug with other cephalosporins that sound alike.

PATIENT TEACHING
• Tell patient to take entire amount of drug exactly as prescribed, even after he feels better.
• Tell patient that drug may be taken with meals. If suspension is used, instruct him to shake container well before measuring dose and to keep the drug refrigerated.

• Advise patient to notify prescriber if rash develops or signs and symptoms of superinfection appear.
• Inform patient not to crush, cut, or chew extended-release tablets and to take them with meals.

---

cefadroxil
sef-a-DROX-ill

Duricef◊

Pharmacologic class: first-generation cephalosporin
Pregnancy risk category B

AVAILABLE FORMS
Capsules: 500 mg
Oral suspension: 125 mg/5 ml, 250 mg/5 ml, 500 mg/5 ml
Tablets: 1 g

INDICATIONS & DOSAGES
➤ **UTIs caused by** *Escherichia coli,* *Proteus mirabilis,* **and** *Klebsiella* **species; skin and soft-tissue infections caused by staphylococci and streptococci; pharyngitis or tonsillitis caused by group A beta-hemolytic streptococci**
Adults: 1 to 2 g P.O. daily, depending on infection being treated. Usually given once daily or in two divided doses.
Children: 30 mg/kg P.O. daily in two divided doses every 12 hours.
Adjust-a-dose: In patients with renal impairment, give first dose of 1 g. Reduce additional doses based on creatinine clearance. If clearance is 25 to 50 ml/minute, give 500 mg P.O. every 12 hours. If clearance is 10 to 25 ml/minute, give 500 mg P.O. every 24 hours; if clearance is less than 10 ml/minute, give 500 mg P.O. every 36 hours.

ADMINISTRATION
P.O.
• Before administration, ask patient if he's allergic to penicillins or cephalosporins.
• Obtain specimen for culture and sensitivity tests before giving first dose. Begin therapy while awaiting results.
• Give drug with food or milk to lessen GI discomfort.

ACTION

Inhibits cell-wall synthesis, promoting osmotic instability; usually bactericidal.

Route	Onset	Peak	Duration
P.O.	Unknown	1–2 hr	Unknown

Half-life: About 1 to 2 hours.

ADVERSE REACTIONS

CNS: *seizures,* fever, dizziness, headache.
GI: *diarrhea, nausea, pseudomembranous colitis,* vomiting, glossitis, abdominal cramps, oral candidiasis.
GU: genital pruritus, candidiasis, vaginitis, renal dysfunction.
Hematologic: *transient neutropenia, leukopenia, agranulocytosis, thrombocytopenia,* anemia, eosinophilia.
Respiratory: dyspnea.
Skin: *maculopapular and erythematous rashes,* urticaria.
Other: *anaphylaxis, angioedema,* hypersensitivity reactions.

INTERACTIONS

Drug-drug. *Aminoglycosides:* May increase risk of nephrotoxicity. Avoid using together.
Probenecid: May inhibit excretion and increase cefadroxil level. Use together cautiously.

EFFECTS ON LAB TEST RESULTS

• May increase alkaline phosphatase, ALT, AST, bilirubin, GGT, and LDH levels. May decrease hemoglobin level.
• May increase eosinophil count. May decrease granulocyte, neutrophil, platelet, and WBC counts.
• May falsely increase serum or urine creatinine level in tests using Jaffe reaction. May cause false-positive results of Coombs' test and urine glucose tests that use cupric sulfate, such as Benedict's reagent and Clinitest.

CONTRAINDICATIONS & CAUTIONS

• Contraindicated in patients hypersensitive to drug or other cephalosporins.
• Use cautiously in patients with a history of sensitivity to penicillin and in breast-feeding women.
• Use cautiously in patients with impaired renal function; adjust dosage as needed.

NURSING CONSIDERATIONS

• If creatinine clearance is less than 50 ml/minute, lengthen dosage interval so drug doesn't accumulate. Monitor renal function in patients with renal dysfunction.
• If large doses are given, therapy is prolonged, or patient is high risk, monitor patient for superinfection.
• *Look alike–sound alike:* Don't confuse drug with other cephalosporins that sound alike.

PATIENT TEACHING

• Instruct patient to take drug with food or milk to lessen GI discomfort.
• Tell patient to take entire amount of drug exactly as prescribed, even after he feels better.
• Advise patient to notify prescriber if rash develops or if signs and symptoms of superinfection appear, such as recurring fever, chills, and malaise.

---

cefazolin sodium
sef-AH-zoe-lin

Ancef, Kefzol

Pharmacologic class: first-generation cephalosporin
Pregnancy risk category B

AVAILABLE FORMS

Infusion: 500 mg/50-ml bag, 1 g/50-ml bag
Injection (parenteral): 500 mg, 1 g

INDICATIONS & DOSAGES

➤ **Perioperative prevention in contaminated surgery**
Adults: 1 g I.M. or I.V. 30 to 60 minutes before surgery; then 0.5 to 1 g I.M. or I.V. every 6 to 8 hours for 24 hours. In operations lasting longer than 2 hours, give another 0.5- to 1-g dose I.M. or I.V. intraoperatively. Continue treatment for 3 to 5 days if life-threatening infection is likely.
➤ **Infections of respiratory, biliary, and GU tracts; skin, soft-tissue, bone, and joint infections; septicemia; endocarditis caused by** *Escherichia coli, Enterobacteriaceae,* **gonococci,** *Haemophilus influenzae,* *Klebsiella* **species,** *Proteus mirabilis,*

Staphylococcus aureus, Streptococcus pneumoniae, and group A beta-hemolytic streptococci
Adults: 250 mg to 500 mg I.M. or I.V. every 8 hours for mild infections or 500 mg to 1.5 g I.M. or I.V. every 6 to 8 hours for moderate to severe or life-threatening infections. Maximum 12 g/day in life-threatening situations.
Children older than age 1 month: 25 to 50 mg/kg/day I.M. or I.V. in three or four divided doses. In severe infections, dose may be increased to 100 mg/kg/day.
Adjust-a-dose: For patients with creatinine clearance of 35 to 54 ml/minute, give full dose every 8 hours; if clearance is 11 to 34 ml/minute, give 50% of usual dose every 12 hours; if clearance is below 10 ml/minute, give 50% of usual dose every 18 to 24 hours.

ADMINISTRATION
I.V.
● Before giving first dose, obtain specimen for culture and sensitivity tests. Begin therapy while awaiting results.
● Before giving drug, ask patient if he's allergic to penicillins or cephalosporins.
● Give commercially available frozen solutions in D_5W only by intermittent or continuous I.V. infusion.
● Reconstitute drug with sterile water, bacteriostatic water, or normal saline solution as follows: Add 2 ml to 500-mg vial or 2.5 ml to 1-g vial, yielding 225 mg/ml or 330 mg/ml, respectively.
● Shake well until dissolved.
● For direct injection, further dilute with 5 ml of sterile water for injection.
● Inject into a large vein or into the tubing of a free-flowing I.V. solution over 3 to 5 minutes.
● For intermittent infusion, add reconstituted drug to 50 to 100 ml of compatible solution or use premixed solution.
● If I.V. therapy lasts longer than 3 days, alternate injection sites. Use of small I.V. needles in larger available veins may be preferable.
● Reconstituted drug is stable 24 hours at room temperature or 10 days refrigerated.
● **Incompatibilities:** Aminoglycosides, amiodarone, amobarbital, ascorbic acid injection, bleomycin, calcium gluconate, cimetidine, colistimethate, hydrocortisone, idarubicin, lidocaine, norepinephrine, oxytetracycline, pentobarbital sodium, polymyxin B, ranitidine, tetracycline, theophylline, vitamin B complex with C.
I.M.
● Before giving first dose, obtain specimen for culture and sensitivity tests. Begin therapy while awaiting results.
● After reconstitution, inject drug I.M. without further dilution. This drug isn't as painful as other cephalosporins. Give injection deep into a large muscle, such as the gluteus maximus or the side of the thigh.

ACTION
Inhibits cell-wall synthesis, promoting osmotic instability; usually bactericidal.

Route	Onset	Peak	Duration
I.V.	Immediate	Immediate	Unknown
I.M.	Unknown	1–2 hr	Unknown

Half-life: About 1 to 2 hours.

ADVERSE REACTIONS
CNS: *seizures,* headache, confusion.
CV: *phlebitis, thrombophlebitis with I.V. injection.*
GI: *diarrhea, pseudomembranous colitis,* nausea, anorexia, vomiting, glossitis, dyspepsia, abdominal cramps, anal pruritus, oral candidiasis.
GU: genital pruritus, candidiasis, vaginitis.
Hematologic: *neutropenia, leukopenia, thrombocytopenia,* eosinophilia.
Skin: *maculopapular and erythematous rashes, urticaria, pruritus, pain, induration, sterile abscesses, tissue sloughing at injection site, Stevens-Johnson syndrome.*
Other: *anaphylaxis,* hypersensitivity reactions, serum sickness, drug fever.

INTERACTIONS
Drug-drug. *Aminoglycosides:* May increase risk of nephrotoxicity. Avoid using together.
Anticoagulants: May increase anticoagulant effects. Monitor PT and INR.
Probenecid: May inhibit excretion and increase cefazolin level. Use together cautiously.

Reactions may be *common,* uncommon, *life-threatening,* or COMMON AND LIFE-THREATENING.
Interaction may have a *rapid onset* or *delayed onset.*

EFFECTS ON LAB TEST RESULTS
• May increase alkaline phosphatase, ALT, AST, bilirubin, GGT, and LDH levels.
• May increase eosinophil count. May decrease neutrophil, platelet, and WBC counts.
• May falsely increase serum or urine creatinine level in tests using Jaffe reaction. May cause false-positive results of Coombs' test and urine glucose tests that use cupric sulfate, such as Benedict's reagent and Clinitest.

CONTRAINDICATIONS & CAUTIONS
• Contraindicated in patients hypersensitive to drug or other cephalosporins.
• Use cautiously in patients hypersensitive to penicillin because of the possibility of cross-sensitivity with other beta-lactam antibiotics.
• Use cautiously in breast-feeding women and in patients with a history of colitis or renal insufficiency.

NURSING CONSIDERATIONS
• If creatinine clearance falls below 55 ml/minute, adjust dosage.
• If large doses are given, therapy is prolonged, or patient is at high risk, monitor patient for signs and symptoms of superinfection.
• *Look alike–sound alike:* Don't confuse drug with other cephalosporins that sound alike.

PATIENT TEACHING
• Instruct patient to report adverse reactions promptly.
• Tell patient to report discomfort at I.V. injection site.
• Advise patient to notify prescriber if a rash develops or if signs and symptoms of superinfection appear, such as recurring fever, chills, and malaise.

cefdinir
sef-DIN-er

Omnicef

Pharmacologic class: third-generation cephalosporin
Pregnancy risk category B

AVAILABLE FORMS
Capsules: 300 mg
Suspension: 125 mg/5 ml, 250 mg/5 ml

INDICATIONS & DOSAGES
➤ **Mild to moderate infections caused by susceptible strains of microorganisms in community-acquired pneumonia, acute worsening of chronic bronchitis, acute maxillary sinusitis, acute bacterial otitis media, and uncomplicated skin and skin-structure infections**
Adults and children age 13 and older: 300 mg P.O. every 12 hours or 600 mg P.O. every 24 hours for 10 days. Give every 12 hours for pneumonia and skin infections.
Children ages 6 months to 12 years: 7 mg/kg P.O. every 12 hours or 14 mg/kg P.O. every 24 hours, for 10 days, up to maximum dose of 600 mg daily. Give every 12 hours for skin infections.
➤ **Pharyngitis, tonsillitis**
Adults and children age 13 and older: 300 mg P.O. every 12 hours for 5 to 10 days or 600 mg P.O. every 24 hours for 10 days.
Children ages 6 months to 12 years: 7 mg/kg P.O. every 12 hours for 5 to 10 days; or 14 mg/kg P.O. every 24 hours, for 10 days.
Adjust-a-dose: If creatinine clearance is less than 30 ml/minute, reduce dosage to 300 mg P.O. once daily for adults and 7 mg/kg up to 300 mg P.O. once daily for children. In patients receiving long-term hemodialysis, give 300 mg or 7 mg/kg P.O. at end of each dialysis session and then every other day.

ADMINISTRATION
P.O.
• Before administration, ask patient if he's allergic to penicillins or cephalosporins.
• Give antacids and iron supplements 2 hours before or after a dose of cefdinir.
• Give drug without regard for meals.

ACTION
Inhibits cell-wall synthesis, promoting osmotic instability; usually bactericidal. Some microorganisms resistant to penicillins and cephalosporins are susceptible to cefdinir. Active against a broad range of gram-positive and gram-negative aerobic microorganisms.

Route	Onset	Peak	Duration
P.O.	Unknown	2–4 hr	Unknown

Half-life: 1¾ hours.

ADVERSE REACTIONS
CNS: headache.
GI: *diarrhea, pseudomembranous colitis,* abdominal pain, nausea, vomiting.
GU: vaginal candidiasis, vaginitis, increased urine proteins, WBCs, and RBCs.
Skin: rash, cutaneous candidiasis.
Other: hypersensitivity reactions, *anaphylaxis.*

INTERACTIONS
Drug-drug. *Aminoglycosides:* May increase risk of nephrotoxicity. Avoid using together.
Antacids containing aluminum and magnesium, iron supplements, multivitamins containing iron: May decrease rate of absorption and bioavailability of cefdinir. Give such preparations 2 hours before or after cefdinir.
Probenecid: May inhibit renal excretion of cefdinir. Monitor patient for adverse reactions.

EFFECTS ON LAB TEST RESULTS
• May increase alkaline phosphatase, GGT, and LDH levels. May decrease bicarbonate levels.
• May increase eosinophil, lymphocyte, and platelet counts.
• May falsely increase serum or urine creatinine level in tests using Jaffe reaction. May cause false-positive results of Coombs' test and urine glucose tests that use cupric sulfate, such as Benedict's reagent and Clinitest.

CONTRAINDICATIONS & CAUTIONS
• Contraindicated in patients hypersensitive to drug or other cephalosporins.
• Use cautiously in patients hypersensitive to penicillin because of the possibility of cross-sensitivity with other beta-lactam antibiotics.
• Use cautiously in patients with history of colitis or renal insufficiency.

NURSING CONSIDERATIONS
• Prolonged drug treatment may result in emergence and overgrowth of resistant or-

ganisms. Monitor patient for signs and symptoms of superinfection.
• Pseudomembranous colitis has been reported with cefdinir and should be considered in patients with diarrhea after antibiotic therapy and in those with history of colitis.
• *Look alike–sound alike:* Don't confuse drug with other cephalosporins that sound alike.

PATIENT TEACHING
• Instruct patient to take antacids and iron supplements 2 hours before or after a dose of cefdinir.
• Inform diabetic patient that each teaspoon of suspension contains 2.86 g of sucrose.
• Tell patient that drug may be taken without regard to meals.
• Tell patient to take drug as prescribed, even after he feels better.
• Advise patient to report severe diarrhea or diarrhea with abdominal pain.
• Tell patient to report adverse reactions or signs and symptoms of superinfection promptly.

cefepime hydrochloride
SEF-ah-peem

Maxipime

Pharmacologic class: fourth-generation cephalosporin
Pregnancy risk category B

AVAILABLE FORMS
Injection: 500-mg vial, 1-g/100-ml piggyback bottle, 1-g ADD-Vantage vial, 1-g vial, 2-g/100-ml piggyback bottle, 2-g ADD-Vantage vial, 2-g vial

INDICATIONS & DOSAGES
➤ **Mild to moderate UTI caused by** *Escherichia coli, Klebsiella pneumoniae,* **or** *Proteus mirabilis,* **including concurrent bacteremia with these microorganisms**
Adults and children age 12 and older: 0.5 to 1 g I.M. or I.V. over 30 minutes every 12 hours for 7 to 10 days. Use I.M. only for *E. coli* infection when I.M. route is considered more appropriate route of administration.

Dosage adjustments for renal impairment

Creatinine clearance (ml/min)	If normal dosage would be			
	500 mg every 12 hr	1 g every 12 hr	2 g every 12 hr	2 g every 8 hr
30–60	500 mg every 24 hr	1 g every 24 hr	2 g every 24 hr	2 g every 12 hr
11–29	500 mg every 24 hr	500 mg every 24 hr	1 g every 24 hr	2 g every 24 hr
< 11	250 mg every 24 hr	250 mg every 24 hr	500 mg every 24 hr	1 g every 24 hr

➤ **Severe UTI, including pyelonephritis, caused by *E. coli* or *K. pneumoniae***
Adults and children age 12 and older: 2 g I.V. over 30 minutes every 12 hours for 10 days.

➤ **Moderate to severe pneumonia caused by *Streptococcus pneumoniae*, *Pseudomonas aeruginosa*, *K. pneumoniae*, or *Enterobacter* species**
Adults and children age 12 and older: 1 to 2 g I.V. over 30 minutes every 12 hours for 10 days.

➤ **Moderate to severe skin infection, uncomplicated skin infection, and skin-structure infection caused by *Streptococcus pyogenes* or methicillin-susceptible strains of *Staphylococcus aureus***
Adults and children age 12 and older: 2 g I.V. over 30 minutes every 12 hours for 10 days.

➤ **Complicated intra-abdominal infection caused by *E. coli*, viridans group streptococci, *P. aeruginosa*, *K. pneumoniae*, *Enterobacter* species, or *Bacteroides fragilis***
Adults: 2 g I.V. over 30 minutes every 12 hours for 7 to 10 days. Give with metronidazole.

➤ **Empiric therapy for febrile neutropenia**
Adults: 2 g I.V. every 8 hours for 7 days or until neutropenia resolves.

➤ **Uncomplicated and complicated UTI (including pyelonephritis), uncomplicated skin and skin-structure infection, pneumonia, empiric therapy for febrile neutropenic children**
Children ages 2 months to 16 years who weigh up to 40 kg (88 lb): 50 mg/kg/dose I.V. over 30 minutes every 12 hours, or every 8 hours for febrile neutropenia, for 7 to 10 days. Don't exceed 2 g/dose.

Adjust-a-dose: Adjust dosage based on creatinine clearance, as shown in the table. For patients receiving hemodialysis, about 68% of drug is removed after a 3-hour dialysis session. Cefepime dosage for patients receiving hemodialysis is 1 g on day 1, followed by 500 mg every 24 hours for treatment of all infections except febrile neutropenia. For patients with febrile neutropenia, give 1 g every 24 hours. Give cefepime after hemodialysis and at the same time each day. For patients receiving continuous ambulatory peritoneal dialysis, give normal dose every 48 hours.

ADMINISTRATION
I.V.
● Before giving drug, ask patient if he's allergic to penicillins or cephalosporins.
● Obtain specimen for culture and sensitivity tests before giving. Begin therapy while awaiting results.
● Follow manufacturer's guidelines closely when reconstituting drug. They vary with concentration of drug ordered and how drug is packaged (piggyback vial, ADD-Vantage vial, or regular vial).
● The type of diluent varies with the product used. Use only solutions recommended by the manufacturer.
● Give intermittent I.V. infusion with a Y-type administration and compatible solutions.
● Stop the main I.V. fluid while infusing.
● Infuse over about 30 minutes.
● **Incompatibilities:** Aminophylline, amphotericin B, amphotericin B cholesteryl sulfate complex, ciprofloxacin, gentamicin, metronidazole, tobramycin, vancomycin.

I.M.
- Before giving drug, ask patient if he's allergic to penicillins or cephalosporins.
- Obtain specimen for culture and sensitivity tests before giving. Begin therapy while awaiting results.
- Reconstitute drug using sterile water for injection, normal saline solution for injection, D_5W injection, 0.5% or 1% lidocaine hydrochloride, or bacteriostatic water for injection with parabens or benzyl alcohol. Follow manufacturer's guidelines for quantity of diluent to use.
- Inspect solution for particulate matter before use. The powder and its solutions tend to darken, depending on storage conditions. If stored as recommended, potency isn't adversely affected.
- Pain may occur at injection site.

ACTION
Inhibits bacterial cell-wall synthesis, promotes osmotic instability, and destroys bacteria.

Route	Onset	Peak	Duration
I.V., I.M.	30 min	1–2 hr	Unknown

Half-life: Adults: 2 to 2½ hours. Children: 1½ to 2 hours.

ADVERSE REACTIONS
CNS: fever, headache.
CV: phlebitis.
GI: colitis, diarrhea, nausea, vomiting, oral candidiasis.
GU: vaginitis.
Skin: rash, pruritus, urticaria.
Other: *anaphylaxis,* pain, inflammation, hypersensitivity reactions.

INTERACTIONS
Drug-drug. *Aminoglycosides:* May increase risk of nephrotoxicity. Monitor renal function closely.
Potent diuretics: May increase risk of nephrotoxicity. Monitor renal function closely.
Probenecid: May inhibit renal excretion of cefepime. Monitor patient for adverse reactions.

EFFECTS ON LAB TEST RESULTS
- May increase ALT and AST levels. May decrease phosphorus level.
- May increase eosinophil count. May alter PT and PTT.
- May falsely increase serum or urine creatinine level in tests using Jaffe reaction. May cause false-positive results of Coombs' test and urine glucose tests that use cupric sulfate, such as Benedict's reagent and Clinitest.

CONTRAINDICATIONS & CAUTIONS
- Contraindicated in patients hypersensitive to drug, cephalosporins, beta-lactam antibiotics, or penicillins.
- Use cautiously in patients hypersensitive to penicillin because of possibility of cross-sensitivity with other beta-lactam antibiotics.
- Use cautiously in breast-feeding women and in patients with history of colitis or renal insufficiency.

NURSING CONSIDERATIONS
- Adjust dosage in patients with impaired renal function. If dosage isn't adjusted, serious adverse reactions, including encephalopathy, myoclonus, seizures, and renal failure may occur.
- Monitor patient for superinfection. Drug may cause overgrowth of nonsusceptible bacteria or fungi.
- Drug may reduce PT activity. Patients at risk include those with renal or hepatic impairment or poor nutrition and those receiving prolonged therapy. Monitor PT and INR in these patients. Give vitamin K, as indicated.
- *Look alike–sound alike:* Don't confuse drug with other cephalosporins that sound alike.

PATIENT TEACHING
- Warn patient receiving drug I.M. that pain may occur at injection site.
- Advise patient to notify prescriber if a rash develops or if signs and symptoms of superinfection appear, such as recurring fever, chills, and malaise.
- Instruct patient to report adverse reactions promptly.

Reactions may be *common,* uncommon, *life-threatening,* or COMMON AND LIFE-THREATENING.
Interaction may have a *rapid onset* or *delayed onset.*

cefotaxime sodium
sef-oh-TAKS-eem

Claforan

Pharmacologic class: third-generation cephalosporin
Pregnancy risk category B

AVAILABLE FORMS
Infusion: 1-g, 2-g premixed package
Injection: 500-mg, 1-g, 2-g vials

INDICATIONS & DOSAGES
➤ **Perioperative prevention in contaminated surgery**
Adults: 1 g I.M. or I.V. 30 to 90 minutes before surgery. In patients undergoing bowel surgery, provide preoperative mechanical bowel cleansing and give a nonabsorbable anti-infective, such as neomycin. In patients undergoing cesarean delivery, give 1 g I.M. or I.V. as soon as the umbilical cord is clamped; then 1 g I.M. or I.V. 6 and 12 hours later.
➤ **Uncomplicated gonorrhea caused by penicillinase-producing strains or non–penicillinase-producing strains of *Neisseria gonorrhoeae***
Adults and adolescents: 500 mg I.M. as a single dose.
➤ **Rectal gonorrhea**
Men: 1 g I.M. as a single dose.
Women: 500 mg I.M. as a single dose.
➤ **Serious infection of the lower respiratory and urinary tract, CNS, skin, bone, and joints; gynecologic and intra-abdominal infection; bacteremia; septicemia caused by susceptible microorganisms, such as streptococci (including *Streptococcus pneumoniae* and *S. pyogenes*, *Staphylococcus aureus* [penicillinase- and non–penicillinase-producing] and *S. epidermidis*), *Escherichia coli*, *Klebsiella*, *Haemophilus influenzae*, *Serratia marcescens*, and species of *Pseudomonas* (including *P. aeruginosa*), *Enterobacter*, *Proteus*, and *Peptostreptococcus***
Adults and children who weigh 50 kg (110 lb) or more: 1 to 2 g I.V. or I.M. every 6 to 8 hours. Up to 12 g daily can be given for life-threatening infections.

Children ages 1 month to 12 years who weigh less than 50 kg: 50 to 180 mg/kg/day I.M. or I.V. in four to six divided doses.
Neonates ages 1 to 4 weeks: 50 mg/kg I.V. every 8 hours.
Neonates to age 1 week: 50 mg/kg I.V. every 12 hours.
Adjust-a-dose: For patients with creatinine clearance less than 20 ml/minute, give half usual dose at usual interval.

ADMINISTRATION
I.V.
● Before giving drug, ask patient if he's allergic to penicillins or cephalosporins.
● Obtain specimen for culture and sensitivity tests before giving. Begin therapy while awaiting results.
● For direct injection, reconstitute drug in 500-mg, 1-g, or 2-g vials with 10 ml of sterile water for injection. Solutions containing 1 g/14 ml are isotonic.
● Inject drug over 3 to 5 minutes into a large vein or into the tubing of a free-flowing I.V. solution.
● For infusion, reconstitute drug in infusion vials with 50 to 100 ml of D_5W or normal saline solution.
● Interrupt flow of primary I.V. solution, and infuse this drug over 20 to 30 minutes.
● **Incompatibilities:** Allopurinol, aminoglycosides, aminophylline, azithromycin, doxapram, filgrastim, fluconazole, hetastarch, pentamidine isethionate, sodium bicarbonate injection, vancomycin.
I.M.
● Before giving drug, ask patient if he's allergic to penicillins or cephalosporins.
● Obtain specimen for culture and sensitivity tests before giving. Begin therapy while awaiting results.
● For doses of 2 g, divide the dose and give at different sites.
● Inject deep into a large muscle, such as the gluteus maximus or the side of the thigh.

ACTION
Inhibits cell-wall synthesis, promoting osmotic instability; usually bactericidal.

Route	Onset	Peak	Duration
I.V.	Immediate	Immediate	Unknown
I.M.	Unknown	30 min	Unknown

Half-life: 1 to 2 hours.

ADVERSE REACTIONS
CNS: fever, headache, dizziness.
CV: *phlebitis, thrombophlebitis.*
GI: *diarrhea, **pseudomembranous colitis,*** nausea, vomiting.
GU: vaginitis, candidiasis, interstitial nephritis.
Hematologic: *agranulocytosis, thrombocytopenia, transient neutropenia,* eosinophilia, hemolytic anemia.
Skin: *maculopapular and erythematous rashes, urticaria, pain, induration, sterile abscesses, temperature elevation, tissue sloughing at I.M. injection site.*
Other: *anaphylaxis,* hypersensitivity reactions, serum sickness.

INTERACTIONS
Drug-drug. *Aminoglycosides:* May increase risk of nephrotoxicity. Monitor patient's renal function tests.
Probenecid: May inhibit excretion and increase cefotaxime. Use together cautiously.

EFFECTS ON LAB TEST RESULTS
• May increase alkaline phosphatase, ALT, AST, bilirubin, GGT, and LDH levels. May decrease hemoglobin level.
• May increase eosinophil count. May decrease granulocyte, neutrophil, and platelet counts.
• May cause positive Coombs' test results.

CONTRAINDICATIONS & CAUTIONS
• Contraindicated in patients hypersensitive to drug or other cephalosporins.
• Use cautiously in patients hypersensitive to penicillin because of possibility of cross-sensitivity with other beta-lactam antibiotics.
• Use cautiously in breast-feeding women and in patients with history of colitis or renal insufficiency.

NURSING CONSIDERATIONS
• If large doses are given, therapy is prolonged, or patient is at high risk, monitor patient for superinfection.
• *Look alike–sound alike:* Don't confuse drug with other cephalosporins that sound alike.

PATIENT TEACHING
• Tell patient to report adverse reactions and signs and symptoms of superinfection promptly.
• Instruct patient to report discomfort at I.V. insertion site.

cefoxitin sodium
se-FOX-i-tin

Mefoxin

Pharmacologic class: second-generation cephalosporin
Pregnancy risk category B

AVAILABLE FORMS
Infusion: 1 g, 2 g in 50-ml or 100-ml container
Injection: 1 g, 2 g

INDICATIONS & DOSAGES
➤ **Serious infection of the respiratory and GU tracts; skin, soft-tissue, bone, or joint infection; bloodstream or intra-abdominal infection caused by susceptible organisms (such as *Escherichia coli* and other coliform bacteria, penicillinase- and non–penicillinase-producing *Staphylococcus aureus, S. epidermidis,* streptococci, *Klebsiella, Haemophilus influenzae,* and *Bacteroides,* including *B. fragilis*)**
Adults: 1 to 2 g I.V. or I.M. every 6 to 8 hours for uncomplicated infections. Up to 12 g daily may be used in life-threatening infections.
Children older than age 3 months: 80 to 160 mg/kg daily I.V. or I.M., given in four to six equally divided doses. Maximum daily dose is 12 g.
➤ **Uncomplicated gonorrhea**
Adults: 2 g I.M. with 1 g probenecid P.O. as a single dose. Give probenecid within 30 minutes before cefoxitin dose.
➤ **Perioperative prevention**
Adults: 2 g I.M. or I.V. 30 to 60 minutes before surgery; then 2 g I.M. or I.V. every 6 hours for up to 24 hours.
Children age 3 months and older: 30 to 40 mg/kg I.M. or I.V. 30 to 60 minutes before surgery; then 30 to 40 mg/kg every 6 hours for up to 24 hours.

Reactions may be *common,* uncommon, *life-threatening,* or COMMON AND LIFE-THREATENING.
Interaction may have a *rapid onset* or *delayed onset.*

Adjust-a-dose: For patients with creatinine clearance of 30 to 50 ml/minute, 1 to 2 g every 8 to 12 hours; if clearance is 10 to 29 ml/minute, 1 to 2 g every 12 to 24 hours; if clearance is 5 to 9 ml/minute, 0.5 to 1 g every 12 to 24 hours; and if clearance is less than 5 ml/minute, 0.5 to 1 g every 24 to 48 hours. For patients receiving hemodialysis, give a loading dose of 1 to 2 g after each hemodialysis session; then give the maintenance dose based on creatinine level.

ADMINISTRATION
I.V.
● Before giving drug, ask patient if he's allergic to penicillins or cephalosporins.
● Obtain specimen for culture and sensitivity tests before giving. Begin therapy while awaiting results.
● Reconstitute 1 g with at least 10 ml of sterile water for injection and 2 g with 10 to 20 ml of sterile water for injection. Solutions of D_5W and normal saline solution for injection also may be used.
● For direct injection, give drug over 3 to 5 minutes into a large vein or into the tubing of a free-flowing I.V. solution.
● For intermittent infusion, add reconstituted drug to 50 or 100 ml of D_5W or normal saline solution for injection.
● Interrupt flow of primary solution during infusion.
● Assess site often to detect evidence of thrombophlebitis.
● **Incompatibilities:** Aminoglycosides, filgrastim, hetastarch, pentamidine isethionate, ranitidine.
I.M.
● Before giving drug, ask patient if he's allergic to penicillins or cephalosporins.
● Obtain specimen for culture and sensitivity tests before giving. Begin therapy while awaiting results.
● Reconstitute each 1 g of drug with 2 ml of sterile water for injection or 0.5% or 1% lidocaine hydrochloride (without epinephrine) to minimize pain. Inject deep into a large muscle, such as the gluteus maximus or the lateral aspect of the thigh.
● After reconstitution, drug may be stored for 24 hours (6 hours for non-ADD-Vantage vials) at room temperature or 1 week under refrigeration.

ACTION
Inhibits cell-wall synthesis, promoting osmotic instability; usually bactericidal.

Route	Onset	Peak	Duration
I.V.	Immediate	Immediate	Unknown
I.M.	Unknown	20–30 min	Unknown

Half-life: About ½ to 1 hours.

ADVERSE REACTIONS
CNS: fever.
CV: *phlebitis, thrombophlebitis,* hypotension.
GI: *diarrhea, pseudomembranous colitis,* nausea, vomiting.
GU: *acute renal failure.*
Hematologic: *thrombocytopenia, transient neutropenia,* eosinophilia, hemolytic anemia, anemia.
Respiratory: dyspnea.
Skin: *maculopapular and erythematous rashes, urticaria, pain, induration, sterile abscesses, tissue sloughing at injection site,* exfoliative dermatitis.
Other: *anaphylaxis,* hypersensitivity reactions, serum sickness.

INTERACTIONS
Drug-drug. *Aminoglycosides:* May increase risk of nephrotoxicity. Monitor patient's renal function tests.
Probenecid: May inhibit excretion and increase cefoxitin level. Probenecid may be used for this effect.

EFFECTS ON LAB TEST RESULTS
● May increase alkaline phosphatase, ALT, AST, bilirubin, and LDH levels. May decrease hemoglobin level.
● May increase eosinophil count. May decrease neutrophil and platelet counts.
● May falsely increase serum or urine creatinine level in tests using Jaffe reaction. May cause false-positive results of Coombs' test and urine glucose tests that use cupric sulfate, such as Benedict's reagent and Clinitest.

CONTRAINDICATIONS & CAUTIONS
● Contraindicated in patients hypersensitive to drug or other cephalosporins.
● Use cautiously in patients hypersensitive to penicillin because of possibility of

cross-sensitivity with other beta-lactam antibiotics.

● Use cautiously in breast-feeding women and in patients with history of colitis or renal insufficiency.

NURSING CONSIDERATIONS

● *Alert:* The premixed frozen product is for I.V. use only.

● If large doses are given, therapy is prolonged, or patient is at high risk, monitor patient for signs and symptoms of superinfection.

● *Look alike–sound alike:* Don't confuse drug with other cephalosporins that sound alike.

PATIENT TEACHING

● Tell patient to report adverse reactions and signs and symptoms of superinfection promptly.

● Instruct patient to report discomfort at I.V. site.

● Advise patient to notify prescriber about loose stools or diarrhea.

cefpodoxime proxetil
SEF-pod-OX-eem

Vantin

Pharmacologic class: third-generation cephalosporin
Pregnancy risk category B

AVAILABLE FORMS

Oral suspension: 50 mg/5 ml or 100 mg/5 ml in 50-, 75-, or 100-ml bottles
Tablets (film-coated): 100 mg, 200 mg

INDICATIONS & DOSAGES

➤ **Acute, community-acquired pneumonia caused by strains of** *Haemophilus influenzae* **or** *Streptococcus pneumoniae*
Adults and children age 12 and older:
200 mg P.O. every 12 hours for 14 days.
➤ **Acute bacterial worsening of chronic bronchitis caused by** *S. pneumoniae* **or** *H. influenzae* **(strains that don't produce beta-lactamase only), or** *Moraxella catarrhalis*
Adults and children age 12 and older:
200 mg P.O. every 12 hours for 10 days.

➤ **Uncomplicated gonorrhea in men and women; rectal gonococcal infections in women**
Adults and children age 12 and older:
200 mg P.O. as a single dose.
➤ **Uncomplicated skin and skin-structure infections caused by** *Staphylococcus aureus* **or** *S. pyogenes*
Adults and children age 12 and older:
400 mg P.O. every 12 hours for 7 to 14 days.
➤ **Acute otitis media caused by** *S. pneumoniae* **(penicillin-susceptible strains only),** *S. pyogenes,* *H. influenzae,* **or** *M. catarrhalis*
Children age 2 months to 12 years:
5 mg/kg P.O. every 12 hours for 5 days. Don't exceed 200 mg per dose.
➤ **Pharyngitis or tonsillitis caused by** *S. pyogenes*
Adults: 100 mg P.O. every 12 hours for 5 to 10 days.
Children ages 2 months to 12 years:
5 mg/kg P.O. every 12 hours for 5 to 10 days. Don't exceed 100 mg per dose.
➤ **Uncomplicated UTIs caused by** *Escherichia coli, Klebsiella pneumoniae, Proteus mirabilis,* **or** *Staphylococcus saprophyticus*
Adults: 100 mg P.O. every 12 hours for 7 days.
➤ **Mild to moderate acute maxillary sinusitis caused by** *H. influenzae, S. pneumoniae,* **or** *M. catarrhalis*
Adults and adolescents age 12 and older:
200 mg P.O. every 12 hours for 10 days.
Children ages 2 months to 12 years:
5 mg/kg P.O. every 12 hours for 10 days; maximum is 200 mg/dose.
Adjust-a-dose: For patients with creatinine clearance less than 30 ml/minute, increase dosage interval to every 24 hours. Give to dialysis patients three times weekly after dialysis.

ADMINISTRATION
P.O.
● Before administration, ask patient if he's allergic to penicillins or cephalosporins.
● Obtain specimen for culture and sensitivity tests before giving. Begin therapy while awaiting results.
● Give drug with food to enhance absorption. Shake suspension well before using.

• Store suspension in the refrigerator (36°
to 46° F [2° to 8° C]). Discard unused portion after 14 days.

ACTION
Inhibits cell-wall synthesis, promoting osmotic instability; usually bactericidal.

Route	Onset	Peak	Duration
P.O.	Unknown	2–3 hr	Unknown

Half-life: 2 to 3 hours.

ADVERSE REACTIONS
CNS: headache.
GI: *diarrhea, pseudomembranous colitis,*
nausea, vomiting, abdominal pain.
GU: vaginal fungal infections.
Skin: rash.
Other: *anaphylaxis,* hypersensitivity
reactions.

INTERACTIONS
Drug-drug. *Aminoglycosides:* May increase risk of nephrotoxicity. Monitor
renal function tests closely.
Antacids, H₂-receptor antagonists: May
decrease absorption of cefpodoxime.
Avoid using together.
Probenecid: May decrease excretion
of cefpodoxime. Monitor patient for
toxicity.
Drug-food. *Any food:* May increase absorption. Give tablets with food to enhance absorption. Oral suspension may be
given without regard to food.

EFFECTS ON LAB TEST RESULTS
• May falsely increase serum or urine creatinine level in tests using Jaffe reaction.
May cause false-positive results of
Coombs' test and urine glucose tests that
use cupric sulfate, such as Benedict's
reagent and Clinitest.

CONTRAINDICATIONS & CAUTIONS
• Contraindicated in patients hypersensitive to drug or other cephalosporins.
• Use cautiously in patients with a history
of penicillin hypersensitivity because of
risk of cross-sensitivity.
• Use cautiously in patients receiving
nephrotoxic drugs because other cephalosporins have been shown to have nephrotoxic potential.

• Use cautiously in breast-feeding women
because drug appears in breast milk.

NURSING CONSIDERATIONS
• Monitor renal function and compare
with baseline.
• Monitor patient for superinfection. Drug
may cause overgrowth of nonsusceptible
bacteria or fungi.
• *Look alike–sound alike:* Don't confuse
drug with other cephalosporins that sound
alike.

PATIENT TEACHING
• Tell patient to take drug as prescribed,
even after he feels better.
• Instruct patient to take drug with
food. If patient is using suspension,
tell him to shake container before
measuring dose and to keep container
refrigerated.
• Tell patient to call prescriber if rash or
signs and symptoms of superinfection
occur.
• Instruct patient to notify prescriber about
loose stools or diarrhea.

---

cefprozil
sef-PRO-zil

Cefzil✐

Pharmacologic class: second-
generation cephalosporin
Pregnancy risk category B

AVAILABLE FORMS
Oral suspension: 125 mg/5 ml,
250 mg/5 ml
Tablets: 250 mg, 500 mg

INDICATIONS & DOSAGES
➤ **Pharyngitis or tonsillitis caused
by** *Streptococcus pyogenes*
*Adults and children age 13 and
older:* 500 mg P.O. daily for at least
10 days.
➤ **Otitis media caused by** *Streptococcus pneumoniae, Haemophilus
influenzae,* **and** *Moraxella
catarrhalis*
*Infants and children ages 6 months to
12 years:* 15 mg/kg P.O. every 12 hours
for 10 days.

➤ Secondary bacterial infections of acute bronchitis and acute bacterial worsening of chronic bronchitis caused by *S. pneumoniae, H. influenzae,* and *M. catarrhalis*
Adults and children age 13 and older: 500 mg P.O. every 12 hours for 10 days.

➤ Uncomplicated skin and skin-structure infections caused by *Staphylococcus aureus* and *S. pyogenes*
Adults and children age 13 and older: 250 or 500 mg P.O. every 12 hours or 500 mg daily for 10 days.

➤ Acute sinusitis caused by *S. pneumoniae, H. influenzae* (beta-lactamase–positive and –negative strains), and *M. catarrhalis* (including strains that produce beta-lactamase)
Adults and children age 13 and older: 250 mg P.O. every 12 hours for 10 days; for moderate to severe infection, 500 mg P.O. every 12 hours for 10 days.
Children ages 6 months to 12 years: 7.5 mg/kg P.O. every 12 hours for 10 days; for moderate to severe infections, 15 mg/kg P.O. every 12 hours for 10 days.
Adjust-a-dose: If creatinine clearance is less than 30 ml/minute, give 50% of standard dose at standard intervals. If patient is receiving dialysis, give dose after hemodialysis is completed; drug is removed by hemodialysis.

ADMINISTRATION
P.O.
● Obtain specimen for culture and sensitivity tests before giving first dose. Start therapy while awaiting results.
● Before giving, ask patient if he's allergic to penicillins or cephalosporins.
● Shake suspension well before using.

ACTION
Inhibits cell-wall synthesis, promoting osmotic instability; usually bactericidal.

Route	Onset	Peak	Duration
P.O.	Unknown	1½ hr	Unknown

Half-life: 1¼ hours in patients with normal renal function; 2 hours in patients with impaired hepatic function; and 5¼ to 6 hours in patients with end-stage renal disease.

ADVERSE REACTIONS
CNS: dizziness, hyperactivity, headache, nervousness, insomnia, confusion, somnolence.
GI: diarrhea, nausea, vomiting, abdominal pain.
GU: genital pruritus, vaginitis.
Hematologic: eosinophilia.
Skin: rash, urticaria, diaper rash.
Other: *anaphylaxis,* superinfection, hypersensitivity reactions, serum sickness.

INTERACTIONS
Drug-drug. *Aminoglycosides:* May increase risk of nephrotoxicity. Monitor renal function tests closely.
Probenecid: May inhibit excretion and increase cefprozil level. Use together cautiously.

EFFECTS ON LAB TEST RESULTS
● May increase alkaline phosphatase, ALT, AST, bilirubin, BUN, creatinine, and LDH levels.
● May increase eosinophil count. May decrease leukocyte, platelet, and WBC counts.
● May falsely increase serum or urine creatinine level in tests using Jaffe reaction. May cause false-positive results of Coombs' test and urine glucose tests that use cupric sulfate, such as Benedict's reagent and Clinitest.

CONTRAINDICATIONS & CAUTIONS
● Contraindicated in patients hypersensitive to drug or other cephalosporins.
● Use cautiously in patients hypersensitive to penicillin because of possibility of cross-sensitivity with other beta-lactam antibiotics.
● Use cautiously in breast-feeding women and in patients with history of colitis and renal insufficiency.

NURSING CONSIDERATIONS
● Monitor renal function and liver function test results.
● Monitor patient for superinfection. May cause overgrowth of nonsusceptible bacteria or fungi.
● ***Look alike–sound alike:*** Don't confuse drug with other cephalosporins that sound alike.

PATIENT TEACHING
- Advise patient to take drug as prescribed, even after he feels better.
- Tell patient to shake suspension well before measuring dose.
- Inform patient or parent that oral suspension is bubble gum–flavored to improve palatability and promote compliance in children. Tell him to refrigerate reconstituted suspension and to discard unused drug after 14 days.
- Instruct patient to notify prescriber if rash or signs and symptoms of superinfection occur.

ceftazidime
sef-TAZ-i-deem

Fortaz, Tazicef

Pharmacologic class: third-generation cephalosporin
Pregnancy risk category B

AVAILABLE FORMS
Infusion: 1 g, 2 g in 50-ml and 100-ml vials (premixed)
Injection (with arginine): 500 mg, 1 g, 2 g
Injection (with sodium carbonate): 500 mg, 1 g, 2 g

INDICATIONS & DOSAGES
➤ **Serious UTI and lower respiratory tract infection; skin, gynecologic, intra-abdominal, and CNS infection; bacteremia; and septicemia caused by susceptible microorganisms, such as streptococci (including *Streptococcus pneumoniae* and *S. pyogenes*), penicillinase- and non–penicillinase-producing *Staphylococcus aureus*, *Escherichia coli*, *Klebsiella*, *Proteus*, *Enterobacter*, *Haemophilus influenzae*, *Pseudomonas*, and some strains of *Bacteroides***
Adults and children age 12 and older: 1 to 2 g I.V. or I.M. every 8 to 12 hours; up to 6 g daily in life-threatening infections.
Children ages 1 month to 12 years: 30 to 50 mg/kg I.V. every 8 hours. Maximum dose is 6 g/day. Use sodium carbonate formulation.

Neonates up to age 4 weeks: 30 mg/kg I.V. every 12 hours. Use sodium carbonate formulation.
➤ **Uncomplicated UTI**
Adults: 250 mg I.V. or I.M. every 12 hours.
➤ **Complicated UTI**
Adults and children age 12 and older: 500 mg to 1 g I.V. or I.M. every 8 to 12 hours.
Adjust-a-dose: If creatinine clearance is 31 to 50 ml/minute, give 1 g every 12 hours; if clearance is 16 to 30 ml/minute, give 1 g every 24 hours; if clearance is 6 to 15 ml/minute, give 500 mg every 24 hours; if clearance is less than 5 ml/minute, give 500 mg every 48 hours. Ceftazidime is removed by hemodialysis; give a loading dose of 1 g, followed by 1 g after each hemodialysis period.

ADMINISTRATION
I.V.
- Before administration, ask patient if he's allergic to penicillins or cephalosporins.
- Obtain specimen for culture and sensitivity tests before giving. Begin therapy while awaiting results.
- Each brand of drug includes specific instructions for reconstitution. Read and follow them carefully.
- To reconstitute solution that contains sodium carbonate, add 5 ml sterile water for injection to a 500-mg vial, or add 10 ml to a 1-g or 2-g vial. Shake well to dissolve drug. Because carbon dioxide is released during dissolution, positive pressure will develop in vial.
- To reconstitute solution that contains arginine, use 10 ml of sterile water for injection. This product won't release gas bubbles.
- Infuse drug over 15 to 30 minutes.
- **Incompatibilities:** Aminoglycosides, aminophylline, amiodarone, amphotericin B cholesteryl sulfate complex, azithromycin, clarithromycin, fluconazole, idarubicin, midazolam, pentamidine isethionate, ranitidine hydrochloride, sargramostim, sodium bicarbonate solutions, vancomycin.
I.M.
- Before administration, ask patient if he's allergic to penicillins or cephalosporins.

• Obtain specimen for culture and sensitivity tests before giving. Begin therapy while awaiting results.
• Inject deep into a large muscle, such as the gluteus maximus or the side of the thigh.

ACTION
Inhibits cell-wall synthesis, promoting osmotic instability; usually bactericidal.

Route	Onset	Peak	Duration
I.V.	Immediate	Immediate	Unknown
I.M.	Unknown	1 hr	Unknown

Half-life: 1½ to 2 hours.

ADVERSE REACTIONS
CNS: *seizures,* headache, dizziness, paresthesia.
CV: *phlebitis, thrombophlebitis.*
GI: *pseudomembranous colitis,* nausea, vomiting, diarrhea, abdominal cramps.
GU: vaginitis, candidiasis.
Hematologic: *agranulocytosis, leukopenia, thrombocytopenia,* eosinophilia, thrombocytosis, hemolytic anemia.
Skin: *maculopapular and erythematous rashes, urticaria, pain, induration, sterile abscesses, tissue sloughing at injection site.*
Other: *anaphylaxis,* hypersensitivity reactions, serum sickness.

INTERACTIONS
Drug-drug. *Aminoglycosides:* May cause additive or synergistic effect against some strains of *Pseudomonas aeruginosa* and *Enterobacteriaceae;* may increase risk of nephrotoxicity. Monitor patient for effects and monitor renal function.
Chloramphenicol: May cause antagonistic effect. Avoid using together.

EFFECTS ON LAB TEST RESULTS
• May increase alkaline phosphatase, ALT, AST, bilirubin, and LDH levels. May decrease hemoglobin level.
• May increase eosinophil count. May decrease granulocyte and WBC counts. May increase or decrease platelet count.
• May falsely increase serum or urine creatinine level in tests using Jaffe reaction. May cause false-positive results of Coombs' test and urine glucose tests that use cupric sulfate, such as Benedict's reagent and Clinitest.

CONTRAINDICATIONS & CAUTIONS
• Contraindicated in patients hypersensitive to drug or other cephalosporins.
• Use cautiously in patients hypersensitive to penicillin because of possibility of cross-sensitivity with other beta-lactam antibiotics.
• Use cautiously in breast-feeding women and in patients with history of colitis or renal insufficiency.

NURSING CONSIDERATIONS
• If large doses are given, therapy is prolonged, or patient is at high risk, monitor patient for signs and symptoms of superinfection.
• *Alert:* Drug contains either sodium carbonate (Fortaz or Tazicef) or arginine to facilitate dissolution of drug. Safety and effectiveness of solutions containing arginine in children younger than age 12 haven't been established.
• *Look alike–sound alike:* Don't confuse drug with other cephalosporins that sound alike.

PATIENT TEACHING
• Tell patient to report adverse reactions or signs and symptoms of superinfection promptly.
• Instruct patient to report discomfort at I.V. insertion site.
• Advise patient to notify prescriber about loose stools or diarrhea.

ceftizoxime sodium
sef-ti-ZOX-eem

Cefizox

Pharmacologic class: third-generation cephalosporin
Pregnancy risk category B

AVAILABLE FORMS
Infusion: 1 g, 2 g in 100-ml vials or in 50-ml containers
Injection: 500 mg, 1 g, 2 g

INDICATIONS & DOSAGES
➤ **Serious UTI, lower respiratory tract infection, gynecologic infection, bacteremia, septicemia, meningitis, intra-abdominal infection, bone or**

---

joint infection, and skin infection caused by susceptible microorganisms, such as streptococci (including *Streptococcus pneumoniae* and *S. pyogenes*), *Staphylococcus aureus, S. epidermidis, Escherichia coli, Haemophilus influenzae,* and *Klebsiella, Enterobacter, Proteus, Peptostreptococcus,* and some *Pseudomonas* species

Adults: 1 to 2 g I.V. or I.M. every 8 to 12 hours. For life-threatening infections, give up to 2 g I.V. every 4 hours, or 3 to 4 g I.V. every 8 hours.

Children older than age 6 months: 50 mg/kg I.V. every 6 to 8 hours. For serious infections, up to 200 mg/kg/day in divided doses may be used. Don't exceed 12 g/day.

➤ **Uncomplicated gonorrhea**
Adults: 1 g I.M. as a single dose.

Adjust-a-dose: If creatinine clearance is 50 to 79 ml/minute, give 500 mg to 1.5 g every 8 hours; if clearance is 5 to 49 ml/minute, give 250 mg to 1 g every 12 hours; if clearance is less than 5 ml/minute or patient undergoes hemodialysis, give 500 mg to 1 g every 48 hours, or 250 to 500 mg every 24 hours.

ADMINISTRATION
I.V.
● Before giving drug, ask patient if he's allergic to penicillins or cephalosporins.
● Obtain specimen for culture and sensitivity tests before giving. Begin therapy while awaiting results.
● To reconstitute powder, add 5 ml of sterile water to a 500-mg vial, 10 ml to a 1-g vial, or 20 ml to a 2-g vial.
● Reconstitute drug in piggyback vials with 50 to 100 ml of normal saline solution or D₅W. Shake well.
● For direct injection, give drug over 3 to 5 minutes or slowly into I.V. tubing of free-flowing compatible solution.
● For infusion, give drug over 15 to 30 minutes.
● **Incompatibilities:** Aminoglycosides, cisatracurium besylate, filgrastim; possibly promethazine hydrochloride and vancomycin hydrochloride.

I.M.
● Before giving drug, ask patient if he's allergic to penicillins or cephalosporins.
● Obtain specimen for culture and sensitivity tests before giving. Begin therapy while awaiting results.
● Mix 1.5 ml of diluent per 500 mg of drug. Inject deep into a large muscle, such as the gluteus maximus or the side of the thigh. Divide doses of more than 2 g and give at two separate sites.

ACTION
Inhibits cell-wall synthesis, promoting osmotic instability; usually bactericidal.

Route	Onset	Peak	Duration
I.V.	Immediate	Immediate	Unknown
I.M.	Unknown	30–90 min	Unknown

Half-life: 1½ to 2 hours.

ADVERSE REACTIONS
CNS: fever.
CV: *phlebitis, thrombophlebitis.*
GI: *diarrhea, pseudomembranous colitis,* nausea, anorexia, vomiting.
GU: vaginitis.
Hematologic: *thrombocytopenia, thrombocytosis, transient neutropenia,* eosinophilia, hemolytic anemia, anemia.
Respiratory: dyspnea.
Skin: *maculopapular and erythematous rashes, urticaria, pain, induration, sterile abscesses, tissue sloughing at injection site.*
Other: *anaphylaxis,* hypersensitivity reactions, serum sickness.

INTERACTIONS
Drug-drug. *Aminoglycosides:* May increase nephrotoxicity. Monitor renal function.
Probenecid: May inhibit excretion and increase ceftizoxime level. Use probenecid for this effect.

EFFECTS ON LAB TEST RESULTS
● May increase alkaline phosphatase, ALT, AST, bilirubin, BUN, creatinine, GGT, and LDH levels. May decrease albumin, hemoglobin, and protein levels.
● May decrease PT and granulocyte, neutrophil, platelet, RBC, and WBC counts.

• May falsely increase serum or urine creatinine level in tests using Jaffe reaction. May cause false-positive results of Coombs' test and urine glucose tests that use cupric sulfate, such as Benedict's reagent and Clinitest.

CONTRAINDICATIONS & CAUTIONS
• Contraindicated in patients hypersensitive to drug or other cephalosporins.
• Use cautiously in patients hypersensitive to penicillin because of possible cross-sensitivity with other beta-lactam antibiotics.
• Use cautiously in breast-feeding women and in patients with history of colitis or renal insufficiency.

NURSING CONSIDERATIONS
• If large doses are given, therapy is prolonged, or patient is at high risk, monitor patient for signs or symptoms of superinfection.
• *Look alike–sound alike:* Don't confuse drug with other cephalosporins that sound alike.

PATIENT TEACHING
• Tell patient to report adverse reactions and signs and symptoms of superinfection promptly.
• Instruct patient to report discomfort at I.V. site.
• Tell patient to notify prescriber about loose stools or diarrhea.

---

ceftriaxone sodium
sef-try-AX-ohn

Rocephin

Pharmacologic class: third-generation cephalosporin
Pregnancy risk category B

AVAILABLE FORMS
Infusion: 1 g, 2-g piggyback; 1 g, 2 g/50 ml premixed
Injection: 250 mg, 500 mg, 1 g, 2 g

INDICATIONS & DOSAGES
➤ **Uncomplicated gonococcal vulvovaginitis**
Adults: 125 mg I.M. as a single dose, plus azithromycin 1 g P.O. as a single dose or doxycycline 100 mg P.O. b.i.d. for 7 days.
➤ **UTI; lower respiratory tract, gynecologic, bone or joint, intra-abdominal, skin, or skin structure infection; septicemia**
Adults and children older than age 12 years: 1 to 2 g I.M. or I.V. daily or in equally divided doses every 12 hours. Total daily dose shouldn't exceed 4 g.
Children age 12 and younger: 50 to 75 mg/kg I.M. or I.V., not to exceed 2 g/day, given in divided doses every 12 hours or given once daily.
➤ **Meningitis**
Adults and children: Initially, 100 mg/kg I.M. or I.V. Don't exceed 4 g; then 100 mg/kg I.M. or I.V., given once daily or in divided doses every 12 hours, not to exceed 4 g, for 7 to 14 days.
➤ **Perioperative prevention**
Adults: 1 g I.V. as a single dose 30 minutes to 2 hours before surgery.
➤ **Acute bacterial otitis media**
Children: 50 mg/kg I.M. as a single dose. Don't exceed 1 g.
➤ **Neurologic complications, carditis, and arthritis from penicillin G–refractory Lyme disease** ◆
Adults: 2 g I.V. daily for 14 to 28 days.

ADMINISTRATION
I.V.
• Before giving drug, ask patient if he's allergic to penicillins or cephalosporins.
• Obtain specimen for culture and sensitivity tests before giving first dose. Begin therapy while awaiting results.
• Reconstitute drug with sterile water for injection, normal saline solution for injection, D_5W, or a combination of normal saline solution and dextrose injection and other compatible solutions.
• Add 2.4 ml of diluent to the 250-mg vial, 4.8 ml to the 500-mg vial, 9.6 ml to the 1-g vial, and 19.2 ml to the 2-g vial. All reconstituted solutions average 100 mg/ml. For intermittent infusion, dilute further to achieve desired concentration, and give over 30 minutes.
• Diluted I.V. preparation is stable for 48 hours at room temperature or 10 days if refrigerated.

Reactions may be *common,* uncommon, *life-threatening,* or COMMON AND LIFE-THREATENING.
Interaction may have a *rapid onset* or *delayed onset.*

- **Alert:** Don't mix or coadminister ceftriaxone with calcium-containing I.V. solutions, including parenteral nutrition. This includes the use of different infusion lines at different sites. Don't administer within 48 hours of each other in any patient.
- **Incompatibilities:** Aminoglycosides, aminophylline, amphotericin B cholesteryl sulfate complex, azithromycin, calcium, clindamycin phosphate, filgrastim, fluconazole, gentamicin, labetalol, lidocaine hydrochloride, linezolid, metronidazole, pentamidine isethionate, theophylline, vancomycin, vinorelbine tartrate.

I.M.
- Before giving drug, ask patient if he's allergic to penicillins or cephalosporins.
- Obtain specimen for culture and sensitivity tests before giving first dose. Begin therapy while awaiting results.
- Inject deep into a large muscle, such as the gluteus maximus or the lateral aspect of the thigh.

ACTION
Inhibits cell-wall synthesis, promoting osmotic instability; usually bactericidal.

Route	Onset	Peak	Duration
I.V.	Immediate	Immediate	Unknown
I.M.	Unknown	1½–4 hr	Unknown

Half-life: 5½ to 11 hours.

ADVERSE REACTIONS
CNS: fever, headache, dizziness.
CV: phlebitis.
GI: *pseudomembranous colitis,* diarrhea.
GU: genital pruritus, candidiasis.
Hematologic: eosinophilia, thrombocytosis, *leukopenia.*
Skin: pain, induration, tenderness at injection site, *rash,* pruritus.
Other: hypersensitivity reactions, serum sickness, *anaphylaxis,* chills.

INTERACTIONS
Drug-drug. *Aminoglycosides:* May cause synergistic effect against some strains of *P. aeruginosa* and *Enterobacteriaceae* species. Monitor patient.
Probenecid: High doses (1 g or 2 g daily) may enhance hepatic clearance of ceftriax-

one and shorten its half-life. Avoid using together.

EFFECTS ON LAB TEST RESULTS
- May increase alkaline phosphatase, ALT, AST, bilirubin, BUN, and LDH levels.
- May increase eosinophil and platelet counts. May decrease WBC count.
- May falsely increase serum or urine creatinine level in tests using Jaffe reaction. May cause false-positive results of Coombs' test and urine glucose tests that use cupric sulfate, such as Benedict's reagent and Clinitest.

CONTRAINDICATIONS & CAUTIONS
- Contraindicated in patients hypersensitive to drug or other cephalosporins.
- Use cautiously in patients hypersensitive to penicillin because of possibility of cross-sensitivity with other beta-lactam antibiotics.
- Use cautiously in breast-feeding women and in patients with history of colitis and renal insufficiency.

NURSING CONSIDERATIONS
- If large doses are given, therapy is prolonged, or patient is at high risk, monitor patient for signs and symptoms of superinfection.
- Monitor PT and INR in patients with impaired vitamin K synthesis or low vitamin K stores. Vitamin K therapy may be needed.
- Drug is commonly used in home antibiotic programs for outpatient treatment of serious infections, such as osteomyelitis and community-acquired pneumonia.
- **Look alike–sound alike:** Don't confuse drug with other cephalosporins that sound alike.

PATIENT TEACHING
- Tell patient to report adverse reactions promptly.
- Instruct patient to report discomfort at I.V. insertion site.
- Teach patient and family receiving home care how to prepare and give drug.
- If home care patient is diabetic and is testing his urine for glucose, tell him drug may affect results of cupric sulfate

tests; he should use an enzymatic test instead.
● Tell patient to notify prescriber about loose stools or diarrhea.

---

cefuroxime axetil
se-fyoor-OX-eem

Ceftin

cefuroxime sodium
Zinacef

Pharmacologic class: second-generation cephalosporin
Pregnancy risk category B

AVAILABLE FORMS
cefuroxime axetil
Suspension: 125 mg/5 ml, 250 mg/5 ml
Tablets: 125 mg, 250 mg, 500 mg
cefuroxime sodium
Infusion: 750-mg, 1.5-g vials, infusion packs, and ADD-Vantage vials
Injection: 750 mg, 1.5 g

INDICATIONS & DOSAGES
➤ **Serious lower respiratory tract infection, UTI, skin or skin-structure infections, bone or joint infection, septicemia, meningitis, and gonorrhea**
Adults and children age 13 and older: 750 mg to 1.5 g cefuroxime sodium I.V. or I.M. every 8 hours for 5 to 10 days. For life-threatening infections and infections caused by less susceptible organisms, 1.5 g I.V. or I.M. every 6 hours; for bacterial meningitis, up to 3 g I.V. every 8 hours.
Children age 3 months to 12 years: 50 to 100 mg/kg/day cefuroxime sodium I.V. or I.M. in equally divided doses every 6 to 8 hours. Use higher dosage of 100 mg/kg/day, not to exceed maximum adult dosage, for more severe or serious infections. For bacterial meningitis, 200 to 240 mg/kg/day cefuroxime sodium I.V. in divided doses every 6 to 8 hours.
➤ **Perioperative prevention**
Adults: 1.5 g I.V. 30 to 60 minutes before surgery; in lengthy operations, 750 mg I.V. or I.M. every 8 hours. For open-heart sur-gery, 1.5 g I.V. at induction of anesthesia and then every 12 hours for a total dose of 6 g.
➤ **Bacterial exacerbations of chronic bronchitis or secondary bacterial infection of acute bronchitis**
Adults and children age 13 and older: 250 or 500 mg P.O. b.i.d. for 10 days (chronic bronchitis) or 5 to 10 days (acute bronchitis).
➤ **Acute bacterial maxillary sinusitis**
Adults and children age 13 and older: 250 mg P.O. b.i.d. for 10 days.
Children ages 3 months to 12 years: 250 mg b.i.d. for 10 days. For children who can't swallow tablets whole, 30 mg/kg/day oral suspension divided b.i.d. for 10 days.
➤ **Pharyngitis and tonsillitis**
Adults and children age 13 and older: 250 mg P.O. b.i.d. for 10 days.
Children ages 3 months to 12 years: 125 mg P.O. b.i.d. for 10 days. For children who can't swallow tablets whole, give 20 mg/kg daily of oral suspension divided b.i.d. for 10 days. Maximum daily dose for suspension is 500 mg.
➤ **Otitis media**
Children ages 3 months to 12 years: 250 mg P.O. b.i.d. for 10 days. For children who can't swallow tablets whole, give 30 mg/kg/day of oral suspension divided b.i.d. for 10 days. Maximum daily dose for suspension is 1,000 mg.
➤ **Uncomplicated skin and skin structure infection**
Adults and children age 13 and older: 250 or 500 mg P.O. b.i.d. for 10 days.
➤ **Uncomplicated UTI**
Adults: 250 mg P.O. b.i.d. for 7 to 10 days.
➤ **Uncomplicated gonorrhea**
Adults: 1.5 g I.M. with 1 g probenecid P.O. for one dose. Or, 1 g P.O. as a single dose.
➤ **Early Lyme disease**
Adults and children age 13 and older: 500 mg P.O. b.i.d. for 20 days.
➤ **Impetigo**
Children ages 3 months to 12 years: 30 mg/kg/day of oral suspension divided b.i.d. for 10 days. Maximum daily dose, 1,000 mg.
Adjust-a-dose: In adults with creatinine clearance of 10 to 20 ml/minute, give

750 mg I.V. or I.M. every 12 hours; if clearance is less than 10 ml/min, give 750 mg I.V. or I.M. every 24 hours.

ADMINISTRATION
P.O.
● Before giving drug, ask patient if he's allergic to penicillins or cephalosporins.
● Obtain specimen for culture and sensitivity tests before giving first dose. Therapy may begin while awaiting results.
● Give tablets without regard for meals; give oral suspension with food.
● Crush tablets, if absolutely necessary, for patients who can't swallow tablets. Tablets may be dissolved in small amounts of apple, orange, or grape juice or chocolate milk. However, the drug has a bitter taste that is difficult to mask, even with food.
I.V.
● Before giving drug, ask patient if he's allergic to penicillins or cephalosporins.
● Obtain specimen for culture and sensitivity tests before giving first dose. Therapy may begin while awaiting results.
● Reconstitute each 750-mg vial with 8 ml and each 1.5-g vial with 16 ml of sterile water for injection.
● Withdraw entire contents of vial for a dose.
● For direct injection, inject over 3 to 5 minutes into a large vein or into the tubing of a free-flowing I.V. solution.
● For intermittent infusion, add reconstituted drug to 100 ml D_5W, normal saline solution for injection, or other compatible I.V. solution.
● Infuse over 15 to 60 minutes.
● **Incompatibilities:** Aminoglycosides, azithromycin, ciprofloxacin, cisatracurium, clarithromycin, cyclophosphamide, doxapram, filgrastim, fluconazole, gentamicin, midazolam, ranitidine, sodium bicarbonate injection, vancomycin, vinorelbine tartrate.
I.M.
● Before giving drug, ask patient if he's allergic to penicillins or cephalosporins.
● Obtain specimen for culture and sensitivity tests before giving first dose. Therapy may begin while awaiting results.
● Inject deep into a large muscle, such as the gluteus maximus or the side of the thigh.

ACTION
Inhibits cell-wall synthesis, promoting osmotic instability; usually bactericidal.

Route	Onset	Peak	Duration
P.O.	Unknown	15–60 min	Unknown
I.V.	Immediate	Immediate	Unknown
I.M.	Unknown	2 hr	Unknown

Half-life: 1 to 2 hours.

ADVERSE REACTIONS
CV: *phlebitis, thrombophlebitis.*
GI: *diarrhea, **pseudomembranous colitis,*** nausea, anorexia, vomiting.
Hematologic: *hemolytic anemia, **thrombocytopenia, transient neutropenia,*** eosinophilia.
Skin: *maculopapular and erythematous rashes, urticaria, pain, induration, sterile abscesses, temperature elevation, tissue sloughing at I.M. injection site.*
Other: ***anaphylaxis,*** hypersensitivity reactions, serum sickness.

INTERACTIONS
Drug-drug. *Aminoglycosides:* May cause synergistic activity against some organisms; may increase nephrotoxicity. Monitor patient's renal function closely.
Loop diuretics: May increase risk of adverse renal reactions. Monitor renal function test results closely.
Probenecid: May inhibit excretion and increase cefuroxime level. Probenecid may be used for this effect.
Drug-food. *Any food:* May increase absorption. Give drug with food.

EFFECTS ON LAB TEST RESULTS
● May increase alkaline phosphatase, ALT, AST, bilirubin, and LDH levels. May decrease hemoglobin level and hematocrit.
● May increase PT and INR and eosinophil count. May decrease neutrophil and platelet counts.
● May falsely increase serum or urine creatinine level in tests using Jaffe reaction. May cause false-positive results of Coombs' test and urine glucose tests that use cupric sulfate, such as Benedict's reagent and Clinitest.

CONTRAINDICATIONS & CAUTIONS
• Contraindicated in patients hypersensitive to drug or other cephalosporins.
• Use cautiously in patients hypersensitive to penicillin because of possibility of cross-sensitivity with other beta-lactam antibiotics.
• Use cautiously in breast-feeding women and in patients with history of colitis or renal insufficiency.

NURSING CONSIDERATIONS
• **Alert:** Tablets and suspension aren't bioequivalent and can't be substituted milligram-for-milligram.
• Monitor patient for signs and symptoms of superinfection.
• **Look alike–sound alike:** Don't confuse drug with other cephalosporins that sound alike.

PATIENT TEACHING
• Tell patient to take drug as prescribed, even after he feels better.
• If patient has difficulty swallowing tablets, show him how to dissolve or crush tablets, but warn him that the bitter taste is hard to mask, even with food.
• Tell parent to shake suspension well before measuring dose. Suspension may be stored at room temperature or refrigerated, but must be discarded after 10 days.
• Instruct caregiver to give oral suspension with food.
• Instruct patient to notify prescriber about rash, loose stools, diarrhea, or evidence of superinfection.
• Advise patient receiving drug I.V. to report discomfort at I.V. insertion site.

---

cephalexin
sef-a-LEX-in

Apo-Cephalex†, Keflex, Novo-Lexin†, Nu-Cephalex†

Pharmacologic class: first-generation cephalosporin
Pregnancy risk category B

AVAILABLE FORMS
Capsules: 250 mg, 333 mg, 500 mg, 750 mg
Oral suspension: 125 mg/5 ml, 250 mg/5 ml
Tablets: 250 mg, 500 mg

INDICATIONS & DOSAGES
➤ **Respiratory tract, GI tract, skin, soft-tissue, bone, and joint infections and otitis media caused by** *Escherichia coli* **and other coliform bacteria, group A beta-hemolytic streptococci,** *Klebsiella* **species,** *Proteus mirabilis, Streptococcus pneumoniae,* **and staphylococci**
Adults: 250 mg to 1 g P.O. every 6 hours or 500 mg every 12 hours. Maximum 4 g daily.
Children: 25 to 50 mg/kg/day P.O. in two to four equally divided doses. In severe infections, dose can be doubled. Don't exceed recommended adult dosage.
Adjust-a-dose: For adults with impaired renal function, initial dose is the same. Then, for those with creatinine clearance of 11 to 40 ml/minute, give 500 mg P.O. every 8 to 12 hours; for clearance of 5 to 10 ml/minute, give 250 mg P.O. every 12 hours; and for clearance of less than 5 ml/minute, give 250 mg P.O. every 12 to 24 hours.

ADMINISTRATION
P.O.
• Before giving, ask patient if he's allergic to penicillins or cephalosporins.
• Obtain specimen for culture and sensitivity tests before giving. Begin therapy while awaiting results.
• To prepare oral suspension, add required amount of water to powder in two portions. Shake well after each addition. After mixing, store in refrigerator. Mixture will remain stable for 14 days. Keep tightly closed and shake well before using.
• Give drug with food or milk to lessen GI discomfort.

ACTION
Inhibits cell-wall synthesis, promoting osmotic instability; usually bactericidal.

Route	Onset	Peak	Duration
P.O.	Unknown	1 hr	Unknown

Half-life: 30 minutes to 1 hour.

Reactions may be *common,* uncommon, *life-threatening,* or COMMON AND LIFE-THREATENING.
Interaction may have a *rapid onset* or **delayed onset.**

ADVERSE REACTIONS
CNS: dizziness, headache, fatigue, agitation, confusion, hallucinations.
GI: *anorexia, diarrhea, nausea, pseudomembranous colitis,* vomiting, gastritis, glossitis, dyspepsia, abdominal pain, anal pruritus, tenesmus, oral candidiasis.
GU: genital pruritus, candidiasis, vaginitis, interstitial nephritis.
Hematologic: *neutropenia, thrombocytopenia,* eosinophilia, anemia.
Musculoskeletal: arthritis, arthralgia, joint pain.
Skin: *maculopapular and erythematous rashes, urticaria.*
Other: *anaphylaxis,* hypersensitivity reactions, serum sickness.

INTERACTIONS
Drug-drug. *Aminoglycosides:* May increase risk of nephrotoxicity. Avoid using together.
Probenecid: May increase cephalosporin level. Use probenecid for this effect.

EFFECTS ON LAB TEST RESULTS
• May increase alkaline phosphatase, ALT, AST, bilirubin, and LDH levels. May decrease hemoglobin level.
• May increase eosinophil count. May decrease neutrophil and platelet counts.
• May falsely increase serum or urine creatinine level in tests using Jaffe reaction. May cause false-positive results of Coombs' test and urine glucose tests that use cupric sulfate, such as Benedict's reagent and Clinitest.

CONTRAINDICATIONS & CAUTIONS
• Contraindicated in patients hypersensitive to cephalosporins.
• Use cautiously in patients hypersensitive to penicillin because of possibility of cross-sensitivity with other beta-lactam antibiotics.
• Use cautiously in breast-feeding women and in patients with history of colitis or renal insufficiency.

NURSING CONSIDERATIONS
• If large doses are given or if therapy is prolonged, monitor patient for superinfection, especially if patient is high risk.
• Treat group A beta-hemolytic streptococcal infections for a minimum of 10 days.

• *Look alike–sound alike:* Don't confuse drug with other cephalosporins that sound alike.

PATIENT TEACHING
• Tell patient to take drug exactly as prescribed, even after he feels better.
• Instruct patient to take drug with food or milk to lessen GI discomfort. If patient is taking suspension form, instruct him to shake container well before measuring dose and to store in refrigerator.
• Tell patient to notify prescriber if rash or signs and symptoms of superinfection develop.

Fluoroquinolones

ciprofloxacin
gemifloxacin mesylate
levofloxacin
moxifloxacin hydrochloride
norfloxacin
ofloxacin

---

ciprofloxacin
si-proe-FLOX-a-sin

Cipro✷, Cipro I.V., Cipro XR,
Proquin XR

Pharmacologic class:
fluoroquinolone
Pregnancy risk category C

AVAILABLE FORMS
Infusion (premixed): 200 mg in 100 ml
D_5W, 400 mg in 200 ml D_5W
Injection: 200 mg, 400 mg
Suspension (oral): 250 mg/5 ml (5%),
500 mg/5 ml (10%)
Tablets (extended-release, film-coated):
500 mg, 1,000 mg
Tablets (film-coated): 100 mg, 250 mg,
500 mg, 750 mg

INDICATIONS & DOSAGES
➤ **Complicated intra-abdominal
infection**
Adults: 500 mg P.O. or 400 mg I.V. every
12 hours for 7 to 14 days. Give with
metronidazole.
➤ **Severe or complicated bone or
joint infection, severe respiratory
tract infection, severe skin or skin-
structure infection**
Adults: 750 mg P.O. every 12 hours or
400 mg I.V. every 8 hours.
➤ **Severe or complicated UTI; mild
to moderate bone or joint infection;
mild to moderate respiratory infection; mild to moderate skin or skin-
structure infection; infectious
diarrhea; typhoid fever**
Adults: 500 mg P.O. or 400 mg I.V. every
12 hours. Or, 1,000 mg extended-release
tablets P.O. every 24 hours.

➤ **Complicated UTI or pyelonephritis**
Adults: 500 mg P.O. every 12 hours for
7 to 14 days.
Children age 1 to 17: 6 to 10 mg/kg I.V.
every 8 hours for 10 to 21 days. Maximum
I.V. dose, 400 mg. Or, 10 to 20 mg/kg P.O.
every 12 hours. Maximum P.O. dose,
750 mg. Don't exceed maximum dose,
even in patients who weigh more than
51 kg (112 lb).
➤ **Nosocomial pneumonia**
Adults: 400 mg I.V. every 8 hours for
10 to 14 days.
➤ **Mild to moderate UTI**
Adults: 250 mg P.O. or 200 mg I.V. every
12 hours for 7 to 14 days.
➤ **Uncomplicated UTI**
Adults: 500 mg extended-release tablet
P.O. once daily for 3 days.
➤ **Chronic bacterial prostatitis**
Adults: 500 mg P.O. every 12 hours
or 400 mg I.V. every 12 hours for
28 days.
➤ **Acute uncomplicated cystitis**
Adults: 100 mg or 250 mg P.O. every
12 hours for 3 days.
➤ **Mild to moderate acute sinusitis**
Adults: 500 mg P.O. or 400 mg I.V. every
12 hours for 10 days.
➤ **Empirical therapy in febrile
neutropenic patients**
Adults: 400 mg I.V. every 8 hours used
with piperacillin 50 mg/kg I.V. every
4 hours (not to exceed 24 g/day).
➤ **Inhalation anthrax (postexposure)**
Adults: 400 mg I.V. every 12 hours initially until susceptibility test results are
known; then 500 mg P.O. b.i.d. Give
drug with one or two additional antimicrobials. Switch to oral therapy when
appropriate. Treat for 60 days (I.V. and
P.O. combined).
Children: 10 mg/kg I.V. every 12 hours;
then 15 mg/kg P.O. every 12 hours.
Don't exceed 800 mg/day I.V. or
1,000 mg/day P.O. Give drug with
one or two additional antimicrobials.
Switch to oral therapy when appropriate.
Treat for 60 days (I.V. and P.O.
combined).

Reactions may be *common,* uncommon, *life-threatening,* or COMMON AND LIFE-THREATENING.
Interaction may have a *rapid onset* or *delayed onset.*

➤ **Cutaneous anthrax ◆**

Adults: 500 mg P.O. b.i.d. for 60 days.
Children: 10 to 15 mg/kg every 12 hours.
Don't exceed 1,000 mg/day. Treat for
60 days.

✸*NEW INDICATION:* **Traveler's**
diarrhea ◆

Adults: 500 mg P.O. b.i.d. for 3 days.

Adjust-a-dose: For patients with a creatinine clearance of 30 to 50 ml/minute, give
250 to 500 mg P.O. every 12 hours or
the usual I.V. dose; if clearance is 5 to
29 ml/minute, give 250 to 500 mg P.O.
every 18 hours or 200 to 400 mg I.V.
every 18 to 24 hours. If patient is receiving hemodialysis, give 250 to 500 mg P.O.
every 24 hours after dialysis.

ADMINISTRATION

P.O.

● Cipro XR, Proquin XR, and immediate-
release oral forms aren't interchangeable.
● Obtain specimen for culture and sensitivity tests before giving first dose. Begin
therapy while awaiting results.
● To avoid decreasing the effects of
ciprofloxacin, separate dosage of certain
drugs by up to 6 hours. Food doesn't affect
absorption but may delay peak levels.
● Caffeine should be avoided during therapy with this drug because of potential for
increased caffeine effects.
● Give drug with plenty of fluids to reduce
risk of urine crystals.
● Don't crush or split the extended-release
tablets.

I.V.

● Obtain specimen for culture and sensitivity tests before giving first dose. Begin
therapy while awaiting results.
● Dilute drug to 1 to 2 mg/ml using D_5W
or normal saline solution for injection.
● If giving drug through a Y-type set,
stop the other I.V. solution while
infusing.
● Infuse over 1 hour into a large vein
to minimize discomfort and vein
irritation.
● **Incompatibilities:** Aminophylline,
ampicillin-sulbactam, azithromycin,
cefepime, clindamycin phosphate,
dexamethasone sodium phosphate,
furosemide, heparin sodium, methylprednisolone sodium succinate, phenytoin
sodium.

ACTION

Inhibits bacterial DNA synthesis, mainly
by blocking DNA gyrase; bactericidal.

Route	Onset	Peak	Duration
P.O.	Unknown	30–120 min	Unknown
P.O. (extended-release)	Unknown	1–4 hr	Unknown
I.V.	Unknown	Immediate	Unknown

Half-life: 4 hours; Cipro XR, 6 hours in adults
with normal renal function.

ADVERSE REACTIONS

CNS: *seizures,* confusion, depression,
dizziness, drowsiness, fatigue, hallucinations, headache, insomnia, light-
headedness, paresthesia, restlessness,
tremor.
CV: chest pain, edema, thrombophlebitis.
GI: *pseudomembranous colitis, diarrhea,
nausea,* abdominal pain or discomfort,
constipation, dyspepsia, flatulence, oral
candidiasis, vomiting.
GU: crystalluria, interstitial nephritis.
Hematologic: *leukopenia, neutropenia,
thrombocytopenia,* eosinophilia.
Musculoskeletal: aching, arthralgia,
arthropathy, joint inflammation, joint or
back pain, joint stiffness, neck pain,
tendon rupture.
Skin: *rash, Stevens-Johnson syndrome,
toxic epidermal necrolysis,* burning,
erythema, exfoliative dermatitis, photosensitivity, pruritus.
Other: hypersensitivity reactions.

INTERACTIONS

Drug-drug. *Aluminum hydroxide,
aluminum-magnesium hydroxide, calcium
carbonate, didanosine (chewable tablets,
buffered tablets, or pediatric powder for
oral solution), magnesium hydroxide,
products containing zinc:* May decrease
ciprofloxacin absorption and effects. Give
ciprofloxacin 2 hours before or 6 hours
after these drugs.
Cyclosporine: May increase risk for cyclosporine toxicity. Monitor cyclosporine
level.
Iron salts: May decrease absorption of
ciprofloxacin, reducing anti-infective
response. Give at least 2 hours apart.
NSAIDs: May increase risk of CNS stimulation. Monitor patient closely.

Probenecid: May elevate level of ciprofloxacin. Monitor patient for toxicity.

■ **Black Box Warning** *Steroids:* May increase risk of tendinitis and tendon rupture. ■

Sucralfate: May decrease ciprofloxacin absorption, reducing anti-infective response. If use together can't be avoided, give at least 6 hours apart.

Theophylline: May increase theophylline level and prolong theophylline half-life. Monitor level of theophylline and watch for adverse effects.

Tizanidine: Increases tizanidine levels, causing low blood pressure, somnolence, dizziness, and slowed psychomotor skills. Avoid using together.

Warfarin: May increase anticoagulant effects. Monitor PT and INR closely.

Drug-herb. *Dong quai, St. John's wort:* May cause photosensitivity. Advise patient to avoid excessive sunlight exposure.

Yerba maté: May decrease clearance of herb's methylxanthines and cause toxicity. Discourage use together.

Drug-food. *Caffeine:* May increase effect of caffeine. Monitor patient closely.

Dairy products, other foods: May delay peak drug levels. Advise patient to take drug on an empty stomach.

Orange juice fortified with calcium: May decrease GI absorption of drug, reducing its effects. Discourage use together.

Drug-lifestyle. *Sun exposure:* May cause photosensitivity reactions. Advise patient to avoid excessive sunlight exposure.

EFFECTS ON LAB TEST RESULTS
● May increase alkaline phosphatase, ALT, AST, bilirubin, BUN, creatinine, LDH, and GGT levels.
● May increase eosinophil count. May decrease WBC, neutrophil, and platelet counts.

CONTRAINDICATIONS & CAUTIONS
● Contraindicated in patients sensitive to fluoroquinolones.
● Use cautiously in patients with CNS disorders, such as severe cerebral arteriosclerosis or seizure disorders, and in those at risk for seizures. Drug may cause CNS stimulation.

■ **Black Box Warning** Drug is associated with increased risk of tendinitis and tendon rupture, especially in patients older than age 60 and those with heart, kidney, or lung transplants. ■

NURSING CONSIDERATIONS
● Monitor patient's intake and output and observe patient for signs of crystalluria.
■ **Black Box Warning** Tendon rupture may occur in patients receiving quinolones. If pain or inflammation occurs or if patient ruptures a tendon, stop drug. ■
● Long-term therapy may result in overgrowth of organisms resistant to drug.
● Cutaneous anthrax patients with signs of systemic involvement, extensive edema, or lesions on the head or neck need I.V. therapy and a multidrug approach.
● Additional antimicrobials for anthrax multidrug regimens can include rifampin, vancomycin, penicillin, ampicillin, chloramphenicol, imipenem, clindamycin, and clarithromycin.
● Steroids may be used as adjunctive therapy for anthrax patients with severe edema and for meningitis.
● Follow current Centers for Disease Control and Prevention (CDC) recommendations for anthrax.
● Pregnant women and immunocompromised patients should receive the usual doses and regimens for anthrax.

PATIENT TEACHING
● Tell patient to take drug as prescribed, even after he feels better.
● Advise patient to drink plenty of fluids to reduce risk of urine crystals.
● Advise patient not to crush, split, or chew the extended-release tablets.
● Warn patient to avoid hazardous tasks that require alertness, such as driving, until effects of drug are known.
● Instruct patient to avoid caffeine while taking drug because of potential for increased caffeine effects.
● Advise patient that hypersensitivity reactions may occur even after first dose. If a rash or other allergic reaction occurs, tell him to stop drug immediately and notify prescriber.

• Tell patient that tendon rupture can occur with drug and to notify prescriber if he experiences pain or inflammation.
• Tell patient to avoid excessive sunlight or artificial ultraviolet light during therapy.
• Because drug appears in breast milk, advise woman to stop breast-feeding during treatment or to consider treatment with another drug.

gemifloxacin mesylate
jem-ah-FLOX-a-sin

Factive

Pharmacologic class:
fluoroquinolone
Pregnancy risk category C

AVAILABLE FORMS
Tablets: 320 mg

INDICATIONS & DOSAGES
➤ **Acute bacterial worsening of chronic bronchitis caused by** *Streptococcus pneumoniae, Haemophilus influenzae, H. parainfluenzae,* **or** *Moraxella catarrhalis*
Adults: 320 mg P.O. once daily for 5 days.
➤ **Mild to moderate community-acquired pneumonia caused by** *S. pneumoniae* **(including multidrug-resistant strains),** *H. influenzae, M. catarrhalis, Mycoplasma pneumoniae, Chlamydia pneumoniae,* **or** *Klebsiella pneumoniae*
Adults: 320 mg P.O. once daily for 7 days.
Adjust-a-dose: If creatinine clearance is 40 ml/minute or less, or if patient receives routine hemodialysis or continuous ambulatory peritoneal dialysis, reduce dosage to 160 mg P.O. once daily.

ADMINISTRATION
P.O.
• Give drug with or without food; however it must be given 2 hours before or 3 hours after an antacid.
• Give plenty of fluids during treatment.

ACTION
Prevents cell growth by inhibiting DNA gyrase and topoisomerase IV, which interferes with DNA synthesis.

Route	Onset	Peak	Duration
P.O.	Unknown	½–2 hr	Unknown

Half-life: 4 to 12 hours.

ADVERSE REACTIONS
CNS: headache.
GI: diarrhea, nausea.
Musculoskeletal: ruptured tendons.
Skin: rash.
Other: *hypersensitivity reactions.*

INTERACTIONS
Drug-drug. *Antacids (magnesium or aluminum), didanosine (chewable tablets, buffered tablets, or pediatric powder for oral solution), ferrous sulfate, multivitamins containing metal cations (such as zinc):* May decrease gemifloxacin level. Give these drugs at least 3 hours before or 2 hours after gemifloxacin.
Antiarrhythmics of class IA (procainamide, quinidine) or class III (amiodarone, sotalol): May increase risk of prolonged QTc interval. Avoid using together.
Antipsychotics, erythromycin, tricyclic antidepressants: May increase risk of prolonged QTc interval. Use together cautiously.
Probenecid: May increase gemifloxacin level. May use with probenecid for this reason.
■ **Black Box Warning** *Steroids:* May increase risk of tendinitis and tendon rupture. Monitor patient for tendon pain or inflammation. ■
Sucralfate: May decrease gemifloxacin level. Use together cautiously.
Warfarin: May increase anticoagulation effect. Monitor PT and INR.
Drug-lifestyle. *Sun exposure:* May increase risk of photosensitivity. Advise patient to avoid excessive sunlight exposure.

EFFECTS ON LAB TEST RESULTS
• May increase alkaline phosphatase, ALT, AST, bilirubin, BUN, CK, creatinine, GGT, and potassium levels. May decrease albumin, protein, and sodium levels. May increase or decrease calcium and hemoglobin levels and hematocrit.
• May increase or decrease neutrophil, platelet, and RBC counts.

CONTRAINDICATIONS & CAUTIONS
■ **Black Box Warning** Drug is associated with increased risk of tendinitis and tendon rupture, especially in patients older than age 60 and those with heart, kidney, or lung transplants. ■

● Contraindicated in patients hypersensitive to fluoroquinolones, gemifloxacin, or their components.

● Contraindicated in patients with a history of prolonged QTc interval, those with uncorrected electrolyte disorders (such as hypokalemia or hypomagnesemia), and those taking a drug that could prolong the QTc interval.

● Use cautiously in patients with a proarrhythmic condition (such as bradycardia or acute myocardial ischemia), epilepsy, or a predisposition to seizures.

● Safety and efficacy haven't been established for children younger than age 18.

NURSING CONSIDERATIONS
● Use drug only for infections caused by susceptible bacteria.

● *Alert:* Don't exceed recommended dosage because this increases the risk of prolonging the QTc interval.

● Mild to moderate maculopapular rash may appear, usually 8 to 10 days after therapy starts. It's more likely in women younger than age 40 and postmenopausal women taking hormone therapy. Stop drug if rash appears.

● *Alert:* Serious, occasionally fatal, hypersensitivity reactions may occur. Stop drug immediately if hypersensitivity reaction occurs.

■ **Black Box Warning** Fluoroquinolones may cause tendon rupture, arthropathy, or osteochondrosis; stop drug if patient reports pain or inflammation or ruptures a tendon. ■

● Stop drug if patient has a photosensitivity reaction.

● Fluoroquinolones may cause CNS effects, such as tremors and anxiety. Monitor patient carefully.

● Serious diarrhea may reflect pseudomembranous colitis; drug may need to be stopped.

● Keep patient adequately hydrated to avoid concentration of urine.

PATIENT TEACHING
● Urge patient to finish full course of treatment, even if symptoms improve.

● Tell patient that drug may be taken with or without food, but that it shouldn't be taken within 3 hours after or 2 hours before an antacid.

● Tell patient to stop drug and seek medical care if evidence of hypersensitivity reaction develops.

● Instruct patient to drink fluids liberally during treatment.

● Warn patient against taking OTC drugs or dietary supplements without consulting his prescriber.

● Tell patient to avoid excessive exposure to sunlight or ultraviolet light.

● Urge patient to report pain, inflammation, or rupture of tendons.

● Warn patient to avoid driving or other hazardous activities until effects of drug are known.

levofloxacin
lee-voe-FLOX-a-sin

Levaquin⊘

Pharmacologic class:
fluoroquinolone
Pregnancy risk category C

AVAILABLE FORMS
Infusion (premixed): 250 mg in 50 ml D_5W, 500 mg in 100 ml D_5W, 750 mg in 150 ml D_5W
Oral solution: 25 mg/ml
Single-use vials: 500 mg, 750 mg
Tablets: 250 mg, 500 mg, 750 mg

INDICATIONS & DOSAGES
➤ **Acute bacterial sinusitis caused by susceptible strains of *Streptococcus pneumoniae*, *Moraxella catarrhalis*, or *Haemophilus influenzae***
Adults: 500 mg P.O. or I.V. infusion over 60 minutes every 24 hours for 10 to 14 days or 750 mg P.O. every 24 hours for 5 days.

➤ **Mild to moderate skin and skin-structure infections caused by *Staphylococcus aureus* or *S. pyogenes***
Adults: 500 mg P.O. or I.V. infusion over 60 minutes every 24 hours for 7 to 10 days.

➤ **Acute bacterial worsening of chronic bronchitis caused by *S. aureus, S. pneumoniae, M. catarrhalis, H. influenzae,* or *H. parainfluenzae***
Adults: 500 mg P.O. or I.V. infusion over 60 minutes every 24 hours for 7 days.

➤ **Community-acquired pneumonia from *S. pneumoniae* (resistant to two or more of the following antibiotics: penicillin, second-generation cephalosporins, macrolides, trimethoprim-sulfamethoxazole, tetracyclines), *S. aureus, M. catarrhalis, H. influenzae, H. parainfluenzae, Klebsiella pneumoniae, Chlamydia pneumoniae, Legionella pneumophila,* or *Mycoplasma pneumoniae***
Adults: 500 mg P.O. or I.V. infusion over 60 minutes every 24 hours for 7 to 14 days.

➤ **To prevent inhalation anthrax after confirmed or suspected exposure to *Bacillus anthracis***
Adults: 500 mg I.V. infusion or P.O. every 24 hours for 60 days.

➤ **Chronic bacterial prostatitis caused by *Escherichia coli, Enterococcus faecalis,* or *Staphylococcus epidermidis***
Adults: 500 mg P.O. or I.V. over 60 minutes every 24 hours for 28 days.

Adjust-a-dose: In patients with a creatinine clearance of 20 to 49 ml/minute, give first dose of 500 mg and then 250 mg daily. If clearance is 10 to 19 ml/minute, give first dose of 500 mg and then 250 mg every 48 hours. For patients receiving dialysis or chronic ambulatory peritoneal dialysis, give first dose of 500 mg and then 250 mg every 48 hours. For patients using the 5-day regimen for acute bacterial sinusitis, use the Adjust-a-dose schedule for nosocomial pneumonia.

➤ **Community-acquired pneumonia from *S. pneumoniae* (excluding multidrug-resistant strains), *H. influenzae, H. parainfluenzae, M. pneumoniae,* and *C. pneumoniae***
Adults: 750 mg P.O. or I.V. over 90 minutes every 24 hours for 5 days.

➤ **Complicated skin and skin-structure infections caused by methicillin-sensitive *S. aureus, E. faecalis, S. pyogenes,* or *Proteus mirabilis***
Adults: 750 mg P.O. or I.V. infusion over 90 minutes every 24 hours for 7 to 14 days.

➤ **Nosocomial pneumonia caused by methicillin-susceptible *S. aureus, Pseudomonas aeruginosa, Serratia marcescens, E. coli, K. pneumoniae, H. influenzae,* or *S. pneumoniae***
Adults: 750 mg P.O. or I.V. infusion over 90 minutes every 24 hours for 7 to 14 days.

Adjust-a-dose: If creatinine clearance is 20 to 49 ml/minute, give 750 mg initially and then 750 mg every 48 hours; if clearance is 10 to 19 ml/minute, or patient is receiving hemodialysis or chronic ambulatory peritoneal dialysis, give 750 mg initially and then 500 mg every 48 hours.

➤ **Complicated UTI caused by *E. faecalis, Enterobacter cloacae, E. coli, K. pneumoniae, P. mirabilis,* or *P. aeruginosa;* acute pyelonephritis caused by *E. coli***
Adults: 250 mg P.O. or I.V. over 60 minutes every 24 hours for 10 days.

Adjust-a-dose: If creatinine clearance is 10 to 19 ml/minute, increase dosage interval to every 48 hours.

➤ **Complicated UTI caused by *E. coli, K. pneumoniae,* or *P. mirabilis;* acute pyelonephritis caused by *E. coli***
Adults: 750 mg P.O. or I.V. over 90 minutes daily for 5 days.

Adjust-a-dose: If creatinine clearance is 20 to 49 ml/minute, increase dosage interval to every 48 hours. If creatinine clearance is 10 to 19 ml/minute or patient is receiving dialysis, give 750 mg P.O. or I.V. initial dose, then 500 mg every 48 hours.

➤ **Mild to moderate uncomplicated UTI caused by *E. coli, K. pneumoniae,* or *S. saprophyticus***
Adults: 250 mg P.O. daily for 3 days.

➤ **Traveler's diarrhea ◆**
Adults: 500 mg P.O. daily for up to 3 days.

➤ **Disseminated gonococcal infection ◆**
Adults: 250 mg I.V. once daily and continued for 24 to 48 hours after patient starts to improve. Therapy may be switched to 500 mg P.O. daily to complete at least 1 week of therapy.

ADMINISTRATION

P.O.
- Obtain specimen for culture and sensitivity tests before therapy and as needed to determine if bacterial resistance has occurred.
- Give drug with plenty of fluids.
- Give 2 hours before or 6 hours after antacids, sucralfate, and products containing iron or zinc.
- Give oral solution 1 hour before or 2 hours after a meal.

I.V.
- Obtain specimen for culture and sensitivity tests before therapy and as needed to determine if bacterial resistance has occurred.
- Give this form only by infusion.
- Dilute drug in single-use vials, according to manufacturer's instructions, with D_5W or normal saline solution for injection to a final concentration of 5 mg/ml.
- Infuse doses of 500 mg or less over 60 minutes and doses of 750 mg over 90 minutes.
- Reconstituted solution should be clear, slightly yellow, and free of particulate matter.
- Reconstituted drug is stable for 72 hours at room temperature, for 14 days when refrigerated in plastic containers, and for 6 months when frozen.
- Thaw at room temperature or in refrigerator.
- **Incompatibilities:** Acyclovir sodium, alprostadil, azithromycin, furosemide, heparin sodium, indomethacin sodium trihydrate, insulin, mannitol 20%, nitroglycerin, propofol, sodium bicarbonate, sodium nitroprusside. The manufacturer recommends not mixing or infusing other drugs with levofloxacin.

ACTION

Inhibits bacterial DNA gyrase and prevents DNA replication, transcription, repair, and recombination in susceptible bacteria.

Route	Onset	Peak	Duration
P.O., I.V.	Unknown	1–2 hr	Unknown

Half-life: About 6 to 8 hours.

ADVERSE REACTIONS

CNS: *encephalopathy, seizures,* dizziness, headache, insomnia, pain, paresthesia.
CV: chest pain, palpitations, vasodilation.
GI: *pseudomembranous colitis,* abdominal pain, constipation, diarrhea, dyspepsia, flatulence, nausea, vomiting.
GU: vaginitis.
Hematologic: *lymphopenia,* eosinophilia, hemolytic anemia.
Metabolic: *hypoglycemia.*
Musculoskeletal: back pain, tendon rupture.
Respiratory: allergic pneumonitis, dyspnea.
Skin: *erythema multiforme, Stevens-Johnson syndrome,* photosensitivity, pruritus, rash.
Other: *anaphylaxis, multisystem organ failure, hypersensitivity reactions.*

INTERACTIONS

Drug-drug. *Aluminum hydroxide, aluminum–magnesium hydroxide, calcium carbonate, didanosine, magnesium hydroxide, products containing zinc, sucralfate:* May interfere with GI absorption of levofloxacin. Give levofloxacin 2 hours before or 6 hours after these products.
Antidiabetics: May alter glucose level. Monitor glucose level closely.
Iron salts: May decrease absorption of levofloxacin, reducing anti-infective response. Separate doses by at least 2 hours.
NSAIDs: May increase CNS stimulation. Monitor patient for seizure activity.
■ **Black Box Warning** *Steroids:* May increase risk of tendinitis and tendon rupture. Monitor patient for tendon pain or inflammation. ■
Theophylline: May decrease clearance of theophylline. Monitor theophylline level.
Warfarin and derivatives: May increase effect of oral anticoagulant. Monitor PT and INR.
Drug-herb. *Dong quai, St. John's wort:* May cause photosensitivity reactions. Advise patient to avoid excessive sunlight exposure.
Drug-lifestyle. *Sun exposure:* May cause photosensitivity reactions. Advise patient to avoid excessive sunlight exposure.

EFFECTS ON LAB TEST RESULTS

- May decrease glucose and hemoglobin levels.

Reactions may be *common,* uncommon, *life-threatening,* or COMMON AND LIFE-THREATENING.
Interaction may have a *rapid onset* or **delayed onset.**

- May increase eosinophil count. May decrease WBC count.
- May produce false-positive opioid assay results.

CONTRAINDICATIONS & CAUTIONS

■ **Black Box Warning** Drug is associated with increased risk of tendinitis and tendon rupture, especially in patients older than age 60 and those with heart, kidney, or lung transplants. ■

- Contraindicated in patients hypersensitive to drug, its components, or other fluoroquinolones.
- Use cautiously in patients with history of seizure disorders or other CNS diseases, such as cerebral arteriosclerosis.
- Use cautiously and with dosage adjustment in patients with renal impairment.
- Safety and efficacy of drug in children younger than age 18 and in pregnant and breast-feeding women haven't been established.

NURSING CONSIDERATIONS

- If patient experiences symptoms of excessive CNS stimulation (restlessness, tremor, confusion, hallucinations), stop drug and notify prescriber. Begin seizure precautions.
- Patients with acute hypersensitivity reactions may need treatment with epinephrine, oxygen, I.V. fluids, antihistamines, corticosteroids, pressor amines, and airway management.
- Most antibacterials can cause pseudomembranous colitis. If diarrhea occurs, notify prescriber; drug may be stopped.
- Drug may cause an abnormal ECG.
- *Alert:* If *P. aeruginosa* is a confirmed or suspected pathogen, use with a beta-lactam.
- Monitor glucose level and results of renal, hepatic, and hematopoietic blood studies.

PATIENT TEACHING

- Tell patient to take drug as prescribed, even if signs and symptoms disappear.
- Advise patient to take drug with plenty of fluids and to space antacids, sucralfate, and products containing iron or zinc.

- Tell patient to take oral solution 1 hour before or 2 hours after eating.
- Warn patient to avoid hazardous tasks until adverse effects of drug are known.
- Advise patient to avoid excessive sunlight, use sunscreen, and wear protective clothing when outdoors.
- Instruct patient to stop drug and notify prescriber if rash or other signs or symptoms of hypersensitivity develop.

■ **Black Box Warning** Tell patient that tendon rupture may occur with drug and to notify prescriber if he experiences pain or inflammation. ■

- Instruct diabetic patient to monitor glucose level and notify prescriber about low-glucose reaction.
- Instruct patient to notify prescriber of loose stools or diarrhea.

---

moxifloxacin hydrochloride
mocks-ah-FLOX-a-sin

Avelox, Avelox I.V.

Pharmacologic class:
fluoroquinolone
Pregnancy risk category C

AVAILABLE FORMS
Injection: 400 mg/250 ml
Tablets (film-coated): 400 mg

INDICATIONS & DOSAGES

➤ **Acute bacterial sinusitis caused by *Streptococcus pneumoniae*, *Haemophilus influenzae*, or *Moraxella catarrhalis***
Adults: 400 mg P.O. or I.V. every 24 hours for 10 days.

➤ **Complicated skin and skin structure infections caused by methicillin-susceptible *Staphylococcus aureus*, *Escherichia coli*, *Klebsiella pneumoniae*, or *Enterobacter cloacae***
Adults: 400 mg P.O. or I.V. every 24 hours for 7 to 21 days.

➤ **Complicated intra-abdominal infection caused by *E. coli*, *Bacteroides fragilis*, *Streptococcus anginosis*, *Streptococcus constellatus*, *Enterococcus faecalis*, *Proteus mirabilis*, *Clostridium perfringens*, *Bacteroides***

thetaiotaomicron, **or** *Peptostrepto-*
coccus species
Adults: 400 mg P.O. or I.V. every 24 hours
for 5 to 14 days. Start with the I.V. form;
switch to P.O. when appropriate.
➤ **Community-acquired pneumonia**
from multidrug-resistant *S. pneumo-*
niae **(resistance to two or more of**
the following antibiotics: penicillin,
second-generation cephalosporins,
macrolides, trimethoprim-
sulfamethoxazole, tetracyclines),
S. aureus, M. catarrhalis, H. influen-
zae, H. parainfluenzae, K. pneumo-
niae, Chlamydia pneumoniae,
Legionella pneumophila, **or**
Mycoplasma pneumoniae
Adults: 400 mg P.O. or I.V. every 24 hours
for 7 to 14 days.
➤ **Acute bacterial worsening of**
chronic bronchitis caused by *S.*
pneumoniae, H. influenzae, H.
parainfluenzae, K. pneumoniae,
S. aureus, **or** *M. catarrhalis*
Adults: 400 mg P.O. or I.V. every 24 hours
for 5 days.
➤ **Uncomplicated skin-structure or**
skin infection caused by *S. aureus* **or**
S. pyogenes
Adults: 400 mg P.O. or I.V. every 24 hours
for 7 days.

ADMINISTRATION
P.O.
• Give drug without regard for food. Give
at same time each day.
• Space doses of antacids, sucralfate,
multivitamins, and products containing
aluminum, magnesium, iron, and zinc to
avoid decreasing drug's therapeutic
effects.
• Store drug at controlled room temperature.
I.V.
• Don't use if particulate matter is visible.
• Flush I.V. line with a compatible solu-
tion such as D_5W, normal saline, or
Ringer's lactate solution before and after
use.
• Give only by infusion over 1 hour. Avoid
rapid or bolus infusion.
• **Incompatibilities:** Other I.V. drugs.

ACTION
Interferes with action of enzymes needed
for bacterial replication. Inhibits topoiso-

merases I (DNA gyrase) and IV, impairing
bacterial DNA replication, transcription,
repair, and recombination.

Route	Onset	Peak	Duration
P.O., I.V.	Unknown	1–3 hr	Unknown

Half-life: About 12 hours.

ADVERSE REACTIONS
CNS: dizziness, headache, asthenia, pain,
malaise, insomnia, nervousness, anxiety,
confusion, somnolence, tremor, vertigo,
paresthesia.
CV: *prolonged QT interval,* chest pain,
hypertension, palpitations, peripheral edema, tachycardia.
GI: *pseudomembranous colitis,* abdominal pain, anorexia, constipation, diarrhea,
dyspepsia, dry mouth, flatulence, GI disorder, glossitis, nausea, oral candidiasis,
stomatitis, taste perversion, vomiting.
GU: vaginal candidiasis, vaginitis.
Hematologic: *leukopenia, thrombo-*
cytopenia, thrombocytosis, eosinophilia.
Hepatic: abnormal liver function,
cholestatic jaundice.
Musculoskeletal: arthralgia, back pain,
leg pain, myalgia, tendon rupture.
Respiratory: dyspnea.
Skin: injection site reaction, pruritus, rash
(maculopapular, purpuric, pustular),
sweating.
Other: allergic reaction, candidiasis.

INTERACTIONS
Drug-drug. *Aluminum hydroxide, alu-*
minum-magnesium hydroxide, calcium
carbonate, didanosine, magnesium
hydroxide, multivitamins, products con-
taining zinc: May interfere with GI
absorption of moxifloxacin. Give moxifloxacin 4 hours before or 8 hours after
these products.
Class IA antiarrhythmics (such as pro-
cainamide, quinidine), class III anti-
arrhythmics (such as amiodarone,
sotalol): May increase risk of cardiac arrhythmias. Avoid using together.
Drugs that prolong QT interval, such as
antipsychotics, erythromycin, tricyclic
antidepressants: May have additive effect.
Avoid using together.
NSAIDs: May increase risk of CNS stimulation and seizures. Avoid using together.

Reactions may be *common,* uncommon, *life-threatening,* or COMMON AND LIFE-THREATENING.
Interaction may have a *rapid onset* or **delayed onset.**

■ **Black Box Warning** *Steroids:* May increase risk of tendinitis and tendon rupture. Monitor patient for tendon pain or inflammation. ■

Sucralfate: May decrease absorption of moxifloxacin, reducing anti-infective response. If use together can't be avoided, give at least 6 hours apart.

Warfarin: May increase anticoagulant effects. Monitor PT and INR closely.

Drug-lifestyle. *Sun exposure:* May cause photosensitivity reactions. Advise patient to avoid excessive sunlight exposure.

EFFECTS ON LAB TEST RESULTS
● May increase GGT, amylase, and LDH levels. May decrease hemoglobin level.
● May increase eosinophil count. May decrease PT and WBC count. May increase or decrease platelet count.

CONTRAINDICATIONS & CAUTIONS
■ **Black Box Warning** Drug is associated with increased risk of tendinitis and tendon rupture, especially in patients older than age 60 and those with heart, kidney, or lung transplants. ■
● Contraindicated in patients hypersensitive to drug or other fluoroquinolones and in those with prolonged QT interval or uncorrected hypokalemia.
● Use cautiously in patients with ongoing proarrhythmic conditions, such as clinically significant bradycardia or acute myocardial ischemia.
● Use cautiously in patients who may have CNS disorders and in those with other risk factors that may lower the seizure threshold or predispose them to seizures.
● Safety and efficacy in children, adolescents younger than age 18, and pregnant or breast-feeding women haven't been established.

NURSING CONSIDERATIONS
● *Alert:* Monitor patient for adverse CNS effects, including seizures, dizziness, confusion, tremors, hallucinations, depression, and suicidal thoughts. If these occur, stop drug and notify prescriber.
● Monitor patient for hypersensitivity reactions, including anaphylaxis.
● If diarrhea develops during therapy, send stool specimen for *Clostridium difficile* test.

■ **Black Box Warning** Rupture of the Achilles and other tendons is linked to fluoroquinolone use. If pain, inflammation, or tendon rupture occurs, stop drug and notify prescriber. ■

PATIENT TEACHING
● Instruct patient to take drug once daily, at the same time each day, without regard to meals.
● Tell patient to finish entire course of therapy, even if symptoms are relieved.
● Advise patient to drink plenty of fluids.
● Tell patient to space antacids, sucralfate, multivitamins, and products containing aluminum, magnesium, iron, and zinc to avoid decreasing drug's therapeutic effects.
● Instruct patient to contact prescriber and stop drug if he experiences allergic reaction, rash, heart palpitations, fainting, or persistent diarrhea.
● Direct patient to contact prescriber, stop drug, rest, and refrain from exercise if he experiences pain, inflammation, or tendon rupture.
● Warn patient that drug may cause dizziness and light-headedness. Tell patient to avoid hazardous activities, such as driving or operating machinery, until effects of drug are known.
● Instruct patient to avoid excessive sunlight exposure and ultraviolet light and to report photosensitivity reactions to prescriber.

norfloxacin
nor-FLOX-a-sin

Noroxin

Pharmacologic class:
fluoroquinolone
Pregnancy risk category C

AVAILABLE FORMS
Tablets (film-coated): 400 mg

INDICATIONS & DOSAGES
✱ *NEW INDICATION:* **Uncomplicated UTI from** *Escherichia coli, Klebsiella pneumoniae,* **or** *Proteus mirabilis*
Adults: 400 mg P.O. every 12 hours for 3 days.

➤ **Complicated or uncomplicated UTI from susceptible strains of** *Enterococcus faecalis, E. cloacae, Enterobacter aerogenes, P. vulgaris, Pseudomonas aeruginosa, Citrobacter freundii, Staphylococcus agalactiae, S. aureus, S. epidermidis, S. saprophyticus,* **or** *Serratia marcescens*

Adults: 400 mg P.O. every 12 hours for 7 to 10 days (uncomplicated infection). Or, 400 mg P.O. every 12 hours for 10 to 21 days (complicated infection).

➤ **Prostatitis**

Adults: 400 mg P.O. every 12 hours for 28 days.

Adjust-a-dose: If creatinine clearance is 30 ml/minute or less, give 400 mg once daily for above indications.

➤ **Acute, uncomplicated urethral and cervical gonorrhea**

Adults: 800 mg P.O. as a single dose, then doxycycline therapy to treat any coexisting chlamydial infection.

➤ **Moderate to severe traveler's diarrhea**

Adults: 400 mg P.O. b.i.d. for 3 days.

ADMINISTRATION
P.O.

• Obtain specimen for culture and sensitivity testing before starting therapy.
• Give drug 1 hour before or 2 hours after meals because food may hinder absorption.
• Space doses of iron products and antacids when taking norfloxacin.
• Make sure that patient drinks several glasses of water throughout the day to maintain hydration and adequate urine output.

ACTION
Inhibits bacterial DNA synthesis, mainly by blocking DNA gyrase; bactericidal.

Route	Onset	Peak	Duration
P.O.	Unknown	15–120 min	Unknown

Half-life: 3 to 4 hours.

ADVERSE REACTIONS
CNS: *seizures,* depression, dizziness, fatigue, fever, headache, insomnia, somnolence.
GI: *pseudomembranous colitis,* abdominal pain, anorexia, constipation, dry mouth, diarrhea, flatulence, heartburn, nausea, vomiting.
GU: crystalluria.
Hematologic: *leukopenia, neutropenia, thrombocytopenia,* eosinophilia.
Musculoskeletal: back pain.
Skin: hyperhidrosis, photosensitivity, rash.
Other: *anaphylaxis,* hypersensitivity reactions.

INTERACTIONS
Drug-drug. *Aluminum hydroxide, calcium carbonate, aluminum–magnesium hydroxide, magnesium hydroxide:* May decrease norfloxacin level. Give antacid at least 6 hours before or 2 hours after norfloxacin.
Iron salts: May decrease absorption of norfloxacin, reducing anti-infective response. Give at least 2 hours apart.
Caffeine: May increase caffeine's effects. Advise patient to avoid caffeine.
Cyclosporine: May increase cyclosporine level. Monitor cyclosporine level.
Nitrofurantoin: May antagonize norfloxacin effect. Monitor patient closely.
Glyburide: May cause severe hypoglycemia. Monitor blood glucose level closely.
Oral anticoagulants: May increase anticoagulant effect. Monitor PT and INR.
Probenecid: May increase norfloxacin level by decreasing its excretion. May give probenecid for this reason, but monitor high-risk patient for toxicity.
■ **Black Box Warning** *Steroids:* May increase risk of tendinitis and tendon rupture. Monitor patient for tendon pain or inflammation. ■
Sucralfate: May decrease absorption of norfloxacin, reducing anti-infective response. If use together can't be avoided, give at least 6 hours apart.
Theophylline: May impair theophylline metabolism, increasing drug level and risk of toxicity. Monitor patient closely.
Drug-herb. *Dong quai, St. John's wort:* May cause photosensitivity reactions. Advise patient to avoid excessive sunlight exposure.

EFFECTS ON LAB TEST RESULTS
• May increase BUN, creatinine, ALT, AST, and alkaline phosphatase levels. May decrease hematocrit.

Reactions may be *common,* uncommon, *life-threatening,* or COMMON AND LIFE-THREATENING.
Interaction may have a *rapid onset* or **delayed onset.**

• May increase eosinophil count. May decrease neutrophil count.

CONTRAINDICATIONS & CAUTIONS
■ **Black Box Warning** Drug is associated with increased risk of tendinitis and tendon rupture, especially in patients older than age 60 and those with heart, kidney, or lung transplants. ■
• Contraindicated in patients hypersensitive to drug or other fluoroquinolones.
• Use cautiously in patients with conditions such as cerebral arteriosclerosis who may be predisposed to seizure disorders.
• Use cautiously and monitor renal function in those with renal impairment.
• Safety and efficacy in children younger than age 18 haven't been established. Use during pregnancy only if potential benefit justifies potential risk to fetus.

NURSING CONSIDERATIONS
■ **Black Box Warning** Tendon rupture may occur in patients receiving quinolones. Stop drug if pain or inflammation occurs or tendon ruptures. ■
• Monitor patient for adverse CNS effects, including dizziness, headache, seizures, or depression. Stop drug and notify prescriber if these effects occur.
• Monitor patient for hypersensitivity reactions. Stop drug and initiate supportive therapy as indicated.
• *Look alike–sound alike:* Don't confuse Noroxin with Neurontin or Floxin.

PATIENT TEACHING
• Tell patient to take drug as prescribed, even after he feels better.
• Advise patient to take drug 1 hour before or 2 hours after meals because food may hinder absorption.
• Advise patient to appropriately space iron products and antacids when taking norfloxacin.
• Warn patient not to exceed the recommended dosages and to drink several glasses of water throughout the day to maintain hydration and adequate urine output.
• Warn patient to avoid hazardous tasks that require alertness until effects of drug are known.
• Instruct patient to avoid exposure to sunlight, wear protective clothing, and use sunscreen while outdoors.

• Tell patient to report pain, inflammation, or tendon rupture, and to refrain from exercise until diagnosis of rupture or tendinitis is excluded.
• Caution patients to limit caffeine intake.

---

ofloxacin
oh-FLOX-a-sin

Floxin⌀

Pharmacologic class:
fluoroquinolone
Pregnancy risk category C

AVAILABLE FORMS
Tablets: 200 mg, 300 mg, 400 mg

INDICATIONS & DOSAGES
➤ **Acute bacterial worsening of chronic bronchitis, uncomplicated skin and skin-structure infections, and community-acquired pneumonia**
Adults: 400 mg P.O. every 12 hours for 10 days.
➤ **Sexually transmitted infections, such as acute uncomplicated urethral and cervical gonorrhea, non-gonococcal urethritis and cervicitis, and mixed infections of urethra and cervix**
Adults: For acute uncomplicated gonorrhea, 400 mg P.O. once as a single dose; for cervicitis and urethritis, 300 mg P.O. every 12 hours for 7 days.
➤ **Cystitis from *Escherichia coli*, *Klebsiella pneumoniae*, or other organisms**
Adults: 200 mg P.O. every 12 hours for 3 days (*E. coli* or *K. pneumoniae*), 200 mg P.O. every 12 hours for 7 days (other organisms).
➤ **Complicated UTI**
Adults: 200 mg P.O. every 12 hours for 10 days.
➤ **Prostatitis from *E. coli***
Adults: 300 mg P.O. every 12 hours for 6 weeks.
➤ **Pelvic inflammatory disease**
Adults: 400 mg P.O. every 12 hours with metronidazole for 10 to 14 days.
➤ **To prevent inhalation anthrax ◆**
Adults: 400 mg P.O. b.i.d. Continue therapy for 60 days if no vaccine is available.

If vaccine is available, continue for 28 to 45 days and until three doses of the vaccine have been given.
➤ **Moderate to severe traveler's diarrhea ♦**
Adults: 300 mg P.O. b.i.d. for 1 to 3 days.
Adjust-a-dose: For patients with creatinine clearance less than 20 ml/minute, give first dose as recommended; then give subsequent doses at 50% of recommended dose every 24 hours. For patients with hepatic impairment, don't exceed 400 mg/day.

ADMINISTRATION
P.O.
● Give drug without regard for meals but not at the same time as antacids and vitamins.
● Give drug with plenty of fluids.

ACTION
Interferes with DNA gyrase, which is needed for synthesis of bacterial DNA. Spectrum of action includes many gram-positive and gram-negative aerobic bacteria, including *Enterobacteriaceae* and *Pseudomonas aeruginosa.*

Route	Onset	Peak	Duration
P.O.	Unknown	15–120 min	Unknown

Half-life: 4 to 7½ hours.

ADVERSE REACTIONS
CNS: *seizures, increased intracranial pressure,* dizziness, drowsiness, fatigue, fever, headache, insomnia, lethargy, malaise, nervousness, sleep disorders, visual disturbances.
CV: chest pain, phlebitis.
GI: *nausea, pseudomembranous colitis,* abdominal pain or discomfort, anorexia, constipation, diarrhea, dry mouth, dysgeusia, flatulence, vomiting.
GU: genital pruritus, glucosuria, hematuria, proteinuria, vaginal discharge, vaginitis.
Hematologic: *leukopenia, neutropenia,* anemia, eosinophilia, leukocytosis.
Metabolic: *hypoglycemia,* hyperglycemia.
Musculoskeletal: body pain, tendon rupture.
Skin: photosensitivity, pruritus, rash.
Other: *anaphylactoid reaction,* hypersensitivity reactions.

INTERACTIONS
Drug-drug. *Aluminum hydroxide, aluminum–magnesium hydroxide, calcium carbonate, magnesium hydroxide:* May decrease effects of ofloxacin. Give antacid at least 6 hours before or 2 hours after ofloxacin.
Antidiabetics: May affect glucose level, causing hypoglycemia or hyperglycemia. Monitor patient closely.
Didanosine (chewable or buffered tablets or pediatric powder for oral solution): May interfere with GI absorption of ofloxacin. Separate doses by 2 hours.
Iron salts: May decrease absorption of ofloxacin, reducing anti-infective response. Separate doses by at least 2 hours.
Hypoglycemic (oral) insulin: Increases hypoglycemic action. Use cautiously.
■ **Black Box Warning** *Steroids:* May increase risk of tendinitis and tendon rupture. Monitor patient for tendon pain or inflammation. ■
Sucralfate: May decrease absorption of ofloxacin, reducing anti-infective response. If use together can't be avoided, separate doses by at least 6 hours.
Theophylline: May increase theophylline level. Monitor patient closely and adjust theophylline dosage as needed.
Warfarin: May prolong PT and INR. Monitor PT and INR.
Drug-lifestyle. *Sun exposure:* May cause photosensitivity reactions. Advise patient to avoid excessive sunlight exposure.

EFFECTS ON LAB TEST RESULTS
● May increase BUN, creatinine, and liver enzyme levels. May decrease hemoglobin level and hematocrit. May increase or decrease glucose level.
● May increase erythrocyte sedimentation rate and eosinophil count. May decrease neutrophil count. May increase or decrease WBC count.
● May produce false-positive opioid assay results.

CONTRAINDICATIONS & CAUTIONS
■ **Black Box Warning** Drug is associated with increased risk of tendinitis and tendon rupture, especially in patients older than age 60 and those with heart, kidney, or lung transplants. ■

Reactions may be *common,* uncommon, *life-threatening,* or COMMON AND LIFE-THREATENING.
Interaction may have a *rapid onset* or *delayed onset.*

- Contraindicated in patients hypersensitive to drug or other fluoroquinolones.
- Use cautiously in pregnant patients and in those with seizure disorders, CNS diseases, such as cerebral arteriosclerosis, hepatic disorders, or renal impairment.
- Ofloxacin appears in breast milk in levels similar to those found in plasma. Safety hasn't been established in breast-feeding or pregnant women.
- Safety and efficacy in children younger than age 18 haven't been established.

NURSING CONSIDERATIONS
■ **Black Box Warning** Rupture of tendons is linked to fluoroquinolone use. If pain, inflammation, or tendon rupture occurs, stop drug and notify prescriber. ■
- *Alert:* Patients treated for gonorrhea should be tested for syphilis. Drug isn't effective against syphilis, and treating gonorrhea may mask or delay syphilis symptoms.
- Periodically assess organ system functions during prolonged therapy.
- Monitor patient for overgrowth of non-susceptible organisms.
- Monitor renal and hepatic studies and CBC in prolonged therapy.
- Monitor blood sugar closely.
- Monitor patient for adverse CNS effects, including dizziness, headache, seizures, or depression. Stop drug and notify prescriber if these effects occur.
- Monitor patient for hypersensitivity reactions. Stop drug and initiate supportive therapy, as indicated.

PATIENT TEACHING
- Tell patient to drink plenty of fluids during drug therapy and to finish the entire prescription, even if he starts feeling better.
- Tell patient drug may be taken without regard to meals, but he shouldn't take antacids and vitamins at the same time as ofloxacin.
- Warn patient that dizziness and light-headedness may occur. Advise caution when driving or operating hazardous machinery until effects of drug are known.
- Warn patient that hypersensitivity reactions may follow first dose; he should stop drug at first sign of rash or other allergic reaction and call prescriber immediately.

- Advise patient to avoid prolonged exposure to direct sunlight and to use a sunscreen when outdoors.

14

Local anti-infectives

acyclovir
azelaic acid
clindamycin phosphate
clotrimazole
econazole nitrate
erythromycin
gentamicin sulfate
ketoconazole
metronidazole
miconazole nitrate
mupirocin
retapamulin
sertaconazole nitrate
silver sulfadiazine
terbinafine hydrochloride
terconazole

---

acyclovir
ay-SYE-kloe-ver

Zovirax

Pharmacologic class: nucleoside
analogue
Pregnancy risk category B

AVAILABLE FORMS
Cream: 5%
Ointment: 5%

INDICATIONS & DOSAGES
➤ **Initial herpes genitalis; limited,
non–life-threatening mucocutaneous herpes simplex virus infections in immunocompromised
patients**
Adults and children 12 years and older:
Cover all lesions every 3 hours six times
daily for 7 days. Although dose varies
depending on total lesion area, use about
½-inch (1.3-cm) ribbon of ointment on
each 4-inch (10-cm) square of surface
area.
➤ **Recurrent herpes labialis (cold
sores)**
Adults and children 12 years and older:
Apply cream five times daily for 4 days.
Start therapy as early as possible after
signs and symptoms start.

ADMINISTRATION
Topical
● Apply drug with a finger cot or rubber
glove to prevent autoinoculation of other
body sites and transmission of infection to
other persons.
● All lesions must be thoroughly covered.
● Drug is for cutaneous use only; don't
apply to eye.

ACTION
Inhibits herpes simplex and varicella
zoster viral DNA synthesis by inhibiting
viral DNA polymerase action.

Route	Onset	Peak	Duration
Topical	Unknown	Unknown	Unknown

Half-life: Unknown.

ADVERSE REACTIONS
Skin: *mild pain, burning or stinging,
eczema, rash, dryness, pruritus, contact
dermatitis, application site reactions.*
Other: *angioedema, anaphylaxis.*

INTERACTIONS
None significant.

EFFECTS ON LAB TEST RESULTS
None reported.

CONTRAINDICATIONS & CAUTIONS
● Contraindicated in patients hypersensitive or chemically intolerant to drug.
● Women who have active herpetic lesions
near or on the breast should avoid breast-
feeding.

NURSING CONSIDERATIONS
● Start therapy as early as possible after
signs or symptoms begin.
● Drug isn't a cure for herpes, but it helps
improve signs and symptoms.

PATIENT TEACHING
● Teach patient that virus transmission can
occur during treatment.
● Tell patient that there may be some discomfort with application.

Reactions may be *common*, uncommon, *life-threatening*, or COMMON AND LIFE-THREATENING.
Interaction may have a *rapid onset* or **delayed onset**.

- Stress importance of compliance for successful therapy.
- Teach patient that therapy should begin as soon as signs and symptoms appear.
- Tell patient to notify prescriber if adverse reactions occur.
- Instruct patient to store drug in a dry place at 59° to 77° F (15° to 25° C).

azelaic acid
aze-eh-LAY-ik

Azelex, Finacea

Pharmacologic class: dicarboxylic acid
Pregnancy risk category B

AVAILABLE FORMS
Cream: 20%
Gel: 15%

INDICATIONS & DOSAGES
➤ **Mild to moderate inflammatory acne vulgaris**
Adults: Apply thin film of cream (Azelex) and gently but thoroughly massage into affected areas b.i.d., in morning and evening.
➤ **Mild to moderate rosacea**
Adults: Apply thin film of gel (Finacea) and gently but thoroughly massage into affected areas b.i.d., in morning and evening.

ADMINISTRATION
Topical
- Wash and pat dry affected areas before applying drug, wear gloves and wash hands well after application.
- Don't apply occlusive dressings or wrappings to affected areas.
- Store drug at 59° to 86° F (15° to 30° C), and protect it from freezing.

ACTION
May inhibit microbial cellular protein synthesis.

Route	Onset	Peak	Duration
Topical	Unknown	Unknown	Unknown

Half-life: 12 hours.

ADVERSE REACTIONS
Skin: pruritus, *burning, stinging, tingling,* dermatitis, peeling, erythema, edema, acne.
Other: allergic reaction.

INTERACTIONS
None significant.

EFFECTS ON LAB TEST RESULTS
None reported.

CONTRAINDICATIONS & CAUTIONS
- Contraindicated in patients hypersensitive to drug or its components.
- Use cautiously in pregnant or breast-feeding women.

NURSING CONSIDERATIONS
- Monitor patient for early signs and symptoms of hypopigmentation, especially patient with dark complexion.
- If sensitivity or severe irritation occurs, notify prescriber, who may stop drug and order appropriate treatment.
- Avoid using occlusive dressings.

PATIENT TEACHING
- Instruct patient to wash and pat dry affected areas before applying drug and to wash hands well after application. Warn him not to apply occlusive dressings or wrappings to affected areas.
- Warn patient that skin irritation may occur, usually at start of therapy, if drug is applied to broken or inflamed skin. Tell him to notify prescriber if irritation persists.
- Advise patient to keep drug away from mouth, eyes, and other mucous membranes. If contact occurs, tell him to rinse thoroughly with water and to notify prescriber if irritation persists.
- Advise patient to report abnormal changes in skin color.
- Urge patient to use drug for full treatment period. In most patients with inflammatory lesions, improvement occurs in 1 to 2 months.
- Warn patients with rosacea to avoid foods and beverages that may cause flushing, such as spicy foods, hot food or drinks, and alcohol.
- Instruct patient to store drug at 59° to 86° F (15° to 30° C) and protect it from freezing.

clindamycin phosphate
klin-da-MYE-sin

Cleocin, Cleocin T, Clinda-
Derm, Clindagel, Clindasol†,
Clindesse, Clindets, Dalacin†,
Evoclin

Pharmacologic class: lincomycin
derivative
Pregnancy risk category B

AVAILABLE FORMS
Foam: 1%
Gel: 1%
Lotion: 1%
Pledget: 1%*
Topical solution: 1%*
Vaginal cream: 2%
Vaginal suppositories: 100 mg

INDICATIONS & DOSAGES
➤ **Inflammatory acne vulgaris**
Adults and adolescents: Apply to
skin b.i.d., morning and evening,
or once daily if using Clindagel or
Evoclin.
➤ **Bacterial vaginosis**
Adults: 1 applicatorful vaginally at bedtime
for 3 to 7 days in nonpregnant women or
7 days in pregnant women, or 1 suppository
vaginally at bedtime for 3 days, or 1 applicatorful of Clindesse vaginally as a single
dose.

ADMINISTRATION
Topical
● Wash area with warm water and soap,
rinse, pat dry, and wait 30 minutes after
washing or shaving to apply.
● Avoid excessive washing of affected area.
● Apply to entire area, but avoid contact
with eyes, nose, mouth, and other mucous
membranes.
Vaginal
● For vaginal treatment, make sure patient
knows how to use applicators that come
with drug.
● Tell patient to remove pledgets from foil
before use.
● Advise patient to use pledgets only
once and then discard. Also, more
than 1 pledget may be used per
application.

ACTION
Bacteriostatic or bactericidal based on
drug level and susceptibility of organism;
suppresses growth of susceptible organisms in sebaceous glands by blocking protein synthesis.

Route	Onset	Peak	Duration
Topical, vaginal	Unknown	Unknown	Unknown

Half-life: 1½ to 2½ hours for topical and vaginal cream; 11 hours for vaginal suppositories.

ADVERSE REACTIONS
CNS: *headache.*
EENT: pharyngitis.
GI: abdominal pain, bloody diarrhea,
colitis including ***pseudomembranous
colitis,*** constipation, diarrhea, GI upset.
GU: Candida albicans *overgrowth, cervicitis, vaginitis, vulvar irritation,* UTI,
vaginal discharge, vaginal moniliasis.
Skin: *dryness, redness,* burning, contact
dermatitis, irritation, rash, pruritus,
swelling.

INTERACTIONS
Drug-drug. *Erythromycin:* May antagonize clindamycin's effect. Separate doses.
Isotretinoin: May cause cumulative dryness, resulting in excessive skin irritation.
Use together cautiously.
Neuromuscular blockers: May increase
action of neuromuscular blocker. Use
together cautiously.
Drug-lifestyle. *Abrasive or medicated
soaps or cleansers, acne products, or
other preparations containing peeling
drugs (benzoyl peroxide, resorcinol, salicylic acid, sulfur, tretinoin), alcohol-
containing products (aftershave, cosmetics, perfumed toiletries, shaving creams or
lotions), astringent soaps or cosmetics,
medicated cosmetics or cover-ups:* May
cause cumulative dryness, resulting in
excessive skin irritation. Urge caution.

EFFECTS ON LAB TEST RESULTS
● May increase liver enzyme levels.

CONTRAINDICATIONS & CAUTIONS
● Contraindicated in patients hypersensitive to clindamycin or lincomycin and in
those with history of ulcerative colitis,

regional enteritis, or antibiotic-related colitis.

NURSING CONSIDERATIONS

• For treating acne, drug may be used with tretinoin or benzoyl peroxide, as well as systemic antibiotics.
• Drug can cause excessive dryness.
• Topical solution and pledgets contain alcohol base, which may irritate eyes.
• Monitor elderly patients for systemic effects.

PATIENT TEACHING

• Tell patient to wash area with warm water and soap, rinse, pat dry, and wait 30 minutes after washing or shaving to apply.
• Warn patient to avoid excessive washing of area. Tell patient to cover entire affected area but to avoid contact with eyes, nose, mouth, and other mucous membranes.
• Instruct patient to use other prescribed acne medicines at a different time.
• Tell patient to use only as prescribed.
• Instruct patient to dab, not roll, applicator-tipped bottle. If tip becomes dry, patient should invert bottle and depress tip several times to moisten.
• Warn patient not to smoke while applying topical solution.
• For vaginal treatment, make sure patient knows how to use applicators that come with drug.
• Advise patient that the vaginal form contains mineral oil, which can weaken latex or rubber products, such as condoms and diaphragms, and that she should use another form of birth control during and within 3 days of therapy.
• Advise patient to avoid sexual intercourse during vaginal treatment.
• Advise patient to avoid use of tampons or douches during vaginal treatment.
• Instruct patient to notify prescriber immediately if abdominal pain or diarrhea occurs. Inform patient that an antidiarrheal may worsen condition and should only be used as directed by prescriber.
• Tell patient to remove pledgets from foil before use.
• Advise patient to use pledgets only once and then discard. Also, more than 1 pledget may be used per application.
• Advise patient to complete entire course of therapy.

clotrimazole
kloe-TRIM-a-zole

Canesten†, Clotrimaderm†, Cruex◊, Desenex◊, Gyne-Lotrimin◊, Lotrimin◊, Lotrimin AF◊, Mycelex, Mycelex-7◊, Mycelex-G, Trivagizole 3◊

Pharmacologic class: imidazole derivative
Pregnancy risk category B; C (for lozenges)

AVAILABLE FORMS

Combination pack: Vaginal tablets 100 mg and vulvar cream 1%◊, vaginal tablets 200 mg and vulvar cream 1%◊
Topical cream: 1%
Topical lotion: 1%
Topical solution: 1%
Troches (lozenges): 10 mg
Vaginal cream: 1%◊, 2%◊
Vaginal suppositories: 100 mg◊, 200 mg◊

INDICATIONS & DOSAGES

➤ **Superficial fungal infections (tinea corporis, tinea cruris, tinea pedis, tinea versicolor, candidiasis)**
Adults and children age 2 and older:
Apply thin film and massage into affected and surrounding area, morning and evening, for 2 to 4 weeks. If improvement doesn't occur after 4 weeks, reevaluate patient.
➤ **Vulvovaginal candidiasis**
Adults: One 100-mg vaginal suppository inserted daily at bedtime for 7 consecutive days. Or, one 200-mg vaginal suppository at bedtime for 3 days. Or, 1 applicatorful of vaginal cream daily at bedtime for 3 days (2%) or 7 days (1%).
➤ **Oropharyngeal candidiasis**
Adults and children age 3 and older:
Dissolve lozenge in mouth over 15 to 30 minutes five times daily for 14 consecutive days.
➤ **To prevent oropharyngeal candidiasis in patients immunocompromised by chemotherapy, radiotherapy, or corticosteroid therapy in the treatment of leukemia, solid tumors, or renal transplantation**

Adults: Dissolve lozenge in mouth over 15 to 30 minutes t.i.d. for duration of chemotherapy or until corticosteroid is reduced to maintenance levels.

ADMINISTRATION
P.O.
● Lozenges should dissolve in mouth and not be chewed, for full benefit.
Topical
● Clean and dry area before applying drug.
● Don't use occlusive wrappings or dressings.
Vaginal
● Insert suppository high into vagina.
● Applicators for cream and some suppositories are disposable. If not disposable, wash with soap and warm water immediately after use. Rinse thoroughly and dry.

ACTION
Fungistatic or fungicidal, depending on level. Alters fungal cell-wall permeability and produces osmotic instability.

Route	Onset	Peak	Duration
P.O.	Unknown	Unknown	3 hr
Topical, vaginal	Unknown	Unknown	Unknown

Half-life: Unknown.

ADVERSE REACTIONS
GI: lower abdominal cramps, nausea and vomiting with lozenges.
GU: *mild vaginal burning or irritation,* urinary frequency.
Skin: *erythema,* blistering, burning, edema, general irritation, peeling, pruritus, skin fissures, stinging, urticaria.

INTERACTIONS
None significant.

EFFECTS ON LAB TEST RESULTS
● May increase liver enzyme levels.

CONTRAINDICATIONS & CAUTIONS
● Contraindicated in patients hypersensitive to drug.
● Contraindicated for ophthalmic use.

NURSING CONSIDERATIONS
● Consult prescriber before using topical preparations in children younger than age 2. Don't use troches in children younger than age 3; don't use vaginal preparations in children younger than age 12.
● Watch for and report irritation or sensitivity; stop if irritation occurs, and notify prescriber.
● Improvement usually occurs within 1 week; if no improvement is seen within 4 weeks, review diagnosis.
● *Look alike–sound alike:* Don't confuse clotrimazole with co-trimoxazole.

PATIENT TEACHING
● Reassure patient that hypopigmentation from tinea versicolor will resolve gradually.
● Warn patient not to use occlusive wrappings or dressings.
● Warn patient to avoid drug contact with eyes.
● Caution patient that frequent or persistent yeast infections may suggest a more serious medical problem.
● Tell patient to refrain from sexual intercourse during vaginal treatment.
● Warn patient that topical preparation may stain clothing.
● Tell patient that using a sanitary napkin protects clothing when using vaginal preparation.
● Stress need to continue use of vaginal preparations, as prescribed, even if menstruation begins.
● Tell patient with athlete's foot to change shoes and cotton socks daily and to dry between the toes after bathing.
● Tell patient to allow lozenges to dissolve in mouth and not to chew, for full benefit.
● Stress need to continue treatment for full course and to notify prescriber if no improvement occurs after 4 weeks.

econazole nitrate
ee-KOE-na-zole

Spectazole

Pharmacologic class: imidazole derivative
Pregnancy risk category C

AVAILABLE FORMS
Cream: 1%

INDICATIONS & DOSAGES
➤ **Tinea corporis, tinea cruris, tinea pedis, tinea versicolor**
Adults and children: Rub into affected areas daily for at least 2 weeks (1 month for tinea pedis).
➤ **Cutaneous candidiasis**
Adults and children: Rub into affected areas b.i.d.

ADMINISTRATION
Topical
● Clean and dry affected area before applying.
● Don't use occlusive dressings.
● Drug isn't for ophthalmic use.

ACTION
Fungistatic, but may be fungicidal depending on level. Appears to alter fungal cell-wall permeability and produce osmotic instability.

Route	Onset	Peak	Duration
Topical	Unknown	Unknown	Unknown

Half-life: Unknown.

ADVERSE REACTIONS
Skin: burning, erythema, pruritus, stinging.

INTERACTIONS
Drug-drug. *Corticosteroids:* May inhibit antifungal activity against certain organisms. Monitor patient for effect.

EFFECTS ON LAB TEST RESULTS
None reported.

CONTRAINDICATIONS & CAUTIONS
● Contraindicated in patients hypersensitive to drug or its components.

NURSING CONSIDERATIONS
● Improvement should be seen after treatment period. If no change is noted, patient should be reevaluated.

PATIENT TEACHING
● Tell patient to use drug for entire treatment period, even if signs and symptoms improve. Instruct him to notify prescriber if no improvement occurs after 2 weeks in fungal infection on hairless skin (tinea corporis), jock itch, or fungal skin infec-

tion (tinea versicolor), or after 4 weeks for athlete's foot.
● Reassure patient that lack of pigmentation from tinea versicolor resolves gradually.
● Tell patient to stop drug and notify prescriber if condition persists or worsens or if irritation occurs.
● Warn patient that drug may stain clothing.
● Tell patient with athlete's foot to change shoes and cotton socks daily and to dry between toes after bathing.
● Tell patient to keep drug out of eyes.

---

erythromycin
er-ith-roe-MYE-sin

Akne-mycin, A/T/S, EryDerm, Ery-Sol†

Pharmacologic class: macrolide
Pregnancy risk category C (topical solution); B (other topical preparations)

AVAILABLE FORMS
Ointment: 2%
Pledgets: 2%
Topical gel: 2%
Topical solution: 2%*

INDICATIONS & DOSAGES
➤ **Inflammatory acne vulgaris**
Adults and children: Apply to affected areas b.i.d., morning and evening.

ADMINISTRATION
Topical
● Wash, rinse, and dry affected areas before application.
● Use pledget once, and then discard.
● Wash hands after each application.

ACTION
Usually bacteriostatic, but may be bactericidal in high concentrations or against highly susceptible organisms. Disrupts protein synthesis in susceptible bacteria.

Route	Onset	Peak	Duration
Topical	Unknown	Unknown	Unknown

Half-life: Unknown.

ADVERSE REACTIONS
GI: *pseudomembranous colitis.*
Skin: *burning, dryness, pruritus,* erythema, irritation, oily skin, peeling, sensitivity reactions.

INTERACTIONS
Drug-drug. *Clindamycin:* May antagonize clindamycin's effect. Avoid using together.
Isotretinoin: May cause cumulative dryness, resulting in excessive skin irritation. Use together cautiously.
Drug-lifestyle. *Abrasive or medicated soaps or cleansers, acne products, or other preparations containing peeling drugs (benzoyl peroxide, resorcinol, salicylic acid, sulfur, tretinoin), alcohol-containing products (aftershave, cosmetics, perfumed toiletries, shaving creams or lotions), astringent soaps or cosmetics, medicated cosmetics or cover-ups:* May cause cumulative dryness, resulting in excessive skin irritation. Urge caution.

EFFECTS ON LAB TEST RESULTS
● May interfere with fluorometric determinations of urine catecholamines.

CONTRAINDICATIONS & CAUTIONS
● Contraindicated in patients hypersensitive to drug or its components.
● Safety and efficacy in children haven't been established.

NURSING CONSIDERATIONS
● Prolonged use may be needed when treating acne vulgaris, which may result in overgrowth of nonsusceptible organisms.

PATIENT TEACHING
● Advise patient to wash, rinse, and dry face thoroughly before each use.
● Advise patient to avoid use near eyes, nose, mouth, or other mucous membranes.
● Tell patient to wash hands after each application.
● Tell patient to stop using drug and notify prescriber if no improvement occurs or if condition worsens in 3 to 12 weeks.
● Advise patient not to share towels or washcloths.
● Instruct patient to use each pledget once, then discard.
● Caution patient to keep drug away from heat and open flame.

gentamicin sulfate
jen-ta-MYE-sin

Pharmacologic class: aminoglycoside
Pregnancy risk category C

AVAILABLE FORMS
Cream: 0.1%
Ointment: 0.1%

INDICATIONS & DOSAGES
➤ **To treat or prevent superficial infections and superficial burns of the skin caused by susceptible bacteria**
Adults and children older than age 1: Rub in small amount gently three or four times daily, with or without gauze dressing.

ADMINISTRATION
Topical
● Clean affected area and remove crusts of impetigo before applying to increase absorption.
● Wash hands after each application.
● Store drug in cool place.

ACTION
Exact mechanism unknown. An aminoglycoside that disrupts bacterial protein synthesis by binding to ribosomes. Susceptible bacteria include sensitive strains of streptococci and *Staphylococcus aureus* and gram-negative bacteria including *Pseudomonas aeruginosa, Aerobacter aerogenes, Escherichia coli, Proteus vulgaris,* and *Klebsiella pneumoniae.*

Route	Onset	Peak	Duration
Topical	Unknown	Unknown	Unknown

Half-life: Unknown.

ADVERSE REACTIONS
Skin: allergic contact dermatitis, erythema, minor skin irritation, photosensitivity.

INTERACTIONS
None significant.

EFFECTS ON LAB TEST RESULTS
None reported.

CONTRAINDICATIONS & CAUTIONS
• Contraindicated in patients hypersensitive to drug or its components and in those who may have cross-sensitivity with other aminoglycosides, such as neomycin.

NURSING CONSIDERATIONS
• *Alert:* Avoid use on large skin lesions or over a wide area because of possible systemic toxic effects.
• Restrict use of drug to selected patients; widespread use may lead to resistant organisms.
• Prolonged use may result in overgrowth of nonsusceptible organisms.

PATIENT TEACHING
• Tell patient to clean affected area and to remove crusts of impetigo before applying to increase absorption.
• Tell patient to wash hands after each application.
• Instruct patient to store drug in cool place.
• Tell patient to stop using drug and notify prescriber immediately if no improvement occurs or if condition worsens.

---

ketoconazole
kee-toe-KOE-na-zole

Ketoderm†, Ketozole, Nizoral, Nizoral A-D ◊

Pharmacologic class: imidazole
Pregnancy risk category C

AVAILABLE FORMS
Cream: 2%
Foam: 2%
Gel: 2%
Shampoo: 1% ◊ , 2%

INDICATIONS & DOSAGES
➤ **Seborrheic dermatitis in immuno-competent patients**
Adults and children age 12 and older: Apply foam to affected area b.i.d. for 4 weeks. Apply gel to affected area once daily for 2 weeks.
➤ **Tinea corporis, tinea cruris, tinea pedis, tinea versicolor from susceptible organisms; seborrheic dermatitis; cutaneous candidiasis**

Adults: Cover affected and immediate surrounding areas daily for at least 2 weeks. For seborrheic dermatitis, apply b.i.d. for 4 weeks. Patients with tinea pedis need 6 weeks of treatment.
➤ **Scaling caused by dandruff**
Adults: Using shampoo, wet hair, lather, and massage for 1 minute. Rinse hair thoroughly with warm water, then repeat. Leave drug on scalp for 3 minutes, then rinse and dry hair with towel or warm air flow. Shampoo twice weekly for 4 weeks, with at least 3 days between shampoos and then intermittently, as needed, to maintain control.

ADMINISTRATION
Topical
• Don't let drug come in contact with eyes.

ACTION
Probably inhibits yeast growth by altering the permeability of the cell membrane.

Route	Onset	Peak	Duration
Topical	Unknown	Unknown	Unknown

Half-life: Unknown.

ADVERSE REACTIONS
Skin: abnormal hair texture, increase in normal hair loss, irritation, pruritus, oiliness, or dryness of hair and scalp with shampoo use, scalp pustules, severe irritation, pruritus, and stinging with cream.

INTERACTIONS
Drug-drug. *Topical corticosteroids:* May cause increased absorption of corticosteroid. Avoid using together.

EFFECTS ON LAB TEST RESULTS
None reported.

CONTRAINDICATIONS & CAUTIONS
• Contraindicated in patients hypersensitive to drug or its components.
• Use cautiously in pregnant and breast-feeding women.
• Ketoconazole cream contains sulfites that may cause allergic reactions, including anaphylaxis, in susceptible patients.

NURSING CONSIDERATIONS
• Most patients show improvement soon after treatment begins.
• Treatment of tinea corporis or tinea cruris should continue for at least 2 weeks to reduce possibility of recurrence.
• *Alert:* Product contains sodium sulfite anhydrous, which may cause severe or life-threatening allergic reactions, including anaphylaxis, in patients with asthma.

PATIENT TEACHING
• Tell patient to stop drug and notify prescriber if hypersensitivity reaction occurs.
• Advise patient to check with prescriber if condition worsens; drug may have to be stopped and diagnosis reevaluated.
• Tell patient to avoid using shampoo on scalp if skin is broken or inflamed.
• Warn patient that shampoo applied to permanent-waved hair removes curl.
• Warn patient to avoid drug contact with eyes.
• Tell patient to continue drug for intended duration of therapy, even if signs and symptoms improve soon after starting treatment.
• Tell patient not to store drug above room temperature (77° F [25° C]) and to protect from light.

metronidazole
me-troe-NI-da-zole

MetroCream, MetroGel, MetroGel Vaginal, MetroLotion, Noritate, Rosasol†

Pharmacologic class: nitroimidazole
Pregnancy risk category B

AVAILABLE FORMS
Topical cream: 0.75%, 1%
Topical gel: 0.75%, 1%
Topical lotion: 0.75%
Vaginal gel: 0.75%

INDICATIONS & DOSAGES
➤ **Inflammatory papules and pustules of acne rosacea**
Adults: If using a 0.75% preparation, apply thin film to affected area b.i.d., morning and evening. If using a 1% preparation, apply thin film to affected area once daily. After response is seen (usually within 3 weeks), adjust frequency and duration of therapy.
➤ **Bacterial vaginosis**
Adults: One applicatorful vaginally daily or b.i.d. for 5 days. For once-daily use, give at bedtime.

ADMINISTRATION
Topical
• Clean area thoroughly before use, and then wait 15 to 20 minutes before applying drug to minimize risk of local irritation. Avoid contact with eyes.
Vaginal
• Screw the end of the applicator onto the tube and squeeze slowly. The plunger will stop when the applicator is full.
• Wash plunger and barrel in warm, soapy water and rinse thoroughly. Dry before reassembling.

ACTION
Unknown. May cause bactericidal effect by interacting with bacterial DNA. Drug is active against many anaerobic gram-negative bacilli, anaerobic gram-positive cocci, *Gardnerella vaginalis*, and *Campylobacter fetus*.

Route	Onset	Peak	Duration
Topical	Unknown	8–12 hr	Unknown
Vaginal	Unknown	6–12 hr	Unknown

Half-life: Unknown.

ADVERSE REACTIONS
Topical form
EENT: lacrimation if applied around eyes.
Skin: *transient redness, dryness, mild burning, stinging,* contact dermatitis, pruritus, rash.
Vaginal form
GI: cramps, nausea, loose stools, metallic or bad taste in mouth, pain.
GU: *cervicitis, vaginitis,* perineal and vulvovaginal itching, vaginal burning.
Skin: *transient redness, dryness, mild burning, stinging.*
Other: overgrowth of nonsusceptible organisms.

INTERACTIONS
Drug-drug. *Disulfiram:* May cause disulfiram-like reaction when used with vaginal form of metronidazole. Avoid

using together, and wait 2 weeks after stopping disulfiram before starting metronidazole vaginal therapy.
Lithium: May increase lithium level. Monitor lithium level.
Oral anticoagulants: May increase anticoagulant effect. Monitor patient for adverse reactions.
Drug-lifestyle. *Alcohol use:* May cause disulfiram-like reaction when used with vaginal form. Discourage use together.

EFFECTS ON LAB TEST RESULTS
• May interfere with AST, ALT, LDH, triglyceride, and glucose levels.
• May increase or decrease WBC count.

CONTRAINDICATIONS & CAUTIONS
• Contraindicated in patients hypersensitive to drug or its ingredients, such as parabens, and other nitroimidazole derivatives.
• Use cautiously in patients with history or evidence of blood dyscrasia and in those with hepatic impairment.
• Use vaginal gel cautiously in patients with history of CNS diseases. Oral form may cause seizures and peripheral neuropathy.
• Use in pregnant and breast-feeding women only if clearly needed.

NURSING CONSIDERATIONS
• Topical therapy hasn't been linked to the adverse effects observed with parenteral or oral therapy, but some drug may be absorbed after topical use.
• Don't use vaginal gel in patients who have taken disulfiram within past 2 weeks.

PATIENT TEACHING
• Instruct patient to avoid use of topical gel around eyes.
• Advise patient to clean area thoroughly before use and to wait 15 to 20 minutes after cleaning skin before applying drug to minimize risk of local irritation. Cosmetics may be used after applying drug.
• If local reactions occur, advise patient to apply drug less frequently or stop using it and notify prescriber.
• Advise patient to avoid sexual intercourse while using vaginal preparation.
• Caution patient to avoid alcohol while being treated with vaginal preparation.

miconazole nitrate
mi-KON-a-zole

Desenex◇, Lotrimin AF◇, Micatin◇, Monistat-Derm, Monistat 3◇, Monistat 7◇, Ting◇, Zeasorb-AF◇

Pharmacologic class: imidazole
Pregnancy risk category C

AVAILABLE FORMS
Aerosol powder: 2%◇
Aerosol spray: 1%, 2%◇
Lotion: 2%◇
Powder: 2%◇
Topical cream: 2%◇
Topical ointment: 2%◇
Topical solution: 2%◇
Vaginal cream: 2%◇, 4%◇
Vaginal suppositories: 100 mg◇, 200 mg◇, 1,200 mg◇

INDICATIONS & DOSAGES
➤ **Tinea corporis, tinea cruris, tinea pedis, cutaneous candidiasis, common dermatophyte infections**
Adults and children older than age 2: Apply sparingly b.i.d. for 2 to 4 weeks. Powder or spray can be used liberally over affected area. In children younger than age 2, use only under the direction and supervision of a physician.
➤ **Tinea versicolor**
Adults and children older than age 2: Apply sparingly daily for 2 weeks. In children younger than age 2, use only under the direction and supervision of a physician.
➤ **Vulvovaginal candidiasis**
Adults: One applicatorful or 100-mg Monistat 7 suppository vaginally at bedtime for 7 days; repeat course, if needed. Or, 200-mg Monistat 3 suppository vaginally at bedtime for 3 days. Or, one 1,200-mg suppository vaginally at bedtime for 1 day. Or, apply topical cream sparingly to affected area b.i.d. for 7 days.

ADMINISTRATION
Topical
• Don't use occlusive dressings.
• Lotion is preferred in skinfolds.

Vaginal
● Suppository is inserted high into vagina with applicator provided.
● Store between 59° and 86° F (15° and 30° C).

ACTION
Fungicidal; disrupts fungal cell membrane permeability.

Route	Onset	Peak	Duration
Topical, vaginal	Unknown	Unknown	Unknown

Half-life: Unknown.

ADVERSE REACTIONS
CNS: headache.
GU: pelvic cramps, pruritus, and irritation with vaginal cream, vulvovaginal burning.
Skin: allergic contact dermatitis, burning, irritation, maceration, pain, edema.

INTERACTIONS
None significant.

EFFECTS ON LAB TEST RESULTS
None reported.

CONTRAINDICATIONS & CAUTIONS
● Contraindicated in patients hypersensitive to drug or its components. Cross-sensitivity to imidazole antifungals may occur.
● Don't use in children younger than age 2.
● Don't use vaginal preparation during the first trimester of pregnancy.
● Use cautiously in breast-feeding women.

NURSING CONSIDERATIONS
● Avoid using within 72 hours of certain vaginal and latex products, such as condoms or vaginal contraceptive diaphragms, because drug causes latex breakdown.

PATIENT TEACHING
● Advise patient that vaginal form of drug is for perineal or vaginal use only and to keep drug out of eyes.
● Caution patient that frequent or persistent yeast infections may suggest a more serious medical problem.

● Tell patient to cautiously insert vaginal form high into the vagina with applicator provided.
● **Alert:** Vaginal preparation shouldn't be used during first trimester of pregnancy. Advise patient to use vaginal preparation during pregnancy only if recommended by prescriber.
● Tell patient that drug may stain clothing.
● Warn patient to stop drug if sensitivity or chemical irritation occurs.
● Tell patient to use drug for full treatment period prescribed and to notify prescriber if signs and symptoms persist or worsen at end of therapy.
● Advise patient to avoid tampons and sexual intercourse during vaginal treatment.
● Instruct patient to apply sparingly in skinfolds and rub in well to prevent skin breakdown.
● Tell patient to store vaginal product between 59° and 86° F (15° and 30° C).

mupirocin
myoo-PIHR-oh-sin

Bactroban, Bactroban Cream, Bactroban Nasal, Centany

Pharmacologic class: antibiotic
Pregnancy risk category B

AVAILABLE FORMS
Intranasal ointment: 2%
Topical cream: 2%
Topical ointment: 2%

INDICATIONS & DOSAGES
➤ **Impetigo**
Adults and children: Apply to affected areas t.i.d. for 1 to 2 weeks. Reevaluate patient in 3 to 5 days; may cover affected area with dressing.
➤ **Traumatic skin lesions infected with *Staphylococcus aureus* or *Streptococcus pyogenes***
Adults and children: Apply thin film t.i.d. for 10 days; may cover with gauze dressing, if needed. Reevaluate patient if improvement doesn't occur in 3 to 5 days.
➤ **To eradicate nasal colonization by methicillin-resistant *S. aureus***

in adult patients and health care workers

Adults and children age 12 and older: Divide ointment in single-use tube between nostrils (½ tube per nostril) b.i.d. for 5 days. After application, close nostrils by pressing together and releasing sides of nose repeatedly for 1 minute to spread ointment throughout nares.

ADMINISTRATION
Topical
● Cosmetics and other skin products shouldn't be used on treated area.
Intranasal
● Other nasal products shouldn't be used with intranasal ointment.

ACTION
Inhibits bacterial protein synthesis by reversibly and specifically binding to bacterial isoleucyl transfer-RNA synthetase.

Route	Onset	Peak	Duration
Topical	Unknown	Unknown	Unknown

Half-life: Unknown.

ADVERSE REACTIONS
CNS: headache.
EENT: rhinitis, pharyngitis, burning or stinging with intranasal use.
GI: taste perversion, nausea, abdominal pain, ulcerative stomatitis.
Respiratory: upper respiratory tract congestion, cough with intranasal use.
Skin: burning, erythema with topical use, pain, pruritus, rash, stinging.

INTERACTIONS
Drug-drug. *Chloramphenicol:* May interfere with the antibacterial action of mupirocin on RNA synthesis. Monitor patient for clinical effect.

EFFECTS ON LAB TEST RESULTS
None reported.

CONTRAINDICATIONS & CAUTIONS
● Contraindicated in patients hypersensitive to drug or its components.
● Use cautiously in patients with burns or large open wounds and in those with impaired renal function because serious renal toxicity may occur.

NURSING CONSIDERATIONS
● Drug isn't for ophthalmic or internal use.
● Prolonged use may cause overgrowth of nonsusceptible bacteria and fungi.
● Local reactions appear to be caused by polyethylene glycol vehicle.
● *Look alike–sound alike:* Don't confuse Bactroban with bacitracin, baclofen, or Bactrim.

PATIENT TEACHING
● Tell patient to notify prescriber immediately if condition doesn't improve or gets worse in 3 to 5 days.
● Tell patient not to use other nasal products with intranasal ointment.
● Warn patient about local adverse reactions related to drug use.
● Caution patient not to use cosmetics or other skin products on treated area.

retapamulin
re-te-PAM-ue-lin

Altabax

Pharmacologic class: pleuromutilin
Pregnancy risk category B

AVAILABLE FORMS
Topical ointment: 1%

INDICATIONS & DOSAGES
➤ **Impetigo**
Adults and children age 9 months and older: Apply a thin layer to affected area b.i.d. for 5 days.

ADMINISTRATION
Topical
● Wash hands before and after application, and use glove if available.
● Affected area may be covered with sterile bandage or gauze if needed.

ACTION
Inhibits bacterial protein synthesis in methicillin-susceptible *Staphylococcus aureus* or *S. pyogenes.*

Route	Onset	Peak	Duration
Topical	Within 24 hr	Unknown	Unknown

Half-life: Unknown.

ADVERSE REACTIONS
CNS: headache, pyrexia.
GI: diarrhea, nausea.
Respiratory: nasopharyngitis.
Skin: application site irritation, eczema, pruritus.

INTERACTIONS
None significant.

EFFECTS ON LAB TEST RESULTS
● May increase creatinine kinase levels.

CONTRAINDICATIONS & CAUTIONS
● Contraindicated in patients hypersensitive to drug or its components.
● Safety and efficacy in children younger than age 9 months haven't been established.
● Safety and efficacy in pregnant and breast-feeding women haven't been established. Use only if benefits outweigh risks.

NURSING CONSIDERATIONS
● To reduce development of resistance or superinfection, treat infection only from organisms proven to be susceptible to this drug.
● Monitor the site for local irritation; if the reaction is severe, wipe the drug off the skin and don't reapply.
● Don't apply drug to mucous membranes.

PATIENT TEACHING
● Tell patient to wash his hands before and after application, and to use a glove if available.
● Tell patient to notify prescriber if his condition doesn't improve in 3 to 4 days, or if a local reaction develops.
● Advise patient to continue using drug for entire prescribed course of therapy.
● Warn patient that drug is for external use only.

---

sertaconazole nitrate
sir-tah-KAHN-uh-zole

Ertaczo

Pharmacologic class: imidazole
Pregnancy risk category C

AVAILABLE FORMS
Topical cream: 2%

INDICATIONS & DOSAGES
➤ **Interdigital tinea pedis caused by *Trichophyton rubrum, Trichophyton mentagrophytes,* or *Epidermophyton floccosum* in immunocompetent patients**
Adults and children age 12 and older:
Apply cream b.i.d. to affected areas between toes and healthy surrounding areas for 4 weeks.

ADMINISTRATION
Topical
● Avoid occlusive coverings on affected area.

ACTION
May inhibit CYP-dependent synthesis of ergosterol. The lack of ergosterol in the cell membrane causes alterations in cell-wall permeability and osmotic instability, leading to fungal cell injury and death.

Route	Onset	Peak	Duration
Topical	Unknown	Unknown	Unknown

Half-life: Unknown.

ADVERSE REACTIONS
Skin: application site reaction, burning, contact dermatitis, dryness, erythema, hyperpigmentation, tenderness.

INTERACTIONS
None known.

EFFECTS ON LAB TEST RESULTS
None reported.

CONTRAINDICATIONS & CAUTIONS
● Contraindicated in patients hypersensitive to drug, its components, or other imidazoles.
● Use cautiously in pregnant or breast-feeding women.
● Efficacy and safety haven't been established for children younger than age 12.

NURSING CONSIDERATIONS
● Before treatment starts, diagnosis should be confirmed by direct microscopic examination of infected tissue in potassium hydroxide

---

Reactions may be *common,* uncommon, *life-threatening,* or COMMON AND LIFE-THREATENING.
Interaction may have a *rapid onset* or **delayed onset**.

solution or by culture on an appropriate medium.
● Use drug only on skin; not for ophthalmic, oral, or vaginal use.
● If condition hasn't improved after 2 weeks, review diagnosis.
● Stop drug if skin irritation or sensitivity develops.

PATIENT TEACHING
● Warn patient to stop using drug if he develops increased irritation, redness, itching, burning, blistering, swelling, or oozing at site of application.
● Caution patient that drug is for external use on skin only. Discourage contact with eyes, nose, mouth, and other mucous membranes.
● If cream is to be applied after bathing, tell patient to dry affected area thoroughly before application.
● Tell patient to wash hands after applying cream.
● Urge patient to use drug for full duration of treatment, even if symptoms have improved.
● Instruct patient to notify prescriber if condition worsens or fails to improve.
● Caution patient to avoid occlusive coverings unless directed by prescriber.
● Teach patient proper foot hygiene.

---

silver sulfadiazine
sul-fa-DYE-a-zeen

Dermazin†, Flamazine†, Silvadene, SSD, SSD AF, Thermazene

Pharmacologic class: broad-spectrum sulfonamide
Pregnancy risk category B

AVAILABLE FORMS
Cream: 1%

INDICATIONS & DOSAGES
➤ **To prevent or treat wound infection in second- and third-degree burns**
Adults: Apply ¹⁄₁₆-inch ribbon of cream to clean, debrided wound daily or b.i.d.

ADMINISTRATION
Topical
● Use sterile application technique to prevent wound contamination.
● Discard darkened cream because drug is ineffective.
● This drug isn't for ophthalmic use.

ACTION
Acts on cell membrane and cell wall; it's bactericidal for many gram-positive and gram-negative organisms.

Route	Onset	Peak	Duration
Topical	Unknown	Unknown	Unknown

Half-life: Unknown.

ADVERSE REACTIONS
GU: interstitial nephritis.
Hematologic: *leukopenia.*
Metabolic: altered serum osmolality.
Skin: *erythema multiforme,* burning, pain, pruritus, rash, skin discoloration, skin necrosis.

INTERACTIONS
Drug-drug. *Topical proteolytic enzymes:* May inactivate enzymes. Avoid using together.
Drug-lifestyle. *Sun exposure:* May cause photosensitivity. Advise patient to avoid excessive sun exposure.

EFFECTS ON LAB TEST RESULTS
● May decrease WBC count.

CONTRAINDICATIONS & CAUTIONS
● Contraindicated in patients hypersensitive to drug and in those with G6PD deficiency.
● Contraindicated in pregnant women at or near term and in premature or full-term neonates during first 2 months after birth. Drug may increase possibility of kernicterus.
● *Alert:* Use cautiously in patients hypersensitive to sulfonamides.

NURSING CONSIDERATIONS
● Use drug only on affected areas. Keep these areas medicated at all times.
● Bathe patient daily, if possible.
● Inspect patient's skin daily, and note any changes. Notify prescriber if burning or excessive pain develops.

• Monitor sulfadiazine levels and renal function, and check urine for sulfa crystals in patients with extensive burns.
• Tell prescriber if hepatic or renal dysfunction occurs; drug may need to be stopped.
• Leukopenia usually resolves without intervention and doesn't always require stopping drug.
• Absorption of propylene glycol (contained in the cream) can interfere with serum osmolality.

PATIENT TEACHING
• Instruct patient to promptly report adverse reactions, especially burning or excessive pain with application.
• Inform patient of need for frequent blood and urine tests to watch for adverse effects.
• Tell patient that he may develop sensitivity to the sun.
• Tell patient to continue treatment until satisfactory healing occurs or until site is ready for grafting.

terbinafine hydrochloride
ter-BIN-ah-fin

Lamisil, Lamisil AT ◇

Pharmacologic class: allylamine derivative
Pregnancy risk category B

AVAILABLE FORMS
Cream: 1% ◇
Gel: 1% ◇
Spray: 1% ◇

INDICATIONS & DOSAGES
➤ **Athlete's foot, tinea versicolor**
Adults and children age 12 and older:
Apply b.i.d. for at least 1 week, but no longer than 4 weeks.
➤ **Jock itch, ringworm**
Adults and children age 12 and older:
Apply once daily for at least 1 week, but no longer than 4 weeks.

ADMINISTRATION
Topical
• Wash affected area with soap and water and dry completely before application.

• Don't apply an occlusive dressing without a specific order.
• This drug isn't for ophthalmic use. Avoid contact with mucous membranes.

ACTION
Fungicidal; selectively inhibits an early step in synthesis of sterols used by fungi for cell-wall synthesis.

Route	Onset	Peak	Duration
Topical	Unknown	Unknown	Unknown

Half-life: About 21 hours.

ADVERSE REACTIONS
Skin: irritation, pruritus, skin exfoliation.

INTERACTIONS
None significant.

EFFECTS ON LAB TEST RESULTS
None reported.

CONTRAINDICATIONS & CAUTIONS
• Contraindicated in patients hypersensitive to drug or its components and in breast-feeding women.

NURSING CONSIDERATIONS
• Observe patient for 2 to 6 weeks after therapy is complete to determine whether treatment was successful; review diagnosis if condition persists.
• Drug isn't intended for oral, ophthalmic, or vaginal use.
• *Look alike–sound alike:* Don't confuse terbinafine with terbutaline. Don't confuse Lamisil with Lamictal.

PATIENT TEACHING
• Teach patient proper use of drug. Tell him to wash affected area with soap and water and dry completely before applying.
• Advise patient to use only as directed for full recommended course, even if signs and symptoms disappear, and not to apply near eyes, mouth, or mucous membranes or to use occlusive dressings unless so directed.
• Instruct patient with athlete's foot to wear well-fitting, ventilated shoes.
• Tell patient to wash hands after applying.
• Tell patient to stop drug and contact prescriber if irritation or sensitivity develops.
• Tell patient to store drug between 41° and 86° F (5° and 30° C).

Reactions may be *common*, uncommon, *life-threatening*, or COMMON AND LIFE-THREATENING.
Interaction may have a *rapid onset* or **delayed onset**.

terconazole
ter-CONE-uh-zole

Terazol 3, Terazol 7

Pharmacologic class: triazole
derivative
Pregnancy risk category C

AVAILABLE FORMS
Vaginal cream: 0.4%, 0.8%
Vaginal suppositories: 80 mg

INDICATIONS & DOSAGES
➤ **Vulvovaginal candidiasis**
Adults: One applicatorful of cream or
1 suppository inserted into vagina at
bedtime; 0.4% cream used for 7 consecutive days; 0.8% cream or 80-mg suppository for 3 consecutive days. Repeat
course, if needed, after reconfirmation by
smear or culture.

ADMINISTRATION
Vaginal
● Insert drug high in vagina (unless patient
is pregnant).
● Store drug at room temperature.

ACTION
May increase *Candida* cell membrane
permeability.

Route	Onset	Peak	Duration
Vaginal	Unknown	Unknown	Unknown

Half-life: Unknown.

ADVERSE REACTIONS
CNS: *headache,* fever.
GI: abdominal pain.
GU: dysmenorrhea, genital pain, vulvo-
vaginal burning.
Skin: pruritus, irritation, photosensitivity.
Other: body aches, chills.

INTERACTIONS
None significant.

EFFECTS ON LAB TEST RESULTS
None reported.

CONTRAINDICATIONS & CAUTIONS
● Contraindicated in patients hypersensitive to drug or its inactive ingredients.

NURSING CONSIDERATIONS
● Therapeutic effect of drug is unaffected
by menstruation or hormonal contraceptive use.
● *Look alike–sound alike:* Don't confuse
terconazole with tioconazole.

PATIENT TEACHING
● Advise patient to continue treatment
during menstrual period. However, tell her
not to use tampons.
● Instruct patient to insert drug high in
vagina (except during pregnancy).
● Tell patient to use drug for full treatment
period prescribed. Explain how to prevent
reinfection.
● Instruct patient to notify prescriber and
stop drug if fever, chills, other flulike signs
and symptoms, or sensitivity develops.
● Caution patient to refrain from sexual
intercourse during treatment.
● Tell patient that drug base may react
with latex, causing decreased effectiveness
of condoms and diaphragms (for up to
72 hours after treatment is completed).
● Instruct patient to store drug at room
temperature.

15

Macrolide anti-infectives

azithromycin
clarithromycin
erythromycin base
erythromycin estolate
erythromycin ethylsuccinate
erythromycin lactobionate
erythromycin stearate

---

azithromycin
ay-zi-thro-MY-sin

Zithromax◆, Zmax

Pharmacologic class: macrolide
Pregnancy risk category B

AVAILABLE FORMS
Injection: 500 mg
Oral suspension (extended-release): 2 g
Powder for oral suspension: 100 mg/5 ml,
200 mg/5 ml; 1,000 mg/packet
Tablets: 250 mg, 500 mg, 600 mg

INDICATIONS & DOSAGES
➤ **Acute bacterial worsening of
COPD caused by** *Haemophilus
influenzae,* **Moraxella catarrhalis, or**
Streptococcus pneumoniae; **uncomplicated skin and skin-structure
infections caused by** *Staphylococcus
aureus,* **Streptococcus pyogenes, or**
Streptococcus agalactiae; **second-line
therapy for pharyngitis or tonsillitis
caused by** *Staphylococcus pyogenes*
Adults and adolescents age 16 and older:
Initially, 500 mg P.O. as a single dose on
day 1, followed by 250 mg daily on days
2 through 5. Total cumulative dose is
1.5 g. Or, for worsening COPD, 500 mg
P.O. daily for 3 days.
➤ **Community-acquired pneumonia
from** *Chlamydia pneumoniae,*
*H. influenzae, Mycoplasma pneumo-
niae,* **or** *S. pneumoniae;* **or caused by**
*Legionella pneumophila, M. catar-
rhalis,* **or** *S. aureus*
Adults and adolescents age 16 and older:
For mild infections, give 500 mg P.O. as a
single dose on day 1; then 250 mg P.O.

daily on days 2 through 5. Total dose is
1.5 g. For more severe infections or those
caused by *S. aureus,* give 500 mg I.V. as a
single daily dose for 2 days; then 500 mg
P.O. as a single daily dose to complete a
7- to 10-day course of therapy. Switch
from I.V. to P.O. therapy based on patient
response.
➤ **Community-acquired pneumonia caused by** *C. pneumoniae,*
H. influenzae, M. pneumoniae,
S. pneumoniae
Children 6 months and older: 10 mg/kg
oral suspension P.O. (maximum of
500 mg) as a single dose on day 1, followed by 5 mg/kg (maximum of 250 mg)
daily on days 2 through 5.
➤ **Single-dose treatment for mild
to moderate acute bacterial sinusitis
caused by** *H. influenzae, M. catarrhalis,* **or** *S. pneumoniae;* **or community-acquired pneumonia
caused by** *C. pneumoniae,*
H. influenzae, M. catarrhalis,
or *S. pneumoniae*
Adults: 2 g Zmax P.O. as a single dose
taken 1 hour before or 2 hours after a
meal.
➤ **Acute bacterial sinusitis caused
by** *H. influenzae, M. catarrhalis,* **or**
S. pneumoniae
Adults: 500 mg P.O. daily for 3 days.
Children age 6 months and older:
10 mg/kg oral suspension P.O. once daily
for 3 days.
➤ **Chancroid**
Adults: 1 g P.O. as a single dose.
Infants and children ◆ : 20 mg/kg
(maximum of 1 g) P.O. as a single dose.
➤ **Nongonococcal urethritis or
cervicitis caused by** *C. trachomatis*
Adults and adolescents age 16 and older:
1 g P.O. as a single dose.
➤ **To prevent disseminated** *Myco-
bacterium avium* **complex in patients
with advanced HIV infection**
Adults and adolescents: 1.2 g P.O. once
weekly alone or with rifabutin.
Infants and children: 20 mg/kg P.O. (max-
imum of 1.2 g) weekly or 5 mg/kg (maxi-

mum of 250 mg) can be given P.O. daily. Children age 6 and older may also receive 300 mg rifabutin P.O. daily.

➤ **M. avium complex in patients with advanced HIV infection**
Adults: 600 mg P.O. daily with ethambutol 15 mg/kg daily.

➤ **Urethritis and cervicitis caused by *Neisseria gonorrhoeae***
Adults: 2 g P.O. as a single dose.

➤ **Pelvic inflammatory disease caused by *C. trachomatis, N. gonorrhoeae,* or *M. hominis* in patients who need initial I.V. therapy**
Adults and adolescents age 16 and older: 500 mg I.V. as a single daily dose for 1 to 2 days; then 250 mg P.O. daily to complete a 7-day course of therapy. Switch from I.V. to P.O. therapy, based on patient response.

➤ **Otitis media**
Children older than age 6 months: 30 mg/kg oral suspension P.O. as a single dose; or, 10 mg/kg P.O. once daily for 3 days; or, 10 mg/kg P.O. on day 1 and then 5 mg/kg once daily on days 2 to 5.

➤ **Pharyngitis, tonsillitis**
Children age 2 and older: 12 mg/kg oral suspension (maximum 500 mg) P.O. daily for 5 days.

ADMINISTRATION
P.O.
• Obtain specimen for culture and sensitivity tests before giving first dose. Begin therapy while awaiting results.
• Give Zmax 1 hour before or 2 hours after a meal. Tablets and single-dose packets for oral suspension can be taken with or without food. Don't give with antacids.
• Reconstitute suspension packet with 2 ounces (60 ml) water. After taking, rinse glass with additional 2 ounces water and have patient drink it to ensure he has taken entire dose. Packets aren't for children.
I.V.
• Reconstitute drug in 500-mg vial with 4.8 ml of sterile water for injection to yield 100 mg/ml.
• Shake well until all drug is dissolved.
• Further dilute in 250- or 500-ml normal saline solution, half-normal saline solution, D₅W, or lactated Ringer's solution to yield a final concentration of 1 or 2 mg/ml, respectively.

• Infuse a 500-mg dose of azithromycin I.V. over 1 hour or longer. Never give it as a bolus or I.M. injection.
• Reconstituted solution and diluted solution are stable for 24 hours when stored below 86° F (30° C). Diluted solution is stable for 7 days when refrigerated at 41° F (5° C).
• **Incompatibilities:** Amikacin sulfate, aztreonam, cefotaxime, ceftazidime, ceftriaxone sodium, cefuroxime, ciprofloxacin, clindamycin phosphate, famotidine, fentanyl citrate, furosemide, gentamicin sulfate, imipenem and cilastatin sodium, ketorolac tromethamine, levofloxacin, morphine sulfate, ondansetron hydrochloride, piperacillin and tazobactam sodium, potassium chloride, ticarcillin disodium and clavulanate potassium, tobramycin sulfate.

ACTION
Binds to the 50S subunit of bacterial ribosomes, blocking protein synthesis; bacteriostatic or bactericidal, depending on concentration.

Route	Onset	Peak	Duration
P.O.	Unknown	2–5 hr	Unknown
I.V.	Unknown	Unknown	Unknown

Half-life: About 3 days.

ADVERSE REACTIONS
CNS: fatigue, headache, somnolence.
CV: chest pain, palpitations.
GI: *abdominal pain,* anorexia, *diarrhea, nausea, vomiting, pseudomembranous colitis,* dyspepsia, flatulence, melena.
GU: candidiasis, nephritis, vaginitis.
Hepatic: cholestatic jaundice.
Skin: photosensitivity reactions, rash, pain at injection site, pruritus.
Other: *angioedema.*

INTERACTIONS
Drug-drug. *Antacids containing aluminum and magnesium:* May lower peak azithromycin level (immediate-release form). Separate doses by at least 2 hours. *Antiarrhythmics (amiodarone, quinidine):* May increase risk of life-threatening arrhythmias, including torsades de pointes. Monitor ECG rhythm carefully.

Carbamazepine, phenytoin: May increase levels of these drugs. Monitor drug levels.

Cyclosporine: May elevate cyclosporine concentrations with increased risk of nephrotoxicity and neurotoxicity. Monitor cyclosporine levels and renal function.

Digoxin: May increase digoxin level. Monitor digoxin level.

Ergotamine: May cause acute ergotamine toxicity. Monitor patient closely.

HMG-CoA reductase inhibitors (atorvastatin, lovastatin): May increase HMG-CoA reductase inhibitor levels, resulting in severe myopathy or rhabdomyolysis. Consider alternative therapy.

Nelfinavir: May increase azithromycin level. Monitor for liver enzyme abnormalities and hearing impairment.

Pimozide: May prolong QT interval and cause ventricular tachycardia. Concurrent use is contraindicated.

Theophylline: May increase theophylline level. Monitor theophylline level carefully.

Triazolam: May decrease triazolam clearance. Monitor patient closely.

Warfarin: May increase INR. Monitor INR carefully.

Drug-food. *Any food:* May decrease absorption of multidose oral suspension form. Advise patient to take drug on empty stomach.

Drug-lifestyle. *Sun exposure:* May cause photosensitivity reactions. Advise patient to avoid excessive sunlight exposure.

EFFECTS ON LAB TEST RESULTS
● May increase ALT, AST, creatinine, LDH, and bilirubin levels.

CONTRAINDICATIONS & CAUTIONS
● Contraindicated in patients hypersensitive to erythromycin or other macrolide or ketolide antibiotics.
● Use cautiously in patients with impaired hepatic function.

NURSING CONSIDERATIONS
● Monitor patient for superinfection. Drug may cause overgrowth of nonsusceptible bacteria or fungi.
● If patient vomits within 60 minutes of taking Zmax, notify prescriber; additional or different therapy may be needed.

PATIENT TEACHING
● Tell patient to take drug as prescribed, even after he feels better.
● Advise patient to avoid excessive sunlight and to wear protective clothing and use sunscreen when outside.
● Tell patient to report adverse reactions promptly.

clarithromycin
klar-ITH-ro-my-sin

Biaxin◊, Biaxin XL◊

Pharmacologic class: macrolide
Pregnancy risk category C

AVAILABLE FORMS
Suspension: 125 mg/5 ml, 250 mg/5 ml
Tablets (extended-release): 500 mg, 1,000 mg
Tablets (film-coated): 250 mg, 500 mg

INDICATIONS & DOSAGES
➤ **Pharyngitis or tonsillitis caused by** *Streptococcus pyogenes*
Adults: 250 mg P.O. every 12 hours for 10 days.
Children: 15 mg/kg/day P.O. divided every 12 hours for 10 days.
➤ **Acute maxillary sinusitis caused by** *S. pneumoniae, Haemophilus influenzae,* **or** *Moraxella catarrhalis*
Adults: 500 mg P.O. every 12 hours for 14 days. Or, if using extended-release form, give two 500-mg tablets or one 1,000-mg tablet P.O. daily for 14 days.
Children: 15 mg/kg/day P.O. divided every 12 hours for 10 days.
➤ **Acute worsening of chronic bronchitis caused by** *M. catarrhalis, S. pneumoniae;* **community-acquired pneumonia caused by** *H. influenzae, S. pneumoniae, Mycoplasma pneumoniae,* **or** *Chlamydia pneumoniae*
Adults: 250 mg P.O. every 12 hours for 7 days (*H. influenzae*) or 7 to 14 days (other bacteria).
➤ **Acute worsening of chronic bronchitis caused by** *H. influenzae* **or** *H. parainfluenzae*
Adults: 500 mg P.O. every 12 hours for 7 days (*H. parainfluenzae*) or 7 to 14 days (*H. influenzae*).

Reactions may be *common,* uncommon, *life-threatening,* or COMMON AND LIFE-THREATENING.
Interaction may have a *rapid onset* or *delayed onset.*

➤ **Acute worsening of chronic bronchitis caused by** *M. catarrhalis, S. pneumoniae, H. parainfluenzae,* **or** *H. influenzae*

Adults: Two 500-mg or one 1,000-mg of the extended-release tablets P.O. daily for 7 days.

➤ **Mild to moderate community-acquired pneumonia, caused by** *H. influenzae, H. parainfluenzae, M. catarrhalis, S. pneumoniae, C. pneumoniae,* **or** *M. pneumoniae*

Adults: Two 500-mg or one 1,000-mg of the extended-release tablets P.O. daily for 7 days.

➤ **Community-acquired pneumonia caused by** *S. pneumoniae, C. pneumoniae,* **and** *M. pneumoniae*

Children: 15 mg/kg/day P.O. divided every 12 hours for 10 days.

➤ **Uncomplicated skin and skin-structure infections caused by** *Staphylococcus aureus* **or** *S. pyogenes*

Adults: 250 mg P.O. every 12 hours for 7 to 14 days.

Children: 15 mg/kg/day P.O. divided every 12 hours for 10 days.

➤ **Acute otitis media caused by** *H. influenzae, M. catarrhalis,* **or** *S. pneumoniae*

Children: 15 mg/kg/day P.O. divided every 12 hours for 10 days.

➤ **To prevent and treat disseminated infection caused by** *Mycobacterium avium* **complex**

Adults: 500 mg P.O. b.i.d.

Children: 7.5 mg/kg P.O. b.i.d., up to 500 mg b.i.d.

➤ *Helicobacter pylori,* **to reduce risk of duodenal ulcer recurrence**

Adults: 500 mg clarithromycin with 30 mg lansoprazole and 1 g amoxicillin, all given every 12 hours for 10 to 14 days. Or, 500 mg clarithromycin with 20 mg omeprazole and 1 g amoxicillin, all given every 12 hours for 10 days. Or, 500 mg clarithromycin b.i.d., 20 mg rabeprazole b.i.d., and 1 g amoxicillin b.i.d., all for 7 days. Or, two-drug regimen with 500 mg clarithromycin every 8 hours and 40 mg omeprazole once daily for 14 days. Continue omeprazole for 14 additional days.

Adjust-a-dose: In patients with creatinine clearance less than 30 ml/minute, cut dose in half or double frequency interval.

ADMINISTRATION
P.O.
● Obtain specimen for culture and sensitivity tests before giving. Begin therapy while awaiting results.
● Give drug with or without food.
● Don't refrigerate the suspension form; discard unused portion after 14 days.

ACTION
Binds to the 50S subunit of bacterial ribosomes, blocking protein synthesis; bacteriostatic or bactericidal, depending on concentration.

Route	Onset	Peak	Duration
P.O.	Unknown	2–4 hr	Unknown
P.O. (extended)	Unknown	5–6 hr	Unknown

Half-life: 5 to 7 hours.

ADVERSE REACTIONS
CNS: headache.
GI: *pseudomembranous colitis,* abdominal pain or discomfort, diarrhea, nausea, taste perversion, vomiting (in children).
Hematologic: coagulation abnormalities.
Skin: rash (in children).

INTERACTIONS
Drug-drug. *Alprazolam, midazolam, triazolam:* May decrease clearance of these drugs, causing adverse reactions. Use together cautiously.
Carbamazepine, phenytoin: May inhibit metabolism of these drugs, increasing serum levels and risk of toxicity. Avoid using together.
Cyclosporine: May increase cyclosporine levels. Monitor cyclosporine level.
Digoxin: May increase digoxin level. Monitor patient for digoxin toxicity.
Dihydroergotamine, ergotamine: May cause acute ergot toxicity. Avoid using together.
Fluconazole: May increase clarithromycin level. Monitor patient closely.
HMG-CoA reductase inhibitors: May increase levels of these drugs; may rarely cause rhabdomyolysis. Use together cautiously.
Other drugs that prolong the QTc interval (amiodarone, antipsychotics, disopyramide, fluoroquinolones, procainamide, quinidine,

sotalol, tricyclic antidepressants): May have additive effects. Monitor ECG for QTc interval prolongation. Avoid using together if possible.

Pimozide: May cause torsades de pointes. Use together is contraindicated.

Rifamycin: May decrease therapeutic effects of macrolide while increasing adverse effects of rifamycin. Monitor patient.

Ritonavir: May increase level of clarithromycin. May need to reduce clarithromycin dosage in renally impaired patients.

Sildenafil: May prolong absorption of sildenafil. May need to reduce sildenafil dosage.

Theophylline: May increase theophylline level. Monitor drug level.

Warfarin: May increase PT and INR. Monitor PT and INR carefully.

Zidovudine: May alter zidovudine level. Monitor patient closely.

Drug-food. _Grapefruit juice:_ May inhibit metabolism, increasing adverse effects. Don't take with grapefruit juice.

EFFECTS ON LAB TEST RESULTS
● May increase BUN level.
● May increase PT and INR.

CONTRAINDICATIONS & CAUTIONS
● Contraindicated in patients hypersensitive to clarithromycin, erythromycin, or other macrolides and in those receiving pimozide or other drugs that prolong QT interval or cause cardiac arrhythmias.
● Use cautiously in patients with hepatic or renal impairment.
● Safety and efficacy in children younger than age 6 months haven't been established.
● Use during pregnancy only if potential benefit justifies potential risk to fetus.

NURSING CONSIDERATIONS
● **Alert:** The safety and effectiveness of the extended-release form haven't been established for treating other infections for which the original form has been approved.
● Monitor patient for superinfection. Drug may cause overgrowth of nonsusceptible bacteria or fungi.
● Giving clarithromycin with a drug metabolized by CYP3A may increase

drug levels and prolong therapeutic and adverse effects.

PATIENT TEACHING
● Tell patient to take drug as prescribed, even after he feels better.
● Advise patient to report persistent adverse reactions.
● Inform patient that drug may be taken with or without food.
● Tell patient not to refrigerate the suspension form, but to discard unused portion after 14 days.

erythromycin base
er-ith-roe-MYE-sin

Apo-Erythro Base†, E-Base, E-Mycin✦, Erybid†, Eryc✦, Ery-Tab✦, Erythromid†, Erythromycin Filmtabs, Erythromycin Delayed-Release, PCE Dispertab

erythromycin ethylsuccinate
Apo-Erythro-ES†, E.E.S., E.E.S. Granules, EryPed, EryPed 200, EryPed 400

erythromycin lactobionate
Erythrocin Lactobionate

erythromycin stearate
Apo-Erythro-S†, Erythrocin Stearate

Pharmacologic class: macrolide
Pregnancy risk category B

AVAILABLE FORMS
erythromycin base
Capsules (delayed-release): 250 mg
Tablets (enteric-coated): 250 mg, 333 mg, 500 mg
Tablets (filmtabs): 250 mg, 500 mg
erythromycin ethylsuccinate
Oral suspension: 100 mg/2.5 ml, 200 mg/5 ml, 400 mg/5 ml (after reconstitution)
Tablets: 400 mg
Powder for oral suspension: 200 mg/5 ml, 400 mg/5 ml
erythromycin lactobionate
Injection: 500-mg, 1-g vials

Reactions may be *common*, uncommon, *life-threatening*, or COMMON AND LIFE-THREATENING.
Interaction may have a *rapid onset* or **delayed onset.**

erythromycin stearate
Tablets (film-coated): 250 mg, 500 mg

INDICATIONS & DOSAGES
➤ **Acute pelvic inflammatory disease caused by** *Neisseria gonorrhoeae*
Adults: 500 mg I.V. every 6 hours for 3 days; then 250 mg P.O. every 6 hours or 333 mg P.O. every 8 hours for 7 days.
➤ **Intestinal amebiasis caused by** *Entamoeba histolytica*
Adults: 250 mg P.O. q.i.d. or 333 mg P.O. every 8 hours, or 500 mg delayed-release tablets P.O. every 12 hours for 10 to 14 days. Or, 400 mg P.O. as ethylsuccinate q.i.d. for 10 to 14 days.
Children: 30 to 50 mg/kg P.O. daily, in divided doses, for 10 to 14 days.
➤ **Erythrasma**
Adults: 250 mg P.O. every 6 hours for 14 days.
➤ **To prevent rheumatic fever recurrence in patients allergic to penicillin and sulfonamides**
Adults: 250 mg base or stearate P.O. b.i.d.; or, 400 mg ethylsuccinate P.O. b.i.d.
➤ **Mild to moderately severe respiratory tract, skin, or soft-tissue infection from sensitive group A beta-hemolytic streptococci,** *Streptococcus pneumoniae, Mycoplasma pneumoniae, Corynebacterium diphtheriae,* **or** *Bordetella pertussis*
Adults: 250 to 500 mg base or stearate P.O. every 6 hours; or 400 to 800 mg ethylsuccinate P.O. every 6 hours; or 15 to 20 mg/kg I.V. daily, as continuous infusion or in divided doses every 6 hours for 10 days (3 weeks for *Mycoplasma* species infection).
Children: 30 to 50 mg/kg P.O. daily, in divided doses every 6 hours; or 15 to 20 mg/kg I.V. daily, in divided doses every 4 to 6 hours for 10 days (3 weeks for *Mycoplasma* species infection).
➤ *Listeria monocytogenes* **infection**
Adults: 250 mg P.O. every 6 hours or 500 mg P.O. every 12 hours.
➤ **Nongonococcal urethritis caused by** *Ureaplasma urealyticum*
Adults: 500 mg P.O. every 6 hours or 666 mg P.O. every 8 hours for at least 7 days.

➤ **Legionnaires' disease**
Adults: 1 to 4 g P.O. daily in divided doses for 10 to 14 days alone or with rifampin. I.V. route may be used initially in severe cases.
➤ **Uncomplicated urethral, endocervical, or rectal infection caused by** *Chlamydia trachomatis,* **when tetracyclines are contraindicated**
Adults: 500 mg base P.O. q.i.d. for at least 7 days, or 666 mg P.O. every 8 hours for at least 7 days, or 250 mg P.O. q.i.d. for 14 days if patient can't tolerate higher doses.
➤ **Urogenital** *C. trachomatis* **infection during pregnancy**
Adults: 500 mg base or stearate P.O. q.i.d. for at least 7 days or 250 mg base or stearate or 400 mg ethylsuccinate P.O. q.i.d. for at least 14 days.
➤ **Pneumonia in infants caused by** *C. trachomatis*
Infants: 50 mg/kg/day base or stearate P.O. in four divided doses for 21 days, or 15 to 20 mg/kg/day lactobionate I.V. as a continuous infusion or in four divided doses.
➤ **Chancroid caused by** *Haemophilus ducreyi* ◆
Adults: 500 mg base P.O. t.i.d. to q.i.d. for 7 days.
➤ **Pertussis**
Adults: 40 to 50 mg/kg/day P.O. in divided doses for 5 to 14 days.
➤ **Preoperative prophylaxis for elective colorectal surgery**
Adults: Two 500-mg tablets, three 333-mg tablets, or four 250-mg tablets P.O. at 1 p.m., 2 p.m., and 11 p.m. on preoperative day 1 before 8 a.m. surgery.

ADMINISTRATION
P.O.
● Obtain urine specimen for culture and sensitivity tests before giving. Begin therapy while awaiting results.
● When giving suspension, note the concentration.
● Give drug with full glass of water 2 hours before or 2 hours after meals for best absorption.
● Give drug with food if GI upset occurs. Don't give drug with fruit juice. Make sure patient doesn't swallow chewable tablets whole.

- Coated tablets or encapsulated pellets cause less GI upset, so they may be better tolerated by patients who have trouble tolerating drug.

I.V.
- Obtain urine specimen for culture and sensitivity tests before giving. Begin therapy while awaiting results.
- Reconstitute drug according to manufacturer's directions.
- Dilute each 250 mg in at least 100 ml of normal saline solution.
- Infuse over 1 hour.
- **Incompatibilities:** Ascorbic acid injection, colistimethate, dextrose 2.5% in half-strength Ringer's lactate, dextrose 5% in lactated Ringer's solution, dextrose 5% in normal saline solution, dextrose 5% in Normosol-M, dextrose 10% in water, D_5W, furosemide, heparin sodium, linezolid, metoclopramide, Normosol-R, Ringer's injection, vitamin B complex with C.

ACTION

Inhibits bacterial protein synthesis by binding to the 50S subunit of the ribosome. Bacteriostatic or bactericidal, depending on concentration.

Route	Onset	Peak	Duration
P.O.	Unknown	1½ hr	Unknown
I.V.	Immediate	1½ hr	Unknown

Half-life: 1½ hours.

ADVERSE REACTIONS

CNS: fever.
CV: *vein irritation or thrombophlebitis after I.V. injection,* **ventricular arrhythmias.**
GI: *pseudomembranous colitis, abdominal pain and cramping, diarrhea, nausea, vomiting.*
Hepatic: hepatocellular or cholestatic hepatitis.
Skin: eczema, rash, urticaria.
Other: *anaphylaxis,* overgrowth of nonsusceptible bacteria or fungi.

INTERACTIONS

Drug-drug. *Carbamazepine:* May inhibit metabolism of carbamazepine, increasing blood level and risk of toxicity. Avoid using together.

Clindamycin, lincomycin: May be antagonistic. Avoid using together.
Cyclosporine: May increase cyclosporine level. Monitor drug level.
Digoxin: May increase digoxin level. Monitor patient for digoxin toxicity.
Disopyramide: May increase disopyramide level, which may cause arrhythmias and prolonged QT intervals. Monitor ECG.
Ergot alkaloids: May cause acute ergot toxicity with severe peripheral vasospasm and dysesthesias. Monitor carefully.
HMG-CoA reductase inhibitors (lovastatin, simvastatin): May increase concentrations of HMG-CoA reductase inhibitors; rhabdomyolysis has occurred rarely. Monitor CK and serum transaminase levels.
Midazolam, triazolam: May increase effects of these drugs. Monitor patient closely.
Oral anticoagulants: May increase anticoagulant effect. Monitor PT and INR closely.
Fluoroquinolones, *other drugs that prolong the QTc interval (amiodarone, antipsychotics, procainamide, quinidine, sotalol, tricyclic antidepressants):* May have additive effects. Monitor ECG for QTc interval prolongation. Avoid using together, if possible.
Rifamycins (rifabutin, rifampin, rifapentine): May decrease therapeutic effects of erythromycin while increasing adverse effects of rifamycin. Monitor patient.
Strong CYP3A inhibitors (such as diltiazem, verapamil, troleandomycin): May increase the risk of sudden death from cardiac causes. Don't use together.
Theophylline: May decrease erythromycin level and increase theophylline toxicity. Use together cautiously.
Drug-herb. *Pill-bearing spurge:* May inhibit CYP3A enzymes, affecting drug metabolism. Urge caution.
Drug-food. *Food, grapefruit juice:* Food can delay absorption; grapefruit juice may inhibit drug's metabolism. Don't give within 2 hours of a meal; caution patient to avoid grapefruit juice during therapy.

EFFECTS ON LAB TEST RESULTS

- May increase alkaline phosphatase, ALT, AST, and bilirubin levels.

Reactions may be *common,* uncommon, *life-threatening,* or COMMON AND LIFE-THREATENING.
Interaction may have a *rapid onset* or **delayed onset.**

• May interfere with fluorometric determination of urine catecholamines and with colorimetric assays.

CONTRAINDICATIONS & CAUTIONS
• Contraindicated in those hypersensitive to drug or other macrolides.
• Use erythromycin salts cautiously in patients with impaired hepatic function.
• Drug appears in breast milk. Use cautiously in breast-feeding women.
• Don't use drug to treat neurosyphilis.

NURSING CONSIDERATIONS
• Monitor patient for superinfection. Drug may cause overgrowth of nonsusceptible bacteria or fungi.
• Monitor hepatic function. Drug may cause hepatotoxicity.

PATIENT TEACHING
• Tell patient to take drug as prescribed, even after he feels better.
• Instruct patient to take oral form of drug with full glass of water 2 hours before or 2 hours after meals for best absorption.
• Drug may be taken with food if GI upset occurs. Tell patient not to take drug with fruit juice or to swallow the chewable tablets whole.
• Instruct patient to report adverse reactions, especially nausea, abdominal pain, vomiting, and fever.

16

Penicillins

amoxicillin and clavulanate potassium
amoxicillin trihydrate
ampicillin
ampicillin sodium
ampicillin sodium and sulbactam sodium
ampicillin trihydrate
nafcillin sodium
penicillin G benzathine
penicillin G potassium
penicillin G procaine
penicillin G sodium
penicillin V potassium
piperacillin sodium and tazobactam sodium
ticarcillin disodium and clavulanate potassium

amoxicillin and clavulanate potassium (amoxycillin and clavulanate potassium)

a-mox-i-SILL-in

Aclavulanate†, Amoxiclav†, Augmentin, Augmentin ES-600, Augmentin XR, Clavamoxin†, Clavulin†

Pharmacologic class: aminopenicillin and beta-lactamase inhibitor
Pregnancy risk category B

AVAILABLE FORMS

Oral suspension: 125 mg amoxicillin trihydrate and 31.25 mg clavulanic acid/5 ml (after reconstitution); 200 mg amoxicillin trihydrate and 28.5 mg clavulanic acid/5 ml (after reconstitution); 250 mg amoxicillin trihydrate and 62.5 mg clavulanic acid/5 ml (after reconstitution); 400 mg amoxicillin trihydrate and 57 mg clavulanic acid/5 ml (after reconstitution); 600 mg amoxicillin trihydrate and 42.9 mg clavulanic acid/5 ml (after reconstitution)
Tablets (chewable): 125 mg amoxicillin trihydrate, 31.25 mg clavulanic acid; 200 mg amoxicillin trihydrate, 28.5 mg clavulanic acid; 250 mg amoxicillin trihydrate, 62.5 mg clavulanic acid; 400 mg amoxicillin trihydrate, 57 mg clavulanic acid
Tablets (extended-release): 1,000 mg amoxicillin trihydrate, 62.5 mg clavulanic acid
Tablets (film-coated): 250 mg amoxicillin trihydrate, 125 mg clavulanic acid; 500 mg amoxicillin trihydrate, 125 mg clavulanic acid; 875 mg amoxicillin trihydrate, 125 mg clavulanic acid

INDICATIONS & DOSAGES

➤ **Recurrent or persistent acute otitis media caused by *Streptococcus pneumoniae, Haemophilus influenzae,* or *Moraxella catarrhalis* in patients exposed to antibiotics within the previous 3 months, who are 2 years old or younger or in day care facilities**
Children age 3 months and older: 90 mg/kg/day Augmentin ES-600 P.O., based on amoxicillin component, every 12 hours for 10 days.
➤ **Lower respiratory tract infections, otitis media, sinusitis, skin and skin-structure infections, and UTIs caused by susceptible strains of gram-positive and gram-negative organisms**
Adults and children weighing 40 kg (88 lb) or more: 250 mg P.O., based on amoxicillin component, every 8 hours; or 500 mg every 12 hours. For more severe infections, 500 mg every 8 hours or 875 mg every 12 hours.
Children age 3 months and older and weighing less than 40 kg: 20 to 45 mg/kg P.O., based on amoxicillin component and severity of infection, daily in divided doses every 8 to 12 hours.
Children younger than age 3 months: 30 mg/kg/day P.O., based on amoxicillin component of the 125-mg/5-ml oral

suspension, in divided doses every 12 hours.

Adjust-a-dose: Don't give the 875-mg tablet to patients with creatinine clearance less than 30 ml/minute. If clearance is 10 to 30 ml/minute, give 250 to 500 mg P.O. every 12 hours. If clearance is less than 10 ml/minute, give 250 to 500 mg P.O. every 24 hours. Give hemodialysis patients 250 to 500 mg P.O. every 24 hours with an additional dose both during and after dialysis.

➤ **Community-acquired pneumonia or acute bacterial sinusitis caused by *H. influenzae, M. catarrhalis, H. parainfluenzae, Klebsiella pneumoniae,* methicillin-susceptible *Staphylococcus aureus,* or *S. pneumoniae* with reduced susceptibility to penicillin**
Adults and children age 16 and older: 2,000 mg/125 mg Augmentin XR tablets every 12 hours for 7 to 10 days for pneumonia; 10 days for sinusitis.
Adjust-a-dose: In patients with creatinine clearance less than 30 ml/minute and patients receiving hemodialysis, don't use Augmentin XR.

ADMINISTRATION
P.O.
• Before giving drug, ask patient about allergic reactions to penicillin. A negative history of penicillin allergy is no guarantee against an allergic reaction.
• Obtain specimen for culture and sensitivity tests before giving first dose. Begin therapy while awaiting results.
• Give drug at the start of a meal to enhance absorption.
• Give drug at least 1 hour before a bacteriostatic antibiotic.
• Avoid use of 250-mg tablet in children weighing less than 40 kg (88 lb). Use chewable form instead.
• After reconstitution, refrigerate the oral suspension; discard after 10 days.

ACTION
Prevents bacterial cell-wall synthesis during replication. Increases amoxicillin's effectiveness by inactivating beta-lactamases, which destroy amoxicillin.

Route	Onset	Peak	Duration
P.O.	Unknown	1–2½ hr	6–8 hr
P.O. (Augmentin ES-600)	Unknown	1–4 hr	Unknown
P.O. (Augmentin XR)	Unknown	1–6 hr	Unknown

Half-life: 1 to 1½ hours. For patients with severe renal impairment, 7½ hours for amoxicillin and 4½ hours for clavulanate.

ADVERSE REACTIONS
CNS: agitation, anxiety, behavioral changes, confusion, dizziness, insomnia.
GI: nausea, vomiting, *diarrhea,* indigestion, gastritis, stomatitis, glossitis, black hairy tongue, enterocolitis, *pseudomembranous colitis,* mucocutaneous candidiasis, abdominal pain.
GU: vaginal candidiasis, vaginitis.
Hematologic: anemia, *thrombocytopenia, thrombocytopenic purpura,* eosinophilia, *leukopenia, agranulocytosis.*
Other: hypersensitivity reactions, *anaphylaxis,* pruritus, rash, urticaria, *angioedema,* overgrowth of nonsusceptible organisms, serum sickness–like reaction.

INTERACTIONS
Drug-drug. *Allopurinol:* May increase risk of rash. Monitor patient for rash.
Hormonal contraceptives: May decrease hormonal contraceptive effectiveness. Advise use of additional form of contraception during penicillin therapy.
Methotrexate: May increase risk of methotrexate toxicity. Monitor methotrexate levels.
Probenecid: May increase levels of amoxicillin and other penicillins. Probenecid may be used for this purpose.
Tetracyclines: May reduce therapeutic action of penicillins. Avoid co-administration.
Drug-herb. *Khat:* May decrease antimicrobial effect of certain penicillins. Discourage khat chewing, or tell patient to take amoxicillin 2 hours after khat chewing.

EFFECTS ON LAB TEST RESULTS
• May increase eosinophil count.
• May falsely decrease aminoglycoside level. May alter results of urine glucose

tests that use cupric sulfate, such as Benedict's reagent and Clinitest.

CONTRAINDICATIONS & CAUTIONS
● Contraindicated in patients hypersensitive to drug or other penicillins and in those with a history of amoxicillin-related cholestatic jaundice or hepatic dysfunction.
● Augmentin XR is contraindicated in patients receiving hemodialysis and those with creatinine clearance less than 30 ml/minute.
● Use cautiously in patients with other drug allergies (especially to cephalosporins) because of possible cross-sensitivity and in those with mononucleosis because of high risk of maculopapular rash.
● Use cautiously in breast-feeding women; it's unknown if drug appears in breast milk.
● Use cautiously in hepatically impaired patients, and monitor the hepatic function of these patients.
● Don't give ampicillin-class antibiotics to patients with mononucleosis due to high incidence of erythematous rash.

NURSING CONSIDERATIONS
● Each Augmentin XR tablet contains 29.3 mg (1.27 mEq) of sodium.
● Augmentin XR isn't indicated for treating infections caused by *S. pneumoniae* with penicillin minimum inhibitory concentration, or MIC, of 4 mcg/ml or greater.
● If large doses are given or therapy is prolonged, bacterial or fungal superinfection may occur, especially in elderly, debilitated, or immunosuppressed patients.
● *Alert:* Don't interchange the oral suspensions because of varying clavulanic acid contents.
● Augmentin ES-600 is intended only for children ages 3 months to 12 years with persistent or recurrent acute otitis media.
● *Alert:* Both 250- and 500-mg film-coated tablets contain the same amount of clavulanic acid (125 mg). Therefore, two 250-mg tablets aren't equivalent to one 500-mg tablet. Regular tablets aren't equivalent to Augmentin XR.
● This drug combination is particularly useful in clinical settings with a high prevalence of amoxicillin-resistant organisms.
● *Look alike–sound alike:* Don't confuse amoxicillin with amoxapine.

PATIENT TEACHING
● Tell patient to take entire quantity of drug exactly as prescribed, even after feeling better.
● Instruct patient to take drug with food to prevent GI upset. If he's taking the oral suspension, tell him to keep drug refrigerated, to shake it well before taking it, and to discard remaining drug after 10 days.
● Tell patient to call prescriber if a rash occurs because rash is a sign of an allergic reaction.

amoxicillin trihydrate (amoxycillin trihydrate)
a-mox-i-SILL-in

Amoxil, Apo-Amoxi†, DisperMox, Moxatag, Novamoxin†, Nu-Amoxi†, Trimox

Pharmacologic class: aminopenicillin
Pregnancy risk category B

AVAILABLE FORMS
Capsules: 250 mg, 500 mg
Oral suspension: 50 mg/ml (pediatric drops), 125 mg/5 ml, 200 mg/5 ml, 250 mg/5 ml, 400 mg/5 ml (after reconstitution)
Tablets (chewable): 125 mg, 200 mg, 250 mg, 400 mg
Tablets (extended-release): 775 mg
Tablets (film-coated): 500 mg, 875 mg
Tablets for oral suspension: 200 mg, 400 mg

INDICATIONS & DOSAGES
➤ **Mild to moderate infections of the ear, nose, and throat; skin and skin structure; or GU tract**
Adults and children who weigh 40 kg (88 lb) or more: 500 mg P.O. every 12 hours or 250 mg P.O. every 8 hours.
Children older than age 3 months who weigh less than 40 kg: 25 mg/kg/day P.O. divided every 12 hours or 20 mg/kg/day P.O. divided every 8 hours.
Neonates and infants up to age 3 months: Up to 30 mg/kg/day P.O. divided every 12 hours.
➤ **Mild to severe infections of the lower respiratory tract and severe**

Reactions may be *common*, uncommon, *life-threatening*, or COMMON AND LIFE-THREATENING.
Interaction may have a *rapid onset* or *delayed onset*.

infections of the ear, nose, and throat; skin and skin structure; or genitourinary tract
Adults and children who weigh 40 kg or more: 875 mg P.O. every 12 hours or 500 mg P.O. every 8 hours.
Children older than age 3 months weighing less than 40 kg: 45 mg/kg/day P.O. divided every 12 hours or 40 mg/kg/day P.O. divided every 8 hours.

✳*NEW INDICATION:* Pharyngitis, tonsillitis, or both secondary to *Streptococcus pyogenes* infection
Adults and children age 12 and older: 775-mg extended-release tablet P.O. once daily with a meal for 10 days.

➤ Uncomplicated gonorrhea
Adults and children who weigh more than 45 kg (99 lb): 3 g P.O. with 1 g probenecid given as a single dose.
Children age 2 and older who weigh less than 45 kg: 50 mg/kg to a maximum of 3 g P.O. with 25 mg/kg of probenecid, to a maximum of 1 g, as a single dose. Don't give probenecid to children younger than age 2.

➤ To prevent endocarditis in patients having dental, oral, or respiratory tract procedures and in moderate-risk patients undergoing GI and GU procedures ♦
Adults: 2 g P.O. 1 hour before procedure.
Children: 50 mg/kg P.O. 1 hour before procedure.

ADMINISTRATION
P.O.
● Before giving, ask patient about allergic reactions to penicillin. A negative history of penicillin allergy is no guarantee against allergic reaction.
● Obtain specimen for culture and sensitivity tests before giving first dose. Begin therapy while awaiting results.
● Give drug with or without food, except for extended-release tablets, which are give with a meal.
● Don't crush or split extended-release tablets.
● For a child, place drops directly on child's tongue for swallowing or add to formula, milk, fruit juice, water, ginger ale, or a cold drink for immediate and complete consumption.
● For a child taking DisperMox, mix one tablet in about 10 ml of water, have the child drink the resulting solution, rinse container with a small amount of water, and have the child drink again to ensure the whole dose is taken. Mix tablet only in water. Don't let child chew tablets, swallow them whole, or let them dissolve in mouth.
● Store Trimox oral suspension in refrigerator, if possible. It also may be stored at room temperature for up to 2 weeks. Be sure to check individual product labels for storage information.

ACTION
Inhibits cell-wall synthesis during bacterial multiplication.

Route	Onset	Peak	Duration
P.O.	Unknown	1–2 hr	6–8 hr

Half-life: 1 to 1½ hours (7½ hours in severe renal impairment).

ADVERSE REACTIONS
CNS: *seizures,* lethargy, hallucinations, anxiety, confusion, agitation, depression, dizziness, fatigue, headache.
GI: *diarrhea, nausea, pseudomembranous colitis,* vomiting, glossitis, stomatitis, gastritis, enterocolitis, abdominal pain, black hairy tongue.
GU: interstitial nephritis, nephropathy, vaginitis.
Hematologic: *agranulocytosis, leukopenia, thrombocytopenia, thrombocytopenic purpura,* anemia, eosinophilia, hemolytic anemia.
Other: *anaphylaxis,* hypersensitivity reactions, overgrowth of nonsusceptible organisms.

INTERACTIONS
Drug-drug. *Allopurinol:* May increase risk of rash. Monitor patient for rash.
Hormonal contraceptives: May decrease contraceptive effectiveness. Advise use of additional form of contraception during penicillin therapy.
Probenecid: May increase levels of amoxicillin and other penicillins. Probenecid may be used for this purpose.
Drug-herb. *Khat:* May decrease antimicrobial effect of certain penicillins. Discourage herb use, or tell patient to take drug 2 hours after herb use.

EFFECTS ON LAB TEST RESULTS
• May decrease hemoglobin level.
• May increase eosinophil count. May decrease granulocyte, platelet, and WBC counts.
• May falsely decrease aminoglycoside level. May alter results of urine glucose tests that use cupric sulfate, such as Benedict's reagent and Clinitest.

CONTRAINDICATIONS & CAUTIONS
• Contraindicated in patients hypersensitive to drug or other penicillins.
• Use cautiously in patients with other drug allergies (especially to cephalosporins) because of possible cross-sensitivity.
• Use cautiously in those with mononucleosis because of high risk of maculopapular rash.

NURSING CONSIDERATIONS
• If large doses are given or if therapy is prolonged, bacterial or fungal superinfection may occur, especially in elderly, debilitated, or immunosuppressed patients.
• *Clostridium difficile*–associated diarrhea, ranging from mild diarrhea to fatal colitis, has been reported with nearly all antibacterial agents, including amoxicillin. Evaluate patient if diarrhea occurs.
• Amoxicillin usually causes fewer cases of diarrhea than ampicillin.
• *Look alike–sound alike:* Don't confuse amoxicillin with amoxapine.

PATIENT TEACHING
• Tell patient to take entire quantity of drug exactly as prescribed, even after he feels better.
• Instruct patient to take drug with or without food, except extended-release tablets, which are taken with a meal.
• Tell patient to swallow extended-release tablets whole and not to chew, crush, or split them.
• Tell patient to notify prescriber if rash, fever, or chills develop. A rash is the most common allergic reaction, especially if allopurinol is also being taken.
• Tell parent to place drops directly on child's tongue for swallowing or add to formula, milk, fruit juice, water, ginger ale, or a cold drink for immediate and complete consumption.
• If child takes DisperMox, tell parent to mix one tablet in about 10 ml of water, to have the child drink the resulting solution, to rinse container with a small amount of water, and to have the child drink again to ensure the whole dose is taken. Parent should mix tablet only in water. Caution parent against allowing child to chew tablets, to swallow them whole, or to let them dissolve in mouth.

---

ampicillin
am-pi-SILL-in

Apo-Ampi†, Nu-Ampi†

ampicillin sodium

ampicillin trihydrate
Principen

Pharmacologic class:
aminopenicillin
Pregnancy risk category B

AVAILABLE FORMS
Capsules: 250 mg, 500 mg
Injection: 250 mg, 500 mg, 1 g, 2 g
Oral suspension: 125 mg/5 ml, 250 mg/5 ml

INDICATIONS & DOSAGES
➤ **Respiratory tract or skin and skin-structure infections**
Adults and children who weigh 40 kg (88 lb) or more: 250 to 500 mg P.O. every 6 hours.
Children who weigh less than 40 kg: 25 to 50 mg/kg/day P.O. in equally divided doses every 6 to 8 hours. Pediatric dosages shouldn't exceed recommended adult dosages.
➤ **GI infections or UTIs**
Adults and children who weigh 40 kg (88 lb) or more: 500 mg P.O. every 6 hours. For severe infections, larger doses may be needed.
Children who weigh less than 40 kg: 50 to 100 mg/kg/day P.O. in equally divided doses every 6 hours.

Reactions may be *common,* uncommon, *life-threatening,* or COMMON AND LIFE-THREATENING.
Interaction may have a *rapid onset* or *delayed onset.*

➤ **Bacterial meningitis or septicemia**
Adults: 150 to 200 mg/kg/day I.V. in divided doses every 3 to 4 hours. May be given I.M. after 3 days of I.V. therapy. Maximum recommended daily dose is 14 g.
Children: 150 to 200 mg/kg I.V. daily in divided doses every 3 to 4 hours. Give I.V. for 3 days; then give I.M.

➤ **Uncomplicated gonorrhea**
Adults and children who weigh more than 45 kg (99 lb): 3.5 g P.O. with 1 g probenecid given as a single dose.
Adjust-a-dose: In patients with creatinine clearance of 10 to 50 ml/minute, use same dose but increase dosing interval to 6 to 12 hours; for those with a clearance less than 10 ml/minute, increase dosing interval to 12 to 24 hours.

ADMINISTRATION
P.O.
● Before giving drug, ask patient about allergic reactions to penicillin. A negative history of penicillin allergy is no guarantee against a future allergic reaction.
● Obtain specimen for culture and sensitivity tests before giving. Begin therapy while awaiting results.
● Give drug 1 to 2 hours before or 2 to 3 hours after meals. When given orally, drug may cause GI disturbances. Food may interfere with absorption.
● Give drug I.M. or I.V. if infection is severe or if patient can't take oral dose.
I.V.
● Before giving drug, ask patient about allergic reactions to penicillin. A negative history of penicillin allergy is no guarantee against a future allergic reaction.
● Obtain specimen for culture and sensitivity tests before giving. Begin therapy while awaiting results.
● Give drug I.M. or I.V. only if infection is severe or if patient can't take oral dose.
● Give drug intermittently to prevent vein irritation. Change site every 48 hours.
● For direct injection, reconstitute with bacteriostatic water for injection. Use 5 ml for 250-mg or 500-mg vials, 7.4 ml for 1-g vials, and 14.8 ml for 2-g vials. Give drug over 10 to 15 minutes to avoid seizures. Don't exceed 100 mg/minute.
● For intermittent infusion, dilute in 50 to 100 ml of normal saline solution for injection. Give drug over 15 to 30 minutes.

● Use first dilution within 1 hour. Follow manufacturer's directions for stability data when drug is further diluted for I.V. infusion.
● **Incompatibilities:** Amikacin, amino acid solutions, chlorpromazine, dextran solutions, dextrose solutions, dopamine, erythromycin lactobionate, 10% fat emulsions, fructose, gentamicin, heparin sodium, hetastarch, hydrocortisone sodium succinate, hydromorphone, kanamycin, lidocaine, lincomycin, polymyxin B, prochlorperazine edisylate, sodium bicarbonate, streptomycin, tobramycin.
I.M.
● Before giving drug, ask patient about allergic reactions to penicillin. A negative history of penicillin allergy is no guarantee against a future allergic reaction.
● Obtain specimen for culture and sensitivity tests before giving. Begin therapy while awaiting results.
● Give drug I.M. or I.V. only if infection is severe or if patient can't take oral dose.

ACTION
Inhibits cell-wall synthesis during bacterial multiplication.

Route	Onset	Peak	Duration
P.O.	Unknown	2 hr	6–8 hr
I.V.	Immediate	Immediate	Unknown
I.M.	Unknown	1 hr	Unknown

Half-life: 1 to 1½ hours (10 to 24 hours in severe renal impairment).

ADVERSE REACTIONS
GI: *diarrhea, nausea, pseudomembranous colitis,* abdominal pain, black hairy tongue, enterocolitis, gastritis, glossitis, stomatitis, vomiting.
GU: interstitial nephritis, nephropathy, vaginitis.
Hematologic: *leukopenia, thrombocytopenia, thrombocytopenic purpura,* anemia, eosinophilia, hemolytic anemia, *agranulocytosis.*
Other: hypersensitivity reactions, overgrowth of nonsusceptible organisms.

INTERACTIONS
Drug-drug. *Allopurinol:* May increase risk of rash. Monitor patient for rash.
H₂ antagonists, proton pump inhibitors: May decrease ampicillin absorption and

level. Separate administration times. Monitor patient for continued antibiotic effectiveness.

Hormonal contraceptives: May decrease hormonal contraceptive effectiveness. Advise use of another form of contraception during therapy.

Oral anticoagulants: May increase risk of bleeding. Monitor PT and INR.

Probenecid: May increase levels of ampicillin and other penicillins. Probenecid may be used for this purpose.

EFFECTS ON LAB TEST RESULTS
• May decrease hemoglobin level.
• May increase eosinophil count. May decrease granulocyte, platelet, and WBC counts.
• May falsely decrease aminoglycoside level. May alter results of urine glucose tests that use cupric sulfate, such as Benedict reagent and Clinitest.

CONTRAINDICATIONS & CAUTIONS
• Contraindicated in patients hypersensitive to drug or other penicillins.
• Use cautiously in patients with other drug allergies (especially to cephalosporins) because of possible cross-sensitivity, and in those with mononucleosis because of high risk of maculopapular rash.

NURSING CONSIDERATIONS
• Monitor sodium level because each gram of ampicillin contains 2.9 mEq of sodium.
• If large doses are given or if therapy is prolonged, bacterial or fungal superinfection may occur, especially in elderly, debilitated, or immunosuppressed patients.
• Watch for signs and symptoms of hypersensitivity, such as erythematous maculopapular rash, urticaria, and anaphylaxis.
• In patients with impaired renal function, decrease dosage.
• In pediatric meningitis, drug may be given with parenteral chloramphenicol for 24 hours, pending cultures.

PATIENT TEACHING
• Tell patient to take entire quantity of drug exactly as prescribed, even after he feels better.
• Instruct patient to take oral form on an empty stomach 1 hour before or 2 hours after meals.

• Inform patient to notify prescriber if rash, fever, or chills develop. A rash is the most common allergic reaction, especially if allopurinol is also being taken.

ampicillin sodium and sulbactam sodium
am-pi-SILL-in

Unasyn

Pharmacologic class: aminopenicillin and beta-lactamase inhibitor
Pregnancy risk category B

AVAILABLE FORMS
Injection: Vials and piggyback vials containing 1.5 g (1 g ampicillin sodium with 0.5 g sulbactam sodium), 3 g (2 g ampicillin sodium with 1 g sulbactam sodium)

INDICATIONS & DOSAGES
➤ **Intra-abdominal, gynecologic, and skin-structure infections caused by susceptible strains**
Adults: 1.5 to 3 g I.M. or I.V. every 6 hours. Don't exceed 4 g/day of sulbactam.
Children age 1 or older (skin and skin-structure infections only): 300 mg/kg/day I.V. in divided doses every 6 hours for no longer than 14 days.
Adjust-a-dose: If creatinine clearance in adults is 15 to 29 ml/minute, give 1.5 to 3 g every 12 hours; if clearance is 5 to 14 ml/minute, give 1.5 to 3 g every 24 hours.

ADMINISTRATION
I.V.
• Before giving drug, ask patient about allergic reactions to penicillin. A negative history of penicillin allergy is no guarantee against future allergic reaction.
• Obtain specimen for culture and sensitivity tests. Begin therapy while awaiting results.
• Reconstitute powder with one of these diluents: normal saline solution, sterile water for injection, D₅W, lactated Ringer's injection, M/6 sodium lactate, dextrose 5% in half-normal saline solution for injection, or 10% invert sugar.

- After reconstitution, let vials stand for a few minutes so foam can dissipate. Inspect solution for particles.
- Give drug at least 1 hour before giving a bacteriostatic antibiotic.
- For infusion, dilute in 50 to 100 ml of compatible diluent and infuse over 15 to 30 minutes.
- Stability varies with diluent, temperature, and concentration of solution.
- **Incompatibilities:** Amikacin, amino acid solutions, amiodarone, amphotericin B, chlorpromazine, ciprofloxacin, dextran solutions, dopamine, erythromycin lactobionate, 10% fat emulsions, fructose, gentamicin, heparin sodium, hetastarch, hydrocortisone sodium succinate, idarubicin, kanamycin, lidocaine, lincomycin, netilmicin, polymyxin B, nicardipine, ondansetron, prochlorperazine edisylate, sargramostim, sodium bicarbonate, streptomycin, tobramycin.

I.M.
- Before giving drug, ask patient about allergic reactions to penicillin. A negative history of penicillin allergy is no guarantee against future allergic reaction.
- Obtain specimen for culture and sensitivity tests. Begin therapy while awaiting results.
- For I.M. injection, reconstitute with sterile water for injection or 0.5% or 2% lidocaine hydrochloride injection. Add 3.2 ml to a 1.5-g vial (or 6.4 ml to a 3-g vial) to yield 375 mg/ml. Give deep into muscle.
- I.M. injection may cause pain at injection site.
- In children, don't use I.M. route.

ACTION
Inhibits cell-wall synthesis during bacterial multiplication.

Route	Onset	Peak	Duration
I.V.	Immediate	15 min	Unknown
I.M.	Unknown	Unknown	Unknown

Half-life: 1 to 1½ hours (10 to 24 in severe renal impairment).

ADVERSE REACTIONS
GI: *diarrhea, nausea, pseudomembranous colitis,* black hairy tongue, enterocolitis, gastritis, glossitis, stomatitis, vomiting.

Hematologic: *agranulocytosis, leukopenia, thrombocytopenia, thrombocytopenic purpura,* anemia, eosinophilia.
Skin: *pain at injection site.*
Other: hypersensitivity reactions, *anaphylaxis,* overgrowth of nonsusceptible organisms.

INTERACTIONS
Drug-drug. *Allopurinol:* May increase risk of rash. Monitor patient for rash.
Hormonal contraceptives: May decrease hormonal contraceptive effectiveness. Strongly advise use of another contraceptive during therapy.
Oral anticoagulants: May increase risk of bleeding. Monitor PT and INR.
Probenecid: May increase ampicillin level. Probenecid may be used for this purpose.

EFFECTS ON LAB TEST RESULTS
- May increase alkaline phosphatase, ALT, AST, bilirubin, BUN, CK, creatinine, GGT, and LDH levels. May decrease hemoglobin level. May transiently decrease conjugated estriol, conjugated estrone, estradiol, and estriol glucuronide levels in pregnant women.
- May increase eosinophil count. May decrease granulocyte, platelet, and WBC counts.
- May alter results of urine glucose tests that use cupric sulfate, such as Benedict's reagent and Clinitest.

CONTRAINDICATIONS & CAUTIONS
- Contraindicated in patients hypersensitive to drug or other penicillins.
- Use cautiously in patients with other drug allergies (especially to cephalosporins) because of possible cross-sensitivity, and in those with mononucleosis because of high risk of maculopapular rash.

NURSING CONSIDERATIONS
- Dosage is expressed as total drug. Each 1.5-g vial contains 1 g ampicillin sodium and 0.5 g sulbactam sodium.
- In patients with impaired renal function, decrease dosage.
- Monitor liver function test results during therapy, especially in patients with impaired liver function.
- If large doses are given or if therapy is prolonged, bacterial or fungal

superinfection may occur, especially in elderly, debilitated, or immunosuppressed patients.

PATIENT TEACHING
● Tell patient to report rash, fever, or chills. A rash is the most common allergic reaction.
● Warn patient that I.M. injection may cause pain at injection site.

---

nafcillin sodium
naf-SIL-in

Pharmacologic class: penicillinase-resistant penicillin
Pregnancy risk category B

AVAILABLE FORMS
Infusion: 1 g, 2 g premixed or Add-Vantage vials

INDICATIONS & DOSAGES
➤ **Systemic infection caused by susceptible organisms (methicillin-sensitive *Staphylococcus aureus*)**
Adults: 500 mg to 1 g I.V. every 4 hours, depending on severity of infection.
Infants and children older than age 1 month: 50 to 200 mg/kg I.V. daily in divided doses every 4 to 6 hours, depending on severity of infection.
Neonates older than 7 days who weigh more than 2 kg (4.4 lb): 25 mg/kg I.V. every 6 hours.
Neonates older than 7 days who weigh 2 kg or less: 25 mg/kg I.V. every 8 hours.
Neonates age 7 days or younger who weigh more than 2 kg: 25 mg/kg I.V. every 8 hours.
Neonates age 7 days or younger who weigh 2 kg or less: 25 mg/kg I.V. every 12 hours.
➤ **Acute or chronic osteomyelitis caused by susceptible organisms**
Adults: 1 to 2 g I.V. every 4 hours for 4 to 8 weeks.
Children older than age 1 month: 100 to 200 mg/kg/day in equally divided doses every 4 to 6 hours for 4 to 8 weeks.
➤ **Native valve endocarditis caused by susceptible organisms**
Adults: 2 g I.V. every 4 hours for 4 to 6 weeks, combined with gentamicin for first 3 to 5 days.

Children older than age 1 month: 100 to 200 mg/kg/day in equally divided doses every 4 to 6 hours for 4 to 8 weeks in combination with gentamicin for first 3 to 5 days.

ADMINISTRATION
I.V.
● Before giving drug, ask patient about allergic reactions to penicillin.
● Obtain specimen for culture and sensitivity tests before giving. Begin therapy while awaiting results.
● Check container for leaks, cloudiness, or precipitate before use. Discard if present.
● Give drug over 30 to 60 minutes.
● Change site every 48 hours to prevent vein irritation.
● Reconstituted vials of 10 to 40 mg/ml are stable for 24 hours at room temperature.
● **Incompatibilities:** Aminoglycosides, aminophylline, ascorbic acid, aztreonam, bleomycin, cytarabine, diltiazem, droperidol, gentamicin, hydrocortisone sodium succinate, insulin, labetalol, meperidine, methylprednisolone sodium succinate, midazolam, nalbuphine, pentazocine lactate, promazine, vancomycin, verapamil hydrochloride, vitamin B complex with C.

ACTION
Inhibits cell-wall synthesis during bacterial multiplication.

Route	Onset	Peak	Duration
I.V.	Immediate	Immediate	Unknown

Half-life: 30 to 90 minutes.

ADVERSE REACTIONS
CNS: *neurotoxicity.*
CV: thrombophlebitis, vein irritation.
GI: *nausea, pseudomembranous colitis,* diarrhea, vomiting.
Hematologic: *agranulocytosis, leukopenia, neutropenia, thrombocytopenia,* anemia, eosinophilia.
Skin: severe tissue necrosis.
Other: *anaphylaxis,* hypersensitivity reactions.

INTERACTIONS
Drug-drug. *Aminoglycosides:* May have synergistic effect; drugs are chemically and physically incompatible. Don't combine in same I.V. solution.

Reactions may be *common*, uncommon, *life-threatening*, or COMMON AND LIFE-THREATENING.
Interaction may have a *rapid onset* or *delayed onset.*

Hormonal contraceptives: May decrease contraceptive effectiveness. Advise use of additional form of contraception during therapy.
Probenecid: May increase nafcillin level. Probenecid may be used for this purpose.
Rifampin: May cause dose-dependent antagonism. Monitor patient closely.
Tetracycline: May decrease nafcillin's effectiveness. Avoid concurrent use.
Warfarin: May decrease effects of warfarin when used with nafcillin. Monitor PT and INR closely.

EFFECTS ON LAB TEST RESULTS
• May decrease hemoglobin level and hematocrit.
• May decrease neutrophil, WBC, eosinophil, granulocyte, and platelet counts.

CONTRAINDICATIONS & CAUTIONS
• Contraindicated in patients hypersensitive to drug or other penicillins.
• Use cautiously in patients with GI distress and in those with other drug allergies (especially to cephalosporins) because of possible cross-sensitivity.
• Skin sloughing from subcutaneous extravasation has been reported.

NURSING CONSIDERATIONS
• If large doses are given or if therapy is prolonged, bacterial or fungal superinfection may occur, especially in elderly, debilitated, or immunosuppressed patients.
• Monitor sodium level because each gram of drug contains 2.9 mEq of sodium.
• Monitor WBC counts twice weekly in patients receiving drug for longer than 2 weeks. Neutropenia commonly occurs in the third week.
• An abnormal urinalysis result may indicate drug-induced interstitial nephritis.

PATIENT TEACHING
• Tell patient to report burning or irritation at the I.V. site.
• Advise patient to notify prescriber if a rash develops or if signs and symptoms of superinfection appear, such as recurring fever, chills, and malaise.

penicillin G benzathine (benzathine benzylpenicillin)
pen-i-SILL-in

Bicillin L-A, Permapen

Pharmacologic class: natural penicillin
Pregnancy risk category B

AVAILABLE FORMS
Injection: 600,000 units/ml; 1.2 million units/2 ml; 2.4 million units/4 ml

INDICATIONS & DOSAGES
➤ **Congenital syphilis**
Children younger than age 2:
50,000 units/kg (up to 2.4 million units) I.M. as a single dose.
➤ **Group A streptococcal upper respiratory tract infections**
Adults: 1.2 million units I.M. as a single injection.
Children who weigh 27 kg (59.5 lb) or more: 900,000 units I.M. as a single injection.
Children who weigh less than 27 kg: 300,000 to 600,000 units I.M. as a single injection.
➤ **To prevent poststreptococcal rheumatic fever**
Adults and children: 1.2 million units I.M. once monthly or 600,000 units I.M. every 2 weeks.
➤ **Syphilis of less than 1 year duration**
Adults: 2.4 million units I.M. as a single dose.
Children: 50,000 units/kg I.M. as a single dose. Don't exceed adult dosage.
➤ **Syphilis of more than 1 year duration**
Adults: 2.4 million units I.M. weekly for 3 weeks.
Children: 50,000 units/kg I.M. weekly for 3 weeks. Don't exceed adult dosage.

ADMINISTRATION
I.M.
• Before giving drug, ask patient about allergic reactions to penicillin.
• Obtain specimen for culture and sensitivity tests before giving first dose. Begin therapy while awaiting results.

- Shake well before injecting.
- Give drug at least 1 hour before a bacteriostatic antibiotic.
- Inject deep into upper outer quadrant of buttocks in adults and in midlateral thigh in infants and small children. Rotate injection sites. Avoid injection into or near major nerves or blood vessels to prevent permanent neurovascular damage.
- Injection may be painful, but ice applied to the site may ease discomfort.

ACTION
Inhibits cell-wall synthesis during bacterial multiplication.

Route	Onset	Peak	Duration
I.M.	Unknown	13–24 hr	1–4 wk

Half-life: 30 to 60 minutes.

ADVERSE REACTIONS
CNS: *seizures,* agitation, anxiety, confusion, depression, dizziness, fatigue, hallucinations, lethargy, neuropathy, pain.
GI: *pseudomembranous colitis,* enterocolitis, nausea, vomiting.
GU: interstitial nephritis, nephropathy.
Hematologic: *agranulocytosis, leukopenia, thrombocytopenia,* anemia, eosinophilia, hemolytic anemia.
Skin: exfoliative dermatitis, maculopapular rash.
Other: *anaphylaxis,* hypersensitivity reactions, sterile abscess at injection site.

INTERACTIONS
Drug-drug. *Aminoglycosides:* Physical and chemical incompatibility. Give separately.
Hormonal contraceptives: May decrease hormonal contraceptive effectiveness. Advise use of additional form of contraception during therapy.
Probenecid: May increase penicillin level. Probenecid may be used for this purpose.
Tetracycline: May antagonize penicillin G benzathine effects. Avoid using together.

EFFECTS ON LAB TEST RESULTS
- May decrease hemoglobin level.
- May increase eosinophil count. May decrease platelet, WBC, and granulocyte counts. May cause positive Coombs' test results.
- May falsely decrease aminoglycoside level. May cause false-positive CSF protein test results. May alter urine glucose testing using cupric sulfate (Benedict's reagent).

CONTRAINDICATIONS & CAUTIONS
- Contraindicated in patients hypersensitive to drug or other penicillins.
- Inadvertent intravascular administration has resulted in severe neurovascular damage, including transverse myelitis with permanent paralysis and gangrene.
- Use cautiously in patients allergic to other drugs, especially to cephalosporins, because of possible cross-sensitivity.

NURSING CONSIDERATIONS
- *Alert:* Bicillin L-A is the only penicillin G benzathine product indicated for sexually transmitted infections. Don't substitute Bicillin C-R because it may not be effective.
- *Alert:* Inadvertent I.V. use may cause cardiac arrest and death. Never give I.V.
- Drug's extremely slow absorption time makes allergic reactions difficult to treat.
- If large doses are given or if therapy is prolonged, bacterial or fungal superinfection may occur, especially in elderly, debilitated, or immunosuppressed patients.
- *Look alike–sound alike:* Don't confuse drug with Polycillin, penicillamine, or the various types of penicillin.

PATIENT TEACHING
- Tell patient to report adverse reactions promptly.
- Inform patient that fever and increased WBC count are the most common reactions.
- Warn patient that I.M. injection may be painful but that ice applied to the site may ease discomfort.

penicillin G potassium (benzylpenicillin potassium)
pen-i-SILL-in

Pfizerpen

Pharmacologic class: natural penicillin
Pregnancy risk category B

AVAILABLE FORMS
Injection: 1 million units, 5 million units, 20 million units

Premixed injection: 1 million units/50 ml, 2 million units/50 ml, 3 million units/ 50 ml

INDICATIONS & DOSAGES
➤ Moderate to severe systemic infection
Adults and children age 12 and older: Highly individualized; 1 to 30 million units I.M. or I.V. daily in divided doses every 2 to 6 hours or via continuous I.V. infusion.
Children younger than age 12: Give 25,000 to 400,000 units/kg I.M. or I.V. daily in divided doses every 4 to 6 hours.
Infants older than 7 days: 75,000 units/ kg/day I.M. or I.V. (preferred route) in divided doses every 8 hours.
Infants younger than 7 days: 50,000 units/ kg/day I.M. or I.V. (preferred route) in divided doses every 12 hours.
➤ Anthrax
Adults: 5 to 20 million units I.V. daily in divided doses every 4 to 6 hours, for at least 14 days after symptoms diminish. The average adult dosage is 4 million units every 4 hours or 2 million units every 2 hours.
Children: 100,000 to 150,000 units/kg/day I.V. in divided doses every 4 to 6 hours for at least 14 days after symptoms diminish.
➤ Meningitis
Infants older than 7 days: 200,000 to 300,000 units/kg/day I.M. or I.V. (preferred route) in divided doses every 6 hours.
Infants younger than 7 days: 100,000 to 150,000 units/kg/day I.M. or I.V. (preferred route) in divided doses every 12 hours.
➤ Group B streptococcus infection
Infants younger than 7 days: 100,000 units/kg/day I.M. or I.V. (preferred route) in divided doses every 12 hours.
Adjust-a-dose: If creatinine clearance is 10 to 50 ml/minute, give the usual dose every 8 to 12 hours. If clearance is less than 10 ml/minute, give 50% of usual dose every 8 to 10 hours or the usual dose every 12 to 18 hours. If patient is uremic and creatinine clearance is more than 10 ml/minute, give full loading dose; then give half the loading dose every 4 to 5 hours for additional doses.

ADMINISTRATION
I.V.
• Before giving drug, ask patient about allergic reactions to penicillin.
• Obtain specimen for culture and sensitivity tests before giving first dose. Begin therapy while awaiting results.
• Reconstitute drug with sterile water for injection, D_5W, or normal saline solution for injection. Volume of diluent varies with manufacturer.
• For intermittent infusion in adults, give drug over 1 to 2 hours. For intermittent infusion in infants, give drug over 15 to 30 minutes.
• For continuous infusion, add reconstituted drug to 1 to 2 L of compatible solution. Determine how much fluid is needed and what the rate should be for a 24-hour period; then, add the drug to this fluid.
• **Incompatibilities:** Alcohol 5%, amikacin, aminoglycosides, aminophylline, amphotericin B sodium, chlorpromazine, dextran, dopamine, heparin sodium, hydroxyzine hydrochloride, lincomycin, metoclopramide, pentobarbital sodium, phenytoin sodium, prochlorperazine mesylate, promethazine hydrochloride, sodium bicarbonate, thiopental, vancomycin, vitamin B complex with C.
I.M.
• Before giving drug, ask patient about allergic reactions to penicillin.
• Obtain specimen for culture and sensitivity tests before giving first dose. Begin therapy while awaiting results.
• Give deep into large muscle; injection may be extremely painful.
• I.M. injection may be painful, but ice applied to the site may help alleviate discomfort.

ACTION
Inhibits cell-wall synthesis during bacterial multiplication.

Route	Onset	Peak	Duration
I.V.	Immediate	Immediate	Unknown
I.M.	Unknown	15–30 min	Unknown

Half-life: 30 to 60 minutes.

ADVERSE REACTIONS
CNS: *seizures,* agitation, anxiety, confusion, depression, dizziness, fatigue, hallucinations, lethargy, neuropathy.

CV: thrombophlebitis, *cardiac arrest, arrhythmias.*
GI: *pseudomembranous colitis,* entero-colitis, nausea, vomiting.
GU: interstitial nephritis, nephropathy.
Hematologic: *agranulocytosis, leukopenia, thrombocytopenia,* anemia, eosino-philia, hemolytic anemia.
Metabolic: *severe potassium poisoning.*
Skin: exfoliative dermatitis, maculopapular eruptions, pain at injection site.
Other: *anaphylaxis,* hypersensitivity reactions, overgrowth of nonsusceptible organisms.

INTERACTIONS
Drug-drug. *Aminoglycosides:* Physically and chemically incompatible. Give separately.
Colestipol: May decrease penicillin G potassium level. Give penicillin G potassium 1 hour before or 4 hours after colestipol.
Hormonal contraceptives: May decrease hormonal contraceptive effectiveness. Advise use of additional form of contraception during therapy.
Oral anticoagulants: May increase risk of bleeding. Monitor PT and INR.
Potassium-sparing diuretics: May increase risk of hyperkalemia. Avoid using together.
Probenecid: May increase penicillin level. Probenecid may be used for this purpose.

EFFECTS ON LAB TEST RESULTS
• May increase potassium level. May decrease hemoglobin level.
• May increase eosinophil count. May decrease platelet, WBC, and granulocyte counts. May cause positive Coombs' test result.
• May falsely decrease aminoglycoside levels. May cause false-positive CSF protein test result. May alter urine glucose testing using cupric sulfate (Benedict's reagent).

CONTRAINDICATIONS & CAUTIONS
• Contraindicated in patients hypersensitive to drug or other penicillins.
• Use cautiously in patients with other drug allergies, especially to cephalosporins, because of possible cross-sensitivity.
• Use cautiously in patients with renal impairment.

NURSING CONSIDERATIONS
• Monitor renal function closely. Patients with poor renal function are predisposed to high levels.
• Due to increased risk of electrolyte imbalances, monitor potassium and sodium levels closely in patients receiving more than 10 million units I.V. daily.
• Observe patient closely. With large doses and prolonged therapy, bacterial or fungal superinfection may occur, especially in elderly, debilitated, or immunosuppressed patients.
• *Look alike–sound alike:* Don't confuse drug with Polycillin, penicillamine, or the various types of penicillin.

PATIENT TEACHING
• Tell patient to notify prescriber if rash, fever, or chills develop. A rash is the most common allergic reaction.
• Warn patient that I.M. injection may be painful but that ice applied to the site may help alleviate discomfort.

---

penicillin G procaine (benzylpenicillin procaine)
pen-i-SILL-in

Pharmacologic class: natural penicillin
Pregnancy risk category B

AVAILABLE FORMS
Injection: 600,000 units/ml; 1.2 million units/ml

INDICATIONS & DOSAGES
➤ **Moderate to severe systemic infection**
Adults: 600,000 to 1.2 million units I.M. daily for a minimum of 10 days.
Children older than age 1 month: 25,000 to 50,000 units/kg I.M. daily in a single dose.
➤ **Anthrax caused by *Bacillus anthracis,* including inhalation anthrax after exposure**
Adults: 1,200,000 units I.M. every 12 hours.
Children: 25,000 units/kg I.M.; not to exceed 1,200,000 units every 12 hours.
➤ **Cutaneous anthrax**
Adults: 600,000 to 1,000,000 units I.M. daily.

Reactions may be *common,* uncommon, *life-threatening,* or COMMON AND LIFE-THREATENING.
Interaction may have a *rapid onset* or **delayed onset.**

➤ **Syphilis (primary, secondary, and latent with negative spinal fluid)**
Adults and children older than age 12:
600,000 units/day I.M. for 8 days.
➤ **Syphilis (tertiary, neurosyphilis, and latent with positive spinal fluid or no spinal fluid examination)**
Adults: 600,000 units/day I.M. for 10 to 15 days.
➤ **Congenital syphilis (under 32 kg [70 lb] body weight)**
Children: 50,000 units/kg/day I.M. for 10 days.

ADMINISTRATION
I.M.
● Before giving drug, ask patient about allergic reactions to penicillin.
● Obtain specimen for culture and sensitivity tests before giving first dose. Begin therapy while awaiting results.
● Give deep in upper outer quadrant of buttocks in adults; in midlateral thigh in small children. Rotate injection sites. Don't give subcutaneously. Don't massage injection site. Avoid injection near major nerves or blood vessels to prevent permanent neurovascular damage and tissue necrosis.
● *Alert:* Inadvertent I.V. use may cause CNS toxicity and death. Toxic reaction may occur after one dose. Never give I.V.
● I.M. injection may be painful, but ice applied to the site may help alleviate discomfort.

ACTION
Inhibits cell-wall synthesis during bacterial multiplication.

Route	Onset	Peak	Duration
I.M.	Unknown	1–4 hr	1–5 days

Half-life: 30 to 60 minutes.

ADVERSE REACTIONS
CNS: *seizures,* agitation, anxiety, confusion, depression, dizziness, fatigue, hallucinations, lethargy.
GI: *pseudomembranous colitis,* enterocolitis, nausea, vomiting.
GU: interstitial nephritis, nephropathy.
Hematologic: *agranulocytosis, thrombocytopenia,* hemolytic anemia, *leukopenia,* anemia, eosinophilia.

Musculoskeletal: arthralgia.
Other: *anaphylaxis,* hypersensitivity reactions, overgrowth of nonsusceptible organisms.

INTERACTIONS
Drug-drug. *Aminoglycosides:* Physically and chemically incompatible. Give separately.
Colestipol: May decrease penicillin G procaine level. Give penicillin G procaine 1 hour before or 4 hours after colestipol.
Hormonal contraceptives: May decrease hormonal contraceptive effectiveness. Advise use of additional form of contraception during therapy.
Probenecid: May increase penicillin level. Probenecid may be used for this purpose.

EFFECTS ON LAB TEST RESULTS
● May decrease hemoglobin level.
● May increase eosinophil count. May decrease platelet, WBC, and granulocyte counts.

CONTRAINDICATIONS & CAUTIONS
● Contraindicated in patients hypersensitive to drug or other penicillins.
● Use cautiously in patients with other drug allergies, especially to cephalosporins, because of possible cross-sensitivity. Some formulations contain sulfites, which may cause allergic reactions in sensitive people.

NURSING CONSIDERATIONS
● *Alert:* Continue postexposure treatment for inhalation anthrax for 60 days. Prescriber should consider the risk-benefit ratio of continuing penicillin longer than 2 weeks, compared with switching to another drug.
● Allergic reactions are hard to treat because of drug's slow absorption rate.
● Monitor renal and hematopoietic function periodically.
● If large doses are given or if therapy is prolonged, bacterial or fungal superinfection may occur, especially in elderly, debilitated, or immunosuppressed patients.
● Treatment duration depends on site and cause of infection.
● *Look alike–sound alike:* Don't confuse drug with Polycillin, penicillamine, or the various types of penicillin.

PATIENT TEACHING
● Tell patient to report adverse reactions promptly. A rash is the most common allergic reaction.
● Warn patient that I.M. injection may be painful but that ice applied to the site may help alleviate discomfort.

---

penicillin G sodium (benzylpenicillin sodium)
pen-i-SILL-in

Pharmacologic class: natural penicillin
Pregnancy risk category B

AVAILABLE FORMS
Injection: 5 million-unit vial

INDICATIONS & DOSAGES
➤ **Moderate to severe systemic infection**
Adults and children age 12 and older:
1.2 to 24 million units daily I.M. or I.V. in divided doses every 4 to 6 hours.
Children younger than age 12: 25,000 to 400,000 units/kg daily I.M. or I.V. in divided doses every 4 to 6 hours.
Infants older than 7 days: 75,000 units/kg/day I.M. or I.V. (preferred route) in divided doses every 8 hours.
Infants younger than 7 days: 50,000 units/kg/day I.M. or I.V. (preferred route) in divided doses every 12 hours.
➤ **Meningitis**
Infants older than 7 days: 200,000 to 300,000 units/kg/day I.M. or I.V. (preferred route) every 6 hours.
Infants younger than 7 days: 100,000 to 150,000 units/kg/day I.M. or I.V. (preferred route) in divided doses every 12 hours.
➤ **Neurosyphilis**
Adults: 18 to 24 million units I.V. daily in divided doses every 4 hours for 10 to 14 days.
Adjust-a-dose: If creatinine clearance is 10 to 50 ml/minute, give the usual dose every 8 to 12 hours. If clearance is less than 10 ml/minute, give 50% of usual dose every 8 to 10 hours or the usual dose every 12 to 18 hours. If patient is uremic and creatinine clearance is more than 10 ml/minute, give full loading dose; then give half the loading dose every 4 to 5 hours for additional doses.

ADMINISTRATION
I.V.
● Before giving drug, ask patient about allergic reactions to penicillin.
● Obtain specimen for culture and sensitivity tests before giving first dose. Begin therapy while awaiting results.
● Reconstitute drug with sterile water for injection, normal saline solution for injection, or D₅W. Check manufacturer's instructions for volume of diluent necessary to produce desired drug level.
● Give by intermittent infusion: Dilute drug in 50 to 100 ml, and give over 30 minutes to 2 hours every 4 to 6 hours.
● In neonates, infants, and children, give divided doses over 15 to 30 minutes.
● **Incompatibilities:** Aminoglycosides, amphotericin B, bleomycin, chlorpromazine, cytarabine, fat emulsions 10%, heparin sodium, hydroxyzine hydrochloride, invert sugar 10%, lincomycin, methylprednisolone sodium succinate, potassium chloride, prochlorperazine mesylate, promethazine hydrochloride.
I.M.
● Before giving drug, ask patient about allergic reactions to penicillin.
● Obtain specimen for culture and sensitivity tests before giving first dose. Begin therapy while awaiting results.
● Injection may be painful, but ice applied to site may help alleviate discomfort.

ACTION
Inhibits cell-wall synthesis during bacterial multiplication.

Route	Onset	Peak	Duration
I.V.	Immediate	Immediate	Unknown
I.M.	Unknown	15–30 min	Unknown

Half-life: 30 to 60 minutes.

ADVERSE REACTIONS
CNS: neuropathy, *seizures,* agitation, anxiety, confusion, depression, dizziness, fatigue, hallucinations, lethargy.
CV: *heart failure,* thrombophlebitis.
GI: enterocolitis, ischemic colitis, nausea, vomiting, *pseudomembranous colitis.*

Reactions may be *common,* uncommon, *life-threatening,* or COMMON AND LIFE-THREATENING.
Interaction may have a *rapid onset* or *delayed onset.*

GU: nephropathy, interstitial nephritis.
Hematologic: hemolytic anemia, *agranulocytosis, leukopenia, thrombocytopenia, anemia,* eosinophilia.
Musculoskeletal: arthralgia.
Other: hypersensitivity reactions, *anaphylaxis,* overgrowth of nonsusceptible organisms, pain at injection site, vein irritation.

INTERACTIONS
Drug-drug. *Aminoglycosides:* Physically and chemically incompatible. Give separately.
Colestipol: May decrease penicillin G sodium level. Give penicillin G sodium 1 hour before or 4 hours after colestipol.
Hormonal contraceptives: May decrease hormonal contraceptive effectiveness. Advise use of additional form of contraception during penicillin therapy.
Oral anticoagulants: May increase risk of bleeding. Monitor PT and INR.
Probenecid: May increase penicillin level. Probenecid may be used for this purpose.

EFFECTS ON LAB TEST RESULTS
● May decrease hemoglobin level.
● May cause positive Coombs' test result. May increase eosinophil count. May decrease platelet, WBC, granulocyte, and RBC counts.
● May cause false-positive CSF protein test result. May falsely decrease aminoglycoside level. May alter urine glucose testing using cupric sulfate (Benedict's reagent).

CONTRAINDICATIONS & CAUTIONS
● Contraindicated in patients hypersensitive to drug or other penicillins and in those on sodium-restricted diets.
● Use cautiously in patients with other drug allergies, especially to cephalosporins, because of possible cross-sensitivity.

NURSING CONSIDERATIONS
● Observe patient closely. With large doses and prolonged therapy, bacterial or fungal superinfection may occur, especially in elderly, debilitated, or immunosuppressed patients.
● *Look alike–sound alike:* Don't confuse drug with Polycillin, penicillamine, or the various types of penicillin.

PATIENT TEACHING
● Tell patient to report adverse reactions promptly.
● Instruct patient to report discomfort at I.V. site.
● Warn patient receiving I.M. injection that the injection may be painful but that ice applied to site may help alleviate discomfort.

penicillin V potassium (phenoxymethyl penicillin potassium)
pen-i-SILL-in

Apo-Pen VK†, Novo-Pen-VK†, Nu-Pen-VK†, Penicillin VK, Veetids

Pharmacologic class: natural penicillin
Pregnancy risk category B

AVAILABLE FORMS
Oral suspension: 125 mg/5 ml, 250 mg/ 5 ml (after reconstitution)
Tablets: 250 mg, 500 mg
Tablets (film-coated): 250 mg, 500 mg

INDICATIONS & DOSAGES
➤ **Mild to moderate systemic infections**
Adults and children age 12 and older: 125 to 500 mg or P.O. every 6 hours.
Children younger than age 12: 15 to 62.5 mg/kg P.O. daily in divided doses every 6 to 8 hours.
➤ **To prevent recurrent rheumatic fever**
Adults and children: 250 mg P.O. b.i.d.
➤ **Erythema migrans in Lyme disease ◆**
Adults: 500 mg P.O. q.i.d. for 10 to 20 days.
➤ **To prevent inhalation anthrax after possible exposure ◆**
Adults: 7.5 mg/kg P.O. q.i.d. Continue treatment until exposure is ruled out. If exposure is confirmed, anthrax vaccine may be indicated. Continue treatment for 60 days.
Children younger than age 9: 50 mg/kg P.O. daily given in four divided doses. Continue treatment until exposure is ruled

out. If exposure is confirmed, anthrax vaccine may be indicated. Continue treatment for 30 to 60 days.

ADMINISTRATION
P.O.
● Before giving drug, ask patient about allergic reactions to penicillins.
● Obtain specimen for culture and sensitivity tests before giving first dose. Begin therapy while awaiting results.
● Give drug with food if patient has stomach upset.

ACTION
Inhibits cell-wall synthesis during bacterial multiplication.

Route	Onset	Peak	Duration
P.O.	Unknown	30–60 min	Unknown

Half-life: 30 minutes.

ADVERSE REACTIONS
CNS: neuropathy.
GI: *epigastric distress, nausea,* diarrhea, black hairy tongue, vomiting.
GU: nephropathy.
Hematologic: *leukopenia, thrombocytopenia,* eosinophilia, hemolytic anemia.
Other: *anaphylaxis,* hypersensitivity reactions, overgrowth of nonsusceptible organisms.

INTERACTIONS
Drug-drug. *Hormonal contraceptives:* May decrease hormonal contraceptive effectiveness. Advise use of another form of contraception during therapy.
Probenecid: May increase penicillin level. Probenecid may be used for this purpose.

EFFECTS ON LAB TEST RESULTS
● May decrease hemoglobin level.
● May increase eosinophil count. May decrease platelet, WBC, and granulocyte counts.
● May alter results of turbidimetric test methods using sulfosalicylic acid, acetic acid, trichloroacetic acid, and nitric acid.

CONTRAINDICATIONS & CAUTIONS
● Contraindicated in patients hypersensitive to drug or other penicillins.
● Use cautiously in patients with GI disturbances and in those with other drug allergies, especially to cephalosporins, because of possible cross-sensitivity.

NURSING CONSIDERATIONS
● Periodically assess renal and hematopoietic function in patients receiving long-term therapy.
● If large doses are given or if therapy is prolonged, bacterial or fungal superinfection may occur, especially in elderly, debilitated, or immunosuppressed patients.
● Amoxicillin is the preferred drug to prevent endocarditis because GI absorption is better and drug levels are sustained longer. Penicillin V is considered an alternate drug.
● *Look alike–sound alike:* Don't confuse drug with Polycillin, penicillamine, or the various types of penicillin.

PATIENT TEACHING
● Instruct patient to take entire quantity of drug exactly as prescribed, even after he feels better.
● Tell patient to take drug with food if stomach upset occurs.
● Advise patient to notify prescriber if rash, fever, or chills develop. A rash is the most common allergic reaction.

---

piperacillin sodium and tazobactam sodium
pie-PER-us-sil-in and taz-oh-BAK-tem

Tazocin†, Zosyn

Pharmacologic class: extended-spectrum penicillin, beta-lactamase inhibitor
Pregnancy risk category B

AVAILABLE FORMS
Powder for injection: 2 g piperacillin and 0.25 g tazobactam per vial, 3 g piperacillin and 0.375 g tazobactam per vial, 4 g piperacillin and 0.5 g tazobactam per vial

INDICATIONS & DOSAGES
➤ **Moderate to severe infections from piperacillin-resistant, piperacillin and tazobactam-susceptible, beta-lactamase–producing strains of microorganisms in appendicitis (complicated by rupture or abscess)**

Reactions may be *common,* uncommon, *life-threatening,* or COMMON AND LIFE-THREATENING.
Interaction may have a *rapid onset* or *delayed onset.*

and peritonitis caused by *Escherichia coli, Bacteroides fragilis, B. ovatus, B. thetaiotaomicron, B. vulgatus;* skin and skin-structure infections caused by *Staphylococcus aureus;* postpartum endometritis or pelvic inflammatory disease caused by *E. coli;* moderately severe community-acquired pneumonia caused by *Haemophilus influenzae*

Adults: 3.375 g (3 g piperacillin/0.375 g tazobactam) every 6 hours as a 30-minute I.V. infusion. Duration of treatment is usually 7 to 10 days.

➤ **Appendicitis, peritonitis**
Children weighing more than 40 kg with normal renal function: 3.375 g (3 g piperacilin/0.375 g tazobactam) every 6 hours by I.V. infusion for 7 to 10 days.
Children age 9 months and older weighing 40 kg (88 lb) or less with normal renal function: 100 mg piperacillin/12.5 mg tazobactam/kg of body weight every 8 hours by I.V. infusion.
Children age 2 to 9 months: 80 mg piperacillin/10 mg tazobactam/kg of body weight every 8 hours by I.V. infusion.
Adjust-a-dose: If creatinine clearance is 20 to 40 ml/minute, give 2.25 g (2 g piperacillin/0.25 g tazobactam) every 6 hours; if less than 20 ml/minute, give 2.25 g (2 g piperacillin/0.25 g tazobactam) every 8 hours. In continuous ambulatory peritoneal dialysis (CAPD) patients, give 2.25 g (2 g piperacillin/0.25 g tazobactam) every 12 hours. In hemodialysis patients, give 2.25 g (2 g piperacillin/0.25 g tazobactam) every 12 hours with a supplemental dose of 0.75 g (0.67 g piperacillin/0.08 g tazobactam) after each dialysis period.

➤ **Moderate to severe nosocomial pneumonia caused by piperacillin-resistant, beta–lactamase-producing strains of *S. aureus* and by piperacillin and tazobactam-susceptible *Acinetobacter baumannii, H. influenzae, Klebsiella pneumoniae,* and *Pseudomonas aeruginosa***
Adults: 4.5 g (4 g piperacillin/0.5 g tazobactam) every 6 hours with aminoglycoside. Patients with *P. aeruginosa* should continue aminoglycoside treatment; if *P. aeruginosa* isn't isolated, aminoglycoside treatment may be

stopped. Duration of treatment is usually 7 to 14 days.
Adjust-a-dose: If creatinine clearance is 20 to 40 ml/minute, give 3.375 g (3 g piperacillin/0.375 g tazobactam) every 6 hours; if less than 20 ml/minute, give 2.25 g (2 g piperacillin/0.25 g tazobactam) every 6 hours. In CAPD patients, give 2.25 g (2 g piperacillin/ 0.25 g tazobactam) every 8 hours. In hemodialysis patients, give 2.25 g (2 g piperacillin/0.25 g tazobactam) every 8 hours with a supplemental dose of 0.75 g (0.67 g piperacillin/0.08 g tazobactam) after each dialysis period.

ADMINISTRATION
I.V.
- Before giving drug, ask patient about allergic reactions to penicillins.
- Obtain specimen for culture and sensitivity tests before giving first dose. Therapy may begin while awaiting results.
- Reconstitute each gram with 5 ml of diluent, such as sterile or bacteriostatic water for injection, normal saline solution for injection, bacteriostatic normal saline solution for injection, D_5W, dextrose 5% in normal saline solution for injection, or dextran 6% in normal saline solution for injection.
- Shake until dissolved.
- Further dilute to 50 to 150 ml before infusion.
- Use drug immediately after reconstitution.
- Stop any primary infusion during administration, if possible.
- Infuse over at least 30 minutes.
- Discard unused drug in single-dose vials after 24 hours if stored at room temperature or 48 hours if refrigerated.
- Change I.V. site every 48 hours.
- Diluted drug is stable in I.V. bags for 24 hours at room temperature or for 1 week refrigerated.
- **Incompatibilities:** Acyclovir sodium, aminoglycosides, amphotericin B, chlorpromazine, cisatracurium, cisplatin, dacarbazine, daunorubicin, dobutamine, doxorubicin, doxycycline hyclate, droperidol, famotidine, ganciclovir, gemcitabine, haloperidol lactate, hydroxyzine hydrochloride, idarubicin, lactated Ringer's solution, minocycline, mitomycin, mitoxantrone, nalbuphine, prochlorperazine

edisylate, promethazine hydrochloride, streptozocin, vancomycin.

ACTION
Inhibits cell-wall synthesis during bacterial multiplication.

Route	Onset	Peak	Duration
I.V.	Immediate	Immediate	Unknown

Half-life. About 1 hour.

ADVERSE REACTIONS
CNS: *headache, insomnia,* fever, *seizures,* agitation, anxiety, dizziness, pain.
CV: chest pain, edema, hypertension, tachycardia.
EENT: rhinitis.
GI: *diarrhea, constipation, nausea, pseudomembranous colitis,* abdominal pain, dyspepsia, stool changes, vomiting.
GU: candidiasis, interstitial nephritis.
Hematologic: *leukopenia, neutropenia, thrombocytopenia,* anemia, eosinophilia.
Respiratory: dyspnea.
Skin: pruritus, rash.
Other: *anaphylaxis,* hypersensitivity reactions, inflammation, phlebitis at I.V. site.

INTERACTIONS
Drug-drug. *Hormonal contraceptives:* May decrease contraceptive effectiveness. Advise use of another form of contraception during therapy.
Oral anticoagulants: May prolong effectiveness. Monitor PT and INR closely.
Probenecid: May increase piperacillin level. Probenecid may be used for this purpose.
Vecuronium: May prolong neuromuscular blockade. Monitor patient closely.

EFFECTS ON LAB TEST RESULTS
● May decrease hemoglobin level.
● May increase eosinophil count. May decrease neutrophil, platelet, and WBC counts.
● May cause false-positive result for urine glucose tests using copper reduction method such as Clinitest.

CONTRAINDICATIONS & CAUTIONS
● Contraindicated in patients hypersensitive to drug or other penicillins.

● Use cautiously in patients with bleeding tendencies, uremia, hypokalemia, and allergies to other drugs, especially cephalosporins, because of possible cross-sensitivity.

NURSING CONSIDERATIONS
● Because peritoneal dialysis removes 6% of the piperacillin dose and 21% of the tazobactam dose, and hemodialysis removes 30% to 40% of a dose in 4 hours, additional doses may be needed after each dialysis period.
● If large doses are given or if therapy is prolonged, bacterial or fungal superinfection may occur, especially in elderly, debilitated, or immunosuppressed patients.
● Drug contains 2.35 mEq sodium/g of piperacillin. Monitor patient's sodium intake and electrolyte levels.
● Monitor hematologic and coagulation parameters.
● Patients with cystic fibrosis may have a higher rate of fever and rash. Monitor these patients closely.

PATIENT TEACHING
● Tell patient to report adverse reactions promptly.
● Tell patient to alert a health care professional about discomfort at the I.V. site.

---

ticarcillin disodium and clavulanate potassium
tie-kar-SIL-in and KLAV-yoo-lan-nayt

Timentin

Pharmacologic class: extended-spectrum penicillin, beta-lactamase inhibitor
Pregnancy risk category B

AVAILABLE FORMS
Injection: 3 g ticarcillin and 100 mg clavulanic acid in 3.1-g vials
Premixed: 3.1 g/100 ml

INDICATIONS & DOSAGES
➤ **Gynecologic infection**
Women who weigh 60 kg (132 lb) or more: For moderate infections, 200 mg/kg (ticarcillin component) I.V. daily in divided doses every 6 hours. For severe infections,

300 mg/kg (ticarcillin component) I.V. daily in divided doses every 4 hours.
Women who weigh less than 60 kg:
200 to 300 mg/kg (ticarcillin component) I.V. daily in divided doses every 4 to 6 hours.

➤ **Lower respiratory tract, urinary tract, bone and joint, intra-abdominal, or skin and skin-structure infection and septicemia caused by beta-lactamase–producing strains of bacteria or by ticarcillin-susceptible organisms**
Adults and children who weigh more than 60 kg (132 lb): 3.1 g (Timentin) by I.V. infusion every 4 to 6 hours.
Adults and children ages 3 months to 16 years who weigh less than 60 kg:
200 mg/kg (ticarcillin component) I.V. daily in divided doses every 6 hours. For severe infections, 300 mg/kg (ticarcillin component) I.V. daily in divided doses every 4 hours.
Adjust-a-dose: If creatinine clearance is 30 to 60 ml/minute, dosage is 2 g I.V. every 4 hours; if clearance is 10 to 29 ml/minute, 2 g I.V. every 8 hours; if clearance is less than 10 ml/minute, 2 g I.V. every 12 hours; if clearance is less than 10 ml/minute and patient has hepatic dysfunction, 2 g I.V. every 24 hours. For patients receiving peritoneal dialysis or hemodialysis, give a loading dose of 3.1 g I.V. and then maintenance doses of 3.1 g I.V. every 12 hours for patients receiving peritoneal dialysis or 2 g I.V. every 12 hours for patients receiving hemodialysis. Supplement with 3.1 g after each hemodialysis session.

ADMINISTRATION
I.V.
• Before giving, ask patient about allergic reactions to penicillin.
• Obtain specimen for culture and sensitivity tests. Begin therapy while awaiting results.
• Give drug at least 1 hour before a bacteriostatic antibiotic.
• Reconstitute drug with 13 ml of sterile water for injection or normal saline solution for injection. Further dilute to a maximum of 10 to 100 mg/ml (based on drug component).
• Infuse over 30 minutes.

• **Incompatibilities:** Aminoglycosides, amphotericin B, azithromycin, cisatracurium, other anti-infectives, sodium bicarbonate, topotecan, vancomycin.

ACTION
Inhibits cell-wall synthesis during bacterial multiplication.

Route	Onset	Peak	Duration
I.V.	Immediate	Immediate	Unknown

Half-life: 1 hour.

ADVERSE REACTIONS
CNS: *seizures,* headache, giddiness, neuromuscular excitability.
CV: phlebitis, vein irritation.
EENT: taste and smell disturbances.
GI: *pseudomembranous colitis,* diarrhea, flatulence, epigastric pain, nausea, stomatitis, vomiting.
Hematologic: *leukopenia, neutropenia, thrombocytopenia,* anemia, eosinophilia, hemolytic anemia.
Metabolic: hypernatremia, hypokalemia.
Skin: *Stevens-Johnson syndrome,* pain at injection site, pruritus, rash.
Other: *anaphylaxis,* hypersensitivity reactions, overgrowth of nonsusceptible organisms.

INTERACTIONS
Drug-drug. *Hormonal contraceptives:* May decrease contraceptive effectiveness. Advise use of another form of contraception during therapy.
Methotrexate: May increase risk of methotrexate toxicity. Monitor methotrexate concentrations twice a week for first 2 weeks.
Oral anticoagulants: May increase risk of bleeding. Monitor PT and INR.
Probenecid: May increase ticarcillin level. Probenecid may be used for this purpose.

EFFECTS ON LAB TEST RESULTS
• May increase ALT, AST, alkaline phosphatase, LDH, and sodium levels. May decrease potassium and hemoglobin levels.
• May increase eosinophil count. May decrease platelet, WBC, and granulocyte counts.
• May alter results of turbidimetric tests that use sulfosalicylic acid, trichloroacetic acid, acetic acid, or nitric acid.

CONTRAINDICATIONS & CAUTIONS
● Contraindicated in patients hypersensitive to drug or other penicillins.
● Use cautiously in patients with other drug allergies, especially to cephalosporins because of possible cross-sensitivity, and in those with impaired renal function, hemorrhagic conditions, hypokalemia, or sodium restriction. Drug contains 4.5 mEq sodium/g.

NURSING CONSIDERATIONS
● Check CBC and platelet counts frequently. Drug may cause thrombo-cytopenia.
● Monitor PT and INR in patients taking oral anticoagulants.
● Monitor potassium and sodium levels.
● If large doses are given or if therapy is prolonged, bacterial or fungal superinfec-tion may occur, especially in elderly, debilitated, or immunosuppressed patients.

PATIENT TEACHING
● Tell patient to report adverse reactions promptly.
● Instruct patient to report discomfort at I.V. site.
● Advise patient to limit salt intake during drug therapy because of high sodium content.

Scabicides and pediculicides

crotamiton
lindane
permethrin
pyrethrins and piperonyl butoxide

crotamiton
kroe-TAM-ih-tuhn

Eurax

Pharmacologic class: scabicide
Pregnancy risk category C

AVAILABLE FORMS
Cream: 10%
Lotion: 10%

INDICATIONS & DOSAGES
➤ **Parasitic infestation (scabies)**
Adults: Scrub entire body with soap and water. Remove scales or crusts. Then apply thin layer of cream over entire body, from chin down (with special attention to skinfolds, creases, interdigital spaces, and genital area). Apply second coat in 24 hours. Change clothing and bed linen the next morning. Wait another 48 hours; then wash off. If retreatment is needed, use an alternative regimen.
➤ **Itching**
Adults: Apply locally, massaging gently into affected area until completely absorbed; repeat p.r.n.

ADMINISTRATION
Topical
• Shake product well before each use.
• Don't apply to face, eyes, mucous membranes, or urethral opening.
• If accidental contact with eyes occurs, flush with water and notify prescriber.

ACTION
Scabicidal and antipruritic actions; mechanism unknown.

Route	Onset	Peak	Duration
Topical	Unknown	Unknown	Unknown

Half-life: Unknown.

ADVERSE REACTIONS
Skin: *irritation,* allergic skin sensitivity.

INTERACTIONS
None significant.

EFFECTS ON LAB TEST RESULTS
None reported.

CONTRAINDICATIONS & CAUTIONS
• Contraindicated in patients hypersensitive to drug or its components and in those whose skin is raw or inflamed.

NURSING CONSIDERATIONS
• Estimate amount of cream needed per application; most patients tend to overuse scabicides. For most adults, a single tube of cream is enough for two applications.
• Don't apply drug to acutely inflamed or raw, weeping areas.
• Apply topical corticosteroids, as prescribed, if dermatitis develops from scratching.
• Make sure hospitalized patients are placed in isolation, with special linen-handling precautions, until treatment is completed.
• Treat sexual contacts simultaneously.
• *** Look alike–sound alike:*** Don't confuse Eurax with Serax or Urex.

PATIENT TEACHING
• Tell patient or family member to shake product well before each use.
• Teach patient or family member how to apply drug. Tell patient not to apply to face, eyes, mucous membranes, or urethral opening. If accidental contact with eyes occurs, tell patient to flush with water and notify prescriber.
• Tell patient to stop using drug, wash it off skin, and notify prescriber immediately if skin irritation or hypersensitivity develops.
• Instruct patient to change all clothing and bed linens the next day and to launder them in hot cycle of washing machine or dry clean them.
• Instruct patient to reapply drug if it's washed off during treatment time.

• Tell patient to warn other family members and sexual contacts about infestation.
• Reassure patient that although itching may continue for several weeks, it will stop; continued itching doesn't indicate that therapy is ineffective.

---

lindane
LIN-dayn

Hexit†

Pharmacologic class:
ectoparasiticide and ovicide
Pregnancy risk category C

AVAILABLE FORMS
Cream: 1%†
Lotion: 1%
Shampoo: 1%

INDICATIONS & DOSAGES
➤ **Parasitic infestation (scabies, pediculosis)**
Adults and children: Centers for Disease Control and Prevention recommend not bathing before applying on skin. If patient does bathe, let skin dry and cool thoroughly before using drug. For scabies, apply thin layer of cream or lotion over entire skin surface from the neck down (with special attention to skinfolds, creases, interdigital spaces, and genital area) and rub in thoroughly; for pediculosis, apply thin layer of cream or lotion to hairy areas. After 8 to 12 hours, wash drug off. Repeat process in 1 week if mites reappear or new lesions develop.

Apply shampoo undiluted to dry hair and work into lather for 4 minutes; small amounts of water may increase lathering. Apply 30 ml of shampoo for short hair, 45 ml for medium-length hair, or 60 ml for long hair. Rinse thoroughly and rub dry with towel. Comb with a fine-tooth comb.
Elderly patients: May need to reduce dosage because of increased skin absorption.

ADMINISTRATION
Topical
• If patient bathes before application, make sure his skin is dry and cool before applying drug.

• Apply thin layer to cover body only once. Use 1 ounce for children younger than age 6 and 1 to 2 ounces for older children and adults.
• Don't leave drug on for longer than 12 hours; remove drug by washing thoroughly.

ACTION
May inhibit neuronal membrane function in arthropods, causing neuronal hyperactivity, seizures, and death after penetrating the parasite's exoskeleton.

Route	Onset	Peak	Duration
Topical	190 min	Unknown	Unknown

Half-life: About 18 hours.

ADVERSE REACTIONS
CNS: *seizures,* dizziness.
Skin: alopecia, dermatitis, pruritus, urticaria.

INTERACTIONS
Drug-drug. *Drugs that lower the seizure threshold (anticholinesterases, antidepressants, antipsychotics, cyclosporine, chloroquine sulfate, imipenem, isoniazid, methocarbamol, meperidine, mofetil, mycophenolate, penicillins, pyrimethamine, quinolones, tacrolimus, theophylline):* May precipitate seizure activity if used together. Monitor patient if used together.
Drug-lifestyle. *Alcohol use:* May lower seizure threshold. Discourage use together.
Oil-based hair products: May increase absorption of drug. If oil-based hair products are used, urge patient to wash and dry hair before using drug.

EFFECTS ON LAB TEST RESULTS
None reported.

CONTRAINDICATIONS & CAUTIONS
■ **Black Box Warning** Contraindicated in premature infants and in those with seizure disorders. Use cautiously in infants, children, elderly patients, patients with skin conditions other than lice infestation, and those who weigh less than 110 lb (50 kg); all are at greater risk for CNS toxicity, including seizures and death. ■

Reactions may be *common,* uncommon, *life-threatening,* or COMMON AND LIFE-THREATENING.
Interaction may have a *rapid onset* or **delayed onset.**

• Contraindicated in patients hypersensitive to drug or its components and in those with inflamed skin.

NURSING CONSIDERATIONS

■ **Black Box Warning** Use lindane products only as second-line treatment of lice infestation or in patients who can't tolerate treatment with safer medications. ■

• Permethrin 1% cream rinse and pyrethrins with piperonyl butoxide are safer than lindane for pubic lice.

• Apply topical corticosteroids or give oral antihistamines, as prescribed, for pruritus.

• Make sure that hospitalized patients are placed in isolation, with special linen-handling precautions, until treatment is completed.

• Intact skin absorbs 6% to 13% of drug. Absorption is increased if applied to face, scalp, axillae, neck, scrotum, or irritated or broken skin.

• Avoid drug contact with eyes.

■ **Black Box Warning** When used correctly, drug is safe and effective. When overused, it can cause adverse reactions. Don't confuse prolonged itching with reinfestation. ■

• Treat sexual partners simultaneously.

PATIENT TEACHING

• Teach patient or family member how to apply drug: Apply thin layer to cover body only once. Use 1 ounce for children younger than age 6 and 1 to 2 ounces for older children and adults. Don't leave drug on for longer than 12 hours; remove drug by washing thoroughly.

• If patient bathes before application, tell him to let skin dry thoroughly and cool before applying drug.

• Inform patient that drug can be poisonous when misused. Warn patient not to apply to open areas, acutely inflamed skin, or to face, eyes, mucous membranes, or urethral opening. If accidental contact with eyes occurs, advise patient to flush with water and notify prescriber.

• Tell patient to avoid inhaling vapors.

• Advise family member to wear gloves when applying drug.

• Tell patient to wash drug off skin and to notify prescriber immediately if skin irritation or hypersensitivity develops.

• Discourage repeated use, which can lead to skin irritation, systemic toxicity, or seizures. Advise patient to repeat use only if live lice or nits are found after 1 week.

• Warn patient not to use other creams or oils during treatment because of potential for increased absorption.

• Advise breast-feeding woman to avoid a lot of skin-to-skin contact with infant while drug is present. Interrupt breast-feeding with expression and discarding of milk for at least 24 hours following use.

• Instruct patient to change all clothing and bed linens and launder them in hot water or dry clean after drug is washed off body.

• After application for lice infestation, tell patient to use fine-tooth comb or tweezers to remove nits from hairy areas.

• Advise patient to use shampoo form to clean combs or brushes and to wash them thoroughly afterward.

• Warn patient that itching may continue for several weeks after effective treatment, especially for scabies.

• Instruct patient to reapply drug if it's washed off during treatment time.

• Tell patient to warn other family members and sexual partners about infestation.

• Advise patient to use product carefully and follow all directions. Overusing product will cause unwanted side effects. Tell him not to confuse prolonged itching with reinfestation.

permethrin
per-METH-rin

Elimite, Kwellada-P†, Nix ◇

Pharmacologic class: pyrethroid
Pregnancy risk category B

AVAILABLE FORMS
Cream: 5%
Lotion: 1%
Topical liquid (cream rinse): 1%

INDICATIONS & DOSAGES
➤ **Infestation with** *Pediculus humanus capitis* **(head louse) and its nits**
Adults and children age 2 and older: Use after hair has been washed with shampoo,

rinsed with water, and towel dried. Apply 25 to 50 ml of liquid to saturate hair and scalp. Allow drug to remain on hair for 10 minutes before rinsing off with water. Remove remaining nits with comb. Usually only one application is needed.

➤ **Infestation with *Sarcoptes scabiei***
Adults and children age 2 months and older: Thoroughly massage into the skin from the head to the soles. Treat infants on hairline, neck, scalp, temple, and forehead. Wash cream off after 8 to 14 hours.

ADMINISTRATION
Topical
• Usually only one application is needed.
• Don't use drug on eyes, eyelashes, eyebrows, nose, mouth, or mucous membranes.

ACTION
Acts on parasites' nerve cells to disrupt the sodium channel current, causing parasitic paralysis.

Route	Onset	Peak	Duration
Topical	10–15 min	Unknown	10 days

Half-life: Unknown.

ADVERSE REACTIONS
Skin: *burning, stinging,* edema, mild erythema, pruritus, scalp numbness or discomfort, scalp rash, tingling.

INTERACTIONS
None significant.

EFFECTS ON LAB TEST RESULTS
None reported.

CONTRAINDICATIONS & CAUTIONS
• Contraindicated in patients hypersensitive to pyrethrins, chrysanthemums, or components of drug.

NURSING CONSIDERATIONS
• Combing of nits isn't needed for effectiveness, but drug package supplies a fine-tooth comb for cosmetic use and to decrease diagnostic confusion that may lead to retreatment.
• Retreat for lice if they are seen 7 days after first application.
• Treat sexual partners simultaneously.

PATIENT TEACHING
• Explain that treatment may temporarily worsen signs and symptoms of head lice infestation, such as itching, redness, and swelling.
• Tell patient to disinfect headgear, comb and brush, scarves, coats, and bed linens by machine washing with hot water and machine drying for at least 20 minutes, using hot cycle. Tell him to seal nonwashable items in plastic bag for 2 weeks or spray with product designed to eliminate lice and their nits.
• Warn patient not to use drug on eyes, eyelashes, eyebrows, nose, mouth, or mucous membranes.
• Tell patient to warn other family members and sexual contacts about infestation.

pyrethrins and piperonyl butoxide
pi-RETH-rinz and PI-per-oh-nel

A-200, Pronto◇, Pyrinyl◇, R & C†◇, RID◇, Tisit◇

Pharmacologic class: pyrethrin
Pregnancy risk category C

AVAILABLE FORMS
Lotion: pyrethrins 0.3% and piperonyl butoxide 2%
Mousse: pyrethrins 0.33% and piperonyl butoxide 4%
Shampoo: pyrethrins 0.33% and piperonyl butoxide 4%
Shampoo and conditioner: pyrethrins 0.33% and piperonyl butoxide 3%
Topical gel: pyrethrins 0.3% and piperonyl butoxide 3%

INDICATIONS & DOSAGES
➤ **Infestations of head, body, and pubic (crab) lice and their eggs**
Adults and children: Apply to hair, scalp, or other infested areas until entirely wet. Allow to remain for 10 minutes but no longer. Wash thoroughly with warm water and soap or shampoo. Remove dead lice and eggs with fine-tooth comb. Repeat treatment in 7 to 10 days to kill newly hatched lice; don't use more than two applications within 24 hours.

Reactions may be *common,* uncommon, ***life-threatening,*** or COMMON AND LIFE-THREATENING.
Interaction may have a *rapid onset* or ***delayed onset.***

ADMINISTRATION
Topical
● Don't apply to open areas, acutely inflamed skin, eyebrows, eyelashes, face, eyes, mucous membranes, or urethral opening. If accidental contact with eyes occurs, flush with water and notify prescriber.
● Stop using drug, wash it off skin, and notify prescriber immediately if skin irritation develops.
● All preparations contain petroleum distillates.

ACTION
Acts as contact poison that disrupts parasite's nervous system, causing parasite's paralysis and death.

Route	Onset	Peak	Duration
Topical	Unknown	Unknown	Unknown

Half-life: Unknown.

ADVERSE REACTIONS
Skin: *irritation with repeated use,* edema, erythema, eczema, pruritus, urticaria.

INTERACTIONS
None significant.

EFFECTS ON LAB TEST RESULTS
None reported.

CONTRAINDICATIONS & CAUTIONS
● Contraindicated in patients hypersensitive to drug, ragweed, or chrysanthemums.
● Use cautiously in infants and small children.

NURSING CONSIDERATIONS
● Apply topical corticosteroids or give oral antihistamines if dermatitis develops from scratching.
● Discard container by wrapping in several layers of newspaper.
● Inspect all family members daily for at least 2 weeks for infestation.
● Drug isn't effective against scabies.
● Treat sexual contacts simultaneously.

PATIENT TEACHING
● Instruct patient not to apply to open areas, acutely inflamed skin, eyebrows, eyelashes, face, eyes, mucous membranes, or urethral opening. If accidental contact with eyes occurs, advise patient to flush with water and notify prescriber.
● Warn patient not to swallow or inhale vapors from the drug.
● Tell patient to stop using drug, wash it off skin, and notify prescriber immediately if skin irritation develops. All preparations contain petroleum distillates.
● Instruct patient to change all clothing and bed linens after drug is washed off body. Tell him to disinfect washable items by machine washing in hot water and drying on hot cycle for at least 20 minutes. Other items can be dry-cleaned and sealed in plastic bags for 2 weeks, or treated with products made for this purpose.
● Teach patient to remove dead parasites with a fine-tooth comb.
● Tell patient to repeat treatment in 7 to 10 days to kill any newly hatched eggs.
● Urge patient to warn other family members and sexual partners so that they can be examined for the presence of lice.

18
Sulfonamides

co-trimoxazole
sulfadiazine
sulfisoxazole
sulfisoxazole acetyl

---

co-trimoxazole
(sulfamethoxazole and trimethoprim)
koh-trye-MOX-a-zole

Apo-Sulfatrim†, Apo-Sulfatrim DS†, Bactrim*, Bactrim DS⌀, Bactrim IV, Cotrim, Cotrim DS, Novo-Trimel†, Novo-Trimel DS†, Nu-Cotrimox†, Protrin DF†, Septra*, Septra DS, Septra IV, Sulfatrim, Sulfatrim Pediatric, Trisulfa DS†

Pharmacologic class: sulfonamide and folate antagonist
Pregnancy risk category C

AVAILABLE FORMS
Injection: trimethoprim 16 mg/ml and sulfamethoxazole 80 mg/ml in 5-ml, 10-ml, 20-ml, and 30-ml vials
Oral suspension: trimethoprim 40 mg and sulfamethoxazole 200 mg/5 ml*
Tablets (double-strength): trimethoprim 160 mg and sulfamethoxazole 800 mg
Tablets (single-strength): trimethoprim 80 mg and sulfamethoxazole 400 mg

INDICATIONS & DOSAGES
➤ **Shigellosis or UTIs caused by susceptible strains of *Escherichia coli, Proteus* (indole positive or negative), *Klebsiella,* or *Enterobacter* species**
Adults: 160 mg trimethoprim/800 mg sulfamethoxazole P.O. every 12 hours for 10 to 14 days in UTIs and for 5 days in shigellosis. If indicated, give I.V. 8 to 10 mg/kg/day, based on trimethoprim component, divided b.i.d. to q.i.d. every 6, 8, or 12 hours for 5 days for shigellosis or up to 14 days for severe UTIs. Maxi-

mum daily dose is 960 mg trimethoprim (as co-trimoxazole).
Children age 2 months and older:
8 mg/kg/day, based on trimethoprim component P.O., in two divided doses every 12 hours for 10 days for UTIs and 5 days for shigellosis. If indicated, give I.V. 8 to 10 mg/kg/day based on trimethoprim component, in two to four divided doses every 6, 8, or 12 hours for up to 14 days for severe UTIs and 5 days for shigellosis. Don't exceed adult dose.
➤ **Otitis media in patients with penicillin allergy or penicillin-resistant infection**
Children age 2 months and older:
8 mg/kg/day, based on trimethoprim component P.O., in two divided doses every 12 hours for 10 days.
➤ **Chronic bronchitis, upper respiratory tract infections**
Adults: 160 mg trimethoprim and 800 mg sulfamethoxazole P.O. every 12 hours for 14 days.
➤ **Traveler's diarrhea**
Adults: 160 mg trimethoprim and 800 mg sulfamethoxazole P.O. b.i.d. for 3 to 5 days. Some patients may only need up to 2 days of therapy.
➤ **To prevent *Pneumocystis jiroveci (carinii)* pneumonia**
Adults: 160 mg of trimethoprim and 800 mg sulfamethoxazole P.O. daily.
Children age 2 months and older:
150 mg/m² trimethoprim and 750 mg/m² sulfamethoxazole P.O. daily in two divided doses on 3 consecutive days each week.
➤ ***P. jiroveci (carinii)* pneumonia**
Adults and children older than age 2 months: 15 to 20 mg/kg/day based on trimethoprim I.V. or P.O. in three or four divided doses for 14 to 21 days.
Adjust-a-dose: For patients with creatinine clearance of 15 to 30 ml/minute, reduce daily dose by 50%. Don't give to those with creatinine clearance less than 15 ml/minute.

ADMINISTRATION

P.O.
- Before giving drug, ask patient if he's allergic to sulfa drugs.
- Obtain specimen for culture and sensitivity tests before giving. Begin therapy while awaiting results.
- Give drug with 8 oz. (240 ml) of water to patient with an empty stomach.

I.V.
- Before giving drug, ask patient if he's allergic to sulfa drugs.
- Obtain specimen for culture and sensitivity tests before giving. Begin therapy while awaiting results.
- Don't give by rapid infusion or bolus injection.
- Dilute each 5 ml of concentrate in 75 to 125 ml of D_5W. Don't mix with other drugs or solutions.
- Infuse slowly over 60 to 90 minutes.
- Don't refrigerate; use within 6 hours if diluted in 125 ml and within 2 hours if diluted in 75 ml.
- Discard solution if it's cloudy or crystallized.
- Never give drug I.M.
- **Incompatibilities:** Cisatracurium, fluconazole, foscarnet, linezolid, midazolam, verapamil, vinorelbine.

ACTION

Sulfamethoxazole inhibits formation of dihydrofolic acid from PABA; trimethoprim inhibits dihydrofolate reductase formation. Both decrease bacterial folic acid synthesis and are bactericidal.

Route	Onset	Peak	Duration
P.O.	Unknown	1–4 hr	Unknown
I.V.	Immediate	1–1½ hr	Unknown

Half-life: Trimethoprim, 8 to 11 hours; sulfamethoxazole, 10 to 13 hours.

ADVERSE REACTIONS

CNS: *seizures,* apathy, aseptic meningitis, ataxia, depression, fatigue, hallucinations, headache, insomnia, nervousness, tinnitus, vertigo.
CV: thrombophlebitis.
GI: *pancreatitis, pseudomembranous colitis,* diarrhea, nausea, vomiting, abdominal pain, anorexia, stomatitis.
GU: *toxic nephrosis with oliguria and anuria,* crystalluria, hematuria, interstitial nephritis.
Hematologic: *agranulocytosis, aplastic anemia, leukopenia, thrombocytopenia,* hemolytic anemia, megaloblastic anemia.
Hepatic: *hepatic necrosis,* jaundice.
Musculoskeletal: arthralgia, muscle weakness, myalgia.
Respiratory: pulmonary infiltrates.
Skin: *generalized skin eruption, erythema multiforme, Stevens-Johnson syndrome, toxic epidermal necrolysis,* exfoliative dermatitis, photosensitivity reactions, pruritus, urticaria.
Other: *anaphylaxis,* drug fever, hypersensitivity reactions, serum sickness.

INTERACTIONS

Drug-drug. *Cyclosporine:* May decrease cyclosporine level and increase nephrotoxicity risk. Avoid using together.
Dofetilide: May increase dofetilide level and effects. May increase risk of prolonged QT-interval syndrome and fatal ventricular arrhythmias. Avoid using together.
Hormonal contraceptives: May decrease contraceptive effectiveness and increase risk of breakthrough bleeding. Advise patient to use a nonhormonal contraceptive.
Methotrexate: May increase methotrexate level. Monitor methotrexate level.
Oral antidiabetics: May increase hypoglycemic effect. Monitor glucose level.
Phenytoin: May inhibit hepatic metabolism of phenytoin. Monitor phenytoin level.
Warfarin: May increase anticoagulant effect. Monitor patient for bleeding; monitor PT and INR.
Drug-herb. *Dong quai, St. John's wort:* May cause photosensitivity reactions. Advise patient to avoid excessive sunlight exposure.
Drug-lifestyle. *Sun exposure:* May cause photosensitivity reactions. Advise patient to avoid excessive sunlight exposure.

EFFECTS ON LAB TEST RESULTS

- May increase aminotransferase, bilirubin, BUN, and creatinine levels. May decrease hemoglobin level.
- May decrease granulocyte, platelet, and WBC counts.

CONTRAINDICATIONS & CAUTIONS
● Contraindicated in patients hypersensitive to trimethoprim or sulfonamides.
● Contraindicated in those with creatinine clearance less than 15 ml/minute, porphyria, or megaloblastic anemia from folate deficiency.
● Contraindicated in pregnant women at term, breast-feeding women, and infants younger than age 2 months.
● Use cautiously and in reduced dosages in patients with creatinine clearance of 15 to 30 ml/minute, severe allergy or bronchial asthma, G6PD deficiency, or blood dyscrasia.

NURSING CONSIDERATIONS
● *Alert:* Double-check dosage, which may be written as trimethoprim component.
● *Alert:* "DS" product means "double strength."
● Monitor renal and liver function test results.
● Promptly report rash, sore throat, fever, cough, mouth sores, or iris lesions—early signs and symptoms of erythema multiforme, which may progress to life-threatening Stevens-Johnson syndrome, or blood dyscrasias.
● Watch for signs and symptoms of super-infection, such as fever, chills, and increased pulse.
● *Alert:* Adverse reactions—especially hypersensitivity reactions, rash, and fever—occur much more frequently in patients with AIDS.

PATIENT TEACHING
● Tell patient to take drug as prescribed, even if he feels better.
● Encourage patient to drink plenty of fluids to prevent crystalluria and kidney stone formation.
● Tell patient to report adverse reactions promptly.
● Instruct patient receiving drug I.V. to report discomfort at I.V. insertion site.
● Advise patient to avoid prolonged sun exposure, wear protective clothing, and use sunscreen.
● Instruct patient to take oral form with 8 ounces (240 ml) of water on an empty stomach.

sulfadiazine
sul-fa-DYE-a-zeen

Pharmacologic class: sulfonamide
Pregnancy risk category C

AVAILABLE FORMS
Tablets: 500 mg

INDICATIONS & DOSAGES
➤ **Asymptomatic meningococcal carrier**
Adults: 1 g P.O. every 12 hours for 2 days.
Children ages 1 to 12: 500 mg P.O. every 12 hours for 2 days.
Children ages 2 to 12 months: 500 mg P.O. daily for 2 days.
➤ **To prevent rheumatic fever, as an alternative to penicillin**
Children who weigh more than 30 kg (66 lb): 1 g P.O. daily.
Children who weigh less than 30 kg: 500 mg P.O. daily.
➤ **Adjunctive treatment for toxoplasmosis**
Adults: Initial loading dose, 2 to 4 g P.O.; then a maintenance dose, 2 to 4 g P.O. daily in three to six divided doses. Maximum, 6 g daily. Usually given with pyrimethamine.
Children: Initial loading dose, 75 mg/kg or 2 g/m^2 P.O.; then maintenance dose, 150 mg/kg/day (4 g/m^2/day) P.O. in four to six divided doses. Maximum, 6 g daily. Usually given with pyrimethamine.
➤ **Nocardiosis**
Adults: 4 to 8 g P.O. daily given in divided doses for at least 6 weeks.

ADMINISTRATION
P.O.
● Before giving drug, ask patient if he's allergic to sulfa drugs.
● Give patient a glass of water with each dose, and encourage him to drink plenty of water each day to prevent urine crystals.

ACTION
Inhibits formation of dihydrofolic acid from PABA, decreasing bacterial folic acid synthesis; bacteriostatic.

Route	Onset	Peak	Duration
P.O.	Unknown	4–6 hr	Unknown

Half-life: Adults, 17 hours; children, 24 hours.

ADVERSE REACTIONS

CNS: *seizures,* depression, hallucinations, headache.

GI: *diarrhea, nausea, vomiting,* abdominal pain, anorexia, stomatitis, pancreatitis.

GU: *toxic nephrosis with oliguria and anuria,* crystalluria, hematuria.

Hematologic: *agranulocytosis, aplastic anemia, leukopenia, thrombocytopenia,* hemolytic anemia, megaloblastic anemia.

Hepatic: jaundice.

Skin: *generalized skin eruption,* **erythema multiforme, Stevens-Johnson syndrome, toxic epidermal necrolysis,** exfoliative dermatitis, photosensitivity reactions, pruritus, urticaria.

Other: *anaphylaxis,* drug fever, hypersensitivity reactions, serum sickness.

INTERACTIONS

Drug-drug. *Cyclosporine:* May decrease cyclosporine level and increase risk of nephrotoxicity. Monitor cyclosporine level.

Drugs containing PABA: May inhibit antibacterial action. Avoid using together.

Hormonal contraceptives: May decrease contraceptive effectiveness and increase risk of breakthrough bleeding. Advise patient to use a nonhormonal contraceptive.

Methotrexate: May increase methotrexate level. Monitor methotrexate level.

Oral antidiabetics: May increase hypoglycemic effect. Monitor glucose level.

Phenytoin: May increase phenytoin level. Monitor phenytoin level.

Thiazide diuretics: May increase diuretic effects. Monitor urine output.

Warfarin: May increase anticoagulant effect. Monitor patient for bleeding; monitor PT and INR.

Drug-herb. *Dong quai, St. John's wort:* May cause photosensitivity reaction. Advise patient to avoid excessive sunlight exposure.

Drug-lifestyle. *Sun exposure:* May cause photosensitivity reaction. Advise patient to avoid excessive sunlight exposure.

EFFECTS ON LAB TEST RESULTS
- May increase bilirubin, BUN, creatinine, and transaminase levels. May decrease hemoglobin level.
- May increase eosinophil count. May decrease PT and fibrinogen, granulocyte, platelet, and WBC counts.
- May alter results of urine glucose tests that use cupric sulfate (Benedict's reagent or Chemstrip uG).

CONTRAINDICATIONS & CAUTIONS
- Contraindicated in patients hypersensitive to sulfonamides, those with porphyria, infants younger than age 2 months (except in congenital toxoplasmosis), pregnant women at term, and breast-feeding women.
- Use cautiously and in reduced doses in patients with impaired hepatic or renal function, bronchial asthma, history of multiple allergies, G6PD deficiency, and blood dyscrasia.

NURSING CONSIDERATIONS
- Give drug on schedule to maintain constant level.
- Monitor patient for signs and symptoms of blood dyscrasia (purpura, ecchymoses, sore throat, fever, and pallor) and report to prescriber immediately.
- Promptly report rash, sore throat, fever, cough, mouth sores, or iris lesions—early signs and symptoms of erythema multiforme, which may progress to life-threatening Stevens-Johnson syndrome, or of blood dyscrasias.
- Monitor urine cultures, CBCs, and urinalyses before and during therapy.
- Monitor renal and liver function test results.
- Watch for signs and symptoms of superinfection, such as fever, chills, and increased pulse.
- Folic or folinic acid may be used during rest periods in toxoplasmosis therapy to reverse hematopoietic depression or anemia caused by pyrimethamine and sulfadiazine.
- Monitor fluid intake and output. Maintain intake between 3,000 and 4,000 ml daily for adults to produce output of 1,500 ml daily. If fluid intake isn't adequate to prevent crystalluria, sodium bicarbonate may be given to alkalinize urine. Monitor urine pH daily.

● *Look alike–sound alike:* Don't confuse sulfadiazine with sulfasalazine. Don't confuse sulfonamides.

PATIENT TEACHING
● Tell patient to take drug as prescribed, even if he feels better.
● Urge patient to drink a glass of water with each dose, plus plenty of water each day to prevent urine crystals.
● Instruct patient to report adverse reactions promptly.
● Warn patient to avoid prolonged exposure to sunlight, wear protective clothing, and use sunscreen.

---

sulfisoxazole
(sulfafurazole, sulphafurazole)
sul-fi-SOZ-a-zole

sulfisoxazole acetyl
Gantrisin Pediatric

Pharmacologic class: sulfonamide
Pregnancy risk category C

AVAILABLE FORMS
sulfisoxazole
Tablets: 500 mg
sulfisoxazole acetyl
Suspension: 500 mg/5 ml*

INDICATIONS & DOSAGES
➤ **UTI, systemic infection**
Adults: Initially, 2 to 4 g P.O.; then 4 to 8 g daily divided in four to six doses.
Children older than age 2 months: Initially, 75 mg/kg P.O. daily or 2 g/m² P.O.; then 150 mg/kg or 4 g/m² P.O. daily in divided doses every 6 hours. Don't exceed total daily dose of 6 g.

ADMINISTRATION
P.O.
● Before giving drug, ask patient if he's allergic to sulfa drugs.
● Obtain specimen for culture and sensitivity tests before giving first dose. Begin therapy while awaiting results.
● Give a glass of water with each dose, and encourage patient to drink plenty of water each day to prevent urine crystals.

ACTION
Inhibits formation of dihydrofolic acid from PABA, decreasing bacterial folic acid synthesis; bacteriostatic.

Route	Onset	Peak	Duration
P.O.	Unknown	1–4 hr	Unknown

Half-life: 4½ to 8 hours.

ADVERSE REACTIONS
CNS: *seizures,* depression, dizziness, hallucinations, headache, syncope, *intracranial hypertension.*
CV: cyanosis, palpitations, tachycardia, angioedema, vasculitis.
GI: *diarrhea, nausea, vomiting, pseudomembranous colitis,* abdominal pain, anorexia, stomatitis, *hemorrhage.*
GU: *acute renal failure, toxic nephrosis with oliguria and anuria,* crystalluria, hematuria.
Hematologic: *agranulocytosis, aplastic anemia, leukopenia, thrombocytopenia,* hemolytic anemia, megaloblastic anemia.
Hepatic: *hepatitis,* jaundice.
Respiratory: cough, dyspnea, pulmonary infiltrates.
Skin: *generalized skin eruption, erythema multiforme, toxic epidermal necrolysis,* exfoliative dermatitis, photosensitivity reactions, pruritus, urticaria.
Other: *anaphylaxis,* drug fever, hypersensitivity reactions, serum sickness, edema.

INTERACTIONS
Drug-drug. *Hormonal contraceptives:* May decrease contraceptive effectiveness and increase risk of breakthrough bleeding. Advise patient to use a nonhormonal contraceptive.
Methotrexate: May increase methotrexate level. Monitor methotrexate level.
Oral antidiabetics: May increase hypoglycemic effect. Monitor glucose level.
Thiopental: Patients may require less thiopental for anesthesia. Reduce thiopental dosage as needed.
Warfarin: May increase anticoagulant effect. Monitor patient for bleeding; monitor PT and INR.
Drug-herb. *Dong quai, St. John's wort:* May cause photosensitivity reactions. Advise patient to avoid excessive sunlight exposure.

Reactions may be *common,* uncommon, *life-threatening,* or COMMON AND LIFE-THREATENING.
Interaction may have a *rapid onset* or *delayed onset.*

Drug-lifestyle. *Sun exposure:* May cause photosensitivity reactions. Advise patient to avoid excessive sunlight exposure.

EFFECTS ON LAB TEST RESULTS
• May increase aminotransferase, bilirubin, BUN, and creatinine levels. May decrease hemoglobin level.
• May increase eosinophil count. May decrease PT and fibrinogen, granulocyte, platelet, and WBC counts.
• May alter results of urine glucose tests that use cupric sulfate (Benedict's reagent or Chemstrip uG).

CONTRAINDICATIONS & CAUTIONS
• Contraindicated in patients hypersensitive to sulfonamides, infants younger than age 2 months (except in congenital toxoplasmosis), pregnant women at term, and breast-feeding women.
• Use cautiously in patients with impaired hepatic or renal function, severe allergy, bronchial asthma, and G6PD deficiency.
• Drug should be discontinued at first appearance of rash or signs of an adverse reaction.

NURSING CONSIDERATIONS
• Monitor urine cultures, CBC, PT, INR, and urinalyses before and during therapy.
• Monitor renal and liver function test results.
• Report moderate to severe diarrhea to prescriber.
• Watch for signs and symptoms of superinfection, such as fever, chills, and increased pulse.
• Monitor fluid intake and output. Maintain intake between 3,000 and 4,000 ml daily for adults to produce output of 1,500 ml daily. If fluid intake isn't adequate to prevent crystalluria, sodium bicarbonate may be given to alkalinize urine. Monitor urine pH daily.
• *Look alike–sound alike:* Don't confuse sulfisoxazole with sulfasalazine. Don't confuse the combination products with sulfisoxazole alone.

PATIENT TEACHING
• Tell patient to take drug as prescribed, even if he feels better.

• Instruct patient to drink a glass of water with each dose, plus plenty of water each day to prevent urine crystals.
• Advise patient to report rash, sore throat, fever, pallor, or yellowed skin or eyes immediately.
• Warn patient to avoid prolonged exposure to sunlight, wear protective clothing, and use sunscreen.

19
Tetracyclines

doxycycline
doxycycline calcium
doxycycline hyclate
doxycycline monohydrate
minocycline hydrochloride
tetracycline hydrochloride
tigecycline

---

doxycycline
dox-i-SYE-kleen

Oracea

doxycycline calcium
Vibramycin

doxycycline hyclate
Apo-Doxy†, Atridox, Doryx,
Doxy 100, Doxy 200, Doxycin†,
Doxytab†, Doxytec†,
Novo-Doxylin†, Periostat,
Vibramycin, Vibra-Tabs

doxycycline monohydrate
Monodox, Vibramycin

Pharmacologic class: tetracycline
Pregnancy risk category D

AVAILABLE FORMS
doxycycline
Capsules: 40 mg (30 mg immediate-
release and 10 mg delayed-release)
doxycycline calcium
Syrup: 50 mg/5 ml
doxycycline hyclate
Capsules: 50 mg, 100 mg
Capsules (coated pellets): 75 mg, 100 mg
Injection: 42.5 mg, 100 mg, 200 mg
Tablets: 20 mg, 100 mg
doxycycline monohydrate
Capsules: 50 mg, 100 mg
Oral suspension: 25 mg/5 ml
Tablets: 50 mg, 75 mg, 100 mg

INDICATIONS & DOSAGES
➤ **Infections caused by susceptible
gram-positive and gram-negative
organisms (including *Haemophilus***
ducreyi, Yersinia pestis, **and** *Campylobacter fetus*), **Rickettsiae** species,
*Mycoplasma pneumoniae, Chlamydia
trachomatis,* **and** *Borrelia burgdorferi*
**(Lyme disease); psittacosis;
granuloma inguinale**
*Adults and children older than age 8 who
weigh at least 45 kg (99 lb):* 100 mg P.O.
every 12 hours on first day; then 100 mg
P.O. daily as a single dose or divided b.i.d.
Or, 200 mg I.V. on first day in one or two
infusions; then 100 to 200 mg I.V. daily.
Daily doses of 200 mg I.V. can be given as
a single dose or divided b.i.d.
*Children older than age 8 who weigh less
than 45 kg:* 4.4 mg/kg P.O. or I.V. daily, in
divided doses every 12 hours on first day;
then 2.2 to 4.4 mg/kg daily given as a
single dose or divided b.i.d.
   Give I.V. infusion slowly (minimum
1 hour). Infusion must be completed within
12 hours (within 6 hours in lactated
Ringer's solution or dextrose 5% in lactated
Ringer's solution).
➤ **Gonorrhea in patients allergic to
penicillin**
Adults: 100 mg P.O. b.i.d. for 7 days. Use
for 10 days for epididymitis.
➤ **Syphilis in patients allergic to
penicillin (except Doryx, Monodox)**
Adults: 100 mg P.O. b.i.d. for 14 days
(early). If more than 1-year duration,
100 mg P.O. daily for 4 weeks.
➤ **Primary or secondary syphilis in
patients allergic to penicillin (Doryx,
Monodox only)**
Adults: 300 mg P.O. daily in divided doses
for at least 10 days.
➤ **Uncomplicated urethral, endocervical, or rectal infections caused
by *C. trachomatis* or *Ureaplasma
urealyticum***
Adults: 100 mg P.O. b.i.d. for at least
7 days. In those with epididymitis, treat for
10 days. In those with lymphogranuloma
venereum, treat for at least 21 days.
➤ **To prevent malaria**
Adults: 100 mg P.O. daily beginning 1 to
2 days before travel to endemic area and
continued for 4 weeks after travel.

Reactions may be *common*, uncommon, *life-threatening*, or COMMON AND LIFE-THREATENING.
Interaction may have a *rapid onset* or *delayed onset*.

Children older than age 8: Give 2 mg/kg P.O. once daily beginning 1 to 2 days before travel to endemic area and continued for 4 weeks after travel. Don't exceed daily dose of 100 mg.

➤ **Pelvic inflammatory disease ◆**
Adults: 100 mg I.V. or P.O. every 12 hours with 2 g cefoxitin I.V. every 6 hours. May stop parenteral doxycycline and cefoxitin after 24 hours and continue with 100 mg doxycycline P.O. every 12 hours for 14 days total.

➤ **Adjunct to other antibiotics for inhalation, GI, and oropharyngeal anthrax**
Adults: 100 mg every 12 hours I.V. initially until susceptibility test results are known. Switch to 100 mg P.O. b.i.d. when appropriate. Treat for 60 days total.
Children older than age 8 who weigh more than 45 kg (99 lb): 100 mg every 12 hours I.V.; then switch to 100 mg P.O. b.i.d. when appropriate. Treat for 60 days total.
Children older than age 8 who weigh 45 kg or less: 2.2 mg/kg every 12 hours I.V.; then switch to 2.2 mg/kg (up to 100 mg) P.O. b.i.d. when appropriate. Treat for 60 days total.
Children age 8 and younger: 2.2 mg/kg every 12 hours I.V.; then switch to 2.2 mg/kg (up to 100 mg) P.O. b.i.d. when appropriate. Treat for 60 days total.

➤ **Cutaneous anthrax**
Adults: 100 mg P.O. every 12 hours for 60 days.
Children older than age 8 who weigh more than 45 kg (99 lb): 100 mg P.O. every 12 hours for 60 days.
Children older than age 8 who weigh 45 kg or less: 2.2 mg/kg (up to 100 mg) every 12 hours P.O. for 60 days.
Children age 8 and younger: 2.2 mg/kg (up to 100 mg) P.O. every 12 hours for 60 days.

➤ **Adjunct to scaling and root planing to improve attachment and reduce pocket depth in periodontitis**
Adults: 20 mg P.O. Periostat b.i.d., more than 1 hour before or 2 hours after the morning and evening meals and after scaling and root planing. Effective for 9 months.

➤ **Inflammatory lesions of rosacea**
Adults: 40 mg Oracea P.O. once daily in the morning, 1 hour before or 2 hours after a meal. Give with a full glass of water.

ADMINISTRATION
P.O.
● Obtain specimen for culture and sensitivity tests before giving. Begin therapy while awaiting results.
● *Alert:* Check expiration date. Outdated or deteriorated tetracyclines may cause reversible nephrotoxicity (Fanconi syndrome).
● Give drug with food or milk if stomach upset occurs.
● Increase fluid intake and don't administer tablets or capsules within 1 hour of bedtime because of possible esophageal irritation or ulceration.
● Give Oracea with a full glass of water.
● Tablets may be crushed and mixed with low-fat or chocolate milk, chocolate pudding, or apple juice mixed equally with sugar. Store mixtures in refrigerator (except apple juice mixture, which can be stored at room temperature) and discard after 24 hours.
I.V.
● Obtain specimen for culture and sensitivity tests before giving. Begin therapy while awaiting results.
● Reconstitute powder for injection with sterile water for injection. Use 10 ml in 100-mg vial and 20 ml in 200-mg vial. Further dilute solution to a concentration of 0.1 mg/ml to 1 mg/ml; don't infuse solution that contains more than 1 mg/ml.
● Don't expose drug to light or heat. Protect it from sunlight during infusion.
● Infusion time varies with dose but usually ranges from 1 to 4 hours. Infusion must be completed within 12 hours.
● Monitor infusion site for evidence of thrombophlebitis.
● Reconstituted injectable solution is stable 72 hours if refrigerated and protected from light.
● **Incompatibilities:** Allopurinol; drugs that are unstable in acidic solutions, such as barbiturates; erythromycin lactobionate; heparin; meropenem; nafcillin; penicillin G potassium; piperacillin with tazobactam; riboflavin; and sulfonamides.

ACTION
May exert bacteriostatic effect by binding to the 30S and possibly 50S ribosomal subunits of microorganisms and inhibiting protein synthesis. May also alter the

cytoplasmic membrane of susceptible microorganisms.

Route	Onset	Peak	Duration
P.O.	Unknown	1½–4 hr	Unknown
I.V.	Immediate	Unknown	Unknown

Half-life: About 1 day after multiple dosing.

ADVERSE REACTIONS
CNS: *intracranial hypertension.*
CV: pericarditis, thrombophlebitis.
GI: *diarrhea, epigastric distress, nausea,* anorexia, glossitis, dysphagia, vomiting, oral candidiasis, enterocolitis, anogenital inflammation.
Hematologic: *neutropenia, thrombocytopenia,* eosinophilia, hemolytic anemia.
Musculoskeletal: bone growth retardation in children younger than age 8.
Skin: *maculopapular and erythematous rashes, photosensitivity reactions, increased pigmentation, urticaria.*
Other: *anaphylaxis,* hypersensitivity reactions, superinfection, permanent discoloration of teeth, enamel defects.

INTERACTIONS
Drug-drug. *Antacids and laxatives containing aluminum, magnesium, or calcium, antidiarrheals:* May decrease antibiotic absorption. Give antibiotic 1 hour before or 2 hours after these drugs.
Carbamazepine, phenobarbital, rifamycins: May decrease antibiotic effect. Avoid using together.
Ferrous sulfate and other iron products, zinc: May decrease antibiotic absorption. Give drug 2 hours before or 3 hours after iron.
Hormonal contraceptives: May decrease contraceptive effectiveness and increase risk of breakthrough bleeding. Advise use of a nonhormonal contraceptive.
Methoxyflurane: May cause nephrotoxicity with tetracyclines. Avoid using together.
Oral anticoagulants: May increase anticoagulant effect. Monitor PT and INR, and adjust dosage.
Penicillins: May interfere with bactericidal action of penicillins. Avoid using together.
Drug-lifestyle. *Alcohol use:* May decrease drug's effect. Discourage use together.
Sun exposure: May cause photosensitivity reactions. Advise patient to avoid excessive sunlight exposure.

EFFECTS ON LAB TEST RESULTS
• May increase BUN and liver enzyme levels. May decrease hemoglobin level.
• May increase eosinophil count. May decrease platelet, neutrophil, and WBC counts.
• May falsely elevate fluorometric tests for urine catecholamines. May cause false-negative results in urine glucose tests using glucose oxidase reagent (Diastix or Chemstrip uG). Parenteral form may cause false-positive Clinitest results.

CONTRAINDICATIONS & CAUTIONS
• Contraindicated in patients hypersensitive to drug or other tetracyclines.
• Use cautiously in patients with impaired renal or hepatic function.
• In a fetus in the last half of gestation or a child younger than age 8, drug may cause permanently discolored teeth, enamel defects, and bone growth retardation.

NURSING CONSIDERATIONS
• If patient receives large doses or prolonged therapy or if patient is at high risk, watch for signs and symptoms of superinfection. If superinfection occurs, drug should be discontinued and appropriate therapy instituted.
• Cutaneous anthrax with signs of systemic involvement, extensive edema, or lesions on the head or neck requires I.V. therapy and a multidrug approach.
• Ciprofloxacin and doxycycline are first-line therapies for anthrax. If anthrax patient also has meningitis, ciprofloxacin is preferred because of better distribution to the CNS.
• In pregnant women and immuno-compromised patients, use the usual dosage schedule for anthrax. In pregnant women, adverse effects on fetal teeth and bones are dose-limited, so drug may be used for 7 to 14 days before the third trimester.
• Check patient's tongue for signs of fungal infection. Emphasize good oral hygiene.
• Photosensitivity reactions may occur within a few minutes to several hours after exposure and may last after therapy ends.
• *Look alike–sound alike:* Don't confuse doxycycline, doxylamine, and dicyclomine.

Reactions may be *common,* uncommon, *life-threatening,* or COMMON AND LIFE-THREATENING.
Interaction may have a *rapid onset* or *delayed onset.*

PATIENT TEACHING

• Tell patient to take entire amount of drug exactly as prescribed, even after he feels better.

• Instruct patient to report adverse reactions promptly. If drug is being given I.V., tell him to report discomfort at I.V. site.

• Advise patient to take oral form of drug with food or milk if stomach upset occurs.

• Advise patient to increase fluid intake and not to take oral tablets or capsules within 1 hour of bedtime because of possible esophageal irritation or ulceration.

• Advise parent giving drug to a child that tablets may be crushed and mixed with low-fat or chocolate milk, chocolate pudding, or apple juice mixed equally with sugar. Tell parent to store mixtures in refrigerator (except apple juice mixture, which can be stored at room temperature) and to discard after 24 hours.

• Warn patient to avoid direct sunlight and ultraviolet light, wear protective clothing, and use sunscreen.

• Tell patient to report signs and symptoms of superinfection to prescriber.

• Tell patient taking Oracea to take drug with a full glass of water.

---

minocycline hydrochloride
mi-noe-SYE-kleen

Dynacin, ENCA†, Minocin, Myrac, Solodyn

Pharmacologic class: tetracycline
Pregnancy risk category D

AVAILABLE FORMS

Capsules: 50 mg, 75 mg, 100 mg
Capsules (pellet-filled): 50 mg, 100 mg
Oral suspension: 50 mg/ml
Tablets: 50 mg, 75 mg, 100 mg
Tablets (extended-release): 45 mg, 90 mg, 135 mg

INDICATIONS & DOSAGES

➤ **Infections caused by susceptible gram-negative and gram-positive organisms (including *Haemophilus ducreyi, Yersinia pestis,* and *Campylobacter fetus*), *Rickettsiae* species, *Mycoplasma pneumoniae,* and**

Chlamydia trachomatis; **psittacosis; granuloma inguinale**
Adults: 200 mg P.O. initially; then 100 mg P.O. every 12 hours. May use 100 or 200 mg P.O. initially; then 50 mg q.i.d.
Children older than age 8: Initially, 4 mg/kg P.O.; then, 2 mg/kg every 12 hours.

➤ **Gonorrhea in patients allergic to penicillin**
Adults: Initially, 200 mg P.O.; then 100 mg every 12 hours for at least 4 days. Obtain samples for follow-up cultures within 2 to 3 days after treatment.

➤ **Syphilis in patients allergic to penicillin**
Adults: Initially, 200 mg P.O.; then 100 mg every 12 hours for 10 to 15 days.

➤ **Meningococcal carrier state**
Adults: 100 mg P.O. every 12 hours for 5 days.

➤ **Uncomplicated urethral, endocervical, or rectal infection caused by *C. trachomatis* or *Ureaplasma urealyticum***
Adults: 100 mg P.O. every 12 hours for at least 7 days.

➤ **Uncomplicated gonococcal urethritis**
Men: 100 mg P.O. every 12 hours for 5 days.

➤ **Treatment of inflammatory lesions of nonnodular moderate to severe acne vulgaris**
Adults: 50 mg P.O. daily to t.i.d.
Adults and children age 12 and older: 1 mg/kg extended release (Solodyn) P.O. once daily for 12 weeks.

➤ **Rheumatoid arthritis** ◆
Adults: 100 mg P.O. twice daily for up to 48 weeks.

Adjust-a-dose: Decrease dosage in patients with renal impairment. Don't exceed 200 mg Minocin in 24 hours.

ADMINISTRATION
P.O.

• Obtain specimen for culture and sensitivity tests before first dose. Begin therapy while awaiting results.

• Give drug with a full glass of water. Drug may be taken with food.

• Drug shouldn't be given within 1 hour of bedtime, to avoid esophageal irritation or ulceration.

• Give Solodyn at the same time each day, with or without food.
• Solodyn tablet must be swallowed whole and not crushed, chewed, or split.

ACTION
May be bacteriostatic by binding to microorganism's ribosomal subunits, inhibiting protein synthesis; may also alter the cytoplasmic membrane of susceptible microorganisms.

Route	Onset	Peak	Duration
P.O.	Unknown	1–4 hr	Unknown
P.O. (extended-release)	Unknown	3½ to 4 hr	Unknown

Half-life: 11 to 26 hours.

ADVERSE REACTIONS
CNS: *intracranial hypertension,* headache, light-headedness, dizziness, vertigo.
CV: *thrombophlebitis,* pericarditis.
GI: *anorexia, diarrhea, nausea,* dysphagia, glossitis, epigastric distress, oral candidiasis, vomiting.
Hematologic: *neutropenia, thrombocytopenia,* eosinophilia, hemolytic anemia.
Hepatic: *hepatotoxicity.*
Musculoskeletal: bone growth retardation in children younger than age 8.
Skin: *increased pigmentation, maculopapular and erythematous rashes, photosensitivity reactions, urticaria.*
Other: *anaphylaxis,* enamel defects, hypersensitivity reactions, permanent discoloration of teeth, superinfection.

INTERACTIONS
Drug-drug. *Antacids (including sodium bicarbonate) and laxatives containing aluminum, magnesium, or calcium, antidiarrheals:* May decrease antibiotic absorption. Give antibiotic 1 hour before or 2 hours after these drugs.
Ferrous sulfate and other iron products, zinc: May decrease antibiotic absorption. Give drug 2 hours before or 3 hours after iron.
Hormonal contraceptives: May decrease contraceptive effectiveness and increase risk of breakthrough bleeding. Advise patient to use nonhormonal contraceptive.
Isotretinoin: May cause pseudomotor cerebri. Avoid giving shortly before,

during, and shortly after minocycline therapy.
Methoxyflurane: May cause nephrotoxicity when given with tetracyclines. Avoid using together.
Oral anticoagulants: May increase anticoagulant effect. Monitor PT and INR, and adjust dosage.
Penicillins: May disrupt bactericidal action of penicillins. Avoid using together.
Drug-lifestyle. *Sun exposure:* May cause photosensitivity reactions. Advise patient to avoid excessive sunlight exposure.

EFFECTS ON LAB TEST RESULTS
• May increase BUN and liver enzyme levels. May decrease hemoglobin level.
• May increase eosinophil count. May decrease platelet and neutrophil counts.
• May falsely elevate fluorometric test results for urine catecholamines. Parenteral form may cause false-positive results of copper sulfate test (Clinitest). May cause false-negative results in urine glucose tests using glucose oxidase reagent (Diastix or Chemstrip uG).

CONTRAINDICATIONS & CAUTIONS
• Contraindicated in patients hypersensitive to drug or other tetracyclines. Solodyn tablets contraindicated in pregnancy, breast-feeding, or by persons of either gender attempting to conceive a child.
• Use cautiously in patients with impaired renal or hepatic function. Use of these drugs during last half of pregnancy and in children younger than age 8 may cause permanent discoloration of teeth, enamel defects, and bone growth retardation.

NURSING CONSIDERATIONS
• Monitor renal and liver function test results.
• **Alert:** Check expiration date. Outdated or deteriorated drug may cause reversible nephrotoxicity (Fanconi syndrome).
• Don't expose drug to light or heat. Keep cap tightly closed.
• If large doses are given, therapy is prolonged, or patient is at high risk, monitor patient for signs and symptoms of superinfection.
• Check patient's tongue for signs of candidal infection. Stress good oral hygiene.

• Drug may discolor teeth in older children and young adults, more commonly when used as long-term treatment. Watch for brown pigmentation, and notify prescriber if it occurs.

• Photosensitivity reactions may occur within a few minutes to several hours after exposure. Photosensitivity lasts after therapy ends.

• *Look alike–sound alike:* Don't confuse Minocin with niacin or Mithracin.

PATIENT TEACHING

• Tell patient to take entire amount of drug exactly as prescribed, even after he feels better.

• Instruct patient to take drug with a full glass of water. Drug may be taken with food. Tell patient not to take within 1 hour of bedtime to avoid esophageal irritation or ulceration.

• Warn patient to avoid driving or other hazardous tasks because of possible adverse CNS effects.

• Caution patient to avoid direct sunlight and ultraviolet light, wear protective clothing, and use sunscreen.

• Tell patient to take Solodyn at the same time each day, with or without food.

• Tell patient to swallow Solodyn tablet whole and not to crush, chew, or split tablet.

• Warn patient not to take more than 1 Solodyn tablet each day.

---

tetracycline hydrochloride
tet-ra-SYE-kleen

Apo-Tetra†, JAA-Tetra†,
Novo-Tetra†, Nu-Tetra†, Sumycin

Pharmacologic class: tetracycline
Pregnancy risk category D

AVAILABLE FORMS
Capsules: 250 mg, 500 mg
Oral suspension: 125 mg/5 ml

INDICATIONS & DOSAGES
➤ **Infections caused by susceptible gram-negative and -positive organisms, including** *Haemophilus ducreyi, Yersinia pestis, Campylobacter fetus, Rickettsiae* **species,**
Mycoplasma pneumoniae, **and** *Chlamydia trachomatis;* **psittacosis; granuloma inguinale**
Adults: 1 g to 2 g/day P.O. divided b.i.d. or q.i.d depending on the severity of infection.
Children older than age 8: 25 to 50 mg/kg P.O. daily, in divided doses every 6 hours.
➤ **Uncomplicated urethral, endocervical, or rectal infections caused by** *C. trachomatis*
Adults: 500 mg P.O. q.i.d. for at least 7 days.
➤ **Brucellosis**
Adults: 500 mg P.O. every 6 hours for 3 weeks with 1 g of streptomycin I.M. every 12 hours for first week; once daily for second week.
➤ **Gonorrhea in patients allergic to penicillin**
Adults: 500 mg P.O. every 6 hours for 7 days.
➤ **Syphilis in patients allergic to penicillin**
Adults and adolescents: 500 mg P.O. q.i.d. for 14 days. If infection has lasted 1 year or longer, treat for 28 days.
➤ **Acne**
Adults and adolescents: Initially, 250 mg P.O. every 6 hours; then 125 to 500 mg daily or every other day.
➤ *Helicobacter pylori* **infection**
Adults: 500 mg P.O. every 6 hours for 10 to 14 days with other drugs, such as metronidazole, bismuth subsalicylate, amoxicillin, or omeprazole.
➤ **Cholera**
Adults: 500 mg P.O. every 6 hours for 48 to 72 hours.
➤ **Malaria caused by** *Plasmodium falciparum*
Adults: 250 to 500 mg P.O. daily for 7 days with quinine sulfate 650 mg P.O. every 8 hours for 3 to 7 days.
➤ **To prevent infection in rape victims**
Adults: 500 mg P.O. q.i.d. for 7 days.

ADMINISTRATION
P.O.
• Obtain specimen for culture and sensitivity tests before giving first dose. Begin therapy while awaiting results.
• Effectiveness is reduced when drug is given with milk or other dairy products,

---

antacids, or iron products. For best drug absorption, give drug with a full glass of water on an empty stomach, at least 1 hour before or 2 hours after meals.
• Give drug at least 1 hour before bedtime to prevent esophageal irritation or ulceration.

ACTION

May exert bacteriostatic effect by binding to the 30S and possibly 50S ribosomal subunits of microorganisms, thus inhibiting protein synthesis. May also alter the cytoplasmic membrane of susceptible microorganisms.

Route	Onset	Peak	Duration
P.O.	Unknown	1–4 hr	Unknown

Half-life: 6 to 11 hours.

ADVERSE REACTIONS

CNS: *intracranial hypertension,* dizziness, headache.
CV: pericarditis.
EENT: sore throat.
GI: *diarrhea, epigastric distress, nausea,* anorexia, dysphagia, enterocolitis, esophagitis, glossitis, oral candidiasis, stomatitis, vomiting.
GU: inflammatory lesions in anogenital region.
Hematologic: *neutropenia, thrombocytopenia,* eosinophilia.
Musculoskeletal: *bone growth retardation in children younger than age 8.*
Skin: *candidal superinfection, increased pigmentation, maculopapular and erythematous rash, photosensitivity reactions,* urticaria.
Other: enamel defects, hypersensitivity reactions, permanent discoloration of teeth.

INTERACTIONS

Drug-drug. *Antacids and laxatives containing aluminum, magnesium, or calcium;* *antidiarrheals containing kaolin, pectin, or bismuth subsalicylate:* May decrease antibiotic absorption. Give antibiotic 1 hour before or 2 hours after these drugs.
Digoxin: May increase digoxin absorption. Monitor digoxin levels and monitor patient for signs of toxicity.

Ferrous sulfate and other iron products, zinc: May decrease antibiotic absorption. Give tetracycline 2 hours before or 3 hours after these products.
Hormonal contraceptives: May decrease contraceptive effectiveness and increase risk of breakthrough bleeding. Advise patient to use nonhormonal contraceptive.
Methoxyflurane: May cause severe nephrotoxicity. Avoid using together.
Oral anticoagulants: May increase anticoagulant effects. Monitor PT and INR, and adjust anticoagulant dosage.
Penicillins: May interfere with bactericidal action of penicillins. Avoid using together.
Drug-food. *Dairy products:* May decrease antibiotic absorption. Give antibiotic 1 hour before or 2 hours after eating or drinking dairy products.
Drug-lifestyle. *Sun exposure:* May cause photosensitivity reactions. Advise patient to avoid excessive sunlight exposure.

EFFECTS ON LAB TEST RESULTS

• May increase BUN and liver enzyme levels.
• May increase eosinophil count. May decrease platelet and neutrophil counts.
• May falsely elevate fluorometric test results for urine catecholamines. May cause false-negative results in urine glucose tests using glucose oxidase reagent (Diastix or Chemstrip uG).

CONTRAINDICATIONS & CAUTIONS

• Contraindicated in patients hypersensitive to drug or other tetracyclines.
• Some tetracyclines may contain sulfites and are contraindicated in patients with sulfite hypersensitivity.
• Use cautiously in patients with renal or hepatic impairment. Avoid using or use cautiously during last half of pregnancy and in children younger than age 8 because drug may cause permanent discoloration of teeth, enamel defects, and bone growth retardation.

NURSING CONSIDERATIONS

• *Alert:* Check expiration date. Using outdated or deteriorated drug has been linked to severe reversible nephrotoxicity (Fanconi syndrome).
• Don't expose drug to light or heat.

Reactions may be *common*, uncommon, *life-threatening*, or COMMON AND LIFE-THREATENING.
Interaction may have a *rapid onset* or *delayed onset*.

- If large doses are given, therapy is prolonged, or patient is at high risk, monitor patient for signs and symptoms of superinfection.
- In patients with renal or hepatic impairment, monitor renal and liver function test results if drug is used.
- Check patient's tongue for signs of candidal infection. Emphasize good oral hygiene.
- Drug isn't indicated for treatment of neurosyphilis.
- Photosensitivity reactions may occur within a few minutes to several hours after sun exposure. Photosensitivity lasts after therapy ends.

PATIENT TEACHING
- Tell patient to take drug exactly as prescribed, even after he feels better, and to take entire amount prescribed.
- Explain that effectiveness is reduced when drug is taken with milk or other dairy products, antacids, or iron products. For best drug absorption, tell patient to take each dose with a full glass of water on an empty stomach, at least 1 hour before or 2 hours after meals. Also tell him to take it at least 1 hour before bedtime to prevent esophageal irritation or ulceration.
- Warn patient to avoid direct sunlight and ultraviolet light, wear protective clothing, and use sunscreen.
- Advise patient to promptly report adverse reactions to prescriber.

---

tigecycline
tye-gah-SYE-klin

Tygacil

Pharmacologic class: glycylcycline antibacterial
Pregnancy risk category D

AVAILABLE FORMS
Lyophilized powder: 50-mg vial

INDICATIONS & DOSAGES
➤ **Complicated skin or skin structure infection; complicated intra-abdominal infection**
Adults: Initially 100 mg I.V.; then 50 mg every 12 hours for 5 to 14 days. Infuse drug over 30 to 60 minutes.

Adjust-a-dose: For patients with severe hepatic impairment, give initial dose of 100 mg I.V. and then 25 mg I.V. every 12 hours.

ADMINISTRATION
I.V.
- Assess patient for tetracycline allergy before therapy.
- Obtain specimen for culture and sensitivity tests before first dose. Begin therapy while awaiting results.
- Reconstitute powder with 5.3 ml of normal saline solution or D_5W to yield 10 mg/ml. Gently swirl the vial until the powder dissolves.
- Immediately withdraw the dose from the vial and add it to 100 ml of normal saline solution or D_5W. The maximum concentration is 1 mg/ml.
- Inspect the solution for particulates and discoloration (green or black) before giving. Reconstituted solution should be yellow or orange.
- Immediately dilute reconstituted drug.
- Use a dedicated I.V. line or a Y-site, and flush the line with normal saline or D_5W before and after infusion.
- Infuse the drug over 30 to 60 minutes.
- Store unopened vials at room temperature in the original package. Store diluted solution at room temperature for up to 6 hours, or refrigerate for up to 24 hours.
- **Incompatibilities:** Amphotericin B, chlorpromazine, methylprednisolone, and voriconazole.

ACTION
Inhibits protein translation in bacteria by binding to the 30S ribosomal unit.

Route	Onset	Peak	Duration
I.V.	Unknown	Unknown	Unknown

Half-life: 27 to 42 hours.

ADVERSE REACTIONS
CNS: asthenia, dizziness, fever, headache, insomnia, pain.
CV: hypertension, hypotension, peripheral edema, phlebitis.
GI: *diarrhea, nausea, vomiting,* abdominal pain, constipation, dyspepsia.
Hematologic: *thrombocytopenia,* anemia, leukocytosis.

Metabolic: hyperglycemia, hypokalemia, hypoproteinemia.
Musculoskeletal: back pain.
Respiratory: cough, dyspnea.
Skin: local reaction, pruritus, rash, sweating.
Other: *sepsis,* abnormal healing, abscess, allergic reaction, infection.

INTERACTIONS
Drug-drug. *Hormonal contraceptives:*
May decrease contraceptive's effectiveness. Advise patient to use nonhormonal form of contraception during treatment.
Warfarin: May increase risk of bleeding. Monitor INR.

EFFECTS ON LAB TEST RESULTS
● May increase alkaline phosphatase, amylase, bilirubin, BUN, creatinine, LDH, and AST and ALT levels. May decrease potassium, protein, calcium, sodium, and hemoglobin levels and hematocrit. May increase or decrease glucose levels.
● May increase WBC count and INR. May prolong activated PTT and PT. May decrease platelet count.

CONTRAINDICATIONS & CAUTIONS
● Contraindicated in patients hypersensitive to drug.
● Use cautiously in patients with severe hepatic impairment and in those hypersensitive to tetracycline antibiotics. Also use cautiously as monotherapy in patients with complicated intra-abdominal infections caused by intestinal perforation.
● Use cautiously in breast-feeding women. Use during pregnancy only if potential benefit justifies potential risk to fetus.

NURSING CONSIDERATIONS
● If patient develops diarrhea, monitor him closely for pseudomembranous colitis.
● If patient has abdominal infection caused by intestinal perforation, monitor for sepsis.
● Monitor patient for symptoms of dangerous toxicities of tetracyclines, such as photosensitivity, pseudotumor cerebri, pancreatitis, and antianabolic action (increased BUN level, azotemia, acidosis, and hypophosphatemia).

PATIENT TEACHING
● Tell patient that drug is used to treat only bacterial infections, not viral.
● Advise patient to take the full course of treatment, even if he feels better after a few days of therapy.
● Tell patient to report burning or pain at the I.V. site.
● Tell woman of childbearing age to avoid becoming pregnant during treatment. Urge those who use hormonal contraception to also use barrier contraception during treatment.
● Advise woman to notify her health care provider if pregnancy is suspected or confirmed.

20

Miscellaneous anti-infectives

aztreonam
chloramphenicol sodium
   succinate
clindamycin hydrochloride
clindamycin palmitate
   hydrochloride
clindamycin phosphate
daptomycin
doripenem
ertapenem sodium
imipenem and cilastatin sodium
linezolid
meropenem
nitrofurantoin macrocrystals
nitrofurantoin microcrystals
quinupristin and dalfopristin
telithromycin
vancomycin hydrochloride

---

aztreonam
AZ-tree-oh-nam

Azactam

Pharmacologic class: monobactam
Pregnancy risk category B

AVAILABLE FORMS
Injection: 500-mg vials, 1-g vials, 2-g vials

INDICATIONS & DOSAGES
➤ **UTI; septicemia; infections of lower respiratory tract, skin, and skin structures; intra-abdominal infections, surgical infections, and gynecologic infections caused by susceptible *Escherichia coli, Klebsiella pneumoniae, Proteus mirabilis, Pseudomonas aeruginosa, Enterobacter cloacae, K. oxytoca, Citrobacter* species, and *Serratia marcescens;* respiratory infections caused by *Haemophilus influenzae***
Adults: 500 mg to 2 g I.V. or I.M. every 8 to 12 hours. For severe systemic or life-threatening infections, 2 g every 6 to 8 hours. Maximum dose is 8 g daily.

Children ages 9 months to 15 years: 30 mg/kg every 6 to 8 hours I.V. Maximum dose is 120 mg/kg/day.
Neonates age 1 to 4 weeks who weigh more than 2 kg (4.4 lb) ♦ *:* 30 mg/kg I.V. every 6 hours.
Neonates age 1 to 4 weeks who weigh 2 kg or less ♦ *:* 30 mg/kg I.V. every 8 hours.
Neonates younger than 7 days who weigh more than 2 kg ♦ *:* 30 mg/kg I.V. every 8 hours.
Neonates younger than 7 days who weigh 2 kg or less ♦ *:* 30 mg/kg I.V. every 12 hours.
Adjust-a-dose: For adults with a creatinine clearance of 10 to 30 ml/minute, give 1 to 2 g; then give 50% of the usual dose at usual interval. If clearance is less than 10 ml/minute, give 500 mg to 2 g; then give 25% of the usual dose at usual interval. For serious infections, add 12½% of the initial dose to maintenance doses after each hemodialysis session. For adults with alcoholic cirrhosis, decrease dose by 20% to 25%.

ADMINISTRATION
I.V.
• Obtain specimen for culture and sensitivity tests before giving first dose. Begin therapy while awaiting results.
• For direct injection, reconstitute with 6 to 10 ml of sterile water for injection and immediately shake vial vigorously. Constituted solutions aren't for multiple-dose use. Discard unused solution.
• To give a bolus, inject drug over 3 to 5 minutes, directly into I.V. tubing.
• For infusion, reconstitute with a compatible I.V. solution to yield 20 mg/ml or less.
• Give infusions over 20 minutes to 1 hour.
• Give thawed solutions only by I.V. infusion.
• **Incompatibilities:** Acyclovir, amphotericin B, ampicillin sodium, azithromycin, chlorpromazine, daunorubicin, ganciclovir,

lorazepam, metronidazole, mitomycin, mitoxantrone, nafcillin, prochlorperazine, streptozocin, vancomycin.

I.M.
● To prepare I.M. injection, add at least 3 ml of one of the following solutions per gram of aztreonam: sterile water for injection, bacteriostatic water for injection, normal saline solution, or bacteriostatic normal saline solution.
● Give I.M. injections deep into a large muscle, such as the upper outer quadrant of the gluteus maximus or the side of the thigh. Give doses more than 1 g by I.V. route.
● *Alert:* Don't give I.M. injection to children.
● Pain and swelling may occur at injection site.

ACTION
Inhibits bacterial cell-wall synthesis, ultimately causing cell-wall destruction; bactericidal.

Route	Onset	Peak	Duration
I.V.	Unknown	Immediate	Unknown
I.M.	Unknown	< 1 hr	Unknown

Half-life: 2 hours.

ADVERSE REACTIONS
CNS: *seizures,* confusion, headache, insomnia.
CV: hypotension, thrombophlebitis.
GI: *pseudomembranous colitis,* diarrhea, nausea, vomiting.
Hematologic: *neutropenia, pancytopenia, thrombocytopenia,* anemia, leukocytosis, thrombocytosis.
Skin: discomfort and swelling at I.M. injection site, rash.
Other: hypersensitivity reactions.

INTERACTIONS
Drug-drug. *Aminoglycosides:* May have synergistic nephrotoxic effects. Monitor renal function.
Cefoxitin, imipenem: May have antagonistic effect. Avoid using together.
Furosemide: May increase aztreonam level. Avoid using together.
Probenecid: May increase aztreonam level. Avoid using together.

EFFECTS ON LAB TEST RESULTS
● May increase ALT, AST, BUN, creatinine, and LDH levels. May decrease hemoglobin level.
● May increase PT, PTT, and INR. May decrease neutrophil and RBC counts. May increase or decrease platelet and WBC counts.
● May cause false-positive Coombs' test result. May alter urine glucose determinations using cupric sulfate (Clinitest or Benedict reagent).

CONTRAINDICATIONS & CAUTIONS
● Contraindicated in patients hypersensitive to drug or any of its components.
● Use cautiously in elderly patients and in those with impaired renal or hepatic function. Dosage adjustment may be needed. Monitor renal function test results.
● Use during pregnancy only if clearly needed. Because aztreonam is excreted in breast milk, consider advising breast-feeding women to temporarily discontinue breast-feeding.

NURSING CONSIDERATIONS
● Observe patient for signs and symptoms of superinfection.
● *Alert:* Because drug is ineffective against gram-positive and anaerobic organisms, combine it with other antibiotics for immediate treatment of life-threatening illnesses.
● *Alert:* Patients allergic to penicillins or cephalosporins may not be allergic to this drug. Monitor closely those who have had an immediate hypersensitivity reaction to these antibiotics, especially to ceftazidime.
● Antibiotics may promote overgrowth of nonsusceptible organisms. Monitor patient for signs of superinfection.

PATIENT TEACHING
● Warn patient receiving I.M. drug that pain and swelling may occur at injection site.
● Tell patient to report discomfort at I.V. insertion site.
● Instruct patient to report adverse reactions and signs and symptoms of superinfection promptly.

Reactions may be *common,* uncommon, *life-threatening,* or COMMON AND LIFE-THREATENING.
Interaction may have a *rapid onset* or *delayed onset.*

chloramphenicol sodium succinate
klor-am-FEN-i-kole

Pentamycetin†

Pharmacologic class: dichloroacetic acid derivative
Pregnancy risk category C

AVAILABLE FORMS
Injection: 1-g vial

INDICATIONS & DOSAGES
➤ **Haemophilus influenzae meningitis, acute *Salmonella typhi* infection, and meningitis, bacteremia, or other severe infections caused by sensitive *Salmonella* species, rickettsia, lymphogranuloma, psittacosis, or various sensitive gram-negative organisms**
Adults: 50 to 100 mg/kg I.V. daily, divided every 6 hours. Maximum dose is 100 mg/kg daily.
Full-term infants older than age 2 weeks with normal metabolic processes: Up to 50 mg/kg I.V. daily, divided every 6 hours. May use up to 100 mg/kg/day in four divided doses for meningitis.
Premature infants, neonates age 2 weeks and younger, and children and infants with immature metabolic processes: 25 mg/kg I.V. once daily.

ADMINISTRATION
I.V.
• Reconstitute 1-g vial of powder for injection with 10 ml of sterile water for injection to yield 100 mg/ml.
• Give slowly over at least 1 minute.
• Check injection site daily for phlebitis and irritation.
• Solution is stable for 30 days at room temperature, but you should refrigerate it.
• Don't use cloudy solution.
• Obtain specimen for culture and sensitivity tests before giving first dose. Begin therapy while awaiting results.
• **Incompatibilities:** Chlorpromazine, fluconazole, glycopyrrolate, hydroxyzine, metoclopramide, polymyxin B sulfate, prochlorperazine, promethazine, vancomycin.

ACTION
Inhibits bacterial protein synthesis by binding to the 50S subunit of the ribosome; bacteriostatic.

Route	Onset	Peak	Duration
I.V.	Unknown	1–3 hr	Unknown

Half-life: 1½ to 4½ hours.

ADVERSE REACTIONS
CNS: confusion, delirium, headache, mild depression, optic and peripheral neuritis with prolonged therapy.
EENT: decreased visual acuity, optic neuritis in patients with cystic fibrosis.
GI: diarrhea, enterocolitis, glossitis, nausea, vomiting, stomatitis.
Hematologic: *aplastic anemia, granulocytopenia, hypoplastic anemia, pancytopenia, thrombocytopenia.*
Hepatic: jaundice.
Other: *anaphylaxis, gray syndrome in neonates,* hypersensitivity reactions.

INTERACTIONS
Drug-drug. *Anticoagulants, barbiturates, hydantoins, iron salts, sulfonylureas:* May increase levels of these drugs. Monitor patient for toxicity.
Penicillins: May have synergistic or antagonistic effects. Monitor patient for change in effectiveness.
Rifampin: May reduce chloramphenicol level. Monitor patient for changes in effectiveness.
Vitamin B_{12}: May decrease response of vitamin B_{12} in patients with pernicious anemia. Monitor patient closely.

EFFECTS ON LAB TEST RESULTS
• May decrease hemoglobin level.
• May decrease granulocyte and platelet counts.
• May falsely elevate urine PABA levels if given during a bentiromide test for pancreatic function. May cause false-positive results in urine glucose tests that use cupric sulfate (Clinitest).

CONTRAINDICATIONS & CAUTIONS
• Contraindicated in patients hypersensitive to drug.
■ **Black Box Warning** Drug has been reported to cause aplastic anemia and other serious and fatal blood dyscrasias. Use for serious infections only. ■
• Use cautiously in patients with impaired hepatic or renal function, acute intermittent porphyria, and G6PD deficiency.
• Use cautiously in those taking other drugs that cause bone marrow suppression or blood disorders.
• *Alert:* Use cautiously in premature infants and neonates because potentially fatal gray syndrome may occur. Symptoms include abdominal distention, gray cyanosis, vasomotor collapse, respiratory distress, and death within a few hours of symptom onset.
• Drug may be toxic to fetus. Give during pregnancy only if potential benefit justifies potential risk to fetus. Consider advising breast-feeding women to temporarily discontinue breast-feeding.

NURSING CONSIDERATIONS
■ **Black Box Warning** To facilitate appropriate studies and observation during therapy, patients taking chloramphenicol should be hospitalized. ■
• Obtain drug level measurement; maintain peak level of 10 to 20 mcg/ml and trough level of 5 to 10 mcg/ml.
• Monitor CBC, iron level, and platelet and reticulocyte counts before and every 2 days during therapy. Stop drug and notify prescriber immediately if anemia, reticulocytopenia, leukopenia, or thrombocytopenia develops.
• Monitor patient for signs and symptoms of superinfection.

PATIENT TEACHING
• Instruct patient to notify prescriber if adverse reactions occur, especially nausea, vomiting, diarrhea, fever, confusion, sore throat, or mouth sores.
• Tell patient receiving drug I.V. to report discomfort at I.V. insertion site.
• Instruct patient to report signs and symptoms of superinfection.

clindamycin hydrochloride
klin-da-MYE-sin

Cleocin, Dalacin C†

clindamycin palmitate hydrochloride
Cleocin Pediatric, Dalacin C Flavored Granules†

clindamycin phosphate
Cleocin Phosphate, Dalacin C Phosphate Sterile Solution†

Pharmacologic class: lincomycin derivative
Pregnancy risk category B

AVAILABLE FORMS
clindamycin hydrochloride
Capsules: 75 mg, 150 mg, 300 mg
clindamycin palmitate hydrochloride
Granules for oral solution: 75 mg/5 ml
clindamycin phosphate
Injectable infusion (in D₅W): 300 mg (50 ml), 600 mg (50 ml), 900 mg (50 ml)
Injection: 150-mg base/ml, 300-mg base/2 ml, 600-mg base/4 ml, 900-mg base/6 ml

INDICATIONS & DOSAGES
➤ **Infections caused by sensitive staphylococci, streptococci, pneumococci, *Bacteroides, Fusobacterium, Clostridium perfringens,* and other sensitive aerobic and anaerobic organisms**
Adults: 150 to 450 mg P.O. every 6 hours; or 300 to 600 mg I.M. or I.V. every 6, 8, or 12 hours. In more severe infections, dosage may be increased to 1,200 to 2,700 mg/day I.M. or I.V. in two, three, or four doses. In life-threatening infections, dosages as high as 4,800 mg daily can be given.
Children ages 1 month to 16 years: 20 to 40 mg/kg/day I.M. or I.V. in three or four equal doses. In beta-hemolytic streptococcal infections, treatment should continue for at least 10 days.
Neonates younger than age 1 month: 15 to 20 mg/kg/day I.M. or I.V. in three or four equal doses.
➤ **Pelvic inflammatory disease**
Adults and adolescents: 900 mg I.V. every 8 hours, with gentamicin. Continue at

least 48 hours after symptoms improve; then switch to oral clindamycin 450 mg q.i.d. for total of 10 to 14 days or doxycycline 100 mg P.O. every 12 hours for total of 10 to 14 days.

➤ *Pneumocystis jiroveci* (carinii) pneumonia◆

Adults: 300 to 450 mg P.O. every 6 to 8 hours or 600 to 900 mg I.V. every 6 to 8 hours with oral primaquine (15 to 30 mg once daily) for 21 days.

➤ **CNS toxoplasmosis in AIDS patients, as alternative to sulfonamides with pyrimethamine◆**

Adults: 1,200 to 2,400 mg/day in divided doses.

ADMINISTRATION

P.O.

● Obtain specimen for culture and sensitivity tests before giving first dose. Begin therapy while awaiting results.

● Give capsule form with a full glass of water to prevent esophageal irritation.

● Don't refrigerate reconstituted oral solution because it will thicken. Drug is stable for 2 weeks at room temperature.

I.V.

● Obtain specimen for culture and sensitivity tests before giving first dose. Begin therapy while awaiting results.

● Never give undiluted as a bolus.

● For infusion, dilute each 300 mg in 50 ml solution and give over 10 to 60 minutes at no more than 30 mg/minute.

● Check site daily for phlebitis and irritation.

● Drug may contain benzyl alcohol. Benzyl alcohol has been associated with a fatal gasping syndrome in premature infants.

● **Incompatibilities:** Allopurinol, aminophylline, ampicillin, azithromycin, barbiturates, calcium gluconate, ceftriaxone, ciprofloxacin hydrochloride, doxapram, filgrastim, fluconazole, gentamicin sulfate with cefazolin sodium, idarubicin, magnesium sulfate, phenytoin sodium, ranitidine, rubber closures such as those on I.V. tubing, tobramycin sulfate.

I.M.

● Obtain specimen for culture and sensitivity tests before giving first dose. Begin therapy while awaiting results.

● Inject deep into muscle. Rotate sites. Don't exceed 600 mg per injection.

ACTION

Inhibits bacterial protein synthesis by binding to the 50S subunit of the ribosome.

Route	Onset	Peak	Duration
P.O.	Unknown	45–60 min	Unknown
I.V.	Immediate	Immediate	Unknown
I.M.	Unknown	3 hr	Unknown

Half-life: 2½ to 3 hours.

ADVERSE REACTIONS

CV: thrombophlebitis.

GI: *nausea, pseudomembranous colitis,* abdominal pain, diarrhea, vomiting.

Hematologic: *thrombocytopenia, transient leukopenia,* eosinophilia.

Hepatic: jaundice.

Skin: maculopapular rash, urticaria.

Other: *anaphylaxis.*

INTERACTIONS

Drug-drug. *Erythromycin:* May block access of clindamycin to its site of action. Avoid using together.

Kaolin: May decrease absorption of oral clindamycin. Separate dosage times.

Neuromuscular blockers: May increase neuromuscular blockade. Monitor patient closely.

Paclitaxel: May increase paclitaxel effects. Observe patient for toxicity.

Drug-food. *Diet foods with sodium cyclamate:* May decrease drug level. Discourage patient from eating these foods.

EFFECTS ON LAB TEST RESULTS

● May increase alkaline phosphatase, AST, and bilirubin levels.

● May increase eosinophil count. May decrease platelet and WBC counts.

CONTRAINDICATIONS & CAUTIONS

● Contraindicated in patients hypersensitive to drug or lincomycin.

● Clindamycin use may result in overgrowth of nonsusceptible organisms, particularly yeasts. Monitor patient for sign of superinfection.

● Use cautiously in neonates and patients with renal or hepatic disease, asthma, history of GI disease, or significant allergies.

■ **Black Box Warning** Clindamycin therapy has been associated with severe, possibly fatal, colitis; its use should be reserved for serious infections. ■

NURSING CONSIDERATIONS
● I.M. injection may raise CK level in response to muscle irritation.
● Monitor renal, hepatic, and hematopoietic functions during prolonged therapy.
● Observe patient for signs and symptoms of superinfection.
● *Alert:* Don't give opioid antidiarrheals to treat drug-induced diarrhea; they may prolong and worsen this condition.
■ **Black Box Warning** Diarrhea, colitis, and pseudomembranous colitis have developed up to several weeks following cessation of drug therapy. ■
● Drug doesn't penetrate blood-brain barrier.

PATIENT TEACHING
● Advise patient to take capsule form with a full glass of water to prevent esophageal irritation.
● Warn patient that I.M. injection may be painful.
● Tell patient to report discomfort at I.V. insertion site.
● Instruct patient to notify prescriber of adverse reactions (especially diarrhea). Warn him not to treat diarrhea himself because drug may cause life-threatening colitis.

---

daptomycin
dap-toe-MYE-sin

Cubicin

Pharmacologic class: cyclic lipopeptide
Pregnancy risk category B

AVAILABLE FORMS
Powder for injection: 500-mg vial

INDICATIONS & DOSAGES
➤ **Bacteremia caused by *Staphylococcus aureus* (including right-sided endocarditis caused by methicillin-** susceptible and methicillin-resistant strains)
Adults: 6 mg/kg I.V. over 30 minutes every 24 hours for at least 2 to 6 weeks based on patient response.
➤ **Complicated skin or skin-structure infection (SSSI) caused by susceptible strains of *S. aureus* (including methicillin-resistant strains), *Streptococcus pyogenes*, *Streptococcus agalactiae*, *Streptococcus dysgalactiae*, and *Enterococcus faecalis* (vancomycin-susceptible strains only)**
Adults: 4 mg/kg I.V. over 30 minutes every 24 hours for 7 to 14 days.
Adjust-a-dose: In patients with SSSI with creatinine clearance less than 30 ml/minute, including those receiving hemodialysis or continuous ambulatory peritoneal dialysis, give 4 mg/kg I.V. every 48 hours. For bacteremic patients with a clearance less than 30 ml/minute, give 6 mg/kg I.V. every 48 hours. When possible, give drug after hemodialysis.

ADMINISTRATION
I.V.
● Obtain specimen for culture and sensitivity tests before giving first dose. Begin therapy while awaiting results.
● Reconstitute 500-mg vial with 10 ml of normal saline solution.
● Further dilute with normal saline solution.
● Infuse over 30 minutes.
● Refrigerate vials at 36° to 46° F (2° to 8° C).
● Vials are for single use; discard excess.
● Reconstituted and diluted solutions are stable 12 hours at room temperature or 48 hours at 36° to 46° F (2° to 8° C).
● **Incompatibilities:** Dextrose-containing solutions and other I.V. drugs. If an I.V. line is used for several drugs, flush the line with normal saline solution or lactated Ringer's injection between drugs.

ACTION
Binds to and depolarizes bacterial membranes to inhibit protein, DNA, and RNA synthesis, thus causing bacterial cell death.

Route	Onset	Peak	Duration
I.V.	Rapid	< 1 hr	Unknown

Half-life: About 8 hours.

Reactions may be *common,* uncommon, *life-threatening,* or COMMON AND LIFE-THREATENING.
Interaction may have a *rapid onset* or *delayed onset.*

ADVERSE REACTIONS
CNS: anxiety, confusion, dizziness, fever, headache, insomnia.
CV: *cardiac failure,* chest pain, edema, hypertension, hypotension.
EENT: sore throat.
GI: *pseudomembranous colitis,* abdominal pain, constipation, decreased appetite, diarrhea, nausea, vomiting.
GU: *renal failure,* urinary tract infection.
Hematologic: anemia.
Metabolic: *hypoglycemia,* hyperglycemia, hypokalemia.
Musculoskeletal: limb and back pain, myopathy.
Respiratory: cough, dyspnea.
Skin: cellulitis, injection site reactions, pruritus, rash.
Other: fungal infections.

INTERACTIONS
Drug-drug. *HMG-CoA reductase inhibitors:* May increase risk of myopathy. Consider stopping these drugs while giving daptomycin.
Tobramycin: May affect levels of both drugs. Use together cautiously.
Warfarin: May alter anticoagulant activity. Monitor PT and INR for the first several days of daptomycin therapy.

EFFECTS ON LAB TEST RESULTS
● May increase alkaline phosphatase and CK levels. May decrease potassium and hemoglobin levels and hematocrit. May increase or decrease glucose level.
● May increase liver function test values.

CONTRAINDICATIONS & CAUTIONS
● Contraindicated in patients hypersensitive to drug.
● Use cautiously in patients with renal insufficiency and those who are older than age 65, pregnant, or breast-feeding.
● Safety and effectiveness haven't been established in patients younger than age 18.

NURSING CONSIDERATIONS
● Monitor CBC and renal and liver function tests periodically.
● *Alert:* Because drug may increase the risk of myopathy, monitor CK level weekly. If CK level rises, monitor it more often. In patients with myopathy and CK elevation over 1,000 units/L or more than 10 times the upper limit of normal, stop drug. Consider stopping all other drugs linked with myopathy (such as HMG-CoA reductase inhibitors) during therapy.
● Monitor patient for superinfection because drug may cause overgrowth of nonsusceptible organisms.
● Watch for evidence of pseudomembranous colitis and treat accordingly.

PATIENT TEACHING
● Advise patient to immediately report muscle weakness and infusion site irritation.
● Tell patient to report severe diarrhea, rash, and infection.
● Inform patient about possible adverse reactions.

doripenem
dor-eh-PEN-em

Doribax

Pharmacologic class: carbapenem
Pregnancy risk category B

AVAILABLE FORMS
Injection: 500-mg vial

INDICATIONS & DOSAGES
➤ **Complicated intra-abdominal infections caused by *Escherichia coli, Klebsiella pneumoniae, Pseudomonas aeruginosa, Bacteroides caccae, B. fragilis, B. thetaiotaomicron, B. uniformis, B. vulgatas, Streptococcus intermedius, S. constellatus,* or *Peptostreptococcus micros***
Adults: 500 mg I.V. every 8 hours for 5 to 14 days.
➤ **Complicated urinary tract infections, including pyelonephritis caused by *E. coli, K. pneumoniae, Proteus mirabilis, Pseudomonas aeruginosa, Acinetobacter baumannii***
Adults: 500 mg I.V. every 8 hours for 10 days. May be given for 14 days to patient with concurrent bacteremia.
Adjust-a-dose: In patients with creatinine clearance of 30 to 50 ml/minute, give 250 mg I.V. every 8 hours; with creatinine clearance of 11 to 29 ml/minute give 250 mg I.V. every 12 hours.

ADMINISTRATION
I.V.
• Assess for history of allergies to beta-lactams (carbapenems, penicillins, cephalosporins).
• Obtain specimen for culture and sensitivity tests before beginning treatment.
• Dilute drug in single-use vials with 10 ml sterile water for injection or normal saline for injection, shake gently to form a concentration of 50 mg/ml.
• Add reconstituted drug to 100 ml normal saline or D₅W for a final concentration of 4.5 mg/ml.
• To prepare a 250-mg dose, remove 55 ml of solution from infusion bag.
• Inspect solution for particulate matter and discoloration. Solution should be clear to slightly yellow.
• Solution prepared with normal saline may be stored at room temperature for 8 hours; D₅W, for 4 hours.
• Give only by infusion over 1 hour.
• **Incompatibilities:** Other I.V. drugs.

ACTION
Inhibits bacterial cell-wall biosynthesis by inactivating multiple penicillin-binding proteins, causing cell death.

Route	Onset	Peak	Duration
I.V.	Rapid	1¼ hr	Unknown

Half-life: 1 hour.

ADVERSE REACTIONS
CNS: *headache, seizures.*
GI: *pseudomembranous colitis,* diarrhea, nausea.
GU: renal insufficiency, *renal failure.*
Hematologic: *anemia.*
Respiratory: interstitial pneumonia.
Skin: phlebitis, pruritus, rash, *Stevens-Johnson syndrome, toxic epidermal necrolysis.*
Other: *anaphylaxis,* infection.

INTERACTIONS
Drug-drug. *Valproic acid:* May decrease valproic acid level, causing seizures. Monitor valproic acid levels. May need to switch to another antibacterial or anticonvulsant if levels can't be maintained.
Probenecid: May increase drug level. Avoid using together.

EFFECTS ON LAB TEST RESULTS
• May increase ALT, AST, transaminase and other hepatic enzyme levels.
• May decrease RBC count.

CONTRAINDICATIONS & CAUTIONS
• Contraindicated in patients hypersensitive to drug, its components, or other beta-lactams.
• Use caution in those with moderate to severe renal impairment.

NURSING CONSIDERATIONS
• Monitor patient closely for pseudomembranous colitis, which can occur up to 2 months after drug administration.
• Monitor renal function.
• *Alert:* If allergic reaction occurs, stop drug, use supportive measures and contact the prescriber.
• To report suspected adverse reactions, contact the FDA at 1-800-FDA-1088 or *www.fda.gov/medwatch.*
• Safety and efficacy haven't been established in pregnant or pediatric patients. It's unknown whether drug is excreted in breast milk.

PATIENT TEACHING
• Tell patient to report any serious adverse effects such as dyspnea, skin reaction, pain at injection site, or diarrhea.
• *Alert:* Severe and life-threatening diarrhea can occur up to 2 months after drug is given; tell patient to report immediately.
• Advise woman to tell prescriber if she's pregnant or breast-feeding.

---

ertapenem sodium
er-tah-PEN-em

Invanz

Pharmacologic class: carbapenem
Pregnancy risk category B

AVAILABLE FORMS
Injection: 1 g

INDICATIONS & DOSAGES
➤ **Complicated intra-abdominal infection caused by** *Escherichia coli,*

Clostridium clostridiforme, Eubacterium lentum, Peptostreptococcus species, *Bacteroides fragilis, B. distasonis, B. ovatus, B. thetaiotaomicron,* or *B. uniformis*
Adults and children age 13 and older: 1 g I.V. or I.M. once daily for 5 to 14 days.
Infants and children ages 3 months to 13 years: 15 mg/kg I.V. or I.M. every 12 hours for 5 to 14 days. Don't exceed 1 g daily.

➤ **Complicated skin or skin-structure infection including diabetic foot infections without osteomyelitis caused by *Staphylococcus aureus* (methicillin-susceptible strains), *Streptococcus agalactiae, S. pyogenes, Escherichia coli, Klebsiella pneumoniae, Proteus mirabilis, Bacteroides fragilis, Peptostreptococcus* species, *Porphyromonas asaccharolytica,* or *Prevotella bivia***
Adults and children age 13 and older: 1 g I.V. or I.M. once daily for 7 to 14 days. Diabetic foot infections may need up to 28 days of treatment.
Infants and children ages 3 months to 13 years: 15 mg/kg I.V. or I.M. every 12 hours for 7 to 14 days. Don't exceed 1 g daily.

➤ **Community-acquired pneumonia from *S. pneumoniae* (penicillin-susceptible strains), *Haemophilus influenzae* (beta-lactamase–negative strains), or *Moraxella catarrhalis;* complicated UTI including pyelonephritis caused by *E. coli* or *K. pneumoniae***
Adults and children age 13 and older: 1 g I.V. or I.M. once daily for 10 to 14 days. If patient improves after at least 3 days of treatment, use appropriate oral therapy to complete the full course of therapy.
Infants and children ages 3 months to 13 years: 15 mg/kg I.V. or I.M. every 12 hours for 10 to 14 days. Don't exceed 1 g daily. If patient improves after at least 3 days of treatment, use appropriate oral therapy to complete the full course of therapy.

➤ **Acute pelvic infection, including postpartum endomyometritis, septic abortion, and postsurgical gynecologic infections caused by *S. agalactiae, E. coli, B. fragilis, P. asaccharolytica, Peptostreptococcus* species, or *P. bivia***
Adults and children age 13 and older: 1 g I.V. or I.M. once daily for 3 to 10 days.
Infants and children ages 3 months to 13 years: 15 mg/kg I.V. or I.M. every 12 hours for 3 to 10 days. Don't exceed 1 g daily.

Adjust-a-dose: In adult patients with creatinine clearance of 30 ml/minute or less, give 500 mg/dose. In hemodialysis patients receiving daily 500-mg dose less than 6 hours before hemodialysis, give supplementary 150-mg dose afterward. In hemodialysis patients receiving dose 6 hours or more before hemodialysis, no supplementary dose is needed.

➤ **Prevention of surgical site infection after elective colorectal surgery**
Adults: 1 g I.V. 1 hour before surgical incision.

ADMINISTRATION
I.V.
● Obtain specimens for culture and sensitivity testing before giving. Begin therapy while awaiting results.
● Before giving first dose, check for previous hypersensitivity to penicillin, cephalosporin, beta-lactam, or local amide-type anesthetics.
● Reconstitute 1-g vial with 10 ml of sterile water for injection, normal saline solution for injection, or bacteriostatic water for injection.
● Shake well to dissolve, and then immediately transfer contents to 50 ml of normal saline solution.
● Infuse over 30 minutes.
● Complete the infusion within 6 hours of reconstitution or refrigerate for up to 24 hours. Infuse within 4 hours once removed from refrigeration. Don't freeze.
● **Incompatibilities:** Diluents containing dextrose (alpha-D-glucose), other I.V. drugs.
I.M.
● Obtain specimens for culture and sensitivity testing before giving. Begin therapy while awaiting results.
● Before giving first dose, check for previous hypersensitivity to penicillin, cephalosporin, beta-lactam, or local amide-type anesthetics.

● Reconstitute 1-g vial with 3.2 ml of 1% lidocaine hydrochloride injection (without epinephrine). Shake vial thoroughly to form solution. Immediately withdraw the contents of the vial and give by deep I.M. injection into a large muscle, such as the gluteal muscles or lateral part of the thigh. Use the reconstituted I.M. solution within 1 hour after preparation. Don't give reconstituted solution I.V.

ACTION

Inhibits cell-wall synthesis through penicillin-binding proteins.

Route	Onset	Peak	Duration
I.V.	Immediate	30 min	24 hr
I.M.	Unknown	2 hr	24 hr

Half-life: 4 hours.

ADVERSE REACTIONS

CNS: altered mental status, anxiety, asthenia, dizziness, fatigue, fever, head-ache, insomnia.
CV: chest pain, edema, hypertension, hypotension, infused vein complication, phlebitis, swelling, tachycardia, thrombo-phlebitis.
EENT: pharyngitis.
GI: *diarrhea,* abdominal pain, acid regur-gitation, constipation, dyspepsia, nausea, oral candidiasis, vomiting.
GU: renal dysfunction, vaginitis.
Hematologic: *leukopenia, neutropenia, thrombocytopenia,* anemia, coagulation abnormalities, eosinophilia, *thrombo-cytosis.*
Hepatic: jaundice.
Metabolic: *hyperkalemia, hypokalemia,* hyperglycemia.
Musculoskeletal: leg pain.
Respiratory: cough, dyspnea, rales, *respiratory distress,* rhonchi.
Skin: erythema, extravasation, infusion site pain and redness, pruritus, rash.
Other: hypersensitivity reactions.

INTERACTIONS

Drug-drug. *Probenecid:* May reduce renal clearance and may increase half-life. Don't give together with probenecid to extend half-life.
Valproic acid: May decrease valproic acid levels, leading to loss of seizure control.

Monitor valproic acid levels, and observe patient for signs of seizure activity.

EFFECTS ON LAB TEST RESULTS

● May increase albumin, ALT, alkaline phosphatase, AST, bilirubin, creatinine, glucose, and potassium levels. May decrease hemoglobin level and hematocrit.
● May increase eosinophil count, PT, and urinary RBC or urine WBC counts. May decrease segmented neutrophil and serum WBC counts. May increase or decrease platelet count.

CONTRAINDICATIONS & CAUTIONS

● Contraindicated in patients hypersensitive to any component of the drug or to other drugs in the same class and in patients who have had anaphylactic reactions to beta-lactams. I.M. use is contraindicated in patients hypersensitive to local anesthetics of the amide type (because of drug's diluent, lidocaine hydrochloride).
● Use cautiously in patients with CNS disorders, compromised renal function, or both, as seizures may occur in these patients.

NURSING CONSIDERATIONS

● If patient has diarrhea during therapy, notify prescriber and collect stool specimen for culture to rule out pseudo-membranous colitis.
● Vomiting occurs more frequently in children than adults. Monitor children closely for signs and symptoms of dehydration and electrolyte imbalance.
● If allergic reaction occurs, stop drug immediately.
● Anaphylactic reactions require immedi-ate emergency treatment with epinephrine, oxygen, I.V. steroids, and airway management.
● Anticonvulsants may continue in patients with seizure disorders. If focal tremors, myoclonus, or seizures occur, notify pre-scriber. Drug may need to be decreased or stopped.
● Monitor renal, hepatic, and hemato-poietic function during prolonged therapy.
● Methicillin-resistant staphylococci and *Enterococcus* species are resistant to drug.
● ***Look alike–sound alike:*** Don't confuse Invanz with Avinza.

PATIENT TEACHING
- Tell patient about adverse reactions.
- Tell patient to alert nurse if discomfort occurs at injection site.

---

imipenem and cilastatin sodium
im-ih-PEN-em and sye-luh-STAT-in

Primaxin I.M., Primaxin I.V.

Pharmacologic class: carbapenem, beta-lactam
Pregnancy risk category C

AVAILABLE FORMS
Powder for injection: 250 mg, 500 mg, 750 mg

INDICATIONS & DOSAGES
➤ **Serious lower respiratory tract, bone, intra-abdominal, gynecologic, joint, skin, and soft-tissue infections; UTIs; endocarditis; and bacterial septicemia, caused by** *Acinetobacter, Enterococcus, Staphylococcus, Streptococcus, Escherichia coli, Haemophilus, Klebsiella, Morganella, Proteus, Enterobacter, Pseudomonas aeruginosa,* **and** *Bacteroides,* **including** *B. fragilis*
Adults who weigh more than 70 kg (154 lb): 250 mg to 1 g by I.V. infusion every 6 to 8 hours. Maximum daily dose is 50 mg/kg/day or 4 g/day, whichever is less. Or, 500 to 750 mg I.M. every 12 hours. Maximum I.M. daily dose is 1,500 mg.
Children age 3 months and older (except for CNS infections): 15 to 25 mg/kg I.V. every 6 hours. Maximum daily dose is 2 to 4 g.
Infants ages 4 weeks to 3 months who weigh 1.5 kg (3.3 lb) or more (except for CNS infections): 25 mg/kg I.V. every 6 hours.
Neonates ages 1 to 4 weeks who weigh 1.5 kg or more (except for CNS infections): 25 mg/kg I.V. every 8 hours.
Neonates younger than age 1 week who weigh 1.5 kg or more (except for CNS infections): 25 mg/kg I.V. every 12 hours.
Adjust-a-dose: If creatinine clearance is less than 70 ml/minute, adjust dosage and monitor renal function test results. Consult manufacturer's package insert for spe-

cific dosage adjustments. For patients on hemodialysis, administer dose after hemodialysis and at 12-hour intervals timed from the end of that dialysis session.

ADMINISTRATION
I.V.
- Obtain specimens for culture and sensitivity testing before giving first dose. Begin therapy while awaiting results.
- Reconstitute piggyback units with 100 ml of compatible I.V. solution to provide solution containing 2.5 to 5 mg/ml.
- When reconstituting powder, shake until the solution is clear. Solutions may be colorless to yellow; variations of color within this range don't affect drug's potency.
- After reconstitution, solution is stable for 4 hours at room temperature and for 24 hours when refrigerated.
- Don't give by direct I.V. bolus injection.
- For adults, give each 250- or 500-mg dose by I.V. infusion over 20 to 30 minutes. Infuse each 750-mg to 1-g dose over 40 to 60 minutes.
- For children, infuse doses of 500 mg or less over 15 to 30 minutes. Infuse doses greater than 500 mg over 40 to 60 minutes. If nausea occurs, the infusion may be slowed.
- **Incompatibilities:** Allopurinol, antibiotics, amiodarone, amphotericin B cholesterol complex, azithromycin, dextrose 5% in lactated Ringer's injection, etoposide, fluconazole, gemcitabine, lorazepam, meperidine, midazolam, milrinone, sargramostim, sodium bicarbonate.
I.M.
- Obtain specimen culture and sensitivity tests before giving first dose. Begin therapy while awaiting results.
- *Alert:* Don't give I.M. solution by I.V. route.

ACTION
Inhibits bacterial cell-wall synthesis; enzymatic breakdown of drug in the kidneys causes adequate antibacterial levels of drug in the urine.

Route	Onset	Peak	Duration
I.V.	Immediate	Immediate	Unknown
I.M.	Unknown	1–2 hr	Unknown

Half-life: 1 hour after I.V. dose; 2 to 3 hours after I.M. dose.

ADVERSE REACTIONS

CNS: *seizures,* dizziness, fever, somnolence.
CV: hypotension, thrombophlebitis.
GI: *pseudomembranous colitis,* diarrhea, nausea, vomiting.
Hematologic: *leukopenia, thrombocytopenia,* eosinophilia.
Skin: injection site pain, pruritus, rash, urticaria.
Other: *anaphylaxis,* hypersensitivity reactions.

INTERACTIONS

Drug-drug. *Beta-lactam antibiotics:* May have antagonistic effect. Avoid using together.
Ganciclovir: May cause seizures. Avoid using together.
Probenecid: May increase cilastatin level. May be used together for this effect.

EFFECTS ON LAB TEST RESULTS

• May increase BUN, creatinine, ALT, AST, alkaline phosphatase, bilirubin, and LDH levels.
• May increase eosinophil count. May decrease WBC and platelet counts.
• May interfere with glucose determination by Benedict's solution or Clinitest.

CONTRAINDICATIONS & CAUTIONS

• Contraindicated in patients hypersensitive to drug, in those with a history of hypersensitivity to local anesthetics of the amide type, and in those with severe shock or heart block.
• Use cautiously in patients allergic to penicillins or cephalosporins because drug has similar properties.
• Use cautiously in patients with history of seizure disorders, especially if they also have compromised renal function.
• Use cautiously in children younger than age 3 months.

NURSING CONSIDERATIONS

• *Alert:* Don't use for CNS infections in children because drug increases the risk of seizures.
• *Alert:* If seizures develop and persist despite anticonvulsant therapy, stop drug and notify prescriber.
• For patients receiving hemodialysis, drug is recommended only when benefits outweigh possible risk of seizures.

• Monitor patient for bacterial or fungal superinfections and resistant infections during and after therapy.

PATIENT TEACHING

• Instruct patient to report adverse reactions promptly.
• Tell patient to report discomfort at I.V. insertion site.
• Urge patient to notify prescriber about loose stools or diarrhea.

---

linezolid
lih-NEH-zoe-lid

Zyvox

Pharmacologic class: oxazolidinone
Pregnancy risk category C

AVAILABLE FORMS

Injection: 2 mg/ml
Powder for oral suspension: 100 mg/5 ml when reconstituted
Tablets: 400 mg, 600 mg

INDICATIONS & DOSAGES

➤ **Vancomycin-resistant *Enterococcus faecium* infections, including those with concurrent bacteremia**
Adults and children age 12 and older: 600 mg I.V. or P.O. every 12 hours for 14 to 28 days.
Neonates age 7 days or older and infants and children through age 11: 10 mg/kg I.V. or P.O. every 8 hours for 14 to 28 days.
Neonates younger than age 7 days: 10 mg/kg I.V. or P.O. every 12 hours for 14 to 28 days. Increase to 10 mg/kg every 8 hours when patient is 7 days old. Consider this dosage increase if neonate has inadequate response.
➤ **Hospital-acquired pneumonia caused by *Staphylococcus aureus* (methicillin-susceptible [MSSA] and methicillin-resistant [MRSA] strains) or *Streptococcus pneumoniae* (including multidrug-resistant strains [MDRSP]); complicated skin and skin-structure infections, including diabetic foot infections without osteomyelitis caused by *S. aureus* (MSSA and MRSA), *S. pyogenes,* or**

S. agalactiae; community-acquired pneumonia caused by *S. pneumoniae* (including MDRSP), including those with concurrent bacteremia, or *S. aureus* (MSSA only)

Adults and children age 12 and older: 600 mg I.V. or P.O. every 12 hours for 10 to 14 days.

Neonates 7 days or older, infants and children through 11 years: 10 mg/kg I.V. or P.O. every 8 hours for 10 to 14 days.

Neonates younger than age 7 days: 10 mg/kg I.V. or P.O. every 12 hours for 10 to 14 days. Increase to 10 mg/kg every 8 hours when patient is 7 days old. Consider this dosage increase if neonate has inadequate response.

➤ Uncomplicated skin and skin-structure infections caused by *S. aureus* (MSSA only) or *S. pyogenes*

Adults: 400 mg P.O. every 12 hours for 10 to 14 days.

Children ages 12 to 18: 600 mg P.O. every 12 hours for 10 to 14 days.

Children ages 5 to 11: 10 mg/kg P.O. every 12 hours for 10 to 14 days.

Neonates age 7 days or older and infants and children younger than age 5: 10 mg/kg P.O. every 8 hours for 10 to 14 days.

Neonates younger than age 7 days: 10 mg/kg P.O. every 12 hours for 10 to 14 days. Increase to 10 mg/kg every 8 hours when patient is 7 days old. Consider this dosage increase if neonate has inadequate response.

ADMINISTRATION

P.O.
● Give tablets and suspension with or without meals.
● Reconstitute suspension according to manufacturer's instructions.
● Store reconstituted suspension at room temperature and use within 21 days.

I.V.
● Inspect solution for particulate matter and leaks.
● Drug is compatible with D₅W injection, normal saline solution for injection, and lactated Ringer's injection.
● Don't inject additives into infusion bag. Give other I.V. drugs separately or via a separate I.V. line to avoid incompatibilities. If single I.V. line is used, flush line

before and after infusion with a compatible solution.
● Infuse over 30 minutes to 2 hours. Don't infuse drug in a series connection.
● Store drug at room temperature in its protective overwrap. Solution may turn yellow over time, but this doesn't affect drug's potency.
● **Incompatibilities:** Amphotericin B, ceftriaxone sodium, chlorpromazine hydrochloride, diazepam, erythromycin lactobionate, pentamidine isethionate, phenytoin sodium, trimethoprim-sulfamethoxazole.

ACTION

Prevents bacterial protein synthesis by interfering with DNA translation in the ribosomes. Also prevents formation of a functional 70S ribosomal subunit by binding to a site on the bacterial 50S ribosomal subunit.

Route	Onset	Peak	Duration
P.O.	Unknown	1 hr	Unknown
I.V.	Unknown	30 min	Unknown

Half-life: 6¼ hours.

ADVERSE REACTIONS

CNS: *headache,* dizziness, fever, insomnia.
GI: *diarrhea, nausea, pseudomembranous colitis,* altered taste, constipation, oral candidiasis, tongue discoloration, vomiting.
GU: vaginal candidiasis.
Hematologic: *leukopenia, myelosuppression, neutropenia, thrombocytopenia,* anemia.
Skin: rash.
Other: fungal infection.

INTERACTIONS

Drug-drug. *Adrenergic drugs (such as dopamine, epinephrine, pseudoephedrine):* May cause hypertension. Monitor blood pressure and heart rate; start continuous infusions of dopamine and epinephrine at lower doses and titrate to response.
Serotoninergic drugs: May cause serotonin syndrome, including confusion, delirium, restlessness, tremors, blushing, diaphoresis, and hyperpyrexia. Notify prescriber immediately of signs and symptoms of serotonin syndrome.

Drug-food. *Foods and beverages high in tyramine (such as aged cheeses, air-dried meats, red wines, sauerkraut, soy sauce, tap beers):* May increase blood pressure. Provide a list of foods containing tyramine and advise patient that tyramine content of meals shouldn't exceed 100 mg.

EFFECTS ON LAB TEST RESULTS
• May increase ALT, AST, bilirubin, alkaline phosphatase, creatinine, amylase, lipase, and BUN levels. May decrease hemoglobin level.
• May decrease WBC, neutrophil, and platelet counts.

CONTRAINDICATIONS & CAUTIONS
• Contraindicated in patients hypersensitive to drug or its components.

NURSING CONSIDERATIONS
• No dosage adjustment is needed when switching from I.V. to P.O. forms.
• *Alert:* Nausea and vomiting may be symptoms of lactic acidosis. Monitor patient for unexplained acidosis or low bicarbonate level and notify prescriber immediately if these occur.
• *Alert:* Drug may cause thrombocytopenia. In patients at increased risk for bleeding, those with existing thrombocytopenia, those taking other drugs that may cause thrombocytopenia, and those receiving this drug for longer than 14 days, monitor platelet count.
• *Alert:* Drug may lead to myelosuppression. Monitor CBC weekly.
• *Alert:* Pseudomembranous colitis or superinfection may occur. Consider these diagnoses and take appropriate measures in patients with persistent diarrhea or secondary infections.
• Inappropriate use of antibiotics may lead to development of resistant organisms; carefully consider other drugs before starting therapy, especially in outpatient setting.
• *Look alike–sound alike:* Don't confuse Zyvox with Zovirax. Both come in a 400-mg strength.

PATIENT TEACHING
• Tell patient that tablets and oral suspension may be taken with or without meals.

• Stress importance of completing entire course of therapy, even if patient feels better.
• Tell patient to alert prescriber if he has high blood pressure, is taking cough or cold preparations, or is being treated with SSRIs or other antidepressants.
• Advise patient to avoid large quantities of tyramine-containing foods (such as aged cheeses, soy sauce, tap beers, red wine) during therapy.
• Inform patient with phenylketonuria that each 5 ml of oral suspension contains 20 mg of phenylalanine. Tablets and injection don't contain phenylalanine.

---

meropenem
mare-oh-PEN-em

Merrem IV

Pharmacologic class: carbapenem
Pregnancy risk category B

AVAILABLE FORMS
Powder for injection: 500 mg, 1 g

INDICATIONS & DOSAGES
➤ **Complicated skin and skin structure infections from *Staphylococcus aureus* (beta-lactamase or non-beta-lactamase–producing, methicillin-susceptible isolates only), *Streptococcus pyogenes*, *S. agalactiae*, viridans group streptococci, *Enterococcus faecalis* (excluding vancomycin-resistant isolates), *Pseudomonas aeruginosa*, *Escherichia coli*, *Proteus mirabilis*, *Bacteroides fragilis*, and *Peptostreptococcus* species**
Adults and children who weigh more than 50 kg (110 lb): 500 mg I.V. every 8 hours over 15 to 30 minutes as I.V. infusion.
Children ages 3 months and older who weigh 50 kg or less: 10 mg/kg I.V. every 8 hours over 15 to 30 minutes as I.V. infusion or over 3 to 5 minutes as I.V. bolus injection (5 to 20 ml); maximum dose is 500 mg I.V. every 8 hours.
➤ **Complicated appendicitis and peritonitis from viridans group streptococci, *E. coli*, *Klebsiella pneu-***

---

moniae, Pseudomonas aeruginosa,
B. fragilis, B. thetaiotaomicron, and
Peptostreptococcus species
Adults and children who weigh more than
50 kg: 1 g I.V. every 8 hours over 15 to
30 minutes as I.V. infusion or over 3 to
5 minutes as I.V. bolus injection (5 to
20 ml).
Children ages 3 months and older, who
weigh 50 kg or less: 20 mg/kg I.V. every
8 hours over 15 to 30 minutes as I.V. infusion or over 3 to 5 minutes as I.V. bolus
injection (5 to 20 ml); maximum dose is
1 g I.V. every 8 hours.
Adjust-a-dose: For adults with creatinine
clearance of 26 to 50 ml/minute, give
usual dose every 12 hours. If clearance is
10 to 25 ml/minute, give half usual dose
every 12 hours; if clearance is less than
10 ml/minute, give half usual dose every
24 hours.

➤ **Bacterial meningitis from**
S. pneumoniae, Haemophilus
influenzae, and *Neisseria*
meningitidis
Children who weigh more than 50 kg:
2 g I.V. every 8 hours.
Children ages 3 months and older, who
weigh 50 kg or less: 40 mg/kg I.V. every
8 hours; maximum dose, 2 g I.V. every
8 hours.

ADMINISTRATION
I.V.
● Obtain specimen for culture and sensitivity tests before giving first dose. Begin
therapy while awaiting results.
● *Alert:* Serious hypersensitivity reactions
may occur in patients receiving beta-
lactams. Before therapy begins,
determine if patient has had previous
hypersensitivity reactions to penicillins,
cephalosporins, betalactams, or other
allergens. If an allergic reaction occurs,
stop drug and notify prescriber. Serious
anaphylactic reactions require emergency
treatment.
● Use freshly prepared solutions of drug
immediately whenever possible. Stability
of drug varies with form of drug used
(injection vial, infusion vial, or ADD-
Vantage container).
● For bolus, add 10 ml of sterile water
for injection to 500 mg/20-ml vial or
20 ml to 1 g/30-ml vial. Shake to dissolve,

and let stand until clear. Give over 3 to
5 minutes.
● For infusion, an infusion vial (500 mg/
100 ml or 1 g/100 ml) may be directly
reconstituted with a compatible infusion
fluid. Or, an injection vial may be
reconstituted and the resulting solution
added to an I.V. container and further
diluted with an appropriate infusion
fluid. Don't use ADD-Vantage vials
for this purpose. Give over 15 to
30 minutes.
● For ADD-Vantage vials, constitute
only with half-normal saline solution
for injection, normal saline solution
for injection, or D₅W in 50-, 100-, or
250-ml Abbott ADD-Vantage flexible
diluent containers. Follow manufacturer's
guidelines closely when using ADD-
Vantage vials.
● **Incompatibilities:** Other I.V. drugs.

ACTION
Inhibits cell-wall synthesis in bacteria.
Readily penetrates cell wall of most
gram-positive and gram-negative bacteria
to reach penicillin-binding protein targets.

Route	Onset	Peak	Duration
I.V.	Unknown	1 hr	Unknown

Half-life: 1 hour.

ADVERSE REACTIONS
CNS: *seizures,* headache, pain.
CV: phlebitis, thrombophlebitis.
GI: *pseudomembranous colitis,* cons-
tipation, diarrhea, glossitis, nausea, oral
candidiasis, vomiting.
GU: RBCs in urine.
Hematologic: anemia.
Respiratory: *apnea,* dyspnea.
Skin: injection site inflammation,
pruritus, rash.
Other: *anaphylaxis,* hypersensitivity
reactions, inflammation.

INTERACTIONS
Drug-drug. *Probenecid:* May decrease
renal excretion of meropenem; probenecid
competes with meropenem for active
tubular secretion, which significantly
increases elimination half-life of
meropenem and extent of systemic
exposure. Avoid using together.

EFFECTS ON LAB TEST RESULTS
- May increase ALT, AST, bilirubin, alkaline phosphatase, LDH, creatinine, and BUN levels. May decrease hemoglobin level and hematocrit.
- May increase eosinophil count. May decrease WBC count. May increase or decrease PT, PTT, and INR, and platelet count.

CONTRAINDICATIONS & CAUTIONS
- Contraindicated in patients hypersensitive to components of drug or other drugs in same class and in patients who have had anaphylactic reactions to beta-lactams.
- Use cautiously in elderly patients and in those with a history of seizure disorders or impaired renal function.
- Safety and effectiveness of drug haven't been established for infants younger than age 3 months.
- Use drug cautiously in breast-feeding women; it's unknown if drug appears in breast milk.

NURSING CONSIDERATIONS
- In patients with CNS disorders, bacterial meningitis, and compromised renal function, drug may cause seizures and other CNS adverse reactions.
- If seizures occur during therapy, stop infusion and notify prescriber. Dosage adjustment may be needed.
- Monitor patient for signs and symptoms of superinfection. Drug may cause overgrowth of nonsusceptible bacteria or fungi.
- Periodic assessment of organ system functions, including renal, hepatic, and hematopoietic function, is recommended during prolonged therapy.
- Monitor patient's fluid balance and weight carefully.

PATIENT TEACHING
- Advise woman not to breast-feed during therapy.
- Instruct patient to report adverse reactions or signs and symptoms of superinfection.
- Advise patient to report loose stools to prescriber.

nitrofurantoin macrocrystals
nye-troh-fyoo-RAN-toyn

Macrobid✔, Macrodantin

nitrofurantoin microcrystals
Furadantin, Novo-Furantoin†

Pharmacologic class: nitrofuran
Pregnancy risk category B

AVAILABLE FORMS
nitrofurantoin macrocrystals
Capsules: 25 mg, 50 mg, 100 mg
nitrofurantoin microcrystals
Oral suspension: 25 mg/5 ml

INDICATIONS & DOSAGES
➤ **UTIs caused by susceptible *Escherichia coli, Staphylococcus aureus, enterococci;* or certain strains of *Klebsiella* and *Enterobacter* species**
Adults and children older than age 12 years: 50 to 100 mg P.O. q.i.d. with meals and at bedtime. Or, 100 mg Macrobid P.O. every 12 hours for 7 days.
Children ages 1 month to 12 years: 5 to 7 mg/kg P.O. daily, divided q.i.d.
➤ **Long-term suppression therapy**
Adults: 50 to 100 mg P.O. daily at bedtime.
Children: 1 mg/kg P.O. daily in a single dose at bedtime or divided into two doses given every 12 hours.

ADMINISTRATION
P.O.
- Obtain urine specimen for culture and sensitivity tests before giving. Repeat as needed. Begin therapy while awaiting results.
- Give drug with food or milk to minimize GI distress and improve absorption.

ACTION
May interfere with bacterial enzyme systems and bacterial cell-wall formation.

Route	Onset	Peak	Duration
P.O.	Unknown	Unknown	Unknown

Half-life: 15 minutes to 1 hour.

Reactions may be *common*, uncommon, *life-threatening*, or COMMON AND LIFE-THREATENING.
Interaction may have a *rapid onset* or *delayed onset.*

ADVERSE REACTIONS
CNS: *ascending polyneuropathy with high doses or renal impairment,* dizziness, drowsiness, headache, peripheral neuropathy.
GI: *anorexia, diarrhea, nausea, vomiting,* abdominal pain.
GU: overgrowth of nonsusceptible organisms in urinary tract.
Hematologic: *agranulocytosis, hemolysis in patients with G6PD deficiency, thrombocytopenia.*
Hepatic: *hepatic necrosis, hepatitis.*
Metabolic: *hypoglycemia.*
Respiratory: *asthmatic attacks, pulmonary sensitivity reactions.*
Skin: *Stevens-Johnson syndrome,* exfoliative dermatitis, maculopapular, erythematous, or eczematous eruption, pruritus, transient alopecia, urticaria.
Other: *anaphylaxis,* drug fever, hypersensitivity reactions.

INTERACTIONS
Drug-drug. *Antacids containing magnesium:* May decrease nitrofurantoin absorption. Separate dosage times by 1 hour.
Probenecid, sulfinpyrazone: May inhibit excretion of nitrofurantoin, increasing drug levels and risk of toxicity. The resulting decreased urinary levels could lessen antibacterial effects. Avoid using together.
Drug-food. *Any food:* May increase absorption. Advise patient to take drug with food or milk.

EFFECTS ON LAB TEST RESULTS
● May increase bilirubin and alkaline phosphatase levels. May decrease glucose level.
● May decrease granulocyte and platelet counts.
● May cause false-positive results in urine glucose tests using cupric sulfate (such as Benedict's reagent, Fehling's solution, or Chemstrip uG).

CONTRAINDICATIONS & CAUTIONS
● Contraindicated in infants age 1 month and younger and in patients with anuria, oliguria, or creatinine clearance less than 60 ml/minute. Also contraindicated in pregnant patients at 38 to 42 weeks' gestation and during labor and delivery.
● Use cautiously in patients with renal impairment, asthma, anemia, diabetes mellitus, electrolyte abnormalities, vitamin B deficiency, debilitating disease, and G6PD deficiency.

NURSING CONSIDERATIONS
● Drug may cause an asthma attack in patients with a history of asthma.
● Monitor fluid intake and output carefully. Treatment may turn urine brown or dark yellow.
● Monitor CBC, renal function, and pulmonary status regularly.
● **Alert:** Monitor patient for signs and symptoms of superinfection. Use of nitrofurantoin may result in growth of nonsusceptible organisms, especially *Pseudomonas* species.
● Monitor patient for pulmonary sensitivity reactions, including cough, chest pain, fever, chills, dyspnea, and pulmonary infiltration with consolidation or effusions.
● **Alert:** Hypersensitivity may develop when drug is used for long-term therapy.
● Some patients may experience fewer adverse GI effects with nitrofurantoin macrocrystals.
● Dual-release capsules (25 mg nitrofurantoin macrocrystals combined with 75 mg nitrofurantoin monohydrate) enable patients to take drug only twice daily.
● Continue treatment for 3 days after sterile urine specimens have been obtained.
● Store drug in amber container. Don't store in metals other than stainless steel or aluminum to avoid precipitation.

PATIENT TEACHING
● Instruct patient to take drug for as long as prescribed, exactly as directed, even after he feels better.
● Tell patient to take drug with food or milk to minimize stomach upset.
● Instruct patient to report adverse reactions, especially peripheral neuropathy, which can become severe or irreversible.
● Alert patient that drug may turn urine dark yellow or brown.
● Warn patient not to store drug in metals other than stainless steel or aluminum.
● Advise patient not to use antacid preparations containing magnesium trisilicate.

quinupristin and dalfopristin
QUIN-uh-pris-tin and
DALF-oh-pris-tin

Synercid

Pharmacologic class: streptogramin
Pregnancy risk category B

AVAILABLE FORMS
Injection: 500 mg/10 ml (150 mg quinupristin and 350 mg dalfopristin)

INDICATIONS & DOSAGES
■ **Black Box Warning** Serious or
life-threatening infections with
vancomycin-resistant *Enterococcus
faecium* bacteremia under the FDA's
accelerated approval regulations for
use in life-threatening conditions when
other therapies aren't available. ■
Adults and adolescents age 16 and older:
7.5 mg/kg I.V. over 1 hour every 8 hours.
Length of treatment depends on site and
severity of infection.
➤ **Complicated skin and skin-
structure infections caused by
methicillin-susceptible *Staphylococcus aureus* or *Streptococcus
pyogenes***
Adults and adolescents age 16 and older:
7.5 mg/kg I.V. over 1 hour every 12 hours
for at least 7 days.

ADMINISTRATION
I.V.
● Reconstitute powder for injection by
adding 5 ml of either sterile water for injection or D_5W and gently swirling vial by
manual rotation to ensure dissolution; avoid
shaking to limit foaming. Reconstituted
solutions must be further diluted within
30 minutes.
● Add appropriate dose of reconstituted
solution to 250 ml of D_5W, according to
patient's weight, to yield no more than
2 mg/ml. This diluted solution is stable for
5 hours at room temperature or 54 hours if
refrigerated.
● Flush line with D_5W before and after
each dose.
● Fluid-restricted patients with a central
venous catheter may receive dose in
100 ml of D_5W. This concentration isn't

recommended for peripheral venous
administration.
● If moderate to severe peripheral venous
irritation occurs, consider increasing
infusion volume to 500 or 750 ml, changing injection site, or infusing by a central
venous catheter.
● Give all doses by I.V. infusion over
1 hour. An infusion pump or device may
be used to control infusion rate.
● **Incompatibilities:** Saline and heparin
solutions.

ACTION
The two antibiotics work synergistically to
inhibit or destroy susceptible bacteria
through combined inhibition of protein
synthesis in bacterial cells. Without the
ability to manufacture new proteins, the
bacterial cells are inactivated or die.

Route	Onset	Peak	Duration
I.V.	Unknown	Unknown	Unknown

Half-life: Quinupristin, 1 hour; dalfopristin,
¾ hour.

ADVERSE REACTIONS
CNS: headache, pain.
CV: thrombophlebitis.
GI: diarrhea, nausea, vomiting.
Musculoskeletal: arthralgia, myalgia.
Skin: *edema at infusion site, inflammation,
infusion site reaction, pain at infusion site,*
pruritus, rash.

INTERACTIONS
Drug-drug. *Cyclosporine:* May lower
metabolism; may increase drug level.
Monitor cyclosporine level.
*Drugs metabolized by CYP3A4, such as
carbamazepine, delavirdine, diazepam,
diltiazem, disopyramide, docetaxel,
indinavir, lidocaine, lovastatin, methylprednisolone, midazolam, nevirapine,
nifedipine, paclitaxel, ritonavir, tacrolimus,
verapamil, vinblastine:* May increase
levels of these drugs, which could increase
both their therapeutic effects and adverse
reactions. Use together cautiously.
*Drugs metabolized by CYP3A4 that may
prolong the QTc interval, such as quinidine:* May decrease metabolism of these
drugs, prolonging QTc interval. Avoid
using together.

Reactions may be *common,* uncommon, *life-threatening,* or COMMON AND LIFE-THREATENING.
Interaction may have a *rapid onset* or **delayed onset.**

EFFECTS ON LAB TEST RESULTS
• May increase AST, ALT, and bilirubin levels.

CONTRAINDICATIONS & CAUTIONS
• Contraindicated in patients hypersensitive to drug or other streptogramin antibiotics.
• Safety and efficacy haven't been established in patients younger than age 16.
• Use only during pregnancy if clearly needed. Use cautiously in breast-feeding women.

NURSING CONSIDERATIONS
• Drug isn't active against *Enterococcus faecalis*. Blood cultures are needed to avoid misidentifying *E. faecalis* as *E. faecium*.
• Because drug may cause mild to life-threatening pseudomembranous colitis, consider this diagnosis in patient who develops diarrhea during or after therapy.
• Adverse reactions, such as arthralgia and myalgia, may be reduced by decreasing dosage interval to every 12 hours.
• Because overgrowth of nonsusceptible organisms may occur, monitor patient closely for signs and symptoms of superinfection.
• Monitor liver function test results during therapy.

PATIENT TEACHING
• Advise patient to immediately report irritation at I.V. site, pain in joints or muscles, and diarrhea.
• Tell patient about importance of reporting persistent or worsening signs and symptoms of infection, such as pain or redness.

---

telithromycin
teh-lith-roh-MY-sin

Ketek

Pharmacologic class: ketolide
Pregnancy risk category C

AVAILABLE FORMS
Tablets: 300 mg, 400 mg

INDICATIONS & DOSAGES
➤ **Mild to moderate community-acquired pneumonia caused by**
S. pneumoniae **(including multi–drug-resistant isolates),** *H. influenzae,* *M. catarrhalis, Chlamydophila pneumoniae,* **or** *Mycoplasma pneumoniae*
Adults: 800 mg P.O. once daily for 7 to 10 days.
Adjust-a-dose: In patients with creatinine clearance less than 30 ml/minute, including those on dialysis, give 600 mg P.O. once daily. On dialysis days, give after session. In patients with clearance less than 30 ml/minute and hepatic impairment, give 400 mg once daily.

ADMINISTRATION
P.O.
• Give drug with or without food.

ACTION
Inhibits bacterial protein synthesis.

Route	Onset	Peak	Duration
P.O.	Unknown	1 hr	Unknown

Half-life: 10 hours.

ADVERSE REACTIONS
CNS: dizziness, headache.
EENT: blurred vision, difficulty focusing, diplopia.
GI: *diarrhea,* loose stools, nausea, taste disturbance, vomiting.

INTERACTIONS
Drug-drug. *Atorvastatin, lovastatin, simvastatin:* May increase levels of these drugs, increasing the risk of myopathy. Avoid using together.
Benzodiazepines (midazolam): May increase benzodiazepine level. Monitor patient closely and adjust benzodiazepine dosage.
CYP3A4 inhibitors (itraconazole, ketoconazole): May increase telithromycin level. Monitor patient closely.
CYP3A4 inducers (carbamazepine, phenobarbital, phenytoin): May decrease telithromycin level. Avoid using together.
Digoxin: May increase digoxin level. Monitor digoxin level.
Drugs metabolized by the cytochrome P-450 system (carbamazepine, cyclosporine, hexobarbital, phenytoin, sirolimus, tacrolimus): May increase levels of these

drugs, increasing or prolonging their effects. Use together cautiously.

Ergot alkaloid derivatives such as ergotamine: May increase the risk of ergot toxicity, characterized by severe peripheral vasospasm and dysesthesia. Avoid using together.

Metoprolol: May increase metoprolol level. Use together cautiously.

Oral anticoagulants: May increase anticoagulant effect. Monitor PT and INR.

Pimozide: May increase pimozide level. Avoid using together.

Rifamycins: May significantly decrease telithromycin level. Avoid using together.

Sotalol: May decrease sotalol level. Monitor patient for lack of effect.

Theophylline: May increase theophylline level and cause nausea and vomiting. Separate doses by 1 hour.

EFFECTS ON LAB TEST RESULTS
• May increase AST and ALT levels.
• May increase platelet count.

CONTRAINDICATIONS & CAUTIONS
• Contraindicated in patients hypersensitive to telithromycin or any macrolide antibiotic. Also contraindicated in patients taking pimozide.

■ **Black Box Warning** Contraindicated in patients with myasthenia gravis due to increased risk of life-threatening respiratory failure. ■

• Don't use in patients with congenitally prolonged QTc interval; those with ongoing proarrhythmic conditions, such as uncorrected hypokalemia, hypomagnesemia, or bradycardia; or those taking class IA antiarrhythmics, such as quinidine or procainamide, or class III antiarrhythmics such as dofetilide.

• Use cautiously in patients with a history of drug-induced hepatitis or jaundice and in breast-feeding women.

NURSING CONSIDERATIONS
• Visual disturbances may occur, particularly in women and patients younger than age 40. Adverse visual effects occur most often after the first or second dose, last several hours, and sometimes return with later doses.

• Monitor patient for signs or symptoms of liver problems, including jaundice, pale stools, darkened urine, and abdominal pain.

• This drug may cause loss of consciousness. Monitor the patient closely.

• Patients with diarrhea may have pseudomembranous colitis.

• This drug may prolong the QTc interval. Rarely, an irregular heartbeat may cause the patient to faint.

PATIENT TEACHING
• Tell patient to take entire amount of drug exactly as directed, even if he feels better.

• Tell patient that drug can be taken with or without food.

• Explain that this drug may cause visual disturbances. Caution patient to avoid hazardous activities.

• Tell patient to report diarrhea or any episodes of fainting that occur while taking this drug.

• Advise patient to immediately report signs of liver problems to prescriber.

vancomycin hydrochloride
van-koh-MYE-sin

Vancocin, Vancoled

Pharmacologic class: glycopeptide
Pregnancy risk category C; B for capsules only

AVAILABLE FORMS
Capsules: 125 mg, 250 mg
Powder for injection: 500-mg vials, 1-g vials, 5-g vials, 10-g vials
Powder for oral solution: 1-g bottles, 10-g bottles

INDICATIONS & DOSAGES
➤ **Serious or severe infections when other antibiotics are ineffective or contraindicated, including those caused by methicillin-resistant *Staphylococcus aureus*, *S. epidermidis*, or diphtheroid organisms**
Adults: 500 mg I.V. every 6 hours or 1 g I.V. every 12 hours.
Children: 10 mg/kg I.V. every 6 hours.

Neonates and young infants: 15 mg/kg I.V. loading dose; then 10 mg/kg I.V. every 12 hours if child is younger than age 1 week or 10 mg/kg I.V. every 8 hours if age is older than 1 week but younger than 1 month.

Elderly patients: 15 mg/kg I.V. loading dose. Subsequent doses are based on renal function and drug levels.

➤ **Antibiotic-related pseudomembranous *Clostridium difficile* and *S. enterocolitis***

Adults: 125 to 500 mg P.O. every 6 hours for 7 to 10 days.

Children: 40 mg/kg P.O. daily, in divided doses every 6 hours for 7 to 10 days. Maximum daily dose is 2 g.

➤ **Endocarditis prophylaxis for dental procedures**

Adults: 1 g I.V. slowly over 1 to 2 hours, completing infusion 30 minutes before procedure.

Children: 20 mg/kg I.V. over 1 to 2 hours, completing infusion 30 minutes before procedure.

Adjust-a-dose: In renal insufficiency, adjust dosage based on degree of renal impairment, drug level, severity of infection, and susceptibility of causative organism. Initially, give 15 mg/kg, and adjust subsequent doses as needed. One possible schedule is as follows: If creatinine level is less than 1.5 mg/dl, give 1 g every 12 hours. If creatinine level is 1.5 to 5 mg/dl, give 1 g every 3 to 6 days. If creatinine level is greater than 5 mg/dl, give 1 g every 10 to 14 days. Or, if GFR is 10 to 50 ml/minute, give usual dose every 3 to 10 days, and if GFR is less than 10 ml/minute, give usual dose every 10 days.

➤ **Bacterial endocarditis from methicillin-resistant or methicillin-susceptible staphylococci in patients with native cardiac valves**

Adults: 30 mg/kg I.V. daily given in two divided doses for 4 to 6 weeks. Doses over 2 g require monitoring of drug level.

ADMINISTRATION

P.O.

● Obtain specimen for culture and sensitivity tests before giving. Because of the emergence of vancomycin-resistant enterococci, reserve use of drug for treatment of serious infections caused by gram-positive bacteria resistant to beta-lactam anti-infectives.

● *Alert:* Oral form is ineffective for systemic infections.

● Oral solution is stable for 2 weeks if refrigerated.

I.V.

● Obtain specimen for culture and sensitivity tests before giving. Because of the emergence of vancomycin-resistant enterococci, reserve use of drug for treatment of serious infections caused by gram-positive bacteria resistant to beta-lactam anti-infectives.

● This form is ineffective for pseudomembranous (*Clostridium difficile*) diarrhea.

● Reconstitute 500-mg vial with 10 ml or 1-g vial with 20 ml sterile water for injection to provide a solution containing 50 mg/ml.

● For infusion, further dilute 500 mg in 100 ml or 1 g in 200 ml normal saline solution for injection or D_5W, and infuse over 60 minutes; if dose is greater than 1 g, infuse over 90 minutes.

● Check site daily for phlebitis and irritation. Severe irritation and necrosis can result from extravasation.

● Refrigerate solution after reconstitution and use within 14 days.

● **Incompatibilities:** Albumin, alkaline solutions, aminophylline, amobarbital, amphotericin B, aztreonam, cephalosporins, chloramphenicol, chlorothiazide, corticosteroids, dexamethasone sodium phosphate, foscarnet, gatifloxacin, heavy metals, heparin, hydrocortisone, idarubicin, methotrexate, nafcillin, omeprazole, penicillin G potassium, pentobarbital, phenobarbital, phenytoin, piperacillin, piperacillin sodium and tazobactam sodium, sargramostim, sodium bicarbonate, ticarcillin disodium, ticarcillin disodium and clavulanate potassium, vitamin B complex with C, warfarin.

ACTION

Hinders bacterial cell-wall synthesis, damaging the bacterial plasma membrane and making the cell more vulnerable to osmotic pressure. Also interferes with RNA synthesis.

Route	Onset	Peak	Duration
P.O.	Unknown	Unknown	Unknown
I.V.	Immediate	Immediate	Unknown

Half-life: 6 hours.

ADVERSE REACTIONS
CNS: fever, pain.
CV: hypotension, thrombophlebitis at injection site.
EENT: ototoxicity, tinnitus.
GI: *pseudomembranous colitis,* nausea.
GU: *nephrotoxicity.*
Hematologic: *leukopenia, neutropenia,* eosinophilia.
Respiratory: dyspnea, wheezing.
Skin: red-man syndrome (with rapid I.V. infusion).
Other: *anaphylaxis,* chills, superinfection.

INTERACTIONS
Drug-drug. *Aminoglycosides, amphotericin B, cisplatin, pentamidine:* May increase risk of nephrotoxicity and ototoxicity. Monitor renal function and hearing function tests.
Nondepolarizing muscle relaxants: May enhance neuromuscular blockade. Monitor patient closely.

EFFECTS ON LAB TEST RESULTS
• May increase BUN and creatinine levels.
• May increase eosinophil counts. May decrease neutrophil and WBC counts.

CONTRAINDICATIONS & CAUTIONS
• Contraindicated in patients hypersensitive to drug.
• Use cautiously in patients receiving other neurotoxic, nephrotoxic, or ototoxic drugs; in patients older than age 60; and in those with impaired hepatic or renal function, hearing loss, or allergies to other antibiotics.

NURSING CONSIDERATIONS
• Patients with renal dysfunction need dosage adjustment. Monitor blood levels to adjust I.V. dosage. Normal therapeutic levels of vancomycin are peak, 30 to 40 mg/L (drawn 1 hour after infusion ends), and trough, 5 to 10 mg/L (drawn just before next dose is given). However, determine the individual facility's therapeutic peak and trough ranges.

• Obtain hearing evaluation and renal function studies before therapy.
• Monitor patient's fluid balance and watch for oliguria and cloudy urine.
• Monitor patient carefully for red-man syndrome, which can occur if drug is infused too rapidly. Signs and symptoms include maculopapular rash on face, neck, trunk, and limbs and pruritus and hypotension caused by histamine release. If wheezing, urticaria, or pain and muscle spasm of the chest and back occur, stop infusion and notify prescriber.
• Don't give drug I.M.
• Monitor renal function (BUN, creatinine and creatinine clearance levels, urinalysis, and urine output) during therapy.
• Monitor patient for signs and symptoms of superinfection.
• Have patient's hearing evaluated during prolonged therapy.
• For staphylococcal endocarditis, give for at least 4 weeks.

PATIENT TEACHING
• Tell patient to take entire amount of drug exactly as directed, even after he feels better.
• Instruct patient receiving drug I.V. to report discomfort at I.V. insertion site.
• Tell patient to report ringing in ears.
• Tell patient to report adverse reactions to prescriber immediately.

Reactions may be *common,* uncommon, *life-threatening,* or COMMON AND LIFE-THREATENING.
Interaction may have a *rapid onset* or *delayed onset.*

21
Antianginals

amlodipine besylate
atenolol
    (See Chapter 23, ANTIHYPERTENSIVES.)
diltiazem hydrochloride
isosorbide dinitrate
isosorbide mononitrate
metoprolol
    (See Chapter 23, ANTIHYPERTENSIVES.)
nadolol
nicardipine hydrochloride
nifedipine
nitroglycerin
propranolol hydrochloride
ranolazine
verapamil hydrochloride

---

amlodipine besylate
am-LOE-di-peen

Norvasc⬚

Pharmacologic class:
calcium channel blocker
Pregnancy risk category C

AVAILABLE FORMS
Tablets: 2.5 mg, 5 mg, 10 mg

INDICATIONS & DOSAGES
➤ **Chronic stable angina, vaso-spastic angina (Prinzmetal's or variant angina)**
Adults: Initially, 5 to 10 mg P.O. daily. Most patients need 10 mg daily.
Elderly patients: Initially, 5 mg P.O. daily.
Adjust-a-dose: For patients who are small or frail or have hepatic insufficiency, initially, 5 mg P.O. daily.
➤ **Hypertension**
Adults: Initially, 2.5 to 5 mg P.O. daily. Dosage adjusted according to patient response and tolerance. Maximum daily dose is 10 mg.
Children ages 6 to 17: 2.5 to 5 mg P.O. once daily. Maximum dosage is 5 mg daily.
Elderly patients: Initially, 2.5 mg P.O. daily.

Adjust-a-dose: For patients who are small or frail, are taking other antihypertensives, or have hepatic insufficiency, initially, 2.5 mg P.O. daily.

ADMINISTRATION
P.O.
• Give drug without regard for food.

ACTION
Inhibits calcium ion influx across cardiac and smooth-muscle cells, dilates coronary arteries and arterioles, and decreases blood pressure and myocardial oxygen demand.

Route	Onset	Peak	Duration
P.O.	Unknown	6–12 hr	24 hr

Half-life: 30 to 50 hours.

ADVERSE REACTIONS
CNS: headache, somnolence, fatigue, dizziness, light-headedness, paresthesia.
CV: *edema,* flushing, palpitations.
GI: nausea, abdominal pain.
GU: sexual difficulties.
Musculoskeletal: muscle pain.
Respiratory: dyspnea.
Skin: rash, pruritus.

INTERACTIONS
None reported.

EFFECTS ON LAB TEST RESULTS
None reported.

CONTRAINDICATIONS & CAUTIONS
• Contraindicated in patients hypersensitive to drug.
• Use cautiously in patients receiving other peripheral vasodilators, especially those with severe aortic stenosis, and in those with heart failure. Because drug is metabolized by the liver, use cautiously and in reduced dosage in patients with severe hepatic disease.

NURSING CONSIDERATIONS
• *Alert:* Monitor patient carefully. Some patients, especially those with

severe obstructive coronary artery disease, have developed increased frequency, duration, or severity of angina or acute MI after initiation of calcium channel blocker therapy or at time of dosage increase.

• Monitor blood pressure frequently during initiation of therapy. Because drug-induced vasodilation has a gradual onset, acute hypotension is rare.

• Notify prescriber if signs of heart failure occur, such as swelling of hands and feet or shortness of breath.

• **Alert:** Abrupt withdrawal of drug may increase frequency and duration of chest pain. Taper dose gradually under medical supervision.

• **Look alike–sound alike:** Don't confuse amlodipine with amiloride.

PATIENT TEACHING

• Caution patient to continue taking drug, even when he feels better.

• Tell patient S.L. nitroglycerin may be taken as needed when angina symptoms are acute. If patient continues nitrate therapy during adjustment of amlodipine dosage, urge continued compliance.

---

diltiazem hydrochloride
dil-TYE-a-zem

Apo-Diltiaz†, Cardizem⊘, Cardizem CD⊘, Cardizem LA⊘, Cartia XT, Dilacor XR, Diltia XT, Dilt-XR, Nu-Diltiaz†, Taztia XT, Tiazac, Tiazac XC†

Pharmacologic class: calcium channel blocker
Pregnancy risk category C

AVAILABLE FORMS

Capsules (extended-release): 60 mg, 90 mg, 120 mg, 180 mg, 240 mg, 300 mg, 360 mg, 420 mg
Injection: 5 mg/ml in 5-, 10-, 25-ml vials
Powder for injection: 25 mg
Tablets: 30 mg, 60 mg, 90 mg, 120 mg
Tablets (extended-release): 120 mg, 180 mg, 240 mg, 300 mg, 360 mg, 420 mg

INDICATIONS & DOSAGES

➤ **To manage Prinzmetal's or variant angina or chronic stable angina pectoris**
Adults: 30 mg P.O. q.i.d. before meals and at bedtime. Increase dose gradually to maximum of 360 mg/day divided into three or four doses, as indicated. Or, give 120- or 180-mg extended-release capsule or 180-mg extended-release tablet P.O. once daily. Adjust over a 7- to 14-day period as needed and tolerated up to a maximum dose of 360 mg/day (Cardizem LA), 480 mg/day (Cardizem CD, Cartia XT, Dilacor XR, Dilacor XT), or 540 mg/day (Tiazac).

➤ **Hypertension**
Adults: 180- to 240-mg extended-release capsule P.O. once daily. Adjust dosage based on patient response to a maximum dose of 480 mg/day. Or, 120 to 240 mg P.O. (Cardizem LA) once daily. Dosage can be adjusted about every 2 weeks to a maximum of 540 mg daily.

➤ **Atrial fibrillation or flutter; paroxysmal supraventricular tachycardia**
Adults: 0.25 mg/kg I.V. as a bolus injection over 2 minutes. Repeat after 15 minutes if response isn't adequate with a dose of 0.35 mg/kg I.V. over 2 minutes. Follow bolus with continuous I.V. infusion at 5 to 15 mg/hour (for up to 24 hours).

ADMINISTRATION

P.O.

• Don't crush or allow patient to chew extended-release tablets; they should be swallowed whole.

• Tiazac extended-release capsules can be opened and the contents sprinkled onto a spoonful of applesauce. The applesauce must be eaten immediately and without chewing, followed by a glass of cool water.

I.V.

• For 100-mg Cardizem Monovials, reconstitute according to manufacturer's directions.

• For direct injection, you need not dilute the 5 mg/ml injection.

• For continuous infusion, add 25 ml of drug to 100 ml solution, 50 ml of drug to 250 ml solution, or 50 ml of drug to 500 ml solution of 5 mg/ml injection to yield 1 mg/ml, 0.83 mg/ml, or

---

Reactions may be *common*, uncommon, *life-threatening*, or COMMON AND LIFE-THREATENING.
Interaction may have a *rapid onset* or *delayed onset*.

0.45 mg/ml, respectively. Compatible solutions include normal saline solution, D₅W, or 5% dextrose and half-normal saline solution.
- For direct injection or continuous infusion; give slowly while monitoring ECG and blood pressure continuously.
- Don't infuse for longer than 24 hours.
- **Incompatibilities:** Acetazolamide, acyclovir, aminophylline, ampicillin, ampicillin sodium and sulbactam sodium, cefoperazone, diazepam, furosemide, heparin, hydrocortisone, insulin, methylprednisolone, nafcillin, phenytoin, rifampin, sodium bicarbonate, thiopental.

ACTION
A calcium channel blocker that inhibits calcium ion influx across cardiac and smooth-muscle cells, decreasing myocardial contractility and oxygen demand. Drug also dilates coronary arteries and arterioles.

Route	Onset	Peak	Duration
P.O.	30–60 min	2–3 hr	6–8 hr
P.O. (extended-release capsule)	2–3 hr	10–14 hr	12–24 hr
P.O. (Cardizem LA)	3–4 hr	11–18 hr	6–9 hr
I.V.	< 3 min	2–7 min	1–10 hr

Half-life: 3 to 9 hours.

ADVERSE REACTIONS
CNS: *headache,* dizziness, asthenia, somnolence.
CV: *edema, arrhythmias, AV block, bradycardia, heart failure,* flushing, hypotension, conduction abnormalities, abnormal ECG.
GI: nausea, constipation, abdominal discomfort.
Hepatic: *acute hepatic injury.*
Skin: rash.

INTERACTIONS
Drug-drug. *Anesthetics:* May increase effects of anesthetics. Monitor patient.
Carbamazepine: May increase level of carbamazepine. Monitor carbamazepine level, and watch for signs and symptoms of toxicity.

Cimetidine: May inhibit diltiazem metabolism, increasing additive AV node conduction slowing. Monitor patient for toxicity.
Cyclosporine: May increase cyclosporine level, possibly by decreasing its metabolism, leading to increased risk of cyclosporine toxicity. Monitor cyclosporine level with each dosage change.
Diazepam, midazolam, triazolam: May increase CNS depression and prolonged effects of these benzodiazepines. Use lower dose of these benzodiazepines.
Digoxin: May increase digoxin level. Monitor patient for digoxin toxicity.
Furosemide: May form a precipitate when mixed with diltiazem injection. Give through separate I.V. lines.
Lithium: May reduce lithium levels, causing loss of mania control, and neurotoxic and psychotic symptoms. Monitor patient for signs of neurotoxicity.
Propranolol, other beta blockers: May precipitate heart failure or prolong conduction time. Use together cautiously.
Sirolimus, tacrolimus: May increase level of these drugs. Monitor drug level and patient for toxicity.
Theophylline: May enhance action of theophylline, causing intoxication. Monitor theophylline levels.

EFFECTS ON LAB TEST RESULTS
None reported.

CONTRAINDICATIONS & CAUTIONS
- Contraindicated in patients hypersensitive to drug and in those with sick sinus syndrome or second- or third-degree AV block in the absence of an artificial pacemaker, cardiogenic shock, ventricular tachycardia, systolic blood pressure below 90 mm Hg, acute MI, or pulmonary congestion (documented by X-ray).
- Contraindicated in I.V. form for patients who have atrial fibrillation or flutter with an accessory bypass tract, as in Wolff-Parkinson-White syndrome or short PR interval syndrome.
- Use cautiously in elderly patients and in those with heart failure or impaired hepatic or renal function.

NURSING CONSIDERATIONS
- Patients controlled on drug alone or with other drugs may be switched to Cardizem

LA tablets once a day at the nearest equivalent total daily dose.
● Monitor blood pressure and heart rate when starting therapy and during dosage adjustments.
● Maximal antihypertensive effect may not be seen for 14 days.
● If systolic blood pressure is below 90 mm Hg or heart rate is below 60 beats/minute, withhold dose and notify prescriber.
● *Look alike–sound alike:* Don't confuse Tiazac with Ziac.

PATIENT TEACHING
● Instruct patient to take drug as prescribed, even when he feels better.
● Advise patient to avoid hazardous activities during start of therapy.
● If nitrate therapy is prescribed during dosage adjustment, stress patient compliance. Tell patient that S.L. nitroglycerin may be taken with drug, as needed, when angina symptoms are acute.
● *Alert:* Tell patient to swallow extended-release tablets whole, and not to crush or chew them.
● If patient is taking Tiazac extended-release capsules, inform him that these capsules can be opened and the contents sprinkled onto a spoonful of applesauce. He must eat the applesauce immediately and without chewing, and then drink a glass of cool water.

---

isosorbide dinitrate
eye-soe-SOR-bide

Apo-ISDN†, Cedocard SR†, Dilatrate-SR, Isordil, Isordil Titradose

isosorbide mononitrate
Apo-ISMN†, Imdur, ISMO, Monoket

Pharmacologic class: nitrate
*Pregnancy risk category C;
B for mononitrate*

AVAILABLE FORMS
isosorbide dinitrate
Capsules (sustained-release): 40 mg
Tablets: 5 mg, 10 mg, 20 mg, 30 mg, 40 mg

Tablets (S.L.): 2.5 mg, 5 mg,
Tablets (sustained-release): 40 mg
isosorbide mononitrate
Tablets: 10 mg, 20 mg
Tablets (extended-release): 30 mg, 60 mg, 120 mg

INDICATIONS & DOSAGES
➤ **Acute anginal attacks (S.L. isosorbide dinitrate only); to prevent situations that may cause anginal attacks**
Adults: 2.5 to 5 mg S.L. tablets for prompt relief of angina, repeated every 5 to 10 minutes (maximum of three doses for each 30-minute period). For prevention, 2.5 to 10 mg every 2 to 3 hours. Or, 5 to 40 mg isosorbide dinitrate P.O. b.i.d. or t.i.d. for prevention only (use smallest effective dose). Or, 30 to 60 mg Imdur P.O. once daily on arising; increase to 120 mg once daily after several days, if needed. Or, 20 mg ISMO or Monoket b.i.d. with the two doses given 7 hours apart.

ADMINISTRATION
P.O.
● Give patient S.L. tablet at first sign of attack. Tell him to wet tablet with saliva and place under his tongue until absorbed. Dose may be repeated every 10 to 15 minutes for a maximum of three doses.
● Tell patient taking P.O. form of isosorbide dinitrate to swallow oral tablet whole on an empty stomach either 30 minutes before or 1 to 2 hours after meals.
● Store drug in a cool place, in a tightly closed container, and away from light.

ACTION
Thought to reduce cardiac oxygen demand by decreasing preload and afterload. Drug also may increase blood flow through the collateral coronary vessels.

Route	Onset	Peak	Duration
P.O.	15–40 min	Unknown	4–8 hr
P.O. (extended-release)	½–4 hr	Unknown	6–12 hr
P.O. (S.L.)	2–5 min	Unknown	1–4 hr

Half-life: dinitrate P.O., 5 to 6 hours; S.L., 2 hours; mononitrate, about 5 hours.

Reactions may be *common*, uncommon, *life-threatening*, or COMMON AND LIFE-THREATENING.
Interaction may have a *rapid onset* or *delayed onset*.

ADVERSE REACTIONS
CNS: *headache,* dizziness, weakness.
CV: *orthostatic hypotension, tachycardia, palpitations, ankle edema, flushing,* fainting.
EENT: S.L. burning.
GI: nausea, vomiting.
Skin: cutaneous vasodilation, rash.

INTERACTIONS
Drug-drug. *Antihypertensives:* May increase hypotensive effects. Monitor patient closely during initial therapy.
Sildenafil, tadalafil, vardenafil: May cause life-threatening hypotension. Use of nitrates in any form with these drugs is contraindicated.
Drug-lifestyle. *Alcohol use:* May increase hypotension. Discourage use together.

EFFECTS ON LAB TEST RESULTS
• May falsely reduce value in cholesterol tests using the Zlatkis-Zak color reaction.

CONTRAINDICATIONS & CAUTIONS
• Contraindicated in patients with hypersensitivity or idiosyncrasy to nitrates and in those with severe hypotension, angle-closure glaucoma, increased intracranial pressure, shock, or acute MI with low left ventricular filling pressure.
• Use cautiously in patients with blood volume depletion (such as from diuretic therapy) or mild hypotension.

NURSING CONSIDERATIONS
• To prevent tolerance, a nitrate-free interval of 10 to 14 hours per day is recommended. The regimen for isosorbide mononitrate (1 tablet on awakening with the second dose in 7 hours, or 1 extended-release tablet daily) is intended to minimize nitrate tolerance by providing a substantial nitrate-free interval.
• Monitor blood pressure and heart rate and intensity and duration of drug response.
• Drug may cause headaches, especially at beginning of therapy. Dosage may be reduced temporarily, but tolerance usually develops. Treat headache with aspirin or acetaminophen.

• Methemoglobinemia has been seen with nitrates. Symptoms are those of impaired oxygen delivery despite adequate cardiac output and adequate arterial partial pressure of oxygen.
• *Look alike–sound alike:* Don't confuse Isordil with Isuprel or Inderal.

PATIENT TEACHING
• Caution patient to take drug regularly, as prescribed, and to keep it accessible at all times.
• *Alert:* Advise patient that stopping drug abruptly may cause spasm of the coronary arteries with increased angina symptoms and potential risk of heart attack.
• Tell patient to take S.L. tablet at first sign of attack. He should wet tablet with saliva and place under his tongue until absorbed; he should sit down and rest. Dose may be repeated every 10 to 15 minutes for a maximum of three doses. If drug doesn't provide relief, tell patient to seek medical help promptly.
• Advise patient who complains of tingling sensation with S.L. drug to try holding tablet in cheek.
• Warn patient not to confuse S.L. with P.O. form.
• Advise patient taking P.O. form of isosorbide dinitrate to take oral tablet on an empty stomach either 30 minutes before or 1 to 2 hours after meals and to swallow oral tablets whole.
• Tell patient to minimize dizziness upon standing up by changing to upright position slowly. Advise him to go up and down stairs carefully and to lie down at first sign of dizziness.
• Caution patient to avoid alcohol because it may worsen low blood pressure effects.
• Advise patient that use of sildenafil, tadalafil, or vardenafil with any nitrate may cause severe low blood pressure. Patient should talk to his prescriber before using these drugs together.
• Instruct patient to store drug in a cool place, in a tightly closed container, and away from light.

nadolol
nay-DOE-lol

Apo-Nadol†, Corgard

Pharmacologic class:
nonselective beta blocker
Pregnancy risk category C

AVAILABLE FORMS
Tablets: 20 mg, 40 mg, 80 mg, 120 mg,
160 mg

INDICATIONS & DOSAGES
➤ **Angina pectoris**
Adults: 40 mg P.O. once daily. Increase in
40- to 80-mg increments at 3- to 7-day
intervals until optimal response occurs.
Usual maintenance dose is 40 to 80 mg
once daily; up to 240 mg once daily may
be needed.
➤ **Hypertension**
Adults: 40 mg P.O. once daily. Increase in
40- to 80-mg increments until optimal
response occurs. Usual maintenance dose
is 40 to 80 mg once daily. Doses of
320 mg may be needed.
Adjust-a-dose: If creatinine clearance is
31 to 50 ml/minute, change dosing interval
to every 24 to 36 hours; if clearance is
10 to 30 ml/minute, every 24 to 48 hours;
and if clearance is less than 10 ml/minute,
every 40 to 60 hours.

ADMINISTRATION
P.O.
● Give drug without regard for food.
● Check apical pulse before giving drug.
If slower than 60 beats/minute, withhold
drug and call prescriber.
● *Alert:* Abruptly stopping drug may
worsen angina and cause an MI. Reduce
dosage gradually over 1 to 2 weeks.

ACTION
Reduces cardiac oxygen demand by
blocking catecholamine-induced increases
in heart rate, blood pressure, and force of
myocardial contraction. Depresses renin
secretion.

Route	Onset	Peak	Duration
P.O.	Unknown	2–4 hr	24 hr

Half-life: About 20 to 24 hours.

ADVERSE REACTIONS
CNS: fatigue, dizziness, fever.
CV: BRADYCARDIA, HEART FAILURE,
hypotension, peripheral vascular disease,
rhythm and conduction disturbances.
GI: nausea, vomiting, diarrhea, abdominal
pain, constipation, anorexia.
Respiratory: *increased airway resistance.*
Skin: rash.

INTERACTIONS
Drug-drug. *Antihypertensives:* May
increase antihypertensive effect. Monitor
blood pressure closely.
Cardiac glycosides: May cause
excessive bradycardia and additive
effects on AV conduction. Use together
cautiously.
Epinephrine: May decrease the patient
response to epinephrine for treatment of
an allergic reaction. Monitor patient
closely for decreased clinical effect.
General anesthetics: May increase
hypotensive effects. Consider stopping
nadolol before surgery.
Insulin: May mask symptoms of
hypoglycemia, as a result of beta
blockade (such as tachycardia). Use
with caution in patients with diabetes.
I.V. lidocaine: May reduce hepatic metabolism of lidocaine, increasing the risk of
toxicity. Give bolus doses of lidocaine at a
slower rate and monitor lidocaine level
closely.
NSAIDs: May decrease antihypertensive
effect. Monitor blood pressure and adjust
dosage.
Oral antidiabetics: May alter dosage
requirements in previously stabilized
diabetic patients. Monitor glucose
closely.
Phenothiazines: May increase hypotensive
effects. Monitor blood pressure.
Prazosin: May increase risk of orthostatic
hypotension in the early phases of use
together. Assist patient to stand slowly
until effects are known.
Reserpine: May increase hypotension or
bradycardia. Monitor patient for adverse
effects, such as dizziness, syncope, and
postural hypotension.
Verapamil: May increase effects of
both drugs. Monitor cardiac function
closely and decrease dosages as
necessary.

Reactions may be *common,* uncommon, ***life-threatening,*** or COMMON AND LIFE-THREATENING.
Interaction may have a *rapid onset* or ***delayed onset.***

EFFECTS ON LAB TEST RESULTS
None reported.

CONTRAINDICATIONS & CAUTIONS
• Contraindicated in patients with bronchial asthma, sinus bradycardia and greater than first-degree heart block, cardiogenic shock, and overt heart failure.
• Use cautiously in patients with heart failure, chronic bronchitis, emphysema, or renal or hepatic impairment and in patients undergoing major surgery involving general anesthesia.
• Use cautiously in diabetic patients because beta blockers may mask certain signs and symptoms of hypoglycemia.
■ **Black Box Warning** Exacerbation of ischemic heart disease may occur following abrupt withdrawal of drug. Exacerbation of angina and, in some cases, myocardial infarction have occurred after abrupt discontinuation of therapy. ■

NURSING CONSIDERATIONS
• Monitor blood pressure frequently. If patient develops severe hypotension, give a vasopressor, as prescribed.
• Drug masks signs and symptoms of shock and hyperthyroidism.
■ **Black Box Warning** If nadolol is to be discontinued after long-term administration, particularly in patients with ischemic heart disease, dosage should be gradually reduced over a period of 1 to 2 weeks and the patient carefully monitored. If angina markedly worsens or acute coronary insufficiency develops after drug cessation, nadolol should be temporarily restarted and other measures taken to appropriately manage unstable angina. Because coronary artery disease is common and may be unrecognized, don't discontinue nadolol therapy abruptly, even in patients treated only for hypertension. ■

PATIENT TEACHING
• Explain importance of taking drug as prescribed, even when patient feels well.
• Teach patient how to check pulse rate and tell him to check it before each dose. If pulse rate is below 60 beats/minute, tell patient to notify prescriber.
■ **Black Box Warning** Warn patient not to stop drug suddenly. ■

nicardipine hydrochloride
nye-KAR-de-peen

Cardene, Cardene I.V., Cardene SR

Pharmacologic class: calcium channel blocker
Pregnancy risk category C

AVAILABLE FORMS
Capsules: 20 mg, 30 mg
Capsules (sustained-release): 30 mg, 45 mg, 60 mg
Injection: 2.5 mg/ml

INDICATIONS & DOSAGES
➤ **Chronic stable angina (used alone or with other antianginals)**
Adults: Initially, 20 mg immediate-release capsule P.O. t.i.d. Adjust dosage based on patient response every 3 days. Usual range, 20 to 40 mg t.i.d.
➤ **Hypertension**
Adults: Initially, 20 mg immediate-release capsule P.O. t.i.d.; range, 20 to 40 mg t.i.d. Or, 30 mg sustained-release capsule b.i.d.; range, 30 to 60 mg b.i.d. Increase dosage based on patient response. Or, for patient who can't take oral form, 5 mg/hour (50 ml/hour) I.V. infusion initially; then, increase by 2.5 mg/hour (25 ml/hour) every 15 minutes to maximum of 15 mg/hour (150 ml/hour).

ADMINISTRATION
P.O.
• Give drug with or without food, but avoid giving with high-fat meal.
• Don't break or crush sustained-release capsules; they must be swallowed whole.
I.V.
• Dilute to a concentration of 0.1 mg/ml with D₅W, dextrose 5% in normal saline solution or half-normal saline solution, and normal saline solution or half-normal saline solution.
• Give by slow infusion.
• Closely monitor blood pressure during and after completion of infusion.
• If hypotension or tachycardia occurs, titrate infusion rate.

- Change peripheral infusion site every 12 hours to minimize risk of venous irritation.
- When switching to oral form, give first dose of t.i.d. regimen 1 hour before stopping infusion. If using a different oral drug, start it when infusion ends.
- If solution is kept at room temperature, use within 24 hours.
- **Incompatibilities:** Ampicillin sodium, ampicillin and sulbactam sodium, cefoperazone, ceftazidime, furosemide, heparin sodium, lactated Ringer's solution, sodium bicarbonate, thiopental.

ACTION
Inhibits calcium ion influx across cardiac and smooth muscle cells but is more selective to vascular smooth muscle than cardiac muscle. Drug also dilates coronary arteries and arterioles.

Route	Onset	Peak	Duration
P.O. (immediate-release)	20 min	1–2 hr	Unknown
P.O. (sustained-release)	20 min	1–4 hr	12 hr
I.V.	Immediate	Immediate	Unknown

Half-life: 2 to 4 hours.

ADVERSE REACTIONS
CNS: *headache,* dizziness, light-headedness, asthenia.
CV: *peripheral edema, palpitations, flushing,* angina, tachycardia.
GI: nausea, abdominal discomfort, dry mouth.
Skin: rash.

INTERACTIONS
Drug-drug. *Antihypertensives:* May increase antihypertensive effect. Monitor blood pressure closely.
Cimetidine: May decrease metabolism of calcium channel blockers. Monitor patient for increased pharmacologic effect.
Cyclosporine: May increase plasma level of cyclosporine. Monitor patient for toxicity.

Drug-food. *Grapefruit and grapefruit juice:* May increase bioavailability of nicardipine. Discourage use together.
High-fat foods: May decrease absorption of nicardipine. Discourage use together.

EFFECTS ON LAB TEST RESULTS
None reported.

CONTRAINDICATIONS & CAUTIONS
- Contraindicated in patients hypersensitive to drug and in those with advanced aortic stenosis.
- Use cautiously in patients with hypotension, heart failure, or impaired hepatic and renal function.

NURSING CONSIDERATIONS
- Measure blood pressure frequently during initial therapy. Maximal response occurs about 1 hour after giving the immediate-release form and 2 to 4 hours after giving the sustained-release form. Check for orthostatic hypotension. Because large swings in blood pressure may occur based on drug level, assess antihypertensive effect 8 hours after dosing.
- Extended-release form is preferred because of improved compliance, fewer fluctuations in blood pressure, and less risk of death than with shorter-acting drugs.
- *Look alike–sound alike:* Don't confuse Cardene with Cardura or codeine.

PATIENT TEACHING
- Tell patient to take oral form exactly as prescribed.
- Advise patient to report chest pain immediately. Some patients may experience increased frequency, severity, or duration of chest pain at beginning of therapy or during dosage adjustments.
- Tell patient to get up from a sitting or lying position slowly to avoid dizziness caused by a decrease in blood pressure.
- Tell patient drug may be taken with or without food but shouldn't be taken with high-fat foods.
- Tell patient to swallow sustained-release capsules whole; don't crush, break, or chew.

Reactions may be *common,* uncommon, **life-threatening**, or COMMON AND LIFE-THREATENING.
Interaction may have a *rapid onset* or **delayed onset.**

nifedipine
nye-FED-i-peen

Adalat CC, Adalat XL†,
Apo-Nifed†, Nifedical XL,
Nu-Nifed†, Procardia XL🔗

Pharmacologic class:
calcium channel blocker
Pregnancy risk category C

AVAILABLE FORMS
Capsules: 10 mg, 20 mg
Tablets (extended-release): 20 mg†,
30 mg, 60 mg, 90 mg

INDICATIONS & DOSAGES
➤ **Vasospastic angina (Prinzmetal's or variant angina), classic chronic stable angina pectoris**
Adults: Initially, 10 mg short-acting capsule P.O. t.i.d. Usual effective dosage range is 10 to 20 mg t.i.d. Some patients may require up to 30 mg q.i.d. Maximum daily dose is 180 mg. Adjust dosage over 7 to 14 days to evaluate response. Or, 30 to 60 mg (extended-release tablets, except Adalat CC) P.O. once daily. Maximum daily dose is 120 mg. Adjust dosage over 7 to 14 days to evaluate response.
➤ **Hypertension**
Adults: 30 or 60 mg P.O. extended-release tablet once daily. Adjusted over 7 to 14 days. Doses larger than 90 mg (Adalat CC) and 120 mg (Procardia XL) aren't recommended.

ADMINISTRATION
P.O.
● Don't give immediate-release capsules within 1 week of acute MI or in acute coronary syndrome.
● *Alert:* Don't use capsules S.L. to rapidly reduce severe high blood pressure because the result may be fatal.
● Give extended-release tablets whole; don't break or crush tablet.
● Don't give drug with grapefruit juice.
● Protect capsules from direct light and moisture and store at room temperature.

ACTION
Thought to inhibit calcium ion influx across cardiac and smooth muscle cells,

decreasing contractility and oxygen demand. Drug may also dilate coronary arteries and arterioles.

Route	Onset	Peak	Duration
P.O.	20 min	30–60 min	4–8 hr
P.O. (extended)	20 min	6 hr	24 hr

Half-life: 2 to 5 hours.

ADVERSE REACTIONS
CNS: *dizziness, light-headedness, headache, weakness,* somnolence, syncope, nervousness.
CV: *flushing, peripheral edema, heart failure, MI,* hypotension, palpitations.
EENT: nasal congestion.
GI: *nausea,* diarrhea, constipation, abdominal discomfort.
Musculoskeletal: muscle cramps.
Respiratory: dyspnea, *pulmonary edema,* cough.
Skin: rash, pruritus.

INTERACTIONS
Drug-drug. *Antiretrovirals, verapamil, cimetidine:* May decrease nifedipine metabolism. Monitor blood pressure closely and adjust nifedipine dosage as needed.
Azole antifungals, erythromycin, quinupristin, and dalfopristin: May increase the effects of nifedipine. Monitor blood pressure closely and decrease nifedipine dosage as needed.
Cyclosporine, tacrolimus: May increase serum levels of these drugs and increase risk of toxicity. Monitor serum levels and adjust dosage as needed.
Digoxin: May cause elevated digoxin level. Monitor digoxin level.
Diltiazem: May increase the effects of nifedipine. Monitor patient closely.
Fentanyl: May cause severe hypotension. Monitor blood pressure.
Phenytoin: May reduce phenytoin metabolism. Monitor phenytoin level.
Propranolol, other beta blockers: May cause hypotension and heart failure. Use together cautiously.
Quinidine: May decrease levels and effects of quinidine while increasing effects of nifedipine. Monitor heart rate and adjust nifedipine dose as needed.

---

†Canada   ◇OTC   ◆Off-label use   🔗Photoguide   *Liquid contains alcohol.

Rifamycins: May decrease nifedipine levels. Monitor patient.

Drug-herb. *Ginkgo:* May increase effects of drug. Discourage use together.

Ginseng: May increase drug levels with possible toxicity. Discourage use together.

Melatonin, St. John's wort: May interfere with antihypertensive effect. Discourage use together.

Drug-food. *Grapefruit juice:* May increase bioavailability of drug. Discourage use together.

EFFECTS ON LAB TEST RESULTS

● May increase ALT, AST, alkaline phosphatase, and LDH levels.

CONTRAINDICATIONS & CAUTIONS

● Contraindicated in patients hypersensitive to drug.

● Use cautiously in patients with heart failure or hypotension and in elderly patients. Use extended-release tablets cautiously in patients with severe GI narrowing.

NURSING CONSIDERATIONS

● Monitor blood pressure and heart rate regularly, especially in patients who take beta blockers or antihypertensives.

● Watch for symptoms of heart failure.

● *Look alike–sound alike:* Don't confuse nifedipine with nimodipine or nicardipine.

PATIENT TEACHING

● If patient is kept on nitrate therapy while nifedipine dosage is being adjusted, urge continued compliance. Patient may take S.L. nitroglycerin, as needed, for acute chest pain.

● Tell patient that chest pain may worsen briefly as therapy starts or dosage increases.

● Instruct patient to swallow extended-release tablets without breaking, crushing, or chewing them.

● Advise patient to avoid taking drug with grapefruit juice.

● Reassure patient taking the extended-release tablet that the wax mold may be passed in the stools. Assure him that drug has already been completely absorbed.

● Tell patient to protect capsules from direct light and moisture and to store at room temperature.

SAFETY ALERT!

nitroglycerin (glyceryl trinitrate)
nye-troe-GLIH-ser-in

Deponit, Minitran, Nitrek, Nitro-Bid, Nitro-Dur, Nitrogard, Nitrolingual, NitroQuick, Nitrostat✛, NitroTab, Nitro-Time, NTS, Trinipatch†

Pharmacologic class: nitrate
Pregnancy risk category C

AVAILABLE FORMS

Aerosol (translingual): 0.4 mg/metered spray
Capsules (sustained-release): 2.5 mg, 6.5 mg, 9 mg
Injection: 5 mg/ml; 100 mcg/ml, 200 mcg/ml, 400 mcg/ml
Tablets (S.L.): 0.3 mg (½₀₀ grain), 0.4 mg (¹⁄₁₅₀ grain), 0.6 mg (¹⁄₁₀₀ grain)
Tablets (sustained-release): 2.6 mg, 6.5 mg, 9 mg
Topical: 2% ointment
Transdermal: 0.1 mg/hour, 0.2 mg/hour, 0.3 mg/hour, 0.4 mg/hour, 0.6 mg/hour, 0.8 mg/hour release rate

INDICATIONS & DOSAGES

➤ **To prevent chronic anginal attacks**

Adults: 2.5 or 2.6 mg sustained-release capsule or tablet every 8 to 12 hours. Increase to an effective dose in 2.5- or 2.6-mg increments b.i.d. to q.i.d. Or, use 2% ointment: Start dosage with ½-inch ointment, increasing by ½-inch increments until desired results are achieved. Range of dosage with ointment is ½ to 5 inches. Usual dose is 1 to 2 inches every 6 to 8 hours. Or, transdermal patch 0.2 to 0.4 mg/hour once daily.

➤ **Acute angina pectoris; to prevent or minimize anginal attacks before stressful events**

Adults: 1 S.L. tablet (¹⁄₂₀₀ grain, ¹⁄₁₅₀ grain, ¹⁄₁₀₀ grain) dissolved under the tongue or in the buccal pouch as soon as angina begins. Repeat every 5 minutes, if needed, for 15 minutes. Or, one or two metered-dose sprays Nitrolingual into mouth, preferably onto or under the tongue.

Reactions may be *common*, uncommon, *life-threatening*, or COMMON AND LIFE-THREATENING.
Interaction may have a *rapid onset* or *delayed onset.*

Repeat every 3 to 5 minutes, if needed, to a maximum of three doses within a 15-minute period.

➤ **Hypertension from surgery, heart failure after MI, angina pectoris in acute situations, to produce controlled hypotension during surgery (by I.V. infusion)**
Adults: Initially, infuse at 5 mcg/minute, increasing as needed by 5 mcg/minute every 3 to 5 minutes until response occurs. If a 20-mcg/minute rate doesn't produce a response, increase dosage by as much as 20 mcg/minute every 3 to 5 minutes. Up to 100 mcg/minute may be needed.

ADMINISTRATION
P.O.
● Give 30 minutes before or 1 to 2 hours after meals.
● Drug must be swallowed whole and not chewed.
I.V.
● Dilute with D₅W or normal saline solution for injection. Concentration shouldn't exceed 400 mcg/ml.
● Always give with an infusion control device and titrate to desired response.
● Regular polyvinyl chloride tubing can bind up to 80% of drug, making it necessary to infuse higher dosages. A special nonabsorbent polyvinyl chloride tubing is available from the manufacturer. Always mix in glass bottles and avoid using a filter.
● Use the same type of infusion set when changing lines.
● When changing the concentration of infusion, flush the administration set with 15 to 20 ml of the new concentration before use. This will clear the line of the old drug solution.
● **Incompatibilities:** Alteplase, bretylium, hydralazine, levofloxacin, phenytoin sodium.
Topical
● To apply ointment, measure the prescribed amount on the application paper; then place the paper on any nonhairy area. Don't rub in. Cover with plastic film to aid absorption and to protect clothing. Remove all excess ointment from previous site before applying the next dose. Avoid getting ointment on fingers.

Transdermal
● Patch can be applied to any nonhairy part of the skin except distal parts of the arms or legs. (Absorption won't be maximal at distal sites.) Patch may cause contact dermatitis.
● Remove patch before defibrillation. Because of the aluminum backing on the patch, the electric current may cause arcing that can damage the paddles and burn the patient.
● When stopping transdermal treatment of angina, gradually reduce the dosage and frequency of application over 4 to 6 weeks.
S.L.
● Give tablet at first sign of attack. Patient should wet the tablet with saliva, place it under tongue until absorbed. Dose may be repeated every 5 minutes for a maximum of three doses. If drug doesn't provide relief, contact prescriber.
Buccal
● The tablet should be placed between the lip and gum above the incisors or between the cheek and gum. Tablets shouldn't be swallowed or chewed.
Translingual
● Patient using translingual aerosol form shouldn't inhale the spray but should release it onto or under the tongue. He should wait about 10 seconds or so before swallowing.

ACTION
A nitrate that reduces cardiac oxygen demand by decreasing left ventricular end-diastolic pressure (preload) and, to a lesser extent, systemic vascular resistance (afterload). Also increases blood flow through the collateral coronary vessels.

Route	Onset	Peak	Duration
P.O.	20–45 min	Unknown	3–8 hr
I.V.	Immediate	Immediate	3–5 min
Topical	30 min	Unknown	2–12 hr
Transdermal	30 min	Unknown	24 hr
S.L.	1–3 min	Unknown	30–60 min
Buccal	3 min	Unknown	3–5 hr
Translingual	2–4 min	Unknown	30–60 min

Half-life: About 1 to 4 minutes.

ADVERSE REACTIONS

CNS: *headache, dizziness,* syncope, weakness.
CV: *orthostatic hypotension, tachycardia, flushing, palpitations.*
EENT: S.L. burning.
GI: nausea, vomiting.
Skin: cutaneous vasodilation, contact dermatitis, rash.
Other: hypersensitivity reactions.

INTERACTIONS

Drug-drug. *Alteplase:* May decrease tissue plasminogen activator-antigen level. Avoid using together; if unavoidable, use lowest effective dose of nitroglycerin.
Antihypertensives: May increase hypotensive effect. Monitor blood pressure closely.
Heparin: I.V. nitroglycerin may interfere with anticoagulant effect of heparin. Monitor PTT.
Sildenafil, tadalafil, vardenafil: May cause severe hypotension. Use of nitrates in any form with these drugs is contraindicated.
Drug-lifestyle. *Alcohol use:* May increase hypotension. Discourage use together.

EFFECTS ON LAB TEST RESULTS

• May falsely decrease values in cholesterol determination tests using the Zlatkis-Zak color reaction.

CONTRAINDICATIONS & CAUTIONS

• Contraindicated in patients with early MI (oral and sublingual), severe anemia, increased intracranial pressure, angle-closure glaucoma, orthostatic hypotension, allergy to adhesives (transdermal), or hypersensitivity to nitrates.
• I.V. nitroglycerin is contraindicated in patients hypersensitive to I.V. form, with cardiac tamponade, restrictive cardiomyopathy, or constrictive pericarditis.
• Use cautiously in patients with hypotension or volume depletion.

NURSING CONSIDERATIONS

• Closely monitor vital signs during infusion, particularly blood pressure, especially in a patient with an MI. Excessive hypotension may worsen the MI.
• Monitor blood pressure and intensity and duration of drug response.

• Drug may cause headaches, especially at beginning of therapy. Dosage may be reduced temporarily, but tolerance usually develops. Treat headache with aspirin or acetaminophen.
• Tolerance to drug can be minimized with a 10- to 12-hour nitrate-free interval. To achieve this, remove the transdermal system in the early evening and apply a new system the next morning or omit the last daily dose of a buccal, sustained-release, or ointment form. Check with the prescriber for alterations in dosage regimen if tolerance is suspected.
• ***Look alike–sound alike:*** Don't confuse Nitro-Bid with Nicobid or nitroglycerin with nitroprusside.

PATIENT TEACHING

• Caution patient to take nitroglycerin regularly, as prescribed, and to have it accessible at all times.
• ***Alert:*** Advise patient that stopping drug abruptly causes spasm of the coronary arteries.
• Teach patient how to give the prescribed form of nitroglycerin.
• Tell patient to take S.L. tablet at first sign of attack. Patient should wet the tablet with saliva, place it under tongue until absorbed, and then sit down and rest. Dose may be repeated every 5 minutes for a maximum of three doses. If drug doesn't provide relief, he should obtain medical help promptly.
• Advise patient who complains of a tingling sensation with S.L. drug to try holding tablet in cheek.
• Tell patient to take oral tablets on an empty stomach either 30 minutes before or 1 to 2 hours after meals, to swallow oral tablets whole, and not to chew tablets.
• Remind patient using translingual aerosol form that he shouldn't inhale the spray but should release it onto or under the tongue. Tell him to wait about 10 seconds or so before swallowing.
• Tell patient to place the buccal tablet between the lip and gum above the incisors or between the cheek and gum. Tablets shouldn't be swallowed or chewed.
• Tell patient to take an additional dose before anticipated stress or at bedtime if chest pain occurs at night.

Reactions may be *common,* uncommon, *life-threatening,* or COMMON AND LIFE-THREATENING.
Interaction may have a *rapid onset* or ***delayed onset.***

- Urge patient using skin patches to dispose of them carefully because enough medication remains after normal use to be hazardous to children and pets.
- Advise patient to avoid alcohol.
- To minimize dizziness when standing up, tell patient to rise slowly. Advise him to go up and down stairs carefully and to lie down at the first sign of dizziness.
- *Alert:* Advise patient that use of sildenafil, tadalafil, or vardenafil with any nitrate may cause life-threatening low blood pressure. Use together is contraindicated.
- Tell patient to store drug in cool, dark place in a tightly closed container. Tell him to remove cotton from container because it absorbs drug.
- Tell patient to store S.L. tablets in original container or other container specifically approved for this use and to carry the container in a jacket pocket or purse, not in a pocket close to the body.

SAFETY ALERT!

propranolol hydrochloride
proe-PRAN-oh-lol

Inderal✒, Inderal LA✒, InnoPran XL, Novopranol†

Pharmacologic class: beta blocker
Pregnancy risk category C

AVAILABLE FORMS
Capsules (extended-release): 60 mg, 80 mg, 120 mg, 160 mg
Injection: 1 mg/ml
Oral solution: 4 mg/ml, 8 mg/ml, 80 mg/ml (concentrate)
Tablets: 10 mg, 20 mg, 40 mg, 60 mg, 80 mg, 90 mg

INDICATIONS & DOSAGES
➤ **Angina pectoris**
Adults: Total daily doses of 80 to 320 mg P.O. when given b.i.d., t.i.d., or q.i.d. Or, one 80-mg extended-release capsule daily. Dosage increased at 3- to 7-day intervals.
➤ **To decrease risk of death after MI**
Adults: 180 to 240 mg P.O. daily in divided doses beginning 5 to 21 days after MI has occurred. Usually given t.i.d. or q.i.d.

➤ **Supraventricular, ventricular, and atrial arrhythmias; tachyarrhythmias caused by excessive catecholamine action during anesthesia, hyperthyroidism, or pheochromocytoma**
Adults: 1 to 3 mg by slow I.V. push, not to exceed 1 mg/minute. After 3 mg have been given, another dose may be given in 2 minutes; subsequent doses, no sooner than every 4 hours. Usual maintenance dose is 10 to 30 mg P.O. t.i.d. or q.i.d.
➤ **Hypertension**
Adults: Initially, 80 mg P.O. daily in two divided doses or extended-release form once daily. Increase at 3- to 7-day intervals to maximum daily dose of 640 mg. Usual maintenance dose is 120 to 240 mg daily or 120 to 160 mg daily as extended-release. For InnoPran XL, dose is 80 mg P.O. once daily at bedtime. Give consistently with or without food. Adjust to maximum of 120 mg daily if needed. Full effects are seen in about 2 to 3 weeks.
Children: 0.5 mg/kg (conventional tablets) P.O. b.i.d. Increase every 3 to 5 days to a maximum dose of 16 mg/kg daily. Usual dose is 2 to 4 mg/kg daily in two equally divided doses.
➤ **To prevent frequent, severe, uncontrollable, or disabling migraine or vascular headache**
Adults: Initially, 80 mg P.O. daily in divided doses or 1 extended-release capsule daily. Usual maintenance dose is 160 to 240 mg daily, t.i.d. or q.i.d.
➤ **Essential tremor**
Adults: 40 mg (tablets or oral solution) P.O. b.i.d. Usual maintenance dose is 120 to 320 mg daily in three divided doses.
➤ **Hypertrophic subaortic stenosis**
Adults: 20 to 40 mg P.O. t.i.d. or q.i.d.; or 80 to 160 mg extended-release capsules once daily.
➤ **Adjunct therapy in pheochromocytoma**
Adults: 60 mg P.O. daily in divided doses with an alpha blocker 3 days before surgery.

ADMINISTRATION
P.O.
- Give drug consistently with meals. Food may increase absorption of propranolol.

• Compliance may be improved by giving drug twice daily or as extended-release capsules. Check with prescriber.

• Check blood pressure and apical pulse before giving drug. If hypotension or extremes in pulse rate occur, withhold drug and notify prescriber.

I.V.

• For direct injection, give into a large vessel or into the tubing of a free-flowing, compatible I.V. solution; don't give by continuous I.V. infusion.

• Drug is compatible with D_5W, half-normal saline solution, normal saline solution, and lactated Ringer's solution.

• Infusion rate shouldn't exceed 1 mg/minute.

• Double-check dose and route. I.V. doses are much smaller than oral doses.

• Monitor blood pressure, ECG, central venous pressure, and heart rate and rhythm frequently, especially during I.V. administration. If patient develops severe hypotension, notify prescriber; a vaso-pressor may be prescribed.

• For overdose, give I.V. isoproterenol, I.V. atropine, or glucagon; refractory cases may require a pacemaker.

• **Incompatibilities:** Amphotericin B, diazoxide.

ACTION

Reduces cardiac oxygen demand by blocking catecholamine-induced increases in heart rate, blood pressure, and force of myocardial contraction. Drug depresses renin secretion and prevents vasodilation of cerebral arteries.

Route	Onset	Peak	Duration
P.O.	30 min	60–90 min	12 hr
P.O. (extended)	Unknown	6–14 hr	24 hr
I.V.	Immediate	1 min	5 min

Half-life: About 4 hours; 8 hours for InnoPran XL.

ADVERSE REACTIONS

CNS: *fatigue, lethargy,* fever, vivid dreams, hallucinations, mental depression, light-headedness, dizziness, insomnia.

CV: *hypotension,* **bradycardia, heart failure, intensification of AV block,** intermittent claudication.

GI: abdominal cramping, constipation, diarrhea, nausea, vomiting.

Hematologic: *agranulocytosis.*

Respiratory: *bronchospasm.*

Skin: rash.

INTERACTIONS

Drug-drug. *Aminophylline:* May antagonize beta-blocking effects of propranolol. Use together cautiously.

Cardiac glycosides: May reduce the positive inotrope effect of the glycoside. Monitor patient for clinical effect.

Cimetidine: May inhibit metabolism of propranolol. Watch for increased beta-blocking effect.

Diltiazem, verapamil: May cause hypotension, bradycardia, and increased depressant effect on myocardium. Use together cautiously.

Epinephrine: May cause severe vasoconstriction. Monitor blood pressure and observe patient carefully.

Glucagon, isoproterenol: May antagonize propranolol effect. May be used therapeutically and in emergencies.

Haloperidol: May cause cardiac arrest. Avoid using together.

Insulin, oral antidiabetics: May alter requirements for these drugs in previously stabilized diabetics. Monitor patient for hypoglycemia.

Phenothiazines (chlorpromazine, thioridazine): May increase risk of serious adverse reactions of either drug. Use with thioridazine is contraindicated. If chlorpromazine must be used, monitor patient's pulse and blood pressure; decrease propranolol dose as needed.

Propafenone: May increase propranolol level. Monitor cardiac function, and adjust propranolol dose as needed.

Drug-herb. *Betel palm:* May decrease temperature-elevating effects and enhanced CNS effects. Discourage use together.

Ma huang: May decrease antihypertensive effects. Discourage use together.

Drug-lifestyle. *Alcohol:* May increase propranolol level. Discourage alcohol use.

Cocaine use: May increase angina-inducing potential of cocaine. Inform patient of this interaction.

Reactions may be *common,* uncommon, *life-threatening,* or COMMON AND LIFE-THREATENING.
Interaction may have a *rapid onset* or **delayed onset.**

EFFECTS ON LAB TEST RESULTS
● May increase BUN, transaminase, alkaline phosphatase, potassium, and LDH levels.
● May decrease granulocyte count.

CONTRAINDICATIONS & CAUTIONS
■ **Black Box Warning** Abrupt withdrawal of drug may cause exacerbation of angina or myocardial infarction. To discontinue drug, gradually reduce dosage over a few weeks. Because coronary artery disease may be unrecognized, don't discontinue drug abruptly, even when taken for other indications. ■
● Contraindicated in patients with bronchial asthma, sinus bradycardia and heart block greater than first-degree, cardiogenic shock, and overt and decompensated heart failure (unless failure is secondary to a tachyarrhythmia that can be treated with propranolol).
● Use cautiously in patients with hepatic or renal impairment, nonallergic bronchospastic diseases, or hepatic disease and in those taking other antihypertensives.
● Use cautiously in patients who have diabetes mellitus because drug masks some symptoms of hypoglycemia.
● In patients with thyrotoxicosis, use drug cautiously because it may mask the signs and symptoms.
● Elderly patients may experience enhanced adverse reactions and may need dosage adjustment.
● Use cautiously in pregnant women because drug may be associated with small placenta and congenital anomalies.

NURSING CONSIDERATIONS
● Drug masks common signs and symptoms of shock and hypoglycemia.
● Monitor black patients for expected therapeutic effects; dosage adjustments may be necessary.
● **Alert:** Don't stop drug before surgery for pheochromocytoma. Before any surgical procedure, tell anesthesiologist that patient is receiving propranolol.
● **Look alike–sound alike:** Don't confuse propranolol with Pravachol. Don't confuse Inderal with Inderide, Isordil, Adderall, or Imuran.

PATIENT TEACHING
● Caution patient to continue taking this drug as prescribed, even when he's feeling well.
● Instruct patient to take drug with food.
● **Alert:** Tell patient not to stop drug suddenly because this can worsen chest pain and trigger a heart attack.

---

ranolazine
ran-OH-lah-zeen

Ranexa◆

Pharmacologic class: cardiovascular drug
Pregnancy risk category C

AVAILABLE FORMS
Tablets (extended-release): 500 mg, 1,000 mg

INDICATIONS & DOSAGES
➤ **Chronic angina, given with amlodipine, beta blockers, or nitrates, in patients who haven't achieved an adequate response with other antianginals**
Adults: Initially, 500 mg P.O. b.i.d. Increase, if needed, to maximum of 1,000 mg b.i.d.

ADMINISTRATION
P.O.
● Give drug without regard for meals.
● Give drug whole; don't crush or cut tablets.
● Don't give drug with grapefruit juice.

ACTION
May result from increased efficiency of myocardial oxygen use when myocardial metabolism is shifted away from fatty acid oxidation toward glucose oxidation. Antianginal and anti-ischemic properties don't decrease heart rate or blood pressure and don't increase myocardial work.

Route	Onset	Peak	Duration
P.O.	Rapid	2–5 hr	Unknown

Half-life: 7 hours.

ADVERSE REACTIONS
CNS: dizziness, headache.
CV: palpitations, peripheral edema, syncope.
EENT: tinnitus, vertigo.
GI: abdominal pain, constipation, dry mouth, nausea, vomiting.
Respiratory: dyspnea.

INTERACTIONS
Drug-drug. *Antipsychotics or tricyclic antidepressants metabolized by CYP2D6:* May increase levels of these drugs. Dosage reduction may be needed.
Cyclosporine, paroxetine, ritonavir: May increase ranolazine level. Use cautiously together, and monitor patient for increased adverse effects.
Digoxin: May increase digoxin level. Monitor digoxin level periodically; digoxin dosage may need to be reduced.
Diltiazem, HIV protease inhibitors, ketoconazole and other azole antifungals, macrolide antibiotics (azithromycin, erythromycin), verapamil: May increase ranolazine level and prolong QT interval. Avoid using together.
Drugs that prolong the QT interval (antiarrhythmics, such as dofetilide, quinidine, and sotalol), antipsychotics, such as Thorazine and ziprasidone: May increase the risk of prolonged QT interval. Avoid using together.
Rifabutin, rifampin, rifapentine, other CYP3A inducers (carbamazepine, pheno-barbital, phenytoin): May reduce plasma concentration of ranolazine to subthera-peutic levels. Don't use together.
Simvastatin: May increase simvastatin level. Monitor patient for adverse effects, and decrease simvastatin dosage as needed.
Drug-herb. *St. John's wort:* May reduce plasma concentration of ranolazine to subtherapeutic levels. Don't use together.
Drug-food. *Grapefruit:* May increase drug level and prolong QT interval. Discourage use together.

EFFECTS ON LAB TEST RESULTS
• May increase creatinine and BUN levels. May decrease hemoglobin level and hematocrit.
• May decrease eosinophil count.

CONTRAINDICATIONS & CAUTIONS
• Contraindicated in patients taking QT interval–prolonging drugs or CYP3A inhibitors (including diltiazem), and in patients with ventricular tachycardia, hepatic impairment, or a prolonged QT interval.
• Use cautiously in patients with renal impairment.
• It isn't known whether drug appears in breast milk. Patient should either stop breast-feeding or stop the drug.

NURSING CONSIDERATIONS
• *Alert:* Drug prolongs the QT interval according to the dose. If drug is given with other drugs that prolong the QTc interval, torsades de pointes or sudden death may occur. Don't exceed maximum dosage.
• Obtain baseline ECG and monitor subsequent ECG for prolonged QT interval. Measure the QTc interval regularly.
• If patient has renal insufficiency, monitor blood pressure closely.

PATIENT TEACHING
• Teach patient about this drug's potential to affect the heart's rhythm. Advise patient to immediately report palpitations or fainting.
• Urge patient to tell prescriber about all other prescription or OTC drugs or herbal supplements he takes.
• Tell patient that he should keep taking other drugs prescribed for angina.
• Tell patient that drug may be taken with or without food.
• Advise patient to avoid grapefruit juice while taking this drug.
• *Alert:* Warn patient that tablets must be swallowed whole and not crushed, broken, or chewed.
• Explain that drug won't stop a sudden anginal attack; advise him to keep other treatments, such as S.L. nitroglycerin, readily available.
• Tell patient to avoid activities that require mental alertness until effects of the drug are known.

Reactions may be *common,* uncommon, *life-threatening,* or COMMON AND LIFE-THREATENING.
Interaction may have a *rapid onset* or *delayed onset.*

verapamil hydrochloride
ver-AP-a-mill

Apo-Verap†, Calan✐, Covera-HS,
Isoptin SR✐, Novo-Veramil†,
Nu-Verap†, Verelan✐, Verelan PM

Pharmacologic class: calcium
channel blocker
Pregnancy risk category C

AVAILABLE FORMS
Capsules (extended-release): 100 mg,
120 mg, 180 mg, 200 mg, 240 mg, 300 mg
Capsules (sustained-release): 120 mg,
180 mg, 240 mg, 360 mg
Injection: 2.5 mg/ml
Tablets: 40 mg, 80 mg, 120 mg
Tablets (extended-release): 120 mg,
180 mg, 240 mg
Tablets (sustained-release): 120 mg,
180 mg, 240 mg

INDICATIONS & DOSAGES
➤ **Vasospastic angina (Prinzmetal's
or variant angina); classic chronic,
stable angina pectoris; chronic atrial
fibrillation**
Adults: Starting dose is 80 to 120 mg P.O.
t.i.d. Increase dosage at daily or weekly
intervals as needed. Some patients may
require up to 480 mg daily.
➤ **To prevent paroxysmal supraventricular tachycardia**
Adults: 80 to 120 mg P.O. t.i.d. or q.i.d.
➤ **Supraventricular arrhythmias**
Adults: 0.075 to 0.15 mg/kg (5 to 10 mg)
by I.V. push over 2 minutes with ECG and
blood pressure monitoring. Repeat dose of
0.15 mg/kg (10 mg) in 30 minutes if no
response occurs.
Children ages 1 to 15: Give 0.1 to
0.3 mg/kg as I.V. bolus over 2 minutes;
not to exceed 5 mg. Repeat dose in
30 minutes if response is inadequate.
Children younger than age 1: Give 0.1 to
0.2 mg/kg as I.V. bolus over 2 minutes
with continuous ECG monitoring.
Repeat dose in 30 minutes if no response
occurs.
➤ **Digitalized patients with chronic
atrial fibrillation or flutter**
Adults: 240 to 320 mg P.O. daily, divided
t.i.d. or q.i.d.

➤ **Hypertension**
Adults: 240 mg extended-release tablet
P.O. once daily in the morning. If response
isn't adequate, give an additional 120 mg
in the evening or 240 mg every 12 hours,
or an 80-mg immediate-release tablet t.i.d.
If using Verelan PM, 200 mg P.O. daily at
bedtime. May increase to 300 mg at bedtime if response is inadequate. Maximum
dose is 400 mg. If using Covera-HS,
180 mg P.O. daily at bedtime. May increase
to 240 mg daily if response is inadequate.
Subsequent dosage adjustments may be
made in 120-mg increments up to a
maximum of 480 mg at bedtime.

ADMINISTRATION
P.O.
● Pellet-filled capsules may be given
by carefully opening the capsule and
sprinkling the pellets on a spoonful of
applesauce. This should be swallowed
immediately without chewing, followed
by a glass of cool water to ensure all the
pellets are swallowed.
● Give long-acting forms of the drug
whole; don't crush or break tablet.
I.V.
● This form is contraindicated in patients
receiving I.V. beta blockers and in those
with ventricular tachycardia.
● Inject directly into a vein or into the
tubing of a free-flowing, compatible solution, such as D_5W, half-normal saline
solution, normal saline solution, Ringer's
solution, or lactated Ringer's solution.
● Give doses over at least 2 minutes
(3 minutes in elderly patients) to minimize
the risk of adverse reactions.
● Monitor ECG and blood pressure
continuously.
● **Incompatibilities:** Albumin, aminophylline, amphotericin B, ampicillin
sodium, co-trimoxazole, dobutamine,
hydralazine, nafcillin, oxacillin, propofol,
sodium bicarbonate, solutions with a pH
greater than 6.

ACTION
Not clearly defined. A calcium channel
blocker that inhibits calcium ion influx
across cardiac and smooth-muscle cells,
thus decreasing myocardial contractility
and oxygen demand; it also dilates
coronary arteries and arterioles.

Route	Onset	Peak	Duration
P.O.	30 min	1–2 hr	8–10 hr
P.O. (extended)	30 min	5–9 hr	24 hr
I.V.	Immediate	1–5 min	1–6 hr

Half-life: 6 to 12 hours.

ADVERSE REACTIONS

CNS: dizziness, headache, asthenia, fatigue, sleep disturbances.
CV: *transient hypotension,* **heart failure, bradycardia, AV block, ventricular asystole, ventricular fibrillation,** peripheral edema.
GI: *constipation,* nausea, diarrhea, dyspepsia.
Respiratory: dyspnea, pharyngitis, **pulmonary edema,** rhinitis, sinusitis, upper respiratory infection.
Skin: rash.

INTERACTIONS

Drug-drug. *Acebutolol, atenolol, betaxolol, carteolol,* **digoxin,** *esmolol, metoprolol, nadolol, penbutolol, pindolol, propranolol, timolol:* May increase effects of both drugs. Monitor cardiac function closely and decrease doses as needed.
Amiodarone: May cause bradycardia and decrease cardiac output. Monitor patient closely.
Antihypertensives, quinidine: May cause hypotension. Monitor blood pressure.
Carbamazepine: May increase levels of carbamazepine. Monitor patient for toxicity and adjust dosage as needed.
Cyclosporine: May increase cyclosporine level. Monitor cyclosporine level.
Disopyramide, flecainide: May cause heart failure. Avoid using together.
Dofetilide: May increase dofetilide level. Avoid using together.
HMG-CoA reductase inhibitors (atorvastatin, lovastatin, simvastatin): May elevate plasma concentrations of these drugs. If coadministration can't be avoided, administer conservative dose of the HMG-CoA reductase inhibitor.
Lithium: May decrease or increase lithium level. Monitor lithium level.
Phenytoin: May decrease effects of verapamil. Monitor patient closely and adjust dose as needed.

Rifampin: May decrease oral bioavailability of verapamil. Monitor patient for lack of effect.
Neuromuscular-blocking drugs: May potentiate the activity of these drugs. Monitor neuromuscular function and adjust dosages of either drug as needed.
Sirolimus, tacrolimus: May increase levels of these drugs. Monitor drug levels closely and adjust dosage as needed.
Drug-herb. *Black catechu:* May cause additive effects. Discourage use together.
St. John's wort: May decrease drug level and effect. Discourage use together.
Yerba maté: May decrease clearance of herb's methylxanthines and cause toxicity. Urge caution.
Drug-food. *Grapefruit juice:* May increase drug level. Discourage use together.
Drug-lifestyle. *Alcohol use:* May enhance the effects of alcohol. Discourage use together.

EFFECTS ON LAB TEST RESULTS
• May increase ALT, AST, alkaline phosphatase, and bilirubin levels.

CONTRAINDICATIONS & CAUTIONS
• Contraindicated in patients hypersensitive to drug and in those with severe left ventricular dysfunction, cardiogenic shock, second- or third-degree AV block or sick sinus syndrome except in presence of functioning pacemaker, atrial flutter or fibrillation and accessory bypass tract syndrome, severe heart failure (unless secondary to therapy), and severe hypotension.
• I.V. form is contraindicated in patients receiving I.V. beta blockers and in those with ventricular tachycardia.
• Use cautiously in elderly patients and in those with increased intracranial pressure or hepatic or renal disease.

NURSING CONSIDERATIONS
• Patients receiving beta blockers should receive lower doses of this drug. Monitor these patients closely.
• When clinically advisable, have the patient perform vagal maneuvers before giving drug.
• Monitor blood pressure at the start of therapy and during dosage adjustments.

Reactions may be *common,* uncommon, *life-threatening,* or **COMMON AND LIFE-THREATENING.**
Interaction may have a *rapid onset* or **delayed onset.**

Assist patient with walking because dizziness may occur.

- If signs and symptoms of heart failure occur, such as swelling of hands and feet and shortness of breath, notify prescriber.
- Monitor liver function test results during prolonged treatment.
- *Look alike–sound alike:* Don't confuse Verelan with Vivarin, Voltaren, or Virilon.

PATIENT TEACHING
- Instruct patient to take oral form of drug exactly as prescribed.
- Tell patient that long-acting forms shouldn't be crushed or chewed.
- Caution patient against abruptly stopping drug.
- If patient continues nitrate therapy during oral verapamil dosage adjustment, urge continued compliance. S.L. nitroglycerin may be taken, as needed, for acute chest pain.
- Encourage patient to increase fluid and fiber intake to combat constipation. Give a stool softener.
- Drug significantly inhibits alcohol elimination. Advise patient to avoid or severely limit alcohol use.
- Inform patient taking Covera-HS that the outer shell of the drug may be excreted in feces.

adenosine
amiodarone hydrochloride
atropine sulfate
digoxin
(See Chapter 26, INOTROPICS.)
disopyramide
disopyramide phosphate
dofetilide
esmolol hydrochloride
flecainide acetate
ibutilide fumarate
isoproterenol hydrochloride
(See Chapter 56, BRONCHODILATORS.)
lidocaine hydrochloride
magnesium sulfate
(See Chapter 37, ANTICONVULSANTS.)
mexiletine hydrochloride
procainamide hydrochloride
propafenone hydrochloride
propranolol hydrochloride
(See Chapter 21, ANTIANGINALS.)
quinidine gluconate
quinidine sulfate
sotalol hydrochloride
verapamil hydrochloride
(See Chapter 21, ANTIANGINALS.)

---

adenosine
a-DEN-oh-seen

Adenocard

Pharmacologic class: nucleoside
Pregnancy risk category C

AVAILABLE FORMS
Injection: 3 mg/ml in 2-ml, 4-ml, and 5-ml vials and syringes

INDICATIONS & DOSAGES
➤ **To convert paroxysmal supraventricular tachycardia (PSVT) to sinus rhythm**
Adults and children who weigh 50 kg (110 lb) or more: 6 mg I.V. by rapid bolus injection over 1 to 2 seconds. If PSVT isn't eliminated in 1 to 2 minutes, give 12 mg by rapid I.V. push and repeat, if needed.

Children who weigh less than 50 kg:
Initially, 0.05 to 0.1 mg/kg I.V. by rapid bolus injection followed by a saline flush. If PSVT isn't eliminated in 1 to 2 minutes, give additional bolus injections, increasing the amount given by 0.05- to 0.1-mg/kg increments, followed by a saline flush. Continue, as needed, until conversion or a maximum single dose of 0.3 mg/kg is given.

ADMINISTRATION
I.V.
● Don't give single doses exceeding 12 mg.
● In adults, avoid giving drug through a central line because more prolonged asystole may occur.
● Give by rapid I.V. injection to ensure drug action.
● Give directly into a vein, if possible. When giving through an I.V. line, use the port closest to the patient.
● Flush immediately and rapidly with normal saline solution to ensure that drug quickly reaches the systemic circulation.
● **Incompatibilities:** Other I.V. drugs.

ACTION
Naturally occurring nucleoside that acts on the AV node to slow conduction and inhibit reentry pathways. Drug is also useful in treating PSVTs, including those with accessory bypass tracts (Wolff-Parkinson-White syndrome).

Route	Onset	Peak	Duration
I.V.	Immediate	Immediate	Unknown

Half-life: Less than 10 seconds.

ADVERSE REACTIONS
CNS: dizziness, light-headedness, numbness, tingling in arms, headache.
CV: chest pressure, *facial flushing.*
GI: nausea.
Respiratory: *dyspnea, shortness of breath.*

Reactions may be common, uncommon, **life-threatening**, or COMMON AND LIFE-THREATENING.
Interaction may have a *rapid onset* or **delayed onset**.

INTERACTIONS

Drug-drug. *Carbamazepine:* May cause high-level heart block. Use together cautiously.

Digoxin, verapamil: May cause ventricular fibrillation. Monitor ECG closely.

Dipyridamole: May increase adenosine's effects. Adenosine dose may need to be reduced. Use together cautiously.

Methylxanthines (caffeine, theophylline): May decrease adenosine's effects. Adenosine dose may need to be increased or patients may not respond to adenosine therapy.

Drug-herb. *Guarana:* May decrease patient's response to drug. Monitor patient.

EFFECTS ON LAB TEST RESULTS
None reported.

CONTRAINDICATIONS & CAUTIONS
• Contraindicated in patients hypersensitive to drug.
• Contraindicated in those with second- or third-degree heart block or sinus node disease (such as sick sinus syndrome and symptomatic bradycardia), except those with a pacemaker.
• Use cautiously in patients with asthma, emphysema, or bronchitis because bronchoconstriction may occur.

NURSING CONSIDERATIONS
• *Alert:* By decreasing conduction through the AV node, drug may produce first-, second-, or third-degree heart block. Patients who develop high-level heart block after a single dose shouldn't receive additional doses.
• *Alert:* New arrhythmias, including heart block and transient asystole, may develop; monitor cardiac rhythm and treat as indicated.
• If solution is cold, crystals may form; gently warm solution to room temperature. Don't use solutions that aren't clear.
• Drug lacks preservatives. Discard unused portion.
• *Alert:* Don't confuse adenosine with adenosine phosphate.

PATIENT TEACHING
• Instruct patient to report adverse reactions promptly.
• Tell patient to report discomfort at I.V. site.

• Inform patient that he may experience flushing or chest pain lasting 1 to 2 minutes.

SAFETY ALERT!

amiodarone hydrochloride
am-ee-OH-dah-rohn

Cordarone✐, Pacerone

Pharmacologic class: benzofuran derivative
Pregnancy risk category D

AVAILABLE FORMS
Injection: 50 mg/ml in 3-ml ampules, vials
Tablets: 100 mg, 200 mg, 400 mg

INDICATIONS & DOSAGES
■ **Black Box Warning** Amiodarone is intended for use only in patients with life-threatening recurrent ventricular fibrillation or recurrent hemodynamically unstable ventricular tachycardia unresponsive to adequate doses of other antiarrhythmics or when alternative drugs can't be tolerated. ■

Adults: Give loading dose of 800 to 1,600 mg P.O. daily divided b.i.d. for 1 to 3 weeks until first therapeutic response occurs; then 600 to 800 mg P.O. daily for 1 month, followed by maintenance dose of 200 to 600 mg P.O. daily for 1 month. Then give 400 mg P.O. daily.

Or, give loading dose of 150 mg I.V. over 10 minutes (15 mg/minute); then 360 mg I.V. over next 6 hours (1 mg/minute), followed by 540 mg I.V. over next 18 hours (0.5 mg/minute). After first 24 hours, continue with maintenance I.V. infusion of 720 mg/24 hours (0.5 mg/minute).

ADMINISTRATION
P.O.
• Divide oral loading dose into two or three equal doses and give with meals to decrease GI intolerance. Give maintenance dose once daily or divide into two doses, with meals to decrease GI intolerance.
I.V.
• Give drug I.V. only if continuous ECG and electrophysiologic monitoring are available.

- Mix first dose of 150 mg in 100 ml of D_5W solution.
- If infusion will last 2 hours or longer, mix solution in glass or polyolefin bottles.
- If concentration is 2 mg/ml or more, give drug through a central line. If possible, use a dedicated line.
- Use an in-line filter.
- Continuously monitor patient's cardiac status. If hypotension occurs, reduce infusion rate.
- Cordarone I.V. leaches out plasticizers from I.V. tubing and adsorbs to polyvinyl chloride (PVC) tubing, which can adversely affect male reproductive tract development in fetuses, infants, and toddlers when used at concentrations or flow rates outside of recommendations.
- **Incompatibilities:** Aminophylline, ampicillin sodium and sulbactam sodium, bivalirudin, cefazolin sodium, ceftazidime, digoxin, furosemide, heparin sodium, imipenem and cilastatin sodium, magnesium sulfate, normal saline solution, piperacillin sodium, piperacillin and tazobactam sodium, quinidine gluconate, sodium bicarbonate, sodium nitroprusside, sodium phosphates.

ACTION
Effects result from blockade of potassium chloride leading to a prolongation of action potential duration.

Route	Onset	Peak	Duration
P.O.	Variable	3–7 hr	Variable
I.V.	Unknown	Unknown	Variable

Half-life: 25 to 110 days (usually 40 to 50 days).

ADVERSE REACTIONS
CNS: *fatigue, malaise, tremor,* peripheral neuropathy, ataxia, paresthesia, insomnia, sleep disturbances, headache.
CV: *hypotension, **bradycardia, arrhythmias, heart failure, heart block, sinus arrest,*** edema.
EENT: *asymptomatic corneal microdeposits, visual disturbances,* optic neuropathy or neuritis resulting in visual impairment, abnormal smell.
GI: *nausea, vomiting,* abnormal taste, anorexia, constipation, abdominal pain.
Hematologic: *coagulation abnormalities.*

Hepatic: ***hepatic failure,*** hepatic dysfunction.
Metabolic: *hypothyroidism,* hyperthyroidism.
Respiratory: ***acute respiratory distress syndrome,*** SEVERE PULMONARY TOXICITY.
Skin: *photosensitivity,* solar dermatitis, blue-gray skin.

INTERACTIONS
Drug-drug. *Antiarrhythmics:* May reduce hepatic or renal clearance of certain antiarrhythmics, especially flecainide, procainamide, and quinidine. Use of amiodarone with other antiarrhythmics, especially mexiletine, propafenone, disopyramide, and procainamide, may induce torsades de pointes. Avoid using together.
Azole antifungals, disopyramide, pimozide: May increase the risk of arrhythmias, including torsades de pointes. Avoid using together.
Beta blockers, calcium channel blockers: May potentiate bradycardia, sinus arrest, and AV block; may increase hypotensive effect. Use together cautiously.
Cimetidine: May increase amiodarone level. Use together cautiously.
Cyclosporine: May increase cyclosporine level, resulting in an increase in the serum creatinine level and renal toxicity. Monitor cyclosporine levels and renal function tests.
Digoxin: May increase digoxin level 70% to 100%. Monitor digoxin level closely and reduce digoxin dosage by half or stop drug completely when starting amiodarone therapy.
Fentanyl: May cause hypotension, bradycardia, and decreased cardiac output. Monitor patient closely.
Fluoroquinolones: May increase risk of arrhythmias, including torsades de pointes. Avoid using together.
Macrolide antibiotics (azithromycin, clarithromycin, erythromycin, telithromycin): May cause additive or prolongation of the QT interval. Use with caution. Avoid use with telithromycin.
Methotrexate: May impair methotrexate metabolism, causing toxicity. Use together cautiously.
Phenytoin: May decrease phenytoin metabolism and amiodarone level. Monitor

---

Reactions may be *common,* uncommon, ***life-threatening***, or COMMON AND LIFE-THREATENING.
Interaction may have a *rapid onset* or ***delayed onset.***

phenytoin level and adjust dosages of drugs if needed.

Protease inhibitors (amprenavir, atazanavir, indinavir, lopinavir and ritonavir, nelfinavir, ritonavir, and saquinavir): May increase the risk of amiodarone toxicity. Use of ritonavir or nelfinavir with amiodarone is contraindicated. Use other protease inhibitors cautiously.

Quinidine: May increase quinidine level, causing life-threatening cardiac arrhythmias. Avoid using together, or monitor quinidine level closely if use together can't be avoided. Adjust quinidine dosage as needed.

Rifamycins: May decrease amiodarone level. Monitor patient closely.

Simvastatin: May cause myopathy and rhabdomyolysis with concomitant use. Simvastatin dosage shouldn't exceed 20 mg daily.

Theophylline: May increase theophylline level and cause toxicity. Monitor theophylline level.

Warfarin: May increase anticoagulant response with the potential for serious or fatal bleeding. Decrease warfarin dosage 33% to 50% when starting amiodarone. Monitor patient closely.

Drug-herb. *Pennyroyal:* May change rate of formation of toxic metabolites of pennyroyal. Discourage use together.

St. John's wort: May decrease amiodarone levels. Discourage use together.

Drug-food. *Grapefruit juice:* May inhibit CYP3A4 metabolism of drug in the intestinal mucosa, causing increased levels and risk of toxicity. Discourage use together.

Drug-lifestyle. *Sun exposure:* May cause photosensitivity reaction. Advise patient to avoid excessive sunlight exposure and to take precautions while in the sun.

EFFECTS ON LAB TEST RESULTS
• May increase alkaline phosphatase, ALT, AST, GGT, reverse T_3, and T_4 levels. May decrease T_3 level.
• May increase total cholesterol and serum lipid levels.
• May increase PT and INR.

CONTRAINDICATIONS & CAUTIONS
• Contraindicated in patients hypersensitive to drug or to iodine.

• Contraindicated in those with cardiogenic shock, second- or third-degree AV block, severe SA node disease resulting in bradycardia unless an artificial pacemaker is present, and in those for whom bradycardia has caused syncope.
• Use cautiously in patients receiving other antiarrhythmics.
• Use cautiously in patients with pulmonary, hepatic, or thyroid disease.

NURSING CONSIDERATIONS
• Be aware of the high risk of adverse reactions.
• Obtain baseline pulmonary, liver, and thyroid function test results and baseline chest X-ray.
■ **Black Box Warning** Give loading doses in a hospital setting and with continuous ECG monitoring because of the slow onset of antiarrhythmic effect and the risk of life-threatening arrhythmias. ■
■ **Black Box Warning** Drug may pose life-threatening management problems in patients at risk for sudden death. Use only in patients with life-threatening, recurrent ventricular arrhythmias unresponsive to or intolerant of other antiarrhythmics or alternative drugs. Amiodarone can cause fatal toxicities, including hepatic and pulmonary toxicity. ■
■ **Black Box Warning** Drug is highly toxic. Watch carefully for pulmonary toxicity. Risk increases in patients receiving doses over 400 mg/day. ■
• Watch for evidence of pneumonitis, exertional dyspnea, nonproductive cough, and pleuritic chest pain. Monitor pulmonary function tests and chest X-ray.
• Monitor liver and thyroid function test results and electrolyte levels, particularly potassium and magnesium.
• Monitor PT and INR if patient takes warfarin and digoxin level if he takes digoxin.
• Instill methylcellulose ophthalmic solution during amiodarone therapy to minimize corneal microdeposits. About 1 to 4 months after starting amiodarone, most patients develop corneal microdeposits, although 10% or less have vision disturbances. Regular ophthalmic examinations are advised.

- Monitor blood pressure and heart rate and rhythm frequently. Perform continuous ECG monitoring when starting or changing dosage. Notify prescriber of significant change in assessment results.
- Safety and efficacy in children haven't been established. Life-threatening gasping syndrome may occur in neonates given I.V. solutions containing benzyl alcohol.
- During or after treatment with I.V. form, patient may be transferred to oral therapy.
- *Look alike–sound alike:* Don't confuse amiodarone with amiloride.

PATIENT TEACHING

- Advise patient to wear sunscreen or protective clothing to prevent sensitivity reaction to the sun. Monitor patient for skin burning or tingling, followed by redness and blistering. Exposed skin may turn blue-gray.
- Tell patient to take oral drug with food if GI reactions occur.
- Inform patient that adverse effects of drug are more common at high doses and become more frequent with treatment lasting longer than 6 months, but are generally reversible when drug is stopped. Resolution of adverse reactions may take up to 4 months.
- Tell patient not to stop taking this medication without consulting with his prescriber.

SAFETY ALERT!

atropine sulfate
AT-troe-peen

AtroPen

Pharmacologic class:
anticholinergic, belladonna alkaloid
Pregnancy risk category C

AVAILABLE FORMS

Injection: 0.05 mg/ml, 0.1 mg/ml, 0.3 mg/ml, 0.4 mg/ml, 0.5 mg/ml, 0.8 mg/ml, 1 mg/ml
Prefilled auto-injectors: 0.5 mg, 1 mg, 2 mg
Tablets: 0.4 mg

INDICATIONS & DOSAGES

➤ **Symptomatic bradycardia, brady-arrhythmia (junctional or escape rhythm)**
Adults: Usually 0.5 to 1 mg I.V. push, repeated every 3 to 5 minutes to maximum of 3 mg.
Children and adolescents: 0.02 mg/kg I.V., with minimum dose of 0.1 mg and maximum single dose of 0.5 mg in children or 1 mg in adolescents. May repeat dose at 5-minute intervals to a maximum total dose of 1 mg in children or 2 mg in adolescents.

➤ **Antidote for anticholinesterase-insecticide poisoning**
Adults: Initially, 1 to 2 mg I.V.; may repeat with 2 mg I.M. or I.V. every 5 to 60 minutes until muscarinic signs and symptoms disappear or signs of atropine toxicity appear. Severe poisoning may require up to 6 mg hourly.
Children: 0.05 mg/kg I.V. or I.M. repeated every 10 to 30 minutes until muscarinic signs and symptoms disappear (may be repeated if they reappear) or until atropine toxicity occurs.

➤ **Preoperatively to diminish secretions and block cardiac vagal reflexes**
Adults and children who weigh 20 kg (44 lb) or more: 0.4 to 0.6 mg I.V., I.M., or subcutaneously 30 to 60 minutes before anesthesia.
Children who weigh less than 20 kg: 0.01 mg/kg I.V., I.M., or subcutaneously up to maximum dose of 0.4 mg 30 to 60 minutes before anesthesia. May repeat every 4 to 6 hours p.r.n.
Infants who weigh more than 5 kg (11 lb): 0.03 mg/kg every 4 to 6 hours p.r.n.
Infants who weigh 5 kg or less: 0.04 mg/kg every 4 to 6 hours p.r.n.

➤ **Adjunct treatment of peptic ulcer disease; functional GI disorders such as irritable bowel syndrome**
Adults: 0.4 to 0.6 mg P.O. every 4 to 6 hours.
Children: 0.01 mg/kg P.O. not to exceed 0.4 mg P.O every 4 to 6 hours.

ADMINISTRATION

P.O.
- Give drug without regard for food.
I.V.
- Give into a large vein or into I.V. tubing over at least 1 minute.

Reactions may be *common,* uncommon, *life-threatening,* or COMMON AND LIFE-THREATENING.
Interaction may have a *rapid onset* or *delayed onset.*

• Slow delivery may cause slowing of the heart rate.
• **Incompatibilities:** Alkalies, bromides, iodides, isoproterenol, methohexital, norepinephrine, pentobarbital sodium, sodium bicarbonate.
I.M.
• Document administration site.
Subcutaneous
• Auto-injection may be given through clothing.
• Firmly jab tip into outer thigh at 90-degree angle.
• Hold auto-injector in place for at least 10 seconds to allow time for complete administration.
• Make sure needle is visible after removing auto-injector. If needle didn't engage, repeat injection, jabbing more firmly.
• Massage injection site for several seconds after removing auto-injector.
• In very thin or young patients, pinch the skin on the thigh together before injection.

ACTION
Inhibits acetylcholine at parasympathetic neuroeffector junction, blocking vagal effects on SA and AV nodes, enhancing conduction through AV node and increasing heart rate.

Route	Onset	Peak	Duration
P.O.	30–120 min	1–2 hr	4 hr
I.V.	Immediate	2–4 min	4 hr
I.M.	5–40 min	20–60 min	4 hr
Subcut.	Unknown	Unknown	Unknown

Half-life: Initial, 2 hours; second phase, 12½ hours.

ADVERSE REACTIONS
CNS: *headache, restlessness, insomnia, dizziness,* ataxia, disorientation, hallucinations, delirium, excitement, agitation, confusion.
CV: *bradycardia,* palpitations, tachycardia.
EENT: *blurred vision, mydriasis,* photophobia, cycloplegia, increased intraocular pressure.
GI: *dry mouth, constipation,* thirst, nausea, vomiting.
GU: urine retention, impotence.
Other: *anaphylaxis.*

INTERACTIONS
Drug-drug. *Antacids:* May decrease absorption of oral anticholinergics. Separate doses by at least 1 hour.
Anticholinergics, drugs with anticholinergic effects (amantadine, antiarrhythmics, antiparkinsonians, glutethimide, meperidine, phenothiazines, tricyclic antidepressants): May increase anticholinergic effects. Use together cautiously.
Ketoconazole, levodopa: May decrease absorption of these drugs. Separate doses by at least 2 hours, and monitor patient for clinical effect.
Potassium chloride wax-matrix tablets: May increase risk of mucosal lesions. Use together cautiously.
Drug-herb. *Jaborandi tree, pill-bearing spurge:* May decrease effectiveness of drug. Discourage use together.
Jimsonweed: May adversely affect CV function. Discourage use together.
Squaw vine: Tannic acid may decrease metabolic breakdown of drug. Monitor patient.

EFFECTS ON LAB TEST RESULTS
None reported.

CONTRAINDICATIONS & CAUTIONS
• Contraindicated in patients hypersensitive to drug.
• Contraindicated in those with acute angle-closure glaucoma, obstructive uropathy, obstructive disease of GI tract, paralytic ileus, toxic megacolon, intestinal atony, unstable CV status in acute hemorrhage, tachycardia, myocardial ischemia, asthma, or myasthenia gravis.
• Use cautiously in patients with Down syndrome because they may be more sensitive to drug.

NURSING CONSIDERATIONS
• In adults, avoid doses less than 0.5 mg because of risk of paradoxical bradycardia.
• **Alert:** Watch for tachycardia in cardiac patients because it may lead to ventricular fibrillation.
• Many adverse reactions (such as dry mouth and constipation) vary with dose.
• Monitor fluid intake and urine output. Drug causes urine retention and urinary hesitancy.

PATIENT TEACHING

● Teach patient receiving oral form of drug how to handle distressing anticholinergic effects such as dry mouth.
● Instruct patient to report serious or persistent adverse reactions promptly.
● Tell patient about potential for sensitivity of the eyes to the sun and suggest use of sunglasses.

---

disopyramide
dye-soe-PEER-a-mide

Rythmodan†

disopyramide phosphate
Norpace, Norpace CR, Rythmodan-LA†

Pharmacologic class: pyridine derivative
Pregnancy risk category C

AVAILABLE FORMS
disopyramide
Capsules: 100 mg†, 150 mg†
disopyramide phosphate
Capsules: 100 mg, 150 mg
Capsules (controlled-release): 100 mg, 150 mg
Tablets (sustained-release): 250 mg†

INDICATIONS & DOSAGES
➤ **Ventricular tachycardia and life-threatening ventricular arrhythmias**
Adults who weigh more than 50 kg (110 lb): 150 mg P.O. every 6 hours with regular-release formulation or 300 mg every 12 hours with extended-release preparations.
Adults who weigh 50 kg or less: 100 mg P.O. every 6 hours with regular-release formulation or 200 mg P.O. every 12 hours with extended-release preparations.
Children ages 12 to 18 years: 6 to 15 mg/kg P.O. daily, divided into four doses (every 6 hours).
Children ages 4 to 12 years: 10 to 15 mg/kg P.O. daily, divided into four doses (every 6 hours).
Children ages 1 to 4 years: 10 to 20 mg/kg P.O. daily, divided into four doses (every 6 hours).

Children younger than age 1 year: 10 to 30 mg/kg P.O. daily, divided into four doses (every 6 hours).
Adjust-a-dose: If creatinine clearance is 30 to 40 ml/minute, give 100 mg every 8 hours; if clearance is 15 to 30 ml/minute, give 100 mg every 12 hours; if clearance is less than 15 ml/minute, give 100 mg every 24 hours. All dosages are for immediate-release form.

Don't use extended-release capsules in patients with a creatinine clearance less than or equal to 40 ml/minute. For patients with creatinine clearance greater than 40 ml/minute or patients with hepatic insufficiency, give 400 mg/day in divided doses (100 mg every 6 hours with immediate-release form or 200 mg every 12 hours with controlled-release form).

ADMINISTRATION
P.O.
● Correct electrolyte abnormalities before starting therapy.
● Check apical pulse before giving drug. Notify prescriber if pulse rate is slower than 60 beats/minute or faster than 120 beats/minute.
● Don't use sustained- or controlled-release preparations to control ventricular arrhythmias when therapeutic drug level must be rapidly attained, in patients with cardiomyopathy or possible cardiac decompensation, or in those with severe renal impairment.
● *Alert:* Don't open the extended-release capsules.
● For use in young children, pharmacist may prepare disopyramide suspension using 100-mg capsules and cherry syrup. Pharmacist should dispense suspension in amber glass bottles. Protect suspension from light.

ACTION
A class IA antiarrhythmic that depresses phase 0, prolongs the action potential, and has membrane-stabilizing effects.

Route	Onset	Peak	Duration
P.O.	½–3½ hr	2–2½ hr	1½–8½ hr

Half-life: 7 hours.

Reactions may be *common*, uncommon, *life-threatening*, or COMMON AND LIFE-THREATENING.
Interaction may have a *rapid onset* or **delayed onset**.

ADVERSE REACTIONS
CNS: *agitation,* dizziness, depression, fatigue, headache, nervousness, acute psychosis, syncope.
CV: *hypotension,* **heart failure, heart block, arrhythmias,** edema, shortness of breath, chest pain.
EENT: blurred vision, dry eyes or nose.
GI: *dry mouth, constipation,* nausea, vomiting, anorexia, bloating, gas, weight gain, abdominal pain, diarrhea.
GU: *urinary hesitancy,* urine retention, urinary frequency, urinary urgency, impotence.
Hepatic: cholestatic jaundice.
Musculoskeletal: muscle weakness, aches, pain.
Skin: rash, pruritus, dermatosis.

INTERACTIONS
Drug-drug. *Antiarrhythmics:* May increase QRS complex or QT interval, which may lead to other arrhythmias. Monitor ECG closely.
Macrolides and related antibiotics (azithromycin, clarithromycin, erythromycin, telithromycin): May prolong the QT interval. Use with caution. Avoid use with telithromycin.
Phenytoin: May increase metabolism of disopyramide. Watch for decreased antiarrhythmic effect.
Quinidine: May increase disopyramide levels and decrease quinidine levels. Monitor patient closely.
Quinolones: May cause life-threatening arrhythmias, including torsades de pointes. Avoid using together.
Rifampin: May decrease disopyramide level. Monitor patient for lack of effect.
Thioridazine: May cause life-threatening arrhythmias, including torsades de pointes. Avoid using together.
Verapamil: May cause additive effects and impairment of left ventricular function. Don't give disopyramide 48 hours before starting verapamil or 24 hours after verapamil is stopped.
Drug-herb. *Jimsonweed:* May adversely affect CV function. Discourage use together.

EFFECTS ON LAB TEST RESULTS
None reported.

CONTRAINDICATIONS & CAUTIONS
● Contraindicated in patients hypersensitive to drug.
■ **Black Box Warning** Because of its proarrhythmic effects, disopyramide should be reserved for patients with life-threatening ventricular arrhythmias. ■
● Contraindicated with ranolazine, sparfloxacin, thioridazine, or ziprasidone because of increased risk of life-threatening arrhythmias.
● Contraindicated in those with sick sinus syndrome, cardiogenic shock, congenital QT interval prolongation, or second- or third-degree heart block in the absence of an artificial pacemaker.
● Use cautiously, or avoid if possible, in patients with heart failure.
● Use cautiously in patients with underlying conduction abnormalities, urinary tract diseases (especially prostatic hyperplasia), hepatic or renal impairment, myasthenia gravis, or acute angle-closure glaucoma.

NURSING CONSIDERATIONS
● Digitalize patients with atrial fibrillation or flutter before starting disopyramide because of the risk of enhancing AV conduction.
● Watch for recurrence of arrhythmias and check for adverse reactions; notify prescriber if any occur.
● Stop drug if heart block develops, if QRS complex widens by more than 25%, or if QT interval lengthens by more than 25% above baseline.
● *Look alike–sound alike:* Don't confuse disopyramide with desipramine or dipyridamole.

PATIENT TEACHING
● Teach patient importance of taking drug on time and exactly as prescribed.
● If transferring patient from immediate-release to sustained-release capsules, advise him to take the first sustained-release capsule 6 hours after taking the last immediate-release capsule.
● Tell patient not to crush or chew sustained-release capsules or tablets.
● If not contraindicated, advise patient to chew gum or hard candy to relieve dry mouth and to increase fiber and fluid intake to relieve constipation.

dofetilide
doe-FE-ti-lyed

Tikosyn

Pharmacologic class:
antiarrhythmic
Pregnancy risk category C

AVAILABLE FORMS
Capsules: 125 mcg, 250 mcg, 500 mcg

INDICATIONS & DOSAGES
➤ **To maintain normal sinus rhythm
in patients with symptomatic
atrial fibrillation or atrial flutter
lasting longer than 1 week who
have been converted to normal
sinus rhythm; to convert atrial
fibrillation and atrial flutter to
normal sinus rhythm**
Adults: Individualized dosage based on
creatinine clearance and baseline QTc
interval (or QT interval if heart rate is
below 60 beats/minute), determined
before first dose; usually 500 mcg P.O.
b.i.d. for patients with creatinine clearance
greater than 60 ml/minute.
Adjust-a-dose: If creatinine clearance is
40 to 60 ml/minute, starting dose is
250 mcg P.O. b.i.d.; if clearance is 20 to
39 ml/minute, starting dose is 125 mcg
P.O. b.i.d. Don't use drug at all if clearance
is less than 20 ml/minute.

Determine QTc interval 2 to 3 hours
after first dose. If QTc interval has
increased by more than 15% above
baseline or if it's more than 500 msec
(550 msec in patients with ventricular
conduction abnormalities), adjust dosage
as follows: If starting dose based on
creatinine clearance was 500 mcg P.O.
b.i.d., give 250 mcg P.O. b.i.d. If starting
dose based on clearance was 250 mcg
b.i.d., give 125 mcg b.i.d. If starting
dose based on clearance was 125 mcg b.i.d.,
give 125 mcg once a day.

Determine QTc interval 2 to 3 hours
after each subsequent dose while
patient is in hospital. If at any time after
second dose the QTc interval exceeds
500 msec (550 msec in patients with
ventricular conduction abnormalities),
stop drug.

ADMINISTRATION
P.O.
• Give drug without regard for food or
antacid administration.
• Don't give drug with grapefruit juice.

ACTION
Prolongs repolarization without affecting
conduction velocity. Drug doesn't affect
sodium channels, alpha-adrenergic
receptors, or beta-adrenergic receptors.

Route	Onset	Peak	Duration
P.O.	Unknown	2–3 hr	Unknown

Half-life: 10 hours.

ADVERSE REACTIONS
CNS: *headache,* **stroke,** dizziness,
insomnia, anxiety, migraine, cerebral
ischemia, asthenia, paresthesia, syncope.
CV: *chest pain,* **ventricular fibrillation,
ventricular tachycardia, torsades
de pointes, AV block, heart block,
bradycardia, cardiac arrest, MI,** bundle-
branch block, angina, atrial fibrillation,
hypertension, palpitations, edema.
GI: nausea, diarrhea, abdominal pain.
GU: UTI.
Hepatic: liver damage.
Musculoskeletal: back pain, arthralgia,
facial paralysis.
Respiratory: respiratory tract infection,
dyspnea, increased cough.
Skin: rash, sweating.
Other: **angioedema,** flu syndrome,
peripheral edema.

INTERACTIONS
Drug-drug. *Antiarrhythmics (classes I
and III):* May increase dofetilide level.
Withhold other antiarrhythmics for at least
three plasma half-lives before giving
dofetilide.
*Drugs secreted by renal tubular cationic
transport (amiloride, metformin, triamterene):* May increase dofetilide level. Use
together cautiously; monitor patient for
adverse effects.
Drugs that prolong QT interval: May
increase risk of QT interval prolongation.
Avoid using together.
*Inhibitors of CYP3A4 including amio-
darone,* **azole antifungals,** *cannabinoids,
diltiazem,* **macrolides,** *nefazodone,*

norfloxacin, protease inhibitors, quinine, SSRIs, zafirlukast: May decrease metabolism and increase dofetilide level. Use together cautiously.

Inhibitors of renal cationic secretion (cimetidine, ketoconazole, megestrol, prochlorperazine, trimethoprim with or without sulfamethoxazole), verapamil: May increase dofetilide level. Use together is contraindicated.

Potassium-depleting diuretics: May increase risk of hypokalemia or hypomagnesemia. Monitor potassium and magnesium levels.

Thiazide diuretics: May cause hypokalemia and arrhythmias. Use together is contraindicated.

Drug-food. *Grapefruit juice:* May decrease hepatic metabolism and increase drug level. Discourage use together.

EFFECTS ON LAB TEST RESULTS
None reported.

CONTRAINDICATIONS & CAUTIONS
• Contraindicated in patients hypersensitive to drug, in those with congenital or acquired long QT interval syndromes or with baseline QTc interval greater than 440 msec (500 msec in patients with ventricular conduction abnormalities), and in those with creatinine clearance less than 20 ml/minute.
• Contraindicated for use with verapamil and with cation transport system inhibitors (cimetidine, ketoconazole, megestrol, prochlorperazine, trimethoprim with or without sulfamethoxazole).
• Use cautiously in patients with severe hepatic impairment.

NURSING CONSIDERATIONS
■ **Black Box Warning** When dofetilide is initiated or reinitiated, patients should be hospitalized for a minimum of 3 days in a facility that can provide calculations of creatinine clearance, continuous electrocardiographic monitoring, and cardiac resuscitation. Dofetilide is available only to hospitals and prescribers who have received appropriate dofetilide dosing and treatment initiation education. ■
• Don't discharge patient within 12 hours of conversion to normal sinus rhythm.

• Monitor patient for prolonged diarrhea, sweating, and vomiting. Report these signs to prescriber because electrolyte imbalance may increase potential for arrhythmia development.
• Monitor renal function and QTc interval every 3 months.
• Use of potassium-depleting diuretics may cause hypokalemia and hypomagnesemia, increasing the risk of torsades de pointes. Give dofetilide after potassium level reaches and stays in normal range.
• If patient doesn't convert to normal sinus rhythm within 24 hours of starting dofetilide, consider electrical conversion.
• Before starting dofetilide, stop previous antiarrhythmics while carefully monitoring patient for a minimum of three plasma half-lives. Don't give drug after amiodarone therapy until amiodarone level falls below 0.3 mcg/ml or until amiodarone has been stopped for at least 3 months.
• If dofetilide must be stopped to allow dosing with interacting drugs, allow at least 2 days before starting other drug therapy.

PATIENT TEACHING
• Tell patient to report any change in OTC or prescription drug use, or supplement or herb use.
• Inform patient that drug can be taken without regard to meals or antacid administration.
• Tell patient to immediately report excessive or prolonged diarrhea, sweating, vomiting, or loss of appetite or thirst.
• Advise patient not to take drug with grapefruit juice.
• Advise patient to use antacids, such as Zantac 75 mg, Pepcid, Prilosec, Axid, or Prevacid, instead of Tagamet HB if needed for ulcers or heartburn.
• Instruct patient to tell prescriber if she becomes pregnant.
• Advise patient not to breast-feed while taking dofetilide because drug appears in breast milk.
• If a dose is missed, tell patient not to double a dose but to skip that dose and take the next regularly scheduled dose.

SAFETY ALERT!

esmolol hydrochloride
ESS-moe-lol

Brevibloc

Pharmacologic class: beta blocker
Pregnancy risk category C

AVAILABLE FORMS
Injection: 10 mg/ml in 10-ml vials,
20 mg/ml in 5-ml vials, 250 mg/ml in
10-ml ampules
Premixed bags in sodium chloride:
10 mg/ml in 250-ml bags; 20 mg/ml in
100-ml bags

INDICATIONS & DOSAGES
➤ **Supraventricular tachycardia;
postoperative tachycardia or hypertension; noncompensatory sinus
tachycardias**
Adults: 500 mcg/kg/minute as loading
dose by I.V. infusion over 1 minute;
then 4-minute maintenance infusion of
50 mcg/kg/minute. If adequate response
doesn't occur within 5 minutes, repeat
loading dose and follow with maintenance
infusion of 100 mcg/kg/minute for 4 minutes. Repeat loading dose and increase
maintenance infusion by increments of
50 mcg/kg/minute. Maximum maintenance infusion for tachycardia is
200 mcg/kg/minute.
➤ **Intraoperative tachycardia or
hypertension**
Adults: For intraoperative treatment
of tachycardia or hypertension,
80 mg (about 1 mg/kg) I.V. bolus
over 30 seconds; then 150 mcg/kg/minute
I.V. infusion, if needed. Titrate infusion
rate, as needed, to maximum of
300 mcg/kg/minute.
➤ **Unstable angina ♦**
Adults ♦ : 2 to 24 mg/minute by continuous I.V. infusion.

ADMINISTRATION
I.V.
● Don't dilute 10-mg/ml single-dose,
ready-to-use vials.
● Before infusion, dilute 250-mg/ml
injection concentrate to maximum
of 10 mg/ml. Remove and discard

20 ml from 500-ml bag of D_5W,
lactated Ringer's solution, or half-
normal or normal saline solution,
and add two ampules of esmolol to
the bag. The final concentration is
10 mg/ml.
● Give with an infusion-control device
rather than by I.V. push.
● If concentration exceeds 10 mg/ml, give
drug through a central line.
● Don't use for longer than 48 hours.
Watch infusion site carefully for signs
of extravasation; if they occur, stop
infusion immediately and call
prescriber.
● **Incompatibilities:** Amphotericin B
cholesteryl sulfate complex, diazepam,
furosemide, procainamide, sodium
bicarbonate 5%, thiopental sodium,
warfarin sodium.

ACTION
A class II antiarrhythmic and ultra–
short-acting selective beta blocker that
decreases heart rate, contractility, and
blood pressure.

Route	Onset	Peak	Duration
I.V.	Immediate	30 min	30 min after infusion

Half-life: About 9 minutes.

ADVERSE REACTIONS
CNS: anxiety, depression, dizziness,
somnolence, headache, agitation, fatigue,
confusion.
CV: *hypotension,* peripheral ischemia.
GI: nausea, vomiting.
Skin: inflammation or induration at
infusion site.

INTERACTIONS
Drug-drug. *Digoxin:* May increase
digoxin level by 10% to 20%. Monitor
digoxin level.
Morphine: May increase esmolol level.
Adjust esmolol dosage carefully.
Prazosin: May increase risk of orthostatic
hypotension. Help patient to stand slowly
until effects are known.
*Reserpine, other catecholamine-depleting
drugs:* May increase bradycardia and
hypotension. Adjust esmolol dosage
carefully.

Reactions may be *common,* uncommon, *life-threatening,* or COMMON AND LIFE-THREATENING.
Interaction may have a *rapid onset* or *delayed onset.*

Succinylcholine: May prolong neuro-muscular blockade. Monitor patient closely.
Verapamil: May increase the effects of both drugs. Monitor cardiac function closely and decrease dosages as necessary.

EFFECTS ON LAB TEST RESULTS
None reported.

CONTRAINDICATIONS & CAUTIONS
• Contraindicated in patients with sinus bradycardia, second- or third-degree heart block, cardiogenic shock, or overt heart failure.
• Use cautiously in patients with renal impairment, diabetes, or broncho-spasm.

NURSING CONSIDERATIONS
• Dosage for postoperative treatment of tachycardia and hypertension is same as for supraventricular tachycardia.
• *Alert:* Monitor ECG and blood pressure continuously during infusion. Nearly half of patients will develop hypotension. Diaphoresis and dizziness may accompany hypotension. Monitor patient closely, especially if he had low blood pressure before treatment.
• Hypotension can usually be reversed within 30 minutes by decreasing the dose or, if needed, by stopping the infusion. Notify prescriber if this becomes necessary.
• If a local reaction develops at the infusion site, change to another site. Avoid using butterfly needles.
• When patient's heart rate becomes stable, replace drug with an alternative antiarrhythmic, such as propranolol, digoxin, or verapamil. Reduce infusion rate by half, 30 minutes after the first dose of the new drug. Monitor patient response and, if heart rate is controlled for 1 hour after administration of the second dose of the replacement drug, stop esmolol infusion.

PATIENT TEACHING
• Instruct patient to report adverse reactions promptly.
• Tell patient to report discomfort at I.V. site.

flecainide acetate
FLEH-kay-nighd

Tambocor

Pharmacologic class: benzamide derivative
Pregnancy risk category C

AVAILABLE FORMS
Tablets: 50 mg, 100 mg, 150 mg

INDICATIONS & DOSAGES
➤ **Prevention of paroxysmal supraventricular tachycardia, including AV nodal reentrant tachycardia and AV reentrant tachycardia or paroxysmal atrial fibrillation or flutter in patients without structural heart disease; life-threatening ventricular arrhythmias such as sustained ventricular tachycardia**
Adults: For paroxysmal supraventricular tachycardia, 50 mg P.O. every 12 hours. Increase in increments of 50 mg b.i.d. every 4 days. Maximum dose is 300 mg/day. For life-threatening ventricular arrhythmias, 100 mg P.O. every 12 hours. Increase in increments of 50 mg b.i.d. every 4 days until desired effect occurs. Maximum dose for most patients is 400 mg/day.
Adjust-a-dose: If creatinine clearance is 35 ml/minute or less, first dose is 100 mg P.O. once daily or 50 mg P.O. b.i.d.

ADMINISTRATION
P.O.
• Give drug exactly as prescribed.
• Give drug without regard for food.

ACTION
A class IC antiarrhythmic that decreases excitability, conduction velocity, and automaticity by slowing atrial, AV node, His-Purkinje system, and intraventricular conduction; prolongs refractory periods in these tissues.

Route	Onset	Peak	Duration
P.O.	Unknown	2–3 hr	Unknown

Half-life: 12 to 27 hours.

ADVERSE REACTIONS

CNS: *dizziness, headache, light-headedness, syncope,* fatigue, fever, tremor, anxiety, insomnia, depression, malaise, paresthesia, ataxia, vertigo, asthenia.

CV: *new or worsened arrhythmias, heart failure, cardiac arrest,* chest pain, palpitations, edema, flushing.

EENT: *blurred vision and other visual disturbances,* eye pain, eye irritation.

GI: nausea, constipation, abdominal pain, dyspepsia, vomiting, diarrhea, anorexia.

Respiratory: *dyspnea.*

Skin: rash.

INTERACTIONS

Drug-drug. *Amiodarone, cimetidine:* May increase level of flecainide. Watch for toxicity. In the presence of amiodarone, reduce usual flecainide dose by 50% and monitor the patient for adverse effects.

Digoxin: May increase digoxin level by 15% to 25%. Monitor digoxin level.

Disopyramide, verapamil: May increase negative inotropic properties. Avoid using together.

Propranolol, other beta blockers: May increase flecainide and propranolol levels by 20% to 30%. Watch for propranolol and flecainide toxicity.

Ritonavir: May significantly increase flecainide levels and toxicity. Use together is contraindicated.

Urine-acidifying and urine-alkalinizing drugs: May cause extremes of urine pH, which may alter flecainide excretion. Monitor patient for flecainide toxicity or decreased effectiveness.

Drug-lifestyle. *Smoking:* May decrease flecainide level. Monitor patient closely.

EFFECTS ON LAB TEST RESULTS

None reported.

CONTRAINDICATIONS & CAUTIONS

• Contraindicated in patients hypersensitive to drug and in those with second- or third-degree AV block or right bundle-branch block with a left hemiblock (in the absence of an artificial pacemaker), recent MI, or cardiogenic shock, and in patients taking ritonavir.

■ **Black Box Warning** Patients who received flecainide for atrial fibrillation or flutter had increased risk of ventricular tachycardia and ventricular fibrillation. Its use for these conditions isn't recommended. ■

• Use cautiously in patients with heart failure, cardiomyopathy, severe renal or hepatic disease, prolonged QT interval, sick sinus syndrome, or blood dyscrasia.

NURSING CONSIDERATIONS

■ **Black Box Warning** When used to prevent ventricular arrhythmias, reserve drug for patients with documented life-threatening arrhythmias. ■

■ **Black Box Warning** Patients treated with flecainide for atrial flutter have a 1:1 atrioventricular conduction due to slowing of the atrial rate. A paradoxical increase in the ventricular rate may occur. Concomitant negative chronotropic therapy with digoxin or beta blockers may lower the risk of this complication. ■

• Check that pacing threshold was determined 1 week before and after starting therapy in a patient with a pacemaker; flecainide can alter endocardial pacing thresholds.

• Correct hypokalemia or hyperkalemia before giving flecainide because these electrolyte disturbances may alter drug's effect.

• Monitor ECG rhythm for proarrhythmic effects.

• Most patients can be adequately maintained on an every-12-hours dosing schedule, but some need to receive flecainide every 8 hours.

• Adjust dosage only once every 3 to 4 days.

• Monitor flecainide level, especially if patient has renal or heart failure. Therapeutic flecainide levels range from 0.2 to 1 mcg/ml. Risk of adverse effects increases when trough blood level exceeds 1 mcg/ml.

PATIENT TEACHING

• Stress importance of taking drug exactly as prescribed.

• Instruct patient to report adverse reactions promptly and to limit fluid and sodium intake to minimize fluid retention.

Reactions may be *common,* uncommon, *life-threatening*, or COMMON AND LIFE-THREATENING.
Interaction may have a *rapid onset* or **delayed onset.**

ibutilide fumarate
eye-BYOO-ti-lyed

Corvert

Pharmacologic class:
methanesulfonanilide derivative
Pregnancy risk category C

AVAILABLE FORMS
Injection: 0.1 mg/ml in 10-ml vials

INDICATIONS & DOSAGES
➤ **Rapid conversion of recent onset atrial fibrillation or atrial flutter to sinus rhythm**
Adults who weigh 60 kg (132 lb) or more:
1 mg I.V. infusion over 10 minutes. May repeat dose if arrhythmia doesn't respond 10 minutes after completing first dose.
Adults who weigh less than 60 kg:
0.01 mg/kg I.V. infusion over 10 minutes. May repeat dose if arrhythmia doesn't respond 10 minutes after completing first dose.

ADMINISTRATION
I.V.
● Give drug undiluted or diluted in 50 ml of diluent, and add to normal saline solution for injection or D₅W before infusion. Add contents of 10-ml vial (0.1 mg/ml) to 50-ml infusion bag to form admixture of about 0.017 mg/ml ibutilide. Use drug with polyvinyl chloride plastic bags or polyolefin bags.
● Give drug over 10 minutes.
● Stop infusion if arrhythmia is terminated or patient develops ventricular tachycardia or marked prolongation of QT or QTc interval. If arrhythmia doesn't respond 10 minutes after infusion ends, may repeat dose.
● Admixtures with approved diluents are stable for 24 hours at room temperature; 48 hours if refrigerated.
● Don't infuse parenteral products that contain particulate matter or are discolored.
● **Incompatibilities:** None reported.

ACTION
Prolongs action potential in isolated cardiac myocyte and increases atrial and ventricular refractoriness, namely class III electrophysiologic effects.

Route	Onset	Peak	Duration
I.V.	Unknown	Unknown	Unknown

Half-life: Averages about 6 hours.

ADVERSE REACTIONS
CNS: headache.
CV: *sustained polymorphic ventricular tachycardia, AV block, bradycardia, heart failure,* ventricular extrasystoles, *nonsustained ventricular tachycardia,* hypotension, bundle-branch block, hypertension, *prolonged QT interval,* palpitations, tachycardia.
GI: nausea.

INTERACTIONS
Drug-drug. *Class IA antiarrhythmics (disopyramide, procainamide, quinidine), other class III drugs (amiodarone, sotalol):* May increase potential for prolonged refractoriness. Don't give these drugs for at least five half-lives before and 4 hours after ibutilide dose.
Digoxin: Supraventricular arrhythmias may mask cardiotoxicity from excessive digoxin level. Use with caution in patients who may have an increased digoxin therapeutic range.
H₁-receptor antagonist antihistamines, phenothiazines, tetracyclic antidepressants, tricyclic antidepressants, other drugs that prolong QT interval: May increase risk for proarrhythmia. Monitor patient closely.

EFFECTS ON LAB TEST RESULTS
None reported.

CONTRAINDICATIONS & CAUTIONS
■ **Black Box Warning** Administer drug only when the benefits of maintaining sinus rhythm outweigh the immediate risks of ibutilide administration and the risks of maintenance therapy. ■
● Contraindicated in patients hypersensitive to drug or its components.
● Contraindicated in patients with history of polymorphic ventricular tachycardia. Use not recommended in breast-feeding women.

- Use cautiously in patients with hepatic or renal dysfunction.
- Safety and effectiveness of drug haven't been established in children.

NURSING CONSIDERATIONS

■ **Black Box Warning** Only skilled personnel trained in identification and treatment of acute ventricular arrhythmias, particularly polymorphic ventricular tachycardia, should give drug. Cardiac monitor, intracardiac pacing, cardioverter or defibrillator, and drugs to treat sustained ventricular tachycardia must be available. ■

- Before therapy, correct hypokalemia and hypomagnesemia to reduce risk of proarrhythmia.

■ **Black Box Warning** Patients with atrial fibrillation lasting longer than 2 to 3 days must be adequately anticoagulated, generally over at least 2 weeks. ■

- Monitor ECG continuously during administration and for at least 4 hours afterward or until QTc interval returns to baseline; drug can induce or worsen ventricular arrhythmias. Longer monitoring is required if ECG shows arrhythmia or patient has hepatic insufficiency.
- Don't give class IA or other class III antiarrhythmics with infusion or for 4 hours afterward.

PATIENT TEACHING

- Tell patient to report adverse reactions promptly.
- Instruct patient to alert nurse of discomfort at injection site.

SAFETY ALERT!

lidocaine hydrochloride (lignocaine hydrochloride)
LYE-doe-kane

LidoPen Auto-Injector, Xylocaine, Xylocard†

Pharmacologic class: amide derivative
Pregnancy risk category B

AVAILABLE FORMS

Infusion (premixed): 0.2% (2 mg/ml), 0.4% (4 mg/ml), 0.8% (8 mg/ml)

Injection (for direct I.V. use): 1% (10 mg/ml), 2% (20 mg/ml)
Injection (for I.M. use): 300 mg/3 ml automatic injection device
Injection (for I.V. admixtures): 4% (40 mg/ml), 10% (100 mg/ml), 20% (200 mg/ml)

INDICATIONS & DOSAGES

➤ **Ventricular arrhythmias caused by MI, cardiac manipulation, or cardiac glycosides**
Adults: 50 to 100 mg (1 to 1.5 mg/kg) by I.V. bolus at 25 to 50 mg/minute. Bolus dose is repeated every 3 to 5 minutes until arrhythmias subside or adverse reactions develop. Don't exceed 300-mg total bolus during a 1-hour period. Simultaneously, constant infusion of 20 to 50 mcg/kg/minute (1 to 4 mg/minute) is begun. If single bolus has been given, smaller bolus dose may be repeated 15 to 20 minutes after start of infusion to maintain therapeutic level.
Children: 1 mg/kg by I.V. or intraosseous bolus. If no response, start infusion of 20 to 50 mcg/kg/minute. Give an additional bolus dose of 0.5 to 1 mg/kg if delay of greater than 15 minutes between initial bolus and starting the infusion. Bolus doses shouldn't exceed 3 to 5 mg/kg.
Elderly patients: Reduce dosage and rate of infusion by 50%.
Adjust-a-dose: For patients with heart failure, with renal or liver disease, or who weigh less than 50 kg (110 lb), reduce dosage.

ADMINISTRATION
I.V.

- Injections (additive syringes and single-use vials) containing 40, 100, or 200 mg/ml are for the preparation of I.V. infusion solutions only and must be diluted before use.
- Prepare I.V. infusion by adding 1 g (using 25 ml of 4% or 5 ml of 20% injection) to 1 L of D₅W injection to provide a solution containing 1 mg/ml.
- Use a more concentrated solution of up to 8 mg/ml in fluid-restricted patient.
- Patients receiving infusions must be on a cardiac monitor and must be attended at all times. Use an infusion control device for giving infusion precisely. Don't exceed

4 mg/minute; faster rate greatly increases risk of toxicity.
● Avoid giving injections containing preservatives.
● **Incompatibilities:** Amphotericin, ampicillin, cefazolin, ceftriaxone, fentanyl citrate (higher pH brands), methohexital sodium, phenytoin sodium, sodium bicarbonate, thiopental sodium.
I.M.
● Give I.M. injections in the deltoid muscle only.
● Drug may cause soreness at injection site.

ACTION
A class IB antiarrhythmic that decreases the depolarization, automaticity, and excitability in the ventricles during the diastolic phase by direct action on the tissues, especially the Purkinje network.

Route	Onset	Peak	Duration
I.V.	Immediate	Immediate	10–20 min
I.M.	5–15 min	10 min	2 hr

Half-life: 1½ to 2 hours (may be prolonged in patients with heart failure or hepatic disease).

ADVERSE REACTIONS
CNS: *confusion, tremor, stupor, restlessness, light-headedness,* **seizures,** lethargy, somnolence, anxiety, hallucinations, nervousness, paresthesia, muscle twitching.
CV: *hypotension,* **bradycardia, new or worsened arrhythmias, cardiac arrest.**
EENT: *tinnitus, blurred or double vision.*
GI: vomiting.
Respiratory: *respiratory depression and arrest.*
Skin: soreness at injection site.
Other: **anaphylaxis,** sensation of cold.

INTERACTIONS
Drug-drug. *Atenolol, metoprolol, nadolol, pindolol, propranolol:* May reduce hepatic metabolism of lidocaine, increasing the risk of toxicity. Give bolus doses of lidocaine at a slower rate, and monitor lidocaine level and patient closely.
Cimetidine: May decrease clearance of lidocaine, increasing the risk of toxicity.

Consider using a different H_2 receptor antagonist if possible. Monitor lidocaine level closely.
Ergot-type oxytocic drugs: May cause severe, persistent hypertension or stroke. Avoid using together.
Mexiletine: May increase pharmacologic effects. Avoid using together.
Phenytoin, procainamide, propranolol, quinidine: May increase cardiac depressant effects. Monitor patient closely.
Succinylcholine: May prolong neuromuscular blockade. Monitor patient closely.
Drug-herb. *Pareira:* May increase the effects of neuromuscular blockade. Discourage use together.
Drug-lifestyle. *Smoking:* May increase metabolism of lidocaine. Monitor patient closely.

EFFECTS ON LAB TEST RESULTS
● May increase CK levels with I.M. use.

CONTRAINDICATIONS & CAUTIONS
● Contraindicated in patients hypersensitive to the amide-type local anesthetics.
● Contraindicated in those with Adams-Stokes syndrome, Wolff-Parkinson-White syndrome, and severe degrees of SA, AV, or intraventricular block in the absence of an artificial pacemaker.
● Use cautiously and at reduced dosages in patients with complete or second-degree heart block or sinus bradycardia, in elderly patients, in those with heart failure or renal or hepatic disease, and in those who weigh less than 50 kg (110 lb).

NURSING CONSIDERATIONS
● Monitor isoenzymes when using I.M. drug for suspected MI. A patient who has received I.M. lidocaine will show a sevenfold increase in CK level. Such an increase originates in the skeletal muscle, not the heart.
● Monitor drug level. Therapeutic levels are 2 to 5 mcg/ml.
● **Alert:** Monitor patient for toxicity. In many severely ill patients, seizures may be the first sign of toxicity, but severe reactions are usually preceded by somnolence, confusion, tremors, and paresthesia. If signs of toxicity occur, stop drug at once and notify prescriber. Continuing could lead to seizures and coma. Give oxygen

through a nasal cannula if not contraindicated. Keep oxygen and cardiopulmonary resuscitation equipment available.
• Monitor patient's response, especially blood pressure and electrolytes, BUN, and creatinine levels. Notify prescriber promptly if abnormalities develop.
• If arrhythmias worsen or ECG changes (for example, QRS complex widens or PR interval substantially prolongs), stop infusion and notify prescriber.

PATIENT TEACHING
• For I.M. form, tell patient that drug may cause soreness at injection site. Tell him to report discomfort at the site.
• Tell patient to report adverse reactions promptly because toxicity can occur.

---

mexiletine hydrochloride
mex-ILL-i-teen

Pharmacologic class: lidocaine analogue
Pregnancy risk category C

AVAILABLE FORMS
Capsules: 100 mg†, 150 mg, 200 mg, 250 mg

INDICATIONS & DOSAGES
➤ **Life-threatening ventricular arrhythmias, including ventricular tachycardia and PVCs**
Adults: Initially, 200 mg P.O. every 8 hours. If satisfactory control isn't obtained at this dosage, increase dosage by 50 to 100 mg every 2 to 3 days up to maximum of 400 mg every 8 hours. If rapid control of ventricular rate is desired, give a loading dose of 400 mg P.O., followed by 200 mg 8 hours later. Patients controlled on 300 mg or less every 8 hours can receive the total daily dose in evenly divided doses every 12 hours. This dosage may be adjusted up to a maximum of 450 mg every 12 hours.

ADMINISTRATION
P.O.
• Give drug with meals or antacids to lessen GI distress.
• When changing from lidocaine to mexiletine, stop the lidocaine infusion

when the first mexiletine dose is given. But keep the infusion line open until the arrhythmia is satisfactorily controlled.
• When switching to mexiletine from another oral class IA antiarrhythmic, begin with a 200-mg dose 6 to 12 hours after the last dose of quinidine sulfate or disopyramide, 3 to 6 hours after the last dose of procainamide, or 8 to 12 hours after the last dose of tocainide.

ACTION
Blocks the fast sodium channel in cardiac tissues without involving the autonomic nervous system. Drug reduces rate of rise, amplitude, and duration of action potential, and automaticity and effective refractory period in the Purkinje fibers.

Route	Onset	Peak	Duration
P.O.	30–120 min	2–3 hr	Unknown

Half-life: 10 to 12 hours.

ADVERSE REACTIONS
CNS: *tremor, dizziness, light-headedness, incoordination, nervousness,* confusion, changes in sleep habits, paresthesia, weakness, fatigue, speech difficulties, depression, headache.
CV: NEW OR WORSENED ARRHYTHMIAS, palpitations, chest pain, nonspecific edema, angina.
EENT: blurred vision, diplopia, tinnitus.
GI: *nausea, vomiting, upper GI distress, heartburn,* diarrhea, constipation, dry mouth, changes in appetite, abdominal pain.
Skin: rash.

INTERACTIONS
Drug-drug. *Antacids, atropine, narcotics:* May slow mexiletine absorption. Monitor patient for effectiveness.
Cimetidine: May alter mexiletine level. Monitor patient.
Fluvoxamine: May decrease mexiletine clearance. Monitor patient for adverse effects and toxicity.
Methylxanthines (such as caffeine, theophylline): May reduce methylxanthine clearance, which may cause toxicity. Monitor drug level.
Metoclopramide: May speed up mexiletine absorption. Monitor patient for toxicity.

Reactions may be *common*, uncommon, *life-threatening*, or COMMON AND LIFE-THREATENING.
Interaction may have a *rapid onset* or **delayed onset**.

Phenobarbital, phenytoin, rifampin, urine acidifiers: May decrease mexiletine level. Monitor patient for effectiveness.
Urine alkalinizers: May increase mexiletine level. Monitor patient for adverse reactions.

EFFECTS ON LAB TEST RESULTS
• May increase AST level.

CONTRAINDICATIONS & CAUTIONS
• Contraindicated in patients with cardiogenic shock or second- or third-degree AV block in the absence of an artificial pacemaker.
• Use cautiously in patients with first-degree heart block, a ventricular pacemaker, sinus node dysfunction, intraventricular conduction disturbances, hypotension, severe heart failure, liver disease, or seizure disorder.

NURSING CONSIDERATIONS
• If patient may be a good candidate for every-12-hours therapy, notify prescriber. Twice-daily dosage enhances compliance.
• Monitor therapeutic drug level, which may range from 0.5 to 2 mcg/ml.
• An early sign of mexiletine toxicity is tremor, usually a fine tremor of the hands, progressing to dizziness and then to ataxia and nystagmus as drug level in the blood increases. Watch for and ask patient about these symptoms.
• Monitor blood pressure and heart rate and rhythm frequently. Notify prescriber of significant change.
• Monitor CBC. If significant hematologic changes occur, consider discontinuing mexiletine. Blood counts usually return to normal within 1 month of discontinuation.

PATIENT TEACHING
• Tell patient to take drug exactly as prescribed.
• Instruct patient to take drug with food or an antacid if GI reactions occur.
• Instruct patient to report adverse reactions promptly.
• Advise patient to notify prescriber if he develops jaundice, fever, or general tiredness; these symptoms may indicate liver damage.

procainamide hydrochloride
proe-KANE-a-myed

Apo-Procainamide†, Procan SR†

Pharmacologic class: procaine derivative
Pregnancy risk category C

AVAILABLE FORMS
Capsules†: 250 mg, 375 mg, 500 mg
Injection: 100 mg/ml, 500 mg/ml
Tablets (extended-release)†: 250 mg, 500 mg, 750 mg

INDICATIONS & DOSAGES
➤ **Symptomatic PVCs, life-threatening ventricular tachycardia**
  For oral therapy, start at 50 mg/kg/day P.O. of conventional capsules in divided doses every 3 hours until therapeutic level is reached. For maintenance, substitute extended-release form to deliver the total daily dose divided every 6 hours or extended-release form at a dose of 50 mg/kg P.O. in two divided doses every 12 hours.
  Adults: 100 mg every 5 minutes by slow I.V. push, no faster than 25 to 50 mg/minute, until arrhythmias disappear, adverse effects develop, or 500 mg has been given. Usual effective loading dose is 500 to 600 mg. Or, give a loading dose of 500 to 600 mg I.V. infusion over 25 to 30 minutes. Maximum total dose is 1 g. When arrhythmias disappear, give continuous infusion of 2 to 6 mg/minute. If arrhythmias recur, repeat bolus as above and increase infusion rate.
  For I.M. administration, give 50 mg/kg divided every 3 to 6 hours; if arrhythmias occur during surgery, give 100 to 500 mg I.M.
  Children ♦ : Dosage not established. Recommendations include 2 to 6 mg/kg I.V., not exceeding 100 mg, repeated as needed at 5- to 10-minute intervals, not exceeding 15 mg/kg in 24 hours or 500 mg in 30 minutes. Or, 15 mg/kg infused over 30 to 60 minutes; then maintenance infusion of 0.02 to 0.08 mg/kg/minute.

➤ **To convert atrial fibrillation or paroxysmal atrial tachycardia** ◆
Adults: 1.25 g P.O. of conventional capsules. If arrhythmias persist after 1 hour, give additional 750 mg. If no change occurs, give 500 mg to 1 g P.O. every 2 hours until arrhythmias disappear or adverse effects occur. Maintenance dose is 1 g extended-release every 6 hours.
Children ◆ . 15 to 50 mg/kg/day P.O. divided every 3 to 6 hours. Maximum dose 4 g daily. Or, 20 to 30 mg/kg/day I.M. Or, loading dose of 3 to 6 mg/kg I.V. over 5 minutes, up to 100 mg/dose; then maintenance dose 20 to 80 mcg/kg/minute as continuous I.V. infusion. Maximum daily dose is 2 g.

➤ **To maintain normal sinus rhythm after conversion of atrial flutter** ◆
Adults: 0.5 to 1 g P.O. of conventional capsules every 4 to 6 hours.
Adjust-a-dose: For patients with renal or hepatic dysfunction, decrease dose or increase dosing interval, as needed.

ADMINISTRATION
P.O.
• *Alert:* Don't crush the extended-release tablets.
I.V.
• Vials for I.V. injection contain 1 g of drug: 100 mg/ml (10 ml) or 500 mg/ml (2 ml).
• Dilute with compatible I.V. solution, such as D_5W injection, and give with the patient supine at a rate not exceeding 25 to 50 mg/minute. Keep patient supine during I.V. administration.
• Attend patient receiving infusion at all times. Use an infusion-control device to give infusion precisely.
• Monitor blood pressure and ECG continuously during I.V. administration. Watch for prolonged QTc intervals and QRS complexes, heart block, or increased arrhythmias. If such reactions occur, withhold drug, obtain rhythm strip, and notify prescriber immediately. If drug is given too rapidly, hypotension can occur. Watch closely for adverse reactions during infusion, and notify prescriber if they occur.
• **Incompatibilities:** Bretylium, esmolol, ethacrynate, milrinone, phenytoin sodium.

I.M.
• I.M. injections are a substitute for oral administration in patients who are not allowed anything by mouth. Oral dosing should be resumed as soon as possible.

ACTION
Decreases excitability, conduction velocity, automaticity, and membrane responsiveness with prolonged refractory period. Larger than usual doses may induce AV block.

Route	Onset	Peak	Duration
P.O.	Unknown	90–120 min	Unknown
I.V.	Immediate	Immediate	Unknown
I.M.	10–30 min	15–60 min	Unknown

Half-life: About 2½ to 4¾ hours.

ADVERSE REACTIONS
CNS: *fever, seizures,* hallucinations, psychosis, giddiness, confusion, depression, dizziness.
CV: *hypotension, bradycardia, AV block, ventricular fibrillation, ventricular asystole.*
GI: abdominal pain, nausea, vomiting, anorexia, diarrhea, bitter taste.
Skin: *maculopapular rash, urticaria, pruritus, flushing.*
Other: *lupuslike syndrome,* ANGIONEUROTIC EDEMA.

INTERACTIONS
Drug-drug. *Amiodarone:* May increase procainamide level and toxicity and have additive effects on QTc interval and QRS complex. Avoid using together.
Anticholinergics: May increase antivagal effects. Monitor patient closely.
Anticholinesterases: May decrease effect of anticholinesterases. Anticholinesterase dosage may need to be increased.
Beta blockers, ranitidine, trimethoprim: May increase procainamide level. Watch for toxicity.
Cimetidine: May increase procainamide level. Avoid using together if possible. Monitor procainamide level closely and adjust the dosage as necessary.
Macrolides and related antibiotics (azithromycin, clarithromycin, erythromycin, telithromycin): May prolong the QT interval. Use with caution. Avoid use with telithromycin.

Reactions may be *common,* uncommon, *life-threatening,* or COMMON AND LIFE-THREATENING.
Interaction may have a *rapid onset* or **delayed onset.**

Neuromuscular blockers: May increase skeletal muscle relaxant effect. Monitor patient closely.

Quinidine, disopyramide: May enhance antiarrhythmic and hypotensive effects. Avoid using together.

Quinolones: Life-threatening arrhythmias, including torsades de pointes, can occur. Avoid using together; sparfloxacin is contraindicated.

Thioridazine, ziprasidone: May prolong QTc interval. Avoid using together.

Drug-herb. *Jimsonweed:* May adversely affect CV function. Discourage use together.

Licorice: May prolong QTc interval. Urge caution.

Drug-lifestyle. *Alcohol use:* May reduce drug level. Discourage use together.

EFFECTS ON LAB TEST RESULTS
• May increase ALT, AST, alkaline phosphatase, LDH, and bilirubin levels.
• May cause positive antinuclear antibody (ANA) titers and positive direct anti-globulin (Coombs) tests.

CONTRAINDICATIONS & CAUTIONS
• Contraindicated in patients hypersensitive to this drug and related drugs.
• Contraindicated in those with complete, second- or third-degree heart block in the absence of an artificial pacemaker. Also contraindicated in those with myasthenia gravis, systemic lupus erythematosus, or atypical ventricular tachycardia (torsades de pointes).
• Use with extreme caution in patients with ventricular tachycardia during coronary occlusion.
• Use cautiously in patients with heart failure or other conduction disturbances, such as bundle-branch heart block, sinus bradycardia, or digoxin intoxication, and in those with hepatic or renal insufficiency.
■ **Black Box Warning** Use cautiously in patients with blood dyscrasias or bone marrow suppression. ■

NURSING CONSIDERATIONS
■ **Black Box Warning** Because of its proarrhythmic effects, procainamide should be reserved for patients with life-threatening ventricular arrhythmias. ■

• Digitalize or cardiovert patients with atrial flutter or fibrillation before therapy with procainamide to prevent ventricular rate acceleration in patient.
• Monitor level of drug and its active metabolite N-acetylprocainamide (NAPA). To suppress ventricular arrhythmias, therapeutic levels of procainamide are 4 to 8 mcg/ml; therapeutic levels of NAPA are 10 to 30 mcg/ml.
• Monitor ECG closely. If QRS widens more than 25% or marked prolongation of the QTc interval occurs, check for overdosage.
• Hypokalemia predisposes patient to arrhythmias. Monitor electrolytes, especially potassium level.
• Elderly patients may be more likely to develop hypotension. Monitor blood pressure carefully.
■ **Black Box Warning** Agranulocytosis, bone marrow depression, neutropenia, hypoplastic anemia, and thrombo-cytopenia have been noted in patients during the first 12 weeks of therapy. It is recommended that CBCs be performed at weekly intervals for the first 3 months of therapy, and periodically thereafter. ■
■ **Black Box Warning** Perform CBCs promptly if patient develops signs of infection, bruising, or bleeding. If hematologic disorder is identified, discontinue drug. Blood counts usually return to normal within 1 month of discontinuation. ■
■ **Black Box Warning** Positive ANA titer is common in about 60% of patients who don't have symptoms of lupuslike syndrome. This response seems to be related to prolonged use, not dosage. May progress to systemic lupus erythematosus if drug isn't stopped. ■
• *Look alike–sound alike:* Don't confuse Procanbid with probenecid.

PATIENT TEACHING
• Stress importance of taking drug exactly as prescribed. This may require use of an alarm clock for nighttime doses.
• Instruct patient to report fever, rash, muscle pain, diarrhea, bleeding, bruises, or pleuritic chest pain.
• Tell patient not to crush or break extended-release tablets.

● Reassure patient who is taking extended-release form that a wax-matrix "ghost" from the tablet may be passed in stools. Drug is completely absorbed before this occurs.

---

propafenone hydrochloride
proe-PAF-a-non

Rythmol, Rythmol SR

Pharmacologic class: sodium channel antagonist
Pregnancy risk category C

AVAILABLE FORMS
Capsules (extended-release): 225 mg, 325 mg, 425 mg
Tablets (immediate-release): 150 mg, 225 mg, 300 mg

INDICATIONS & DOSAGES
➤ **To suppress life-threatening ventricular arrhythmias such as sustained ventricular tachycardia; to prevent paroxysmal supraventricular tachycardia (PSVT) and paroxysmal atrial fibrillation or flutter**
Adults: Initially, 150 mg immediate-release tablet P.O. every 8 hours. May increase dosage every 3 or 4 days to 225 mg every 8 hours. If needed, increase dosage to 300 mg every 8 hours. Maximum daily dose, 900 mg.
➤ **To prolong time until recurrence of symptomatic atrial fibrillation**
Adults: Initially, 225 mg extended-release capsule P.O. every 12 hours. May increase dose after 5 days to 325 mg P.O. every 12 hours. May increase dose to 425 mg every 12 hours.
Adjust-a-dose: For patients with hepatic impairment, reduce initial dose of immediate-release tablets by 70% to 80%.

ADMINISTRATION
P.O.
● Give drug with food, to minimize adverse GI reactions.
● Don't crush or open the extended-release capsules.

ACTION
Reduces inward sodium current in cardiac cells, prolongs refractory period in AV node, and decreases excitability, conduction velocity, and automaticity in cardiac tissue.

Route	Onset	Peak	Duration
P.O. (immediate-release)	Unknown	3½ hr	Unknown
P.O. (extended-release)	Unknown	3–8 hr	Unknown

Half-life: Estimated at 10 to 32 hours.

ADVERSE REACTIONS
CNS: *dizziness,* anxiety, ataxia, drowsiness, fatigue, headache, insomnia, syncope, tremor, weakness.
CV: ***heart failure, bradycardia, arrhythmias, ventricular tachycardia, premature ventricular contractions, ventricular fibrillation,*** atrial fibrillation, bundle-branch block, angina, chest pain, edema, first-degree AV block, hypotension, increased QRS complex, intraventricular conduction delay, palpitations.
EENT: blurred vision.
GI: *nausea, vomiting,* abdominal pain or cramps, constipation, diarrhea, dyspepsia, anorexia, flatulence, dry mouth, unusual taste.
Musculoskeletal: arthralgia.
Respiratory: dyspnea.
Skin: rash, diaphoresis.

INTERACTIONS
Drug-drug. *Antiarrhythmics:* May increase risk of prolonged QTc interval. Monitor patient closely.
Beta blockers (metoprolol, propranolol): May decrease metabolism of these drugs. Adjust dosage of beta blocker as needed.
Cimetidine: May increase propafenone levels. Monitor patient for adverse effects and toxicity.
Cyclosporine, **digoxin:** May increase levels of these drugs, causing toxicity. Monitor patient closely; dosage adjustment may be necessary.
Desipramine: May decrease desipramine metabolism. Monitor patient closely.
Lidocaine: May decrease lidocaine metabolism. Monitor patient for increased CNS adverse effects and lidocaine toxicity.

Reactions may be *common,* uncommon, *life-threatening,* or COMMON AND LIFE-THREATENING.
Interaction may have a *rapid onset* or *delayed onset.*

Local anesthetics: May increase risk of
CNS toxicity. Monitor patient closely.
Mexiletine: May decrease mexiletine
metabolism, increasing level and adverse
reactions. Monitor mexiletine level and
patient closely.
Phenobarbital, rifampin: May increase
propafenone clearance. Watch for
decreased antiarrhythmic effect.
Quinidine: May decrease propafenone
metabolism; may be useful in certain
patients refractory to propafenone and
quinidine monotherapy. Monitor patient
closely.
Ritonavir: May increase propafenone level,
causing life-threatening arrhythmias.
Avoid using together.
Theophylline: May decrease theophylline
metabolism. Monitor theophylline level
and ECG closely.
Warfarin: May increase warfarin level.
Monitor PT and INR closely, and adjust
warfarin dose as needed.

EFFECTS ON LAB TEST RESULTS
• May increase alkaline phosphatase, ALT,
and AST levels.
• May cause positive ANA titers.

CONTRAINDICATIONS & CAUTIONS
• Contraindicated in patients hypersensitive to drug and in those with severe or
uncontrolled heart failure; cardiogenic
shock; SA, AV, or intraventricular disorders
of impulse conduction without a pacemaker; bradycardia; marked hypotension;
bronchospastic disorders; or electrolyte
imbalances.
• Use cautiously in patients with a history
of heart failure because drug may weaken
the contraction of the heart.
• Use cautiously in patients taking other
cardiac depressants and in those with
hepatic or renal impairment.
• Use cautiously in patients with myasthenia gravis; may cause exacerbation.

NURSING CONSIDERATIONS
■ **Black Box Warning** Because of its
proarrhythmic effects, propafenone should
be reserved for patients with life-
threatening ventricular arrhythmias. ■
• *Alert:* Perform continuous cardiac
monitoring at start of therapy and during
dosage adjustments. If PR interval or QRS

complex increases by more than 25%,
reduce dosage.
• If using with digoxin, frequently monitor
ECG and digoxin level.
• Pacing and sensing thresholds of artificial pacemakers may change; monitor
pacemaker function.
• Agranulocytosis may develop during the
first 2 to 3 months of therapy. If patient
has an unexplained fever, monitor leukocyte count.

PATIENT TEACHING
• Stress importance of taking drug exactly
as prescribed.
• Tell patient not to double the dose if he
misses one, but to take the next dose at the
usual time.
• Tell patient to report adverse reactions
promptly, including fever, sore throat,
chills, and other signs and symptoms of
infection.
• Instruct patient to notify prescriber if
prolonged diarrhea, sweating, vomiting, or
loss of appetite or thirst occurs; these may
cause an electrolyte imbalance.
• Tell patient not to crush, chew, or open
the extended-release capsules.

quinidine gluconate
KWIN-i-deen

Apo-Quin-G†

quinidine sulfate
Apo-Quinidine†

Pharmacologic class: cinchona
alkaloid
Pregnancy risk category C

AVAILABLE FORMS
quinidine gluconate (62% quinidine base)
Injection: 80 mg/ml
Tablets (extended-release): 324 mg, 325 mg†
quinidine sulfate (83% quinidine base)
Injection: 190 mg/ml†
Tablets: 200 mg, 300 mg
Tablets (extended-release): 300 mg

INDICATIONS & DOSAGES
➤ **Atrial flutter or fibrillation**
Adults: 300 to 400 mg quinidine sulfate
or equivalent base P.O. every 6 hours.

Or, 200 mg P.O. every 2 to 3 hours for five to eight doses, increased daily until sinus rhythm is restored or toxic effects develop. Maximum, 3 to 4 g daily.
Children ♦ : 30 mg/kg or 900 mg/m² P.O. (sulfate) or I.V. or I.M. (gluconate) daily in five divided doses.

➤ **Paroxysmal supraventricular tachycardia**
Adults: 400 to 600 mg P.O. gluconate every 2 to 3 hours until toxic adverse reactions develop or arrhythmia subsides.
Children ♦ : 30 mg/kg or 900 mg/m² P.O. (sulfate) or I.V. or I.M. (gluconate) daily in five divided doses.

➤ **Premature atrial and ventricular contractions, paroxysmal AV junctional rhythm, paroxysmal atrial tachycardia, paroxysmal ventricular tachycardia, maintenance after cardioversion of atrial fibrillation or flutter**
Adults: Test dose is 200 mg P.O. or I.M. Quinidine sulfate or equivalent base 200 to 400 mg P.O. every 4 to 6 hours or 600 mg quinidine sulfate extended-release every 8 to 12 hours; or 324 mg quinidine gluconate extended-release tablets every 8 to 12 hours; or quinidine gluconate 800 mg (10 ml of commercially available solution) added to 40 ml of D₅W, infused I.V. at 0.25 mg/kg/minute.
Children ♦ : 30 mg/kg or 900 mg/m² P.O. (sulfate) or I.V. or I.M. (gluconate) daily in five divided doses.

➤ **Severe** *Plasmodium falciparum* **malaria**
Adults: 10 mg/kg gluconate I.V. diluted in 250 ml normal saline solution and infused over 1 to 2 hours; then begin a continuous infusion of 0.02 mg/kg/minute for at least 24 hours, and until parasitemia is reduced to less than 1% and oral therapy can be started. Or, give a loading dose of 24 mg/kg of quinidine gluconate I.V. diluted in 250 ml of normal saline and infused over 4 hours; then 4 hours later, give maintenance dose of 12 mg/kg of quinidine gluconate given by I.V. infusion over 4 hours at 8-hour intervals until three maintenance doses have been given and parasitemia is reduced to less than 1% and oral quinidine sulfate can be initiated.

Children ♦ : 10 mg/kg gluconate I.V. over 1 to 2 hours; then continuous infusion of 0.02 mg/kg/minute.
Adjust-a-dose: In patients with hepatic impairment or heart failure, reduce dosage.

ADMINISTRATION
P.O.
● Give drug with food to avoid adverse GI reactions.
● Don't crush or open extended-release tablets. If necessary, scored tablets may be broken in half to adjust quinidine dose.
● Don't give drug with grapefruit juice.
I.V.
● For quinidine gluconate infusion to treat atrial fibrillation or flutter in adults, dilute 800 mg (10 ml of injection) with 40 ml D₅W and infuse at up to 0.25 mg/kg/minute.
● For quinidine gluconate infusion to treat malaria, dilute in 5 ml/kg (usually 250 ml) normal saline solution and infuse over 1 to 2 hours, followed by a continuous maintenance infusion.
● During infusion, continuously monitor patient's blood pressure and ECG.
● Adjust rate so that the arrhythmia is corrected without disturbing the normal mechanism of the heartbeat.
● Never use discolored (brownish) quinidine solution.
● Store drug away from heat and direct light.
● **Incompatibilities:** Alkalies, amiodarone, atracurium besylate, furosemide, heparin sodium, iodides.
I.M.
● Never use discolored (brownish) quinidine solution.
● Quinidine gluconate I.M. is no longer recommended for arrhythmias because of erratic absorption.
● Store drug away from heat and direct light.

ACTION
A class IA antiarrhythmic with direct and indirect (anticholinergic) effects on cardiac tissue. Decreases automaticity, conduction velocity, and membrane responsiveness; prolongs effective refractory period; and reduces vagal tone.

Reactions may be *common,* uncommon, *life-threatening,* or COMMON AND LIFE-THREATENING.
Interaction may have a *rapid onset* or *delayed onset.*

Route	Onset	Peak	Duration
P.O.	1–3 hr	1–6 hr	6–8 hr
I.V.	Immediate	Immediate	Unknown
I.M.	Unknown	30–90 min	Unknown

Half-life: 5 to 12 hours.

ADVERSE REACTIONS
CNS: *vertigo, fever, headache, light-headedness,* ataxia, confusion, depression, dementia.
CV: *ECG changes, tachycardia, **PVCs, ventricular tachycardia, atypical ventric-ular tachycardia, complete AV block, aggravated heart failure,*** hypotension.
EENT: *tinnitus,* blurred vision, diplopia, photophobia.
GI: *diarrhea, nausea, vomiting,* anorexia, excessive salivation, abdominal pain.
Hematologic: ***thrombocytopenia, agranulocytosis,*** hemolytic anemia.
Hepatic: *hepatotoxicity.*
Respiratory: ***acute asthmatic attack, respiratory arrest.***
Skin: rash, petechial hemorrhage of buccal mucosa, pruritus, urticaria, photosensitivity reactions.
Other: *cinchonism,* **angioedema,** lupus erythematosus.

INTERACTIONS
Drug-drug. *Antacids, sodium bicarbonate:* May increase quinidine level. Monitor patient for increased effect.
Amiloride: May increase the risk of arrhythmias. If use together can't be avoided, monitor ECG closely.
Amiodarone: May increase quinidine level, producing life-threatening cardiac arrhythmias. Monitor quinidine level closely if use together can't be avoided. Adjust quinidine as needed.
Azole antifungals: May increase the risk of cardiovascular events. Use together is contraindicated.
Barbiturates, phenytoin, rifampin: May decrease quinidine level. Monitor patient for decreased effect.
Cimetidine: May increase quinidine level. Monitor patient for increased arrhythmias.
Digoxin: May increase digoxin level after starting quinidine therapy. Monitor digoxin level.
Drugs that prolong the QT interval (anti-psychotics, disopyramide, procainamide,

tricyclic antidepressants, sotalol): May have additive effect with quinidine and cause life-threatening cardiac arrhythmias. Avoid using together when possible.
Fluvoxamine, nefazodone, tricyclic anti-depressants: May increase antidepressant level, thus increasing its effect. Monitor patient for adverse reactions.
Macrolides and related antibiotics (azithromycin, clarithromycin, erythromycin, telithromycin): May cause additive effects or prolongation of the QT interval. Use with caution. Avoid use with telithromycin.
Neuromuscular blockers: May potentiate effects of these drugs. Avoid use of quinidine immediately after surgery.
Nifedipine: May decrease quinidine level. May need to adjust dosage.
Other antiarrhythmics (such as lidocaine, procainamide, propranolol): May increase risk of toxicity. Use together cautiously.
Protease inhibitors (nelfinavir, ritonavir): May significantly increase quinidine levels and toxicity. Use together is contraindicated.
Quinolones: Life-threatening arrhythmias, including torsades de pointes, can occur. Avoid using together.
Verapamil: May decrease quinidine clearance and cause hypotension, bradycardia, AV block, or pulmonary edema. Monitor blood pressure and heart rate.
Warfarin: May increase anticoagulant effect. Monitor patient closely.
Drug-herb. *Jimsonweed:* May adversely affect CV function. Discourage use together.
Licorice: May have additive effect and prolong QT interval. Urge caution.
Drug-food. *Grapefruit:* May delay absorption and onset of action of drug. Discourage use together.

EFFECTS ON LAB TEST RESULTS
● May decrease hemoglobin level.
● May decrease platelet and granulocyte counts.

CONTRAINDICATIONS & CAUTIONS
● Contraindicated in patients with idiosyncrasy or hypersensitivity to quinidine or related cinchona derivatives.
● Contraindicated in those with myasthenia gravis, intraventricular conduction

defects, digoxin toxicity when AV conduction is grossly impaired, abnormal rhythms caused by escape mechanisms, complete AV block, history of drug-induced torsades de pointes, and history of prolonged QT interval syndrome.

• Contraindicated in patients who developed thrombocytopenia after exposure to quinidine or quinine.

• Use cautiously in patients with asthma, muscle weakness, or infection accompanied by fever because hypersensitivity reactions to drug may be masked.

• Use cautiously in patients with hepatic or renal impairment because systemic accumulation may occur.

NURSING CONSIDERATIONS

• Check apical pulse rate and blood pressure before therapy. If extremes in pulse rate are detected, withhold drug and notify prescriber at once.

• *Alert:* For atrial fibrillation or flutter, give quinidine only after AV node has been blocked with a beta blocker, digoxin, or a calcium channel blocker to avoid increasing AV conduction.

• Anticoagulant therapy is commonly advised before quinidine therapy in long-standing atrial fibrillation because restoration of normal sinus rhythm may result in thromboembolism caused by dislodgment of thrombi from atrial wall.

• Monitor patient for atypical ventricular tachycardia, such as torsades de pointes and ECG changes, particularly widening of QRS complex, widened QT and PR intervals.

• *Alert:* When changing route of administration or oral salt form, prescriber should alter dosage to compensate for variations in quinidine base content.

• *Alert:* Hospitalize patients with severe malaria in an intensive care setting, with continuous monitoring. Decrease infusion rate if quinidine level exceeds 6 mcg/ml, uncorrected QT interval exceeds 0.6 seconds, or QRS complex widening exceeds 25% of baseline.

• Monitor liver function test results during first 4 to 8 weeks of therapy.

• Monitor quinidine level. Therapeutic levels for antiarrhythmic effects are 4 to 8 mcg/ml.

• Monitor patient response carefully. If adverse GI reactions occur, especially diarrhea, notify prescriber. Check quinidine level, which is increasingly toxic when greater than 10 mcg/ml. GI symptoms may be decreased by giving drug with meals or aluminum hydroxide antacids.

• *Look alike–sound alike:* Don't confuse quinidine with quinine or clonidine.

PATIENT TEACHING

• Stress importance of taking drug exactly as prescribed and taking it with food if adverse GI reactions occur.

• *Alert:* Instruct patient not to crush or chew extended-release tablets. If necessary, he may break scored tablets in half to adjust quinidine dose.

• Tell patient to avoid grapefruit juice because it may delay drug absorption and inhibit drug metabolism.

• Advise patient to report persistent or serious adverse reactions promptly, especially signs and symptoms of quinidine toxicity (ringing in the ears, visual disturbances, dizziness, headache, nausea).

---

sotalol hydrochloride
SOH-ta-lol

Betapace, Betapace AF, Rylosol†

Pharmacologic class: nonselective beta blocker
Pregnancy risk category B

AVAILABLE FORMS
Betapace
Tablets: 80 mg, 120 mg, 160 mg, 240 mg
Betapace AF
Tablets: 80 mg, 120 mg, 160 mg

INDICATIONS & DOSAGES
➤ **Documented, life-threatening ventricular arrhythmias**
Adults: Initially, 80 mg Betapace P.O. b.i.d. Increase dosage every 3 days as needed and tolerated. Most patients respond to 160 to 320 mg/day, although some patients with refractory arrhythmias need up to 640 mg/day.
Adjust-a-dose: If creatinine clearance is 30 to 60 ml/minute, increase dosage interval to every 24 hours; if clearance is 10 to

---

29 ml/minute, increase interval to every 36 to 48 hours; and if clearance is less than 10 ml/minute, individualize dosage.

➤ **To maintain normal sinus rhythm or to delay recurrence of atrial fibrillation or atrial flutter in patients with symptomatic atrial fibrillation or flutter who are currently in sinus rhythm**

Adults: 80 mg Betapace AF P.O. b.i.d. Increase dosage as needed to 120 mg P.O. b.i.d. after 3 days if the QTc interval is less than 500 msec. Maximum dose is 160 mg P.O. b.i.d.

Adjust-a-dose: If creatinine clearance is 40 to 60 ml/minute, increase dosage interval to every 24 hours. If clearance is less than 40 ml/minute, Betapace AF is contra-indicated.

ADMINISTRATION

P.O.

● Give 1 hour before or 2 hours after meals or antacids.

ACTION

Depresses sinus heart rate, slows AV conduction, decreases cardiac output, and lowers systolic and diastolic blood pressure. Drug also has class III anti-arrhythmic action potential's duration and prolongation.

Route	Onset	Peak	Duration
P.O.	Unknown	2½–4 hr	Unknown

Half-life: 12 hours.

ADVERSE REACTIONS

CNS: *asthenia, headache, dizziness, weakness, fatigue, light-headedness,* sleep problems.

CV: *chest pain, palpitations, **bradycardia, arrhythmias, heart failure, AV block, proarrhythmic events (including poly-morphic ventricular tachycardia, PVCs, ventricular fibrillation),** edema, ECG abnormalities, hypotension.*

GI: *nausea, vomiting,* diarrhea, dyspepsia.

Metabolic: hyperglycemia.

Respiratory: *dyspnea, **bronchospasm.***

INTERACTIONS

Drug-drug. *Antiarrhythmics:* May increase drug effects. Avoid using together.

Antihypertensives, catecholamine-depleting drugs (such as guanethidine, reserpine): May increase hypotensive effects or cause marked bradycardia. Monitor blood pressure and pulse closely.

Calcium channel blockers: May increase myocardial depression. Avoid using together.

Clonidine: May enhance rebound effect after withdrawal of clonidine. Stop sotalol several days before withdrawing clonidine.

Drugs that prolong the QT interval (Class I and III antiarrhythmics, bepridil, phenothiazines, tricyclics): May cause excessive QT prolongation. Monitor QT interval.

General anesthetics: May increase myocardial depression. Monitor patient closely.

Insulin, oral antidiabetics: May cause hyperglycemia and may mask signs and symptoms of hypoglycemia. Adjust dosage accordingly.

Macrolides and related antibiotics (azithromycin, clarithromycin, erythromycin, telithromycin): May cause additive effects or prolong the QT inter-val. Use with caution. Avoid use with telithromycin.

Prazosin: May increase the risk of ortho-static hypotension. Assist patient to stand slowly until effects are known.

Quinolones: May cause life-threatening arrhythmias, including torsades de pointes. Avoid using together.

Drug-food. *Any food:* May decrease absorption by 20%. Advise patient to take on empty stomach.

EFFECTS ON LAB TEST RESULTS

● May increase glucose level.
● May cause false-positive catecholamine level.

CONTRAINDICATIONS & CAUTIONS

● Contraindicated in patients hypersensitive to drug.
● Contraindicated in those with severe sinus node dysfunction, sinus bradycardia, second- and third-degree AV block unless patient has a pacemaker, congenital or acquired long QT-interval syndrome, cardiogenic shock, uncontrolled heart failure, and bronchial asthma.

• Use cautiously in patients with renal impairment or diabetes mellitus (beta blockers may mask signs and symptoms of hypoglycemia).

NURSING CONSIDERATIONS
■ **Black Box Warning** Because pro-arrhythmic events may occur at the start of therapy and during dosage adjustments, patients should be hospitalized for a minimum of 3 days in a facility that can provide calculations of creatinine clearance, continuous electrocardiographic monitoring, and cardiac resuscitation. Calculate creatinine clearance prior to dosing. ■
• The baseline QTc interval must be less than or equal to 450 msec before starting Betapace AF.
• Assess patient for new or worsened symptoms of heart failure.
• Although patients receiving I.V. lidocaine may start sotalol therapy without ill effects, withdraw other antiarrhythmics before therapy begins. Sotalol therapy typically is delayed until two or three half-lives of the withdrawn drug have elapsed. After withdrawing amiodarone, give sotalol only after QT interval normalizes.
• Adjust dosage slowly, allowing 3 days between dosage increments for adequate monitoring of QT intervals and for drug levels to reach a steady-state level.
■ **Black Box Warning** Don't substitute Betapace for Betapace AF. ■
• Monitor electrolytes regularly, especially if patient is receiving diuretics. Electrolyte imbalances, such as hypokalemia or hypomagnesemia, may enhance QT-interval prolongation and increase the risk of serious arrhythmias such as torsades de pointes.
• *Look alike–sound alike:* Don't confuse sotalol with Stadol.

PATIENT TEACHING
• Explain to patient that he will need to be hospitalized for initiation of drug therapy.
• Stress need to take drug as prescribed, even when he is feeling well. Caution patient against stopping drug suddenly.
• Caution patient against using OTC drugs and decongestants while taking drug.
• Because food and antacids can interfere with absorption, tell patient to take drug on an empty stomach, 1 hour before or 2 hours after meals or antacids.

Reactions may be *common*, uncommon, *life-threatening*, or COMMON AND LIFE-THREATENING.
Interaction may have a *rapid onset* or **delayed onset.**

23

Antihypertensives

aliskiren
amlodipine
(See Chapter 21, ANTIANGINALS.)
atenolol
benazepril hydrochloride
candesartan cilexetil
captopril
carvedilol
carvedilol phosphate
clonidine hydrochloride
diltiazem hydrochloride
(See Chapter 21, ANTIANGINALS.)
doxazosin mesylate
enalaprilat
enalapril maleate
eplerenone
eprosartan mesylate
ethacrynate sodium
(See Chapter 25, DIURETICS.)
felodipine
fosinopril sodium
furosemide
(See Chapter 25, DIURETICS.)
guanfacine hydrochloride
hydralazine hydrochloride
hydrochlorothiazide
(See Chapter 25, DIURETICS.)
indapamide
(See Chapter 25, DIURETICS.)
irbesartan
labetalol hydrochloride
lisinopril
losartan potassium
methyldopa
methyldopate hydrochloride
metolazone
(See Chapter 25, DIURETICS.)
metoprolol succinate
metoprolol tartrate
nadolol
(See Chapter 21, ANTIANGINALS.)
nebivolol
nicardipine
(See Chapter 21, ANTIANGINALS.)
nifedipine
(See Chapter 21, ANTIANGINALS.)
nisoldipine
nitroglycerin
(See Chapter 21, ANTIANGINALS.)
nitroprusside sodium

olmesartan medoxomil
perindopril erbumine
phentolamine mesylate
prazosin hydrochloride
propranolol hydrochloride
(See Chapter 21, ANTIANGINALS.)
quinapril hydrochloride
ramipril
spironolactone
(See Chapter 25, DIURETICS.)
telmisartan
terazosin hydrochloride
torsemide
(See Chapter 25, DIURETICS.)
trandolapril
valsartan
verapamil hydrochloride
(See Chapter 21, ANTIANGINALS.)

---

aliskiren
a-LIS-ke-ren

Tekturna

Pharmacologic class: renin
inhibitor
*Pregnancy risk category C for
1st trimester; D for 2nd and
3rd trimesters*

AVAILABLE FORMS
Tablets: 150 mg, 300 mg

INDICATIONS & DOSAGES
➤ **Hypertension, alone or with other
antihypertensives**
Adults: 150 mg P.O. daily; may increase to
300 mg P.O. daily.

ADMINISTRATION
P.O.
• Don't give drug with high-fat meal
because this may decrease the drug's
effectiveness.

ACTION
Inhibits conversion of angiotensin I to
angiotensin II, decreasing vasoconstriction
and lowering blood pressure.

Route	Onset	Peak	Duration
P.O.	Unknown	1–3 hr	Unknown

Half-life: Unknown.

ADVERSE REACTIONS
CNS: *headache,* dizziness, fatigue, *seizures.*
CV: *hypotension.*
EENT: nasopharyngitis.
GI: abdominal pain, diarrhea, dyspepsia, gastroesophageal reflux.
Metabolic: hyperuricemia, *hyperkalemia.*
Musculoskeletal: back pain.
Respiratory: cough, upper respiratory tract infection.
Skin: rash.
Other: *angioedema.*

INTERACTIONS
Drug-drug. *Atorvastatin:* May increase aliskiren levels. Use cautiously together.
Cyclosporine: May increase aliskiren levels. Avoid concomitant use.
Ketoconazole: May significantly increase aliskiren levels. Use cautiously together.
Irbesartan: May decrease aliskiren levels. Monitor patient for effectiveness.
Furosemide: May reduce furosemide peak levels. Monitor patient for effectiveness.
Drug-food. *High fat meals:* May substantially decrease plasma levels of drug. Monitor patient for effectiveness.

EFFECTS ON LAB TEST RESULTS
• May increase potassium, creatine kinase, BUN, and serum creatinine levels.

CONTRAINDICATIONS & CAUTIONS
• Contraindicated in patients hypersensitive to drug or its components.
■ **Black Box Warning** Contraindicated in pregnant women. Because of risk of fetal toxicity, stop drug as soon as possible if patient becomes pregnant. ■
• Contraindicated in breast-feeding patients and patients taking cyclosporine.
• Use cautiously in patients with history of angioedema, severe renal dysfunction (creatinine of 1.7 mg/dl in women and 2 mg/dl in men, or GFR <30 ml/minute), history of dialysis, nephrotic syndrome, or renovascular hypertension.

NURSING CONSIDERATIONS
• Monitor blood pressure for hypotension, especially if used in combination with other antihypertensives.
• Monitor potassium levels, especially in patients also taking ACE inhibitors.
• *Alert:* Rarely, angioedema occurs. Supportive measures may include antihistamines, steroids, and epinephrine.
• Monitor renal function. It's unknown how patients with significant renal disorders will respond to the use of this drug.
• Effect of any dose is usually seen within 2 weeks.

PATIENT TEACHING
• Instruct patient not to take drug with a high-fat meal because this may decrease the drug's effectiveness.
• Instruct patient to monitor blood pressure daily, if possible, and to report low readings, dizziness, and headaches to prescriber.
• Tell patient to immediately report swelling of the face or neck or difficulty breathing.
• Advise patient of need for regular laboratory tests to monitor for adverse effects.

SAFETY ALERT!

atenolol
a-TEN-o-loll

Tenormin⊘

Pharmacologic class: beta blocker
Pregnancy risk category D

AVAILABLE FORMS
Tablets: 25 mg, 50 mg, 100 mg

INDICATIONS & DOSAGES
➤ **Hypertension**
Adults: Initially, 50 mg P.O. daily alone or in combination with a diuretic as a single dose, increased to 100 mg once daily after 7 to 14 days. Dosages of more than 100 mg daily are unlikely to produce further benefit.
➤ **Angina pectoris**
Adults: 50 mg P.O. once daily, increased as needed to 100 mg daily after 7 days

---

Reactions may be *common,* uncommon, *life-threatening,* or COMMON AND LIFE-THREATENING.
Interaction may have a *rapid onset* or **delayed onset.**

for optimal effect. Maximum, 200 mg daily.

➤ **Migraine prophylaxis** ◆
Adults: 50 to 200 mg P.O. daily.
Adjust-a-dose: If creatinine clearance is 15 to 35 ml/minute, maximum dose is 50 mg daily; if clearance is below 15 ml/minute, maximum dose is 25 mg daily. Hemodialysis patients need 25 to 50 mg after each dialysis session.

ADMINISTRATION
P.O.
● Check apical pulse before giving drug; if slower than 60 beats/minute, withhold drug and call prescriber.
● Give drug exactly as prescribed, at the same time each day.

ACTION
Selectively blocks beta$_1$ beta-adrenergic receptors, decreases cardiac output and cardiac oxygen consumption, and depresses renin secretion.

Route	Onset	Peak	Duration
P.O.	1 hr	2–4 hr	24 hr

Half-life: 6 to 7 hours.

ADVERSE REACTIONS
CNS: *dizziness, fatigue,* lethargy, vertigo, drowsiness, fever.
CV: *hypotension, bradycardia, heart failure,* intermittent claudication.
GI: nausea, diarrhea.
Musculoskeletal: leg pain.
Respiratory: *bronchospasm,* dyspnea.
Skin: rash.

INTERACTIONS
Drug-drug. *Amiodarone:* May increase risk of bradycardia, AV block, and myocardial depression. Monitor ECG and vital signs.
Antihypertensives: May increase hypotensive effect. Use together cautiously.
Calcium channel blockers, hydralazine, methyldopa: May cause additive hypotension and bradycardia. Adjust dosage as needed.
Cardiac glycosides, diltiazem, verapamil: May cause excessive bradycardia and increased depressant effect on myocardium. Use together cautiously.

Clonidine: May exacerbate rebound hypertension if clonidine is withdrawn. Atenolol should be withdrawn before clonidine by several days or added several days after clonidine is stopped.
Dolasetron: May decrease clearance of dolasetron and increase risk of toxicity. Monitor patient for toxicity.
Insulin, oral antidiabetics: May alter dosage requirements in previously stabilized diabetic patient. Observe patient carefully.
I.V. lidocaine: May reduce hepatic metabolism of lidocaine, increasing risk of toxicity. Give bolus doses of lidocaine at a slower rate and monitor lidocaine level closely.
NSAIDs: May decrease antihypertensive effects. Monitor blood pressure.
Prazosin: May increase the risk of orthostatic hypotension in the early phases of use together. Help patient stand slowly until effects are known.
Reserpine: May cause hypotension or marked bradycardia. Use together cautiously.

EFFECTS ON LAB TEST RESULTS
● May increase alkaline phosphatase, BUN, creatinine, glucose, LDH, potassium, transaminase, and uric acid levels. May decrease glucose level.
● May increase platelet count.

CONTRAINDICATIONS & CAUTIONS
● Contraindicated in patients with sinus bradycardia, heart block greater than first degree, overt cardiac failure, untreated pheochromocytoma, or cardiogenic shock.
● Use cautiously in patients at risk for heart failure and in those with bronchospastic disease, diabetes, hyperthyroidism, and impaired renal or hepatic function.

NURSING CONSIDERATIONS
● Monitor patient's blood pressure.
● Monitor hemodialysis patients closely because of hypotension risk.
● Beta blockers may mask tachycardia caused by hyperthyroidism. In patients with suspected thyrotoxicosis, withdraw beta blocker gradually to avoid thyroid storm.

• Drug may mask signs and symptoms of hypoglycemia in diabetic patients.

• Drug may cause changes in exercise tolerance and ECG.

■ **Black Box Warning** Avoid abrupt discontinuation of therapy. Withdraw drug gradually to avoid serious adverse reactions, such as severe exacerbations of angina, myocardial infarction, and ventricular arrhythmias even in patients treated only for hypertension. ■

• *Look alike–sound alike:* Don't confuse atenolol with timolol or albuterol.

PATIENT TEACHING

• Instruct patient to take drug exactly as prescribed, at the same time every day.

• Caution patient not to stop drug suddenly, but to notify prescriber if unpleasant adverse reactions occur.

• Teach patient how to take his pulse. Tell him to withhold drug and call prescriber if pulse rate is below 60 beats/minute.

• Tell woman of childbearing age to notify prescriber about planned, suspected, or known pregnancy. Drug will need to be stopped.

• Advise breast-feeding mother to contact prescriber; drug isn't recommended for breast-feeding women.

---

benazepril hydrochloride
ben-A-za-pril

Lotensin✲

Pharmacologic class: ACE inhibitor
Pregnancy risk category C; D in 2nd and 3rd trimesters

AVAILABLE FORMS
Tablets: 5 mg, 10 mg, 20 mg, 40 mg

INDICATIONS & DOSAGES
➤ **Hypertension**
Adults: For patients not receiving a diuretic, 10 mg P.O. daily initially. Adjust dosage as needed and tolerated; usually 20 to 40 mg daily in one or two divided doses. For patients receiving a diuretic, 5 mg P.O. daily initially.
Children age 6 and older: 0.2 mg/kg (up to 10 mg) P.O. daily. Adjust as needed up to 0.6 mg/kg (maximum 40 mg) P.O. daily.

➤ **Nephropathy (nondiabetic)** ◆
Adults: 1.25 to 20 mg P.O. daily.
Adjust-a-dose: If creatinine clearance is below 30 ml/minute, give 5 mg P.O. daily. Daily dose may be adjusted up to 40 mg.

ADMINISTRATION
P.O.
• Request oral suspension for patients who can't swallow tablets.

ACTION
Inhibits ACE, preventing conversion of angiotensin I to angiotensin II, a potent vasoconstrictor. Less angiotensin II decreases peripheral arterial resistance, decreasing aldosterone secretion, which reduces sodium and water retention and lowers blood pressure. Drug also acts as antihypertensive in patients with low-renin hypertension.

Route	Onset	Peak	Duration
P.O.	1 hr	2–4 hr	24 hr

Half-life: benazepril, 0.6 hour.

ADVERSE REACTIONS
CNS: headache, dizziness, drowsiness, fatigue, somnolence.
CV: symptomatic hypotension.
GI: nausea.
GU: impotence.
Metabolic: *hyperkalemia.*
Musculoskeletal: arthralgia, arthritis, myalgia.
Respiratory: dry, persistent, nonproductive cough.
Skin: increased diaphoresis.
Other: hypersensitivity reactions, *angioedema.*

INTERACTIONS
Drug-drug. *Azathioprine:* May increase risk of anemia or leukopenia. Monitor hematologic study results if used together.
Diuretics, other antihypertensives: May cause excessive hypotension. Stop diuretic or lower dosage of benazepril, as needed.
Lithium: May increase lithium level and toxicity. Use together cautiously; monitor lithium level.
Nesiritide: May increase risk of hypotension. Monitor blood pressure.

Reactions may be *common*, uncommon, *life-threatening*, or COMMON AND LIFE-THREATENING.
Interaction may have a *rapid onset* or *delayed onset.*

NSAIDs: May decrease antihypertensive effects. Monitor blood pressure.
Potassium-sparing diuretics, potassium supplements: May cause hyperkalemia. Monitor potassium level and renal function.
Drug-herb. *Capsaicin:* May cause cough. Discourage use together.
Ma huang: May decrease antihypertensive effects. Discourage use together.
Drug-food. *Salt substitutes containing potassium:* May cause hyperkalemia. Monitor potassium level and renal function.

EFFECTS ON LAB TEST RESULTS
• May increase BUN, creatinine, and potassium levels.

CONTRAINDICATIONS & CAUTIONS
• Contraindicated in patients hypersensitive to ACE inhibitors.
■ **Black Box Warning** ACE inhibitors can cause injury and even death to the developing fetus when used during the second and third trimesters. When pregnancy is detected, discontinue drug as soon as possible. ■
• Use cautiously in patients with impaired hepatic or renal function.

NURSING CONSIDERATIONS
• Monitor patient for hypotension. Excessive hypotension can occur when drug is given with diuretics. If possible, diuretic therapy should be stopped 2 to 3 days before starting benazepril to decrease potential for excessive hypotensive response. If drug doesn't adequately control blood pressure, diuretic may be cautiously reinstituted.
• Although ACE inhibitors reduce blood pressure in all races, they reduce it less in blacks taking the ACE inhibitor alone. Black patients should take drug with a thiazide diuretic for a more favorable response.
• Drug may increase risk of angioedema in black patients.
• Measure blood pressure when drug level is at peak (2 to 6 hours after administration) and at trough (just before a dose) to verify adequate blood pressure control.
• Assess renal and hepatic function before and periodically during therapy. Monitor potassium level.

• **Look alike–sound alike:** Don't confuse benazepril with Benadryl or Lotensin with Loniten or lovastatin.

PATIENT TEACHING
• Instruct patient to avoid salt substitutes because they may contain potassium, which can cause high potassium level in patients taking drug.
• Inform patient that light-headedness can occur, especially during first few days of therapy. Tell him to rise slowly to minimize this effect and to report dizziness to prescriber. If fainting occurs, he should stop drug and call prescriber immediately.
• Warn patient to use caution in hot weather and during exercise. Inadequate fluid intake, vomiting, diarrhea, and excessive perspiration can lead to light-headedness and fainting.
• Advise patient to report signs of infection, such as fever and sore throat. Tell him to call prescriber if he develops easy bruising or bleeding; swelling of tongue, lips, face, eyes, mucous membranes, or extremities; difficulty swallowing or breathing; or hoarseness.
• Tell woman of childbearing age to notify prescriber if she becomes pregnant. Drug will need to be stopped.

---

candesartan cilexetil
kan-dah-SAR-tan

Atacand

Pharmacologic class: angiotensin II receptor antagonist
Pregnancy risk category C; D in 2nd and 3rd trimesters

AVAILABLE FORMS
Tablets: 4 mg, 8 mg, 16 mg, 32 mg

INDICATIONS & DOSAGES
➤ **Hypertension (used alone or with other antihypertensives)**
Adults: Initially, 16 mg P.O. once daily when used alone; usual range is 8 to 32 mg P.O. daily as a single dose or divided b.i.d.
➤ **Heart failure**
Adults: Initially, 4 mg P.O. once daily. Double the dose about every 2 weeks as

tolerated to a target dose of 32 mg once daily.
Adjust-a-dose: If patient takes a diuretic, consider a lower starting dose.

ADMINISTRATION
P.O.
● Give drug without regard for food.

ACTION
Inhibits vasoconstrictive action of angiotensin II by blocking angiotensin II receptor on the surface of vascular smooth muscle and other tissue cells.

Route	Onset	Peak	Duration
P.O.	Unknown	3–4 hr	24 hr

Half-life: 9 hours.

ADVERSE REACTIONS
CNS: dizziness, fatigue, headache.
CV: chest pain, peripheral edema.
EENT: pharyngitis, rhinitis, sinusitis.
GI: abdominal pain, diarrhea, nausea, vomiting.
GU: albuminuria.
Musculoskeletal: arthralgia, back pain.
Respiratory: coughing, bronchitis, upper respiratory tract infection.
Other: *angioedema.*

INTERACTIONS
Drug-drug. *Lithium:* May increase lithium concentration. Monitor lithium levels closely.
Potassium-sparing diuretics, potassium supplements: May cause hyperkalemia. Monitor patient closely.
Drug-herb. *Ma huang:* May decrease antihypertensive effects. Discourage use together.
Drug-food. *Salt substitutes containing potassium:* May cause hyperkalemia. Monitor patient closely.

EFFECTS ON LAB TEST RESULTS
● May increase potassium, BUN, and serum creatinine levels.

CONTRAINDICATIONS & CAUTIONS
● Contraindicated in patients hypersensitive to drug or its components.
● Use cautiously in patients whose renal function depends on the renin-angiotensin-aldosterone system (such as patients with heart failure) because of risk of oliguria and progressive azotemia with acute renal failure or death.
● **Black Box Warning** Contraindicated in pregnant patients, especially in the second and third trimesters. ■
● Use cautiously in patients who are volume or salt depleted because they could develop symptoms of hypotension. Start therapy with a lower dosage range, and monitor blood pressure carefully.

NURSING CONSIDERATIONS
■ **Black Box Warning** Drugs such as candesartan that act directly on the renin-angiotensin system can cause fetal and neonatal illness and death when given to pregnant women. If pregnancy is detected, discontinue candesartan as soon as possible. ■
● If hypotension occurs after a dose of candesartan, place patient in the supine position and, if needed, give an I.V. infusion of normal saline solution.
● Most of drug's antihypertensive effect occurs within 2 weeks. Maximal effect may take 4 to 6 weeks. Diuretic may be added if blood pressure isn't controlled by drug alone.
● Carefully monitor elderly patients and those with renal disease for therapeutic response and adverse reactions.

PATIENT TEACHING
● Inform woman of childbearing age of the consequences of second and third trimester exposure to drug. Prescriber should be notified immediately if pregnancy is suspected.
● Advise breast-feeding woman of the risk of adverse effects on the infant and the need to stop either breast-feeding or drug.
● Instruct patient to store drug at room temperature and to keep container tightly sealed.
● Inform patient to report adverse reactions without delay.
● Tell patient that drug may be taken without regard to meals.

Reactions may be *common*, uncommon, *life-threatening*, or COMMON AND LIFE-THREATENING.
Interaction may have a *rapid onset* or *delayed onset.*

captopril
KAP-toe-pril

Capoten◆

Pharmacologic class: ACE inhibitor
*Pregnancy risk category C; D in 2nd
and 3rd trimesters*

AVAILABLE FORMS
Tablets: 12.5 mg, 25 mg, 50 mg, 100 mg

INDICATIONS & DOSAGES
➤ **Hypertension**
Adults: Initially, 25 mg P.O. b.i.d. or t.i.d.
If dosage doesn't control blood pressure
satisfactorily in 1 or 2 weeks, increase it
to 50 mg b.i.d. or t.i.d. If that dosage
doesn't control blood pressure satisfactorily after another 1 or 2 weeks, expect to
add a diuretic. If patient needs further
blood pressure reduction, dosage may be
raised to 150 mg t.i.d. while continuing diuretic. Maximum daily dose is
450 mg.
➤ **Diabetic nephropathy**
Adults: 25 mg P.O. t.i.d.
➤ **Heart failure**
Adults: Initially, 25 mg P.O. t.i.d. Patients
with normal or low blood pressure who
have been vigorously treated with diuretics
and who may be hyponatremic or hypovolemic may start with 6.25 or 12.5 mg
P.O. t.i.d.; starting dosage may be adjusted
over several days. Gradually increase
dosage to 50 mg P.O. t.i.d.; once patient
reaches this dosage, delay further dosage
increases for at least 2 weeks. Maximum
dosage is 450 mg daily.
Elderly patients: Initially, 6.25 mg P.O.
b.i.d. Increase gradually as needed.
➤ **Left ventricular dysfunction after
acute MI**
Adults: Start therapy as early as 3 days
after MI with 6.25 mg P.O. for one dose,
followed by 12.5 mg P.O. t.i.d. Increase
over several days to 25 mg P.O. t.i.d.; then
increase to 50 mg P.O. t.i.d. over several
weeks.

ADMINISTRATION
P.O.
● Give 1 hour before meals to enhance
drug absorption.

ACTION
Inhibits ACE, preventing conversion of
angiotensin I to angiotensin II, a potent
vasoconstrictor. Less angiotensin II
decreases peripheral arterial resistance,
decreasing aldosterone secretion, which
reduces sodium and water retention and
lowers blood pressure.

Route	Onset	Peak	Duration
P.O.	15–60 min	60–90 min	6–12 hr

Half-life: Less than 2 hours.

ADVERSE REACTIONS
CNS: dizziness, fainting, headache,
malaise, fatigue, fever.
CV: tachycardia, hypotension, angina
pectoris.
GI: abdominal pain, anorexia, constipation, diarrhea, dry mouth, dysgeusia,
nausea, vomiting.
Hematologic: *leukopenia, agranulocytosis, thrombocytopenia, pancytopenia,*
anemia.
Metabolic: hyperkalemia.
Respiratory: *dry, persistent, nonproductive cough,* dyspnea.
Skin: *urticarial rash, maculopapular
rash,* pruritus, alopecia.
Other: *angioedema.*

INTERACTIONS
Drug-drug. *Antacids:* May decrease captopril effect. Separate dosage times.
Digoxin: May increase digoxin level by
15% to 30%. Monitor digoxin level,
and observe patient for signs of digoxin
toxicity.
Diuretics, other antihypertensives: May
cause excessive hypotension. May need
to stop diuretic or reduce captopril
dosage.
Insulin, oral antidiabetics: May cause
hypoglycemia when captopril therapy is
started. Monitor patient closely.
Lithium: May increase lithium level;
symptoms of toxicity possible. Monitor
patient closely.
NSAIDs: May reduce antihypertensive
effect. Monitor blood pressure.
*Potassium-sparing diuretics, potassium
supplements:* May cause hyperkalemia.
Avoid using together unless hypokalemia
is confirmed.

---

†Canada   ◇OTC   ◆Off-label use   ◆Photoguide   *Liquid contains alcohol.

Drug-herb. *Black catechu:* May cause additional hypotensive effect. Discourage use together.
Capsaicin: May worsen cough. Discourage use together.
Drug-food. *Salt substitutes containing potassium:* May cause hyperkalemia. Monitor patient closely.

EFFECTS ON LAB TEST RESULTS
● May increase alkaline phosphatase, bilirubin, and potassium levels. May decrease hemoglobin level and hematocrit.
● May decrease granulocyte, platelet, RBC, and WBC counts.
● May cause false-positive urine acetone test results.

CONTRAINDICATIONS & CAUTIONS
● Contraindicated in patients hypersensitive to drug or other ACE inhibitors.
■ **Black Box Warning** Use during pregnancy can cause injury and death to the developing fetus. When pregnancy is detected, stop drug as soon as possible. ■
● Use cautiously in patients with impaired renal function or serious autoimmune disease, especially systemic lupus erythematosus, and in those who have been exposed to other drugs that affect WBC counts or immune response.

NURSING CONSIDERATIONS
● Monitor patient's blood pressure and pulse rate frequently.
● *Alert:* Elderly patients may be more sensitive to drug's hypotensive effects.
● Assess patient for signs of angioedema.
● Drug causes the most frequent occurrence of cough, compared with other ACE inhibitors.
● In patients with impaired renal function or collagen vascular disease, monitor WBC and differential counts before starting treatment, every 2 weeks for the first 3 months of therapy, and periodically thereafter.
● *Look alike–sound alike:* Don't confuse captopril with Capitrol.

PATIENT TEACHING
● Instruct patient to take drug 1 hour before meals; food in the GI tract may reduce absorption.

● Inform patient that light-headedness is possible, especially during first few days of therapy. Tell him to rise slowly to minimize this effect and to report occurrence to prescriber. If fainting occurs, he should stop drug and call prescriber immediately.
● Tell patient to use caution in hot weather and during exercise. Lack of fluids, vomiting, diarrhea, and excessive perspiration can lead to light-headedness and syncope.
● Advise patient to report signs and symptoms of infection, such as fever and sore throat.
● Tell women to notify prescriber if pregnancy occurs. Drug will need to be stopped.
● Urge patient to promptly report swelling of the face, lips, or mouth; or difficulty breathing.

carvedilol
kar-VAH-da-lol

Coreg

carvedilol phosphate
Coreg CR

Pharmacologic class: alpha-nonselective beta blocker
Pregnancy risk category C

AVAILABLE FORMS
Capsules (extended-release): 10 mg, 20 mg, 40 mg, 80 mg
Tablets: 3.125 mg, 6.25 mg, 12.5 mg, 25 mg

INDICATIONS & DOSAGES
➤ **Hypertension**
Adults: Dosage highly individualized. Initially, 6.25 mg P.O. b.i.d. Measure standing blood pressure 1 hour after first dose. If tolerated, continue dosage for 7 to 14 days. May increase to 12.5 mg P.O. b.i.d. for 7 to 14 days, following same blood pressure monitoring protocol as before. Maximum dose is 25 mg P.O. b.i.d. as tolerated. May be switched to extended-release capsule after controlled on immediate-release tablets.

Reactions may be *common,* uncommon, *life-threatening,* or COMMON AND LIFE-THREATENING.
Interaction may have a *rapid onset* or **delayed onset.**

> **Left ventricular dysfunction after MI**

Adults: Dosage individualized. Start therapy after patient is hemodynamically stable and fluid retention has been minimized. Initially, 6.25 mg P.O. b.i.d. Increase after 3 to 10 days to 12.5 mg b.i.d., then again to a target dose of 25 mg b.i.d. Or start with 3.25 mg b.i.d., or adjust dosage slower if indicated. May be switched to extended-release capsule after controlled on immediate-release tablets.

> **Mild to severe heart failure**

Adults: Dosage highly individualized. Initially, 3.125 mg P.O. b.i.d. for 2 weeks; if tolerated, may increase to 6.25 mg P.O. b.i.d. Dosage may be doubled every 2 weeks, as tolerated. Maximum dose for patients who weigh less than 85 kg (187 lb) is 25 mg P.O. b.i.d.; for those weighing more than 85 kg, dose is 50 mg P.O. b.i.d. May be switched to extended-release capsule after controlled on immediate-release tablets.

Adjust-a-dose: In patient with pulse rate below 55 beats/minute, reduce dosage.

> **Angina pectoris ♦**

Adults: 25 to 50 mg P.O. b.i.d. May be switched to extended-release capsule after controlled on immediate-release tablets.

> **Idiopathic cardiomyopathy ♦**

Adults: 6.25 to 25 mg P.O. b.i.d. May be switched to extended-release capsule after controlled on immediate-release tablets.

ADMINISTRATION

P.O.
- Give drug with food.
- Capsules may be opened, mixed in cool applesauce, and taken immediately; don't store.
- Give capsules in the morning.
- Extended-release equivalent of 3.125 mg immediate-release b.i.d. is 10 mg; 6.25 mg immediate-release b.i.d. is 20 mg; 12.5 mg immediate-release b.i.d. is 40 mg; and 25 mg immediate-release b.i.d. is 80 mg. Dosage may be further titrated based on clinical response.

ACTION

Nonselective beta blocker with alpha-blocking activity.

Route	Onset	Peak	Duration
P.O.	Rapid	1–2 hr	7–10 hr
P.O. (extended-release)	30 min	5 hr	Unknown

Half-life: Immediate release: 7 to 10 hours; extended-release: unknown.

ADVERSE REACTIONS

CNS: *asthenia, dizziness, fatigue, stroke,* pain, headache, malaise, fever, hypesthesia, paresthesia, vertigo, somnolence, depression, insomnia.

CV: *hypotension, postural hypertension, AV block, bradycardia,* edema, syncope, angina pectoris, peripheral edema, hypovolemia, fluid overload, hypertension, palpitations, peripheral vascular disorder, chest pain.

EENT: sinusitis, abnormal vision, blurred vision, pharyngitis, rhinitis.

GI: *diarrhea,* vomiting, nausea, melena, periodontitis, abdominal pain, dyspepsia.

GU: impotence, abnormal renal function, albuminuria, hematuria, UTI.

Hematologic: *thrombocytopenia,* purpura, anemia.

Metabolic: *hyperglycemia, weight gain, hyperkalemia, hypoglycemia,* weight loss, hypercholesterolemia, hyperuricemia, hyponatremia, glycosuria, hypervolemia, diabetes mellitus, gout, hypertriglyceridemia.

Musculoskeletal: arthralgia, back pain, muscle cramps, hypotonia, arthritis.

Respiratory: *upper respiratory tract infection, lung edema,* bronchitis, cough, rales, dyspnea.

Other: *hypersensitivity reactions,* infection, flulike syndrome, viral infection, injury.

INTERACTIONS

Drug-drug. *Amiodarone:* May increase risk of bradycardia, AV block, and myocardial depression. Monitor patient's ECG and vital signs.

Catecholamine-depleting drugs such as MAO inhibitors, reserpine: May cause bradycardia or severe hypotension. Monitor patient closely.

Cimetidine: May increase bioavailability of carvedilol. Monitor vital signs closely.

Clonidine: May increase blood pressure- and heart rate-lowering effects. Monitor vital signs closely.

Cyclosporine: May increase cyclosporine level. Monitor cyclosporine level.

Digoxin: May increase digoxin level by about 15% when given together. Monitor digoxin level.

Diltiazem, verapamil: May cause isolated conduction disturbances. Monitor patient's heart rhythm and blood pressure.

Fluoxetine, paroxetine, propafenone, quinidine: May increase level of carvedilol. Monitor patient for hypotension and dizziness.

Insulin, oral antidiabetics: May enhance hypoglycemic properties. Monitor glucose level.

NSAIDs: May decrease antihypertensive effects. Monitor blood pressure.

Rifampin: May reduce carvedilol level by 70%. Monitor vital signs closely.

Drug-herb. *Ma huang:* May decrease antihypertensive effects. Discourage use together.

Drug-food. *Any food:* May delay rate of absorption of carvedilol with no change in bioavailability. Advise patient to take drug with food to minimize orthostatic effects.

EFFECTS ON LAB TEST RESULTS
• May increase alkaline phosphatase, ALT, AST, BUN, cholesterol, creatinine, GGT, nonprotein nitrogen, potassium, triglyceride, sodium, and uric acid levels. May increase or decrease glucose level.
• May decrease PT and platelet count.

CONTRAINDICATIONS & CAUTIONS
• Contraindicated in patients hypersensitive to drug and in those with New York Heart Association class IV decompensated cardiac failure requiring I.V. inotropic therapy.
• Contraindicated in those with bronchial asthma or related bronchospastic conditions, second- or third-degree AV block, sick sinus syndrome (unless a permanent pacemaker is in place), cardiogenic shock, severe bradycardia, or symptomatic hepatic impairment.
• Use cautiously in hypertensive patients with left-sided heart failure, perioperative patients who receive anesthetics that depress myocardial function (such as cyclopropane and trichloroethylene), and diabetic patients receiving insulin or oral antidiabetics, and in those subject to spontaneous hypoglycemia.
• Use cautiously in patients with thyroid disease (may mask hyperthyroidism; withdrawal may precipitate thyroid storm or exacerbation of hyperthyroidism), pheochromocytoma, Prinzmetal's or variant angina, bronchospastic disease (in those who can't tolerate other antihypertensives), or peripheral vascular disease (may precipitate or aggravate symptoms of arterial insufficiency).
• Use cautiously in breast-feeding women.
• Safety and effectiveness in children younger than age 18 haven't been established.

NURSING CONSIDERATIONS
• *Alert:* Patients who have a history of severe anaphylactic reaction to several allergens may be more reactive to repeated challenge (accidental, diagnostic, or therapeutic). They may be unresponsive to dosages of epinephrine typically used to treat allergic reactions.
• Mild hepatocellular injury may occur during therapy. At first sign of hepatic dysfunction, perform tests for hepatic injury or jaundice; if present, stop drug.
• If drug must be stopped, do so gradually over 1 to 2 weeks, if possible.
• Patient should be stable on maximum immediate-release dose before switching to extended-release form.
• Monitor patient with heart failure for worsened condition, renal dysfunction, or fluid retention; diuretics may need to be increased.
• Monitor diabetic patient closely; drug may mask signs of hypoglycemia, or hyperglycemia may be worsened.
• Observe patient for dizziness or lightheadedness for 1 hour after giving each new dose.
• Monitor elderly patients carefully; drug levels are about 50% higher in elderly patients than in younger patients.

PATIENT TEACHING
• Tell patient not to interrupt or stop drug without medical approval.

Reactions may be *common,* uncommon, *life-threatening,* or COMMON AND LIFE-THREATENING.
Interaction may have a *rapid onset* or **delayed onset.**

- Inform patient that improvement of heart failure symptoms might take several weeks of drug therapy.
- Advise patient with heart failure to call prescriber if weight gain or shortness of breath occurs.
- Inform patient that he may experience low blood pressure when standing. If dizziness or fainting occurs (rare), advise him to sit or lie down and to notify prescriber if symptoms persist.
- Caution patient against performing hazardous tasks during start of therapy.
- Advise diabetic patient to promptly report changes in glucose level.
- Inform patient who wears contact lenses that his eyes may feel dry.
- Tell patient to take drug with food. Extended-release capsule may be opened and contents mixed with cool applesauce and taken immediately; don't store.
- Advise patient that capsules shouldn't be crushed, chewed, or contents divided.

clonidine hydrochloride
KLOE-ni-deen

Catapres, Catapres-TTS, Dixarit†, Duraclon

Pharmacologic class: centrally acting alpha agonist
Pregnancy risk category C

AVAILABLE FORMS
Transdermal: TTS-1 (releases 0.1 mg/ 24 hours), TTS-2 (releases 0.2 mg/ 24 hours), TTS-3 (releases 0.3 mg/ 24 hours)
Injection for epidural use: 100 mcg/ml
Injection for epidural use, concentrate: 500 mcg/ml
Tablets: 0.025 mg†, 0.1 mg, 0.2 mg, 0.3 mg

INDICATIONS & DOSAGES
➤ **Essential and renal hypertension**
Adults and children age 12 and older: Initially, 0.1 mg P.O. b.i.d.; then increased by 0.1 to 0.2 mg daily on a weekly basis. Usual range is 0.2 to 0.6 mg daily in divided doses; infrequently, dosages as high as 2.4 mg daily are used.

Or, apply transdermal patch once every 7 days, starting with 0.1-mg system and adjusted with another 0.1-mg or larger system.
➤ **Severe cancer pain that is unresponsive to epidural or spinal opiate analgesia or other more conventional methods of analgesia**
Adults: Initially, 30 mcg/hour by continuous epidural infusion. Experience with rates greater than 40 mcg/hour is limited.
Children: Initially, 0.5 mcg/kg/hour by epidural infusion. Dosage should be cautiously adjusted, based on response.
➤ **Pheochromocytoma diagnosis** ◆
Adults: 0.3 mg P.O. for a single dose.
➤ **Vasomotor symptoms of menopause** ◆
Adults: 0.05 to 0.4 mg P.O. b.i.d. or 0.1-mg/24-hour patch applied once every 7 days.
➤ **Opiate dependence** ◆
Adults: Initially, 0.005 or 0.006 mg/kg test dose, followed by 0.017 mg/kg P.O. daily in three or four divided doses for 10 days. Or, initially, 0.1 mg P.O. three or four times daily, with dosage adjusted by 0.1 to 0.2 mg daily. Dosage range is 0.3 to 1.2 mg P.O. daily. Stop drug gradually. Follow protocols.
➤ **Smoking cessation** ◆
Adults: Initially, 0.1 mg P.O. b.i.d., beginning on or shortly before the day of smoking cessation. Increase dosage every 7 days by 0.1 mg daily, if needed. Or, 0.2-mg/24-hour transdermal patch applied every 7 days. Therapy should begin on or shortly before the day of smoking cessation. Increase dosage by 0.1 mg/24 hours at weekly intervals, if needed.
➤ **Attention deficit hyperactivity disorder** ◆
Children: Initially, 0.05 mg P.O. at bedtime. May increase dosage cautiously over 2 to 4 weeks. Maintenance dosage is 0.05 to 0.4 mg P.O. daily.

ADMINISTRATION
P.O.
- Give last dose immediately before bedtime.
Transdermal
- Apply patch to nonhairy area of intact skin on upper arm or torso.

Epidural
• **Alert:** The injection form is for epidural use only.
■ **Black Box Warning** The injection form concentrate containing 500 mcg/ml must be diluted in normal saline injection before use to yield 100 mcg/ml. ■

ACTION

Unknown. Thought to stimulate alpha$_2$ receptors and inhibit the central vasomotor centers, decreasing sympathetic outflow to the heart, kidneys, and peripheral vasculature, and lowering peripheral vascular resistance, blood pressure, and heart rate.

Route	Onset	Peak	Duration
P.O.	30–60 min	2–4 hr	12–24 hr
Trans-dermal	2–3 days	2–3 days	7–8 days
Epidural	Unknown	30–60 min	Unknown

Half-life: 6 to 20 hours.

ADVERSE REACTIONS

CNS: *drowsiness, dizziness, sedation, weakness,* fatigue, malaise, agitation, depression.
CV: *bradycardia, severe rebound hypertension,* orthostatic hypotension.
GI: *constipation, dry mouth,* nausea, vomiting, anorexia.
GU: urine retention, impotence.
Metabolic: weight gain.
Skin: *pruritus, dermatitis with transdermal patch,* rash.
Other: loss of libido.

INTERACTIONS

Drug-drug. *Amitriptyline, amoxapine, clomipramine, desipramine, doxepin, imipramine, nortriptyline, protriptyline, trimipramine:* May cause loss of blood pressure control with life-threatening elevations in blood pressure. Avoid using together.
CNS depressants: May increase CNS depression. Use together cautiously.
Digoxin, verapamil: May cause AV block and severe hypotension. Monitor BP and ECG.
Diuretics, other antihypertensives: May increase hypotensive effect. Monitor patient closely.

Beta blockers: May cause life-threatening hypertension. Closely monitor blood pressure.
Levodopa: May reduce effectiveness of levodopa. Monitor patient.
MAO inhibitors, prazosin: May decrease antihypertensive effect. Use together cautiously.
Propranolol, other beta blockers: May cause paradoxical hypertensive response. Monitor patient carefully.
Drug-herb. *Capsicum:* May reduce antihypertensive effectiveness. Discourage use together.
Ma huang: May decrease antihypertensive effects. Discourage use together.

EFFECTS ON LAB TEST RESULTS

• May decrease urinary excretion of vanillylmandelic acid and catecholamines. May cause a weakly positive Coombs' test result.

CONTRAINDICATIONS & CAUTIONS

• Contraindicated in patients hypersensitive to drug.
• Transdermal form is contraindicated in patients hypersensitive to any component of the adhesive layer of transdermal system.
• Epidural form is contraindicated in patients receiving anticoagulant therapy, in those with bleeding diathesis, in those with an injection site infection, and in those who are hemodynamically unstable or have severe CV disease.
• Use cautiously in patients with severe coronary insufficiency, conduction disturbances, recent MI, cerebrovascular disease, chronic renal failure, or impaired liver function.

NURSING CONSIDERATIONS

• Drug may be given to lower blood pressure rapidly in some hypertensive emergencies.
• Monitor blood pressure and pulse rate frequently. Dosage is usually adjusted to patient's blood pressure and tolerance.
• Elderly patients may be more sensitive than younger ones to drug's hypotensive effects.
• Observe patient for tolerance to drug's therapeutic effects, which may require increased dosage.

Reactions may be *common,* uncommon, *life-threatening,* or COMMON AND LIFE-THREATENING.
Interaction may have a *rapid onset* or *delayed onset.*

• Noticeable antihypertensive effects of transdermal clonidine may take 2 to 3 days. Oral antihypertensive therapy may have to be continued in the interim.

• **Alert:** Remove transdermal patch before defibrillation to prevent arcing.

• Stop drug gradually by reducing dosage over 2 to 4 days to avoid rapid rise in blood pressure, agitation, headache, and tremor. When stopping therapy in patients receiving both clonidine and a beta blocker, gradually withdraw the beta blocker several days before gradually stopping clonidine to minimize adverse reactions.

• Don't stop drug before surgery.

• When drug is given epidurally, carefully monitor infusion pump, and inspect catheter tubing for obstruction or dislodgment.

■ **Black Box Warning** Epidural clonidine isn't recommended for obstetric, postpartum, or perioperative pain management due to the risk of hemodynamic instability. ■

• **Look alike–sound alike:** Don't confuse clonidine with quinidine or clomiphene; or Catapres with Cetapred or Combipres.

PATIENT TEACHING

• Instruct patient to take drug exactly as prescribed.

• Advise patient that stopping drug abruptly may cause severe rebound high blood pressure. Tell him dosage must be reduced gradually over 2 to 4 days, as instructed by prescriber.

• Tell patient to take the last dose immediately before bedtime.

• Reassure patient that the transdermal patch usually remains attached despite showering and other routine daily activities. Instruct him on the use of the adhesive overlay to provide additional skin adherence, if needed. Also tell him to place patch at a different site each week.

• Caution patient that drug may cause drowsiness but that this adverse effect usually diminishes over 4 to 6 weeks.

• Inform patient that dizziness upon standing can be minimized by rising slowly from a sitting or lying position and avoiding sudden position changes.

doxazosin mesylate
dox-AY-zo-sin

Cardura✔, Cardura XL

Pharmacologic class: alpha blocker
Pregnancy risk category C

AVAILABLE FORMS
Tablets: 1 mg, 2 mg, 4 mg, 8 mg
Tablets (extended-release): 4 mg, 8 mg

INDICATIONS & DOSAGES
➤ **Essential hypertension**
Adults: Initially, 1 mg P.O. daily; determine effect on standing and supine blood pressure at 2 to 6 hours and 24 hours after dose. May increase at 2-week intervals to 2 mg and, thereafter, 4 mg and 8 mg once daily, if needed. Maximum daily dose is 16 mg, but doses over 4 mg daily increase the risk of adverse reactions. Don't use extended-release formulation to treat hypertension.
➤ **BPH**
Adults: Initially, 1 mg P.O. once daily in the morning or evening; may increase at 1- or 2-week intervals to 2 mg and, thereafter, 4 mg and 8 mg once daily, if needed.

ADMINISTRATION
P.O.
• Swallow extended-release tablets whole: don't chew, divide, cut, or crush.
• Give extended-release tablet with breakfast.
• Don't give evening dose the night before switching to extended-release from immediate-release formula.

ACTION
An alpha blocker that acts on the peripheral vasculature to reduce peripheral vascular resistance and produce vasodilation. Drug also decreases smooth muscle tone in the prostate and bladder neck.

Route	Onset	Peak	Duration
P.O.	1–2 hr	2–3 hr	24 hr

Half-life: 19 to 22 hours.

ADVERSE REACTIONS
CNS: *dizziness, asthenia, headache,* vertigo, somnolence, drowsiness, pain.

CV: *orthostatic hypotension,* **arrhythmias,** hypotension, edema, palpitations, tachycardia.
EENT: rhinitis, pharyngitis, abnormal vision.
GI: nausea, vomiting, diarrhea, constipation.
Hematologic: *leukopenia, neutropenia.*
Musculoskeletal: arthralgia, myalgia.
Respiratory: dyspnea.
Skin: rash, pruritus.

INTERACTIONS
Drug-drug. *Midodrine:* May decrease the effectiveness of midodrine. Monitor patient for therapeutic effect.
Drug-herb. *Butcher's broom:* May decrease effect of doxazosin. Discourage use together.
Ma huang: May decrease antihypertensive effects. Discourage use together.

EFFECTS ON LAB TEST RESULTS
• May decrease WBC and neutrophil counts.

CONTRAINDICATIONS & CAUTIONS
• Contraindicated in patients hypersensitive to drug and quinazoline derivatives (including prazosin and terazosin).
• Use cautiously in patients with impaired hepatic function.

NURSING CONSIDERATIONS
• Monitor blood pressure closely.
• If syncope occurs, place patient in a recumbent position and treat supportively. A transient hypotensive response isn't considered a contraindication to continued therapy.
• Initial extended-release dose is 4 mg. If patient stops medication briefly, he should resume at 4-mg dose and titrate back to 8 mg if appropriate.
• Wait 3 to 4 weeks before increasing extended-release dose.
• *Look alike–sound alike:* Don't confuse doxazosin with doxapram, doxorubicin, or doxepin. Don't confuse Cardura with Coumadin, K-Dur, Cardene, or Cordarone.

PATIENT TEACHING
• Instruct patient to take drug exactly as prescribed.
• *Alert:* Advise patient that he is susceptible to a first-dose effect (marked low blood pressure on standing up with dizziness or fainting). This is most common after first dose but also can occur during dosage adjustment or interruption of therapy.
• Advise patient to consult prescriber if dizziness or palpitations are bothersome.
• Advise patient to rise slowly from sitting or lying position.
• Advise patient to avoid driving and other hazardous activities until drug's effects are known.

enalaprilat
eh-NAH-leh-prel-at

enalapril maleate
Vasotec✦

Pharmacologic class: ACE inhibitor
Pregnancy risk category C; D in 2nd and 3rd trimesters

AVAILABLE FORMS
enalaprilat
Injection: 1.25 mg/ml
enalapril maleate
Tablets: 2.5 mg, 5 mg, 10 mg, 20 mg

INDICATIONS & DOSAGES
➤ **Hypertension**
Adults: In patients not taking diuretics, initially, 5 mg P.O. once daily; then adjusted based on response. Usual dosage range is 10 to 40 mg daily as a single dose or two divided doses. Or, 1.25 mg I.V. infusion over 5 minutes every 6 hours.
Children ages 1 month to 16 years: 0.08 mg/kg (up to 5 mg) P.O. once daily; dosage should be adjusted as needed up to 0.58 mg/kg (maximum 40 mg). Don't use if creatinine clearance is less than 30 ml/minute.
Adjust-a-dose: If patient is taking diuretics or creatinine clearance is 30 ml/minute or less, initially, 2.5 mg P.O. once daily. Or, 0.625 mg I.V. over 5 minutes, and repeat in 1 hour, if needed; then 1.25 mg I.V. every 6 hours.
➤ **To convert from I.V. therapy to oral therapy in patients receiving diuretics**
Adults: Initially, 2.5 mg P.O. once daily; if patient was receiving 0.625 mg I.V. every

6 hours, then 2.5 mg P.O. once daily.
Adjust dosage based on response.

➤ **To convert from oral therapy to I.V. therapy**
Adults: 1.25 mg I.V. over 5 minutes every 6 hours.

Adjust-a-dose: If creatinine level is more than 1.6 mg/dl or sodium level below 130 mEq/L, initially, 2.5 mg P.O. daily and adjust slowly.

➤ **To manage symptomatic heart failure**
Adults: Initially, 2.5 mg P.O. daily or b.i.d., increased gradually over several weeks. Maintenance is 5 to 20 mg daily in two divided doses. Maximum daily dose is 40 mg in two divided doses.

➤ **Asymptomatic left ventricular dysfunction**
Adults: Initially, 2.5 mg P.O. b.i.d. Increase as tolerated to target daily dose of 20 mg P.O. in divided doses.

ADMINISTRATION
P.O.
● Give drug without regard for food.
● Request oral suspension for patient who has difficulty swallowing.
I.V.
● Compatible solutions include D₅W, normal saline solution for injection, dextrose 5% in lactated Ringer's injection, dextrose 5% in normal saline solution for injection, and Isolyte E.
● Inject drug slowly over at least 5 minutes, or dilute in 50 ml of a compatible solution and infuse over 15 minutes.
● Incompatibilities: Amphotericin B, cefepime hydrochloride, phenytoin sodium.

ACTION
May inhibit ACE, preventing conversion of angiotensin I to angiotensin II, a potent vasoconstrictor. Less angiotensin II decreases peripheral arterial resistance, decreasing aldosterone secretion, reducing sodium and water retention, and lowering blood pressure.

Route	Onset	Peak	Duration
P.O.	1 hr	4–6 hr	24 hr
I.V.	15 min	1–4 hr	6 hr

Half-life: 12 hours.

ADVERSE REACTIONS
CNS: *asthenia,* headache, dizziness, fatigue, vertigo, syncope.
CV: hypotension, chest pain, angina pectoris.
GI: diarrhea, nausea, abdominal pain, vomiting.
GU: decreased renal function (in patients with bilateral renal artery stenosis or heart failure).
Hematologic: bone marrow depression.
Respiratory: *dry, persistent, tickling, nonproductive cough,* dyspnea.
Skin: rash.
Other: *angioedema.*

INTERACTIONS
Drug-drug. *Azathioprine:* May increase risk of anemia or leukopenia. Monitor hematologic study results if used together.
Diuretics: May excessively reduce blood pressure. Use together cautiously.
Insulin, oral antidiabetics: May cause hypoglycemia, especially at start of enalapril therapy. Monitor patient closely.
Lithium: May cause lithium toxicity. Monitor lithium level.
NSAIDs: May reduce antihypertensive effect. Monitor blood pressure.
Potassium-sparing diuretics, potassium supplements: May cause hyperkalemia. Avoid using together unless hypokalemia is confirmed.
Drug-herb. *Capsaicin:* May cause cough. Discourage use together.
Ma huang: May decrease antihypertensive effects. Discourage use together.
Drug-food. *Salt substitutes containing potassium:* May cause hyperkalemia. Monitor patient closely.

EFFECTS ON LAB TEST RESULTS
● May increase bilirubin, BUN, creatinine, and potassium levels. May decrease sodium and hemoglobin levels and hematocrit.
● May increase liver function test values.

CONTRAINDICATIONS & CAUTIONS
● Contraindicated in patients hypersensitive to drug and in those with a history of angioedema related to previous treatment with an ACE inhibitor.
■ **Black Box Warning** Use during pregnancy can cause injury and death to the

developing fetus. When pregnancy is detected, stop drug as soon as possible. ■
• Use cautiously in renally impaired patients or those with aortic stenosis or hypertrophic cardiomyopathy.

NURSING CONSIDERATIONS
• Closely monitor blood pressure response to drug.
• *Look alike–sound alike:* Similar packaging and labeling of enalaprilat injection and pancuronium, a neuromuscular-blocking drug, could result in a fatal medication error. Check all labels carefully.
• Monitor CBC with differential counts before and during therapy.
• Diabetic patients, those with impaired renal function or heart failure, and those receiving drugs that can increase potassium level may develop hyperkalemia. Monitor potassium intake and potassium level.
• *Look alike–sound alike:* Don't confuse enalapril with Anafranil or Eldepryl.

PATIENT TEACHING
• Instruct patient to report breathing difficulty or swelling of face, eyes, lips, or tongue. Swelling of the face and throat (including swelling of the larynx) may occur, especially after first dose.
• Advise patient to report signs of infection, such as fever and sore throat.
• Inform patient that light-headedness can occur, especially during first few days of therapy. Tell him to rise slowly to minimize this effect and to notify prescriber if symptoms develop. If he faints, he should stop taking drug and call prescriber immediately.
• Tell patient to use caution in hot weather and during exercise. Inadequate fluid intake, vomiting, diarrhea, and excessive perspiration can lead to light-headedness and fainting.
• Advise patient to avoid salt substitutes; these products may contain potassium, which can cause high potassium levels in patients taking this drug.
• Tell woman of childbearing age to notify prescriber if pregnancy occurs. Drug will need to be stopped.

eplerenone
ep-LER-eh-nown

Inspra

Pharmacologic class: selective aldosterone receptor antagonist
Pregnancy risk category B

AVAILABLE FORMS
Tablets: 25 mg, 50 mg

INDICATIONS & DOSAGES
➤ **Hypertension**
Adults: 50 mg P.O. once daily. If response is inadequate after 4 weeks, increase dosage to 50 mg P.O. b.i.d. Maximum daily dose, 100 mg.
Adjust-a-dose: In patients taking weak CYP3A4 inhibitors (erythromycin, fluconazole, saquinavir, verapamil), reduce eplerenone starting dose to 25 mg P.O. once daily.
➤ **Heart failure after an MI**
Adults: Initially, 25 mg P.O. once daily. Increase within 4 weeks, as tolerated and according to potassium level, to 50 mg P.O. once daily.
Adjust-a-dose: If potassium level is less than 5 mEq/L, increase dosage from 25 mg every other day to 25 mg daily; or increase dosage from 25 mg daily to 50 mg daily. If potassium level is 5 to 5.4 mEq/L, don't adjust dosage. If potassium level is 5.5 to 5.9 mEq/L, decrease dosage from 50 mg daily to 25 mg daily; or decrease dosage from 25 mg daily to 25 mg every other day; or if dosage was 25 mg every other day, withhold drug. If potassium level is greater than 6 mEq/L, withhold drug. May restart drug at 25 mg every other day when potassium level is less than 5.5 mEq/L. In patients taking weak CYP3A4 inhibitors (erythromycin, fluconazole, saquinavir, verapamil), reduce eplerenone starting dose to 25 mg P.O. once daily.

ADMINISTRATION
P.O.
• Give drug without regard for meals.

ACTION
Binds to mineralocorticoid receptors and blocks aldosterone, which increases blood

---

Reactions may be *common*, uncommon, *life-threatening*, or COMMON AND LIFE-THREATENING.
Interaction may have a *rapid onset* or *delayed onset*.

pressure through induction of sodium reabsorption and possibly other mechanisms.

Route	Onset	Peak	Duration
P.O.	Unknown	90 min	Unknown

Half-life: 4 to 6 hours.

ADVERSE REACTIONS
CNS: dizziness, fatigue.
GI: diarrhea, abdominal pain.
GU: albuminuria, abnormal vaginal bleeding.
Metabolic: *hyperkalemia.*
Respiratory: cough.
Other: flulike syndrome, gynecomastia.

INTERACTIONS
Drug-drug. *ACE inhibitors, angiotensin II receptor antagonists:* May increase risk of hyperkalemia. Use together cautiously.
Azole antifungals (itraconazole, ketoconazole), macrolides (clarithromycin), nefazodone, protease inhibitors (nelfinavir, ritonavir): Inhibits the CYP3A4 metabolism of eplerenone. Use together is contraindicated.
Lithium: May increase risk of lithium toxicity. Monitor lithium level.
NSAIDs: May reduce the antihypertensive effect and cause severe hyperkalemia in patients with impaired renal function. Monitor blood pressure and potassium level.
Potassium supplements, potassium-sparing diuretics (amiloride, spironolactone, triamterene): May increase risk of hyperkalemia and sometimes-fatal arrhythmias. Use together is contraindicated.
Weak CYP3A4 inhibitors (erythromycin, fluconazole, saquinavir, verapamil): May increase eplerenone level. Reduce eplerenone starting dose to 25 mg P.O. once daily.
Drug-herb. *St. John's wort:* May decrease eplerenone level over time. Discourage use together.

EFFECTS ON LAB TEST RESULTS
• May increase ALT, BUN, cholesterol, creatinine, GGT, potassium, triglyceride, and uric acid levels. May decrease sodium level.

CONTRAINDICATIONS & CAUTIONS
• When used for hypertension, contraindicated in patients with type 2 diabetes with microalbuminuria, creatinine level greater than 2 mg/dl in men or greater than 1.8 mg/dl in women, or creatinine clearance less than 50 ml/minute and in patients taking potassium supplements or potassium-sparing diuretics (amiloride, spironolactone, or triamterene).
• Contraindicated in patients with potassium level greater than 5.5 mEq/ml or creatinine clearance 30 ml/minute or less and in patients taking strong CYP3A4 inhibitors, such as ketoconazole, clarithromycin, ritonavir, nelfinavir, nefazodone, or itraconazole.
• Use cautiously in patient with mild to moderate hepatic impairment.
• Use in pregnant woman only if the potential benefits justify the potential risk to the fetus. Use cautiously in breast-feeding women; it's unknown if drug appears in breast milk.

NURSING CONSIDERATIONS
• Drug may be used alone or with other antihypertensives.
• Full therapeutic effect of the drug occurs in 4 weeks.
• In patients with heart failure, measure potassium level at baseline, within the first week, at 1 month after starting therapy, and periodically thereafter.
• Monitor patient for signs and symptoms of hyperkalemia.
• *Look alike–sound alike:* Don't confuse Inspra with Spiriva.

PATIENT TEACHING
• Inform patient that drug may be taken with or without food.
• Advise patient to avoid potassium supplements and salt substitutes during treatment.
• Tell patient to report adverse reactions.

eprosartan mesylate
ep-row-SAR-tan

Teveten

Pharmacologic class: angiotensin II
receptor antagonist
*Pregnancy risk category C; D in 2nd
and 3rd trimesters*

AVAILABLE FORMS
Tablets: 400 mg, 600 mg

INDICATIONS & DOSAGES
➤ **Hypertension (alone or with other
antihypertensives)**
Adults: Initially, 600 mg P.O. daily.
Dosage ranges from 400 to 800 mg daily,
given as single daily dose or two divided
doses.

ADMINISTRATION
P.O.
• Give drug without regard for meals.

ACTION
An angiotensin II receptor antagonist that
reduces blood pressure by blocking the
vasoconstrictor and aldosterone-secreting
effects of angiotensin II. Drug selectively
blocks the binding of angiotensin II to its
receptor sites found in many tissues, such
as vascular smooth muscle and the adrenal
gland.

Route	Onset	Peak	Duration
P.O.	1–2 hr	1–3 hr	24 hr

Half-life: 5 to 9 hours.

ADVERSE REACTIONS
CNS: depression, fatigue, headache,
dizziness.
CV: chest pain, dependent edema.
EENT: pharyngitis, rhinitis, sinusitis.
GI: abdominal pain, dyspepsia,
diarrhea.
GU: UTI.
Hematologic: *neutropenia.*
Musculoskeletal: arthralgia, myalgia.
Respiratory: cough, upper respiratory
tract infection, bronchitis.
Other: injury, viral infection.

INTERACTIONS
Drug-drug. *NSAIDs:* May decrease
antihypertensive effects. Monitor blood
pressure.
Drug-herb. *Ma huang:* May decrease
antihypertensive effects. Discourage use
together.

EFFECTS ON LAB TEST RESULTS
• May increase BUN and triglyceride levels.

CONTRAINDICATIONS & CAUTIONS
• Contraindicated in patients hypersensitive to eprosartan or its components.
• Use cautiously in patients with renal
artery stenosis; in patients with an activated
renin-angiotensin system, such as
volume- or salt-depleted patients; and in
patients whose renal function may depend
on the renin-angiotensin-aldosterone
system, such as those with severe heart
failure.
• Safety and effectiveness in children
haven't been established.
■ **Black Box Warning** Use during
pregnancy can cause injury and death
to the developing fetus. When pregnancy
is detected, stop drug as soon as
possible. ■

NURSING CONSIDERATIONS
• Correct hypovolemia and hyponatremia
before starting therapy to reduce risk of
symptomatic hypotension.
• Monitor blood pressure closely for
2 hours at start of treatment. If hypotension occurs, place patient in a supine
position and, if needed, give an I.V. infusion of normal saline solution.
• A transient episode of hypotension
isn't a contraindication to continued
treatment. Drug may be restarted once
patient's blood pressure has stabilized.
• Drug may be used alone or with other
antihypertensives, such as diuretics and
calcium channel blockers. Maximal
blood pressure response may take
2 or 3 weeks.
• Monitor patient for facial or lip swelling
because angioedema has occurred with
other angiotensin II antagonists.
• Closely observe infants exposed to
eprosartan in utero for hypotension,
oliguria, and hyperkalemia.

Reactions may be *common,* uncommon, *life-threatening,* or COMMON AND LIFE-THREATENING.
Interaction may have a *rapid onset* or **delayed onset.**

PATIENT TEACHING
• Advise woman of childbearing age to use a reliable form of contraception and to notify her prescriber immediately if pregnancy is suspected. Treatment may need to be stopped under medical supervision.
• Advise patient to report facial or lip swelling and signs and symptoms of infection, such as fever and sore throat.
• Tell patient to notify prescriber before taking OTC medication to treat a dry cough.
• Inform patient that drug may be taken without regard to meals.
• Advise breast-feeding woman to stop either therapy or breast-feeding because of potential for adverse reactions in infant.

---

felodipine
fell-OH-di-peen

Plendil, Renedil†

Pharmacologic class: calcium channel blocker
Pregnancy risk category C

AVAILABLE FORMS
Tablets (extended-release): 2.5 mg, 5 mg, 10 mg

INDICATIONS & DOSAGES
➤ **Hypertension**
Adults: Initially, 5 mg P.O. daily. Adjust dosage based on patient response, usually at intervals not less than 2 weeks. Usual dose is 2.5 to 10 mg daily; maximum dosage is 10 mg daily.
Elderly patients: 2.5 mg P.O. daily; adjust dosage as for adults. Maximum dosage is 10 mg daily.
Adjust-a-dose: For patients with impaired hepatic function, 2.5 mg P.O. daily; adjust dosage as for adults. Maximum daily dose is 10 mg.

ADMINISTRATION
P.O.
• Give drug whole; don't crush or cut tablets.
• Give drug without food or with a light meal.
• Don't give drug with grapefruit juice.

ACTION
Unknown. A dihydropyridine-derivative calcium channel blocker that prevents entry of calcium ions into vascular smooth muscle and cardiac cells; shows some selectivity for smooth muscle compared with cardiac muscle.

Route	Onset	Peak	Duration
P.O.	2–5 hr	2½–5 hr	24 hr

Half-life: 11 to 16 hours.

ADVERSE REACTIONS
CNS: *headache,* dizziness, paresthesia, asthenia.
CV: *peripheral edema,* chest pain, palpitations, flushing.
EENT: rhinorrhea, pharyngitis.
GI: abdominal pain, nausea, constipation, diarrhea.
Musculoskeletal: muscle cramps, back pain.
Respiratory: upper respiratory tract infection, cough.
Skin: rash.

INTERACTIONS
Drug-drug. *Anticonvulsants:* May decrease felodipine level. Avoid using together.
CYP3A4 inhibitors such as azole antifungals, cimetidine, erythromycin: May decrease clearance of felodipine. Reduce doses of felodipine; monitor patient for toxicity.
Metoprolol: May alter pharmacokinetics of metoprolol. Monitor patient for adverse reactions.
NSAIDs: May decrease antihypertensive effects. Monitor blood pressure.
Tacrolimus: May increase tacrolimus level. Monitor patient closely.
Theophylline: May slightly decrease theophylline level. Monitor patient response closely.
Drug-herb. *Ma huang:* May decrease antihypertensive effects. Discourage use together.
Drug-food. *Grapefruit, lime:* May increase drug level and adverse effects. Discourage use together.

EFFECTS ON LAB TEST RESULTS
None reported.

CONTRAINDICATIONS & CAUTIONS
• Contraindicated in patients hypersensitive to drug.
• Use cautiously in patients with heart failure, particularly those receiving beta blockers, and in patients with impaired hepatic function.

NURSING CONSIDERATIONS
• Monitor blood pressure for response.
• Monitor patient for peripheral edema, which appears to be both dose- and age-related. It's more common in patients taking higher doses, especially those older than age 60.
• *Look alike–sound alike:* Don't confuse Plendil with pindolol.

PATIENT TEACHING
• Tell patient to swallow tablets whole and not to crush or chew them.
• Tell patient to take drug without food or with a light meal.
• Advise patient not to take drug with grapefruit juice.
• Advise patient to continue taking drug even when he feels better, to watch his diet, and to check with prescriber or pharmacist before taking other drugs, including OTC drugs, nutritional supplements, or herbal remedies.
• Advise patient to observe good oral hygiene and to see a dentist regularly; use of drug may cause mild gum problems.

---

fosinopril sodium
foh-SIN-oh-pril

Monopril♦

Pharmacologic class: ACE inhibitor
Pregnancy risk category C; D in 2nd and 3rd trimesters

AVAILABLE FORMS
Tablets: 10 mg, 20 mg, 40 mg

INDICATIONS & DOSAGES
➤ **Hypertension**
Adults: Initially, 10 mg P.O. daily; adjust dosage based on blood pressure response at peak and trough levels. Usual dosage is 20 to 40 mg daily; maximum is 80 mg daily. Dosage may be divided.

➤ **Heart failure**
Adults: Initially, 10 mg P.O. once daily. Increase dosage over several weeks to a maximum of 40 mg P.O. daily, if needed.
Adjust-a-dose: For patients with moderate to severe renal failure or vigorous diuresis, start with 5 mg P.O. once daily.

ADMINISTRATION
P.O.
• Give drug without regard for meals.

ACTION
Inhibits ACE, preventing conversion of angiotensin I to angiotensin II, a potent vasoconstrictor. Less angiotensin II decreases peripheral arterial resistance, thus decreasing aldosterone secretion, which reduces sodium and water retention and lowers blood pressure.

Route	Onset	Peak	Duration
P.O.	1 hr	3 hr	24 hr

Half-life: 11½ hours.

ADVERSE REACTIONS
CNS: *dizziness, stroke,* headache, fatigue, syncope, paresthesia, sleep disturbance.
CV: *MI,* chest pain, angina pectoris, rhythm disturbances, palpitations, hypotension, orthostatic hypotension.
EENT: tinnitus, sinusitis.
GI: *pancreatitis,* nausea, vomiting, diarrhea, dry mouth, abdominal distention, abdominal pain, constipation.
GU: sexual dysfunction, renal insufficiency.
Hepatic: *hepatitis.*
Metabolic: *hyperkalemia.*
Musculoskeletal: arthralgia, musculoskeletal pain, myalgia.
Respiratory: *dry, persistent, tickling, nonproductive cough,* **bronchospasm.**
Skin: urticaria, rash, photosensitivity reactions, pruritus.
Other: *angioedema,* decreased libido, gout.

INTERACTIONS
Drug-drug. *Antacids:* May impair absorption. Separate dosage times by at least 2 hours.
Azathioprine: May increase risk of anemia or leukopenia. Monitor hematologic studies if used together.

Reactions may be *common,* uncommon, *life-threatening,* or COMMON AND LIFE-THREATENING.
Interaction may have a *rapid onset* or *delayed onset.*

Diuretics, other antihypertensives: May cause excessive hypotension. Stop diuretic or lower fosinopril dosage.
Lithium: May increase lithium level and lithium toxicity. Monitor lithium level.
Nesiritide: May increase hypotensive effects. Monitor blood pressure.
NSAIDs: May decrease antihypertensive effects. Monitor blood pressure.
Potassium-sparing diuretics, potassium supplements: May cause risk of hyperkalemia. Monitor patient closely.
Drug-herb. *Capsaicin:* May cause cough. Discourage use together.
Ma huang: May decrease antihypertensive effects. Discourage use together.
Drug-food. *Salt substitutes containing potassium:* May cause hyperkalemia. Discourage use together.

EFFECTS ON LAB TEST RESULTS
● May increase BUN, creatinine, potassium, and hemoglobin levels and hematocrit.
● May increase liver function test values.
● May cause falsely low digoxin level with the Digi-Tab radioimmunoassay kit for digoxin.

CONTRAINDICATIONS & CAUTIONS
● Contraindicated in patients hypersensitive to drug or other ACE inhibitors and in breast-feeding women.
● Use cautiously in patients with impaired renal or hepatic function.
■ **Black Box Warning** Use during pregnancy can cause injury and death to the developing fetus. When pregnancy is detected, stop drug as soon as possible. ■

NURSING CONSIDERATIONS
● Monitor blood pressure for drug effect.
● Although ACE inhibitors reduce blood pressure in all races, they reduce it less in blacks taking the ACE inhibitor alone. Black patients should take drug with a thiazide diuretic for a more favorable response.
● ACE inhibitors appear to cause a higher risk of angioedema in black patients.
● Monitor potassium intake and potassium level. Diabetic patients, those with impaired renal function, and those receiving drugs that can increase potassium level may develop hyperkalemia.

● Other ACE inhibitors may cause agranulocytosis and neutropenia. Monitor CBC with differential counts before therapy and periodically thereafter.
● Assess renal and hepatic function before and periodically throughout therapy.
● **Look alike–sound alike:** Don't confuse fosinopril with lisinopril. Don't confuse Monopril with Monurol.

PATIENT TEACHING
● Tell patient to avoid salt substitutes; these products may contain potassium, which can cause high potassium level in patients taking drug.
● Instruct patient to contact prescriber if light-headedness or fainting occurs.
● Advise patient to report evidence of infection, such as fever and sore throat.
● Instruct patient to call prescriber if he develops easy bruising or bleeding; swelling of tongue, lips, face, eyes, mucous membranes, arms, or legs; difficulty swallowing or breathing; and hoarseness.
● Urge patient to use caution in hot weather and during exercise. Inadequate fluid intake, vomiting, diarrhea, and excessive perspiration can lead to light-headedness and fainting.
● Tell woman of childbearing age to notify prescriber if pregnancy occurs. Drug will need to be stopped.

---

guanfacine hydrochloride
GWAHN-fa-seen

Tenex

Pharmacologic class: centrally acting antiadrenergic
Pregnancy risk category B

AVAILABLE FORMS
Tablets: 1 mg, 2 mg

INDICATIONS & DOSAGES
➤ **Hypertension**
Adults: Initially, 1 mg P.O. once daily at bedtime. If response isn't adequate after 3 to 4 weeks, increase dosage to 2 mg daily. Dosage may be further increased to 3 mg P.O. after an additional 3 to 4 weeks.
➤ **Migraine** ◆
Adults: 1 mg P.O. once daily for 12 weeks.

ADMINISTRATION
P.O.
● When given with another antihypertensive, give dose at bedtime to reduce somnolence.

ACTION
Reduces sympathetic outflow from the vasomotor center to the heart and blood vessels, resulting in a decrease in peripheral vascular resistance and a reduction in heart rate.

Route	Onset	Peak	Duration
P.O.	Unknown	1–4 hr	24 hr

Half-life: About 17 hours.

ADVERSE REACTIONS
CNS: *dizziness, somnolence,* fatigue, headache, insomnia, asthenia.
CV: *bradycardia.*
GI: *constipation, dry mouth,* diarrhea, nausea.
GU: impotence.
Skin: dermatitis, pruritus.

INTERACTIONS
Drug-drug. *CNS depressants:* May increase sedation. Use together cautiously.
Tricyclic antidepressants: May inhibit antihypertensive effects. Monitor blood pressure.
Drug-lifestyle. *Alcohol:* May increase sedation. Discourage alcohol use.

EFFECTS ON LAB TEST RESULTS
None reported.

CONTRAINDICATIONS & CAUTIONS
● Contraindicated in patients hypersensitive to drug.
● Use cautiously in patients with severe coronary insufficiency, recent MI, cerebrovascular disease, or chronic renal or hepatic insufficiency.

NURSING CONSIDERATIONS
● Monitor blood pressure frequently.
● Risk and severity of adverse reactions increase with higher dosages.
● Drug may be used alone or with a diuretic.

● Rebound hypertension may occur and, if it occurs, will be noticeable within 2 to 4 days after therapy ends.
● ***Look alike–sound alike:*** Don't confuse guanfacine with guanidine, guaifenesin, or guanabenz. Don't confuse Tenex with Xanax, Entex, or Ten-K.

PATIENT TEACHING
● Tell patient not to stop therapy abruptly. Rebound high blood pressure may occur but is less common than that which occurs with similar drugs.
● Advise patient to avoid activities that require alertness before drug's effects are known; drowsiness may occur.
● Warn patient that he may have a lower tolerance to alcohol and other CNS depressants during therapy.

---

hydralazine hydrochloride
hye-DRAL-a-zeen

Novo-Hylazin†

Pharmacologic class: peripheral dilator
Pregnancy risk category C

AVAILABLE FORMS
Injection: 20 mg/ml in 1-ml vial
Tablets: 10 mg, 25 mg, 50 mg, 100 mg

INDICATIONS & DOSAGES
➤ **Hypertension**
Adults: Initially, 10 mg P.O. q.i.d.; gradually increase over 2 weeks to 50 mg q.i.d., based on patient tolerance and response. Once stabilized, maintenance dosage can be divided b.i.d. Recommended range is 12.5 to 50 mg b.i.d.
Children: Initially, 0.75 mg/kg daily P.O. divided into four doses; gradually increased over 3 to 4 weeks to maximum of 7.5 mg/kg or 200 mg daily. Maximum first P.O. dose is 25 mg.
➤ **Hypertensive crisis**
Adults: 10 to 20 mg I.V. slowly or 10 to 50 mg I.M.; repeat as needed. Switch to oral form as soon as possible.
➤ **Severe heart failure ♦**
Adults: Initially, 50 to 75 mg P.O. daily. Maintenance doses range from 200 to

---

600 mg P.O. daily in divided doses every 6 to 12 hours.

ADMINISTRATION
P.O.
● Give drug with food to increase absorption.
I.V.
● Give drug slowly and repeat p.r.n., generally every 4 to 6 hours. Hydralazine changes color in most infusion solutions; these color changes don't indicate loss of potency.
● Drug is compatible with normal saline, Ringer's, lactated Ringer's, and several other common I.V. solutions.
● Replace parenteral therapy with oral therapy as soon as possible.
● **Incompatibilities:** Aminophylline, ampicillin sodium, chlorothiazide, D_5W, dextrose 10% in lactated Ringer's solution, dextrose 10% in normal saline solution, diazoxide, doxapram, edetate calcium disodium, ethacrynate, fructose 10% in normal saline solution, fructose 10% in water, furosemide, hydrocortisone sodium succinate, mephentermine, metaraminol bitartrate, methohexital, nitroglycerin, phenobarbital sodium, verapamil.
I.M.
● Switch to oral form as soon as possible.

ACTION
Unknown. A direct-acting peripheral vasodilator that relaxes arteriolar smooth muscle.

Route	Onset	Peak	Duration
P.O.	20–30 min	1–2 hr	2–4 hr
I.V.	5–20 min	10–80 min	2–6 hr
I.M.	10–30 min	1 hr	2–6 hr

Half-life: 3 to 7 hours.

ADVERSE REACTIONS
CNS: *headache,* peripheral neuritis, dizziness.
CV: *angina pectoris, palpitations, tachycardia,* orthostatic hypotension, edema, flushing.
EENT: nasal congestion.
GI: *nausea, vomiting, diarrhea, anorexia,* constipation.
Hematologic: *neutropenia, leukopenia, agranulocytopenia, agranulocytosis, thrombocytopenia with or without purpura.*
Skin: rash.
Other: *lupuslike syndrome.*

INTERACTIONS
Drug-drug. *Diazoxide, MAO inhibitors:* May cause severe hypotension. Use together cautiously.
Diuretics, other hypotensive drugs: May cause excessive hypotension. Dosage adjustment may be needed.
Indomethacin: May decrease effects of hydralazine. Monitor blood pressure.
Metoprolol, propranolol: May increase levels and effects of these beta blockers. Monitor patient closely. May need to adjust dosage of either drug.

EFFECTS ON LAB TEST RESULTS
● May decrease hemoglobin level.
● May decrease neutrophil, WBC, granulocyte, platelet, and RBC counts.
● May cause positive ANA titers.

CONTRAINDICATIONS & CAUTIONS
● Contraindicated in patients hypersensitive to drug.
● Contraindicated in those with coronary artery disease or mitral valvular rheumatic heart disease.
● Use cautiously in patients with suspected cardiac disease, stroke, or severe renal impairment and in those taking other antihypertensives.

NURSING CONSIDERATIONS
● Monitor patient's blood pressure, pulse rate, and body weight frequently. Drug may be given with diuretics and beta blockers to decrease sodium retention and tachycardia and to prevent angina attacks.
● Elderly patients may be more sensitive to drug's hypotensive effects.
● Monitor CBC, lupus erythematosus cell preparation, and antinuclear antibody titer determination before therapy and periodically during long-term therapy.
● *Alert:* Monitor patient closely for signs and symptoms of lupuslike syndrome (sore throat, fever, muscle and joint aches, rash), and notify prescriber immediately if they develop.

• Improve patient compliance by giving drug b.i.d. Check with prescriber.

• *Look alike–sound alike:* Don't confuse hydralazine with hydroxyzine or Apresoline with Apresazide.

• Apresoline may contain tartrazine.

PATIENT TEACHING
• Instruct patient to take oral form with meals to increase absorption.

• Inform patient that low blood pressure and dizziness upon standing can be minimized by rising slowly and avoiding sudden position changes.

• Tell woman of childbearing age to notify prescriber if she suspects pregnancy. Drug will need to be stopped.

• Tell patient to notify prescriber of unexplained prolonged general tiredness or fever, muscle or joint aching, or chest pain.

---

irbesartan
er-bah-SAR-tan

Avapro

Pharmacologic class: angiotensin II receptor antagonist
Pregnancy risk category C; D in 2nd and 3rd trimesters

AVAILABLE FORMS
Tablets: 75 mg, 150 mg, 300 mg

INDICATIONS & DOSAGES
➤ **Hypertension**
Adults and children age 13 and older: Initially, 150 mg P.O. daily, increased to maximum of 300 mg daily, if needed.
Children ages 6 to 12: Initially, 75 mg P.O. once daily, increased to maximum of 150 mg daily, if needed.
Adjust-a-dose: For volume- and sodium-depleted patients, initially, 75 mg P.O. daily.
➤ **Nephropathy in patients with type 2 diabetes**
Adults: Target maintenance dose is 300 mg P.O. once daily.

ADMINISTRATION
P.O.
• Give drug without regard for meals.

ACTION
Produces antihypertensive effect by competitive antagonist activity at the angiotensin II receptor.

Route	Onset	Peak	Duration
P.O.	Unknown	½–2 hr	24 hr

Half-life: 11 to 15 hours.

ADVERSE REACTIONS
CNS: fatigue, anxiety, dizziness, headache.
CV: chest pain, edema, tachycardia.
EENT: pharyngitis, rhinitis, sinus abnormality.
GI: diarrhea, dyspepsia, abdominal pain, nausea, vomiting.
GU: UTI.
Musculoskeletal: musculoskeletal trauma or pain.
Respiratory: upper respiratory tract infection, cough.
Skin: rash.

INTERACTIONS
None reported.

EFFECTS ON LAB TEST RESULTS
None reported.

CONTRAINDICATIONS & CAUTIONS
• Contraindicated in patients hypersensitive to drug or its components.

• Use cautiously in patients with impaired renal function, heart failure, and renal artery stenosis and in breast-feeding women.

■ **Black Box Warning** Use during pregnancy can cause injury and death to the developing fetus. When pregnancy is detected, stop drug as soon as possible. ■

NURSING CONSIDERATIONS
• Drug may be given with a diuretic or other antihypertensive, if needed, for control of hypertension.

• Symptomatic hypotension may occur in volume- or sodium-depleted patients (vigorous diuretic use or dialysis). Correct the cause of volume depletion before administration or before a lower dose is used.

• If hypotension occurs, place patient in a supine position and give an I.V. infusion

---

Reactions may be *common,* uncommon, *life-threatening,* or COMMON AND LIFE-THREATENING.
Interaction may have a *rapid onset* or **delayed onset.**

of normal saline solution, if needed. Once blood pressure has stabilized after a transient hypotensive episode, drug may be continued.
• Dizziness and orthostatic hypotension may occur more frequently in patients with type 2 diabetes and renal disease.

PATIENT TEACHING
• Warn woman of childbearing age of consequences of drug exposure to fetus. Tell her to call prescriber immediately if pregnancy is suspected.
• Tell patient that drug may be taken without regard for food.

SAFETY ALERT!

labetalol hydrochloride
la-BET-ah-loll

Trandate

Pharmacologic class: alpha and beta blocker
Pregnancy risk category C

AVAILABLE FORMS
Injection: 5 mg/ml in 20- and 40-ml multiple-dose vials
Tablets: 100 mg, 200 mg, 300 mg

INDICATIONS & DOSAGES
➤ **Hypertension**
Adults: 100 mg P.O. b.i.d. with or without a diuretic. If needed, dosage is increased to 200 mg b.i.d. after 2 days. Further increases may be made every 2 to 3 days until optimal response is reached. Usual maintenance dosage is 100 to 400 mg b.i.d. Maximum dose is 2.4 g daily in two divided doses given alone or with a diuretic.
➤ **Severe hypertension, hypertensive emergencies**
Adults: 200 mg diluted in 160 ml of D₅W, infused at 2 mg/minute until satisfactory response is obtained; then infusion is stopped. May be repeated every 6 to 12 hours.
   Or, give by repeated I.V. injection; initially, 20 mg I.V. slowly over 2 minutes. Repeat injections of 40 to 80 mg every 10 minutes until maximum dose of 300 mg is reached, as needed.

ADMINISTRATION
P.O.
• When switching from I.V. to P.O. form, begin P.O. regimen at 200 mg after blood pressure begins to rise; repeat dose with 200 to 400 mg in 6 to 12 hours. Adjust dosage according to blood pressure response.
• If dizziness occurs, give dose at bedtime or in smaller doses t.i.d.
I.V.
• Give by slow, direct I.V. injection over 2 minutes at 10-minute intervals.
• For I.V. infusion, prepare by diluting with D₅W or normal saline solutions; for example, 200 mg of drug to 160 ml D₅W to yield 1 mg/ml.
• Give labetalol infusion with an infusion-control device.
• Monitor blood pressure closely every 5 minutes for 30 minutes; then every 30 minutes for 2 hours. Then, monitor hourly for 6 hours.
• Patient should remain supine for 3 hours after infusion. When given I.V. for hypertensive emergencies, drug produces a rapid, predictable fall in blood pressure within 5 to 10 minutes.
• Store at room temperature. Protect from light.
• **Incompatibilities:** Alkali solutions, amphotericin B, cefoperazone, ceftriaxone, furosemide, heparin, nafcillin, sodium bicarbonate, thiopental, warfarin.

ACTION
May be related to reduced peripheral vascular resistance, as a result of alpha and beta blockade.

Route	Onset	Peak	Duration
P.O.	20 min	2–4 hr	8–12 hr
I.V.	2–5 min	5 min	2–4 hr

Half-life: About 5½ hours after I.V. use; 6 to 8 hours after P.O. use.

ADVERSE REACTIONS
CNS: *dizziness,* vivid dreams, fatigue, headache, paresthesia, transient scalp tingling, syncope.
CV: *orthostatic hypotension,* **ventricular arrhythmias.**
EENT: nasal congestion.
GI: nausea, vomiting.

GU: sexual dysfunction, urine retention.
Respiratory: *bronchospasm,* dyspnea.
Skin: rash.

INTERACTIONS
Drug-drug. *Beta agonists:* May blunt bronchodilator effect of these drugs in patients with bronchospasm. May need to increase dosages of these drugs.
Cimetidine: May enhance labetalol's effect. Use together cautiously.
Halothane: May increase hypotensive effect. Monitor blood pressure closely.
Insulin, oral antidiabetics: May alter dosage requirements in previously stabilized diabetic patient. Monitor patient closely.
Nitroglycerin: May blunt reflex tachycardia produced by nitroglycerin but not the hypotension. Monitor BP if used together.
NSAIDs: May decrease antihypertensive effects. Monitor blood pressure.
Tricyclic antidepressants: May increase incidence of tremor. Monitor patient for tremor.
Drug-herb. *Ma huang:* May decrease antihypertensive effects. Discourage use together.

EFFECTS ON LAB TEST RESULTS
● May increase transaminase and urea levels.
● May cause false-positive increase of urine free and total catecholamine levels when measured by a nonspecific trihydroxyindole fluorometric method. May cause false-positive test result for amphetamines when screening urine for drugs.

CONTRAINDICATIONS & CAUTIONS
● Contraindicated in patients hypersensitive to drug and in those with bronchial asthma, overt cardiac failure, greater than first-degree heart block, cardiogenic shock, severe bradycardia, and other conditions that may cause severe and prolonged hypotension.
● Use cautiously in patients with heart failure, hepatic failure, chronic bronchitis, emphysema, peripheral vascular disease, and pheochromocytoma.

NURSING CONSIDERATIONS
● Monitor blood pressure frequently. Drug masks common signs and symptoms of shock.

● In diabetic patients, monitor glucose level closely because beta blockers may mask certain signs and symptoms of hypoglycemia.
● *Look alike–sound alike:* Don't confuse Trandate with Trental or Tridrate.

PATIENT TEACHING
● *Alert:* Tell patient that stopping drug abruptly can worsen chest pain and trigger a heart attack.
● Advise patient that dizziness is the most troublesome adverse reaction and tends to occur in the early stages of treatment, in patients taking diuretics, and with higher dosages. Inform patient that dizziness can be minimized by rising slowly and avoiding sudden position changes.
● Warn patient that occasional, harmless scalp tingling may occur, especially when therapy begins.

lisinopril
lye-SIN-oh-pril

Prinivil◆, Zestril◆

Pharmacologic class: ACE inhibitor
Pregnancy risk category C; D in 2nd and 3rd trimesters

AVAILABLE FORMS
Tablets: 2.5 mg, 5 mg, 10 mg, 20 mg, 30 mg, 40 mg

INDICATIONS & DOSAGES
➤ **Hypertension**
Adults: Initially, 10 mg P.O. daily for patients not taking a diuretic. Most patients are well controlled on 20 to 40 mg daily as a single dose. For patients taking a diuretic, initially, 5 mg P.O. daily.
Children age 6 and older: Initially, 0.07 mg/kg (up to 5 mg) P.O. once daily. Increase dosage based on patient response and tolerance. Maximum dose, 0.61 mg/kg (don't exceed 40 mg). Don't use in children with a creatinine clearance less than 30 ml/minute.
Adjust-a-dose: In adults, if creatinine clearance is 10 to 30 ml/minute, give 5 mg P.O. daily; if clearance is less than 10 ml/minute, give 2.5 mg P.O. daily.

Reactions may be *common,* uncommon, *life-threatening,* or COMMON AND LIFE-THREATENING.
Interaction may have a *rapid onset* or *delayed onset.*

➤ **Adjunct treatment (with diuretics and cardiac glycosides) for heart failure**
Adults: Initially, 5 mg P.O. daily; increased as needed to maximum of 20 mg P.O. daily.
Adjust-a-dose: If sodium level is less than 130 mEq/L or creatinine clearance less than 30 ml/minute, start treatment at 2.5 mg daily.

➤ **Hemodynamically stable patients within 24 hours of acute MI to improve survival**
Adults: Initially, 5 mg P.O.; then 5 mg after 24 hours, 10 mg after 48 hours, followed by 10 mg once daily for 6 weeks.
Adjust-a-dose: For patients with systolic blood pressure 120 mm Hg or less when treatment is started or during first 3 days after an infarct, decrease dosage to 2.5 mg P.O. If systolic blood pressure drops to 100 mm Hg or less, reduce daily maintenance dose of 5 mg to 2.5 mg, if needed. If prolonged systolic blood pressure stays under 90 mm Hg for longer than 1 hour, withdraw drug.

ADMINISTRATION
P.O.
● Give drug without regard for food.
● If made into a suspension by pharmacist, shake before each use.

ACTION
Causes decreased production of angiotensin II and suppression of the renin-angiotensin-aldosterone system.

Route	Onset	Peak	Duration
P.O.	1 hr	7 hr	24 hr

Half-life: 12 hours.

ADVERSE REACTIONS
CNS: *dizziness,* headache, fatigue, paresthesia.
CV: *orthostatic hypotension,* hypotension, chest pain.
EENT: *nasal congestion.*
GI: *diarrhea,* nausea, dyspepsia.
GU: impaired renal function, impotence.
Metabolic: *hyperkalemia.*
Respiratory: dyspnea, dry, persistent, tickling, nonproductive cough.
Skin: rash.
Other: *angioedema.*

INTERACTIONS
Drug-drug. *Allopurinol:* May cause hypersensitivity reaction. Use together cautiously.
Azathioprine: May increase risk of anemia or leukopenia. Monitor hematologic studies if used together.
Diuretics, thiazide diuretics: May cause excessive hypotension with diuretics. Monitor blood pressure closely.
Indomethacin, NSAIDs: May reduce hypotensive effects of drug. Adjust dose as needed.
Insulin, oral antidiabetics: May cause hypoglycemia, especially at start of lisinopril therapy. Monitor glucose level.
Lithium: May cause lithium toxicity. Monitor lithium levels.
Phenothiazines: May increase hypotensive effects. Monitor blood pressure closely.
Potassium-sparing diuretics, potassium supplements: May cause hyperkalemia. Monitor laboratory values.
Tizanidine: May cause severe hypotension. Monitor patient.
Drug-herb. *Capsaicin:* May cause ACE inhibitor-induced cough. Discourage use together.
Ma huang: May decrease antihypertensive effects. Discourage use together.
Drug-food. *Potassium-containing salt substitutes:* May cause hyperkalemia. Monitor laboratory values.

EFFECTS ON LAB TEST RESULTS
● May increase BUN, creatinine, potassium, and bilirubin levels.
● May increase liver function test values.

CONTRAINDICATIONS & CAUTIONS
● Contraindicated in patients hypersensitive to ACE inhibitors and in those with a history of angioedema related to previous treatment with ACE inhibitor.
■ **Black Box Warning** Use during pregnancy can cause injury and death to the developing fetus. When pregnancy is detected, stop drug as soon as possible. ■
● Use cautiously in patients with impaired renal function; adjust dosage.
● Use cautiously in patients at risk for hyperkalemia and in those with aortic stenosis or hypertrophic cardiomyopathy. The safety and efficacy of lisinopril on blood pressure in children younger than

age 6 or in children with GFR less than 30 ml/minute hasn't been established.

NURSING CONSIDERATIONS
- When using drug in acute MI, give patient the appropriate and standard recommended treatment, such as thrombolytics, aspirin, and beta blockers.
- Although ACE inhibitors reduce blood pressure in all races, blood pressure reduction is less in blacks taking the ACE inhibitor alone. Black patients should take drug with a thiazide diuretic for a more favorable response.
- ACE inhibitors appear to increase risk of angioedema in black patients.
- Monitor blood pressure frequently. If drug doesn't adequately control blood pressure, diuretics may be added.
- Monitor WBC with differential counts before therapy, every 2 weeks for first 3 months of therapy, and periodically thereafter.
- *Look alike–sound alike:* Don't confuse lisinopril with fosinopril or Lioresal. Don't confuse Zestril with Zostrix, Zetia, Zebeta, or Zyrtec. Don't confuse Prinivil with Proventil or Prilosec.

PATIENT TEACHING
- *Alert:* Rarely, facial and throat swelling (including swelling of the larynx) may occur, especially after first dose. Advise patient to report signs or symptoms of breathing problems or swelling of face, eyes, lips, or tongue.
- Inform patient that light-headedness can occur, especially during first few days of therapy. Tell him to rise slowly to minimize this effect and to report symptoms to prescriber. If he faints, advise patient to stop taking drug and call prescriber immediately.
- If unpleasant adverse reactions occur, tell patient not to stop drug suddenly but to notify prescriber.
- Advise patient to report signs and symptoms of infection, such as fever and sore throat.
- Tell woman of childbearing age to notify prescriber if pregnancy occurs. Drug will need to be stopped.
- Instruct patient not to use salt substitutes that contain potassium without first consulting prescriber.

losartan potassium
low-SAR-tan

Cozaar◆

Pharmacologic class: angiotensin II receptor antagonist
Pregnancy risk category C; D in 2nd and 3rd trimesters

AVAILABLE FORMS
Tablets: 25 mg, 50 mg, 100 mg

INDICATIONS & DOSAGES
➤ **Hypertension**
Adults: Initially, 25 to 50 mg P.O. daily. Maximum daily dose is 100 mg in one or two divided doses.
Children age 6 and older: 0.7 mg/kg (up to 50 mg) P.O. daily, adjust as needed up to 1.4 mg/kg/day (maximum 100 mg).
Adjust-a-dose: For adults who are hepatically impaired or intravascularly volume depleted (such as those taking diuretics), initially, 25 mg.
➤ **Nephropathy in type 2 diabetic patients**
Adults: 50 mg P.O. once daily. Increase dosage to 100 mg once daily based on blood pressure response.
➤ **To reduce risk of stroke in patients with hypertension and left ventricular hypertrophy**
Adults: Initially, 50 mg P.O. once daily. Adjust dosage based on blood pressure response, adding hydrochlorothiazide 12.5 mg once daily, increasing losartan to 100 mg daily, or both. If further adjustments are required, may increase the daily dosage of hydrochlorothiazide to 25 mg.

ADMINISTRATION
P.O.
- Give drug without regard for meals.
- If made into suspension by pharmacist, store in refrigerator and shake well before each use.

ACTION
Inhibits vasoconstrictive and aldosterone-secreting action of angiotensin II by blocking angiotensin II receptor on the surface of vascular smooth muscle and other tissue cells.

Reactions may be *common*, uncommon, *life-threatening*, or COMMON AND LIFE-THREATENING.
Interaction may have a *rapid onset* or *delayed onset*.

Route	Onset	Peak	Duration
P.O.	Unknown	1 hr	Unknown

Half-life: 2 hours.

ADVERSE REACTIONS

Patients with hypertension or left ventricular hypertrophy

CNS: dizziness, asthenia, fatigue, headache, insomnia.

CV: edema, chest pain.

EENT: nasal congestion, sinusitis, pharyngitis, sinus disorder.

GI: abdominal pain, nausea, diarrhea, dyspepsia.

Musculoskeletal: muscle cramps, myalgia, back or leg pain.

Respiratory: cough, upper respiratory infection.

Other: *angioedema.*

Patients with nephropathy

CNS: *asthenia, fatigue,* fever, hypesthesia.

CV: *chest pain,* hypotension, orthostatic hypotension.

EENT: sinusitis, cataract.

GI: *diarrhea,* dyspepsia, gastritis.

GU: *UTI.*

Hematologic: *anemia.*

Metabolic: *hyperkalemia, hypoglycemia,* weight gain.

Musculoskeletal: *back pain,* leg or knee pain, muscle weakness.

Respiratory: *cough, bronchitis.*

Skin: cellulitis.

Other: *flulike syndrome, diabetic vascular disease, angioedema,* infection, trauma, diabetic neuropathy.

INTERACTIONS

Drug-drug. *Lithium:* May increase lithium level. Monitor lithium level and patient for toxicity.

NSAIDs: May decrease antihypertensive effects. Monitor blood pressure.

Potassium-sparing diuretics, potassium supplements: May cause hyperkalemia. Monitor patient closely.

Drug-herb. *Ma huang:* May decrease antihypertensive effects. Discourage use together.

Drug-food. *Salt substitutes containing potassium:* May cause hyperkalemia. Monitor patient closely.

EFFECTS ON LAB TEST RESULTS

None reported.

CONTRAINDICATIONS & CAUTIONS

● Contraindicated in patients hypersensitive to drug. Breast-feeding isn't recommended during losartan therapy.

● Use cautiously in patients with impaired renal or hepatic function.

■ **Black Box Warning** Drugs that act directly on the renin-angiotensin system (such as losartan) can cause fetal and neonatal morbidity and death when given to women in the second or third trimester of pregnancy. These problems haven't been detected when exposure was limited to the first trimester. If pregnancy is suspected, notify prescriber because drug should be stopped. ■

NURSING CONSIDERATIONS

● Drug can be used alone or with other antihypertensives.

● If antihypertensive effect is inadequate using once-daily doses, a twice-daily regimen using the same or increased total daily dose may give a more satisfactory response.

● Monitor patient's blood pressure closely to evaluate effectiveness of therapy. When used alone, drug has less of an effect on blood pressure in black patients than in patients of other races.

● Monitor patients who are also taking diuretics for symptomatic hypotension.

● Regularly assess the patient's renal function (via creatinine and BUN levels).

● Patients with severe heart failure whose renal function depends on the angiotensin-aldosterone system may develop acute renal failure during therapy. Closely monitor patient, especially during first few weeks of therapy.

● *Look alike–sound alike:* Don't confuse Cozaar with Zocor.

PATIENT TEACHING

● Tell patient to avoid salt substitutes; these products may contain potassium, which can cause high potassium level in patients taking losartan.

● Inform woman of childbearing age about consequences of second and third trimester exposure to drug. Prescriber

should be notified immediately if pregnancy is suspected.
• Advise patient to immediately report swelling of face, eyes, lips, or tongue or any breathing difficulty.

SAFETY ALERT!

methyldopa
meth-ill-DOE-pa

Novo-Medopa†, Nu-Medopa†

methyldopate hydrochloride

Pharmacologic class: centrally acting antiadrenergic
Pregnancy risk category B for P.O.; C for I.V.

AVAILABLE FORMS
methyldopa
Tablets: 250 mg, 500 mg
methyldopate hydrochloride
Injection: 50 mg/ml

INDICATIONS & DOSAGES
➤ **Hypertension, hypertensive crisis**
Adults: Initially, 250 mg P.O. b.i.d. to t.i.d. in first 48 hours. Increase if needed every 2 days. May give entire daily dose in evening or at bedtime. Adjust dosages if other antihypertensives are added to or deleted from therapy. Maintenance dosage is 500 mg to 2 g daily in two to four divided doses. Maximum recommended daily dose is 3 g. Or, 250 to 500 mg I.V. every 6 hours. Maximum dosage is 1 g every 6 hours. Switch to oral antihypertensives as soon as possible.
Children: Initially, 10 mg/kg P.O. daily in two to four divided doses; or, 20 to 40 mg/kg I.V. daily in four divided doses. Increase dose daily until desired response occurs. Maximum daily dose is 65 mg/kg or 3 g, whichever is less.

ADMINISTRATION
P.O.
• If unpleasant adverse reactions occur, patient shouldn't suddenly stop taking drug but should notify his prescriber.
I.V.
• Dilute appropriate dose in 100 ml D_5W. Infuse slowly over 30 to 60 minutes.

• **Incompatibilities:** Amphotericin B; drugs with poor solubility in acidic media, such as barbiturates and sulfonamides; methohexital; some total parenteral nutrition solutions.

ACTION
May inhibit the central vasomotor centers, decreasing sympathetic outflow to the heart, kidneys, and peripheral vasculature.

Route	Onset	Peak	Duration
P.O.	4–6 hr	Unknown	12–48 hr
I.V.	4–6 hr	Unknown	10–16 hr

Half-life: About 2 hours.

ADVERSE REACTIONS
CNS: *decreased mental acuity, sedation, headache,* weakness, dizziness, paresthesia, parkinsonism, involuntary choreoathetoid movements, psychic disturbances, depression, nightmares.
CV: *orthostatic hypotension, edema,* **bradycardia, myocarditis,** aggravated angina.
EENT: *nasal congestion.*
GI: *dry mouth, pancreatitis,* nausea, vomiting, diarrhea, constipation.
GU: galactorrhea.
Hematologic: **thrombocytopenia, leukopenia, bone marrow depression,** hemolytic anemia.
Hepatic: **hepatic necrosis, hepatitis.**
Musculoskeletal: arthralgia.
Skin: rash.
Other: drug-induced fever, gynecomastia.

INTERACTIONS
Drug-drug. *Amphetamines, nonselective beta blockers, norepinephrine, phenothiazines, tricyclic antidepressants:* May cause hypertensive effects. Monitor patient closely.
Anesthetics: May need lower doses of anesthetics. Use together cautiously.
Barbiturates: May decrease actions of methyldopa. Monitor patient closely.
Ferrous sulfate: May decrease bioavailability of methyldopa. Separate doses.
Haloperidol: May increase antipsychotic effects of haloperidol or cause psychosis. Use together cautiously.

Reactions may be *common,* uncommon, *life-threatening,* or COMMON AND LIFE-THREATENING.
Interaction may have a *rapid onset* or **delayed onset.**

Levodopa: May increase hypotensive effects, which may increase adverse CNS reactions. Monitor patient closely.

Lithium: May increase lithium level. Watch for increased lithium level and signs and symptoms of toxicity.

MAO inhibitors: May cause excessive sympathetic stimulation. Avoid using together.

Tolbutamide: May impair metabolism of tolbutamide. Monitor patient for hypoglycemic effect.

Drug-herb. *Capsicum:* May reduce antihypertensive effect. Discourage use together.

EFFECTS ON LAB TEST RESULTS

- May increase creatinine level. May decrease hemoglobin level and hematocrit.
- May increase liver function test values. May decrease platelet and WBC counts.
- May interfere with results of urinary uric acid testing, serum creatinine test, and AST test. May cause positive Coombs' test result. May falsely increase urine catecholamine level, interfering with the diagnosis of pheochromocytoma.

CONTRAINDICATIONS & CAUTIONS

- Contraindicated in patients hypersensitive to drug and in those with active hepatic disease (such as acute hepatitis) or active cirrhosis.
- Contraindicated in those whose previous methyldopa therapy caused liver problems and in those taking MAO inhibitors.
- Use cautiously in patients with history of impaired hepatic function or sulfite sensitivity and in breast-feeding women.

NURSING CONSIDERATIONS

- Monitor patient's blood pressure regularly. Elderly patients are more likely to experience hypotension and sedation.
- Occasionally, tolerance may occur, usually between the second and third months of therapy. Adding a diuretic or adjusting dosage may be needed. If patient's response changes significantly, notify prescriber.
- After dialysis, monitor patient for hypertension and notify prescriber, if needed. Patient may need an extra dose of drug.
- Monitor CBC with differential counts before therapy and periodically thereafter.

- Patients who need blood transfusions should have direct and indirect Coombs' tests to prevent crossmatching problems.
- Monitor patient's Coombs' test results. In patients who have received drug for several months, positive reaction to direct Coombs' test indicates hemolytic anemia.
- Report involuntary choreoathetoid movements. Drug may be stopped.

PATIENT TEACHING

- If unpleasant adverse reactions occur, advise patient not to suddenly stop taking drug but to notify prescriber.
- Instruct patient to report signs and symptoms of infection.
- Tell patient to check his weight daily and to notify prescriber if he gains 2 or more pounds in 1 day or 5 pounds in 1 week. Sodium and water retention may occur but can be relieved with diuretics.
- Warn patient that, particularly at the start of therapy, drug may impair ability to perform tasks that require mental alertness. A once-daily dose at bedtime minimizes daytime drowsiness.
- Inform patient that low blood pressure and dizziness upon rising can be minimized by rising slowly and avoiding sudden position changes and that dry mouth can be relieved by chewing gum or sucking on hard candy or ice chips.
- Tell patient that urine may turn dark if left sitting in toilet bowl or if toilet bowl has been treated with bleach.

---

metoprolol succinate
meh-TOH-pruh-lol

Toprol-XL⬦

metoprolol tartrate
Betaloc Durules†, Lopresor†, Lopresor SR†, Lopressor, Novo-Metoprol†, Nu-Metop†

Pharmacologic class: beta blocker
Pregnancy risk category C

AVAILABLE FORMS
metoprolol succinate
Tablets (extended-release): 25 mg, 50 mg, 100 mg, 200 mg

metoprolol tartrate
Injection: 1 mg/ml in 5-ml ampules
Tablets: 25 mg, 50 mg, 100 mg
Tablets (extended-release): 100 mg†,
200 mg†

INDICATIONS & DOSAGES
➤ **Hypertension**
Adults: Initially, 50 mg P.O. b.i.d. or
100 mg P.O. once daily; then up to 100 to
400 mg daily in two or three divided doses.
Or, 50 to 100 mg of extended-release
tablets (tartrate equivalent) once daily.
Adjust dosage as needed and tolerated
at intervals of not less than 1 week to
maximum of 400 mg daily.
➤ **Early intervention in acute MI**
Adults: 5 mg metoprolol tartrate I.V. bolus
every 2 minutes for three doses. Then,
15 minutes after the last I.V. dose, give
25 to 50 mg P.O. every 6 hours for
48 hours. Maintenance dosage is 100 mg
P.O. b.i.d.
➤ **Angina pectoris**
Adults: Initially, 100 mg P.O. daily as a
single dose or in two equally divided
doses; increased at weekly intervals
until an adequate response or a pronounced decrease in heart rate is seen.
Effects of daily dose beyond 400 mg
aren't known. Or, give 100 mg of
extended-release tablets (tartrate equivalent) once daily. Adjust dosage as needed
and tolerated at intervals of not less than
1 week to maximum of 400 mg daily.
➤ **Stable symptomatic heart failure
(New York Heart Association class
II) resulting from ischemia, hypertension, or cardiomyopathy**
Adults: 25 mg Toprol-XL P.O. once daily
for 2 weeks. Double the dose every
2 weeks, as tolerated, to a maximum of
200 mg daily.
Adjust-a-dose: In patients with more
severe heart failure, start with 12.5 mg
Toprol-XL P.O. once daily for 2 weeks.

ADMINISTRATION
P.O.
● Give drug with or immediately after
meal.
I.V.
● Give drug undiluted by direct injection.
● Although best avoided, drug can be
mixed with meperidine hydrochloride or

morphine sulfate or given with an
alteplase infusion at a Y-site connection.
● Store drug at room temperature and
protect from light. Discard solution if it's
discolored or contains particles.
● **Incompatibilities:** Amphotericin B.

ACTION
Unknown. A selective beta blocker
that selectively blocks beta$_1$ receptors;
decreases cardiac output, peripheral
resistance, and cardiac oxygen
consumption; and depresses renin
secretion.

Route	Onset	Peak	Duration
P.O.	15 min	1 hr	6–12 hr
P.O. (extended-release)	15 min	6–12 hr	24 hr
I.V.	5 min	20 min	5–8 hr

Half-life: 3 to 7 hours.

ADVERSE REACTIONS
CNS: *fatigue, dizziness,* depression.
CV: *hypotension,* **bradycardia, heart
failure, AV block,** edema.
GI: nausea, diarrhea.
Respiratory: dyspnea.
Skin: rash.

INTERACTIONS
Drug-drug. *Amobarbital, butabarbital,
butalbital, pentobarbital, phenobarbital,
primidone, secobarbital:* May reduce
metoprolol effect. May need to increase
metoprolol dose.
Cardiac glycosides, diltiazem: May cause
excessive bradycardia and increased
depressant effect on myocardium. Use
together cautiously.
*Catecholamine-depleting drugs such as
MAO inhibitors, reserpine:* May have
additive effect. Monitor patient for
hypotension and bradycardia.
Chlorpromazine: May decrease hepatic
clearance. Watch for greater beta-blocking
effect.
Cimetidine: May increase metoprolol
effects. Give another H$_2$ agonist or
decrease dose of metoprolol.
*Fluoxetine, paroxetine, propafenone,
quinidine:* May increase metoprolol level.
Monitor vital signs.

Reactions may be *common,* uncommon, *life-threatening,* or COMMON AND LIFE-THREATENING.
Interaction may have a *rapid onset* or **delayed onset.**

Hydralazine: May increase levels and effects of both drugs. Monitor patient closely. May need to adjust dosage.

Indomethacin, NSAIDs: May decrease antihypertensive effect. Monitor blood pressure and adjust dosage.

Insulin, oral antidiabetics: May alter dosage requirements in previously stabilized diabetic patients. Monitor patient closely.

I.V. lidocaine: May reduce hepatic metabolism of lidocaine, increasing risk of toxicity. Give bolus doses of lidocaine at a slower rate, and monitor lidocaine level closely.

Prazosin: May increase risk of orthostatic hypotension in the early phases of use together. Assist patient to stand slowly until effects are known.

Rifampin: May increase metoprolol metabolism. Watch for decreased effect.

Terbutaline: May antagonize bronchodilatory effects of terbutaline. Monitor patient.

Verapamil: May increase effects of both drugs. Monitor cardiac function closely, and decrease dosages as needed.

Drug-herb. *Ma huang:* May decrease antihypertensive effects. Discourage use together.

Drug-food. *Food:* May increase absorption. Encourage patient to take drug with food.

EFFECTS ON LAB TEST RESULTS

● May increase transaminase, alkaline phosphatase, LDH, and uric acid levels.

CONTRAINDICATIONS & CAUTIONS

● Contraindicated in patients hypersensitive to drug or other beta blockers.

● Contraindicated in patients with sinus bradycardia, greater than first-degree heart block, cardiogenic shock, or overt cardiac failure when used to treat hypertension or angina. When used to treat MI, drug is contraindicated in patients with heart rate less than 45 beats/minute, greater than first-degree heart block, PR interval of 0.24 second or longer with first-degree heart block, systolic blood pressure less than 100 mm Hg, or moderate to severe cardiac failure.

● Use cautiously in patients with heart failure, diabetes, or respiratory or hepatic disease.

NURSING CONSIDERATIONS

● Always check patient's apical pulse rate before giving drug. If it's slower than 60 beats/minute, withhold drug and call prescriber immediately.

● In diabetic patients, monitor glucose level closely because drug masks common signs and symptoms of hypoglycemia.

● Monitor blood pressure frequently; drug masks common signs and symptoms of shock.

● Beta blockers may mask tachycardia caused by hyperthyroidism. In patients with suspected thyrotoxicosis, taper off beta blocker to avoid thyroid storm.

■ **Black Box Warning** When stopping therapy, taper dosage over 1 to 2 weeks. Abrupt discontinuation may cause exacerbations of angina or myocardial infarction. Don't discontinue therapy abruptly even in patients treated only for hypertension. ■

● Beta selectivity is lost at higher doses. Watch for peripheral side effects.

● *Look alike–sound alike:* Don't confuse metoprolol with metaproterenol misoprostol, or metolazone. Don't confuse Toprol-XL with Topamax, Tegretol, or Tegretol-XR.

PATIENT TEACHING

● Instruct patient to take drug exactly as prescribed and with meals.

● Caution patient to avoid driving and other tasks requiring mental alertness until response to therapy has been established.

● Advise patient to inform dentist or prescriber about use of this drug before procedures or surgery.

● Tell patient to alert prescriber if shortness of breath occurs.

● Instruct patient not to stop drug suddenly but to notify prescriber about unpleasant adverse reactions. Inform him that drug must be withdrawn gradually over 1 or 2 weeks.

● Inform patient that use isn't advisable in breast-feeding women.

* NEW DRUG

nebivolol
neh-BIH-voh-lawl

Bystolic

Pharmacologic class: beta blocker
Pregnancy risk category C

AVAILABLE FORMS
Tablets: 2.5 mg, 5 mg, 10 mg

INDICATIONS & DOSAGES
➤ **Hypertension**
Adults: Initially, 5 mg P.O. once daily.
Increase at 2-week intervals to a maximum
dose of 40 mg, if needed.
Adjust-a-dose: For patients with severe
renal impairment or moderate hepatic
impairment, start with 2.5 mg P.O. once
daily. Increase dose cautiously, if
needed.

ACTION
Selectively blocks beta$_1$-adrenergic receptors, reducing heart rate, myocardial contractility, and sympathetic tone. Nebivolol
also reduces blood pressure by suppressing
renin activity and decreasing peripheral
vascular resistance.

Route	Onset	Peak	Duration
P.O.	Unknown	1½–4 hr	Unknown

Half-life: 12 to 19 hours.

ADVERSE REACTIONS
CNS: asthenia, dizziness, fatigue, head-
ache, insomnia, paresthesia.
CV: *bradycardia,* chest pain, peripheral
edema.
GI: abdominal pain, diarrhea, nausea.
Metabolic: hypercholesterolemia, hyper-
uricemia.
Respiratory: dyspnea.
Skin: rash.

INTERACTIONS
Drug-drug. *CYP2D6 inhibitors, such
as fluoxetine, paroxetine, propafenone,
quinidine:* May increase nebivolol level.
Monitor blood pressure closely, and adjust
nebivolol dose as needed.
*Digoxin, diltiazem, disopyramide, vera-
pamil:* May increase the risk of brady-

cardia. Monitor patient's ECG and vital
signs.
*Catecholamine-depleting drugs, such as,
guanethidine, reserpine:* May cause
bradycardia or severe hypotension. Monitor patient closely.

EFFECTS ON LAB TEST RESULTS
● May increase BUN, uric acid, and
triglyceride levels. May decrease HDL
and cholesterol levels.
● May decrease platelet count.

CONTRAINDICATIONS & CAUTIONS
● Contraindicated in patients hypersensitive to drug and those with decompensated cardiac failure, severe bradycardia,
second- or third-degree AV block, sick
sinus syndrome (unless a permanent
pacemaker is in place), cardiogenic
shock, bronchial asthma or related bronchospastic conditions, severe renal
impairment, or severe hepatic impairment
(greater than Child-Pugh B).
    Use cautiously in patients with com-
pensated heart failure, in perioperative
patients receiving anesthetics that
depress myocardial function (such as
cyclopropane and trichloroethylene), in
diabetic patients receiving insulin or oral
antidiabetics or subject to spontaneous
hypoglycemia, and in patients with thyroid disease (use may mask hyperthyroidism and withdrawal may worsen it), pheochromocytoma, or peripheral vascular
disease (may cause or worsen symptoms
of arterial insufficiency).

NURSING CONSIDERATIONS
● *Alert:* Patients with a history of severe
anaphylactic reaction to several allergens
may be more reactive to repeated exposure
to nebivolol (accidental, diagnostic, or
therapeutic), and they may not respond to
amounts of epinephrine typically used to
treat allergic reactions.
● Check patient's blood pressure and heart
rate often.
● Monitor hepatic and renal function test
results.
● If nebivolol must be stopped, do so gradually over 1 to 2 weeks.
● Because beta blockers may mask tachycardia caused by hyperthyroidism, be sure
to withdraw nebivolol gradually in patients

Reactions may be *common,* uncommon, *life-threatening,* or **COMMON AND LIFE-THREATENING.**
Interaction may have a *rapid onset* or **delayed onset.**

with suspected thyrotoxicosis to avoid thyroid storm.
• Observe a diabetic patient closely because drug may mask evidence of hypoglycemia.
• If patient has heart failure, watch for worsening symptoms, renal dysfunction, or fluid retention. His diuretic dosage may need to be increased.
• Store drug at room temperature in a light-resistant container.

PATIENT TEACHING
• Instruct patient not to stop drug suddenly but to notify prescriber about unpleasant adverse reactions. Explain that drug must be withdrawn gradually over 1 or 2 weeks.
• Caution patient to avoid driving and other tasks requiring alertness until his response to therapy is known.
• Tell patient to alert prescriber if he develops shortness of breath.
• Urge women not to breast-feed during therapy.

nisoldipine
nye-SOHL-di-peen

Sular

Pharmacologic class: calcium channel blocker
Pregnancy risk category C

AVAILABLE FORMS
Tablets (extended-release): 8.5 mg, 17 mg, 25.5 mg, 34 mg

INDICATIONS & DOSAGES
➤ **Hypertension**
Adults: Initially, 17 mg P.O. once daily, increased by 8.5 mg/week or at longer intervals, as needed. Usual maintenance dose is 17 to 34 mg daily. Doses of more than 34 mg daily aren't recommended.
Patients older than age 65: Initially, 8.5 mg P.O. once daily; adjust dosage as for other adults.
Adjust-a-dose: For patients with impaired liver function, initially, 8.5 mg P.O. once daily; dosage is adjusted as for adults.

ADMINISTRATION
P.O.
• Give drug whole; don't crush or split tablet.
• Don't give with high-fat meal or grapefruit products.

ACTION
Prevents calcium ions from entering vascular smooth muscle cells, causing dilation of arterioles, which decreases peripheral vascular resistance.

Route	Onset	Peak	Duration
P.O.	Unknown	6–12 hr	24 hr

Half-life: 7 to 12 hours.

ADVERSE REACTIONS
CNS: *headache,* dizziness.
CV: *peripheral edema,* vasodilation, palpitations, chest pain.
EENT: sinusitis, pharyngitis.
GI: nausea.
Skin: rash.

INTERACTIONS
Drug-drug. *Cimetidine:* May increase bioavailability and peak nisoldipine level. Monitor blood pressure closely.
CYP3A4 inducers such as phenytoin: May decrease nisoldipine level. Avoid using together; consider alternative antihypertensive therapy.
Quinidine: May decrease bioavailability of nisoldipine. Adjust dosage accordingly.
Drug-herb. *Ma huang:* May decrease antihypertensive effects. Discourage use together.
Peppermint oil: May decrease drug effect. Discourage use together.
Drug-food. *Grapefruit products:* May increase drug level, increasing adverse reactions. Discourage use together.
High-fat foods: May increase peak drug level. Discourage use together.

EFFECTS ON LAB TEST RESULTS
None reported.

CONTRAINDICATIONS & CAUTIONS
• Contraindicated in patients hypersensitive to dihydropyridine calcium channel blockers.

• Contraindicated in breast-feeding women.
• Use cautiously in patients with heart failure or compromised ventricular function, particularly those receiving beta blockers and those with severe hepatic dysfunction.

NURSING CONSIDERATIONS
• Monitor frequency, duration, or severity of angina after starting calcium channel blocker therapy or at time of dosage increase. Report worsening of symptoms to prescriber immediately.
• Monitor blood pressure regularly, especially when starting therapy and during dosage adjustment.

PATIENT TEACHING
• Tell patient to take drug as prescribed, even if he feels better.
• Advise patient to swallow tablet whole and not to chew, divide, or crush it.
• Remind patient not to take drug with a high-fat meal or with grapefruit products. Both may increase drug level in the body beyond intended amount.

SAFETY ALERT!

nitroprusside sodium
nye-troe-PRUSS-ide

Nipride†, Nitropress

Pharmacologic class: vasodilator
Pregnancy risk category C

AVAILABLE FORMS
Injection: 50 mg/vial in 2-ml and 5-ml vials

INDICATIONS & DOSAGES
➤ **To lower blood pressure quickly in hypertensive emergencies, to produce controlled hypotension during anesthesia, to reduce preload and afterload in cardiac pump failure or cardiogenic shock (may be used with or without dopamine)**
Adults and children: Begin infusion at 0.3 mcg/kg/minute I.V. and gradually titrate every few minutes to a maximum infusion rate of 10 mcg/kg/minute.
Adjust-a-dose: Patients also taking other antihypertensives are extremely sen-

sitive to nitroprusside. Titrate dosage accordingly. Use with caution in patients with severe renal impairment or hepatic insufficiency; use minimum effective dose.

ADMINISTRATION
I.V.
• Prepare solution by dissolving 50 mg in 2 to 3 ml of D₅W injection or according to manufacturer's instructions.
■ **Black Box Warning** Further dilute concentration in 250, 500, or 1,000 ml of D₅W to provide solutions with 200, 100, or 50 mcg/ml, respectively. ■
• Reconstitute ADD-Vantage vials labeled as containing 50 mg of drug according to manufacturer's directions.
• Because drug is sensitive to light, wrap solution in foil or other opaque material; it's not necessary to wrap the tubing. Fresh solution has a faint brownish tint. Discard if highly discolored after 24 hours.
• Use an infusion pump. Drug is best given via piggyback through a peripheral line with no other drug. Don't titrate rate of main I.V. line while drug is being infused. Even a small bolus can cause severe hypotension.
• Check blood pressure every 5 minutes during titration at start of infusion and every 15 minutes thereafter.
• If severe hypotension occurs, stop infusion; effects of drug quickly reverse. Notify prescriber.
• If possible, start an arterial pressure line. Regulate drug flow to desired blood pressure response.
• **Incompatibilities:** Amiodarone, atracurium besylate, bacteriostatic water for injection, levofloxacin. Don't mix with other I.V. drugs or preservatives.

ACTION
Relaxes arteriolar and venous smooth muscle.

Route	Onset	Peak	Duration
I.V.	Immediate	1–2 min	10 min

Half-life: 2 minutes.

ADVERSE REACTIONS
CNS: *headache, dizziness, increased intracranial pressure,* loss of consciousness, apprehension, restlessness.

Reactions may be *common,* uncommon, *life-threatening,* or COMMON AND LIFE-THREATENING.
Interaction may have a *rapid onset* or *delayed onset.*

CV: *bradycardia,* hypotension, tachycardia, palpitations, ECG changes, flushing.
GI: *nausea, abdominal pain,* ileus.
Hematologic: *methemoglobinemia.*
Metabolic: acidosis, hypothyroidism.
Musculoskeletal: *muscle twitching.*
Skin: *diaphoresis,* pink color, rash.
Other: *thiocyanate toxicity, cyanide toxicity,* venous streaking, irritation at infusion site.

INTERACTIONS
Drug-drug. *Antihypertensives:* May cause sensitivity to nitroprusside. Adjust dosage. *Ganglionic-blocking drugs, general anesthetics, negative inotropic drugs, other antihypertensives:* May cause additive effects. Monitor blood pressure closely. *Sildenafil, vardenafil:* May increase hypotensive effects. Avoid use together.

EFFECTS ON LAB TEST RESULTS
● May increase creatinine level.
● May decrease RBC and WBC counts.

CONTRAINDICATIONS & CAUTIONS
● Contraindicated in patients hypersensitive to drug.
● Contraindicated in those with compensatory hypertension (such as in arteriovenous shunt or coarctation of the aorta), inadequate cerebral circulation, acute heart failure with reduced peripheral vascular resistance, congenital optic atrophy, or tobacco-induced amblyopia.
● Use with extreme caution in patients with increased intracranial pressure.
● Use cautiously in patients with hypothyroidism, hepatic or renal disease, hyponatremia, or low vitamin B level.

NURSING CONSIDERATIONS
■ **Black Box Warning** Use drug only when available equipment and personnel allow blood pressure to be continuously monitored. ■
● Obtain baseline vital signs before giving drug; find out parameters prescriber wants to achieve.
● Keep patient in supine position when starting therapy or titrating drug.
■ **Black Box Warning** Giving excessive doses of 500 mcg/kg delivered faster than 2 mcg/kg/minute or using maximum infusion rate of 10 mcg/kg/minute for more than 10 minutes can cause cyanide toxicity. ■
● *Alert:* If patient is at risk, check thiocyanate level every 72 hours. Level higher than 100 mcg/ml may be toxic. If profound hypotension, metabolic acidosis, dyspnea, headache, loss of consciousness, ataxia, or vomiting occurs, stop drug immediately and notify prescriber.
● *Look alike–sound alike:* Don't confuse nitroprusside with nitroglycerin.

PATIENT TEACHING
● Instruct patient to report adverse reactions promptly.
● Tell patient to alert nurse if discomfort occurs at I.V. insertion site.

---

olmesartan medoxomil
ol-ma-SAR-tan

Benicar✐

Pharmacologic class: angiotensin II receptor antagonist
Pregnancy risk category C; D in 2nd and 3rd trimesters

AVAILABLE FORMS
Tablets: 5 mg, 20 mg, 40 mg

INDICATIONS & DOSAGES
➤ **Hypertension**
Adults: 20 mg P.O. once daily if patient has no volume depletion. May increase dosage to 40 mg P.O. once daily if blood pressure isn't reduced after 2 weeks of therapy.
Adjust-a-dose: In patients with possible depletion of intravascular volume (those with impaired renal function who are taking diuretics), consider using lower starting dose.

ADMINISTRATION
P.O.
● Give drug without regard for food.

ACTION
Blocks vasoconstrictor and aldosterone-secreting effects of angiotensin II by selectively blocking the binding of angiotensin II to the angiotensin I, or AT_1, receptor in the vascular smooth muscle.

Route	Onset	Peak	Duration
P.O.	Rapid	1–2 hr	24 hr

Half-life: 13 hours.

ADVERSE REACTIONS
CNS: headache.
EENT: pharyngitis, rhinitis, sinusitis.
GI: diarrhea.
GU: hematuria.
Metabolic: hyperglycemia, hypertriglyceridemia.
Musculoskeletal: back pain.
Respiratory: bronchitis, upper respiratory tract infection.
Other: flulike symptoms, accidental injury.

INTERACTIONS
Drug-herb. *Ma huang:* May decrease antihypertensive effects. Discourage use together.

EFFECTS ON LAB TEST RESULTS
• May increase glucose, triglyceride, uric acid, liver enzyme, bilirubin, and CK levels. May decrease hemoglobin level and hematocrit.

CONTRAINDICATIONS & CAUTIONS
• Contraindicated in patients hypersensitive to the drug or any of its components and in patients who are pregnant.
■ **Black Box Warning** Drug may cause fetal and neonatal complications and death when given to pregnant women after the first trimester. If patient taking drug becomes pregnant, stop drug immediately. ■
• Use cautiously in patients who are volume- or sodium-depleted, those whose renal function depends on the renin-angiotensin-aldosterone system (such as patients with severe heart failure), and those with unilateral and bilateral renal artery stenosis.
• It's unknown if drug appears in breast milk. Patient should stop either breast-feeding or using drug.
• Safety and efficacy in children haven't been established.

NURSING CONSIDERATIONS
• Symptomatic hypotension may occur in patients who are volume- or sodium-depleted, especially those being treated with high doses of a diuretic. If hypotension occurs, place patient supine and treat supportively. Treatment may continue once blood pressure is stabilized.
• If blood pressure isn't adequately controlled, a diuretic or other antihypertensive drugs also may be prescribed.
• Overdose may cause hypotension and tachycardia, along with bradycardia from parasympathetic (vagal) stimulation. Treatment should be supportive.
• Closely monitor patients with heart failure for oliguria, azotemia, and acute renal failure.
• Monitor BUN and creatinine level in patients with unilateral or bilateral renal artery stenosis.

PATIENT TEACHING
• Tell patient to take drug exactly as prescribed and not to stop taking it, even if he feels better.
• Tell patient to take drug without regard to meals.
• Tell patient to report to health care provider any adverse reactions promptly, especially light-headedness and fainting.
• Advise woman of childbearing age to immediately report pregnancy to health care provider.
• Inform diabetic patients that glucose readings may rise and that the dosage of their diabetes drugs may need adjustment.
• Warn patients that inadequate fluid intake, excessive perspiration, diarrhea, or vomiting may lead to an excessive drop in blood pressure, light-headedness, and possibly fainting.
• Instruct patients that other antihypertensives can have additive effects. Patient should inform his prescriber of all medications he's taking, including OTC drugs.

perindopril erbumine
pur-IN-doh-pril

Aceon, Coversyl†

Pharmacologic class: ACE inhibitor
Pregnancy risk category C; D in 2nd and 3rd trimesters

AVAILABLE FORMS
Tablets: 2 mg, 4 mg, 8 mg

INDICATIONS & DOSAGES
➤ **To reduce the risk of CV death or nonfatal MI in patients with stable coronary artery disease**
Adults age 70 or younger: 4 mg P.O. once daily for 2 weeks; then, increase as tolerated to 8 mg once daily.
Elderly adults older than age 70: Initially, 2 mg P.O. once daily for the first week; then, 4 mg once daily for the second week and 8 mg once daily after that, if tolerated.
➤ **Essential hypertension**
Adults: Initially, 4 mg P.O. once daily. Increase dosage until blood pressure is controlled or to maximum of 16 mg/day; usual maintenance dosage is 4 to 8 mg once daily; may be given in two divided doses.
Patients older than age 65: Initially, 4 mg P.O. daily as one dose or in two divided doses. Dosage may be increased by more than 8 mg/day only under close medical supervision.
Adjust-a-dose: For renally insufficient patients with creatinine clearance 30 ml/minute or greater, initially 2 mg P.O. daily. Maximum daily maintenance dose is 8 mg. In patients taking diuretics, initially 2 to 4 mg P.O. daily as single dose or in two divided doses, with close medical supervision for several hours and until blood pressure has stabilized. Adjust dosage based on patient's blood pressure response.

ADMINISTRATION
P.O.
● Give drug without regard for food.

ACTION
Prevents conversion of angiotensin I to angiotensin II, a potent vasoconstrictor. Less angiotensin II decreases peripheral arterial resistance, decreasing aldosterone secretion, which reduces sodium and water retention and lowers blood pressure.

Route	Onset	Peak	Duration
P.O.	Unknown	1 hr	Unknown

Half-life: About 1 hour for perindopril; mean half-life, 3 to 10 hours, and terminal elimination half-life, 30 to 120 hours for perindoprilat.

ADVERSE REACTIONS
CNS: *headache,* dizziness, asthenia, sleep disorder, paresthesia, depression, somnolence, nervousness, fever.
CV: palpitations, edema, chest pain, hypotension, abnormal ECG.
EENT: rhinitis, sinusitis, ear infection, pharyngitis, tinnitus.
GI: dyspepsia, diarrhea, abdominal pain, nausea, vomiting, flatulence.
GU: proteinuria, UTI, male sexual dysfunction, menstrual disorder.
Metabolic: *hyperkalemia.*
Musculoskeletal: back pain, hypertonia, neck pain, joint pain, myalgia, arthritis, arm or leg pain.
Respiratory: *cough,* upper respiratory tract infection.
Skin: rash.
Other: viral infection, injury, seasonal allergy.

INTERACTIONS
Drug-drug. *Diuretics:* May increase hypotensive effect. Monitor patient closely.
Lithium: May increase lithium level and risk of lithium toxicity. Use together cautiously; monitor lithium level.
NSAIDs: May decrease antihypertensive effects. Monitor blood pressure.
Potassium-sparing diuretics (amiloride, spironolactone, triamterene), potassium supplements, other drugs capable of increasing potassium level (cyclosporine, heparin, indomethacin): May increase hyperkalemic effect. Use together cautiously; monitor potassium level.
Drug-herb. *Capsaicin:* May cause cough. Discourage use together.
Drug-food. *Salt substitutes containing potassium:* May cause hyperkalemia. Discourage use together.

EFFECTS ON LAB TEST RESULTS
● May increase ALT, alkaline phosphatase, uric acid, cholesterol, and creatinine levels. May increase potassium level.

CONTRAINDICATIONS & CAUTIONS
● Contraindicated in patients hypersensitive to drug or other ACE inhibitors and in those with a history of angioedema caused by ACE inhibitor use.
■ **Black Box Warning** Use during pregnancy can cause injury and death to the developing fetus. When pregnancy is detected, stop drug as soon as possible. ■

• Use cautiously in patients with a history of angioedema unrelated to ACE inhibitor use.

• Use cautiously in patients with renal impairment, heart failure, ischemic heart disease, cerebrovascular disease, or renal artery stenosis and in those with collagen vascular disease, such as systemic lupus erythematosus or scleroderma.

NURSING CONSIDERATIONS

• When used alone in black patients, drug affects blood pressure less than in other patients. Monitor blood pressure closely.

• Patients with a history of angioedema unrelated to ACE inhibitor use may be at increased risk for angioedema during therapy. Black patients are at a higher risk for angioedema regardless of prior ACE inhibitor use.

• *Alert:* If angioedema occurs, stop drug and observe patient until swelling disappears. Antihistamines may relieve swelling of the face and lips. Swelling of the tongue, glottis, or throat may cause life-threatening airway obstruction. Give prompt treatment, such as epinephrine.

• Monitor CBC with differential for agranulocytosis and neutropenia before therapy, especially in renally impaired patients with lupus or scleroderma.

• Monitor patient for hypotension when starting therapy and when adjusting dosage. If severe hypotension occurs, place patient in supine position and treat symptomatically.

• Severe hypotension can occur when drug is given with diuretics. If possible, stop diuretic 2 to 3 days before starting this drug. If impossible, use lower doses of either drug.

• In patient who is volume- or sodium-depleted from prolonged diuretic therapy, dietary sodium restriction, dialysis, diarrhea, or vomiting, correct fluid and sodium deficits before starting drug.

• Monitor renal function before and periodically throughout therapy.

• Monitor potassium level closely.

PATIENT TEACHING

• Inform patient that throat and facial swelling, including swelling of the throat, can occur during therapy, especially with the first dose. Advise patient to stop taking

drug and immediately report any signs or symptoms of swelling of face, extremities, eyes, lips, or tongue; hoarseness; or difficulty in swallowing or breathing.

• Advise patient to report promptly any sign or symptom of infection (sore throat, fever) or jaundice (yellowing of eyes or skin).

• Advise patient to avoid salt substitutes containing potassium unless instructed otherwise by prescriber.

• Caution patient that light-headedness may occur, especially during first few days of therapy. Advise patient to report light-headedness and, if fainting occurs, to stop drug and consult prescriber promptly.

• Caution patient that inadequate fluid intake or excessive perspiration, diarrhea, or vomiting can lead to an excessive drop in blood pressure.

• Advise woman of childbearing age of the consequences of second- and third-trimester exposure to drug. Advise her to notify prescriber immediately if she suspects pregnancy.

phentolamine mesylate
fen-TOLE-a-meen

Rogitine†

Pharmacologic class: alpha blocker
Pregnancy risk category C

AVAILABLE FORMS
Injection: 5 mg/ml, 10 mg/ml†

INDICATIONS & DOSAGES
➤ **To aid in diagnosis of pheochromocytoma, to control or prevent hypertension before or during pheochromocytomectomy**
Adults: I.V. or I.M. diagnostic dose is 5 mg with close monitoring of blood pressure. Give 5 mg I.V. or I.M 1 to 2 hours before surgical removal of tumor. During surgery, patient may need an additional 5 mg I.V.
Children: I.V. diagnostic dose is 1 mg, and I.M. diagnostic dose is 3 mg with close monitoring of blood pressure. Give 1 mg I.V. or I.M 1 to 2 hours before surgical removal of tumor. During surgery, patient may need an additional 1 mg I.V.

➤ **To prevent dermal necrosis from norepinephrine extravasation**
Adults: Add 10 mg of phentolamine to each liter of solution containing norepinephrine; the pressor effect of norepinephrine is unaffected.

➤ **Dermal necrosis and sloughing after I.V. extravasation of norepinephrine or dopamine**
Adults: Infiltrate area with 5 to 10 mg phentolamine in 10 to 15 ml of normal saline solution. Must be done within 12 hours of extravasation.
Children: Inject 0.1 to 0.2 mg/kg up to a maximum of 10 mg in the extravasation area.

ADMINISTRATION
I.V.
● Reconstitute drug by adding 1 ml of sterile water for injection to vial containing 5 mg of drug; resulting solution contains 5 mg/ml of drug.
● Delay injection until effect of venipuncture on blood pressure has passed, then inject drug rapidly.
● For pheochromocytoma diagnosis, inject drug rapidly. Test result is positive if severe hypotension develops.
● **Incompatibilities:** None reported.
I.M.
● Reconstitute drug by adding 1 ml of sterile water for injection to vial containing 5 mg of drug.
● Document injection site.

ACTION
Competitively blocks the effects of catecholamines on alpha-adrenergic receptors.

Route	Onset	Peak	Duration
I.V.	Immediate	<2 min	15–30 min
I.M.	Unknown	<20 min	30–45 min

Half-life: 19 minutes (I.V.).

ADVERSE REACTIONS
CNS: *dizziness, weakness, flushing,* **cerebrovascular occlusion,** *cerebrovascular spasm.*
CV: *hypotension, tachycardia,* **shock, arrhythmias, MI.**
EENT: *nasal congestion.*
GI: *diarrhea, nausea, vomiting.*

INTERACTIONS
Drug-drug. *Ephedrine, epinephrine:* May cause excessive hypotension. Don't use together.

EFFECTS ON LAB TEST RESULTS
None reported.

CONTRAINDICATIONS & CAUTIONS
● Contraindicated in patients with hypersensitivity to drug and in those with angina, coronary artery disease, or MI or history of MI.
● Use cautiously in patients with gastritis or peptic ulcer.

NURSING CONSIDERATIONS
● When drug is given as a diagnostic test for pheochromocytoma, check patient's blood pressure first; monitor blood pressure frequently during administration.
● *Alert:* Don't give epinephrine to treat phentolamine-induced hypotension because it may cause additional fall in blood pressure ("epinephrine reversal"). Use norepinephrine instead.
● *Look alike–sound alike:* Don't confuse phentolamine with phentermine.

PATIENT TEACHING
● Explain use and administration of drug.
● Tell patient to report adverse reactions promptly.

prazosin hydrochloride
PRA-zo-sin

Minipress

Pharmacologic class: alpha blocker
Pregnancy risk category C

AVAILABLE FORMS
Capsules: 1 mg, 2 mg, 5 mg

INDICATIONS & DOSAGES
➤ **Mild to moderate hypertension**
Adults: Test dose is 1 mg P.O. at bedtime to prevent first-dose syncope (severe syncope with loss of consciousness). First dosage is 1 mg P.O. b.i.d. or t.i.d. Dosage may be increased slowly. Maximum daily dose is 20 mg. Maintenance dosage is 6 to 15 mg daily in divided doses. Some

patients need larger dosages (up to 40 mg daily).

If other antihypertensives or diuretics are added to therapy, decrease prazosin dosage to 1 to 2 mg t.i.d. and readjust to maintenance dosage.

➤ **Benign prostatic hyperplasia ◆**
Adults: 2 mg P.O. b.i.d. Dose range is 1 to 9 mg P.O. daily.

ADMINISTRATION
P.O.
● Give drug without regard for meals.

ACTION
Unknown. Thought to act by blocking alpha-adrenergic receptors.

Route	Onset	Peak	Duration
P.O.	30–90 min	2–4 hr	7–10 hr

Half-life: 2 to 4 hours.

ADVERSE REACTIONS
CNS: *dizziness, first-dose syncope,* headache, drowsiness, nervousness, paresthesia, weakness, depression, fever.
CV: orthostatic hypotension, palpitations, edema.
EENT: blurred vision, tinnitus, conjunctivitis, epistaxis, nasal congestion.
GI: vomiting, diarrhea, abdominal cramps, nausea.
GU: priapism, impotence, urinary frequency, incontinence.
Musculoskeletal: arthralgia, myalgia.
Respiratory: dyspnea.
Skin: pruritus.

INTERACTIONS
Drug-drug. *Acebutolol, atenolol, betaxolol, carteolol, esmolol, metoprolol, nadolol, pindolol, propranolol, sotalol, timolol:* May increase the risk of orthostatic hypotension in the early phases of use together. Help patient stand slowly until effects are known.
Diuretics: May increase frequency of syncope with loss of consciousness. Advise patient to sit or lie down if dizziness occurs.
Verapamil: May increase prazosin level. Monitor patient closely.
Drug-herb. *Butcher's broom:* May reduce effect. Discourage use together.

Ma huang: May decrease antihypertensive effects. Discourage use together.

EFFECTS ON LAB TEST RESULTS
● May increase levels of BUN, uric acid, and urinary metabolite of norepinephrine and vanillylmandelic acid.
● May increase liver function test values. May alter results of screening tests for pheochromocytoma.
● May cause positive antinuclear antibody titer.

CONTRAINDICATIONS & CAUTIONS
● Contraindicated in patients hypersensitive to drug or other alpha blockers.
● Use cautiously in patients receiving other antihypertensives.

NURSING CONSIDERATIONS
● Monitor patient's blood pressure and pulse rate frequently.
● Elderly patients may be more sensitive to drug's hypotensive effects.
● Compliance might be improved with twice-daily dosing. Discuss dosing change with prescriber if compliance problems are suspected.
● *Alert:* If first dose is more than 1 mg, first-dose syncope may occur.

PATIENT TEACHING
● Warn patient that dizziness may occur with first dose. If he experiences dizziness, tell him to sit or lie down. Reassure him that this effect disappears with continued dosing.
● Caution patient to avoid driving or performing hazardous tasks for the first 24 hours after starting this drug or increasing the dose.
● Tell patient not to suddenly stop taking drug, but to notify prescriber if unpleasant adverse reactions occur.
● Advise patient to minimize low blood pressure and dizziness upon standing by rising slowly and avoiding sudden position changes. Dry mouth can be relieved by chewing gum or sucking on hard candy or ice chips.

Reactions may be *common*, uncommon, *life-threatening*, or **COMMON AND LIFE-THREATENING**.
Interaction may have a *rapid onset* or *delayed onset*.

quinapril hydrochloride
KWIN-ah-pril

Accupril◢

Pharmacologic class: ACE inhibitor
Pregnancy risk category C; D in 2nd and 3rd trimesters

AVAILABLE FORMS
Tablets: 5 mg, 10 mg, 20 mg, 40 mg

INDICATIONS & DOSAGES
➤ **Hypertension**
Adults: Initially, 10 to 20 mg P.O. daily. Dosage may be adjusted based on patient response at intervals of about 2 weeks. Most patients are controlled at 20, 40, or 80 mg daily as a single dose or in two divided doses. If patient is taking a diuretic, start therapy with 5 mg daily.
Elderly patients: For patients older than age 65, start therapy at 10 mg P.O. daily.
Adjust-a-dose: For adults with creatinine clearance over 60 ml/minute, initially, 10 mg maximum daily; for clearance of 30 to 60 ml/minute, 5 mg; for clearance of 10 to 30 ml/minute, 2.5 mg.
➤ **Heart failure**
Adults: If patient is taking a diuretic, give 5 mg P.O. b.i.d. initially. If patient isn't taking a diuretic, give 10 to 20 mg P.O. b.i.d. Dosage may be increased at weekly intervals. Usual effective dose is 20 to 40 mg daily in two equally divided doses.
Adjust-a-dose: For patients with creatinine clearance over 30 ml/minute, first dose is 5 mg daily; if clearance is 10 to 30 ml/minute, 2.5 mg.

ADMINISTRATION
P.O.
● Give drug 1 hour before or 2 hours after meals, or with a light meal.
● Don't give drug with a high-fat meal because this may decrease absorption of drug.

ACTION
Prevents conversion of angiotensin I to angiotensin II, a potent vasoconstrictor. Less angiotensin II decreases peripheral arterial resistance, decreasing aldosterone secretion, which reduces sodium and water retention and lowers blood pressure.

Route	Onset	Peak	Duration
P.O.	1 hr	2–6 hr	24 hr

Half-life: 25 hours.

ADVERSE REACTIONS
CNS: somnolence, vertigo, nervousness, headache, dizziness, fatigue, depression.
CV: *hypertensive crisis,* palpitations, tachycardia, angina pectoris, orthostatic hypotension, rhythm disturbances.
GI: *hemorrhage,* dry mouth, abdominal pain, constipation, vomiting, nausea, diarrhea.
Metabolic: *hyperkalemia.*
Respiratory: dry, persistent, tickling, nonproductive cough.
Skin: pruritus, photosensitivity reactions, diaphoresis.

INTERACTIONS
Drug-drug. *Diuretics, other antihypertensives:* May cause excessive hypotension. Stop diuretic or reduce dose of quinapril, as needed.
Lithium: May increase lithium level and lithium toxicity. Monitor lithium level.
NSAIDs: May decrease antihypertensive effects. Monitor blood pressure.
Potassium-sparing diuretics, potassium supplements: May cause hyperkalemia. Monitor patient closely.
Tetracycline: May decrease absorption if taken with quinapril. Avoid using together.
Drug-herb. *Capsaicin:* May cause cough. Discourage use together.
Ma huang: May decrease antihypertensive effects. Discourage use together.
Drug-food. *Salt substitutes containing potassium:* May cause hyperkalemia. Discourage use together.

EFFECTS ON LAB TEST RESULTS
● May increase potassium, BUN, and creatinine levels.
● May increase liver function test values.

CONTRAINDICATIONS & CAUTIONS
● Contraindicated in patients hypersensitive to ACE inhibitors and in those with a history of angioedema related to treatment with an ACE inhibitor.

■ **Black Box Warning** Use during pregnancy can cause injury and death to the developing fetus. When pregnancy is detected, stop drug as soon as possible. ■
● Use cautiously in patients with impaired renal function.

NURSING CONSIDERATIONS
● Assess renal and hepatic function before and periodically throughout therapy.
● Monitor blood pressure for effectiveness of therapy.
● Monitor potassium level. Risk factors for the development of hyperkalemia include renal insufficiency, diabetes, and concomitant use of drugs that raise potassium level.
● Although ACE inhibitors reduce blood pressure in all races, they reduce it less in blacks taking the ACE inhibitor alone. Black patients should take drug with a thiazide diuretic for a better response.
● ACE inhibitors appear to increase risk of angioedema in black patients.
● Other ACE inhibitors have caused agranulocytosis and neutropenia. Monitor CBC with differential counts before therapy and periodically thereafter.

PATIENT TEACHING
● Advise patient to report signs of infection, such as fever and sore throat.
● **Alert:** Facial and throat swelling (including swelling of the larynx) may occur, especially after first dose. Advise patient to report signs or symptoms of breathing difficulty or swelling of face, eyes, lips, or tongue.
● Light-headedness can occur, especially during first few days of therapy. Tell patient to rise slowly to minimize effect and to report signs and symptoms to prescriber. If he faints, patient should stop taking drug and call prescriber immediately.
● Inform patient that inadequate fluid intake, vomiting, diarrhea, and excessive perspiration can lead to light-headedness and fainting. Tell him to use caution in hot weather and during exercise.
● Tell patient to avoid salt substitutes. These products may contain potassium, which can cause high potassium level in patients taking quinapril.

● Advise woman of childbearing age to notify prescriber if pregnancy occurs. Drug will need to be stopped.
● Tell patient to avoid taking with a high-fat meal because this may decrease absorption of drug.

ramipril
ra-MI-pril

Altace

Pharmacologic class: ACE inhibitor
Pregnancy risk category C; D in 2nd and 3rd trimesters

AVAILABLE FORMS
Capsules: 1.25 mg, 2.5 mg, 5 mg, 10 mg
Tablets: 1.25 mg, 2.5 mg, 5 mg, 10 mg

INDICATIONS & DOSAGES
➤ **Hypertension**
Adults: Initially, 2.5 mg P.O. once daily for patients not taking a diuretic, and 1.25 mg P.O. once daily for patients taking a diuretic. Increase dosage, if needed, based on patient response. Maintenance dose is 2.5 to 20 mg daily as a single dose or in divided doses.
Adjust-a-dose: For patients with creatinine clearance less than 40 ml/minute, give 1.25 mg P.O. daily. Adjust dosage gradually based on response. Maximum daily dose is 5 mg.
➤ **Heart failure after an MI**
Adults: Initially, 2.5 mg P.O. b.i.d. If hypotension occurs; decrease dosage to 1.25 mg P.O. b.i.d. Adjust as tolerated to target dosage of 5 mg P.O. b.i.d.
Adjust-a-dose: For patients with creatinine clearance less than 40 ml/minute, give 1.25 mg P.O. daily. Adjust dosage gradually based on response. Maximum dosage is 2.5 mg b.i.d.
➤ **To reduce risk of MI, stroke, and death from CV causes**
Adults age 55 and older: 2.5 mg P.O. once daily for 1 week, then 5 mg P.O. once daily for 3 weeks. Increase as tolerated to a maintenance dose of 10 mg P.O. once daily.
Adjust-a-dose: In patients who are hypertensive or who have recently had an MI, daily dose may be divided.

ADMINISTRATION
P.O.
● Give drug without regard for meals.
● Open capsule and sprinkle contents on a small amount of applesauce or mix with 4 oz of water or apple juice. Give to patient immediately.

ACTION
Prevents conversion of angiotensin I to angiotensin II, a potent vasoconstrictor. Less angiotensin II decreases peripheral arterial resistance, decreasing aldosterone secretion, which reduces sodium and water retention and lowers blood pressure.

Route	Onset	Peak	Duration
P.O.	1–2 hr	1–3 hr	24 hr

Half-life: 13 to 17 hours.

ADVERSE REACTIONS
CNS: headache, dizziness, fatigue, asthenia, malaise, light-headedness, anxiety, amnesia, depression, insomnia, nervousness, neuralgia, neuropathy, paresthesia, somnolence, tremor, vertigo, syncope.
CV: *hypotension, heart failure, MI,* postural hypotension, angina pectoris, chest pain, palpitations, edema.
EENT: epistaxis, tinnitus.
GI: nausea, vomiting, abdominal pain, anorexia, constipation, diarrhea, dyspepsia, dry mouth, gastroenteritis.
GU: impotence.
Metabolic: *hyperkalemia,* hyperglycemia, weight gain.
Musculoskeletal: arthralgia, arthritis, myalgia.
Respiratory: dyspnea, dry, persistent, tickling, nonproductive cough.
Skin: rash, dermatitis, pruritus, photosensitivity reactions, increased diaphoresis.
Other: hypersensitivity reactions.

INTERACTIONS
Drug-drug. *Diuretics:* May cause excessive hypotension, especially at start of therapy. Stop diuretic at least 3 days before therapy begins, increase sodium intake, or reduce starting dose of ramipril.
Insulin, oral antidiabetics: May cause hypoglycemia, especially at start of ramipril therapy. Monitor glucose level closely.

Lithium: May increase lithium level. Use together cautiously and monitor lithium level.
Nesiritide: May increase hypotensive effects. Monitor blood pressure.
NSAIDs: May decrease antihypertensive effects. Monitor blood pressure.
Potassium-sparing diuretics, potassium supplements: May cause hyperkalemia; ramipril attenuates potassium loss. Monitor potassium level closely.
Drug-herb. *Capsaicin:* May cause cough. Discourage use together.
Ma huang: May decrease antihypertensive effects. Discourage use together.
Drug-food. *Salt substitutes containing potassium:* May cause hyperkalemia; ramipril attenuates potassium loss. Discourage use of salt substitutes during therapy.

EFFECTS ON LAB TEST RESULTS
● May increase BUN, creatinine, bilirubin, liver enzymes, glucose, and potassium levels. May decrease hemoglobin level and hematocrit.
● May decrease RBC and platelet counts.

CONTRAINDICATIONS & CAUTIONS
● Contraindicated in patients hypersensitive to ACE inhibitors and in those with a history of angioedema related to treatment with an ACE inhibitor.
■ **Black Box Warning** Use during pregnancy can cause injury and death to the developing fetus. When pregnancy is detected, stop drug as soon as possible. ■
● Use cautiously in patients with renal impairment.

NURSING CONSIDERATIONS
● Monitor blood pressure regularly for drug effectiveness.
● Closely assess renal function in patients during first few weeks of therapy. Regular assessment of renal function is advisable. Patients with severe heart failure whose renal function depends on the renin-angiotensin-aldosterone system may have experienced acute renal failure during ACE inhibitor therapy. Hypertensive patients with unilateral or bilateral renal artery stenosis also may show signs of worsening renal function during first few

days of therapy. Dose reduction or drug stoppage may be necessary.
• Although ACE inhibitors reduce blood pressure in all races, they reduce it less in blacks taking the ACE inhibitor alone. Black patients should take drug with a thiazide diuretic for a more favorable response.
• ACE inhibitors appear to increase risk of angioedema in black patients.
• Monitor CBC with differential counts before therapy and periodically thereafter.
• Drug may reduce hemoglobin and WBC, RBC, and platelet counts, especially in patients with impaired renal function or collagen vascular diseases (systemic lupus erythematosus or scleroderma).
• Monitor potassium level. Risk factors for the development of hyperkalemia include renal insufficiency, diabetes, and concomitant use of drugs that raise potassium level.

PATIENT TEACHING
• Tell patient to notify prescriber if any adverse reactions occur. Dosage adjustment or stoppage of drug may be needed.
• *Alert:* Rarely, swelling of the face and throat (including swelling of the larynx) may occur, especially after first dose. Advise patient to report signs or symptoms of breathing difficulty or swelling of face, eyes, lips, or tongue.
• Inform patient that light-headedness can occur, especially during the first few days of therapy. Tell him to rise slowly to minimize this effect and to report signs and symptoms to prescriber. If he faints, patient should stop taking drug and call prescriber immediately.
• Tell patient that if he has difficulty swallowing capsules, he can open drug and sprinkle contents on a small amount of applesauce.
• Advise patient to report signs and symptoms of infection, such as fever and sore throat.
• Tell patient to avoid salt substitutes. These products may contain potassium, which can cause high potassium level in patients taking ramipril.
• Tell woman of childbearing age to notify prescriber if pregnancy occurs. Drug will need to be stopped.

telmisartan
tell-mah-SAR-tan

Micardis

Pharmacologic class: angiotensin II receptor antagonist
Pregnancy risk category C; D in 2nd and 3rd trimesters

AVAILABLE FORMS
Tablets: 20 mg, 40 mg, 80 mg

INDICATIONS & DOSAGES
➤ **Hypertension (used alone or with other antihypertensives)**
Adults: 40 mg P.O. daily. Blood pressure response is dose-related over a range of 20 to 80 mg daily.

ADMINISTRATION
P.O.
• Give drug without regard to meals.

ACTION
Blocks vasoconstricting and aldosterone-secreting effects of angiotensin II by preventing angiotensin II from binding to the angiotensin I receptor.

Route	Onset	Peak	Duration
P.O.	Unknown	30–60 min	24 hr

Half-life: 24 hours.

ADVERSE REACTIONS
CNS: dizziness, pain, fatigue, headache.
CV: chest pain, hypertension, peripheral edema.
EENT: pharyngitis, sinusitis.
GI: *nausea,* abdominal pain, diarrhea, dyspepsia.
GU: UTI.
Musculoskeletal: back pain, myalgia.
Respiratory: cough, upper respiratory tract infection.
Other: flulike symptoms.

INTERACTIONS
Drug-drug. *Digoxin:* May increase digoxin level. Monitor digoxin level closely.
Warfarin: May decrease warfarin level. Monitor INR.

Reactions may be *common,* uncommon, *life-threatening,* or COMMON AND LIFE-THREATENING.
Interaction may have a *rapid onset* or *delayed onset.*

Drug-herb. *Ma huang:* May decrease antihypertensive effects. Discourage use together.

Drug-food. *Salt substitutes containing potassium:* May cause hyperkalemia. Discourage use together.

EFFECTS ON LAB TEST RESULTS
● May increase liver enzyme levels.

CONTRAINDICATIONS & CAUTIONS
● Contraindicated in patients hypersensitive to drug or its components.
● Use cautiously in patients with biliary obstruction disorders or renal and hepatic insufficiency and in those with an activated renin-angiotensin system, such as volume- or sodium-depleted patients (for example, those being treated with high doses of diuretics).
■ **Black Box Warning** Use during pregnancy can cause injury and death to the developing fetus. When pregnancy is detected, stop drug as soon as possible. ■

NURSING CONSIDERATIONS
● Monitor patient for hypotension after starting drug. Place patient supine if hypotension occurs, and give I.V. normal saline, if needed.
● Most of the antihypertensive effect occurs within 2 weeks. Maximal blood pressure reduction is usually reached after 4 weeks. Diuretic may be added if blood pressure isn't controlled by drug alone.
● *Alert:* In patients whose renal function may depend on the activity of the renin-angiotensin-aldosterone system (such as those with severe heart failure), drug may cause oliguria or progressive azotemia and (rarely) acute renal failure or death.
● Drug isn't removed by hemodialysis. Patients undergoing dialysis may develop orthostatic hypotension. Closely monitor blood pressure.

PATIENT TEACHING
● Instruct patient to report suspected pregnancy to prescriber immediately.
● Inform woman of childbearing age of the consequences of second and third trimester exposure to drug.
● Advise breast-feeding woman about risk of adverse drug effects in infants and the need to stop either drug or breast-feeding.

● Tell patient that if he feels dizzy or has low blood pressure on standing, he should lie down, rise slowly from a lying to standing position, and climb stairs slowly.
● Tell patient that drug may be taken without regard to meals.
● Tell patient not to remove drug from blister-sealed packet until immediately before use.

---

terazosin hydrochloride
ter-AY-zoe-sin

Hytrin✒

Pharmacologic class: alpha blocker
Pregnancy risk category C

AVAILABLE FORMS
Capsules: 1 mg, 2 mg, 5 mg, 10 mg
Tablets: 1 mg, 2 mg, 5 mg, 10 mg

INDICATIONS & DOSAGES
➤ **Hypertension**
Adults: Initially, 1 mg P.O. at bedtime. Dosage may be increased gradually based on response. Usual dosage range is 1 to 5 mg daily. Maximum recommended dose is 20 mg daily.
➤ **Symptomatic BPH**
Adults: Initially, 1 mg P.O. at bedtime. Dosage may be titrated to 2, 5, or 10 mg once daily to achieve optimal response. Most patients need 10 mg daily for optimal response.

ADMINISTRATION
P.O.
● Give drug without regard for meals.

ACTION
Improves urine flow in patients with BPH by blocking alpha-adrenergic receptors in the bladder neck and prostate, relieving urethral pressure. Drug also reduces peripheral vascular resistance and blood pressure via arterial and venous dilation.

Route	Onset	Peak	Duration
P.O.	15 min	2–3 hr	24 hr

Half-life: About 12 hours.

ADVERSE REACTIONS
CNS: *headache, dizziness,* asthenia, first-dose syncope, nervousness, paresthesia, somnolence.
CV: *peripheral edema,* palpitations, orthostatic hypotension, tachycardia, atrial fibrillation.
EENT: *nasal congestion,* sinusitis, blurred vision.
GI: nausea.
GU: impotence, priapism.
Hematologic: *thrombocytopenia.*
Musculoskeletal: back pain, muscle pain.
Respiratory: dyspnea.

INTERACTIONS
Drug-drug. *Antihypertensives:* May cause excessive hypotension. Use together cautiously.
Drug-herb. *Butcher's broom:* May decrease drug effect. Discourage use together.
Ma huang: May decrease antihypertensive effects. Discourage use together.

EFFECTS ON LAB TEST RESULTS
• May decrease total protein and albumin levels. May decrease hemoglobin level and hematocrit.
• May decrease WBC and platelet counts.

CONTRAINDICATIONS & CAUTIONS
• Contraindicated in patients hypersensitive to drug.

NURSING CONSIDERATIONS
• Monitor blood pressure frequently.
• *Alert:* If terazosin is stopped for several days, readjust dosage using first dosing regimen (1 mg P.O. at bedtime).

PATIENT TEACHING
• Tell patient not to stop drug suddenly, but to notify prescriber if adverse reactions occur.
• Warn patient to avoid hazardous activities that require mental alertness, such as driving or operating heavy machinery, for 12 hours after first dose.
• Tell patient that light-headedness can occur, especially during the first few days of therapy. Advise him to rise slowly to minimize this effect and to report signs and symptoms to prescriber.

trandolapril
tran-DOLE-ah-pril

Mavik

Pharmacologic class: ACE inhibitor
Pregnancy risk category C; D in 2nd and 3rd trimesters

AVAILABLE FORMS
Tablets: 1 mg, 2 mg, 4 mg

INDICATIONS & DOSAGES
➤ **Hypertension**
Adults: For patients not taking a diuretic, initially 2 mg P.O. for a black patient and 1 mg P.O. for all other races, once daily. If control isn't adequate, increase dosage at intervals of at least 1 week. Maintenance doses for most patients range from 2 to 4 mg daily. Some patients taking once-daily doses of 4 mg may need b.i.d. doses. For patients also taking a diuretic, initially, 0.5 mg P.O. once daily. Subsequent dosage adjustment is based on blood pressure response.
➤ **Heart failure or ventricular dysfunction after MI**
Adults: Initially, 1 mg P.O. daily, adjusted to 4 mg P.O. daily. If patient can't tolerate 4 mg, continue at highest tolerated dose.
Adjust-a-dose: If creatinine clearance is below 30 ml/minute or patient has hepatic cirrhosis, first dose is 0.5 mg daily.

ADMINISTRATION
P.O.
• Give drug without regard for food.
• Don't give antacid 1 hour before or up to 2 hours after dose.

ACTION
Thought to inhibit ACE, reducing angiotensin II formation, which decreases peripheral arterial resistance, decreases aldosterone secretion, reduces sodium and water retention, and lowers blood pressure. Drug is converted in the liver to the prodrug, trandolaprilat.

Route	Onset	Peak	Duration
P.O.	4 hr	1–10 hr	24 hr

Half-life: 5 to 10 hours; longer in patients with renal impairment.

ADVERSE REACTIONS

CNS: *dizziness,* headache, fatigue, drowsiness, insomnia, paresthesia, vertigo, anxiety.

CV: *hypotension, bradycardia,* chest pain, first-degree AV block, edema, flushing, palpitations.

EENT: epistaxis, throat irritation.

GI: *pancreatitis,* diarrhea, dyspepsia, abdominal distention, abdominal pain or cramps, constipation, vomiting.

GU: urinary frequency, impotence.

Hematologic: *neutropenia, leukopenia.*

Metabolic: *hyperkalemia,* hyponatremia.

Respiratory: *persistent, nonproductive cough,* dyspnea, upper respiratory tract infection.

Skin: rash, pruritus, pemphigus.

Other: decreased libido.

INTERACTIONS

Drug-drug. *Azathioprine:* May increase risk of anemia or leukopenia. Monitor hematologic studies.

Diuretics: May cause excessive hypotension. Stop diuretic or reduce first dosage of trandolapril.

Lithium: May increase lithium level and lithium toxicity. Avoid using together; monitor lithium level.

NSAIDs: May decrease antihypertensive effects. Monitor blood pressure.

Potassium-sparing diuretics, potassium supplements: May cause hyperkalemia. Monitor potassium level closely.

Drug-herb. *Capsaicin:* May cause cough. Discourage use together.

Ma huang: May decrease antihypertensive effects. Discourage use together.

Drug-food. *Salt substitutes containing potassium:* May cause hyperkalemia. Discourage use of salt substitutes.

EFFECTS ON LAB TEST RESULTS

● May increase BUN, creatinine, potassium, and liver enzyme levels. May decrease sodium level.

● May decrease neutrophil and WBC counts.

CONTRAINDICATIONS & CAUTIONS

● Contraindicated in patients hypersensitive to drug and in those with a history of angioedema related to previous treatment with an ACE inhibitor.

■ **Black Box Warning** Use during pregnancy can cause injury and death to the developing fetus. When pregnancy is detected, stop drug as soon as possible. ■

● Use cautiously in patients with impaired renal function, heart failure, or renal artery stenosis.

● Safety and effectiveness of drug in children haven't been established.

● Don't use drug in breast-feeding women.

NURSING CONSIDERATIONS

● Monitor potassium level closely.

● Watch for hypotension. Excessive hypotension can occur when drug is given with diuretics. If possible, stop diuretic therapy 2 to 3 days before starting trandolapril to decrease potential for excessive hypotension response. If drug doesn't adequately control blood pressure, diuretic therapy may be started again cautiously.

● Assess patient's renal function before and periodically throughout therapy.

● Other ACE inhibitors have been reported to cause agranulocytosis and neutropenia. Monitor CBC with differential before therapy, especially in patients with collagen vascular disease and impaired renal function.

● Although drug reduces blood pressure in patients of all races, drug reduces pressure less in blacks taking this drug alone. Blacks should take drug with a thiazide diuretic for a more favorable response.

● *Alert:* Angioedema involving the tongue, glottis, or larynx may be fatal because of airway obstruction. Give appropriate therapy, including epinephrine 1:1,000 (0.3 to 0.5 ml) subcutaneously; have resuscitation equipment for maintaining a patent airway readily available. The risk of angioedema is higher in blacks.

● If patient develops jaundice, stop drug under prescriber's advice because, although rare, ACE inhibitors have been linked to a syndrome of cholestatic jaundice, fulminant hepatic necrosis, and death.

PATIENT TEACHING

● Instruct patient to report yellowing of skin or eyes.

● Advise patient to report fever and sore throat (signs of infection), easy bruising or bleeding; swelling of the tongue, lips, face, eyes, mucous membranes, or

extremities; difficulty swallowing or breathing; hoarseness; and nonproductive, persistent cough.

• Tell patient to avoid salt substitutes during drug therapy. These products may contain potassium, which can cause high potassium level in patients taking drug.

• Tell patient that light-headedness can occur, especially during first few days of therapy. Advise him to rise slowly to minimize this effect and to report it immediately.

• Advise patient to use caution in hot weather and during exercise. Inadequate fluid intake, vomiting, diarrhea, and excessive perspiration can lead to light-headedness and fainting.

• Tell woman of childbearing age to report suspected pregnancy immediately. Drug will need to be stopped.

• Advise patient planning to undergo surgery or receive anesthesia to inform prescriber that he is taking this drug.

• Tell patient drug may be taken with or without food.

• Instruct patient not to take an antacid 1 hour before or up to 2 hours after dose.

---

valsartan
val-SAR-tan

Diovan♦

Pharmacologic class: angiotensin II receptor antagonist
Pregnancy risk category C; D in 2nd and 3rd trimesters

AVAILABLE FORMS
Tablets: 40 mg, 80 mg, 160 mg, 320 mg

INDICATIONS & DOSAGES
➤ **Hypertension (used alone or with other antihypertensives)**
Adults: Initially, 80 mg P.O. once daily. Expect to see a reduction in blood pressure in 2 to 4 weeks. If additional antihypertensive effect is needed, dose may be increased to 160 or 320 mg daily, or a diuretic may be added. (Addition of a diuretic has a greater effect than dosage increases beyond 80 mg.) Usual dosage range is 80 to 320 mg daily.

Children ages 6 to 16: Initially, 1.3 mg/kg P.O. daily. Adjust according to patient response up to 40 mg.
➤ **New York Heart Association class II to IV heart failure**
Adults: Initially, 40 mg P.O. b.i.d.; increase as tolerated to 80 mg b.i.d., and then to target dose of 160 mg b.i.d.
➤ **To reduce CV death in stable post-MI patients with left-ventricular failure or dysfunction**
Adults: 20 mg P.O. b.i.d. Initial dose may be given as soon as 12 hours after MI. Increase dose to 40 mg b.i.d. within 7 days. Increase subsequent doses, as tolerated, to target dose of 160 mg b.i.d.

ADMINISTRATION
P.O.
• Give drug without regard for food.
• Pharmacists may prepare suspension for children unable to swallow pills.
• Shake suspension at least 10 seconds before pouring. Store suspension at room temperature for 30 days or in refrigerator for 75 days.

ACTION
Blocks the binding of angiotensin II to receptor sites in vascular smooth muscle and the adrenal gland, which inhibits the pressor effects of the renin-angiotensin-aldosterone system.

Route	Onset	Peak	Duration
P.O.	2 hr	2–4 hr	24 hr

Half-life: 6 hours.

ADVERSE REACTIONS
CNS: *dizziness,* headache, insomnia, fatigue, vertigo.
CV: edema, hypotension, orthostatic hypotension, syncope.
EENT: rhinitis, sinusitis, pharyngitis, blurred vision.
GI: abdominal pain, diarrhea, nausea, dyspepsia.
GU: renal impairment.
Hematologic: *neutropenia.*
Metabolic: hyperkalemia.
Musculoskeletal: arthralgia, back pain.
Respiratory: upper respiratory tract infection, cough.
Other: *angioedema,* viral infection.

Reactions may be *common,* uncommon, *life-threatening,* or COMMON AND LIFE-THREATENING.
Interaction may have a *rapid onset* or **delayed onset.**

INTERACTIONS

Drug-drug. *Lithium:* May increase lithium level. Monitor lithium level and patient for toxicity.

Potassium supplements, potassium-sparing diuretics, other angiotensin II blockers: May increase potassium level. May also increase creatinine level in heart failure patients. Avoid using together.

Drug-herb. *Ma huang:* May decrease antihypertensive effects. Discourage use together.

Drug-food. *Salt substitutes containing potassium:* May increase potassium level. May also increase creatinine level in heart failure patients. Discourage use together.

EFFECTS ON LAB TEST RESULTS

• May increase potassium, BUN, and creatinine levels.

• May decrease neutrophil count.

CONTRAINDICATIONS & CAUTIONS

• Contraindicated in patients hypersensitive to drug.

• Contraindicated in breast-feeding women.

■ **Black Box Warning** Drugs that act directly on the renin-angiotensin system can cause injury and even death to the developing fetus. When pregnancy is detected, stop drug as soon as possible. ■

• Use cautiously in patients with renal or hepatic disease.

• Safety and efficacy of drug haven't been established in children less than age 6 and children of any age with GFR less than 30 ml/minute/1.73 m^2.

NURSING CONSIDERATIONS

• Watch for hypotension. Excessive hypotension can occur when drug is given with high doses of diuretics.

• Correct volume and sodium depletions before starting drug.

• Suspension has 1.6 times greater exposure than tablets. Patients may require a higher dose if switched to tablets.

PATIENT TEACHING

• Tell woman of childbearing age to notify prescriber if pregnancy occurs. Drug will need to be stopped.

• Advise patient that drug may be taken without regard for food.

---

†Canada   ◇ OTC   ◆ Off-label use   ✐Photoguide   *Liquid contains alcohol.

atorvastatin calcium
cholestyramine
colesevelam hydrochloride
ezetimibe
fenofibrate
fluvastatin sodium
gemfibrozil
lovastatin
niacin
(See Appendix.)
omega-3-acid ethyl esters
pravastatin sodium
rosuvastatin calcium
simvastatin

---

atorvastatin calcium
ah-TOR-va-stah-tin

Lipitor◆

Pharmacologic class: HMG-CoA
reductase inhibitor
Pregnancy risk category X

AVAILABLE FORMS
Tablets: 10 mg, 20 mg, 40 mg, 80 mg

INDICATIONS & DOSAGES
➤ **In patients with clinically evident coronary heart disease, to reduce the risk of nonfatal MI, fatal and nonfatal strokes, angina, heart failure, and revascularization procedures**
Adults: Initially, 10 to 20 mg P.O. daily. May increase based on patient response and tolerance; usual dosage, 10 to 80 mg P.O. daily.
➤ **To reduce the risk of MI, stroke, angina, or revascularization procedures in patients with multiple risk factors for CAD but who don't yet have the disease**
Adults: 10 mg P.O. daily.
➤ **Adjunct to diet to reduce LDL, total cholesterol, apolipoprotein B, and triglyceride levels and to increase HDL levels in patients with primary hypercholesterolemia**
(heterozygous familial and non-familial) and mixed dyslipidemia (Fredrickson types IIa and IIb); adjunct to diet to reduce triglyceride level (Fredrickson type IV); primary dysbetalipoproteinemia (Fredrickson type III) in patients who don't respond adequately to diet
Adults: Initially, 10 or 20 mg P.O. once daily. Patient who requires a reduction of more than 45% in LDL level may be started at 40 mg once daily. Increase dose, as needed, to maximum of 80 mg daily as single dose. Dosage based on lipid levels drawn within 2 to 4 weeks of starting therapy and after dosage adjustment.
➤ **Alone or as an adjunct to lipid-lowering treatments, such as LDL apheresis, to reduce total and LDL cholesterol in patients with homozygous familial hypercholesterolemia**
Adults: 10 to 80 mg P.O. once daily.
➤ **Heterozygous familial hypercholesterolemia**
Children ages 10 to 17 (girls should be 1 year postmenarche): Initially, 10 mg P.O. once daily. Adjustment intervals should be at least 4 weeks. Maximum daily dose is 20 mg.

ADMINISTRATION
P.O.
● Give drug without regard for meals.

ACTION
Inhibits HMG-CoA reductase, an early (and rate-limiting) step in cholesterol biosynthesis.

Route	Onset	Peak	Duration
P.O.	Unknown	1–2 hr	Unknown

Half-life: 14 hours.

ADVERSE REACTIONS
CNS: *headache,* asthenia, insomnia.
CV: peripheral edema.

EENT: pharyngitis, rhinitis, sinusitis.
GI: abdominal pain, constipation, diarrhea, dyspepsia, flatulence, nausea.
GU: UTI.
Musculoskeletal: *rhabdomyolysis,* arthritis, arthralgia, myalgia.
Respiratory: bronchitis.
Skin: rash.
Other: allergic reactions, flulike syndrome, infection.

INTERACTIONS

Drug-drug. *Antacids, cholestyramine, colestipol:* May decrease atorvastatin level. Separate administration times.
Cyclosporine, diltiazem, *fibric acid derivatives,* **macrolides (azithromycin, clarithromycin, erythromycin, telithromycin),** *nefazodone, niacin, protease inhibitors, tacrolimus,* **verapamil:** May decrease metabolism of HMG-CoA reductase inhibitors, increasing toxicity. Monitor patient for adverse effects and report unexplained muscle pain.
Digoxin: May increase digoxin level. Monitor digoxin level and patient for evidence of toxicity.
Fluconazole, itraconazole, ketoconazole, voriconazole: May increase atorvastatin level and adverse effects. Avoid using together; or if unavoidable, reduce dose of atorvastatin.
Hormonal contraceptives: May increase norethindrone and ethinyl estradiol levels. Consider increased drug levels when selecting an oral contraceptive.
Drug-herb. *Eucalyptus, jin bu huan, kava:* May increase risk of hepatotoxicity. Discourage use together.
Red yeast rice: May increase risk of adverse reactions because herb contains compounds similar to those in drug. Discourage use together.
Drug-food. *Grapefruit juice:* May increase drug levels, increasing risk of adverse reactions. Discourage use together.

EFFECTS ON LAB TEST RESULTS
● May increase ALT, AST, and CK levels.

CONTRAINDICATIONS & CAUTIONS
● Contraindicated in patients hypersensitive to drug and in those with active liver disease or unexplained persistent elevations of transaminase levels.
● Contraindicated in pregnant and breast-feeding women and in women of childbearing age.
● Use cautiously in patients with history of liver disease or heavy alcohol use.
● Withhold or stop drug in patients at risk for renal failure caused by rhabdomyolysis resulting from trauma; in serious, acute conditions that suggest myopathy; and in major surgery, severe acute infection, hypotension, uncontrolled seizures, or severe metabolic, endocrine, or electrolyte disorders.
● Limit use in children to those older than age 9 with homozygous familial hypercholesterolemia.

NURSING CONSIDERATIONS
● Patient should follow a standard cholesterol-lowering diet before and during therapy.
● Before treatment, assess patient for underlying causes for hypercholesterolemia and obtain a baseline lipid profile. Obtain periodic liver function test results and lipid levels before starting treatment and at 6 and 12 weeks after initiation, or after an increase in dosage and periodically thereafter.
● Watch for signs of myositis.
● *Look alike–sound alike:* Don't confuse Lipitor with Levatol.

PATIENT TEACHING
● Teach patient about proper dietary management, weight control, and exercise. Explain their importance in controlling high fat levels.
● Warn patient to avoid alcohol.
● Tell patient to inform prescriber of adverse reactions, such as muscle pain, malaise, and fever.
● Advise patient that drug can be taken at any time of day, without regard for meals.
● *Alert:* Tell woman to stop drug and notify prescriber immediately if she is or may be pregnant or if she's breast-feeding.

cholestyramine
koe-LESS-tir-a-meen

Prevalite, Questran, Questran
Light

Pharmacologic class: bile acid
sequestrant
Pregnancy risk category C

AVAILABLE FORMS
Powder: 378-g cans, 9-g single-dose
packets; each scoop of powder or
single-dose packet contains 4 g of
cholestyramine resin

INDICATIONS & DOSAGES
➤ **Primary hyperlipidemia or
pruritus caused by partial bile
obstruction, adjunct for reduction
of increased cholesterol level in
patients with primary hyper
cholesterolemia**
Adults: 4 g once or twice daily. Maintenance dose is 8 to 16 g daily divided into
two doses. Maximum daily dose is 24 g.
Children: 240 mg/kg daily in two to three
divided doses, not to exceed 8 g/day.

ADMINISTRATION
P.O.
• Mix thoroughly with 60 to 180 ml of
water or other noncarbonated beverage.
• Give drug with a meal.
• Give other drugs 1 hour before or at
least 4 hours after cholestyramine to avoid
impeding absorption.

ACTION
Binds bile acids in the intestinal tract, impeding their absorption and causing their
elimination in feces. In response to this
bile acid depletion, LDL cholesterol levels
decrease as the liver uses LDL cholesterol
to replenish reduced bile acid stores.

Route	Onset	Peak	Duration
P.O.	Unknown	Unknown	2–4 wk

Half-life: Unknown.

ADVERSE REACTIONS
CNS: *dizziness, headache, vertigo,* anxiety,
fatigue, insomnia, syncope, tinnitus.
GI: *abdominal discomfort, constipation,
fecal impaction, nausea,* anorexia,
diarrhea, flatulence, ***GI bleeding,***
hemorrhoids, steatorrhea, vomiting.
GU: dysuria, hematuria.
Hematologic: anemia, bleeding tendencies, ecchymoses.
Metabolic: hyperchloremic acidosis.
Musculoskeletal: backache, muscle and
joint pains, osteoporosis.
Skin: *rash,* irritation of skin, tongue, and
perianal area.
Other: *vitamin A, D, E, and K deficiencies
from decreased absorption.*

INTERACTIONS
Drug-drug. *Acetaminophen, beta
blockers, cardiac glycosides, corticosteroids, estrogens, fat-soluble vitamins
(A, D, E, and K), iron preparations,
niacin, penicillin G, phenobarbital,
progestins, tetracycline, thiazide
diuretics, thyroid hormones, warfarin
and other coumarin derivatives:* May
decrease absorption of these drugs.
Give other drugs 1 hour before or 4 to
6 hours after cholestyramine.

EFFECTS ON LAB TEST RESULTS
• May increase alkaline phosphatase and
triglyceride levels. May decrease hemoglobin level and hematocrit.
• May increase PT.
• May cause abnormal results in chole-
cystography that uses iopanoic acid
because iopanoic acid is also bound by
cholestyramine.

CONTRAINDICATIONS & CAUTIONS
• Contraindicated in patients hypersensitive to bile-acid sequestering resins
and in those with complete biliary
obstruction.
• Use cautiously in patients predisposed
to constipation and in those with conditions aggravated by constipation, such
as severe, symptomatic coronary artery
disease.

NURSING CONSIDERATIONS
• Monitor cholesterol and triglyceride
levels regularly during therapy.
• Monitor levels of cardiac glycosides in
patients receiving cardiac glycosides and
cholestyramine together. If cholestyramine

therapy is stopped, adjust dosage of cardiac glycosides, if necessary, to avoid toxicity.
• Monitor bowel habits. Encourage a diet high in fiber and fluids. If severe constipation develops, decrease dosage, add a stool softener, or stop drug.
• Watch for hyperchloremic acidosis with long-term use or very high doses.
• Long-term use may lead to deficiencies of vitamins A, D, E, and K, and folic acid.
• For patients with phenylketonuria, light form contains 28.1 mg of phenylalanine per 6.4-g dose.
• *Look alike–sound alike:* Don't confuse Questran with Quarzan.

PATIENT TEACHING
• *Alert:* Tell patient never to take drug in its dry form because it may irritate the esophagus or cause severe constipation.
• Tell patient to prepare drug in a large glass containing water, milk, or juice (especially pulpy fruit juice). Tell him to sprinkle powder on the surface of the beverage, let the mixture stand for a few minutes, and then stir thoroughly. Discourage mixing with carbonated beverages because of excessive foaming. After drinking preparation, patient should swirl a small additional amount of liquid in the same glass and then drink again to make sure he has taken the entire dose.
• Tell patient to avoid sipping or holding the suspension in the mouth because drug may damage tooth surfaces. Advise patient to maintain good oral hygiene.
• Advise patient to take at mealtime, if possible.
• Advise patient to take all other drugs at least 1 hour before or 4 to 6 hours after cholestyramine to avoid blocking their absorption.
• Teach patient about proper dietary management of fats. When appropriate, recommend weight control, exercise, and smoking cessation programs.
• Tell patient that drug may deplete body stores of vitamins A, D, E, and K, and folic acid. Patient should discuss need for supplements with prescriber.

colesevelam hydrochloride
koe-leh-SEVE-eh-lam

WelChol

Pharmacologic class: bile acid sequestrant
Pregnancy risk category B

AVAILABLE FORMS
Tablets: 625 mg

INDICATIONS & DOSAGES
➤ **Adjunct to diet and exercise, either alone or with an HMG-CoA reductase inhibitor, to reduce elevated LDL cholesterol in patients with primary hypercholesterolemia (Fredrickson type IIa)**
Adults: 3 tablets (1,875 mg) P.O. b.i.d. or 6 tablets (3,750 mg) once daily.
✳*NEW INDICATION:* **Adjunct to diet and exercise to improve glycemic control in type 2 diabetes mellitus**
Adults: 3 tablets (1,875 mg) P.O. b.i.d. or 6 tablets (3,750 mg) P.O. once daily.

ADMINISTRATION
P.O.
• Give drug with a meal and plenty of fluids.
• Store tablets at room temperature and protect them from moisture.

ACTION
Binds bile acids in the intestinal tract, impeding their absorption and causing their elimination in feces. In response to this bile acid depletion, LDL cholesterol levels decrease as the liver uses LDL cholesterol to replenish reduced bile acid stores.

Route	Onset	Peak	Duration
P.O.	Unknown	2 wk	Unknown

Half-life: Unknown.

ADVERSE REACTIONS
CNS: *headache,* asthenia, pain.
EENT: pharyngitis, rhinitis, sinusitis.
GI: *constipation, flatulence,* abdominal pain, diarrhea, dyspepsia, nausea.
Musculoskeletal: back pain, myalgia.

Respiratory: increased cough.
Other: *infection,* accidental injury, flulike syndrome.

INTERACTIONS
Glyburide: May decrease glyburide level. Administer glyburide at least 4 hours prior to colesevelam.
Hormonal contraceptives containing ethinyl estradiol and norethindrone: May decrease levels of these contraceptives. Administer hormonal contraceptive at least 4 hours prior to colesevelam.
Phenytoin: May decrease phenytoin level and increase seizure activity. Administer phenytoin 4 hours prior to colesevelam and monitor phenytoin level.
Thyroid hormones: Coadministration may increase thyroid-stimulating hormone level. Administer thyroid hormone replacement 4 hours prior to colesevelam.
Warfarin: May decrease INR. Monitor INR and patient closely.

EFFECTS ON LAB TEST RESULTS
• May increase triglyceride levels.

CONTRAINDICATIONS & CAUTIONS
• Contraindicated in patients hypersensitive to drug or any of its components and in patients with bowel obstruction.
• Use cautiously in patients susceptible to vitamin K or fat-soluble vitamin deficiencies and in patients with swallowing disorders, severe GI motility disorders, or major GI tract surgery.
• Use cautiously in patients with triglyceride levels greater than 300 mg/dl.

NURSING CONSIDERATIONS
• Before starting drug, assess patient for underlying causes of hypercholesterolemia, such as poorly controlled diabetes, hypothyroidism, nephrotic syndrome, dysproteinemias, obstructive liver disease, other drug therapy, and alcoholism.
• Monitor patient's bowel habits. If severe constipation develops, decrease dosage, add a stool softener, or stop drug.
• Monitor the effects of patient's other drugs to identify drug interactions.
• Monitor total and LDL cholesterol and triglyceride levels periodically during therapy.

• Use only when clearly needed in breast-feeding women because it's not known if drug appears in breast milk.

PATIENT TEACHING
• Instruct patient to take drug with a meal and plenty of fluids.
• Teach patient to monitor bowel habits. Encourage a diet high in fiber and fluids. Instruct patient to notify prescriber promptly if severe constipation develops.
• Encourage patient to follow prescribed diet, exercise, and monitoring of cholesterol and triglyceride levels.
• Tell patient to notify prescriber if she's pregnant or breast-feeding.

---

ezetimibe
ee-ZET-ah-mibe

Zetia♥

Pharmacologic class: selective cholesterol absorption inhibitor
Pregnancy risk category C

AVAILABLE FORMS
Tablets: 10 mg

INDICATIONS & DOSAGES
➤ **Adjunct to diet and exercise to reduce total-cholesterol (C), LDL-C, and apolipoprotein B (Apo B) levels in patients with primary hypercholesterolemia, alone or combined with HMG-CoA reductase inhibitors (statins) or bile acid sequestrants; adjunct to other lipid-lowering drugs (combined with atorvastatin or simvastatin) in patients with homozygous familial hypercholesterolemia; adjunct to diet in patients with homozygous sitosterolemia to reduce sitosterol and campesterol levels; adjunct to fenofibrate and diet to reduce total-C, LDL-C, Apo B, and non–HDL-C levels in patients with mixed hyperlipidemia**
Adults and children age 10 and older: 10 mg P.O. daily.

ADMINISTRATION
P.O.
• Give drug without regard for meals.

ACTION

Inhibits absorption of cholesterol by the small intestine, unlike other drugs used for cholesterol reduction; causes reduced hepatic cholesterol stores and increased cholesterol clearance from the blood.

Route	Onset	Peak	Duration
P.O.	Unknown	4–12 hr	Unknown

Half-life: 22 hours.

ADVERSE REACTIONS

CNS: dizziness, fatigue, headache.
CV: chest pain.
EENT: pharyngitis, sinusitis.
GI: abdominal pain, diarrhea.
Musculoskeletal: arthralgia, back pain, myalgia.
Respiratory: *upper respiratory tract infection,* cough.
Other: viral infection.

INTERACTIONS

Drug-drug. *Bile acid sequestrant (cholestyramine):* May decrease ezetimibe level. Give ezetimibe at least 2 hours before or 4 hours after cholestyramine. *Cyclosporine, fenofibrate, gemfibrozil:* May increase ezetimibe level. Monitor patient for adverse reactions. *Fibrates:* May increase excretion of cholesterol into the gallbladder bile. Avoid using together.

EFFECTS ON LAB TEST RESULTS

• May increase liver function test values.

CONTRAINDICATIONS & CAUTIONS

• Contraindicated in patients allergic to any component of the drug.
• Contraindicated with HMG-CoA reductase inhibitor in pregnant or breast-feeding women and in patients with active hepatic disease or unexplained increased transaminase level.
• Use cautiously in elderly patients.

NURSING CONSIDERATIONS

• Before starting treatment, assess patient for underlying causes of dyslipidemia.
• Obtain baseline triglyceride and total, LDL, and HDL cholesterol levels.
• Using drug with an HMG-CoA reductase inhibitor significantly decreases total and LDL cholesterol, apolipoprotein B, and triglyceride levels and (except with pravastatin) increases HDL cholesterol level more than use of an HMG-CoA reductase inhibitor alone. Check liver function test values when therapy starts and thereafter according to the HMG-CoA reductase inhibitor manufacturer's recommendations.
• Patient should maintain a cholesterol-lowering diet during treatment.

PATIENT TEACHING

• Emphasize importance of following a cholesterol-lowering diet during drug therapy.
• Tell patient he may take drug without regard for meals.
• Advise patient to notify prescriber of unexplained muscle pain, weakness, or tenderness.
• Urge patient to tell his prescriber about any herbal or dietary supplements he's taking.
• Advise patient to visit his prescriber for routine follow-ups and blood tests.
• Tell woman to notify prescriber if she becomes pregnant.

fenofibrate
fee-no-FYE-brate

Antara, Lipofen, Lofibra, TriCor, Triglide

Pharmacologic class: fibric acid derivative
Pregnancy risk category C

AVAILABLE FORMS

Capsules: 50 mg, 100 mg, 150 mg
Capsules (micronized): 43 mg, 67 mg, 130 mg, 134 mg, 200 mg
Tablets: 48 mg, 50 mg, 54 mg, 145 mg, 160 mg

INDICATIONS & DOSAGES

➤ **Hypertriglyceridemia (Fredrickson types IV and V hyperlipidemia) in patients who don't respond adequately to diet alone**
Adults: For Antara, initial dose is 43 to 130 mg P.O. daily. Maximum dose,

130 mg daily. For Lipofen, initial dose is 50 to 150 mg daily. Maximum dose, 150 mg daily. For Lofibra capsules, initial dose is 67 to 200 mg daily. Maximum dose, 200 mg daily. For Lofibra tablets, initial dose is 54 to 160 mg daily. Maximum dose, 160 mg daily. For TriCor, initial dose is 48 to 145 mg daily. Maximum dose, 145 mg daily. For Triglide, initial dose is 50 to 160 mg daily. Maximum dose, 160 mg daily. For all forms, adjust dose based on patient response and repeat lipid determinations every 4 to 8 weeks.

➤ **Primary hypercholesterolemia or mixed dyslipidemia (Fredrickson types IIa and IIb) in patients who don't respond adequately to diet alone**

Adults: For Antara, initial dose is 130 mg P.O. daily. For Lipofen, initial dose is 150 mg daily. For Lofibra, initial dose is 200 mg (capsules) or 160 mg (tablets) daily. For TriCor, initial dose is 145 mg daily. For Triglide, initial dose is 160 mg daily. May reduce dose if lipid levels fall significantly below the target range.

➤ **Hyperuricemia ◆**

Adults: 200 mg/day (micronized formulation) P.O. for up to 12 months or 100 mg t.i.d. for 6 weeks.

Adjust-a-dose: If creatinine clearance is less than 50 ml/minute or in elderly patients, initially 43 mg daily for Antara, 50 mg daily for Lipofen, 67 mg daily for Lofibra capsules or 54 mg daily for Lofibra tablets, 48 mg daily for TriCor, or 50 mg daily for Triglide. Increase only after evaluating effects on renal function and triglyceride level at this dose.

ADMINISTRATION
P.O.
● Give Lipofen or Lofibra capsules with food to enhance absorption; give other preparations without regard for food.

ACTION
May lower triglyceride levels by inhibiting triglyceride synthesis with less very–low-density lipoproteins released into circulation. Drug may also stimulate breakdown of triglyceride-rich protein.

Route	Onset	Peak	Duration
P.O.	Unknown	6–8 hr	Unknown

Half-life: 20 hours.

ADVERSE REACTIONS
CNS: *dizziness, headache,* asthenia, fatigue, insomnia, localized pain, paresthesia.
CV: *arrhythmias.*
EENT: blurred vision, conjunctivitis, earache, eye discomfort, eye floaters, rhinitis, sinusitis.
GI: abdominal pain, constipation, diarrhea, dyspepsia, eructation, flatulence, increased appetite, nausea, vomiting.
GU: polyuria, vaginitis.
Musculoskeletal: arthralgia.
Respiratory: cough.
Skin: pruritus, rash.
Other: *infection,* decreased libido, flulike syndrome, hypersensitivity reactions.

INTERACTIONS
Drug-drug. *Bile-acid sequestrants:* May bind and inhibit absorption of fenofibrate. Give drug 1 hour before or 4 to 6 hours after bile-acid sequestrants.
Coumarin-type anticoagulants: May potentiate anticoagulant effect, prolonging PT and INR. Monitor PT and INR closely. May need to reduce anticoagulant dosage.
Cyclosporine, immunosuppressants, nephrotoxic drugs: May induce renal dysfunction that may affect fenofibrate elimination. Use together cautiously.
HMG-CoA reductase inhibitors: May increase risk of adverse musculoskeletal effects. Avoid using together, unless potential benefit outweighs risk.
Drug-food. *Any food:* May increase capsule absorption. Advise patient to take capsule with meals.
Drug-lifestyle. *Alcohol use:* May increase triglyceride levels. Discourage use together.

EFFECTS ON LAB TEST RESULTS
● May increase ALT, AST, BUN, CK, and creatinine levels. May decrease uric acid and hemoglobin levels and hematocrit.
● May decrease WBC count.

Reactions may be *common,* uncommon, *life-threatening,* or COMMON AND LIFE-THREATENING.
Interaction may have a *rapid onset* or **delayed onset.**

CONTRAINDICATIONS & CAUTIONS
• Contraindicated in patients hypersensitive to drug and in those with gallbladder disease, hepatic dysfunction, primary biliary cirrhosis, severe renal dysfunction, or unexplained persistent liver function abnormalities.
• Use cautiously in patients with a history of pancreatitis.

NURSING CONSIDERATIONS
• Obtain baseline lipid levels and liver function test results before therapy, and monitor liver function periodically during therapy. Stop drug if enzyme levels persist above three times normal.
• Watch for signs and symptoms of pancreatitis, myositis, rhabdomyolysis, cholelithiasis, and renal failure. Monitor patient for muscle pain, tenderness, or weakness, especially with malaise or fever.
• If an adequate response isn't obtained after 2 months of treatment with maximum daily dose, stop therapy.
• Drug lowers uric acid level by increasing uric acid excretion in patients with or without hyperuricemia.
• Beta blockers, estrogens, and thiazide diuretics may increase triglyceride levels; evaluate need for continued use of these drugs.
• Hemoglobin level, hematocrit, and WBC count may decrease when therapy starts but will stabilize with long-term administration.

PATIENT TEACHING
• Inform patient that drug therapy doesn't reduce need for following a triglyceride-lowering diet.
• Advise patient to promptly report unexplained muscle weakness, pain, or tenderness, especially with malaise or fever.
• Tell patient to take capsules with meals for best drug absorption.
• Advise patient to continue weight control measures, including diet and exercise, and to limit alcohol before therapy.
• Instruct patient who is also taking a bile-acid resin to take fenofibrate 1 hour before or 4 to 6 hours after resin.
• Advise patient about risk of tumor growth.
• Tell breast-feeding woman to either stop breast-feeding or stop taking drug.

fluvastatin sodium
flue-va-STA-tin

Lescol✍, Lescol XL

Pharmacologic class: HMG-CoA reductase inhibitor
Pregnancy risk category X

AVAILABLE FORMS
Capsules: 20 mg, 40 mg
Tablets (extended-release): 80 mg

INDICATIONS & DOSAGES
➤ To reduce LDL and total cholesterol levels in patients with primary hypercholesterolemia (types IIa and IIb); to slow progression of coronary atherosclerosis in patients with coronary artery disease; elevated triglyceride and apolipoprotein B (apoB) levels in patients with primary hypercholesterolemia and mixed dyslipidemia whose response to dietary restriction and other nonpharmacologic measures has been inadequate
Adults: Initially, 20 to 40 mg P.O. at bedtime, increasing if needed to maximum of 80 mg daily in divided doses or 80 mg Lescol XL P.O. at bedtime.
✱ *NEW INDICATION:* Adjunct to diet to reduce LDL, total cholesterol, and apoB levels in patients with heterozygous familial hypercholesterolemia whose response to dietary restriction hasn't been adequate and for whom the following findings are present: LDL-C remains at 190 mg/dl or more; or LDL-C remains at 160 mg/dl or more and there's a positive family history of premature cardiovascular disease or two or more other cardiovascular disease risk factors are present
Adolescent boys and girls (who are at least 1 year postmenarche) ages 10 to 16: 20 mg P.O. once daily at bedtime. Dosage adjustments may be made at 6-week intervals up to maximum of 40 mg (capsule) P.O. b.i.d. or 80 mg extended-release tablet P.O. once daily.

➤ **To reduce the risk of undergoing coronary revascularization procedures**
Adults: In patients who must reduce LDL cholesterol level by at least 25%, initially, 40 mg P.O. once daily or b.i.d.; or one 80-mg extended-release tablet as a single dose in the evening. In patients who must reduce LDL cholesterol level by less than 25%, initially, 20 mg P.O. daily. Dosages range from 20 to 80 mg daily.

ADMINISTRATION
P.O.
● Give drug without regard for meals.
● For once-daily dosage, give immediate-release capsules in the evening.
● Don't crush or break tablets; don't open capsules.

ACTION
Inhibits HMG-CoA reductase, an early (and rate-limiting) step in the synthetic pathway of cholesterol.

Route	Onset	Peak	Duration
P.O.	Unknown	1 hr	Unknown

Half-life: Less than 1 hour.

ADVERSE REACTIONS
CNS: dizziness, fatigue, headache, insomnia.
EENT: pharyngitis, rhinitis, sinusitis.
GI: abdominal pain, constipation, diarrhea, dyspepsia, flatulence, nausea, vomiting.
Hematologic: *leukopenia, thrombo-cytopenia,* hemolytic anemia.
Musculoskeletal: *rhabdomyolysis,* arthralgia, back pain, myalgia.
Respiratory: *upper respiratory tract infection,* bronchitis, cough.
Other: hypersensitivity reactions.

INTERACTIONS
Drug-drug. *Cholestyramine, colestipol:* May bind with fluvastatin in the GI tract and decrease absorption. Separate doses by at least 4 hours.
Cimetidine, omeprazole, ranitidine: May decrease fluvastatin metabolism. Monitor patient for enhanced effects.
Cyclosporine and other immuno-suppressants, erythromycin, gemfibrozil, niacin: May increase risk of poly-myositis and rhabdomyolysis. Avoid using together.
Digoxin: May alter digoxin pharmacokinetics. Monitor digoxin level carefully.
Fluconazole, itraconazole, ketoconazole: May increase fluvastatin level and adverse effects. Use cautiously together, or, if given together, reduce dose of fluvastatin.
Glyburide: May increase levels of both drugs. Monitor serum glucose and signs and symptoms of toxicity.
Phenytoin: May increase phenytoin levels. Monitor phenytoin levels.
Rifampin: May enhance fluvastatin metabolism and decrease levels. Monitor patient for lack of effect.
Warfarin: May increase anticoagulant effect with bleeding. Monitor PT and INR.
Drug-herb. *Eucalyptus, jin bu huan, kava:* May increase risk of hepatotoxicity. Discourage use together.
Red yeast rice: May increase risk of adverse reactions because herb contains compounds similar to those in drug. Discourage use together.
Drug-lifestyle. *Alcohol use:* May increase risk of hepatotoxicity. Discourage use together.

EFFECTS ON LAB TEST RESULTS
● May increase ALT, AST, and CK levels. May decrease hemoglobin level and hematocrit.
● May decrease platelet and WBC counts.

CONTRAINDICATIONS & CAUTIONS
● Contraindicated in patients hypersensitive to drug and in those with active liver disease or unexplained persistent elevations of transaminase levels; also contraindicated in pregnant and breast-feeding women and in women of childbearing age.
● Use cautiously in patients with severe renal impairment and history of liver disease or heavy alcohol use.

NURSING CONSIDERATIONS
● Patient should follow a diet restricted in saturated fat and cholesterol during therapy.
● Test liver function at start of therapy, at 12 weeks after start of therapy,

---

Reactions may be *common,* uncommon, ***life-threatening,*** or COMMON AND LIFE-THREATENING.
Interaction may have a *rapid onset* or ***delayed onset.***

12 weeks after an increase in dose, and then periodically. Stop drug if there is a persistent increase in ALT or AST levels of at least three times the upper limit of normal.
• Watch for signs of myositis.
• *Look alike–sound alike:* Don't confuse fluvastatin with fluoxetine.

PATIENT TEACHING
• Tell patient that drug may be taken without regard for meals; if taken once daily, immediate-release capsules are taken in the evening.
• Advise the patient who is also taking a bile-acid resin such as cholestyramine to take fluvastatin at bedtime, at least 4 hours after taking the resin.
• Teach patient about proper dietary management, weight control, and exercise. Explain their importance in controlling elevated cholesterol and triglyceride levels.
• Warn patient to avoid alcohol.
• Tell patient to notify prescriber of adverse reactions, especially muscle aches and pains.
• Advise patient that it may take up to 4 weeks for the drug to be completely effective.
• *Alert:* Tell woman of childbearing age to stop drug and notify prescriber immediately if she is or may be pregnant or if she's breast-feeding.

---

gemfibrozil
jem-FI-broe-zil

Lopid◆

Pharmacologic class: fibric acid derivative
Pregnancy risk category C

AVAILABLE FORMS
Tablets: 600 mg

INDICATIONS & DOSAGES
➤ **Types IV and V hyperlipidemia unresponsive to diet and other drugs; to reduce risk of coronary heart disease in patients with type IIb hyperlipidemia who can't tolerate or who are refractory to treatment with bile-acid sequestrants or niacin**
Adults: 1,200 mg P.O. daily in two divided doses, 30 minutes before morning and evening meals.

ADMINISTRATION
P.O.
• Give drug 30 minutes before breakfast and dinner.

ACTION
Inhibits peripheral lipolysis and reduces triglyceride synthesis in the liver; lowers triglyceride levels and increases HDL cholesterol levels.

Route	Onset	Peak	Duration
P.O.	2–5 days	4 wk	Unknown

Half-life: 1¼ hours.

ADVERSE REACTIONS
CNS: fatigue, headache, vertigo.
CV: atrial fibrillation.
GI: *abdominal and epigastric pain,* dyspepsia, acute appendicitis, constipation, diarrhea, nausea, vomiting.
Hematologic: *leukopenia, thrombocytopenia,* anemia, eosinophilia.
Hepatic: bile duct obstruction.
Metabolic: hypokalemia.
Skin: dermatitis, eczema, pruritus, rash.

INTERACTIONS
Drug-drug. *Cyclosporine:* May decrease cyclosporine levels. Monitor cyclosporine levels and adjust dose as needed.
Glyburide: May increase hypoglycemic effects. Monitor glucose level, and watch for signs of hypoglycemia.
HMG-CoA reductase inhibitors: May cause myopathy with rhabdomyolysis. Avoid using together.
Oral anticoagulants: May enhance effects of oral anticoagulants. Monitor patient closely.
Repaglinide: May increase repaglinide level. Avoid using together if possible. If already taking both drugs, monitor glucose levels and adjust repaglinide dosage.

EFFECTS ON LAB TEST RESULTS

● May increase ALT, AST, and CK levels. May decrease potassium and hemoglobin levels and hematocrit.
● May decrease eosinophil, WBC, and platelet counts.

CONTRAINDICATIONS & CAUTIONS

● Contraindicated in patients hypersensitive to drug and in those with hepatic or severe renal dysfunction (including primary biliary cirrhosis) or gallbladder disease.

NURSING CONSIDERATIONS

● Check CBC and test liver function periodically during the first 12 months of therapy.
● If drug has no benefits after 3 months of therapy, stop drug.
● Patient shouldn't take drug together with repaglinide or itraconazole.

PATIENT TEACHING

● Instruct patient to take drug 30 minutes before breakfast and dinner.
● Teach patient about proper dietary management of cholesterol and triglycerides. When appropriate, recommend weight control, exercise, and smoking cessation programs.
● Because of possible dizziness and blurred vision, advise patient to avoid driving and other hazardous activities until effects of drug are known.
● Tell patient to observe bowel movements and to report evidence of excess fat in feces or other signs of bile duct obstruction.
● Advise patient to report muscle pain to prescriber if occurs during therapy.

---

lovastatin (mevinolin)
loe-va-STA-tin

Altoprev, Mevacor⬦

Pharmacologic class: HMG-CoA reductase inhibitor
Pregnancy risk category X

AVAILABLE FORMS
Tablets: 10 mg, 20 mg, 40 mg
Tablets (extended-release): 10 mg, 20 mg, 40 mg, 60 mg

INDICATIONS & DOSAGES
➤ **To prevent and treat coronary heart disease; hyperlipidemia**
Adults: Initially, 20 mg P.O. once daily with evening meal. Recommended range is 10 to 80 mg as a single dose or in two divided doses; maximum daily recommended dose is 80 mg.
Or, 20 to 60 mg extended-release tablets P.O. at bedtime. Starting dose of 10 mg can be used for patients requiring smaller reductions; usual dosage range is 10 to 60 mg daily.
➤ **Heterozygous familial hypercholesterolemia in adolescents**
Adolescents ages 10 to 17: Give 10 to 40 mg daily P.O. with evening meal. Patients requiring reductions in LDL cholesterol level of 20% or more should start with 20 mg daily.
Adjust-a-dose: For patients also taking cyclosporine, give 10 mg P.O. daily, not to exceed 20 mg daily. Avoid use of lovastatin with fibrates or niacin; if combined with either, the dosage of lovastatin shouldn't exceed 20 mg daily. For patients also taking amiodarone or verapamil, the dosage of lovastatin shouldn't exceed 40 mg daily. For patients with creatinine clearance less than 30 ml/minute, carefully consider dosage increase greater than 20 mg daily and implement cautiously if necessary.

ADMINISTRATION
P.O.
● Give drug with evening meal, which improves absorption and cholesterol biosynthesis.
● Don't crush or split extended-release tablets.

ACTION
Inhibits HMG-CoA reductase, an early (and rate-limiting) step in cholesterol biosynthesis.

Route	Onset	Peak	Duration
P.O.	Unknown	2 hr	Unknown
P.O. (extended-release)	Unknown	14 hr	Unknown

Half-life: 3 hours.

Reactions may be *common*, uncommon, *life-threatening*, or COMMON AND LIFE-THREATENING.
Interaction may have a *rapid onset* or *delayed onset*.

ADVERSE REACTIONS

CNS: *headache,* dizziness, insomnia, peripheral neuropathy.

CV: chest pain.

EENT: blurred vision.

GI: abdominal pain or cramps, constipation, diarrhea, dyspepsia, flatulence, heartburn, nausea, vomiting.

Musculoskeletal: muscle cramps, myalgia, myositis, *rhabdomyolysis.*

Skin: alopecia, rash, pruritus.

INTERACTIONS

Drug-drug. *Amiodarone,* **verapamil:** May cause myopathy and rhabdomyolysis. Don't exceed 40 mg lovastatin daily.

Azole antifungals, **protease inhibitors:** May cause myopathy and rhabdomyolysis. Avoid using together.

Cyclosporine, *danazol, gemfibrozil or other fibrates, niacin:* May cause myopathy and rhabdomyolysis. Don't exceed 20 mg lovastatin daily.

Diltiazem, macrolides (azithromycin, clarithromycin, erythromycin, telithromycin), nefazodone: May decrease metabolism of HMG-CoA reductase inhibitor, increasing toxicity. Monitor patient for adverse effects and report unexplained muscle pain.

Oral anticoagulants: May increase oral anticoagulant effect. Monitor patient closely.

Drug-herb. *Eucalyptus, jin bu huan, kava:* May increase risk of hepatotoxicity. Discourage use together.

Pectin: May decrease drug effect. Discourage use together.

Red yeast rice: May increase risk of adverse reactions because herb contains compounds similar to those in drug. Discourage use together.

Drug-food. *Grapefruit juice:* May increase drug level, increasing risk of adverse effects. Discourage use together.

Drug-lifestyle. *Alcohol use:* May increase risk of hepatotoxicity. Discourage use together.

EFFECTS ON LAB TEST RESULTS

● May increase ALT, AST, and CK levels.

CONTRAINDICATIONS & CAUTIONS

● Contraindicated in patients hypersensitive to drug and in those with active liver disease or unexplained persistently increased transaminase level.

● Contraindicated in pregnant and breast-feeding women and in women of childbearing age.

● Use cautiously in patients who consume substantial quantities of alcohol or have a history of liver disease.

NURSING CONSIDERATIONS

● Have patient follow a diet restricted in saturated fat and cholesterol during therapy.

● Obtain liver function test results at the start of therapy, at 6 and 12 weeks after the start of therapy, and when increasing dose; then monitor results periodically.

● Heterozygous familial hypercholesterolemia can be diagnosed in adolescent boys and in girls who are at least 1 year postmenarche and are 10 to 17 years old; if after an adequate trial of diet therapy LDL cholesterol level remains over 189 mg/dl or LDL cholesterol over 160 mg/dl and patient has a positive family history of premature CV disease or two or more other CV disease risk factors.

● *Look alike–sound alike:* Don't confuse lovastatin with Lotensin, Leustatin, or Livostin. Don't confuse Mevacor with Mivacron.

PATIENT TEACHING

● Instruct patient to take drug with the evening meal.

● Teach patient about proper dietary management of cholesterol and triglycerides. When appropriate, recommend weight control, exercise, and smoking cessation programs.

● Advise patient to have periodic eye examinations; related compounds cause cataracts.

● Instruct patient to store tablets at room temperature in a light-resistant container.

● Advise patient to promptly report unexplained muscle pain, tenderness, or weakness, particularly when accompanied by malaise or fever.

● *Alert:* Tell woman to stop drug and notify prescriber immediately if she is or may be pregnant or if she's breast-feeding.

● *Alert:* Advise patient not to crush or chew extended-release tablets.

omega-3–acid ethyl esters
oh-may-gah-three-ASS-id

Lovaza

Pharmacologic class: ethyl ester
Pregnancy risk category C

AVAILABLE FORMS
Capsules: 1 g

INDICATIONS & DOSAGES
➤ **Adjunct to diet to reduce triglyceride levels 500 mg/dl or higher**
Adults: 4 g P.O. once daily or divided as 2 g b.i.d.

ADMINISTRATION
P.O.
● Give drug without regard for meals.

ACTION
May reduce hepatic formation of triglycerides because two components of drug are poor substrates for the necessary enzymes. These components also block formation of other fatty acids.

Route	Onset	Peak	Duration
P.O.	Unknown	Unknown	Unknown

Half-life: Unknown.

ADVERSE REACTIONS
CNS: pain.
CV: angina pectoris.
GI: altered taste, belching, dyspepsia.
Musculoskeletal: back pain.
Skin: rash.
Other: flulike syndrome, infection.

INTERACTIONS
Drug-drug. *Anticoagulants:* May prolong bleeding time. Monitor patient.

EFFECTS ON LAB TEST RESULTS
● May increase ALT and LDL cholesterol levels.

CONTRAINDICATIONS & CAUTIONS
● Contraindicated in patients hypersensitive to drug or its components.
● Use cautiously in patients sensitive to fish.

NURSING CONSIDERATIONS
● Assess patient for conditions that contribute to increased triglycerides, such as diabetes and hypothyroidism, before treatment.
● Evaluate patient's current drug regimen for any drugs known to sharply increase triglyceride levels, including estrogen therapy, thiazide diuretics, and beta blockers. Stopping these drugs, if appropriate, may negate the need for drug.
● Continue diet and lifestyle modifications during treatment.
● Obtain baseline triglyceride levels to confirm that they're consistently abnormal before therapy; then recheck periodically during treatment. If patient has an inadequate response after 2 months, stop drug.
● Monitor LDL level to make sure it doesn't increase excessively during treatment.
● *Look alike–sound alike:* Don't confuse Lovaza with lorazepam or lovastatin.

PATIENT TEACHING
● Explain that taking drug doesn't reduce the importance of following the recommended diet and exercise plan.
● Remind patient of the need for follow-up blood work to evaluate progress.
● Advise patient to notify prescriber about bothersome side effects.
● Tell patient to report planned or suspected pregnancy.

pravastatin sodium (eptastatin)
prah-va-STA-tin

Pravachol⬩

Pharmacologic class: HMG-CoA reductase inhibitor
Pregnancy risk category X

AVAILABLE FORMS
Tablets: 10 mg, 20 mg, 40 mg, 80 mg

INDICATIONS & DOSAGES
➤ **Primary and secondary prevention of coronary events; hyperlipidemia**
Adults: Initially, 40 mg P.O. once daily at the same time each day, with or without food. Adjust dosage every 4 weeks, based

---

Reactions may be *common*, uncommon, *life-threatening*, or COMMON AND LIFE-THREATENING.
Interaction may have a *rapid onset* or **delayed onset.**

on patient tolerance and response; maximum daily dose is 80 mg.
➤ **Heterozygous familial hypercholesterolemia**
Adolescents ages 14 to 18: Give 40 mg P.O. once daily.
Children ages 8 to 13: Give 20 mg P.O. once daily.
Adjust-a-dose: In patients with renal or hepatic dysfunction, start with 10 mg P.O. daily. In patients taking immunosuppressants, begin with 10 mg P.O. at bedtime and adjust to higher dosages with caution. Most patients treated with the combination of immunosuppressants and pravastatin receive up to 20 mg pravastatin daily.

ADMINISTRATION
P.O.
● Give drug without regard for meals.

ACTION
Inhibits HMG-CoA reductase, an early (and rate-limiting) step in cholesterol biosynthesis.

Route	Onset	Peak	Duration
P.O.	Unknown	60–90 min	Unknown

Half-life: 1¼ to 2¼ hours.

ADVERSE REACTIONS
CNS: dizziness, fatigue, headache.
CV: chest pain.
EENT: rhinitis.
GI: *nausea,* abdominal pain, constipation, diarrhea, flatulence, heartburn, vomiting.
GU: *renal failure caused by myoglobinuria,* urinary abnormality.
Musculoskeletal: *localized muscle pain, rhabdomyolysis,* myalgia, myopathy, myositis.
Respiratory: common cold, cough.
Skin: rash.
Other: flulike symptoms, influenza.

INTERACTIONS
Drug-drug. *Cholestyramine, colestipol:* May decrease pravastatin level. Give pravastatin 1 hour before or 4 hours after these drugs.
Cyclosporine: May decrease metabolism of HMG-CoA reductase inhibitor, increasing toxicity. Monitor patient for adverse effects and report unexplained muscle pain.

Erythromycin, fibric acid derivatives (such as clofibrate, gemfibrozil), immunosuppressants, high doses (1 g or more daily) of niacin (nicotinic acid): May cause rhabdomyolysis. Avoid using together; if unavoidable, monitor patient closely.
Fluconazole, itraconazole, ketoconazole: May increase pravastatin level and adverse effects. Avoid using together; if unavoidable, reduce dose of pravastatin.
Gemfibrozil: May decrease protein-binding and urinary clearance of pravastatin. Avoid using together.
Hepatotoxic drugs: May increase risk of hepatotoxicity. Avoid using together.
Drug-herb. *Eucalyptus, jin bu huan, kava:* May increase the risk of hepatotoxicity. Discourage use together.
Red yeast rice: May increase risk of adverse reactions because herb contains compounds similar to those in drug. Discourage use together.
Drug-lifestyle. *Alcohol use:* May increase risk of hepatotoxicity. Discourage use together.

EFFECTS ON LAB TEST RESULTS
● May increase ALT, AST, CK, alkaline phosphatase, and bilirubin levels.
● May alter thyroid function test values.

CONTRAINDICATIONS & CAUTIONS
● Contraindicated in patients hypersensitive to drug and in those with active liver disease or conditions that cause unexplained, persistent elevations of transaminase levels.
● Contraindicated in pregnant and breastfeeding women and in women of childbearing age.
● Use cautiously in patients who consume large quantities of alcohol or have history of liver disease.
● Safety and efficacy in children younger than age 8 haven't been established.

NURSING CONSIDERATIONS
● Patient should follow a diet restricted in saturated fat and cholesterol during therapy.
● Use in children with heterozygous familial hypercholesterolemia if LDL cholesterol level is at least 190 mg/dl, or if LDL cholesterol is at least 160 mg/dl and patient has either a positive family history of premature CV disease or two or more other CV disease risk factors.

● Obtain liver function test results at start of therapy and then periodically. A liver biopsy may be performed if elevated liver enzyme levels persist.
● *Look alike–sound alike:* Don't confuse Pravachol with Prevacid or propranolol.

PATIENT TEACHING
● Advise patient who is also taking a bile-acid resin such as cholestyramine to take pravastatin at least 1 hour before or 4 hours after taking resin.
● Tell patient to notify prescriber of adverse reactions, particularly muscle aches and pains.
● Teach patient about proper dietary management of cholesterol and triglycerides. When appropriate, recommend weight control, exercise, and smoking cessation programs.
● Inform patient that it will take up to 4 weeks to achieve full therapeutic effect.
● *Alert:* Tell woman of childbearing age to stop drug and notify prescriber immediately if she is or may be pregnant or if she's breast-feeding.

---

rosuvastatin calcium
row-SUE-va-sta-tin

Crestor⧫

Pharmacologic class: HMG-CoA reductase inhibitor
Pregnancy risk category X

AVAILABLE FORMS
Tablets: 5 mg, 10 mg, 20 mg, 40 mg

INDICATIONS & DOSAGES
➤ **Adjunct to diet to reduce LDL cholesterol, total cholesterol, apolipoprotein B, non-HDL cholesterol, and triglyceride (TG) levels and to increase HDL cholesterol level in patients with primary hypercholesterolemia (heterozygous familial and nonfamilial) and mixed dyslipidemia (Fredrickson types IIa and IIb); adjunct to diet to treat elevated TG level (Fredrickson type IV)**
Adults: Initially, 10 mg P.O. once daily; 5 mg P.O. once daily in patients needing

less aggressive LDL cholesterol level reduction or those predisposed to myopathy. For aggressive lipid lowering, initially, 20 mg P.O. once daily. Increase as needed to maximum of 40 mg P.O. daily. Dosage may be increased every 2 to 4 weeks, based on lipid levels.
➤ **Adjunct to diet to slow atherosclerosis progression in patients with elevated cholesterol**
Adults: Initially, 10 mg P.O. daily. Increase as needed every 2 to 4 weeks based on lipid levels, to maximum of 40 mg daily.
➤ **Adjunct to lipid-lowering therapies; to reduce LDL cholesterol, apolipoprotein B, and total cholesterol levels in homozygous familial hypercholesterolemia**
Adults: Initially, 20 mg P.O. once daily. Maximum, 40 mg once daily.
Adjust-a-dose: If creatinine clearance is less than 30 ml/minute, initially, 5 mg once daily; don't exceed 10 mg once daily. For Asian patients, initial dose is 5 mg. For patients also taking cyclosporine, limit rosuvastatin dose to 5 mg once daily. For patients taking combination of lopinavir and ritonavir, limit rosuvastatin dose to 10 mg once daily.

ADMINISTRATION
P.O.
● Give drug without regard for meals.
● Wait 2 hours after giving dose to give aluminum- or magnesium-containing antacid.

ACTION
Inhibits HMG-CoA reductase, increases LDL receptors on liver cells, and inhibits hepatic synthesis of very–low-density lipoprotein.

Route	Onset	Peak	Duration
P.O.	Unknown	3–5 hr	Unknown

Half-life: About 19 hours.

ADVERSE REACTIONS
CNS: anxiety, asthenia, depression, dizziness, headache, insomnia, neuralgia, pain, paresthesia, vertigo.
CV: angina pectoris, chest pain, hypertension, palpitations, peripheral edema, vasodilation.

Reactions may be *common*, uncommon, *life-threatening*, or COMMON AND LIFE-THREATENING.
Interaction may have a *rapid onset* or *delayed onset.*

EENT: pharyngitis, rhinitis, sinusitis.
GI: abdominal pain, constipation, diarrhea, dyspepsia, flatulence, gastritis, gastroenteritis, nausea, periodontal abscess, vomiting.
GU: UTI.
Hematologic: anemia, ecchymosis.
Metabolic: diabetes mellitus.
Musculoskeletal: arthralgia, arthritis, back pain, hypertonia, myalgia, neck pain, pathologic fracture, pelvic pain.
Respiratory: asthma, bronchitis, dyspnea, increased cough, pneumonia.
Skin: pruritus, rash.
Other: accidental injury, flulike syndrome, infection.

INTERACTIONS
Drug-drug. *Antacids:* May decrease rosuvastatin level. Give antacids at least 2 hours after rosuvastatin.
Cimetidine, ketoconazole, spironolactone: May decrease level or effect of endogenous steroid hormones. Use together cautiously.
Cyclosporine: May increase rosuvastatin level and risk of myopathy or rhabdomyolysis. Don't exceed 5 mg of rosuvastatin daily. Watch for evidence of toxicity.
Gemfibrozil: May increase rosuvastatin level and risk of myopathy or rhabdomyolysis. Don't exceed 10 mg of rosuvastatin once daily. Watch for evidence of toxicity.
Hormonal contraceptives: May increase ethinyl estradiol and norgestrel levels. Watch for adverse effects.
Lopinavir/ritonavir: This drug combination increases exposure to rosuvastatin. Limit dose of rosuvastatin to 10 mg once daily.
Warfarin: May increase INR and risk of bleeding. Monitor INR, and watch for evidence of increased bleeding.
Drug-lifestyle. *Alcohol use:* May increase risk of hepatotoxicity. Discourage use together.

EFFECTS ON LAB TEST RESULTS
• May increase CK, transaminase, glucose, glutamyl transpeptidase, alkaline phosphatase, and bilirubin levels. May decrease hemoglobin level and hematocrit.
• May cause thyroid function abnormalities, dipstick-positive proteinuria, and microscopic hematuria.

CONTRAINDICATIONS & CAUTIONS
• Contraindicated in patients hypersensitive to rosuvastatin or its components, pregnant patients, patients with active liver disease, and those with unexplained persistently increased transaminases.
• Use cautiously in patients who drink substantial amounts of alcohol or have a history of liver disease and in those at increased risk for myopathies, such as those with renal impairment, advanced age, or hypothyroidism.
• Use cautiously in Asian patients because they have a greater risk of elevated drug levels.

NURSING CONSIDERATIONS
• Before therapy starts, assess patient for underlying causes of hypercholesterolemia, including poorly controlled diabetes, hypothyroidism, nephrotic syndrome, dyslipoproteinemias, obstructive liver disease, drug interaction, and alcoholism.
• Before therapy starts, advise patient to control hypercholesterolemia with diet, exercise, and weight reduction.
• Test liver function before therapy starts, 12 weeks afterward, 12 weeks after any increase in dosage, and twice a year routinely. If AST or ALT level persists at more than three times the upper limit of normal, decrease dose or stop drug.
• **Alert:** Rarely, rhabdomyolysis with acute renal failure has developed in patients taking drugs in this class, including rosuvastatin.
• Patients who are 65 or older, have hypothyroidism, or have renal insufficiency may be at a greater risk for developing myopathy while receiving a statin.
• Notify prescriber if CK level becomes markedly elevated or myopathy is suspected, or if routine urinalysis shows persistent proteinuria and patient is taking 40 mg daily.
• Withhold drug temporarily if patient becomes predisposed to myopathy or rhabdomyolysis because of sepsis, hypotension, major surgery, trauma, uncontrolled seizures, or severe metabolic, endocrine, or electrolyte disorders.

PATIENT TEACHING
• Instruct patient to take drug exactly as prescribed.

- Teach patient about diet, exercise, and weight control.
- Tell patient to immediately report unexplained muscle pain, tenderness, or weakness, especially if accompanied by malaise or fever.
- Instruct patient to take drug at least 2 hours before taking aluminum- or magnesium-containing antacids.

---

simvastatin (synvinolin)
sim-va-STAH-tin

Zocor♦

Pharmacologic class: HMG-CoA reductase inhibitor
Pregnancy risk category X

AVAILABLE FORMS
Tablets: 5 mg, 10 mg, 20 mg, 40 mg, 80 mg

INDICATIONS & DOSAGES
➤ **To reduce risk of death from CV disease and CV events in patients at high risk for coronary events**
Adults: Initially, 20 to 40 mg P.O. daily in evening. In patients at high risk for a coronary heart disease event due to existing coronary heart disease, diabetes, peripheral vascular disease, or history of stroke, the recommended initial dose is 40 mg P.O. daily. Adjust dosage every 4 weeks based on patient tolerance and response. Maximum, 80 mg daily.
➤ **To reduce total and LDL cholesterol levels in patients with homozygous familial hypercholesterolemia**
Adults: 40 mg daily in evening; or, 80 mg daily in three divided doses of 20 mg in morning, 20 mg in afternoon, and 40 mg in evening.
➤ **Heterozygous familial hypercholesterolemia**
Children ages 10 to 17: Give 10 mg P.O. once daily in the evening. Maximum, 40 mg daily.
Adjust-a-dose: For patients taking cyclosporine, begin with 5 mg P.O. simvastatin daily; don't exceed 10 mg P.O. simvastatin daily. In patients taking fibrates or niacin, maximum is 10 mg P.O. simvastatin daily. In patients taking amiodarone or verapamil, maximum is 20 mg P.O. simvastatin daily.

In patients with severe renal insufficiency, start with 5 mg P.O. daily.

ADMINISTRATION
P.O.
- Give drug in the evening.

ACTION
Inhibits HMG-CoA reductase, an early (and rate-limiting) step in cholesterol biosynthesis.

Route	Onset	Peak	Duration
P.O.	Unknown	1–2 hr	Unknown

Half-life: 3 hours.

ADVERSE REACTIONS
CNS: asthenia, headache.
GI: abdominal pain, constipation, diarrhea, dyspepsia, flatulence, *nausea, vomiting.*
Respiratory: upper respiratory tract infection.

INTERACTIONS
Drug-drug. *Amiodarone, verapamil:* May increase risk of myopathy and rhabdomyolysis. Don't exceed 20 mg simvastatin daily.
Cyclosporine, fibrates, niacin: May increase risk of myopathy and rhabdomyolysis. Avoid using together; if unavoidable, monitor patient closely and don't exceed 10 mg simvastatin daily.
Digoxin: May slightly increase digoxin level. Closely monitor digoxin levels at the start of simvastatin therapy.
Diltiazem, macrolides (azithromycin, clarithromycin, erythromycin, telithromycin), nefazodone: May decrease metabolism of HMG-CoA reductase inhibitor, increasing toxicity. Monitor patient for adverse effects and report unexplained muscle pain.
Fluconazole, itraconazole, ketoconazole: May increase simvastatin level and adverse effects. Avoid using together or, if it can't be avoided, reduce dose of simvastatin.
Hepatotoxic drugs: May increase risk for hepatotoxicity. Avoid using together.
Protease inhibitors (amprenavir, atazanavir, indinavir, lopinavir and ritonavir, nelfinavir, ritonavir, saquinavir): May inhibit metabolism of simvastatin and

---

Reactions may be *common,* uncommon, *life-threatening,* or COMMON AND LIFE-THREATENING.
Interaction may have a *rapid onset* or **delayed onset.**

increase the risk of adverse effects, including rhabdomyolysis. Avoid using together.
Warfarin: May slightly enhance anticoagulant effect. Monitor PT and INR when therapy starts or dose is adjusted.
Drug-herb. *Eucalyptus, jin bu huan, kava:* May increase risk of hepatotoxicity. Discourage use together.
Red yeast rice: May increase risk of adverse events or toxicity because it contains similar components to those in drugs. Discourage use together.
Drug-food. *Grapefruit juice:* May increase drug levels, increasing risk of adverse effects including myopathy and rhabdomyolysis. Discourage use together.
Drug-lifestyle. *Alcohol use:* May increase risk of hepatotoxicity. Discourage use together.

EFFECTS ON LAB TEST RESULTS
• May increase ALT, AST, and CK levels.

CONTRAINDICATIONS & CAUTIONS
• Contraindicated in patients hypersensitive to drug and in those with active liver disease or conditions that cause unexplained persistent elevations of transaminase levels.
• Contraindicated in pregnant and breast-feeding women and in women of childbearing age.
• Use cautiously in patients who consume large amounts of alcohol or have a history of liver disease.

NURSING CONSIDERATIONS
• Patient should follow a diet restricted in saturated fat and cholesterol during therapy.
• Obtain liver function test results at start of therapy and then periodically. A liver biopsy may be performed if enzyme elevations persist.
• A daily dose of 40 mg significantly reduces risk of death from coronary heart disease, nonfatal MIs, stroke, and revascularization procedures.
• *Look alike–sound alike:* Don't confuse Zocor with Cozaar.

PATIENT TEACHING
• Instruct patient to take drug in the evening.
• Teach patient about proper dietary management of cholesterol and triglycerides.

When appropriate, recommend weight control, exercise, and smoking cessation programs.
• Tell patient to inform prescriber if adverse reactions occur, particularly muscle aches and pains.
• *Alert:* Tell woman to stop drug and notify prescriber immediately if she is or may be pregnant or if she's breast-feeding.

25
Diuretics

acetazolamide
acetazolamide sodium
bumetanide
ethacrynate sodium
ethacrynic acid
furosemide
hydrochlorothiazide
indapamide
mannitol
metolazone
spironolactone
torsemide
triamterene

---

acetazolamide
ah-set-a-ZOLE-ah-mide

Acetazolam†, Diamox Sequels

acetazolamide sodium

Pharmacologic class: carbonic
anhydrase inhibitor
Pregnancy risk category C

AVAILABLE FORMS
acetazolamide
Capsules (extended-release): 500 mg
Tablets: 125 mg, 250 mg
acetazolamide sodium
Powder for injection: 500-mg vial

INDICATIONS & DOSAGES
➤ **Secondary glaucoma; preoperative treatment of acute angle-closure glaucoma**
Adults: 250 mg P.O. every 4 hours or
250 mg P.O. b.i.d. for short-term therapy.
In acute cases, 500 mg P.O.; then 125 to
250 mg P.O. every 4 hours. To rapidly
lower intraocular pressure (IOP), initially,
500 mg I.V.; may repeat in 2 to 4 hours, if
needed, followed by 125 to 250 mg P.O.
every 4 to 6 hours.
Children: 10 to 15 mg/kg P.O. daily in
divided doses every 6 to 8 hours. For acute
angle-closure glaucoma, 5 to 10 mg/kg
I.V. every 6 hours.

➤ **Chronic open-angle glaucoma**
Adults: 250 mg to 1 g P.O. daily in divided
doses q.i.d., or 500 mg extended-release
P.O. b.i.d.
➤ **To prevent or treat acute mountain sickness (high-altitude sickness)**
Adults: 500 mg to 1 g (regular or extended-release) P.O. daily in divided doses every
12 hours. Start 24 to 48 hours before
ascent and continue for 48 hours while
at high altitude. When rapid ascent is
required, start with 1,000 mg P.O. daily.
➤ **Adjunct for epilepsy and myoclonic, refractory, generalized tonic-clonic, absence, or mixed seizures**
Adults and children: 8 to 30 mg/kg P.O.
daily in divided doses. For adults, 375 mg
to 1 g daily is ideal. If given with other
anticonvulsants, start at 250 mg P.O. once
daily, and increase to 375 mg to 1 g daily.
➤ **Edema caused by heart failure; drug-induced edema**
Adults: 250 mg to 375 mg (5 mg/kg) P.O.
daily in the morning. For best results, use
every other day or 2 days on followed by
1 to 2 days off.
Children: 5 mg/kg or 150 mg/m^2 P.O. or
I.V. daily in the morning.

ADMINISTRATION
P.O.
● Give drug with food to minimize GI
upset.
● Don't crush or open extended-release
capsules.
● If patient can't swallow oral form, pharmacist may make a suspension using
crushed tablets in a highly flavored syrup,
such as cherry, raspberry, or chocolate to
mask the bitter flavor. Although concentrations up to 500 mg/5 ml are possible,
concentrations of 250 mg/5 ml are more
palatable.
● Refrigeration improves palatability but
doesn't improve stability. Suspensions are
stable for 1 week.
I.V.
● Reconstitute drug in 500-mg vial with at
least 5 ml of sterile water for injection.
Use within 12 hours of reconstitution.

Reactions may be *common*, uncommon, *life-threatening*, or COMMON AND LIFE-THREATENING.
Interaction may have a *rapid* onset or *delayed onset.*

- Inject 100 to 500 mg/minute into a large vein using a 21G or 23G needle.
- Direct I.V. injection is the preferred route.
- Intermittent and continuous infusions aren't recommended.
- **Incompatibilities:** Multivitamins.

ACTION
Promotes renal excretion of sodium, potassium, bicarbonate, and water. As anticonvulsant, drug normalizes neuronal discharge. In mountain sickness, drug stimulates ventilation and increases cerebral blood flow. In glaucoma, drug reduces intraocular pressure (IOP).

Route	Onset	Peak	Duration
P.O.	60–90 min	1–4 hr	8–12 hr
P.O. (extended-release)	2 hr	3–6 hr	18–24 hr
I.V.	2 min	15 min	4–5 hr

Half-life: 10 to 15 hours.

ADVERSE REACTIONS
CNS: *seizures,* drowsiness, paresthesia, confusion, depression, weakness, ataxia.
EENT: transient myopia, hearing dysfunction, tinnitus.
GI: nausea, vomiting, anorexia, metallic taste, diarrhea, black tarry stools, constipation.
GU: polyuria, hematuria, crystalluria, glycosuria, phosphaturia, renal calculus.
Hematologic: *aplastic anemia, leukopenia, thrombocytopenia,* hemolytic anemia.
Metabolic: hypokalemia, asymptomatic hyperuricemia, hyperchloremic acidosis.
Skin: *pain at injection site, Stevens-Johnson syndrome,* rash, urticaria.
Other: sterile abscesses.

INTERACTIONS
Drug-drug. *Amphetamines, anticholinergics, mecamylamine, procainamide, quinidine:* May decrease renal clearance of these drugs, increasing toxicity. Monitor patient for toxicity.
Cyclosporine: May increase cyclosporine level, causing nephrotoxicity and neurotoxicity. Monitor patient for toxicity.

Diflunisal: May increase acetazolamide adverse effects; may significantly decrease IOP. Use together cautiously.
Lithium: May increase lithium excretion, decreasing its effect. Monitor lithium level.
Methenamine: May reduce methenamine effect. Avoid using together.
Primidone: May decrease serum and urine primidone levels. Monitor patient closely.
Salicylates: May cause accumulation and toxicity of acetazolamide, including CNS depression and metabolic acidosis. Monitor patient for toxicity.
Drug-lifestyle. *Sun exposure:* May increase risk of photosensitivity reactions. Advise patient to avoid excessive sunlight exposure.

EFFECTS ON LAB TEST RESULTS
- May increase uric acid level. May decrease potassium and hemoglobin levels and hematocrit.
- May decrease WBC and platelet counts.
- May decrease iodine uptake by the thyroid in hyperthyroid and euthyroid patients. May cause false-positive urine protein test result.

CONTRAINDICATIONS & CAUTIONS
- Contraindicated in patients hypersensitive to drug and in those with hyponatremia or hypokalemia, renal or hepatic disease or dysfunction, renal calculi, adrenal gland failure, hyperchloremic acidosis, or severe pulmonary obstruction.
- Contraindicated in those receiving long-term treatment for chronic noncongestive angle-closure glaucoma.
- Use cautiously in patients receiving other diuretics and in those with respiratory acidosis or COPD.

NURSING CONSIDERATIONS
- Cross-sensitivity between antibacterial sulfonamides and sulfonamide-derivative diuretics such as acetazolamide has been reported.
- Monitor fluid intake and output, glucose, and electrolytes, especially potassium, bicarbonate, and chloride. When drug is used in diuretic therapy, consult prescriber and dietitian about providing a high-potassium diet.

• Monitor elderly patients closely because they are especially susceptible to excessive diuresis.

• Weigh patient daily. Rapid or excessive fluid loss may cause weight loss and hypotension.

• Diuretic effect decreases when acidosis occurs but can be reestablished by using intermittent administration schedules.

• Monitor patient for signs of hemolytic anemia (pallor, weakness, and palpitations).

• Drug may increase glucose level and cause glycosuria.

• **Look alike–sound alike:** Don't confuse acetazolamide with acetaminophen or acyclovir.

PATIENT TEACHING

• Tell patient to take oral form with food to minimize GI upset.

• Tell patient not to crush, chew, or open capsules.

• Caution patient not to perform hazardous activities if adverse CNS reactions occur.

• Instruct patient to avoid prolonged exposure to sunlight because drug may cause phototoxicity.

• Instruct patient to notify prescriber of any unusual bleeding, bruising, tingling, or tremors.

---

bumetanide
byoo-MET-a-nide

Bumex◆

Pharmacologic class: loop diuretic
Pregnancy risk category C

AVAILABLE FORMS
Injection: 0.25 mg/ml
Tablets: 0.5 mg, 1 mg, 2 mg

INDICATIONS & DOSAGES
➤ **Edema caused by heart failure or hepatic or renal disease**
Adults: 0.5 to 2 mg P.O. once daily. If diuretic response isn't adequate, a second or third dose may be given at 4- to 5-hour intervals. Maximum dose is 10 mg daily. May be given parenterally if oral route isn't possible. Usual first dose is 0.5 to

1 mg given I.V. or I.M. If response isn't adequate, a second or third dose may be given at 2- to 3-hour intervals. Maximum, 10 mg daily.

ADMINISTRATION
P.O.
• Give drug with food to minimize GI upset.
• To prevent nocturia, give drug in morning. If second dose is needed, give in early afternoon.
I.V.
• For direct injection, give drug over 1 to 2 minutes using a 21G or 23G needle.
• For intermittent infusion, give diluted drug through an intermittent infusion device or piggyback into an I.V. line containing a free-flowing, compatible solution.
• **Incompatibilities:** Dobutamine, fenoldopam, midazolam.
I.M.
• Document injection site.

ACTION
Inhibits sodium and chloride reabsorption in the ascending loop of Henle.

Route	Onset	Peak	Duration
P.O.	30–60 min	1–2 hr	4–6 hr
I.V.	Within min	15–30 min	30–60 min
I.M.	40 min	Unknown	5–6 hr

Half-life: 1 to 1½ hours.

ADVERSE REACTIONS
CNS: *weakness,* dizziness, headache, vertigo.
CV: orthostatic hypotension, ECG changes, chest pain.
EENT: transient deafness.
GI: nausea, vomiting, upset stomach, dry mouth, diarrhea.
GU: premature ejaculation, difficulty maintaining erection, oliguria.
Hematologic: *thrombocytopenia,* azotemia.
Metabolic: volume depletion and dehydration, hypokalemia, hypochloremic alkalosis, *hypomagnesemia,* asymptomatic hyperuricemia.
Musculoskeletal: arthritic pain, muscle cramps and pain.
Skin: rash, pruritus, diaphoresis.

Reactions may be *common,* uncommon, *life-threatening,* or COMMON AND LIFE-THREATENING.
Interaction may have a *rapid onset* or **delayed onset.**

INTERACTIONS

Drug-drug. *Aminoglycoside antibiotics:* May increase ototoxicity. Avoid using together if possible.

Antidiabetics: May decrease hypo-glycemic effects. Monitor glucose level.

Antihypertensives: May increase hypotensive effects. Consider dosage adjustment.

Cardiac glycosides: May increase risk of digoxin toxicity from bumetanide-induced hypokalemia. Monitor potassium and digoxin levels.

Chlorothiazide, chlorthalidone, hydro-chlorothiazide, indapamide, metolazone: May cause excessive diuretic response, causing serious electrolyte abnormalities or dehydration. Adjust doses carefully, and monitor patient closely for signs and symptoms of excessive diuretic response.

Cisplatin: May increase risk of ototoxicity. Monitor patient closely.

Lithium: May decrease lithium clearance, increasing risk of lithium toxicity. Monitor lithium level.

Neuromuscular blockers: May prolong neuromuscular blockade. Monitor patient closely.

NSAIDs, probenecid: May inhibit diuretic response. Use together cautiously.

Other potassium-wasting drugs (such as amphotericin B, corticosteroids): May increase risk of hypokalemia. Use together cautiously.

Warfarin: May increase anticoagulant effect. Use together cautiously.

Drug-herb. *Dandelion:* May interfere with drug activity. Discourage use together.

Licorice: May cause unexpected, rapid potassium loss. Discourage use together.

EFFECTS ON LAB TEST RESULTS

● May increase alkaline phosphatase, ALT, AST, bilirubin, cholesterol, creatinine, glucose, LDH, and urine urea levels. May decrease calcium, magnesium, potassium, sodium, and chloride levels.

● May decrease platelet count.

CONTRAINDICATIONS & CAUTIONS

● Contraindicated in patients hypersensitive to drug or sulfonamides (possible cross-sensitivity) and in patients with anuria, hepatic coma, or severe electrolyte depletion.

● Use cautiously in patients with hepatic cirrhosis and ascites, in elderly patients, and in those with decreased renal function.

NURSING CONSIDERATIONS

● Safest and most effective dosage schedule is alternate days or 3 or 4 consecutive days with 1 or 2 days off between cycles.

● Monitor fluid intake and output, weight, and electrolyte, BUN, creatinine, and carbon dioxide levels frequently.

● Watch for evidence of hypokalemia, such as muscle weakness and cramps. Instruct patient to report these symptoms.

● Consult prescriber and dietitian about a high-potassium diet. Foods rich in potassium include citrus fruits, tomatoes, bananas, dates, and apricots.

● Monitor glucose level in diabetic patients.

● Monitor uric acid level, especially in patients with history of gout.

■ **Black Box Warning** Monitor blood pressure and pulse rate during rapid diuresis. Profound water and electrolyte depletion may occur. ■

● If oliguria or azotemia develops or increases, prescriber may stop drug.

● Drug can be safely used in patients allergic to furosemide; 1 mg of bumetanide equals about 40 mg of furosemide.

● *Look alike–sound alike:* Don't confuse Bumex with Buprenex.

PATIENT TEACHING

● Instruct patient to take drug with food to minimize GI upset.

● Advise patient to take drug in morning to avoid need to urinate at night; if patient needs second dose, have him take it in early afternoon.

● Advise patient to avoid sudden posture changes and to rise slowly to avoid dizziness upon standing quickly.

● Instruct patient to notify prescriber about extreme thirst, muscle weakness, cramps, nausea, or dizziness.

● Instruct patient to weigh himself daily to monitor fluid status.

ethacrynate sodium
eth-uh-KRIH-nayt

Edecrin Sodium

ethacrynic acid
Edecrin

Pharmacologic class: loop diuretic
Pregnancy risk category B

AVAILABLE FORMS
ethacrynate sodium
Injection: 50 mg
ethacrynic acid
Tablets: 25 mg

INDICATIONS & DOSAGES
➤ **Acute pulmonary edema**
Adults: 50 mg or 0.5 to 1 mg/kg I.V.
Usually only one dose is needed, although
a second dose may be needed.
➤ **Edema**
Adults: 50 to 200 mg P.O. daily. May
increase to 200 mg b.i.d. for desired
effect.
Children: First dose is 25 mg P.O., increase
cautiously by 25 mg daily until desired
effect is achieved. Dosage for infants
hasn't been established.
Adjust-a-dose: If added to an existing
diuretic regimen, first dose is 25 mg and
dosage adjustments are made in 25-mg
increments.

ADMINISTRATION
P.O.
● Give drug in morning to prevent
nocturia.
I.V.
● Add to vial 50 ml of D$_5$W or normal
saline solution.
● Don't use cloudy or opalescent solution.
● Give over several minutes through
tubing of running infusion.
● If more than one I.V. dose is needed,
use a new injection site to avoid thrombo-
phlebitis.
● Discard unused solution after 24 hours.
● **Incompatibilities:** Hydralazine,
Normosol-M, procainamide, ranitidine,
reserpine, solutions or drugs with pH
below 5, tolazoline, triflupromazine,
whole blood, and its derivatives.

ACTION
Potent loop diuretic; inhibits sodium and
chloride reabsorption at the proximal and
distal tubules and the ascending loop of
Henle.

Route	Onset	Peak	Duration
P.O.	30 min	2 hr	6–8 hr
I.V.	5 min	15–30 min	2 hr

ADVERSE REACTIONS
CNS: malaise, confusion, fatigue, vertigo,
headache, nervousness, fever.
CV: orthostatic hypotension.
EENT: transient or permanent deafness
with over-rapid I.V. injection, blurred
vision, tinnitus, hearing loss.
GI: cramping, diarrhea, anorexia, nausea,
vomiting, *GI bleeding, pancreatitis.*
GU: oliguria, hematuria, nocturia,
polyuria, frequent urination.
Hematologic: *agranulocytosis, neutropenia, thrombocytopenia,* azotemia.
Metabolic: asymptomatic hyperuricemia,
hypokalemia, hypochloremic alkalosis,
fluid and electrolyte imbalances, including
dilutional hyponatremia, hypocalcemia
and hypomagnesemia, hyperglycemia
and impaired glucose tolerance, volume
depletion and dehydration.
Skin: rash.
Other: chills.

INTERACTIONS
Drug-drug. *Aminoglycoside antibiotics:*
May increase ototoxic adverse reactions of
both drugs. Use together cautiously.
Antidiabetics: May decrease hypoglycemic effects. Monitor glucose level.
Antihypertensives: May increase risk of
hypotension. Use together cautiously.
Cardiac glycosides: May increase risk of
digoxin toxicity from ethacrynate-induced
hypokalemia. Monitor potassium and
digoxin levels.
*Chlorothiazide, chlorthalidone,
hydrochlorothiazide, indapamide,
metolazone:* May cause excessive diuretic
response, causing serious electrolyte
abnormalities or dehydration. Adjust
doses carefully, and monitor patient
closely for signs and symptoms of excessive diuretic response.
Cisplatin: May increase risk of ototoxicity.
Avoid using together.

Reactions may be *common*, uncommon, *life-threatening*, or COMMON AND LIFE-THREATENING.
Interaction may have a *rapid onset* or *delayed onset.*

Lithium: May decrease lithium clearance, increasing risk of lithium toxicity. Monitor lithium level.

Neuromuscular blockers: May enhance neuromuscular blockade. Monitor patient closely.

NSAIDs: May decrease diuretic effect. Use together cautiously.

Other potassium-wasting drugs (amphotericin B, corticosteroids): May increase risk of hypocalcemia. Use together cautiously.

Probenecid: May decrease diuretic effect. Avoid using together.

Warfarin: May increase anticoagulant effect. Use together cautiously.

Drug-herb. *Dandelion:* May interfere with diuretic activity. Discourage use together.

Licorice: May cause unexpected rapid potassium loss. Discourage use together.

EFFECTS ON LAB TEST RESULTS
• May increase glucose and uric acid levels. May decrease calcium, magnesium, potassium, and sodium levels.
• May decrease granulocyte, neutrophil, and platelet counts.

CONTRAINDICATIONS & CAUTIONS
• Contraindicated in infants, patients hypersensitive to drug, and patients with anuria.
■ **Black Box Warning** Drug is potent diuretic and can cause severe diuresis with water and electrolyte depletion. Monitor patient closely. ■
• Use cautiously in patients with electrolyte abnormalities or hepatic impairment.

NURSING CONSIDERATIONS
• Monitor fluid intake and output, weight, blood pressure, and electrolyte levels.
• Watch for signs of hypokalemia, such as muscle weakness and cramps.
• Monitor glucose level in diabetic patients.
• Consult prescriber and dietitian about providing a high-potassium diet. Foods rich in potassium include citrus fruits, tomatoes, bananas, dates, and apricots. Potassium chloride and sodium supplements may be needed.
• Drug may increase risk of gastric hemorrhage caused by steroid treatment.
• Monitor elderly patients, who are especially susceptible to excessive diuresis.

• Monitor uric acid level, especially in patients with history of gout.
• **Alert:** If patient develops severe diarrhea, stop drug. Patient shouldn't receive drug again after diarrhea has resolved.

PATIENT TEACHING
• Instruct patient to take drug with food to minimize GI upset.
• Advise patient to take drug in morning to avoid need to urinate at night; if patient needs second dose, have him take it in early afternoon.
• Advise patient to avoid sudden posture changes and to rise slowly to avoid dizziness upon standing quickly.
• Tell patient to notify prescriber about muscle weakness, cramps, nausea, or dizziness.
• Caution patient not to perform hazardous activities if drug causes drowsiness.
• Advise diabetic patient to closely monitor glucose level.

---

furosemide
fur-OH-se-mide

Furosemide Special†, Lasix*✐, Novo-semide†

Pharmacologic class: loop diuretic
Pregnancy risk category C

AVAILABLE FORMS
Injection: 10 mg/ml
Oral solution: 10 mg/ml, 40 mg/5 ml
Tablets: 20 mg, 40 mg, 80 mg

INDICATIONS & DOSAGES
➤ **Acute pulmonary edema**
Adults: 40 mg I.V. injected slowly over 1 to 2 minutes; then 80 mg I.V. in 60 to 90 minutes if needed.
➤ **Edema**
Adults: 20 to 80 mg P.O. daily in the morning. If response is inadequate, give a second dose, and each succeeding dose, every 6 to 8 hours. Carefully increase dose in 20- to 40-mg increments up to 600 mg daily. Once effective dose is attained, may give once or twice daily. Or, 20 to 40 mg I.V. or I.M., increased by 20 mg every 2 hours until desired effect achieved.

Infants and children: 2 mg/kg P.O. daily, increased by 1 to 2 mg/kg in 6 to 8 hours if needed; carefully adjusted up to 6 mg/kg daily if needed.

➤ **Hypertension**
Adults: 40 mg P.O. b.i.d. Dosage adjusted based on response. May be used as adjunct to other antihypertensives if needed.
Children ◆ : 0.5 to 2 mg/kg P.O. once or twice daily. Increase dose as needed up to 6 mg/kg daily.

ADMINISTRATION
P.O.
• To prevent nocturia, give in the morning. Give second dose if ordered in early afternoon, 6 to 8 hours after morning dose.
• Give drug with food to prevent GI upset.
• Store tablets in light-resistant container to prevent discoloration (doesn't affect potency). Refrigerate oral solution to ensure drug stability.
I.V.
• If discolored yellow, don't use.
• For direct injection, give over 1 to 2 minutes.
• For infusion, dilute with D_5W, normal saline solution, or lactated Ringer's solution.
• To avoid ototoxicity, infuse no more than 4 mg/minute.
• Use prepared infusion solution within 24 hours.
• **Incompatibilities:** Acidic solutions, aminoglycosides, amiodarone, ascorbic acid, azithromycin, bleomycin, buprenorphine, chlorpromazine, ciprofloxacin, diazepam, diltiazem, dobutamine, doxapram, doxorubicin, droperidol, epinephrine, erythromycin, esmolol, filgrastim, fluconazole, fructose 10% in water, gentamicin, hydralazine, idarubicin, invert sugar 10% in electrolyte #2, isoproterenol, levofloxacin, mannitol, meperidine, methocarbamol, metoclopramide, midazolam, milrinone, morphine, netilmicin, norepinephrine, ondansetron, oxytetracycline, prochlorperazine, promethazine, protamine, quinidine, tetracycline, thiamine, vinblastine, vincristine, vitamins B and C.
I.M.
• To prevent nocturia, give in the morning. Give second dose if ordered in early afternoon, 6 to 8 hours after morning dose.
• Record administration site.

ACTION
Inhibits sodium and chloride reabsorption at the proximal and distal tubules and the ascending loop of Henle.

Route	Onset	Peak	Duration
P.O.	20–60 min	1–2 hr	6–8 hr
I.V.	Within 5 min	30 min	2 hr
I.M.	Unknown	30 min	2 hr

Half-life: 30 minutes.

ADVERSE REACTIONS
CNS: vertigo, headache, dizziness, paresthesia, weakness, restlessness, fever.
CV: orthostatic hypotension, thrombophlebitis with I.V. administration.
EENT: transient deafness, blurred or yellowed vision, tinnitus.
GI: abdominal discomfort and pain, diarrhea, anorexia, nausea, vomiting, constipation, *pancreatitis.*
GU: azotemia, nocturia, polyuria, frequent urination, oliguria.
Hematologic: *agranulocytosis, aplastic anemia, leukopenia, thrombocytopenia,* anemia.
Hepatic: hepatic dysfunction, jaundice.
Metabolic: volume depletion and dehydration, asymptomatic hyperuricemia, impaired glucose tolerance, hypokalemia, hypochloremic alkalosis, hyperglycemia, dilutional hyponatremia, hypocalcemia, hypomagnesemia.
Musculoskeletal: muscle spasm.
Skin: dermatitis, purpura, photosensitivity reactions, transient pain at I.M. injection site.
Other: gout.

INTERACTIONS
Drug-drug. *Aminoglycoside antibiotics, cisplatin:* May increase ototoxicity. Use together cautiously.
Amphotericin B, corticosteroids, corticotropin, metolazone: May increase risk of hypokalemia. Monitor potassium level closely.
Antidiabetics: May decrease hypoglycemic effects. Monitor glucose level.
Antihypertensives: May increase risk of hypotension. Use together cautiously. Decrease antihypertensive dose if needed.
Cardiac glycosides, neuromuscular blockers: May increase toxicity of these drugs

---

Reactions may be *common*, uncommon, *life-threatening*, or **COMMON AND LIFE-THREATENING.**
Interaction may have a *rapid onset* or **delayed onset.**

from furosemide-induced hypokalemia. Monitor potassium level.

Chlorothiazide, chlorthalidone, hydrochlorothiazide, indapamide, metolazone: May cause excessive diuretic response, causing serious electrolyte abnormalities or dehydration. Adjust doses carefully, and monitor patient closely for signs and symptoms of excessive diuretic response.

Ethacrynic acid: May increase risk of ototoxicity. Avoid using together.

Lithium: May decrease lithium excretion, resulting in lithium toxicity. Monitor lithium level.

NSAIDs: May inhibit diuretic response. Use together cautiously.

Phenytoin: May decrease diuretic effects of furosemide. Use together cautiously.

Propranolol: May increase propranolol level. Monitor patient closely.

Salicylates: May cause salicylate toxicity. Use together cautiously.

Sucralfate: May reduce diuretic and antihypertensive effect. Separate doses by 2 hours.

Drug-herb. *Aloe:* May increase drug effect. Discourage use together.

Dandelion: May interfere with drug activity. Discourage use together.

Ginseng: May decrease drug effect. Discourage use together.

Licorice: May cause unexpected rapid potassium loss. Discourage use together.

Drug-lifestyle. *Sun exposure:* May increase risk for photosensitivity reactions. Advise patient to avoid excessive sunlight exposure.

EFFECTS ON LAB TEST RESULTS
● May increase cholesterol, glucose, BUN, creatinine, and uric acid levels. May decrease calcium, hemoglobin, magnesium, potassium, and sodium levels.
● May decrease granulocyte, platelet, and WBC counts.

CONTRAINDICATIONS & CAUTIONS
● Contraindicated in patients hypersensitive to drug and in those with anuria.
● Use cautiously in patients with hepatic cirrhosis and in those allergic to sulfonamides. Use during pregnancy only if potential benefits to mother clearly outweigh risks to fetus.

NURSING CONSIDERATIONS
● *Alert:* Monitor weight, blood pressure, and pulse rate routinely with long-term use.
■ **Black Box Warning** Drug is potent diuretic and can cause severe diuresis with water and electrolyte depletion. Monitor patient closely. ■
● If oliguria or azotemia develops or increases, drug may need to be stopped.
● Monitor fluid intake and output and electrolyte, BUN, and carbon dioxide levels frequently.
● Watch for signs of hypokalemia, such as muscle weakness and cramps.
● Consult prescriber and dietitian about a high-potassium diet or potassium supplements. Foods rich in potassium include citrus fruits, tomatoes, bananas, dates, and apricots.
● Monitor glucose level in diabetic patients.
● Drug may not be well absorbed orally in patient with severe heart failure. Drug may need to be given I.V. even if patient is taking other oral drugs.
● Monitor uric acid level, especially in patients with a history of gout.
● Monitor elderly patients, who are especially susceptible to excessive diuresis, because circulatory collapse and thromboembolic complications are possible.
● *Look alike–sound alike:* Don't confuse furosemide with torsemide or Lasix with Lonox, Lidex, or Luvox.

PATIENT TEACHING
● Advise patient to take drug with food to prevent GI upset, and to take drug in morning to prevent need to urinate at night. If patient needs second dose, tell him to take it in early afternoon, 6 to 8 hours after morning dose.
● Inform patient of possible need for potassium or magnesium supplements.
● Instruct patient to stand slowly to prevent dizziness and to limit alcohol intake and strenuous exercise in hot weather to avoid worsening dizziness upon standing quickly.
● Advise patient to immediately report ringing in ears, severe abdominal pain, or sore throat and fever; these symptoms may indicate toxicity.

- *Alert:* Discourage patient from storing different types of drugs in the same container, increasing the risk of drug errors. The most popular strengths of this drug and digoxin are white tablets about equal in size.
- Tell patient to check with prescriber or pharmacist before taking OTC drugs.
- Teach patient to avoid direct sunlight and to use protective clothing and a sunblock because of risk of photosensitivity reactions.

---

hydrochlorothiazide
hye-droe-klor-oh-THYE-a-zide

Apo-Hydro†, Esidrix, Ezide, HydroDIURIL, Hydro-Par, Microzide, Novo-Hydrazide†, Nu-hydro†, Oretic, Urozide†

Pharmacologic class: thiazide diuretic
Pregnancy risk category B

AVAILABLE FORMS
Capsules: 12.5 mg
Oral solution: 50 mg/5 ml
Tablets: 25 mg, 50 mg, 100 mg

INDICATIONS & DOSAGES
➤ **Edema**
Adults: 25 to 100 mg P.O. daily or intermittently; up to 200 mg initially for several days until nonedematous weight is attained.
➤ **Hypertension**
Adults: 12.5 to 50 mg P.O. once daily. Increase or decrease daily dose based on blood pressure.
Children ages 6 months to 12 years: 1 to 2 mg/kg P.O. daily in a single dose or two divided doses. The total daily dose shouldn't exceed 37.5 mg for children up to age 2 or 100 mg in children ages 2 to 12.
Children younger than age 6 months: Up to 3 mg/kg P.O. daily in two divided doses.
Adjust-a-dose: In patients older than age 65 initially, 12.5 mg daily. Adjust in increments of 12.5 mg, if needed.

ADMINISTRATION
P.O.
- Give drug with food to minimize GI upset.

- To prevent nocturia, give drug in morning. If second dose is needed, give in early afternoon.

ACTION
Increases sodium and water excretion by inhibiting sodium and chloride reabsorption in distal segment of the nephron.

Route	Onset	Peak	Duration
P.O.	2 hr	4–6 hr	6–12 hr

Half-life: 5½ to 15 hours.

ADVERSE REACTIONS
CNS: dizziness, vertigo, headache, paresthesia, weakness, restlessness.
CV: orthostatic hypotension, allergic myocarditis, vasculitis.
GI: *pancreatitis,* anorexia, nausea, epigastric distress, vomiting, abdominal pain, diarrhea, constipation.
GU: *renal failure,* polyuria, frequent urination, interstitial nephritis.
Hematologic: *aplastic anemia, agranulocytosis, leukopenia, thrombocytopenia,* hemolytic anemia.
Hepatic: jaundice.
Metabolic: asymptomatic hyperuricemia, hypokalemia, hyperglycemia and impaired glucose tolerance, fluid and electrolyte imbalances, including dilutional hyponatremia and hypochloremia, metabolic alkalosis, hypercalcemia, volume depletion and dehydration.
Musculoskeletal: muscle cramps.
Respiratory: *respiratory distress,* pneumonitis.
Skin: dermatitis, photosensitivity reactions, rash, purpura, alopecia.
Other: *anaphylactic reactions,* hypersensitivity reactions, gout.

INTERACTIONS
Drug-drug. *Amphotericin B, corticosteroids:* May increase risk of hypokalemia. Monitor potassium level closely.
Antidiabetics: May decrease hypoglycemic effects. Adjust dosage if needed. Monitor glucose level.
Antihypertensives: May have additive antihypertensive effect. Use together cautiously.
Barbiturates, opioids: May increase orthostatic hypotensive effect. Monitor patient closely.

Reactions may be *common,* uncommon, *life-threatening,* or COMMON AND LIFE-THREATENING.
Interaction may have a *rapid onset* or *delayed onset.*

Bumetanide, ethacrynic acid, furosemide, torsemide: May cause excessive diuretic response, causing serious electrolyte abnormalities or dehydration. Adjust doses carefully, and monitor patient closely for signs and symptoms of excessive diuretic response.

Cardiac glycosides: May increase risk of digoxin toxicity from diuretic-induced hypokalemia. Monitor potassium and digoxin levels.

Cholestyramine, colestipol: May decrease intestinal absorption of thiazides. Separate doses by 2 hours.

Diazoxide: May increase antihypertensive, hyperglycemic, and hyperuricemic effects. Use together cautiously.

Lithium: May decrease lithium excretion, increasing risk of lithium toxicity. Monitor lithium level.

NSAIDs: May increase risk of renal failure. May decrease diuretic and antihypertensive effects. Monitor renal function and blood pressure.

Drug-herb. *Dandelion:* May interfere with diuretic activity. Discourage use together.

Licorice: May cause unexpected rapid potassium loss. Discourage use together.

Drug-lifestyle. *Alcohol use:* May increase orthostatic hypotensive effect. Discourage use together.

EFFECTS ON LAB TEST RESULTS

• May increase glucose, cholesterol, triglyceride, calcium, and uric acid levels. May decrease potassium, sodium, chloride, and hemoglobin levels.
• May decrease granulocyte, WBC, and platelet counts.

CONTRAINDICATIONS & CAUTIONS

• Contraindicated in patients with anuria and patients hypersensitive to other thiazides or other sulfonamide derivatives.
• Use cautiously in children and in patients with severe renal disease, impaired hepatic function, or progressive hepatic disease.

NURSING CONSIDERATIONS

• Monitor fluid intake and output, weight, blood pressure, and electrolyte levels.

• Watch for signs and symptoms of hypokalemia, such as muscle weakness and cramps.
• Drug may be used with potassium-sparing diuretic to prevent potassium loss.
• Consult prescriber and dietitian about a high-potassium diet or potassium supplement. Foods rich in potassium include citrus fruits, tomatoes, bananas, dates, and apricots.
• Monitor creatinine and BUN levels regularly. Cumulative effects of drug may occur with impaired renal function.
• Monitor uric acid level, especially in patients with history of gout.
• Monitor glucose level, especially in diabetic patients.
• Monitor elderly patients, who are especially susceptible to excessive diuresis.
• Stop thiazides and thiazide-like diuretics before parathyroid function tests.
• In patients with hypertension, therapeutic response may be delayed several weeks.

PATIENT TEACHING

• Instruct patient to take drug with food to minimize GI upset.
• Advise patient to take drug in morning to avoid need to urinate at night; if patient needs second dose, have him take it in early afternoon.
• Advise patient to avoid sudden posture changes and to rise slowly to avoid dizziness upon standing quickly.
• Encourage patient to use a sunblock to prevent photosensitivity reactions.
• Tell patient to check with prescriber or pharmacist before using OTC drugs.

---

indapamide
in-DAP-a-mide

Lozide†

Pharmacologic class: thiazide-like diuretic
Pregnancy risk category B

AVAILABLE FORMS
Tablets: 1.25 mg, 2.5 mg

INDICATIONS & DOSAGES
➤ **Edema**
Adults: Initially, 2.5 mg P.O. daily in the morning. Increased to 5 mg daily after 1 week, if needed.
➤ **Hypertension**
Adults: Initially, 1.25 mg P.O. daily in the morning. Increased to 2.5 mg daily after 4 weeks, if needed. Increased to 5 mg daily after 4 more weeks, if needed. If response is inadequate, a second antihypertensive, given at 50% of the usual starting dose, may be needed.

ADMINISTRATION
P.O.
● Give drug with food to minimize GI upset.
● To prevent nocturia, give drug in the morning.

ACTION
Enhances excretion of sodium chloride and water by interfering with sodium transport in the distal tubule.

Route	Onset	Peak	Duration
P.O.	1–2 hr	Within 2 hr	Up to 36 hr

Half-life: About 14 hours.

ADVERSE REACTIONS
CNS: headache, nervousness, dizziness, light-headedness, weakness, vertigo, restlessness, drowsiness, fatigue, anxiety, depression, numbness of limbs, irritability, agitation, lethargy.
CV: orthostatic hypotension, palpitations, PVCs, irregular heartbeat, vasculitis, flushing.
EENT: rhinorrhea, blurred vision.
GI: anorexia, nausea, epigastric distress, vomiting, abdominal pain or cramps, diarrhea, constipation.
GU: nocturia, polyuria, frequent urination, impotence.
Metabolic: asymptomatic hyperuricemia, fluid and electrolyte imbalances, including dilutional hyponatremia, hypochloremia, metabolic alkalosis and hypokalemia, weight loss, volume depletion and dehydration, hyperglycemia.
Musculoskeletal: muscle cramps and spasms.
Skin: rash, pruritus, urticaria.
Other: gout.

INTERACTIONS
Drug-drug. *Amphotericin B, corticosteroids:* May increase risk of hypokalemia. Monitor potassium level closely.
Antidiabetics: May decrease hypoglycemic effect of sulfonylureas, causing elevated glucose levels. Adjust dosage, if needed. Monitor glucose level.
Barbiturates, opioids: May increase orthostasis. Monitor patient closely.
Bumetanide, ethacrynic acid, furosemide, torsemide: May cause excessive diuretic response, causing serious electrolyte abnormalities or dehydration. Adjust doses carefully, and monitor patient closely for signs and symptoms of excessive diuretic response.
Cardiac glycosides: May increase risk of digoxin toxicity from indapamide-induced hypokalemia. Monitor potassium and digoxin levels.
Cholestyramine, colestipol: May decrease absorption of thiazides. Separate doses by 2 hours.
Diazoxide: May increase antihypertensive, hyperglycemic, and hyperuricemic effects. Use together cautiously.
Lithium: May decrease lithium clearance that may increase lithium toxicity. Avoid using together.
NSAIDs: May increase risk of NSAID-induced renal failure. Monitor patient for signs and symptoms of renal failure.
Drug-herb. *Dandelion:* May interfere with drug activity. Discourage use together.
Licorice: May cause unexpected rapid potassium loss. Discourage use together.
Drug-lifestyle. *Alcohol use:* May increase orthostatic hypotensive effect. Discourage use together.

EFFECTS ON LAB TEST RESULTS
● May increase BUN, creatinine, glucose, cholesterol, triglyceride, calcium, and uric acid levels. May decrease potassium, sodium, phosphate, and chloride levels.

CONTRAINDICATIONS & CAUTIONS
● Contraindicated in patients hypersensitive to other sulfonamide-derived drugs and in those with anuria.

• Use cautiously in patients with severe renal disease, impaired hepatic function, or progressive hepatic disease.

NURSING CONSIDERATIONS

• Monitor fluid intake and output, weight, blood pressure, and electrolyte levels.
• Watch for signs of hypokalemia, such as muscle weakness and cramps. Drug may be used with potassium-sparing diuretic to prevent potassium loss.
• Consult prescriber and dietitian about a high-potassium diet or potassium supplement. Foods rich in potassium include citrus fruits, tomatoes, bananas, dates, and apricots.
• Monitor creatinine and BUN levels regularly. Cumulative effects of drug may occur in patients with impaired renal function.
• Monitor uric acid level, especially in patients with history of gout.
• Monitor glucose level, especially in diabetic patients.
• Monitor elderly patients, who are especially susceptible to excessive diuresis.
• Stop thiazides and thiazide-like diuretics before parathyroid function tests.
• Therapeutic response may be delayed several weeks in hypertensive patients.

PATIENT TEACHING

• Instruct patient to take drug in morning to prevent need to urinate at night.
• Tell patient to take drug with food to minimize GI upset.
• Advise patient to avoid sudden posture changes and to rise slowly to avoid dizziness upon standing quickly.

---

mannitol
MAN-i-tole

Osmitrol

Pharmacologic class:
osmotic diuretic
Pregnancy risk category B

AVAILABLE FORMS
Injection: 5%, 10%, 15%, 20%, 25%

INDICATIONS & DOSAGES
➤ **Test dose for marked oliguria or suspected inadequate renal function**
Adults and children older than age 12: 200 mg/kg or 12.5 g as a 15% to 20% I.V. solution over 3 to 5 minutes. Response is adequate if 30 to 50 ml of urine/hour is excreted over 2 to 3 hours; if response is inadequate, a second test dose is given. If still no response after second dose, stop drug.
➤ **Oliguria**
Adults and children older than age 12: 50 to 100 g I.V. as a 15% to 25% solution over 90 minutes to several hours.
➤ **To prevent oliguria or acute renal failure**
Adults and children older than age 12: 50 to 100 g I.V. of a 5% to 25% solution. Determine exact concentration by fluid requirements.
➤ **To reduce intraocular or intracranial pressure or cerebral edema**
Adults and children older than age 12: 1.5 to 2 g/kg as a 15%, 20%, or 25% I.V. solution over 30 to 60 minutes. For maximum intraocular pressure reduction before surgery, give 60 to 90 minutes preoperatively.
➤ **Diuresis in drug intoxication**
Adults and children older than age 12: 5% to 25% solution continuously up to 200 g I.V., while maintaining 100 to 500 ml urine output/hour and a positive fluid balance.
➤ **Irrigating solution during transurethral resection of prostate gland**
Adults: 2.5% to 5% solution.

ADMINISTRATION
I.V.
• Change I.V. administration apparatus every 24 hours.
• To redissolve crystallized solution (crystallization occurs at low temperatures or in concentrations higher than 15%), warm bottle or bag in a hot water bath with occasional shaking. Cool to body temperature before giving. Don't use solution with undissolved crystals.
• Give as intermittent or continuous infusion at prescribed rate, using an inline filter and an infusion pump. Don't give as direct injection.

- Check patency at infusion site before and during administration.
- Monitor patient for signs and symptoms of infiltration; if it occurs, watch for inflammation, edema, and necrosis.
- **Incompatibilities:** Blood products, cefepime, doxorubicin liposomal, filgrastim, imipenem-cilastatin, meropenem, potassium chloride, sodium chloride, strongly acidic or alkaline solutions.

ACTION
Increases osmotic pressure of glomerular filtrate, thus inhibiting tubular reabsorption of water and electrolytes. Drug elevates plasma osmolality and increases water flow into extracellular fluid.

Route	Onset	Peak	Duration
I.V.	30–60 min	1 hr	6–8 hr

Half-life: About 1½ hours.

ADVERSE REACTIONS
CNS: *seizures,* dizziness, headache, fever.
CV: edema, thrombophlebitis, hypotension, hypertension, *heart failure,* tachycardia, angina-like chest pain, vascular overload.
EENT: blurred vision, rhinitis.
GI: thirst, dry mouth, nausea, vomiting, *diarrhea.*
GU: urine retention.
Metabolic: dehydration.
Skin: local pain, urticaria.
Other: chills, thirst.

INTERACTIONS
Drug-drug. *Lithium:* May increase urinary excretion of lithium. Monitor lithium level closely.

EFFECTS ON LAB TEST RESULTS
- May increase or decrease electrolyte levels.
- May interfere with tests for inorganic phosphorus or ethylene glycol level.

CONTRAINDICATIONS & CAUTIONS
- Contraindicated in patients hypersensitive to drug.
- Contraindicated in patients with anuria; severe pulmonary congestion; frank pulmonary edema; active intracranial bleeding (except during craniotomy); severe dehydration; metabolic edema; previous progressive renal disease or dysfunction after starting drug, including increasing azotemia and oliguria; or previous progressive heart failure or pulmonary congestion after drug.

NURSING CONSIDERATIONS
- Monitor vital signs, including central venous pressure and fluid intake and output hourly. Report increasing oliguria. Check weight, renal function, fluid balance, and serum and urine sodium and potassium levels daily.
- In comatose or incontinent patient, use urinary catheter because therapy is based on strict evaluation of fluid intake and output. If patient has urinary catheter, use an hourly urometer collection bag to evaluate output accurately and easily.
- To relieve thirst, give frequent mouth care or fluids.
- Drug is commonly used in chemotherapy regimens to enhance diuresis of renally toxic drugs.
- Don't give electrolyte-free solutions with blood. If blood is given simultaneously, add at least 20 mEq of sodium chloride to each liter of drug solution to avoid pseudoagglutination.

PATIENT TEACHING
- Tell patient that he may feel thirsty or have a dry mouth, and emphasize importance of drinking only the amount of fluids ordered.
- Instruct patient to promptly report adverse reactions and discomfort at I.V. site.

---

metolazone
me-TOLE-a-zone

Zaroxolyn

Pharmacologic class: thiazide-like diuretic
Pregnancy risk category B

AVAILABLE FORMS
Tablets (extended-release): 2.5 mg, 5 mg, 10 mg

INDICATIONS & DOSAGES
➤ **Edema in heart failure or renal disease**
Adults: 5 to 20 mg P.O. once daily.
➤ **Hypertension**
Adults: 2.5 to 5 mg P.O. once daily. Base maintenance dosage on blood pressure.

ADMINISTRATION
P.O.
● Give drug without regard for meals.
● To prevent nocturia, give drug in the morning.
■ **Black Box Warning** Don't interchange Zaroxolyn tablets and other formulations of metolazone that share its slow and incomplete bioavailability. ■

ACTION
Increases sodium and water excretion by inhibiting sodium reabsorption in ascending loop of Henle.

Route	Onset	Peak	Duration
P.O.	1 hr	2–8 hr	12–24 hr

Half-life: About 14 hours.

ADVERSE REACTIONS
CNS: *dizziness,* headache, fatigue, vertigo, paresthesia, weakness, restlessness, drowsiness, anxiety, depression, nervousness, blurred vision.
CV: orthostatic hypotension, palpitations, vasculitis.
GI: *pancreatitis,* anorexia, nausea, epigastric distress, vomiting, abdominal pain, diarrhea, constipation, dry mouth.
GU: nocturia, polyuria, impotence.
Hematologic: *aplastic anemia, agranulocytosis, leukopenia,* purpura.
Hepatic: jaundice, *hepatitis.*
Metabolic: hyperglycemia and impaired glucose tolerance, fluid and electrolyte imbalances, including hypokalemia, hypomagnesemia, dilutional hyponatremia and hypochloremia, metabolic alkalosis, and hypercalcemia, volume depletion and dehydration.
Musculoskeletal: muscle cramps.
Skin: dermatitis, photosensitivity reactions, rash, pruritus, urticaria.

INTERACTIONS
Drug-drug. *Amphotericin B, corticosteroids:* May increase risk of hypokalemia. Monitor potassium level closely.
Anticoagulants: May decrease anticoagulant response. Monitor PT and INR.
Antidiabetics: May alter glucose level and require dosage adjustment of antidiabetics. Monitor glucose level.
Barbiturates, opioids: May increase orthostatic hypotensive effect. Monitor patient closely.
Bumetanide, ethacrynic acid, furosemide, torsemide: May cause excessive diuretic response, causing serious electrolyte abnormalities or dehydration. Adjust doses carefully, and monitor patient closely for signs and symptoms of excessive diuretic response.
Cardiac glycosides: May increase risk of digoxin toxicity from metolazone-induced hypokalemia. Monitor potassium and digoxin levels.
Cholestyramine, colestipol: May decrease intestinal absorption of thiazides. Separate doses.
Diazoxide: May increase antihypertensive, hyperglycemic, and hyperuricemic effects. Use together cautiously.
Lithium: May decrease lithium clearance, increasing risk of lithium toxicity. Monitor lithium level.
NSAIDs: May increase risk of renal failure. May decrease diuretic and antihypertensive effects. Monitor renal function and blood pressure.
Other antihypertensives: May have additive effects. Use together cautiously.
Drug-herb. *Dandelion:* May interfere with diuretic activity. Discourage use together.
Licorice: May cause unexpected rapid potassium loss. Discourage use together.
Drug-lifestyle. *Alcohol use:* May increase orthostatic hypotensive effect. Discourage use together.
Sun exposure: May increase risk for photosensitivity reaction. Advise patient to avoid excessive sunlight exposure.

EFFECTS ON LAB TEST RESULTS
● May increase glucose, calcium, cholesterol, and triglyceride levels.

May decrease potassium, sodium, magnesium, chloride, and hemoglobin levels.
● May decrease granulocyte and WBC counts.

CONTRAINDICATIONS & CAUTIONS
● Contraindicated in patients hypersensitive to thiazides or other sulfonamide-derived drugs and in those with anuria, hepatic coma, or precoma.
● Use cautiously in patients with impaired renal or hepatic function.

NURSING CONSIDERATIONS
● Monitor fluid intake and output, weight, blood pressure, and electrolyte levels.
● Watch for signs and symptoms of hypokalemia, such as muscle weakness and cramps. Drug may be used with potassium-sparing diuretic to prevent potassium loss.
● Consult prescriber and dietitian about a high-potassium diet. Foods rich in potassium include citrus fruits, tomatoes, bananas, dates, and apricots.
● Monitor glucose level, especially in diabetic patients.
● Monitor uric acid level, especially in patients with history of gout.
● Monitor elderly patients, who are especially susceptible to excessive diuresis.
● In hypertensive patients, therapeutic response may be delayed several weeks.
● Monitor blood pressure. If response is inadequate, another antihypertensive may be added.
● Metolazone and furosemide may be used together to enhance diuretic effect.
● Unlike thiazide diuretics, metolazone is effective in patients with decreased renal function.
● Stop thiazides and thiazide-like diuretics before parathyroid function tests.
● *Look alike–sound alike:* Don't confuse Zaroxolyn with Zarontin.

PATIENT TEACHING
● Tell patient to take drug in morning to prevent need to urinate at night.
● Advise patient to avoid sudden posture changes and to rise slowly to avoid effects of dizziness upon standing quickly.
● Instruct patient to use a sunblock to prevent photosensitivity reactions.

---

spironolactone
speer-on-oh-LAK-tone

Aldactone, Novospiroton†

Pharmacologic class: potassium-sparing diuretic; aldosterone receptor antagonist
Pregnancy risk category C

AVAILABLE FORMS
Tablets: 25 mg, 50 mg, 100 mg

INDICATIONS & DOSAGES
■ **Black Box Warning** Use spironolactone only for those conditions for which it's indicated. ■
➤ **Edema**
Adults: Initially, 100 mg P.O. daily given as a single dose or in divided doses. Usual range is 25 to 200 mg P.O. daily.
Children: Give 3.3 mg/kg P.O. daily or in divided doses.
➤ **Hypertension**
Adults: 50 to 100 mg P.O. daily or in divided doses. Some practitioners use a lower dose range of 25 to 50 mg daily and add another antihypertensive to the regimen, rather than continually increasing this drug.
Children ◆: Give 1 to 3.3 mg/kg P.O. (up to 100 mg daily) as a single dose or divided b.i.d.
➤ **Diuretic-induced hypokalemia**
Adults: 25 to 100 mg P.O. daily.
➤ **To detect primary hyper-aldosteronism**
Adults: 400 mg P.O. daily for 4 days (short test) or 3 to 4 weeks (long test). If hypokalemia and hypertension are corrected, a presumptive diagnosis of primary hyperaldosteronism is made.
➤ **To manage primary hyper-aldosteronism**
Adults: 100 to 400 mg P.O. daily. Use lowest effective dose.

Reactions may be *common*, uncommon, *life-threatening*, or COMMON AND LIFE-THREATENING.
Interaction may have a *rapid onset* or *delayed onset*.

➤ **Heart failure, as adjunct to ACE inhibitor or loop diuretic, with or without cardiac glycoside)** ◆
Adults: 12.5 to 25 mg P.O. daily. May increase to 50 mg daily after 8 weeks.
➤ **Hirsutism** ◆
Women: 50 to 200 mg P.O. daily.

ADMINISTRATION
P.O.
● To enhance absorption, give drug with meals.
● Give drug in morning to prevent nocturia. If second dose is needed, give it with food in early afternoon.
● Protect tablets from light.

ACTION
Antagonizes aldosterone in the distal tubules, increasing sodium and water excretion.

Route	Onset	Peak	Duration
P.O.	1–2 days	2–3 days	2–3 days

Half-life: 1¼ to 2 hours.

ADVERSE REACTIONS
CNS: headache, drowsiness, lethargy, confusion, ataxia.
GI: diarrhea, *gastric bleeding,* ulceration, cramping, gastritis, vomiting.
GU: inability to maintain erection, menstrual disturbances.
Hematologic: *agranulocytosis.*
Metabolic: *hyperkalemia,* dehydration, hyponatremia, mild acidosis.
Skin: urticaria, hirsutism, maculopapular eruptions.
Other: *anaphylaxis,* gynecomastia, breast soreness, drug fever.

INTERACTIONS
Drug-drug. *ACE inhibitors, indomethacin, other potassium-sparing diuretics, potassium supplements:* May increase risk of hyperkalemia. Use together cautiously, especially in patients with renal impairment. Monitor potassium level.
Anticoagulants: May decrease anticoagulant effects. Monitor PT and INR.
Aspirin and other salicylates: May block diuretic effect of spironolactone. Watch for diminished spironolactone response.

Digoxin: May alter digoxin clearance, increasing risk of toxicity. Monitor digoxin level.
Drug-herb. *Licorice:* May block ulcer-healing and aldosterone-like effects of herb; may increase risk of hypokalemia. Discourage use together.
Drug-food. *Potassium-rich foods, such as citrus fruits and tomatoes, salt substitutes containing potassium:* May increase risk of hyperkalemia. Urge caution.

EFFECTS ON LAB TEST RESULTS
● May increase BUN and potassium levels. May decrease sodium level.
● May decrease granulocyte count.
● May alter fluorometric determinations of plasma and urinary 17-hydroxycortico-steroid levels.

CONTRAINDICATIONS & CAUTIONS
● Contraindicated in patients hypersensitive to drug and in those with anuria, acute or progressive renal insufficiency, or hyperkalemia.
● Use cautiously in patients with fluid or electrolyte imbalances, impaired renal function, or hepatic disease, or in pregnant women.

NURSING CONSIDERATIONS
● Monitor electrolyte levels, fluid intake and output, weight, and blood pressure.
● Monitor elderly patients closely, who are more susceptible to excessive diuresis.
● Inform laboratory that patient is taking spironolactone because drug may interfere with tests that measure digoxin level.
● Drug is less potent than thiazide and loop diuretics and is useful as an adjunct to other diuretic therapy. Diuretic effect is delayed 2 to 3 days when used alone.
● Maximum antihypertensive response may be delayed for up to 2 weeks.
● Watch for hyperchloremic metabolic acidosis, especially in patients with hepatic cirrhosis.
● *Look alike–sound alike:* Don't confuse Aldactone with Aldactazide.

PATIENT TEACHING
● Instruct patient to take drug in morning to prevent need to urinate at

night. If second dose is needed, tell him to take it with food in early afternoon.

● *Alert:* To prevent serious hyperkalemia, warn patient to avoid excessive ingestion of potassium-rich foods (such as citrus fruits, tomatoes, bananas, dates, and apricots), salt substitutes containing potassium, and potassium supplements.

● Caution patient not to perform hazardous activities if adverse CNS reactions occur.

● Advise men about possible breast tenderness or enlargement.

torsemide
TOR-seh-mide

Demadex

Pharmacologic class: loop diuretic
Pregnancy risk category B

AVAILABLE FORMS
Injection: 10 mg/ml
Tablets: 5 mg, 10 mg, 20 mg, 100 mg

INDICATIONS & DOSAGES
➤ **Diuresis in patients with heart failure**
Adults: Initially, 10 to 20 mg P.O. or I.V. once daily. If response is inadequate, double dose until desired effect is achieved. Maximum, 200 mg daily.
➤ **Diuresis in patients with chronic renal failure**
Adults: Initially, 20 mg P.O. or I.V. once daily. If response is inadequate, double dose until response is obtained. Maximum, 200 mg daily.
➤ **Diuresis in patients with hepatic cirrhosis**
Adults: Initially, 5 to 10 mg P.O. or I.V. once daily with an aldosterone antagonist or a potassium-sparing diuretic. If response is inadequate, double dose until desired effect is achieved. Maximum, 40 mg daily.
➤ **Hypertension**
Adults: Initially, 5 mg P.O. daily. Increased to 10 mg if needed and tolerated. Add another antihypertensive if response is still inadequate.

ADMINISTRATION
P.O.
● To prevent nocturia, give drug in the morning.
I.V.
● Inspect ampules for precipitate or discoloration before use.
● Give by direct injection over at least 2 minutes. Rapid injection may cause ototoxicity. Don't give more than 200 mg at a time.
● Drug may be given as a continuous infusion.
● Drug remains stable for 24 hours at room temperature when mixed in D₅W, normal saline solution, or half-normal saline solution.
● **Incompatibilities:** Solutions with pH below 8.3. Flush line with normal saline before and after administration to avoid incompatibility.

ACTION
Enhances excretion of sodium, chloride, and water by acting on the ascending loop of Henle.

Route	Onset	Peak	Duration
P.O.	1 hr	1–2 hr	6–8 hr
I.V.	10 min	1 hr	6–8 hr

Half-life: 3½ hours.

ADVERSE REACTIONS
CNS: asthenia, dizziness, headache, nervousness, insomnia, syncope.
CV: ECG abnormalities, chest pain, edema, orthostatic hypotension.
EENT: rhinitis, sore throat.
GI: *excessive thirst, hemorrhage,* diarrhea, constipation, nausea, dyspepsia.
GU: excessive urination, impotence.
Metabolic: *electrolyte imbalances including hypokalemia and, hypomagnesemia, dehydration,* hypochloremic alkalosis, hyperuricemia, hypercholesterolemia.
Musculoskeletal: arthralgia, myalgia.
Respiratory: cough.
Skin: rash.

INTERACTIONS
Drug-drug. *Aminoglycoside antibiotics, cisplatin:* May increase ototoxicity. Use together cautiously.

Reactions may be *common,* uncommon, *life-threatening,* or COMMON AND LIFE-THREATENING.
Interaction may have a *rapid onset* or **delayed onset.**

Amphotericin B, corticosteroids, metolazone: May increase risk of hypokalemia. Monitor potassium level.

Anticoagulants: May enhance anticoagulant activity. Use together cautiously.

Antidiabetics: May decrease hypoglycemic effect, resulting in higher glucose level. Monitor glucose level.

Chlorothiazide, chlorthalidone, hydrochlorothiazide, indapamide, metolazone: May cause excessive diuretic response, resulting in serious electrolyte abnormalities or dehydration. Adjust doses carefully, and monitor patient closely for signs and symptoms of excessive diuretic response.

Cholestyramine: May decrease absorption of torsemide. Separate doses by at least 3 hours.

Digoxin: Electrolyte imbalance caused by diuretic may lead to digoxin-induced arrhythmia. Use together cautiously.

Lithium: May increase lithium level and cause toxicity. Use together cautiously and monitor lithium level.

NSAIDs: May decrease effects of loop diuretics. Use together cautiously.

Probenecid: May decrease diuretic effect. Avoid using together.

Salicylates: May decrease excretion, possibly leading to salicylate toxicity. Avoid using together.

Spironolactone: May decrease renal clearance of spironolactone. Use together cautiously.

Drug-herb. *Dandelion:* May interfere with drug activity. Discourage use together.

Licorice: May cause unexpected rapid potassium loss. Discourage use together.

Drug-lifestyle. *Sun exposure:* May cause photosensitivity. Advise patient to take precautions.

EFFECTS ON LAB TEST RESULTS
● May increase BUN, creatinine, cholesterol, glucose, and uric acid levels. May decrease potassium and magnesium levels.

CONTRAINDICATIONS & CAUTIONS
● Contraindicated in patients hypersensitive to drug or other sulfonamide derivatives and in those with anuria.
● Use cautiously in patients with hepatic disease and related cirrhosis and ascites;

sudden changes in fluid and electrolyte balance may precipitate hepatic coma in these patients.

NURSING CONSIDERATIONS
● Monitor fluid intake and output, electrolyte levels, blood pressure, weight, and pulse rate during rapid diuresis and routinely with long-term use. Drug can cause profound diuresis and water and electrolyte depletion.
● Watch for signs of hypokalemia, such as muscle weakness and cramps.
● Consult prescriber and dietitian about providing a high-potassium diet or potassium supplement. Foods rich in potassium include citrus fruits, tomatoes, bananas, dates, and apricots.
● Monitor elderly patients, who are especially susceptible to excessive diuresis with potential for circulatory collapse and thromboembolic complications.
● *Look alike–sound alike:* Don't confuse torsemide with furosemide.

PATIENT TEACHING
● Tell patient to take drug in morning to prevent the need to urinate at night.
● Advise patient to change positions slowly to prevent dizziness and to limit alcohol intake and strenuous exercise in hot weather to prevent dizziness.
● Advise patient to immediately report ringing in ears because it may indicate toxicity.
● Tell patient to report weakness, cramping, nausea, and dizziness.
● Tell patient to check with prescriber or pharmacist before taking OTC drugs.
● Advise patient that drug may cause photosensitivity, and tell him to take precautions with sun exposure.

---

triamterene
try-AM-ter-een

Dyrenium

Pharmacologic class: potassium-sparing diuretic
Pregnancy risk category C

AVAILABLE FORMS
Capsules: 50 mg, 100 mg

INDICATIONS & DOSAGES
➤ **Edema**
Adults: Initially, 100 mg P.O. b.i.d. after meals. Maximum, 300 mg daily.

ADMINISTRATION
P.O.
- Give drug after meals to minimize nausea.
- If a single daily dose is prescribed, give it in the morning to prevent nocturia.

ACTION
Inhibits sodium reabsorption and potassium and hydrogen excretion by direct action on the distal tubules.

Route	Onset	Peak	Duration
P.O.	2–4 hr	6–8 hr	12–16 hr

Half-life: 3 hours.

ADVERSE REACTIONS
CNS: dizziness, weakness, fatigue, headache.
GI: dry mouth, nausea, vomiting, diarrhea.
GU: interstitial nephritis, nephrolithiasis.
Hematologic: *thrombocytopenia, agranulocytosis,* megaloblastic anemia from low folic acid level.
Hepatic: jaundice.
Metabolic: *hyperkalemia,* azotemia, hypokalemia, hyponatremia, hyperglycemia, acidosis.
Musculoskeletal: muscle cramps.
Skin: photosensitivity reactions, rash.
Other: *anaphylaxis.*

INTERACTIONS
Drug-drug. *ACE inhibitors, potassium supplements:* May increase risk of hyperkalemia. If used together, monitor potassium level.
Amantadine: May increase risk of amantadine toxicity. Avoid using together.
Chlorpropamide: May increase risk of hyponatremia. Monitor sodium level.
Cimetidine: May increase bioavailability and decrease renal clearance of triamterene. Monitor potassium level and blood pressure closely.
Lithium: May decrease lithium clearance, increasing risk of lithium toxicity. Monitor lithium level.

NSAIDs: May enhance risk of nephrotoxicity. Use together cautiously.
Quinidine: May interfere with some laboratory tests that measure quinidine level. Inform laboratory that patient is taking triamterene.
Drug-herb. *Licorice:* May increase risk of hypokalemia. Discourage use together.
Drug-food. *Potassium-containing salt substitutes, potassium-rich foods:* May increase risk of hyperkalemia. Urge caution, and monitor potassium level.
Drug-lifestyle. *Sun exposure:* May increase risk for photosensitivity reactions. Advise patient to avoid excessive sunlight exposure.

EFFECTS ON LAB TEST RESULTS
- May increase BUN, creatinine, glucose, and uric acid levels. May decrease sodium and hemoglobin levels. May increase or decrease potassium level.
- May decrease granulocyte and platelet counts. May increase liver function test values.
- May interfere with enzyme assays that use fluorometry, such as quinidine determinations.

CONTRAINDICATIONS & CAUTIONS
- Contraindicated in patients hypersensitive to drug and in those with anuria, severe or progressive renal disease or dysfunction, severe hepatic disease, or hyperkalemia.
- Use cautiously in elderly or debilitated patients and in those with hepatic impairment or diabetes mellitus.

NURSING CONSIDERATIONS
- Monitor blood pressure, uric acid, CBC, and glucose, BUN, and electrolyte levels.
- Monitor potassium levels frequently, especially with dosage changes or with illness that may affect renal function.
- Obtain an ECG if hyperkalemia is present or suspected.
- Stop potassium supplements when therapy starts.
- Watch for blood dyscrasia.
- To minimize excessive rebound potassium excretion, withdraw drug gradually.
- Drug is less potent than thiazides and loop diuretics and is useful as an adjunct to other diuretic therapy. It's usually used with potassium-wasting diuretics; full

---

effect is delayed 2 to 3 days when used alone.
• *Look alike–sound alike:* Don't confuse triamterene with trimipramine.

PATIENT TEACHING
• Tell patient to take drug after meals to minimize nausea.
• If a single daily dose is prescribed, instruct patient to take it in the morning to prevent need to urinate at night.
• *Alert:* Warn patient to avoid excessive ingestion of potassium-rich foods (such as citrus fruits, tomatoes, bananas, dates, and apricots), potassium-containing salt substitutes, and potassium supplements to prevent serious hyperkalemia.
• Teach patient to avoid direct sunlight, wear protective clothing, and use sunblock to prevent photosensitivity reactions.
• Tell patient that urine may turn blue.

Inotropics

dobutamine hydrochloride
  (See Chapter 28, VASOPRESSORS.)
dopamine hydrochloride
  (See Chapter 28, VASOPRESSORS.)
digoxin
ephedrine sulfate
  (See Chapter 28, VASOPRESSORS.)
epinephrine
  (See Chapter 56, BRONCHODILATORS.)
inamrinone lactate
milrinone lactate
ephedrine sulfate
  (See Chapter 28, VASOPRESSORS.)

SAFETY ALERT!

digoxin
di-JOX-in

Digitek, Digoxin, Lanoxicaps,
Lanoxin*

Pharmacologic class: cardiac
glycoside
Pregnancy risk category C

AVAILABLE FORMS
Capsules: 0.05 mg, 0.1 mg, 0.2 mg
Elixir: 0.05 mg/ml (pediatric)
Injection: 0.05 mg/ml†, 0.1 mg/ml
(pediatric), 0.25 mg/ml
Tablets: 0.125 mg, 0.25 mg

INDICATIONS & DOSAGES
➤ **Heart failure, paroxysmal supra-ventricular tachycardia, atrial fibrillation and flutter**
Capsules
Adults: For rapid digitalization, give 0.4 to 0.6 mg P.O. initially, followed by 0.1 to 0.3 mg every 6 to 8 hours, as needed and tolerated, for 24 hours. For slow digitalization, give 0.05 to 0.35 mg daily in two divided doses. Therapeutic levels are reached in 7 to 22 days. Maintenance dose is 0.05 to 0.35 mg daily in one or two divided doses.
Children: Digitalizing dose is based on child's age and is given in three or more divided doses over the first 24 hours. First

dose is 50% of the total dose; subsequent doses are given as 25% of total dose for two doses every 6 to 8 hours as needed and tolerated.
Children age 10 and older: For rapid digitalization, give 8 to 12 mcg/kg P.O. over 24 hours, divided as described previously. Maintenance dose is 25% to 35% of total digitalizing dose, given daily as a single dose.
Children ages 5 to 10: For rapid digitalization, give 15 to 30 mcg/kg P.O. over 24 hours, divided as described previously. Maintenance dose is 25% to 35% of total digitalizing dose, divided and given in two or three equal portions daily.
Children ages 2 to 5: For rapid digitalization, give 25 to 35 mcg/kg P.O. over 24 hours, divided as described previously. Maintenance dose is 25% to 35% of total digitalizing dose, divided and given in two or three equal portions daily.
Elixir, tablets
Adults: For rapid digitalization, give 0.75 to 1.25 mg P.O. over 24 hours in two or more divided doses every 6 to 8 hours. For slow digitalization, give 0.0625 to 0.5 mg daily. Titrate every 2 weeks as needed. Maintenance dose is 0.0625 to 0.5 mg daily.
Children age 10 and older: 10 to 15 mcg/kg P.O. over 24 hours in two or more divided doses every 6 to 8 hours. Maintenance dose is 25% to 35% of total digitalizing dose.
Children ages 5 to 10: 20 to 35 mcg/kg P.O. over 24 hours in two or more divided doses every 6 to 8 hours. Maintenance dose is 25% to 35% of total digitalizing dose.
Children ages 2 to 5: 30 to 40 mcg/kg P.O. over 24 hours in two or more divided doses every 6 to 8 hours. Maintenance dose is 25% to 35% of total digitalizing dose.
Infants ages 1 month to 2 years: 35 to 60 mcg/kg P.O. over 24 hours in two or more divided doses every 6 to 8 hours. Maintenance dose is 25% to 35% of total digitalizing dose.
Neonates: 25 to 35 mcg/kg P.O. over 24 hours in two or more divided doses every 6 to 8 hours. Maintenance dose is 25% to 35% of total digitalizing dose.

Premature infants: 20 to 30 mcg/kg P.O. over 24 hours in two or more divided doses every 6 to 8 hours. Maintenance dose is 20% to 30% of total digitalizing dose.

Injection

Adults: For rapid digitalization, give 0.4 to 0.6 mg I.V. initially, followed by 0.1 to 0.3 mg I.V. every 6 to 8 hours, as needed and tolerated, for 24 hours. For slow digitalization, give appropriate daily maintenance dose for 7 to 22 days until therapeutic levels are reached. Maintenance dose is 0.075 to 0.35 mg I.V. daily in one or two divided doses.

Children: Digitalizing dose is based on child's age; give in three or more divided doses over the first 24 hours. First dose is 50% of total dose; subsequent doses are given every 6 to 8 hours as needed and tolerated.

Children age 10 and older: For rapid digitalization, give 8 to 12 mcg/kg I.V. over 24 hours, divided as described previously. Maintenance dose is 25% to 35% of total digitalizing dose, given daily as a single dose.

Children ages 5 to 10: For rapid digitalization, give 15 to 30 mcg/kg I.V. over 24 hours, divided as described previously. Maintenance dose is 25% to 35% of total digitalizing dose, divided and given in two or three equal portions daily.

Children ages 2 to 5: For rapid digitalization, give 25 to 35 mcg/kg I.V. over 24 hours, divided as described previously. Maintenance dose is 25% to 35% of total digitalizing dose, divided and given in two or three equal portions daily.

Infants ages 1 month to 2 years: For rapid digitalization, give 30 to 50 mcg/kg I.V. over 24 hours, divided as described previously. Maintenance dose is 25% to 35% of total digitalizing dose, divided and given in two or three equal portions daily.

Neonates: For rapid digitalization, give 20 to 30 mcg/kg I.V. over 24 hours, divided as described previously. Maintenance dose is 25% to 35% of the total digitalizing dose, divided and given in two or three equal portions daily.

Premature infants: For rapid digitalization, give 15 to 25 mcg/kg I.V. over 24 hours, divided as described previously. Maintenance dose is 20% to 30% of the total digitalizing dose, divided and

given in two or three equal portions daily.

Adjust-a-dose: For patients with impaired renal function, give smaller loading and maintenance doses; extended dosing intervals may be needed.

ADMINISTRATION

P.O.
● Before giving loading dose, obtain baseline data (heart rate and rhythm, blood pressure, and electrolytes) and ask patient about use of cardiac glycosides within the previous 2 to 3 weeks.
● Before giving drug, take apical-radial pulse for 1 minute. Record and notify prescriber of significant changes (sudden increase or decrease in pulse rate, pulse deficit, irregular beats and, particularly, regularization of a previously irregular rhythm). If these occur, check blood pressure and obtain a 12-lead ECG.

I.V.
● Before giving loading dose, obtain baseline data (heart rate and rhythm, blood pressure, and electrolytes) and ask patient about use of cardiac glycosides within the previous 2 to 3 weeks.
● Before giving drug, take apical-radial pulse for 1 minute. Record and notify prescriber of significant changes (sudden increase or decrease in pulse rate, pulse deficit, irregular beats and, particularly, regularization of a previously irregular rhythm). If these occur, check blood pressure and obtain a 12-lead ECG.
● Dilute fourfold with D_5W, normal saline solution, or sterile water for injection to reduce the chance of precipitation.
● Infuse drug slowly over at least 5 minutes.
● Protect solution from light.
● **Incompatibilities:** Amiodarone, amphotericin B cholesteryl sulfate complex, dobutamine, doxapram, fluconazole, foscarnet, propofol, remifentanil. Mixing with other drugs isn't recommended.

ACTION

Inhibits sodium-potassium–activated adenosine triphosphatase, promoting movement of calcium from extracellular to intracellular cytoplasm and strengthening myocardial contraction. Also acts on CNS to enhance vagal tone, slowing conduction through the SA and AV nodes.

Route	Onset	Peak	Duration
P.O.	30–120 min	2–6 hr	3–4 days
I.V.	5–30 min	1–4 hr	3–4 days

Half-life: 30 to 40 hours.

ADVERSE REACTIONS

CNS: *agitation, fatigue, generalized muscle weakness, hallucinations,* dizziness, headache, malaise, paresthesia, stupor, vertigo.
CV: *arrhythmias, heart block.*
EENT: blurred vision, diplopia, light flashes, photophobia, yellow-green halos around visual images.
GI: *anorexia, nausea,* diarrhea, vomiting.

INTERACTIONS

Drug-drug. *Amiloride:* May decrease digoxin effect and increase renal clearance of digoxin. Monitor patient for altered digoxin effect.
Amiodarone, *diltiazem, indomethacin, nifedipine,* **quinidine, verapamil:** May increase digoxin level. Monitor patient for toxicity.
Amphotericin B, carbenicillin, cortico-steroids, **diuretics (such as chlorthalidone, loop diuretics, metolazone, thiazides),** *ticarcillin:* May cause hypokalemia, predisposing patient to digitalis toxicity. Monitor potassium level.
Antacids, kaolin-pectin: May decrease absorption of oral digoxin. Separate doses as much as possible.
Antibiotics (azole antifungals, macrolides, telithromycin, tetracyclines), propafenone, ritonavir: May increase risk of toxicity. Monitor patient for toxicity.
Anticholinergics: May increase digoxin absorption of oral digoxin tablets. Monitor drug level and observe for toxicity.
Beta blockers, calcium channel blockers: May have additive effects on AV node conduction causing advanced or complete heart block. Use cautiously.
Cholestyramine, colestipol, metoclo-pramide: May decrease absorption of oral digoxin. Monitor patient for decreased digoxin level and effect. Give digoxin 1½ hours before or 2 hours after other drugs.
Parenteral calcium, thiazides: May cause hypercalcemia and hypomagnesemia, predisposing patient to digitalis

toxicity. Monitor calcium and magnesium levels.
Drug-herb. *Betel palm, Foxglove, fumitory, goldenseal, hawthorn, lily of the valley, motherwort, rue, shepherd's purse:* May increase cardiac effects. Discourage use together.
Gossypol, horsetail, licorice, oleander, Siberian ginseng, squill: May increase toxicity. Monitor patient closely.
Plantain, St. John's wort: May decrease effectiveness of drug. Discourage use together.

EFFECTS ON LAB TEST RESULTS
● May prolong PR interval or depress ST segment.

CONTRAINDICATIONS & CAUTIONS
● Contraindicated in patients hypersensitive to drug and in those with digitalis-induced toxicity, ventricular fibrillation, or ventricular tachycardia unless caused by heart failure.
● Don't use in patients with Wolff-Parkinson-White syndrome unless the conduction accessory pathway has been pharmacologically or surgically disabled.
● Use with extreme caution in elderly patients and in those with acute MI, incomplete AV block, sinus bradycardia, PVCs, chronic constrictive pericarditis, hypertrophic cardiomyopathy, renal insufficiency, severe pulmonary disease, or hypothyroidism.

NURSING CONSIDERATIONS
● Drug-induced arrhythmias may increase the severity of heart failure and hypotension.
● In children, cardiac arrhythmias, including sinus bradycardia, are usually early signs of toxicity.
● Patients with hypothyroidism are extremely sensitive to cardiac glycosides and may need lower doses.
● Loading dose is usually divided over the first 24 hours with about half the loading dose given in the first dose.
● Toxic effects on the heart may be life-threatening and require immediate attention.
● Absorption of digoxin from liquid-filled capsules is superior to absorption from tablets or elixir. Expect dosage reduction

---

Reactions may be *common,* uncommon, *life-threatening,* or COMMON AND LIFE-THREATENING.
Interaction may have a *rapid onset* or **delayed onset.**

of 20% to 25% when changing from tablets or elixir to liquid-filled capsules or parenteral therapy.
• Monitor digoxin level. Therapeutic level ranges from 0.8 to 2 nanogram/ml. Obtain blood for digoxin level at least 6 to 8 hours after last oral dose, preferably just before next scheduled dose.
• *Alert:* Excessively slow pulse rate (60 beats/minute or less) may be a sign of digitalis toxicity. Withhold drug and notify prescriber.
• Monitor potassium level carefully. Take corrective action before hypokalemia occurs. Hyperkalemia may result from digoxin toxicity.
• Reduce drug dose for 1 or 2 days before elective cardioversion. Adjust dosage after cardioversion.
• *Look alike–sound alike:* Don't confuse digoxin with doxepin.

PATIENT TEACHING
• Teach patient and a responsible family member about drug action, dosage regimen, how to take pulse, reportable signs, and follow-up care.
• Tell patient to report pulse less than 60 beats/minute or more than 110 beats/minute, or skipped beats or other rhythm changes.
• Instruct patient to report adverse reactions promptly. Nausea, vomiting, diarrhea, appetite loss, and visual disturbances may be indicators of toxicity.
• Encourage patient to eat a consistent amount of potassium-rich foods.
• Tell patient not to substitute one brand for another.
• Advise patient to avoid the use of herbal drugs or to consult his prescriber before taking one.

SAFETY ALERT!

inamrinone lactate
in-AM-ri-none

Pharmacologic class: bipyridine phosphodiesterase inhibitor
Pregnancy risk category C

AVAILABLE FORMS
Injection: 5 mg/ml in 20-ml ampules

INDICATIONS & DOSAGES
➤ **Short-term management of heart failure**
Adults: Initially, 0.75 mg/kg I.V. bolus over 2 to 3 minutes. Then begin maintenance infusion of 5 to 10 mcg/kg/minute. May give additional bolus of 0.75 mg/kg after 30 minutes. Don't exceed total daily dose of 10 mg/kg.

ADMINISTRATION
I.V.
• Give drug with an infusion pump. Use drug as supplied or dilute in half-normal saline solution or normal saline solution to a concentration of 1 to 3 mg/ml. Use diluted solution within 24 hours.
• Don't dilute with solutions containing dextrose because a slow chemical reaction occurs over 24 hours. Inamrinone can be injected into free-flowing dextrose infusions through a Y-connector or directly into tubing.
• Monitor blood pressure and heart rate throughout the infusion. If patient's blood pressure falls, slow or stop infusion and notify prescriber.
• **Incompatibilities:** Bicarbonate, dextrose-containing solutions such as D_5W, furosemide, glucose, procainamide, sodium bicarbonate, torsemide.

ACTION
Produces inotropic action by increasing cellular levels of cAMP. Produces vasodilation through a direct relaxant effect on vascular smooth muscle.

Route	Onset	Peak	Duration
I.V.	2–5 min	10 min	30–120 min

Half-life: About 4 hours.

ADVERSE REACTIONS
CNS: fever.
CV: *arrhythmias,* chest pain, hypotension.
GI: abdominal pain, anorexia, nausea, vomiting.
Hematologic: *thrombocytopenia.*
Hepatic: *hepatotoxicity.*
Metabolic: hypokalemia.
Skin: burning at injection site.
Other: hypersensitivity reactions.

INTERACTIONS
Drug-drug. *Cardiac glycosides:* May increase inotropic effect, which is a beneficial drug interaction. Monitor patient.
Disopyramide: May cause excessive hypotension. Monitor blood pressure.

EFFECTS ON LAB TEST RESULTS
● May increase liver enzyme level. May decrease potassium level.
● May increase sedimentation rate. May decrease platelet count.

CONTRAINDICATIONS & CAUTIONS
● Contraindicated in patients hypersensitive to inamrinone or bisulfites.
● Contraindicated in patients with severe aortic or pulmonic valvular disease in place of surgery or during acute phase of MI.
● Use cautiously in patients with hypertrophic cardiomyopathy.
● Safety and effectiveness haven't been established in children, although drug has been used in preterm infants for heart failure.

NURSING CONSIDERATIONS
● Drug is prescribed primarily for patients who haven't responded to cardiac glycosides, diuretics, and vasodilators.
● Dosage depends on clinical response, including assessment of pulmonary wedge pressure and cardiac output, as well as lessening of dyspnea, orthopnea, and fatigue.
● In patients with atrial fibrillation and flutter, drug may be added to cardiac glycoside therapy because it slightly enhances AV conduction and increases ventricular response rate.
● Correct hypokalemia before or during therapy.
● Monitor platelet count. If it falls below 150,000/mm^3, decrease dosage or stop drug if risk outweighs benefit.
● Monitor patient for hypersensitivity reactions, such as pericarditis, ascites, myositis, vasculitis, and pleuritis.
● Monitor intake and output and daily weight.
● Patients with end-stage cardiac disease may receive home treatment while awaiting heart transplantation.

● *Look alike–sound alike:* Because of confusion with amiodarone, "amrinone" was changed to "inamrinone."

PATIENT TEACHING
● Warn patient that burning may occur at injection site.
● Instruct home care patient and family about drug administration; tell them to report adverse reactions promptly.

SAFETY ALERT!

milrinone lactate
MILL-ri-none

Primacor

Pharmacologic class: bipyridine phosphodiesterase inhibitor
Pregnancy risk category C

AVAILABLE FORMS
Injection: 1 mg/ml
Injection (premixed): 200 mcg/ml in D_5W

INDICATIONS & DOSAGES
➤ **Short-term treatment of acutely decompensated heart failure**
Adults: Give first loading dose of 50 mcg/kg I.V. slowly over 10 minutes; then give continuous I.V. infusion of 0.375 to 0.75 mcg/kg/minute. Titrate infusion dose based on clinical and hemodynamic responses. Don't exceed 1.13 mg/kg/day.
Adjust-a-dose: If creatinine clearance is 50 ml/minute, infusion rate is 0.43 mcg/kg/minute; if 40 ml/minute, infusion rate is 0.38 mcg/kg/minute; if 30 ml/minute, infusion rate is 0.33 mcg/kg/minute; if 20 ml/minute, infusion rate is 0.28 mcg/kg/minute; if 10 ml/minute, infusion rate is 0.23 mcg/kg/minute; and if 5 ml/minute, infusion rate is 0.2 mcg/kg/minute. Don't exceed 1.13 mg/kg/day.

ADMINISTRATION
I.V.
● Give loading dose undiluted as a direct injection over 10 minutes.
● Prepare I.V. infusion solution using half-normal saline solution, normal saline

Reactions may be *common*, uncommon, *life-threatening*, or COMMON AND LIFE-THREATENING.
Interaction may have a *rapid onset* or **delayed onset.**

solution, or D$_5$W. Prepare the 100-mcg/ml solution by adding 180 ml of diluent per 20-mg (20-ml) vial, the 150-mcg/ml solution by adding 113 ml of diluent per 20-mg (20-ml) vial, and the 200-mcg/ml solution by adding 80 ml of diluent per 20-mg (20-ml) vial.

● **Incompatibilities:** Bumetanide, furosemide, imipenem and cilastatin sodium, procainamide, torsemide.

ACTION
Produces inotropic action by increasing cellular levels of cAMP and vasodilation by relaxing vascular smooth muscle.

Route	Onset	Peak	Duration
I.V.	5–15 min	1–2 hr	3–6 hr

Half-life: 2½ to 3¾ hours.

ADVERSE REACTIONS
CNS: headache.
CV: VENTRICULAR ARRHYTHMIAS, *ventricular ectopic activity,* **sustained ventricular tachycardia, ventricular fibrillation,** hypotension, nonsustained ventricular tachycardia.

INTERACTIONS
None significant.

EFFECTS ON LAB TEST RESULTS
● May cause abnormal liver function test results.

CONTRAINDICATIONS & CAUTIONS
● Contraindicated in patients hypersensitive to drug.
● Contraindicated for use in patients with severe aortic or pulmonic valvular disease in place of surgery and during acute phase of MI.
● Use cautiously in patients with atrial flutter or fibrillation because drug slightly shortens AV node conduction time and may increase ventricular response rate.

NURSING CONSIDERATIONS
● In patients with atrial flutter or fibrillation, give digoxin before milrinone therapy. Drug is typically given with digoxin and diuretics.
● Improved cardiac output may increase urine output. Reduce diuretic dosage when

heart failure improves. Potassium loss may cause digitalis toxicity.
● Monitor fluid and electrolyte status, blood pressure, heart rate, and renal function during therapy. Excessive decrease in blood pressure requires stopping or slowing rate of infusion.
● Correct hypoxemia.

PATIENT TEACHING
● Instruct patient to report adverse reactions to prescriber promptly, especially angina.
● Tell patient that drug may cause headache, which can be treated with analgesics.
● Tell patient to report discomfort at I.V. insertion site.

ambrisentan
bosentan
hydralazine hydrochloride
  (See Chapter 23, ANTIHYPERTENSIVES.)
iloprost
isosorbide dinitrate
  (See Chapter 21, ANTIANGINALS.)
isosorbide mononitrate
  (See Chapter 21, ANTIANGINALS.)
minoxidil
  (See Chapter 23, ANTIHYPERTENSIVES.)
nesiritide
nimodipine
nitroglycerine
  (See Chapter 21, ANTIANGINALS.)
nitroprusside sodium
  (See Chapter 23, ANTIHYPERTENSIVES.)
sildenafil citrate
treprostinil sodium

SAFETY ALERT!

---

ambrisentan
am-bree-SEN-tan

Letairis

Pharmacologic class: endothelin-
receptor antagonist
Pregnancy risk category X

AVAILABLE FORMS
Tablets: 5 mg, 10 mg

INDICATIONS & DOSAGES
➤ **Pulmonary arterial hypertension
in patients with World Health Organization class II (with significant
exertion) or III (with mild exertion)
symptoms to improve exercise tolerance and decrease rate of clinical
worsening**
Adults: 5 mg P.O. once daily; may increase
to 10 mg P.O. once daily if tolerated.
Adjust-a-dose: Don't start therapy in
patients with elevated aminotransferase
levels (ALT and AST) of more than three
times the upper limit of normal (ULN)
at baseline. If ALT elevations during
therapy are between three and five times

the ULN, remeasure. If confirmed level
is in the same range, reduce dose or stop
therapy and remeasure every 2 weeks
until levels are less than three times
ULN. If ALT and AST are between five
and eight times the ULN, stop therapy
and monitor until the levels are less than
three times ULN. Restart therapy with
more frequent monitoring. If ALT and
AST exceed eight times the ULN, stop
therapy and don't restart.

ADMINISTRATION
P.O.
● Give drug without regard for food.
● Give drug whole; don't crush or split
tablets.

ACTION
Blocks endothelin-1 receptors on vascular
endothelin and smooth muscle. Stimulation of these receptors in smooth muscle
cells is associated with vasoconstriction
and PAH.

Route	Onset	Peak	Duration
P.O.	Rapid	2 hr	Unknown

Half-life: 9 hours.

ADVERSE REACTIONS
CNS: *headache.*
CV: *peripheral edema,* flushing, palpitations.
EENT: nasal congestion, sinusitis,
nasopharyngitis.
GI: abdominal pain, constipation.
Hematologic: anemia.
Hepatic: hepatic impairment.
Respiratory: dyspnea.

INTERACTIONS
Drug-drug. *CYP enzyme inducers, such
as carbamazepine, phenobarbital,
phenytoin, and rifampin:* May decrease
effects of ambrisentan. Use together
cautiously.
*CYP enzyme inhibitors, such as atanaza-
vir, clarithromycin, fluvoxamine, fluconazole, indinavir, itraconazole, ketoconazole,
nefazodone, nelfinavir, omeprazole, riton-*

Reactions may be *common,* uncommon, *life-threatening,* or COMMON AND LIFE-THREATENING.
Interaction may have a *rapid onset* or *delayed onset.*

avir, saquinavir, telithromycin, and ticlopidine: May increase the effects of ambrisentan. Use together cautiously.
Cyclosporine: May increase ambrisentan levels. Use together cautiously and monitor patient for increased adverse effects.

EFFECTS ON LAB TEST RESULTS
■ **Black Box Warning** May increase AST, ALT, and bilirubin levels. ■
● May decrease hemoglobin level and hematocrit.

CONTRAINDICATIONS & CAUTIONS
● Contraindicated in patients hypersensitive to drug or its components.
■ **Black Box Warning** Contraindicated in pregnant women because it may harm the fetus. ■
■ **Black Box Warning** Contraindicated in those with moderate to severe hepatic impairment; don't begin therapy in those with elevated baseline ALT and AST levels of more than three times the ULN. ■
● Use cautiously in those with mild hepatic impairment.
● Use cautiously in those with renal impairment; drug hasn't been studied in those with severe renal impairment.

PATIENT TEACHING
■ **Black Box Warning** Inform female patient that she'll need to have a pregnancy test done monthly and to report suspected pregnancy to her prescriber immediately. ■
■ **Black Box Warning** Teach woman of childbearing age to use two reliable birth control methods unless she has had tubal sterilization or has a Copper T 380A intrauterine device (IUD) or an LNg 20 IUD inserted. ■
● Tell patient that monthly blood tests will be done to monitor for adverse effects.
● Advise patient to take the pill whole and not to split, crush, or chew the tablet.
● *Alert:* Teach patient to notify prescriber immediately of signs or symptoms of liver injury, including anorexia, nausea, vomiting, fever, malaise, fatigue, right upper quadrant abdominal discomfort, itching, and jaundice.
● Tell the patient to report edema and weight gain.

bosentan
bow-SEN-tan

Tracleer

Pharmacologic class: endothelin-receptor antagonist
Pregnancy risk category X

AVAILABLE FORMS
Tablets: 62.5 mg, 125 mg

INDICATIONS & DOSAGES
➤ **Pulmonary arterial hypertension in patients with World Health Organization class III (with mild exertion) or IV (at rest) symptoms, to improve exercise ability and decrease rate of clinical worsening**
Adults: 62.5 mg P.O. b.i.d. in the morning and evening for 4 weeks. Increase to maintenance dosage of 125 mg P.O. b.i.d. in the morning and evening.
Adjust-a-dose: For patients who develop ALT and AST abnormalities, the dose may need to be decreased or the therapy stopped until ALT and AST levels return to normal. If therapy is resumed, begin with initial dose. Test levels within 3 days; then give using the following table. If liver function abnormalities are accompanied by symptoms of liver injury or if bilirubin level is at least twice the upper limit of normal (ULN), stop treatment and don't restart. In patients who weigh less than 40 kg (88 lb), the initial and maintenance dosage is 62.5 mg b.i.d.

ALT and AST levels	Treatment and monitoring recommendations
> 3 and < 5 times upper limit of normal (ULN)	Confirm with repeat test; if confirmed, reduce dose or interrupt treatment and retest every 2 wk. Once ALT and AST levels return to pretreatment levels, continue or reintroduce treatment at starting dose.
> 5 and < 8 times ULN	Confirm with repeat test; if confirmed, stop treatment and retest at least every 2 wk. Once levels return to pretreatment levels, consider reintroduction of treatment.
> 8 times ULN	Stop treatment; don't consider restarting drug.

ADMINISTRATION
P.O.
- Give drug in morning and evening without regard for meals.

ACTION
Specific and competitive antagonist for endothelin-1 (ET-1). ET-1 levels are elevated in patients with pulmonary arterial hypertension, suggesting a pathogenic role for ET-1 in this disease.

Route	Onset	Peak	Duration
P.O.	Unknown	3–5 hr	Unknown

Half-life: About 5 hours.

ADVERSE REACTIONS
CNS: *headache,* fatigue.
CV: edema, flushing, hypotension, palpitations.
EENT: *nasopharyngitis.*
GI: dyspepsia.
Hematologic: *anemia.*
Hepatic: HEPATOTOXICITY.
Skin: pruritus.
Other: leg edema.

INTERACTIONS
Drug-drug. *Cyclosporine A:* May increase bosentan level and decrease cyclosporine level. Use together is contraindicated.
Glyburide: May increase risk of elevated liver function test values and decrease levels of both drugs. Use together is contraindicated.
Hormonal contraceptives: May cause contraceptive failure. Advise use of an additional method of birth control.
Ketoconazole: May increase bosentan effect. Watch for adverse effects.
Simvastatin, other statins: May decrease levels of these drugs. Monitor cholesterol levels to assess need to adjust statin dose.
Tacrolimus: May increase bosentan levels. Use together cautiously.

EFFECTS ON LAB TEST RESULTS
■ **Black Box Warning** May increase AST, ALT, and bilirubin levels. ■
- May decrease hemoglobin level and hematocrit.

CONTRAINDICATIONS & CAUTIONS
- Contraindicated in patients hypersensitive to drug and in those taking cyclosporine A or glyburide.
■ **Black Box Warning** Generally avoid using in patients with moderate to severe liver impairment or in those with elevated aminotransferase levels greater than three times the ULN. ■
■ **Black Box Warning** Contraindicated in pregnant women. ■
- Use cautiously in patients with mild liver impairment.
- Because it's unknown whether drug appears in breast milk, drug isn't recommended for breast-feeding women.
- Safety and efficacy in children haven't been established.

NURSING CONSIDERATIONS
■ **Black Box Warning** Use of this drug can cause serious liver injury. AST and ALT level elevations may be dose dependent and reversible, so measure these levels before treatment and monthly thereafter, adjusting dosage accordingly. If elevations are accompanied by symptoms of liver injury (nausea, vomiting, fever, abdominal pain, jaundice, or unusual lethargy or fatigue) or if bilirubin level increases by greater than twice the ULN, notify prescriber immediately. ■
- Fluid retention and heart failure may occur. Patient may require diuretics, fluid management, or hospitalization for decompensating heart failure.
- Monitor hemoglobin level after 1 and 3 months of therapy; then every 3 months.
- Gradually reduce dose before stopping drug.

PATIENT TEACHING
- Advise patient to take doses in the morning and evening, with or without food.
■ **Black Box Warning** Warn patient to avoid becoming pregnant while taking this drug. Hormonal contraceptives, including oral, implantable, and injectable methods, may not be effective when used with this drug. Advise patient to use a backup method of contraception. A monthly pregnancy test must be performed. ■
- Advise patient to have liver function tests and blood counts performed regularly.

Reactions may be *common,* uncommon, *life-threatening,* or COMMON AND LIFE-THREATENING.
Interaction may have a *rapid onset* or **delayed onset.**

iloprost
EYE-loe-prost

Ventavis

Pharmacologic class: prostacyclin analog
Pregnancy risk category C

AVAILABLE FORMS
Inhalation solution: 10 mcg/ml in 1- and 2-ml single-dose ampules

INDICATIONS & DOSAGES
➤ **Pulmonary arterial hypertension in patients with New York Heart Association (NYHA) Class III or IV symptoms**
Adults: Initially, 2.5 mcg inhaled using the I-neb or the Prodose Adaptive Aerosol Delivery (AAD) systems. As tolerated, increase to 5 mcg inhaled six to nine times daily while patient is awake, as needed, but to no more than every 2 hours. Maximum, 5 mcg nine times daily.

ADMINISTRATION
Inhalational
• Use only I-neb AAD or Prodose AAD delivery devices, per manufacturer's instructions.

ACTION
Lowers pulmonary arterial pressure by dilating systemic and pulmonary arterial beds. Drug also affects platelet aggregation, although effect in pulmonary hypertension treatment isn't known.

Route	Onset	Peak	Duration
Inhalation	Unknown	Unknown	30–60 min

Half-life: 20 to 30 minutes.

ADVERSE REACTIONS
CNS: *headache,* insomnia, syncope.
CV: *hypotension, vasodilation, chest pain, heart failure, supraventricular tachycardia,* palpitations, peripheral edema.
GI: *nausea,* tongue pain, vomiting.
GU: *renal failure.*
Musculoskeletal: *trismus,* back pain, muscle cramps.
Respiratory: *cough,* dyspnea, hemoptysis, pneumonia.
Other: *flulike syndrome.*

INTERACTIONS
Drug-drug. *Anticoagulants:* May increase risk of bleeding. Monitor patient closely.
Antihypertensives, vasodilators: May increase effects of these drugs. Monitor patient's blood pressure.

EFFECTS ON LAB TEST RESULTS
• May increase alkaline phosphatase and GGT levels.

CONTRAINDICATIONS & CAUTIONS
• No contraindications known. Avoid using in patients whose systolic blood pressure is less than 85 mm Hg.
• Use cautiously in elderly patients, patients with hepatic or renal impairment, and patients with COPD, severe asthma, or acute pulmonary infection.

NURSING CONSIDERATIONS
• Keep drug away from skin and eyes.
• The 2-ml ampule must be used with the Prodose AAD System and may be used with the I-neb AAD System. The 1-ml ampule must be used only with the I-neb AAD System.
• Take care not to inhale drug while providing treatment.
• Monitor patient's vital signs carefully at start of treatment.
• Watch for syncope.
• If patient develops evidence of pulmonary edema, stop treatment immediately.

PATIENT TEACHING
• Advise patient to take drug exactly as prescribed and using Prodose AAD or I-neb AAD.
• Urge patient to follow manufacturer's instructions for preparing and inhaling drug.
• Advise patient to keep a backup Prodose AAD or I-neb AAD in case the original malfunctions.
• Tell patient to keep drug away from skin and eyes and to rinse the area immediately if contact occurs.
• Caution patient not to ingest drug solution.
• Inform patient that drug may cause dizziness and fainting. Urge him to stand

up slowly from a sitting or lying position and to report to prescriber worsening of symptoms.
● Tell patient to take drug before physical exertion but no more than every 2 hours.
● Tell patient not to expose others, especially pregnant women and infants, to drug.
● Teach patient how to clean equipment and safely dispose of used ampules after each treatment. Caution patient not to save or use leftover solution.

nesiritide
neh-SIR-ih-tide

Natrecor

Pharmacologic class: human B-type natriuretic peptide
Pregnancy risk category C

AVAILABLE FORMS
Injection: Single-dose vials of 1.5 mg sterile, lyophilized powder

INDICATIONS & DOSAGES
➤ **Acutely decompensated heart failure in patients with dyspnea at rest or with minimal activity**
Adults: 2 mcg/kg by I.V. bolus over 60 seconds, followed by continuous infusion of 0.01 mcg/kg/minute.
Adjust-a-dose: If hypotension develops during administration, reduce dosage or stop drug. Restart drug at dosage reduced by 30% with no bolus doses.

ADMINISTRATION
I.V.
● Reconstitute one 1.5-mg vial with 5 ml of diluent (such as D_5W, normal saline solution, 5% dextrose and 0.2% saline solution injection, or 5% dextrose and half-normal saline solution) from a prefilled 250-ml I.V. bag.
● Gently rock (don't shake) vial until solution becomes clear and colorless.
● Withdraw contents of vial and add back to the 250-ml I.V. bag to yield 6 mcg/ml. Invert the bag several times to ensure

complete mixing, and use the solution within 24 hours.
● Use the formulas below to calculate bolus volume (2 mcg/kg) and infusion flow rate (0.01 mcg/kg/minute):

$$\text{Bolus volume} = 0.33 \times \text{patient weight}$$
$$\text{(ml)} \qquad\qquad \text{(kg)}$$

$$\text{Infusion flow rate} = 0.1 \times \text{patient weight}$$
$$\text{(ml/hr)} \qquad\qquad \text{(kg)}$$

● Before giving bolus dose, prime the I.V. tubing. Withdraw the bolus and give over 60 seconds through an I.V. port in the tubing.
● Immediately after giving bolus, infuse drug at 0.1 ml/kg/hour to deliver 0.01 mcg/kg/minute.
● Store drug at 68° to 77° F (20° to 25° C).
● **Incompatibilities:** Bumetanide, enalaprilat, ethacrynate sodium, furosemide, heparin, hydralazine, insulin, sodium metabisulfite.

ACTION
Increases cyclic guanosine monophosphate (cGMP) level, relaxes smooth muscle, and dilates veins and arteries. Drug reduces pulmonary capillary wedge pressure and systemic arterial pressure in patients with heart failure.

Route	Onset	Peak	Duration
I.V.	15 min	1 hr	3 hr

Half-life: 18 minutes.

ADVERSE REACTIONS
CNS: anxiety, confusion, dizziness, fever, headache, insomnia, paresthesia, somnolence, tremor.
CV: *hypotension, bradycardia, ventricular tachycardia,* angina, atrial fibrillation, AV node conduction abnormalities, ventricular extrasystoles.
GI: abdominal pain, nausea, vomiting.
Hematologic: anemia.
Musculoskeletal: back pain, leg cramps.
Respiratory: *apnea,* cough.
Skin: injection site reactions, rash, pruritus, sweating.

Reactions may be *common,* uncommon, *life-threatening,* or COMMON AND LIFE-THREATENING.
Interaction may have a *rapid onset* or **delayed onset.**

INTERACTIONS
Drug-drug. *ACE inhibitors:* May increase hypotension symptoms. Monitor blood pressure closely.

EFFECTS ON LAB TEST RESULTS
● May increase creatinine level more than 0.5 mg/dl above baseline. May decrease hemoglobin level and hematocrit.

CONTRAINDICATIONS & CAUTIONS
● Contraindicated in patients hypersensitive to drug or its components.
● Contraindicated in patients with cardiogenic shock, systolic blood pressure below 90 mm Hg, low cardiac filling pressures, conditions in which cardiac output depends on venous return, or conditions that make vasodilators inappropriate, such as valvular stenosis, restrictive or obstructive cardiomyopathy, constrictive pericarditis, and pericardial tamponade.

NURSING CONSIDERATIONS
● Don't start drug at higher-than-recommended dosage because this may cause hypotension and may increase creatinine level.
● *Alert:* This drug may cause hypotension. Monitor patient's blood pressure closely, particularly if he also takes an ACE inhibitor.
● *Alert:* Drug binds to heparin, including the heparin lining of a coated catheter, decreasing the amount of nesiritide delivered. Don't give nesiritide through a central heparin-coated catheter.
● Drug may affect renal function. In patients with severe heart failure whose renal function depends on the renin-angiotensin-aldosterone system, treatment may lead to azotemia.
● Results of giving this drug for longer than 48 hours are unknown.

PATIENT TEACHING
● Tell patient to report discomfort at I.V. site.
● Urge patient to report to prescriber symptoms of hypotension, such as dizziness, light-headedness, blurred vision, or sweating.

● Tell patient to report to prescriber other adverse effects promptly.

---

nimodipine
nye-MOE-dih-peen

Nimotop

Pharmacologic class: calcium channel blocker
Pregnancy risk category C

AVAILABLE FORMS
Capsules: 30 mg

INDICATIONS & DOSAGES
➤ **To improve neurologic deficits after subarachnoid hemorrhage from ruptured intracranial berry aneurysm**
Adults: 60 mg P.O. every 4 hours for 21 days. Begin therapy within 96 hours after subarachnoid hemorrhage.
Adjust-a-dose: For patients with hepatic failure, 30 mg P.O. every 4 hours for 21 days.

ADMINISTRATION
P.O.
● If drug needs to be given via nasogastric (NG) tube, make a hole in each end of capsule with an 18G needle and extract contents into syringe. Empty syringe into patient's NG tube. Flush tube with 30 ml of normal saline solution according to manufacturer's directions.
■ **Black Box Warning** If using a needle to extract contents of capsule, make sure that drug isn't then given I.V. instead of P.O. Label the syringe "for oral use only" before withdrawing the contents of the capsule. ■
● Administer drug not less than 1 hour before or 2 hours after a meal.

ACTION
Inhibits calcium ion influx across cardiac and smooth-muscle cells, decreasing myocardial contractility and oxygen demand; also dilates coronary and cerebral arteries and arterioles.

Route	Onset	Peak	Duration
P.O.	Unknown	1 hr	Unknown

Half-life: 8 to 9 hours; may be 1 to 2 hours.

ADVERSE REACTIONS
CNS: headache, psychic disturbances.
CV: hypotension, flushing, edema, tachycardia.
GI: nausea, diarrhea, abdominal discomfort.
Musculoskeletal: muscle cramps.
Respiratory: dyspnea, wheezing.
Skin: dermatitis, rash.

INTERACTIONS
Drug-drug. *Antihypertensives:* May increase hypotensive effect. Monitor blood pressure.
Calcium channel blockers: May increase CV effects. Monitor patient closely.
Cimetidine: May increase nimodipine bioavailability. Monitor patient for adverse effects.
Drug-food. *Any food:* May decrease drug absorption. Advise patient to take drug on empty stomach.

EFFECTS ON LAB TEST RESULTS
None reported.

CONTRAINDICATIONS & CAUTIONS
● No known contraindications.
● Use cautiously in patients with hepatic failure.

NURSING CONSIDERATIONS
● Monitor blood pressure and heart rate in all patients, especially at start of therapy.

PATIENT TEACHING
● Explain use of drug and review administration schedule with patient and family. Stress importance of compliance for maximum drug effectiveness.
● Instruct patient to report persistent or severe adverse reactions promptly.
● Tell patient not to drink grapefruit juice while taking this drug.

sildenafil citrate
sill-DEN-ah-fill

Revatio

Pharmacologic class: cyclic guanosine monophosphate (cGMP)-specific phosphodiesterase type-5, or PDE5, inhibitor
Pregnancy risk category B

AVAILABLE FORMS
Tablets: 20 mg

INDICATIONS & DOSAGES
➤ **To improve exercise ability in patients with World Health Organization group I pulmonary arterial hypertension (PAH)**
Adults: 20 mg P.O. t.i.d., 4 to 6 hours apart.

ADMINISTRATION
P.O.
● Give drug without regard for food.
● Don't give to patients taking nitrates.

ACTION
Increases cGMP level by preventing its breakdown by phosphodiesterase, prolonging smooth muscle relaxation of the pulmonary vasculature, which leads to vasodilation.

Route	Onset	Peak	Duration
P.O.	15–30 min	30–120 min	4 hr

Half-life: 4 hours.

ADVERSE REACTIONS
CNS: *headache,* dizziness, fever.
CV: *flushing,* hypotension.
EENT: blurred vision, burning, epistaxis, impaired color discrimination, photophobia, rhinitis, sinusitis.
GI: *dyspepsia,* diarrhea, gastritis.
Musculoskeletal: myalgia.
Skin: erythema.

INTERACTIONS
Drug-drug. *Alpha blockers:* May cause symptomatic hypotension. Consider dosage reduction.

Amlodipine: May further reduce blood pressure. Monitor blood pressure closely.
Bosentan: May decrease sildenafil level. Monitor patient.
Cytochrome P-4503A4 and 2C9 inducers, rifampin: May reduce sildenafil level. Monitor effect.
Hepatic isoenzyme inhibitors (such as cimetidine, erythromycin, itraconazole, ketoconazole): May increase sildenafil level. Avoid using together.
Isosorbide, nitroglycerin: May cause severe hypotension. Use of nitrates in any form is contraindicated during therapy.
Protease inhibitors (ritonavir): May significantly increase sildenafil level. Don't use together.
Vitamin K antagonists: May increase risk of bleeding (primarily epistaxis). Monitor patient.
Drug-food. *Grapefruit:* May increase drug level, while delaying absorption. Discourage use together.

EFFECTS ON LAB TEST RESULTS
None reported.

CONTRAINDICATIONS & CAUTIONS
● Contraindicated in patients hypersensitive to drug or its components and in those taking organic nitrates.
● Don't use in patients with pulmonary veno-occlusive disease.
● Use cautiously in patients with resting hypotension, severe left ventricular outflow obstruction, autonomic dysfunction, and volume depletion.
● Use cautiously in elderly patients; in patients with hepatic or severe renal impairment, retinitis pigmentosa, bleeding disorders, or active peptic ulcer disease; in those who have suffered an MI, stroke, or life-threatening arrhythmia in last 6 months; in those with history of coronary artery disease causing unstable angina or of uncontrolled high or low blood pressure; in those with deformation of the penis or with conditions that may cause priapism (such as sickle cell anemia, multiple myeloma, or leukemia); and in those taking bosentan.
● It's unknown if drug appears in breast milk. Use cautiously in breast-feeding women.
● Safety and efficacy in children haven't been established.

NURSING CONSIDERATIONS
● The serious CV events linked to this drug's use in erectile dysfunction mainly involve patients with underlying CV disease who are at increased risk for cardiac effects related to sexual activity.
● Patients with PAH caused by connective tissue disease are more prone to epistaxis during therapy than those with primary pulmonary hypertension.
● *Alert:* Don't substitute Viagra for Revatio because there isn't an equivalent dose.

PATIENT TEACHING
● Warn patient that drug should never be used with nitrates.
● Advise patient to rise slowly from lying down.
● Inform patient that drug can be taken with or without food.
● Warn patient that discrimination between colors, such as blue and green, may become impaired during therapy; warn him to avoid hazardous activities that rely on color discrimination.
● Instruct patient to notify prescriber of visual changes, dizziness, or fainting.
● Caution patient to take drug only as prescribed.

treprostinil sodium
tra-PROS-tin-ill

Remodulin

Pharmacologic class: vasodilator
Pregnancy risk category B

AVAILABLE FORMS
Injection: 1 mg/ml, 2.5 mg/ml, 5 mg/ml, 10 mg/ml in 20-ml vials

INDICATIONS & DOSAGES
➤ **To reduce symptoms caused by exercise in patients with New York Heart Association class II to IV pulmonary arterial hypertension (PAH)**
Adults: Initially, 1.25 nanogram/kg/minute by continuous subcutaneous infusion. If patient doesn't tolerate initial dose, reduce infusion rate to 0.625 nanogram/kg/minute. Increase by 1.25 nanogram/kg/minute each week for the first 4 weeks and then by no more than 2.5 nanogram/kg/minute

each week for the remaining duration of infusion. Experience with treprostinil dosages exceeding 40 nanogram/kg/minute is limited. May be given I.V. through a central catheter if subcutaneous route isn't tolerated.

Adjust-a-dose: In patients with mild or moderate hepatic insufficiency, initially, 0.625 nanogram/kg ideal body weight per minute, and increase cautiously.

➤ **To decrease the rate of clinical deterioration in patients requiring transition from epoprostenol sodium (Flolan)**

Adults: Start treprostinil at 10% of the current epoprostenol dose; increase dose as the epoprostenol dose is reduced. Decrease epoprostenol dose in 20% increments and increase treprostinil in 20% increments, always maintaining a total dose of 110% of epoprostenol starting dose. Once epoprostenol is at 20% of starting dose and treprostinil is at 90%, decrease epoprostenol to 5% and increase treprostinil to 110%. Finally, stop epoprostenol and maintain treprostinil dose at 110% of epoprostenol starting dose plus an additional 5% to 10% as needed. Change rate based on individual patient response. Treat worsening of PAH symptoms with increases in treprostinil dose. Treat adverse effects associated with prostacyclin and prostacyclin analogs with decreases in epoprostenol dose.

ADMINISTRATION
I.V.
- Give I.V. through a central venous catheter only if subcutaneous route isn't tolerated.
- Dilute with either sterile water for injection or normal saline solution.
- Inspect for particulate matter and discoloration before giving.
- Give by continuous infusion through a surgically placed indwelling central venous catheter, using an infusion pump designed for I.V. drug delivery.
- To avoid potential interruptions in drug delivery, make sure patient has immediate access to a backup infusion pump and infusion sets.
- Diluted drug is stable at room temperature for up to 48 hours.

- **Incompatibilities:** Other I.V. drugs.
Subcutaneous
- Preferred route is continuous subcutaneous infusion via a self-inserted subcutaneous catheter, using an infusion pump designed for subcutaneous drug delivery.
- The infusion pump should be small and lightweight; adjustable to about 0.002 ml/hour; have occlusion/no delivery, low-battery, programming-error, and motor-malfunction alarms; have delivery accuracy of ± 6% or better; and be positive-pressure driven.
- The reservoir should be made of polyvinyl chloride, polypropylene, or glass.

ACTION
Directly vasodilates pulmonary and systemic arterial vascular beds and inhibits platelet aggregation.

Route	Onset	Peak	Duration
I.V.	Unknown	Unknown	Unknown
Subcut.	Rapid	Unknown	Unknown

Half-life: 2 to 4 hours.

ADVERSE REACTIONS
CNS: dizziness, fatigue, *headache.*
CV: *vasodilation,* **right ventricular heart failure,** chest pain, edema, hypotension.
GI: *diarrhea, nausea.*
Musculoskeletal: *jaw pain.*
Respiratory: dyspnea.
Skin: *infusion site pain, infusion site reaction, rash,* pallor, pruritus.

INTERACTIONS
Drug-drug. *Antihypertensives, diuretics, vasodilators:* May worsen reduction in blood pressure. Monitor blood pressure.
Anticoagulants: May increase risk of bleeding. Monitor patient closely for bleeding.

EFFECTS ON LAB TEST RESULTS
None reported.

CONTRAINDICATIONS & CAUTIONS
- Contraindicated in patients hypersensitive to drug or structurally related compounds.
- Use cautiously in patients with hepatic or renal impairment and in elderly patients.

Reactions may be *common,* uncommon, *life-threatening,* or COMMON AND LIFE-THREATENING.
Interaction may have a *rapid onset* or **delayed onset.**

• Use cautiously in pregnant and breast-feeding women. Use only if clearly needed.

NURSING CONSIDERATIONS

• Assess the patient's ability to accept, place, and care for a subcutaneous catheter and to use an infusion pump.
• During use, a single reservoir syringe can be given for up to 72 hours at 98.6° F (37° C).
• Don't use a single vial longer than 14 days after the initial introduction to the vial.
• Start treatment in setting where adequate monitoring and emergency care are available.
• Increase dose if patient doesn't improve or symptoms worsen, and decrease if drug effects become excessive or unacceptable infusion site symptoms develop.
• Avoid abrupt withdrawal or sudden large dose reductions because PAH symptoms may worsen.

PATIENT TEACHING

• Inform patient that he'll need to continue therapy for a prolonged period, possibly years.
• Tell patient that subsequent disease management may require I.V. therapy.
• Inform patient that many side effects, such as labored breathing, fatigue, and chest pain, may be related to the underlying disease.
• Tell patient that the most common local reactions are pain, redness, tissue hardening, and rash at the infusion site.
• Tell patient that a backup infusion pump must be available to avoid interruption in therapy.

**dobutamine hydrochloride
dopamine hydrochloride
ephedrine sulfate
epinephrine**
(See Chapter 56, BRONCHODILATORS.)
**norepinephrine bitartrate
phenylephrine hydrochloride**

SAFETY ALERT!

dobutamine hydrochloride
DOE-byoo-ta-meen

Pharmacologic class: adrenergic,
beta$_1$ agonist
Pregnancy risk category B

AVAILABLE FORMS
Injection: 12.5 mg/ml in 20-ml vials
(parenteral)
Dobutamine in 5% dextrose: 0.5 mg/ml
(125 or 250 mg); 1 mg/ml (250 or
500 mg); 2 mg/ml (500 mg); 4 mg/ml
(1,000 mg)

INDICATIONS & DOSAGES
➤ **Increased cardiac output in short-
term treatment of cardiac decompensation caused by depressed contractility, such as during refractory
heart failure; adjunctive therapy in
cardiac surgery**
Adults: 0.5 to 1 mcg/kg/minute I.V. infusion, titrating to optimum dosage of 2 to
20 mcg/kg/minute. Usual effective range
to increase cardiac output is 2.5 to 10 mcg/
kg/minute. Rarely, rates up to 40 mcg/kg/
minute may be needed.

ADMINISTRATION
I.V.
● Before starting therapy, give a plasma
volume expander to correct hypovolemia
and a cardiac glycoside.
● Dilute concentrate before injecting.
Compatible solutions include D$_5$W, D$_{10}$W,
half-normal or normal saline solution for
injection, lactated Ringer's injection,
Isolyte-M with D$_5$W, Normosol-M in
D$_5$W, and 20% Osmitrol.

● Diluting one vial (250 mg) with 1,000 ml
of solution yields 250 mcg/ml. Diluting
with 500 ml yields 500 mcg/ml. Diluting
with 250 ml yields 1,000 mcg/ml.
● Oxidation may slightly discolor admixture. This doesn't indicate a significant
loss of potency, provided drug is used
within 24 hours of reconstitution.
● Give through a central venous catheter
or large peripheral vein using an infusion
pump.
● Titrate rate according to patient's condition. Don't exceed 5 mg/ml.
● Infusions lasting up to 72 hours produce
no more adverse effects than shorter
infusions.
● Watch for irritation and infiltration;
extravasation can cause tissue damage and
necrosis. Change I.V. sites regularly to
avoid phlebitis.
● Solution remains stable for 24 hours.
Don't freeze.
● **Incompatibilities:** Acyclovir, alkaline
solutions, alteplase, aminophylline,
bretylium, bumetanide, calcium chloride,
calcium gluconate, cefamandole, cefazolin,
cefepime, diazepam, digoxin, ethacrynate,
furosemide, heparin, hydrocortisone
sodium succinate, indomethacin, insulin,
magnesium sulfate, midazolam, penicillin,
phenytoin, phytonadione, piperacillin with
tazobactam, potassium chloride, sodium
bicarbonate, thiopental, verapamil,
warfarin. Don't give through same line
with other drugs.

ACTION
Stimulates heart's beta$_1$ receptors to
increase myocardial contractility and
stroke volume. At therapeutic dosages,
drug increases cardiac output by decreasing
peripheral vascular resistance, reducing
ventricular filling pressure, and facilitating
AV node conduction.

Route	Onset	Peak	Duration
I.V.	1–2 min	10 min	< 5 min after infusion

Half-life: 2 minutes.

Reactions may be *common,* uncommon, *life-threatening,* or COMMON AND LIFE-THREATENING.
Interaction may have a *rapid onset* or *delayed onset.*

ADVERSE REACTIONS
CNS: headache.
CV: *hypertension, increased heart rate,* angina, PVCs, phlebitis, nonspecific chest pain, palpitations, ventricular ectopy, hypotension.
GI: nausea, vomiting.
Respiratory: *asthma attack,* shortness of breath.
Other: *anaphylaxis,* hypersensitivity reactions.

INTERACTIONS
Drug-drug. *Beta blockers:* May antagonize dobutamine effects. Avoid using together.
Bretylium: May increase risk of arrhythmias. Monitor ECG.
General anesthetics: May have greater risk of ventricular arrhythmias. Monitor ECG closely.
Guanethidine, oxytocic drugs: May increase pressor response, causing severe hypertension. Monitor blood pressure closely.
Tricyclic antidepressants: May potentiate pressor response and cause arrhythmias. Use together cautiously.
Drug-herb. *Rue:* May increase inotropic potential. Discourage use together.

EFFECTS ON LAB TEST RESULTS
● May decrease potassium level.
● May decrease platelet count.

CONTRAINDICATIONS & CAUTIONS
● Contraindicated in patients hypersensitive to drug or its components and in those with idiopathic hypertrophic subaortic stenosis.
● Use cautiously in patients with history of hypertension because drug may increase pressor response.
● Use cautiously after acute MI.
● Use cautiously in patients with history of sulfite sensitivity.

NURSING CONSIDERATIONS
● *Alert:* Because drug increases AV node conduction, patients with atrial fibrillation may develop a rapid ventricular rate.
● Continuously monitor ECG, blood pressure, pulmonary artery wedge pressure, cardiac output, and urine output.

● Monitor electrolyte levels. Drug may lower potassium level.
● *Look alike–sound alike:* Don't confuse dobutamine with dopamine.

PATIENT TEACHING
● Tell patient to report adverse reactions promptly, especially labored breathing and drug-induced headache.
● Instruct patient to report discomfort at I.V. insertion site.

SAFETY ALERT!

dopamine hydrochloride
DOE-pa-meen

Pharmacologic class: adrenergic
Pregnancy risk category C

AVAILABLE FORMS
Injection: 40 mg/ml, 80 mg/ml, 160 mg/ml parenteral concentrate for injection for I.V. infusion; 0.8 mg/ml (200 or 400 mg) in D_5W; 1.6 mg/ml (400 or 800 mg) in D_5W; 3.2 mg/ml (800 mg) in D_5W parenteral injection for I.V. infusion

INDICATIONS & DOSAGES
➤ **To treat shock and correct hemodynamic imbalances; to improve perfusion to vital organs; to increase cardiac output; to correct hypotension**
Adults: Initially, 2 to 5 mcg/kg/minute by I.V. infusion. Titrate dosage to desired hemodynamic or renal response. Increase by 1 to 4 mcg/kg/minute at 10- to 30-minute intervals. In seriously ill patients, start with 5 mcg/kg/minute and increase gradually in increments of 5 to 10 mcg/kg/minute to a rate of 20 to 50 mcg/kg/minute, as needed.
Adjust-a-dose: In patients with occlusive vascular disease, initial dose is 1 mcg/kg/minute or less.

ADMINISTRATION
I.V.
● Dilute with D_5W, normal saline solution, D_5W in normal saline or 0.45% saline, lactated Ringer's, or D_5W in lactated Ringer's. Mix just before use.

• Use a central line or large vein, as in the antecubital fossa, to minimize risk of extravasation.

• Use a continuous infusion pump to regulate flow rate. Avoid inadvertent administration of a bolus of the drug.

■ **Black Box Warning** Watch infusion site carefully for extravasation; if it occurs, stop infusion immediately and call prescriber. To prevent sloughing and necrosis in ischemic areas, you may need to infiltrate area with 5 to 10 mg phentolamine in 10 to 15 ml normal saline solution. ■

• Because solution will deteriorate rapidly, discard after 24 hours or earlier if it's discolored.

• **Incompatibilities:** Acyclovir sodium, additives with a dopamine and dextrose solution, alteplase, amphotericin B, cefepime, furosemide, gentamicin, indomethacin sodium trihydrate, iron salts, insulin, oxidizing agents, penicillin G potassium, sodium bicarbonate or other alkaline solutions, thiopental. Don't mix other drugs in I.V. container with dopamine.

ACTION

Stimulates dopaminergic and alpha and beta receptors of the sympathetic nervous system resulting in a positive inotropic effect and increased cardiac output. Action is dose-related; large doses cause mainly alpha stimulation.

Route	Onset	Peak	Duration
I.V.	5 min	Unknown	< 10 min after infusion

Half-life: 2 minutes.

ADVERSE REACTIONS

CNS: headache, anxiety.
CV: *hypotension, **ventricular arrhythmias (high doses)***, ectopic beats, tachycardia, angina, palpitations, vasoconstriction.
GI: nausea, vomiting.
Metabolic: azotemia, hyperglycemia.
Respiratory: *asthmatic episodes,* dyspnea.
Skin: necrosis and tissue sloughing with extravasation, piloerection.
Other: *anaphylactic reactions.*

INTERACTIONS

Drug-drug. *Alpha and beta blockers:* May antagonize dopamine effects. Monitor patient closely.
Ergot alkaloids: May cause extremely high blood pressure. Avoid using together.
Inhaled anesthetics: May increase risk of arrhythmias or hypertension. Monitor patient closely.
MAO inhibitors (phenelzine, tranyl-cypromine): May cause fever, hypertensive crisis, or severe headache. Avoid using together; if patient received an MAO inhibitor in the past 2 to 3 weeks, initial dopamine dose is less than or equal to 10% of the usual dose.
Oxytocics: May cause severe, persistent hypertension. Use together cautiously.
Phenytoin: May cause severe hypotension, bradycardia, and cardiac arrest. Monitor patient carefully.
Tricyclic antidepressants: May decrease pressor response. Monitor patient closely.

EFFECTS ON LAB TEST RESULTS

• May increase catecholamine, glucose, and urine urea levels.

CONTRAINDICATIONS & CAUTIONS

• Contraindicated in patients with uncorrected tachyarrhythmias, pheochromocytoma, or ventricular fibrillation.

• Use cautiously in patients with occlusive vascular disease, cold injuries, diabetic endarteritis, and arterial embolism; in pregnant or breast-feeding women; in those with a history of sulfite sensitivity; and in those taking MAO inhibitors.

NURSING CONSIDERATIONS

• Most patients receive less than 20 mcg/kg/minute. Doses of 0.5 to 2 mcg/kg/minute mainly stimulate dopamine receptors and dilate the renal vasculature. Doses of 2 to 10 mcg/kg/minute stimulate beta receptors for a positive inotropic effect. Higher doses also stimulate alpha receptors, constricting blood vessels and increasing blood pressure.

• Drug isn't a substitute for blood or fluid volume deficit. If deficit exists, replace fluid before giving vasopressors.

• During infusion, frequently monitor ECG, blood pressure, cardiac output,

---

Reactions may be *common*, uncommon, *life-threatening*, or COMMON AND LIFE-THREATENING.
Interaction may have a *rapid onset* or *delayed onset.*

central venous pressure, pulmonary artery wedge pressure, pulse rate, urine output, and color and temperature of limbs.

• If diastolic pressure rises disproportionately with a significant decrease in pulse pressure, decrease infusion rate, and watch carefully for further evidence of predominant vasoconstrictor activity, unless such an effect is desired.

• Observe patient closely for adverse reactions; dosage may need to be adjusted or drug stopped.

• Check urine output often. If urine flow decreases without hypotension, notify prescriber because dosage may need to be reduced.

• **Alert:** After drug is stopped, watch closely for sudden drop in blood pressure. Taper dosage slowly to evaluate stability of blood pressure.

• Acidosis decreases effectiveness of drug.

• **Look alike–sound alike:** Don't confuse dopamine with dobutamine.

PATIENT TEACHING
• Tell patient to report adverse reactions promptly.
• Instruct patient to report discomfort at I.V. insertion site.

SAFETY ALERT!

ephedrine sulfate
e-FED-rin

Pharmacologic class: adrenergic
Pregnancy risk category C

AVAILABLE FORMS
Capsules: 25 mg, 50 mg
Injection: 25 mg/ml, 50 mg/ml

INDICATIONS & DOSAGES
➤ **Hypotension**
Adults: 25 mg P.O. once daily to q.i.d. Or, 5 to 25 mg I.V., p.r.n., to maximum of 150 mg/24 hours. Or, 25 to 50 mg I.M. or subcutaneously.
Children: 3 mg/kg P.O. or 0.5 mg/kg or 16.7 mg/m² subcutaneously or I.M. every 4 to 6 hours.
➤ **Bronchodilation**
Adults and children older than age 12: 12.5 to 25 mg P.O. every 4 hours, as needed, not to exceed 150 mg in 24 hours.

Children age 2 to 12: 2 to 3 mg/kg or 100 mg/m² P.O. daily in four to six divided doses. Or, for children ages 6 to 12, 6.25 to 12.5 mg P.O. every 4 hours, not to exceed 75 mg in 24 hours.

ADMINISTRATION
P.O.
• Give last dose of the day at least 2 hours before bedtime, to prevent insomnia.
I.V.
• Drug is compatible with most common solutions.
• Give slowly by direct injection.
• If needed, repeat in 5 to 10 minutes.
• **Incompatibilities:** Fructose 10% in normal saline solution; hydrocortisone sodium succinate; Ionosol B, D-CM, and D solutions; pentobarbital sodium; phenobarbital sodium; thiopental.
I.M.
• Don't use solution with particulate matter or discoloration.
• Document injection site.
Subcutaneous
• Don't use solution with particulate matter or discoloration.
• Document injection site.

ACTION
Relaxes bronchial smooth muscle by stimulating beta₂ receptors; also stimulates alpha and beta receptors and is a direct- and indirect-acting sympathomimetic.

Route	Onset	Peak	Duration
P.O.	15–60 min	Unknown	3–5 hr
I.V.	5 min	Unknown	60 min
I.M., Subcut.	10–20 min	Unknown	30–60 min

Half-life: 3 to 6 hours.

ADVERSE REACTIONS
CNS: *insomnia, nervousness, cerebral hemorrhage,* dizziness, headache, muscle weakness, euphoria, confusion, delirium, tremor.
CV: *palpitations, arrhythmias,* tachycardia, hypertension, precordial pain.
EENT: dry nose and throat.
GI: nausea, vomiting, anorexia.
GU: urine retention, painful urination from visceral sphincter spasm.
Skin: diaphoresis.

INTERACTIONS
Drug-drug. *Acetazolamide:* May increase ephedrine level. Monitor patient for toxicity.
Alpha blockers: May reduce vasopressor response. Monitor patient closely.
Antihypertensives: May decrease effects. Monitor blood pressure.
Beta blockers: May block the effects of ephedrine. Monitor patient closely.
Cardiac glycosides, general anesthetics (halogenated hydrocarbons): May increase risk of ventricular arrhythmias. Monitor ECG closely.
Guanethidine: May decrease pressor effects of ephedrine. Monitor patient closely.
MAO inhibitors (phenelzine, tranylcypromine): May cause severe headache, hypertension, fever, and hypertensive crisis. Avoid using together.
Methyldopa, reserpine: May inhibit ephedrine effects. Use together cautiously.
Oxytocics: May cause severe hypertension. Avoid using together.
Tricyclic antidepressants: May decrease pressor response. Monitor patient closely.

EFFECTS ON LAB TEST RESULTS
None reported.

CONTRAINDICATIONS & CAUTIONS
• Contraindicated in patients hypersensitive to ephedrine and other sympathomimetics and in those with porphyria, severe coronary artery disease, arrhythmias, angle-closure glaucoma, psychoneurosis, angina pectoris, substantial organic heart disease, or CV disease.
• Contraindicated in those receiving MAO inhibitors or general anesthesia with cyclopropane or halothane.
• Use with caution in elderly patients and in those with hypertension, hyperthyroidism, nervous or excitable states, diabetes, or prostatic hyperplasia.

NURSING CONSIDERATIONS
• *Alert:* Hypoxia, hypercapnia, and acidosis must be identified and corrected before or during therapy because they may reduce effectiveness or increase adverse reactions.
• Drug isn't a substitute for blood or fluid volume replenishment. Volume deficit must be corrected before giving vasopressors.

• Effectiveness decreases after 2 to 3 weeks as tolerance develops. Prescriber may increase dosage. Drug isn't addictive.
• ***Look alike–sound alike:*** Don't confuse ephedrine with epinephrine.

PATIENT TEACHING
• Tell patient taking oral form of drug at home to take last dose of day at least 2 hours before bedtime to prevent insomnia.
• Warn patient not to take OTC drugs or herbs that contain ephedrine without consulting prescriber.

SAFETY ALERT!

norepinephrine bitartrate (levarterenol bitartrate, noradrenaline acid tartrate)
nor-ep-i-NEF-rin

Levophed

Pharmacologic class: direct-acting adrenergic
Pregnancy risk category C

AVAILABLE FORMS
Injection: 1 mg/ml

INDICATIONS & DOSAGES
➤ **To restore blood pressure in acute hypotension; severe hypotension during cardiac arrest**
Adults: Initially, 8 to 12 mcg/minute by I.V. infusion; then titrate to maintain systolic blood pressure at 80 to 100 mm Hg in previously normotensive patients and 30 to 40 mm Hg below preexisting systolic blood pressure in previously hypertensive patients. Average maintenance dose is 2 to 4 mcg/minute.

ADMINISTRATION
I.V.
• Use a central venous catheter or large vein, such as the antecubital fossa, to minimize risk of extravasation. Give in D_5W alone or D_5W in normal saline solution for injection. Use continuous infusion pump to regulate infusion flow rate and a piggyback setup so I.V. line stays open if norepinephrine is stopped.

Reactions may be *common,* uncommon, *life-threatening*, or COMMON AND LIFE-THREATENING.
Interaction may have a *rapid onset* or ***delayed onset***.

• Never leave patient unattended during infusion. Check blood pressure every 2 minutes until stabilized; then check every 5 minutes.

• During infusion, frequently monitor ECG, cardiac output, central venous pressure, pulmonary artery wedge pressure, pulse rate, urine output, and color and temperature of limbs. Titrate infusion rate based on findings and prescriber guidelines.

■ **Black Box Warning** Check site frequently for signs and symptoms of extravasation. If they appear, stop infusion immediately and call prescriber. To prevent sloughing and necrosis, use a fine hypodermic needle to infiltrate area with 5 to 10 mg phentolamine in 10 to 15 ml of normal saline solution. Also, check for blanching along course of infused vein, which may progress to superficial sloughing. ■

• Protect drug from light. Discard discolored solution or solution that contains precipitate. Solution will deteriorate after 24 hours.

• If prolonged therapy is needed, change injection site frequently.

• Avoid mixing with alkaline solutions, oxidizing drugs, or iron salts. The use of normal saline solution alone isn't recommended because of the lack of oxidation protection.

• **Incompatibilities:** Alkaline-buffered antibiotics, aminophylline, amobarbital, chlorothiazide, chlorpheniramine, insulin, lidocaine, pentobarbital sodium, phenobarbital sodium, phenytoin sodium, ranitidine hydrochloride, sodium bicarbonate, streptomycin, thiopental, whole blood.

ACTION
Stimulates alpha and beta₁ receptors in the sympathetic nervous system, causing vasoconstriction and cardiac stimulation.

Route	Onset	Peak	Duration
I.V.	Immediate	Immediate	1–2 min after infusion

Half-life: About 1 minute.

ADVERSE REACTIONS
CNS: *headache,* anxiety, weakness, dizziness, tremor, restlessness, insomnia.

CV: *bradycardia, severe hypertension, arrhythmias.*
Respiratory: *asthma attacks,* respiratory difficulties.
Skin: irritation with extravasation, necrosis and gangrene secondary to extravasation.
Other: *anaphylaxis.*

INTERACTIONS
Drug-drug. *Alpha blockers:* May antagonize drug effects. Avoid using together.
Antihistamines, atropine, ergot alkaloids, guanethidine, MAO inhibitors, methyldopa, oxytocics: When given with sympathomimetics, may cause severe hypertension (hypertensive crisis). Avoid using together.
Inhaled anesthetics: May increase risk of arrhythmias. Monitor ECG.
Tricyclic antidepressants: May potentiate the pressor response and cause arrhythmias. Use together cautiously.

EFFECTS ON LAB TEST RESULTS
None reported.

CONTRAINDICATIONS & CAUTIONS
• Contraindicated in patients with mesenteric or peripheral vascular thrombosis, profound hypoxia, hypercarbia, or hypotension resulting from blood volume deficit.

• Contraindicated during cyclopropane and halothane anesthesia.

• Use cautiously in patients taking MAO inhibitors or tricyclic or imipramine-type antidepressants.

• Use cautiously in patients with sulfite sensitivity.

NURSING CONSIDERATIONS
• Drug isn't a substitute for blood or fluid replacement therapy. If patient has volume deficit, replace fluids before giving vasopressors.

• Keep emergency drugs on hand to reverse effects of drug: atropine for reflex bradycardia, phentolamine to decrease vasopressor effects, and propranolol for arrhythmias.

• Notify prescriber immediately of decreased urine output.

• When stopping drug, gradually slow infusion rate. Continue monitoring vital signs, watching for possible severe drop in blood pressure.

ext######

f begin.

• *Look alike–sound alike:* Don't confuse norepinephrine with epinephrine.

PATIENT TEACHING
• Tell patient to report adverse reactions promptly.
• Advise patient to report discomfort at I.V. insertion site.

SAFETY ALERT!

phenylephrine hydrochloride
fen-ill-EF-rin

Neo-Synephrine

Pharmacologic class: adrenergic
Pregnancy risk category C

AVAILABLE FORMS
Injection: 10 mg/ml (1%)

INDICATIONS & DOSAGES
➤ **Hypotensive emergencies during spinal anesthesia**
Adults: 0.2 mg I.V.; subsequent doses should be no more than 0.1 to 0.2 mg over the previous dose; don't exceed 0.5 mg in a single dose.
Children: 0.044 to 0.088 mg/kg I.M. or subcutaneously.
➤ **Prevention of hypotension during spinal anesthesia**
Adults: 2 to 3 mg I.M. or subcutaneously 3 to 4 minutes before injection of spinal anesthesia.
Children: 0.5 to 1 mg per 11 kg (25 lb) body weight I.M. or subcutaneously 3 to 4 minutes before injection of spinal anesthesia.
➤ **To prolong spinal anesthesia**
Adults: 2 to 5 mg added to anesthetic solution.
➤ **Vasoconstrictor for regional anesthesia**
Adults: 1 mg phenylephrine added to each 20 ml local anesthetic.
➤ **Mild to moderate hypotension**
Adults: 2 to 5 mg I.M. (dose ranges from 1 to 10 mg) or subcutaneously; repeat in 1 or 2 hours as needed and tolerated. First dose shouldn't exceed 5 mg. Or, 0.1 to 0.5 mg slow I.V., not to be repeated more often than 10 to 15 minutes.
Children: 0.1 mg/kg or 3 mg/m² I.M. or subcutaneously; repeat in 1 or 2 hours as needed and tolerated.
➤ **Severe hypotension and shock (including drug-induced)**
Adults: 10 mg in 250 to 500 ml of D_5W or normal saline solution for injection. I.V. infusion started at 100 to 180 mcg/minute; then decrease to maintenance infusion of 40 to 60 mcg/minute when blood pressure stabilizes.
➤ **Paroxysmal supraventricular tachycardia**
Adults: Initially, 0.5 mg rapid I.V.; increase in increments of 0.1 to 0.2 mg. Use cautiously. Maximum single dose is 1 mg.

ADMINISTRATION
■ **Black Box Warning** Practitioners should be completely familiar with drug before prescribing. ■
I.V.
• For direct injection, dilute 10 mg (1 ml) with 9 ml sterile water for injection to provide 1 mg/ml. Infusions are usually prepared by adding 10 mg of drug to 500 ml of D_5W or normal saline solution for injection. The first I.V. infusion rate is usually 100 to 180 mcg/minute; maintenance rate is usually 40 to 60 mcg/minute.
• Use a central venous catheter or large vein, as in the antecubital fossa, to minimize risk of extravasation. Use a continuous infusion pump to regulate infusion flow rate.
• During infusion, frequently monitor ECG, blood pressure, cardiac output, central venous pressure, pulmonary artery wedge pressure, pulse rate, urine output, and color and temperature of limbs. Titrate infusion rate according to findings and prescriber guidelines. Maintain blood pressure slightly below patient's normal level. In previously normotensive patients, maintain systolic blood pressure at 80 to 100 mm Hg; in previously hypertensive patients, maintain systolic blood pressure at 30 to 40 mm Hg below usual level.
• Avoid abrupt withdrawal after prolonged I.V. infusions.
• *Alert:* To treat extravasation and prevent sloughing and necrosis, infiltrate site promptly with 10 to 15 ml of normal saline solution for injection containing 5 to 10 mg phentolamine. Use a fine needle.

• **Incompatibilities:** Alkaline solutions, iron salts, other metals, phenytoin sodium, thiopental sodium.
I.M.
• Don't give drug if solution is discolored or has particulate matter.
• Document injection site.
• Discard unused solution.
Subcutaneous
• Don't give drug if solution is discolored or has particulate matter.
• Document injection site.
• Discard unused solution.

ACTION
Stimulates alpha receptors in the sympathetic nervous system, causing vasoconstriction.

Route	Onset	Peak	Duration
I.V.	Immediate	Unknown	15–20 min
I.M.	10–15 min	Unknown	30–120 min
Subcut.	10–15 min	Unknown	50–60 min

Half-life: 2 to 3 hours.

ADVERSE REACTIONS
CNS: *headache,* excitability, restlessness, anxiety, nervousness, dizziness, weakness.
CV: *bradycardia, arrhythmias,* hypertension.
Respiratory: *asthmatic episodes.*
Skin: tissue sloughing with extravasation.
Other: *anaphylaxis,* tachyphylaxis and decreased organ perfusion with continued use.

INTERACTIONS
Drug-drug. *Alpha blockers, phenothiazines:* May decrease pressor response. Monitor patient closely.
Atropine, guanethidine, oxytocics: May increase pressor response. Monitor patient.
Beta blockers: May block cardiostimulation. Monitor patient closely.
Halogenated hydrocarbon anesthetics, sympathomimetics: May cause serious arrhythmias. Use together with caution.
MAO inhibitors (phenelzine, tranylcypromine): May cause severe headache, hypertension, fever, and hypertensive crisis. Avoid using together.
Tricyclic antidepressants: May potentiate pressor response and cause arrhythmias. Use together cautiously.

EFFECTS ON LAB TEST RESULTS
• May cause false-normal tonometry reading.

CONTRAINDICATIONS & CAUTIONS
• Contraindicated in patients hypersensitive to drug and in those with severe hypertension or ventricular tachycardia.
• Use with caution in elderly patients and in patients with heart disease, hyperthyroidism, severe atherosclerosis, bradycardia, partial heart block, myocardial disease, or sulfite sensitivity.

NURSING CONSIDERATIONS
• Drug causes little or no CNS stimulation.
• Drug may lower intraocular pressure in normal eyes or in open-angle glaucoma.
• Drug is used in OTC eyedrops and cold preparations for decongestant effects.

PATIENT TEACHING
• Tell patient to report adverse reactions promptly.
• Instruct patient to report discomfort at I.V. insertion site.

Miscellaneous cardiovascular drugs

alprostadil
midodrine hydrochloride
pentoxifylline

alprostadil
al-PROSS-ta-dil

Prostin VR Pediatric

Pharmacologic class: prostaglandin
Pregnancy risk category NR

AVAILABLE FORMS
Injection: 500 mcg/ml

INDICATIONS & DOSAGES
➤ **Palliative therapy for temporary maintenance of patency of ductus arteriosus until surgery can be performed**
Neonates: 0.05 to 0.1 mcg/kg/minute by I.V. infusion. When therapeutic response is achieved, reduce infusion rate to lowest dose that will maintain response. Maximum dose is 0.4 mcg/kg/minute. Or, give drug through umbilical artery catheter placed at ductal opening.

ADMINISTRATION
I.V.
● Dilute drug before giving. Prepare fresh solution daily; discard solution after 24 hours.
● For infusion, dilute 1 ml of concentrate labeled as containing 500 mcg in normal saline solution or D$_5$W injection to yield a solution containing 2 to 20 mcg/ml.
● When using a device with a volumetric infusion chamber, add appropriate volume of diluent to the chamber; then add 1 ml of alprostadil concentrate.
● During dilution, avoid direct contact between concentrate and wall of plastic volumetric infusion chamber because solution may become hazy. If this occurs, discard solution.

● Don't use diluents that contain benzyl alcohol. Fatal toxic syndrome may occur.
● Drug isn't recommended for direct injection or intermittent infusion. Give by continuous infusion using an infusion pump. Infuse through a large peripheral or central vein or through an umbilical artery catheter placed at the level of the ductus arteriosus. If flushing from peripheral vasodilation occurs, reposition catheter.
● Reduce infusion rate if patient develops fever or significant hypotension.
● **Incompatibilities:** None reported.

ACTION
Relaxes smooth muscle of ductus arteriosus.

Route	Onset	Peak	Duration
I.V.	20 min	1–2 hr	Length of infusion

Half-life: About 5 to 10 minutes.

ADVERSE REACTIONS
CNS: *fever, seizures.*
CV: *flushing, bradycardia, cardiac arrest,* edema, hypotension, tachycardia.
GI: diarrhea.
Hematologic: *DIC.*
Metabolic: hypokalemia.
Respiratory: APNEA.
Other: *sepsis.*

INTERACTIONS
None significant.

EFFECTS ON LAB TEST RESULTS
● May decrease potassium level.

CONTRAINDICATIONS & CAUTIONS
● Contraindicated in neonates before making differential diagnosis between respiratory distress syndrome and cyanotic heart disease and in those with respiratory distress syndrome.
● Use cautiously in neonates with bleeding tendencies because drug inhibits platelet aggregation.

NURSING CONSIDERATIONS

■ **Black Box Warning** Apnea is most often seen in neonates weighing less than 2 kg (4.5 lb) at birth and usually appears during the first hour of drug infusion. Monitor respiratory status and keep emergency respiratory support available. ■

• In infants with restricted pulmonary blood flow, measure drug's effectiveness by monitoring blood oxygenation. In infants with restricted systemic blood flow, measure drug's effectiveness by monitoring systemic blood pressure and blood pH.

• Monitor arterial pressure by umbilical artery catheter, auscultation, or Doppler transducer. If arterial pressure falls significantly, slow infusion rate.

• Carefully monitor neonates receiving drug at recommended doses for longer than 120 hours for gastric outlet obstruction and antral hyperplasia.

• *Alert:* CV and CNS adverse reactions occur more often in infants weighing less than 2 kg and in those receiving infusions for longer than 48 hours.

• *Alert:* Apnea and bradycardia may reflect drug overdose; if either occurs, stop infusion immediately.

• *Look alike–sound alike:* Don't confuse alprostadil with alprazolam.

PATIENT TEACHING

• Tell parents why this drug is needed, and explain its use.

• Encourage parents to ask questions and express concerns.

midodrine hydrochloride
MID-oh-dryn

Orvaten, ProAmatine

Pharmacologic class: synthetic sympathomimetic amine
Pregnancy risk category C

AVAILABLE FORMS
Tablets: 2.5 mg, 5 mg, 10 mg

INDICATIONS & DOSAGES

➤ **Symptomatic orthostatic hypotension unresponsive to standard clinical care**

Adults: 10 mg P.O. t.i.d. The patient takes the first dose upon arising in the morning, the second dose at noon, and the third dose in late afternoon but no later than 6 p.m. or 4 hours before bedtime.

Adjust-a-dose: For patients with renal impairment, initially, 2.5 mg.

ADMINISTRATION
P.O.
• Space doses at least 3 hours apart.
• Give drug during the day when patient can be upright and performing activities of daily living. Don't give drug after the evening meal or within 4 hours of bedtime to reduce risk of supine hypertension during sleep.

ACTION
Forms an active metabolite, desglymidodrine, which is an alpha$_1$ agonist. It increases blood pressure by activating alpha-adrenergic receptors in arteriolar and venous vasculature.

Route	Onset	Peak	Duration
P.O.	Unknown	1–2 hr	Unknown

Half-life: 3 to 4 hours.

ADVERSE REACTIONS
CNS: *paresthesia,* anxiety, pain, confusion, headache.
CV: *vasodilation,* **supine and sitting hypertension.**
GI: abdominal pain, dry mouth.
GU: *dysuria,* frequency and urgency, urine retention.
Skin: *piloerection, pruritus,* rash.
Other: chills.

INTERACTIONS
Drug-drug. *Alpha agonists:* May enhance vasopressor effects. Monitor blood pressure closely.
Alpha blockers: May antagonize drug effects. Avoid using together.
Beta blockers, cardiac glycosides: May cause or worsen bradycardia, AV block, or arrhythmias. Avoid using together.

Fludrocortisone: May increase risk of supine hypertension and lead to increased intraocular pressure and worsened glaucoma. Monitor patient closely.

EFFECTS ON LAB TEST RESULTS
None reported.

CONTRAINDICATIONS & CAUTIONS
• Contraindicated in patients with severe organic heart disease, persistent and excessive supine hypertension, acute renal disease, urine retention, pheochromocytoma, or thyrotoxicosis.
• Use cautiously in patients with history of urine retention, visual problems, diabetes, or renal or hepatic impairment, and in breast-feeding women.
• Safety and effectiveness of drug in children haven't been established.
• Give drug to pregnant woman only if potential benefit outweighs fetal risk.

NURSING CONSIDERATIONS
• Perform renal and hepatic tests before and during drug therapy.
• Monitor supine and sitting blood pressures closely, and notify prescriber if supine blood pressure increases excessively.
• Monitor patient for signs and symptoms of bradycardia, such as slowed pulse, syncope or dizziness, especially after giving the drug.
■ **Black Box Warning** Use drug only in patients whose lives are impaired despite standard clinical care because of the risk of marked elevation of supine blood pressure. Continue drug only if symptoms improve during initial therapy. ■
• *Look alike–sound alike:* Don't confuse ProAmatine with protamine.

PATIENT TEACHING
• Instruct patient to separate doses by 3 to 4 hours; tell him to take last dose of the day 4 hours before bedtime.
• Instruct patient to stop drug and immediately notify prescriber about signs and symptoms of supine hypertension (cardiac awareness, pounding in ears, headache, blurred vision).
• Tell patient to consult prescriber before taking OTC drugs.

pentoxifylline
pen-tox-IH-fi-leen

Trental◆

Pharmacologic class: xanthine derivative
Pregnancy risk category C

AVAILABLE FORMS
Tablets (extended-release): 400 mg

INDICATIONS & DOSAGES
➤ **Intermittent claudication from chronic occlusive vascular disease**
Adults: 400 mg P.O. t.i.d. with meals. May decrease to 400 mg b.i.d. if GI and CNS adverse effects occur.

ADMINISTRATION
P.O.
• Give drug whole; don't crush or split tablet.
• Give drug with meals to minimize GI upset.

ACTION
Unknown. Improves capillary blood flow, probably by increasing RBC flexibility and lowering blood viscosity.

Route	Onset	Peak	Duration
P.O.	Unknown	1 hr	Unknown

Half-life: About 30 to 45 minutes.

ADVERSE REACTIONS
CNS: dizziness, headache.
GI: dyspepsia, nausea, vomiting.

INTERACTIONS
Drug-drug. *Anticoagulants:* May increase anticoagulant effect. Monitor PT.
Antihypertensives: May increase hypotensive effect. May need to adjust dosage.
Theophylline: May increase theophylline level. Monitor patient closely.
Drug-lifestyle. *Smoking:* May cause vasoconstriction. Advise patient to avoid smoking.

EFFECTS ON LAB TEST RESULTS
None reported.

Reactions may be *common,* uncommon, *life-threatening,* or COMMON AND LIFE-THREATENING.
Interaction may have a *rapid onset* or **delayed onset.**

CONTRAINDICATIONS & CAUTIONS
• Contraindicated in patients intolerant to this drug or to methylxanthines, such as caffeine, theophylline, and theobromine, and in those with recent cerebral or retinal hemorrhage.

NURSING CONSIDERATIONS
• Drug is useful in patients who aren't good surgical candidates.
• Elderly patients may be more sensitive to drug's effects.
• *Look alike–sound alike:* Don't confuse Trental with Trandate.

PATIENT TEACHING
• Advise patient to take drug with meals to minimize GI upset.
• Instruct patient to swallow tablet whole, without breaking, crushing, or chewing.
• Tell patient to report GI or CNS adverse reactions; prescriber may reduce dosage.
• Urge patient not to stop drug during the first 8 weeks of therapy unless directed by prescriber.

30
Antianemics

darbepoetin alfa
epoetin alfa
ferrous fumarate
ferrous gluconate
ferrous sulfate
ferrous sulfate, dried
folic acid
iron dextran
iron sucrose injection
methoxy polyethylene glycol-epoetin beta
sodium ferric gluconate complex

SAFETY ALERT!

darbepoetin alfa
dar-bah-poe-E-tin

Aranesp

Pharmacologic class: recombinant human erythropoietin
Pregnancy risk category C

AVAILABLE FORMS
Injection (with albumin or polysorbate solution): 25 mcg/ml, 40 mcg/ml, 60 mcg/ml, 100 mcg/ml, 150 mcg/0.75 ml, 200 mcg/ml, 300 mcg/ml, and 500 mcg/ml in single-dose vials
Prefilled syringe or autoinjector (with albumin or polysorbate solution): 25 mcg/0.42 ml, 40 mcg/0.4 ml, 60 mcg/0.3 ml, 100 mcg/0.5 ml, 150 mcg/0.3 ml, 200 mcg/0.4 ml, 300 mcg/0.6 ml, and 500 mcg/ml

INDICATIONS & DOSAGES
➤ **Anemia from chronic renal failure**
Adults: 0.45 mcg/kg I.V. or subcutaneously once weekly. The I.V. route is preferred for patients on dialysis. Give the lowest effective dose to gradually increase hemoglobin to a level where blood transfusion isn't necessary. Adjust dose so hemoglobin level doesn't exceed 12 g/dl. Don't increase dose more often than once a month. In adults and children older than age 1 converting from epoetin alfa, base starting dose on the previous epoetin alfa dose (see table). Don't use as initial treatment of anemia in children with chronic renal failure.

Previous epoetin alfa dose (units/wk)	Darbepoetin alfa dose (mcg/wk): Adults	Darbepoetin alfa dose (mcg/wk): Children
< 1,500	6.25	Unknown
1,500–2,499	6.25	6.25
2,500–4,999	12.5	10
5,000–10,999	25	20
11,000–17,999	40	40
18,000–33,999	60	60
34,000–89,999	100	100
≥ 90,000	200	200

Give darbepoetin alfa less often than epoetin alfa. If patient was receiving epoetin alfa two to three times weekly, give darbepoetin alfa once weekly. If patient was receiving epoetin alfa once weekly, give darbepoetin alfa once every 2 weeks.
Adjust-a-dose: If increasing hemoglobin level approaches 12 g/dl, reduce dose by 25%. If hemoglobin level continues to increase, withhold dose until hemoglobin level begins to decrease; then restart therapy at a dose 25% below the previous dose. If hemoglobin level increases more than 1 g/dl over 2 weeks, decrease dose by 25%. If hemoglobin level increases less than 1 g/dl over 4 weeks and iron stores are adequate, increase dose by 25% of previous dose. Make further increases at 4-week intervals until target hemoglobin level is reached. Patients who don't need dialysis may need lower maintenance doses.
➤ **Anemia from chemotherapy in patients with nonmyeloid malignancies**
Adults: 2.25 mcg/kg subcutaneously once weekly or 500 mcg subcutaneously once every 3 weeks.
Adjust-a-dose: For either dosing schedule, adjust dose to maintain a target hemoglobin below 12 g/dl. Give the lowest effective dose to gradually increase hemoglobin to a level where blood transfusion isn't

necessary. If hemoglobin exceeds 12 g/dl, hold drug until hemoglobin drops to 11 g/dl, then resume at 40% of previous dose. If hemoglobin increases more than 1 g/dl in a 2-week period, or when hemoglobin exceeds 11 g/dl, reduce dose by 40%. For patients receiving the drug on a once-a-week schedule, if hemoglobin level increases less than 1 g/dl after 6 weeks of therapy, increase dose up to 4.5 mcg/kg.

ADMINISTRATION
I.V.
• Don't shake. Shaking can denature drug.
• If drug contains particles or is discolored, don't use.
• Give undiluted by I.V. injection.
• Single-dose vials contain no preservatives; don't pool unused portions.
• Store drug in refrigerator; don't freeze. Protect drug from light.
• **Incompatibilities:** Other I.V. drugs or solutions.
Subcutaneous
• Don't give subcutaneously in patients with chronic renal failure on dialysis.
• Don't shake. Shaking can denature drug.
• Store drug in refrigerator; don't freeze. Protect drug from light.

ACTION
Mimics effects of erythropoietin. Functions as a growth factor and as a differentiating factor, enhancing RBC production.

Route	Onset	Peak	Duration
I.V.	Unknown	Unknown	Unknown
Subcut.	Unknown	34 hr	Unknown

Half-life: 21 hours (I.V.); 49 hours (subcutaneous).

ADVERSE REACTIONS
CNS: *seizures, dizziness, fatigue, fever, headache,* asthenia.
CV: CARDIAC ARREST, CARDIAC ARRHYTHMIA, *edema, hypertension, hypotension, peripheral edema, acute MI, heart failure, stroke, thrombosis,* angina, chest pain, TIA, vascular access thrombosis.
GI: *abdominal pain, constipation, diarrhea, nausea, vomiting, GI hemorrhage.*
Metabolic: dehydration.

Musculoskeletal: *arthralgia, limb pain, myalgia,* back pain.
Respiratory: *cough, dyspnea, upper respiratory tract infection, pulmonary embolism,* bronchitis, pneumonia.
Skin: pruritus, rash.
Other: *infection, bacteremia, hemorrhage at access site, peritonitis, sepsis,* abscess, access infection, fluid overload, flulike symptoms, injection site pain.

INTERACTIONS
None reported.

EFFECTS ON LAB TEST RESULTS
None reported.

CONTRAINDICATIONS & CAUTIONS
• Contraindicated in patients hypersensitive to drug or its components and in those with uncontrolled hypertension.
• Safety and efficacy haven't been established in patients with underlying hematologic disease, such as hemolytic anemia, sickle cell anemia, thalassemia, or porphyria. Use with caution.

NURSING CONSIDERATIONS
■ **Black Box Warning** In patients with renal failure, drug may increase risk of serious CV events, including death, when target hemoglobin is greater than 12 g/dl. Monitor hemoglobin level weekly until stabilized. Hemoglobin shouldn't exceed 12 g/dl, and rate of hemoglobin increase shouldn't exceed 1 g/dl in 2 weeks. ■
■ **Black Box Warning** In patients with non-small-cell lung cancer and breast, head and neck, lymphoid, and cervical cancers, there is a risk of tumor growth and shortened survival when hemoglobin levels of 12 g/dl are achieved. Target dosage to achieve hemoglobin level of less than 12 g/dl. Use the lowest dosage needed to avoid RBC transfusions. Use only for treatment of anemia due to concomitant myelosuppressive chemotherapy and discontinue drug following chemotherapy course. ■
• Hemoglobin level may not increase until 2 to 6 weeks after starting therapy.
• If patient has a minimal response or lack of response at recommended dose, check for deficiencies in folic acid, iron,

or vitamin B_{12}. Other contributing factors include infection, malignancy, and occult blood loss.

• *Alert:* If patient develops a sudden loss of response with severe anemia and low reticulocyte count, withhold drug and test patient for antierythropoietin antibodies. If antibodies are present, stop treatment. Don't switch to another erythropoietic protein because a cross-reaction is possible.

• *Alert:* Give I.V., not subcutaneously, in patients with chronic renal failure on dialysis.

• Control blood pressure and monitor it carefully.

• Monitor renal function and electrolytes in predialysis patients.

• Patients who are marginally dialyzed may need adjustments in dialysis prescriptions.

• Serious allergic reactions, including skin rash and urticaria, may occur. If an anaphylactic reaction occurs, stop the drug and give appropriate therapy.

PATIENT TEACHING

• Instruct patients on proper administration and use and disposal of needles.

• Advise patient of possible side effects and allergic reactions.

• Inform patient of the need for frequent monitoring of blood pressure and hemoglobin level; stress compliance with his treatment for high blood pressure.

• Instruct patient how to take drug correctly at home, including how to store drug and dispose of supplies properly.

SAFETY ALERT!

epoetin alfa (erythropoietin)
e-poe-E-tin

Epogen, Eprex†, Procrit

Pharmacologic class: recombinant human erythropoietin
Pregnancy risk category C

AVAILABLE FORMS

Injection: 2,000 units/ml, 3,000 units/ml, 4,000 units/ml, 10,000 units/ml; multidose vials of 10,000 units/ml, 20,000 units/ml, 40,000 units/ml

INDICATIONS & DOSAGES
➤ **Anemia caused by chronic renal failure**
Adults: Dosage is individualized. Starting dose is 50 to 100 units/kg subcutaneously or I.V. three times weekly. Maintenance dosage is highly individualized. Give the lowest effective dose to gradually increase hemoglobin to a level where blood transfusion isn't necessary.

Infants and children ages 1 month to 16 years who are on dialysis: Initially, 50 units/kg I.V. or subcutaneously three times weekly. Maintenance dosage is highly individualized to keep hemoglobin level within target range. Give the lowest effective dose to gradually increase hemoglobin to a level where blood transfusion isn't necessary.

Infants and children ages 3 to 20 months who aren't on dialysis ♦: 50 to 250 units/kg subcutaneously or I.V once to three times per week.

Adjust-a-dose: Reduce dosage by 25% when target hemoglobin level approaches 12 g/dl or if it rises more than 1 g/dl in any 2-week period. If hemoglobin level continues to increase, hold dose until hemoglobin level begins to decrease; then restart at 25% below previous dose. Increase dosage if hemoglobin level doesn't increase by 2 g/dl after 8 weeks of therapy and is below the target range.

➤ **Anemia from zidovudine therapy (less than or equal to 4,200 mg/week) in HIV-infected patients**
Adults: Initially, 100 units/kg I.V. or subcutaneously three times weekly for 8 weeks or until target hemoglobin level is reached. If response isn't satisfactory after 8 weeks, increase dosage by 50 to 100 units/kg I.V. or subcutaneously three times weekly. After 4 to 8 weeks, further increase dosage in increments of 50 to 100 units/kg three times weekly, up to maximum of 300 units/kg I.V. or subcutaneously three times weekly. Give the lowest effective dose to gradually increase hemoglobin to a level where blood transfusion isn't necessary.

Infants and children ages 8 months to 17 years ♦: 50 to 400 units/kg subcutaneously or I.V. two to three times per week.

Reactions may be *common*, uncommon, *life-threatening*, or COMMON AND LIFE-THREATENING.
Interaction may have a *rapid onset* or *delayed onset*.

➤ **Anemia from chemotherapy**

Adults: Initially, 150 units/kg subcutaneously three times weekly for 8 weeks or until target hemoglobin level is reached. If response isn't satisfactory after 8 weeks, increase dosage up to 300 units/kg subcutaneously three times weekly. Or, 40,000 units subcutaneously once weekly. If hemoglobin level hasn't increased by at least 1 g/dl (in the absence of RBC transfusion), increase dose to 60,000 units weekly. Give the lowest effective dose to gradually increase hemoglobin to a level where blood transfusion isn't necessary. *Children ages 5 to 18:* 600 units/kg (maximum 40,000 units) I.V. once weekly.

Adjust-a-dose: Withhold drug if hemoglobin level exceeds 12 g/dl. Reduce dose by 25% and resume therapy when hemoglobin level is less than 11 g/dl. If hemoglobin level increases by more than 1 g/dl in any 2-week period, reduce dose by 25%.

➤ **Reduce need for allogenic blood transfusion in anemic patients scheduled to have elective, non-cardiac, nonvascular surgery**

Adults: 300 units/kg daily subcutaneously daily for 10 days before surgery, on day of surgery, and for 4 days after surgery. Or, 600 units/kg subcutaneously in once-weekly doses (21, 14, and 7 days before surgery), plus a fourth dose on day of surgery.

ADMINISTRATION
I.V.
● Store in refrigerator.
● Don't shake.
● Give by direct injection without dilution.
● If patient is having dialysis, drug may be given into venous return line after dialysis session. To keep drug from adhering to tubing, inject drug with blood still in the line. Then flush with normal saline solution.
● Single-dose vials contain no preservatives. Discard unused portion.
● *Alert:* Multidose vials contain benzyl alcohol, which has been associated with sometimes fatal neurologic and other complications in premature infants.
● **Incompatibilities:** Other I.V. drugs.
Subcutaneous
● Store in refrigerator
● Don't shake.

● Don't use if solution is discolored or has particulate matter.
● Give in upper arm, abdomen, mid-thigh or outer buttocks.
● Single use vial without preservative may be admixed in a syringe with bacteriostatic sodium chloride 0.9% injection with benzyl alcohol 0.9% (bacteriostatic saline) at a 1:1 ratio to provide local anesthetic.
● Rotate injection sites and document.

ACTION
Mimics effects of erythropoietin. Functions as a growth factor and as a differentiating factor, enhancing RBC production.

Route	Onset	Peak	Duration
I.V.	Immediate	Immediate	Unknown
Subcut.	Unknown	5–24 hr	Unknown

Half-life: 4 to 13 hours.

ADVERSE REACTIONS
CNS: *asthenia, dizziness, fatigue, headache, paresthesia, seizures.*
CV: *edema, hypertension,* increased clotting of arteriovenous grafts.
EENT: *pharyngitis.*
GI: *abdominal pain and constipation (in children), diarrhea, nausea, vomiting.*
Metabolic: *hyperkalemia,* hyperphosphatemia, hyperuricemia.
Musculoskeletal: *arthralgia.*
Respiratory: *cough, shortness of breath.*
Skin: *injection site reactions, rash,* urticaria.
Other: *pyrexia.*

INTERACTIONS
None significant.

EFFECTS ON LAB TEST RESULTS
● May increase BUN, creatinine, phosphate, potassium, and uric acid levels.

CONTRAINDICATIONS & CAUTIONS
● Contraindicated in patients hypersensitive to products derived from mammal cells or albumin (human) and in those with uncontrolled hypertension.
● Use cautiously in breast-feeding women.

NURSING CONSIDERATIONS
■ **Black Box Warning** In patients with renal failure, drug may increase risk of serious CV events, including death, when

target hemoglobin is greater than 12 g/dl. Monitor hemoglobin level weekly until stabilized. Hemoglobin shouldn't exceed 12 g/dl, and rate of hemoglobin increase shouldn't exceed 1 g/dl in 2 weeks. ∎
● Before starting therapy, evaluate patient's iron status. Patient should receive adequate iron supplementation beginning no later than when epoetin alfa treatment starts and continuing throughout therapy. Patient also may need vitamin B₁₂ and folic acid.
● Monitor blood pressure before therapy. Most patients with chronic renal failure have hypertension. Blood pressure may increase, especially when hematocrit increases in the early part of therapy.
∎ **Black Box Warning** In patients with non-small-cell lung cancer and breast, head and neck, lymphoid, and cervical cancers, there is a risk of tumor growth and shortened survival when hemoglobin levels of 12 g/dl are achieved. Target dosage to achieve hemoglobin level of less than 12 g/dl. Use the lowest dosage needed to avoid RBC transfusions. Use only for treatment of anemia due to concomitant myelosuppressive chemotherapy and discontinue drug following chemotherapy course. ∎
● Institute diet restrictions or drug therapy to control blood pressure.
● Monitor hemoglobin level twice weekly until it stabilizes in the target range (10 to 12 g/dl for most patients) and maintenance dose is achieved, then continue to monitor at regular intervals. Resume twice weekly testing following any dosage adjustments.
● When used in HIV-infected adults, dosage recommendations are for those with endogenous erythropoietin levels of 500 units/L or less and cumulative zidovudine doses of 4.2 g/week or less.
● Monitor blood counts; elevated hematocrit may cause excessive clotting.
● Patient may need additional heparin to prevent clotting during dialysis treatments.
∎ **Black Box Warning** Due to increased risk of deep vein thrombosis, consider prophylaxis. ∎
● *Alert:* Evaluate patient who experiences a lack or loss of effect for pure red cell aplasia.
● *Look alike–sound alike:* Don't confuse Epogen with Neupogen.

PATIENT TEACHING
● Inform patient that pain or discomfort in limbs (long bones) and pelvis, and coldness and sweating may occur after injection (usually within 2 hours). Symptoms may last for 12 hours and then disappear.
● Advise patient to avoid driving or operating heavy machinery at start of therapy. There may be a relationship between too-rapid increase in hematocrit and seizures.
● Tell patient to monitor blood pressure at home and to adhere to dietary restrictions.
● Advise women that they may resume menstruating after therapy and to consider the need for contraception.

ferrous fumarate
FAIR-us

Euro-Fer† ◊ , Femiron ◊ ,
Feostat ◊ , Ferrate† ◊ ,
Hemocyte ◊ , Ircon ◊ , Neo-Fer† ◊ ,
Nephro-Fer ◊ , Palafer† ◊

Pharmacologic class: hematinic
Pregnancy risk category A

AVAILABLE FORMS
Each 100 mg of ferrous fumarate provides 33 mg of elemental iron.
Capsule: 100 mg† ◊ , 300 mg† ◊
Tablets: 90 mg ◊ , 200 mg ◊ , 300 mg† ◊ , 324 mg ◊ , 325 mg ◊ , 350 mg ◊
Tablets (chewable): 100 mg ◊

INDICATIONS & DOSAGES
➤ **Iron deficiency**
Adults: 150 to 300 mg P.O. elemental iron daily in three divided doses.
Children: 3 to 6 mg/kg P.O. daily in three divided doses.
➤ **As a supplement during pregnancy**
Women: 15 to 30 mg elemental iron P.O. daily during last two trimesters.

ADMINISTRATION
P.O.
● Between-meal doses are preferable. Drug can be given with some foods, although absorption may be decreased.
● Give tablets with juice (preferably orange juice) or water but not with milk or antacids.

Reactions may be *common,* uncommon, *life-threatening,* or COMMON AND LIFE-THREATENING.
Interaction may have a *rapid onset* or *delayed onset.*

- Have patient drink suspension with straw and place drops at back of throat to avoid staining teeth.
- Don't crush tablets.

ACTION
Provides elemental iron, an essential component in the formation of hemoglobin.

Route	Onset	Peak	Duration
P.O.	4 days	7–10 days	2–4 mo

Half-life: Unknown.

ADVERSE REACTIONS
GI: *nausea,* epigastric pain, vomiting, *constipation,* diarrhea, *black stools,* anorexia.
Other: temporarily stained teeth from suspension and drops.

INTERACTIONS
Drug-drug. *Antacids, cholestyramine resin, H₂ antagonists, proton pump inhibitors:* May decrease iron absorption. Separate doses by at least 2 hours.
Chloramphenicol: May delay response to iron therapy. Monitor patient.
Fluoroquinolones, penicillamine, tetracyclines: May decrease GI absorption of these drugs, possibly causing decreased levels or effect. Separate doses by 2 to 4 hours.
Levodopa, methyldopa: May decrease absorption and effectiveness of levodopa and methyldopa. Watch for decreased effect of these drugs.
Mycophenolate mofetil: May decrease absorption of mycophenolate. Avoid simultaneous administration.
Penicillamine: May decrease absorption and effect of penicillamine. Separate doses by 2 hours.
L-thyroxine: May decrease L-thyroxine absorption. Separate doses by at least 2 hours. Monitor thyroid function.
Vitamin C: May increase iron absorption. Use together for therapeutic effect.
Drug-herb. *Black cohosh, chamomile, feverfew, gossypol, hawthorn, nettle, plantain, St. John's wort:* May decrease iron absorption. Discourage use together.
Oregano: May decrease iron absorption. Tell patient to separate ingestion of herb from ingestion of food containing iron or iron supplement by at least 2 hours.
Drug-food. *Cereals, cheese, coffee, eggs, milk, tea, whole-grain breads, yogurt:* May decrease iron absorption. Discourage use together.

EFFECTS ON LAB TEST RESULTS
- May yield false-positive guaiac test results. May decrease uptake of technetium-99m and interfere with skeletal imaging.

CONTRAINDICATIONS & CAUTIONS
- Contraindicated in patients with primary hemochromatosis or hemosiderosis, hemolytic anemia (unless patient also has iron deficiency anemia), peptic ulcer disease, regional enteritis, or ulcerative colitis.
- Contraindicated in those receiving repeated blood transfusions.
- Use cautiously on long-term basis.

NURSING CONSIDERATIONS
- GI upset may be related to dose.
- Enteric-coated products reduce GI upset but also reduce amount of iron absorbed.
- Check for constipation; record color and amount of stools.
- **Alert:** Oral iron may turn stools black. Although this unabsorbed iron is harmless, it could mask presence of melena.
- Monitor hemoglobin level, hematocrit, and reticulocyte count during therapy.
- Combination products such as Ferro-Sequels contain stool softeners, which help prevent constipation—a common adverse reaction.

PATIENT TEACHING
- **Black Box Warning** Inform parents that as few as 5 or 6 tablets of a high-potency form can cause fatal poisoning in children. Tell parents to keep iron-containing products out of the reach of children and to immediately call prescriber or poison control center if an accidental overdose occurs. ■
- Tell patient to take tablets with juice (preferably orange juice) or water but not with milk or antacids.
- Tell patient to take suspension with straw and place drops at back of throat to avoid staining teeth.

- Caution patient not to crush tablets.
- Advise patient not to substitute one iron salt for another; the amount of elemental iron may vary.
- Advise patient to report constipation and change in stool color or consistency.

---

ferrous gluconate
FAIR-us

Fergon◇, Fertinic†,
Novo-ferrogluc† ◇

Pharmacologic class: hematinic
Pregnancy risk category A

AVAILABLE FORMS
Each 100 mg of ferrous gluconate provides 11.6 mg of elemental iron.
Tablets: 225 mg ◇, 324 mg ◇, 325 mg ◇

INDICATIONS & DOSAGES
➤ Iron deficiency
Adults: 150 to 300 mg P.O. elemental iron daily in three divided doses.
Children: 3 to 6 mg/kg P.O. daily in three divided doses.
➤ As a supplement during pregnancy
Adults: 15 to 30 mg elemental iron P.O. daily during last two trimesters.

ADMINISTRATION
P.O.
- Between-meal doses are preferable. Drug can be given with some foods, although absorption may be decreased.
- Give tablets with juice (preferably orange juice) or water but not with milk or antacids.

ACTION
Provides elemental iron, an essential component in the formation of hemoglobin.

Route	Onset	Peak	Duration
P.O.	4 days	7–10 days	2–4 mo

Half-life: Unknown.

ADVERSE REACTIONS
GI: *nausea,* epigastric pain, vomiting, *constipation,* diarrhea, *black stools,* anorexia.

INTERACTIONS
Drug-drug. *Antacids, cholestyramine resin, H_2 antagonists, proton pump inhibitors:* May decrease iron absorption. Separate doses by at least 2 hours.
Chloramphenicol: Delays response to iron therapy. Monitor patient.
Fluoroquinolones, penicillamine, tetracyclines: May decrease GI absorption of these drugs, possibly causing decreased level or effect. Separate doses by 2 to 4 hours.
Levodopa, methyldopa: May decrease levodopa and methyldopa absorption and effect. Watch for decreased effect of these drugs.
L-thyroxine: May decrease L-thyroxine absorption. Separate doses by at least 2 hours. Monitor thyroid function.
Mycophenolate mofetil: May decrease absorption of mycophenolate. Avoid simultaneous administration.
Penicillamine: May decrease absorption and effect of penicillamine. Separate doses by 2 hours.
Vitamin C: May increase iron absorption. Use together for therapeutic effect.
Drug-herb. *Black cohosh, chamomile, feverfew, gossypol, hawthorn, nettle, plantain, St. John's wort:* May decrease iron absorption. Discourage use together.
Oregano: May decrease iron absorption. Tell patient to separate ingestion of herb from ingestion of food containing iron or iron supplement by at least 2 hours.
Drug-food. *Cereals, cheese, coffee, eggs, milk, tea, whole-grain breads, yogurt:* May decrease iron absorption. Discourage using together.

EFFECTS ON LAB TEST RESULTS
- May yield false-positive guaiac test results. May decrease uptake of technetium-99m and interfere with skeletal imaging.

CONTRAINDICATIONS & CAUTIONS
- Contraindicated in patients with peptic ulceration, regional enteritis, ulcerative colitis, hemosiderosis, primary hemochromatosis, or hemolytic anemia (unless patient also has iron deficiency anemia) and in those receiving repeated blood transfusions.
- Use cautiously on long-term basis.

Reactions may be *common,* uncommon, *life-threatening,* or COMMON AND LIFE-THREATENING.
Interaction may have a *rapid onset* or ***delayed onset.***

NURSING CONSIDERATIONS
- GI upset may be related to dose.
- Enteric-coated products reduce GI upset but also reduce amount of iron absorbed.
- Check for constipation; record color and amount of stools.
- *Alert:* Oral iron may turn stools black. Although this unabsorbed iron is harmless, it could mask melena.
- Monitor hemoglobin level, hematocrit, and reticulocyte count during therapy.

PATIENT TEACHING
■ **Black Box Warning** Inform parents that as few as 5 or 6 high-potency tablets can cause fatal poisoning in children. Tell parents to keep all iron-containing products out of the reach of children and to immediately call prescriber or poison control center if an accidental overdose occurs. ■
- Tell patient to take tablets with juice (preferably orange juice) or water, but not with milk or antacids.
- Caution patient not to substitute one iron salt for another because the amounts of elemental iron vary.
- Advise patient to report constipation and change in stool color or consistency.

---

ferrous sulfate
FAIR-us

Feosol* ◊ , Fer-Gen-Sol* ◊ ,
Fer-In-Sol* ◊ , Fer-Iron* ◊ ,
FeroSul, Mol-Iron ◊

ferrous sulfate, dried
Fe⁵⁰ ◊ , Feosol ◊ , Feratab ◊ ,
Novo-ferrosulfate† ◊ , Slow FE ◊

Pharmacologic class: hematinic
Pregnancy risk category A

AVAILABLE FORMS
Each 100 mg of ferrous sulfate provides 20 mg of elemental iron, about 30 mg of elemental iron in ferrous sulfate dried products.
Caplets (extended-release) ◊ : 160 mg (dried)
Capsules: 190 mg (dried)
Drops ◊ : 125 mg/ml
Elixir ◊ : 220 mg/5 ml* ◊
Liquid ◊ : 150 mg/5 ml†, 300 mg/5 ml

Tablets ◊ : 195 mg, 200 mg (dried), 300 mg (dried), 325 mg
Tablets (slow-release) ◊ : 160 mg (dried)

INDICATIONS & DOSAGES
➤ **Iron deficiency**
Adults: 150 to 300 mg P.O. elemental iron daily in three divided doses.
Children: 3 to 6 mg/kg P.O. daily in three divided doses.
➤ **As a supplement during pregnancy**
Adults: 15 to 30 mg elemental iron P.O. daily during last two trimesters.
➤ **Prevention of iron deficiency**
Children (birth to 1 year): 1 mg/kg/day P.O. in one to three divided doses. Maximum is 15 mg/day.
Premature infants: 2 to 4 mg/kg/day P.O. in one to three divided doses. Maximum is 15 mg/day.

ADMINISTRATION
P.O.
- Between-meal doses are preferable. Drug can be given with some foods, although absorption may be decreased.
- Give tablets with juice (preferably orange juice) or water, but not with milk or antacids.
- Don't crush extended-release form.

ACTION
Provides elemental iron, an essential component in the formation of hemoglobin.

Route	Onset	Peak	Duration
P.O.	4 days	7–10 days	2–4 mo

Half-life: Unknown.

ADVERSE REACTIONS
GI: *nausea,* epigastric pain, vomiting, *constipation, black stools,* diarrhea, anorexia.
Other: temporarily stained teeth from liquid forms.

INTERACTIONS
Drug-drug. *Antacids, cholestyramine resin, H₂ antagonists, proton pump inhibitors:* May decrease iron absorption. Separate doses if possible.
Chloramphenicol: May delay response to iron therapy. Monitor patient.

Fluoroquinolones, penicillamine, tetracyclines: May decrease GI absorption of these drugs, possibly resulting in decreased levels or effect. Separate doses by 2 to 4 hours.

Levodopa, methyldopa: May decrease absorption and effect of levodopa and methyldopa. Watch for decreased effect of these drugs.

L thyroxine: May decrease L-thyroxine absorption. Separate doses by at least 2 hours. Monitor thyroid function.

Mycophenolate mofetil: May decrease absorption of mycophenolate. Avoid simultaneous administration.

Penicillamine: May decrease absorption and effect of penicillamine. Separate doses by 2 hours.

Vitamin C: May increase iron absorption. Use together for therapeutic effect.

Drug-herb. *Black cohosh, chamomile, feverfew, gossypol, hawthorn, nettle, plantain, St. John's wort:* May decrease iron absorption. Discourage use together.

Oregano: May decrease iron absorption. Tell patient to separate ingestion of herb from ingestion of food containing iron or iron supplement by at least 2 hours.

Drug-food. *Cereals, cheese, coffee, eggs, milk, tea, whole-grain breads, yogurt:* May decrease iron absorption. Discourage use together.

EFFECTS ON LAB TEST RESULTS
● May yield false-positive guaiac test results. May decrease uptake of technetium-99m and interfere with skeletal imaging.

CONTRAINDICATIONS & CAUTIONS
● Contraindicated in patients with hemosiderosis, primary hemochromatosis, hemolytic anemia (unless patient also has iron deficiency anemia), peptic ulceration, ulcerative colitis, or regional enteritis and in those receiving repeated blood transfusions.
● Use cautiously on long-term basis.

NURSING CONSIDERATIONS
● GI upset may be related to dose.
● Enteric-coated products reduce GI upset but also reduce amount of iron absorbed.
● *Alert:* Oral iron may turn stools black. Although this unabsorbed iron is harmless, it could mask melena.

● Monitor hemoglobin level, hematocrit, and reticulocyte count during therapy.
● *Look alike–sound alike:* Don't confuse different iron salts; elemental content may vary.

PATIENT TEACHING
● Tell patient to take tablets with juice (preferably orange juice) or water, but not with milk or antacids.
● Instruct patient not to crush or chew extended-release form.
■ **Black Box Warning** Inform parents that as few as 5 to 6 high-potency tablets can cause fatal poisoning in a child. Tell parents to keep all iron-containing products out of the reach of children and to call prescriber or poison control center immediately if an accidental overdose occurs. ■
● Caution patient not to substitute one iron salt for another because amounts of elemental iron vary.
● Advise patient to report constipation and change in stool color or consistency.

folic acid (vitamin B₉)
FOE-lik

Novo-Folacid†

Pharmacologic class: folic acid derivative
Pregnancy risk category A

AVAILABLE FORMS
Injection: 10-ml vials (5 mg/ml with 1.5% benzyl alcohol, 5 mg/ml with 1.5% benzyl alcohol and 0.2% ethylenediaminetetraacetic acid)
Tablets: 0.4 mg, 0.8 mg, 1 mg, 5 mg†

INDICATIONS & DOSAGES
➤ **RDA**
Adults and children age 14 and older: 400 mcg.
Children ages 9 to 13: 300 mcg.
Children ages 4 to 8: 200 mcg.
Children ages 1 to 3: 150 mcg.
Infants ages 6 months to 1 year: 80 mcg.
Neonates and infants younger than age 6 months: 65 mcg.
Pregnant women: 600 mcg.
Breast-feeding women: 500 mcg.

➤ **Megaloblastic or macrocytic anemia from folic acid or other nutritional deficiency, hepatic disease, alcoholism, intestinal obstruction, or excessive hemolysis**

Adults and children age 4 and older: 0.4 to 1 mg P.O., I.V., I.M., or subcutaneously daily. After anemia caused by folic acid deficiency is corrected, proper diet and RDA supplements are needed to prevent recurrence.

Children younger than age 4: Up to 0.3 mg P.O., I.V., I.M., or subcutaneously daily.

Pregnant and breast-feeding women: 0.8 mg P.O., I.V., I.M., or subcutaneously daily.

➤ **To prevent fetal neural tube defects during pregnancy**

Adults: 0.4 mg P.O. daily.

➤ **To prevent megaloblastic anemia during pregnancy to prevent fetal damage**

Adults: Up to 1 mg P.O., I.V., I.M., or subcutaneously daily throughout pregnancy.

➤ **Tropical sprue**

Adults: 3 to 15 mg P.O. daily.

ADMINISTRATION

P.O.
● Give drug without regard for food.

I.V.
● Protect from light and heat; store at room temperature.

I.M.
● Don't mix with other drugs in same syringe for I.M. injections.
● Protect drug from light and heat; store at room temperature.

Subcutaneous
● Protect drug from light and heat; store at room temperature.

ACTION

Stimulates normal erythropoiesis and nucleoprotein synthesis.

Route	Onset	Peak	Duration
P.O., I.M., Subcut.	Unknown	30–60 min	Unknown

Half-life: Unknown.

ADVERSE REACTIONS

CNS: altered sleep pattern, general malaise, difficulty concentrating, confusion, impaired judgment, irritability, hyperactivity.
GI: anorexia, nausea, flatulence, bitter taste.
Respiratory: *bronchospasm.*
Skin: allergic reactions including rash, pruritus, and erythema.

INTERACTIONS

Drug-drug. *Aminosalicylic acid, chloramphenicol, hormonal contraceptives, methotrexate, sulfasalazine, trimethoprim:* May antagonize folic acid. Watch for decreased folic acid effect. Use together cautiously.
Phenytoin: May increase anticonvulsant metabolism, which decreases anticonvulsant level. Monitor phenytoin level closely.

EFFECTS ON LAB TEST RESULTS

● May decrease serum and RBC folate levels.

CONTRAINDICATIONS & CAUTIONS

● Contraindicated in patients with undiagnosed anemia (it may mask pernicious anemia) and in those with vitamin B_{12} deficiency.

NURSING CONSIDERATIONS

● The U.S. Public Health Service recommends use of folic acid during pregnancy to decrease fetal neural tube defects. Patients with history of fetal neural tube defects in pregnancy should increase folic acid intake for 1 month before and 3 months after conception.
● Patients with small-bowel resections and intestinal malabsorption may need parenteral administration.
● Most CNS and GI adverse reactions occur at higher doses, such as 15 mg daily for 1 month.
● *Look alike–sound alike:* Don't confuse folic acid with folinic acid.

PATIENT TEACHING

● Teach patient about proper nutrition to prevent recurrence of anemia.
● Stress importance of follow-up visits and laboratory studies.
● Teach patient about foods that contain folic acid: liver, oranges, whole wheat, broccoli, and Brussels sprouts.

iron dextran
DexFerrum, InFeD

Pharmacologic class: hematinic
Pregnancy risk category C

AVAILABLE FORMS
1 ml iron dextran provides 50 mg elemental iron.
Injection: 50 mg elemental iron/ml in 1-ml and 2-ml single-dose vials

INDICATIONS & DOSAGES
➤ **Iron deficiency anemia**
Adults and children weighing more than 15 kg (33 lb): I.V. or I.M. test dose is required. Total dose may be calculated using dosage table in package insert or by using the following formula:

$$\text{Dose (ml)} = \frac{0.0442}{(\text{desired Hb} - \text{observed Hb})} \times \text{LBW} + (0.26 \times \text{LBW})$$

Note: LBW = lean body weight in kg. For males, LBW = 50 kg + 2.3 kg for each inch of patient's height over 5 feet. For females, LBW = 45.5 kg + 2.3 kg for each inch of patient's height over 5 feet.

Children weighing 5 to 15 kg (11 to 33 lb): Use dosage table in package insert or calculate dose as follows:

$$\text{Dose (ml)} = \frac{0.0442}{(\text{desired Hb} - \text{observed Hb})} \times \text{weight} + (0.26 \times \text{weight})$$

I.V.
Adults and children: Inject 0.5-ml test dose over at least 5 minutes. If no reaction occurs in 1 hour, give remainder of therapeutic I.V. dose. Repeat therapeutic I.V. dose daily. Single daily dose shouldn't exceed 100 mg. Give slowly (1 ml/minute). Don't give drug in the first 4 months of life.
I.M. (by Z-track method)
Adults and children: Inject 0.5-ml test dose. If no reaction occurs in 1 hour, give remainder of dose. Daily dose ordinarily shouldn't exceed 0.5 ml (25 mg) for infants who weigh less than 5 kg (11 lb); 1 ml (50 mg) for those who weigh less than 10 kg (22 lb); and 2 ml (100 mg) for heavier children and adults. Don't give drug in the first 4 months of life.

ADMINISTRATION
I.V.
• Check hospital policy before giving I.V.
• After completing I.V. dose, flush the vein with 10 ml of normal saline solution.
• Patient should rest for 15 to 30 minutes after I.V. administration.
• **Incompatibilities:** Other I.V. drugs, parenteral nutrition solutions for I.V. infusion.
I.M.
• Inject I.M. deep into upper outer quadrant of buttock—never into the arm or other exposed area—with a 2- to 3-inch 19G or 20G needle.
• Use Z-track method to avoid leakage into subcutaneous tissue and staining of skin.
• After drawing up drug, use a new sterile needle to give injection.

ACTION
Provides elemental iron, an essential component in the formation of hemoglobin.

Route	Onset	Peak	Duration
I.V.	Unknown	Unknown	Unknown
I.M.	72 hr	Unknown	3–4 wk

Half-life: 6 hours.

ADVERSE REACTIONS
CNS: headache, transitory paresthesia, dizziness, malaise, fever, chills.
CV: chest pain, tachycardia, ***bradycardia,*** hypotensive reaction, peripheral vascular flushing.
GI: nausea, anorexia.
Musculoskeletal: arthralgia, myalgia.
Respiratory: *bronchospasm,* dyspnea.
Skin: rash, urticaria, *soreness, inflammation, brown skin discoloration at I.M. injection site, local phlebitis at I.V. injection site,* sterile abscess, necrosis, atrophy.
Other: fibrosis, ***anaphylaxis, delayed sensitivity reactions.***

INTERACTIONS
Drug-drug. *Chloramphenicol:* May increase iron level. Monitor patient closely.

EFFECTS ON LAB TEST RESULTS
• May cause false increase in bilirubin level and false decrease in calcium level. Use of more than 250 mg iron may color

the serum brown. Drug may alter measurement of iron level and total iron-binding capacity for up to 3 weeks; I.M. injection may cause dense areas of activity for 1 to 6 days on bone scans using technetium-99m diphosphonate.

CONTRAINDICATIONS & CAUTIONS
■ **Black Box Warning** Fatal anaphylactic reactions have been reported. Give only when indications have been clearly established and for iron deficiencies not amenable to oral iron therapy. Keep emergency equipment readily available. ■
● Contraindicated in patients hypersensitive to drug, in those with acute infectious renal disease, and in those with any anemia except iron deficiency anemia.
● Use cautiously in patients who have serious hepatic impairment, rheumatoid arthritis, or other inflammatory diseases because these patients may be at higher risk for certain delays and reactions.
● Use cautiously in patients with history of significant allergies or asthma.

NURSING CONSIDERATIONS
● Have epinephrine immediately available in event of acute hypersensitivity reaction.
● Don't give iron dextran with oral iron preparations.
● I.V. or I.M. injections of iron are advisable only for patients in whom oral administration is impossible or ineffective.
● Monitor hemoglobin level, hematocrit, and reticulocyte count.
● Maximum daily dose should not exceed 2 ml undiluted iron dextran.

PATIENT TEACHING
● Teach patient signs and symptoms of hypersensitivity and iron toxicity, and tell him to report them to prescriber.
● Inform patient that drug may stain skin.

---

iron sucrose injection
Venofer

Pharmacologic class: hematinic
Pregnancy risk category B

AVAILABLE FORMS
Injection: 20 mg/ml of elemental iron in 5-ml and 10-ml single-dose vials

INDICATIONS & DOSAGES
➤ **Iron deficiency anemia in patients who are hemodialysis dependent and receiving erythropoietin therapy**
Adults: 100 mg (5 ml) of elemental iron I.V. directly in the dialysis line, either by slow injection over 5 minutes or by infusion over 15 minutes during the dialysis session one to three times a week to a total of 1,000 mg in 10 doses; repeat as needed.
➤ **Iron deficiency anemia in chronic kidney disease patients not on dialysis**
Adults: 200 mg by undiluted slow I.V. injection over 5 minutes on five separate occasions in a 14-day period to a total cumulative dose of 1,000 mg.
➤ **Iron deficiency anemia in peritoneal dialysis-dependent chronic kidney disease patients**
Adults: 300 mg I.V. infusion over 90 minutes on two separate occasions 14 days apart, followed by one 400-mg infusion over 2½ hours 14 days later.

ADMINISTRATION
I.V.
● Inspect drug for particulate matter and discoloration before giving.
● For infusion, dilute 100 mg elemental iron in a maximum of 100 ml normal saline solution immediately before infusion, and infuse over at least 15 minutes. Dilute dose 300 mg or greater in a maximum of 250 ml normal saline solution.
● **Incompatibilities:** Other I.V. drugs, parenteral nutrition solutions.

ACTION
Exogenous source of iron that replenishes depleted body iron stores and is essential for hemoglobin synthesis.

Route	Onset	Peak	Duration
I.V.	Unknown	Unknown	Variable

Half-life: 6 hours.

ADVERSE REACTIONS
CNS: headache, asthenia, malaise, dizziness, fever.

CV: *heart failure,* *hypotension,* chest pain, hypertension, fluid retention.
GI: nausea, vomiting, diarrhea, abdominal pain, taste perversion.
Metabolic: gout, hyperglycemia.
Musculoskeletal: *leg cramps,* bone and muscle pain.
Respiratory: dyspnea, wheezing, pneumonia, cough.
Skin: rash, pruritus, application site reaction.
Other: accidental injury, pain, *sepsis, hypersensitivity reactions.*

INTERACTIONS
Drug-drug. *Oral iron preparations:* May reduce absorption of oral iron preparations. Avoid using together.

EFFECTS ON LAB TEST RESULTS
● May increase blood glucose, uric acid, and liver enzyme levels.

CONTRAINDICATIONS & CAUTIONS
● Contraindicated in patients with hypersensitivity to drug or its components, evidence of iron overload, or anemia not caused by iron deficiency.
● Use cautiously in breast-feeding women.

NURSING CONSIDERATIONS
● *Alert:* Rare but fatal hypersensitivity reactions, characterized by anaphylactic shock, loss of consciousness, collapse, hypotension, dyspnea, or seizures, may occur. Have epinephrine readily available.
● Mild to moderate hypersensitivity reactions, with wheezing, dyspnea, hypotension, rash, or pruritus, may occur.
● Giving drug by infusion may reduce the risk of hypotension.
● *Alert:* Symptoms associated with overdose or too-rapid drug infusion include hypotension, dyspnea, headache, vomiting, nausea, dizziness, joint aches, paresthesia, abdominal and muscle pain, edema, and cardiovascular collapse.
● Transferrin saturation level increases rapidly after I.V. administration of drug. Obtain iron level 48 hours after I.V. use.

● Monitor ferritin level, transferrin saturation, hemoglobin level, and hematocrit.
● Withhold dose in patient with signs and symptoms of iron overload.
● Keep dose selection in elderly patients conservative because of decreased hepatic, renal, or cardiac function; other disease; and other drug therapy.

PATIENT TEACHING
● Instruct patient to notify prescriber if symptoms of overdose (headache, nausea, dizziness, joint aches, tingling, or abdominal and muscle pain) or allergic reaction (labored breathing, collapse, or loss of consciousness) occur.

✳ NEW DRUG
methoxy polyethylene glycol-epoetin beta
meh-THOCKS-ee paw-lee-ETH-ah-leen GLIGH-call eh-poe-EH-tin BAY-tah

Mircera

Pharmacologic class: erythropoietin receptor activator
Pregnancy risk category C

AVAILABLE FORMS
Injection: 50 mcg/ml, 100 mcg/ml, 200 mcg/ml, 300 mcg/ml, 400 mcg/ml, 600 mcg/ml, 1,000 mcg/ml in single-dose vials
Prefilled syringe: 50 mcg/0.3 ml, 75 mcg/0.3 ml, 100 mcg/0.3 ml, 150 mcg/0.3 ml, 200 mcg/0.3 ml, 250 mcg/0.3 ml, 400 mcg/0.6 ml, 600 mcg/0.6 ml, 800 mcg/0.6 ml

INDICATIONS & DOSAGES
➤ **Anemia caused by chronic renal failure**
Adults: 0.6 mcg/kg I.V. (preferred for patient on hemodialysis) or subcutaneously once every 2 weeks to keep hemoglobin level at 10 to 12 g/dl. When hemoglobin reaches maintenance level, give 0.12 mcg/kg I.V or subcutaneously once monthly, and adjust as needed. Don't increase dosage more often than once monthly.

If patient is converting from epoetin alfa or darbepoetin, use this dosage table:

Previous epoetin alfa dose (units/wk)	Previous darbepoetin alfa dose (mcg/wk)	methoxy polyethylene glycol-epoetin beta (mcg/ 2 wk)	(mcg/ month)
Less than 8,000	Less than 40	60	120
8,000–16,000	40–80	100	200
More than 16,000	More than 80	180	360

Adjust-a-dose: If increasing hemoglobin level approaches 12 g/dl, reduce dosage by 25%. If level continues to increase, withhold dose until hemoglobin level begins to decrease; then restart therapy at a dosage 25% below the previous dose. If hemoglobin level increases more than 1 g/dl over 2 weeks, decrease dosage by 25%. If hemoglobin level increases less than 1 g/dl over 4 weeks, increase dosage by 25%. Dosage shouldn't be increased more often than every 4 weeks

PHARMACODYNAMICS
Antianemic action: Activates erythropoietin receptors to stimulate erythropoietin production.

PHARMACOKINETICS
Absorption: Not reported.
Distribution: Not reported.
Metabolism: Not reported.
Excretion: Terminal half-life is 3 to 8 days. Drug isn't dialyzable.

ADMINISTRATION
I.V.
• Don't shake drug; doing so may denature it.
• Don't give drug if it contains particles or is discolored.
• Give drug undiluted.
• Don't pool unused portions of drug because it contains no preservatives.
• Plunger must be fully depressed in order for the needle guard to activate.

• Store drug in original carton, in refrigerator, and protect from light.
• **Incompatibilities:** Don't give with other I.V. drugs or solutions.

Route	Onset	Peak	Duration
I.V.	Unknown	Unknown	Unknown
Subcut.	Unknown	72 br	Unknown

ADVERSE REACTIONS
CNS: headache, *seizures, stroke.*
CV: *heart failure,* hypertension, hypotension, *myocardial infarction,* procedural hypotension.
EENT: *nasopharyngitis.*
GI: constipation, *diarrhea,* vomiting.
GU: urinary tract infection.
Hematologic: arteriovenous (AV) fistula site complication, AV fistula thrombosis, *pure red cell aplasia.*
Metabolic: fluid overload.
Musculoskeletal: back pain, limb pain, muscle spasms.
Respiratory: cough, upper respiratory tract infection.
Other: allergic reactions, *increased risk of death, tumor progression.*

INTERACTIONS
None reported.

EFFECTS ON LAB TEST RESULTS
• May increase hemoglobin level.
• May decrease platelet count.

CONTRAINDICATIONS & CAUTIONS
• Contraindicated in patients hypersensitive to drug or its components, patients with anemia from chemotherapy, and patients with uncontrolled hypertension.
• Use cautiously in patients with history of hypertension and in breast-feeding women.

NURSING CONSIDERATIONS
• Check hemoglobin level often until it's stabilized. Don't allow hemoglobin level to exceed 12 g/dl.
• Monitor patient for signs and symptoms of allergic reaction, such as tachycardia, pruritus, and rash.
• Assess ferritin level and transferrin saturation before and during treatment.

Provide iron supplement if patient's ferritin level is less than 100 mcg/L or serum transferrin saturation is less than 20%.

• Drug may increase risk of cardiovascular events. Control patient's blood pressure, and monitor it carefully.

• Assess renal function and fluid and electrolyte balance.

• Store drug in refrigerator at 36° to 46° F (2° to 8° C).

• Protect drug from light, and avoid shaking it.

Pregnant patients

• Use drug during pregnancy only if potential benefit to mother outweighs risk to fetus.

Breast-feeding patients

• Use cautiously in breast-feeding women. It isn't known whether drug appears in breast milk

Pediatric patients

• Safety and effectiveness haven't been established.

Geriatric patients

• Start drug at lowest recommended dosage, and adjust as appropriate.

PATIENT TEACHING

• Teach patient how to inject drug and safely dispose of used needles.

• Tell patient how to store drug at home.

• Explain possible side effects and allergic reactions, and urge patient to report them to health care provider immediately.

• Inform patient about the need for frequent monitoring of blood pressure and iron and hemoglobin levels. Urge patient to comply with treatment for hypertension.

---

sodium ferric gluconate complex
Ferrlecit

Pharmacologic class:
macromolecular iron complex;
hematinic
Pregnancy risk category B

AVAILABLE FORMS

Injection: 62.5 mg elemental iron (12.5 mg/ml) in 5-ml ampules

INDICATIONS & DOSAGES

➤ **Iron deficiency anemia in patients receiving long-term hemodialysis and supplemental erythropoietin**
Adults: 10 ml (125 mg elemental iron) I.V. over 1 hour. Most patients need minimum cumulative dose of 1 g elemental iron given over more than eight sequential dialysis treatments to achieve a favorable hemoglobin or hematocrit response.
Children age 6 and older: 1.5 mg/kg (maximum 125 mg) I.V. over 1 hour during 8 consecutive hemodialysis treatments.

ADMINISTRATION

I.V.

• Drug contains benzyl alcohol. Don't use in neonates.

• For adults, dilute in 100 ml normal saline solution; for children, dilute in 25 ml normal saline solution. Give immediately over 1 hour.

• Alternatively, give undiluted at a rate not to exceed 1 ml/minute (12.5 mg/minute) at the end of dialysis.

• Life-threatening hypersensitivity reactions, such as CV collapse, cardiac arrest, bronchospasm, oral or pharyngeal edema, dyspnea, angioedema, urticaria, and pruritus—sometimes linked to pain and muscle spasm of chest or back—may occur during infusion. Have adequate supportive measures readily available. Monitor patient closely during infusion.

• After rapid administration, profound hypotension with flushing, light-headedness, malaise, fatigue, weakness, or severe chest, back, flank, or groin pain may occur; these symptoms aren't hypersensitivity reactions. Don't exceed 2.1 mg/minute. Monitor patient closely during infusion.

• **Incompatibilities:** Other I.V. drugs. Don't add drug to parenteral nutrition solutions for infusion.

ACTION

Restores total body iron content, which is critical for normal hemoglobin synthesis and oxygen transport.

Route	Onset	Peak	Duration
I.V.	Unknown	Varies	Unknown

Half-life: 1 hour in healthy, iron-deficient people.

Reactions may be *common*, uncommon, *life-threatening*, or COMMON AND LIFE-THREATENING.
Interaction may have a *rapid onset* or **delayed onset**.

ADVERSE REACTIONS
CNS: asthenia, headache, fatigue, malaise, *dizziness,* paresthesia, agitation, insomnia, somnolence, syncope, pain, chills, fever.
CV: *hypotension, hypertension,* tachycardia, **bradycardia,** angina, chest pain, *MI,* edema, flushing.
EENT: conjunctivitis, abnormal vision, rhinitis.
GI: *nausea, vomiting, diarrhea,* rectal disorder, dyspepsia, eructation, flatulence, melena, abdominal pain.
GU: urinary tract infection.
Hematologic: anemia.
Metabolic: *hyperkalemia, hypoglycemia,* hypokalemia, hypervolemia.
Musculoskeletal: myalgia, arthralgia, back pain, arm pain, *cramps.*
Respiratory: *dyspnea,* coughing, upper respiratory tract infection, pneumonia, pulmonary edema.
Skin: pruritus, increased sweating, rash, *injection site reaction.*
Other: infection, rigors, flu syndrome, *sepsis, carcinoma,* hypersensitivity reactions, lymphadenopathy.

INTERACTIONS
Drug-drug. *ACE inhibitors:* May cause sensitivity reactions. Stop I.V. iron if sensitivity reactions occur.
Oral iron preparations: May reduce absorption of oral iron preparations. Avoid using together.

EFFECTS ON LAB TEST RESULTS
● May decrease glucose and hemoglobin levels. May increase or decrease potassium level.

CONTRAINDICATIONS & CAUTIONS
● Contraindicated in patients hypersensitive to drug or its components (such as benzyl alcohol) and in those with iron overload or anemias not related to iron deficiency.
● Don't use in patients with ferritin levels greater than 1,000 nanograms/ml.
● Use cautiously in elderly patients.

NURSING CONSIDERATIONS
● *Alert:* Dosage is expressed in milligrams of elemental iron.
● Drug shouldn't be used in patients with iron overload, which often occurs in hemoglobinopathies and other refractory anemias.

● Monitor ferritin level, iron saturation, hemoglobin level, and hematocrit.
● In hemodialysis patients, adverse reactions may be related to dialysis itself or to chronic renal failure.
● Check with patient about other potential sources of iron, such as OTC iron preparations and iron-containing multiple vitamins with minerals.

PATIENT TEACHING
● Abdominal pain, diarrhea, vomiting, drowsiness, and rapid breathing may indicate iron poisoning. Urge patient to notify prescriber immediately.

31
Anticoagulants

argatroban
bivalirudin
dalteparin sodium
desirudin
enoxaparin sodium
fondaparinux sodium
heparin sodium
tinzaparin sodium
warfarin sodium

argatroban
ahr-GAH-troh-ban

Pharmacologic class: direct
thrombin inhibitor
Pregnancy risk category B

AVAILABLE FORMS
Injection: 100 mg/ml

INDICATIONS & DOSAGES
➤ **To prevent or treat thrombosis in patients with heparin-induced thrombocytopenia**
Adults without hepatic impairment:
2 mcg/kg/minute, given as a continuous
I.V. infusion; adjust dose until the
steady-state activated PTT is 1½ to
3 times the initial baseline value, not
to exceed 100 seconds; maximum dose
10 mcg/kg/minute. See current manufacturer's label for recommended doses
and infusion rates.
Adjust-a-dose: For patients with moderate
hepatic impairment, reduce first dose to
0.5 mcg/kg/minute, given as a continuous
infusion. Monitor PTT closely and adjust
dosage as needed.
➤ **Anticoagulation in patients with or at risk for heparin-induced thrombocytopenia during percutaneous coronary intervention (PCI)**
Adults: 350 mcg/kg I.V. bolus over 3 to
5 minutes. Start a continuous I.V. infusion
at 25 mcg/kg/minute. Check activated
clotting time (ACT) 5 to 10 minutes after
the bolus dose is completed.

Adjust-a-dose: Use the following table to
adjust the dosage.

Activated clotting time	Additional I.V. bolus	Continuous I.V. infusion
< 300 sec	150 mcg/kg	30 mcg/kg/min
300–450 sec	None needed	25 mcg/kg/min
> 450 sec	None needed	15 mcg/kg/min*

*Check ACT again after 5 to 10 minutes.

In case of dissection, impending abrupt
closure, thrombus formation during the
procedure, or inability to achieve or maintain an ACT exceeding 300 seconds, give
an additional bolus of 150 mcg/kg and increase infusion rate to 40 mcg/kg/minute.
Check ACT again after 5 to 10 minutes.

ADMINISTRATION
I.V.
● Before starting therapy, obtain a complete list of patient's prescription and
OTC drugs and supplements, including
herbs.
● Stop all parenteral anticoagulants before
giving drug. Giving with antiplatelets,
thrombolytics, and other anticoagulants
may increase risk of bleeding.
● Before starting drug, get results of
baseline coagulation tests, platelet count,
hemoglobin level, and hematocrit, and
report any abnormalities to prescriber.
● Dilute in normal saline solution, D₅W,
or lactated Ringer's injection to a final
concentration of 1 mg/ml.
● Dilute each 2.5-ml vial 100-fold by
mixing it with 250 ml of diluent.
● Mix the solution by repeated inversion
of the diluent bag for 10 minutes.
● Don't expose solution to direct sunlight.
● Prepared solutions are stable for up to
24 hours at 77° F (25° C).
● **Incompatibilities:** Other I.V. drugs.

ACTION
Reversibly binds to the thrombin-active
site and inhibits thrombin-catalyzed or
-induced reactions: fibrin formation;
coagulation factor V, VIII, and XIII activation; protein C activation; and platelet

---

Reactions may be *common*, uncommon, *life-threatening*, or COMMON AND LIFE-THREATENING.
Interaction may have a *rapid onset* or *delayed onset*.

aggregation. May inhibit the action of free and clot-associated thrombin.

Route	Onset	Peak	Duration
I.V.	Rapid	1–3 hr	Duration of infusion

Half-life: 39 to 51 minutes.

ADVERSE REACTIONS

CNS: *cerebrovascular disorder, hemorrhage,* fever, pain.
CV: *atrial fibrillation, cardiac arrest,* hypotension, *ventricular tachycardia.*
GI: abdominal pain, diarrhea, *GI bleeding,* nausea, vomiting.
GU: abnormal renal function, groin bleeding, *hematuria,* UTI.
Respiratory: cough, dyspnea, pneumonia, hemoptysis.
Other: allergic reactions, brachial bleeding, infection, *sepsis.*

INTERACTIONS

Drug-drug. *Antiplatelet drugs (clopidogrel, NSAIDs, salicylates), heparin, thrombolytics:* May increase risk of intracranial bleeding. Avoid using together.
Oral anticoagulants: May prolong PT and INR and may increase risk of bleeding. Monitor patient closely.
Drug-herb. *Angelica (dong quai), boldo, bromelains, capsicum, chamomile, dandelion, danshen, devil's claw, fenugreek, feverfew, garlic, ginger, ginkgo, ginseng, horse chestnut, licorice, meadowsweet, onion, passion flower, red clover, willow:* May increase risk of bleeding. Discourage use together.

EFFECTS ON LAB TEST RESULTS

● May decrease hemoglobin level and hematocrit.

CONTRAINDICATIONS & CAUTIONS

● Contraindicated in patients who have overt major bleeding who are hypersensitive to drug or any of its components.
● Use cautiously in patients with hepatic disease or conditions that increase the risk of hemorrhage, such as severe hypertension.
● Use cautiously in patients who have just had lumbar puncture, spinal anesthesia, or major surgery, especially of the brain, spinal cord, or eye; patients with hematologic conditions causing increased bleeding tendencies, such as congenital or acquired bleeding disorders; and patients with GI ulcers or other lesions.

NURSING CONSIDERATIONS

● Check activated PTT 2 hours after giving drug; dose adjustments may be required to get a targeted activated PTT of 1.5 to 3 times the baseline, no longer than 100 seconds. Steady state is achieved 1 to 3 hours after starting drug.
● Draw blood for additional ACT about every 20 to 30 minutes during prolonged PCI.
● *Alert:* Patients can hemorrhage from any site in the body. Any unexplained decrease in hematocrit or blood pressure or any other unexplained symptoms may signify a hemorrhagic event.
● To convert to oral anticoagulant therapy, give warfarin P.O. with argatroban at up to 2 mcg/kg/minute until the INR exceeds 4 on combined therapy. After argatroban is stopped, repeat the INR in 4 to 6 hours. If the repeat INR is less than the desired therapeutic range, resume the I.V. argatroban infusion. Repeat the procedure daily until the desired therapeutic range on warfarin alone is reached.
● Use cautiously in breast-feeding women; it's unknown if drug appears in breast milk.
● *Look alike–sound alike:* Don't confuse argatroban with Aggrastat.

PATIENT TEACHING

● Tell patient that this drug can cause bleeding, and ask him to report any unusual bruising or bleeding (nosebleeds, bleeding gums) or tarry stools to the prescriber immediately.
● Advise patient to avoid activities that carry a risk of injury, and to use a soft toothbrush and an electric razor during therapy.
● Advise patient to consult with prescriber before initiating any herbal therapy; many herbs have anticoagulant, antiplatelet, and fibrinolytic properties.
● Instruct patient to notify prescriber if he has wheezing, trouble breathing, or skin rash.
● Instruct woman who is pregnant, has recently delivered, or is breast-feeding to notify her prescriber.

• Tell patient to notify prescriber if he has GI ulcers or liver disease, or has had recent surgery, radiation treatment, falling episodes, or injury.

bivalirudin
bye-VAL-ih-roo-din

Angiomax

Pharmacologic class: direct thrombin inhibitor
Pregnancy risk category B

AVAILABLE FORMS
Injection: 250-mg vial

INDICATIONS & DOSAGES
➤ **Anticoagulation in patients with unstable angina undergoing percutaneous transluminal coronary angioplasty (PTCA); anticoagulation in patients with unstable angina undergoing percutaneous coronary intervention (PCI), with provisional use of a platelet glycoprotein IIb/IIIa inhibitor (GPI)**
Adults: 0.75 mg/kg I.V. bolus followed by a continuous infusion of 1.75 mg/kg/hour during the procedure. Check activated clotting time 5 minutes after bolus dose is given. May give additional 0.3 mg/kg bolus dose if needed. Infusion may continue for up to 4 hours after procedure. After 4-hour infusion, may give an additional infusion of 0.2 mg/kg/hour for up to 20 hours, if needed. Use with 300 to 325 mg aspirin.
➤ **Patients undergoing PCI who have or are at risk for heparin-induced thrombocytopenia (HIT) or heparin-induced thrombocytopenia and thrombosis syndrome (HITTS)**
Adults: 0.75 mg/kg I.V. bolus, followed by a continuous infusion of 1.75 mg/kg/hour throughout the procedure. Consult prescriber about continuing the infusion after PCI.
Adjust-a-dose: For patients with creatinine clearance of 30 ml/minute or less, decrease infusion rate to 1 mg/kg/hour. For patients on hemodialysis, reduce infusion rate to

0.25 mg/kg/hour. No reduction of bolus dose is needed.

ADMINISTRATION
I.V.
• Reconstitute each 250-mg vial with 5 ml of sterile water for injection.
• Dilute each reconstituted vial in 50 ml D_5W or normal saline solution to yield a final concentration of 5 mg/ml.
• To prepare low-rate infusion, further dilute each reconstituted vial in 500 ml D_5W or normal saline solution to yield a final concentration of 0.5 mg/ml.
• Solutions with concentrations of 0.5 to 5 mg/ml are stable at room temperature for 24 hours.
• **Incompatibilities:** Alteplase, amiodarone, amphotericin B, chlorpromazine, diazepam, prochlorperazine, reteplase, streptokinase, vancomycin. *Note:* Compatible with dobutamine at concentrations up to 4 mg/ml, but incompatible at concentration of 12.5 mg/ml.

ACTION
Binds specifically and rapidly to thrombin to produce an anticoagulant effect.

Route	Onset	Peak	Duration
I.V.	Rapid	Immediate	1–2 hr

Half-life: 25 minutes in patients with normal renal function.

ADVERSE REACTIONS
CNS: anxiety, *headache,* insomnia, nervousness, fever, *pain.*
CV: *bradycardia,* hypertension, *hypotension.*
GI: abdominal pain, dyspepsia, *nausea,* vomiting.
GU: urine retention.
Hematologic: *severe, spontaneous bleeding (cerebral, retroperitoneal, GU, GI).*
Musculoskeletal: *back pain,* pelvic pain.
Skin: pain at injection site.

INTERACTIONS
Drug-drug. *GPIIb/IIIa inhibitors, heparin, thrombolytics, warfarin:* May increase risk of hemorrhage. Use together cautiously.
Drug-herb. *Angelica (dong quai), boldo, bromelains, capsicum, chamomile, dandelion, danshen, devil's claw, fenugreek, feverfew, garlic, ginger, ginkgo, ginseng,*

horse chestnut, licorice, meadowsweet, onion, passion flower, red clover, willow: May increase risk of bleeding. Discourage use together.

EFFECTS ON LAB TEST RESULTS
None reported.

CONTRAINDICATIONS & CAUTIONS
• Contraindicated in patients hypersensitive to drug or its components and in those with active major bleeding. Avoid using in patients with unstable angina who aren't undergoing PTCA or PCI or in patients with other acute coronary syndromes.
• Use cautiously in patients with HIT or HITTS and in those with diseases linked to increased risk of bleeding.
• Use cautiously in breast-feeding women; it's unknown if drug appears in breast milk.

NURSING CONSIDERATIONS
• Monitor coagulation test results, hemoglobin level, and hematocrit before starting therapy and periodically thereafter.
• Circumstances for provisional use of a GPI during PCI include decreased thrombolysis-in-MI, flow; slow reflow; dissection with decreased flow; new or suspected thrombus; persistent residual stenosis; distal embolization; unplanned stent; suboptimal stenting; side-branch closure; abrupt closure; instability; and prolonged ischemia.
• Obtain a complete list of patient's prescription and OTC drugs and supplements, including herbs.
• **Alert:** Hemorrhage can occur at any site in the body. If patient has unexplained decrease in hematocrit, decrease in blood pressure, or other unexplained symptoms, suspect hemorrhage.
• Monitor venipuncture sites for bleeding, hematoma, or inflammation.
• Puncture-site hemorrhage and catheterization-site hematoma may occur in patients age 65 and older more often than in younger patients.
• Don't give drug I.M.

PATIENT TEACHING
• Advise patient that drug can cause bleeding and tell him to report unusual bruising or bleeding (nosebleeds, bleeding gums) or tarry stools immediately.

• Counsel patient that drug is given with aspirin and caution him to avoid other aspirin-containing drugs or NSAIDs while receiving this drug.
• Advise patient to consult with prescriber before initiating any herbal therapy; many herbs have anticoagulant, antiplatelet, and fibrinolytic properties.
• Advise patient to avoid activities that carry a risk of injury and instruct him to use a soft toothbrush and electric razor while on drug.

SAFETY ALERT!

dalteparin sodium
DAHL-tep-ah-rin

Fragmin

*Pharmacologic class:
low–molecular-weight heparin
Pregnancy risk category B*

AVAILABLE FORMS
Injection: 2,500 antifactor Xa international units/0.2 ml syringe, 5,000 antifactor Xa international units/0.2 ml syringe, 7,500 antifactor Xa international units/0.3 ml syringe, 10,000 antifactor Xa international units/0.4 ml syringe, 10,000 antifactor Xa international units/ml syringe, 10,000 antifactor Xa international units/ml in 9.5-ml multidose vial, 12,500 antifactor Xa international units/0.5 ml syringe, 15,000 antifactor Xa international units/ 0.6 ml syringe, 18,000 antifactor Xa international units/0.72 ml syringe, 25,000 antifactor Xa international units/ml in 3.8-ml multidose vial. Each multidose vial contains 14 mg/ml of benzyl alcohol.

INDICATIONS & DOSAGES
➤ **To prevent deep vein thrombosis (DVT) in patients undergoing abdominal surgery who are at moderate to high risk for thromboembolic complications**
Adults: 2,500 international units subcutaneously daily, starting 1 to 2 hours before surgery and repeated once daily for 5 to 10 days postoperatively. Or, for patients at high risk, give 5,000 international units subcutaneously the evening before surgery,

then once daily postoperatively for 5 to 10 days. Or, in patients with malignancy, give 2,500 international units subcutaneously 1 to 2 hours before surgery followed by 2,500 international units subcutaneously 12 hours later, then 5,000 international units subcutaneously once daily for 5 to 10 days postoperatively.

➤ **To prevent DVT in patients undergoing hip replacement surgery**
Adults: 2,500 international units subcutaneously within 2 hours before surgery and second dose 2,500 international units subcutaneously in the evening after surgery (at least 6 hours after first dose). If surgery is performed in the evening, omit second dose on day of surgery. Starting on first postoperative day, give 5,000 international units subcutaneously once daily for 5 to 10 days. Or, give 5,000 international units subcutaneously on the evening before surgery; then 5,000 international units subcutaneously once daily starting in the evening of surgery for 5 to 10 days postoperatively.

➤ **Unstable angina non–Q-wave MI**
Adults: 120 international units/kg subcutaneously every 12 hours with aspirin (75 to 165 mg daily) P.O., unless contraindicated. Maximum dose, 10,000 international units. Treatment usually lasts 5 to 8 days.

➤ **To prevent DVT in patients at risk for thromboembolic complications because of severely restricted mobility during acute illness**
Adults: 5,000 international units subcutaneously once daily for 12 to 14 days.

➤ **Symptomatic venous thromboembolism in cancer patients**
Adults: Initially, 200 international units/kg (maximum, 18,000 international units) subcutaneously daily for 30 days; then 150 international units/kg (maximum, 18,000 international units) subcutaneously daily months 2 through 6.
Adjust-a-dose: In patients with platelet count 50,000 to 100,000/mm³, reduce dose by 2,500 international units until platelet count exceeds 100,000/mm³. In patients with platelet count less than 50,000/mm³, stop drug until platelet count exceeds 50,000/mm³. For patients with creatinine clearance of 30 ml/minute or less, monitor anti-Xa levels to determine appropriate dose. Target anti-Xa range is

0.5 to 1.5 international units/ml. Draw anti-Xa 4 to 6 hours after dose and only after the patient has received three to four doses.

ADMINISTRATION
Subcutaneous
● Before giving injection, obtain complete list of all prescribed and OTC medications, and supplements, including herbs.
● Have patient sit or lie supine when giving drug.
● Injection sites include a U-shaped area around the navel, upper outer side of thigh, and upper outer quadrangle of buttock. Rotate sites daily.
● When area around the navel or thigh is used, use thumb and forefinger to lift up a fold of skin while giving injection.
● Give subcutaneous injection deeply, inserting the entire length of needle at a 45- to 90-degree angle.

ACTION
Enhances inhibition of factor Xa and thrombin by antithrombin.

Route	Onset	Peak	Duration
Subcut.	Unknown	4 hr	Unknown

Half-life: 3 to 5 hours.

ADVERSE REACTIONS
CNS: fever.
GU: hematuria.
Hematologic: *thrombocytopenia, hemorrhage,* ecchymoses, bleeding complications.
Skin: pruritus, rash, *hematoma at injection site,* injection site pain.
Other: *anaphylaxis.*

INTERACTIONS
Drug-drug. *Antiplatelet drugs (aspirin, NSAIDs, clopidogrel, dipyridamole, ticlodipine), oral anticoagulants, thrombolytics:* May increase risk of bleeding. Use together cautiously.
Drug-herb. *Angelica (dong quai), boldo, bromelains, capsicum, chamomile, dandelion, danshen, devil's claw, fenugreek, feverfew, garlic, ginger, ginkgo, ginseng, horse chestnut, licorice, meadowsweet, onion, passion flower, red clover, willow:* May increase risk of bleeding. Discourage use together.

Reactions may be *common,* uncommon, *life-threatening,* or COMMON AND LIFE-THREATENING.
Interaction may have a *rapid onset* or **delayed onset.**

EFFECTS ON LAB TEST RESULTS
- May increase ALT and AST levels.
- May decrease platelet count.

CONTRAINDICATIONS & CAUTIONS
- Contraindicated in patients hypersensitive to drug, heparin, or pork products; in those with active major bleeding; and in those with thrombocytopenia and antiplatelet antibodies in presence of drug.
- Contraindicated in patients with unstable angina or non-Q-wave MI who are undergoing regional anesthesia because of an increased risk of bleeding associated with the dose of dalteparin recommended for these indications.
- Use with caution in patients with history of heparin-induced thrombocytopenia and in patients at increased risk for hemorrhage, such as those with severe uncontrolled hypertension, bacterial endocarditis, congenital or acquired bleeding disorders, active ulceration, angiodysplastic GI disease, or hemorrhagic stroke; also use with caution shortly after brain, spinal, or ophthalmic surgery. Monitor vital signs.
- Use with caution in patients with bleeding diathesis, thrombocytopenia, platelet defects, severe hepatic or renal insufficiency, hypertensive or diabetic retinopathy, or recent GI bleeding.

NURSING CONSIDERATIONS
■ **Black Box Warning** Patients who have received epidural or spinal anesthesia or spinal puncture are at increased risk for developing an epidural or spinal hematoma, which may result in long-term or permanent paralysis. Monitor these patients closely for neurologic impairment. ■
- DVT is a risk factor in patients who are candidates for therapy, including those older than age 40, those who are obese, those undergoing surgery under general anesthesia lasting longer than 30 minutes, and those who have additional risk factors (such as malignancy or history of DVT or pulmonary embolism).
- Never give drug I.M.
- Don't mix with other injections or infusions unless specific compatibility data support such mixing.
- Multidose vial shouldn't be used in pregnant women because of benzyl alcohol content. Benzyl alcohol has been associated with fatal "gasping syndrome" in premature neonates.
- *Alert:* Drug isn't interchangeable (unit for unit) with unfractionated heparin or other low–molecular-weight heparin.
- Periodic, routine CBC and fecal occult blood tests are recommended during therapy. Patients don't need regular monitoring of PT or activated PTT.
- Monitor patient closely for thrombocytopenia.
- Stop drug if a thromboembolic event occurs despite dalteparin prophylaxis. May use alternative therapy, or may have been inadequate dose.
- Obtain a complete list of patient's prescription and OTC drugs and supplements, including herbs.

PATIENT TEACHING
- Instruct patient and family to watch for and report signs of bleeding (bruising and blood in stools).
- Tell patient to avoid OTC drugs containing aspirin or other salicylates unless ordered by prescriber.
- Advise patient to consult with prescriber prior to initiating any herbal therapy; many herbs have anticoagulant, antiplatelet, and fibrinolytic properties.
- Tell patient to use a soft toothbrush and electric razor during treatment.

SAFETY ALERT!

desirudin
deh-SIHR-uh-din

Iprivask

Pharmacologic class: thrombin inhibitor
Pregnancy risk category C

AVAILABLE FORMS
Injection: 15.75 mg desirudin lyophilized powder and 0.6 ml mannitol (3%) diluent

INDICATIONS & DOSAGES
➤ **To prevent deep vein thrombosis in patients undergoing hip replacement surgery**

Adults: 15 mg subcutaneously every 12 hours for 9 to 12 days. Give first injection 5 to 15 minutes before surgery, after induction of regional block anesthesia, if used.

Adjust-a-dose: If creatinine clearance is 31 to 60 ml/minute, give 5 mg subcutaneously every 12 hours. If creatinine clearance is less than 31 ml/minute, give 1.7 mg subcutaneously every 12 hours. Check activated PTT and creatinine daily. If activated PTT exceeds two times control, stop therapy until it's within two times control; then resume at a reduced dose.

ADMINISTRATION

Subcutaneous

● Reconstitute each 15-mg vial with 0.5 ml of provided diluent (mannitol 3%).
● Shake vial gently until powder is dissolved. Once reconstituted, each 0.5 ml contains 15.75 mg of desirudin.
● Inspect vial. If solution contains visible particles, don't use it.
● Use reconstituted solution immediately or store it at room temperature for up to 24 hours protected from light.
● Use a syringe with a ½-inch 26G or 27G needle to withdraw all the reconstituted solution.
● With the patient lying down, inject entire contents of syringe by deep subcutaneous injection. Insert entire length of needle into a skinfold held between thumb and forefinger.
● Rotate sites between the right and left thigh or right and left anterolateral and posterolateral abdominal walls.
● **Incompatibilities:** Don't mix with any other drugs.

ACTION

Selectively inhibits free and clot-bound thrombin, which prolongs plasma clotting time.

Route	Onset	Peak	Duration
Subcut.	30 min	60–180 min	Unknown

Half-life: 2 to 3 hours.

ADVERSE REACTIONS

CNS: cerebrovascular disorder, dizziness, fever.
CV: *thrombosis,* deep thrombophlebitis, hypotension.

EENT: epistaxis.
GI: *hematemesis,* nausea, vomiting.
GU: hematuria.
Hematologic: *hemorrhage,* anemia.
Other: *anaphylaxis,* impaired healing, injection site mass, leg edema, leg pain, wound seeping.

INTERACTIONS

Drug-drug. *Abciximab, acetylsalicylic acid, clopidogrel, dipyridamole, glycoprotein IIb/IIIa antagonists, ketorolac, salicylates, sulfinpyrazone, ticlopidine:* May increase the risk of bleeding. Use together cautiously.
Anticoagulants, dextran 40, glucocorticoids, thrombolytics: May increase the risk of bleeding. Avoid using together.
Epidural or spinal anesthesia: May increase risk of neuraxial hematoma and paralysis. Catheter may be placed before desirudin is started and removed when anticoagulant effect is low.
Drug-herb. *Alfalfa, angelica (dong quai), anise, boldo, bromelains, capsicum, chamomile, dandelion, danshen, devil's claw, fenugreek, feverfew, garlic, ginger, ginkgo, ginseng, horse chestnut, licorice, meadowsweet, onion, passion flower, red clover, willow:* May increase the risk of bleeding. Discourage use together.

EFFECTS ON LAB TEST RESULTS

● May decrease hemoglobin level and hematocrit.

CONTRAINDICATIONS & CAUTIONS

● Contraindicated in patients hypersensitive to natural or recombinant hirudins and in patients with active bleeding or irreversible coagulation disorders.
● Use cautiously in patients with a creatinine clearance less than 60 ml/minute; patients undergoing spinal or epidural anesthesia; patients with hepatic insufficiency or injury; patients with GI or pulmonary bleeding within 3 months; patients with severe uncontrolled hypertension, bacterial endocarditis, or a hemostatic disorder; and patients with an increased risk of bleeding, such as those with recent major surgery, organ biopsy, puncture of a noncompressible vessel (within 1 month), intracranial or intraocular bleeding, or hemorrhagic or ischemic stroke.

Reactions may be *common,* uncommon, *life-threatening,* or COMMON AND LIFE-THREATENING.
Interaction may have a *rapid onset* or *delayed onset.*

NURSING CONSIDERATIONS

- Don't give this drug I.M.
- **Alert:** If the patient has either an unexplained decline in hematocrit or blood pressure or other unexplained symptoms, consider the possibility of hemorrhage.
- Monitor coagulation tests, hemoglobin level, hematocrit, and renal function throughout therapy.
- Watch venipuncture sites for bleeding, hematoma, or inflammation.
- ■ **Black Box Warning** Patients who receive epidural or spinal anesthesia or spinal puncture are at increased risk of an epidural or spinal hematoma, which may result in long-term or permanent paralysis. Monitor these patients closely for neurologic impairment. ■

PATIENT TEACHING

- Advise patient that this drug can cause bleeding. Stress the need to report unusual bruising or bleeding (nosebleeds, blood in urine, tarry stools) immediately.
- Caution patient not to take any other drugs that increase the risk of bleeding, such as aspirin or NSAIDs, while receiving desirudin.
- Advise patient to consult with prescriber before starting any herbal therapy; many herbs have anticoagulant, antiplatelet, or fibrinolytic properties.
- Advise against activities that risk injury.
- Tell patient to use a soft toothbrush and electric razor during therapy.

SAFETY ALERT!

enoxaparin sodium
en-OCKS-a-par-in

Lovenox

Pharmacologic class:
low–molecular-weight heparin
Pregnancy risk category B

AVAILABLE FORMS

Syringes (graduated prefilled): 60 mg/ 0.6 ml, 80 mg/0.8 ml, 100 mg/ml, 120 mg/ 0.8 ml, 150 mg/ml
Syringes (prefilled): 30 mg/0.3 ml, 40 mg/ 0.4 ml
Vial (multidose): 300 mg/3 ml (contains 15 mg/ml of benzyl alcohol)

INDICATIONS & DOSAGES

➤ **To prevent pulmonary embolism and deep vein thrombosis (DVT) after hip or knee replacement surgery**
Adults: 30 mg subcutaneously every 12 hours for 7 to 10 days. Give initial dose between 12 and 24 hours postoperatively, as long as hemostasis has been established. Continue treatment during postoperative period until risk of DVT has diminished. Hip replacement patients may receive 40 mg subcutaneously given 12 hours preoperatively. After initial phase of therapy, hip replacement patients should continue with 40 mg subcutaneously daily for 3 weeks.

➤ **To prevent pulmonary embolism and DVT after abdominal surgery**
Adults: 40 mg subcutaneously daily with initial dose 2 hours before surgery. Give subsequent dose, as long as hemostasis has been established, 24 hours after initial preoperative dose and continue once daily for 7 to 10 days. Continue treatment during postoperative period until risk of DVT has diminished.

➤ **To prevent pulmonary embolism and DVT in patients with acute illness who are at increased risk because of decreased mobility**
Adults: 40 mg once daily subcutaneously for 6 to 11 days. Treatment for up to 14 days has been well tolerated.
Adjust-a-dose: In patients with creatinine clearance less than 30 ml/minute receiving drug as prophylaxis after abdominal surgery or hip or knee replacement surgery, and in medical patients for prophylaxis during acute illness, give 30 mg subcutaneously once daily.

➤ **To prevent ischemic complications of unstable angina and non–Q-wave MI with oral aspirin therapy**
Adults: 1 mg/kg subcutaneously every 12 hours until clinical stabilization (minimum 2 days) with aspirin 100 to 325 mg P.O. once daily. Usual duration of treatment is 2 to 8 days.

➤ **Acute ST-segment elevation MI**
Adults younger than age 75: 30 mg single I.V. bolus plus 1 mg/kg subcutaneously followed by 1 mg/kg subcutaneously every 12 hours (maximum of 100 mg for the first two doses only) with aspirin.

When given with a thrombolytic, give enoxaparin from 15 minutes before to 30 minutes after the start of fibrinolytic therapy. For patients with percutaneous coronary intervention (PCI), if the last subcutaneous dose was given less than 8 hours before balloon inflation, no additional dose is needed. If the last dose was given more than 8 hours before balloon inflation, give 0.3 mg/kg I.V. bolus.

Adults age 75 and older: 0.75 mg/kg subcutaneously every 12 hours (maximum 75 mg for the first two doses only).

Adjust-a-dose: In adults younger than age 75 with severe renal impairment, 30 mg single I.V. bolus plus 1 mg/kg subcutaneously followed by 1 mg/kg subcutaneously once daily. In adults age 75 and older with severe renal impairment, 1 mg/kg subcutaneously once daily with no initial bolus.

➤ **Inpatient treatment of acute DVT with and without pulmonary embolism when given with warfarin sodium**

Adults: 1 mg/kg subcutaneously every 12 hours. Or, 1.5 mg/kg subcutaneously once daily (at same time daily) for 5 to 7 days until therapeutic oral anticoagulant effect (INR 2 to 3) is achieved. Warfarin sodium therapy is usually started within 72 hours of enoxaparin injection.

➤ **Outpatient treatment of acute DVT without pulmonary embolism when given with warfarin sodium**

Adults: 1 mg/kg subcutaneously every 12 hours for 5 to 7 days until therapeutic oral anticoagulant effect (INR 2 to 3) is achieved. Warfarin sodium therapy usually is started within 72 hours of enoxaparin injection.

Adjust-a-dose: In patients with creatinine clearance less than 30 ml/minute receiving drug for acute DVT or prophylaxis of ischemic complications of unstable angina and non–Q-wave MI, give 1 mg/kg subcutaneously once daily.

ADMINISTRATION

Subcutaneous

• With patient lying down, give by deep subcutaneous injection, alternating doses between left and right anterolateral and posterolateral abdominal walls.

• Don't massage after subcutaneous injection. Watch for signs of bleeding at site. Rotate sites and keep record.

ACTION

Accelerates formation of antithrombin III–thrombin complex and deactivates thrombin, preventing conversion of fibrinogen to fibrin. Drug has a higher antifactor-Xa-to-antifactor-IIa activity ratio than heparin.

Route	Onset	Peak	Duration
Subcut.	Unknown	4 hr	Unknown

Half-life: 4½ hours.

ADVERSE REACTIONS

CNS: confusion, fever, pain.
CV: edema, peripheral edema.
GI: nausea, diarrhea.
Hematologic: *thrombocytopenia, hemorrhage,* ecchymoses, bleeding complications, hypochromic anemia.
Skin: irritation, pain, hematoma, and erythema at injection site, *rash, urticaria.*
Other: *angioedema, anaphylaxis.*

INTERACTIONS

Drug-drug. *Anticoagulants, antiplatelet drugs, NSAIDs:* May increase risk of bleeding. Use together cautiously. Monitor PT and INR.
SSRIs: May increase risk of severe bleeding. Monitor PT, INR, and patient. Adjust therapy as needed.
Drug-herb. *Angelica (dong quai), boldo, bromelains, capsicum, chamomile, dandelion, danshen, devil's claw, fenugreek, feverfew, garlic, ginger, ginkgo, ginseng, horse chestnut, licorice, meadowsweet, onion, passion flower, red clover, willow:* May increase risk of bleeding. Discourage use together.

EFFECTS ON LAB TEST RESULTS

• May increase ALT and AST levels. May decrease hemoglobin level.
• May decrease platelet count.

CONTRAINDICATIONS & CAUTIONS

• Contraindicated in patients hypersensitive to drug, heparin, or pork products; in those with active major bleeding; and in those with thrombocytopenia

---

and antiplatelet antibodies in presence of drug.
- Use cautiously in patients with history of heparin-induced thrombocytopenia, aneurysms, cerebrovascular hemorrhage, spinal or epidural punctures (as with anesthesia), uncontrolled hypertension, or threatened abortion.
- Use cautiously in elderly patients and in those with conditions that place them at increased risk for hemorrhage, such as bacterial endocarditis, congenital or acquired bleeding disorders, ulcer disease, angiodysplastic GI disease, hemorrhagic stroke, or recent spinal, eye, or brain surgery.
- Use cautiously in patients with prosthetic heart valves, with regional or lumbar block anesthesia, blood dyscrasias, recent childbirth, pericarditis or pericardial effusion, renal insufficiency, or severe CNS trauma.

NURSING CONSIDERATIONS
- It's important to achieve hemostasis at the puncture site after PCI. The vascular access sheath for instrumentation should remain in place for 6 hours after a dose if manual compression method is used; give next dose no sooner than 6 to 8 hours after sheath removal. Monitor vital signs and site for hematoma and bleeding.
- Monitor pregnant women closely. Warn pregnant women and women of childbearing age about the potential risk of therapy to her and the fetus.
- Multidose vial shouldn't be used in pregnant women because of benzyl alcohol content.
- Monitor anti-Xa levels in pregnant women with mechanical heart valves.
- ■ **Black Box Warning** Patients who receive epidural or spinal anesthesia or spinal puncture during therapy are at increased risk for developing an epidural or spinal hematoma, which may result in long-term or permanent paralysis. Monitor these patients closely for neurologic impairment. ■
- Draw blood to establish baseline coagulation parameters before therapy.
- Never give drug I.M.
- *Alert:* Don't try to expel the air bubble from the 30- or 40-mg prefilled syringes. This may lead to loss of drug and an incorrect dose.

- Avoid I.M. injections of other drugs to prevent or minimize hematoma.
- Monitor platelet counts regularly. Patients with normal coagulation won't need close monitoring of PT or PTT.
- Regularly inspect patient for bleeding gums, bruises on arms or legs, petechiae, nosebleeds, melena, tarry stools, hematuria, hematemesis.
- To treat severe overdose, give protamine sulfate (a heparin antagonist) by slow I.V. infusion at concentration of 1% to equal dose of drug injected.
- *Alert:* Drug isn't interchangeable with heparin or other low–molecular-weight heparins.

PATIENT TEACHING
- Instruct patient and family to watch for signs of bleeding or abnormal bruising and to notify prescriber immediately if any occur.
- Tell patient to avoid OTC drugs containing aspirin or other salicylates unless ordered by prescriber.
- Advise patient to consult with prescriber before initiating any herbal therapy; many herbs have anticoagulant, antiplatelet, or fibrinolytic properties.

SAFETY ALERT!

fondaparinux sodium
fon-dah-PEAR-ah-nucks

Arixtra

Pharmacologic class: activated factor X inhibitor
Pregnancy risk category B

AVAILABLE FORMS
Injection: 2.5 mg/0.5 ml, 5 mg/0.4 ml, 7.5 mg/0.6 ml, 10 mg/0.8 ml single-dose prefilled syringe

INDICATIONS & DOSAGES
➤ **To prevent deep vein thrombosis (DVT), which may lead to pulmonary embolism, in patients undergoing surgery for hip fracture, hip replacement, knee replacement, or abdominal surgery**
Adults who weigh 50 kg (110 lb) or more: 2.5 mg subcutaneously once daily for 5 to

9 days. Give first dose after hemostasis is established, 6 to 8 hours after surgery. Giving the dose earlier than 6 hours after surgery increases the risk of major bleeding. Patients undergoing hip fracture surgery should receive an extended prophylaxis course of up to 24 additional days; a total of 32 days (perioperative and extended prophylaxis) has been tolerated.

➤ **Acute DVT (with warfarin); acute pulmonary embolism (with warfarin) when treatment is started in the hospital**

Adults who weigh more than 100 kg (220 lb): 10 mg subcutaneously daily for 5 to 9 days, and until INR level is 2 to 3. Begin warfarin therapy as soon as possible, usually within 72 hours.

Adults who weigh 50 to 100 kg: 7.5 mg subcutaneously daily for 5 to 9 days, and until INR level is 2 to 3. Begin warfarin therapy as soon as possible, usually within 72 hours.

Adults who weigh less than 50 kg: 5 mg subcutaneously daily for 5 to 9 days, and until INR level is 2 to 3. Begin warfarin therapy as soon as possible, usually within 72 hours.

ADMINISTRATION
Subcutaneous
● Give subcutaneously only, never I.M. Inspect the single-dose, prefilled syringe for particulate matter and discoloration before giving.
● Give the drug in fatty tissue, rotating injection sites. If the drug has been properly injected, the needle will pull back into the syringe security sleeve and the white safety indicator will appear above the blue upper body. A soft click may be heard or felt when the syringe plunger is fully released. After injection of the syringe contents, the plunger automatically rises while the needle withdraws from the skin and retracts into the security sleeve. Don't recap the needle.
● **Incompatibilities:** Other injections or infusions.

ACTION
Binds to antithrombin III (AT-III) and potentiates the neutralization of factor Xa by AT-III, which interrupts coagulation and inhibits formation of thrombin and blood clots.

Route	Onset	Peak	Duration
Subcut.	Unknown	2–3 hr	Unknown

Half-life: 17 to 21 hours.

ADVERSE REACTIONS
CNS: *fever,* insomnia, dizziness, confusion, headache, pain.
CV: hypotension, edema.
GI: *nausea,* constipation, vomiting, diarrhea, dyspepsia.
GU: UTI, urine retention.
Hematologic: *hemorrhage, anemia,* hematoma, *postoperative hemorrhage, thrombocytopenia.*
Metabolic: hypokalemia.
Skin: mild local irritation (injection site bleeding, rash, pruritus), bullous eruption, purpura, rash, increased wound drainage.

INTERACTIONS
Drug-drug. *Drugs that increase risk of bleeding (NSAIDs, platelet inhibitors, anticoagulants):* May increase risk of hemorrhage. Stop these drugs before starting fondaparinux. If use together is unavoidable, monitor patient closely.
Drug-herb. *Angelica (dong quai), boldo, bromelains, capsicum, chamomile, dandelion, danshen, devil's claw, fenugreek, feverfew, garlic, ginger, ginkgo, ginseng, horse chestnut, licorice, meadowsweet, onion, passion flower, red clover, willow:* May increase risk of bleeding. Discourage use together.

EFFECTS ON LAB TEST RESULTS
● May increase AST, ALT, and bilirubin levels. May decrease potassium and hemoglobin levels and hematocrit.
● May decrease platelet count.

CONTRAINDICATIONS & CAUTIONS
● Contraindicated in patients with creatinine clearance less than 30 ml/minute and in those who are hypersensitive to the drug.
● Contraindicated for prophylaxis in patients who weigh less than 50 kg who are undergoing hip fracture, hip replacement, knee replacement, or abdominal surgery.
● Contraindicated in patients with active major bleeding, bacterial endocarditis, or thrombocytopenia with a positive test result for antiplatelet antibody after taking fondaparinux.

Reactions may be *common,* uncommon, *life-threatening,* or COMMON AND LIFE-THREATENING.
Interaction may have a *rapid onset* or *delayed onset.*

• Use cautiously in patients being treated with platelet inhibitors; in those at increased risk for bleeding, such as congenital or acquired bleeding disorders; in those with active ulcerative and angiodysplastic GI disease; in those with hemorrhagic stroke; and in patients shortly after brain, spinal, or ophthalmologic surgery.

• Use cautiously in patients who have had epidural or spinal anesthesia or spinal puncture; they are at increased risk for developing an epidural or spinal hematoma (which may cause paralysis).

• Use cautiously in elderly patients, in patients with creatinine clearance of 30 to 50 ml/minute, and in those with a history of heparin-induced thrombocytopenia, a bleeding diathesis, uncontrolled arterial hypertension, or a history of recent GI ulceration, diabetic retinopathy, or hemorrhage.

NURSING CONSIDERATIONS
• Don't use interchangeably with heparin, low–molecular-weight heparins, or heparinoids.

• *Alert:* To avoid loss of drug, don't expel air bubble from the syringe.

■ **Black Box Warning** Patients who receive epidural or spinal anesthesia or spinal puncture are at increased risk for developing an epidural or spinal hematoma, which may result in long-term or permanent paralysis. Monitor these patients closely for neurologic impairment. ■

• Monitor renal function periodically and stop drug in patients who develop unstable renal function or severe renal impairment while receiving therapy.

• Routinely assess patient for signs and symptoms of bleeding, and regularly monitor CBC, platelet count, creatinine level, and stool occult blood test results. Stop use if platelet count is less than 100,000/mm^3.

• Anticoagulant effects may last for 2 to 4 days after stopping drug in patients with normal renal function.

• PT and activated PTT aren't suitable monitoring tests to measure drug activity. If coagulation parameters change unexpectedly or patient develops major bleeding, stop drug.

PATIENT TEACHING
• Tell patient to report signs and symptoms of bleeding.

• Instruct patient to avoid OTC products that contain aspirin or other salicylates.

• Advise patient to consult with prescriber before starting herbal therapy; many herbs have anticoagulant, antiplatelet, or fibrinolytic properties.

• Teach patient the correct technique for subcutaneous use, if needed.

SAFETY ALERT!

heparin sodium
HEP-ah-rin

Hepalean†, Heparin Lock Flush Solution (with Tubex), Heparin Sodium Injection, Hep-Lock, Hep-Pak

Pharmacologic class: anticoagulant
Pregnancy risk category C

AVAILABLE FORMS
Products are derived from beef lung or pork intestinal mucosa.
heparin sodium
Carpuject: 5,000 units/ml
Premixed I.V. solutions: 1,000 units in 500 ml of normal saline solution; 2,000 units in 1,000 ml of normal saline solution; 12,500 units in 250 ml of half-normal saline solution; 25,000 units in 250 ml of half-normal saline solution; 25,000 units in 500 ml of half-normal saline solution; 10,000 units in 100 ml of D$_5$W; 12,500 units in 250 ml of D$_5$W; 20,000 units in 500 ml of D$_5$W; 25,000 units in 250 ml D$_5$W; 25,000 units in 500 ml D$_5$W
Single-dose ampules and vials: 1,000 units/ml, 5,000 units/ml, 10,000 units/ml, 20,000 units/ml, 40,000 units/ml
Syringes: 1,000 units/ml, 2,500 units/ml, 5,000 units/ml, 7,500 units/ml, 10,000 units/ml, 20,000 units/ml
Unit-dose vials: 1,000 units/ml, 2,500 units/ml, 5,000 units/ml, 7,500 units/ml, 10,000 units/ml, 20,000 units/ml
Vials (multidose): 1,000 units/ml, 2,000 units/ml, 2,500 units/ml,

5,000 units/ml, 10,000 units/ml,
20,000 units/ml, 40,000 units/ml
heparin sodium flush
Syringes: 10 units/ml, 100 units/ml
Vials: 10 units/ml, 100 units/ml

INDICATIONS & DOSAGES
➤ **Full-dose continuous I.V. infusion
therapy for deep vein thrombosis
(DVT), MI, pulmonary embolism**
Adults: Initially, 5,000 units by I.V. bolus;
then 20,000 to 40,000 units/day by I.V.
infusion with pump. Titrate hourly rate
based on PTT results (every 4 to 6 hours
in the early stages of treatment).
Children: Initially, 50 units/kg I.V.; then
25 units/kg/hour or 20,000 units/m^2 daily
by I.V. infusion pump. Titrate dosage
based on PTT.
➤ **Full-dose subcutaneous therapy
for DVT, MI, pulmonary embolism**
Adults: Initially, 5,000 units I.V. bolus and
10,000 to 20,000 units in a concentrated
solution subcutaneously; then 8,000 to
10,000 units subcutaneously every 8 hours
or 15,000 to 20,000 units in a concentrated
solution every 12 hours.
➤ **Full-dose intermittent I.V. therapy
for DVT, MI, pulmonary embolism**
Adults: Initially, 10,000 units by I.V.
bolus; then titrated according to PTT, and
5,000 to 10,000 units I.V. every 4 to
6 hours.
Children: Initially, 100 units/kg by I.V.
bolus; then 50 to 100 units/kg every
4 hours.
➤ **Fixed low-dose therapy for prevention of venous thrombosis, pulmonary embolism, embolism associated
with atrial fibrillation, and postoperative DVT**
Adults: 5,000 units subcutaneously every
12 hours. In surgical patients, give first
dose 2 hours before procedure; then
5,000 units subcutaneously every 8 to
12 hours for 5 to 7 days or until patient
can walk.
➤ **Consumptive coagulopathy
(such as disseminated intravascular
coagulation)**
Adults: 50 to 100 units/kg by I.V. bolus
or continuous I.V. infusion every
4 hours.
Children: 25 to 50 units/kg by I.V. bolus
or continuous I.V. infusion every 4 hours.

If no improvement within 4 to 8 hours,
stop heparin.
➤ **Open-heart surgery**
Adults: For total body perfusion, 150 to
400 units/kg continuous I.V. infusion.
➤ **Patency maintenance of I.V. indwelling catheters**
Adults: 10 to 100 units I.V. flush. Use sufficient volume to fill device. Not intended
for therapeutic use.

ADMINISTRATION
I.V.
● Draw blood to establish baseline coagulation parameters before therapy.
● Use an infusion pump to provide maximum safety. Check constant infusions regularly, even when pumps are in good
working order, to ensure correct dosing.
Place notice above patient's bed to caution
I.V. team or laboratory personnel to apply
pressure dressings after taking blood.
● During intermittent infusion, always
draw blood 30 minutes before next
scheduled dose to avoid falsely elevated
PTT. Blood for PTT may be drawn 4 hours
after continuous I.V. heparin therapy
starts. Never draw blood for PTT from
the tubing of the heparin infusion or
from the infused vein, because falsely
elevated PTT will result. Always draw
blood from the opposite arm.
● Don't skip a dose or try to "catch up"
with a solution containing heparin. If solution runs out, restart it as soon as possible,
and reschedule bolus dose immediately.
Monitor PTT.
● Concentrated heparin solutions (more
than 100 units/ml) can irritate blood
vessels.
● Never piggyback other drugs into an
infusion line while heparin infusion is running. Never mix another drug and heparin
in same syringe when giving a bolus.
● **Incompatibilities:** Alteplase; amikacin;
amiodarone; amphotericin B cholesteryl;
ampicillin sodium; atracurium; caspofungin; chlorpromazine; ciprofloxacin;
codeine phosphate; cytarabine; dacarbazine; dantrolene; daunorubicin; dextrose
4.3% in sodium chloride solution 0.18%;
diazepam; diltiazem; dobutamine; doxorubicin; doxycycline hyclate; droperidol;
ergotamine; erythromycin gluceptate or
lactobionate; filgrastim; gentamicin;

Reactions may be *common*, uncommon, *life-threatening*, or COMMON AND LIFE-THREATENING.
Interaction may have a *rapid onset* or **delayed onset.**

haloperidol lactate; hydrocortisone sodium succinate; hydroxyzine hydrochloride; idarubicin; kanamycin; labetalol; levofloxacin; levorphanol; meperidine; methadone; methylprednisolone sodium succinate; morphine sulfate; nesiritide; netilmicin; nicardipine; penicillin G potassium; penicillin G sodium; pentazocine lactate; phenytoin sodium; polymyxin B sulfate; prochlorperazine edisylate; promethazine hydrochloride; quinidine gluconate; reteplase; 1/6 M sodium lactate; solutions containing a phosphate buffer, sodium carbonate, or sodium oxalate; streptomycin; sulfamethoxazole and trimethoprim; tobramycin sulfate; trifluoperazine; triflupromazine; vancomycin; vinblastine; warfarin.

Subcutaneous
● Give low-dose injections sequentially between iliac crests in lower abdomen deep into subcutaneous fat. Inject drug subcutaneously slowly into fat pad.
● Don't massage injection site; watch for signs of bleeding there.
● Alternate sites every 12 hours—right for morning, left for evening. Record location.

ACTION
Accelerates formation of antithrombin III-thrombin complex and deactivates thrombin, preventing conversion of fibrinogen to fibrin.

Route	Onset	Peak	Duration
I.V.	Immediate	Unknown	Variable
Subcut.	20–60 min	2–4 hr	Variable

Half-life: 1 to 2 hours. Half-life is dose-dependent and nonlinear and may be disproportionately prolonged at higher doses.

ADVERSE REACTIONS
CNS: fever.
EENT: rhinitis.
Hematologic: *hemorrhage, overly prolonged clotting time, thrombocytopenia, white clot syndrome.*
Metabolic: *hyperkalemia,* hypoaldosteronism.
Skin: irritation, mild pain, hematoma, ulceration, cutaneous or subcutaneous necrosis, pruritus, urticaria.
Other: hypersensitivity reactions, including chills, *anaphylactoid reactions.*

INTERACTIONS
Drug-drug. *Antihistamines, digoxin, quinine, tetracycline:* May interfere with anticoagulant effect of heparin. Monitor patient for therapeutic effect.
Antiplatelet drugs, salicylates: May increase anticoagulant effect. Use together cautiously. Monitor coagulation studies and patient closely.
Cephalosporins, penicillins: May increase risk of bleeding. Monitor patient closely.
Nitroglycerin: May decrease effects of heparin. Monitor patient closely.
Oral anticoagulants: May increase additive anticoagulation. Monitor PT, INR, and PTT.
Thrombolytics: May increase risk of hemorrhage. Monitor patient closely.
Drug-herb. *Angelica (dong quai), boldo, bromelains, capsicum, chamomile, dandelion, danshen, devil's claw, fenugreek, feverfew, garlic, ginger, ginkgo, ginseng, horse chestnut, licorice, meadowsweet, motherwort, onion, passion flower, red clover, white willow:* May increase risk of bleeding. Discourage herb use.
Drug-lifestyle. *Smoking:* May interfere with anticoagulant effect of heparin. Discourage smoking.

EFFECTS ON LAB TEST RESULTS
● May increase ALT, AST, and potassium levels.
● May increase INR, PT, and PTT. May decrease platelet count.
● Drug may cause false elevations in some tests for thyroxine level.

CONTRAINDICATIONS & CAUTIONS
● Contraindicated in patients hypersensitive to drug. Conditionally contraindicated in patients with active bleeding, blood dyscrasia, or bleeding tendencies, such as hemophilia, thrombocytopenia, or hepatic disease with hypoprothrombinemia; suspected intracranial hemorrhage; suppurative thrombophlebitis; inaccessible ulcerative lesions (especially of GI tract) and open ulcerative wounds; extensive denudation of skin; ascorbic acid deficiency and other conditions that cause increased capillary permeability.
● Conditionally contraindicated during or after brain, eye, or spinal cord surgery; during spinal tap or spinal anesthesia;

during continuous tube drainage of stomach or small intestine; and in sub-acute bacterial endocarditis, shock, advanced renal disease, threatened abortion, or severe hypertension.

• Use cautiously in women during menses or after childbirth and in patients with mild hepatic or renal disease, alcoholism, occupations with high risk of physical injury, or history of allergies, asthma, or GI ulcerations.

NURSING CONSIDERATIONS

• Although heparin use is clearly hazardous in certain conditions, its risks and benefits must be evaluated.

• If a woman needs anticoagulation during pregnancy, most prescribers use heparin.

• *Alert:* Some commercially available heparin injections contain benzyl alcohol. Avoid using these products in neonates and pregnant women if possible.

• Drug requirements are higher in early phases of thrombogenic diseases and febrile states; they are lower when patient's condition stabilizes.

• Elderly patients should usually start at lower dosage.

• Check order and vial carefully; heparin comes in various concentrations.

• *Alert:* USP and international units aren't equivalent for heparin.

• *Alert:* Heparin, low–molecular-weight heparins, and danaparoid aren't inter-changeable.

• *Alert:* Don't change concentrations of infusions unless absolutely necessary. This is a common source of dosage errors.

• *Alert:* There is the potential for delayed onset of heparin-induced thrombocytopenia (HIT), a serious antibody-mediated re-action resulting from irreversible aggre-gation of platelets. HIT may progress to the development of venous and arterial thromboses, a condition referred to as heparin-induced thrombocytopenia and thrombosis (HITT). Thrombotic events may be the initial presentation for HITT, which can occur up to several weeks after stopping heparin therapy. Evaluate patients presenting with thrombocytope-nia or thrombosis after stopping heparin for HIT and HITT

• Draw blood for PTT 4 to 6 hours after dose given subcutaneously.

• Avoid I.M. injections of other drugs to prevent or minimize hematoma.

• Measure PTT carefully and regularly. Anticoagulation is present when PTT values are 1½ to 2 times the control values.

• Monitor platelet count regularly. When new thrombosis accompanies thrombo-cytopenia (white clot syndrome), stop heparin.

• Regularly inspect patient for bleeding gums, bruises on arms or legs, petechiae, nosebleeds, melena, tarry stools, hema-turia, and hematemesis.

• Monitor vital signs.

• *Alert:* To treat severe overdose, use protamine sulfate (1% solution), a heparin antagonist. Dosage is based on the dose of heparin, its route of administration, and the time since it was given. Generally, 1 to 1.5 mg of prota-mine per 100 units of heparin is given if only a few minutes have elapsed; 0.5 to 0.75 mg protamine per 100 units heparin, if 30 to 60 minutes have elapsed; and 0.25 to 0.375 mg prota-mine per 100 units heparin, if 2 hours or more have elapsed. Don't give more than 50 mg protamine in a 10-minute period.

• Abrupt withdrawal may cause increased coagulability; warfarin therapy usually overlaps heparin therapy for continuation of prophylaxis or treatment.

• *Look alike–sound alike:* Don't confuse heparin with Hespan.

• *Look alike–sound alike:* Don't confuse heparin sodium injection 10,000 units/ml and Hep-Lock 10 units/ml.

PATIENT TEACHING

• Instruct patient and family to watch for signs of bleeding or bruising and to notify prescriber immediately if any occur.

• Tell patient to avoid OTC drugs contain-ing aspirin, other salicylates, or drugs that may interact with heparin unless ordered by prescriber.

• Advise patient to consult with prescriber before starting herbal therapy; many herbs have anticoagulant, antiplatelet, or fibri-nolytic properties.

tinzaparin sodium
ten-ZAH-pear-in

Innohep

Pharmacologic class:
low–molecular-weight heparin
Pregnancy risk category B

AVAILABLE FORMS
Injection: 20,000 anti-factor Xa international units/ml in 2-ml multidose vials. Each vial contains 3.1 mg/ml sodium metabisulfite and 10 mg/ml benzyl alcohol.

INDICATIONS & DOSAGES
➤ **Symptomatic deep vein thrombosis with or without pulmonary embolism**
Adults: 175 anti-factor Xa international units/kg of body weight subcutaneously once daily for at least 6 days and until patient is adequately anticoagulated with warfarin sodium (INR of at least 2) for 2 consecutive days. Start warfarin sodium therapy when appropriate, usually within 1 to 3 days of tinzaparin initiation. Volume of dose to be given may be calculated as follows:

$$\text{Patient's weight in kg} \times 0.00875 \text{ ml/kg} = \text{Volume to be given in ml}$$

ADMINISTRATION
Subcutaneous
- Use an appropriate calibrated syringe to ensure correct withdrawal of volume of drug from vials.
- When giving drug, have patient lie or sit down. Give by deep subcutaneous injection into abdominal wall. Introduce whole length of needle into skinfold held between thumb and forefinger. Make sure to hold skinfold throughout injection.
- Alternate injection sites between right and left anterolateral and posterolateral abdominal wall. Record location.
- To minimize bruising, don't rub injection site after administration.

ACTION
Inhibits reactions that lead to blood clotting, including formation of fibrin clots, and helps to inactivate coagulation factor Xa and thrombin. Drug also induces release of tissue factor pathway inhibitor, which may contribute to the antithrombotic effect.

Route	Onset	Peak	Duration
Subcut.	2–3 hr	4–5 hr	18–24 hr

Half-life: 3 to 4 hours.

ADVERSE REACTIONS
CNS: *cerebral or intracranial bleeding,* headache, dizziness, insomnia, confusion, fever, pain.
CV: *arrhythmias, MI, thromboembolism,* chest pain, hypotension, hypertension, tachycardia, dependent edema, angina pectoris.
EENT: epistaxis, ocular hemorrhage.
GI: *GI hemorrhage,* anorectal bleeding, constipation, flatulence, hematemesis, nausea, vomiting, dyspepsia, retroperitoneal or intra-abdominal bleeding, melena.
GU: *vaginal hemorrhage,* dysuria, hematuria, UTI, urine retention.
Hematologic: *granulocytopenia, thrombocytopenia, agranulocytosis, pancytopenia, hemorrhage,* anemia.
Musculoskeletal: back pain, hemarthrosis.
Respiratory: *pulmonary embolism,* pneumonia, respiratory disorder, dyspnea.
Skin: bullous eruption, cellulitis, *injection site hematoma,* pruritus, purpura, rash, skin necrosis, wound hematoma, bullous eruption.
Other: *allergic reaction, fetal death, spinal or epidural hematoma,* hypersensitivity reaction, infection, impaired healing, congenital anomaly, *fetal distress.*

INTERACTIONS
Drug-drug. *Oral anticoagulants, platelet inhibitors (such as dextran, dipyridamole, NSAIDs, salicylates, sulfinpyrazone), thrombolytics:* May increase risk of bleeding. Use together cautiously. If drugs must be given together, monitor patient.
Drug-herb. *Angelica (dong quai), boldo, bromelains, capsicum, chamomile, dandelion, danshen, devil's claw, fenugreek, feverfew, garlic, ginger, ginkgo, ginseng,*

horse chestnut, licorice, meadowsweet, onion, passion flower, red clover, willow: May increase risk of bleeding. Discourage use together.

EFFECTS ON LAB TEST RESULTS
● May increase AST and ALT levels. May decrease hemoglobin level.
● May decrease granulocyte, platelet, RDC, and WDC counts.

CONTRAINDICATIONS & CAUTIONS
● Contraindicated in patients hypersensitive to tinzaparin sodium or other low–molecular-weight heparins, heparin, sulfites, benzyl alcohol, or pork products.
● Contraindicated in patients with active major bleeding and in those with history of heparin-induced thrombocytopenia.
● Use cautiously in patients with increased risk of hemorrhage, such as those with bacterial endocarditis; uncontrolled hypertension; diabetic retinopathy; congenital or acquired bleeding disorders, including hepatic failure and amyloidosis; GI ulceration; or hemorrhagic stroke.
● Use cautiously in patients who have recently undergone brain, spinal, or ophthalmologic surgery, and in those being treated with platelet inhibitors.
● Use drug with care in elderly patients and patients with renal insufficiency, whose elimination of the drug may be reduced.
● Use cautiously in breast-feeding women; it's unknown if drug appears in breast milk.

NURSING CONSIDERATIONS
● Drug isn't intended for I.M. or I.V. administration, nor should it be mixed with other injections or infusions.
● Don't interchange drug (unit to unit) with heparin or other low–molecular-weight heparins.
● Monitor platelet count during therapy. Stop drug if platelet count goes below 100,000/mm^3.
● Periodically monitor CBC count and stool tests for occult blood during treatment.
● Drug may affect PT and INR levels. Patient also receiving warfarin should have blood for PT and INR drawn just before next scheduled dose of tinzaparin.
● Drug contains sodium metabisulfite, which may cause allergic reactions in susceptible people.

■ **Black Box Warning** Patients who receive epidural or spinal anesthesia or spinal puncture are at increased risk of epidural or spinal hematoma, which may result in long-term or permanent paralysis. Monitor these patients closely for neurologic impairment. ■
● If woman becomes pregnant while taking drug, warn her of potential risks to the fetus. Cases of fatal "gasping syndrome" may occur in premature neonates when large amounts of benzyl alcohol are given.
● Store drug at room temperature.

PATIENT TEACHING
● Explain to patient importance of laboratory monitoring to ensure effectiveness of drug while maintaining safety.
● Teach patient warning signs of bleeding and instruct him to report these signs immediately.
● Advise patient to consult with prescriber before starting any herbal therapy; many herbs have anticoagulant, antiplatelet, or fibrinolytic properties.
● Caution patient to use soft toothbrush and electric razor to prevent cuts and bruises.
● Instruct patient that warfarin will be started when appropriate, within 1 to 3 days of therapy. Explain importance of warfarin and the monitoring for safety and effectiveness.

SAFETY ALERT!

warfarin sodium
WAR-far-in

Coumadin⌀, Jantoven

Pharmacologic class: coumarin derivative
Pregnancy risk category X

AVAILABLE FORMS
Powder for injection: 2 mg/ml
Tablets: 1 mg, 2 mg, 2.5 mg, 3 mg, 4 mg, 5 mg, 6 mg, 7.5 mg, 10 mg

INDICATIONS & DOSAGES
➤ **Pulmonary embolism, deep vein thrombosis, MI, rheumatic heart disease with heart valve damage, prosthetic heart valves, chronic atrial fibrillation**

Adults: 2 to 5 mg P.O. or I.V. daily for 2 to 4 days; then dosage based on daily PT and INR. Usual maintenance dosage is 2 to 10 mg P.O. or I.V. daily.

ADMINISTRATION

P.O.

• Draw blood to establish baseline coagulation parameters before therapy. PT and INR determinations are essential for proper control. INR range for chronic atrial fibrillation is usually 2 to 3.
• Give drug at same time daily.

I.V.

• Draw blood to establish baseline coagulation parameters before therapy. PT and INR determinations are essential for proper control. INR range for chronic atrial fibrillation is usually 2 to 3.
• I.V. form may be ordered in rare instances when oral therapy can't be given.
• Reconstitute powder with 2.7 ml sterile water, or as instructed in manufacturer guidelines.
• Give as a slow bolus injection over 1 to 2 minutes into a peripheral vein.
• Because onset of action is delayed, heparin sodium is often given during the first few days of treatment of embolic disease. Blood for PT and INR may be drawn at any time during continuous heparin infusion.
• **Incompatibilities:** Aminophylline, ammonium chloride, bretylium tosylate, ceftazidime, cimetidine, ciprofloxacin, dobutamine, esmolol, gentamicin, heparin sodium, labetalol, lactated Ringer's injection, metronidazole, promazine, Ringer's injection, vancomycin.

ACTION

Inhibits vitamin K–dependent activation of clotting factors II, VII, IX, and X, formed in the liver.

Route	Onset	Peak	Duration
P.O.	Within 24 hr	4 hr	2–5 days
I.V.	Within 24 hr	< 4 hr	2–5 days

Half-life: 20 to 60 hours.

ADVERSE REACTIONS

CNS: *fever,* headache.
GI: *diarrhea,* anorexia, nausea, vomiting, cramps, mouth ulcerations, sore mouth, melena.

GU: enhanced uric acid excretion, hematuria, excessive menstrual bleeding.
Hematologic: *hemorrhage.*
Hepatic: *hepatitis,* jaundice.
Skin: dermatitis, urticaria, necrosis, gangrene, alopecia, *rash.*

INTERACTIONS

Drug-drug. *Acetaminophen:* May increase bleeding with long-term therapy (more than 2 weeks) at high doses (more than 2 g/day) of acetaminophen. Monitor patient very carefully.

Allopurinol, **amiodarone, anabolic steroids,** *anticoagulants (argatroban, bivalirudin), antidepressants,* **azole antifungals,** *aspirin, beta blockers (atenolol, propranolol), cephalosporins, chloramphenicol, cimetidine,* **danazol,** *diazoxide, diflunisal, disulfiram, erythromycin, ethacrynic acid, felbamate,* **fibric acids, fluoxymesterone, fluoroquinolones,** *furosemide, glucagon, heparin, influenza virus vaccine, isoniazid,* **lansoprazole,** *meclofenamate, methimazole, methyldopa, methylphenidate,* **methyltestosterone, metronidazole, nalidixic acid,** *neomycin (oral),* **NSAIDs,** *omeprazole,* **oxandrolone,** *pentoxifylline, propafenone, propoxyphene, propylthiouracil, quinidine,* **salicylates,** *selective COX-2 inhibitors (celecoxib, rofecoxib, valdecoxib), SSRIs,* **sulfinpyrazone,** *sulfamethoxazole and trimethoprim,* **sulfonamides,** *tamoxifen, tetracyclines, thiazides, thrombolytics,* **thyroid drugs,** *ticlopidine, tramadol, vitamin E, valproic acid, zafirlukast:* May increase anticoagulant effect. Monitor patient carefully for bleeding. Reduce anticoagulant dosage as directed.
Anticonvulsants: May increase levels of phenytoin and phenobarbital. Monitor drug levels closely.
Aprepitant, ascorbic acid, **barbiturates,** *bosentan, carbamazepine, clozapine, corticosteroids, corticotropin, cyclosporine, dicloxacillin, ethchlorvynol, griseofulvin, haloperidol, meprobamate, mercaptopurine, nafcillin, oral contraceptives containing estrogen, protease inhibitors (indinavir, ritonavir), raloxifene, ribavirin, rifampin, spironolactone, sucralfate, thiazide diuretics, trazodone, vitamin K:* May decrease PT and INR with reduced anticoagulant effect. Monitor PT and INR

carefully. Increase warfarin dosage, as needed.

Chloral hydrate, cyclophosphamide, HMG-CoA reductase inhibitors, phenytoin, propylthiouracil, ranitidine: May increase or decrease PT and INR. Monitor PT and INR carefully.

Cholestyramine: May decrease response when given too closely together. Give 6 hours after oral anticoagulants.

Sulfonylureas (oral antidiabetics): May increase hypoglycemic response. Monitor glucose levels.

Drug-herb. *Agrimony, anise, arnica flower, asafoetida, bogbean, boldo, bromelain, buchu, capsicum, celery, chamomile, clove, dandelion, danshen, devil's claw, dong quai, fenugreek, feverfew, garlic, ginger,* **ginkgo, ginseng,** *horse chestnut, horseradish, licorice, meadowsweet, motherwort, onion, papain, parsley, passion flower, quassia, red clover, Reishi mushroom, rue, sweet clover, turmeric, white willow:* May increase risk of bleeding. Discourage use together.

Angelica (dong quai): May significantly prolong PT and INR. Discourage use together.

Coenzyme Q10, ginseng, St. John's wort: May reduce action of drug. Ask patient about use of herbal remedies, and advise caution.

Green tea: May decrease anticoagulant effect caused by vitamin K content of green tea. Advise patient to minimize variable consumption of green tea and other foods or nutritional supplements containing vitamin K.

Drug-food. *Foods, multivitamins, and other enteral products containing vitamin K:* May impair anticoagulation. Tell patient to maintain consistent daily intake of foods containing vitamin K.

Cranberry juice: May increase risk of severe bleeding. Discourage use together.

Drug-lifestyle. *Alcohol use:* May enhance anticoagulant effects. Tell patient to avoid large amounts of alcohol.

EFFECTS ON LAB TEST RESULTS
• May increase ALT and AST levels.
• May increase INR, PT, and PTT.
• May falsely decrease theophylline level.

CONTRAINDICATIONS & CAUTIONS
• Contraindicated in patients hypersensitive to drug and in those with bleeding from the GI, GU, or respiratory tract; aneurysm; cerebrovascular hemorrhage; severe or malignant hypertension; severe renal or hepatic disease; subacute bacterial endocarditis, pericarditis, or pericardial effusion; or blood dyscrasias or hemorrhagic tendencies.
• Contraindicated during pregnancy, threatened abortion, eclampsia, or preeclampsia, and after recent surgery involving large open areas, eye, brain, or spinal cord; recent prostatectomy; major regional lumbar block anesthesia, spinal puncture, or diagnostic or therapeutic invasive procedures.
• Avoid using in patients with a history of warfarin-induced necrosis; in unsupervised patients with senility, alcoholism, or psychosis; or in situations in which there are inadequate laboratory facilities for coagulation testing.
• Use cautiously in patients with diverticulitis, colitis, mild or moderate hypertension, or mild or moderate hepatic or renal disease; with drainage tubes in any orifice; with regional or lumbar block anesthesia; with heparin-induced thrombocytopenia and deep venous thrombosis; or in conditions that increase risk of hemorrhage.
• Use cautiously in breast-feeding women.

NURSING CONSIDERATIONS
■ **Black Box Warning** Warfarin can cause major or fatal bleeding, which is more likely to occur during the starting period and with a higher dose. Regularly monitor INR in all patients. Consider more frequent INR monitoring in those at high risk for bleeding. ■
• Avoid all I.M. injections.
• Regularly inspect patient for bleeding gums, bruises on arms or legs, petechiae, nosebleeds, melena, tarry stools, hematuria, and hematemesis.
• Check for unexpected bleeding in breast-fed children of women who take this drug.
• Monitor patient for purple-toes syndrome, characterized by a dark purple or mottled color of the toes; may occur 3 to 10 weeks, or even later after start of therapy.

Reactions may be *common*, uncommon, *life-threatening*, or COMMON AND LIFE-THREATENING.
Interaction may have a *rapid onset* or **delayed onset.**

• *Alert:* Withhold drug and call prescriber at once in the event of fever or rash (signs of severe adverse reactions).

• Effect can be neutralized by oral or parenteral vitamin K.

• Elderly patients and patients with renal or hepatic failure are especially sensitive to drug's effect.

• *Look alike–sound alike:* Don't confuse Coumadin with Arandia, Cordura, or Kemadrin.

PATIENT TEACHING

• Stress importance of complying with prescribed dosage and follow-up appointments. Tell patient to carry a card that identifies his increased risk of bleeding.

■ **Black Box Warning** Tell patient and family to watch for signs of bleeding or abnormal bruising and to call prescriber at once if they occur. ■

• Warn patient to avoid OTC products containing aspirin, other salicylates, or drugs that may interact with warfarin unless ordered by prescriber.

• Advise patient to consult with prescriber before initiating any herbal therapy; many herbs have anticoagulant, antiplatelet, or fibrinolytic properties.

• Tell patient to consult a prescriber before using miconazole vaginal cream or suppositories. Abnormal bleeding and bruising have occurred.

• Instruct woman to notify prescriber if menstruation is heavier than usual; she may need dosage adjustment.

• Tell patient to use electric razor when shaving and to use a soft toothbrush.

• Tell patient to read food labels. Food, nutritional supplements, and multivitamins that contain vitamin K may impair anticoagulation.

• Tell patient to eat a daily, consistent diet of food and drinks containing vitamin K, because eating varied amounts may alter anticoagulant effects.

32

Blood derivatives

albumin 5%
albumin 25%
antihemophilic factor
anti-inhibitor coagulant complex
eculizumab
factor IX complex
factor IX (human)
factor IX (recombinant)
plasma protein fractions
protein C concentrate

---

albumin 5%
al-BYOO-min

Albumarc, Albuminar-5, Albutein
5%, Buminate 5%, Plasbumin-5

albumin 25%
Albuminar-25, Albutein 25%,
Buminate 25%, Plasbumin-25

Pharmacologic class: blood
derivative
Pregnancy risk category C

AVAILABLE FORMS
albumin 5%
Injection: 50 mg/ml in 50-ml, 250-ml,
500-ml, 1,000-ml vials
albumin 25%
Injection: 250 mg/ml in 20-ml, 50-ml,
100-ml vials

INDICATIONS & DOSAGES
➤ **Hypovolemic shock**
Adults: Initially, 500 to 750 ml of 5% solution by I.V. infusion, repeated every
30 minutes, as needed. As plasma volume
approaches normal, rate of infusion of 5%
solution shouldn't exceed 2 to 4 ml/minute.
Or, 100 to 200 ml I.V. of 25% solution,
repeated after 10 to 30 minutes, if needed.
Dosage varies with patient's condition and
response. As plasma volume approaches
normal, rate of infusion of 25% solution
shouldn't exceed 1 ml/minute.
Children: 12 to 20 ml of 5% solution/kg
by I.V. infusion, repeated in 15 to 30 minutes if response is inadequate.

➤ **Burns**
Adults: 25% or 20% solution infused no
faster than 2 to 3 ml/minute to maintain
plasma albumin concentration at approximately 2.5 plus or minus 0.5 g/100 ml with
a plasma oncotic pressure of 20 mm Hg
(equal to a total plasma protein concentration of 5.2 g/100 ml). The duration of therapy is determined by the loss of protein
from burned areas and in the urine.
➤ **Hypoproteinemia**
Adults: 200 to 300 ml of 25% albumin.
Dosage varies with patient's condition and
response. Usual daily dose is 50 to 75 g.
Rate of infusion shouldn't exceed 2 to
3 ml/minute.
Children: Usual daily dosage is 25 g.
➤ **Hyperbilirubinemia**
Infants: 1 g albumin (4 ml of 25%) per kg
1 to 2 hours before exchange transfusion;
or 50 ml of 25% albumin substituted for
50 ml of donor plasma.

ADMINISTRATION
I.V.
• Make sure patient is properly hydrated
before infusion.
• Minimize waste when preparing and
giving drug. This product is expensive,
and supply shortages are common.
• Albumin 5% is infused undiluted; albumin
25% may be infused undiluted or diluted with
normal saline solution or D₅W injection.
• Avoid rapid I.V. infusion in stable patient. Specific rate is based on patient's
age, condition, and diagnosis.
• Don't give more than 250 g in 48 hours.
• Use solution promptly. Discard unused
solution.
• Make sure solution is a clear amber
color. Don't use cloudy or sediment-filled
solutions.
• Follow storage instructions on bottle.
Freezing may cause bottle to break.
• **Incompatibilities:** Midazolam, vancomycin, verapamil hydrochloride.

ACTION
Albumin 5% supplies colloid to the blood
and expands plasma volume. Albumin

Reactions may be *common*, uncommon, *life-threatening*, or COMMON AND LIFE-THREATENING.
Interaction may have a *rapid onset* or *delayed onset*.

25% provides intravascular oncotic pressure in a 5:1 ratio, shifting fluid from interstitial spaces to the circulation and slightly increasing plasma protein level.

Route	Onset	Peak	Duration
I.V.	< 15 min	< 15 min	Several hr

Half-life: 15 to 20 days.

ADVERSE REACTIONS
CNS: headache, fever.
CV: *vascular overload after rapid infusion,* hypotension, tachycardia.
GI: increased salivation, nausea, vomiting.
Musculoskeletal: back pain.
Respiratory: altered respiration, dyspnea, *pulmonary edema.*
Skin: urticaria, rash.
Other: chills.

INTERACTIONS
Drug-drug. *ACE inhibitors:* May increase risk of atypical reactions, such as flushing and hypotension. Withhold ACE inhibitors 24 hours before giving albumin, if possible.

EFFECTS ON LAB TEST RESULTS
• May increase albumin level.

CONTRAINDICATIONS & CAUTIONS
• Contraindicated in patients hypersensitive to drug and in those with severe anemia, pulmonary edema, or cardiac failure.
• Use with extreme caution in patients with hypertension, low cardiac reserve, hypervolemia, pulmonary edema, or hypoalbuminemia with peripheral edema.
• Use cautiously in patients with hepatic or renal failure because of increased protein load.

NURSING CONSIDERATIONS
• **Alert:** Watch for hemorrhage or shock after surgery or injury. Rapid increase in blood pressure may cause bleeding from sites that aren't apparent at lower pressures.
• Monitor vital signs carefully.
• Watch for signs of vascular overload (heart failure or pulmonary edema).
• Monitor fluid intake and output; protein, electrolyte, and hemoglobin levels; and hematocrit during therapy.

PATIENT TEACHING
• Explain use and administration to patient and family.
• Tell patient to report adverse reactions promptly.

antihemophilic factor (AHF, Factor VIII)
an-tye-he-mo-FILL-ik

Advate, Alphanate, Helixate FS, Hemofil M, Hyate:C, Koate-DVI, Kogenate FS, Monarc-M, Monoclate-P, Recombinate, ReFacto, Xyntha

Pharmacologic class: plasma protein
Pregnancy risk category C

AVAILABLE FORMS
Injection: Vials, with diluent; units specified on label

INDICATIONS & DOSAGES
Drug provides hemostasis in factor VIII deficiency, hemophilia A. Specific dosage depends on patient's weight, severity of hemorrhage, and presence of inhibitors. Mild bleeding episodes require a circulating factor VIII level 20% to 40% of normal; moderate to major bleeding episodes and minor surgery, a level 30% to 60% of normal; severe bleeding or major surgery, a level 60% to 100% of normal. The following dosages provide guidelines. Refer to specific brand for actual dosage.
The dose (international units/kg) can be calculated by dividing the desired level (as a percent of normal) by 2. For example, if a peak level of 50% is the goal, divide 50 by 2 to get 25 international units/kg.
➤ **Mild bleeding in patients with hemophilia**
Adults and children: 10 to 20 international units/kg daily.
➤ **Moderate bleeding and minor surgery in patients with hemophilia**
Adults and children: Initially, 15 to 30 international units/kg, then repeat one dose at 12 to 24 hours if needed.
➤ **Severe bleeding and bleeding near vital organs in patients with hemophilia**

Adults and children: Initially, 40 to 50 international units/kg, then 20 to 25 international units/kg every 8 to 12 hours, as needed.

➤ **Major surgery in patients with hemophilia**

Adults and children: 50 international units/kg 1 hour before surgery, then repeat as needed 6 to 12 hours after first dose. Maintain circulating factor levels at 30% to 60% of normal for 10 to 14 days after surgery.

ADMINISTRATION
I.V.
- Refrigerate concentrate until ready to use.
- Warm concentrate and diluent bottles to room temperature before reconstituting.
- Follow manufacturer's instructions for reconstituting.
- To mix drug, gently roll vial between hands. Don't shake.
- Use reconstituted solution within 3 hours.
- Filter solution before giving it.
- Use plastic syringe; drug may bind to glass syringe.
- Take baseline pulse rate before administration.
- Give at 2 ml/minute; may be given up to 10 ml/minute, depending on the preparation being used.
- If pulse rate increases significantly, reduce flow rate or stop administration.
- **Incompatibilities:** Protein precipitants, other I.V. solutions.

ACTION
Directly replaces deficient clotting factor.

Route	Onset	Peak	Duration
I.V.	Immediate	1–2 hr	Unknown

Half-life: 10 to 18 hours.

ADVERSE REACTIONS
CNS: headache, somnolence, lethargy, dizziness, tingling, asthenia, *fever.*
CV: tightness in chest, *thrombosis,* hypotension, tachycardia, angina pectoris.
GI: nausea.
Hematologic: *hemolytic anemia, thrombocytopenia.*
Hepatic: *risk of hepatitis B, risk of hepatitis C.*
Musculoskeletal: myalgias, muscle weakness, joint swelling.

Respiratory: wheezing.
Skin: *urticaria,* stinging at injection site.
Other: *chills,* hypersensitivity reactions, *anaphylaxis, risk of HIV infection.*

INTERACTIONS
None significant.

EFFECTS ON LAB TEST RESULTS
- May decrease hemoglobin level.
- May decrease platelet count.

CONTRAINDICATIONS & CAUTIONS
- For monoclonally prepared drug, contraindicated in patients hypersensitive to drug or murine (mouse) protein.
- For porcine-derived Hyate:C, don't give to patients hypersensitive to pork products.
- Don't use Alphanate in patients with severe von Willebrand's disease (VWD) (type 3) who are undergoing major surgery.
- Use cautiously in neonates, infants, and patients with hepatic disease because of their susceptibility to hepatitis, which may be transmitted in drug.

NURSING CONSIDERATIONS
- Monitor coagulation studies before therapy.
- Monitor patients with blood types A, B, and AB for possible hemolysis.
- Orange or red urine discoloration may signify a hemolytic reaction.
- Determine if patient has received vaccinations for hepatitis A and B before administering drug. Give vaccines if necessary.
- Don't give drug I.M. or subcutaneously.
- Monitor vital signs regularly.
- Monitor coagulation studies and platelets frequently during therapy.
- Monitor patient for allergic reactions.
- Patient may develop inhibitors to factor VIII, resulting in decreased response to drug.
- Risk of hepatitis must be weighed against risk of patient not receiving drug.
- When using Alphanate for surgical prophylaxis in VWD patients, be aware that the ratio of factor VIII to von Willebrand factor:ristocetin cofactor (VWF:Rco) varies by lot; recalculate the dosage when lot selection is changed.
- Because of manufacturing process, risk of HIV, hepatitis, and West Nile virus transmission is extremely low.

Reactions may be *common,* uncommon, *life-threatening,* or COMMON AND LIFE-THREATENING.
Interaction may have a *rapid onset* or **delayed onset.**

PATIENT TEACHING
• Explain use and administration of drug to patient and family.
• Advise patient to report adverse reactions promptly.
• Advise patient to carry medical identification.
• Tell patient to notify prescriber if drug begins to seem less effective; a change may signify the development of antibodies.

---

anti-inhibitor coagulant complex
Feiba VH Immuno

Pharmacologic class: plasma protein
Pregnancy risk category C

AVAILABLE FORMS
Injection: Number of units of factor VIII correctional activity indicated on label of vial

INDICATIONS & DOSAGES
➤ **To prevent or control hemorrhagic episodes in some patients with hemophilia A and B in whom inhibitor antibodies to antihemophilic factor have developed; to manage bleeding in patients with acquired hemophilia who have spontaneously acquired inhibitors to factor VIII, XI and XII**
Adults and children: Drug controls hemorrhage in hemophilia A patients who have a factor VIII inhibitor level above 10 Bethesda units. Patients with a level of 2 to 10 Bethesda units may receive the drug if they have severe hemorrhage or respond poorly to factor VIII infusion.
Adults and children: Dosage is highly individualized and varies among manufacturers. For Feiba VH Immuno, give 50 to 100 units/kg I.V. every 6 or 12 hours until patient shows signs of improvement. Maximum daily dose of Feiba VH Immuno is 200 units/kg.
➤ **Joint hemorrhage**
Adults and children: 50 to 100 units/kg Feiba VH Immuno every 12 hours until patient's condition improves.

➤ **Mucous membrane hemorrhage**
Adults and children: 50 units/kg Feiba VH Immuno every 6 hours, increasing to 100 units/kg every 6 hours if hemorrhage continues. Maximum daily dose, 200 units/kg.
➤ **Soft-tissue hemorrhage**
Adults and children: 100 units/kg Feiba VH Immuno every 12 hours. Maximum daily dose, 200 units/kg.
➤ **Other severe hemorrhage**
Adults and children: 100 units/kg Feiba VH Immuno every 12 hours (occasionally, every 6 hours).

ADMINISTRATION
I.V.
• Dosages of the two available products aren't equivalent.
• Warm drug and diluent to room temperature before reconstitution. Reconstitute according to manufacturer's directions. Give drug as soon as possible.
• Use filter needle provided by manufacturer to withdraw reconstituted solution from vial into syringe; then replace filter needle with a sterile injection needle for administration.
• For infusion, use administration set with filter.
• Individualize rate of administration based on patient's response. Autoplex T infusion may start at 2 ml/minute; if well tolerated, increase gradually to 10 ml/minute. Feiba VH Immuno infusion shouldn't exceed 2 units/kg/minute.
• Complete Feiba VH Immuno infusion within 3 hours.
• If flushing, lethargy, headache, transient chest discomfort, or changes in blood pressure or pulse rate develop because of a rapid infusion, stop drug and notify prescriber. These problems usually disappear when infusion stops. Resume at a slower rate.
• **Incompatibilities:** Other I.V. drugs or solutions.

ACTION
May be related to presence of activated factors, which leads to more complete factor X activation with tissue factor, phospholipid, and ionic calcium to extend the coagulation process beyond stages in which factor VIII is needed.

Route	Onset	Peak	Duration
I.V.	10–30 min	Unknown	Unknown

Half-life: Unknown.

ADVERSE REACTIONS
CNS: headache, lethargy, fever.
CV: changes in blood pressure, flushing, *acute MI, thromboembolic events.*
GI: nausea, vomiting.
Hematologic: *DIC.*
Hepatic: *risk of hepatitis C infection.*
Skin: rash, urticaria.
Other: chills, hypersensitivity reactions, *anaphylaxis, risk of HIV infection.*

INTERACTIONS
Drug-drug. *Antifibrinolytic drugs:* May alter effects of anti-inhibitor coagulant complex. Avoid using together.

EFFECTS ON LAB TEST RESULTS
None reported.

CONTRAINDICATIONS & CAUTIONS
• Contraindicated in patients hypersensitive to drug, in those with DIC or a normal coagulation mechanism, and in those showing signs of fibrinolysis.
• Don't give to patients with severe latex allergies. Some packaging components (vial closures, needle covers, syringe plungers) contain natural latex proteins.
• Feiba VH Immuno is contraindicated in neonates.
• Use cautiously in patients with hepatic disease.
• Use Autoplex T cautiously in neonates.

NURSING CONSIDERATIONS
• Determine if patient has received vaccinations for hepatitis A and B before administering drug. Give vaccines if necessary.
• Keep epinephrine available to treat anaphylaxis. Monitor patient closely for hypersensitivity reactions.
• Monitor vital signs regularly, and report significant changes to prescriber.
• Observe patient closely for signs of thromboembolic events.
• Reassure patient that, because of the manufacturing process, his risk of HIV, hepatitis, or West Nile virus transmission is extremely low.

PATIENT TEACHING
• Explain use and administration of anti-inhibitor coagulant complex to patient and family.
• Tell patient to report adverse reactions promptly.

SAFETY ALERT!

eculizumab
eck-u-LIZ-uh-mob

Soliris

Pharmacologic class: monoclonal IgG antibody
Pregnancy risk category C

AVAILABLE FORMS
Injection: 10 mg/ml in 300-mg single-use vial

INDICATIONS & DOSAGES
■ **Black Box Warning** Meningococcal vaccine is required at least 2 weeks before administration of eculizumab. ■
➤ **Hemolysis in patients with paroxysmal nocturnal hemoglobinuria (PNH)**
Adults: 600 mg I.V. every 7 days for 4 weeks, 900 mg 7 days later, then 900 mg every 14 days thereafter.

ADMINISTRATION
I.V.
• Dilute to a final concentration of 5 mg/ml with 0.9% or 0.45% NaCl, D_5W or Ringer's solution (equal volume of diluent to drug volume).
• Don't give as I.V. push or bolus injection.
• Solution should be clear and at room temperature before giving.
• Discard any unused portion left in vial; solution contains no preservatives.
• Reconstituted solution remains stable for 24 hours refrigerated or at room temperature.
• Infuse over 35 minutes. Don't exceed 2 hours total infusion time if infusion is slowed.
• Monitor the patient for adverse reactions, including anaphylaxis or hypersensitivity during and 1 hour after infusion.
• Store vials in refrigerator and protect from light. Don't freeze or shake.
• **Incompatibilities:** Other drugs.

Reactions may be *common,* uncommon, *life-threatening,* or COMMON AND LIFE-THREATENING.
Interaction may have a *rapid onset* or *delayed onset.*

ACTION

Antibody binds to complement protein C5 to reduce intravascular hemolysis.

Route	Onset	Peak	Duration
I.V.	Immediate	Unknown	Unknown

Half-life: 272 hours.

ADVERSE REACTIONS

CNS: *headache, fatigue,* fever.
EENT: *nasopharyngitis, cough,* sinusitis, respiratory tract infection, influenza-like illness.
GI: *nausea,* constipation.
Musculoskeletal: *back pain,* myalgia, pain in arm or leg.
Hematologic: anemia.
Other: ***meningococcal infection/sepsis,*** herpes simplex infection.

INTERACTIONS

Drug interaction studies haven't been performed.

EFFECTS ON LAB TEST RESULTS

• May decrease LDH level if hemolysis declines.
• May increase RBC count.

CONTRAINDICATIONS & CAUTIONS

• Contraindicated in patient with unresolved serious *Neisseria meningitidis* infection or in patients who aren't vaccinated against *N meningitidis*.
• Use cautiously in patients with any systemic infection.
• Use during pregnancy only if benefits outweigh risks to fetus.
• Use cautiously in breast-feeding woman because drug may appear in breast milk.
• Safety and efficacy in patients younger than age 18 haven't been established.

NURSING CONSIDERATIONS

■ **Black Box Warning** Eculizumab increases the risk of meningococcal infections. Give meningococcal vaccine at least 2 weeks before infusing eculizumab; revaccinate according to guidelines. Monitor patient for early signs of meningococcal infections. Evaluate immediately if infection is suspected and treat with antibiotics if necessary. ■
• Give infusion at recommended intervals.

• Monitor the patient for hemolysis after therapy is stopped. Signs of hemolysis include increased LDH levels greater than pretreatment level; greater than 25% absolute decrease in PNH red blood cell clone size within a week; hemoglobin of less than 5 g/dl or a decrease of more than 4 g/dl in less than 7 days; angina; mental status changes; 50% increase in serum creatinine; or thrombosis.
• Watch for hemolysis for 8 weeks after stopping drug.
• If hemolysis occurs, treatment may include blood transfusion, anticoagulation, corticosteroids, or restarting eculizumab.

PATIENT TEACHING

• Tell patient that meningococcal vaccine is required at least 2 weeks before eculizumab infusion; revaccination may also be required, according to guidelines.
• *Alert:* Advise patient that vaccination won't prevent all meningococcal infection and to report moderate to severe headache accompanied by nausea or vomiting, fever, or stiff neck or back.
• Advise patient to report high fever, fever with rash, confusion, severe muscle aches with flulike symptoms, and sensitivity to light.
• Tell patient he will need periodic blood tests during treatment and continued monitoring for at least 8 weeks after therapy is stopped.
• Advise patient to carry the provided Patient Safety Card at all times and to show the card to any health care provider who treats him.

factor IX complex
Bebulin VH, Profilnine SD, Proplex T

factor IX (human)
AlphaNine SD, Mononine

factor IX (recombinant)
BeneFIX

Pharmacologic class: plasma protein
Pregnancy risk category C

AVAILABLE FORMS

Injection: Vials, with diluent; International units specified on label

INDICATIONS & DOSAGES
➤ **Factor IX deficiency (also called hemophilia B or Christmas disease), anticoagulant overdosage; factor VII deficiency (Proplex T only)**
Adults and children: To calculate international units of factor IX needed, use the following equations:

Human product

$$1 \text{ international unit/kg} \times \text{body weight in kg} \times \text{percentage of desired increase of factor IX level}$$

Recombinant product

$$1.2 \text{ international unit/kg} \times \text{body weight in kg} \times \text{percentage of desired increase of factor IX level}$$

Proplex T

$$0.5 \text{ international unit/kg} \times \text{body weight in kg} \times \text{percentage of desired increase of factor VII level}$$

➤ **Factor IX deficiency, anticoagulant overdosage**
Adults and children: Infusion rates vary with product and patient comfort. Dosage is highly individualized, depending on degree of deficiency, level of factor VII or IX desired, patient weight, and severity of bleeding.

ADMINISTRATION
I.V.
- Warm to room temperature before reconstituting.
- Reconstitute each vial of lyophilized drug with sterile water for injection according to manufacturer's directions.
- Don't shake, refrigerate, or mix with other solutions.
- Use factor IX (human) within 3 hours after reconstitution. Factor IX complex is stable 12 hours after reconstitution, although delivery should start within 3 hours of reconstitution.
- Filter drug before giving.
- The rate of administration varies between each product; infuse slowly at suggested rate of 2 to 3 ml/minute and adapt to patient response.
- Avoid rapid infusion. If tingling sensation, fever, chills, or headache develop, decrease flow rate and notify prescriber.
- Store away from heat.
- **Incompatibilities:** All I.V. drugs and solutions, except normal saline solution.

ACTION
Directly replaces deficient clotting factor.

Route	Onset	Peak	Duration
I.V.	Immediate	10–30 min	Unknown

Half-life: 20 to 25 hours.

ADVERSE REACTIONS
CNS: headache, *transient fever, chills.*
CV: *thromboembolic reactions, MI, pulmonary embolism,* changes in blood pressure, *flushing.*
GI: nausea, vomiting.
Hematologic: *DIC.*
Hepatic: Hepatitis B or C.
Skin: urticaria.
Other: *tingling, anaphylaxis.*

INTERACTIONS
Drug-drug. *Aminocaproic acid:* May increase risk of thrombosis. Avoid using together.

EFFECTS ON LAB TEST RESULTS
None reported.

CONTRAINDICATIONS & CAUTIONS
- Contraindicated in patients hypersensitive to murine (mouse) protein (Mononine) or hamster protein (BeneFIX).
- Use cautiously in neonates and infants because of susceptibility to hepatitis, which may be transmitted with factor.

NURSING CONSIDERATIONS
- Determine if patient has been vaccinated against hepatitis A and B. If necessary, give hepatitis A and B vaccines before giving factor.
- Observe patient for allergic reactions and monitor vital signs regularly.
- Observe patient closely for signs and symptoms of thromboembolic events.
- Risk of hepatitis must be weighed against risk of not receiving drug.

PATIENT TEACHING
- Explain use and administration of factor to patient and family.

Reactions may be *common,* uncommon, *life-threatening,* or COMMON AND LIFE-THREATENING.
Interaction may have a *rapid onset* or **delayed onset.**

• Tell patient to report adverse reactions promptly and to stop using drug if they occur.
• Advise patient to report chest tightness, wheezing, respiratory distress, cough, or low blood pressure.
• Tell patient that risk of HIV, hepatitis, or West Nile virus transmission is extremely low because of manufacturing process.

Route	Onset	Peak	Duration
I.V.	Immediate	Immediate	Unknown

Half-life: Unknown.

plasma protein fractions
Plasmanate, Plasma-Plex, Plasmatein, Protenate

Pharmacologic class: plasma protein
Pregnancy risk category C

AVAILABLE FORMS
Injection: 5% (50 mg/ml) solution in 50-ml, 250-ml, 500-ml vials

INDICATIONS & DOSAGES
➤ **Shock**
Adults: Varies with patient's condition and response, but usual dose is 250 to 500 ml I.V. (12.5 to 25 g protein), usually no faster than 10 ml/minute.
Infants and children: 6.6 to 33 ml/kg (0.33 to 1.65 g/kg of protein) I.V., 5 to 10 ml/minute.

ADMINISTRATION
I.V.
• Check expiration date before using. Don't use solutions that are cloudy, contain sediment, or have been frozen. Discard solutions in containers that have been open for longer than 4 hours because solution contains no preservatives.
• Don't give more than 250 g or 5,000 ml in 48 hours.
• If patient is dehydrated, give additional fluids P.O. or I.V.
• Store at room temperature—no more than 86° F (30° C). Don't freeze.
• **Incompatibilities:** Protein hydrolysates, solutions containing alcohol, norepinephrine bitartrate.

ACTION
Supplies colloid to the blood and expands plasma volume. Primary constituent is albumin.

ADVERSE REACTIONS
CNS: headache, fever.
CV: hypotension, *vascular overload,* tachycardia, flushing.
GI: nausea, vomiting, hypersalivation.
Hepatic: Hepatitis B or C.
Musculoskeletal: back pain.
Respiratory: dyspnea, *pulmonary edema.*
Skin: rash, erythema.
Other: chills.

INTERACTIONS
None significant.

EFFECTS ON LAB TEST RESULTS
None reported.

CONTRAINDICATIONS & CAUTIONS
• Contraindicated in patients with severe anemia or heart failure and in those undergoing cardiac bypass.
• Use cautiously in patients with hepatic or renal failure, low cardiac reserve, or restricted sodium intake.

NURSING CONSIDERATIONS
• Hypotension risk is greater when infusion rate exceeds 10 ml/minute.
• Monitor blood pressure. Be prepared to slow or stop infusion if hypotension suddenly occurs. Vital signs should return to normal gradually; assess them hourly.
• Watch for signs of vascular overload (heart failure or pulmonary edema).
• *Alert:* Watch for hemorrhage or shock after surgery or injury. A rapid increase in blood pressure may cause bleeding that isn't apparent at lower pressures.
• Report decreased urine output.
• Drug contains 130 to 160 mEq of sodium per liter.

PATIENT TEACHING
• Explain use of drug to patient and family.
• Tell patient to report adverse reactions promptly.
• Reassure patient that, because of manufacturing process, risk of HIV, hepatitis, Creutzfeldt-Jacob disease or West Nile virus transmission is extremely low.

protein C concentrate
Ceprotin

Pharmacologic class: protein C
replacement
Pregnancy risk category C

AVAILABLE FORMS
Vials: 500 international units, 1,000 international units

INDICATIONS & DOSAGES
➤ **Venous thrombosis and purpura fulminans in patients with severe congenital protein C deficiency**
Adults, neonates and pediatric patients:
Initially for acute episodes and short-term prophylaxis, 100 to 120 international units/kg IV; then, 60 to 80 international units/kg I.V. every 6 hours for subsequent three doses to maintain peak protein C activity of 100%. Maintenance dose of 45 to 60 international units/kg I.V. every 6 to 12 hours to maintain trough protein C activity levels above 25%.
➤ **Long-term prevention of venous thrombosis and purpura fulminans**
Adults, neonates, and pediatric patients:
45 to 60 international units/kg I.V. every 12 hours to maintain trough protein C activity levels above 25%.
Adjust-a-dose: Dose is adjusted based on severity of protein C deficiency, plasma level of protein C, and the patient's age and condition.

ADMINISTRATION
I.V.
● Refrigerate drug and diluent until ready for use; don't use drug unless a vacuum is present in vial. If no vacuum is present, contact Baxter at 1-888-CEPROTIN (237-7684).
● Reconstitute drug with provided sterile water for injection using double-ended transfer needle; remove transfer needle and gently swirl vial until all powder is dissolved.
● After reconstitution, solution is colorless to slightly yellowish and clear; don't use if discolored, or if particles are visible.
● Use within 3 hours of reconstitution.

● Withdraw contents of vial using a filter needle and then change to a suitable needle or infusion set to give.
● Give I.V. at a maximum rate of 2 ml/minute; in children with body weight of less than 10 kg, injection rate shouldn't exceed 0.2 ml/kg/minute.
● **Incompatibilities:** None.

ACTION
Temporarily increases protein C plasma levels in deficient patients; replacement of protein C in protein C–deficient patients controls or prevents thrombotic complications.

Route	Onset	Peak	Duration
I.V.	Immediate	30 to 60 min	Unknown

Half-life: 9.8 hours.

ADVERSE REACTIONS
CNS: *fever,* light-headedness, restlessness.
CV: *hypotension.*
Hematologic: heparin-induced thrombocytopenia.
Hepatic: Hepatitis B or C.
Metabolic: hyperhidrosis.
Respiratory: *hemothorax.*
Skin: itching, rash.
Other: hypersensitivity reaction.

INTERACTIONS
Drug-drug. *Tissue plasminogen activator:* Use together may increase bleeding risk. Avoid using together.
Oral anticoagulants (vitamin K antagonists): May suppress Protein C activity. Continue protein C replacement until adequate anticoagulation occurs; start with lower dose of oral anticoagulant and adjust incrementally. Monitor patient closely.

EFFECTS ON LAB TEST RESULTS
None reported.

CONTRAINDICATIONS & CAUTIONS
● Use cautiously in patients with allergies to mouse protein or heparin.

NURSING CONSIDERATIONS
● Only prescribers experienced in using coagulation factors or inhibitors should initiate treatment.

Reactions may be *common*, uncommon, *life-threatening*, or COMMON AND LIFE-THREATENING.
Interaction may have a *rapid onset* or *delayed onset.*

• Monitor protein C levels regularly to achieve desired therapeutic effect.

• As a plasma product, this drug may potentially transmit disease; report any signs or symptoms of infection to prescriber and to the Baxter Corporation at 1-866-888-2472.

• Vaccinate patient against hepatitis A and B if he will need repeated courses of protein C replacement.

• Drug contains heparin; monitor patient's platelet count for signs of heparin-induced thrombocytopenia.

• Drug contains up to 200 mg sodium per dose; monitor sodium level in patients with renal impairment or on a low-sodium diet.

• Perform serum coagulation studies and check protein C levels routinely throughout treatment.

PATIENT TEACHING

• Instruct patient to alert prescriber of signs or symptom of infection, bleeding, or hypersensitivity.

• Inform patient on a low-sodium diet that the maximum daily dose contains more than 200 mg of sodium.

• Reassure patient that, because of manufacturing process, risk of HIV, hepatitis, Creutzfeldt-Jacob disease, or West Nile virus transmission is extremely low.

33

Neutropenia drugs

filgrastim
pegfilgrastim
sargramostim

SAFETY ALERT!

filgrastim (G-CSF; granulocyte-colony stimulating factor)
fill-GRASS-tim

Neupogen

Pharmacologic class:
hematopoietic
Pregnancy risk category C

AVAILABLE FORMS
Injection: 300 mcg/ml, 600 mcg/ml

INDICATIONS & DOSAGES
➤ **To decrease risk of infection in patients with nonmyeloid malignant disease receiving myelosuppressive antineoplastics**
Adults and children: 5 mcg/kg daily I.V. (as continuous or intermittent infusion), subcutaneous infusion, or subcutaneously as a single dose given no sooner than 24 hours after cytotoxic chemotherapy. Doses may be increased in increments of 5 mcg/kg for each chemotherapy cycle depending on duration and severity of the nadir of absolute neutrophil count (ANC).

➤ **To decrease risk of infection in patients with nonmyeloid malignant disease receiving myelosuppressive antineoplastics followed by bone marrow transplantation**
Adults and children: 10 mcg/kg daily I.V. infusion of 4 or 24 hours or as continuous 24-hour subcutaneous infusion at least 24 hours after cytotoxic chemotherapy and bone marrow infusion. Adjust subsequent dosages based on neutrophil response.
Adjust-a-dose: For patients with ANC over 1,000/mm³ for 3 consecutive days, reduce dosage to 5 mcg/kg daily; if ANC remains over 1,000/mm³ for 3 more con-

secutive days, stop drug. If ANC decreases to below 1,000/mm³, resume therapy at 5 mcg/kg daily.

➤ **Congenital neutropenia**
Adults: 6 mcg/kg subcutaneously b.i.d. Adjust dosage based on patient response.
Adjust-a-dose: For patients with an ANC persistently above 10,000/mm³, reduce dosage, as directed.

➤ **Idiopathic or cyclic neutropenia**
Adults: 5 mcg/kg subcutaneously daily. Adjust dosage based on patient response.

➤ **Peripheral blood progenitor cell collection and therapy in cancer patients**
Adults: 10 mcg/kg subcutaneously (as bolus or continuous infusion) daily. Give 4 days before leukapheresis and continue until last leukapheresis.
Adjust-a-dose: Patients with WBC count over 100,000/mm³ may need dosage adjustment.

➤ **To reduce the risk of bacterial infection in patients with HIV ◆**
Adults and adolescents: 5 to 10 mcg/kg subcutaneously once daily for 2 to 4 weeks.

ADMINISTRATION
I.V.
• Dilute in 50 to 100 ml of D₅W. Dilution to less than 5 mcg/ml isn't recommended.
• Don't dilute with normal saline solution.
• If drug yield is 5 to 15 mcg/ml, add albumin at 2 mg/ml (0.2%) to minimize binding of drug to plastic containers or tubing.
• Give by intermittent infusion over 15 to 60 minutes or by continuous infusion over 24 hours.
• **Incompatibilities:** Amphotericin B, cefepime, cefonicid, cefotaxime, cefoxitin, ceftizoxime, ceftriaxone, cefuroxime, clindamycin, dactinomycin, etoposide, fluorouracil, furosemide, heparin sodium, mannitol, methylprednisolone sodium succinate, metronidazole, mitomycin, piperacillin, prochlorperazine edisylate, sodium solutions, thiotepa.
Subcutaneous
• Rotate administration sites and record.

Reactions may be *common*, uncommon, *life-threatening*, or COMMON AND LIFE-THREATENING.
Interaction may have a *rapid onset* or *delayed onset*.

ACTION
Binds cell receptors to stimulate proliferation, differentiation, commitment, and end-cell function of neutrophils.

Route	Onset	Peak	Duration
I.V.	5–60 min	24 hr	1–7 days
Subcut.	5–60 min	2–8 hr	1–7 days

Half-life: 3½ hours.

ADVERSE REACTIONS
CNS: *fever,* headache, weakness, *fatigue.*
CV: *MI, arrhythmias,* chest pain, hypotension.
GI: *nausea, vomiting, diarrhea, mucositis,* stomatitis, constipation.
Hematologic: *thrombocytopenia,* leukocytosis, NEUTROPENIC FEVER.
Metabolic: hyperuricemia.
Musculoskeletal: *bone pain.*
Respiratory: dyspnea, cough.
Skin: *alopecia,* rash, cutaneous vasculitis.
Other: hypersensitivity reactions.

INTERACTIONS
Drug-drug. *Chemotherapeutic drugs:* Rapidly dividing myeloid cells may be sensitive to cytotoxic drugs. Don't use within 24 hours before or after a dose of one of these drugs.
Lithium: May potentiate release of neutrophils, causing a greater increase in WBC count than expected. Use together cautiously.

EFFECTS ON LAB TEST RESULTS
• May increase alkaline phosphatase, creatinine, LDH, and uric acid levels.
• May increase WBC count. May decrease platelet count.

CONTRAINDICATIONS & CAUTIONS
• Contraindicated in patients hypersensitive to drug or its components or to proteins derived from *Escherichia coli.*
• Use cautiously in breast-feeding women.

NURSING CONSIDERATIONS
• Obtain baseline CBC and platelet count before therapy.
• Once a dose is withdrawn, don't reuse vial. Discard unused portion. Vials are for single-dose use and contain no preservatives.

• Obtain CBC and platelet count two to three times weekly during therapy. Patients who receive drug also may receive high doses of chemotherapy, which may increase risk of toxicities.
• A transiently increased neutrophil count is common 1 or 2 days after therapy starts. Give daily for up to 2 weeks or until ANC has returned to 10,000/mm³ after the expected chemotherapy-induced neutrophil nadir.
• *Look alike–sound alike:* Don't confuse Neupogen with Epogen or Neumega.

PATIENT TEACHING
• If patient will give drug, teach him how to do so and how to dispose of used needles, syringes, drug containers, and unused medicine.
• *Alert:* Rarely, splenic rupture may occur. Advise patient to immediately report upper left abdominal or shoulder tip pain.
• Instruct patient to report persistent or serious adverse reactions promptly.

SAFETY ALERT!

pegfilgrastim
peg-fill-GRASS-tim

Neulasta

Pharmacologic class: hematopoietic
Pregnancy risk category C

AVAILABLE FORMS
Injection: 6-mg/0.6-ml single-use, preservative-free, prefilled syringes

INDICATIONS & DOSAGES
➤ **To reduce frequency of infection in patients with nonmyeloid malignancies receiving myelosuppressive chemotherapy that may cause febrile neutropenia**
Adults: 6 mg subcutaneously once per chemotherapy cycle. Don't give in period between 14 days before and 24 hours after administration of cytotoxic chemotherapy.

ADMINISTRATION
Subcutaneous
• Let drug come to room temperature before giving.

- Don't shake.
- Don't use if discoloration or particulate matter is seen.
- Discard drug if left at room temperature for more than 48 hours.

ACTION
Binds cell receptors to stimulate proliferation, differentiation, commitment, and end-cell function of neutrophils.

Route	Onset	Peak	Duration
Subcut.	Unknown	Unknown	Unknown

Half-life: 15 to 80 hours.

ADVERSE REACTIONS
CNS: *dizziness, fatigue, fever, headache, insomnia.*
GI: *abdominal pain, anorexia, constipation, diarrhea, dyspepsia, mucositis, nausea, stomatitis, taste perversion, vomiting.*
Hematologic: GRANULOCYTOPENIA, NEUTROPENIC FEVER.
Musculoskeletal: *arthralgia, bone pain, generalized weakness, myalgia, skeletal pain.*
Respiratory: *acute respiratory distress syndrome (ARDS).*
Skin: *alopecia.*
Other: *splenic rupture, peripheral edema.*

INTERACTIONS
Drug-drug. *Lithium:* May increase the release of neutrophils. Monitor neutrophil counts closely.

EFFECTS ON LAB TEST RESULTS
- May increase LDH, alkaline phosphatase, and uric acid levels.
- May decrease granulocyte count.

CONTRAINDICATIONS & CAUTIONS
- Contraindicated in patients hypersensitive to *Escherichia coli*–derived proteins, filgrastim, or any component of the drug. Don't use for peripheral blood progenitor cell mobilization.
- Use cautiously in patients with sickle cell disease, those receiving chemotherapy causing delayed myelosuppression, or those receiving radiation therapy.
- Infants, children, and adolescents who weigh less than 45 kg (99 lb) shouldn't receive the 6-mg single-use syringe dose. Safety and efficacy in children haven't been established.

NURSING CONSIDERATIONS
- *Alert:* Splenic rupture may occur rarely. Assess patient who experiences signs or symptoms of left upper abdominal or shoulder pain for an enlarged spleen or splenic rupture.
- Obtain CBC and platelet count before therapy.
- Monitor patient's hemoglobin level, hematocrit, CBC, and platelet count, as well as LDH, alkaline phosphatase, and uric acid levels during therapy.
- Monitor patient for allergic-type reactions, including anaphylaxis, skin rash, and urticaria, which can occur with first or subsequent treatment.
- Evaluate patient with fever, lung infiltrates, or respiratory distress for ARDS. Notify prescriber if respiratory status worsens.
- Keep patient with sickle cell disease well hydrated, and monitor him for symptoms of sickle cell crisis.
- Pegfilgrastim may act as a growth factor for tumors.
- *Look alike–sound alike:* Don't confuse Neulasta with Neumega.

PATIENT TEACHING
- Inform patient of the potential side effects of the drug.
- Tell patient to report signs and symptoms of allergic reactions, fever, or breathing problems.
- *Alert:* Rarely, splenic rupture may occur. Advise patient to immediately report upper left abdominal or shoulder tip pain.
- Tell patient with sickle cell disease to keep drinking fluids and report signs or symptoms of sickle cell crisis.
- Instruct patient or caregiver how to give drug if it's to be given at home.

Reactions may be *common*, uncommon, *life-threatening*, or COMMON AND LIFE-THREATENING.
Interaction may have a *rapid* onset or *delayed* onset.

SAFETY ALERT!

sargramostim (GM-CSF; granulocyte-macrophage colony-stimulating factor)
sar-GRAM-oh-stim

Leukine, Leukine Liquid*

Pharmacologic class:
hematopoietic
Pregnancy risk category C

AVAILABLE FORMS
Powder for injection: 250 mcg
Solution for injection: 500 mcg/ml*

INDICATIONS & DOSAGES
➤ **To accelerate hematopoietic reconstitution after autologous or allogenic bone marrow transplantation in patients with malignant lymphoma or acute lymphoblastic leukemia or in patients with Hodgkin lymphoma**
Adults: 250 mcg/m² daily given as 2-hour I.V. infusion beginning 2 to 4 hours after bone marrow transplantation. Continue until absolute neutrophil count (ANC) is more than 1,500/mm³ for 3 consecutive days.
➤ **Neutrophil recovery following chemotherapy in acute myelogenous leukemia**
Adults age 55 and older: Initially, 250 mcg/m² I.V. once daily over 4 hours beginning day 11 or 4 days following completion of induction therapy; initiate only if bone marrow is hypoplastic with less than 5% blasts on day 10. If a second induction cycle is needed, begin sargramostim 4 days after completing chemotherapy and only if bone marrow is hypoplastic with less than 5% blasts. Continue until the ANC is more than 1,500/mm³ for 3 consecutive days or for a maximum of 42 days.
➤ **Mobilization of peripheral blood progenitor cells (PBPC)**
Adults: 250 mcg/m² by continuous I.V. infusion over 24 hours or by subcutaneous injection once daily. Continue through PBPC collection.

➤ **Post-PBPC transplantation**
Adults: 250 mcg/m² by continuous I.V. infusion over 24 hours or by subcutaneous injection once daily beginning immediately following PBPC infusion; continue until ANC is more than 1,500/mm³ for 3 consecutive days.
➤ **Bone marrow transplantation failure or engraftment delay**
Adults: 250 mcg/m² as a 2-hour I.V. infusion daily for 14 days. This course of therapy may be repeated after 7 days of no therapy. If engraftment still hasn't occurred, a third course of 500 mcg/m² daily I.V. for 14 days may be attempted after another therapy-free 7 days.
Adjust-a-dose: Stimulation of marrow precursors may result in rapid rise of WBC count. If blast cells appear or increase to 10% or more of WBC count or if the underlying disease progresses, stop therapy. If ANC is above 20,000/mm³ or if platelet count is above 500,000/mm³, temporarily stop drug or reduce dose by 50%.

ADMINISTRATION
I.V.
● Reconstitute with 1 ml of sterile or bacteriostatic water for injection. Direct stream of sterile water against side of vial and gently swirl contents to minimize foaming. Avoid excessive or vigorous agitation or shaking.
● Dilute in normal saline solution. If drug yield is below 10 mcg/ml, add human albumin at final concentration of 0.1% to saline solution before adding sargramostim to prevent adsorption to components of the delivery system. To yield 0.1% human albumin, add 1 mg human albumin to each milliliter of saline solution (dilute 1 ml of 5% human albumin in 50 ml of saline solution).
● Don't use in-line filter.
● Give as soon as possible after mixing and no later than 6 hours after reconstituting.
● **Incompatibilities:** Other I.V. drugs, unless specific compatibility data are available.
Subcutaneous
● Further dilution of injection or reconstituted solution isn't needed.

ACTION
Induces cellular responses by binding to specific receptors on surfaces of target cells.

Route	Onset	Peak	Duration
I.V.	15 min	1–3 hr	Unknown
Subcut.	15 min	2–4 hr	Unknown

Half-life: About 1 hour (I.V.); about 3 hours (Subcut.).

ADVERSE REACTIONS
CNS: *asthenia, CNS disorders, fever, headache, malaise.*
CV: HEMORRHAGE, *edema, peripheral edema, hypertension,* **supraventricular arrhythmias,** *pericardial effusion.*
GI: *anorexia, diarrhea, GI disorders, nausea, stomatitis, vomiting,* **GI hemorrhage.**
GU: *urinary tract disorder,* abnormal kidney function.
Hematologic: *blood dyscrasias.*
Hepatic: *liver damage.*
Musculoskeletal: *arthralgias.*
Respiratory: *dyspnea, lung disorders, pleural effusion.*
Skin: *alopecia, pruritus, rash.*
Other: SEPSIS, *mucous membrane disorder.*

INTERACTIONS
Drug-drug. *Corticosteroids, lithium:*
May increase myeloproliferative effects of sargramostim. Use cautiously together.

EFFECTS ON LAB TEST RESULTS
● May increase BUN, creatinine, AST, ALT, alkaline phosphatase, bilirubin, glucose, and cholesterol levels. May decrease calcium and albumin levels.

CONTRAINDICATIONS & CAUTIONS
● Contraindicated in patients hypersensitive to drug or its components or to yeast-derived products and in those with excessive leukemic myeloid blasts in bone marrow or peripheral blood.
● Giving within 24 hours of chemotherapy or radiation is contraindicated.
● Use cautiously in patients with cardiac disease, hypoxia, fluid retention, pulmonary infiltrates, heart failure, or impaired renal or hepatic function because these conditions may be worsened.

● Safety and efficacy haven't been established in children.

NURSING CONSIDERATIONS
● If severe adverse reactions occur, reduce dose by 50% or temporarily stop drug and notify prescriber. Resume therapy when reactions decrease. Transient rash and local reactions at injection site may occur.
● Solution for injection contains benzyl alcohol, which has been associated with fatal "gasping syndrome" in neonates. Don't administer to neonates.
● Rapidly dividing progenitor cells may be sensitive to cytotoxic therapies, making the drug ineffective; don't give within 24 hours of last dose of chemotherapy or within 12 hours of last dose of radiotherapy.
● Monitor CBC with differential, including examination for presence of blast cells, biweekly.
● Drug accelerates myeloid recovery in patients receiving bone marrow that is either unpurged or purged by anti-B cell monoclonal antibodies more than in those who receive bone marrow that is chemically purged.
● Drug may produce a limited response in transplant patients who have received extensive radiotherapy or who have received other myelotoxic drugs.
● Drug can act as a growth factor for any tumor type, particularly myeloid malignant disease.

PATIENT TEACHING
● Review administration schedule with patient and caregivers, and address their concerns.
● Urge patient to report adverse reactions promptly.

Reactions may be *common,* uncommon, *life-threatening,* or COMMON AND LIFE-THREATENING.
Interaction may have a *rapid onset* or **delayed onset.**

Platelet drugs

abciximab
cilostazol
clopidogrel bisulfate
dipyridamole
eptifibatide
oprelvekin
ticlopidine hydrochloride
tirofiban hydrochloride

---

abciximab
ab-SIX-ah-mab

ReoPro

Pharmacologic class: antiplatelet aggregator
Pregnancy risk category C

AVAILABLE FORMS
Injection: 2 mg/ml

INDICATIONS & DOSAGES
➤ **Adjunct to percutaneous coronary intervention (PCI) to prevent acute cardiac ischemic complications**
Adults: 0.25 mg/kg as an I.V. bolus given 10 to 60 minutes before start of PCI; then, a continuous I.V. infusion of 0.125 mcg/ kg/minute to maximum 10 mcg/minute for 12 hours.
➤ **Unstable angina not responding to conventional medical therapy in patients scheduled for PCI within 24 hours**
Adults: 0.25 mg/kg as an I.V. bolus; then an 18- to 24-hour infusion of 10 mcg/ minute concluding 1 hour after PCI.

ADMINISTRATION
I.V.
● Give drug in a separate I.V. line. Don't add other drugs to infusion solution.
● Inspect solution for particulate matter before administration. If opaque particles are visible, discard solution and obtain new vial.
● For bolus, withdraw needed amount of drug through a low–protein-binding 0.2- or 5-micron syringe filter.

● Give bolus 10 to 60 minutes before procedure.
● For continuous infusion, filter drug either by withdrawing needed amount of drug through a low–protein-binding 0.2- or 5-micron syringe filter into a syringe or by infusing with a continuous infusion set equipped with a low–protein-binding 0.2 or 0.22-micron in-line filter. Use normal saline solution or D_5W.
● Infuse at 0.125 mcg/kg/minute (maximum, 10 mcg/minute) for 12 hours via a continuous infusion pump.
● Discard unused portion after 12-hour infusion.
● **Incompatibilities:** None reported.

ACTION
Binds to the glycoprotein IIb/IIIa (GPIIb/IIIa) receptor of human platelets and inhibits platelet aggregation.

Route	Onset	Peak	Duration
I.V.	Immediate	Immediate	48 hr

Half-life: 10 to 30 minutes.

ADVERSE REACTIONS
CNS: confusion, headache, hyperesthesia, hypoesthesia, pain.
CV: *hypotension, bradycardia, chest pain,* peripheral edema.
EENT: abnormal vision.
GI: *nausea,* abdominal pain, vomiting.
Hematologic: *bleeding, thrombocytope- nia,* anemia, leukocytosis.
Musculoskeletal: *back pain.*
Respiratory: pleural effusion, pleurisy, pneumonia.

INTERACTIONS
Drug-drug. *Antiplatelet drugs, dipyrid- amole, heparin, NSAIDs, other anticoagu- lants, thrombolytics, ticlopidine:* May increase risk of bleeding. Monitor patient closely.

EFFECTS ON LAB TEST RESULTS
● May decrease hemoglobin level.

• May increase WBC count. May decrease platelet count.

CONTRAINDICATIONS & CAUTIONS
• Contraindicated in patients hypersensitive to drug, its ingredients, or murine proteins.
• Contraindicated in those with active internal bleeding, significant GI or GU bleeding within 6 weeks, stroke within past 2 years, or significant residual neurologic deficit, bleeding diathesis, thrombocytopenia (platelet count lower than 100,000/mm³), major surgery or trauma within 6 weeks, intracranial neoplasm, intracranial arteriovenous malformation, intracranial aneurysm, severe uncontrolled hypertension, or history of vasculitis.
• Contraindicated when oral anticoagulants have been given within past 7 days unless PT is 1.2 times control or less, or when I.V. dextran is used before or during PCI.
• Use with caution in patients at increased risk for bleeding, including those who weigh less than 75 kg (165 lb) or who are older than age 65, those who have a history of GI disease, and those who are receiving thrombolytics. Conditions that increase patient's risk of bleeding include PCI within 12 hours of onset of symptoms for acute MI, prolonged PCI (lasting longer than 70 minutes), or failed PCI. Heparin use may also increase the risk of bleeding.

NURSING CONSIDERATIONS
• The risk of bleeding is reduced by using low-dose, weight-adjusted heparin, early sheath removal, and careful maintenance of access site immobility.
• Drug is intended for use with aspirin and heparin; review and monitor other drugs patient is taking.
• **Alert:** Keep epinephrine, dopamine, theophylline, antihistamines, and corticosteroids readily available in case of anaphylaxis.
• Monitor patient closely for bleeding at the arterial access site used for cardiac catheterization and internal bleeding involving the GI or GU tract or retroperitoneal sites.

• Institute bleeding precautions. Keep patient on bed rest for 6 to 8 hours after sheath removal or end of drug infusion, whichever is later. Minimize arterial and venous punctures, I.M. injections, urinary catheters, nasogastric tubes, automatic blood pressure cuffs, and nasotracheal intubation; avoid, if possible.
• During infusion, remove sheath only after heparin has been stopped and its effects largely reversed.
• Before treatment, obtain platelet count, PT, ACT, and activated PTT.
• Monitor platelet count closely. Obtain levels 2 to 4 hours after bolus dose, and 24 hours after bolus dose or before discharge, whichever is first.
• Anticipate stopping drug and giving platelets for severe bleeding or thrombocytopenia.
• **Look alike–sound alike:** Don't confuse abciximab with infliximab.

PATIENT TEACHING
• Explain use and administration of drug to patient and family.
• Instruct patient to report adverse reactions immediately.

---

cilostazol
sill-AHS-tah-zoll

Pletal

Pharmacologic class: quinolone phosphodiesterase inhibitor
Pregnancy risk category C

AVAILABLE FORMS
Tablets: 50 mg, 100 mg

INDICATIONS & DOSAGES
➤ **To reduce symptoms of intermittent claudication**
Adults: 100 mg P.O. b.i.d., at least 30 minutes before or 2 hours after breakfast and dinner.
Adjust-a-dose: Decrease dose to 50 mg P.O. b.i.d. when giving with drugs that may interact to cause an increase in cilostazol level.

ADMINISTRATION
P.O.
- Give drug at least 30 minutes before or 2 hours after breakfast and dinner.
- Don't give drug with grapefruit juice.

ACTION
Thought to inhibit the enzyme phosphodiesterase III, thus inhibiting platelet aggregation and causing vasodilation.

Route	Onset	Peak	Duration
P.O.	Unknown	2–4 hr	Unknown

Half-life: 11 to 13 hours.

ADVERSE REACTIONS
CNS: *dizziness, headache,* vertigo.
CV: *palpitations,* peripheral edema, tachycardia.
EENT: *pharyngitis, rhinitis.*
GI: *abnormal stools, diarrhea,* abdominal pain, dyspepsia, flatulence, nausea.
Musculoskeletal: back pain, myalgia.
Respiratory: increased cough.
Other: *infection,* bleeding.

INTERACTIONS
Drug-drug. *Diltiazem:* May increase cilostazol level. Reduce cilostazol dosage to 50 mg b.i.d.
Erythromycin, other macrolides: May increase level of cilostazol and its metabolites. Reduce cilostazol dosage to 50 mg b.i.d.
Omeprazole: May increase level of cilostazol metabolite. Reduce cilostazol dosage to 50 mg b.i.d.
Strong inhibitors of CYP3A4 (such as fluconazole, fluoxetine, fluvoxamine, itraconazole, ketoconazole, miconazole, nefazodone, sertraline): May increase level of cilostazol and its metabolites. Reduce cilostazol dosage to 50 mg b.i.d.
Drug-food. *Grapefruit juice:* May increase drug level. Discourage use together.
Drug-lifestyle. *Smoking:* May decrease drug exposure. Discourage smoking.

EFFECTS ON LAB TEST RESULTS
- May reduce triglyceride levels. May increase HDL level.

CONTRAINDICATIONS & CAUTIONS
- Contraindicated in patients hypersensitive to drug or its components.
- ■ **Black Box Warning** Contraindicated in patients with heart failure of any severity. ■
- Contraindicated in patients with hemostatic disorders or active bleeding, such as bleeding peptic ulcer and intracranial bleeding.
- Use cautiously in patients with severe underlying heart disease; also use cautiously with other drugs having antiplatelet activity.
- Use cautiously in patients with severe renal impairment (creatinine clearance less than 25 ml/minute) and in those with moderate to severe hepatic impairment.

NURSING CONSIDERATIONS
- Beneficial effects may not be seen for up to 12 weeks after therapy starts.
- *Alert:* Cilostazol and similar drugs that inhibit the enzyme phosphodiesterase decrease the likelihood of survival in patients with class III and IV heart failure.
- *Alert:* CV risk is unknown in patients who use drug on long-term basis and in those with severe underlying heart disease.
- Dosage can be reduced or stopped without such rebound effects as platelet hyperaggregation.

PATIENT TEACHING
- Instruct patient to take drug on an empty stomach, at least 30 minutes before or 2 hours after breakfast and dinner.
- Tell patient that beneficial effect of drug on cramping pain isn't likely to be noticed for 2 to 4 weeks and that it may take as long as 12 weeks.
- Advise patient to avoid drinking grapefruit juice during drug therapy.
- Inform patient that CV risk is unknown in patients who use drug on a long-term basis and in those with severe underlying heart disease.
- Tell patient that drug may cause dizziness. Caution patient not to drive or perform other activities that require alertness until response to drug is known.

clopidogrel bisulfate
cloe-PID-oh-grel

Plavix

Pharmacologic class: inhibitor of adenosine diphosphate-induced platelet aggregation
Pregnancy risk category B

AVAILABLE FORMS
Tablets: 75 mg, 300 mg

INDICATIONS & DOSAGES
➤ **To reduce thrombotic events in patients with atherosclerosis documented by recent stroke, MI, or peripheral arterial disease**
Adults: 75 mg P.O. daily.
➤ **To reduce thrombotic events in patients with acute coronary syndrome (unstable angina and non–Q-wave MI), including those receiving drugs and those having percutaneous coronary intervention (with or without stent) or coronary artery bypass graft**
Adults: Initially, a single 300-mg P.O. loading dose; then 75 mg P.O. once daily. Start and continue aspirin (75 to 325 mg once daily) with clopidogrel.
➤ **ST-segment elevation acute MI**
Adults: 75 mg P.O. once daily, with aspirin, with or without thrombolytics. A 300-mg loading dose is optional.

ADMINISTRATION
P.O.
• Give drug without regard to meals.

ACTION
Inhibits the binding of adenosine diphosphate (ADP) to its platelet receptor, impeding ADP-mediated activation and subsequent platelet aggregation, and irreversibly modifies the platelet ADP receptor.

Route	Onset	Peak	Duration
P.O.	2 hr	Unknown	5 days

Half-life: 8 hours.

ADVERSE REACTIONS
CNS: depression, dizziness, fatigue, headache, pain.
CV: edema, hypertension.
EENT: epistaxis, rhinitis.
GI: *hemorrhage,* abdominal pain, constipation, diarrhea, dyspepsia, gastritis, ulcers.
GU: UTI.
Hematologic: purpura.
Musculoskeletal: arthralgia.
Respiratory: bronchitis, coughing, dyspnea, upper respiratory tract infection.
Skin: *rash,* pruritus.
Other: flulike syndrome.

INTERACTIONS
Drug-drug. *Aspirin, NSAIDs:* May increase risk of GI bleeding. Monitor patient.
Warfarin: May increase risk of bleeding. Use together cautiously.
Salicylates: May increase the risk of serious bleeding in patients with TIA or ischemic stroke. Avoid use together.
Drug-herb. *Red clover:* May increase risk of bleeding. Discourage use together.

EFFECTS ON LAB TEST RESULTS
• May decrease platelet count.

CONTRAINDICATIONS & CAUTIONS
• Contraindicated in patients hypersensitive to drug or its components and in those with pathologic bleeding (such as peptic ulcer or intracranial hemorrhage).
• Use cautiously in patients at risk for increased bleeding from trauma, surgery, or other pathologic conditions and in those with renal or hepatic impairment.

NURSING CONSIDERATIONS
• Platelet aggregation won't return to normal for at least 5 days after drug has been stopped.
• *Alert:* Drug may cause fatal thrombotic thrombocytopenic purpura (thrombocytopenia, hemolytic anemia, neurologic findings, renal dysfunction, and fever) that requires urgent treatment, including plasmapheresis.
• *Look alike–sound alike:* Don't confuse Plavix with Paxil.

Reactions may be *common*, uncommon, *life-threatening*, or COMMON AND LIFE-THREATENING.
Interaction may have a *rapid onset* or *delayed onset*.

PATIENT TEACHING
• Advise patient it may take longer than usual to stop bleeding. Tell him to refrain from activities in which trauma and bleeding may occur, and encourage him to wear a seat belt when in a car.
• Instruct patient to notify prescriber if unusual bleeding or bruising occurs.
• Tell patient to inform all health care providers, including dentists, before undergoing procedures or starting new drug therapy, that he is taking drug.
• Inform patient that drug may be taken without regard to meals.

---

dipyridamole
dye-peer-IH-duh-mohl

Persantine

Pharmacologic class: pyrimidine analogue
Pregnancy risk category B

AVAILABLE FORMS
Injection: 5 mg/ml in 2- and 10-ml vials
Tablets: 25 mg, 50 mg, 75 mg

INDICATIONS & DOSAGES
➤ **To inhibit platelet adhesion in prosthetic heart valves (given together with warfarin)**
Adults: 75 to 100 mg P.O. q.i.d.
➤ **Alternative to exercise in evaluation of coronary artery disease during thallium myocardial perfusion scintigraphy**
Adults: 0.57 mg/kg as an I.V. infusion at a constant rate over 4 minutes (0.142 mg/kg/minute).

ADMINISTRATION
P.O.
• If GI distress develops, give drug 1 hour before meals or with meals.
I.V.
• For use as a diagnostic drug, dilute in half-normal or normal saline solution or D_5W in at least a 1:2 ratio for a total volume of 20 to 50 ml.
• Inject thallium-201 within 5 minutes after completing the 4-minute dipyridamole infusion.

• Don't mix in same syringe or infusion container with other drugs.
• **Incompatibilities:** Other drugs.

ACTION
May involve drug's ability to increase adenosine, which is a coronary vasodilator and platelet aggregation inhibitor.

Route	Onset	Peak	Duration
P.O.	Unknown	75 min	Unknown
I.V.	Unknown	2 min	Unknown

Half-life: 1 to 12 hours.

ADVERSE REACTIONS
CNS: *dizziness, headache,* paresthesia, syncope.
CV: *angina pectoris, chest pain,* **ECG abnormalities,** blood pressure lability, flushing, hypertension, hypotension.
GI: *nausea,* abdominal distress, diarrhea, vomiting.
Other: pain.

INTERACTIONS
Drug-drug. *Adenosine:* May increase levels and cardiac effects of adenosine. Adjust adenosine dose as needed.
Cholinesterase inhibitors: May counteract anticholinesterase effects and aggravate myasthenia gravis. Monitor patient.
Heparin: May increase risk of bleeding. Monitor patient closely.
Theophylline: May prevent coronary vasodilation by I.V. dipyridamole, causing a false-negative thallium-imaging result. Avoid using together.

EFFECTS ON LAB TEST RESULTS
• May increase liver enzyme levels.

CONTRAINDICATIONS & CAUTIONS
• Contraindicated in patients hypersensitive to drug.
• Use cautiously in patients with hypotension and those with severe coronary artery disease.

NURSING CONSIDERATIONS
• Observe for adverse reactions, especially with large doses. Monitor blood pressure.

• Observe for signs and symptoms of bleeding; note prolonged bleeding time (especially with large doses or long-term therapy).
• The value of drug as part of an anti-thrombotic regimen is controversial; its use may not provide significantly better results than aspirin alone.
• Dipyridamole injection may contain tartrazine, which may cause allergic reactions in some patients.
• *Look alike–sound alike:* Don't confuse dipyridamole with disopyramide. Don't confuse Persantine with Periactin or Bosentan.

PATIENT TEACHING
• Instruct patient to take drug exactly as prescribed.
• Tell patient to report adverse reactions promptly.
• Tell patient receiving drug I.V. to report discomfort at insertion site.

eptifibatide
ep-tiff-IB-ah-tide

Integrilin

Pharmacologic class: glycoprotein IIb/IIIa (GPIIb/IIIa) inhibitor
Pregnancy risk category B

AVAILABLE FORMS
Injection: 10-ml (2 mg/ml), 100-ml (0.75 mg/ml and 2 mg/ml) vials

INDICATIONS & DOSAGES
➤ **Acute coronary syndrome (unstable angina or non–ST-segment elevation MI) in patients receiving drug therapy and in those having a percutaneous coronary intervention (PCI)**
Adults: 180 mcg/kg I.V. bolus as soon as possible after diagnosis, followed by a continuous I.V. infusion at a rate of 2 mcg/kg/minute until hospital discharge or start of coronary artery bypass graft (CABG) surgery, for up to 72 hours. If patient is having a PCI, continue infusion until hospital discharge or for 18 to 24 hours after the procedure, whichever comes first, for up to 96 hours. Patients who

weigh more than 121 kg (266 lb) should receive a bolus not to exceed 22.6 mg, followed by a maximum infusion rate of 15 mg/hour.
Adjust-a-dose: If creatinine clearance is less than 50 ml/minute or creatinine level is greater than 2 mg/dl, give 180 mcg/kg I.V. bolus as soon as possible after diagnosis, followed by a continuous I.V. infusion at 1 mcg/kg/minute. Patients with this creatinine clearance who weigh more than 121 kg should receive a bolus not to exceed 22.6 mg, followed by a maximum infusion rate of 7.5 mg/hour.
➤ **PCI**
Adults: 180 mcg/kg I.V. bolus given just before the procedure, immediately followed by an infusion of 2 mcg/kg/minute and a second I.V. bolus of 180 mcg/kg given 10 minutes after the first bolus. Continue infusion until hospital discharge or for 18 to 24 hours, whichever comes first; the minimum duration of infusion is 12 hours. Patients weighing more than 121 kg should receive a bolus not to exceed 22.6 mg, followed by a maximum infusion rate of 15 mg/hour.
Adjust-a-dose: If creatinine clearance is less than 50 ml/minute or creatinine level is greater than 2 mg/dl, give 180 mcg/kg I.V. bolus just before the procedure, immediately followed by a continuous I.V. infusion at 1 mcg/kg/minute and a second bolus of 180 mcg/kg given 10 minutes after the first bolus. Patients with this creatinine clearance who weigh more than 121 kg should receive a bolus not to exceed 22.6 mg, followed by a maximum infusion rate of 7.5 mg/hour.

ADMINISTRATION
I.V.
• Inspect solution for particles before use; if they appear, drug may not be sterile. Discard it.
• Protect drug from light before giving.
• Drug may be given in same line with normal saline solution, D$_5$W, alteplase, atropine, dobutamine, heparin, lidocaine, meperidine, metoprolol, midazolam, morphine, nitroglycerin, or verapamil. Main infusion may also contain up to 60 mEq/L of potassium chloride.

Reactions may be *common*, uncommon, *life-threatening*, or COMMON AND LIFE-THREATENING.
Interaction may have a *rapid onset* or **delayed onset**.

• For I.V. push, withdraw bolus dose from 10-ml vial into a syringe and give over 1 or 2 minutes.
• For infusion, give undiluted drug directly from 100-ml vial using an infusion pump.
• If patient needs thrombolytics, stop infusion.
• Refrigerate vials at 36° to 46° F (2° to 8° C). Store vials at room temperature for no longer than 2 months; afterward, discard them.
• **Incompatibilities:** Furosemide.

ACTION
Reversibly binds to the GP IIb/IIIa receptor on human platelets and inhibits platelet aggregation.

Route	Onset	Peak	Duration
I.V.	Immediate	Immediate	4–6 hr

Half-life: 2½ hours.

ADVERSE REACTIONS
CV: hypotension.
GU: hematuria.
Hematologic: *bleeding, thrombocytopenia.*
Other: bleeding at femoral artery access site.

INTERACTIONS
Drug-drug. *Clopidogrel, dipyridamole, NSAIDs, oral anticoagulants (warfarin), thrombolytics, ticlopidine:* May increase risk of bleeding. Monitor patient closely for signs of bleeding.
Other inhibitors of platelet receptor IIb/IIIa: May cause serious bleeding. Avoid using together.

EFFECTS ON LAB TEST RESULTS
• May decrease platelet count.

CONTRAINDICATIONS & CAUTIONS
• Contraindicated in patients hypersensitive to drug or its ingredients and in those with history of bleeding diathesis or evidence of active abnormal bleeding within previous 30 days; severe hypertension (systolic blood pressure higher than 200 mm Hg or diastolic blood pressure higher than 110 mm Hg) not adequately controlled with antihypertensives; major

surgery within previous 6 weeks; history of stroke within 30 days or history of hemorrhagic stroke; current or planned use of another parenteral GP IIb/IIIa inhibitor; or platelet count less than 100,000/mm³.
• Contraindicated in patients with creatinine level 4 mg/dl or higher and in patients dependent on renal dialysis.
• Use cautiously in patients at increased risk for bleeding, in those with platelet count less than 150,000/mm³, in those with hemorrhagic retinopathy, and in those weighing more than 143 kg (315 lb).

NURSING CONSIDERATIONS
• Drug is intended for use with heparin and aspirin.
• At least 4 hours before hospital discharge, stop this drug and heparin and achieve sheath hemostasis by standard compressive techniques.
• Remove sheath during infusion only after heparin has been stopped and its effects largely reversed.
• If patient is to have a CABG, stop infusion before surgery.
• Minimize use of arterial and venous punctures, I.M. injections, urinary catheters, and nasotracheal and nasogastric tubes.
• When obtaining I.V. access, avoid use of noncompressible sites (such as subclavian or jugular veins).
• Monitor patient for bleeding.
• *Alert:* If patient's platelet count is less than 100,000/mm³, stop this drug and heparin.
• Perform baseline laboratory tests before start of drug therapy; also determine hemoglobin level, hematocrit, PT, INR, activated PTT, platelet count, and creatinine level.

PATIENT TEACHING
• Explain that drug is a blood thinner used to prevent chest pain and heart attack.
• Explain that benefits of drug far outweigh risk of serious bleeding.
• Tell patient to report to prescriber chest discomfort or other adverse effects immediately.

SAFETY ALERT!

oprelvekin
oh-PRELL-veh-kin

Neumega

Pharmacologic class: recombinant human interleukin
Pregnancy risk category C

AVAILABLE FORMS
Injection: 5-mg single-dose vial with diluent

INDICATIONS & DOSAGES
➤ **To prevent severe thrombocytopenia and reduce need for platelet transfusions after myelosuppressive chemotherapy with nonmyeloid malignancies**
Adults: 50 mcg/kg as single daily subcutaneous injection until postnadir platelet count is at least 50,000/mm³. Treatment beyond 21 days per course isn't recommended.
Adjust-a-dose: In patients with severe renal impairment (creatinine clearance less than 30 ml/minute), the recommended dosage is 25 mcg/kg.

ADMINISTRATION
Subcutaneous
• Give drug in the abdomen, thigh, hip, or upper arm. Don't inject I.D. or intravascularly.
• Dosing should begin 6 to 24 hours after completing chemotherapy and end at least 2 days before starting next cycle of chemotherapy.
• Reconstitute each single-dose vial with 1 ml of supplied diluent. Avoid excessive or vigorous agitation. Discard unused portions.
• Use reconstituted drug within 3 hours.
• Store drug and diluent in refrigerator until ready to use. Don't freeze.

ACTION
Directly stimulates proliferation of hematopoietic stem cells and megakaryocyte progenitor cells. Also induces megakaryocyte maturation, resulting in increased platelet production.

Route	Onset	Peak	Duration
Subcut.	Unknown	3–5 hr	Unknown

Half-life: 7 hours.

ADVERSE REACTIONS
CNS: *asthenia, fever, headache, insomnia, dizziness,* paresthesia, *syncope.*
CV: ATRIAL FLUTTER OR FIBRILLATION, *tachycardia, palpitations, edema.*
EENT: *conjunctival injection,* blurred vision, eye hemorrhage, pharyngitis.
GI: *oral candidiasis, nausea, vomiting, diarrhea.*
Hematologic: anemia, *neutropenic fever.*
Metabolic: dehydration, hypocalcemia.
Respiratory: dyspnea, cough, pleural effusions.
Skin: *rash,* skin discoloration, exfoliative dermatitis.
Other: hypersensitivity reactions, allergic reaction, ***anaphylaxis.***

INTERACTIONS
Drug-drug. *Diuretics, ifosfamide:* May cause life-threatening hypokalemia. Avoid using together.

EFFECTS ON LAB TEST RESULTS
• May increase fibrinogen and von Willebrand factor.
• May decrease calcium and hemoglobin levels and hematocrit.

CONTRAINDICATIONS & CAUTIONS
• Contraindicated in patients hypersensitive to drug or its components.
• Use drug cautiously in patients with heart failure because of fluid retention.

NURSING CONSIDERATIONS
• Closely monitor fluid and electrolyte status in patients receiving long-term diuretic therapy.
• Fluid retention can be severe; monitor patient closely.
• Obtain a CBC before chemotherapy and at regular intervals during drug therapy.
• **Black Box Warning** Oprelvekin has caused allergic or hypersensitivity reactions, including anaphylaxis. Discontinue drug permanently in patients

---

Reactions may be *common*, uncommon, *life-threatening*, or COMMON AND LIFE-THREATENING.
Interaction may have a *rapid onset* or *delayed onset*.

who develop allergic or hypersensitivity reaction. ■

PATIENT TEACHING
• Instruct patient about appropriate preparation and administration of drug if he is going to self-administer.
• Warn patient about potential adverse reactions. Tell him to report any occurrence.
• Tell patient to keep drug refrigerated and not to reconstitute until just before use.
• Urge patient to call prescriber immediately if swelling, rapid heartbeat, or difficulty breathing occurs.
• Tell patient to report signs and symptoms of increased bleeding or bruising.

ticlopidine hydrochloride
tye-KLOH-pih-deen

Ticlid◊

Pharmacologic class: platelet aggregation inhibitor
Pregnancy risk category B

AVAILABLE FORMS
Tablets: 250 mg

INDICATIONS & DOSAGES
➤ **To reduce risk of thrombotic stroke in patients who have had a stroke or stroke precursors**
Adults: 250 mg P.O. b.i.d. with meals.
➤ **Adjunct to aspirin to prevent subacute stent thrombosis in patients having coronary stent placement**
Adults: 250 mg P.O. b.i.d., combined with antiplatelet doses of aspirin. Start therapy after stent placement and continue for up to 30 days. If prescribed longer than 30 days, use is off-label.

ADMINISTRATION
P.O.
• Give drug with meals.

ACTION
Unknown. An antiplatelet that probably blocks adenosine diphosphate–induced

platelet-to-fibrinogen and platelet-to-platelet binding.

Route	Onset	Peak	Duration
P.O.	Unknown	2 hr	Unknown

Half-life: 1½ hours after single dose; 4 to 5 days after multiple doses.

ADVERSE REACTIONS
CNS: *intracranial bleeding,* dizziness, peripheral neuropathy.
CV: vasculitis.
EENT: conjunctival hemorrhage.
GI: *diarrhea,* abdominal pain, anorexia, bleeding, dyspepsia, flatulence, nausea, vomiting.
GU: dark urine, hematuria.
Hematologic: *agranulocytosis, aplastic anemia, immune thrombocytopenia, neutropenia, pancytopenia.*
Musculoskeletal: arthropathy, myositis.
Respiratory: *allergic pneumonitis.*
Skin: *thrombocytopenic purpura,* ecchymoses, maculopapular rash, pruritus, rash, urticaria.
Other: hypersensitivity reactions, postoperative bleeding.

INTERACTIONS
Drug-drug. *Antacids:* May decrease ticlopidine level. Separate doses by at least 2 hours.
Aspirin: May increase effect of aspirin on platelets. Use together cautiously.
Cimetidine: May decrease clearance of ticlopidine and increase risk of toxicity. Avoid using together.
Digoxin: May decrease digoxin level. Monitor digoxin level.
Phenytoin: May increase phenytoin level. Monitor patient closely.
Theophylline: May decrease theophylline clearance and risk of toxicity. Monitor patient closely and adjust theophylline dosage.
Drug-herb. *Red clover:* May cause bleeding. Discourage use together.

EFFECTS ON LAB TEST RESULTS
• May increase ALT, AST, alkaline phosphatase, cholesterol, and triglyceride levels.
• May decrease neutrophil, WBC, RBC, platelet, and granulocyte counts.

CONTRAINDICATIONS & CAUTIONS
• Contraindicated in patients hypersensitive to drug and in those with severe hepatic impairment, hematopoietic disorders, active pathologic bleeding from peptic ulceration, or active intracranial bleeding.
• Use cautiously and with close monitoring of CBC and WBC differentials, watching for signs and symptoms of neutropenia and agranulocytosis.

NURSING CONSIDERATIONS
• Because of life-threatening adverse reactions, use drug only in patients who are allergic to, can't tolerate, or have failed aspirin therapy.
• Obtain baseline liver function test results before therapy.
■ **Black Box Warning** Ticlopidine can cause life-threatening hematologic adverse reactions, including neutropenia/agranulocytosis, thrombotic thrombocytopenic purpura (TTP), and aplastic anemia. Severe hematologic adverse reactions may occur within a few days of the start of therapy. During first 3 months of treatment, monitor patient for symptoms of neutropenia or TTP; discontinue drug immediately if they occur. ■
• Determine CBC and WBC differentials prior to initiating therapy and repeat every 2 weeks until end of third month.
• Monitor liver function test results and repeat if dysfunction is suspected.
• Thrombocytopenia has occurred rarely. Stop drug in patients with platelet count of 80,000/mm³ or less. If needed, give methylprednisolone 20 mg I.V. to normalize bleeding time within 2 hours.
• When used preoperatively, drug may decrease risk of graft occlusion in patients receiving coronary artery bypass grafts and reduce severity of drop in platelet count in patients receiving extracorporeal hemoperfusion during open heart surgery.

PATIENT TEACHING
• Tell patient to take drug with meals.
• Warn patient to avoid aspirin and aspirin-containing products unless directed to by prescriber and to check with prescriber or pharmacist before taking OTC drugs.

• Explain that drug will prolong bleeding time and that patient should report unusual or prolonged bleeding. Advise patient to tell dentists and other health care providers that he takes ticlopidine.
• Stress importance of regular blood tests. Because neutropenia can result with increased risk of infection, tell patient to immediately report signs and symptoms of infection, such as fever, chills, or sore throat.
• If drug is being substituted for a fibrinolytic or anticoagulant, tell patient to stop those drugs before starting ticlopidine therapy.
• Advise patient to stop drug 10 to 14 days before undergoing elective surgery.
• Tell patient to immediately report to prescriber yellow skin or sclera, severe or persistent diarrhea, rashes, bleeding under the skin, light-colored stools, or dark urine.

SAFETY ALERT!

tirofiban hydrochloride
tye-row-FYE-ban

Aggrastat

Pharmacologic class: glycoprotein (GP) IIb/IIIa receptor antagonist
Pregnancy risk category B

AVAILABLE FORMS
Injection: 25-ml and 50-ml vials (250 mcg/ml), 250-ml and 500-ml premixed vials (50 mcg/ml)

INDICATIONS & DOSAGES
➤ **Acute coronary syndrome, with heparin or aspirin, including patients who are to be managed medically and those undergoing percutaneous transluminal coronary angioplasty (PTCA) or atherectomy**
Adults: I.V. loading dose of 0.4 mcg/kg/minute for 30 minutes; then continuous I.V. infusion of 0.1 mcg/kg/minute. Continue infusion through angiography and for 12 to 24 hours after PTCA or atherectomy.
Adjust-a-dose: If creatinine clearance is less than 30 ml/minute, use a loading dose

of 0.2 mcg/kg/minute for 30 minutes; then continuous infusion of 0.05 mcg/kg/minute. Continue infusion through angiography and for 12 to 24 hours after PTCA or atherectomy.

ADMINISTRATION

I.V.
● Dilute injections of 250 mcg/ml to same strength as 500-ml premixed vials (50 mcg/ml) as follows: Withdraw and discard 100 ml from a 500-ml bag of sterile normal saline solution or D_5W and replace this volume with 100 ml of tirofiban injection (from four 25-ml vials or two 50-ml vials); or withdraw 50 ml from a 250-ml bag of sterile normal saline solution or D_5W and replace this volume with 50 ml of tirofiban injection (from two 25-ml vials or one 50-ml vial), to yield 50 mcg/ml.
● Inspect solution for particulate matter before giving, and check for leaks by squeezing the inner bag firmly. If bag leaks or particles are visible, discard solution.
● Avoid use of noncompressible sites (such as subclavian or jugular veins).
● Heparin and tirofiban may be given through the same I.V. catheter. Tirofiban may be given through the same I.V. line as dopamine, lidocaine, potassium chloride, and famotidine.
● Discard unused solution 24 hours after the start of infusion.
● Store drug at room temperature. Protect from light.
● **Incompatibilities:** Diazepam.

ACTION

Reversibly binds to the GP IIb/IIIa receptor on human platelets and inhibits platelet aggregation.

Route	Onset	Peak	Duration
I.V.	Immediate	Immediate	4–6 hr

Half-life: About 2 hours.

ADVERSE REACTIONS

CNS: dizziness, fever, headache.
CV: *bradycardia, coronary artery dissection,* edema, vasovagal reaction.
GI: *occult bleeding,* nausea.
Hematologic: *bleeding, thrombocytopenia.*

Musculoskeletal: leg pain.
Skin: sweating.
Other: *bleeding at arterial access site,* pelvic pain.

INTERACTIONS

Drug-drug. *Anticoagulants such as warfarin, aspirin, clopidogrel, dipyridamole, heparin, NSAIDs, thrombolytics, ticlopidine:* May increase risk of bleeding. Monitor patient closely.
Levothyroxine, omeprazole: May increase tirofiban renal clearance. Monitor patient.

EFFECTS ON LAB TEST RESULTS

● May decrease hemoglobin level and hematocrit.
● May decrease platelet count.

CONTRAINDICATIONS & CAUTIONS

● Contraindicated in patients hypersensitive to drug or its components.
● Contraindicated in those with active internal bleeding or history of bleeding diathesis within the previous 30 days and in those with history of intracranial hemorrhage, intracranial neoplasm, arteriovenous malformation, aneurysm, thrombocytopenia after previous exposure to drug, stroke within 30 days, or hemorrhagic stroke.
● Contraindicated in those with history, symptoms, or findings suggestive of aortic dissection; severe hypertension (systolic blood pressure higher than 180 mm Hg or diastolic blood pressure higher than 110 mm Hg); acute pericarditis; major surgical procedure or severe physical trauma within previous month; or concomitant use of another parenteral GP IIb/IIIa inhibitor.
● Use cautiously in patients with increased risk of bleeding, including those with hemorrhagic retinopathy or platelet count less than 150,000/mm³.
● Safety and efficacy of drug haven't been studied in patients younger than age 18.

NURSING CONSIDERATIONS

● Monitor hemoglobin level, hematocrit, and platelet count before starting therapy, 6 hours after loading dose, and at least daily during therapy. If thrombocytopenia occurs, notify prescriber.

- Give drug with aspirin and heparin.
- Monitor patient for bleeding.
- *Alert:* The most common adverse effect is bleeding at the arterial access site for cardiac catheterization.
- The risk of bleeding may decrease with early sheath removal and by keeping the access site immobile. The sheath may be removed during infusion, but only after heparin has been stopped and its effects largely reversed.
- Minimize use of arterial and venous punctures, I.M. injections, urinary catheters, and nasotracheal and nasogastric tubes.
- Elderly patients have a higher risk of bleeding complications.
- *Look alike–sound alike:* Don't confuse Aggrastat with argatroban.

PATIENT TEACHING
- Explain that drug is a blood thinner used to prevent chest pain and heart attack.
- Explain that risk of serious bleeding is far outweighed by the benefits of drug.
- Instruct patient to report chest discomfort or other adverse effects immediately.
- Tell patient that frequent blood sampling may be needed to evaluate therapy.

Thrombolytic enzymes

alteplase
drotrecogin alfa (activated)
reteplase, recombinant
streptokinase
tenecteplase
urokinase

alteplase (tissue plasminogen activator, recombinant; t-PA)
al-ti-PLAZE

Activase, Cathflo Activase

Pharmacologic class: enzyme
Pregnancy risk category C

AVAILABLE FORMS
Cathflo Activase injection: 2-mg single-patient vials
Injection: 50-mg (29 million international units), 100-mg (58 million international units) vials

INDICATIONS & DOSAGES
➤ **Lysis of thrombi obstructing coronary arteries in acute MI**
3-hour infusion
Adults who weigh 65 kg (143 lb) or more:
100 mg by I.V. infusion over 3 hours, as follows: 60 mg in first hour, 6 to 10 mg of which is given as a bolus over first 1 to 2 minutes. Then 20 mg/hour infused for 2 hours.
Adults who weigh less than 65 kg:
1.25 mg/kg in a similar fashion: 60% in first hour, 10% of which is given as a bolus; then 20% of total dose per hour for 2 hours. Don't exceed total dose of 100 mg.
Accelerated infusion
Adults who weigh more than 67 kg (147 lb): 100 mg maximum total dose. Give 15 mg I.V. bolus over 1 to 2 minutes, followed by 50 mg infused over the next 30 minutes; then 35 mg infused over the next hour. Don't exceed total dose of 100 mg.

Adults who weigh 67 kg or less: 15 mg I.V. bolus over 1 to 2 minutes, followed by 0.75 mg/kg (not to exceed 50 mg) infused over the next 30 minutes; then 0.5 mg/kg (not to exceed 35 mg) infused over the next hour. Don't exceed total dose of 100 mg.
➤ **To manage acute massive pulmonary embolism**
Adults: 100 mg by I.V. infusion over 2 hours. Begin heparin at end of infusion when PTT or thrombin time returns to twice normal or less. Don't exceed 100-mg dose. Higher doses may increase risk of intracranial bleeding.
➤ **Acute ischemic stroke**
Adults: 0.9 mg/kg by I.V. infusion over 1 hour with 10% of total dose given as an initial I.V. bolus over 1 minute. Maximum total dose is 90 mg.
➤ **To restore function to central venous access devices**
Cathflo Activase
Adults and children older than age 2:
For patients who weigh more than 30 kg (66 lb), instill 2 mg in 2 ml sterile water into catheter. For patients who weigh 10 kg (22 lb) to less than 30 kg, instill 110% of the internal lumen volume of the catheter, not to exceed 2 mg in 2 ml sterile water. After 30 minutes of dwell time, assess catheter function by aspirating blood. If function is restored, aspirate 4 ml to 5 ml of blood to remove drug and residual clot, and gently irrigate the catheter with normal saline solution. If catheter function isn't restored after 120 minutes, instill a second dose.
➤ **Lysis of arterial occlusion in a peripheral vessel or bypass graft ◆**
Adults: 0.05 to 0.1 mg/kg/hour infused intra-arterially for 1 to 8 hours.

ADMINISTRATION
I.V.
● Immediately before use, reconstitute solution with unpreserved sterile water

for injection. Check manufacturer's labeling for specific information.
• Don't use 50-mg vial if vacuum isn't present; 100-mg vials don't have a vacuum.
• Using an 18G needle, direct stream of sterile water at lyophilized cake. Don't shake.
• Slight foaming is common. Let it settle before giving drug. Solution should be colorless or pale yellow.
• Drug may be given reconstituted (at 1 mg/ml) or diluted with an equal volume of normal saline solution or D_5W to yield 0.5 mg/ml.
• Give drug using a controlled infusion device.
• Discard any unused drug after 8 hours.

Cathflo Activase
• Assess the cause of catheter dysfunction before using drug. Possible causes of occlusion include catheter malposition, mechanical failure, constriction by a suture, and lipid deposits or drug precipitates in the catheter lumen. Don't try to suction the catheter because you risk damaging the vessel wall or collapsing a soft-walled catheter.
• Reconstitute Cathflo Activase with 2.2 ml sterile water to yield 1 mg/ml. Dissolve completely to produce a colorless to pale yellow solution. Don't shake.
• Don't use excessive pressure while instilling drug into catheter; doing so could rupture the catheter or expel a clot into circulation.
• Solution is stable up to 8 hours at room temperature.
• **Incompatibilities:** None reported, but don't mix with other drugs.

ACTION
Converts plasminogen to plasmin by directly cleaving peptide bonds at two sites, causing fibrinolysis.

Route	Onset	Peak	Duration
I.V.	Unknown	Unknown	Unknown

Half-life: Less than 10 minutes.

ADVERSE REACTIONS
CNS: *cerebral hemorrhage,* fever.
CV: *arrhythmias,* hypotension, edema, *cholesterol embolization, venous thrombosis.*
GI: *bleeding (Cathflo Activase),* nausea, vomiting.
GU: *bleeding.*
Hematologic: *spontaneous bleeding.*
Skin: ecchymosis.
Other: *anaphylaxis, sepsis (Cathflo Activase),* bleeding at puncture sites, hypersensitivity reactions.

INTERACTIONS
Drug-drug. *Aspirin, clopidogrel, dipyridamole, drugs affecting platelet activity (abciximab), heparin, warfarin anticoagulants:* May increase risk of bleeding. Monitor patient carefully.
Nitroglycerin: May decrease alteplase antigen level. Avoid using together. If use together is unavoidable, use the lowest effective dose of nitroglycerin.

EFFECTS ON LAB TEST RESULTS
• May alter coagulation and fibrinolytic test results.

CONTRAINDICATIONS & CAUTIONS
• Contraindicated in patients with active internal bleeding, intracranial neoplasm, arteriovenous malformation, aneurysm, severe uncontrolled hypertension, or history or current evidence of intracranial hemorrhage, suspicion of subarachnoid hemorrhage, or seizure at onset of stroke when used for acute ischemic stroke.
• Contraindicated in patients with history of stroke, intraspinal or intracranial trauma or surgery within 2 months, or known bleeding diathesis.
• Use cautiously in patients having major surgery within 10 days (when bleeding is difficult to control because of its location); organ biopsy; trauma (including cardiopulmonary resuscitation); GI or GU bleeding; cerebrovascular disease; systolic pressure of 180 mm Hg or higher or diastolic pressure of 110 mm Hg or higher; mitral stenosis, atrial fibrillation, or other conditions that may lead to left heart thrombus; acute pericarditis or subacute bacterial endocarditis; hemostatic defects caused

by hepatic or renal impairment; septic thrombophlebitis; or diabetic hemorrhagic retinopathy.
• Use cautiously in patients receiving anticoagulants, in patients age 75 and older, and during pregnancy and the first 10 days postpartum.

NURSING CONSIDERATIONS
• *Alert:* When used for acute ischemic stroke, give drug within 3 hours after symptoms occur and only when intracranial bleeding has been ruled out.
• Drug may be given to menstruating women.
• To recanalize occluded coronary arteries and to improve heart function, begin treatment as soon as possible after symptoms start.
• Anticoagulant and antiplatelet therapy is commonly started during or after treatment, to decrease risk of another thrombosis.
• Monitor vital signs and neurologic status carefully. Keep patient on strict bed rest.
• Coronary thrombolysis is linked with arrhythmias caused by reperfusion of ischemic myocardium. Such arrhythmias don't differ from those commonly linked with MI. Have antiarrhythmics readily available, and carefully monitor ECG.
• Avoid invasive procedures during thrombolytic therapy. Closely monitor patient for signs of internal bleeding, and frequently check all puncture sites. Bleeding is the most common adverse effect and may occur internally and at external puncture sites.
• If uncontrollable bleeding occurs, stop infusion (and heparin) and notify prescriber.
• Avoid I.M. injections.

PATIENT TEACHING
• Explain use and administration of drug to patient and family.
• Tell patient to report adverse reactions promptly.

SAFETY ALERT!

drotrecogin alfa (activated)
drow-tra-COH-gin

Xigris

Pharmacologic class: recombinant human activated protein C
Pregnancy risk category C

AVAILABLE FORMS
Injection (preservative-free): 5-mg vial, 20-mg vial

INDICATIONS & DOSAGES
➤ **To reduce the risk of death in patients with severe sepsis from acute organ dysfunction**
Adults: 24 mcg/kg/hour I.V. infusion for a total of 96 hours.

ADMINISTRATION
I.V.
• Avoid exposing drug to heat or direct sunlight.
• Use aseptic technique during preparation.
• Reconstitute 5-mg vial with 2.5 ml or 20-mg vial with 10 ml sterile water for injection. Swirl vial gently until powder is completely dissolved. Don't invert or shake vial.
• Use reconstituted solution immediately.
• Dilute with sterile normal saline for injection by adding drug to infusion bag. Direct the stream to the side of the bag to avoid agitating solution.
• When using an infusion pump, dilute drug to between 100 mcg/ml and 200 mcg/ml.
• When using a syringe pump, dilute drug to between 100 mcg/ml and 1,000 mcg/ml.
• Gently invert the infusion bag to mix.
• Don't transport the infusion bag between locations using a mechanical delivery system.
• Inspect solution for particulates and discoloration before giving drug.
• If drug is diluted to less than 200 mcg/ml and flow rate is less than 5 ml/hour, prime the infusion set for about 15 minutes at 5 ml/hour.
• Give through a dedicated I.V. line or lumen of a multilumen central venous catheter. The only other solutions that can

---

be given through the same line are normal saline solution, lactated Ringer's injection, D_5W, or dextrose in saline mixtures.
• If the infusion is interrupted, restart at the 24-mcg/kg/hour infusion rate.
• Complete infusion within 12 hours after preparing solution.
• Store in refrigerator at 35° to 46° F (2° to 8° C). Don't freeze.
• If needed, reconstituted vial may be stored at 59° to 86° F (15° to 30° C) for up to 3 hours.
• **Incompatibilities:** Other I.V. drugs.

ACTION
May produce dose-dependent reductions in D-dimer and interleukin (IL)-6. Activated protein C exerts an antithrombotic effect by inhibiting factors Va and VIIIa.

Route	Onset	Peak	Duration
I.V.	Immediate	Unknown	Unknown

Half-life: Unknown.

ADVERSE REACTIONS
Hematologic: *hemorrhage.*

INTERACTIONS
Drug-drug. *Drugs that affect hemostasis:* May increase risk of bleeding. Use together cautiously.

EFFECTS ON LAB TEST RESULTS
• May prolong PT and PTT.

CONTRAINDICATIONS & CAUTIONS
• Contraindicated in patients hypersensitive to drug or any of its components, those with active internal bleeding, and those who have had hemorrhagic stroke in the past 3 months or intracranial or intraspinal surgery in the past 2 months.
• Contraindicated in patients with severe head trauma, trauma with increased risk of life-threatening bleeding, an epidural catheter, intracranial neoplasm or mass lesion, or cerebral herniation.
• *Alert:* Use only after assessing the risk versus benefit in patients with single organ dysfunction and recent surgery because these patients may not be at a high risk of death.
• Use cautiously in patients taking other drugs that affect hemostasis such as heparin (at least 15 units/kg/hour) and in those with

a platelet count less than $30,000 \times 10^6$/L (even if the platelet count is increased after transfusions) or an INR greater than 3.
• Use cautiously in patients who have had GI bleeding in the past 6 weeks; thrombolytic therapy in the past 3 days; oral anticoagulants, glycoprotein IIb/IIIa inhibitors, or aspirin (more than 650 mg/day) or other platelet inhibitors in the past week; ischemic stroke in the past 3 months; or intracranial arteriovenous malformation or aneurysm, bleeding diathesis, chronic severe hepatic disease, or any condition in which bleeding poses a significant hazard or would be difficult to manage because of its location.

NURSING CONSIDERATIONS
• *Alert:* Monitor patient closely for bleeding. If clinically important bleeding occurs, stop infusion immediately.
• Stop drug 2 hours before an invasive surgical procedure. After hemostasis has been achieved, drug may be restarted 12 hours after major invasive procedure or immediately after uncomplicated less invasive procedure.
• Because drug has minimal effect on the PT, this value can be used to monitor the patient's coagulopathy status.

PATIENT TEACHING
• Inform patient of the potential adverse reactions.
• Instruct patient to promptly report signs of bleeding.
• Advise patient that bleeding may occur for up to 28 days after treatment.

SAFETY ALERT!

reteplase, recombinant
RET-ah-place

Retavase

Pharmacologic class: tissue plasminogen activator
Pregnancy risk category C

AVAILABLE FORMS
Injection: 10.4 units (18.1 mg)/vial. Supplied in a kit with components for reconstitution for two single-use vials

---

Reactions may be *common,* uncommon, *life-threatening,* or COMMON AND LIFE-THREATENING.
Interaction may have a *rapid onset* or *delayed onset.*

INDICATIONS & DOSAGES
➤ **To manage acute MI**
Adults: Double-bolus injection of 10 +
10 units. Give each bolus I.V. over 2 minutes. If complications, such as serious
bleeding or anaphylactoid reaction, don't
occur after first bolus, give second bolus
30 minutes after start of first.

ADMINISTRATION
I.V.
● Reconstitute drug according to manufacturer's instructions using items provided in
kit and sterile water for injection, without
preservatives. Make sure reconstituted solution is colorless; resulting concentration
is 1 unit/ml. If foaming occurs, let vial
stand for several minutes. Inspect for precipitation. Use within 4 hours of reconstitution; discard unused portions.
● Give as a double-bolus injection. If
bleeding or anaphylactoid reaction occurs
after first bolus, notify prescriber; second
bolus may be withheld.
● **Incompatibilities:** Other I.V. drugs.

ACTION
Enhances cleavage of plasminogen to generate plasmin, which leads to fibrinolysis.

Route	Onset	Peak	Duration
I.V.	Unknown	Unknown	Unknown

Half-life: 13 to 16 minutes.

ADVERSE REACTIONS
CNS: *intracranial hemorrhage.*
CV: *arrhythmias, cholesterol emboliza-
tion, hemorrhage.*
GI: *hemorrhage.*
GU: hematuria.
Hematologic: *bleeding tendency,* anemia.
Other: bleeding at puncture sites, hyper-
sensitivity reactions.

INTERACTIONS
Drug-drug. *Heparin, oral anticoagulants,
platelet inhibitors (abciximab, aspirin,
dipyridamole, eptifibatide, tirofiban):* May
increase risk of bleeding. Use together
cautiously.

EFFECTS ON LAB TEST RESULTS
● May increase PT, PTT, and INR.
● May alter coagulation study results.

CONTRAINDICATIONS & CAUTIONS
● Contraindicated in patients with active
internal bleeding, known bleeding diathesis, history of stroke, recent intracranial or
intraspinal surgery or trauma, severe uncontrolled hypertension, intracranial neoplasm, arteriovenous malformation, or
aneurysm.
● Use cautiously in patients with previous
puncture of noncompressible vessels; in
those with recent (within 10 days) major
surgery, obstetric delivery, organ biopsy,
GI or GU bleeding, or trauma; in those
with cerebrovascular disease, systolic
blood pressure 180 mm Hg or higher or
diastolic pressure 110 mm Hg or higher,
and conditions that may lead to left heart
thrombus, including mitral stenosis, acute
pericarditis, subacute bacterial endocarditis, and hemostatic defects.
● Use cautiously in those with diabetic
hemorrhagic retinopathy, septic thrombophlebitis, and other conditions in which
bleeding would be difficult to manage.
● Use cautiously in patients age 75 and
older and in breast-feeding women.

NURSING CONSIDERATIONS
● Drug remains active in vitro and can
lead to degradation of fibrinogen in
sample, changing coagulation study
results. Collect blood samples with
chloromethylketone at 2-micromolar
concentrations.
● Drug may be given to menstruating
women.
● Carefully monitor ECG during treatment. Coronary thrombolysis may cause
arrhythmias linked with reperfusion. Be
prepared to treat bradycardia or ventricular irritability.
● Closely monitor patient for bleeding.
Avoid I.M. injections, invasive procedures,
and nonessential handling of patient.
Bleeding is the most common adverse reaction and may occur internally or at external puncture sites. If local measures
don't control serious bleeding, stop anticoagulant and notify prescriber. Withhold
second bolus of reteplase.
● Potency is expressed in units specific to
reteplase and isn't comparable with other
thrombolytics.
● Avoid use of noncompressible puncture
sites during therapy. If an arterial puncture

is needed, use an arm vessel that can be compressed manually. Apply pressure for at least 30 minutes; then apply a pressure dressing. Check site frequently.

PATIENT TEACHING
● Explain use and administration of drug to patient and family.
● Tell patient to report adverse reactions immediately.

streptokinase
strep-to-KIN-ase

Streptase

Pharmacologic class: plasminogen activator
Pregnancy risk category C

AVAILABLE FORMS
Injection: 250,000 international units; 750,000 international units; 1.5 million international units in vials for reconstitution

INDICATIONS & DOSAGES
➤ **Arteriovenous-cannula occlusion**
Adults: 250,000 international units in 2 ml I.V. solution by I.V. pump infusion into each occluded limb of the cannula over 25 to 35 minutes. Clamp off cannula for 2 hours. Then aspirate contents of cannula, flush with normal saline solution, and reconnect.
➤ **Venous thrombosis, pulmonary embolism, arterial thrombosis, and embolism**
Adults: Loading dose is 250,000 international units by I.V. infusion over 30 minutes. Sustaining dose is 100,000 international units/hour I.V. infusion for 72 hours for deep vein thrombosis (DVT) and 100,000 international units/hour over 24 to 72 hours by I.V. infusion pump for pulmonary embolism (72 hours if concurrent DVT is suspected), and arterial thrombosis or embolism.
➤ **Lysis of coronary artery thrombi following acute MI**
Adults: Infuse 1.5 million international units I.V. over 30 to 60 minutes. For intracoronary infusion, give 20,000 interna-

tional units over 1 to 2 minutes (bolus) followed by 2,000 international units/minute for 60 minutes (for total dose of 140,000 international units).

ADMINISTRATION
I.V.
● Reconstitute drug in each vial with 5 ml of normal saline solution for injection or D₅W solution. Further dilute to 45 ml (if needed, total volume may be increased to 500 ml in a glass or 50 ml in a plastic container). Don't shake; roll gently to mix. Solution may precipitate after reconstituting; discard if large amounts are present.
● Filter solution with 0.8-micron or larger filter.
● Use immediately after reconstitution. If refrigerated, solution can be used for direct I.V. administration within 8 hours.
● Use an infusion pump to start a continuous infusion of heparin 1 to 4 hours after stopping streptokinase. Starting heparin 12 hours after intracoronary streptokinase may minimize bleeding risk.
● Store powder at room temperature.
● **Incompatibilities:** Dextrans. Don't mix with other drugs or give other drugs through the same I.V. line.

ACTION
Converts plasminogen to plasmin by directly cleaving peptide bonds at two sites, causing fibrinolysis.

Route	Onset	Peak	Duration
I.V.	Immediate	20 min–2 hr	4–24 hr

Half-life: First phase, 18 minutes; second phase, 83 minutes.

ADVERSE REACTIONS
CNS: polyradiculoneuropathy, headache, *fever.*
CV: ***reperfusion arrhythmias,*** *hypotension,* vasculitis, flushing.
EENT: periorbital edema.
GI: nausea.
GU: interstitial nephritis.
Hematologic: *bleeding,* moderately decreased hematocrit.
Respiratory: minor breathing difficulty, ***bronchospasm, pulmonary edema.***
Skin: urticaria, pruritus.

Other: phlebitis at injection site, hypersensitivity reactions, *anaphylaxis,* delayed hypersensitivity reactions, *angioedema,* shivering.

INTERACTIONS
Drug-drug. *Anticoagulants:* May increase risk of bleeding. Monitor patient closely.
Antifibrinolytic drugs (such as aminocaproic acid): May inhibit and reverse streptokinase activity. Avoid using together.
Aspirin, dipyridamole, drugs affecting platelet activity (abciximab, eptifibatide, tirofiban), indomethacin, NSAIDs, phenylbutazone: May increase risk of bleeding. Monitor patient closely.

EFFECTS ON LAB TEST RESULTS
- May increase AST and ALT levels.
- May increase PT, PTT, and INR.
- May decrease hematocrit, plasminogen, and fibrinogen levels.

CONTRAINDICATIONS & CAUTIONS
- Contraindicated in patients with active internal bleeding; recent (within 2 months) cerebrovascular accident, or intracranial or intraspinal surgery; intracranial neoplasm; severe uncontrolled hypertension, or any patient with a history of an allergic reaction to the drug.
- Contraindicated with I.M. injections and other invasive procedures.
- Use cautiously in patients with recent (within 10 days) major surgery, obstetric delivery, organ biopsy, previous puncture of noncompressible vessels, serious GI bleeding, or trauma including cardiopulmonary resuscitation.
- Use cautiously in patients with a systolic blood pressure of 180 mm Hg or greater or a diastolic blood pressure of 110 mm Hg or greater, a high likelihood of left heart thrombus (mitral stenosis with atrial fibrillation), subacute bacterial endocarditis, hemostatic defects including those secondary to severe hepatic or renal disease, age older than 75 years, pregnancy, cerebrovascular disease, diabetic hemorrhagic retinopathy, septic thrombophlebitis or occluded AV cannula at seriously infected site, or any other condition in which bleeding constitutes a significant

hazard or would be particularly difficult to manage because of its location.

NURSING CONSIDERATIONS
- For acute MI, give as soon as possible after symptom onset. The greatest benefit in mortality reduction was observed when streptokinase was given within 4 hours, but significant benefit has been reported up to 24 hours.
- For pulmonary embolism, deep vein thrombosis, arterial thrombosis, or embolism, institute treatment as soon as possible after thrombotic event onset, preferably within 7 days.
- Drug may be given to menstruating women.
- Only prescribers with experience managing thrombotic disease should give drug and only where clinical and laboratory monitoring can be performed.
- Before using drug to clear an occluded AV cannula, try flushing with heparinized saline solution.
- Keep aminocaproic acid available to treat bleeding and corticosteroids to treat allergic reactions.
- Before starting therapy, draw blood for coagulation studies, hematocrit, platelet count, and type and crossmatching. Rate of infusion depends on thrombin time and drug resistance.
- To check for hypersensitivity in acutely ill patients or patients with known allergies, give 100 international units I.D.; a wheal-and-flare response within 20 minutes means patient is probably allergic. Monitor vital signs frequently.
- For patient who has had a streptococcal infection or has been treated with streptokinase or anistreplase in the last 2 years, use a different thrombolytic.
- Combined therapy with low-dose aspirin (162.5 mg) or dipyridamole has improved short- and long-term results.
- Monitor patient for excessive bleeding every 15 minutes for first hour, every 30 minutes for second through eighth hours, and then every 4 hours. If bleeding is evident, stop therapy and notify prescriber. Pretreatment with heparin or drugs that affect platelets causes high risk of bleeding but may improve long-term results.

• Monitor pulse, color, and sensation of arms and legs every hour.
• Keep involved limb in straight alignment to prevent bleeding from infusion site.
• Monitor blood pressure closely.
• Avoid unnecessary handling of patient; pad side rails. Bruising is more likely during therapy.
• Keep a laboratory flow sheet on patient's chart to monitor PTT, PT, thrombin time, hemoglobin level, and hematocrit. Monitor vital signs and neurologic status.
• Avoid I.M. injection. Keep venipuncture sites to a minimum; use pressure dressing on puncture sites for at least 15 minutes.
• **Alert:** Watch for signs of hypersensitivity and notify prescriber immediately if any occur. Antihistamines or corticosteroids may be used for mild allergic reactions. If a severe reaction occurs, stop infusion immediately and notify prescriber.

PATIENT TEACHING
• Explain use and administration of drug to patient and family.
• Tell patient to promptly report adverse reactions, such as bleeding and bruising.

SAFETY ALERT!

tenecteplase
teh-NEK-ti-plaze

TNKase

Pharmacologic class: recombinant tissue plasminogen activator
Pregnancy risk category C

AVAILABLE FORMS
Injection: 50 mg

INDICATIONS & DOSAGES
➤ **To reduce risk of death from an acute MI**
Adults who weigh 90 kg (198 lb) or more: 50 mg (10 ml) by I.V. bolus over 5 seconds.
Adults who weigh 80 to less than 90 kg (176 to 198 lb): 45 mg (9 ml) by I.V. bolus over 5 seconds.
Adults who weigh 70 to just under 80 kg (154 to 176 lb): 40 mg (8 ml) by I.V. bolus over 5 seconds.

Adults who weigh 60 to just under 70 kg (132 to 154 lb): 35 mg (7 ml) by I.V. bolus over 5 seconds.
Adults who weigh less than 60 kg (132 lb): 30 mg (6 ml) by I.V. bolus over 5 seconds. Maximum dose is 50 mg.

ADMINISTRATION
I.V.
• Use syringe prefilled with sterile water for injection, and inject the entire contents into drug vial. Gently swirl solution once mixed. Don't shake. Visually inspect product for particulate matter before administration.
• Draw up the appropriate dose needed from the reconstituted vial with the syringe and discard any unused portion. Give drug immediately, or refrigerate and use within 8 hours.
• Give drug in a designated line. Flush dextrose-containing lines with normal saline solution before administration.
• Give the drug rapidly over 5 seconds.
• **Incompatibilities:** Solutions containing dextrose, other I.V. drugs.

ACTION
Binds to fibrin and converts plasminogen to plasmin. The specificity to fibrin decreases systemic activation of plasminogen and the resulting breakdown of circulating fibrinogen.

Route	Onset	Peak	Duration
I.V.	Immediate	Immediate	Unknown

Half-life: 20 minutes to 2 hours.

ADVERSE REACTIONS
CNS: *stroke, intracranial hemorrhage,* fever.
CV: *arrhythmias, cardiogenic shock, myocardial reinfarction, thrombosis, embolism,* hypotension.
EENT: pharyngeal bleeding, epistaxis.
GI: *GI bleeding,* nausea, vomiting.
GU: hematuria.
Respiratory: *pulmonary edema.*
Skin: *hematoma.*
Other: bleeding at puncture site, hypersensitivity reactions.

INTERACTIONS
Drug-drug. *Anticoagulants (heparin, vitamin K antagonists), drugs that alter*

Reactions may be *common*, uncommon, *life-threatening*, or COMMON AND LIFE-THREATENING.
Interaction may have a *rapid onset* or **delayed onset**.

platelet function (acetylsalicylic acid, dipyridamole, glycoprotein IIb/IIIa inhibitors, NSAIDs): May increase risk of bleeding when used before, during, or after tenecteplase use. Use together cautiously.

EFFECTS ON LAB TEST RESULTS
• May increase PT, PTT, and INR.

CONTRAINDICATIONS & CAUTIONS
• Contraindicated in patients with active internal bleeding; history of stroke; intracranial or intraspinal surgery or trauma during previous 2 months; intracranial neoplasm, aneurysm, or arteriovenous malformation; severe uncontrolled hypertension; or bleeding diathesis.
• Use cautiously in patients who have had recent major surgery (such as coronary artery bypass graft), organ biopsy, obstetric delivery, or previous puncture of non-compressible vessels.
• Use cautiously in pregnant women, patients age 75 and older, and patients with recent trauma, recent GI or GU bleeding, high risk of left ventricular thrombus, acute pericarditis, systolic blood pressure 180 mm Hg or higher or diastolic pressure 110 mm Hg or higher, severe hepatic dysfunction, hemostatic defects, subacute bacterial endocarditis, septic thrombophlebitis, diabetic hemorrhagic retinopathy, or cerebrovascular disease.

NURSING CONSIDERATIONS
• Begin therapy as soon as possible after onset of MI symptoms.
• Avoid noncompressible arterial punctures and internal jugular and subclavian venous punctures. Minimize all arterial and venous punctures during treatment.
• Avoid I.M. use.
• Give heparin but not in the same I.V. line.
• Monitor patient for bleeding. If serious bleeding occurs, stop heparin and antiplatelet drugs immediately.
• *Alert:* Use exact patient weight for dosage. An overestimation in patient weight can lead to significant increase in bleeding or intracerebral hemorrhage.

• Monitor ECG for reperfusion arrhythmias.
• A life-threatening cholesterol embolism is rarely caused by thrombolytics. Signs and symptoms may include livedo reticularis (blue toe syndrome), acute renal failure, gangrenous digits, hypertension, pancreatitis, MI, cerebral infarction, spinal cord infarction, retinal artery occlusion, bowel infarction, and rhabdomyolysis.

PATIENT TEACHING
• Advise patient about proper dental care to avoid excessive gum bleeding.
• Tell patient to report any adverse effects or excessive bleeding immediately.
• Explain use of drug to patient and family.

SAFETY ALERT!

urokinase
yoor-oh-KIN-ase

Kinlytic

Pharmacologic class: enzyme
Pregnancy risk category B

AVAILABLE FORMS
Injection: 250,000 international units/vial

INDICATIONS & DOSAGES
➤ **Lysis of acute massive pulmonary embolism and of pulmonary embolism with unstable hemodynamics**
Adults: For I.V. infusion only by constant infusion pump. For priming dose, give 4,400 international units/kg with normal saline solution or D₅W solution, over 10 minutes, followed by 4,400 international units/kg/hour for 12 hours. Then give continuous I.V. infusion of heparin and oral anticoagulants.
➤ **Lysis of coronary artery thrombi following an acute MI**
Adults: After bolus dose of heparin ranging from 2,500 to 10,000 units, infuse 6,000 international units/minute urokinase into occluded artery for up to 2 hours. Average total dose is 500,000 international units. Start drug within 6 hours after symptoms start.

ADMINISTRATION
I.V.
• Reconstitute according to manufacturer's directions using sterile water for injection. Gently roll vial; don't shake. Don't use bacteriostatic water for injection to reconstitute; it contains preservatives. Dilute further with normal saline solution or D$_5$W solution before infusion. Filter urokinase solutions through a 0.45-micron or smaller cellulose-membrane filter before administration. Discard unused solution. Total volume of fluid given by I.V. infusion shouldn't exceed 195 ml.
• Heparin by continuous infusion may be started concurrently or within 3 to 4 hours after urokinase has been stopped to prevent recurrent thrombosis.
• **Incompatibilities:** Other I.V. drugs.

ACTION
Converts plasminogen to plasmin by directly cleaving peptide bonds at two different sites, causing fibrinolysis.

Route	Onset	Peak	Duration
I.V.	Immediate	20 min–4 hr	12–24 hr

Half-life: 10 to 20 minutes.

ADVERSE REACTIONS
CNS: fever.
CV: *reperfusion arrhythmias,* tachycardia, transient hypotension or hypertension.
GI: nausea, vomiting.
Hematologic: *bleeding.*
Respiratory: *bronchospasm,* minor breathing difficulties.
Skin: phlebitis at injection site, rash.
Other: *anaphylaxis,* chills.

INTERACTIONS
Drug-drug. *Anticoagulants, aspirin, dipyridamole, indomethacin, NSAIDs, phenylbutazone, other drugs affecting platelet activity:* May increase risk of bleeding. Monitor patient.

EFFECTS ON LAB TEST RESULTS
• May decrease hematocrit.
• May increase PT, PTT, and INR.

CONTRAINDICATIONS & CAUTIONS
• Contraindicated in patients with a history of hypersensitivity to the drug; active internal bleeding; recent (within 2 months) cerebrovascular accident, or intracranial or intraspinal surgery; recent trauma including cardiopulmonary resuscitation; intracranial neoplasm, arteriovenous malformation, or aneurysm; severe uncontrolled hypertension, or known bleeding diatheses.
• Contraindicated with I.M. injections and other invasive procedures.
• Use cautiously in patients with recent (within 10 days) major surgery, obstetric delivery, organ biopsy, previous puncture of noncompressible vessels, or serious GI bleeding. Also use cautiously in patients with a high likelihood of left heart thrombus (mitral stenosis with atrial fibrillation), subacute bacterial endocarditis, hemostatic defects including those secondary to severe hepatic or renal disease, pregnancy, cerebrovascular disease, diabetic hemorrhagic retinopathy, or any other condition in which bleeding constitutes a significant hazard or would be particularly difficult to manage because of its location.
■ **Black Box Warning** Thrombolytic therapy should be considered in all situations in which the benefits to be achieved outweigh the risk of potentially serious hemorrhage. When internal bleeding does occur, it may be more difficult to manage than that which occurs with conventional anticoagulant therapy. ■

NURSING CONSIDERATIONS
■ **Black Box Warning** Urokinase therapy should be instituted as soon as possible after onset of pulmonary embolism, preferably no later than 7 days after onset. For treatment of coronary artery thrombosis associated with evolving transmural MI, therapy should be instituted within 6 hours of symptom onset. Any delay in instituting lytic therapy to evaluate the effect of heparin decreases the potential for optimal efficacy. ■
• Give other drugs through separate I.V. line.
• Have aminocaproic acid and crossmatched and crosstyped RBCs, whole blood, plasma expanders (other than dextran) available for bleeding. Keep corticosteroids, epinephrine, and antihistamines available for allergic reactions.

Reactions may be *common,* uncommon, *life-threatening,* or COMMON AND LIFE-THREATENING.
Interaction may have a *rapid onset* or *delayed onset.*

• Drug may be given to menstruating women.
• Only prescribers with extensive experience in thrombotic disease management should use drug and only in facilities where clinical and laboratory monitoring can be performed.
• Monitor patient for excessive bleeding every 15 minutes for first hour; every 30 minutes for second through eighth hours; then once every 4 hours. Pretreatment with drugs affecting platelets places patient at high risk of bleeding.
• Monitor pulse, color, and sensation of arms and legs every hour.
• Although risk of hypersensitivity reactions is low, monitor patient.
• Keep a laboratory flow sheet on patient's chart to monitor PTT, PT, thrombin time, hemoglobin level, and hematocrit.
• Monitor vital signs and neurologic status. Don't take blood pressure in legs because doing so could dislodge a clot.
• Keep venipuncture sites to a minimum; use pressure dressing on puncture sites for at least 15 minutes.
• Avoid I.M. injections.
• Keep involved limb in straight alignment to prevent bleeding from infusion site.
• Because bruising is more likely during therapy, avoid unnecessary handling of patient, and pad side rails.
• Rarely, orolingual edema, urticaria, cholesterol embolization, and infusion reactions causing hypoxia, cyanosis, acidosis, and back pain may occur.

PATIENT TEACHING
• Explain use and administration of drug to patient and family.
• Instruct patient to report adverse reactions promptly.

Alzheimer disease drugs

donepezil hydrochloride
galantamine hydrobromide
memantine hydrochloride
rivastigmine tartrate

---

donepezil hydrochloride
doe-NEP-ah-zill

Aricept, Aricept ODT

Pharmacologic class:
cholinesterase inhibitor
Pregnancy risk category C

AVAILABLE FORMS
Orally disintegrating tablets (ODTs):
5 mg, 10 mg
Tablets: 5 mg, 10 mg

INDICATIONS & DOSAGES
➤ **Mild to severe Alzheimer dementia**
Adults: Initially, 5 mg P.O. daily at bedtime. After 4 to 6 weeks, increase to 10 mg daily, if needed.

ADMINISTRATION
P.O.
• Allow ODT to dissolve on tongue; then follow with water.
• Give drug at bedtime, without regard for food.

ACTION
Thought to increase acetylcholine level by inhibiting cholinesterase enzyme, which causes acetylcholine hydrolysis.

Route	Onset	Peak	Duration
P.O.	Unknown	3–4 hr	Unknown

Half-life: 70 hours.

ADVERSE REACTIONS
CNS: *headache, insomnia, seizures,* dizziness, fatigue, depression, abnormal dreams, somnolence, tremor, irritability, paresthesia, aggression, vertigo, ataxia, restlessness, abnormal crying, nervousness, aphasia, syncope, pain.
CV: chest pain, hypertension, vasodilation, atrial fibrillation, hot flashes, hypotension, *bradycardia, heart block.*
EENT: cataract, blurred vision, eye irritation, sore throat.
GI: *nausea, diarrhea,* vomiting, anorexia, fecal incontinence, *GI bleeding,* bloating, epigastric pain.
GU: urinary frequency.
Metabolic: weight loss, dehydration.
Musculoskeletal: muscle cramps, arthritis, bone fracture.
Respiratory: dyspnea, bronchitis.
Skin: pruritus, urticaria, diaphoresis, ecchymoses.
Other: toothache, influenza, increased libido.

INTERACTIONS
Drug-drug. *Anticholinergics:* May decrease donepezil effects. Avoid using together.
Anticholinesterases, cholinomimetics: May have synergistic effect. Monitor patient closely.
Bethanechol, succinylcholine: May have additive effects. Monitor patient closely.
Carbamazepine, dexamethasone, phenobarbital, phenytoin, rifampin: May increase rate of donepezil elimination. Monitor patient.
NSAIDs: May increase gastric acid secretions. Monitor for active or occult GI bleeding.

EFFECTS ON LAB TEST RESULTS
• May increase CK level.

CONTRAINDICATIONS & CAUTIONS
• Contraindicated in patients hypersensitive to drug or piperidine derivatives and in breast-feeding women.
• Use cautiously in pregnant women and in patients who take NSAIDs or have CV disease, asthma, obstructive pulmonary disease, urinary outflow impairment, or history of ulcer disease.

Reactions may be *common,* uncommon, *life-threatening,* or COMMON AND LIFE-THREATENING.
Interaction may have a *rapid onset* or *delayed onset.*

NURSING CONSIDERATIONS
• Monitor patient for evidence of active or occult GI bleeding.
• **Look alike–sound alike:** Don't confuse Aricept with Ascriptin.

PATIENT TEACHING
• Stress that drug doesn't alter underlying degenerative disease but can temporarily stabilize or relieve symptoms. Effectiveness depends on taking drug at regular intervals.
• Tell caregiver to give drug just before patient's bedtime.
• ODTs may be taken with or without food. Have patient allow tablet to dissolve on his tongue, then swallow with a sip of water.
• Advise patient and caregiver to report immediately significant adverse effects or changes in overall health status and to inform health care team that patient is taking drug before he receives anesthesia.
• Tell patient to avoid OTC cold or sleep remedies because of risk of increased anticholinergic effects.

---

galantamine hydrobromide
gah-LAN-tah-meen

Razadyne, Razadyne ER

Pharmacologic class:
cholinesterase inhibitor
Pregnancy risk category B

AVAILABLE FORMS
Capsules (extended-release): 8 mg, 16 mg, 24 mg
Oral solution: 4 mg/ml
Tablets: 4 mg, 8 mg, 12 mg

INDICATIONS & DOSAGES
➤ **Mild to moderate Alzheimer dementia**
Adults: Initially, 4 mg b.i.d., preferably with morning and evening meals. If dose is well tolerated after minimum of 4 weeks of therapy, increase dosage to 8 mg b.i.d. A further increase to 12 mg b.i.d. may be attempted, but only after at least 4 weeks of therapy at the previous dosage. Dosage range

is 16 to 24 mg daily in two divided doses.
Or, 8 mg extended-release capsule P.O. once daily in the morning with food. Increase to 16 mg P.O. once daily after a minimum of 4 weeks. May further increase to 24 mg once daily after a minimum of 4 weeks, based upon patient response and tolerability.
Adjust-a-dose: For patients with Child-Pugh score of 7 to 9, dosage usually shouldn't exceed 16 mg daily. Drug isn't recommended for patients with Child-Pugh score of 10 to 15. For patients with moderate renal impairment, dosage usually shouldn't exceed 16 mg daily. For patients with creatinine clearance less than 9 ml/minute, drug isn't recommended.

ADMINISTRATION
P.O.
• **Alert:** Give Razadyne tablets twice daily; give Razadyne ER capsules once daily. To avoid dosing errors, verify any prescription that suggests a different dosing schedule.
• Give drug with food and antiemetics, and ensure adequate fluid intake to decrease the risk of nausea and vomiting.
• Use proper technique when dispensing the oral solution with the pipette. Dispense measured amount into a beverage and give to patient right away.

ACTION
Thought to enhance cholinergic function by increasing acetylcholine level in brain.

Route	Onset	Peak	Duration
P.O.	Unknown	1 hr	Unknown

Half-life: About 7 hours.

ADVERSE REACTIONS
CNS: depression, dizziness, headache, tremor, insomnia, somnolence, fatigue, syncope.
CV: *bradycardia, AV block.*
EENT: rhinitis.
GI: *diarrhea, nausea, vomiting,* anorexia, abdominal pain, dyspepsia, anorexia.
GU: UTI, hematuria.
Hematologic: anemia.
Metabolic: weight loss.

INTERACTIONS

Drug-drug. *Amitriptyline, fluoxetine, fluvoxamine, quinidine:* May decrease galantamine clearance. Monitor patient closely.

Anticholinergics: May antagonize anticholinergic activity. Monitor patient.

Cholinergics (such as bethanechol, succinylcholine): May have synergistic effect. Monitor patient closely. May need to avoid use before procedures using general anesthesia with succinylcholine-type neuromuscular blockers.

Cimetidine, clarithromycin, erythromycin, ketoconazole, paroxetine: May increase galantamine bioavailability. Monitor patient closely.

NSAIDs: May increase risk of bleeding due to increased gastric acid secretion. Monitor patient for symptoms of active or occult GI bleeding.

EFFECTS ON LAB TEST RESULTS
● None reported.

CONTRAINDICATIONS & CAUTIONS
● Contraindicated in patients hypersensitive to drug or its components.
● Use cautiously in patients with supraventricular cardiac conduction disorders and in those taking other drugs that significantly slow heart rate.
● Use cautiously during or before procedures involving anesthesia using succinylcholine-type or similar neuromuscular blockers.
● Use cautiously in patients with history of peptic ulcer disease and in those taking NSAIDs. Because of the potential for cholinomimetic effects, use cautiously in patients with bladder outflow obstruction, seizures, asthma, or COPD.

NURSING CONSIDERATIONS
● Drug may cause bradycardia and heart block. Consider all patients at risk for adverse effects on cardiac conduction.
● *Alert:* The original trade name for galantamine, "Reminyl," was changed to "Razadyne" because of name confusion with the antidiabetic Amaryl.
● If drug is stopped for several days or longer, restart at the lowest dose and gradually increase, at 4-week or longer intervals, to the previous dosage level.
● Because of the risk of increased gastric acid secretion, monitor patients closely for symptoms of active or occult GI bleeding, especially those with an increased risk of developing ulcers.

PATIENT TEACHING
● Advise caregiver to give drug with morning and evening meals (for the conventional form), or only in the morning (for the extended-release form).
● Inform patient that nausea and vomiting are common adverse effects.
● Teach caregiver the proper technique when measuring the oral solution with the pipette. Tell her to place measured amount in a nonalcoholic beverage and have patient drink right away.
● Urge patient or caregiver to report slow heartbeat immediately.
● Advise patient and caregiver that although drug may improve cognitive function, it doesn't alter the underlying disease process.

---

memantine hydrochloride
meh-MAN-teen

Namenda

Pharmacologic class: N-methyl-D-aspartate (NMDA) receptor antagonist
Pregnancy risk category B

AVAILABLE FORMS
Oral solution: 2 mg/ml
Tablets: 5 mg, 10 mg

INDICATIONS & DOSAGES
➤ **Moderate to severe Alzheimer dementia**
Adults: Initially, 5 mg P.O. once daily. Increase by 5 mg/day every week until target dose is reached. Maximum, 10 mg P.O. b.i.d. Doses greater than 5 mg should be divided b.i.d.
Adjust-a-dose: Reduce dosage in patients with moderate renal impairment. Drug isn't recommended for patients with severe renal impairment.

Reactions may be *common*, uncommon, *life-threatening*, or COMMON AND LIFE-THREATENING.
Interaction may have a *rapid onset* or **delayed onset**.

ADMINISTRATION
P.O.
● Give drug without regard for food.

ACTION
Antagonizes NMDA receptors, the persistent activation of which seems to increase Alzheimer symptoms.

Route	Onset	Peak	Duration
P.O.	Unknown	3–7 hr	Unknown

Half-life: 60 to 80 hours.

ADVERSE REACTIONS
CNS: *stroke,* aggressiveness, agitation, anxiety, ataxia, confusion, depression, dizziness, fatigue, hallucinations, headache, hypokinesia, insomnia, pain, somnolence, syncope, transient ischemic attack, vertigo.
CV: *heart failure,* edema, hypertension.
EENT: cataracts, conjunctivitis.
GI: anorexia, constipation, diarrhea, nausea, vomiting.
GU: incontinence, urinary frequency, UTI.
Hematologic: anemia.
Metabolic: weight loss.
Musculoskeletal: arthralgia, back pain.
Respiratory: bronchitis, coughing, dyspnea, flulike symptoms, pneumonia, upper respiratory tract infection.
Skin: rash.
Other: abnormal gait, falls, injury.

INTERACTIONS
Drug-drug. *Cimetidine, hydrochlorothiazide, quinidine, ranitidine, triamterene:* May alter levels of both drugs. Monitor patient.
NMDA antagonists (amantadine, dextromethorphan, ketamine): Combined use unknown. Use together cautiously.
Urine alkalinizers (carbonic anhydrase inhibitors, sodium bicarbonate): May decrease memantine clearance. Monitor patient for adverse effects.
Drug-herb. *Herbs that alkalinize urine:* May increase drug level and adverse effects. Use together cautiously.
Drug-food. *Foods that alkalinize urine:* May increase drug level and adverse effects. Use together cautiously.

Drug-lifestyle. *Alcohol use:* May alter drug adherence, decrease its effectiveness, or increase adverse effects. Discourage use together.
Nicotine: May alter levels of drug and nicotine. Discourage use together.

EFFECTS ON LAB TEST RESULTS
● May increase alkaline phosphatase level. May decrease hemoglobin level and hematocrit.

CONTRAINDICATIONS & CAUTIONS
● Contraindicated in patients allergic to drug or its components.
● Contraindicated for mild Alzheimer disease or other types of dementia.
● Drug isn't recommended for patients with severe renal impairment.
● Use cautiously in patients with seizures, hepatic impairment, or moderate renal impairment.
● Use cautiously in patients who may have an increased urine pH (from drugs, diet, renal tubular acidosis, or severe UTI, for example).

NURSING CONSIDERATIONS
● In elderly patients, even those with a normal creatinine level, use of this drug may impair renal function. Estimate creatinine clearance; reduce dosage in patients with moderate renal impairment. Don't give drug to patients with severe renal impairment.
● Monitor patient carefully for adverse reactions as he may not be able to recognize changes or communicate effectively.

PATIENT TEACHING
● Explain that drug doesn't cure Alzheimer disease but may aid patient to maintain function for a longer period of time.
● Tell patient or caregiver to report adverse effects.
● Urge patient to avoid alcohol during treatment.
● To avoid possible interactions, advise patient not to take herbal or OTC products without consulting prescriber.

rivastigmine tartrate
riv-ah-STIG-meen

Exelon, Exelon Patch

Pharmacologic class:
cholinesterase inhibitor
Pregnancy risk category B

AVAILABLE FORMS
Capsules: 1.5 mg, 3 mg, 4.5 mg, 6 mg
Patch, transdermal: 4.6 mg/24 hours,
9.5 mg/24 hours
Solution: 2 mg/ml

INDICATIONS & DOSAGES
➤ **Mild to moderate Alzheimer dementia**
Adults: Initially, 1.5 mg P.O. b.i.d. with food. If tolerated, may increase to 3 mg b.i.d. after 2 weeks. After 2 weeks at this dose, may increase to 4.5 mg b.i.d. and 6 mg b.i.d., as tolerated. Effective dosage range is 6 to 12 mg daily; maximum, 12 mg daily. Or, 4.6 mg/24 hours transdermal patch. After 4 weeks, if tolerated, increase to 9.5 mg/24 hours transdermal patch.
➤ **Mild to moderate dementia associated with Parkinson disease**
Adults: Initially, 1.5 mg P.O. b.i.d. May increase, as tolerated, to 3 mg b.i.d., then 4.5 mg b.i.d., and finally to 6 mg b.i.d. after a minimum of 4 weeks at each dose. Or, 4.6 mg/24 hours transdermal patch. After 4 weeks, if tolerated, increase to 9.5 mg/24 hours transdermal patch.

ADMINISTRATION
P.O.
● Give drug with food in the morning and evening.
● Solution may be taken directly or mixed with small glass of water, cold fruit juice, or soda.
● Capsule and solution doses are interchangeable.
Transdermal
● Apply patch once daily to clean, dry, hairless skin on the upper or lower back, upper arm, or chest, in a place not rubbed by tight clothing.
● Change the site daily, and don't use the same site within 14 days.

● Press patch firmly into place until the edges stick well.

ACTION
Thought to increase acetylcholine level by inhibiting cholinesterase enzyme, which causes acetylcholine hydrolysis.

Route	Onset	Peak	Duration
P.O.	Unknown	1 hr	12 hr
Transdermal	Unknown	8 hr	24 hr

Half-life: 1½ hours (oral); 3 hours (transdermal).

ADVERSE REACTIONS
CNS: *headache, dizziness,* syncope, fatigue, asthenia, malaise, somnolence, tremor, insomnia, confusion, depression, anxiety, hallucinations, aggressive reaction, vertigo, agitation, nervousness, delusion, paranoid reaction, pain.
CV: hypertension, chest pain, peripheral edema, ***bradycardia.***
EENT: rhinitis, pharyngitis.
GI: *nausea, vomiting, diarrhea, anorexia, abdominal pain,* dyspepsia, constipation, flatulence, eructation.
GU: UTI, incontinence.
Metabolic: weight loss.
Musculoskeletal: back pain, arthralgia, bone fracture.
Respiratory: upper respiratory tract infection, cough, bronchitis.
Skin: increased sweating, rash.
Other: *accidental trauma,* flulike symptoms.

INTERACTIONS
Drug-drug. *Anticholinergics:* May decrease effectiveness of anticholinergic. Monitor patient for expected therapeutic effects.
Bethanechol, succinylcholine, other neuromuscular-blocking drugs or cholinergic antagonists: May have synergistic effect. Monitor patient closely.
NSAIDs: May increase gastric acid secretions. Monitor patient for symptoms of active or occult GI bleeding.
Drug-lifestyle. *Smoking:* May increase drug clearance. Discourage smoking.

EFFECTS ON LAB TEST RESULTS
None reported.

Reactions may be *common*, uncommon, ***life-threatening***, or **COMMON AND LIFE-THREATENING**.
Interaction may have a *rapid onset* or ***delayed onset***.

CONTRAINDICATIONS & CAUTIONS

• Contraindicated in patients hypersensitive to drug, other carbamate derivatives, or other components of the drug.
• Use cautiously in patients with history of cardiovascular disease, GI bleeding, seizure disorder, genitourinary conditions, asthma, or obstructive pulmonary disease.

NURSING CONSIDERATIONS

• Expect significant GI adverse effects (such as nausea, vomiting, anorexia, and weight loss). These effects are less common during maintenance doses.
• Monitor patient for evidence of active or occult GI bleeding.
• Dramatic memory improvement is unlikely. As disease progresses, the benefits of drug may decline.
• Monitor patient for severe nausea, vomiting, and diarrhea, which may lead to dehydration and weight loss.
• Carefully monitor patient with a history of GI bleeding, NSAID use, arrhythmias, seizures, or pulmonary conditions for adverse effects.
• If adverse reactions, such as diarrhea, loss of appetite, nausea, or vomiting, occur with patch, stop use for several days, then restart at the same or lower dose. If treatment is interrupted for more than several days, restart patch at the lowest dose and retitrate.
• Patients weighing less than 50 kg (110 lb) may experience more adverse reactions when using the transdermal patch.
• When switching from an oral form to the transdermal patch, patients on a total daily dose of less than 6 mg can be switched to 4.6 mg/24 hours. Patients taking 6 to 12 mg orally can switch to the 9.5 mg/24 hour patch. The patch should be applied on the day after the last oral dose.

PATIENT TEACHING

• Tell caregiver to give drug with food in the morning and evening.
• Advise patient that memory improvement may be subtle and that drug more likely slows future memory loss.
• Tell patient to report nausea, vomiting, or diarrhea.
• Tell patient to consult prescriber before using OTC drugs.
• Tell patient to apply patch once daily to clean, dry, hairless skin in a place not rubbed by tight clothing.
• Teach patient that the recommended sites for patch placement include the upper or lower back, upper arm, or chest.
• Tell patient to change the site daily and not to use the same site within 14 days.
• Tell patient to press the patch firmly into place until the edges stick well.

37

Anticonvulsants

acetazolamide sodium
(See Chapter 25, DIURETICS.)
carbamazepine
clonazepam
diazepam
(See Chapter 42, ANXIOLYTICS.)
divalproex sodium
fosphenytoin sodium
gabapentin
lamotrigine
levetiracetam
magnesium sulfate
oxcarbazepine
phenobarbital
phenobarbital sodium
phenytoin
phenytoin sodium (prompt)
phenytoin sodium (extended)
primidone
tiagabine hydrochloride
topiramate
valproate sodium
valproic acid
zonisamide

---

carbamazepine
kar-ba-MAZ-e-peen

Carbatrol, Epitol, Equetro,
Novo-Carbamaz†, Tegretol,
Tegretol CR†, Tegretol-XR, Teril

Pharmacologic class: iminostilbene
derivative
Pregnancy risk category D

AVAILABLE FORMS
Capsules (extended-release): 100 mg,
200 mg, 300 mg
Oral suspension: 100 mg/5 ml
Tablets: 200 mg
Tablets (chewable): 100 mg, 200 mg
Tablets (extended-release): 100 mg,
200 mg, 300 mg, 400 mg†

INDICATIONS & DOSAGES
➤ **Generalized tonic-clonic and
complex partial seizures, mixed
seizure patterns (except Carbatrol)**
Adults and children older than age 12:
Initially, 200 mg P.O. b.i.d. (conventional
or extended-release tablets), or 100 mg
P.O. q.i.d. of suspension with meals. May
be increased weekly by 200 mg P.O. daily
in divided doses at 12-hour intervals for
extended-release tablets or 6- to 8-hour intervals for conventional tablets or suspension, adjusted to minimum effective level.
Maximum, 1,000 mg daily in children
ages 12 to 15, and 1,200 mg daily in patients older than age 15. Usual maintenance dosage is 800 to 1,200 mg daily.
Children ages 6 to 12: Initially, 100 mg
P.O. b.i.d. (conventional or extended-
release tablets) or 50 mg of suspension
P.O. q.i.d. with meals, increased at weekly
intervals by up to 100 mg P.O. divided in
three to four doses daily (divided b.i.d.
for extended-release form). Maximum,
1,000 mg daily. Usual maintenance
dosage is 400 to 800 mg daily; or, 20 to
30 mg/kg in divided doses three to four
times daily.
Children younger than age 6: 10 to
20 mg/kg in two to three divided doses
(conventional tablets) or four divided
doses (suspension). Maximum dosage is
35 mg/kg in 24 hours.
➤ **Epilepsy (Carbatrol only)**
Adults and children older than age 12:
200 mg P.O. b.i.d. Increase at weekly intervals by adding up to 200 mg daily until
optimal response is obtained. Dosage
shouldn't exceed 1,000 mg daily in children ages 12 to 15 and 1,200 mg daily in
patients older than age 15. Usual effective
maintenance level is 800 to 1,200 mg
daily.
➤ **Acute manic and mixed episodes
associated with bipolar I disorder**
Adults: Initially, 200 mg Equetro P.O.
b.i.d. Increase by 200 mg daily to
achieve therapeutic response. Doses
higher than 1,600 mg daily haven't
been studied.

Reactions may be *common*, uncommon, *life-threatening*, or COMMON AND LIFE-THREATENING.
Interaction may have a *rapid onset* or *delayed onset.*

➤ **Trigeminal neuralgia (except Carbatrol)**
Adults: Initially, 100 mg P.O. b.i.d. (conventional or extended-release tablets) or 50 mg of suspension q.i.d. with meals, increased by 100 mg every 12 hours for tablets or 50 mg of suspension q.i.d. until pain is relieved. Maximum, 1,200 mg daily. Maintenance dosage is usually 200 to 400 mg P.O. b.i.d.

➤ **Trigeminal neuralgia (Carbatrol only)**
Adults: Initially, 200-mg capsule P.O. daily. Daily dosage may be increased by up to 200 mg/day every 12 hours, only as needed to achieve freedom from pain. Don't exceed 1,200 mg daily.

➤ **Restless legs syndrome** ✦
Adults: 100 to 600 mg P.O. daily for up to 5 weeks.

➤ **Alcohol withdrawal** ✦
Adults: 600 to 1,200 mg P.O. on day 1, tapered to 0 mg over 5 to 10 days.

ADMINISTRATION
P.O.
• Shake oral suspension well before measuring dose.
• Contents of extended-release capsules may be sprinkled over applesauce if patient has difficulty swallowing capsules. Capsules and tablets shouldn't be crushed or chewed, unless labeled as chewable form.
• When giving by nasogastric tube, mix dose with an equal volume of water, normal saline solution, or D₅W. Flush tube with 100 ml of diluent after giving dose.
• Don't crush or split extended-release form or give broken or chipped tablets.

ACTION
Thought to stabilize neuronal membranes and limit seizure activity by either increasing efflux or decreasing influx of sodium ions across cell membranes in the motor cortex during generation of nerve impulses.

Route	Onset	Peak	Duration
P.O.	Unknown	1½–12 hr	Unknown
P.O. (extended-release)	Unknown	4–8 hr	Unknown

Half-life: 25 to 65 hours with single dose; 8 to 29 hours with long-term use.

ADVERSE REACTIONS
CNS: *ataxia, dizziness, drowsiness, vertigo,* **worsening of seizures,** confusion, fatigue, fever, headache, syncope.
CV: **arrhythmias, AV block, heart failure,** aggravation of coronary artery disease, hypertension, hypotension.
EENT: blurred vision, conjunctivitis, diplopia, dry pharynx, nystagmus.
GI: *nausea, vomiting,* abdominal pain, anorexia, diarrhea, dry mouth, glossitis, stomatitis.
GU: albuminuria, glycosuria, impotence, urinary frequency, urine retention.
Hematologic: *agranulocytosis, aplastic anemia, thrombocytopenia,* eosinophilia, leukocytosis.
Hepatic: *hepatitis.*
Metabolic: hyponatremia, SIADH.
Respiratory: pulmonary hypersensitivity.
Skin: *erythema multiforme, Stevens-Johnson syndrome,* excessive diaphoresis, rash, urticaria.
Other: chills.

INTERACTIONS
Drug-drug. *Atracurium, cisatracurium, pancuronium, rocuronium, vecuronium:* May decrease the effects of nondepolarizing muscle relaxant, causing it to be less effective. May need to increase the dose of the nondepolarizing muscle relaxant.
Cimetidine, danazol, diltiazem, fluoxetine, fluvoxamine, isoniazid, macrolides, propoxyphene, valproic acid, verapamil: May increase carbamazepine level. Use together cautiously.
Clarithromycin, erythromycin, troleandomycin: May inhibit metabolism of carbamazepine, increasing carbamazepine level and risk of toxicity. Avoid using together.
Doxycycline, felbamate, haloperidol, hormonal contraceptives, phenytoin, theophylline, tiagabine, topiramate, valproate, warfarin: May decrease levels of these drugs. Watch for decreased effect.
Lamotrigine: May decrease lamotrigine level and increase carbamazepine level. Monitor patient for clinical effects and toxicity.
Lithium: May increase CNS toxicity of lithium. Avoid using together.

MAO inhibitors: May increase depressant and anticholinergic effects. Avoid using together.

Phenobarbital, phenytoin, primidone: May decrease carbamazepine level. Watch for decreased effect.

Nefazodone: May increase carbamazepine levels and toxicity while reducing nefazodone levels and therapeutic benefits. Use together is contraindicated.

Drug-herb. *Plantains (psyllium seed):* May inhibit GI absorption of drug. Discourage use together.

EFFECTS ON LAB TEST RESULTS
● May increase BUN level. May decrease hemoglobin level and hematocrit.
● May increase liver function test values and eosinophil and WBC counts. May decrease thyroid function test values and granulocyte and platelet counts.
● May cause false pregnancy test results.

CONTRAINDICATIONS & CAUTIONS
● Contraindicated in patients hypersensitive to this drug or tricyclic antidepressants and in those with a history of bone marrow suppression; also contraindicated in those who have taken an MAO inhibitor within 14 days.
● Use cautiously in patients with mixed seizure disorders because they may experience an increased risk of seizures. Also, use with caution in patients with hepatic dysfunction.

NURSING CONSIDERATIONS
● *Alert:* Patients of Asian ancestry should get a genetic blood test to identify their risk for rare, but serious skin reactions (toxic epidermal necrolysis, Stevens-Johnson syndrome). Screen for HLA-B*1502 allele before starting treatment with carbamazepine.
● Watch for worsening of seizures, especially in patients with mixed seizure disorders, including atypical absence seizures.
● *Alert:* Closely monitor all patients taking or starting antiepileptic drugs for changes in behavior indicating worsening of suicidal thoughts or behavior or depression. Symptoms such as anxiety, agitation, hostility, mania, and hypo-

mania may be precursors to emerging suicidality.
● Obtain baseline determinations of urinalysis, BUN and iron levels, liver function, CBC, and platelet and reticulocyte counts. Monitor these values periodically thereafter.
■ **Black Box Warning** Aplastic anemia and agranulocytosis have been reported in association with carbamazepine therapy. Obtain complete pretreatment hematologic testing as a baseline. If patient in the course of treatment exhibits low or decreased WBC or platelet counts, monitor patient closely. Consider discontinuing drug if evidence of significant bone marrow depression develops. ■
● Never stop drug suddenly when treating seizures. Notify prescriber immediately if adverse reactions occur.
● Adverse reactions may be minimized by gradually increasing dosage.
● Therapeutic level is 4 to 12 mcg/ml. Monitor level and effects closely. Ask patient when last dose was taken to better evaluate drug level.
● When managing seizures, take appropriate precautions.
● *Alert:* Watch for signs of anorexia or subtle appetite changes, which may indicate excessive drug level.
● *Look alike–sound alike:* Don't confuse Tegretol or Tegretol-XR with Topamax, Toprol-XL, or Toradol. Don't confuse Carbatrol with carvedilol.

PATIENT TEACHING
● Instruct patient to take drug with food to minimize GI distress. Tell patient taking suspension form to shake container well before measuring dose.
● Tell patient not to crush or chew extended-release form and not to take broken or chipped tablets.
● Tell patient that Tegretol-XR tablet coating may appear in stool because it isn't absorbed.
● Advise patient to keep tablets in the original container and to keep the container tightly closed and away from moisture. Some formulations may harden when exposed to excessive moisture, so that less is available in the body, decreasing seizure control.

Reactions may be *common*, uncommon, *life-threatening*, or COMMON AND LIFE-THREATENING.
Interaction may have a *rapid onset* or *delayed onset.*

- Inform patient that when drug is used for trigeminal neuralgia, an attempt to decrease dosage or withdraw drug is usually made every 3 months.
- Advise patient to notify prescriber immediately if fever, sore throat, mouth ulcers, or easy bruising or bleeding occurs.
- Tell patient that drug may cause mild to moderate dizziness and drowsiness when first taken. Advise him to avoid hazardous activities until effects disappear, usually within 3 to 4 days.
- Advise patient that periodic eye examinations are recommended.
- Advise woman of risks to fetus if pregnancy occurs while taking carbamazepine.
- Advise woman that breast-feeding isn't recommended during therapy.

SAFETY ALERT!

clonazepam
kloe-NAZ-e-pam

Klonopin✔, Klonopin wafers

Pharmacologic class:
benzodiazepine
Pregnancy risk category D
Controlled substance schedule IV

AVAILABLE FORMS
Tablets: 0.5 mg, 1 mg, 2 mg
Tablets (orally disintegrating): 0.125 mg, 0.25 mg, 0.5 mg, 1 mg, 2 mg

INDICATIONS & DOSAGES
➤ **Lennox-Gastaut syndrome, atypical absence seizures, akinetic and myoclonic seizures**
Adults: Initially, no more than 1.5 mg P.O. daily in three divided doses. May be increased by 0.5 to 1 mg every 3 days until seizures are controlled. If given in unequal doses, give largest dose at bedtime. Maximum recommended daily dose is 20 mg.
Children up to age 10 or 30 kg (66 lb): Initially, 0.01 to 0.03 mg/kg P.O. daily (not to exceed 0.05 mg/kg daily) in two or three divided doses. Increase by 0.25 to 0.5 mg every third day to maximum main-

tenance dose of 0.1 to 0.2 mg/kg daily, as needed.
➤ **Panic disorder**
Adults: Initially, 0.25 mg P.O. b.i.d.; increase to target dose of 1 mg daily after 3 days. Some patients may benefit from dosages up to maximum of 4 mg daily. To achieve 4 mg daily, increase dosage in increments of 0.125 to 0.25 mg b.i.d. every 3 days, as tolerated, until panic disorder is controlled. Taper drug with decrease of 0.125 mg b.i.d. every 3 days until drug is stopped.

ADMINISTRATION
P.O.
- Peel back the foil of the orally disintegrating tablet (ODT) pouch carefully. Don't push ODT through foil.
- Give ODT to patient with or without water.

ACTION
Unknown. Probably acts by facilitating the effects of the inhibitory neurotransmitter GABA.

Route	Onset	Peak	Duration
P.O.	Unknown	1–2 hr	Unknown

Half-life: 18 to 50 hours.

ADVERSE REACTIONS
CNS: *drowsiness,* agitation, ataxia, behavioral disturbances, confusion, depression, slurred speech, tremor.
CV: palpitations.
EENT: abnormal eye movements, nystagmus.
GI: anorexia, change in appetite, constipation, diarrhea, gastritis, nausea, sore gums, vomiting.
GU: dysuria, enuresis, nocturia, urine retention.
Hematologic: *leukopenia, thrombocytopenia,* eosinophilia.
Respiratory: *respiratory depression,* chest congestion, shortness of breath.
Skin: rash.

INTERACTIONS
Drug-drug. *Carbamazepine, phenobarbital, phenytoin:* May lower clonazepam levels. Monitor patient closely.
CNS depressants: May increase CNS depression. Avoid using together.

Fluconazole, itraconazole, ketoconazole, miconazole: May increase and prolong drug levels, CNS depression, and psychomotor impairment. Avoid using together.

Drug-lifestyle. *Alcohol use:* May cause additive CNS effects. Discourage use together.

Smoking: May increase clearance of clonazepam. Monitor patient for decreased drug effects.

EFFECTS ON LAB TEST RESULTS
• May increase liver function test values and eosinophil count. May decrease platelet and WBC counts.

CONTRAINDICATIONS & CAUTIONS
• Contraindicated in patients hypersensitive to benzodiazepines and in those with significant hepatic disease or acute angle-closure glaucoma.
• Use cautiously in patients with mixed-type seizures because drug may cause generalized tonic-clonic seizures.
• Use cautiously in children and in patients with chronic respiratory disease, open-angle glaucoma, or a history of drug or alcohol addiction.
• Use cautiously in elderly patients. Drug may accumulate due to potential decrease in hepatic and renal function.

NURSING CONSIDERATIONS
• Watch for behavioral disturbances, especially in children.
• Don't stop drug abruptly because this may worsen seizures. Call prescriber at once if adverse reactions develop.
• Assess elderly patient's response closely. Elderly patients are more sensitive to drug's CNS effects.
• Monitor patient for oversedation.
• Monitor CBC and liver function tests.
• Withdrawal symptoms are similar to those of barbiturates.
• To reduce inconvenience of somnolence when drug is used for panic disorder, giving one dose at bedtime may be desirable.

PATIENT TEACHING
• Advise patient to avoid driving and other hazardous activities that require mental alertness until drug's CNS effects are known.

• Instruct parent to monitor child's school performance because drug may interfere with attentiveness.
• Warn patient and parents not to stop drug abruptly because seizures may occur.
• Advise patient that drug isn't for use during pregnancy or breast-feeding.
• Tell patients to open pouch of ODTs and peel back the foil. He shouldn't push the tablet *through* the foil.
• Tell patient to use dry hands when removing the ODT.
• Tell patient that ODTs can be taken with or without water.

---

fosphenytoin sodium
faws-FEN-i-toe-in

Cerebyx

Pharmacologic class: hydantoin derivative
Pregnancy risk category D

AVAILABLE FORMS
Injection: 2 ml (150 mg fosphenytoin sodium equivalent to 100 mg phenytoin sodium), 10 ml (750 mg fosphenytoin sodium equivalent to 500 mg phenytoin sodium)

INDICATIONS & DOSAGES
➤ **Status epilepticus**
Adults: 15 to 20 mg phenytoin sodium equivalent (PE)/kg I.V. at 100 to 150 mg PE/minute as loading dose; then 4 to 6 mg PE/kg daily I.V. as maintenance dose.
➤ **To prevent and treat seizures during neurosurgery (nonemergent loading or maintenance dosing)**
Adults: Loading dose of 10 to 20 mg PE/kg I.M. or I.V. at infusion rate not exceeding 150 mg PE/minute. Maintenance dose is 4 to 6 mg PE/kg daily I.V. or I.M.
➤ **Short-term substitution for oral phenytoin therapy**
Adults: Same total daily dose equivalent as oral phenytoin sodium therapy given as a single daily dose I.M. or I.V. at infusion rate not exceeding 150 mg PE/minute. Some patients may need more frequent dosing.

Elderly patients: Phenytoin clearance is decreased slightly in elderly patients; lower or less-frequent dosing may be required.

ADMINISTRATION

I.V.
● If rapid phenytoin loading is a main goal, this form is preferred.
● For status epilepticus, give I.V. rather than I.M. because therapeutic phenytoin level occurs more rapidly.
● For infusion, dilute in D_5W or normal saline solution for injection to yield 1.5 to 25 mg PE/ml.
● Don't give more than 150 mg PE/minute. For a 50-kg (110-lb) patient, infusion should take 5 to 7 minutes. (Infusion of identical molar dose of phenytoin takes at least 15 minutes, because giving phenytoin I.V. at more than 50 mg/minute causes adverse CV effects.)
● Patients receiving 20 mg PE/kg at 150 mg PE/minute typically feel discomfort, usually in the groin. To reduce discomfort, slow or temporarily stop infusion.
● Monitor patient's ECG, blood pressure, and respirations continuously during maximum phenytoin level—about 10 to 20 minutes after end of fosphenytoin infusion. Severe CV complications are most common in elderly or gravely ill patients. If needed, decrease rate or stop infusion.
● Store drug under refrigeration. Don't store at room temperature longer than 48 hours. Discard vials that develop particulate matter.
● **Incompatibilities:** Other I.V. drugs.
I.M.
● Depending on dose ordered, may require two separate I.M. injections.
● I.M. administration generates systemic phenytoin levels similar enough to oral phenytoin sodium to allow essentially interchangeable use.
● Store drug under refrigeration. Don't store at room temperature longer than 48 hours. Discard vials that develop particulate matter.

ACTION

May stabilize neuronal membranes and limit seizure activity either by increasing efflux or decreasing influx of sodium ions across cell membranes in the motor cortex during generation of nerve impulses.

Route	Onset	Peak	Duration
I.V.	Unknown	End of infusion	Unknown
I.M.	Unknown	30 min	Unknown

Half-life: 15 minutes.

ADVERSE REACTIONS

CNS: *ataxia, dizziness, somnolence, **brain edema, intracranial hypertension,*** agitation, asthenia, dysarthria, extrapyramidal syndrome, fever, headache, hypesthesia, incoordination, increased or decreased reflexes, nervousness, paresthesia, speech disorders, stupor, thinking abnormalities, tremor, vertigo.
CV: hypertension, hypotension, tachycardia, vasodilation.
EENT: *nystagmus,* amblyopia, deafness, diplopia, tinnitus.
GI: constipation, dry mouth, taste perversion, tongue disorder, vomiting.
GU: pelvic pain.
Metabolic: hypokalemia.
Musculoskeletal: back pain, myasthenia.
Respiratory: pneumonia.
Skin: *pruritus,* ecchymoses, injection site reaction and pain, rash.
Other: accidental injury, chills, facial edema, infection.

INTERACTIONS

Drug-drug. *Amiodarone, chloramphenicol, chlordiazepoxide, cimetidine, diazepam, disulfiram, estrogens, ethosuximide, fluoxetine, H_2 antagonists, halothane, isoniazid, methylphenidate, phenothiazines, phenylbutazone, salicylates, succinimides, sulfonamides, tolbutamide, trazodone:* May increase phenytoin level and effect. Use together cautiously.
Carbamazepine, reserpine: May decrease phenytoin level. Monitor patient.
Corticosteroids, doxycycline, estrogens, furosemide, hormonal contraceptives, quinidine, rifampin, theophylline, vitamin D, warfarin: May decrease effects of these drugs because of increased hepatic metabolism. Monitor patient closely.
Lithium: May increase lithium toxicity. Monitor patient's neurologic status closely.

Marked neurologic symptoms have been reported despite normal lithium level.

Phenobarbital, valproate sodium, valproic acid: May increase or decrease phenytoin level. May increase or decrease levels of these drugs. Monitor patient.

Tricyclic antidepressants: May lower seizure threshold and require adjustments in phenytoin dosage. Use together cautiously.

Drug-lifestyle. *Alcohol use:* Acute intoxication may increase phenytoin level and effect. Discourage use together.

Long-term alcohol use: May decrease phenytoin level. Monitor patient and strongly discourage use together.

EFFECTS ON LAB TEST RESULTS

● May increase alkaline phosphatase, GGT, and glucose levels. May decrease folate, potassium, and T_4 levels.
● May cause falsely low dexamethasone and metyrapone test results.

CONTRAINDICATIONS & CAUTIONS

● Contraindicated in patients hypersensitive to drug or its components, phenytoin, or other hydantoins.
● Contraindicated in those with sinus bradycardia, SA block, second- or third-degree AV block, or Adams-Stokes syndrome.
● Use cautiously in patients with porphyria and in those with history of hypersensitivity to similarly structured drugs, such as barbiturates, oxazolidinediones, and succinimide.

NURSING CONSIDERATIONS

● Most significant drug interactions are those commonly seen with phenytoin.
● *Alert:* Drug should always be prescribed and dispensed in phenytoin sodium equivalent units (PE). Don't make adjustments in the recommended doses when substituting fosphenytoin for phenytoin, and vice versa.
● In status epilepticus, phenytoin may be used instead of fosphenytoin as maintenance, using the appropriate dose.
● Phosphate load provided by fosphenytoin (0.0037 millimole phosphate/mg PE fosphenytoin) must be taken into consideration when treating patients who need

phosphate restriction, such as those with severe renal impairment. Monitor laboratory values.

● If patient gets exfoliative, purpuric, or bullous rash or signs and symptoms of lupus erythematosus, Stevens-Johnson syndrome, or toxic epidermal necrolysis, stop drug and notify prescriber. If rash is mild (measleslike or scarlatiniform), therapy may resume after rash disappears. If rash recurs when therapy is resumed, further fosphenytoin or phenytoin administration is contraindicated. Document that patient is allergic to drug.
● Stop drug in patients with acute hepatotoxicity.
● After administration, phenytoin levels shouldn't be monitored until conversion to phenytoin is essentially complete—about 2 hours after the end of an I.V. infusion or 4 hours after I.M. administration.
● Interpret total phenytoin levels cautiously in patients with renal or hepatic disease or hypoalbuminemia caused by an increased fraction in unbound phenytoin. It may be more useful to monitor unbound phenytoin levels in these patients. When giving drug I.V., monitor patients with renal and hepatic disease because they are at increased risk for more frequent and severe adverse reactions.
● Monitor glucose level closely in diabetic patients; drug may cause hyperglycemia.
● Abrupt withdrawal of drug may precipitate status epilepticus.
● *Look alike–sound alike:* Don't confuse Cerebyx with Cerezyme, Celexa, or Celebrex.

PATIENT TEACHING

● Warn patient that sensory disturbances may occur with I.V. administration.
● Instruct patient to immediately report adverse reactions, especially rash.
● Warn patient not to stop drug abruptly or adjust dosage without discussing with prescriber.
● Advise woman of childbearing age to discuss drug therapy with prescriber if she's considering pregnancy.
● Advise woman of childbearing age that breast-feeding isn't recommended during therapy.

gabapentin
gab-ah-PEN-tin

Neurontin✍, Gabarone

Pharmacologic class: gamma-
aminobutyric acid (GABA)
structural analog
Pregnancy risk category C

AVAILABLE FORMS
Capsules: 100 mg, 300 mg, 400 mg
Oral solution: 250 mg/5 ml
Tablets: 100 mg, 300 mg, 400 mg,
600 mg, 800 mg

INDICATIONS & DOSAGES
➤ **Adjunctive treatment of partial
seizures with or without secondary
generalization in patients with
epilepsy**
Adults and children older than age 12:
Initially, 300 mg P.O. t.i.d. Increase dosage
as needed and tolerated to 1,800 mg daily
in divided doses. Dosages up to 3,600 mg
daily have been well tolerated.
➤ **Adjunctive treatment to control
partial seizures in children**
Starting dosage, children ages 3 to 12:
10 to 15 mg/kg daily P.O. in three divided
doses, adjusting over 3 days to reach
effective dosage.
Effective dosage, children ages 5 to 12:
25 to 35 mg/kg daily P.O. in three divided
doses.
Effective dosage, children ages 3 to 4:
40 mg/kg daily P.O. in three divided doses.
➤ **Postherpetic neuralgia**
Adults: 300 mg P.O. once daily on first
day, 300 mg b.i.d. on day 2, and 300 mg
t.i.d. on day 3. Adjust as needed for pain
to a maximum daily dose of 1,800 mg in
three divided doses.
Adjust-a-dose: In patients age 12 and
older with creatinine clearance of 30 to
59 ml/minute, give 400 to 1,400 mg daily,
divided into two doses. For clearance of
15 to 29 ml/minute, give 200 to 700 mg
daily in single dose. For clearance less
than 15 ml/minute, give 100 to 300 mg
daily, in single dose. Reduce daily dose in
proportion to creatinine clearance (patients with a clearance of 7.5 ml/minute
should receive one-half the daily dose of

those with a clearance of 15 ml/minute).
For patients receiving hemodialysis, maintenance dose is based on estimates of creatinine clearance. Give supplemental dose
of 125 to 350 mg after each 4 hours of
hemodialysis.
➤ **Pain from diabetic neuropathy ◆**
Adults: 3.6 g P.O. daily in divided doses.
➤ **Vasomotor symptoms in women
with breast cancer and in postmenopausal women ◆**
Women: 300 mg P.O. once daily at bedtime. May increase to 300 mg P.O. b.i.d.,
then 300 mg P.O. t.i.d. at 3- to 4-day
intervals.

ADMINISTRATION
P.O.
● Give drug without regard for food.
● Refrigerate oral solution.

ACTION
Unknown. Structurally related to GABA
but doesn't interact with GABA receptors,
isn't converted into GABA or GABA agonist, doesn't inhibit GABA reuptake, and
doesn't prevent degradation.

Route	Onset	Peak	Duration
P.O.	Unknown	Unknown	Unknown

Half-life: 5 to 7 hours.

ADVERSE REACTIONS
CNS: *ataxia, dizziness, fatigue, somno-
lence,* abnormal thinking, amnesia, de-
pression, dysarthria, incoordination, ner-
vousness, nystagmus, tremor, twitching.
CV: peripheral edema, vasodilation.
EENT: amblyopia, diplopia, dry throat,
pharyngitis, rhinitis.
GI: constipation, dry mouth, dyspepsia,
increased appetite, nausea, vomiting.
GU: impotence.
Hematologic: *leukopenia.*
Metabolic: weight gain.
Musculoskeletal: back pain, fractures,
myalgia.
Respiratory: coughing.
Skin: abrasion, pruritus.
Other: dental abnormalities.

INTERACTIONS
Drug-drug. *Antacids:* May decrease absorption of gabapentin. Separate dosage
times by at least 2 hours.

Hydrocodone: May increase gabapentin level and decrease hydrocodone level. Monitor patient for increased adverse effects or loss of clinical effect.

EFFECTS ON LAB TEST RESULTS
• May decrease WBC count.
• May cause false-positive results with the Ames-N-Multistix SG dipstick test for urine protein when used with other antiepileptics.

CONTRAINDICATIONS & CAUTIONS
• Contraindicated in patients hypersensitive to drug.
• In elderly patients, adjust dosage based on creatinine clearance values due to potentially decreased renal function.

NURSING CONSIDERATIONS
• Give first dose at bedtime to minimize drowsiness, dizziness, fatigue, and ataxia.
• *Alert:* Closely monitor all patients taking or starting antiepileptic drugs for changes in behavior indicating worsening of suicidal thoughts or behavior or depression. Symptoms such as anxiety, agitation, hostility, mania, and hypomania may be precursors to emerging suicidality.
• If drug is to be stopped or an alternative drug substituted, do so gradually over at least 1 week to minimize risk of precipitating seizures.
• *Alert:* Don't suddenly withdraw other anticonvulsants in patients starting gabapentin therapy.
• Routine monitoring of drug levels isn't necessary. Drug doesn't appear to alter levels of other anticonvulsants.
• *Look alike–sound alike:* Don't confuse Neurontin with Noroxin.

PATIENT TEACHING
• Advise patient that drug may be taken without regard for meals.
• Instruct patient to take first dose at bedtime to minimize adverse reactions.
• Tell patient with seizures the maximum time interval between doses shouldn't exceed 12 hours.
• Warn patient to avoid driving and operating heavy machinery until drug's CNS effects are known.
• Advise patient not to stop drug abruptly.

• Advise woman to discuss drug therapy with prescriber if she's considering pregnancy.
• Tell patient to keep oral solution refrigerated.

---

lamotrigine
la-MO-tri-geen

Lamictal, Lamictal CD

Pharmacologic class: phenyltriazine
Pregnancy risk category C

AVAILABLE FORMS
Tablets: 25 mg, 100 mg, 150 mg, 200 mg
Tablets (chewable dispersible): 2 mg, 5 mg, 25 mg

INDICATIONS & DOSAGES
➤ **Adjunct treatment of partial seizures or primary generalized tonic-clonic seizures caused by epilepsy or generalized seizures of Lennox-Gastaut syndrome**
Adults and children older than age 12 taking other enzyme-inducing anticonvulsants with valproic acid: 25 mg P.O. every other day for 2 weeks; then 25 mg P.O. daily for 2 weeks. Continue to increase, as needed, by 25 to 50 mg daily every 1 to 2 weeks until an effective maintenance dosage of 100 to 400 mg daily given in one or two divided doses is reached. When added to valproic acid alone, the usual daily maintenance dose is 100 to 200 mg.
Adults and children older than age 12 taking other enzyme-inducing anticonvulsants but not valproic acid: 50 mg P.O. daily for 2 weeks; then 100 mg P.O. daily in two divided doses for 2 weeks. Increase, as needed, by 100 mg daily every 1 to 2 weeks. Usual maintenance dosage is 300 to 500 mg P.O. daily in two divided doses.
Children ages 2 to 12 weighing 6.7 to 40 kg (15 to 88 lb) taking other enzyme-inducing anticonvulsants with valproic acid: 0.15 mg/kg P.O. daily in one or two divided doses (rounded down to nearest whole tablet) for 2 weeks, followed by 0.3 mg/kg daily in one or two divided doses for another 2 weeks. Thereafter,

---

Reactions may be *common,* uncommon, *life-threatening,* or COMMON AND LIFE-THREATENING.
Interaction may have a *rapid onset* or *delayed onset.*

usual maintenance dosage is 1 to 5 mg/kg daily (maximum, 200 mg daily in one to two divided doses).

Children ages 2 to 12 weighing 6.7 to 40 kg (15 to 88 lb) taking other enzyme-inducing anticonvulsants but not valproic acid: 0.6 mg/kg P.O. daily in two divided doses (rounded down to nearest whole tablet) for 2 weeks; then 1.2 mg/kg daily in two divided doses for another 2 weeks. Usual maintenance dosage is 5 to 15 mg/kg P.O. daily (maximum 400 mg daily in two divided doses).

➤ **To convert patients from therapy with a hepatic enzyme-inducing anticonvulsant alone to lamotrigine therapy**

Adults and children age 16 and older: Add lamotrigine 50 mg P.O. once daily to current drug regimen for 2 weeks, followed by 100 mg P.O. daily in two divided doses for 2 weeks. Then increase daily dosage by 100 mg every 1 to 2 weeks until maintenance dose of 500 mg daily in two divided doses is reached. The concomitant hepatic enzyme-inducing anticonvulsant can then be gradually reduced by 20% decrements weekly for 4 weeks.

Adjust-a-dose: For patients with severe renal impairment, use lower maintenance dosage.

➤ **To convert patients with partial seizures from adjunctive therapy with valproate to therapy with lamotrigine alone**

Adults and children age 16 and older: Add lamotrigine until 200 mg daily is achieved; then gradually decrease valproate to 500 mg daily by decrements of no more than 500 mg daily per week. Maintain these dosages for 1 week, then increase lamotrigine to 300 mg daily while decreasing valproate to 250 mg daily. Maintain these dosages for 1 week, then stop valproate completely while increasing lamotrigine by 100 mg daily every week until a dose of 500 mg daily is reached.

➤ **Bipolar disorder**

Adults: Initially, 25 mg P.O. once daily for 2 weeks; then 50 mg P.O. once daily for 2 weeks. Dosage may then be doubled at weekly intervals, to maintenance dosage of 200 mg daily.

Adults taking carbamazepine or other hepatic enzyme-inducing drugs without valproic acid: Initially, 50 mg P.O. once daily for 2 weeks; then 100 mg daily in two divided doses for 2 weeks. Dosage is then increased by 100 mg weekly to maintenance dosage of 400 mg daily, given in two divided doses.

Adults taking valproic acid: Initially, 25 mg P.O. every other day for 2 weeks; then 25 mg P.O. once daily for 2 weeks. Dosage may then be doubled at weekly intervals to maintenance dosage of 100 mg daily.

ADMINISTRATION
P.O.
● Chewable dispersible tablets may be swallowed whole, chewed, or dispersed in water or diluted fruit juice.
● If tablets are chewed, give a small amount of water or diluted fruit juice to aid in swallowing.

ACTION
Unknown. May inhibit release of glutamate and aspartate (excitatory neurotransmitters) in the brain via an action at voltage-sensitive sodium channels.

Route	Onset	Peak	Duration
P.O.	Unknown	1–5 hr	Unknown

Half-life: 14½ to 70¼ hours, depending on dosage schedule and use of other anticonvulsants.

ADVERSE REACTIONS
CNS: *ataxia, dizziness, headache, somnolence, **seizures,*** aggravated reaction, anxiety, concentration disturbance, decreased memory, depression, dysarthria, emotional lability, fever, incoordination, insomnia, irritability, malaise, mind racing, speech disorder, sleep disorder, tremor, vertigo.
CV: palpitations.
EENT: *blurred vision, diplopia, rhinitis,* nystagmus, pharyngitis, vision abnormality.
GI: *nausea, vomiting,* abdominal pain, anorexia, constipation, diarrhea, dry mouth, dyspepsia.
GU: amenorrhea, dysmenorrhea, vaginitis.
Musculoskeletal: muscle spasm, neck pain.
Respiratory: cough, dyspnea.

Skin: *rash,* ***Stevens-Johnson syndrome, toxic epidermal necrolysis,*** acne, alopecia, hot flashes, pruritus.
Other: chills, flulike syndrome, infection, tooth disorder.

INTERACTIONS
Drug-drug. *Acetaminophen:* May decrease therapeutic effects of lamotrigine. Monitor patient
Carbamazepine: May decrease effects of lamotrigine while increasing toxicity of carbamazepine. Adjust doses and monitor patient.
Ethosuximide, oxcarbazepine, phenobarbital, phenytoin, primidone: May decrease lamotrigine level. Monitor patient closely.
Folate inhibitors, such as co-trimoxazole and methotrexate: May have additive effect because lamotrigine inhibits dihydrofolate reductase, an enzyme involved in folic acid synthesis. Monitor patient.
Hormonal contraceptives containing estrogen, rifampin: May decrease lamotrigine levels. Adjust dosage. By the end of the "pill-free" week, lamotrigine levels may double.
Valproic acid: May decrease clearance of lamotrigine, which increases lamotrigine level; also decreases valproic acid level. Monitor patient for toxicity.
Drug-lifestyle. *Sun exposure:* May cause photosensitivity reactions. Advise patient to avoid excessive sun exposure.

EFFECTS ON LAB TEST RESULTS
None reported.

CONTRAINDICATIONS & CAUTIONS
● Contraindicated in patients hypersensitive to drug or its components.
● Use cautiously in patients with renal, hepatic, or cardiac impairment.

NURSING CONSIDERATIONS
● *Alert:* Closely monitor all patients taking or starting antiepileptic drugs for changes in behavior indicating worsening of suicidal thoughts or behavior or depression. Symptoms such as anxiety, agitation, hostility, mania, and hypomania may be precursors to emerging suicidality.
● Don't stop drug abruptly because this may increase seizure frequency. Instead, taper drug over at least 2 weeks.

■ **Black Box Warning** Serious rashes requiring hospitalization and discontinuation of treatment have been reported in association with lamotrigine therapy. Stop drug at first sign of rash, unless rash is clearly not drug-related. ■
● Reduce lamotrigine dose if drug is added to a multidrug regimen that includes valproic acid.
● Evaluate patients for changes in seizure activity. Check adjunct anticonvulsant level.
● *Look alike–sound alike:* Don't confuse lamotrigine with lamivudine or Lamictal with Lamisil, Ludiomil, labetalol, or Lomotil.

PATIENT TEACHING
● Inform patient that drug may cause rash. Combination therapy of valproic acid and lamotrigine may cause a serious rash. Tell patient to report rash or signs or symptoms of hypersensitivity promptly to prescriber because they may warrant stopping drug.
● Warn patient not to engage in hazardous activity until drug's CNS effects are known.
● Warn patient that the drug may trigger sensitivity to the sun and to take precautions until tolerance is determined.
● Warn patient not to stop drug abruptly.
● *Alert:* Advise woman of childbearing age to discuss drug therapy with prescriber if she's considering pregnancy. Babies exposed to drug during the first trimester have a greater risk of cleft lip or palate.
● Advise woman of childbearing age that breast-feeding isn't recommended during therapy.

---

levetiracetam
lee-vah-tih-RACE-ah-tam

Keppra

Pharmacologic class: pyrrolidine derivative
Pregnancy risk category C

AVAILABLE FORMS
Injection: 500 mg/5 ml single-use vial
Oral solution: 100 mg/ml
Tablets: 250 mg, 500 mg, 750 mg, 1,000 mg

INDICATIONS & DOSAGES
➤ **Adjunctive therapy for myoclonic seizures of juvenile myoclonic epilepsy**
Adults and adolescents age 12 and older:
Initially, 500 mg P.O. b.i.d. Increase by 1,000 mg/day every 2 weeks to daily dose of 3,000 mg.
➤ **Adjunctive therapy for primary generalized tonic-clonic seizures**
Adults and adolescents age 16 and older:
Initially, 500 mg P.O. b.i.d. Increase dose by 500 mg b.i.d. every 2 weeks to dose of 1,500 mg b.i.d.
Children ages 6 to 16: Initially, 10 mg/kg P.O. b.i.d. Increase dose by 10 mg/kg b.i.d. at 2-week intervals to dose of 30 mg/kg b.i.d. For children who weigh more than 20 kg (44 lb), use either tablets or oral solution. For children who weigh 20 kg or less, use the oral solution.
➤ **Adjunctive treatment for partial-onset seizures in patients with epilepsy**
Adults and adolescents age 16 or older:
Initially, 500 mg P.O. or I.V. b.i.d. Increase dosage by 500 mg b.i.d., as needed, for seizure control at 2-week intervals to maximum of 1,500 mg b.i.d.
Children ages 4 to 16: Initially, 10 mg/kg P.O. b.i.d. Increase dose by 10 mg/kg b.i.d. at 2-week intervals to recommended dose of 30 mg/kg b.i.d. If patient can't tolerate this dose, reduce it. For children who weigh 20 kg or less, use the oral solution.
Adjust-a-dose: For adults with creatinine clearance of 50 to 80 ml/minute, give 500 to 1,000 mg every 12 hours; if clearance is 30 to 50 ml/minute, give 250 to 750 mg every 12 hours; if clearance is less than 30 ml/minute, give 250 to 500 mg every 12 hours. For dialysis patients, give 500 to 1,000 mg every 24 hours. Give a 250- to 500-mg dose after dialysis.

ADMINISTRATION
P.O.
● Give drug without regard for food.
● P.O. and I.V. forms are bioequivalent.
I.V.
● Dilute drug before giving.
● Dilute 500-mg, 1,000-mg, or 1,500-mg dose in 100 ml normal saline, D₅W, or lactated Ringer's injection and infuse over 15 minutes.

● Drug is compatible with diazepam, lorazepam, and valproate sodium for 24 hours at a controlled room temperature.
● **Incompatibilities:** Unknown with other antiepileptics besides diazepam, lorazepam, and valproate sodium.

ACTION
May act by inhibiting simultaneous neuronal firing that leads to seizure activity.

Route	Onset	Peak	Duration
P.O., I.V.	1 hr	1 hr	12 hr

Half-life: About 7 hours in patients with normal renal function.

ADVERSE REACTIONS
CNS: *asthenia, headache, somnolence,* amnesia, anxiety, ataxia, depression, dizziness, emotional lability, hostility, nervousness, paresthesia, pain, vertigo.
EENT: diplopia, pharyngitis, rhinitis, sinusitis.
GI: anorexia.
Hematologic: *leukopenia, neutropenia.*
Respiratory: cough, infection.

INTERACTIONS
Drug-drug. *Antihistamines, benzodiazepines, opioids, other drugs that cause drowsiness, tricyclic antidepressants:* May lead to severe sedation. Avoid using together.
Drug-lifestyle. *Alcohol use:* May lead to severe sedation. Discourage use together.

EFFECTS ON LAB TEST RESULTS
● May alter liver function test results. May decrease hemoglobin and hematocrit.
● May decrease WBC, RBC, and neutrophil counts.

CONTRAINDICATIONS & CAUTIONS
● Contraindicated in patients hypersensitive to drug.
● Use cautiously in immunocompromised patients, such as those with cancer or HIV infection. Leukopenia and neutropenia have been reported with drug use.
● Use cautiously in patients with history of psychiatric symptoms, especially psychotic symptoms and behaviors.

NURSING CONSIDERATIONS
• *Look alike–sound alike:* Don't confuse Keppra with Kaletra.
• Use drug only with other anticonvulsants; it's not recommended for monotherapy.
• Seizures can occur if drug is stopped abruptly. Tapering is recommended.
• Monitor patients closely for such adverse reactions as dizziness, which may lead to falls.
• *Alert:* Closely monitor all patients taking or starting antiepileptic drugs for changes in behavior indicating worsening of suicidal thoughts or behavior or depression. Symptoms such as anxiety, agitation, hostility, mania, and hypomania may be precursors to emerging suicidality.

PATIENT TEACHING
• Warn patient to use extra care when sitting or standing to avoid falling.
• Advise patient to call prescriber and not to stop drug suddenly if adverse reactions occur.
• Tell patient to take with other prescribed seizure drugs.
• For the oral solution, tell patient or parent to use a calibrated measuring device, not a household spoon.
• Warn patient that drug may cause dizziness and somnolence and that he should avoid driving, bike riding, or other hazardous activities until he knows how the drug will affect him.
• Inform patient that drug can be taken with or without food.

SAFETY ALERT!

magnesium sulfate
mag-NEE-zee-um

Pharmacologic class: mineral; electrolyte
Pregnancy risk category A

AVAILABLE FORMS
Injection: 4%, 8%, 10%, 12.5%, 25%, 50%
Injection solution: 1% in D_5W, 2% in D_5W

INDICATIONS & DOSAGES
➤ **To prevent or control seizures in preeclampsia or eclampsia**
Women: Initially, 4 g I.V. in 250 ml D_5W or normal saline and 4 to 5 g deep I.M. into each buttock; then 4 to 5 g deep I.M. into alternate buttock every 4 hours, as needed. Or, 4 g I.V. loading dose; then 1 to 3 g hourly as I.V. infusion. Total dose shouldn't exceed 30 or 40 g daily.
➤ **Hypomagnesemia**
Adults: For mild deficiency, 1 g I.M. every 6 hours for four doses; for severe deficiency, 5 g in 1,000 ml D_5W or normal saline solution infused over 3 hours.
➤ **Seizures, hypertension, and encephalopathy with acute nephritis in children**
Children: 20 to 40 mg/kg I.M. as needed to control seizures. Dilute the 50% concentration to a 20% solution and give 0.1 to 0.2 ml/kg of the 20% solution.
➤ **To manage paroxysmal atrial tachycardia**
Adults: 3 to 4 g I.V. over 30 seconds, with extreme caution.
➤ **To manage life-threatening ventricular arrhythmias, such as sustained ventricular tachycardia or torsades de pointes ♦**
Adults: 1 to 6 g I.V. over several minutes; then continuous I.V. infusion of 3 to 20 mg/minute for 5 to 48 hours. Base dosage and duration of therapy on patient response and magnesium level.
➤ **To manage preterm labor ♦**
Adults: 4 to 6 g I.V. over 20 minutes, followed by 2 to 4 g/hour I.V. infusion for 12 to 24 hours, as tolerated, after contractions have stopped.

ADMINISTRATION
I.V.
• If necessary, dilute to maximum level of 20%. Infuse no faster than 150 mg/minute (1.5 ml/minute of a 10% solution or 0.75 ml/minute of a 20% solution). Drug is compatible with D_5W and normal saline solution.

Reactions may be *common,* uncommon, *life-threatening,* or COMMON AND LIFE-THREATENING.
Interaction may have a *rapid onset* or *delayed onset.*

• Maximum infusion rate is 150 mg/ minute. Too-rapid infusion produces uncomfortable feeling of heat.
• Monitor vital signs every 15 minutes when giving drug I.V.
• **Incompatibilities:** Alkali carbonates and bicarbonates, amiodarone, amphotericin B, calcium gluconate, cefepime, ciprofloxacin, clindamycin, cyclosporine, dobutamine, heavy metals, I.V. fat emulsion 10%, polymyxin B, procaine, salicylates, sodium bicarbonate, soluble phosphates.
I.M.
• For adults, give undiluted 50% concentration by deep injection.
• For children, dilute to concentration of 20% or less with D_5W or normal saline for injection.

ACTION
May decrease acetylcholine released by nerve impulses, but anticonvulsant mechanism is unknown.

Route	Onset	Peak	Duration
I.V.	1–2 min	Rapid	30 min
I.M.	1 hr	Unknown	3–4 hr

Half-life: Unknown.

ADVERSE REACTIONS
CNS: *depressed reflexes,* drowsiness, flaccid paralysis, hypothermia.
CV: *flushing, hypotension,* **bradycardia, circulatory collapse,** depressed cardiac function.
EENT: diplopia.
Metabolic: hypocalcemia.
Respiratory: *respiratory paralysis.*
Skin: diaphoresis.

INTERACTIONS
Drug-drug. *Anesthetics, CNS depressants:* May cause additive CNS depression. Use together cautiously.
Cardiac glycosides: May worsen arrhythmias. Use together cautiously.
Neuromuscular blockers: May cause increased neuromuscular blockade. Use together cautiously.

EFFECTS ON LAB TEST RESULTS
• May increase magnesium level. May decrease calcium level.

CONTRAINDICATIONS & CAUTIONS
• Parenteral administration contraindicated in patients with heart block or myocardial damage.
• Contraindicated in patients with toxemia of pregnancy during 2 hours preceding delivery.
• Use cautiously in patients with impaired renal function.
• Use cautiously in pregnant women during labor.

NURSING CONSIDERATIONS
• If used to treat seizures, take appropriate seizure precautions.
• ***Alert:*** Watch for respiratory depression and signs and symptoms of heart block.
• Keep I.V. calcium gluconate available to reverse magnesium intoxication, but use cautiously in digitalized patients because of danger of arrhythmias.
• Check magnesium level after repeated doses. Disappearance of knee-jerk and patellar reflexes is sign of impending magnesium toxicity.
• Signs of hypermagnesemia begin to appear at levels of 4 mEq/L.
• Effective anticonvulsant level ranges from 2.5 to 7.5 mEq/L.
• Monitor fluid intake and output. Make sure urine output is 100 ml or more in 4-hour period before each dose.
• Observe neonates for signs of magnesium toxicity, including neuromuscular or respiratory depression, when giving I.V. form of drug to toxemic mothers within 24 hours before delivery.
• ***Look alike–sound alike:*** Don't confuse magnesium sulfate with manganese sulfate.

PATIENT TEACHING
• Inform patient of short-term need for drug and answer any questions and address concerns.
• Review potential adverse reactions and instruct patient to promptly report any occurrences. Reassure patient that, although adverse reactions can occur, vital signs, reflexes, and drug level will be monitored frequently to ensure safety.

---

†Canada   ◇OTC   ♦Off-label use   ℰPhotoguide   *Liquid contains alcohol.

oxcarbazepine
oks-car-BAZ-e-peen

Trileptal

Pharmacologic class: carboxamide derivative
Pregnancy risk category C

AVAILABLE FORMS
Oral suspension: 300 mg/5 ml (60 mg/ml)
Tablets (film-coated): 150 mg, 300 mg, 600 mg

INDICATIONS & DOSAGES
➤ **Adjunctive treatment of partial seizures in patients with epilepsy**
Adults: Initially, 300 mg P.O. b.i.d. Increase by a maximum of 600 mg daily (300 mg P.O. b.i.d.) at weekly intervals. Recommended daily dose is 1,200 mg P.O. divided b.i.d.
Children ages 4 to 16: Initially, 8 to 10 mg/kg daily P.O. divided b.i.d., not to exceed 600 mg daily. The target maintenance dose depends on patient's weight and should be divided b.i.d. If patient weighs between 20 and 29 kg (44 and 64 lb), target maintenance dose is 900 mg daily. If patient weighs between 29 and 39 kg (64 and 86 lb), target maintenance dose is 1,200 mg daily. If patient weighs more than 39 kg (86 lb), target maintenance dose is 1,800 mg daily. Target doses should be achieved over 2 weeks.
➤ **To change from multidrug to single-drug treatment of partial seizures in patients with epilepsy**
Adults: Initially, 300 mg P.O. b.i.d. while reducing dose of concomitant anticonvulsant. Increase oxcarbazepine by a maximum of 600 mg daily at weekly intervals over 2 to 4 weeks. Recommended daily dose is 2,400 mg P.O. divided b.i.d. Withdraw other anticonvulsant completely over 3 to 6 weeks.
Children ages 4 to 16: Initially, 8 to 10 mg/kg daily P.O. divided b.i.d., while reducing dose of concomitant anticonvulsant. Increase oxcarbazepine by a maximum of 10 mg/kg daily at weekly intervals. Withdraw other anticonvulsant completely over 3 to 6 weeks.

➤ **To start single-drug treatment of partial seizures in patients with epilepsy**
Adults: Initially, 300 mg P.O. b.i.d. Increase dosage by 300 mg daily every third day to a daily dose of 1,200 mg divided b.i.d.
Children ages 4 to 16: Initially, 8 to 10 mg/kg daily P.O. divided b.i.d., increasing the dosage by 5 mg/kg daily every third day to the recommended daily dose range shown in the table.

Weight (kg)	Dose (mg/day)
20	600–900
25	900–1,200
30	900–1,200
35	900–1,500
40	900–1,500
45	1,200–1,500
50	1,200–1,800
55	1,200–1,800
60	1,200–2,100
65	1,200–2,100
70	1,500–2,100

Adjust-a-dose: If creatinine clearance is less than 30 ml/minute, start therapy at 150 mg P.O. b.i.d. (one-half usual starting dose) and increase slowly to achieve desired response.

ADMINISTRATION
P.O.
• Shake suspension well.
• Mix suspension with water or give directly from syringe.
• Suspension and tablets may be interchanged at equal doses.
• Give drug without regard for food.

ACTION
Thought to prevent seizure spread in the brain by blocking voltage-sensitive sodium channels, and to produce anticonvulsant effects by increasing potassium conduction and modulating high-voltage activated calcium channels.

Route	Onset	Peak	Duration
P.O.	Unknown	Variable	Unknown

Half-life: About 2 hours for the drug; about 9 hours for the active metabolite. Children younger than age 8 have a 30% to 40% increase in clearance.

ADVERSE REACTIONS

CNS: *abnormal gait, ataxia, dizziness, fatigue, headache, somnolence, tremor, vertigo, aggravated seizures,* abnormal coordination, agitation, amnesia, anxiety, asthenia, confusion, emotional lability, feeling abnormal, fever, hypesthesia, impaired concentration, insomnia, nervousness, speech disorder.

CV: chest pain, edema, hypotension.

EENT: *abnormal vision, diplopia, nystagmus,* abnormal accommodation, ear pain, epistaxis, pharyngitis, rhinitis, sinusitis.

GI: *abdominal pain, nausea, vomiting, rectal hemorrhage,* anorexia, constipation, diarrhea, dry mouth, dyspepsia, gastritis, taste perversion, thirst.

GU: urinary frequency, UTI, vaginitis.

Metabolic: hyponatremia, weight increase.

Musculoskeletal: back pain, muscular weakness.

Respiratory: *upper respiratory tract infection,* bronchitis, chest infection, coughing.

Skin: acne, bruising, hot flashes, increased sweating, purpura, rash.

Other: allergic reaction, infection, lymphadenopathy, toothache.

INTERACTIONS

Drug-drug. *Carbamazepine, valproic acid, verapamil:* May decrease level of active metabolite of oxcarbazepine. Monitor patient and level closely.

Felodipine: May decrease felodipine level. Monitor patient closely.

Hormonal contraceptives: May decrease levels of ethinyl estradiol and levonorgestrel, reducing hormonal contraceptive effectiveness. Caution women of childbearing age to use alternative forms of contraception.

Phenobarbital: May decrease level of active metabolite of oxcarbazepine; may increase phenobarbital level. Monitor patient closely.

Phenytoin: May decrease level of active metabolite of oxcarbazepine; may increase phenytoin level in adults receiving high doses of oxcarbazepine. Monitor phenytoin level closely when starting therapy in these patients.

Drug-lifestyle. *Alcohol use:* May increase CNS depression. Discourage use together.

EFFECTS ON LAB TEST RESULTS

● May decrease sodium and thyroxine levels.

CONTRAINDICATIONS & CAUTIONS

● Contraindicated in patients hypersensitive to drug or its components.

NURSING CONSIDERATIONS

● *Alert:* Between 25% and 30% of patients with history of hypersensitivity reaction to carbamazepine may develop hypersensitivities to oxcarbazepine. Ask patient about carbamazepine hypersensitivity and stop drug immediately if signs or symptoms of hypersensitivity occur.

● *Alert:* Closely monitor all patients taking or starting antiepileptic drugs for changes in behavior indicating worsening of suicidal thoughts or behavior or depression. Symptoms such as anxiety, agitation, hostility, mania, and hypomania may be precursors to emerging suicidality.

● *Alert:* Withdraw drug gradually to minimize potential for increased seizure frequency.

● Watch for signs and symptoms of hyponatremia, including nausea, malaise, headache, lethargy, confusion, and decreased sensation.

● Monitor sodium level in patients receiving oxcarbazepine for maintenance treatment, especially patients receiving other therapies that may decrease sodium levels.

● Oxcarbazepine use has been linked to several nervous system–related adverse reactions, including psychomotor slowing, difficulty with concentration, speech or language problems, somnolence, fatigue, and coordination abnormalities, such as ataxia and gait disturbances.

PATIENT TEACHING

● Tell patient to take drug with or without food.

● Tell patient to contact prescriber before interrupting or stopping drug.

● Advise patient to report signs and symptoms of low sodium in the blood, such as nausea, malaise, headache, lethargy, and confusion.

● *Alert:* Multiorgan hypersensitivity reactions may occur. Tell patient to report fever and swollen lymph nodes to his prescriber.

• *Alert:* Serious skin reactions, including Stevens-Johnson syndrome and toxic epidermal necrosis, can occur. Advise patient to immediately report skin rashes to his prescriber.

• Caution patient to avoid driving and other potentially hazardous activities that require mental alertness until effects of drug are known.

• Instruct woman using hormonal contraceptives to use alternative form of contraception while taking drug.

• Tell patient to avoid alcohol while taking drug.

• Advise patient to inform prescriber if he has ever experienced hypersensitivity reaction to carbamazepine.

SAFETY ALERT!

phenobarbital (phenobarbitone)
fee-noe-BAR-bi-tal

Solfoton

phenobarbital sodium
Luminal Sodium

Pharmacologic class: barbiturate
Pregnancy risk category D
Controlled substance schedule IV

AVAILABLE FORMS
Elixir: 15 mg/5 ml*, 20 mg/5 ml*
Injection: 30 mg/ml, 60 mg/ml, 65 mg/ml, 130 mg/ml
Tablets: 15 mg, 16 mg, 30 mg, 60 mg, 100 mg

INDICATIONS & DOSAGES
➤ **Anticonvulsant, febrile seizures**
Adults: 60 to 200 mg P.O. daily. For acute seizures, 200 to 320 mg I.M. or I.V., repeat in 6 hours as necessary.
Children: 3 to 6 mg/kg P.O. daily, usually divided every 12 hours. Drug can be given once daily, usually at bedtime. Or, 10 to 15 mg/kg daily I.V. or I.M.
➤ **Status epilepticus**
Adults: 200 to 600 mg I.V.
Children: 15 to 20 mg/kg I.V. over 10 to 15 minutes.

➤ **Sedation**
Adults: 30 to 120 mg P.O., I.V., or I.M. daily in two or three divided doses. Maximum dose is 400 mg/24 hours.
Children: 6 mg/kg daily P.O. in three divided doses.
➤ **Short-term treatment of insomnia**
Adults: 100 to 200 mg P.O. or 100 to 320 mg I.M. or I.V. at bedtime.
➤ **Preoperative sedation**
Adults: 100 to 200 mg I.M. 60 to 90 minutes before surgery.
Children: 1 to 3 mg/kg I.V. or I.M. 60 to 90 minutes before surgery.
➤ **Prevention and treatment of hyperbilirubinemia ◆**
Neonates: 7 mg/kg P.O. daily from days 1 to 5 of life. Or, 5 mg/kg I.M. on day 1 of life, then 5 mg/kg P.O. on days 2 to 7 of life.
➤ **To lower serum bilirubin or serum lipid levels in the treatment of chronic cholestasis ◆**
Adults: 90 to 180 mg P.O. daily in two or three divided doses.
Children younger than age 12: 3 to 12 mg/kg P.O. daily in two to three divided doses.

ADMINISTRATION
P.O.
• Give drug without regard for food.
I.V.
• I.V. route is used for emergency treatment only.
• Dilute drug in half-normal or normal saline, D_5W, lactated Ringer's, or Ringer's solution.
• If solution contains precipitate, don't use.
• Give slowly (no more than 60 mg/minute) under close supervision. Have resuscitation equipment available.
• Monitor respirations closely.
• Inadvertent intra-arterial injection can cause spasm of the artery and severe pain and may lead to gangrene.
• Up to 30 minutes may be required for maximum effect; allow time for anticonvulsant effect to develop to avoid overdose.
• **Incompatibilities:** Acidic solutions, amphotericin B, chlorpromazine, dimenhydrinate, diphenhydramine, ephedrine, hydralazine, hydrocortisone sodium succinate, hydromorphone,

---

insulin, kanamycin, levorphanol, meperidine, morphine, norepinephrine, pentazocine lactate, phenytoin, prochlorperazine mesylate, promethazine hydrochloride, ranitidine hydrochloride, streptomycin, vancomycin.

I.M.
● Give I.M. injection deeply into large muscles. Superficial injection may cause pain, sterile abscess, and tissue sloughing.

ACTION

As a barbiturate, may depress CNS and increase seizure threshold. As a sedative, may interfere with transmission of impulses from thalamus to cortex of brain.

Route	Onset	Peak	Duration
P.O.	1 hr	8–12 hr	10–12 hr
I.V.	5 min	30 min	4–10 hr
I.M.	> 5 min	> 30 min	4–10 hr

Half-life: 5 to 7 days.

ADVERSE REACTIONS

CNS: *drowsiness, lethargy, hangover,* paradoxical excitement in elderly patients, somnolence, changes in EEG patterns, physical and psychological dependence, pain.
CV: bradycardia, hypotension, syncope.
GI: nausea, vomiting.
Hematologic: exacerbation of porphyria.
Respiratory: respiratory depression, apnea.
Skin: rash, **erythema multiforme, Stevens-Johnson syndrome,** urticaria, swelling, thrombophlebitis, necrosis, nerve injury at injection site.
Other: injection site pain, **angioedema.**

INTERACTIONS

Drug-drug. *Chloramphenicol, MAO inhibitors:* May potentiate barbiturate effect. Monitor patient for increased CNS and respiratory depression.
CNS depressants including opioid analgesics: Excessive CNS depression. Monitor patient closely.
Corticosteroids, doxycycline, estrogens and hormonal contraceptives, oral anticoagulants, tricyclic antidepressants: May enhance metabolism of these drugs. Watch for decreased effect.

Diazepam: May increase effects of both drugs. Use together cautiously.
Griseofulvin: May decrease absorption of griseofulvin. Monitor effectiveness of griseofulvin.
Mephobarbital, primidone: May cause excessive phenobarbital level. Monitor patient closely.
Metoprolol, propranolol: May reduce the effects of these drugs. Consider an increased beta-blocker dose.
Rifampin: May decrease barbiturate level. Watch for decreased effect.
Valproic acid: May increase phenobarbital level. Watch for toxicity.
Warfarin: May increase warfarin metabolism and decrease effect. Monitor patient for decreased warfarin effect.
Drug-herb. *Evening primrose oil:* May increase anticonvulsant dosage requirement. Discourage use together.
Drug-lifestyle. *Alcohol use:* May impair coordination, increase CNS effects, and lead to death. Strongly discourage use together.

EFFECTS ON LAB TEST RESULTS
● May decrease bilirubin level.
● May cause false-positive phentolamine test result.

CONTRAINDICATIONS & CAUTIONS
● Contraindicated in patients hypersensitive to barbiturates and in those with history of manifest or latent porphyria.
● Contraindicated in patients with hepatic or renal dysfunction, respiratory disease with dyspnea or obstruction, or nephritis.
● Use cautiously in patients with acute or chronic pain, depression, suicidal tendencies, history of drug abuse, fever, hyperthyroidism, diabetes mellitus, severe anemia, blood pressure alterations, CV disease, shock, or uremia, and in elderly or debilitated patients.

NURSING CONSIDERATIONS
● **Alert:** Watch for signs of barbiturate toxicity, such as coma, cyanosis, asthmatic breathing, clammy skin, and hypotension. Overdose can be fatal.

- Therapeutic level is 15 to 40 mcg/ml.
- Elderly patients are more sensitive to drug's effects; drug may produce paradoxical excitement.
- Don't stop drug abruptly because this may worsen seizures. Call prescriber immediately if adverse reactions develop.
- First withdrawal symptoms occur within 8 to 12 hours and include anxiety, muscle twitching, tremor of hands and fingers, progressive weakness, dizziness, visual distortion, nausea, vomiting, insomnia, and orthostatic hypotension. Seizures and delirium may occur within 16 hours and last up to 5 days after abruptly stopping drug.
- Use for insomnia isn't recommended, and treatment shouldn't last longer than 14 days.
- Some products contain tartrazine; use cautiously in patients with aspirin sensitivity.
- EEG patterns show a change in low-voltage fast activity. Changes persist after therapy ends.
- Drug may decrease bilirubin level in neonates, patients with epilepsy, and those with congenital nonhemolytic, unconjugated hyperbilirubinemia.
- The physiologic effects of drug may impair the absorption of cyanocobalamin Co 57.
- *Look alike–sound alike:* Don't confuse phenobarbital with pentobarbital.

PATIENT TEACHING
- Ensure that patient is aware that drug is available in different milligram strengths and sizes. Advise him to check prescription and refills closely.
- Inform patient that full therapeutic effects aren't seen for 2 to 3 weeks, except when loading dose is used.
- Advise patient to avoid driving and other potentially hazardous activities that require mental alertness until drug's CNS effects are known.
- Warn patient and parents not to stop drug abruptly.
- Tell woman using hormonal contraceptives to consider a nonhormonal form of birth control because drug may decrease effectiveness.

phenytoin (diphenylhydantoin)
FEN-i-toe-in

Dilantin 125, Dilantin Infatabs

phenytoin sodium (prompt)
Dilantin

phenytoin sodium (extended)
Dilantin Kapseals⬥, Phenytek

Pharmacologic class: hydantoin derivative
Pregnancy risk category D

AVAILABLE FORMS
phenytoin
Oral suspension: 125 mg/5 ml
Tablets (chewable): 50 mg
phenytoin sodium (extended)
Capsules: 30 mg (27.6 mg base), 100 mg (92 mg base), 200 mg (184 mg base), 300 mg (276 mg base)
phenytoin sodium (prompt)
Capsules: 100 mg (92 mg base)
Injection: 50 mg/ml (46 mg base)

INDICATIONS & DOSAGES
➤ **To control tonic-clonic (grand mal) and complex partial (temporal lobe) seizures**
Adults: Highly individualized. Initially, 100 mg P.O. t.i.d., increasing by 100 mg P.O. every 2 to 4 weeks until desired response is obtained. Usual range is 300 to 600 mg daily. If patient is stabilized with extended-release capsules, once-daily dosing with 300-mg extended-release capsules is possible as an alternative.
Children: 5 mg/kg or 250 mg/m² P.O. divided b.i.d. or t.i.d. Usual dose range is 4 to 8 mg/kg daily. Maximum daily dose is 300 mg.
➤ **For patient requiring a loading dose**
Adults: Initially, 1 g P.O. daily divided into three doses and given at 2-hour intervals. Or, 10 to 15 mg/kg I.V. at a rate not exceeding 50 mg/minute. Normal maintenance dosage is started 24 hours after loading dose.

Reactions may be *common*, uncommon, *life-threatening*, or COMMON AND LIFE-THREATENING.
Interaction may have a *rapid onset* or *delayed onset*.

Children: 500 to 600 mg P.O. in divided doses, followed by maintenance dosage 24 hours after loading dose.

➤ **To prevent and treat seizures occurring during neurosurgery**
Adults: 100 to 200 mg I.M. every 4 hours during and after surgery.

➤ **Status epilepticus**
Adults: Loading dose of 10 to 15 mg/kg I.V. (1 to 1.5 g may be needed) at a rate not exceeding 50 mg/minute; then maintenance dosage of 100 mg P.O. or I.V. every 6 to 8 hours.
Children: Loading dose of 15 to 20 mg/kg I.V., at a rate not exceeding 1 to 3 mg/kg/minute; then highly individualized maintenance dosages.
Elderly patients: May need lower dosages.

ADMINISTRATION
P.O.
● Give divided doses with or after meals to decrease adverse GI reactions.
I.V.
● Clear tubing with normal saline solution. Use only clear solution for injection. A slight yellow color is acceptable.
● Mix with normal saline solution, if needed, and give as an infusion over 30 minutes to 1 hour, when possible.
● Infusion must begin within 1 hour after preparation and should run through an in-line filter.
● Check patency of catheter before giving. Monitor site for extravasation because it can cause severe tissue damage.
■ **Black Box Warning** Drug must be administered slowly. In adults, don't exceed 50 mg/minute I.V. In neonates, administer drug at a rate not exceeding 1 to 3 mg/kg/minute. ■
● If possible, don't give by I.V. push into veins on back of hand to avoid purple glove syndrome. Inject into larger veins or central venous catheter, if available.
● Check vital signs, blood pressure, and ECG during I.V. administration.
● Discard 4 hours after preparation. Don't refrigerate.
● **Incompatibilities:** Amikacin, aminophylline, amphotericin B, bretylium, cephapirin, ciprofloxacin, D₅W, diltiazem, dobutamine, enalaprilat, fat emulsions, hydromorphone, insulin (regular), levor-

phanol, lidocaine, lincomycin, meperidine, morphine sulfate, nitroglycerin, norepinephrine, other I.V. drugs or infusion solutions, pentobarbital sodium, potassium chloride, procaine, propofol, streptomycin, sufentanil citrate, theophylline, vitamin B complex with C. If giving as an infusion, don't mix drug with D₅W because it will precipitate.
I.M.
● Give I.M. only if dosage adjustments are made; I.M. dose is 50% greater than oral dose.
● Be aware that drug may precipitate at injection site, cause pain, and be absorbed erratically.

ACTION
May stabilize neuronal membranes and limit seizure activity either by increasing efflux or decreasing influx of sodium ions across cell membranes in the motor cortex during generation of nerve impulses.

Route	Onset	Peak	Duration
P.O.	Unknown	1½–12 hr	Unknown
P.O. (Phenytek)	Unknown	4–12 hr	Unknown
I.V.	Immediate	1–2 hr	Unknown
I.M.	Unknown	Unknown	Unknown

Half-life: Varies with dose and concentration changes.

ADVERSE REACTIONS
CNS: *ataxia, decreased coordination, mental confusion, slurred speech,* dizziness, headache, insomnia, nervousness, twitching.
CV: periarteritis nodosa.
EENT: *diplopia, nystagmus,* blurred vision.
GI: *gingival hyperplasia, nausea, vomiting,* constipation.
Hematologic: *agranulocytosis, leukopenia, pancytopenia, thrombocytopenia,* macrocythemia, megaloblastic anemia.
Hepatic: *toxic hepatitis.*
Metabolic: hyperglycemia.
Musculoskeletal: osteomalacia.
Skin: *Stevens-Johnson syndrome, toxic epidermal necrolysis,* bullous or purpuric dermatitis, discoloration of skin if given by I.V. push in back of hand,

Central nervous system drugs

exfoliative dermatitis, hypertrichosis,
inflammation at injection site, lupus
erythematosus, necrosis, pain, photosensitivity reactions, scarlatiniform or
morbilliform rash.
Other: *hirsutism,* lymphadenopathy.

INTERACTIONS
Drug-drug. *Acetaminophen:* May
decrease the therapeutic effects of acetaminophen and increase the incidence of
hepatotoxicity. Monitor for toxicity.
*Amiodarone, antihistamines, chloram-
phenicol,* **cimetidine,** *cycloserine,
diazepam,* **fluconazole, isoniazid,**
*metronidazole, omeprazole, phenyl-
butazone, salicylates,* **sulfonamides,
ticlodipine,** *valproate:* May increase
phenytoin activity and toxicity. Monitor
patient for toxicity and adjust dose as
needed.
*Atracurium, cisatracurium, pancuronium,
rocuronium, vecuronium:* May decrease
the effects of nondepolarizing muscle
relaxant. May need to increase the
nondepolarizing muscle relaxant dose.
*Barbiturates, carbamazepine, dexametha-
sone, diazoxide, folic acid, rifampin:* May
decrease phenytoin activity. Monitor
phenytoin level.
*Carbamazepine, cardiac glycosides,
doxycycline, hormonal contraceptives,
quinidine, theophylline, valproic acid:*
May decrease effects of these drugs.
Monitor patient.
Cyclosporine: May decrease cyclosporine
levels, risking organ rejection. Monitor
cyclosporine levels closely and adjust
dose as needed.
Disulfiram: May increase toxic
effects of phenytoin. Monitor phenytoin
level closely and adjust dose as
needed.
Lithium: May increase toxicity of lithium,
despite normal lithium levels. Monitor
patient for adverse effects.
Warfarin: May increase effects of warfarin. Monitor patient for bleeding.
Drug-food. *Enteral tube feedings:* May
interfere with absorption of oral drug.
Stop enteral feedings for 2 hours before
and 2 hours after drug use.
Drug-lifestyle. *Long-term alcohol use:*
May decrease drug's activity. Strongly
discourage use together.

EFFECTS ON LAB TEST RESULTS
● May increase alkaline phosphatase,
GGT, and glucose levels. May decrease
urinary 17-hydroxysteroid, 17-ketosteroid,
and hemoglobin levels and hematocrit.
● May decrease platelet, WBC, RBC, and
granulocyte counts.
● May increase urine 6-hydroxycortisol
excretion. May decrease dexamethasone
suppression and metyrapone test
results.
● May falsely reduce protein-bound iodine
or free T_4 level test results.

CONTRAINDICATIONS & CAUTIONS
● Contraindicated in patients hypersensitive to hydantoin and in those with sinus
bradycardia, SA block, second- or third-
degree AV block, or Adams-Stokes
syndrome.
● Use cautiously in patients with hepatic
dysfunction, hypotension, myocardial
insufficiency, diabetes, or respiratory
depression; in elderly or debilitated
patients; and in those receiving other
hydantoin derivatives.
● Elderly patients tend to metabolize
drug slowly and may need reduced
dosages.

NURSING CONSIDERATIONS
● Therapeutic dose usually increases
during pregnancy.
● If rash appears, stop drug. If rash
is scarlatiniform or morbilliform,
resume drug after rash clears. If rash
reappears, stop therapy. If rash is
exfoliative, purpuric, or bullous, don't
resume drug.
● Don't stop drug suddenly because
this may worsen seizures. Call prescriber
immediately if adverse reactions
develop.
● Monitor drug level. Therapeutic level is
10 to 20 mcg/ml.
● Allow at least 7 to 10 days to elapse between dosage changes.
● Monitor CBC and calcium level every
6 months, and periodically monitor hepatic
function. If megaloblastic anemia is evident, prescriber may order folic acid and
vitamin B_{12}.
● Maintain seizure precautions, as needed.
● Mononucleosis may decrease level.
Watch for increased seizures.

Reactions may be *common,* uncommon, *life-threatening,* or COMMON AND LIFE-THREATENING.
Interaction may have a *rapid onset* or **delayed onset.**

• Watch for gingival hyperplasia, especially in children.

• *Alert:* Doubling the dose doesn't double the level but may cause toxicity. Consult pharmacist for specific dosing recommendations.

• If seizure control is established with divided doses, once-daily dosing may be considered.

• *Look alike–sound alike:* Don't confuse phenytoin with mephenytoin or fosphenytoin or Dilantin with Dilaudid.

PATIENT TEACHING

• Tell patient to notify prescriber if skin rash develops.

• Advise patient to avoid driving and other potentially hazardous activities that require mental alertness until drug's CNS effects are known.

• Advise patient not to change brands or dosage forms once he's stabilized on therapy.

• Dilantin capsules are the only oral form that can be given once daily. Toxic levels may result if any other brand or form is given once daily. Dilantin tablets and oral suspension should never be taken once daily.

• Tell patient not to use capsules that are discolored.

• Advise patient to avoid alcohol.

• Warn patient and parents not to stop drug abruptly.

• Stress importance of good oral hygiene and regular dental examinations. Surgical removal of excess gum tissue may be needed periodically if dental hygiene is poor.

• Caution patient that drug may color urine pink, red, or reddish brown.

---

primidone
PRI-mi-done

Mysoline, Sertan†

Pharmacologic class: barbiturate analogue
Pregnancy risk category D

AVAILABLE FORMS

Tablets: 50 mg, 250 mg

INDICATIONS & DOSAGES

➤ **Tonic-clonic, complex partial, and simple partial seizures**

Adults and children age 8 and older: Initially, 100 to 125 mg P.O. at bedtime on days 1 to 3; then 100 to 125 mg P.O. b.i.d. on days 4 to 6; then 100 to 125 mg P.O. t.i.d. on days 7 to 9, followed by maintenance dose of 250 mg P.O. t.i.d. Maintenance dose may be increased to 250 mg q.i.d., if needed. Dosage may be increased to maximum of 2 g daily in divided doses.

Children younger than age 8: Initially, 50 mg P.O. at bedtime for 3 days; then 50 mg P.O. b.i.d. for days 4 to 6; then 100 mg P.O. b.i.d. for days 7 to 9, followed by maintenance dose of 125 to 250 mg P.O. t.i.d. or 10 to 25 mg/kg daily in divided doses.

➤ **Essential tremor ♦**

Adults: 750 mg P.O. daily.

ADMINISTRATION

P.O.

• Give drug without regard for food.

ACTION

Unknown. Some activity may be caused by phenylethylmalonamide and phenobarbital, which are active metabolites.

Route	Onset	Peak	Duration
P.O.	Unknown	3–4 hr	Unknown

Half-life: 5 to 15 hours.

ADVERSE REACTIONS

CNS: *ataxia, drowsiness,* emotional disturbances, fatigue, hyperirritability, paranoid symptoms, vertigo.
EENT: *diplopia,* nystagmus.
GI: *nausea, vomiting,* anorexia.
GU: impotence, polyuria.
Hematologic: megaloblastic anemia, *thrombocytopenia.*
Skin: morbilliform rash.

INTERACTIONS

Drug-drug. *Acetazolamide, succinimide:* May decrease primidone level. Monitor level.
Anticoagulants, felodipine: May decrease the effects of these drugs. Adjust doses as needed.

Carbamazepine: May increase carbamazepine level and decrease primidone and phenobarbital levels. Watch for toxicity.

CNS depressants: May cause additive CNS depression. Avoid using together.

Corticosteroids, doxycycline: May decrease the effects of these drugs. Avoid using together, if possible.

Hormonal contraceptives: May decrease the effectiveness of contraceptives. Recommend alternative birth control method.

Isoniazid: May increase primidone level. Monitor level.

Metoprolol, propranolol, **other beta blockers:** May reduce effects of these drugs. Consider increasing beta-blocker dose.

Phenytoin: May stimulate conversion of primidone to phenobarbital. Watch for increased phenobarbital effect.

Valproic acid: May increase primidone levels. Decrease primidone dose as needed.

Drug-lifestyle. *Alcohol use:* May impair coordination, increase CNS effects, and cause death. Strongly discourage alcohol use with this drug.

EFFECTS ON LAB TEST RESULTS
• May decrease hemoglobin level.
• May alter liver function test values. May decrease platelet count.

CONTRAINDICATIONS & CAUTIONS
• Contraindicated in patients hypersensitive to phenobarbital and in those with porphyria.

NURSING CONSIDERATIONS
• Don't withdraw drug suddenly because seizures may worsen. Notify prescriber immediately if adverse reactions develop.
• Therapeutic level of primidone is 5 to 12 mcg/ml. Therapeutic level of phenobarbital is 15 to 40 mcg/ml.
• Monitor CBC and routine blood chemistry every 6 months.
• Brand interchange isn't recommended because of documented bioequivalence problems for primidone products marketed by different manufacturers.

• **Look alike–sound alike:** Don't confuse primidone with prednisone or Prinivil.

PATIENT TEACHING
• Advise patient to avoid driving and other potentially hazardous activities that require mental alertness until drug's CNS effects are known.
• Warn patient and parents not to stop taking drug suddenly.
• Tell patient that full therapeutic response may take 2 weeks or longer.
• Advise woman of childbearing age to discuss drug therapy with prescriber if she's considering pregnancy.
• Caution woman of childbearing age that breast-feeding is contraindicated while taking this drug.

tiagabine hydrochloride
tye-AG-ah-been

Gabitril Filmtabs

Pharmacologic class: gamma aminobutyric acid (GABA) enhancer
Pregnancy risk category C

AVAILABLE FORMS
Tablets: 2 mg, 4 mg, 12 mg, 16 mg

INDICATIONS & DOSAGES
➤ **Adjunctive treatment of partial seizures**
Adults: Initially, 4 mg P.O. once daily. Total daily dose may be increased by 4 to 8 mg at weekly intervals until clinical response or up to 56 mg daily. Give total daily dose in divided doses b.i.d. to q.i.d.
Children ages 12 to 18: Initially, 4 mg P.O. once daily. Total daily dose may be increased by 4 mg at beginning of week 2 and thereafter by 4 to 8 mg per week until clinical response or up to 32 mg daily. Give total daily dose in divided doses b.i.d. to q.i.d.
Adjust-a-dose: For patients with hepatic impairment, reduce first and maintenance doses or increase dosing intervals.

ADMINISTRATION
P.O.
- Give drug with food.

ACTION
Unknown. May act by facilitating the effects of the inhibitory neurotransmitter GABA. By binding to recognition sites linked to GABA uptake carrier, drug may make more GABA available.

Route	Onset	Peak	Duration
P.O.	Rapid	45 min	7–9 hr

Half-life: 7 to 9 hours.

ADVERSE REACTIONS
CNS: *asthenia, dizziness, nervousness, somnolence,* abnormal gait, agitation, ataxia, confusion, depression, difficulty with concentration and attention, difficulty with memory, emotional lability, hostility, insomnia, language problems, paresthesia, speech disorder, tremor, pain.
CV: vasodilation.
EENT: nystagmus, pharyngitis.
GI: *nausea,* abdominal pain, diarrhea, increased appetite, mouth ulceration, vomiting.
Musculoskeletal: generalized weakness, myasthenia.
Respiratory: increased cough.
Skin: pruritus, rash.

INTERACTIONS
Drug-drug. *Carbamazepine, phenobarbital, phenytoin:* May increase tiagabine clearance. Monitor patient closely.
CNS depressants: May enhance CNS effects. Use together cautiously.
Drug-lifestyle. *Alcohol use:* May enhance CNS effects. Discourage use together.

EFFECTS ON LAB TEST RESULTS
None reported.

CONTRAINDICATIONS & CAUTIONS
- Contraindicated in patients hypersensitive to drug or its components.
- *Alert:* Drug may cause new-onset seizures and status epilepticus in patients without a history of epilepsy. In these patients, stop drug and evaluate for underlying seizure disorder. Drug shouldn't be used for off-label uses.
- Use cautiously in patients with psychiatric symptoms.
- Use cautiously in breast-feeding women.

NURSING CONSIDERATIONS
- *Alert:* Closely monitor all patients taking or starting antiepileptic drugs for changes in behavior indicating worsening of suicidal thoughts or behavior or depression. Symptoms such as anxiety, agitation, hostility, mania, and hypomania may be precursors to emerging suicidality.
- Withdraw drug gradually unless safety concerns require a more rapid withdrawal because sudden withdrawal may cause more frequent seizures.
- *Alert:* Use of anticonvulsants, including tiagabine, may cause status epilepticus and sudden unexpected death in patients with epilepsy.
- *Look alike–sound alike:* Don't confuse tiagabine with tizanidine; both have 4-mg starting doses.
- Patients who aren't receiving at least one enzyme-inducing anticonvulsant when starting tiagabine may need lower doses or slower dosage adjustment.
- Monitor patient for cognitive and neuropsychiatric symptoms, including impaired concentration, speech or language problems, confusion, somnolence, and fatigue.
- Drug may cause moderately severe to incapacitating generalized weakness, which resolves after dosage is reduced or drug stopped.

PATIENT TEACHING
- Advise patient to take drug only as prescribed.
- Tell patient to take drug with food.
- Warn patient that drug may cause dizziness, somnolence, and other signs and symptoms of CNS depression. Advise patient to avoid driving and other potentially hazardous activities that require mental alertness until drug's CNS effects are known.
- Tell woman of childbearing age to call prescriber if she becomes pregnant or plans to become pregnant during therapy.
- Instruct woman of childbearing age to notify prescriber if she's planning to breast-feed because drug may appear in breast milk.

topiramate
toe-PIE-rah-mate

Topamax

Pharmacologic class: sulfamate-
substituted monosaccharide
Pregnancy risk category C

AVAILABLE FORMS
Capsules, sprinkles: 15 mg, 25 mg
Tablets: 25 mg, 50 mg, 100 mg, 200 mg

INDICATIONS & DOSAGES
➤ **Initial monotherapy for partial-
onset or primary generalized tonic-
clonic seizures**
Adults and children age 10 or older:
Recommended daily dose is 400 mg
P.O. divided b.i.d. (morning and
evening). To achieve this dosage,
adjust as follows: first week, 25 mg
P.O. b.i.d.; second week, 50 mg P.O.
b.i.d.; third week, 75 mg P.O. b.i.d.;
fourth week, 100 mg P.O. b.i.d.; fifth
week, 150 mg P.O. b.i.d.; and sixth
week, 200 mg P.O. b.i.d.
➤ **Adjunct treatment for partial-
onset or primary generalized tonic-
clonic seizures**
Adults: Initially, 25 to 50 mg P.O. daily;
increase gradually by 25 to 50 mg/week
until an effective daily dose is reached.
Adjust to recommended daily dose of
200 to 400 mg P.O. in two divided doses
for adults with partial seizures or 400 mg
P.O. in two divided doses for adults
with primary generalized tonic-clonic
seizures.
Children ages 2 to 16: Initially, 1 to 3 mg/
kg daily given at bedtime for 1 week. Increase at 1- or 2-week intervals by 1 to
3 mg/kg daily in two divided doses to
achieve optimal response. Recommended
daily dose is 5 to 9 mg/kg, in two divided
doses.
➤ **Lennox-Gastaut syndrome**
Children ages 2 to 16: Initially, 1 to 3 mg/
kg daily given at bedtime for 1 week. Increase at 1- or 2-week intervals by 1 to
3 mg/kg daily in two divided doses to
achieve optimal response. Recommended
daily dose is 5 to 9 mg/kg, in two divided
doses.

➤ **To prevent migraine headache**
Adults: Initially, 25 mg P.O. daily in
evening for first week. Then, 25 mg P.O.
b.i.d. in morning and evening for second
week. For third week, 25 mg P.O. in morning and 50 mg P.O. in evening. For fourth
week, 50 mg P.O. b.i.d. in morning and
evening.
Adjust-a-dose: If creatinine clearance is
less than 70 ml/minute, reduce dosage by
50%. For hemodialysis patients, supplemental doses may be needed to avoid
rapid drops in drug level during prolonged
dialysis treatment.

ADMINISTRATION
P.O.
● Give drug without regard for food.
● Crushed or broken tablets have a bitter
taste.
● Capsules may be opened and contents
sprinkled on a teaspoon of soft food. Patient should swallow immediately without
chewing.

ACTION
Unknown. May block a sodium channel,
potentiate the activity of GABA, and inhibit kainate's ability to activate an amino
acid receptor.

Route	Onset	Peak	Duration
P.O.	Unknown	2 hr	Unknown

Half-life: 21 hours.

ADVERSE REACTIONS
CNS: *ataxia, confusion, difficulty with
memory, dizziness, fatigue, nervousness,
paresthesia, psychomotor slowing, somnolence, speech disorders, tremor, generalized tonic-clonic seizures, suicide attempts,* abnormal coordination, aggressive
reaction, agitation, apathy, asthenia, depression, depersonalization, difficulty with
concentration, attention, or language,
emotional lability, euphoria, fever, hallucination, hyperkinesia, hypertonia, hypoesthesia, hypokinesia, insomnia, malaise,
mood problems, personality disorder, psychosis, stupor, vertigo.
CV: chest pain, edema, palpitations, vasodilation.
EENT: *abnormal vision, diplopia, nystagmus,* conjunctivitis, epistaxis, eye pain,

---

Reactions may be *common,* uncommon, *life-threatening,* or COMMON AND LIFE-THREATENING.
Interaction may have a *rapid onset* or **delayed onset.**

hearing problems, pharyngitis, sinusitis, tinnitus.

GI: *anorexia, nausea,* abdominal pain, constipation, diarrhea, dry mouth, dyspepsia, flatulence, gastroenteritis, gingivitis, taste perversion, vomiting.

GU: amenorrhea, dysuria, dysmenorrhea, hematuria, impotence, intermenstrual bleeding, leukorrhea, menstrual disorder, menorrhagia, urinary frequency, renal calculi, urinary incontinence, UTI, vaginitis.

Hematologic: *leukopenia,* anemia.

Metabolic: *decreased weight,* increased weight.

Musculoskeletal: arthralgia, back or leg pain, muscle weakness, myalgia, rigors.

Respiratory: *upper respiratory tract infection,* bronchitis, coughing, dyspnea.

Skin: acne, alopecia, increased sweating, pruritus, rash.

Other: body odor, breast pain, decreased libido, flulike syndrome, hot flashes, lymphadenopathy.

INTERACTIONS

Drug-drug. *Carbamazepine:* May decrease topiramate level. Monitor patient.

Carbonic anhydrase inhibitors (acetazolamide, dichlorphenamide): May cause renal calculus formation. Avoid using together.

CNS depressants: May cause CNS depression and other adverse cognitive and neuropsychiatric events. Use together cautiously.

Hormonal contraceptives: May decrease efficacy. Report changes in menstrual patterns. Advise patient to use another contraceptive method.

Phenytoin: May decrease topiramate level and increase phenytoin level. Monitor levels.

Valproic acid: May decrease valproic acid and topiramate level. Monitor patient.

Drug-lifestyle. *Alcohol use:* May cause CNS depression and other adverse cognitive and neuropsychiatric events. Discourage use together.

EFFECTS ON LAB TEST RESULTS

● May increase liver enzyme levels. May decrease bicarbonate and hemoglobin levels and hematocrit.

● May decrease WBC count.

CONTRAINDICATIONS & CAUTIONS

● Contraindicated in patients hypersensitive to drug or its components.

● Use cautiously in breast-feeding or pregnant women and in those with hepatic impairment.

● Use cautiously with other drugs that predispose patients to heat-related disorders, including other carbonic anhydrase inhibitors and anticholinergics.

NURSING CONSIDERATIONS

● *Alert:* Closely monitor all patients taking or starting antiepileptic drugs for changes in behavior indicating worsening of suicidal thoughts or behavior or depression. Symptoms such as anxiety, agitation, hostility, mania, and hypomania may be precursors to emerging suicidality.

● If needed, withdraw anticonvulsant (including topiramate) gradually to minimize risk of increased seizure activity.

● Monitoring topiramate level isn't necessary.

● Drug may infrequently cause oligohidrosis and hyperthermia, mainly in children. Monitor patient closely, especially in hot weather.

● Drug may cause hyperchloremic, non-anion gap metabolic acidosis from renal bicarbonate loss. Factors that may predispose patients to acidosis, such as renal disease, severe respiratory disorders, status epilepticus, diarrhea, surgery, ketogenic diet, or drugs, may add to topiramate's bicarbonate-lowering effects.

● Measure baseline and periodic bicarbonate levels. If metabolic acidosis develops and persists, consider reducing the dose, gradually stopping the drug, or alkali treatment.

● Drug is rapidly cleared by dialysis. A prolonged period of dialysis may cause low drug level and seizures. A supplemental dose may be needed.

● Stop drug if patient experiences acute myopia and secondary angle-closure glaucoma.

● *Look alike–sound alike:* Don't confuse Topamax with Toprol-XL, Tegretol, or Tegretol-XR.

PATIENT TEACHING
• Tell patient to drink plenty of fluids during therapy to minimize risk of forming kidney stones.
• Advise patient not to drive or operate hazardous machinery until CNS effects of drug are known. Drug can cause sleepiness, dizziness, confusion, and concentration problems.
• Tell woman of childbearing age that drug may decrease effectiveness of hormonal contraceptives. Advise woman using hormonal contraceptives to report change in menstrual patterns.
• Tell patient to avoid crushing or breaking tablets because of bitter taste.
• Inform patient that drug can be taken without regard to food.
• Tell patient that capsules may either be swallowed whole or carefully opened and contents sprinkled on a teaspoonful of soft food. Tell patient to swallow immediately without chewing.
• Tell patient to notify prescriber immediately if he experiences changes in vision.

---

valproate sodium
val-PROH-ayt

Depacon, Depakene

valproic acid
Depakene, Stavzor

divalproex sodium
Depakote✒, Depakote ER, Depakote Sprinkle✒, Epival†

Pharmacologic class: carboxylic acid derivative
Pregnancy risk category D

AVAILABLE FORMS
valproate sodium
Injection: 100 mg/ml
Syrup: 250 mg/5 ml
valproic acid
Capsules: 250 mg
Capsules (delayed-release): 125 mg, 250 mg, 500 mg
Syrup: 200 mg/5 ml
Tablets (enteric-coated): 200 mg, 500 mg
divalproex sodium
Capsules (sprinkle): 125 mg
Tablets (delayed-release): 125 mg, 250 mg, 500 mg
Tablets (extended-release): 250 mg, 500 mg

INDICATIONS & DOSAGES
➤ **Simple and complex absence seizures, mixed seizure types (including absence seizures)**
Adults and children: Initially, 15 mg/kg P.O. or I.V. daily; then increase by 5 to 10 mg/kg daily at weekly intervals up to maximum of 60 mg/kg daily. Don't use Depakote ER in children younger than age 10.
➤ **Complex partial seizures**
Adults and children age 10 and older: 10 to 15 mg/kg Depakote or Depakote ER P.O. or valproate sodium I.V. daily; then increase by 5 to 10 mg/kg daily at weekly intervals, up to 60 mg/kg daily.
➤ **Mania**
Adults: Initially, 750 mg Depakote daily P.O. in divided doses, or 25 mg/kg Depakote ER once daily. Adjust dosage based on patient's response; maximum dose for either form is 60 mg/kg daily. Or, give Stavzor 750 mg P.O. daily in divided doses. Maximum recommended dosage is 60 mg/kg/day.
➤ **To prevent migraine headache**
Adults: Initially, 250 mg delayed-release divalproex sodium P.O. b.i.d. Some patients may need up to 1,000 mg daily. Or, 500 mg Depakote ER P.O. daily for 1 week; then 1,000 mg P.O. daily. Or, give Stavzor 250 mg P.O. b.i.d. Some patients may benefit from 1,000 mg/day. Maximum recommended dosage is 60 mg/kg/day.
Adjust-a-dose: For elderly patients, start at lower dosage. Increase dosage more slowly and with regular monitoring of fluid and nutritional intake, and watch for dehydration, somnolence, and other adverse reactions.

ADMINISTRATION
P.O.
• Give drug with food or milk to reduce adverse GI effects.
• Don't mix syrup with carbonated beverages; mixture may be irritating to oral mucosa.

Reactions may be *common,* uncommon, *life-threatening,* or COMMON AND LIFE-THREATENING.
Interaction may have a *rapid onset* or **delayed onset.**

• Don't give syrup to patients who need sodium restriction. Check with prescriber.
• Capsules may be swallowed whole or opened and contents sprinkled on a teaspoonful of soft food. Patient should swallow immediately without chewing.

I.V.

• I.V. use is indicated only in patients who can't take drug orally. Switch patient to oral form as soon as feasible; effects of I.V. use for longer than 14 days are unknown.
• Dilute valproate sodium injection with at least 50 ml of a compatible diluent. It's physically compatible and chemically stable in D_5W, normal saline, and lactated Ringer's solution for 24 hours.
• Infuse drug over 60 minutes at no more than 20 mg/minute and at the same frequency as oral dosage.
• Monitor drug level, and adjust dosage as needed.
• **Incompatibilities:** None reported.

ACTION

Unknown. Probably facilitates the effects of the inhibitory neurotransmitter GABA.

Route	Onset	Peak	Duration
P.O.	Unknown	15 min–4 hr	Unknown
I.V.	Unknown	1 hr	Unknown

Half-life: 6 to 16 hours.

ADVERSE REACTIONS

CNS: *asthenia, dizziness, headache, insomnia, nervousness, somnolence, tremor,* abnormal thinking, amnesia, ataxia, depression, emotional upset, fever.
CV: chest pain, edema, hypertension, hypotension, tachycardia.
EENT: *blurred vision, diplopia,* nystagmus, pharyngitis, rhinitis, tinnitus.
GI: *abdominal pain, anorexia, diarrhea, dyspepsia, nausea, vomiting, pancreatitis,* constipation, increased appetite.
Hematologic: *bone marrow suppression, hemorrhage, thrombocytopenia,* bruising, petechiae.
Hepatic: *hepatotoxicity.*
Metabolic: hyperammonemia, weight gain or loss.
Musculoskeletal: back and neck pain.
Respiratory: bronchitis, dyspnea.

Skin: *alopecia, flu syndrome, infection, erythema multiforme, hypersensitivity reactions, Stevens-Johnson syndrome,* rash, photosensitivity reactions, pruritus.

INTERACTIONS

Drug-drug. *Aspirin, chlorpromazine, cimetidine, erythromycin, felbamate:* May cause valproic acid toxicity. Use together cautiously and monitor drug level.
Benzodiazepines, other CNS depressants: May cause excessive CNS depression. Avoid using together.
Carbamazepine: May cause carbamazepine CNS toxicity; may decrease valproic acid level and cause loss of seizure control. Use together cautiously, if at all. Monitor patient for seizure activity and toxicity during therapy and for at least 1 month after stopping either drug.
Lamotrigine: May increase lamotrigine level; may decrease valproate level. Monitor levels closely.
Phenobarbital: May increase phenobarbital level; may increase clearance of valproate. Monitor patient closely.
Phenytoin: May increase or decrease phenytoin level; may decrease valproate level. Monitor patient closely.
Rifampin: May decrease valproate level. Monitor level of valproate.
Warfarin: May displace warfarin from binding sites. Monitor PT and INR.
Zidovudine: May decrease zidovudine clearance. Avoid using together.
Drug-lifestyle. *Alcohol use:* May cause excessive CNS depression. Discourage use together.

EFFECTS ON LAB TEST RESULTS

• May increase ammonia, ALT, AST, and bilirubin levels.
• May increase eosinophil count and bleeding time. May decrease platelet, RBC, and WBC counts.
• May cause false-positive results for urine ketone levels.

CONTRAINDICATIONS & CAUTIONS

• Contraindicated in patients hypersensitive to drug and in those with hepatic disease or significant hepatic dysfunction, and in patients with a urea cycle disorder (UCD).

■ **Black Box Warning** Avoid use in women who may become pregnant. Valproate can cause teratogenic effects such as neural tube defects. ■

● Safety and efficacy of Depakote ER in children younger than age 10 haven't been established.

NURSING CONSIDERATIONS

● Obtain liver function test results, platelet count, and PT and INR before starting therapy, and monitor these values periodically.

● *Alert:* Closely monitor all patients taking or starting antiepileptic drugs for changes in behavior indicating worsening of suicidal thoughts or behavior or depression. Symptoms such as anxiety, agitation, hostility, mania, and hypomania may be precursors to emerging suicidality.

● Adverse reactions may not be caused by valproic acid alone because it's usually used with other anticonvulsants.

● When converting adults and children age 10 and older with seizures from Depakote to Depakote ER, make sure the extended-release dose is 8% to 20% higher than the regular dose taken previously. See manufacturer's package insert for more details.

● Divalproex sodium has a lower risk of adverse GI reactions.

● Never withdraw drug suddenly because sudden withdrawal may worsen seizures. Call prescriber at once if adverse reactions develop.

■ **Black Box Warning** Fatal hepatotoxicity may follow nonspecific symptoms, such as malaise, fever, anorexia, facial edema, vomiting, weakness, and lethargy. If these symptoms occur during therapy, notify prescriber at once because patient who might be developing hepatic dysfunction must stop taking drug. Perform liver function tests prior to therapy and at frequent intervals, especially during the first 6 months. ■

■ **Black Box Warning** Patients at high risk for hepatotoxicity include those with congenital metabolic disorders, mental retardation, or organic brain disease; those taking multiple anticonvulsants; and children younger than age 2. ■

● Notify prescriber if tremors occur; a dosage reduction may be needed.

● Monitor drug level. Therapeutic level is 50 to 100 mcg/ml.

● When converting patients from a brand-name drug to a generic drug, use caution because breakthrough seizures may occur.

● *Alert:* Sometimes fatal, hyperammonemic encephalopathy may occur when starting valproate therapy in patients with UCD. Evaluate patients with UCD risk factors before starting valproate therapy. Patients who develop symptoms of unexplained hyperammonemic encephalopathy during valproate therapy should stop drug, undergo prompt appropriate treatment, and be evaluated for underlying UCD.

● *Look alike–sound alike:* Don't confuse Depakote with Depakote ER.

PATIENT TEACHING

● Tell patient to take drug with food or milk to reduce adverse GI effects.

● Advise patient not to chew capsules; irritation of mouth and throat may result.

● Tell patient that capsules may be either swallowed whole or carefully opened and contents sprinkled on a teaspoonful of soft food. Tell patient to swallow immediately without chewing.

● Tell patient and parents that syrup shouldn't be mixed with carbonated beverages; mixture may be irritating to mouth and throat.

● Tell patient and parents to keep drug out of children's reach.

● Warn patient and parents not to stop drug therapy abruptly.

■ **Black Box Warning** Cases of life-threatening pancreatitis have been reported in children and adults receiving valproate shortly after initial use, as well as after several years of use. Warn patients and guardians that abdominal pain, nausea, vomiting, and anorexia can be symptoms of pancreatitis that require prompt medical evaluation. ■

● Advise patient to avoid driving and other potentially hazardous activities that require mental alertness until drug's CNS effects are known.

● Instruct patient or parents to call prescriber if malaise, weakness, lethargy, facial swelling, loss of appetite, or vomiting occurs.

Reactions may be *common,* uncommon, *life-threatening,* or COMMON AND LIFE-THREATENING.
Interaction may have a *rapid onset* or *delayed onset.*

• Tell woman to call prescriber if she becomes pregnant or plans to become pregnant during therapy.

zonisamide
zoh-NISS-a-mide

Zonegran

Pharmacologic class: sulfonamide
Pregnancy risk category C

AVAILABLE FORMS
Capsules: 25 mg, 50 mg, 100 mg

INDICATIONS & DOSAGES
➤ **Adjunct therapy for partial seizures in adults with epilepsy**
Adults and children older than age 16: Initially, 100 mg P.O. as a single daily dose for 2 weeks. Then, dosage may be increased to 200 mg daily for at least 2 weeks. Dosage can be increased to 300 mg and 400 mg P.O. daily, with the dose stable for at least 2 weeks to achieve steady state at each level. Doses can be given once or twice daily, except for the daily dose of 100 mg at start of therapy. Maximum recommended dose is 600 mg daily.
Adjust-a-dose: For patients with renal or hepatic impairment, titrate dosages more slowly and monitor patients more frequently.

ADMINISTRATION
P.O.
• Give drug without regard for food.
• Don't crush or open capsule.

ACTION
May stabilize neuronal membranes and suppress neuronal hypersynchronization, which prevents seizures.

Route	Onset	Peak	Duration
P.O.	Unknown	2–6 hr	Unknown

Half-life: 63 hours.

ADVERSE REACTIONS
CNS: *dizziness, headache, somnolence, seizures, status epilepticus,* agitation or irritability, anxiety, asthenia, ataxia, confusion, depression, difficulties in concentra-

tion or memory, difficulties in verbal expression, fatigue, hyperesthesia, incoordination, insomnia, mental slowing, nervousness, nystagmus, paresthesia, schizophrenic or schizophreniform behavior, speech disorders, tremor.
EENT: amblyopia, diplopia, pharyngitis, rhinitis, taste perversion, tinnitus.
GI: *anorexia,* abdominal pain, constipation, diarrhea, dry mouth, dyspepsia, nausea, vomiting.
GU: kidney stones.
Hematologic: ecchymoses.
Metabolic: weight loss.
Respiratory: cough.
Skin: pruritus, rash.
Other: accidental injury, flulike syndrome.

INTERACTIONS
Drug-drug. *Drugs that induce or inhibit CYP3A4:* May change zonisamide level; phenytoin, carbamazepine, phenobarbital, and valproate increase zonisamide clearance. Monitor patient closely.

EFFECTS ON LAB TEST RESULTS
• May increase BUN and creatinine levels.

CONTRAINDICATIONS & CAUTIONS
• Contraindicated in patients hypersensitive to drug or to sulfonamides.
• Contraindicated in those with glomerular filtration rate less than 50 ml/minute.
• Use cautiously in patients with renal and hepatic dysfunction or kidney stones.
• Use cautiously in patients with history of psychiatric symptoms.
• Use cautiously with other drugs that predispose patients to heat-related disorders, including but not limited to carbonic anhydrase inhibitors and drugs with anticholinergic activity.
• Safety and efficacy in children younger than age 16 haven't been established; children are at increased risk for oligohidrosis and hyperthermia caused by zonisamide.

NURSING CONSIDERATIONS
• *Alert:* Rarely, patients receiving sulfonamides have died because of severe reactions, such as Stevens-Johnson syndrome, fulminant hepatic necrosis, aplastic anemia, otherwise unexplained rashes, and agranulocytosis. If signs and symptoms of

hypersensitivity or other serious reactions occur, stop drug immediately and notify prescriber.
• **Alert:** Closely monitor all patients taking or starting antiepileptic drugs for changes in behavior indicating worsening of suicidal thoughts or behavior or depression. Symptoms such as anxiety, agitation, hostility, mania, and hypomania may be precursors to emerging suicidality.
• If patient develops acute renal failure or a significant sustained increase in creatinine or BUN level, stop drug and notify prescriber.
• Don't stop drug abruptly because this may cause increased seizures or status epilepticus; reduce dosage or stop drug gradually.
• Achieving steady-state levels may take 2 weeks.
• Monitor patient for signs and symptoms of hypersensitivity.
• Increase fluid intake and urine output to help prevent kidney stones, especially in patients with predisposing factors.
• Monitor renal function periodically.
• Monitor patient for cognitive and neuropsychiatric adverse reactions, including psychomotor slowing, difficulty with concentration, speech or language problems (especially word-finding difficulties), somnolence or fatigue, depression, and psychosis.

PATIENT TEACHING
• Tell patient to take drug with or without food and not to bite or break capsule.
• Advise patient to call prescriber immediately if rash develops or seizures worsen.
• Tell patient to contact prescriber immediately if he develops sudden back or abdominal pain, pain when urinating, bloody or dark urine, fever, sore throat, mouth sores or easy bruising, decreased sweating, fever, depression, or speech or language problems.
• Tell patient to drink 6 to 8 glasses of water a day.
• Caution patient that this drug can cause drowsiness and not to drive or operate dangerous machinery until drug's effects are known.
• Advise patient not to stop taking drug without prescriber's approval.

• Instruct woman of childbearing age to call prescriber if she is pregnant or breast-feeding or plans to become pregnant or breast-feed.
• Advise woman of childbearing age to use contraceptives while taking drug.

Reactions may be *common*, uncommon, *life-threatening*, or COMMON AND LIFE-THREATENING.
Interaction may have a *rapid onset* or **delayed onset**.

38

Antidepressants

amitriptyline hydrochloride
bupropion hydrochloride
citalopram hydrobromide
clomipramine hydrochloride
desipramine hydrochloride
desvenlafaxine succinate
doxepin hydrochloride
duloxetine hydrochloride
escitalopram oxalate
fluoxetine hydrochloride
fluvoxamine maleate
imipramine hydrochloride
imipramine pamoate
mirtazapine
nortriptyline hydrochloride
paroxetine hydrochloride
sertraline hydrochloride
trazodone hydrochloride
venlafaxine hydrochloride

---

amitriptyline hydrochloride
a-mee-TRIP-ti-leen

Pharmacologic class: tricyclic
antidepressant
Pregnancy risk category C

AVAILABLE FORMS
amitriptyline hydrochloride
Injection: 10 mg/ml
Tablets: 10 mg, 25 mg, 50 mg, 75 mg,
100 mg, 150 mg

INDICATIONS & DOSAGES
➤ **Depression (outpatients)**
Adults: Initially, 50 to 100 mg P.O.
at bedtime, increasing to 150 mg
daily. Maximum, 300 mg daily, if
needed. Maintenance, 50 to 100 mg
daily.
Elderly patients and adolescents:
10 mg P.O. t.i.d. and 20 mg at bedtime
daily
■ **Black Box Warning** Drug isn't
approved for use in children. ■

ADMINISTRATION
P.O.
● Give drug without regard for food.

I.M.
● *Alert:* Parenteral form of drug is for I.M.
administration only. Drug shouldn't be
given I.V.

ACTION
Unknown. A tricyclic antidepressant that
increases the amount of norepinephrine,
serotonin, or both in the CNS by blocking
their reuptake by the presynaptic
neurons.

Route	Onset	Peak	Duration
P.O., I.M.	Unknown	2–12 hr	Unknown

Half-life: Not established, varies widely.

ADVERSE REACTIONS
CNS: *stroke, seizures, coma,* ataxia,
tremor, peripheral neuropathy, anxiety,
insomnia, restlessness, drowsiness,
dizziness, weakness, fatigue, headache,
extrapyramidal reactions, hallucinations,
delusions, disorientation.
CV: *orthostatic hypotension, tachycardia,
heart block, arrhythmias, MI,* ECG
changes, hypertension, edema.
EENT: blurred vision, tinnitus, mydriasis,
increased intraocular pressure.
GI: *dry mouth,* nausea, vomiting,
anorexia, epigastric pain, diarrhea,
constipation, paralytic ileus.
GU: urine retention, altered libido,
impotence.
Hematologic: *agranulocytosis, thrombocytopenia, leukopenia,* eosinophilia.
Metabolic: *hypoglycemia,* hyperglycemia.
Skin: rash, urticaria, photosensitivity
reactions, diaphoresis.
Other: hypersensitivity reactions.

INTERACTIONS
Drug-drug. *Barbiturates, CNS depressants:* May enhance CNS depression.
Avoid using together.
Cimetidine, **fluoxetine, fluvoxamine,**
hormonal contraceptives, **paroxetine,
sertraline:** May increase tricyclic antidepressant level. Monitor drug levels
and patient for signs of toxicity.

Clonidine: May cause life-threatening hypertension. Avoid using together.

Epinephrine, norepinephrine: May increase hypertensive effect. Use together cautiously.

MAO inhibitors: May cause severe excitation, hyperpyrexia, or seizures, usually with high doses. Avoid using within 14 days of MAO inhibitor therapy.

Quinolones: May increase the risk of life-threatening arrhythmias. Avoid using together.

Drug-herb. *Evening primrose:* May cause additive or synergistic effect, resulting in lower seizure threshold and increasing the risk of seizures. Discourage use together.

St. John's wort, SAM-e, yohimbe: May cause serotonin syndrome and decrease amitriptyline level. Discourage use together.

Drug-lifestyle. *Alcohol use:* May enhance CNS depression. Discourage use together.

Smoking: May lower drug level. Watch for lack of effect.

Sun exposure: May increase risk of photosensitivity reactions. Advise patient to avoid excessive sunlight exposure.

EFFECTS ON LAB TEST RESULTS
• May increase or decrease glucose level.
• May increase eosinophil count and liver function test values. May decrease granulocyte, platelet, and WBC counts.

CONTRAINDICATIONS & CAUTIONS
• Contraindicated in patients hypersensitive to drug and in those who have received an MAO inhibitor within the past 14 days.
• Contraindicated during acute recovery phase of MI.
• Use cautiously in patients with history of seizures, urine retention, angle-closure glaucoma, or increased intraocular pressure; in those with hyperthyroidism, CV disease, diabetes, or impaired liver function; and in those receiving thyroid drugs.
• Use cautiously in elderly patients and in patients with suicidal ideation.
• Use cautiously in those receiving electroconvulsive therapy.

NURSING CONSIDERATIONS
■ **Black Box Warning** Drug may increase the risk of suicidal thinking and behavior in children and adolescents with major depressive disorder or other psychiatric disorder. Don't use in children younger than age 12. ■

■ **Black Box Warning** Drug may increase the risk of suicidal thinking and behavior in young adults ages 18 to 24 during the first 2 months of treatment. ■

• Amitriptyline has strong anticholinergic effects and is one of the most sedating tricyclic antidepressants. Anticholinergic effects have rapid onset even though therapeutic effect is delayed even weeks.
• Elderly patients may have an increased sensitivity to anticholinergic effects of drug; sedating effects of drug may increase the risk of falls in this population.
• If signs or symptoms of psychosis occur or increase, expect prescriber to reduce dosage. Record mood changes. Monitor patient for suicidal tendencies and allow only minimum supply of drug.
• Because patients using tricyclic antidepressants may suffer hypertensive episodes during surgery, stop drug gradually several days before surgery.
• Monitor glucose level.
• Watch for nausea, headache, and malaise after abrupt withdrawal of long-term therapy; these symptoms don't indicate addiction.
• Don't withdraw drug abruptly.
• *Look alike–sound alike:* Don't confuse amitriptyline with nortriptyline or aminophylline.

PATIENT TEACHING
• Whenever possible, advise patient to take full dose at bedtime, but warn him of possible morning orthostatic hypotension.
• Tell patient to avoid alcohol during drug therapy.
• Advise patient to consult prescriber before taking other drugs.
• Warn patient to avoid activities that require alertness and good psychomotor coordination until CNS effects of drug are known. Drowsiness and dizziness usually subside after a few weeks.
• Inform patient that dry mouth may be relieved with sugarless hard candy or gum. Saliva substitutes may be useful.
• To prevent photosensitivity reactions, advise patient to use a sunblock, wear pro-

tective clothing, and avoid prolonged exposure to strong sunlight.
• Warn patient not to stop drug abruptly.
• Advise patient that it may take as long as 30 days to achieve full therapeutic effect.

---

bupropion hydrobromide
Aplenzin

bupropion hydrochloride
byoo-PROE-pee-on

Wellbutrin✔, Wellbutrin SR✔, Wellbutrin XL, Zyban✔

Pharmacologic class: aminoketone
Pregnancy risk category B

AVAILABLE FORMS
bupropion hydrobromide
Tablets (extended-release): 174 mg, 348 mg, 522 mg
bupropion hydrochloride
Tablets (extended-release): 150 mg, 300 mg
Tablets (immediate-release): 75 mg, 100 mg
Tablets (sustained-release): 100 mg, 150 mg, 200 mg

INDICATIONS & DOSAGES
✳*NEW INDICATION:* **Major depressive disorder (Aplenzin only)**
Adults: Initially, 174 mg P.O. (equivalent to 150 mg/day bupropion HCl) given as a single daily dose in the morning. If the 174-mg initial dose is adequately tolerated, increase to the 348-mg/day target dose as early as day 4 of dosing. There should be an interval of at least 24 hours between successive doses. The full antidepressant effect may not be evident until after 4 weeks of treatment or longer. Consider increasing dosage to the maximum of 522 mg P.O. daily, given as a single dose, for patients in whom no clinical improvement is noted after several weeks of treatment at 348 mg/day. When switching patients from Wellbutrin, Wellbutrin SR, or Wellbutrin XL to Aplenzin, give the equivalent total daily dose when possible (522 mg bupropion HBr is equivalent to 450 mg bupropion HCl; 348 mg bupropion HBr is equivalent to 300 mg bupro-

pion HCl; 174 mg bupropion HBr is equivalent to 150 mg bupropion HCl).
Adjust-a-dose: In patients with renal impairment or mild to moderate hepatic impairment, including hepatic cirrhosis, reduced frequency or dose should be considered. In patients with severe hepatic cirrhosis, don't exceed 174 mg every other day.

➤ **Seasonal affective disorder**
Adults: Start treatment in autumn before depressive symptoms appear. Initially, 150 mg extended-release P.O. once daily in the morning. After 1 week, increase to 300 mg once daily, if tolerated. Continue 300 mg daily during the autumn and winter and taper to 150 mg daily for 2 weeks before stopping the drug in the early spring.

➤ **Depression**
Adults: For immediate-release, initially, 100 mg P.O. b.i.d.; increase after 3 days to 100 mg P.O. t.i.d., if needed. If patient doesn't improve after several weeks of therapy, increase dosage to 150 mg t.i.d. No single dose should exceed 150 mg. Allow at least 6 hours between successive doses. Maximum dose is 450 mg daily. For sustained-release, initially, 150 mg P.O. every morning; increase to target dose of 150 mg P.O. b.i.d., as tolerated, as early as day 4 of dosing. Allow at least 8 hours between successive doses. Maximum dose is 400 mg daily. For extended-release, initially, 150 mg P.O. every morning; increase to target dosage of 300 mg P.O. daily, as tolerated, as early as day 4 of dosing. Allow at least 24 hours between successive doses. Maximum is 450 mg daily.

➤ **Aid to smoking-cessation treatment**
Adults: 150 mg Zyban P.O. daily for 3 days; increased to maximum of 300 mg daily in two divided doses at least 8 hours apart.
Adjust-a-dose: In patients with mild to moderate hepatic cirrhosis or renal impairment, reduce frequency and dose. In patients with severe hepatic cirrhosis, don't exceed 75 mg immediate-release P.O. daily, 100 mg sustained-release P.O. daily, 150 mg (sustained-release) P.O. every other day, or 150 mg extended-release P.O. every other day.

ADMINISTRATION
P.O.
• Don't crush or split tablets.
• When switching patients from regular- or sustained-release tablets to extended-release tablets, give the same total daily dose (when possible) as the once-daily dosage provided.

ACTION
Unknown. Drug doesn't inhibit MAO, but it weakly inhibits norepinephrine, dopamine, and serotonin reuptake. Noradrenergic or dopaminergic mechanisms, or both, may cause drug's effect.

Route	Onset	Peak	Duration
P.O. (extended-release)	Unknown	5 hr	Unknown
P.O. (immediate-release)	Unknown	2 hr	Unknown
P.O. (sustained-release)	Unknown	3 hr	Unknown

Half-life: 8 to 24 hours.

ADVERSE REACTIONS
CNS: *abnormal dreams, insomnia, headache, sedation, tremor, agitation, dizziness,* **seizures, suicidal behavior,** anxiety, confusion, delusions, euphoria, fever, hostility, impaired concentration, impaired sleep quality, akinesia, akathisia, fatigue, syncope.
CV: *tachycardia,* **arrhythmias,** hypertension, hypotension, palpitations, chest pain.
EENT: *blurred vision, rhinitis,* auditory disturbances, epistaxis, pharyngitis, sinusitis, *dry mouth.*
GI: *constipation, nausea, vomiting, anorexia, dry mouth,* taste disturbance, dyspepsia, diarrhea, abdominal pain.
GU: impotence, menstrual complaints, urinary frequency, urine retention.
Metabolic: increased appetite, *weight loss, weight gain.*
Musculoskeletal: arthritis, myalgia, arthralgia, muscle spasm or twitch.
Respiratory: upper respiratory complaints, increase in coughing.
Skin: *excessive sweating,* pruritus, rash, cutaneous temperature disturbance, urticaria.

Other: fever and chills, decreased libido, accidental injury.

INTERACTIONS
Drug-drug. *Amantadine, levodopa:* May increase risk of adverse reactions. If used together, give small first doses of bupropion and increase dosage gradually.
Antidepressants (desipramine, fluoxetine, imipramine, nortriptyline, sertraline), antipsychotics (haloperidol, risperidone, thioridazine), systemic corticosteroids, theophylline: May lower seizure threshold. Use cautiously together.
Beta blockers, class IC antiarrhythmics: May increase levels of these drugs and adverse reactions. Use a reduced dose if used with bupropion.
Carbamazepine, phenobarbital, phenytoin: May enhance metabolism of bupropion and decrease its effect. Monitor patient closely.
CYP2B6 substrates or inhibitors (cyclophosphamide, orphenadrine, thiotepa), efavirenz, fluvoxamine, nelfinavir, norfluoxetine, paroxetine, ritonavir, sertraline: May increase bupropion activity. Monitor patient for expected therapeutic effects and adverse effects.
MAO inhibitors: May increase the risk of bupropion toxicity. Don't use drugs within 14 days of each other.
Nicotine replacement agents: May cause hypertension. Monitor blood pressure.
Ritonavir: May increase bupropion level. Monitor patient closely for adverse reactions.
Drug-lifestyle. *Alcohol use:* May alter seizure threshold. Discourage use together.
Sun exposure: May increase risk of photosensitivity reactions. Advise patient to avoid excessive sunlight exposure.

EFFECTS ON LAB TEST RESULTS
• May increase liver function test values.

CONTRAINDICATIONS & CAUTIONS
• Contraindicated in patients hypersensitive to drug, in those who have taken MAO inhibitors within previous 14 days, and in those with seizure disorders or history of bulimia or anorexia

nervosa because of a higher risk of seizures.

• Contraindicated in patients abruptly stopping use of alcohol or sedatives (including benzodiazepines).

• Don't use with other drugs containing bupropion.

■ **Black Box Warning** Bupropion isn't approved for use in children. ■

• Use cautiously in patients with recent history of MI, unstable heart disease, renal or hepatic impairment, a history of seizures, head trauma, or other predisposition to seizures, and in those being treated with drugs that lower seizure threshold.

NURSING CONSIDERATIONS

• Many patients experience a period of increased restlessness, including agitation, insomnia, and anxiety, especially at start of therapy.

• *Alert:* To minimize the risk of seizures, don't exceed maximum recommended dose.

• *Alert:* Patient with major depressive disorder may experience a worsening of depression and suicidal thoughts. Carefully monitor patient for worsening depression or suicidal thoughts, especially at the beginning of therapy and during dosage changes.

■ **Black Box Warning** Drug may increase the risk of suicidal thinking and behavior in children and adolescents with major depressive disorder or other psychiatric disorder. ■

■ **Black Box Warning** Drug may increase the risk of suicidal thinking and behavior in young adults ages 18 to 24 during the first 2 months of treatment. ■

• Closely monitor patient with history of bipolar disorder. Antidepressants can cause manic episodes during the depressed phase of bipolar disorder. This may be less likely to occur with bupropion than with other antidepressants.

• Begin smoking-cessation treatment while patient is still smoking; about 1 week is needed to achieve steady-state drug levels.

• Stop smoking-cessation treatment if patient hasn't progressed toward abstinence by week 7. Treatment usually lasts

up to 12 weeks. Patient can stop taking drug without tapering off.

■ **Black Box Warning** Zyban isn't indicated for treatment of depression. ■

• *Look alike–sound alike:* Don't confuse bupropion with buspirone or Wellbutrin with Wellcovorin.

PATIENT TEACHING

• *Alert:* Explain that excessive use of alcohol, abrupt withdrawal from alcohol or other sedatives, and addiction to cocaine, opiates, or stimulants during therapy may increase risk of seizures. Seizure risk is also increased in those using OTC stimulants, in anorectics, and in diabetic patients using oral antidiabetics or insulin.

• Tell patient not to chew, crush, or divide tablets.

• Advise patient to consult prescriber before taking other prescription or OTC drugs.

• Advise patient to avoid hazardous activities that require alertness and good psychomotor coordination until effects of drug are known.

• *Alert:* Advise patient that Zyban and Wellbutrin contain the same active ingredient and shouldn't be used together.

• Tell patient that it may take 4 weeks to reach full antidepressant effect.

• *Alert:* Advise patient to report mood swings or suicidal thoughts immediately.

• Inform patient that tablets may have an odor.

---

citalopram hydrobromide
si-TAL-oh-pram

Celexa◆

Pharmacologic class: SSRI
Pregnancy risk category C

AVAILABLE FORMS
Solution: 10 mg/5 ml
Tablets: 10 mg, 20 mg, 40 mg
Tablets (orally disintegrating): 40 mg

INDICATIONS & DOSAGES
➤ **Depression**
Adults: Initially, 20 mg P.O. once daily, increasing to 40 mg daily after no less

than 1 week. Maximum recommended dose is 40 mg daily.

Elderly patients: 20 mg daily P.O. with adjustment to 40 mg daily only for unresponsive patients.

Adjust-a-dose: For patients with hepatic impairment, use 20 mg daily P.O. with adjustment to 40 mg daily only for unresponsive patients.

➤ **Premenstrual disorders** ◆

Adults: Intermittent dosing consists of initiating treatment on the estimated day of ovulation. Give 5 mg P.O. Each day increase dose by 5 mg to a maximum dose of 30 mg P.O. daily until first day of menstruation. On first day of menstruation, reduce dose to 20 mg P.O. daily. On second day, reduce dose to 10 mg P.O. daily. No drug is given from menstruation day 3 until estimated ovulation begins.

ADMINISTRATION
P.O.
- Allow orally disintegrating tablet (ODT) to dissolve on the patient's tongue, then be swallowed, with or without water.
- Don't cut, break, or crush ODTs.
- Give drug without regard for food.

ACTION
Probably linked to potentiation of serotonergic activity in the CNS resulting from inhibition of neuronal reuptake of serotonin.

Route	Onset	Peak	Duration
P.O.	Unknown	4 hr	Unknown

Half-life: 35 hours.

ADVERSE REACTIONS
CNS: *somnolence, insomnia,* **suicide attempt,** anxiety, agitation, dizziness, paresthesia, migraine, impaired concentration, amnesia, depression, apathy, tremor, confusion, fatigue, fever.
CV: tachycardia, orthostatic hypotension, hypotension.
EENT: rhinitis, sinusitis, abnormal accommodation.
GI: *dry mouth, nausea,* diarrhea, anorexia, dyspepsia, vomiting, abdominal pain, taste perversion, increased saliva, flatulence, increased appetite.

GU: dysmenorrhea, amenorrhea, ejaculation disorder, impotence, anorgasmia, polyuria.
Metabolic: decreased or increased weight.
Musculoskeletal: arthralgia, myalgia.
Respiratory: upper respiratory tract infection, coughing.
Skin: rash, pruritus.
Other: *increased sweating,* yawning, decreased libido.

INTERACTIONS
Drug-drug. *Amphetamines, buspirone, dextromethorphan, dihydroergotamine, meperidine, other SSRIs or SSNRIs (duloxetine, venlafaxine),* **tramadol,** *trazodone, tricyclic antidepressants, tryptophan:* May increase the risk of serotonin syndrome. Avoid other drugs that increase the availability of serotonin in the CNS; monitor patient closely if used together.
Carbamazepine: May increase citalopram clearance. Monitor patient for effects.
CNS drugs: May cause additive effects. Use together cautiously.
Drugs that inhibit cytochrome P-450 isoenzymes 3A4 and 2C19: May cause decreased clearance of citalopram. Monitor patient for increased adverse effects.
Imipramine, other tricyclic antidepressants: May increase level of imipramine metabolite desipramine by about 50%. Use together cautiously.
Lithium: May enhance serotonergic effect of citalopram. Use together cautiously, and monitor lithium level.
MAO inhibitors (phenelzine, selegiline, tranylcypromine): May cause serotonin syndrome. Avoid using within 14 days of MAO inhibitor therapy.
Sumatriptan: May cause weakness, hyperreflexia, and incoordination. Monitor patient closely.
Drug-herb. *St. John's wort:* May increase the risk of serotonin syndrome. Discourage use together.
Drug-lifestyle. *Alcohol use:* May increase CNS effects. Discourage use together.

EFFECTS ON LAB TEST RESULTS
None reported.

CONTRAINDICATIONS & CAUTIONS
- Contraindicated in patients hypersensitive to drug or its inactive components,

within 14 days of MAO inhibitor therapy, and in patients taking pimozide.
- Use cautiously in patients with history of mania, seizures, suicidal thoughts, or hepatic or renal impairment.
- Use in third trimester of pregnancy may be linked to neonatal complications at birth. Consider the risk versus benefit of treatment during this time.
- **Black Box Warning** Safety and efficacy of drug haven't been established in children. ▪

NURSING CONSIDERATIONS
- Although drug hasn't been shown to impair psychomotor performance, any psychoactive drug has the potential to impair judgment, thinking, or motor skills.
- The possibility of a suicide attempt is inherent in depression and may persist until significant remission occurs. Closely supervise high-risk patients at start of drug therapy. Reduce risk of overdose by limiting amount of drug available per refill.
- **Black Box Warning** Drug may increase the risk of suicidal thinking and behavior in children and adolescents with major depressive disorder or other psychiatric disorders. ▪
- **Black Box Warning** Drug may increase the risk of suicidal thinking and behavior in young adults ages 18 to 24 during the first 2 months of treatment. ▪
- At least 14 days should elapse between MAO inhibitor therapy and citalopram therapy.
- *Alert:* Combining triptans with an SSRI or an SSNRI may cause serotonin syndrome. Signs and symptoms may include restlessness, hallucinations, loss of coordination, fast heartbeat, rapid changes in blood pressure, increased body temperature, overactive reflexes, nausea, vomiting, and diarrhea. Serotonin syndrome may be more likely to occur when starting or increasing the dose of triptan, SSRI, or SNRI.
- *Look alike–sound alike:* Don't confuse Celexa with Celebrex or Cerebyx.

PATIENT TEACHING
- Caution patient against use of MAO inhibitors while taking citalopram.

- Inform patient that, although improvement may take 1 to 4 weeks, he should continue therapy as prescribed.
- Advise patient not to stop drug abruptly.
- Tell patient that drug may be taken in the morning or evening without regard to meals. If drowsiness occurs, he should take drug in evening.
- Tell patient to allow orally disintegrating tablet to dissolve on his tongue then swallow, with or without water. Tell him not to cut, crush, or chew.
- Instruct patient to exercise caution when driving or operating hazardous machinery; drug may impair judgment, thinking, and motor skills.
- Advise patient to consult prescriber before taking other prescription or OTC drugs.
- Advise woman of childbearing age to consult prescriber before breast-feeding.
- Warn patient to avoid alcohol during drug therapy.
- Instruct woman of childbearing age to use contraceptives during drug therapy and to notify prescriber immediately if pregnancy is suspected.

clomipramine hydrochloride
kloe-MI-pra-meen

Anafranil

Pharmacologic class: tricyclic antidepressant (TCA)
Pregnancy risk category C

AVAILABLE FORMS
Capsules: 25 mg, 50 mg, 75 mg

INDICATIONS & DOSAGES
➤ **Obsessive-compulsive disorder**
Adults: Initially, 25 mg P.O. daily with meals, gradually increased to 100 mg daily in divided doses during first 2 weeks. Thereafter, increase to maximum dose of 250 mg daily in divided doses with meals, as needed. After adjustment, give total daily dose at bedtime.
Children and adolescents: Initially, 25 mg P.O. daily with meals, gradually increased over first 2 weeks to daily maximum of 3 mg/kg or 100 mg P.O. in divided doses, whichever is smaller. Maximum daily

dose is 3 mg/kg or 200 mg, whichever is smaller; give at bedtime after adjustment. Reassess and adjust dosage periodically.

➤ **To manage panic disorder with or without agoraphobia**
Adults: 12.5 to 150 mg P.O. daily (maximum 200 mg).

➤ **Depression, chronic pain** ◆
Adults: 100 to 250 mg P.O. daily.

➤ **Cataplexy and related narcolepsy** ◆
Adults: 25 to 200 mg P.O. daily.

ADMINISTRATION
P.O.
● Give drug without regard for food.

ACTION
Unknown. Inhibits reuptake of serotonin and norepinephrine at the presynaptic neuron.

Route	Onset	Peak	Duration
P.O.	Unknown	2–6 hr	Unknown

Half-life: Parent compound, 32 hours; active metabolite, 69 hours.

ADVERSE REACTIONS
CNS: *somnolence, tremor, dizziness, headache, insomnia, nervousness, myoclonus, fatigue,* **seizures,** *EEG changes.*
CV: *orthostatic hypotension, palpitations,* tachycardia.
EENT: *pharyngitis, rhinitis, visual changes.*
GI: *dry mouth, constipation, nausea, dyspepsia, increased appetite, anorexia, abdominal pain,* diarrhea.
GU: *urinary hesitancy, UTI, dysmenorrhea, ejaculation failure, impotence.*
Hematologic: purpura.
Metabolic: *weight gain.*
Musculoskeletal: *myalgia.*
Skin: *diaphoresis,* rash, pruritus, dry skin.
Other: *altered libido.*

INTERACTIONS
Drug-drug. *Barbiturates:* May decrease TCA level. Watch for decreased antidepressant effect.
Cimetidine, **fluoxetine, fluvoxamine, paroxetine, sertraline:** May increase TCA level. Monitor drug level and patient for signs of toxicity.

Clonidine: May cause life-threatening hypertension. Avoid using together.
CNS depressants: May enhance CNS depression. Avoid using together.
Epinephrine, norepinephrine: May increase hypertensive effect. Use together cautiously.
MAO inhibitors: May cause hyperpyretic crisis, seizures, coma, or death. Avoid using within 14 days of MAO inhibitor therapy.
Quinolones: May increase the risk of life-threatening arrhythmias. Avoid using together.
Drug-herb. *Evening primrose oil:* May cause additive or synergistic effect, resulting in lower seizure threshold and increasing the risk of seizure. Discourage use together.
St. John's wort, SAM-e, yohimbe: May cause serotonin syndrome. Discourage use together.
Drug-lifestyle. *Alcohol use:* May enhance CNS depression. Discourage use together.
Sun exposure: May increase risk of photosensitivity reactions. Advise patient to avoid excessive sunlight exposure.

EFFECTS ON LAB TEST RESULTS
None reported.

CONTRAINDICATIONS & CAUTIONS
● Contraindicated in patients hypersensitive to drug or other tricyclic antidepressants, in those who have taken MAO inhibitors within previous 14 days, and in patients in acute recovery period after MI.
● Use cautiously in patients with history of seizure disorders or with brain damage of varying cause; in patients receiving other seizure threshold–lowering drugs; in patients at risk for suicide; in patients with history of urine retention or angle-closure glaucoma, increased intraocular pressure, CV disease, impaired hepatic or renal function, or hyperthyroidism; in patients with tumors of the adrenal medulla; in patients receiving thyroid drug or electroconvulsive therapy; and in those undergoing elective surgery.
■ **Black Box Warning** Clomipramine isn't approved for use in children except for those with obsessive compulsive disorder. ■

Reactions may be *common,* uncommon, *life-threatening,* or COMMON AND LIFE-THREATENING.
Interaction may have a *rapid onset* or **delayed onset.**

NURSING CONSIDERATIONS
• Monitor mood and watch for suicidal tendencies. Allow patient to have only the minimum amount of drug.
■ **Black Box Warning** Drug may increase risk of suicidal thinking and behavior in children, adolescents, and young adults ages 18 to 24 during the first 2 months of treatment, especially in those with major depressive disorder or other psychiatric disorder. ■
• Don't withdraw drug abruptly.
• Because patients may suffer hypertensive episodes during surgery, stop drug gradually several days before surgery.
• Relieve dry mouth with sugarless candy or gum. Saliva substitutes may be needed.
• *Look alike–sound alike:* Don't confuse clomipramine with chlorpromazine or clomiphene, or Anafranil with enalapril, nafarelin, or alfentanil.

PATIENT TEACHING
• Warn patient to avoid hazardous activities requiring alertness and good coordination, especially during adjustment. Daytime sedation and dizziness may occur.
• Tell patient to avoid alcohol during drug therapy.
• Warn patient not to stop drug suddenly.
• Advise patient to use sunblock, wear protective clothing, and avoid prolonged exposure to strong sunlight to prevent oversensitivity to the sun.

---

desipramine hydrochloride
dess-IP-ra-meen

Norpramin

Pharmacologic class: tricyclic antidepressant (TCA)
Pregnancy risk category NR

AVAILABLE FORMS
Tablets: 10 mg, 25 mg, 50 mg, 75 mg, 100 mg, 150 mg

INDICATIONS & DOSAGES
➤ **Depression**
Adults: 100 to 200 mg P.O. daily in divided doses; increase to maximum of 300 mg daily. Or, give entire dose at bedtime.

Adolescents and elderly patients: 25 to 100 mg P.O. daily in divided doses; increase gradually to maximum of 150 mg daily, if needed.

ADMINISTRATION
P.O.
• Give drug without regard for food.

ACTION
Unknown. Increases the amount of norepinephrine, serotonin, or both in the CNS by blocking their reuptake by the presynaptic neurons.

Route	Onset	Peak	Duration
P.O.	Unknown	4–6 hr	Unknown

Half-life: Unknown.

ADVERSE REACTIONS
CNS: *drowsiness, dizziness, seizures,* excitation, tremor, weakness, confusion, anxiety, restlessness, agitation, headache, nervousness, EEG changes, extrapyramidal reactions.
CV: *tachycardia,* orthostatic hypotension, ECG changes, hypertension.
EENT: *blurred vision,* tinnitus, mydriasis.
GI: *dry mouth,* constipation, nausea, vomiting, anorexia, paralytic ileus.
GU: urine retention.
Metabolic: *hypoglycemia,* hyperglycemia.
Skin: rash, urticaria, photosensitivity reactions, diaphoresis.
Other: *sudden death in children,* hypersensitivity reactions.

INTERACTIONS
Drug-drug. *Barbiturates, CNS depressants:* May enhance CNS depression. Avoid using together.
Cimetidine, **fluoxetine, fluvoxamine, paroxetine, sertraline:** May increase desipramine level. Monitor drug levels and patient for signs of toxicity.
Clonidine: May cause life-threatening blood pressure elevations. Avoid using together.
Epinephrine, norepinephrine: May increase hypertensive effect. Use together cautiously.
MAO inhibitors: May cause severe excitation, hyperpyrexia, or seizures, usually

with high doses. Avoid using within 14 days of MAO inhibitor therapy.

Quinolones: May increase the risk of life-threatening arrhythmias. Avoid using together.

Drug-herb. *Evening primrose oil:* May cause additive or synergistic effect, resulting in lower seizure threshold and increasing the risk of seizure. Discourage use together.

St. John's wort, SAM-e, yohimbe. May cause serotonin syndrome. Discourage use together.

Drug-lifestyle. *Alcohol use:* May enhance CNS depression. Discourage use together.

Smoking: May lower drug level. Monitor patient for lack of effect.

Sun exposure: May increase risk of photosensitivity reactions. Advise patient to avoid excessive sunlight exposure.

EFFECTS ON LAB TEST RESULTS
- May increase or decrease glucose level.
- May increase liver function test values.

CONTRAINDICATIONS & CAUTIONS
- Contraindicated in patients hypersensitive to drug and in those who have taken MAO inhibitors within previous 14 days.
- Contraindicated during acute recovery phase after MI.
- ■ **Black Box Warning** Desipramine isn't approved for use in children. ■
- Use with extreme caution in patients with CV disease; in those with history of urine retention, glaucoma, seizure disorders, or thyroid disease; and in those taking thyroid drug.
- *Alert:* Treatment of patients who require as much as 300 mg desipramine should be initiated in hospitals where access to skilled health care providers and frequent electrocardiograms is available. High doses may cause prolongation of the QRS or QT interval.

NURSING CONSIDERATIONS
- Monitor patient for nausea, headache, and malaise after abrupt withdrawal of long-term therapy; these symptoms don't indicate addiction.

- Don't withdraw drug abruptly.
- Because patients may suffer hypertensive episodes during surgery, stop drug gradually several days before surgery.
- If signs or symptoms of psychosis occur or increase, notify prescriber. Record mood changes. Monitor patient for suicidal tendencies.
- ■ **Black Box Warning** Drug may increase risk of suicidal thinking and behavior in children, adolescents, and young adults ages 18 to 24 during the first 2 months of treatment, especially in those with major depressive disorder or other psychiatric disorder. ■
- Because drug produces fewer anticholinergic effects than other TCAs, it's often prescribed for cardiac patients.
- Recommend sugarless hard candy or gum to relieve dry mouth. Saliva substitutes may be needed.
- *Alert:* Norpramin may contain tartrazine.
- *Look alike–sound alike:* Don't confuse desipramine with disopyramide or imipramine.

PATIENT TEACHING
- Advise patient to take full dose at bedtime to avoid daytime sedation; if insomnia occurs, tell him to take drug in the morning.
- Warn patient to avoid hazardous activities that require alertness and good coordination until effects of drug are known. Drowsiness and dizziness usually subside after a few weeks.
- Advise patient to call prescriber if fever and sore throat occur. Blood counts may need to be obtained.
- Tell patient to avoid alcohol during therapy because it may antagonize effects of drug.
- Tell patient to consult prescriber before taking other prescription or OTC drugs.
- Warn patient not to stop drug suddenly.
- To prevent sensitivity to the sun, advise patient to use sunblock, wear protective clothing, and avoid prolonged exposure to strong sunlight.

Reactions may be *common*, uncommon, *life-threatening*, or COMMON AND LIFE-THREATENING.
Interaction may have a *rapid* onset or **delayed onset.**

✳ NEW DRUG

desvenlafaxine succinate
des-ven-lah-FAX-in

Pristiq

Pharmacologic class: selective serotonin and selective norepinephrine reuptake inhibitor (SNRI)
Pregnancy risk category C

AVAILABLE FORMS
Tablets (extended-release): 50 mg, 100 mg

INDICATIONS & DOSAGES
➤ **Major depressive disorder**
Adults: 50 mg P.O. once daily.
Adjust-a-dose: For patients with creatinine clearance less than 30 ml/minute, give 50 mg P.O. every other day. For patients with hepatic impairment, maximum dosage is 100 mg/day.

ACTION
Thought to stimulate receptors, increasing the release of serotonin and norepinephrine.
Absorption: Steady-state plasma concentrations are reached within 4 to 5 days.
Distribution: 30% protein-bound.
Metabolism: TBy CYP3A4 pathway in the liver.
Excretion: 45% excreted unchanged in urine.

Route	Onset	Peak	Duration
P.O.	Unknown	7.5 hr	Unknown

Half-life: About 11 hours.

ADVERSE REACTIONS
CNS: abnormal dreams, anxiety, asthenia, chills, *dizziness,* fatigue, jittery feeling, *headache, insomnia,* irritability, paresthesia, somnolence, tremor.
CV: hot flashes, hypertension, palpitations, tachycardia.
EENT: blurred vision, mydriasis, tinnitus.
GI: constipation, *diarrhea, dry mouth,* dysgeusia, *GI bleeding, nausea,* vomiting.
GU: proteinuria.
Metabolic: *decreased appetite,* weight loss.

Respiratory: yawning.
Skin: *hyperhidrosis,* rash.
Other: *sexual dysfunction.*

INTERACTIONS
Drug-drug. *Aspirin, NSAIDs, warfarin, other drugs that affect coagulation:* May increase risk of bleeding. Use together cautiously.
CNS drugs: Drug may cause additive effect. Avoid using together.
CYP3A4 inhibitors (ketoconazole): May increase desvenlafaxine levels. Use together cautiously.
Desipramine, other drugs metabolized by CYP2D6: May increase levels of these drugs. Use together cautiously.
MAO inhibitors: May cause serotonin syndrome. Avoid using within 7 days of MAO inhibitor therapy.
Midazolam, other drugs metabolized by CYP3A4: May decrease levels of these drugs. Use together cautiously.
SSRIs, SNRIs: May increase risk of serotonin syndrome. Monitor patient closely if used together.
Venlafaxine: Drug is a major active metabolite of venlafaxine. Avoid using together.
Drug-lifestyle. *Alcohol use:* May enhance CNS depression. Discourage use together.

EFFECTS ON LAB TEST RESULTS
● May increase total cholesterol, LDL, triglyceride, and sodium levels.

CONTRAINDICATIONS & CAUTIONS
● Contraindicated in patients hypersensitive to drug or within 14 days of MAO inhibitor therapy.
● Use cautiously in patients with renal impairment, diseases or conditions that could affect hemodynamic responses or metabolism, and in those with a history of mania or seizures. Use only in pregnant or breast-feeding women when the benefits outweigh the possible risks to the fetus.
■ **Black Box Warning** Desvenlafaxine isn't approved for use in children. ■

OVERDOSE AND TREATMENT
Doses over 600 mg may cause headache, vomiting, agitation, dizziness, nausea, constipation, diarrhea, dry mouth, paresthesia, and tachycardia. Provide support-

ive care and monitor vital signs and cardiac rhythm. Perform gastric lavage and administer activated charcoal, as needed.

NURSING CONSIDERATIONS

■ **Black Box Warning** Closely monitor patient being treated for depression for signs and symptoms of clinical worsening and suicidal ideation, especially at the beginning of therapy and with dosage adjustments. Symptoms may include agitation, insomnia, anxiety, aggressiveness, or panic attacks. ■

• Carefully monitor blood pressure. Drug may cause dose-related increases in blood pressure.
• Monitor intraocular pressure in patients at risk for angle-closure glaucoma.
• Record mood changes. Monitor patient for suicidal tendencies and allow patient only a minimum supply of the drug.
• Monitor patient for signs and symptoms of bleeding.
• Monitor lipid and sodium levels before and during therapy.
• *Alert:* Don't stop drug abruptly. Withdrawal or discontinuation syndrome may occur if drug is stopped abruptly. Signs and symptoms of withdrawal syndrome include dizziness, nausea, headache, irritability, insomnia, diarrhea, anxiety, fatigue, abnormal dreams, and hyperhidrosis. Taper drug slowly.
• Monitor respiratory status. Drug may cause interstitial lung disease or eosinophilic pneumonia. If patient develops dyspnea, cough, or chest discomfort, discontinue drug.

Pregnant patients
• Use in third trimester of pregnancy may be associated with neonatal complications at birth. Consider risk versus benefit of treatment during this time.

Pediatric patients
• Safety and effectiveness haven't been established.

Geriatric patients
• Use cautiously in elderly patients.

PATIENT TEACHING

• Advise a woman of childbearing age to contact prescriber if she becomes pregnant, intends to become pregnant during therapy, or is breast-feeding.

• Warn family members to closely monitor patient for signs and symptoms of worsening condition or suicidal ideation.
• Tell patient to avoid alcohol and to consult prescriber before taking other prescription or OTC drugs.
• Warn patient to avoid hazardous activities that require alertness and good coordination until effects of drug are known.
• If medication is to be stopped, tell patient to stop drug gradually by tapering the dosage as instructed by prescriber and not to abruptly stop taking drug.
• Tell patient not to divide, crush, chew, or dissolve tablets.

---

doxepin hydrochloride
DOKS-eh-pin

Sinequan

Pharmacologic class: tricyclic antidepressant (TCA)
Pregnancy risk category C

AVAILABLE FORMS
Capsules: 10 mg, 25 mg, 50 mg, 75 mg, 100 mg, 150 mg
Oral concentrate: 10 mg/ml

INDICATIONS & DOSAGES
➤ **Depression; anxiety**
Adults: Initially, 75 mg P.O. daily. Usual dosage range is 75 to 150 mg daily to maximum of 300 mg daily in divided doses. Or, entire maintenance dose may be given once daily with maximum dose of 150 mg.

ADMINISTRATION
P.O.
• Dilute oral concentrate with 4 ounces (120 ml) of water, milk, or juice (orange, grapefruit, tomato, prune, or pineapple, but not grape); don't mix preparation with carbonated beverages.
• Give at bedtime, if possible, because it may cause drowsiness and dizziness.

ACTION
Unknown. Increases amount of norepinephrine, serotonin, or both in the CNS by blocking their reuptake by the presynaptic neurons.

Reactions may be *common,* uncommon, *life-threatening,* or COMMON AND LIFE-THREATENING.
Interaction may have a *rapid onset* or *delayed onset.*

Route	Onset	Peak	Duration
P.O.	Unknown	2 hr	Unknown

Half-life: 6 to 8 hours.

ADVERSE REACTIONS

CNS: *drowsiness, dizziness, seizures,* confusion, numbness, hallucinations, paresthesia, ataxia, weakness, headache, extrapyramidal reactions.
CV: *orthostatic hypotension, tachycardia,* ECG changes.
EENT: *blurred vision,* tinnitus.
GI: *dry mouth, constipation,* nausea, vomiting, anorexia.
GU: urine retention.
Metabolic: *hypoglycemia,* hyperglycemia.
Skin: *diaphoresis,* rash, urticaria, photosensitivity reactions.
Other: hypersensitivity reactions.

INTERACTIONS

Drug-drug. *Barbiturates, CNS depressants:* May enhance CNS depression. Avoid using together.
Cimetidine, **fluoxetine, fluvoxamine, paroxetine, sertraline:** May increase doxepin level. Monitor drug levels and patient for signs of toxicity.
Clonidine: May cause life-threatening hypertension. Avoid using together.
Epinephrine, norepinephrine: May increase hypertensive effect. Use together cautiously.
MAO inhibitors: May cause severe excitation, hyperpyrexia, or seizures, usually with high dosage. Avoid using within 14 days of MAO inhibitor therapy.
Quinolones: May increase the risk of life-threatening arrhythmias. Avoid using together.
Drug-herb. *Evening primrose oil:* May cause additive or synergistic effect, resulting in lower seizure threshold and increasing the risk of seizure. Discourage use together.
St. John's wort, SAM-e, yohimbe: May cause serotonin syndrome. Discourage use together.
Drug-lifestyle. *Alcohol use:* May enhance CNS depression. Discourage use together.
Sun exposure: May increase risk of photosensitivity reactions. Advise patient to avoid excessive sunlight exposure.

EFFECTS ON LAB TEST RESULTS
● May increase or decrease glucose level.
● May increase liver function test values.

CONTRAINDICATIONS & CAUTIONS
● Contraindicated in patients hypersensitive to drug and in those with glaucoma or tendency toward urine retention; also contraindicated in those who have received an MAO inhibitor within past 14 days and during acute recovery phase of an MI.
■ **Black Box Warning** Doxepin isn't approved for use in children. ■

NURSING CONSIDERATIONS
● Don't withdraw drug abruptly.
● Monitor patient for nausea, headache, and malaise after abrupt withdrawal of long-term therapy; these symptoms don't indicate addiction.
● *Alert:* Because hypertensive episodes may occur during surgery in patients receiving drug, stop it gradually several days before surgery.
● If signs or symptoms of psychosis occur or increase, expect prescriber to reduce dosage. Record mood changes. Monitor patient for suicidal tendencies and allow only a minimum supply of drug.
■ **Black Box Warning** Drug may increase risk of suicidal thinking and behavior in children, adolescents, and young adults ages 18 to 24 during the first 2 months of treatment, especially in those with major depressive disorder or other psychiatric disorder. ■
● Drug has strong anticholinergic effects and is one of the most sedating TCAs. Adverse anticholinergic effects can occur rapidly.
● Recommend use of sugarless hard candy or gum to relieve dry mouth.
● *Look alike–sound alike:* Don't confuse doxepin with doxazosin, digoxin, doxapram, or Doxidan; don't confuse Sinequan with saquinavir.

PATIENT TEACHING
● Tell patient to dilute oral concentrate with 4 ounces (120 ml) of water, milk, or juice (orange, grapefruit, tomato, prune, or pineapple, but not grape); preparation shouldn't be mixed with carbonated beverages.

- Tell patient to take full dose at bedtime whenever he can, but warn him of possible morning dizziness on standing up quickly.
- Advise patient to consult prescriber before taking other prescription or OTC drugs.
- Warn patient to avoid hazardous activities that require alertness and good psychomotor coordination until effects of drug are known. Drowsiness and dizziness usually subside after a few weeks.
- Tell patient to avoid alcohol during drug therapy.
- Tell patient that maximal effect may not be evident for 2 to 3 weeks.
- Warn patient not to stop drug suddenly.
- To prevent sensitivity to the sun, advise patient to use sunblock, wear protective clothing, and avoid prolonged exposure to strong sunlight.

duloxetine hydrochloride
do-LOCKS-ah-teen

Cymbalta♪

Pharmacologic class: SSNRI
Pregnancy risk category C

AVAILABLE FORMS
Capsules (delayed-release): 20 mg, 30 mg, 60 mg

INDICATIONS & DOSAGES
➤ **Major depressive disorder**
Adults: Initially, 20 mg P.O. b.i.d.; then, 60 mg P.O. once daily or divided in two equal doses. Maximum, 60 mg daily.
➤ **Generalized anxiety disorder**
Adults: 60 mg P.O. daily. Or, 30 mg P.O. daily for 1 week; then increase to 60 mg P.O. daily.
✳ *NEW INDICATION:* **Fibromyalgia**
Adults: Initially, 30 mg P.O. once daily for 1 week; increase to 60 mg P.O. once daily after a week. Some patients may respond to the starting dose. Maximum dose is 60 mg/day. Base continued treatment on individual patient response.
➤ **Neuropathic pain related to diabetic peripheral neuropathy**
Adults: 60 mg P.O. once daily.
Adjust-a-dose: Duloxetine isn't recommended for patients with end-stage renal disease, severe renal dysfunction, or hepatic dysfunction.

ADMINISTRATION
P.O.
- Give drug whole; don't crush or open capsule.

ACTION
May inhibit serotonin and norepinephrine reuptake in the CNS.

Route	Onset	Peak	Duration
P.O.	Unknown	6 hr	Unknown

Half-life: 12 hours.

ADVERSE REACTIONS
CNS: *dizziness, fatigue, headache, insomnia, somnolence,* **suicidal thoughts,** fever, hypoesthesia, initial insomnia, irritability, lethargy, nervousness, nightmares, restlessness, sleep disorder, anxiety, asthenia, tremor.
CV: hot flashes, hypertension, increased heart rate.
EENT: blurred vision, nasopharyngitis, pharyngolaryngeal pain.
GI: *constipation, diarrhea, dry mouth, nausea,* dyspepsia, gastritis, vomiting.
GU: abnormal orgasm, abnormally increased frequency of urinating, delayed or dysfunctional ejaculation, dysuria, erectile dysfunction, urinary hesitation.
Metabolic: *decreased appetite,* **hypoglycemia,** increased appetite, weight gain or loss.
Musculoskeletal: muscle cramps, myalgia.
Respiratory: cough.
Skin: increased sweating, night sweats, pruritus, rash.
Other: decreased libido, rigors.

INTERACTIONS
Drug-drug. *Antiarrhythmics of type 1C (flecainide, propafenone), phenothiazines:* May increase levels of these drugs. Use together cautiously.
CNS drugs: May increase adverse effects. Use together cautiously.
CYP1A2 inhibitors (cimetidine, fluvoxamine, certain quinolones): May increase duloxetine level. Avoid using together.

Reactions may be *common,* uncommon, *life-threatening,* or COMMON AND LIFE-THREATENING.
Interaction may have a *rapid onset* or **delayed onset.**

CYP2D6 inhibitors (fluoxetine, paroxetine, quinidine): May increase duloxetine level. Use together cautiously.

Drugs that reduce gastric acidity: May cause premature breakdown of duloxetine's protective coating and early release of the drug. Monitor patient for effects.

MAO inhibitors: May cause hyperthermia, rigidity, myoclonus, autonomic instability, rapid fluctuations of vital signs, agitation, delirium, and coma. Avoid use within 2 weeks after MAO inhibitor therapy; wait at least 5 days after stopping duloxetine before starting MAO inhibitor.

Thioridazine: May prolong the QT interval and increase risk of serious ventricular arrhythmias and sudden death. Avoid using together.

Tricyclic antidepressants (amitriptyline, nortriptyline, imipramine): May increase levels of these drugs. Reduce tricyclic antidepressant dose, and monitor drug levels closely.

Triptans: May cause serotonin syndrome (restlessness, hallucinations, loss of coordination, fast heartbeat, rapid changes in blood pressure, increased body temperature, hyperreflexia, nausea, vomiting, and diarrhea). Use cautiously and with increased monitoring, especially when starting or increasing dosages.

Drug-lifestyle. *Alcohol use:* May increase risk of liver damage. Discourage use together.

EFFECTS ON LAB TEST RESULTS
• May increase alkaline phosphatase, ALT, AST, bilirubin, and CK levels.

CONTRAINDICATIONS & CAUTIONS
• Contraindicated in patients hypersensitive to drug or its ingredients, patients taking MAO inhibitors, patients with uncontrolled angle-closure glaucoma, and patients with a creatinine clearance less than 30 ml/minute. Drug isn't recommended for patients with hepatic dysfunction or end-stage renal disease.

■ **Black Box Warning** Duloxetine isn't approved for use in children. ■

• Use cautiously in patients with a history of mania or seizures, patients who drink substantial amounts of alcohol, patients with hypertension, patients with con-

trolled angle-closure glaucoma, and those with conditions that slow gastric emptying.

NURSING CONSIDERATIONS
• Monitor patient for worsening of depression or suicidal behavior, especially when therapy starts or dosage changes.

■ **Black Box Warning** Drug may increase risk of suicidal thinking and behavior in children, adolescents, and young adults ages 18 to 24 during the first 2 months of treatment, especially in those with major depressive disorder or other psychiatric disorder. ■

• Treatment of overdose is symptomatic. Don't induce emesis; gastric lavage or activated charcoal may be performed soon after ingestion or if patient is still symptomatic. Because drug undergoes extensive distribution, forced diuresis, dialysis, hemoperfusion, and exchange transfusion aren't useful. Contact a poison control center for information.

• If taken with tricyclic antidepressants, duloxetine metabolism will be prolonged, and patient will need extended monitoring.

• Periodically reassess patient to determine the need for continued therapy.

• Decrease dosage gradually, and watch for symptoms that may arise when drug is stopped, such as dizziness, nausea, headache, paresthesia, vomiting, irritability, and nightmares.

• If intolerable symptoms arise when decreasing or stopping drug, restart at previous dose and decrease even more gradually.

• Monitor blood pressure periodically during treatment.

• Use during the third trimester of pregnancy may cause neonatal complications including respiratory distress, cyanosis, apnea, seizures, vomiting, hypoglycemia, and hyperreflexia, which may require prolonged hospitalization, respiratory support, and tube feeding. Consider potential benefit of drug to the mother versus risks to the fetus.

• Older patients may be more sensitive to drug effects than younger adults.

• *Alert:* Combining triptans with an SSRI or an SSNRI may cause serotonin syndrome. Signs and symptoms may include restlessness, hallucinations, loss of coordination, fast heartbeat, rapid changes in

blood pressure, increased body temperature, overactive reflexes, nausea, vomiting, and diarrhea. Serotonin syndrome may be more likely to occur when starting or increasing the dose of triptan, SSRI, or SSNRI.

PATIENT TEACHING

• *Alert:* Warn families or caregivers to report signs of worsening depression (such as agitation, irritability, insomnia, hostility, impulsivity) and signs of suicidal behavior to prescriber immediately.
• Tell patient to consult his prescriber or pharmacist if he plans to take other prescription or OTC drugs or an herbal or other dietary supplement.
• Instruct patient to swallow capsules whole and not to chew, crush, or open them because they have an enteric coating.
• Urge patient to avoid activities that are hazardous or require mental alertness until he knows how the drug affects him.
• Warn against drinking alcohol during therapy.
• If patient takes drug for depression, explain that it may take 1 to 4 weeks to notice an effect.

---

escitalopram oxalate
ess-si-TAL-oh-pram

Lexapro◆

Pharmacologic class: SSRI
Pregnancy risk category C

AVAILABLE FORMS
Oral solution: 5 mg/5 ml
Tablets: 5 mg, 10 mg, 20 mg

INDICATIONS & DOSAGES
➤ **Treatment and maintenance therapy for patients with major depressive disorder; general anxiety disorder**
Adults: Initially, 10 mg P.O. once daily, increasing to 20 mg if needed after at least 1 week.
Adjust-a-dose: For elderly patients and those with hepatic impairment, 10 mg P.O. daily, initially and as maintenance dosages.

ADMINISTRATION
P.O.
• Give drug without regard for food.

ACTION
Action may be linked to increase of serotonergic activity in the CNS from inhibition of neuronal reuptake of serotonin. Drug is closely related to citalopram, which may be the active component.

Route	Onset	Peak	Duration
P.O.	Unknown	5 hr	Unknown

Half-life: 27 to 32 hours.

ADVERSE REACTIONS
CNS: *suicidal behavior,* fever, insomnia, dizziness, somnolence, paresthesia, light-headedness, migraine, tremor, vertigo, abnormal dreams, irritability, impaired concentration, fatigue, lethargy.
CV: palpitations, hypertension, flushing, chest pain.
EENT: rhinitis, sinusitis, blurred vision, tinnitus, earache.
GI: *nausea,* diarrhea, constipation, indigestion, abdominal pain, vomiting, increased or decreased appetite, dry mouth, flatulence, heartburn, cramps, gastroesophageal reflux.
GU: ejaculation disorder, impotence, anorgasmia, menstrual cramps, UTI, urinary frequency.
Metabolic: weight gain or loss.
Musculoskeletal: arthralgia, myalgia, muscle cramps, pain in arms or legs.
Respiratory: bronchitis, cough.
Skin: rash, increased sweating.
Other: decreased libido, yawning, flulike symptoms.

INTERACTIONS
Drug-drug. *Aspirin, NSAIDs, other drugs known to affect coagulation:* May increase the risk of bleeding. Use together cautiously.
Carbamazepine: May increase escitalopram clearance. Monitor patient for expected antidepressant effect and adjust dose as needed.
Cimetidine: May increase escitalopram level. Monitor patient for increased adverse reactions to escitalopram.

Reactions may be *common*, uncommon, *life-threatening*, or COMMON AND LIFE-THREATENING.
Interaction may have a *rapid onset* or **delayed onset**.

Citalopram: May cause additive effects. Using together is contraindicated.
CNS drugs: May cause additive effects. Use together cautiously.
Desipramine, other drugs metabolized by CYP2D6: May increase levels of these drugs. Use together cautiously.
Lithium: May enhance serotonergic effect of escitalopram. Use together cautiously, and monitor lithium level.
MAO inhibitors: May cause fatal serotonin syndrome. Avoid using within 14 days of MAO inhibitor therapy.
Triptans: May increase serotonergic effects, leading to weakness, hyperreflexia, incoordination, rapid changes in blood pressure, nausea, and diarrhea. Use together cautiously, especially at the start of therapy or at dosage increases.
Tramadol: May cause serotonin syndrome. Monitor patient closely.
Drug-lifestyle. *Alcohol use:* May increase CNS effects. Discourage use together.

EFFECTS ON LAB TEST RESULTS
None reported.

CONTRAINDICATIONS & CAUTIONS
● Contraindicated in patients taking pimozide, MAO inhibitors, or within 14 days of MAO inhibitor therapy and in those hypersensitive to escitalopram, citalopram, or any of its inactive ingredients.
■ **Black Box Warning** Escitalopram isn't approved for use in children. ■
● Use cautiously in patients with a history of mania, seizure disorders, suicidal thoughts, or renal or hepatic impairment.
● Use cautiously in patients with diseases that produce altered metabolism or hemodynamic responses.
● Use with caution in elderly patients because they may have greater sensitivity to drug.
● Use in third trimester of pregnancy may cause complications at birth. Consider the risk versus benefit of treatment during this time.
● Drug appears in breast milk. Patient should either stop breast-feeding or stop taking drug.

NURSING CONSIDERATIONS
● Closely monitor patients at high risk of suicide.

■ **Black Box Warning** Drug may increase risk of suicidal thinking and behavior in children, adolescents, and young adults ages 18 to 24 during the first 2 months of treatment, especially in those with major depressive disorder or other psychiatric disorder. ■
● *Look alike–sound alike:* Don't confuse escitalopram with estazolam.
● Evaluate patient for history of drug abuse and observe for signs of misuse or abuse.
● Periodically reassess patient to determine need for maintenance treatment and appropriate dosing.
● *Alert:* Combining triptans with an SSRI or an SSNRI may cause serotonin syndrome. Signs and symptoms may include restlessness, hallucinations, loss of coordination, fast heart beat, rapid changes in blood pressure, increased body temperature, overactive reflexes, nausea, vomiting, and diarrhea. Serotonin syndrome may be more likely to occur when starting or increasing the dose of triptan, SSRI, or SSNRI.

PATIENT TEACHING
● Inform patient that symptoms should improve gradually over several weeks, rather than immediately.
● Tell patient that although improvement may occur within 1 to 4 weeks, he should continue drug as prescribed.
● *Alert:* Caution patient and patient's family to report signs of worsening depression (such as agitation, irritability, insomnia, hostility, impulsivity) and signs of suicidal behavior to prescriber immediately.
● Tell patient to use caution while driving or operating hazardous machinery because of drug's potential to impair judgment, thinking, and motor skills.
● Advise patient to consult health care provider before taking other prescription or OTC drugs.
● Tell patient that drug may be taken in the morning or evening without regard to meals.
● Encourage patient to avoid alcohol while taking drug.
● Tell woman to notify health care provider if she's pregnant or breast-feeding.

---

fluoxetine hydrochloride
floo-OX-e-teen

Prozac✒, Prozac Weekly,
Sarafem✒

Pharmacologic class: SSRI
Pregnancy risk category C

AVAILABLE FORMS
Capsules (delayed-release): 90 mg
Capsules (pulvules): 10 mg, 20 mg,
40 mg
Oral solution: 20 mg/5 ml
Tablets: 10 mg, 20 mg

INDICATIONS & DOSAGES
➤ **Depression, obsessive-compulsive disorder (OCD) (excluding Sarafem)**
Adults: Initially, 20 mg P.O. in the morning; increase dosage based on patient response. Maximum daily dose is 80 mg.
Children ages 7 to 17 (OCD): 10 mg P.O. daily. After 2 weeks, increase to 20 mg daily. Dosage is 20 to 60 mg daily.
Children ages 8 to 18 (depression): 10 mg P.O. once daily for 1 week; then increase to 20 mg daily.
➤ **Depression in elderly patients (excluding Sarafem)**
Adults age 65 and older: Initially, 20 mg P.O. daily in the morning. Increase dose based on response. Doses may be given b.i.d., morning and noon. Maximum daily dose is 80 mg. Consider using a lower dosage or less-frequent doses in these patients, especially those with systemic illness and those who are receiving drugs for other illnesses.
➤ **Maintenance therapy for depression (excluding Sarafem) in stabilized patients (not for newly diagnosed depression)**
Adults: 90 mg Prozac Weekly P.O. once weekly. Start once-weekly doses 7 days after the last daily dose of Prozac 20 mg.
➤ **Short-term and long-term treatment of bulimia nervosa (excluding Sarafem)**
Adults: 60 mg P.O. daily in the morning.

➤ **Short-term treatment of panic disorder with or without agoraphobia**
Adults: 10 mg P.O. once daily for 1 week; then increase dose as needed to 20 mg daily. Maximum daily dose is 60 mg.
Adjust-a-dose: For patients with renal or hepatic impairment, reduce dose or increase interval.
➤ **Anorexia nervosa in weight-restored patients ♦**
Adults: 40 mg P.O. daily.
➤ **Depression caused by bipolar disorder ♦**
Adults: 20 to 60 mg P.O. daily.
➤ **Cataplexy ♦**
Adults: 20 mg P.O. once or twice daily with CNS stimulant therapy.
➤ **Alcohol dependence ♦**
Adults: 60 mg P.O. daily. Use in conjunction with CNS stimulant therapy.
➤ **Premenstrual dysphoric disorder**
Adults: 20 mg Sarafem P.O. daily continuously (every day of the menstrual cycle) or intermittently (daily dose starting 14 days before the anticipated onset of menstruation through the first full day of menses and repeating with each new cycle). Maximum daily dose is 80 mg P.O.
➤ **Raynaud phenomenon ♦**
Adults: 20 to 60 mg P.O. daily.
Adjust-a-dose: For patients with renal or hepatic impairment and those taking several drugs at the same time, reduce dose or increase dosing interval.

ADMINISTRATION
P.O.
● Give drug without regard for food.
● Avoid giving drug in the afternoon, whenever possible, because doing so commonly causes nervousness and insomnia.
● Delayed-release capsules must be swallowed whole; don't crush or open.

ACTION
Thought to be linked to drug's inhibition of CNS neuronal uptake of serotonin.

Route	Onset	Peak	Duration
P.O.	Unknown	6–8 hr	Unknown

Half-life: Fluoxetine, 2 to 3 days; norfluoxetine, 7 to 9 days.

Reactions may be *common,* uncommon, *life-threatening,* or COMMON AND LIFE-THREATENING.
Interaction may have a *rapid onset* or **delayed onset.**

ADVERSE REACTIONS

CNS: *nervousness, somnolence, anxiety, insomnia, headache, drowsiness, tremor, dizziness, asthenia,* **suicidal behavior,** fatigue, fever.

CV: palpitations, hot flashes.

EENT: nasal congestion, pharyngitis, sinusitis.

GI: *nausea, diarrhea, dry mouth, anorexia,* dyspepsia, constipation, abdominal pain, vomiting, flatulence, increased appetite.

GU: sexual dysfunction.

Metabolic: weight loss.

Musculoskeletal: muscle pain.

Respiratory: upper respiratory tract infection, cough, *respiratory distress.*

Skin: rash, pruritus, diaphoresis.

Other: flulike syndrome.

INTERACTIONS

Drug-drug. *Amphetamines, buspirone, dextromethorphan, dihydroergotamine, lithium salts, meperidine, other SSRIs or SSNRIs (duloxetine, venlafaxine),* **tramadol,** *trazodone, tricyclic antidepressants, tryptophan:* May increase the risk of serotonin syndrome. Avoid combinations of drugs that increase the availability of serotonin in the CNS; monitor patient closely if used together.

Benzodiazepines, lithium, tricyclic antidepressants: May increase CNS effects. Monitor patient closely.

Beta blockers, carbamazepine, flecainide, vinblastine: May increase levels of these drugs. Monitor drug levels and monitor patient for adverse reactions.

Cyproheptadine: May reverse or decrease fluoxetine effect. Monitor patient closely.

Dextromethorphan: May cause unusual side effects such as visual hallucinations. Advise use of cough suppressant that doesn't contain dextromethorphan while taking fluoxetine.

Highly protein-bound drugs: May increase level of fluoxetine or other highly protein-bound drugs. Monitor patient closely.

Insulin, oral antidiabetics: May alter glucose level and antidiabetic requirements. Adjust dosage.

MAO inhibitors (phenelzine, selegiline, tranylcypromine): May cause serotonin syndrome. Avoid using at the same time and for at least 5 weeks after stopping.

Phenytoin: May increase phenytoin level and risk of toxicity. Monitor phenytoin level and adjust dosage.

Triptans: May cause weakness, hyperreflexia, incoordination, rapid changes in blood pressure, nausea, and diarrhea. Monitor patient closely, especially at the start of treatment and when dosage increases.

Thioridazine: May increase thioridazine level, increasing risk of serious ventricular arrhythmias and sudden death. Avoid using at the same time and for at least 5 weeks after stopping.

Warfarin: May increase risk for bleeding. Monitor PT and INR.

Drug-herb. *St. John's wort:* May increase sedative and hypnotic effects; may cause serotonin syndrome. Discourage use together.

Drug-lifestyle. *Alcohol use:* May increase CNS depression. Discourage use together.

EFFECTS ON LAB TEST RESULTS
None reported.

CONTRAINDICATIONS & CAUTIONS

● Contraindicated in patients hypersensitive to drug and in those taking MAO inhibitors within 14 days of starting therapy. MAO inhibitors shouldn't be started within 5 weeks of stopping fluoxetine. Avoid using thioridazine with fluoxetine or within 5 weeks after stopping fluoxetine.

● Use cautiously in patients at high risk for suicide and in those with history of diabetes mellitus, seizures, mania, or hepatic, renal, or CV disease.

● Use in third trimester of pregnancy may be associated with neonatal complications at birth. Consider the risk versus benefit of treatment during this time.

■ **Black Box Warning** Fluoxetine is approved for use in children with manic depressive disorder and obsessive-compulsive disorder. Sarafem isn't approved for use in children. ■

NURSING CONSIDERATIONS

● Use antihistamines or topical corticosteroids to treat rashes or pruritus.

• Watch for weight change during therapy, particularly in underweight or bulimic patients.

• Record mood changes. Watch for suicidal tendencies.

■ **Black Box Warning** Drug may increase the risk of suicidal thinking and behavior in children and adolescents with major depressive disorder or other psychiatric disorder. ■

■ **Black Box Warning** Drug may increase the risk of suicidal thinking and behavior in young adults ages 18 to 24 during the first 2 months of treatment. ■

• Drug has a long half-life; monitor patient for adverse effects for up to 2 weeks after drug is stopped.

• *Alert:* Combining triptans with an SSRI or an SSNRI may cause serotonin syndrome. Signs and symptoms may include restlessness, hallucinations, loss of coordination, fast heartbeat, rapid changes in blood pressure, increased body temperature, overactive reflexes, nausea, vomiting, and diarrhea. Serotonin syndrome may be more likely to occur when starting or increasing the dose of triptan, SSRI, or SSNRI.

• *Look alike–sound alike:* Don't confuse fluoxetine with fluvoxamine or fluvastatin. Don't confuse Prozac with Proscar, Prilosec, or ProSom.

PATIENT TEACHING
• Tell patient to avoid taking drug in the afternoon whenever possible because doing so commonly causes nervousness and insomnia.

• Drug may cause dizziness or drowsiness. Warn patient to avoid driving and other hazardous activities that require alertness and good psychomotor coordination until effects of drug are known.

• Tell patient to consult prescriber before taking other prescription or OTC drugs.

• Advise patient that full therapeutic effect may not be seen for 4 weeks or longer.

fluvoxamine maleate
floo-VOX-a-meen

Luvox, Luvox CR

Pharmacologic class: SSRI
Pregnancy risk category C

AVAILABLE FORMS
Capsules (extended-release): 100 mg, 150 mg
Tablets: 25 mg, 50 mg, 100 mg

INDICATIONS & DOSAGES
➤ **Obsessive-compulsive disorder (OCD)**
Adults: Initially, 50 mg (tablet) P.O. daily at bedtime; increase by 50 mg every 4 to 7 days. Maximum, 300 mg daily. Give total daily amounts above 100 mg in two divided doses. Or, 100-mg extended-release capsule P.O. once per day as a single daily dose at bedtime. Increase in 50-mg increments every week, as tolerated, until maximum therapeutic benefit is achieved. Maximum dose is 300 mg/day.
Children ages 8 to 17: Initially, 25 mg P.O. daily at bedtime; increase by 25 mg every 4 to 7 days. Maximum, 200 mg daily for children ages 8 to less than 11 and 300 mg daily for children ages 11 to 17. Give total daily amounts over 50 mg in two divided doses.

✱ *NEW INDICATION:* **Social anxiety disorder (capsules only)**
Adults: Initially, 100-mg extended-release capsule P.O. once per day as a single daily dose at bedtime. Increase in 50 mg increments every week, as tolerated, until maximum therapeutic benefit is achieved. Maximum dose is 300 mg/day.
Adjust-a-dose: In elderly patients and those with hepatic impairment, give lower first dose and adjust dose more slowly. When using Luvox CR capsules, titrate dosage more slowly after initial 100-mg dose.

ADMINISTRATION
P.O.
• Give drug without regard for food.
• Capsules shouldn't be crushed or chewed.
• Give extended-release capsules at bedtime.

ACTION

Unknown. Selectively inhibits the pre-synaptic neuronal uptake of serotonin, which may improve OCD.

Route	Onset	Peak	Duration
P.O. (capsules)	Unknown	Unknown	Unknown
P.O. (tablets)	Unknown	3–8 hr	Unknown

Half-life: 15–17 hours.

ADVERSE REACTIONS

CNS: *agitation, headache, asthenia, somnolence, insomnia, nervousness, dizziness,* tremor, anxiety, hypertonia, depression, CNS stimulation.
CV: palpitations, vasodilation.
EENT: amblyopia.
GI: *nausea, diarrhea, constipation, dyspepsia, vomiting, dry mouth,* anorexia, flatulence, dysphagia, taste perversion.
GU: abnormal ejaculation, urinary frequency, impotence, anorgasmia, urine retention.
Respiratory: upper respiratory tract infection, dyspnea.
Skin: sweating.
Other: tooth disorder, flulike syndrome, chills, decreased libido, yawning.

INTERACTIONS

Drug-drug. *Benzodiazepines, theophylline, warfarin:* May reduce clearance of these drugs. Use together cautiously (except for diazepam, which shouldn't be used with fluvoxamine). Adjust dosage as needed.
Carbamazepine, clozapine, methadone, metoprolol, propranolol, theophylline, tricyclic antidepressants: May increase levels of these drugs. Use together cautiously, and monitor patient closely for adverse reactions. Dosage adjustments may be needed.
Diltiazem: May cause bradycardia. Monitor heart rate.
Lithium, tryptophan: May enhance effects of fluvoxamine. Use together cautiously.
MAO inhibitors (phenelzine, selegiline, tranylcypromine): May cause serotonin syndrome (CNS irritability, shivering, and altered consciousness). Avoid using within 2 weeks of MAO inhibitor.

Pimozide, thioridazine: May prolong QTc interval. Avoid using together.
Sumatriptan: May cause weakness, hyper-reflexia, and incoordination. Monitor patient closely. May cause serotonin syndrome. Avoid using within 2 weeks of MAO inhibitor.
Tramadol: May cause serotonin syndrome. Monitor patient closely.
Drug-lifestyle. *Alcohol use:* May increase CNS effects. Discourage use together.
Smoking: May decrease drug's effectiveness. Urge patient to stop smoking.

EFFECTS ON LAB TEST RESULTS
None reported.

CONTRAINDICATIONS & CAUTIONS

● Contraindicated in patients hypersensitive to drug or to other phenyl piperazine antidepressants, in those receiving pimozide, alosetron, tizanidine, or thioridazine therapy, and within 2 weeks of MAO inhibitor.
● Use cautiously in patients with hepatic dysfunction, other conditions that may affect hemodynamic responses or metabolism, or history of mania or seizures.
■ **Black Box Warning** Fluvoxamine tablets aren't approved for use in children, except for those with obsessive-compulsive disorder. Fluvoxamine extended-release capsules shouldn't be used in children. ■

NURSING CONSIDERATIONS

● Record mood changes. Monitor patient for suicidal tendencies.
■ **Black Box Warning** Don't use for the treatment of major depressive disorders in children younger than age 18 because of an increased risk of suicidal behavior. ■
■ **Black Box Warning** Drug may increase the risk of suicidal thinking and behavior in young adults ages 18 to 24 during the first 2 months of treatment. ■
● *Alert:* Combining an SSRI with a triptan may cause serotonin syndrome. Signs and symptoms may include restlessness, hallucinations, loss of coordination, fast heartbeat, rapid changes in blood pressure, increased body temperature, hyperreflexia, nausea, vomiting, and diarrhea. Serotonin syndrome is more likely to occur when starting or increasing the dose of a triptan.

● **Look alike–sound alike:** Don't confuse fluvoxamine with fluoxetine.

● Patients shouldn't stop drug without first consulting prescriber; abruptly stopping drug may cause withdrawal syndrome, including headache, muscle ache, and flu-like symptoms.

PATIENT TEACHING

● Warn patient to avoid hazardous activities until CNS effects of drug are known.

● Tell woman to notify prescriber about planned, suspected, or known pregnancy.

● Tell patient who develops a rash, hives, or a related allergic reaction to notify prescriber.

● Inform patient that several weeks of therapy may be needed to obtain full therapeutic effect. Once improvement occurs, advise patient not to stop drug until directed by prescriber.

● Suggest that patient keep a diary of changes in mood or behavior. Tell patient to report suicidal thoughts immediately.

● Advise patient to check with prescriber before taking OTC drugs; drug interactions can occur.

● Tell patient drug can be taken with or without food.

---

imipramine hydrochloride
im-IP-ra-meen

Novo-pramine†, Tofranil

imipramine pamoate
Tofranil-PM

Pharmacologic class: tricyclic antidepressant (TCA)
Pregnancy risk category D

AVAILABLE FORMS
imipramine hydrochloride
Tablets: 10 mg, 25 mg, 50 mg
imipramine pamoate
Capsules: 75 mg, 100 mg, 125 mg, 150 mg

INDICATIONS & DOSAGES
➤ **Depression**
Adults: 75 to 100 mg P.O. daily in divided doses, increased by 25 to 50 mg. Maximum daily dose is 200 mg for outpatients

and 300 mg for hospitalized patients. Give entire dose at bedtime.
Adolescents and elderly patients:
Initially, 30 to 40 mg daily; maximum shouldn't exceed 100 mg daily.
➤ **Childhood enuresis**
Children age 5 and older: 25 mg P.O. 1 hour before bedtime. If patient doesn't improve within 1 week, increase dose to 50 mg if child is younger than age 12; increase dose to 75 mg for children age 12 and older. In either case, maximum daily dose is 2.5 mg/kg.

ADMINISTRATION
P.O.
● Give drug without regard for food.
● Give full dose at bedtime if possible.

ACTION
Unknown. Increases norepinephrine, serotonin, or both in the CNS by blocking their reuptake by the presynaptic neurons.

Route	Onset	Peak	Duration
P.O.	Unknown	1–2 hr	Unknown

Half-life: 11 to 25 hours.

ADVERSE REACTIONS
CNS: *drowsiness, dizziness, **seizures, stroke,*** excitation, tremor, confusion, hallucinations, anxiety, ataxia, paresthesia, nervousness, EEG changes, extrapyramidal reactions.
CV: *orthostatic hypotension, tachycardia, ECG changes, **MI, arrhythmias, heart block,*** hypertension, ***precipitation of heart failure.***
EENT: *blurred vision,* tinnitus, mydriasis.
GI: *dry mouth, constipation,* nausea, vomiting, anorexia, paralytic ileus, abdominal cramps.
GU: *urine retention.*
Metabolic: *hypoglycemia,* hyperglycemia.
Skin: rash, urticaria, photosensitivity reactions, pruritus, diaphoresis.
Other: hypersensitivity reactions.

INTERACTIONS
Drug-drug. *Barbiturates, CNS depressants:* May enhance CNS depression. Avoid using together.

Reactions may be *common,* uncommon, *life-threatening,* or COMMON AND LIFE-THREATENING.
Interaction may have a *rapid onset* or ***delayed onset.***

Cimetidine, **fluoxetine, fluvoxamine, paroxetine, sertraline:** May increase imipramine level. Monitor drug levels and patient for signs of toxicity.

Clonidine: May cause life-threatening hypertension. Avoid using together.

Epinephrine, norepinephrine: May increase hypertensive effect. Use together cautiously.

MAO inhibitors: May cause hyperpyretic crisis, severe seizures, and death. Avoid using within 14 days of MAO inhibitor therapy.

Quinolones: May increase the risk of life-threatening arrhythmias. Avoid using together.

Drug-herb. *Evening primrose oil:* May cause additive or synergistic effect, lowering the seizure threshold and increasing the risk of seizure. Discourage use together.

St. John's wort, SAM-e, yohimbe: May cause serotonin syndrome. Discourage use together.

Drug-lifestyle. *Alcohol use:* May enhance CNS depression. Discourage use together.

Smoking: May lower level of drug. Monitor patient for lack of effect.

Sun exposure: May increase risk of photosensitivity reactions. Advise patient to avoid excessive sunlight exposure.

EFFECTS ON LAB TEST RESULTS
• May increase or decrease glucose level.
• May increase liver function test values.

CONTRAINDICATIONS & CAUTIONS
• Contraindicated in patients hypersensitive to drug and in those receiving MAO inhibitors; also contraindicated during acute recovery phase of MI.
• Use with extreme caution in patients at risk for suicide; in patients with history of urine retention, angle-closure glaucoma, or seizure disorders; in patients with increased intraocular pressure, CV disease, impaired hepatic function, hyperthyroidism, or impaired renal function; and in patients receiving thyroid drugs. Injectable form contains sulfites, which may cause allergic reactions in hypersensitive patients.

■ **Black Box Warning** Imipramine isn't approved for use in children except for those with nocturnal enuresis. ■

NURSING CONSIDERATIONS
• Monitor patient for nausea, headache, and malaise after abrupt withdrawal of long-term therapy; these symptoms don't indicate addiction.
• Don't withdraw drug abruptly.
• Because of hypertensive episodes during surgery in patients receiving TCAs, stop drug gradually several days before surgery.
• If signs or symptoms of psychosis occur or increase, expect prescriber to reduce dosage. Record mood changes. Monitor patient for suicidal tendencies, and allow only a minimum supply of drug.

■ **Black Box Warning** Drug may increase the risk of suicidal thinking and behavior in children and adolescents with major depressive disorder or other psychiatric disorder. ■

■ **Black Box Warning** Drug may increase the risk of suicidal thinking and behavior in young adults ages 18 to 24 during the first 2 months of treatment. ■

• To prevent relapse in children receiving drug for enuresis, withdraw drug gradually.
• Recommend sugarless hard candy or gum to relieve dry mouth. Saliva substitutes may be useful.
• *Alert:* Tofranil and Tofranil-PM may contain tartrazine.
• *Look alike–sound alike:* Don't confuse imipramine with desipramine.

PATIENT TEACHING
• Tell patient to take full dose at bedtime whenever possible, but warn him of possible morning dizziness upon standing up quickly.
• If child is an early-night bed-wetter, tell parents it may be more effective to divide dose and give the first dose earlier in day.
• Tell patient to avoid alcohol while taking this drug.
• Advise patient to consult prescriber before taking other prescription or OTC drugs.
• Warn patient to avoid hazardous activities that require alertness and good coordination until effects of the drug are known.

Drowsiness and dizziness usually subside after a few weeks.
• Warn patient not to stop drug suddenly.
• To prevent oversensitivity to the sun, advise patient to use sunblock, wear protective clothing, and avoid prolonged exposure to strong sunlight.

mirtazapine
mer-TAH-zah-peen

Remeron, Remeron Soltab

Pharmacologic class: tetracyclic antidepressant
Pregnancy risk category C

AVAILABLE FORMS
Orally disintegrating tablets (ODTs): 15 mg, 30 mg, 45 mg
Tablets: 15 mg, 30 mg, 45 mg

INDICATIONS & DOSAGES
➤ **Depression**
Adults: Initially, 15 mg P.O. at bedtime. Maintenance dose is 15 to 45 mg daily. Adjust dosage at intervals of at least 1 week.

ADMINISTRATION
P.O.
• Give drug without regard for food.
• Remove ODT from blister pack and immediately place on patient's tongue.
• ODT may be given with or without water.
• Don't split or crush ODT.

ACTION
Thought to enhance central noradrenergic and serotonergic activity.

Route	Onset	Peak	Duration
P.O.	Unknown	2 hr	Unknown

Half-life: About 20 to 40 hours.

ADVERSE REACTIONS
CNS: *somnolence,* **suicidal behavior,** dizziness, asthenia, abnormal dreams, abnormal thinking, tremors, confusion.
CV: edema, peripheral edema.
GI: *increased appetite, dry mouth, constipation,* nausea.

GU: urinary frequency.
Metabolic: *weight gain.*
Musculoskeletal: back pain, myalgia.
Respiratory: dyspnea.
Other: flulike syndrome.

INTERACTIONS
Drug-drug. *Diazepam, other CNS depressants:* May cause additive CNS effects. Avoid using together.
MAO inhibitors: May sometimes cause fatal reactions. Avoid using within 14 days of MAO inhibitor therapy.
Drug-lifestyle. *Alcohol use:* May cause additive CNS effects. Discourage use together.

EFFECTS ON LAB TEST RESULTS
• May increase ALT, cholesterol and triglyceride levels.

CONTRAINDICATIONS & CAUTIONS
• Contraindicated in patients hypersensitive to drug and within 14 days of MAO inhibitor therapy.
■ **Black Box Warning** Mirtazapine isn't approved for use in children. ■
• Use cautiously in patients with CV or cerebrovascular disease, seizure disorders, suicidal thoughts, hepatic or renal impairment, or history of mania or hypomania.
• Use cautiously in patients with conditions that predispose them to hypotension, such as dehydration, hypovolemia, or antihypertensive therapy.
• Give drug cautiously to elderly patients; decreased clearance has occurred in this age group.

NURSING CONSIDERATIONS
• Don't use within 14 days of MAOI therapy.
• Record mood changes. Watch for suicidal tendencies.
■ **Black Box Warning** Drug may increase risk of suicidal thinking and behavior in children, adolescents, and young adults ages 18 to 24 with major depressive or other psychiatric disorder. ■
• Although agranulocytosis occurs rarely, stop drug and monitor patient closely if he develops a sore throat, fever, stomatitis, or other signs and symptoms of infection with a low WBC count.

Reactions may be *common,* uncommon, *life-threatening,* or COMMON AND LIFE-THREATENING.
Interaction may have a *rapid onset* or **delayed onset.**

• Lower dosages tend to be more sedating than higher dosages.

PATIENT TEACHING
• Caution patient not to perform hazardous activities if he gets too sleepy.
• Tell patient to report signs and symptoms of infection, such as fever, chills, sore throat, mucous membrane irritation, or flulike syndrome.
• Instruct patient not to use alcohol or other CNS depressants while taking drug.
• Stress importance of following prescriber's orders.
• Instruct patient not to take other drugs without prescriber's approval.
• Tell woman of childbearing age to report suspected pregnancy immediately and to notify prescriber if she is breast-feeding.
• Instruct patient to remove ODTs from blister pack and place immediately on tongue. Tell the patient to be sure his hands are clean and dry if he touches the tablet.
• Advise patient not to break or split tablet.

---

nortriptyline hydrochloride
nor-TRIP-ti-leen

Aventyl, Pamelor*✐

Pharmacologic class: tricyclic antidepressant
Pregnancy risk category D

AVAILABLE FORMS
Capsules: 10 mg, 25 mg, 50 mg, 75 mg
Oral solution: 10 mg/5 ml*

INDICATIONS & DOSAGES
➤ **Depression**
Adults: 25 mg P.O. t.i.d. or q.i.d., gradually increased to maximum of 150 mg daily. Give entire dose at bedtime. Monitor level when doses above 100 mg daily are given.
Adolescents and elderly patients: 30 to 50 mg daily given once or in divided doses.

ADMINISTRATION
P.O.
• Give drug without regard for food.
• Whenever possible, give full dose at bedtime.

ACTION
Unknown. Increases the amount of norepinephrine, serotonin, or both in the CNS by blocking reuptake by the presynaptic neurons.

Route	Onset	Peak	Duration
P.O.	Unknown	7–8½ hr	Unknown

Half-life: 18 to 24 hours.

ADVERSE REACTIONS
CNS: *drowsiness, dizziness, seizures, stroke,* tremor, weakness, confusion, headache, nervousness, EEG changes, extrapyramidal syndrome, insomnia, nightmares, hallucinations, paresthesia, ataxia, agitation.
CV: *tachycardia, heart block, MI,* ECG changes, hypertension, hypotension.
EENT: *blurred vision,* tinnitus, mydriasis.
GI: *constipation,* dry mouth, nausea, vomiting, anorexia, paralytic ileus.
GU: *urine retention.*
Hematologic: *agranulocytosis, thrombocytopenia,* bone marrow depression, eosinophilia.
Metabolic: *hypoglycemia,* hyperglycemia.
Skin: rash, urticaria, photosensitivity reactions, diaphoresis.
Other: hypersensitivity reactions.

INTERACTIONS
Drug-drug. *Barbiturates, CNS depressants:* May enhance CNS depression. Avoid using together.
Cimetidine, **fluoxetine, fluvoxamine, paroxetine, sertraline:** May increase nortriptyline level. Monitor drug levels and patient for signs of toxicity.
Clonidine: May cause life-threatening hypertension. Avoid using together.
Epinephrine, norepinephrine: May increase hypertensive effect. Use together cautiously.
MAO inhibitors: May cause severe excitation, hyperpyrexia, or seizures, usually with high doses. Avoid using within 14 days of MAO inhibitor therapy.
Quinolones: May increase the risk of life-threatening arrhythmias. Avoid using together.
Drug-herb. *Evening primrose oil:* May cause additive or synergistic effect, lowering seizure threshold and increasing

---

the risk of seizure. Discourage use together.

St. John's wort, SAM-e, yohimbe: May cause serotonin syndrome and reduced drug level. Discourage use together.

Drug-lifestyle. *Alcohol use:* May enhance CNS depression. Discourage use together.

Smoking: May decrease drug level. Monitor patient for lack of effect.

Sun exposure: May increase risk of photosensitivity reactions. Advise patient to avoid excessive sunlight exposure.

EFFECTS ON LAB TEST RESULTS
● May increase or decrease glucose level.
● May increase eosinophil count and liver function test values. May decrease WBC, RBC, granulocyte, and platelet counts.

CONTRAINDICATIONS & CAUTIONS
● Contraindicated in patients hypersensitive to drug and during acute recovery phase of MI; also contraindicated within 14 days of MAO inhibitor therapy.
■ **Black Box Warning** Nortriptyline isn't approved for use in children. ■
● Use with extreme caution in patients with glaucoma, suicidal tendency, history of urine retention or seizures, CV disease, or hyperthyroidism and in those receiving thyroid drugs.

NURSING CONSIDERATIONS
● Monitor patient for nausea, headache, and malaise after abrupt withdrawal of long-term therapy; these symptoms don't indicate addiction.
● Because patients using tricyclic antidepressants may suffer hypertensive episodes during surgery, stop drug gradually several days before surgery.
● If signs or symptoms of psychosis occur or increase, expect to reduce dosage. Record mood changes. Monitor patient for suicidal tendencies and allow him only a minimum supply of drug.
■ **Black Box Warning** Drug may increase the risk of suicidal thinking and behavior in children and adolescents with major depressive disorder or other psychiatric disorder. ■
■ **Black Box Warning** Drug may increase the risk of suicidal thinking and behavior in young adults ages 18 to 24 during the first 2 months of treatment. ■

● *Look alike–sound alike:* Don't confuse nortriptyline with amitriptyline.

PATIENT TEACHING
● Advise patient to take full dose at bedtime whenever possible to reduce risk of dizziness upon standing quickly.
● Warn patient to avoid activities that require alertness and good coordination until effects of drug are known. Drowsiness and dizziness usually subside after a few weeks.
● Recommend use of sugarless hard candy or gum to relieve dry mouth. Saliva substitutes may be needed.
● Tell patient to consult prescriber before taking other prescription or OTC drugs.
● Warn patient not to stop drug suddenly.
● To prevent oversensitivity to the sun, advise patient to use sunblock, wear protective clothing, and avoid prolonged exposure to strong sunlight.

paroxetine hydrochloride
pah-ROX-a-teen

Paxil, Paxil CR

Pharmacologic class: SSRI
Pregnancy risk category D

AVAILABLE FORMS
Suspension: 10 mg/5 ml
Tablets: 10 mg, 20 mg, 30 mg, 40 mg
Tablets (controlled-release): 12.5 mg, 25 mg, 37.5 mg

INDICATIONS & DOSAGES
➤ **Depression**
Adults: Initially, 20 mg P.O. daily, preferably in morning, as indicated. If patient doesn't improve, increase dose by 10 mg daily at intervals of at least 1 week to a maximum of 50 mg daily. If using controlled-release form, initially, 25 mg P.O. daily. Increase dose by 12.5 mg daily at weekly intervals to a maximum of 62.5 mg daily.
Elderly patients: Initially, 10 mg P.O. daily, preferably in morning, as indicated. If patient doesn't improve, increase dose by 10 mg daily at weekly intervals, to a maximum of 40 mg daily. If using controlled-

release form, start therapy at 12.5 mg P.O. daily. Don't exceed 50 mg daily.

➤ **Obsessive-compulsive disorder (OCD)**
Adults: Initially, 20 mg P.O. daily, preferably in morning. Increase dose by 10 mg daily at weekly intervals. Recommended daily dose is 40 mg. Maximum daily dose is 60 mg.

➤ **Panic disorder**
Adults: Initially, 10 mg P.O. daily. Increase dose by 10 mg at no less than weekly intervals to maximum of 60 mg daily. Or, 12.5 mg Paxil CR P.O. as a single daily dose, usually in the morning, with or without food; increase dose at intervals of at least 1 week by 12.5 mg daily, up to a maximum of 75 mg daily.
Adjust-a-dose: In elderly or debilitated patients and in those with severe renal or hepatic impairment, the first dose of Paxil CR is 12.5 mg daily; increase if indicated. Dosage shouldn't exceed 50 mg daily.

➤ **Social anxiety disorder**
Adults: Initially, 20 mg P.O. daily, preferably in morning. Dosage range is 20 to 60 mg daily. Adjust dosage to maintain patient on lowest effective dose. Or, 12.5 mg Paxil CR P.O. as a single daily dose, usually in the morning, with or without food. Increase dosage at weekly intervals in increments of 12.5 mg daily, up to a maximum of 37.5 mg daily.

➤ **Generalized anxiety disorder**
Adults: 20 mg P.O. daily initially, increasing by 10 mg per day weekly up to 50 mg daily.
Adjust-a-dose: For debilitated patients or those with renal or hepatic impairment taking immediate-release form, initially, 10 mg P.O. daily, preferably in morning. If patient doesn't respond after full antidepressant effect has occurred, increase dose by 10 mg per day at weekly intervals to a maximum of 40 mg daily. If using controlled-release form, start therapy at 12.5 mg daily. Don't exceed 50 mg daily.

➤ **Posttraumatic stress disorder**
Adults: Initially, 20 mg P.O. daily. Increase dose by 10 mg daily at intervals of at least 1 week. Maximum daily dose is 50 mg P.O.

➤ **Premenstrual dysphoric disorder (PMDD)**
Adults: Initially, 12.5 mg Paxil CR P.O. as a single daily dose, usually in the morning, with or without food, daily or during the luteal phase of the menstrual cycle. Dose changes should occur at intervals of at least 1 week. Maximum dose is 25 mg P.O. daily.

➤ **Hot flashes (breast cancer)**
Adults: 20 mg P.O. daily or nightly.

➤ **Hot flashes (menopausal)**
Adults: 10 or 20 mg P.O. daily (immediate release) or 12.5 or 25 mg P.O. daily (controlled-release).

➤ **Premature ejaculation ◆**
Adults: 10 to 40 mg P.O. daily. Or, 20 mg P.O. as needed 3 to 4 hours before planned intercourse.

➤ **Diabetic neuropathy ◆**
Adults: 40 mg P.O. daily.

ADMINISTRATION
P.O.
● Give drug without regard for food.
● Don't split or crush controlled-release tablets.

ACTION
Thought to be linked to drug's inhibition of CNS neuronal uptake of serotonin.

Route	Onset	Peak	Duration
P.O.	Unknown	2–8 hr	Unknown
P.O. (controlled-release)	Unknown	6–10 hr	Unknown

Half-life: About 24 hours.

ADVERSE REACTIONS
CNS: *asthenia, dizziness, headache, insomnia, somnolence, tremor, nervousness, suicidal behavior,* anxiety, paresthesia, confusion, agitation.
CV: palpitations, vasodilation, orthostatic hypotension.
EENT: lump or tightness in throat.
GI: *dry mouth, nausea, constipation, diarrhea,* flatulence, vomiting, dyspepsia, dysgeusia, increased or decreased appetite, abdominal pain.
GU: *ejaculatory disturbances, sexual dysfunction,* urinary frequency, other urinary disorders.

Musculoskeletal: myopathy, myalgia, myasthenia.
Skin: *diaphoresis*, rash, pruritus.
Other: *decreased libido*, yawning.

INTERACTIONS

Drug-drug. *Amphetamines, buspirone, dextromethorphan, dihydroergotamine, lithium salts, meperidine, other SSRIs or SSNRIs (duloxetine, venlafaxine),* **tramadol,** *trazodone, tricyclic antidepressants, tryptophan:* May increase the risk of serotonin syndrome. Avoid combining drugs that increase the availability of serotonin in the CNS; monitor patient closely if used together.
Cimetidine: May decrease hepatic metabolism of paroxetine, leading to risk of adverse reactions. Dosage adjustments may be needed.
Digoxin: May decrease digoxin level. Use together cautiously.
MAO inhibitors, such as phenelzine, selegiline, tranylcypromine: May cause serotonin syndrome. Avoid using within 14 days of MAO inhibitor therapy.
Phenobarbital, phenytoin: May alter pharmacokinetics of both drugs. Dosage adjustments may be needed.
Procyclidine: May increase procyclidine level. Watch for excessive anticholinergic effects.
Sumatriptan: May cause weakness, hyperreflexia, and incoordination. Monitor patient closely.
Theophylline: May decrease theophylline clearance. Monitor theophylline level.
Thioridazine: May prolong QTc interval and increase risk of serious ventricular arrhythmias, such as torsades de pointes, and sudden death. Avoid using together.
Tricyclic antidepressants: May inhibit tricyclic antidepressant metabolism. Dose of tricyclic antidepressant may need to be reduced. Monitor patient closely.
Triptans: May cause serotonin syndrome (restlessness, hallucinations, loss of coordination, fast heartbeat, rapid changes in blood pressure, increased body temperature, overactive reflexes, nausea, vomiting, and diarrhea). Use cautiously, especially at the start of therapy and at dosage increases.
Warfarin: May cause bleeding. Use together cautiously.

Drug-herb. *St. John's wort:* May increase sedative-hypnotic effects. Discourage use together.
Drug-lifestyle. *Alcohol use:* May alter psychomotor function. Discourage use together.

EFFECTS ON LAB TEST RESULTS
None reported.

CONTRAINDICATIONS & CAUTIONS
● Contraindicated in patients hypersensitive to drug, within 14 days of MAO inhibitor therapy, and in those taking thioridazine.
● Contraindicated in children and adolescents younger than age 18.
● Use cautiously in patients with history of seizure disorders or mania and in those with other severe, systemic illness.
● Use cautiously in patients at risk for volume depletion and monitor them appropriately.
● Using drug in the first trimester may increase the risk of congenital fetal malformations; using drug in the third trimester may cause neonatal complications at birth. Consider the risk versus benefit of therapy.

NURSING CONSIDERATIONS
● Patients taking drug may be at increased risk for developing suicidal behavior, but this hasn't been definitively attributed to use of the drug.
● Patients taking Paxil CR for PMDD should be periodically reassessed to determine the need for continued treatment.
● If signs or symptoms of psychosis occur or increase, expect prescriber to reduce dosage. Record mood changes. Monitor patient for suicidal tendencies, and allow only a minimum supply of drug.
■ **Black Box Warning** Drug may increase the risk of suicidal thinking and behavior in children, adolescents, and young adults ages 18 to 24 during the first 2 months of treatment, especially in those with major depressive disorder or other psychiatric disorder. ■
● Monitor patient for complaints of sexual dysfunction. In men, they include anorgasmy, erectile difficulties, delayed ejaculation or orgasm, or impotence; in women,

---

Reactions may be *common*, uncommon, *life-threatening*, or COMMON AND LIFE-THREATENING.
Interaction may have a *rapid onset* or *delayed onset*.

they include anorgasmia or difficulty with orgasm.

• *Alert:* Don't stop drug abruptly. Withdrawal or discontinuation syndrome may occur if drug is stopped abruptly. Symptoms include headache, myalgia, lethargy, and general flulike symptoms. Taper drug slowly over 1 to 2 weeks.

• *Alert:* Combining triptans with an SSRI or an SSNRI may cause serotonin syndrome. Signs and symptoms may include restlessness, hallucinations, loss of coordination, fast heartbeat, rapid changes in blood pressure, increased body temperature, overactive reflexes, nausea, vomiting, and diarrhea. Serotonin syndrome may be more likely to occur when starting or increasing the dose of triptan, SSRI, or SSNRI.

• *Look alike–sound alike:* Don't confuse paroxetine with paclitaxel, or Paxil with Doxil, paclitaxel, Plavix, or Taxol.

PATIENT TEACHING
• Tell patient that drug may be taken with or without food, usually in morning.
• Tell patient not to break, crush, or chew controlled-release tablets.
• Warn patient to avoid activities that require alertness and good coordination until effects of drug are known.
• Advise woman of childbearing age to contact prescriber if she becomes pregnant or plans to become pregnant during therapy or if she's currently breast-feeding.
• Tell patient to avoid alcohol and to consult prescriber before taking other prescription or OTC drugs or herbal medicines.
• Instruct patient not to stop taking drug abruptly.

---

sertraline hydrochloride
SIR-trah-leen

Apo-Sertraline†, Zoloft⌀

Pharmacologic class: SSRI
Pregnancy risk category C

AVAILABLE FORMS
Capsules†: 25 mg, 50 mg, 100 mg
Oral concentrate: 20 mg/ml
Tablets: 25 mg, 50 mg, 100 mg

INDICATIONS & DOSAGES
➤ **Depression**
Adults: 50 mg P.O. daily. Adjust dosage as needed and tolerated; dosage range is 50 to 200 mg daily.
➤ **Obsessive-compulsive disorder**
Adults: 50 mg P.O. once daily. If patient doesn't improve, increase dosage, up to 200 mg daily.
Children ages 6 to 17: Initially, 25 mg P.O. daily in children ages 6 to 12, or 50 mg P.O. daily in adolescents ages 13 to 17. Increase dosage, as needed, up to 200 mg daily at intervals of no less than 1 week.
➤ **Panic disorder**
Adults: Initially, 25 mg P.O. daily. After 1 week, increase dose to 50 mg P.O. daily. If patient doesn't improve, increase dose to maximum of 200 mg daily.
➤ **Posttraumatic stress disorder**
Adults: Initially, 25 mg P.O. once daily. Increase dosage to 50 mg P.O. once daily after 1 week. Increase at weekly intervals to a maximum of 200 mg daily. Maintain patient on lowest effective dose.
➤ **Premenstrual dysphoric disorder**
Adults: Initially, 50 mg daily P.O. either continuously or only during the luteal phase of the menstrual cycle. If patient doesn't respond, dose may be increased 50 mg per menstrual cycle, up to 150 mg daily for use throughout the menstrual cycle or 100 mg daily for luteal-phase doses. If a 100-mg daily dose has been established with luteal-phase dose, use a 50-mg daily adjustment for 3 days at the beginning of each luteal phase.
➤ **Social anxiety disorder**
Adults: Initially, 25 mg P.O. once daily. Increase dosage to 50 mg P.O. once daily after 1 week of therapy. Dose range is 50 to 200 mg daily. Adjust to the lowest effective dosage and periodically reassess patient to determine the need for long-term treatment.
➤ **Premature ejaculation ◆**
Adults: 25 to 50 mg P.O. daily or as needed.
Adjust-a-dose: For patients with hepatic disease, use lower or less-frequent doses.

ADMINISTRATION
P.O.
• Give drug without regard for food.

- Don't use oral concentrate dropper, which is made of rubber, for a patient with latex allergy.
- Mix oral concentrate with 4 oz (118 ml) of water, ginger ale, lemon-lime soda, lemonade, or orange juice only, and give immediately.

ACTION
Thought to be linked to drug's inhibition of CNS neuronal uptake of serotonin.

Route	Onset	Peak	Duration
P.O.	Unknown	4–8 hr	Unknown

Half-life: 26 hours.

ADVERSE REACTIONS
CNS: *fatigue, headache, tremor, dizziness, insomnia, somnolence,* **suicidal behavior,** paresthesia, hypesthesia, nervousness, anxiety, agitation, hypertonia, twitching, confusion.
CV: palpitations, chest pain, hot flashes.
GI: *dry mouth, nausea, diarrhea, loose stools, dyspepsia,* vomiting, constipation, thirst, flatulence, anorexia, abdominal pain, increased appetite.
GU: *male sexual dysfunction.*
Musculoskeletal: myalgia.
Skin: rash, pruritus, diaphoresis.

INTERACTIONS
Drug-drug. *Amphetamines, buspirone, dextromethorphan, dihydroergotamine, lithium salts, meperidine, other SSRIs or SSNRIs (duloxetine, venlafaxine), sumatriptan,* **tramadol,** *trazodone, tricyclic antidepressants, tryptophan:* May increase the risk of serotonin syndrome. Avoid combinations of drugs that increase the availability of serotonin in the CNS; monitor patient closely if used together.
Benzodiazepines, tolbutamide: May decrease clearance of these drugs. Significance unknown; monitor patient for increased drug effects.
Cimetidine: May decrease clearance of sertraline. Monitor patient closely.
Disulfiram: Oral concentrate contains alcohol, which may react with drug. Avoid using together.
MAO inhibitors, such as phenelzine, selegiline, tranylcypromine: May cause serotonin syndrome. Avoid using within 14 days of MAO inhibitor therapy.

Pimozide: May increase pimozide level. Avoid using together.
Triptans: May cause serotonin syndrome (restlessness, hallucinations, loss of coordination, fast heartbeat, rapid changes in blood pressure, increased body temperature, hyperreflexia, nausea, vomiting, and diarrhea). Use cautiously, with close monitoring, especially at the start of treatment and during dosage adjustments.
Warfarin, other highly protein-bound drugs: May increase level of sertraline or other highly protein-bound drug. May increase PT, or INR may increase by 8%. Monitor patient closely; monitor PT and INR.
Drug-herb. *St. John's wort:* May cause additive effects and serotonin syndrome. Discourage use together.

EFFECTS ON LAB TEST RESULTS
- May increase ALT and AST levels.

CONTRAINDICATIONS & CAUTIONS
- Contraindicated in patients hypersensitive to drug or its components.
- Contraindicated in patients taking pimozide or MAO inhibitors or within 14 days of MAO inhibitor therapy.
- Use cautiously in patients at risk for suicide and in those with seizure disorders, major affective disorder, or diseases or conditions that affect metabolism or hemodynamic responses.
- Use in third trimester of pregnancy may cause neonatal complications at birth. Consider the risk versus benefit of treatment during this time.
- ■ **Black Box Warning** Sertraline isn't approved for use in children except those with obsessive-compulsive disorder. ■

NURSING CONSIDERATIONS
- Give sertraline once daily, either in morning or evening, with or without food.
- Make dosage adjustments at intervals of no less than 1 week.
- Record mood changes. Monitor patient for suicidal tendencies and allow only a minimum supply of drug.
- ■ **Black Box Warning** Drug may increase the risk of suicidal thinking and behavior in children and adolescents with major depressive disorder or other psychiatric disorder. ■

Reactions may be *common*, uncommon, *life-threatening*, or COMMON AND LIFE-THREATENING.
Interaction may have a *rapid onset* or **delayed onset.**

■ **Black Box Warning** Drug may increase the risk of suicidal thinking and behavior in young adults ages 18 to 24 during the first 2 months of treatment. ■

● Don't use the oral concentrate dropper, which is made of rubber, for a patient with latex allergy.

● *Alert:* Combining triptans with an SSRI or an SSNRI may cause serotonin syndrome. Signs and symptoms may include restlessness, hallucinations, loss of coordination, fast heart beat, rapid changes in blood pressure, increased body temperature, overactive reflexes, nausea, vomiting, and diarrhea. Serotonin syndrome may be more likely to occur when starting or increasing the dose of triptan, SSRI, or SSNRI.

PATIENT TEACHING

● Advise patient to use caution when performing hazardous tasks that require alertness.

● Tell patient to avoid alcohol and to consult prescriber before taking OTC drugs.

● Advise patient to mix the oral concentrate with 4 oz (½ cup) of water, ginger ale, lemon-lime soda, lemonade, or orange juice only, and to take the dose right away.

● Instruct patient to avoid stopping drug abruptly.

---

trazodone hydrochloride
TRAYZ-oh-dohn

Pharmacologic class:
triazolopyridine derivative
Pregnancy risk category C

AVAILABLE FORMS
Tablets: 50 mg, 100 mg, 150 mg, 300 mg

INDICATIONS & DOSAGES
➤ **Depression**
Adults: Initially, 150 mg P.O. daily in divided doses; then increased by 50 mg daily every 3 to 4 days, as needed. Dose ranges from 150 to 400 mg daily. Maximum, 600 mg daily for inpatients and 400 mg daily for outpatients.
➤ **Insomnia** ◆
Adults: 50 to 100 mg P.O. daily.

ADMINISTRATION
P.O.
● Give drug after meals or a light snack for optimal absorption and to decrease risk of dizziness.

ACTION
Unknown. Inhibits CNS neuronal uptake of serotonin; not a tricyclic derivative.

Route	Onset	Peak	Duration
P.O.	Unknown	1–2 hr	Unknown

Half-life: First phase, 3 to 6 hours; second phase, 5 to 9 hours.

ADVERSE REACTIONS
CNS: *drowsiness, dizziness,* nervousness, fatigue, confusion, tremor, weakness, hostility, anger, nightmares, vivid dreams, headache, insomnia, syncope.
CV: orthostatic hypotension, tachycardia, hypertension, shortness of breath, ECG changes.
EENT: blurred vision, tinnitus, nasal congestion.
GI: dry mouth, dysgeusia, constipation, nausea, vomiting, anorexia.
GU: urine retention, priapism possibly leading to impotence, hematuria.
Hematologic: anemia.
Skin: rash, urticaria, diaphoresis.
Other: decreased libido.

INTERACTIONS
Drug-drug. *Amphetamines, buspirone, dextromethorphan, dihydroergotamine, lithium salts, meperidine, SSRIs or SSNRIs (duloxetine, venlafaxine), sumatriptan, tramadol, tricyclic antidepressants, tryptophan:* May increase the risk of serotonin syndrome. Avoid combining drugs that increase the availability of serotonin in the CNS; monitor patient closely if used together.
Antihypertensives: May increase hypotensive effect of trazodone. Antihypertensive dosage may need to be decreased.
Clonidine, CNS depressants: May enhance CNS depression. Avoid using together.
CYP3A4 inducers (carbamazepine): May reduce trazodone level. Monitor patient closely; may need to increase trazodone dose.

CYP3A4 inhibitors (ketoconazole):
May slow the clearance of trazodone
and increase trazodone level. May
cause nausea, hypotension, and fainting.
Consider decreasing trazodone dose.
Digoxin, phenytoin: May increase levels
of these drugs. Watch for toxicity.
MAO inhibitors: Effects unknown. Use
together with extreme caution.
**Protease inhibitors (amprenavir,
atazanavir, fosamprenavir, Indinavir,
lopinavir and ritonavir, nelfinavir, ritonavir,
saquinavir):** May increase trazodone levels
and adverse effects. Monitor patient and
adjust trazodone dose, as needed.
Drug-herb. *Ginkgo biloba:* May cause
sedation. Discourage use together.
St. John's wort: May cause serotonin
syndrome. Discourage use together.
Drug-lifestyle. *Alcohol use:* May
enhance CNS depression. Discourage
use together.

EFFECTS ON LAB TEST RESULTS
• May increase ALT and AST levels. May
decrease hemoglobin level.

CONTRAINDICATIONS & CAUTIONS
• Contraindicated in patients hypersensitive to drug.
■ **Black Box Warning** Trazodone isn't
approved for use in children. ■
• Use cautiously in patients with
cardiac disease or in the initial recovery
phase of MI and in patients at risk for
suicide.

NURSING CONSIDERATIONS
• Record mood changes. Monitor patient
for suicidal tendencies and allow only
minimum supply of drug.
■ **Black Box Warning** Drug may increase
the risk of suicidal thinking and behavior
in children, adolescents, and young adults
ages 18 to 24 during the first 2 months of
treatment, especially those with major
depressive disorder or other psychiatric
disorder. ■
• *Look alike–sound alike:* Don't confuse
trazodone hydrochloride with tramadol
hydrochloride.

PATIENT TEACHING
• *Alert:* Tell patient to report a persistent,
painful erection (priapism) right away

because he may need immediate
intervention.
• Warn patient to avoid activities that
require alertness and good coordination
until effects of drug are known. Drowsiness and dizziness usually subside after
first few weeks.
• Teach caregivers how to recognize signs
and symptoms of suicidal tendency or
suicidal thoughts.

venlafaxine hydrochloride
vin-lah-FACKS-in

Effexor✒, Effexor XR✒

Pharmacologic class: SSNRI
Pregnancy risk category C

AVAILABLE FORMS
Capsules (extended-release): 37.5 mg,
75 mg, 150 mg
Tablets: 25 mg, 37.5 mg, 50 mg, 75 mg,
100 mg
Tablets (extended-release): 37.5 mg,
75 mg, 150 mg, 225 mg

INDICATIONS & DOSAGES
➤ **Depression**
Adults: Initially, 75 mg P.O. daily in two or
three divided doses with food. Increase as
tolerated and needed by 75 mg daily every
4 days. For moderately depressed outpatients, usual maximum is 225 mg daily;
in certain severely depressed patients,
dose may be as high as 375 mg daily. For
extended-release capsules, 75 mg P.O.
daily in a single dose. For some patients, it
may be desirable to start at 37.5 mg P.O.
daily for 4 to 7 days before increasing to
75 mg daily. Dosage may be increased by
75 mg daily every 4 days to maximum of
225 mg daily.
➤ **Generalized anxiety disorder**
Adults: Initially, 75 mg extended-release
capsule P.O. daily in a single dose. For
some patients, it may be desirable to start
at 37.5 mg P.O. daily for 4 to 7 days before
increasing to 75 mg daily. Dosage may be
increased by 75 mg daily every 4 days to
maximum of 225 mg daily.
➤ **Panic disorder**
Adults: Initially, 37.5 mg extended-release
capsule P.O. daily for 1 week, then increase

dose to 75 mg daily. If patient isn't
responding, may increase dose by up to
75 mg/day in no less than weekly intervals, as needed, to a maximum dose of
225 mg daily.
➤ **Social anxiety disorder**
Adults: Initially, 75 mg extended-release
capsule daily as a single dose. For some
patients, it may be desirable to start at
37.5 mg P.O. daily for 4 to 7 days before
increasing to 75 mg daily. Increase dosage
as needed by 75 mg daily every 4 days.
Maximum dose is 225 mg daily.
Adjust-a-dose: For patients with
renal impairment, reduce daily amount
by 25%. For those undergoing hemodialysis, reduce daily amount by 50%
and withhold dose until dialysis is
completed. For patients with hepatic
impairment, reduce daily amount
by 50%.
➤ **To prevent major depressive
disorder relapse** ♦
Adults: 100 to 200 mg daily P.O. regular-
release tablets or 75 to 225 mg daily P.O.
extended-release capsules.
➤ **Hot flashes** ♦
Adults: 12.5 mg (immediate-release) P.O.
b.i.d. for 4 weeks. Or, 37.5 to 150 mg
(extended-release) P.O. daily for up to
3 months.

ADMINISTRATION
P.O.
● Give drug with food and a full glass of
water.
● Give capsule whole; if patient can't
swallow whole, open and sprinkle contents on spoonful of applesauce; mix and
give immediately. Follow with a full glass
of water.

ACTION
May increase the amount of norepinephrine, serotonin, or both in the CNS by
blocking their reuptake by the presynaptic
neurons.

Route	Onset	Peak	Duration
P.O.	Unknown	1–2 hr	Unknown

Half-life: 5 hours.

ADVERSE REACTIONS
CNS: *asthenia, headache, somnolence,
dizziness, nervousness, insomnia,* **suicidal
behavior,** anxiety, tremor, abnormal
dreams, paresthesia, agitation.
CV: hypertension, tachycardia,
vasodilation.
EENT: blurred vision.
GI: *nausea, constipation, dry mouth,
anorexia,* vomiting, diarrhea, dyspepsia,
flatulence.
GU: *abnormal ejaculation,* impotence,
urinary frequency, impaired urination.
Metabolic: weight loss.
Skin: *diaphoresis,* rash.
Other: yawning, chills, infection.

INTERACTIONS
Drug-drug. *MAO inhibitors, such as
phenelzine, selegiline, tranylcypromine:*
May cause serotonin syndrome. Avoid
using within 14 days of MAO inhibitor
therapy.
Tramadol, *sibutramine, sumatriptan, trazodone:* May cause serotonin syndrome.
Monitor patient closely.
Triptans: May cause serotonin syndrome
(restlessness, hallucinations, loss of coordination, fast heartbeat, rapid changes in
blood pressure, increased body temperature, hyperreflexia, nausea, vomiting,
and diarrhea). Use cautiously and with
increased monitoring at the start of therapy and with dose increase.
Warfarin: May increase PT, PTT, or INR.
Monitor these lab values and patient
closely.
Drug-herb. *Yohimbe:* May cause additive
stimulation. Urge caution.

EFFECTS ON LAB TEST RESULTS
None reported.

CONTRAINDICATIONS & CAUTIONS
● Contraindicated in patients hypersensitive to drug or within 14 days of MAO
inhibitor therapy.
■ **Black Box Warning** Venlafaxine isn't
approved for use in children. ■
● Use cautiously in patients with renal
impairment, diseases or conditions that
could affect hemodynamic responses or
metabolism, and in those with history of
mania or seizures.
● Use in third trimester of pregnancy may
be associated with neonatal complications
at birth. Consider the risk versus benefit of
treatment during this time.

NURSING CONSIDERATIONS

● *Alert:* Closely monitor patients being treated for depression for signs and symptoms of clinical worsening and suicidal ideation, especially at the beginning of therapy and with dosage adjustments. Symptoms may include agitation, insomnia, anxiety, aggressiveness, or panic attacks.

■ **Black Box Warning** Drug may increase the risk of suicidal thinking and behavior in children, adolescents, and young adults ages 18 to 24 during the first 2 months of treatment, especially those with major depressive disorder or other psychiatric disorder. ■

● Carefully monitor blood pressure. Drug therapy may cause sustained, dose-dependent increases in blood pressure. Greatest increases (averaging about 7 mm Hg above baseline) occur in patients taking 375 mg daily.

● Monitor patient's weight, particularly underweight, depressed patients.

● *Alert:* Combining triptans with an SSRI or an SSNRI may cause serotonin syndrome. Signs and symptoms may include restlessness, hallucinations, loss of coordination, fast heartbeat, rapid changes in blood pressure, increased body temperature, overactive reflexes, nausea, vomiting, and diarrhea. Serotonin syndrome may be more likely to occur when starting or increasing the dose of triptan, SSRI, or SSNRI.

PATIENT TEACHING

● If medication is to be stopped, inform patient who has received drug for 6 weeks or longer that drug will be stopped gradually by tapering dosage over a 2-week period, as instructed by prescriber. Patient shouldn't abruptly stop taking the drug.

● *Alert:* Warn family members to closely monitor patient for signs of worsening condition or suicidal ideation.

● Warn patient to avoid hazardous activities that require alertness and good coordination until effects of drug are known.

● Tell patient to avoid alcohol and to consult prescriber before taking other prescription or OTC drugs.

● Advise woman of childbearing age to contact prescriber if she becomes pregnant or intends to become pregnant during therapy or if she's breast-feeding.

● Tell patient to take each dose with food and a full glass of water.

● Tell patient that if he can't swallow capsule whole, he may carefully open it and sprinkle contents on a spoonful of applesauce, mix, and take immediately. Follow with a full glass of water.

Reactions may be *common,* uncommon, *life-threatening,* or COMMON AND LIFE-THREATENING.
Interaction may have a *rapid onset* or **delayed onset**.

39

Antimigraine drugs

almotriptan malate
eletriptan hydrobromide
frovatriptan succinate
naratriptan hydrochloride
rizatriptan benzoate
sumatriptan succinate
zolmitriptan

---

almotriptan malate
al-moh-TRIP-tan

Axert

Pharmacologic class: serotonin
5-HT$_1$ receptor agonist
Pregnancy risk category C

AVAILABLE FORMS
Tablets: 6.25 mg, 12.5 mg

INDICATIONS & DOSAGES
➤ **Acute migraine with or without
aura**
Adults: 6.25-mg or 12.5-mg tablet P.O.,
with one additional dose after 2 hours
if headache is unresolved or recurs.
Maximum, two doses within 24 hours.
Adjust-a-dose: For patients with hepatic
or renal impairment, initially 6.25 mg,
with maximum daily dose of 12.5 mg.

ADMINISTRATION
P.O.
• Give drug without regard for food.
• Give only one repeat dose within
24 hours, no sooner than 2 hours after first
dose.

ACTION
May act as an agonist at serotonin receptors
on extracerebral intracranial blood vessels,
which constricts the affected vessels, inhibits neuropeptide release, and reduces pain
transmission in the trigeminal pathways.

Route	Onset	Peak	Duration
P.O.	1–3 hr	1–3 hr	3–4 hr

Half-life: 3 to 4 hours.

ADVERSE REACTIONS
CNS: paresthesia, headache, dizziness,
somnolence.
CV: *coronary artery vasospasm,
transient myocardial ischemia, MI,
ventricular tachycardia, ventricular
fibrillation.*
GI: nausea, dry mouth.

INTERACTIONS
Drug-drug. *MAO inhibitors, verapamil:*
May increase almotriptan level. No dose
adjustment is necessary.
CYP3A4 inhibitors such as ketoconazole:
May increase almotriptan level. Monitor
patient for potential adverse reaction.
May need to reduce dosage.
*Ergot-containing drugs, serotonin
5-HT$_{1B/1D}$ agonists:* May cause additive
effects. Avoid using within 24 hours of
almotriptan.
SSRIs: May cause additive serotonin
effects, resulting in weakness, hyperreflexia, or incoordination. Monitor
patient closely if given together.

EFFECTS ON LAB TEST RESULTS
None reported.

CONTRAINDICATIONS & CAUTIONS
• Contraindicated in patients hypersensitive to drug.
• Contraindicated in those with
angina pectoris, history of MI,
silent ischemia, coronary artery
vasospasm, or Prinzmetal's variant
angina, or other CV disease; uncontrolled hypertension; and hemiplegic
or basilar migraine.
• Don't give within 24 hours after treatment with other 5-HT$_{1B/1D}$ agonists or
ergot derivatives.
• Use cautiously in patients with renal or
hepatic impairment and in those with
cataracts because of the potential for
corneal opacities.
• Use cautiously in patients with risk
factors for coronary artery disease
(CAD), such as obesity, diabetes, and
family history of CAD.

NURSING CONSIDERATIONS
● Patients with poor renal or hepatic function should receive a reduced dosage.
● Repeat dose after 2 hours, if needed and don't give more than two doses in 24 hours.
● *Alert:* Combining triptans with SSRIs or SSNRIs may cause serotonin syndrome. Signs and symptoms include restlessness, hallucinations, loss of coordination, rapid heartbeat, rapid changes in blood pressure, increased body temperature, overactive reflexes, nausea, vomiting, and diarrhea. Serotonin syndrome occurs more often when starting or increasing the dose of a triptan, SSRI, or SSNRI.
● *Look alike–sound alike:* Don't confuse Axert with Antivert.

PATIENT TEACHING
● Tell patient that drug can be taken with or without food.
● Advise patient to take drug only when he's having a migraine; explain that drug isn't taken on a regular schedule.
● Advise patient to use only one repeat dose within 24 hours, no sooner than 2 hours after first dose.
● Advise patient that other commonly prescribed migraine drugs can interact with almotriptan.
● Advise patient to report chest or throat tightness, pain, or heaviness.
● Teach patient to avoid possible migraine triggers, such as cheese, chocolate, citrus fruits, caffeine, and alcohol.

eletriptan hydrobromide
ell-ah-TRIP-tan

Relpax⧗

Pharmacologic class: serotonin 5-HT$_1$ receptor agonist
Pregnancy risk category C

AVAILABLE FORMS
Tablets: 20 mg, 40 mg

INDICATIONS & DOSAGES
➤ **Acute migraine with or without aura**
Adults: 20 to 40 mg P.O. at first migraine symptom. If headache recurs, dose may be repeated at least 2 hours later to a maximum of 80 mg daily.

ADMINISTRATION
P.O.
● Give drug without regard for food.
● Give drug whole; don't crush or break tablet.
● Give drug with a full glass of water.
● If headache returns after first dose, give a second dose after 2 hours. Don't give more than 80 mg in 24 hours.

ACTION
Binds to 5-HT$_1$ receptors and may constrict intracranial blood vessels and inhibit proinflammatory neuropeptide release.

Route	Onset	Peak	Duration
P.O.	½ hr	1½–2 hr	Unknown

Half-life: About 4 hours.

ADVERSE REACTIONS
CNS: *asthenia,* dizziness, headache, hypertonia, hypesthesia, pain, paresthesia, somnolence, vertigo.
CV: chest tightness, pain, and pressure, flushing, palpitations.
EENT: pharyngitis.
GI: abdominal pain, discomfort or cramps, dry mouth, dyspepsia, dysphagia, nausea.
Musculoskeletal: back pain.
Skin: increased sweating.
Other: chills.

INTERACTIONS
Drug-drug. *CYP3A4 inhibitors (such as clarithromycin, itraconazole, ketoconazole, nefazodone, nelfinavir, ritonavir, troleandomycin):* May decrease eletriptan metabolism. Avoid use within 72 hours of these drugs.
Ergotamine-containing or ergot-type drugs (such as dihydroergotamine or methysergide), other triptans: May prolong vasospastic reactions. Avoid use within 24 hours of these drugs.
SSRIs: May increase the risk of serotonin syndrome (weakness, hyperreflexia, and incoordination). If used together, observe patient closely.

EFFECTS ON LAB TEST RESULTS
None known.

Reactions may be *common,* uncommon, *life-threatening,* or COMMON AND LIFE-THREATENING.
Interaction may have a *rapid onset* or *delayed onset.*

CONTRAINDICATIONS & CAUTIONS
• Contraindicated in patients hypersensitive to drug or its components and in those with severe hepatic impairment; ischemic heart disease, such as angina pectoris, a history of MI, or silent ischemia; coronary artery vasospasm, including Prinzmetal's variant angina; and other significant CV conditions.
• Contraindicated in patients with cerebrovascular syndromes, such as stroke or transient ischemic attack; peripheral vascular disease, including ischemic bowel disease; uncontrolled hypertension; or hemiplegic or basilar migraine.
• Contraindicated within 24 hours of another 5-HT₁ agonist, drugs containing ergotamine, or ergot-type drug.
• Contraindicated in patients with risk factors for coronary artery disease (CAD), such as hypertension, hypercholesterolemia, smoking, obesity, diabetes, strong family history of CAD, postmenopausal women, or men older than age 40, unless patient is free from cardiac disease. Monitor patient closely after first dose.
• Safety of treating more than three migraine headaches in 30 days hasn't been established.

NURSING CONSIDERATIONS
• Drug isn't intended for migraine prevention.
• **Alert:** Combining a triptan with an SSRI or an SSNRI may cause serotonin syndrome. Signs and symptoms may include restlessness, hallucinations, loss of coordination, fast heartbeat, rapid changes in blood pressure, increased body temperature, hyperreflexia, nausea, vomiting, and diarrhea. Serotonin syndrome may be more likely to occur when starting or increasing the dose of a triptan, SSRI, or SSNRI.
• Use drug only when patient has a clear diagnosis of migraine. If the first use produces no response, reconsider the migraine diagnosis.
• **Alert:** Serious cardiac events including acute MI, arrhythmias, and death occur rarely within a few hours after use of 5-HT₁ agonists.

• Ophthalmologic effects may occur with long-term use.
• Older patients may develop higher blood pressure than younger patients after taking drug.

PATIENT TEACHING
• Instruct patient to take dose at the first sign of a migraine headache. If the headache comes back after the first dose, he may take a second dose after 2 hours. Caution patient not to take more than 80 mg in 24 hours.
• Warn patient to avoid driving and operating machinery if he feels dizzy or fatigued after taking the drug.
• Tell patient to immediately report pain, tightness, heaviness, or pressure in the chest, throat, neck, or jaw.
• Tell patient to swallow tablet whole and not to split, crush, or chew.
• Instruct patient to take each dose with a full glass of water.

---

frovatriptan succinate
frow-vah-TRIP-tan

Frova⊘

Pharmacologic class: serotonin 5-HT₁ receptor agonist
Pregnancy risk category C

AVAILABLE FORMS
Tablets: 2.5 mg

INDICATIONS & DOSAGES
➤ **Acute treatment of migraine attacks with or without aura**
Adults: 2.5 mg P.O. taken at the first sign of migraine attack. If the headache recurs, a second tablet may be taken at least 2 hours after the first dose. The total daily dose shouldn't exceed 7.5 mg.

ADMINISTRATION
P.O.
• Give drug without regard for food.
• Give drug with a full glass of water.
• If headache returns after first dose, give a second dose after 2 hours. Don't give more than 3 tablets in 24 hours.

ACTION
May inhibit excessive dilation of extra-cerebral and intracranial arteries during migraine headaches.

Route	Onset	Peak	Duration
P.O.	Unknown	2–4 hr	Unknown

Half-life: 26 hours.

ADVERSE REACTIONS
CNS: dizziness, headache, fatigue, paresthesia, insomnia, anxiety, somnolence, dysesthesia, hypoesthesia, hot or cold sensation, pain.
CV: *coronary artery vasospasm, transient myocardial ischemia, MI, ventricular tachycardia, ventricular fibrillation,* chest pain, palpitations, flushing.
EENT: abnormal vision, tinnitus, sinusitis, rhinitis.
GI: dry mouth, dyspepsia, vomiting, abdominal pain, diarrhea, nausea.
Musculoskeletal: skeletal pain.
Skin: increased sweating.

INTERACTIONS
Drug-drug. *5-HT₁ agonists:* May cause additive effects. Separate doses by 24 hours.
Ergotamine-containing or ergot-type drugs (such as dihydroergotamine or methysergide): May cause prolonged vasospastic reactions. Separate doses by 24 hours.
SSRIs (such as citalopram, fluoxetine, fluvoxamine, paroxetine, sertraline): May cause weakness, hyperreflexia, and incoordination. Monitor patient closely.

EFFECTS ON LAB TEST RESULTS
None reported.

CONTRAINDICATIONS & CAUTIONS
• Contraindicated in patients hypersensitive to drug or any of its components.
• Contraindicated in patients with history or symptoms of ischemic heart disease or coronary artery vasospasm, including Prinzmetal's variant angina; in those with cerebrovascular or peripheral vascular disease, including ischemic bowel disease; in those with uncontrolled hypertension; and in those with hemiplegic or basilar migraine.

• Contraindicated within 24 hours of another triptan, drug containing ergotamine, or ergot-type drug.
• Contraindicated in patients with risk factors for coronary artery disease (CAD), such as hypertension, hypercholesterolemia, smoking, obesity, diabetes, strong family history of CAD, postmenopausal women, or men older than age 40, unless patient is free from cardiac disease. If drug is used in such a patient, monitor patient closely and consider obtaining an ECG after the first dose. Intermittent, long-term users of triptans or those with risk factors should undergo periodic cardiac evaluation while using drug.
• Use cautiously in breast-feeding women. It's unknown if drug appears in breast milk.
• The safety of treating an average of more than four migraine headaches in a 30-day period hasn't been established.

NURSING CONSIDERATIONS
• *Alert:* Serious cardiac events, including acute MI, life-threatening cardiac arrhythmias, and death may occur within a few hours of taking a triptan.
• Use drug only when patient has a clear diagnosis of migraine. If a patient has no response for the first migraine attack treated with frovatriptan, reconsider the diagnosis of migraine.
• *Alert:* Combining a triptan with an SSRI or an SSNRI may cause serotonin syndrome. Symptoms may include restlessness, hallucinations, loss of coordination, fast heartbeat, rapid changes in blood pressure, increased body temperature, hyperreflexia, nausea, vomiting, and diarrhea. Serotonin syndrome is more likely to occur when starting or increasing the dose of a triptan, SSRI, or SSNRI.

PATIENT TEACHING
• Instruct patient to take dose at first sign of migraine headache. If headache comes back after first dose, he may take a second dose after 2 hours. Tell patient not to take more than 3 tablets in 24 hours.
• Caution patient to take extra care or avoid driving and operating machinery if dizziness or fatigue develops after taking drug.

Reactions may be *common,* uncommon, *life-threatening,* or COMMON AND LIFE-THREATENING.
Interaction may have a *rapid onset* or **delayed onset.**

• Stress importance of immediately reporting pain, tightness, heaviness, or pressure in chest, throat, neck, or jaw, or rash or itching after taking drug.
• Instruct the patient not to take drug within 24 hours of taking another serotonin-receptor agonist or ergot-type drug.
• Tell patient dose may be taken with or without food, but to take with a full glass of fluid.

naratriptan hydrochloride
nar-ah-TRIP-tan

Amerge

Pharmacologic class: serotonin 5-HT₁ receptor agonist
Pregnancy risk category C

AVAILABLE FORMS
Tablets: 1 mg, 2.5 mg

INDICATIONS & DOSAGES
➤ **Acute migraine attacks with or without aura**
Adults: 1 or 2.5 mg P.O. as a single dose. If headache returns or responds only partially, dose may be repeated after 4 hours. Maximum, 5 mg in 24 hours.
Adjust-a-dose: For patients with mild to moderate renal or hepatic impairment, reduce dosage. Maximum, 2.5 mg in 24 hours.

ADMINISTRATION
P.O.
• Give drug without regard for food.
• Give drug whole; don't split or crush tablet.
• If no response occurs with first tablet, prescriber should be consulted before giving second tablet. If more relief is needed after first tablet (if a partial response occurs or headache returns), and prescriber has approved a second dose, give a second tablet (but not sooner than 4 hours after first tablet).

ACTION
May act as an agonist at serotonin receptors on extracerebral intracranial blood vessels, which constricts the affected vessels, inhibits neuropeptide release, and reduces pain transmission in the trigeminal pathways.

Route	Onset	Peak	Duration
P.O.	Unknown	2–3 hr	Unknown

Half-life: 6 hours.

ADVERSE REACTIONS
CNS: paresthesia, dizziness, drowsiness, malaise, fatigue, vertigo, syncope.
CV: *tachyarrhythmias, abnormal ECG changes, coronary artery vasospasm, transient myocardial ischemia, MI, ventricular tachycardia, ventricular fibrillation,* palpitations, hypertension.
EENT: ear, nose, and throat infections, photophobia.
GI: nausea, hyposalivation, vomiting.
Other: sensations of warmth, cold, pressure, tightness, or heaviness.

INTERACTIONS
Drug-drug. *Ergot-containing or ergot-type drugs (dihydroergotamine, methy-sergide), other 5-HT₁ agonists:* May prolong vasospastic reactions. Avoid using within 24 hours of naratriptan.
Hormonal contraceptives: May slightly increase naratriptan level. Monitor patient.
SSRIs (fluoxetine, fluvoxamine, paroxetine, sertraline): May cause weakness, hyper-reflexia, and incoordination. Monitor patient.
Drug-herb. *St. John's wort:* May increase serotonergic effect. Discourage use together.
Drug-lifestyle. *Smoking:* May increase naratriptan clearance. Discourage smoking.

EFFECTS ON LAB TEST RESULTS
None reported.

CONTRAINDICATIONS & CAUTIONS
• Contraindicated in patients hypersensitive to drug or its components, in those with prior or current cardiac ischemia, in those with cerebrovascular or peripheral vascular syndromes, and in those with uncontrolled hypertension.
• Contraindicated in elderly patients, patients with creatinine clearance below 15 ml/minute, patients with Child-Pugh grade C, and patients who have used

ergot-containing, ergot-type, or other 5-HT₁ agonists within 24 hours.

- Use cautiously in patients with risk factors for coronary artery disease (CAD), such as hypertension, hypercholesterolemia, obesity, diabetes, smoking, strong family history of CAD, postmenopausal women, and men older than age 40, unless patient is free from cardiac disease. Monitor patient closely after first dose.
- Use cautiously in patients with renal or hepatic impairment.
- Safety and efficacy of treating cluster headaches or more than four headaches in a 30-day period haven't been established.

NURSING CONSIDERATIONS
- Assess cardiac status in patients who develop risk factors for CAD.
- **Alert:** Drug can cause coronary artery vasospasm and increased risk of cerebrovascular events.
- Drug isn't intended to prevent migraines or manage hemiplegic or basilar migraine.
- Use drug only when patient has a clear diagnosis of migraine.
- **Alert:** Combining drug with an SSRI or an SSNRI may cause serotonin syndrome. Symptoms include restlessness, hallucinations, loss of coordination, fast heartbeat, rapid changes in blood pressure, increased body temperature, hyperreflexia, nausea, vomiting, and diarrhea. Serotonin syndrome is more likely to occur when starting or increasing the dose of naratriptan, the SSRI, or the SSNRI.

PATIENT TEACHING
- Instruct patient to take drug only as prescribed and to read the accompanying patient instruction leaflet before using drug.
- Tell patient that drug is intended to relieve, not prevent, migraines.
- Instruct patient to take dose soon after headache starts. If no response occurs with first tablet, tell him to seek medical approval before taking second tablet. Tell patient that if more relief is needed after first tablet (if a partial response occurs or headache returns), and prescriber has approved a second dose, he may take a second tablet (but not sooner than 4 hours after first tablet). Tell him not to exceed 2 tablets within 24 hours.

- Advise patient to increase fluid intake.
- Advise patient not to use drug if she suspects or knows that she's pregnant.
- Tell patient to alert prescriber about bothersome adverse effects.
- Tell patient to swallow tablet whole, and not to split, crush, or chew tablet.

rizatriptan benzoate
rih-zah-TRIP-tan

Maxalt, Maxalt-MLT

Pharmacologic class: serotonin 5-HT₁ receptor agonist
Pregnancy risk category C

AVAILABLE FORMS
Orally disintegrating tablets (ODTs): 5 mg, 10 mg
Tablets: 5 mg, 10 mg

INDICATIONS & DOSAGES
➤ **Acute migraine headaches with or without aura**
Adults: Initially, 5 or 10 mg P.O. If first dose is ineffective, may give another dose at least 2 hours after first dose; maximum, 30 mg in 24 hours. For patients receiving propranolol, 5 mg P.O.; maximum, 15 mg in 24 hours.

ADMINISTRATION
P.O.
- Give drug with or without food, although food may delay onset of drug action.
- Give tablet with plenty of fluid.
- Give ODT with or without fluid.
- For Maxalt-MLT, remove blister pack from pouch and remove drug from blister pack immediately before use. Tablet shouldn't be popped out of blister pack; carefully peel away package with dry hands, place tablet on patient's tongue, and let tablet dissolve until it can be swallowed with saliva.

ACTION
May act as an agonist at serotonin receptors on extracerebral intracranial blood vessels, which constricts the affected vessels, inhibits neuropeptide release,

and reduces pain transmission in the trigeminal pathways.

Route	Onset	Peak	Duration
P.O.	Unknown	60–90 min	Unknown

Half-life: 2 to 3 hours.

ADVERSE REACTIONS

CNS: dizziness, headache, somnolence, paresthesia, asthenia, fatigue, decreased mental acuity, euphoria, tremor, pain.
CV: *coronary artery vasospasm, transient myocardial ischemia, MI, ventricular tachycardia, ventricular fibrillation,* chest pain, pressure, or heaviness, palpitations, flushing.
EENT: neck, throat, and jaw pain.
GI: dry mouth, nausea, diarrhea, vomiting.
Respiratory: dyspnea.
Other: hot flashes, warm or cold feelings.

INTERACTIONS

Drug-drug. *Ergot-containing or ergot-type drugs (dihydroergotamine, methysergide), other 5-HT$_1$ agonists:* May prolong vasospastic reactions. Avoid using within 24 hours of rizatriptan.
MAO inhibitors: May increase rizatriptan level. Avoid using within 2 weeks of MAO inhibitor.
Propranolol: May increase rizatriptan level. Reduce rizatriptan dose to 5 mg.
SSRIs (fluoxetine, fluvoxamine, paroxetine, sertraline): May cause weakness, hyperreflexia, and incoordination. Monitor patient.

EFFECTS ON LAB TEST RESULTS

None reported.

CONTRAINDICATIONS & CAUTIONS

• Contraindicated in patients hypersensitive to drug or its components and in those with a history or symptoms of ischemic heart disease, coronary artery vasospasm (Prinzmetal's variant angina), or other significant underlying CV disease.
• Contraindicated in patients with uncontrolled hypertension; within 24 hours of another 5-HT$_1$ agonist, drug containing ergotamine, or ergot-type drug, such as dihydroergotamine or methysergide; or within 2 weeks of MAO inhibitor.
• Contraindicated in patients with hemiplegic or basilar migraine.

• Use cautiously in patients with risk factors for coronary artery disease (CAD), such as hypertension, hypercholesterolemia, smoking, obesity, diabetes, strong family history of CAD, postmenopausal women, or men older than age 40, unless patient is free from cardiac disease. Monitor patient closely after first dose.
• Use cautiously in patients with hepatic or renal impairment.
• Safety and efficacy in children are unknown.
• Safety of treating more than four headaches in 30 days hasn't been established.

NURSING CONSIDERATIONS

• Assess CV status in patients who develop risk factors for CAD during treatment.
• Use drug only when patient has a clear diagnosis of migraine.
• Don't use drug to prevent migraines or to treat hemiplegic or basilar migraine or cluster headaches.
• **Alert:** Combining drug with an SSRI or an SSNRI may cause serotonin syndrome. Symptoms include restlessness, hallucinations, loss of coordination, fast heartbeat, rapid changes in blood pressure, increased body temperature, hyperreflexia, nausea, vomiting, and diarrhea. Serotonin syndrome is more likely to occur when starting or increasing the dose of this drug, the SSRI, or the SSNRI.
• The ODTs contain phenylalanine.

PATIENT TEACHING

• Inform patient that drug doesn't prevent migraine headache.
• For Maxalt-MLT, tell patient to remove blister pack from pouch and remove drug from blister pack immediately before use. Tablet shouldn't be popped out of blister pack; tell patient to carefully peel away package with dry hands, place tablet on tongue, and allow tablet to dissolve. Tablet is then swallowed with saliva. No water is needed or recommended. Tell patient that ODT doesn't relieve headache more quickly.
• Instruct patient to take regular tablets with plenty of fluid.
• Advise patient that, if headache returns after first dose, he may take a second dose at least 2 hours after the first dose. Warn

against taking more than 30 mg in a 24-hour period.
● Inform patient that drug may cause sleepiness and dizziness, and warn him to avoid hazardous activities until effects are known.
● Tell patient that food may delay onset of drug action.
● Advise patient to notify prescriber about suspected or known pregnancy.
● Instruct patient not to breast-feed during therapy because effects on the infant are unknown.

sumatriptan succinate
sue-mah-TRIP-tan

Imitrex◆

Pharmacologic class: serotonin 5-HT$_1$ receptor agonist
Pregnancy risk category C

AVAILABLE FORMS
Injection: 6 mg/0.5 ml (12 mg/ml) in 0.5-ml prefilled syringes and vials
Nasal solution: 5 mg/0.1 ml, 20 mg/0.1 ml
Tablets: 25 mg, 50 mg, 100 mg (base)†

INDICATIONS & DOSAGES
➤ **Acute migraine attacks (with or without aura)**
Adults: For injection, 6 mg subcutaneously; maximum dose is two 6-mg injections in 24 hours, separated by at least 1 hour.
  For tablets, 25 to 100 mg P.O., initially. If desired response isn't achieved in 2 hours, may give second dose of 25 to 100 mg. Additional doses may be used in at least 2-hour intervals. Maximum daily dose, 200 mg.
  For nasal spray, give 5 mg, 10 mg, or 20 mg once in one nostril; may repeat once after 2 hours, for maximum daily dose of 40 mg. A 10-mg dose may be achieved by giving a 5-mg dose in each nostril.
➤ **Cluster headache**
Adults: 6 mg subcutaneously. Maximum recommended dose is two 6-mg injections in 24 hours, separated by at least 1 hour.
Adjust-a-dose: In patients with hepatic impairment, the maximum single oral dose shouldn't exceed 50 mg.

ADMINISTRATION
P.O.
● Give drug without regard for food.
● Give drug whole; don't crush or break tablet.
Subcutaneous
● Redness or pain at injection site should subside within 1 hour after injection.
Intranasal
● Have patient blow his nose before use.
● Give medication on inhalation in one nostril, while blocking the other nostril.

ACTION
May act as an agonist at serotonin receptors on extracerebral intracranial blood vessels, which constricts the affected vessels, inhibits neuropeptide release, and reduces pain transmission in the trigeminal pathways.

Route	Onset	Peak	Duration
P.O.	30 min	90 min	Unknown
Subcut.	10 min	12 min	Unknown
Intranasal	Rapid	1–2 hr	Unknown

Half-life: About 2 hours.

ADVERSE REACTIONS
CNS: *dizziness, vertigo,* drowsiness, headache, anxiety, malaise, fatigue.
CV: *atrial fibrillation, ventricular fibrillation, ventricular tachycardia, coronary artery vasospasm, transient myocardial ischemia, MI,* pressure or tightness in chest.
EENT: discomfort of throat, nasal cavity or sinus, mouth, jaw, or tongue, altered vision.
GI: abdominal discomfort, dysphagia, diarrhea, nausea, vomiting, unusual or bad taste (nasal spray).
Musculoskeletal: myalgia, muscle cramps, neck pain.
Respiratory: upper respiratory inflammation and dyspnea (P.O.).
Skin: *injection site reaction, tingling,* diaphoresis, flushing.
Other: *warm or hot sensation, burning sensation,* heaviness, pressure or tightness, tight feeling in head, cold sensation, numbness.

INTERACTIONS
Drug-drug. *Ergot and ergot derivatives, other 5-HT$_1$ agonists:* May prolong vaso-

spastic effects. Don't use within 24 hours of sumatriptan therapy.
MAO inhibitors: May reduce sumatriptan clearance. Avoid using within 2 weeks of MAO inhibitor. Use injection cautiously and decrease sumatriptan dose.
SSRIs: May cause weakness, hyper-reflexia, and incoordination. Monitor patient closely if use together can't be avoided.
Drug-herb. *Horehound:* May enhance serotonergic effects. Discourage use together.

EFFECTS ON LAB TEST RESULTS
● May increase liver enzyme levels.

CONTRAINDICATIONS & CAUTIONS
● Contraindicated in patients with hyper-sensitivity to drug or its components; those with history, symptoms, or signs of ischemic cardiac, cerebrovascular (such as stroke or transient ischemic attack), or peripheral vascular syndromes (such as ischemic bowel disease); significant underlying CV diseases, including angina pectoris, MI, and silent myocardial ischemia; uncontrolled hypertension; or severe hepatic impairment.
● Contraindicated within 24 hours of another 5-HT agonist or drug containing ergotamine and within 2 weeks of MAO inhibitor.
● Use cautiously in woman who is or may become pregnant.
● Use cautiously in patient with risk factors for coronary artery disease (CAD), such as postmenopausal women, men older than age 40, or patients with hypertension, hypercholesterolemia, obesity, diabetes, smoking, or family history of CAD.

NURSING CONSIDERATIONS
● *Alert:* When giving drug to patient at risk for CAD, give first dose in presence of other medical personnel. Rarely, serious adverse cardiac effects can follow admin-istration.
● *Alert:* Combining drug with an SSRI or an SSNRI may cause serotonin syndrome. Symptoms include restlessness, hallucina-tions, loss of coordination, fast heartbeat, rapid changes in blood pressure, increased body temperature, hyperreflexia, nausea,

vomiting, and diarrhea. Serotonin syn-drome may occur when starting or increasing the dose of drug, SSRI, or SSNRI.
● After subcutaneous injection, most patients experience relief in 1 to 2 hours.
● *Look alike–sound alike:* Don't confuse sumatriptan with somatropin.

PATIENT TEACHING
● Inform patient that drug is intended only to treat migraine attacks, not to prevent them or reduce their occurrence.
● If patient is pregnant or may become pregnant, tell her not to use drug but to discuss with prescriber the risks and bene-fits of using drug during pregnancy.
● Tell patient that drug may be taken any time during a migraine attack, as soon as signs or symptoms appear.
● Review information about drug's injectable form, which is available in a spring-loaded injector system for easier patient use. Make sure patient understands how to load the injector, give the injection, and dispose of used syringes.
● *Alert:* Tell patient to tell prescriber im-mediately about persistent or severe chest pain. Warn him to stop using drug and to call prescriber if he develops pain or tight-ness in the throat, wheezing, heart throb-bing, rash, lumps, hives, or swollen eye-lids, face, or lips.
● Teach patient to blow his nose before use. The patient should block other nostril while inhaling gently during administra-tion. He should keep his head upright and breathe gently for 10 to 20 seconds after dose is given.

zolmitriptan
zohl-mah-TRIP-tan

Zomig, Zomig ZMT

Pharmacologic class: serotonin 5-HT$_1$ receptor agonist
Pregnancy risk category C

AVAILABLE FORMS
Nasal spray: 5 mg
Tablets (immediate-release): 2.5 mg, 5 mg
Tablets (oral disintegrating): 2.5 mg, 5 mg

INDICATIONS & DOSAGES
➤ **Acute migraine headaches**
Adults: Initially, 2.5 mg or less P.O. Break a 2.5-mg immediate-release tablet in half if a lower dose is needed. Increase to 5 mg per dosage, as needed. If using orally disintegrating tablets (ODTs), initially, 2.5 mg P.O. Or, 1 spray (5 mg) into nostril. If headache returns after first dose, give a second dose at least 2 hours after the first dose. Maximum dosage is 10 mg in 24 hours.
Adjust-a-dose: In patients with hepatic disease, use doses less than 2.5 mg. Don't use ODTs because they shouldn't be broken in half, or nasal spray because 5 mg is the lowest deliverable dose.

ADMINISTRATION
P.O.
● Give ODT immediately after opening.
● Don't break or crush ODT.
● ODT dissolves on tongue and is swallowed with saliva; fluid isn't needed.
Intranasal
● Don't test the spray before use.

ACTION
May act as an agonist at serotonin receptors on extracerebral intracranial blood vessels, which constricts the affected vessels, inhibits neuropeptide release, and reduces pain transmission in the trigeminal pathways.

Route	Onset	Peak	Duration
P.O.	Unknown	2 hr	3 hr
Intranasal	5 min	3 hr	Unknown

Half-life: 3 hours.

ADVERSE REACTIONS
CNS: *dizziness,* somnolence, vertigo, hypesthesia, paresthesia, asthenia, pain.
CV: *coronary artery vasospasm, transient myocardial ischemia, MI, ventricular tachycardia, ventricular fibrillation,* palpitations, pain, tightness, pressure, or heaviness in chest.
EENT: *pain, tightness, or pressure in the neck, throat, or jaw.*
GI: dry mouth, dyspepsia, dysphagia, nausea.
Musculoskeletal: myalgia, myasthenia.
Skin: sweating.
Other: warm or cold sensations.

INTERACTIONS
Drug-drug. *Cimetidine:* May double half-life of zolmitriptan. Monitor patient closely.
Ergot-containing drugs, other triptans: May cause additive effects. Avoid using within 24 hours of almotriptan.
Hormonal contraceptives, propranolol: May increase zolmitriptan level. Monitor patient closely.
MAO inhibitors: May increase zolmitriptan level. Avoid using within 2 weeks of MAO inhibitor.
SSRIs: May cause additive serotonin effects, resulting in weakness, hyperreflexia, or incoordination. Monitor patient closely if given together.

EFFECTS ON LAB TEST RESULTS
● May increase glucose levels.

CONTRAINDICATIONS & CAUTIONS
● Contraindicated in patients hypersensitive to drug or its components, pregnant or breast-feeding patients, and those with uncontrolled hypertension, hemiplegic or basilar migraine, ischemic heart disease (angina pectoris, history of MI or documented silent ischemia), symptoms of ischemic heart disease (coronary artery vasospasm, including Prinzmetal's variant angina), or other significant heart disease.
● Contraindicated within 24 hours of other triptans or drugs containing ergot or within 2 weeks of stopping MAO inhibitor.
● Use cautiously in patients with liver disease and in those who may be at risk for coronary artery disease (such as postmenopausal women or men older than age 40) or those with risk factors, such as hypertension, hypercholesterolemia, obesity, diabetes, smoking, or family history.

NURSING CONSIDERATIONS
● Drug isn't intended for preventing migraines or treating hemiplegic or basilar migraines.
● Safety of drug hasn't been established for cluster headaches.
● *Alert:* Combining drug with an SSRI or an SSNRI may cause serotonin syndrome. Signs and symptoms may include restlessness, hallucinations, loss of coordination, fast heartbeat, rapid changes in blood pressure, increased body temperature,

overactive reflexes, nausea, vomiting, and diarrhea. Serotonin syndrome may be more likely to occur when starting or increasing the dose of drug, SSRI, or SSNRI.

PATIENT TEACHING
• Tell patient that drug is intended to relieve, not prevent, signs and symptoms of migraine.
• Advise patient to take drug as prescribed and not to take a second dose unless instructed by prescriber. Tell patient if a second dose is indicated and permitted, he should take it 2 hours after first dose.
• Instruct patient to release the ODTs from the blister pack just before taking; tablet should dissolve on tongue.
• Advise patient not to break the ODTs in half.
• Advise patient to immediately report pain or tightness in the chest or throat, heart throbbing, rash, skin lumps, or swelling of the face, lips, or eyelids.
• Tell woman not to take drug if she is or may become pregnant.

Antiparkinsonians

amantadine hydrochloride
apomorphine hydrochloride
benztropine mesylate
bromocriptine mesylate
entacapone
levodopa and carbidopa
levodopa, carbidopa, and
   entacapone
pramipexole dihydrochloride
rasagiline mesylate
ropinirole hydrochloride
selegiline
selegiline hydrochloride
tolcapone

---

amantadine hydrochloride
a-MAN-ta-deen

Symmetrel

Pharmacologic class: synthetic
cyclic primary amine
Pregnancy risk category C

AVAILABLE FORMS
Capsules: 100 mg
Syrup: 50 mg/5 ml
Tablets: 100 mg

INDICATIONS & DOSAGES
➤ **Parkinson disease**
Adults: Initially, if used as monotherapy,
100 mg P.O. b.i.d. In patients with serious
illness or in those already receiving high
doses of other antiparkinsonians, begin
dose at 100 mg P.O. once daily. Increase
to 100 mg b.i.d. if needed after at least
1 week. Some patients may benefit from
400 mg daily in divided doses.
➤ **To prevent or treat symptoms of
influenza type A virus and respiratory tract illnesses**
*Children age 13 or older and adults up to
age 65:* 200 mg P.O. daily in a single dose
or 100 mg P.O. b.i.d.
Children ages 9 to 12: 100 mg P.O. b.i.d.
*Children ages 1 to 8 or who weigh less
than 45 kg (99 lb):* 4.4 to 8.8 mg/kg P.O.
as a total daily dose given once daily or

divided equally b.i.d. Maximum daily
dose is 150 mg.
Elderly patients: 100 mg P.O. once daily
in patients older than age 65 with normal
renal function.

  Begin treatment within 24 to 48 hours
after symptoms appear and continue for
24 to 48 hours after symptoms disappear
(usually 2 to 7 days). Start prophylaxis as
soon as possible after exposure and continue for at least 10 days after exposure.
May continue prophylactic treatment up to
90 days for repeated or suspected exposures if influenza vaccine is unavailable. If
used with influenza vaccine, continue dose
for 2 to 3 weeks until antibody response to
vaccine has developed.
Adjust-a-dose: For patients with creatinine clearance of 30 to 50 ml/minute,
200 mg the first day and 100 mg thereafter; if clearance is 15 to 29 ml/minute,
200 mg the first day and then 100 mg on
alternate days; if clearance is less than
15 ml/minute or if patient is receiving
hemodialysis, 200 mg every 7 days.
➤ **Drug-induced extrapyramidal
reactions**
Adults: 100 mg P.O. b.i.d. May increase to
300 mg daily in divided doses.

ADMINISTRATION
P.O.
● Give drug without regard for food.

ACTION
May exert its antiparkinsonian effect by
causing the release of dopamine in the
substantia nigra. As an antiviral, may prevent release of viral nucleic acid into the
host cell, reducing duration of fever and
other systemic symptoms.

Route	Onset	Peak	Duration
P.O.	Unknown	1–4 hr	Unknown

Half-life: About 24 hours; with renal dysfunction, as long as 10 days.

ADVERSE REACTIONS
CNS: *dizziness, insomnia, irritability,
light-headedness,* depression, fatigue,

---

confusion, hallucinations, anxiety, ataxia, headache.
CV: *heart failure,* peripheral edema, orthostatic hypotension.
EENT: blurred vision.
GI: *nausea,* anorexia, constipation, vomiting, dry mouth.
Skin: livedo reticularis.

INTERACTIONS
Drug-drug. *Anticholinergics:* May increase anticholinergic effects. Use together cautiously; reduce dosage of anticholinergic before starting amantadine.
CNS stimulants: May increase CNS stimulation. Use together cautiously.
Co-trimoxazole, quinidine, thiazide diuretics, triamterene: May increase amantadine level, increasing the risk of toxicity. Use together cautiously.
Thioridazine: May worsen Parkinson disease tremor. Monitor patient closely.
Drug-herb. *Jimsonweed:* May adversely affect CV function. Discourage use together.
Drug-lifestyle. *Alcohol use:* May increase CNS effects, including dizziness, confusion, and orthostatic hypotension. Discourage use together.

EFFECTS ON LAB TEST RESULTS
● May increase CK, BUN, creatinine, alkaline phosphatase, LDH, bilirubin, GGT, AST, and ALT levels.

CONTRAINDICATIONS & CAUTIONS
● Contraindicated in patients hypersensitive to drug.
● Use cautiously in elderly patients and in patients with seizure disorders, heart failure, peripheral edema, hepatic disease, mental illness, eczematoid rash, renal impairment, orthostatic hypotension, and CV disease. Monitor renal and liver function tests.

NURSING CONSIDERATIONS
● Patients with Parkinson disease who don't respond to anticholinergics may respond to this drug.
● Begin treatment for influenza within 24 to 48 hours after symptoms appear and continue for 24 to 48 hours after symptoms disappear (usually 2 to 7 days of therapy).
● Start influenza prophylaxis as soon as possible after first exposure and continue

for at least 10 days after exposure. For repeated or suspected exposures, if influenza vaccine is unavailable, may continue prophylaxis for up to 90 days. If used with influenza vaccine, continue dose for 2 to 3 weeks until antibody response to vaccine has developed.
● *Alert:* Elderly patients are more susceptible to adverse neurologic effects. Monitor patient for mental status changes.
● Suicidal ideation and attempts may occur in any patient, regardless of psychiatric history.
● Drug can worsen mental problems in patients with a history of psychiatric disorders or substance abuse.
● *Look alike–sound alike:* Don't confuse amantadine with rimantadine.

PATIENT TEACHING
● *Alert:* Tell patient to take drug exactly as prescribed because not doing so may result in serious adverse reactions or death.
● If insomnia occurs, tell patient to take drug several hours before bedtime.
● If patient gets dizzy when he stands up, instruct him not to stand or change positions too quickly.
● Instruct patient to notify prescriber of adverse reactions, especially dizziness, depression, anxiety, nausea, and urine retention.
● Caution patient to avoid activities that require mental alertness until effects of drug are known.
● Encourage patient with Parkinson disease to gradually increase his physical activity as his symptoms improve.
● Advise patient to avoid alcohol while taking drug.

apomorphine hydrochloride
ah-poe-MORE-feen

Apokyn

Pharmacologic class: nonergot-derivative dopamine agonist
Pregnancy risk category C

AVAILABLE FORMS
Solution for injection: 10 mg/ml (contains benzyl alcohol)

INDICATIONS & DOSAGES

➤ **Intermittent hypomobility, "off" episodes caused by advanced Parkinson disease (given with an antiemetic)**

Adults: Initially, give a 0.2-ml subcutaneous test dose. Measure supine and standing blood pressure every 20 minutes for the first hour. If patient tolerates and responds to drug, start with 0.2 ml subcutaneously as needed as outpatient. Separate doses by at least 2 hours. Increase by 0.1 ml every few days, as needed.

If initial 0.2-ml dose is ineffective but tolerated, give 0.4 ml at next "off" period, measuring supine and standing blood pressure every 20 minutes for the first hour. If drug is tolerated, start with 0.3 ml subcutaneously as outpatient. If needed, increase by 0.1 ml every few days.

If patient doesn't tolerate 0.4-ml dose, give 0.3 ml as a test dose at the next "off" period, measuring supine and standing blood pressure every 20 minutes for the first hour. If drug is tolerated, give 0.2 ml as outpatient. Increase by 0.1 ml every few days, as needed; doses higher than 0.4 ml usually aren't tolerated if 0.2 ml is the starting dose.

Maximum recommended dose is usually 0.6 ml as needed. Most patients use drug t.i.d. Experience is limited at more than five times daily or more than 2 ml daily.

Adjust-a-dose: In patients with mild to moderate renal impairment, give test and starting doses of 0.1 ml subcutaneously.

ADMINISTRATION

Subcutaneous

● Give with an antiemetic to avoid severe nausea and vomiting. Start with trimethobenzamide 300 mg P.O. t.i.d. 3 days before starting apomorphine, and continue antiemetic at least 2 months.

● When programming the dosing pen, it's possible to select the appropriate dose even though insufficient drug remains in the pen. To avoid insufficient dosing, track the amount of drug received at each dose and change the cartridge before drug runs out.

● Rotate injection sites and record.

● *Alert:* Drug is for subcutaneous injection only. Avoid I.V. use.

ACTION

Thought to improve motor function by stimulating dopamine D2 receptors in the brain.

Route	Onset	Peak	Duration
Subcut.	20 min	10–60 min	2 hr

Half-life: About 30 to 60 minutes in patients with normal or impaired renal function.

ADVERSE REACTIONS

CNS: *confusion, dizziness, drowsiness, hallucinations, somnolence,* aggravated Parkinson disease, anxiety, depression, fatigue, headache, insomnia, syncope, weakness.

CV: *angina, chest pain, chest pressure, edema, hypotension, orthostatic hypotension,* **cardiac arrest, heart failure, MI,** flushing.

EENT: *rhinorrhea.*

GI: *nausea, vomiting,* constipation, diarrhea.

GU: UTI.

Respiratory: dyspnea, pneumonia.

Metabolic: dehydration.

Musculoskeletal: *dyskinesias,* arthralgia, back pain, limb pain.

Skin: bruising, injection site reaction, pallor, sweating.

Other: *falls, yawning.*

INTERACTIONS

Drug-drug. *Antihypertensives, vasodilators:* May increase risk of hypotension, MI, pneumonia, falls, and joint injury. Use together cautiously.

Dopamine antagonists, metoclopramide: May reduce apomorphine's effectiveness. Use together cautiously.

Drugs that prolong the QTc interval: May further prolong the QTc interval. Use together cautiously.

5-HT$_3$ antagonists (alosetron, dolasetron, granisetron, ondansetron, palonosetron): May cause serious hypotension and loss of consciousness. Don't use together.

Drug-lifestyle. *Alcohol use:* May increase risk of sedation and hypotension. Discourage use together.

EFFECTS ON LAB TEST RESULTS

None reported.

Reactions may be *common,* uncommon, *life-threatening,* or COMMON AND LIFE-THREATENING.
Interaction may have a *rapid onset* or *delayed onset.*

CONTRAINDICATIONS & CAUTIONS
• Contraindicated in patients allergic to apomorphine or its ingredients, including sulfites, and in patients who take 5-HT₃ antagonists.
• Use cautiously in patients at risk for prolonged QTc interval, such as those with hypokalemia, hypomagnesemia, bradycardia, or genetic predisposition.
• Use cautiously in patients with CV or cerebrovascular disease and in those with renal or hepatic impairment.

NURSING CONSIDERATIONS
• *Alert:* The prescribed dose should always be specified in milliliters rather than milligrams to avoid confusion; the dosing pen is marked in milliliters.
• Give test dose in a medically supervised setting to determine tolerability and effect.
• Monitor supine and standing blood pressure every 20 minutes for the first hour after starting doses or dosage changes.
• *Alert:* Monitor patient for drowsiness or sleepiness, which may occur well after treatment starts. Stop drug if patient develops significant daytime sleepiness that interferes with activities of daily living.
• Watch for evidence of coronary or cerebral ischemia, and stop drug if it occurs.
• Adverse effects are more likely in elderly patients, particularly hallucinations, falls, CV events, respiratory problems, and GI effects.

PATIENT TEACHING
• Tell patient to avoid sudden position changes, especially rising too quickly from lying down. A sudden drop in blood pressure, dizziness, or fainting can occur.
• Urge patient to keep taking the prescribed antiemetic because nausea and vomiting are likely.
• Instruct patient or caregiver to document each dose to make sure enough drug remains in the cartridge to provide a full next dose.
• Tell patient or caregiver to wait at least 2 hours between doses.
• *Alert:* Show patient or caregiver how to read the dosing pen, and make sure he understands that it's marked in milliliters and not milligrams.

• Tell patient or caregiver to rotate injection sites and to wash hands before each injection. Applying ice to the site before and after the injection may reduce soreness, redness, pain, itching, swelling, or bruising at the site.
• Explain that hallucinations (either visual or auditory) may occur, and urge patient or caregiver to report them immediately.
• Explain that headaches may occur and tell patient to notify prescriber if they become severe or don't go away.
• Advise patient to avoid hazardous activities that require alertness until drug effects are known.
• Caution patient to avoid consuming alcohol.

benztropine mesylate
BENZ-troe-peen

Cogentin

Pharmacologic class:
anticholinergic
Pregnancy risk category C

AVAILABLE FORMS
Injection: 1 mg/ml in 2-ml ampules
Tablets: 0.5 mg, 1 mg, 2 mg

INDICATIONS & DOSAGES
➤ **Drug-induced extrapyramidal disorders (except tardive dyskinesia)**
Adults: 1 to 4 mg P.O. or I.M. once or twice daily.
➤ **Acute dystonic reaction**
Adults: 1 to 2 mg I.V. or I.M.; then 1 to 2 mg P.O. b.i.d. to prevent recurrence.
➤ **Parkinsonism**
Adults: 0.5 to 6 mg P.O. or I.M. daily. First dosage is 0.5 mg to 1 mg, increased by 0.5 mg every 5 to 6 days. Adjust dosage to meet individual requirements. Maximum, 6 mg daily.

ADMINISTRATION
P.O.
• Drug may be given before or after meals depending on patient reaction. If patient is prone to excessive salivation, give drug after meal. If his mouth dries excessively, give drug before meals unless it causes nausea.

I.V.
- Reserve I.V. delivery for emergencies, such as acute dystonic reactions.
- The I.V. form is seldom used because no significant difference exists between it and the I.M. form.
- **Incompatibilities:** Haloperidol lactate.

I.M.
- Use filtered needle to draw up solution from ampule.

ACTION
Unknown. May block central cholinergic receptors, helping to balance cholinergic activity in the basal ganglia.

Route	Onset	Peak	Duration
P.O.	1–2 hr	Unknown	24 hr
I.V., I.M.	15 min	Unknown	24 hr

Half-life: Unknown.

ADVERSE REACTIONS
CNS: confusion, memory impairment, nervousness, depression, disorientation, hallucinations, toxic psychosis.
CV: tachycardia.
EENT: dilated pupils, blurred vision.
GI: *dry mouth, constipation,* nausea, vomiting, paralytic ileus.
GU: urine retention, dysuria.
Skin: decreased sweating.

INTERACTIONS
Drug-drug. *Amantadine, pheno-thiazines, tricyclic antidepressants:* May cause additive anticholinergic adverse reactions, such as confusion and hallucinations. Reduce dosage before giving.
Cholinergics (donepezil, galantamine, rivastigmine, tacrine): May antagonize the therapeutic effects of these drugs. If used together, monitor patient for therapeutic effect.

EFFECTS ON LAB TEST RESULTS
None reported.

CONTRAINDICATIONS & CAUTIONS
- Contraindicated in patients hypersensitive to drug or its components, in those with angle-closure glaucoma, and in children younger than age 3.

- Use cautiously in hot weather, in patients with mental disorders, in elderly patients, and in children age 3 and older.
- Use cautiously in patients with prostatic hyperplasia, arrhythmias, or seizure disorders.

NURSING CONSIDERATIONS
- Monitor vital signs carefully. Watch closely for adverse reactions, especially in elderly or debilitated patients. Call prescriber promptly if adverse reactions occur.
- At certain doses, drug produces atropine-like toxicity, which may aggravate tardive dyskinesia.
- Watch for intermittent constipation and abdominal distention and pain, which may indicate onset of paralytic ileus.
- Monitor elderly patients closely as they are more prone to severe adverse effects.
- *Alert:* Never stop drug abruptly. Reduce dosage gradually.
- *Look alike–sound alike:* Don't confuse benztropine with bromocriptine.

PATIENT TEACHING
- Warn patient to avoid activities that require alertness until CNS effects of drug are known.
- If patient takes a single daily dose, tell him to do so at bedtime.
- Advise patient to report signs and symptoms of urinary hesitancy or urine retention.
- Tell patient to relieve dry mouth with cool drinks, ice chips, sugarless gum, or hard candy.
- Advise patient to limit hot weather activities because drug-induced lack of sweating may cause overheating.

---

bromocriptine mesylate
broe-moe-KRIP-teen

Parlodel

Pharmacologic class: dopamine receptor agonist
Pregnancy risk category B

AVAILABLE FORMS
Capsules: 5 mg
Tablets: 2.5 mg

Reactions may be *common,* uncommon, *life-threatening,* or COMMON AND LIFE-THREATENING.
Interaction may have a *rapid onset* or *delayed onset.*

INDICATIONS & DOSAGES
➤ **Parkinson disease**
Adults: 1.25 mg P.O. b.i.d. with meals. Increase dosage by 2.5 mg/day every 14 to 28 days, up to 100 mg daily.
➤ **Amenorrhea and galactorrhea from hyperprolactinemia; hypogonadism, infertility**
Adults: 0.5 to 2.5 mg P.O. daily, increased by 2.5 mg daily at 3- to 7-day intervals until desired effect occurs. Therapeutic daily dose is 2.5 to 15 mg.
➤ **Acromegaly**
Adults: 1.25 to 2.5 mg P.O. with bedtime snack for 3 days. Another 1.25 to 2.5 mg may be added every 3 to 7 days until therapeutic benefit occurs. Maximum, 100 mg daily.
➤ **Neuroleptic malignant syndrome ◆**
Adults: 2.5 to 5 mg P.O. two to six times daily.

ADMINISTRATION
P.O.
● Give drug in the evening with food to minimize adverse reactions.

ACTION
Inhibits secretion of prolactin and acts as a dopamine-receptor agonist by activating postsynaptic dopamine receptors.

Route	Onset	Peak	Duration
P.O.	2 hr	8 hr	24 hr

Half-life: 15 hours.

ADVERSE REACTIONS
CNS: *dizziness, headache, fatigue,* **seizures, stroke,** mania, light-headedness, drowsiness, delusions, nervousness, insomnia, depression.
CV: *hypotension,* **acute MI.**
EENT: nasal congestion, blurred vision.
GI: *nausea, abdominal cramps, constipation,* diarrhea, vomiting, anorexia.
GU: urine retention, urinary frequency.
Skin: coolness and pallor of fingers and toes.

INTERACTIONS
Drug-drug. *Amitriptyline, haloperidol, imipramine, loxapine, MAO inhibitors, methyldopa, metoclopramide, pheno-*

thiazines, reserpine: May interfere with bromocriptine's effects. Bromocriptine dosage may need to be increased.
Antihypertensives: May increase hypotensive effects. Adjust dosage of antihypertensive.
Erythromycin: May increase bromocriptine level and risk of adverse reactions. Use together cautiously.
Estrogens, hormonal contraceptives, progestins: May interfere with effects of bromocriptine. Avoid using together.
Levodopa: May have additive effects. Adjust dosage of levodopa, if needed.
Drug-lifestyle. *Alcohol use:* May cause disulfiram-like reaction. Discourage use together.

EFFECTS ON LAB TEST RESULTS
● May increase alkaline phosphatase, ALT, AST, BUN, CK, and uric acid levels.

CONTRAINDICATIONS & CAUTIONS
● Contraindicated in patients hypersensitive to ergot derivatives and in those with uncontrolled hypertension, toxemia of pregnancy, severe ischemic heart disease, or peripheral vascular disease.
● Use cautiously in patients with impaired renal or hepatic function and in those with a history of MI with residual arrhythmias.

NURSING CONSIDERATIONS
● For Parkinson disease, bromocriptine usually is given with levodopa or levodopa and carbidopa. The levodopa and carbidopa may need to be reduced.
● *Alert:* Monitor patient for adverse reactions, which occur in 68% of patients, particularly at start of therapy. Most reactions are mild to moderate; nausea is most common. Minimize adverse reactions by gradually adjusting dosages to effective levels. Adverse reactions are more common when drug is used for Parkinson disease.
● Baseline and periodic evaluations of cardiac, hepatic, renal, and hematopoietic function are recommended during prolonged therapy.
● Drug may lead to early postpartum conception. After menses resumes, test for pregnancy every 4 weeks or as soon as a period is missed.

● **Look alike–sound alike:** Don't confuse bromocriptine with benztropine or brimonidine, or Parlodel with pindolol.

PATIENT TEACHING
● Instruct patient to take drug with meals.
● Advise patient to use contraceptive methods during treatment other than oral contraceptives or subdermal implants.
● Instruct patient to avoid dizziness and fainting by rising slowly to an upright position and avoiding sudden position changes.
● Inform patient that it may take 8 weeks or longer for menses to resume and excess production of milk to slow down.
● Advise patient to avoid alcohol while taking drug.

entacapone
en-tah-KAP-own

Comtan

Pharmacologic class: catechol-O-methyltransferase (COMT) inhibitor
Pregnancy risk category C

AVAILABLE FORMS
Tablets: 200 mg

INDICATIONS & DOSAGES
➤ **Adjunct to levodopa and carbidopa for treatment of idiopathic Parkinson disease in patients with signs and symptoms of end-of-dose wearing off**
Adults: 200 mg P.O. with each dose of levodopa and carbidopa, up to eight times daily. Maximum, 1,600 mg daily. May need to reduce daily levodopa dose or extend the interval between doses to optimize patient's response.

ADMINISTRATION
P.O.
● Give drug with immediate- or sustained-release levodopa and carbidopa.
● Give drug without regard for food.

ACTION
A reversible COMT inhibitor given with levodopa and carbidopa. The combination is thought to cause higher levels of levodopa and optimal control of parkinsonian symptoms.

Route	Onset	Peak	Duration
P.O.	1 hr	1 hr	6 hr

Half-life: About ½ to ¾ hour for first phase and about 2½ hours for second phase.

ADVERSE REACTIONS
CNS: *dyskinesia, hyperkinesia,* hypokinesia, dizziness, anxiety, somnolence, agitation, fatigue, asthenia, hallucinations.
GI: *nausea, diarrhea,* abdominal pain, constipation, vomiting, dry mouth, dyspepsia, flatulence, gastritis, taste perversion.
GU: *urine discoloration.*
Hematologic: purpura.
Musculoskeletal: back pain.
Respiratory: dyspnea.
Skin: sweating.
Other: bacterial infection.

INTERACTIONS
Drug-drug. *Ampicillin, chloramphenicol, cholestyramine, erythromycin, probenecid:* May block biliary excretion, resulting in higher levels of entacapone. Use together cautiously.
CNS depressants: May cause additive effect. Use together cautiously.
Drugs metabolized by COMT (dobutamine, dopamine, epinephrine, isoetharine, isoproterenol, norepinephrine): May cause higher levels of these drugs, resulting in increased heart rate, changes in blood pressure, or arrhythmias. Use together cautiously.
Nonselective MAO inhibitors (such as phenelzine, tranylcypromine): May inhibit normal catecholamine metabolism. Avoid using together.
Drug-lifestyle. *Alcohol use:* May cause additive CNS effects. Discourage use together.

EFFECTS ON LAB TEST RESULTS
None reported.

CONTRAINDICATIONS & CAUTIONS
● Contraindicated in patients hypersensitive to drug.
● Use cautiously in patients with hepatic impairment, biliary obstruction, or orthostatic hypotension.

Reactions may be *common,* uncommon, *life-threatening,* or COMMON AND LIFE-THREATENING.
Interaction may have a *rapid onset* or **delayed onset.**

NURSING CONSIDERATIONS

- Use drug only with levodopa and car-bidopa; no antiparkinsonian effects occur when drug is given as monotherapy.
- Levodopa and carbidopa dosage requirements are usually lower when drug is given with entacapone; lower levodopa and carbidopa dose or increase dosing interval to avoid adverse effects.
- Drug may cause or worsen dyskinesia, even if levodopa dose is lowered.
- Hallucinations may occur or worsen during therapy with this drug.
- Monitor blood pressure closely, and watch for orthostatic hypotension.
- Diarrhea most often begins within 4 to 12 weeks of starting therapy but may begin as early as 1 week or as late as many months after starting treatment.
- Drug may discolor urine.
- Rarely, rhabdomyolysis has occurred with drug use.
- Rapid withdrawal or abrupt reduction in dose could lead to signs and symptoms of Parkinson disease; it may also lead to hyperpyrexia and confusion, a group of symptoms resembling neuroleptic malig-nant syndrome. Stop drug gradually, and monitor patient closely. Adjust other dopaminergic treatments, as needed.

PATIENT TEACHING

- Instruct patient not to crush or break tablet and to take it at same time as levo-dopa and carbidopa.
- Warn patient to avoid hazardous activi-ties until CNS effects of drug are known.
- Advise patient to avoid alcohol during treatment.
- Instruct patient to use caution when standing after a prolonged period of sit-ting or lying down because dizziness may occur. This effect is more common during initial therapy.
- Warn patient that hallucinations, increased difficulty with voluntary movements, nausea, and diarrhea could occur.
- Inform patient that drug may turn urine brownish orange.
- Advise patient to notify prescriber about planned, suspected, or known pregnancy, and to notify prescriber if she's breast-feeding.

levodopa and carbidopa
lee-voe-DOE-pa and kar-bih-DOE-pa

Parcopa, Sinemet✔,
Sinemet CR✔

Pharmacologic class:
decarboxylase inhibitor and
dopamine precursor
Pregnancy risk category C

AVAILABLE FORMS

Tablets: 100 mg levodopa with 10 mg car-bidopa (Sinemet 10–100), 100 mg levo-dopa with 25 mg carbidopa (Sinemet 25–100), 250 mg levodopa with 25 mg carbidopa (Sinemet 25–250)
Tablets (extended-release): 200 mg levo-dopa with 50 mg carbidopa (Sinemet CR), 100 mg levodopa with 25 mg carbidopa
Tablets (orally disintegrating): 100 mg levodopa with 10 mg carbidopa, 100 mg levodopa with 25 mg carbidopa, 250 mg levodopa with 25 mg carbidopa

INDICATIONS & DOSAGES

➤ **Idiopathic Parkinson disease, postencephalitic parkinsonism, and symptomatic parkinsonism resulting from carbon monoxide or man-ganese intoxication**
Adults: 1 tablet of 100 mg levodopa with 25 mg carbidopa P.O. t.i.d.; then increased by 1 tablet daily or every other day, as needed, to maximum daily dose of 8 tablets. May use 250 mg levodopa with 25 mg carbidopa or 100 mg levodopa with 10 mg carbidopa tablets, as directed, to obtain maximal response. Optimum daily dose must be determined by careful adjustment for each patient.

Patients given conventional tablets may receive extended-release tablets; dosage is calculated on current levodopa intake. Extended-release tablets should provide 10% more levodopa daily, increased as needed and as tolerated to 30% more levo-dopa daily. Give in divided doses at inter-vals of 4 to 8 hours.

ADMINISTRATION
P.O.
- Give drug with food to decrease GI upset, but avoid giving with high-protein

meals, which can impair absorption and reduce effectiveness.
● Don't crush or break extended-release form.
● Give orally disintegrating tablet (ODT) immediately after removing from bottle. Place tablet on patient's tongue, where it will dissolve in seconds and be swallowed with saliva. No additional fluid is needed.

ACTION
Levodopa, a dopamine precursor, relieves parkinsonian symptoms by being converted to dopamine in the brain. Carbidopa inhibits the decarboxylation of peripheral levodopa, which allows more intact levodopa to travel to the brain.

Route	Onset	Peak	Duration
P.O.	Unknown	40–150 min	Unknown

Half-life: 1 to 2 hours.

ADVERSE REACTIONS
CNS: *choreiform, dystonic, dyskinetic movements, involuntary grimacing, head movements, myoclonic body jerks, ataxia,* **suicidal tendencies,** tremor, muscle twitching, bradykinetic episodes, psychiatric disturbances, anxiety, disturbing dreams, euphoria, malaise, fatigue, severe depression, dementia, delirium, hallucinations, confusion, insomnia, agitation.
CV: *orthostatic hypotension,* cardiac irregularities, phlebitis.
EENT: blepharospasm, blurred vision, diplopia, mydriasis or miosis, oculogyric crises, excessive salivation.
GI: *dry mouth, nausea, vomiting, anorexia,* bitter taste, constipation, flatulence, diarrhea, abdominal pain.
GU: urinary frequency, urine retention, urinary incontinence, darkened urine, priapism.
Hematologic: ***thrombocytopenia, leukopenia, agranulocytosis,*** hemolytic anemia.
Hepatic: *hepatotoxicity.*
Metabolic: weight loss.
Respiratory: hiccups, hyperventilation.
Skin: dark perspiration.

INTERACTIONS
Drug-drug. *Antihypertensives:* May cause additive hypotensive effects. Use together cautiously.

Iron salts: May reduce bioavailability of levodopa and carbidopa. Give iron 1 hour before or 2 hours after Sinemet.
MAO inhibitors: May cause risk of severe hypertension. Avoid using together.
Papaverine, phenytoin: May antagonize antiparkinsonian actions. Avoid using together.
Phenothiazines, other antipsychotics: May antagonize antiparkinsonian actions. Use together cautiously.
Drug-herb. *Kava:* May decrease action of drug. Discourage kava use altogether.
Octacosanol: May worsen dyskinesias. Discourage use together.
Drug-food. *Foods high in protein:* May decrease levodopa absorption. Don't give levodopa with high-protein foods.

EFFECTS ON LAB TEST RESULTS
● May increase uric acid, ALT, AST, alkaline phosphatase, LDH, and bilirubin levels. May decrease hemoglobin level and hematocrit.
● May decrease WBC, granulocyte, and platelet counts.
● May falsely increase urinary catecholamine level and serum and urinary uric acid levels in colorimetric tests. May falsely decrease urinary vanillylmandelic acid level. May cause false-positive results in urine ketone tests using sodium nitroprusside reagent and in urinary glucose tests using cupric sulfate reagent. May cause false-negative results in tests using glucose oxidase. May alter results of urine screening tests for phenylketonuria.

CONTRAINDICATIONS & CAUTIONS
● Contraindicated in patients hypersensitive to drug and in those with angle-closure glaucoma, melanoma, or undiagnosed skin lesions.
● Contraindicated within 14 days of MAO inhibitor therapy.
● Use cautiously in patients with severe CV, renal, hepatic, endocrine, or pulmonary disorders; history of peptic ulcer; psychiatric illness; MI with residual arrhythmias; bronchial asthma; emphysema; or well-controlled, chronic open-angle glaucoma.

NURSING CONSIDERATIONS
• If patient takes levodopa, stop drug at least 8 hours before starting levodopa-carbidopa.
• Giving levodopa and carbidopa together typically decreases amount of levodopa needed by 75%, reducing risk of adverse reactions.
• Therapeutic and adverse reactions occur more rapidly with levodopa and carbidopa than with levodopa alone. Observe patient and monitor vital signs, especially while adjusting dosage. Report significant changes.
• *Alert:* Because of risk of precipitating a symptom complex resembling neuroleptic malignant syndrome, observe patient closely if levodopa dosage is reduced abruptly or stopped.
• Hallucinations may require reduction or withdrawal of drug.
• *Alert:* Muscle twitching and blepharospasm may be early signs of drug overdose; report immediately.
• Test patients receiving long-term therapy regularly for diabetes and acromegaly, and periodically for hepatic, renal, and hematopoietic function.

PATIENT TEACHING
• Tell patient to take drug with food to minimize GI upset; however, high-protein meals can impair absorption and reduce effectiveness.
• Tell patient not to chew or crush extended-release form.
• Warn patient and caregivers not to increase dosage without prescriber's orders.
• Caution patient about possible dizziness when standing up quickly, especially at start of therapy. Tell him to change positions slowly and dangle his legs before getting out of bed. Elastic stockings may control these adverse reactions in some patients.
• Instruct patient to report adverse reactions and therapeutic effects.
• Inform patient that pyridoxine (vitamin B₆) doesn't reverse beneficial effects of levodopa and carbidopa. Multivitamins can be taken without reversing levodopa's effects.
• Teach patient to take ODT immediately after taking from bottle and to place on

top of tongue. Tablet will dissolve in seconds and will be swallowed with saliva. No additional fluid is needed.

---

levodopa, carbidopa, and entacapone
lee-voe-DOE-pa, kar-bih-DOE-pa, and en-ta-KAP-own

Stalevo♪

Pharmacologic class: dopamine precursor, decarboxylase inhibitor, and catecholamine-*O*-methyltransferase (COMT) inhibitor
Pregnancy risk category C

AVAILABLE FORMS
Tablets (film-coated): 50 mg levodopa, 12.5 mg carbidopa, 200 mg entacapone; 75 mg levodopa, 18.75 mg carbidopa, 200 mg entacapone; 100 mg levodopa, 25 mg carbidopa, 200 mg entacapone; 125 mg levodopa, 31.25 mg carbidopa, 200 mg entacapone; 150 mg levodopa, 37.5 mg carbidopa, 200 mg entacapone; 200 mg levodopa, 50 mg carbidopa, 200 mg entacapone

INDICATIONS & DOSAGES
➤ **Idiopathic Parkinson disease, to replace (with equivalent strengths) levodopa, carbidopa, and entacapone given individually or to replace immediate-release levodopa and carbidopa for a patient who has end-of-dose "wearing off," who's taking a total daily levodopa dose of 600 mg or less and who has no dyskinesia**
Adults: 1 tablet P.O.; determine dose and interval by therapeutic response. Maximum, 8 tablets daily.

ADMINISTRATION
P.O.
• Don't cut tablets.
• Give only 1 tablet at each dosing interval.
• Give drug with food to decrease GI upset, but avoid giving with high-protein meal, which can decrease absorption.

ACTION
Levodopa, a dopamine precursor, relieves parkinsonian symptoms by converting to dopamine in the brain. Carbidopa inhibits the decarboxylation of peripheral levodopa, which allows more intact levodopa to travel to the brain. Entacapone is a reversible COMT inhibitor that increases levodopa level.

Route	Onset	Peak	Duration
P.O.	Unknown	1½ hr	Unknown

Half-life: 1½ to 2 hours carbidopa, 1 to 5 hours levodopa, and 1 to 4 hours entacapone.

ADVERSE REACTIONS
levodopa and carbidopa
CNS: *neuroleptic malignant syndrome,* agitation, asthenia, confusion, delusions, dementia, depression, dizziness, dyskinesia, hallucinations, headache, increased libido, insomnia, nightmares, paranoid ideation, paresthesias, psychosis, somnolence, syncope.
CV: cardiac irregularities, chest pain, hypertension, hypotension, orthostatic hypotension, palpitations, phlebitis.
GI: anorexia, constipation, dark saliva, diarrhea, dry mouth, duodenal ulcer, dyspepsia, *GI bleeding,* nausea, taste alterations, vomiting.
GU: dark urine, urinary frequency, UTI.
Hematologic: *agranulocytosis, leukopenia, thrombocytopenia,* anemia.
Musculoskeletal: back pain, muscle cramps, shoulder pain.
Respiratory: dyspnea, upper respiratory infection.
Skin: alopecia, bullous lesions, dark sweat, Henoch-Schönlein purpura, increased sweating, pruritus, rash, urticaria.
Other: *angioedema.*
entacapone
CNS: *dyskinesia, hyperkinesia,* agitation, anxiety, asthenia, dizziness, fatigue, hypokinesia, somnolence.
GI: *diarrhea, nausea,* abdominal pain, constipation, dry mouth, dyspepsia, flatulence, gastritis, taste perversion, vomiting.
GU: *urine discoloration.*
Musculoskeletal: back pain.
Respiratory: dyspnea.
Skin: increased sweating, purpura.
Other: bacterial infection.

INTERACTIONS
Drug-drug. *Ampicillin, chloramphenicol, cholestyramine, erythromycin, probenecid, rifampicin:* May interfere with entacapone excretion. Use together cautiously.
Antihypertensives: May cause orthostatic hypotension. Adjust antihypertensive dosage as needed.
CNS depressants: Additive effects. Use together cautiously.
Dopamine (D2) receptor antagonists such as butyrophenones, iron salts, isoniazid, metoclopramide, phenothiazines, phenytoin, risperidone: May decrease levodopa, carbidopa, and entacapone effects. Monitor patient for effectiveness.
Drugs metabolized by COMT, such as alpha-methyldopa, apomorphine, dobutamine, dopamine, epinephrine, isoproterenol, isoetharine, norepinephrine: May increase heart rate, arrhythmias, and excessive blood pressure changes. Use together cautiously.
Metoclopramide: May increase availability of levodopa and carbidopa by increasing gastric emptying. Monitor patient for adverse effects.
Nonselective MAO inhibitor: May disrupt catecholamine metabolism. Avoid using together.
Selegiline: May cause severe hypotension. Use together cautiously, and monitor blood pressure.
Tricyclic antidepressants: May increase risk of hypertension and dyskinesia. Monitor patient closely.

EFFECTS ON LAB TEST RESULTS
● May increase alkaline phosphatase, AST, ALT, LDH, glucose, BUN, and bilirubin levels. May decrease hemoglobin level and hematocrit.
● May decrease platelet and WBC counts.
● May cause false-positive reaction for urinary ketone bodies on a test tape. May cause false-negative result for glucosuria with glucose oxidase testing methods.

CONTRAINDICATIONS & CAUTIONS
● Contraindicated in patients hypersensitive to drug or its ingredients.
● Contraindicated in patients with angle-closure glaucoma, suspicious undiagnosed skin lesions, or a history of melanoma.

Reactions may be *common,* uncommon, *life-threatening,* or **COMMON AND LIFE-THREATENING.**
Interaction may have a *rapid onset* or *delayed onset.*

- Contraindicated within 2 weeks of MAO inhibitor therapy.
- Use cautiously in patients with past or current psychosis and in patients with severe CV or pulmonary disease; bronchial asthma; biliary obstruction; or renal, hepatic, or endocrine disease.
- Use cautiously in patients with chronic open-angle glaucoma or a history of MI and residual atrial, nodal, or ventricular arrhythmias.

NURSING CONSIDERATIONS
- Certain CNS effects, such as dyskinesia, may occur at lower dosages and sooner with levodopa, carbidopa, and entacapone than with levodopa alone. Dyskinesia may require a reduced dosage.
- During the first adjustment period, monitor patient with CV disease carefully and in a facility equipped to provide intensive cardiac care.
- Neuroleptic malignant syndrome may develop when levodopa and carbidopa are reduced or stopped, especially in patients taking antipsychotic drugs. Watch patient carefully for fever, hyperthermia, muscle rigidity, involuntary movements, altered consciousness, mental status changes, and autonomic dysfunction.
- During extended therapy, periodically monitor hepatic, hematopoietic, CV, and renal function.
- Diarrhea is common; it usually develops 4 to 12 weeks after treatment starts but may appear as early as the first week or as late as many months after treatment starts.
- *Alert:* Monitor patient for hallucinations, depression, and suicidal tendencies.

PATIENT TEACHING
- Advise patient to take drug exactly as prescribed.
- Tell patient to report a "wearing-off" effect, which may occur at the end of the dosing interval.
- Tell patient that urine, sweat, and saliva may turn dark (red, brown, or black) during treatment.
- Advise patient to notify the prescriber if problems making voluntary movements increase.
- Tell patient that diarrhea is common with this treatment.

- Inform patient that hallucinations may occur.
- Urge patient to immediately report depression or suicidal thoughts.
- Explain that he may become dizzy if he rises quickly. Urge patient to use caution when rising.
- Tell patient that a high-protein diet, excessive acidity, and iron salts may reduce the drug's effectiveness.
- Urge patient to avoid hazardous activities until the CNS effects of the drug are known.
- Advise patient to notify prescriber if she becomes pregnant.

pramipexole dihydrochloride
pram-ah-PEX-ole

Mirapex

Pharmacologic class: nonergot dopamine agonist
Pregnancy risk category C

AVAILABLE FORMS
Tablets: 0.125 mg, 0.25 mg, 0.5 mg, 1 mg, 1.5 mg

INDICATIONS & DOSAGES
➤ **Signs and symptoms of idiopathic Parkinson disease**
Adults: Initially, 0.375 mg P.O. daily in three divided doses. Adjust doses slowly (not more often than every 5 to 7 days) over several weeks until desired therapeutic effect is achieved. Maintenance dosage is 1.5 to 4.5 mg daily in three divided doses.
Adjust-a-dose: For patients with creatinine clearance over 60 ml/minute, first dosage is 0.125 mg P.O. t.i.d., up to 1.5 mg t.i.d. For those with clearance of 35 to 59 ml/minute, first dosage is 0.125 mg P.O. b.i.d., up to 1.5 mg b.i.d. For those with clearance of 15 to 34 ml/minute, first dosage is 0.125 mg P.O. daily, up to 1.5 mg daily.
➤ **Moderate to severe primary restless leg syndrome**
Adults: 0.125 mg P.O. daily, 2 to 3 hours before bedtime. May increase after 4 to 7 days to 0.25 mg P.O. daily, as needed. May increase again after

4 to 7 days to 0.5 mg P.O. daily, if needed.
Adjust-a-dose: For patients with creatinine clearance 20 to 60 mg/minute, increase the duration between titration steps to 14 days.

ADMINISTRATION
P.O.
● Give drug with or without food; giving with food may reduce nausea.

ACTION
Thought to stimulate dopamine receptors.

Route	Onset	Peak	Duration
P.O.	Rapid	2 hr	8–12 hr

Half-life: 8 to 12 hours.

ADVERSE REACTIONS
CNS: *asthenia, confusion, dizziness, dream abnormalities, dyskinesia, extrapyramidal syndrome, hallucinations, insomnia, somnolence,* amnesia, akathisia, drowsiness, delusions, dystonia, gait abnormalities, hypoesthesia, hypertonia, myoclonus, paranoid reaction, malaise, sleep disorders, thought abnormalities, fever.
CV: *orthostatic hypotension,* chest pain, peripheral edema.
EENT: accommodation abnormalities, diplopia, rhinitis, vision abnormalities.
GI: *constipation, nausea,* dry mouth, anorexia, dysphagia.
GU: impotence, urinary frequency, UTI, urinary incontinence.
Metabolic: weight loss.
Musculoskeletal: arthritis, bursitis, myasthenia, twitching.
Respiratory: dyspnea, pneumonia.
Skin: skin disorders.
Other: *accidental injury,* decreased libido, general edema.

INTERACTIONS
Drug-drug. *Cimetidine, diltiazem, quinidine, quinine, ranitidine, triamterene, verapamil:* May decrease pramipexole clearance. Adjust dosage as needed.
Dopamine antagonists: May reduce pramipexole effectiveness. Monitor patient closely.

EFFECTS ON LAB TEST RESULTS
None reported.

CONTRAINDICATIONS & CAUTIONS
● Contraindicated in patients hypersensitive to drug or its components.
● Use cautiously in renally impaired patients.
● Use cautiously in breast-feeding women. It's unknown if drug appears in breast milk.

NURSING CONSIDERATIONS
● If drug must be stopped, withdraw over 1 week.
● Drug may cause orthostatic hypotension, especially during dosage increases. Monitor patient carefully.
● Adjust dosage gradually to achieve maximal therapeutic effect, balanced against the main adverse effects of dyskinesia, hallucinations, somnolence, and dry mouth.

PATIENT TEACHING
● Instruct patient not to rise rapidly after sitting or lying down because of risk of dizziness.
● Caution patient to avoid hazardous activities until CNS response to drug is known.
● Tell patient to use caution before taking drug with other CNS depressants.
● Tell patient (especially elderly patient) that hallucinations may occur.
● Advise patient to take drug with food if nausea develops.
● Tell woman to notify prescriber if she is or will be breast-feeding.
● Advise patient that it may take 4 weeks for effects of drug to be noticed because of slow adjustment schedule.

rasagiline mesylate
reh-SAH-jih-leen

Azilect✷

Pharmacologic class: irreversible, selective MAO inhibitor type B
Pregnancy risk category C

AVAILABLE FORMS
Tablets: 0.5 mg, 1 mg

Reactions may be *common,* uncommon, ***life-threatening,*** or COMMON AND LIFE-THREATENING.
Interaction may have a *rapid onset* or *delayed onset.*

INDICATIONS & DOSAGES
➤ **Idiopathic Parkinson disease, as monotherapy or with levodopa**
Adults: As monotherapy, 1 mg P.O. once daily.
Adjust-a-dose: If patient has mild hepatic impairment or takes a CYP1A2 inhibitor such as ciprofloxacin, give 0.5 mg once daily.

ADMINISTRATION
P.O.
● Give drug without regard for food.

ACTION
Unknown. May increase extracellular dopamine level in the CNS, improving neurotransmission and relieving signs and symptoms of Parkinson disease.

Route	Onset	Peak	Duration
P.O.	Variable	1 hr	1 wk

Half-life: 3 hours.

ADVERSE REACTIONS
Monotherapy
CNS: *dizziness, falls, headache,* depression, fever, hallucinations, malaise, paresthesia, syncope, vertigo.
CV: *chest pain,* angina pectoris, postural hypotension.
EENT: gingivitis.
GI: anorexia, diarrhea, dyspepsia, gastroenteritis, vomiting.
GU: albuminuria, impotence.
Hematologic: *leukopenia.*
Musculoskeletal: arthralgia, arthritis, neck pain.
Respiratory: asthma, flu syndrome, rhinitis.
Skin: alopecia, *carcinoma,* ecchymosis, vesiculobullous rash.
Other: allergic reaction, decreased libido.
Combined with levodopa
CNS: *confusion, falls, headache,* abnormal dreams, amnesia, ataxia, dyskinesia, dystonia, hallucinations, paresthesia, somnolence, sweating.
EENT: epistaxis, gingivitis.
GI: *nausea,* abdominal pain, anorexia, constipation, diarrhea, dry mouth, dyspepsia, dysphagia, vomiting, weight loss.
GU: albuminuria.
Hematologic: *hemorrhage,* anemia.

Musculoskeletal: arthralgia, arthritis, bursitis, hernia, leg cramps, myasthenia, neck pain, tenosynovitis.
Respiratory: dyspnea.
Skin: *carcinoma,* ecchymosis, pruritus, rash, ulcer.
Other: infection.

INTERACTIONS
Drug-drug. *Ciprofloxacin and other CYP1A2 inhibitors:* May double rasagiline level. Decrease rasagiline dosage to 0.5 mg daily.
Levodopa: May increase rasagiline level. Watch for dyskinesia, dystonia, hallucinations, and hypotension, and reduce levodopa dosage if needed.
SSRIs, SSNRIs, tricyclic antidepressants: May cause severe or fatal CNS toxicity. Stop rasagiline for at least 14 days before starting an antidepressant. Stop fluoxetine for 5 weeks before starting rasagiline.
Drug-herb. *St. John's wort:* May cause severe reaction. Strongly discourage use together.
Drug-food. *Tyramine-rich foods and supplements:* May cause hypertensive crisis. Urge patient to avoid tyramine-rich foods, such as aged meat, salami, pickled herring, aged cheese, unpasteurized beer, red wine, fava beans, sauerkraut, soybean products, and concentrated yeast extract.

EFFECTS ON LAB TEST RESULTS
● May increase liver enzyme levels.
● May decrease WBC count.

CONTRAINDICATIONS & CAUTIONS
● Contraindicated in patients with pheochromocytoma, those with moderate to severe hepatic impairment, and those taking amphetamines, cold products, dextromethorphan, ephedrine, MAO inhibitors, meperidine, methadone, phenylephrine, propoxyphene, pseudoephedrine, sympathomimetic amines, or tramadol.
● Use cautiously in patients with mild hepatic impairment and in pregnant or breast-feeding women.

NURSING CONSIDERATIONS
● Orthostatic hypotension may occur during first 2 months of therapy; help patient to rise from a reclining position.

• Notify prescriber if patient experiences adverse effects; levodopa dose may need to be reduced.
• Examine the patient's skin periodically for possible melanoma because of drug's associated risk of skin cancer.
• Notify prescriber if patient is having elective surgery, drug should be stopped at least 2 weeks before.

PATIENT TEACHING
• Explain the risk of hypertensive crisis if patient ingests tyramine while taking rasagiline. Give patient a list of foods and products containing tyramine.
• Tell patient to contact prescriber if hallucinations occur.
• Urge patient to watch for skin changes that could suggest melanoma and to have periodic skin examinations by a health professional.
• Instruct patient to maintain his usual dosage schedule if he misses a dose and not to double the next dose to make up for a missed one.

---

ropinirole hydrochloride
row-PIN-ah-roll

Requip, Requip XL

Pharmacologic class: nonergot dopamine agonist
Pregnancy risk category C

AVAILABLE FORMS
Tablets: 0.25 mg, 0.5 mg, 1 mg, 2 mg, 3 mg, 4 mg, 5 mg.
Tablets (extended-release): 2 mg, 3 mg, 4 mg, 8 mg

INDICATIONS & DOSAGES
➤ **Idiopathic Parkinson disease**
Adults: Initially, 0.25 mg P.O., t.i.d. Increase dose by 0.25 mg t.i.d. at weekly intervals for 4 weeks. After week 4, dosage may be increased by 1.5 mg daily divided t.i.d.; at weekly intervals, up to 9 mg daily divided t.i.d.; then dosage may be increased by up to 3 mg daily divided t.i.d.; at weekly intervals, up to 24 mg daily divided t.i.d.
Elderly patients: Adjust dosages individually, according to patient response; clearance is reduced in these patients.

➤ **Moderate to severe restless leg syndrome (immediate-release)**
Adults: Initially, 0.25 mg P.O. 1 to 3 hours before bedtime. May increase dose as needed and tolerated after 2 days to 0.5 mg, then to 1 mg by the end of the first week. May further increase dose as needed and tolerated as follows: week 2, give 1 mg once daily. Week 3, give 1.5 mg once daily. Week 4, give 2 mg once daily. Week 5, give 2.5 mg once daily. Week 6, give 3 mg once daily. And week 7, give 4 mg once daily. All doses should be taken 1 to 2 hours before bedtime.

ADMINISTRATION
P.O.
• Give drug with food if nausea occurs.

ACTION
Thought to stimulate dopamine (D2) receptors.

Route	Onset	Peak	Duration
P.O.	Unknown	1–2 hr	6 hr

Half-life: 6 hours.

ADVERSE REACTIONS
Early Parkinson disease (without levodopa)
CNS: *dizziness, fatigue, somnolence, syncope,* hallucinations, aggravated Parkinson disease, headache, confusion, hyperkinesia, hypoesthesia, vertigo, amnesia, impaired concentration, malaise, asthenia, pain.
CV: orthostatic hypotension, orthostatic symptoms, hypertension, edema, chest pain, extrasystoles, atrial fibrillation, palpitations, tachycardia, flushing.
EENT: pharyngitis, abnormal vision, eye abnormality, xerophthalmia, rhinitis, sinusitis.
GI: *nausea, vomiting, dyspepsia,* dry mouth, flatulence, abdominal pain, anorexia, constipation.
GU: UTI, impotence.
Respiratory: bronchitis, dyspnea, yawning.
Other: *viral infection,* increased sweating, peripheral ischemia.
Advanced Parkinson disease (with levodopa)

CNS: *dizziness, somnolence, headache, hallucinations,* aggravated parkinsonism, insomnia, abnormal dreaming, confusion, tremor, anxiety, nervousness, amnesia, paresis, paresthesia, syncope, pain.
CV: hypotension.
EENT: diplopia.
GI: *nausea,* abdominal pain, dry mouth, vomiting, constipation, diarrhea, dysphagia, flatulence, increased saliva.
GU: UTI, pyuria, urinary incontinence.
Hematologic: anemia.
Metabolic: weight decrease, suppressed prolactin.
Musculoskeletal: *dyskinesia,* arthralgia, arthritis, hypokinesia.
Respiratory: upper respiratory tract infection, dyspnea.
Skin: increased sweating.
Other: *falls,* injury, viral infection.
Restless leg syndrome
CNS: *fatigue, somnolence, dizziness,* vertigo, paresthesia.
CV: peripheral edema.
EENT: *nasopharyngitis,* nasal congestion.
GI: *nausea, vomiting,* diarrhea, dyspepsia, dry mouth.
Musculoskeletal: arthralgia, muscle cramps, extremity pain.
Respiratory: cough.
Skin: increased sweating.
Other: influenza.

INTERACTIONS
Drug-drug. *Cimetidine, ciprofloxacin, fluvoxamine, inhibitors or substrates of CYP1A2, ritonavir:* May alter ropinirole clearance. Adjust ropinirole dose if other drugs are started or stopped during treatment.
CNS depressants: May increase CNS effects. Use together cautiously.
Dopamine antagonists (neuroleptics), metoclopramide: May decrease ropinirole effects. Avoid using together.
Estrogens: May decrease ropinirole clearance. Adjust ropinirole dosage if estrogen therapy is started or stopped during treatment.
Drug-lifestyle. *Alcohol use:* May increase sedative effect. Discourage use together.
Smoking: May increase drug clearance. Discourage use together.

EFFECTS ON LAB TEST RESULTS
● May increase BUN and alkaline phosphatase levels. May decrease hemoglobin level.

CONTRAINDICATIONS & CAUTIONS
● Contraindicated in patients hypersensitive to drug.
● Use cautiously in patients with severe hepatic or renal impairment.

NURSING CONSIDERATIONS
● *Alert:* Monitor patient carefully for orthostatic hypotension, especially during dosage increases.
● Drug may potentiate the adverse effects of levodopa and may cause or worsen dyskinesia. Dosage may be decreased.
● Although not reported with ropinirole, other adverse reactions reported with dopaminergic therapy include hyperpyrexia, fibrotic complications, and confusion, which may occur with rapid dosage reduction or withdrawal of drug.
● Patient may have syncope, with or without bradycardia. Monitor patient carefully, especially for 4 weeks after start of therapy and with dosage increases.
● When used for Parkinson disease, withdraw drug gradually over 7 days.
● When used for restless leg syndrome, stop drug without tapering.

PATIENT TEACHING
● Advise patient to take drug with food if nausea occurs.
● Inform patient (especially elderly patient) that hallucinations can occur.
● Instruct patient not to rise rapidly after sitting or lying down because of risk of dizziness, which may occur more frequently early in therapy or when dosage increases.
● Sleepiness can occur early in therapy. Warn patient to minimize hazardous activities until CNS effects of drug are known.
● Advise patient to avoid alcohol.
● Tell woman to notify prescriber about planned, suspected, or known pregnancy; also tell her to inform prescriber if she's breast-feeding.

---

selegiline
se-LEH-ge-leen

Emsam

selegiline hydrochloride (L-deprenyl hydrochloride)
Eldepryl, Zelapar

Pharmacologic class: MAO inhibitor
Pregnancy risk category C

AVAILABLE FORMS
selegiline
Transdermal system: 6 mg/24 hours,
9 mg/24 hours, 12 mg/24 hours
selegiline hydrochloride
Capsules: 5 mg
Orally disintegrating tablets (ODTs):
1.25 mg
Tablets: 5 mg

INDICATIONS & DOSAGES
➤ **Adjunctive treatment with levodopa and carbidopa in managing signs and symptoms of Parkinson disease**
Adults: 10 mg P.O. daily divided
as 5 mg at breakfast and 5 mg at lunch.
After 2 or 3 days, gradual decrease of
levodopa and carbidopa dosage may
be needed. Or, if using ODTs, start
with 1.25 mg P.O. once daily before
breakfast and without liquid. Increase
to 2.5 mg daily after at least 6 weeks,
if needed.
➤ **Major depressive disorder**
Adults: Apply one patch daily to dry
intact skin on the upper torso, upper
thigh, or upper arm. Initially, use
6 mg/day. Increase, if needed, in
increments of 3 mg/day at intervals
of 2 or more weeks. Maximum daily
dose, 12 mg.
Elderly patients: 6 mg daily.

ADMINISTRATION
P.O.
● Don't give food or liquids for
5 minutes before and after giving
ODTs.
● Don't push ODTs through the
foil backing; peel the backing off
and gently remove the tablet.

Transdermal
● Apply patch to dry, intact skin on the
upper torso, upper thigh, or outer surface
of the upper arm once every 24 hours.
● Don't cut the transdermal patch into
smaller pieces.

ACTION
May inhibit MAO type B (mainly found in
the brain) and dopamine metabolism. At
higher-than-recommended doses, drug
nonselectively inhibits MAO, including
MAO type A (mainly found in the intestine). May also directly increase dopaminergic activity by decreasing the reuptake
of dopamine into nerve cells.

Route	Onset	Peak	Duration
P.O.	Unknown	30–120 min	Unknown
Trans-dermal	Unknown	Unknown	24 hr

Half-life: selegiline, 2 to 10 hours;
N-desmethyldeprenyl, 2 hours;
L-amphetamine, 17¾ hours;
L-methamphetamine, 20½ hours.

ADVERSE REACTIONS
Transdermal form
CNS: *headache, insomnia.*
CV: chest pain, hypotension, orthostatic
blood pressure.
GI: diarrhea, dry mouth, dyspepsia.
Metabolic: weight gain, weight loss.
Respiratory: pharyngitis, sinusitis.
Skin: *application site reaction,* rash.
oral form
CNS: *dizziness,* agitation, delusions, loss
of balance, depression, increased bradykinesia, involuntary movements, headache,
confusion, hallucinations, vivid dreams,
insomnia, syncope.
CV: *arrhythmias,* orthostatic hypotension,
hypertension, new or increased angina.
GI: *nausea,* dry mouth, abdominal pain.

INTERACTIONS
Drug-drug. *Citalopram, duloxetine, fluoxetine, fluvoxamine, nefazodone, paroxetine, sertraline, venlafaxine:* May cause
serotonin syndrome (CNS irritability,
shivering, and altered consciousness).
Separate use by at least 2 weeks (5 weeks
if switching to or from fluoxetine).
Bupropion; cyclobenzaprine; dextromethorphan; meperidine; methadone;

Reactions may be *common,* uncommon, *life-threatening,* or COMMON AND LIFE-THREATENING.
Interaction may have a *rapid onset* or **delayed onset.**

mirtazapine; MAO inhibitors; propoxyphene, sympathomimetic amines, including amphetamines, cold products, and weight-loss preparations containing vasoconstrictors; tramadol; tricyclic antidepressants: May cause hypertensive crisis. Separate use by at least 2 weeks. *Carbamazepine, oxcarbazepine:* May increase selegiline levels. Use together is contraindicated.

Drug-herb. *Ginseng:* May cause headache, tremors, or mania. Discourage use together.

St. John's wort: May cause increased serotonergic effects. Warn patient against use together.

Drug-food. *Foods high in tyramine:* May cause hypertensive crisis especially at increased doses. Provide patient with a list of foods to avoid.

EFFECTS ON LAB TEST RESULTS
● May cause positive result for amphetamine on urine drug screen.

CONTRAINDICATIONS & CAUTIONS
● Contraindicated in patients hypersensitive to drug, in patients with pheochromocytoma, and in those taking bupropion, carbamazepine, cyclobenzaprine, dextromethorphan, duloxetine, methadone, meperidine, mirtazapine, MAO inhibitors, oxcarbazepine, propoxyphene, SSRIs, sympathomimetics, tramadol, tricyclic antidepressants, venlafaxine.
● Don't use oral drug with the transdermal system.
■ **Black Box Warning** Selegiline isn't approved for use in children. Emsam shouldn't be used in children under age 12, even when administered with dietary modifications. ■

NURSING CONSIDERATIONS
● **Alert:** Some patients experience increased levodopa adverse reactions when it's used with selegiline and need a 10% to 30% reduction of levodopa and carbidopa dosage.
■ **Black Box Warning** Drug may increase the risk of suicidal thinking and behavior in children, adolescents, and young adults ages 18 to 24 during the first 2 months of treatment, especially in those with major depressive or other psychiatric disorder. ■

● Monitor patients with major depressive disorder for worsening of symptoms and of suicidal behavior, especially during the first few weeks of treatment and during dosage changes.
● *Look alike–sound alike:* Don't confuse selegiline with Stelazine or Eldepryl with enalapril.

PATIENT TEACHING
● Warn patient to move cautiously or change positions slowly at start of therapy because he may become dizzy or lightheaded.
● Caution patient to avoid driving and other hazardous activities that require mental alertness until the drug's effects are known.
● Advise patient not to take drug in the evening because doing so may cause insomnia.
● Advise patient not to overindulge in tyramine-rich foods or beverages. If using a 9 mg/day or higher transdermal system, avoid these products all together.
● Advise patient to avoid liquids for 5 minutes before and after taking ODTs.
● *Alert:* Warn patient about the many drugs, including OTC drugs, that may interact with this drug and about the need to consult a pharmacist or his prescriber before using them.
● Teach patient and family the signs and symptoms of hypertensive crisis including severe headache, sore or stiff neck, nausea, vomiting, sweating, rapid heartbeat, dilated pupils, and photophobia.
■ **Black Box Warning** Advise family members to watch patient for anxiety, agitation, insomnia, irritability, hostility, and aggressiveness and to report these immediately to prescriber. ■
● Tell patient to avoid exposing transdermal system to direct external heat sources, such as heating pads, electric blankets, hot tubs, heated water beds, and prolonged sunlight.
● Tell patient to stop using the transdermal system 10 days before having surgery requiring general anesthesia.
● Tell patient not to cut the transdermal system into smaller pieces.
● Advise woman planning pregnancy or breast-feeding to first contact her prescriber.

tolcapone
toll-KAP-own

Tasmar

Pharmacologic class: catechol-O-methyltransferase (COMT) inhibitor
Pregnancy risk category C

AVAILABLE FORMS
Tablets: 100 mg, 200 mg

INDICATIONS & DOSAGES
➤ **Adjunct to levodopa and carbidopa for signs and symptoms of idiopathic Parkinson disease in patients who have symptom fluctuation or haven't responded to other adjunctive treatment**
Adults: Initially, 100 mg P.O. t.i.d. with levodopa and carbidopa. Recommended daily dosage is 100 mg P.O. t.i.d. Levodopa dosage may need to be reduced by 20% to 30% to minimize risk of dyskinesias. Maximum, 600 mg daily. Stop drug if patient shows no benefit within 3 weeks.

ADMINISTRATION
P.O.
• Give drug without regard for food.
• Give first dose of the day with first daily dose of levodopa and carbidopa.

ACTION
May reversibly inhibit COMT when given with levodopa and carbidopa, increasing levodopa bioavailability. This causes a more constant dopaminergic stimulation in the brain.

Route	Onset	Peak	Duration
P.O.	Unknown	2 hr	Unknown

Half-life: 2 to 3 hours.

ADVERSE REACTIONS
CNS: *dyskinesia, sleep disorder, dystonia, excessive dreaming, somnolence, confusion, headache, hallucinations,* dizziness, fever, hyperkinesia, hypertonia, fatigue, falling, syncope, balance loss, depression, tremor, speech disorder, paresthesia, agitation, irritability, mental deficiency, hyperactivity, hypokinesia.

CV: *orthostatic complaints,* chest pain, chest discomfort, palpitations, hypotension.
EENT: pharyngitis, tinnitus, sinus congestion.
GI: *nausea, anorexia, diarrhea, vomiting,* flatulence, constipation, abdominal pain, dyspepsia, dry mouth.
GU: UTI, urine discoloration, hematuria, micturition disorder, urinary incontinence, impotence.
Hematologic: *bleeding.*
Hepatic: *hepatotoxicity.*
Musculoskeletal: *muscle cramps,* stiffness, arthritis, neck pain.
Respiratory: bronchitis, dyspnea, upper respiratory tract infection.
Skin: increased sweating, rash.
Other: influenza.

INTERACTIONS
Drug-drug. *CNS depressants:* May cause additive effects. Monitor patient closely.
Desipramine, SSRIs, tricyclic antidepressants: May increase risk of adverse effects. Use together cautiously.
Nonselective MAO inhibitors (phenelzine, tranylcypromine): May cause hypertensive crisis. Avoid using together.
Warfarin: May cause increased warfarin level. Monitor INR and adjust warfarin dosage as needed.

EFFECTS ON LAB TEST RESULTS
• May increase liver function test values.

CONTRAINDICATIONS & CAUTIONS
• Contraindicated in patients hypersensitive to drug or its components and in those with history of drug-related confusion and nontraumatic rhabdomyolysis or hyperpyrexia.
■ **Black Box Warning** Tolcapone therapy shouldn't be initiated if patient exhibits clinical evidence of liver disease or two ALT or AST values greater than the upper limit of normal. Drug is contraindicated in those previously withdrawn from drug because of drug-induced hepatocellular injury. ■
■ **Black Box Warning** Use cautiously in patients with severe dyskinesia or dystonia. ■
• Use cautiously in patients with severe renal impairment and in breast-feeding women.

Reactions may be *common,* uncommon, *life-threatening,* or **COMMON AND LIFE-THREATENING.**
Interaction may have a *rapid onset* or *delayed onset.*

NURSING CONSIDERATIONS
■ **Black Box Warning** Because of risk of liver toxicity, stop treatment if patient shows no benefit within 3 weeks. ■

■ **Black Box Warning** Because of fatal hepatic failure risk, use drug only in patients taking levodopa and carbidopa who don't respond to or who aren't appropriate candidates for other adjunctive therapies. ■

■ **Black Box Warning** Make sure patient provides written informed consent before taking drug. ■

• Monitor liver function test results before starting drug, every 2 weeks for the first year of therapy, every 4 weeks for the next 6 months, and then every 8 weeks thereafter. If the dose is increased to 200 mg t.i.d., obtain liver enzyme levels before increasing dose and then resume monitoring as described. Stop drug if AST or ALT exceeds two times the upper limit of normal or if patient shows signs or symptoms of hepatic dysfunction.

• Because drug is highly protein bound, it isn't significantly removed during dialysis.

• Monitor patient for orthostatic hypotension and syncope.

PATIENT TEACHING
• Advise patient to take drug exactly as prescribed.

■ **Black Box Warning** Teach patient to immediately report the signs and symptoms of liver injury (yellow eyes or skin, fatigue, loss of appetite, persistent nausea, itching, dark urine, or right upper abdominal tenderness). ■

• Warn patient about risk of dizziness upon standing up quickly; tell him to stand up cautiously.

• Advise patient to avoid hazardous activities until CNS effects of drug are known.

• Tell patient that nausea may occur early in therapy.

• Inform patient that diarrhea is common, sometimes occurring 2 to 12 weeks after therapy begins, and usually resolves when therapy stops.

• Advise patient about risk of increased problems making voluntary movements or impaired muscle tone.

• Inform patient that hallucinations may occur.

• Tell woman to notify prescriber about planned, suspected, or known pregnancy.

• Inform patient that drug may be taken without regard to meals.

41

Antipsychotics

aripiprazole
carbamazepine
(See Chapter 37, ANTICONVULSANTS.)
chlorpromazine hydrochloride
clonazepam
(See Chapter 37, ANTICONVULSANTS.)
clozapine
divalproex sodium
(See Chapter 37, ANTICONVULSANTS.)
fluphenazine decanoate
fluphenazine hydrochloride
gabapentin
(See Chapter 37, ANTICONVULSANTS.)
haloperidol
haloperidol decanoate
haloperidol lactate
lithium carbonate
lithium citrate
loxapine succinate
olanzapine
paliperidone
perphenazine
prochlorperazine
(See Chapter 60, ANTIEMETICS.)
quetiapine fumarate
risperidone
thioridazine hydrochloride
thiothixene
thiothixene hydrochloride
trifluoperazine hydrochloride
ziprasidone

---

aripiprazole
air-eh-PIP-rah-zole

Abilify✐, Abilify Discmelt

Pharmacologic class: quinolone
derivative
Pregnancy risk category C

AVAILABLE FORMS
Injection: 9.75 mg/1.3 ml (7.5 mg/ml)
single-dose vial
Oral solution: 1 mg/ml
Orally disintegrating tablets (ODTs):
10 mg, 15 mg
Tablets: 2 mg, 5 mg, 10 mg, 15 mg,
20 mg, 30 mg

INDICATIONS & DOSAGES
➤ **Schizophrenia**
Adults: Initially, 10 to 15 mg P.O. daily;
increase to maximum daily dose of 30 mg
if needed, after at least 2 weeks. Responding patients should be continued on the
lowest dosage needed to maintain remission. Patients should be periodically reassessed to determine the need for maintenance treatment.
Adolescents age 13 to 17: Initially,
2 mg P.O. daily; increase to 5 mg after
2 days, then to recommended dose of
10 mg in 2 more days. May titrate to
maximum daily dose of 30 mg in 5-mg
increments. Responding patients should
be continued on the lowest dosage
needed to maintain remission. Patients
should be periodically reassessed to
determine the need for maintenance
treatment.
➤ **Bipolar mania, including
manic and mixed episodes, with
or without psychotic features;
adjunctive therapy to either lithium
or valproate for treatment
of manic and mixed episodes
associated with bipolar I disorder
with or without psychotic features
(acute treatment only)**
Adults: Initial and target dose is 15 mg
P.O. once daily. Dose can be increased
to maximum of 30 mg/day based on
clinical response. For maintenance,
responding patients on monotherapy
should be continued on the lowest dose
needed to maintain remission. Patients
should be periodically reassessed to
determine the long-term usefulness of
maintenance treatment.
Children ages 10 to 17: Initially,
2 mg P.O. daily; increase to 5 mg
P.O. daily after 2 days then to recommended dose of 10 mg in two more
days. May titrate to maximum daily
dose of 30 mg in 5-mg increments
every 5 days. For maintenance,
responding patients on monotherapy
should be continued on the lowest
dose needed to maintain remission.

Reactions may be *common*, uncommon, *life-threatening*, or COMMON AND LIFE-THREATENING.
Interaction may have a *rapid onset* or **delayed onset**.

Patients should be periodically reassessed to determine the need for maintenance treatment.

✱NEW INDICATION:Adjunctive treatment of major depressive disorder
Adults: Initially, 2 to 5 mg P.O. daily. Dose range is 2 to 15 mg/day. Dosage adjustments of up to 5 mg/day should occur gradually, at intervals of no less than 1 week.

➤ **Agitation associated with schizophrenia or bipolar 1 disorder, mixed or manic**
Adults: 5.25 to 15 mg by deep I.M. injection. Recommended dose is 9.75 mg. May give a second dose after 2 hours, if needed. Safety of giving more frequently than every 2 hours or a total daily dose more than 30 mg isn't known. Switch to oral form as soon as possible.

Adjust-a-dose: When using with CYP3A4 inhibitors, such as ketoconazole or clarithromycin, or CYP2D6 inhibitors, such as quinidine, fluoxetine, or paroxetine, give half the aripiprazole dose. When using with CYP3A4 inducers such as carbamazepine, double the aripiprazole dose. Return to original dosing after the other drugs are stopped.

ADMINISTRATION
P.O.
● Give drug without regard for food.
● Substitute the oral solution on a milligram-by-milligram basis for the 5-, 10-, 15-, or 20-mg tablets, up to 25 mg. Give patients taking 30-mg tablets 25 mg of solution.
● Keep ODTs in blister package until ready to use. Use dry hands to carefully peel open the foil backing and remove the tablet. Don't split tablet.
● Store oral solution in refrigerator; it can be used up to 6 months after opening.
I.M.
● Inject slowly and deep into the muscle mass.
● Don't give I.V. or subcutaneously.

ACTION
Thought to exert partial agonist activity at D2 and serotonin 1A receptors and antagonist activity at serotonin 2A receptors.

Route	Onset	Peak	Duration
P.O.	Unknown	3–5 hr	Unknown
I.M.	Unknown	1–3 hr	Unknown

Half-life: About 75 hours in patients with normal metabolism; about 6 days in those who can't metabolize the drug through CYP2D6.

ADVERSE REACTIONS
CNS: *headache, anxiety, insomnia, light-headedness, somnolence, akathisia, increased suicide risk, neuroleptic malignant syndrome, seizures, suicidal thoughts,* tremor, asthenia, depression, fatigue, dizziness, nervousness, hostility, manic behavior, confusion, abnormal gait, cogwheel rigidity, fever, tardive dyskinesia.
CV: peripheral edema, chest pain, hypertension, tachycardia, orthostatic hypotension, *bradycardia.*
EENT: rhinitis, blurred vision, increased salivation, conjunctivitis, ear pain.
GI: *nausea, vomiting, constipation,* anorexia, dry mouth, dyspepsia, diarrhea, abdominal pain, esophageal dysmotility.
GU: urinary incontinence.
Hematologic: ecchymosis, anemia.
Metabolic: weight gain, weight loss, hyperglycemia, hypercholesterolemia.
Musculoskeletal: neck pain, neck stiffness, muscle cramps.
Respiratory: dyspnea, pneumonia, cough.
Skin: rash, dry skin, pruritus, sweating, ulcer.
Other: flulike syndrome.

INTERACTIONS
Drug-drug. *Antihypertensives:* May enhance antihypertensive effects. Monitor blood pressure.
Carbamazepine and other CYP3A4 inducers: May decrease levels and effectiveness of aripiprazole. Double the usual dose of aripiprazole, and monitor the patient closely.
Ketoconazole and other CYP3A4 inhibitors: May increase risk of serious toxic effects. Start treatment with half the usual dose of aripiprazole, and monitor patient closely.
Potential CYP2D6 inhibitors (fluoxetine, paroxetine, quinidine): May increase

levels and toxicity of aripiprazole. Give half the usual dose of aripiprazole.
Drug-food. *Grapefruit juice:* May increase drug level. Tell patient not to take drug with grapefruit juice.
Drug-lifestyle. *Alcohol use:* May increase CNS effects. Discourage use together.

EFFECTS ON LAB TEST RESULTS
• May increase CK and glucose levels.

CONTRAINDICATIONS & CAUTIONS
• Contraindicated in patients hypersensitive to drug.
• Use cautiously in patients with CV disease, cerebrovascular disease, or conditions that could predispose the patient to hypotension, such as dehydration or hypovolemia.
• Use cautiously in patients with history of seizures or with conditions that lower the seizure threshold.
• Use cautiously in patients who engage in strenuous exercise, are exposed to extreme heat, take anticholinergics, or are susceptible to dehydration.
• Use cautiously in patients at risk for aspiration pneumonia, such as those with Alzheimer disease.
• Use cautiously in pregnant and breast-feeding women.
■ **Black Box Warning** Abilify isn't approved for use in children with depression. ■
■ **Black Box Warning** Elderly patients with dementia-related psychosis treated with atypical antipsychotics are at an increased risk for death. Ability isn't approved for the treatment of patients with dementia-related psychosis. ■

NURSING CONSIDERATIONS
• *Alert:* Neuroleptic malignant syndrome may occur. Monitor patient for hyperpyrexia, muscle rigidity, altered mental status, irregular pulse or blood pressure, tachycardia, diaphoresis, and cardiac dysrhythmias.
• If signs and symptoms of neuroleptic malignant syndrome occur, immediately stop drug and notify prescriber.
• Monitor patient for signs and symptoms of tardive dyskinesia. Elderly patients, especially women, are at highest risk of developing this adverse effect.

• *Alert:* Fatal cerebrovascular adverse events (stroke, transient ischemic attack) may occur in elderly patients with dementia. Drug isn't safe or effective in these patients.
■ **Black Box Warning** Drug may increase the risk of suicidal thinking and behavior in children, adolescents, and young adults ages 18 to 24 during the first 2 months of treatment, especially in those with major depressive or other psychiatric disorder. ■
• *Alert:* Hyperglycemia may occur. Monitor patient with diabetes regularly. Patient with risk factors for diabetes should undergo fasting blood glucose testing at baseline and periodically. Monitor all patients for symptoms of hyperglycemia including increased hunger, thirst, frequent urination, and weakness. Hyperglycemia may resolve when patient stops taking drug.
• *Alert:* Monitor patient for symptoms of metabolic syndrome (significant weight gain and increased body mass index, hypertension, hyperglycemia, hypercholesterolemia, and hypertriglyceridemia).
• Treat patient with the smallest dose for the shortest time and periodically reevaluate for need to continue.
• Give prescriptions only for small quantities of drug, to reduce risk of overdose.
• Don't give I.V. or subcutaneously.

PATIENT TEACHING
• Tell patient to use caution while driving or operating hazardous machinery because psychoactive drugs may impair judgment, thinking, or motor skills.
• Tell patient that drug may be taken without regard to meals.
• Advise patients that grapefruit juice may interact with aripiprazole and to limit or avoid its use.
• Advise patient that gradual improvement in symptoms should occur over several weeks rather than immediately.
• Tell patients to avoid alcohol use while taking drug.
• Advise patients to limit strenuous activity while taking drug to avoid dehydration.
• Tell patient to keep ODT in blister package until ready to use. Using dry hands, he should carefully peel open the foil backing

Reactions may be *common*, uncommon, *life-threatening*, or COMMON AND LIFE-THREATENING.
Interaction may have a *rapid onset* or *delayed onset*.

and place tablet on the tongue. Tell him not to split tablet.

● Tell patient to store oral solution in refrigerator, and that the solution can be used for up to 6 months after opening.

---

chlorpromazine hydrochloride
klor-PROE-ma-zeen

Pharmacologic class: phenothiazine
Pregnancy risk category C

AVAILABLE FORMS
Injection: 25 mg/ml
Tablets: 10 mg, 25 mg, 50 mg, 100 mg, 200 mg

INDICATIONS & DOSAGES
➤ **Psychosis, mania**
Adults: For hospitalized patients with acute disease, 25 mg I.M.; may give an additional 25 to 50 mg I.M. in 1 hour if needed. Increase over several days to 400 mg every 4 to 6 hours. Switch to oral therapy as soon as possible. Or, 25 mg P.O. t.i.d. initially; then gradually increase to 400 mg daily in divided doses. For outpatients, 30 to 75 mg daily in two to four divided doses. Increase dosage by 20 to 50 mg twice weekly until symptoms are controlled.
Children age 6 months and older: 0.5 mg/kg P.O. every 4 to 6 hours or I.M. every 6 to 8 hours. Maximum I.M. dose in children younger than age 5 or who weigh less than 22.7 kg (50 lb) is 40 mg. Maximum I.M. dose in children ages 5 to 12 or who weigh 22.7 to 45.4 kg (50 to 100 lb) is 75 mg.

➤ **Nausea and vomiting**
Adults: 10 to 25 mg P.O. every 4 to 6 hours, p.r.n. Or, 25 mg I.M. initially. If no hypotension occurs, 25 to 50 mg I.M. every 3 to 4 hours may be given, p.r.n., until vomiting stops.
Children age 6 months and older: 0.55 mg/kg P.O. every 4 to 6 hours or I.M. every 6 to 8 hours. Maximum I.M. dose in children younger than age 5 or who weigh less than 22.7 kg (50 lb) is 40 mg. Maximum I.M. dose in children ages 5 to 12 or who weigh 22.7 to 45.4 kg (50 to 100 lb) is 75 mg.

➤ **Acute intermittent porphyria, intractable hiccups**
Adults: 25 to 50 mg P.O. t.i.d. or q.i.d. If symptoms persist for 2 to 3 days, 25 to 50 mg I.M. For hiccups, if symptoms still persist, 25 to 50 mg diluted in 500 to 1,000 ml of normal saline solution and infused slowly with patient in supine position.

➤ **Tetanus**
Adults: 25 to 50 mg I.V. or I.M. t.i.d. or q.i.d.
Children age 6 months and older: 0.5 mg/kg I.M. or I.V. every 6 to 8 hours. Maximum parenteral dosage in children who weigh less than 22.7 kg (50 lb) is 40 mg daily; for children who weigh 22.7 to 45.4 kg (50 to 100 lb), 75 mg, except in severe cases. If giving I.V., dilute to 1 mg/ml with normal saline and give at a rate of 0.5 mg/minute.

➤ **Behavioral disorders; hyperactivity**
Children older than 6 months to 12 years: For outpatients: 0.5 mg/kg P.O. every 4 to 6 hours or I.M. every 6 to 8 hours, as needed. For hospitalized patients, start with low oral doses and increase gradually. In severe behavior disorders, 50 to 100 mg P.O. or P.R. daily or, in older children, 200 mg/day or more P.O. may be necessary. There is little evidence that improvement in severely disturbed mentally retarded patients is enhanced by doses beyond 500 mg/day. In hospitalized patients age 5 or younger or weighing less than 23 kg (50 lb), don't exceed 40 mg/day I.M. In children ages 5 to 12 weighing 23 to 45 kg (50 to 100 lb), don't exceed 75 mg/day I.M., except in unmanageable cases.

➤ **Surgery**
Adults: Preoperatively, 25 to 50 mg P.O. 2 to 3 hours before surgery or 12.5 to 25 mg I.M. 1 to 2 hours before surgery; during surgery, 12.5 mg I.M., repeated in 30 minutes, if needed, or fractional 2-mg doses I.V. at 2-minute intervals to maximum dose of 25 mg; postoperatively, 10 to 25 mg P.O. every 4 to 6 hours or 12.5 to 25 mg I.M., repeated in 1 hour, if needed.
Children age 6 months and older: Preoperatively, 0.5 mg/kg P.O. 2 to 3 hours before surgery or I.M. 1 to 2 hours before surgery. During surgery, 0.25 mg/kg I.M.,

repeated in 30 minutes if needed, or fractional 1-mg doses I.V. at 2-minute intervals to maximum of 0.25 mg/kg. May repeat fractional I.V. regimen in 30 minutes if needed. Postoperatively, 0.55 mg/kg P.O. or I.M. every 4 to 6 hours (oral dose) or 1 hour (I.M. dose), if needed and if hypotension doesn't occur.

Elderly patients: Lower dosages are sufficient; dosage increments should be more gradual than in adults.

ADMINISTRATION
P.O.
● Wear gloves when preparing solutions and avoid contact with skin and clothing. Oral liquid forms can cause contact dermatitis.
● Slight yellowing of concentrate is common and doesn't affect potency. Discard markedly discolored solutions.
● Protect liquid concentrate from light. Dilute with fruit juice, milk, or semisolid food just before giving.
● Don't crush or break extended-release capsules.
I.V.
● Wear gloves when preparing solutions and avoid contact with skin and clothing. Parenteral forms can cause contact dermatitis.
● Drug is compatible with most common I.V. solutions, including D_5W, Ringer's injection, lactated Ringer's injection, and normal saline solution for injection.
● For direct injection, dilute with normal saline solution for injection and give into a large vein or through the tubing of a free-flowing I.V. solution.
● Don't exceed 1 mg/minute for adults or 0.5 mg/minute for children.
● For intermittent infusion, dilute with 50 or 100 ml of a compatible solution.
● Infuse over 30 minutes.
● **Incompatibilities:** Aminophylline, amphotericin B, ampicillin, chloramphenicol sodium succinate, chlorothiazide, cimetidine, dimenhydrinate, furosemide, heparin sodium, linezolid, melphalan, methohexital, paclitaxel, penicillin, pentobarbital, phenobarbital, solutions with a pH of 4 to 5, thiopental.
I.M.
● Wear gloves when preparing solutions and avoid contact with skin and clothing.

Parenteral forms can cause contact dermatitis.
● Slight yellowing of injection is common and doesn't affect potency. Discard markedly discolored solutions.
● Monitor blood pressure before and after I.M. administration; keep patient supine for 1 hour afterward and have him get up slowly.
● Give deep I.M. only in upper outer quadrant of buttocks. Consider giving injection by Z-track method. Massage slowly afterward to prevent sterile abscess. Injection stings. Rotate injection sites.
Rectal
● Store suppositories in well-closed containers between 15° and 30° C (59° and 86° F).

ACTION
A piperidine phenothiazine that may block postsynaptic dopamine receptors in the brain.

Route	Onset	Peak	Duration
P.O.	30–60 min	Unknown	4–6 hr
P.O. (extended)	30–60 min	Unknown	10–12 hr
I.V., I.M.	Unknown	Unknown	Unknown
P.R.	> 1 hr	Unknown	3–4 hr

Half-life: 20 to 24 hours.

ADVERSE REACTIONS
CNS: *extrapyramidal reactions, sedation, tardive dyskinesia, pseudoparkinsonism,* **neuroleptic malignant syndrome, seizures,** dizziness, drowsiness.
CV: *orthostatic hypotension,* tachycardia, quinidine-like ECG effects.
EENT: ocular changes, blurred vision, nasal congestion.
GI: *dry mouth, constipation,* nausea.
GU: *urine retention,* menstrual irregularities, inhibited ejaculation, priapism.
Hematologic: *leukopenia, agranulocytosis, aplastic anemia, thrombocytopenia,* eosinophilia, hemolytic anemia.
Hepatic: jaundice.
Skin: *mild photosensitivity reactions, pain at I.M. injection site,* allergic reactions, sterile abscess, skin pigmentation changes.
Other: gynecomastia, lactation, galactorrhea.

Reactions may be *common,* uncommon, *life-threatening,* or COMMON AND LIFE-THREATENING.
Interaction may have a *rapid onset* or **delayed onset.**

INTERACTIONS

Drug-drug. *Antacids:* May inhibit absorption of oral phenothiazines. Separate antacid and phenothiazine doses by at least 2 hours.

Anticholinergics such as tricyclic antidepressants, antiparkinsonians: May increase anticholinergic activity, aggravated parkinsonian symptoms. Use together cautiously.

Anticonvulsants: May lower seizure threshold. Monitor patient closely.

Barbiturates, lithium: May decrease phenothiazine effect. Monitor patient.

Centrally acting antihypertensives: May decrease antihypertensive effect. Monitor blood pressure.

CNS depressants: May increase CNS depression. Use together cautiously.

Electroconvulsive therapy, insulin: May cause severe reactions. Monitor patient closely.

Lithium: May increase neurologic effects. Monitor patient closely.

Meperidine: May cause excessive sedation and hypotension. Don't use together.

Propranolol: May increase levels of both propranolol and chlorpromazine. Monitor patient closely.

Warfarin: May decrease effect of oral anticoagulants. Monitor PT and INR.

Drug-herb. *St. John's wort:* May cause photosensitivity reactions. Advise patient to avoid excessive sunlight exposure.

Drug-lifestyle. *Alcohol use:* May increase CNS depression, particularly psychomotor skills. Strongly discourage alcohol use.

Sun exposure: May increase risk of photosensitivity reactions. Advise patient to avoid excessive sunlight exposure.

EFFECTS ON LAB TEST RESULTS

● May decrease hemoglobin level and hematocrit.

● May increase liver function test values and eosinophil count. May decrease granulocyte, platelet, and WBC counts.

● May cause false-positive results for urinary porphyrin, urobilinogen, amylase, and 5-hydroxyindoleacetic acid tests and for urine pregnancy tests that use human chorionic gonadotropin.

CONTRAINDICATIONS & CAUTIONS

● Contraindicated in patients hypersensitive to drug; in those with CNS depression, bone marrow suppression, or subcortical damage, and in those in coma.

● Use cautiously in elderly or debilitated patients and in patients with hepatic or renal disease, severe CV disease (may suddenly decrease blood pressure), respiratory disorders, hypocalcemia, glaucoma, or prostatic hyperplasia. Also use cautiously in those exposed to extreme heat or cold (including antipyretic therapy) or organophosphate insecticides.

● Use cautiously in acutely ill or dehydrated children.

NURSING CONSIDERATIONS

● Obtain baseline blood pressure measurements before therapy, and monitor regularly. Watch for orthostatic hypotension, especially with parenteral administration.

● Monitor patient for tardive dyskinesia, which may occur after prolonged use. It may not appear until months or years later and may disappear spontaneously or persist for life, despite stopping drug.

● After abrupt withdrawal of long-term therapy, gastritis, nausea, vomiting, dizziness, or tremor may occur.

● **Alert:** Watch for evidence of neuroleptic malignant syndrome (extrapyramidal effects, hyperthermia, autonomic disturbance), which is rare but usually fatal. It may not be related to length of drug use or type of neuroleptic; more than 60% of affected patients are men.

● If jaundice, symptoms of blood dyscrasia (fever, sore throat, infection, cellulitis, weakness), or persistent extrapyramidal reactions (longer than a few hours) develop, or if such reactions occur in children or pregnant women, withhold dose and notify prescriber.

● Don't withdraw drug abruptly unless required by severe adverse reactions.

■ **Black Box Warning** Elderly patients with dementia-related psychosis treated with atypical or conventional antipsychotics are at increased risk for death. Antipsychotics aren't approved for the treatment of dementia-related psychosis. ■

● **Look alike–sound alike:** Don't confuse chlorpromazine with clomipramine or with chlorpropamide, a hypoglycemic.

PATIENT TEACHING
• Warn patient to avoid activities that require alertness or good coordination until effects of drug are known. Drowsiness and dizziness usually subside after first few weeks.
• *Alert:* Advise patient not to crush, chew, or break extended-release capsule before swallowing.
• Tell patient to avoid alcohol while taking drug.
• Have patient report signs of urine retention or constipation.
• Tell patient to use sunblock and to wear protective clothing to avoid oversensitivity to the sun. This drug is more likely to cause sun sensitivity than other drugs in its class.
• Tell patient to relieve dry mouth with sugarless gum or hard candy.
• Advise patient receiving drug by any method other than by mouth to remain lying down for 1 hour afterward and to rise slowly.

SAFETY ALERT!

clozapine
KLOE-za-peen

Clozaril, FazaClo

Pharmacologic class: dibenzapine derivative
Pregnancy risk category B

AVAILABLE FORMS
Orally disintegrating tablets (ODTs): 12.5 mg, 25 mg, 100 mg
Tablets: 12.5 mg, 25 mg, 100 mg, 200 mg

INDICATIONS & DOSAGES
➤ **Schizophrenia in severely ill patients unresponsive to other therapies; to reduce risk of recurrent suicidal behavior in schizophrenia or schizoaffective disorders**
Adults: Initially, 12.5 mg P.O. once daily or b.i.d. If using the ODT, cut in half and discard the unused half. Adjust dose upward by 25 to 50 mg daily (if tolerated) to 300 to 450 mg daily by end of 2 weeks. Individual dosage is based on clinical response, patient tolerance, and adverse reactions. Subsequent dosage shouldn't be increased more than once or twice weekly and shouldn't exceed 50- to 100-mg increments. Many patients respond to dosages of 200 to 600 mg daily, but some may need as much as 900 mg daily. Don't exceed 900 mg daily.

ADMINISTRATION
P.O.
• Peel the foil from the ODT blister and gently remove the tablet immediately before giving.
• Give ODT with or without water.

ACTION
Unknown. Binds selectively to dopaminergic receptors in the CNS and may interfere with adrenergic, cholinergic, histaminergic, and serotonergic receptors.

Route	Onset	Peak	Duration
P.O.	Unknown	2½ hr	4–12 hr

Half-life: Proportional to dose; may range from 8 to 12 hours.

ADVERSE REACTIONS
CNS: *drowsiness, sedation, dizziness, vertigo, headache,* **seizures,** *syncope, tremor, disturbed sleep or nightmares, restlessness, hypokinesia or akinesia, agitation, rigidity, akathisia, confusion, fatigue, insomnia, hyperkinesia, weakness, lethargy, ataxia, slurred speech, depression, myoclonus, anxiety, fever.*
CV: *tachycardia,* **cardiomyopathy, myocarditis, pulmonary embolism, cardiac arrest,** *hypotension, hypertension, chest pain, ECG changes, orthostatic hypotension.*
EENT: *visual disturbances.*
GI: *constipation, excessive salivation,* dry mouth, nausea, vomiting, heartburn, diarrhea.
GU: urinary frequency or urgency, urine retention, incontinence, abnormal ejaculation.
Hematologic: *leukopenia, agranulocytosis, granulocytopenia,* eosinophilia.
Metabolic: *hyperglycemia,* weight gain, hypercholesterolemia, hypertriglyceridemia.

Reactions may be *common*, uncommon, *life-threatening*, or COMMON AND LIFE-THREATENING.
Interaction may have a *rapid onset* or *delayed onset.*

Musculoskeletal: muscle pain or spasm, muscle weakness.
Respiratory: *respiratory arrest.*
Skin: rash, diaphoresis.

INTERACTIONS
Drug-drug. *Anticholinergics:* May potentiate anticholinergic effects of clozapine. Use together cautiously.
Antihypertensives: May potentiate hypotensive effects. Monitor blood pressure.
■ **Black Box Warning** *Benzodiazepines, other psychotropic drugs:* May increase risk of sedation and CV and respiratory arrest. Use together cautiously. ■
Bone marrow suppressants: May increase bone marrow toxicity. Avoid using together.
Citalopram, *fluoroquinolones,* **fluoxetine, fluvoxamine,** *paroxetine,* **sertraline:** May increase clozapine levels and toxicity. Adjust clozapine dose as needed.
Digoxin, other highly protein-bound drugs, warfarin: May increase levels of these drugs. Monitor patient closely for adverse reactions.
Phenytoin: May decrease clozapine level and cause breakthrough psychosis. Monitor patient for psychosis and adjust clozapine dosage.
Psychoactive drugs: May cause additive effects. Use together cautiously.
Ritonavir: May increase clozapine levels and toxicity. Avoid using together.
Drug-herb. *St. John's wort:* May decrease drug level. Discourage use together.
Drug-lifestyle. *Alcohol use:* May increase CNS depression. Discourage use together.
Smoking: May decrease drug level. Urge patient to quit smoking. Monitor patient for effectiveness and adjust dosage.

EFFECTS ON LAB TEST RESULTS
● May increase glucose, cholesterol, and triglyceride levels.
● May increase eosinophil count. May decrease granulocyte and WBC counts.

CONTRAINDICATIONS & CAUTIONS
● Contraindicated in patients with uncontrolled epilepsy, history of clozapine-induced agranulocytosis, WBC count below 3,500/mm³, severe CNS depression or coma, paralytic ileus, and myelo-suppressive disorders.
● Contraindicated in patients taking other drugs that suppress bone marrow function.
● Use cautiously in patients with prostatic hyperplasia or angle-closure glaucoma because drug has potent anticholinergic effects.

NURSING CONSIDERATIONS
● ODTs contain phenylalanine.
■ **Black Box Warning** Drug carries significant risk of agranulocytosis. If possible, give patient at least two trials of standard antipsychotic before starting clozapine. Obtain baseline WBC and differential counts before clozapine therapy. Baseline WBC count must be at least 3,500/mm³ and baseline antineutrophil cytoplasmic antibody (ANCA) at least 2,000/mm³. Monitor WBC and ANCA values weekly for at least 4 weeks after stopping drug, regardless of how often you were monitoring when therapy stopped. ■
● During the first 6 months of therapy, monitor patient weekly and dispense no more than a 1-week supply of drug. If acceptable WBC and ANCA values [WBC 3,500/mm³ or higher and ANCA 2,000/mm³ or higher] are maintained during the first 6 months of continuous therapy, reduce monitoring to every other week. After 6 months of every-other-week monitoring without interruption by leukopenia, reduce frequency of monitoring WBC and ANCA to monthly.
● If WBC count drops below 3,500/mm³ after therapy begins or if it drops substantially from baseline, monitor patient closely for signs and symptoms of infection. If WBC count is 3,000 to 3,500/mm³ and granulocyte count is above 1,500/mm³, perform WBC and differential count twice weekly. If WBC count drops to 2,000/mm³ to 3,000/mm³ or granulocyte count drops to 1,000/mm³ to 1,500/mm³, interrupt therapy and notify prescriber. Monitor WBC and differential daily until WBC exceeds 3,000/mm³ and ANCA exceeds 1,500/mm³, and monitor patient for signs and symptoms of infection. Continue monitoring WBC and differential counts twice weekly until WBC count exceeds

3,500/mm³ and ANCA exceeds 2,000/mm³. Then, restart therapy with weekly monitoring for 1 year before returning to the usual monitoring schedule of every 2 weeks for 6 months and then every 4 weeks.
• If WBC count drops below 2,000/mm³ and granulocyte count drops below 1,000/mm³, patient may need protective isolation. Bone marrow aspiration may be needed to assess bone marrow function. Future clozapine therapy is contraindicated in these patients.

■ **Black Box Warning** Drug increases the risk of fatal myocarditis, especially during, but not limited to, the first month of therapy. In patients in whom myocarditis is suspected (unexplained fatigue, dyspnea, tachypnea, chest pain, tachycardia, fever, palpitations, and other signs or symptoms of heart failure or ECG abnormalities, such as ST-T wave abnormalities or arrhythmias), stop therapy immediately and don't restart. ■

• *Alert:* Drug may cause hyperglycemia. Monitor patients with diabetes regularly. In patients with risk factors for diabetes, obtain fasting blood glucose test results at baseline and periodically.

• *Alert:* Monitor patient for metabolic syndrome, including significant weight gain and increased body mass index, hypertension, hyperglycemia, hypercholesterolemia, and hypertriglyceridemia.

• Monitor patient for signs and symptoms of cardiomyopathy.

■ **Black Box Warning** Orthostatic hypotension, with or without syncope, can occur. Rarely, collapse can be profound and be accompanied by respiratory or cardiac arrest. Orthostatic hypotension is more likely to occur during initial titration with rapid dose escalation. In patients who have had even a brief interval off clozapine (2 or more days since the last dose), start treatment with 12.5 mg once or twice daily. ■

■ **Black Box Warning** Seizures may occur, especially in patients receiving high doses. ■

• Some patients experience transient fever with temperature higher than 100.4° F (38° C), especially in the first 3 weeks of therapy. Monitor these patients closely.

■ **Black Box Warning** Drug isn't indicated for use in elderly patients with dementia-related psychoses because of an increased risk for death from CV disease or infection. ■

• After abrupt withdrawal of long-term therapy, abrupt recurrence of psychosis is possible.

• If therapy must be stopped, withdraw drug gradually over 1 or 2 weeks. If changes in patient's medical condition (including development of leukopenia) require that drug be stopped immediately, monitor patient closely for recurrence of psychosis.

• If therapy is reinstated in patients withdrawn from drug, follow usual guidelines for dosage increase. Reexposure of patient to drug may increase severity and risk of adverse reactions. If therapy was stopped because WBC counts were below 2,000/mm³ or granulocyte counts were below 1,000/mm³, don't restart.

• *Look alike–sound alike:* Don't confuse clozapine with clonidine, clofazimine, or Klonopin.

PATIENT TEACHING
• Tell patient about need for weekly blood tests to check for blood-cell deficiency. Advise him to report flulike symptoms, fever, sore throat, lethargy, malaise, or other signs of infection.

• Warn patient to avoid hazardous activities that require alertness and good coordination while taking drug.

• Tell patient to check with prescriber before taking alcohol or OTC drugs.

• Advise patient that smoking may decrease drug effectiveness.

• Tell patient to rise slowly to avoid dizziness.

• Tell patient to keep ODTs in the blister package until ready to take it.

• Inform patient that ice chips or sugarless candy or gum may help relieve dry mouth.

Reactions may be *common*, uncommon, *life-threatening*, or COMMON AND LIFE-THREATENING.
Interaction may have a *rapid onset* or *delayed onset*.

fluphenazine decanoate
floo-FEN-a-zeen

Modecate†, Modecate
Concentrate†

fluphenazine hydrochloride
Pharmacologic class:
phenothiazine
Pregnancy risk category C

AVAILABLE FORMS
fluphenazine decanoate
Depot injection: 25 mg/ml
fluphenazine hydrochloride
Elixir: 2.5 mg/5 ml*
I.M. injection: 2.5 mg/ml, 25 mg/ml
Oral concentrate: 5 mg/ml*
Tablets: 1 mg, 2.5 mg, 5 mg, 10 mg

INDICATIONS & DOSAGES
➤ **Psychotic disorders**
Adults: Initially, 2.5 to 10 mg
fluphenazine hydrochloride P.O.
daily in divided doses every 6 to
8 hours; may increase cautiously to
20 mg. Maintenance dose is 1 to 5 mg
P.O. daily. I.M. doses are one-third to
one-half of P.O. doses. Usual I.M. dose
is 1.25 mg. Give more than 10 mg daily
with caution.
   Or, 12.5 to 25 mg of fluphenazine
decanoate I.M. or subcutaneously every
1 to 6 weeks; maintenance dose is 25 to
100 mg, as needed.
Elderly patients: 1 to 2.5 mg fluphenazine
hydrochloride P.O. daily.

ADMINISTRATION
P.O.
● Oral liquid forms can cause contact
dermatitis. Wear gloves when preparing
solutions, and avoid contact with skin and
clothing.
● Protect drug from light. Slight yellowing
of concentrate is common and doesn't
affect potency. Discard markedly discolored solutions.
● Dilute liquid concentrate with water,
fruit juice, milk, or semisolid food just
before administration.
I.M.
● Parenteral forms can cause contact
dermatitis. Wear gloves when preparing

solutions, and avoid contact with skin and
clothing.
● Protect drug from light. Slight yellowing
of injection is common and doesn't affect
potency. Discard markedly discolored
solutions.
● For long-acting form (decanoate), which
is an oil preparation, use a dry needle of at
least 21G.
Subcutaneous
● Long-acting form (decanoate) is indicated
for subcutaneous administration.
● Use a dry needle of at least 21G.

ACTION
A piperazine phenothiazine that probably
blocks postsynaptic dopamine receptors in
the brain.

Route	Onset	Peak	Duration
P.O.	< 1 hr	30 min	6–8 hr
I.M. (deca-noate)	24–72 hr	Unknown	1–6 wk
I.M. (hydro-chloride)	< 1 hr	90–120 min	6–8 hr
Subcut.	Unknown	Unknown	Unknown

Half-life: Hydrochloride, 15 hours;
decanoate, 7 to 10 days.

ADVERSE REACTIONS
CNS: *extrapyramidal reactions,*
tardive dyskinesia, pseudoparkinsonism,
seizures, neuroleptic malignant
syndrome, sedation, EEG changes,
drowsiness, dizziness.
CV: orthostatic hypotension, tachycardia,
ECG changes.
EENT: *blurred vision,* ocular changes,
nasal congestion.
GI: *dry mouth, constipation,* increased
appetite.
GU: *urine retention,* dark urine,
menstrual irregularities, inhibited
ejaculation.
Hematologic: **leukopenia, agranulo-**
cytosis, aplastic anemia, thrombo-
cytopenia, eosinophilia, hemolytic
anemia.
Hepatic: cholestatic jaundice.
Metabolic: weight gain.
Skin: *mild photosensitivity reactions,*
allergic reactions.
Other: gynecomastia, galactorrhea.

INTERACTIONS
Drug-drug. *Antacids:* May inhibit absorption of oral phenothiazines. Separate antacid and phenothiazine doses by at least 2 hours.
Anticholinergics: May increase anticholinergic effects. Use together cautiously.
Barbiturates, lithium: May decrease phenothiazine effect and increase neurologic adverse effects. Monitor patient.
Centrally acting antihypertensives: May decrease antihypertensive effect. Monitor blood pressure.
CNS depressants: May increase CNS depression. Use together cautiously.
Drug-herb. *St. John's wort:* May increase risk of photosensitivity reactions. Advise patient to avoid excessive sunlight exposure.
Drug-lifestyle. *Alcohol use:* May increase CNS depression, especially that involving psychomotor skills. Strongly discourage alcohol use.
Sun exposure: May increase risk of photosensitivity reactions. Advise patient to avoid excessive sunlight exposure.

EFFECTS ON LAB TEST RESULTS
● May increase liver function test values. May decrease hemoglobin level and hematocrit.
● May increase eosinophil count. May decrease granulocyte, platelet, and WBC counts.
● May cause false-positive results for amylase, 5-hydroxyindoleacetic acid, urinary porphyrin, and urobilinogen tests and for urine pregnancy tests that use human chorionic gonadotropin.

CONTRAINDICATIONS & CAUTIONS
● Contraindicated in patients hypersensitive to drug and in those with coma, CNS depression, bone marrow suppression or other blood dyscrasia, subcortical damage, or liver damage.
● Use cautiously in elderly or debilitated patients and in those with pheochromocytoma, severe CV disease (may cause sudden drop in blood pressure), peptic ulcer, respiratory disorder, hypocalcemia, seizure disorder (may lower seizure threshold), severe reactions to insulin or electroconvulsive therapy, mitral insufficiency, glaucoma, or prostatic hyperplasia.

● Use cautiously in those exposed to extreme heat or cold (including antipyretic therapy) or phosphorus insecticides.
● Use parenteral form cautiously in patients who have asthma or are allergic to sulfites.

NURSING CONSIDERATIONS
● Monitor patient for tardive dyskinesia, which may occur after prolonged use. It may not appear until months or years later and may disappear spontaneously or persist for life, despite ending drug.
● **Alert:** Watch for signs and symptoms of neuroleptic malignant syndrome (extrapyramidal effects, hyperthermia, autonomic disturbance), which is rare but often fatal. It may not be related to length of drug use or type of neuroleptic; more than 60% of affected patients are men.
● Withhold dose and notify prescriber if patient, especially child or pregnant woman, develops signs or symptoms of blood dyscrasia (fever, sore throat, infection, cellulitis, weakness) or extrapyramidal reactions persisting longer than a few hours.
■ **Black Box Warning** Elderly patients with dementia-related psychosis treated with atypical or conventional antipsychotics are at increased risk for death. Antipsychotics aren't approved for the treatment of dementia-related psychosis. ■
● Don't withdraw drug abruptly unless serious adverse reactions occur.
● Abrupt withdrawal of long-term therapy may cause gastritis, nausea, vomiting, dizziness, tremor, feeling of warmth or cold, diaphoresis, tachycardia, headache, or insomnia.

PATIENT TEACHING
● Warn patient to avoid activities that require alertness and good coordination until effects of drug are known. Drowsiness and dizziness usually subside after first few weeks.
● Warn patient to avoid alcohol while taking drug.
● Tell patient to relieve dry mouth with sugarless gum or hard candy.
● Have patient report signs of urine retention or constipation.
● Advise patient to use sunblock and wear protective clothing to avoid sensitivity to the sun.
● Tell patient that drug may discolor urine.

haloperidol
ha-loe-PER-i-dole

Haldol, Novo-Peridol†

haloperidol decanoate
Haldol Decanoate, Haloperidol
LA†

haloperidol lactate
Haldol, Haldol Concentrate

Pharmacologic class:
phenylbutylpiperadine derivative
Pregnancy risk category C

AVAILABLE FORMS
haloperidol
Tablets: 0.5 mg, 1 mg, 2 mg, 5 mg, 10 mg,
20 mg
haloperidol decanoate
Injection: 50 mg/ml, 100 mg/ml
haloperidol lactate
Injection: 5 mg/ml
Oral concentrate: 2 mg/ml

INDICATIONS & DOSAGES
➤ **Psychotic disorders**
Adults and children older than age 12:
Dosage varies for each patient. Initially,
0.5 to 5 mg P.O. b.i.d. or t.i.d. Or, 2 to
5 mg I.M. lactate every 4 to 8 hours,
although hourly administration may be
needed until control is obtained. Maximum,
100 mg P.O. daily.
*Children ages 3 to 12 who weigh 15 to
40 kg (33 to 88 lb):* Initially, 0.5 mg P.O.
daily divided b.i.d. or t.i.d. May increase
dose by 0.5 mg at 5- to 7-day intervals,
depending on therapeutic response and
patient tolerance. Maintenance dose,
0.05 mg/kg to 0.15 mg/kg P.O. daily
given in two or three divided doses.
Severely disturbed children may need
higher doses.
➤ **Chronic psychosis requiring prolonged therapy**
Adults: 50 to 100 mg I.M. decanoate
every 4 weeks.
➤ **Nonpsychotic behavior
disorders**
Children ages 3 to 12: 0.05 to 0.075 mg/kg
P.O. daily, in two or three divided doses.
Maximum, 6 mg daily.

➤ **Tourette syndrome**
Adults: 0.5 to 5 mg P.O. b.i.d., t.i.d., or as
needed.
Children ages 3 to 12: 0.05 to 0.075 mg/kg
P.O. daily, in two or three divided doses.
Elderly patients: 0.5 to 2 mg P.O.
b.i.d. or t.i.d.; increase gradually,
as needed.
Adjust-a-dose: For debilitated patients,
initially, 0.5 to 2 mg P.O. b.i.d. or t.i.d.;
increase gradually, as needed.
➤ **Delirium ◆**
Adults: 1 to 2 mg I.V. lactate every 2 to
4 hours. Severely agitated patients may
require higher doses.
Elderly patients: 0.25 to 0.5 mg I.V. every
4 hours.

ADMINISTRATION
P.O.
● Protect drug from light. Slight yellowing
of concentrate is common and doesn't
affect potency. Discard very discolored
solutions.
● Dilute oral dose with water or a beverage, such as orange juice, apple juice,
tomato juice, or cola, immediately before
administration.
I.V.
● Only the lactate form can be given I.V.
● Monitor patient receiving single doses
higher than 50 mg or total daily doses
greater than 500 mg closely for prolonged QTc interval and torsades de
pointes.
● Store at controlled room temperature,
and protect from light.
● **Incompatibilities:** Allopurinol, amphotericin B cholesteryl sulfate complex,
benztropine, cefepime, diphenhydramine,
fluconazole, foscarnet, heparin, hydromorphone, hydroxyzine, ketorolac,
morphine, nitroprusside sodium,
piperacillin and tazobactam sodium,
sargramostim.
I.M.
● Protect drug from light. Slight yellowing
of injection is common and doesn't
affect potency. Discard very discolored
solutions.
● When switching from tablets to
decanoate injection, give 10 to 15 times
the oral dose once a month (maximum
100 mg).
● **Alert:** Don't give decanoate form I.V.

ACTION

A butyrophenone that probably exerts antipsychotic effects by blocking post-synaptic dopamine receptors in the brain.

Route	Onset	Peak	Duration
P.O.	Unknown	3–6 hr	Unknown
I.V.	Unknown	Unknown	Unknown
I.M. (decanoate)	Unknown	3–9 days	Unknown
I.M. (lactate)	Unknown	10–20 min	Unknown

Half-life: P.O., 24 hours; I.M., 21 hours.

ADVERSE REACTIONS

CNS: *severe extrapyramidal reactions, tardive dyskinesia,* **neuroleptic malignant syndrome, seizures,** sedation, drowsiness, lethargy, headache, insomnia, confusion, vertigo.
CV: tachycardia, hypotension, hypertension, ECG changes, ***torsades de pointes,*** with I.V. use.
EENT: blurred vision.
GI: dry mouth, anorexia, constipation, diarrhea, nausea, vomiting, dyspepsia.
GU: urine retention, menstrual irregularities, priapism.
Hematologic: *leukopenia,* leukocytosis.
Hepatic: jaundice.
Skin: rash, other skin reactions, diaphoresis.
Other: gynecomastia.

INTERACTIONS

Drug-drug. *Anticholinergics:* May increase anticholinergic effects and glaucoma. Use together cautiously.
Azole antifungals, buspirone, macrolides: May increase haloperidol level. Monitor patient for increased adverse reactions; haloperidol dose may need to be adjusted.
Carbamazepine: May decrease haloperidol level. Monitor patient.
CNS depressants: May increase CNS depression. Use together cautiously.
Lithium: May cause lethargy and confusion after high doses. Monitor patient.
Methyldopa: May cause dementia. Monitor patient closely.
Rifampin: May decrease haloperidol level. Monitor patient for clinical effect.
Drug-lifestyle. *Alcohol use:* May increase CNS depression. Discourage use together.

EFFECTS ON LAB TEST RESULTS

● May increase liver function test values.
● May increase or decrease WBC count.

CONTRAINDICATIONS & CAUTIONS

● Contraindicated in patients hypersensitive to drug and in those with parkinsonism, coma, or CNS depression.
● Use cautiously in elderly and debilitated patients; in patients with history of seizures or EEG abnormalities, severe CV disorders, allergies, glaucoma, or urine retention; and in those taking anticonvulsants, anticoagulants, antiparkinsonians, or lithium.

NURSING CONSIDERATIONS

● Monitor patient for tardive dyskinesia, which may occur after prolonged use. It may not appear until months or years later and may disappear spontaneously or persist for life, despite ending drug.
● *Alert:* Watch for signs and symptoms of neuroleptic malignant syndrome (extrapyramidal effects, hyperthermia, autonomic disturbance), which is rare but commonly fatal.
■ **Black Box Warning** Elderly patients with dementia-related psychosis treated with atypical or conventional antipsychotics are at increased risk for death. Antipsychotics aren't approved for the treatment of dementia-related psychosis. ■
● Don't withdraw drug abruptly unless required by severe adverse reactions.
● *Alert:* Haldol may contain tartrazine.
● *Look alike–sound alike:* Don't confuse Haldol with Halcion or Halog.

PATIENT TEACHING

● Although drug is the least sedating of the antipsychotics, warn patient to avoid activities that require alertness and good coordination until effects of drug are known. Drowsiness and dizziness usually subside after a few weeks.
● Warn patient to avoid alcohol during therapy.
● Tell patient to relieve dry mouth with sugarless gum or hard candy.

Reactions may be *common,* uncommon, *life-threatening,* or COMMON AND LIFE-THREATENING.
Interaction may have a *rapid onset* or *delayed onset.*

lithium carbonate
LITH-ee-um

Carbolith†, Duralith†, Eskalith, Lithane†, Lithobid

lithium citrate
Cibalith-S*

Pharmacologic class: alkali metal
Pregnancy risk category D

AVAILABLE FORMS
lithium carbonate
Capsules: 150 mg, 300 mg, 600 mg
Tablets: 300 mg (300 mg equals 8.12 mEq lithium)
Tablets (extended-release): 300 mg, 450 mg
lithium citrate
Syrup (sugarless): 8 mEq lithium/5 ml;
5 ml lithium citrate liquid contains 8 mEq lithium, equal to 300 mg lithium carbonate

INDICATIONS & DOSAGES
➤ **To prevent or control mania**
Adults: 600 mg P.O. t.i.d. Or, 900-mg controlled-release tablets P.O. every 12 hours. Increase dosage based on blood levels to achieve optimum dosage. Recommended therapeutic lithium levels are 1 to 1.5 mEq/L for acute mania and 0.6 to 1.2 mEq/L for maintenance therapy.

ADMINISTRATION
P.O.
● Give drug after meals with plenty of water to minimize GI upset.
● Don't crush controlled-release tablets.

ACTION
Probably alters chemical transmitters in the CNS, possibly by interfering with ionic pump mechanisms in brain cells, and may compete with or replace sodium ions.

Route	Onset	Peak	Duration
P.O.	Unknown	30 min–3 hr	Unknown

Half-life: 18 hours (adolescents) to 36 hours (elderly).

ADVERSE REACTIONS
CNS: *fatigue, lethargy,* **coma, epileptiform seizures,** tremors, drowsiness, headache, confusion, restlessness, dizziness, psychomotor retardation, blackouts, EEG changes, worsened organic mental syndrome, impaired speech, ataxia, incoordination.
CV: **arrhythmias, bradycardia,** reversible ECG changes, hypotension.
EENT: tinnitus, blurred vision.
GI: *vomiting, anorexia, diarrhea, thirst,* nausea, metallic taste, dry mouth, abdominal pain, flatulence, indigestion.
GU: *polyuria,* **renal toxicity with long-term use,** glycosuria, decreased creatinine clearance, albuminuria.
Hematologic: *leukocytosis with leukocyte count of 14,000 to 18,000/mm³.*
Metabolic: transient hyperglycemia, goiter, hypothyroidism, hyponatremia.
Musculoskeletal: *muscle weakness.*
Skin: pruritus, rash, diminished or absent sensation, drying and thinning of hair, psoriasis, acne, alopecia.
Other: ankle and wrist edema.

INTERACTIONS
Drug-drug. *ACE inhibitors:* May increase lithium level. Monitor lithium level; adjust lithium dosage, as needed.
Aminophylline, sodium bicarbonate, urine alkalinizers: May increase lithium excretion. Avoid excessive salt, and monitor lithium levels.
Calcium channel blockers (verapamil): May decrease lithium levels and may increase risk of neurotoxicity. Use together cautiously.
Carbamazepine, fluoxetine, methyldopa, NSAIDs, probenecid: May increase effect of lithium. Monitor patient for lithium toxicity.
Neuromuscular blockers: May cause prolonged paralysis or weakness. Monitor patient closely.
Thiazide diuretics: May increase reabsorption of lithium by kidneys, with possible toxic effect. Use with caution, and monitor lithium and electrolyte levels (especially sodium).
Drug-food. *Caffeine:* May decrease lithium level and drug effect. Advise patient who ingests large amounts of caffeine to tell prescriber before stopping caffeine. Adjust lithium dosage, as needed.

EFFECTS ON LAB TEST RESULTS
● May increase glucose and creatinine and TSH levels. May decrease sodium, T_3, T_4, and protein-bound iodine levels.
● May increase ^{131}I uptake and WBC and neutrophil counts.

CONTRAINDICATIONS & CAUTIONS
● Contraindicated if therapy can't be closely monitored
● Avoid using in pregnant patient unless benefits outweigh risks.
● Use with caution in patients receiving neuromuscular blockers and diuretics; in elderly or debilitated patients; and in patients with thyroid disease, seizure disorder, infection, renal or CV disease, severe debilitation or dehydration, or sodium depletion.

NURSING CONSIDERATIONS
■ **Black Box Warning** Drug has a narrow therapeutic margin of safety. Determining drug level is crucial to safe use of drug. Don't use drug in patients who can't have regular tests. Monitor level 8 to 12 hours after first dose, the morning before second dose is given, two or three times weekly for the first month, and then weekly to monthly during maintenance therapy. ■
● When drug level is less than 1.5 mEq/L, adverse reactions are usually mild.
● Monitor baseline ECG, thyroid studies, renal studies, and electrolyte levels.
● Check fluid intake and output, especially when surgery is scheduled.
● Weigh patient daily; check for edema or sudden weight gain.
● Adjust fluid and salt ingestion to compensate if excessive loss occurs from protracted diaphoresis or diarrhea. Under normal conditions, patient fluid intake should be 2½ to 3 L daily, and he should follow a balanced diet with adequate salt intake.
● Check urine specific gravity and report level below 1.005, which may indicate diabetes insipidus.
● Drug alters glucose tolerance in diabetics. Monitor glucose level closely.
● Perform outpatient follow-up of thyroid and renal functions every 6 to 12 months. Palpate thyroid to check for enlargement.
● *Look alike–sound alike:* Don't confuse Lithobid with Levbid.

PATIENT TEACHING
● Tell patient to take drug with plenty of water and after meals to minimize GI upset.
● Explain the importance of having regular blood tests to determine drug levels; even slightly high values can be dangerous.
● Warn patient and caregivers to expect transient nausea, large amounts of urine, thirst, and discomfort during first few days of therapy and to watch for evidence of toxicity (diarrhea, vomiting, tremor, drowsiness, muscle weakness, incoordination).
● Instruct patient to withhold one dose and call prescriber if signs and symptoms of toxicity appear, but not to stop drug abruptly.
● Warn patient to avoid hazardous activities that require alertness and good psychomotor coordination until CNS effects of drug are known.
● Tell patient not to switch brands or take other prescription or OTC drugs without prescriber's guidance.
● Tell patient to wear or carry medical identification at all times.

loxapine succinate
LOX-a-peen

Pharmacologic class: dibenzapine derivative
Pregnancy risk category NR

AVAILABLE FORMS
Capsules: 5 mg, 10 mg, 25 mg, 50 mg

INDICATIONS & DOSAGES
➤ **Psychotic disorders**
Adults: 10 mg P.O. b.i.d. to q.i.d., rapidly increasing to 60 to 100 mg P.O. daily for most patients; dosage varies.
Elderly patients: Initially, 5 mg P.O. b.i.d. Adjust dosage as needed and as tolerated.

ADMINISTRATION
P.O.
● Give drug without regard for food.

ACTION
Unknown. Probably exerts antipsychotic effects by blocking postsynaptic dopamine receptors in the brain.

Route	Onset	Peak	Duration
P.O.	30 min	90 min–3 hr	12 hr

Half-life: 8 hours.

ADVERSE REACTIONS

CNS: *extrapyramidal reactions, sedation, tardive dyskinesia,* **neuroleptic malignant syndrome, seizures,** drowsiness, numbness, confusion, syncope, pseudoparkinsonism, EEG changes, dizziness.
CV: orthostatic hypotension, tachycardia, ECG changes, hypertension.
EENT: *blurred vision,* nasal congestion.
GI: *dry mouth, constipation,* nausea, vomiting, paralytic ileus.
GU: *urine retention,* menstrual irregularities.
Hematologic: *leukopenia, agranulocytosis, thrombocytopenia.*
Hepatic: jaundice.
Metabolic: weight gain.
Skin: allergic reactions, rash, pruritus.
Other: gynecomastia, galactorrhea.

INTERACTIONS

Drug-drug. *Anticholinergics:* May increase anticholinergic effect. Use together cautiously.
CNS depressants: May increase CNS depression. Use together cautiously.
Epinephrine: May inhibit vasopressor effect of epinephrine. Avoid using together.
Drug-lifestyle. *Alcohol use:* May increase CNS depression. Discourage use together.

EFFECTS ON LAB TEST RESULTS

• May increase liver function test values. May decrease WBC, granulocyte, and platelet counts.
• May cause false-positive results for urinary porphyrin, urobilinogen, amylase, and 5-hydroxyindoleacetic acid tests and for urine pregnancy tests that use human chorionic gonadotropin.

CONTRAINDICATIONS & CAUTIONS

• Contraindicated in patients hypersensitive to dibenzapines, in those in a coma, and in those with severe CNS depression or drug-induced depressed states.
• Use cautiously in patients with seizure disorder, CV disorder, glaucoma, or history of urine retention.

NURSING CONSIDERATIONS

• Obtain baseline blood pressure measurements before starting therapy and monitor pressure regularly.
• Monitor patient for tardive dyskinesia, which may occur after prolonged use. It may not appear until months or years later and may disappear spontaneously or persist for life, despite ending drug.
• *Alert:* Watch for evidence of neuroleptic malignant syndrome (extrapyramidal effects, hyperthermia, autonomic disturbance), a rare but deadly disorder.
■ **Black Box Warning** Elderly patients with dementia-related psychosis treated with atypical or conventional antipsychotics are at increased risk for death. Antipsychotics aren't approved for the treatment of dementia-related psychosis. ■

PATIENT TEACHING

• Warn patient to avoid activities that require alertness and good coordination until effects of drug are known. Drowsiness and dizziness usually subside after first few weeks.
• Advise patient to report bruising, fever, or sore throat immediately.
• Tell patient to avoid alcohol while taking drug.
• Advise patient to get up slowly to avoid dizziness upon standing quickly.
• Tell patient to relieve dry mouth with sugarless gum or hard candy.
• Recommend periodic eye examinations.

olanzapine
oh-LAN-za-peen

Zyprexa, Zyprexa Zydis

Pharmacologic class: dibenzapine derivative
Pregnancy risk category C

AVAILABLE FORMS
Injection: 10 mg
Tablets: 2.5 mg, 5 mg, 7.5 mg, 10 mg, 15 mg, 20 mg
Tablets (orally disintegrating): 5 mg, 10 mg, 15 mg, 20 mg

INDICATIONS & DOSAGES

➤ **Schizophrenia**
Adults: Initially, 5 to 10 mg P.O. once daily with the goal to be at 10 mg daily within several days of starting therapy. Adjust dose in 5-mg increments at intervals of 1 week or more. Most patients respond to 10 to 15 mg daily. Safety of dosages greater than 20 mg daily hasn't been established.

➤ **Short-term treatment of acute manic episodes linked to bipolar I disorder**
Adults: Initially, 10 to 15 mg P.O. daily. Adjust dosage as needed in 5-mg daily increments at intervals of 24 hours or more. Maximum, 20 mg P.O. daily. Duration of treatment is 3 to 4 weeks.

➤ **Short-term treatment, with lithium or valproate, of acute manic episodes linked to bipolar I disorder**
Adults: 10 mg P.O. once daily. Dosage range is 5 to 20 mg daily. Duration of treatment is 6 weeks.

➤ **Long-term treatment of bipolar I disorder**
Adults: 5 to 20 mg P.O. daily.

➤ **Adjunct to lithium or valproate to treat bipolar mania**
Adults: 10 mg P.O. daily. Usual range 5 to 20 mg daily.

Adjust-a-dose: In elderly or debilitated patients, those predisposed to hypotensive reactions, patients who may metabolize olanzapine more slowly than usual (nonsmoking women older than age 65) or may be more pharmacodynamically sensitive to olanzapine, initially, 5 mg P.O. Increase dose cautiously.

➤ **Agitation caused by schizophrenia and bipolar I mania**
Adults: 10 mg I.M. (range 2.5 to 10 mg). Subsequent doses of up to 10 mg may be given 2 hours after the first dose or 4 hours after the second dose, up to 30 mg I.M. daily. If maintenance therapy is required, convert patient to 5 to 20 mg P.O. daily.

Adjust-a-dose: In elderly patients, give 5 mg I.M. In debilitated patients, in those predisposed to hypotension, and in patients sensitive to effects of drug, give 2.5 mg I.M.

ADMINISTRATION
P.O.
● Give drug without regard for food.

● Don't crush or break orally disintegrating tablet (ODT).
● Place immediately on patient's tongue after opening package.
● ODT may be given without water.
I.M.
● Inspect I.M. solution for particulate matter and discoloration before administration.
● To reconstitute I.M. injection, dissolve contents of one vial with 2.1 ml of sterile water for injection to yield a clear yellow 5 mg/ml solution. Store at room temperature and give within 1 hour of reconstitution. Discard any unused solution.

ACTION
May block dopamine and 5-HT$_2$ receptors.

Route	Onset	Peak	Duration
P.O.	Unknown	6 hr	Unknown
I.M.	Rapid	15–45 min	Unknown

Half-life: 21 to 54 hours.

ADVERSE REACTIONS
CNS: *somnolence, insomnia, parkinsonism, dizziness,* **neuroleptic malignant syndrome, suicide attempt,** abnormal gait, asthenia, personality disorder, akathisia, tremor, articulation impairment, tardive dyskinesia, fever, extrapyramidal events (I.M.).
CV: orthostatic hypotension, tachycardia, chest pain, hypertension, ecchymosis, peripheral edema, hypotension (I.M.).
EENT: amblyopia, rhinitis, pharyngitis, conjunctivitis.
GI: *constipation, dry mouth, dyspepsia,* increased appetite, increased salivation, vomiting, thirst.
GU: hematuria, metrorrhagia, urinary incontinence, UTI, amenorrhea, vaginitis.
Hematologic: *leukopenia.*
Metabolic: *hyperglycemia,* weight gain.
Musculoskeletal: joint pain, extremity pain, back pain, neck rigidity, twitching, hypertonia.
Respiratory: increased cough, dyspnea.
Skin: sweating, injection site pain (I.M.).
Other: flulike syndrome, injury.

INTERACTIONS
Drug-drug. *Antihypertensives:* May potentiate hypotensive effects. Monitor blood pressure closely.

Reactions may be *common,* uncommon, *life-threatening,* or COMMON AND LIFE-THREATENING.
Interaction may have a *rapid onset* or *delayed onset.*

Carbamazepine, omeprazole, rifampin: May increase clearance of olanzapine. Monitor patient.

Ciprofloxacin: May increase olanzapine level. Monitor patient for increased adverse effects.

Diazepam: May increase CNS effects. Monitor patient.

Dopamine agonists, levodopa: May cause antagonized activity of these drugs. Monitor patient.

Fluoxetine: May increase olanzapine level. Use together cautiously.

Fluvoxamine: May increase olanzapine level. May need to reduce olanzapine dose.

Drug-herb. *St. John's wort:* May decrease drug level. Discourage use together.

Drug-lifestyle. *Alcohol use:* May increase CNS effects. Discourage use together.

Smoking: May increase drug clearance. Urge patient to quit smoking.

EFFECTS ON LAB TEST RESULTS
• May increase AST, ALT, GGT, CK, triglyceride, and prolactin levels.
• May increase eosinophil count. May decrease WBC count.

CONTRAINDICATIONS & CAUTIONS
• Contraindicated in patients hypersensitive to drug.
• Use cautiously in patients with heart disease, cerebrovascular disease, conditions that predispose patient to hypotension, history of seizures or conditions that might lower the seizure threshold, and hepatic impairment.
• Use cautiously in elderly patients, those with a history of paralytic ileus, and those at risk for aspiration pneumonia, prostatic hyperplasia, or angle-closure glaucoma.

NURSING CONSIDERATIONS
• ODTs contain phenylalanine.
• Monitor patient for abnormal body temperature regulation, especially if he exercises, is exposed to extreme heat, takes anticholinergics, or is dehydrated.
• Obtain baseline and periodic liver function test results.
• Monitor patient for weight gain.
• *Alert:* Watch for evidence of neuroleptic malignant syndrome (hyperpyrexia, muscle rigidity, altered mental status, autonomic

instability), which is rare but commonly fatal. Stop drug immediately; monitor and treat patient as needed.
• *Alert:* Drug may cause hyperglycemia. Monitor patients with diabetes regularly. In patients with risk factors for diabetes, obtain fasting blood glucose test results at baseline and periodically.
• *Alert:* Monitor patient for symptoms of metabolic syndrome (significant weight gain and increased body mass index, hypertension, hyperglycemia, hypercholesterolemia, and hypertriglyceridemia).
• Monitor patient for tardive dyskinesia, which may occur after prolonged use. It may not appear until months or years later and may disappear spontaneously or persist for life, despite stopping drug.
• Periodically reevaluate the long-term usefulness of olanzapine.
■ **Black Box Warning** Drug may increase risk of cardiovascular or infection-related death in elderly patients with dementia. Olanzapine isn't approved to treat patients with dementia-related psychosis. ■
• A patient who feels dizzy or drowsy after an I.M. injection should remain recumbent until he can be assessed for orthostatic hypotension and bradycardia. He should rest until the feeling passes.
• *Alert:* Drug may increase the risk of suicidal thinking and behavior in young adults ages 18 to 24 during the first 2 months of treatment.
• *Look alike–sound alike:* Don't confuse olanzapine with olsalazine or Zyprexa with Zyrtec.

PATIENT TEACHING
• Warn patient to avoid hazardous tasks until full effects of drug are known.
• Warn patient against exposure to extreme heat; drug may impair body's ability to reduce temperature.
• Inform patient that he may gain weight.
• Advise patient to avoid alcohol.
• Tell patient to rise slowly to avoid dizziness upon standing up quickly.
• Inform patient that ODTs contain phenylalanine.
• Tell patient to peel foil away from ODT, not to push tablet through. Have patient take tablet immediately, allowing tablet to dissolve on tongue and be swallowed with saliva; no additional fluid is needed.

- Tell patient to take drug with or without food.
- Urge woman of childbearing age to notify prescriber if she becomes pregnant or plans or suspects pregnancy. Tell her not to breast-feed during therapy.

paliperidone
pahl-ee-PEHR-ih-dohn

Invega

Pharmacologic class:
benzisoxazole derivative
Pregnancy risk category C

AVAILABLE FORMS
Tablets (extended-release): 1.5 mg, 3 mg, 6 mg, 9 mg

INDICATIONS & DOSAGES
➤ **Schizophrenia**
Adults: 6 mg P.O. once daily in the morning; may increase or decrease dose by 3-mg increments to a range of 3 mg to 12 mg daily; don't exceed 12 mg per day.
Adjust-a-dose: In patients with creatinine clearance of 50 to 80 ml/minute, maximum dosage is 6 mg once daily; for patients with creatinine clearance of 10 to 49 ml/minute, maximum dosage is 3 mg once daily.

ADMINISTRATION
P.O.
- Don't crush or break tablets.

ACTION
May antagonize both central dopamine (D_2) and serotonin type 2 receptors; also alpha-1, alpha-2, and histamine-1 receptors. Drug is a major active metabolite of risperidone.

Route	Onset	Peak	Duration
P.O.	Unknown	24 hr	Unknown

Half-life: 23 hours.

ADVERSE REACTIONS
CNS: *akathisia, headache, parkinsonism, somnolence,* anxiety, asthenia, dizziness, dystonia, extrapyramidal disorder, fatigue, hypertonia, pyrexia, tremor, dyskinesia, hyperkinesia.

CV: abnormal T waves, hypertension, orthostatic hypotension, palpitations, sinus arrhythmia, tachycardia, AV BLOCK, *bundle branch block,* PROLONGED QTc INTERVAL.
EENT: blurred vision.
GI: abdominal pain, dry mouth, dyspepsia, nausea, salivary hypersecretion.
Metabolic: blood insulin increases, hyperprolactinemia.
Musculoskeletal: back pain, extremity pain.
Respiratory: cough.

INTERACTIONS
Drug-drug. *Drugs that prolong QTc intervals, such as antiarrhythmics (quinidine, procainamide, amiodarone, sotalol), antipsychotics (chlorpromazine, thioridazine), quinolone antibiotics (moxifloxacin):* May further prolong QTc interval. Avoid using together.
Levodopa, dopamine agonists: May antagonize effects of these drugs. Use cautiously together.
Central-acting drugs: May worsen CNS side effects. Use cautiously together.
Anticholinergics: May worsen side effects. Use cautiously together.
Antihypertensives: May worsen orthostatic hypotension. Avoid using together.
Drug-lifestyle. *Alcohol use:* May worsen CNS side effects. Discourage use together.

EFFECTS ON LAB TEST RESULTS
- May increase insulin and prolactin levels.

CONTRAINDICATIONS & CAUTIONS
- Contraindicated in patients hypersensitive to paliperidone or risperidone.
- ■ **Black Box Warning** Elderly patients with dementia-related psychosis treated with atypical or conventional antipsychotics are at increased risk for death. Antipsychotics aren't approved for the treatment of dementia-related psychosis. ■
- Contraindicated in dementia-related psychosis.
- Contraindicated in patients with congenital long QT syndrome or history of cardiac arrhythmias.
- Contraindicated in patients with preexisting severe GI narrowing (esophageal

motility disorders, small bowel inflammatory disease, short gut syndrome).
• Use cautiously in patients with a history of seizures or diabetes; those at risk for aspiration pneumonia; and those with bradycardia, hypokalemia, hypomagnesemia, CV disease, cerebrovascular disease, dehydration, or hypovolemia.
• Use cautiously in patients taking antihypertensives and drugs that lower the seizure threshold.
• Use cautiously in patients with history of suicide attempts.

NURSING CONSIDERATIONS
• *Alert:* Monitor patient for atypical ventricular tachycardia, such as torsades de pointes, and ECG changes, particularly lengthening of the QT interval.
• Obtain baseline blood pressure before starting therapy and monitor pressure regularly. Watch for orthostatic hypotension.
• *Alert:* Watch for evidence of neuroleptic malignant syndrome (extrapyramidal effects, hyperthermia, autonomic disturbance), which is rare but deadly.
• Monitor patient for tardive dyskinesia; it may disappear spontaneously or persist for life, despite ending drug. Seek smallest dosage and shortest duration of treatment that produce a satisfactory clinical response. Periodically reassess need for continued treatment.
• *Alert:* Drug may cause hyperglycemia. Monitor patient with diabetes regularly. In patient with risk factors for diabetes, obtain fasting blood glucose test results at baseline and periodically.
• Monitor patient for seizure activity, especially if patient has conditions that lower the seizure threshold.
• Monitor patient for dysphagia that can lead to aspiration and aspiration pneumonia.
• Monitor patient for abnormal body temperature regulation, especially if he exercises, is exposed to extreme heat, takes anticholinergics, or is dehydrated.
• Monitor patient for somnolence and sedation. Antipsychotics, including paliperidone, have the potential to impair judgment, thinking, or motor skills.
• Dispense lowest appropriate quantity of drug, to reduce risk of overdose.

PATIENT TEACHING
• Tell patient that remains of the tablet may appear in feces.
• Tell patient to swallow whole with liquids and not to chew, crush, or break tablets.
• Instruct the patient not to perform activities that require mental alertness until effects of drug are known.
• Warn patient to use caution in performing excessively strenuous activities because his body temperature may be disrupted.
• Advise patient that drug may lower blood pressure and to change positions slowly.
• Instruct patient to contact prescriber before taking any other drugs to avoid potential interactions.
• Advise patient to avoid alcohol while taking this medication.
• Advise patient to contact prescriber if she becomes pregnant or wants to breast-feed.

---

perphenazine
per-FEN-uh-zeen

Pharmacologic class:
phenothiazine
Pregnancy risk category C

AVAILABLE FORMS
Oral concentrate: 16 mg/5 ml
Tablets: 2 mg, 4 mg, 8 mg, 16 mg

INDICATIONS & DOSAGES
➤ **Psychosis in nonhospitalized patients**
Adults and children older than age 12: Initially, 4 to 8 mg P.O. t.i.d.; reduce as soon as possible to minimum effective dose.
➤ **Psychosis in hospitalized patients**
Adults and children older than age 12: Initially, 8 to 16 mg P.O. b.i.d., t.i.d., or q.i.d.; increase to 64 mg daily, as needed.
➤ **Severe nausea and vomiting, intractable hiccups**
Adults: 8 to 16 mg P.O. daily in divided doses to maximum of 24 mg.

ADMINISTRATION
P.O.
• Dilute liquid concentrate with fruit juice, milk, carbonated beverage, or semisolid food just before giving. Don't use colas,

---

black coffee, grape juice, apple juice, or tea because turbidity or precipitation may result.

● Protect drug from light. Slight yellowing of concentrate is common and doesn't affect potency. Discard markedly discolored solutions.

ACTION
May exert antipsychotic effects by blocking postsynaptic dopamine receptors in the brain.

Route	Onset	Peak	Duration
P.O.	Unknown	Unknown	Unknown

Half-life: 9 to 12 hours.

ADVERSE REACTIONS
CNS: *extrapyramidal reactions, tardive dyskinesia,* **seizures, neuroleptic malignant syndrome,** sedation, pseudoparkinsonism, dizziness, drowsiness.
CV: *orthostatic hypotension,* tachycardia, ECG changes.
EENT: *blurred vision,* ocular changes, nasal congestion.
GI: *dry mouth, constipation,* nausea, vomiting, diarrhea.
GU: *urine retention,* dark urine, menstrual irregularities, inhibited ejaculation.
Hematologic: *leukopenia, agranulo-cytosis, thrombocytopenia,* eosinophilia, hemolytic anemia.
Hepatic: cholestatic jaundice.
Metabolic: weight gain.
Skin: *mild photosensitivity reactions,* allergic reactions, sterile abscess.
Other: gynecomastia.

INTERACTIONS
Drug-drug. *Antacids:* May inhibit absorption of oral phenothiazines. Separate antacid and phenothiazine doses by at least 2 hours.
Barbiturates: May decrease phenothiazine effect. Monitor patient.
CNS depressants: May increase CNS depression. Use together cautiously.
Fluoxetine, paroxetine, sertraline, tricyclic antidepressants: May increase phenothiazine level. Monitor patient for increased adverse effects.
Lithium: May increase neurologic adverse effects. Monitor patient closely.

Drug-herb. *St. John's wort:* May cause photosensitivity reactions. Advise patient to avoid excessive sunlight exposure.
Drug-lifestyle. *Alcohol use:* May increase CNS depression, particularly psychomotor skills. Strongly discourage alcohol use.
Sun exposure: May increase risk of photosensitivity reactions. Advise patient to avoid excessive sunlight exposure.

EFFECTS ON LAB TEST RESULTS
● May decrease hemoglobin level and hematocrit.
● May increase liver function test values and eosinophil count. May decrease WBC, granulocyte, and platelet counts.
● May cause false-positive results for urinary porphyrin, urobilinogen, amylase, and 5-hydroxyindoleacetic acid tests and for urine pregnancy tests that use human chorionic gonadotropin.

CONTRAINDICATIONS & CAUTIONS
● Contraindicated in patients hypersensitive to drug and in those with CNS depression, blood dyscrasia, bone marrow depression, liver damage, or subcortical damage; also contraindicated in those experiencing coma or receiving large doses of CNS depressants.
● Use cautiously in elderly or debilitated patients and in those taking other CNS depressants or anticholinergics.
● Use cautiously in patients with alcohol withdrawal, psychotic depression, suicidal tendency, severe adverse reactions to other phenothiazines, renal impairment, CV disease, or respiratory disorders.

NURSING CONSIDERATIONS
● Obtain baseline blood pressure measurements before starting therapy and monitor pressure regularly. Watch for orthostatic hypotension, especially with parenteral administration.
● Monitor patient for tardive dyskinesia, which may occur after prolonged use. It may not appear until months or years later and may disappear spontaneously or persist for life, despite ending drug.
● *Alert:* Watch for evidence of neuroleptic malignant syndrome (extrapyramidal effects, hyperthermia, autonomic disturbance), which is rare but deadly.

Reactions may be *common,* uncommon, *life-threatening,* or COMMON AND LIFE-THREATENING.
Interaction may have a *rapid onset* or **delayed onset.**

• Monitor therapy with weekly bilirubin tests during first month, periodic blood tests (CBCs and liver function tests), and ophthalmic tests (long-term use).
• Withhold dose and notify prescriber if jaundice, symptoms of blood dyscrasia (fever, sore throat, infection, cellulitis, weakness), or persistent extrapyramidal reactions (longer than a few hours) develop.

■ **Black Box Warning** Elderly patients with dementia-related psychosis treated with atypical or conventional antipsychotics are at increased risk for death. Antipsychotics aren't approved for the treatment of dementia-related psychosis. ■

• Don't withdraw drug abruptly unless severe adverse reactions occur.
• After abrupt withdrawal of long-term therapy, gastritis, nausea, vomiting, dizziness, tremor, feeling of warmth or cold, diaphoresis, tachycardia, headache, or insomnia may occur.

PATIENT TEACHING
• Tell patient which beverages he may use to dilute oral concentrate.
• Warn patient to avoid activities that require alertness or good coordination until effects of drug are known. Drowsiness and dizziness usually subside after a few weeks.
• Tell patient to avoid alcohol while taking drug.
• Advise patient to report signs of urine retention or constipation.
• Tell patient to use sunblock and wear protective clothing to avoid oversensitivity to the sun.
• Advise patient to relieve dry mouth with sugarless gum or hard candy.

---

quetiapine fumarate
kwe-TIE-ah-peen

Seroquel, Seroquel XR

Pharmacologic class:
dibenzothiazepine derivative
Pregnancy risk category C

AVAILABLE FORMS
Tablets: 25 mg, 50 mg, 100 mg, 200 mg, 300 mg, 400 mg

Tablets (extended-release): 50 mg, 150 mg, 200 mg, 300 mg, 400 mg

INDICATIONS & DOSAGES
➤ **Schizophrenia**
Adults: Initially, 25 mg P.O. b.i.d., with increases in increments of 25 to 50 mg b.i.d. or t.i.d. on days 2 and 3, as tolerated. Target range is 300 to 400 mg daily divided into two or three doses by day 4. Further dosage adjustments, if indicated, should occur at intervals of not less than 2 days. Dosage can be increased or decreased by 25 to 50 mg b.i.d. Effect generally occurs at 150 to 750 mg daily. Safety of dosages over 800 mg daily hasn't been evaluated.
Or, 300 mg/day extended-release tablets P.O. once daily, preferably in the evening. Titrate within a dose range of 400 to 800 mg/day, depending on the response and tolerance of the individual. Increase at intervals as short as 1 day and in increments of 300 mg/day.
Adjust-a-dose: Elderly patients: Titrate on immediate-release formula, starting at 25 mg/day. Use slow titration and regular monitoring; may be switched to extended-release formulation when stabilized on 200 mg/day. In patients with hepatic impairment, initial dose is 25 mg daily. Increase daily in increments of 25 to 50 mg daily to an effective dose; may be switched to extended-release formulation when stabilized on 200 mg/day. For debilitated patients and those with hypotension, consider lower dosages and slower adjustment.
➤ **Monotherapy and adjunct therapy with lithium or divalproex for the short-term treatment of acute manic episodes associated with bipolar I disorder; adjunct maintenance therapy with lithium or divalproex**
Adults: Initially, 50 mg P.O. b.i.d. Increase dosage in increments of 100 mg daily in two divided doses up to 200 mg P.O. b.i.d. on day 4. May increase dosage in increments no greater than 200 mg daily up to 800 mg daily by day 6. Usual dose is 400 to 800 mg daily. For maintenance therapy with lithium or divalproex, continue treatment at the dosage required to maintain symptom remission.

Adjust-a-dose: Elderly patients: Titrate on immediate release formula, starting at 25 mg/day. Use slow titration and regular monitoring. In patients with hepatic impairment, initial dose is 25 mg daily. Increase daily in increments of 25 to 50 mg daily in an effective dose. For debilitated patients and those with hypotension, consider lower dosages and slower adjustment.

➤ **Depression associated with bipolar disorder**

Adults: Initially, 50 mg P.O. once daily at bedtime; increase on day 2 to 100 mg; increase on day 3 to 200 mg; increase on day 4 to maintenance dose of 300 mg.

Adjust-a-dose: Elderly patients: Titrate on immediate-release formula, starting at 25 mg/day. Use slow titration and regular monitoring. In patients with hepatic impairment, initial dose is 25 mg daily. Increase daily in increments of 25 to 50 mg daily to an effective dose. For debilitated patients and those with hypotension, consider lower dosages and slower adjustment.

ADMINISTRATION
P.O.
- Don't break or crush extended-release tablets.
- Give drug without regard for food; give extended-release tablets without food or with a light meal (about 300 calories).
- Schizophrenic patients who are currently being treated with divided doses of the immediate-release form may be switched to extended-release tablets at the equivalent total daily dose taken once daily. Individual dosage adjustments may be necessary. Those requiring less than 200 mg/dose should remain on the immediate-release form.

ACTION
Blocks dopamine and serotonin 5-HT$_2$ receptors. Its action may be mediated through this antagonism.

Route	Onset	Peak	Duration
P.O.	Unknown	1½ hr	Unknown
P.O. extended-release	Unknown	6 hr	Unknown

Half-life: 6 hours, extended-release 7 to 12 hours.

ADVERSE REACTIONS
CNS: *dizziness, headache, somnolence,* **neuroleptic malignant syndrome,** **seizures,** hypertonia, dysarthria, asthenia.
CV: orthostatic hypotension, tachycardia, palpitations, peripheral edema.
EENT: ear pain, pharyngitis, rhinitis.
GI: dry mouth, dyspepsia, abdominal pain, constipation, anorexia.
Hematologic: *leukopenia.*
Metabolic: *weight gain,* hyperglycemia.
Musculoskeletal: back pain.
Respiratory: increased cough, dyspnea.
Skin: rash, diaphoresis.
Other: flulike syndrome.

INTERACTIONS
Drug-drug. *Antihypertensives:* May increase effects of antihypertensives. Monitor blood pressure.
Carbamazepine, glucocorticoids, phenobarbital, phenytoin, rifampin, thioridazine: May increase quetiapine clearance. May need to adjust quetiapine dosage.
CNS depressants: May increase CNS effects. Use together cautiously.
Dopamine agonists, levodopa: May antagonize the effects of these drugs. Monitor patient.
Erythromycin, fluconazole, itraconazole, ketoconazole: May decrease quetiapine clearance. Use together cautiously.
Lorazepam: May decrease lorazepam clearance. Monitor patient for increased CNS effects.
Drug-lifestyle. *Alcohol use:* May increase CNS effects. Discourage use together.

EFFECTS ON LAB TEST RESULTS
- May increase liver enzyme, cholesterol, triglyceride, and glucose levels. May decrease T$_4$ and thyroid-stimulating hormone levels.
- May decrease WBC count.

CONTRAINDICATIONS & CAUTIONS
- Contraindicated in patients hypersensitive to drug or its ingredients.
- Use cautiously in patients with CV disease, cerebrovascular disease, conditions that predispose to hypotension, a history of seizures or conditions that lower the seizure threshold, and conditions in which core body temperature may be elevated.

• Use cautiously in patients at risk for aspiration pneumonia.

■ **Black Box Warning** Drug isn't approved for use in children. ■

NURSING CONSIDERATIONS

• Dispense lowest appropriate quantity of drug to reduce risk of overdose.

■ **Black Box Warning** Drug isn't indicated for use in elderly patients with dementia-related psychosis because of increased risk of death from CV disease or infection. ■

• *Alert:* Watch for evidence of neuroleptic malignant syndrome (extrapyramidal effects, hyperthermia, autonomic disturbance), which is rare but deadly.

• Monitor patient for tardive dyskinesia, which may occur after prolonged use. It may not appear until months or years later and may disappear spontaneously or persist for life, despite ending drug.

• Hyperglycemia may occur in patients taking drug. Monitor patients with diabetes regularly.

• Monitor patient for weight gain.

• *Alert:* Monitor patient for symptoms of metabolic syndrome (significant weight gain and increased body mass index, hypertension, hyperglycemia, hyper-cholesterolemia, and hypertriglyceridemia).

• Drug use may cause cataract formation. Obtain baseline ophthalmologic examination and reassess every 6 months.

■ **Black Box Warning** Drug (immediate-release tablets) may increase the risk of suicidal thinking and behavior in children, adolescents, and young adults ages 18 to 24 during the first 2 months of treatment, especially in those with major depressive or other psychiatric disorder. ■

PATIENT TEACHING

• Warn patient about risk of dizziness when standing up quickly. The risk is greatest during the 3- to 5-day period of first dosage adjustment, when resuming treatment, and when increasing dosages.

• Tell patient to avoid becoming over-heated or dehydrated.

• Warn patient to avoid activities that require mental alertness until effects of drug are known, especially during first dosage adjustment or dosage increases.

• Remind patient to have an eye examination at start of therapy and every 6 months during therapy to check for cataracts.

• Tell patient to notify prescriber about other prescription or OTC drugs he's taking or plans to take.

• Tell woman of childbearing age to notify prescriber about planned, suspected, or known pregnancy.

• Advise her not to breast-feed during therapy.

• Advise patient to avoid alcohol while taking drug.

• Tell patient to take drug with or without food.

• Tell patient not to crush, chew, or break extended-release tablets.

• Tell patient to take extended-release tablets without food or with a light meal.

---

risperidone
ris-PEER-i-dohn

Risperdal*, Risperdal Consta

Pharmacologic class:
benzisoxazole derivative
Pregnancy risk category C

AVAILABLE FORMS

Injection: 12.5 mg, 25 mg, 37.5 mg, 50 mg
Solution: 1 mg/ml
Tablets: 0.25 mg, 0.5 mg, 1 mg, 2 mg, 3 mg, 4 mg
Tablets (orally disintegrating): 0.5 mg, 1 mg, 2 mg, 3 mg, 4 mg

INDICATIONS & DOSAGES

➤ **Schizophrenia**

Adults: Drug may be given once or twice daily. Initial dosing is generally 2 mg/day. Increase dosage at intervals not less than 24 hours, in increments of 1 to 2 mg/day, as tolerated, to a recommended dose of 4 to 8 mg/day. Periodically reassess to determine the need for maintenance treatment with an appropriate dose.

Adolescents ages 13 to 17: Start treatment with 0.5 mg once daily, given as a single daily dose in either the morning or evening. Adjust dose, if indicated, at intervals not less than 24 hours, in increments of 0.5 or 1 mg/day, as tolerated, to a

recommended dose of 3 mg/day. There are no data to support use beyond 8 weeks.

➤ **12-week parenteral therapy for schizophrenia**

Adults: Establish tolerance to oral risperidone before giving I.M. Give 25 mg deep I.M. into the buttock every 2 weeks, alternating injections between the two buttocks. Adjust dose no sooner than every 4 weeks. Maximum, 50 mg I.M. every 2 weeks. Continue oral antipsychotic for 3 weeks after first I.M. injection, then stop oral therapy.

Adjust-a-dose: Patients with hepatic or renal impairment: Titrate slowly to 2 mg P.O.; if tolerated, give 25 mg I.M. every 2 weeks, or give initial dose of 12.5 mg I.M. Continue oral form of risperidone (or another antipsychotic drug) with the first injection and for 3 subsequent weeks to maintain therapeutic drug levels.

➤ **Monotherapy or combination therapy with lithium or valproate for 3-week treatment of acute manic or mixed episodes from bipolar I disorder**

Adults: 2 to 3 mg P.O. once daily. Adjust dose by 1 mg daily. Dosage range is 1 to 6 mg daily.

Adjust-a-dose: In elderly or debilitated patients, hypotensive patients, or those with severe renal or hepatic impairment, start with 0.5 mg P.O. b.i.d. Increase dosage by 0.5 mg b.i.d. Increase in dosages above 1.5 mg b.i.d. should occur at least 1 week apart. Subsequent switches to once-daily dosing may be made after patient is on a twice-daily regimen for 2 to 3 days at the target dose.

Children and adolescents ages 10 to 17: 0.5 mg P.O. as a single daily dose in either the morning or evening. Adjust dose, if indicated, at intervals not less than 24 hours, in increments of 0.5 or 1 mg/day, as tolerated, to a recommended dose of 2.5 mg/day.

➤ **Irritability, including aggression, self-injury, and temper tantrums, associated with an autistic disorder**

Adolescents and children age 5 and older who weigh 20 kg (44 lb) or more: Initially, 0.5 mg P.O. once daily or divided b.i.d. After 4 days, increase dose to 1 mg. Increase dosage further in 0.5-mg increments at intervals of at least 2 weeks.

Children age 5 and older who weigh less than 20 kg: Initially, 0.25 mg P.O. once daily or divided b.i.d. After 4 days, increase dose to 0.5 mg. Increase dosage further in 0.25-mg increments at intervals of at least 2 weeks. Increase cautiously in children who weigh less than 15 kg (33 lb).

➤ **Tourette syndrome ◆**

Adults and children: Initially, 0.5 to 1 mg P.O. daily. Titrate by 0.5 or 1 mg every 5 days. Average dose is less than 4 mg daily; maximum dose 6 to 9 mg daily.

ADMINISTRATION
P.O.
● Give drug without regard for meals.
● Open package for orally disintegrating tablets (ODTs) immediately before giving by peeling off foil backing with dry hands. Don't push tablets through the foil.
● Phenylalanine contents of ODTs are as follows: 0.5-mg tablet contains 0.14 mg phenylalanine; 1-mg tablet contains 0.28 mg phenylalanine; 2-mg tablet contains 0.56 mg phenylalanine; 3-mg tablet contains 0.63 mg phenylalanine; 4-mg tablet contains 0.84 mg phenylalanine.

I.M.
● Continue oral therapy for the first 3 weeks of I.M. injection therapy until injections take effect, then stop oral therapy.
● To reconstitute I.M. injection, inject premeasured diluent into vial and shake vigorously for at least 10 seconds. Suspension appears uniform, thick, and milky; particles are visible, but no dry particles remain. Use drug immediately, or refrigerate for up to 6 hours after reconstitution. If more than 2 minutes pass before injection, shake vigorously again. See manufacturer's package insert for more detailed instructions.
● Refrigerate I.M. injection kit and protect it from light. Drug can be stored at temperature less than 77° F (25° C) for no more than 7 days before administration.

ACTION
Blocks dopamine and 5-HT$_2$ receptors in the brain.

Route	Onset	Peak	Duration
P.O.	Unknown	1 hr	Unknown
I.M.	3 wk	4–6 wk	7 wk

Half-life: 3 to 20 hours.

ADVERSE REACTIONS

CNS: *akathisia, somnolence, dystonia, headache, insomnia, agitation, anxiety, pain, parkinsonism,* **neuroleptic malignant syndrome, suicide attempt,** dizziness, fever, hallucination, mania, impaired concentration, abnormal thinking and dreaming, tremor, hypoesthesia, fatigue, depression, nervousness.
CV: tachycardia, chest pain, orthostatic hypotension, peripheral edema, syncope, hypertension.
EENT: *rhinitis,* sinusitis, pharyngitis, abnormal vision, ear disorder (I.M.).
GI: *constipation, nausea, vomiting, dyspepsia, abdominal pain,* anorexia, dry mouth, increased saliva, diarrhea.
GU: urinary incontinence, increased urination, abnormal orgasm, vaginal dryness.
Metabolic: *weight gain, hyperglycemia,* weight loss.
Musculoskeletal: arthralgia, back pain, leg pain, myalgia.
Respiratory: coughing, dyspnea, upper respiratory infection.
Skin: rash, dry skin, photosensitivity reactions, acne, injection site pain (I.M.).
Other: tooth disorder, toothache, injury, decreased libido.

INTERACTIONS

Drug-drug. *Antihypertensives:* May enhance hypotensive effects. Monitor blood pressure.
Carbamazepine: May increase risperidone clearance and decrease effectiveness. Monitor patient closely.
Clozapine: May decrease risperidone clearance, increasing toxicity. Monitor patient closely.
CNS depressants: May cause additive CNS depression. Use together cautiously.
Dopamine agonists, levodopa: May antagonize effects of these drugs. Use together cautiously and monitor patient.
Fluoxetine, paroxetine: May increase the risk of risperidone's adverse effects, including serotonin syndrome. Monitor patient closely and adjust risperidone dose, as needed.
Drug-lifestyle. *Alcohol use:* May cause additive CNS depression. Discourage use together.

Sun exposure: May increase risk of photosensitivity reactions. Advise patient to avoid excessive sunlight exposure.

EFFECTS ON LAB TEST RESULTS

● May increase prolactin level. May decrease hemoglobin level and hematocrit.

CONTRAINDICATIONS & CAUTIONS

● Contraindicated in patients hypersensitive to drug and in breast-feeding women.
● Use cautiously in patients with prolonged QT interval, CV disease, cerebrovascular disease, dehydration, hypovolemia, history of seizures, or conditions that could affect metabolism or hemodynamic responses.
● Use cautiously in patients exposed to extreme heat.
● Use caution in patients at risk for aspiration pneumonia.
● Use I.M. injection cautiously in those with hepatic or renal impairment.

NURSING CONSIDERATIONS

● **Alert:** Obtain baseline blood pressure measurements before starting therapy, and monitor pressure regularly. Watch for orthostatic hypotension, especially during first dosage adjustment.
■ **Black Box Warning** Fatal cardiovascular or infectious adverse events may occur in elderly patients with dementia. Drug isn't safe or effective in these patients. ■
● Monitor patient for tardive dyskinesia, which may occur after prolonged use. It may not appear until months or years later and may disappear spontaneously or persist for life, despite stopping drug.
● **Alert:** Watch for evidence of neuroleptic malignant syndrome (extrapyramidal effects, hyperthermia, autonomic disturbance), which is rare but can be fatal.
● Life-threatening hyperglycemia may occur in patients taking atypical antipsychotics. Monitor patients with diabetes regularly.
● **Alert:** Monitor patient for symptoms of metabolic syndrome (significant weight gain and increased body mass index, hypertension, hyperglycemia, hypercholesterolemia, and hypertriglyceridemia).
● Periodically reevaluate drug's risks and benefits, especially during prolonged use.
● Monitor patient for weight gain.

- **Look alike–sound alike:** Don't confuse risperidone with reserpine.

PATIENT TEACHING
- Warn patient to avoid activities that require alertness until effects of drug are known.
- Warn patient to rise slowly, avoid hot showers, and use other precautions to avoid fainting when starting therapy.
- Advise patient to use caution in hot weather to prevent heatstroke.
- Tell patient to take drug with or without food.
- Instruct patient to keep the ODT in the blister pack until just before taking it. After opening the pack, dissolve the tablet on tongue without cutting or chewing. Use dry hands to peel apart the foil to expose the tablet; don't attempt to push it through the foil.
- Tell patient to use sunblock and wear protective clothing outdoors.
- Advise women not to become pregnant or to breast-feed for 12 weeks after the last I.M. injection.
- Advise patient to avoid alcohol during therapy.

---

thioridazine hydrochloride
thye-oh-RYE-da-zeen

Pharmacologic class:
phenothiazine
Pregnancy risk category C

AVAILABLE FORMS
Oral concentrate: 30 mg/ml, 100 mg/ml (3% to 4.2% alcohol)
Tablets: 10 mg, 15 mg, 25 mg, 50 mg, 100 mg

INDICATIONS & DOSAGES
➤ **Schizophrenia in patients who don't respond to treatment with at least two other anti-psychotic drugs**
Adults: Initially, 50 to 100 mg P.O. t.i.d., increase gradually to 800 mg daily in divided doses, as needed.
Children age 2 to 12: Initially, 0.5 mg/kg daily in divided doses. Increase gradually to optimal therapeutic effect; maximum dose is 3 mg/kg daily.

ADMINISTRATION
P.O.
- **Alert:** Different liquid formulations have different concentrations. Check dosage carefully.
- Prevent contact dermatitis by keeping drug away from skin and clothes. Wear gloves when preparing liquid forms.
- Dilute liquid concentrate with water or fruit juice just before giving.
- Shake suspension well before using.

ACTION
Unknown. A piperidine phenothiazine that probably blocks postsynaptic dopamine receptors in the brain.

Route	Onset	Peak	Duration
P.O.	Unknown	Unknown	Unknown

Half-life: 20 to 40 hours.

ADVERSE REACTIONS
CNS: *tardive dyskinesia, sedation,* **neuroleptic malignant syndrome,** EEG changes, dizziness.
CV: *orthostatic hypotension,* **prolonged QTc interval, torsades de pointes,** ECG changes, tachycardia.
EENT: *ocular changes, blurred vision,* retinitis pigmentosa.
GI: *dry mouth, constipation,* increased appetite.
GU: *urine retention,* dark urine, menstrual irregularities, inhibited ejaculation.
Hematologic: *transient leukopenia,* **agranulocytosis,** hyperprolactinemia.
Hepatic: cholestatic jaundice.
Metabolic: weight gain.
Skin: *mild photosensitivity reactions,* allergic reactions.
Other: gynecomastia, galactorrhea.

INTERACTIONS
Drug-drug. *Antacids:* May inhibit absorption of oral phenothiazines. Separate dosages by at least 2 hours.
antiarrhythmics (amiodarone, bretylium, disopyramide, dofetilide, procainamide, quinidine, sotalol), duloxetine, fluoxetine, fluvoxamine, paroxetine, pimozide, pindolol, propranolol, other drugs that inhibit CYP2D6 enzyme, *quinolones:* May inhibit metabolism of thioridazine; may cause arrhythmias resulting from QTc interval

---

Reactions may be *common,* uncommon, *life-threatening,* or COMMON AND LIFE-THREATENING.
Interaction may have a *rapid onset* or **delayed onset.**

prolongation. Use together is contraindicated.
Barbiturates: May decrease phenothiazine
effect. Monitor patient.
Centrally acting antihypertensives: May
decrease antihypertensive effect. Monitor
blood pressure.
Lithium: May decrease phenothiazine
effect and increase neurologic adverse
effects. Monitor patient closely.
Other CNS depressants: May increase
CNS depression. Use together cautiously.
Drug-herb. *St. John's wort:* May
cause photosensitivity reactions. Advise
patient to avoid excessive sunlight
exposure.
Drug-lifestyle. *Alcohol use:* May increase
CNS depression, particularly psychomotor
skills. Strongly discourage use together.
Sun exposure: May increase risk of photosensitivity reactions. Advise patient to
avoid excessive sunlight exposure.

EFFECTS ON LAB TEST RESULTS
• May increase liver enzyme levels.
• May decrease granulocyte and WBC
counts.
• May cause false-positive results for
urinary porphyrin, urobilinogen, amylase,
and 5-hydroxyindoleacetic acid tests and
for urine pregnancy tests that use human
chorionic gonadotropin.

CONTRAINDICATIONS & CAUTIONS
• Contraindicated in patients hypersensitive
to drug and in those with CNS depression,
coma, or severe hypertensive or hypotensive cardiac disease.
• Contraindicated in patients taking
fluvoxamine, propranolol, pindolol, fluoxetine, drugs that inhibit CYP2D6 enzyme,
or drugs that prolong the QTc interval.
• Contraindicated in patients with reduced
levels of CYP2D6 enzyme, those with
congenital long QT interval syndrome, or
those with history of cardiac arrhythmias.
• Use cautiously in elderly or debilitated
patients and in patients with hepatic disease, CV disease, respiratory disorders,
hypocalcemia, seizure disorders, or severe
reactions to insulin or electroconvulsive
therapy.
• Use cautiously in those exposed to extreme heat or cold (including antipyretic
therapy) or organophosphate insecticides.

NURSING CONSIDERATIONS
• *Alert:* Before therapy, obtain baseline
ECG and potassium level. Patients with
a QTc interval greater than 450 msec
shouldn't receive drug. Patients with a
QTc interval greater than 500 msec should
stop drug.
■ **Black Box Warning** Thioridazine has
been shown to prolong the QTc interval
and may cause torsade de pointes–type
arrhythmias and sudden death. Reserve
thioridazine for the treatment of schizophrenic patients who fail to show an
acceptable response to adequate courses
of treatment with other antipsychotics. ■
• Monitor patient for tardive dyskinesia,
which may occur after prolonged use.
It may not appear until months or
years later and may disappear spontaneously or persist for life, despite
ending drug.
■ **Black Box Warning** Elderly patients
with dementia-related psychosis treated
with atypical or conventional antipsychotics are at increased risk for
death. Antipsychotics aren't approved
for the treatment of dementia-related
psychosis. ■
• *Alert:* Watch for evidence of neuroleptic
malignant syndrome (extrapyramidal
effects, hyperthermia, autonomic disturbance), which is rare but commonly
deadly.
• Monitor periodic blood tests (CBCs and
liver function tests) and ophthalmic tests
(long-term use).
• Withhold dose and notify prescriber if
jaundice, blood dyscrasia (fever, sore
throat, infection, cellulitis, weakness),
or persistent extrapyramidal reactions
develop, especially in children or pregnant
women.
• Don't stop drug abruptly unless required
by severe adverse reactions.
• After abrupt withdrawal of long-term
therapy, gastritis, nausea, vomiting, dizziness, tremor, feeling of warmth or cold,
diaphoresis, tachycardia, headache, or
insomnia may occur.
• *Look alike–sound alike:* Don't confuse
thioridazine with Thorazine.

PATIENT TEACHING
• Tell patient to shake suspension before
use.

- Warn patient to avoid activities that require alertness until effects of drug are known.
- Tell patient to watch for dizziness when standing quickly. Advise patient to change positions slowly.
- Instruct patient to report symptoms of dizziness, palpitations, or fainting to prescriber.
- Tell patient to avoid alcohol use.
- Have patient report signs of urine retention, constipation, or blurred vision.
- Tell patient that drug may discolor the urine.
- Advise patient to relieve dry mouth with sugarless gum or hard candy.
- Instruct patient to use sunblock and to wear protective clothing outdoors.

thiothixene
thye-oh-THIX-een

Navane

thiothixene hydrochloride
Navane*

Pharmacologic class: thioxanthene
Pregnancy risk category C

AVAILABLE FORMS
thiothixene
Capsules: 1 mg, 2 mg, 5 mg, 10 mg, 20 mg
thiothixene hydrochloride
Oral concentrate: 5 mg/ml*

INDICATIONS & DOSAGES
➤ **Mild to moderate psychosis**
Adults: Initially, 2 mg P.O. t.i.d. Increase gradually to 15 mg daily, as needed.
➤ **Severe psychosis**
Adults: Initially, 5 mg P.O. b.i.d. Increase gradually to 20 to 30 mg daily, as needed. Maximum dose is 60 mg daily.

ADMINISTRATION
P.O.
- Prevent contact dermatitis by keeping drug off skin and clothes. Wear gloves when preparing liquid forms.
- Dilute liquid concentrate with fruit juice, milk, or semisolid food just before giving.

- Slight yellowing of injection or concentrate is common and doesn't affect potency. Discard markedly discolored solutions.

ACTION
Unknown. Probably blocks dopamine receptors in the brain.

Route	Onset	Peak	Duration
P.O.	Unknown	Unknown	Unknown

Half-life: 20 to 40 hours.

ADVERSE REACTIONS
CNS: *extrapyramidal reactions, drowsiness, tardive dyskinesia,* **neuroleptic malignant syndrome,** restlessness, agitation, insomnia, sedation, EEG changes, pseudoparkinsonism, dizziness.
CV: *hypotension,* tachycardia, ECG changes.
EENT: *blurred vision,* ocular changes, nasal congestion.
GI: *dry mouth, constipation.*
GU: *urine retention,* menstrual irregularities, inhibited ejaculation.
Hematologic: **agranulocytosis, transient leukopenia,** leukocytosis.
Hepatic: jaundice.
Metabolic: weight gain.
Skin: *mild photosensitivity reactions,* allergic reactions, exfoliative dermatitis.
Other: gynecomastia.

INTERACTIONS
Drug-drug. *CNS depressants:* May increase CNS depression. Use together cautiously.
Drug-lifestyle. *Alcohol use:* May increase CNS depression. Discourage use together.
Sun exposure: May increase risk of photosensitivity reactions. Advise patient to avoid excessive sunlight exposure.

EFFECTS ON LAB TEST RESULTS
- May increase liver enzyme levels.
- May increase or decrease WBC counts. May decrease granulocyte counts.
- May cause false-positive results for urinary porphyrin, urobilinogen, amylase, and 5-hydroxyindoleacetic acid tests and for urine pregnancy tests that use human chorionic gonadotropin.

Reactions may be *common,* uncommon, *life-threatening,* or COMMON AND LIFE-THREATENING.
Interaction may have a *rapid onset* or *delayed onset.*

CONTRAINDICATIONS & CAUTIONS
- Contraindicated in patients hypersensitive to drug and in those with CNS depression, circulatory collapse, coma, or blood dyscrasia.
- Use with caution in patients with history of seizure disorder and in those undergoing alcohol withdrawal.
- Use cautiously in elderly or debilitated patients and in those with CV disease (may cause sudden drop in blood pressure), hepatic disease, heat exposure, glaucoma, or prostatic hyperplasia.
- Drug isn't recommended for use in children younger than age 12.

NURSING CONSIDERATIONS
- Monitor patient for tardive dyskinesia, which may occur after prolonged use; it may not appear until months or years later, and may disappear spontaneously or persist for life, despite stopping drug.
- *Alert:* Watch for evidence of neuroleptic malignant syndrome (extrapyramidal effects, hyperthermia, autonomic disturbance), which is rare but deadly.
- Monitor periodic CBCs, liver function tests, and renal function tests; and ophthalmic tests for long-term use.
- Watch for orthostatic hypotension. Keep patient supine for 1 hour after drug administration, and tell him to change positions slowly.
- Withhold dose and notify prescriber if jaundice, blood dyscrasia (fever, sore throat, infection, cellulitis, weakness), or persistent extrapyramidal reactions develop, especially in pregnant women.
- ■ **Black Box Warning** Elderly patients with dementia-related psychosis treated with atypical or conventional antipsychotics are at increased risk for death. Antipsychotics aren't approved for the treatment of dementia-related psychosis. ■
- Don't withdraw drug abruptly unless severe adverse reactions occur.
- After abrupt withdrawal of long-term therapy, gastritis, nausea, vomiting, dizziness, tremor, feeling of warmth or cold, diaphoresis, tachycardia, headache, or insomnia may occur.
- *Look alike–sound alike:* Don't confuse Navane with Nubain or Norvasc.

PATIENT TEACHING
- Warn patient to avoid activities that require alertness until effects of drug are known.
- Tell patient to watch for dizziness upon standing quickly. Advise him to change positions slowly.
- Instruct patient to dilute liquid appropriately.
- Tell patient to avoid alcohol use during therapy.
- Have patient report signs of urine retention, constipation, or blurred vision.
- Instruct patient to use sunblock and to wear protective clothing outdoors.

---

trifluoperazine hydrochloride
trye-floo-oh-PER-eh-zeen

Pharmacologic class:
phenothiazine
Pregnancy risk category NR

AVAILABLE FORMS
Tablets (regular and film-coated): 1 mg, 2 mg, 5 mg, 10 mg

INDICATIONS & DOSAGES
➤ **Anxiety states**
Adults: 1 to 2 mg P.O. b.i.d. Maximum, 6 mg daily. Don't give drug for longer than 12 weeks for anxiety.
➤ **Schizophrenia, other psychotic disorders**
Adults: In outpatients, 1 to 2 mg P.O. b.i.d. In hospitalized patients, 2 to 5 mg P.O. b.i.d., gradually increased until therapeutic response occurs. Most patients respond to 15 to 20 mg P.O. daily, although some may need 40 mg daily or more.
Children ages 6 to 12: For hospitalized or closely supervised patients, 1 mg P.O. daily or b.i.d.; may increase gradually to 15 mg daily, if needed.

ADMINISTRATION
P.O.
- Give drug without regard for meals.

ACTION
Unknown. A piperazine phenothiazine that probably blocks dopamine receptors in the brain.

Route	Onset	Peak	Duration
P.O.	Unknown	Unknown	Unknown

Half-life: 20 to 40 hours.

ADVERSE REACTIONS

CNS: *extrapyramidal reactions, tardive dyskinesia,* **neuroleptic malignant syndrome,** pseudoparkinsonism, dizziness, drowsiness, insomnia, fatigue, headache.
CV: *orthostatic hypotension,* tachycardia, ECG changes.
EENT: *blurred vision,* ocular changes.
GI: *dry mouth, constipation,* nausea.
GU: *urine retention,* menstrual irregularities, inhibited ejaculation.
Hematologic: *transient leukopenia, agranulocytosis.*
Hepatic: cholestatic jaundice.
Metabolic: weight gain.
Skin: *photosensitivity reactions,* allergic reactions, rash.
Other: gynecomastia.

INTERACTIONS

Drug-drug. *Antacids:* May inhibit absorption of oral phenothiazines. Separate antacid and phenothiazine doses by at least 2 hours.
Barbiturates, lithium: May decrease phenothiazine effect. Monitor patient.
Centrally acting antihypertensives: May decrease antihypertensive effect. Monitor blood pressure.
CNS depressants: May increase CNS depression. Use together cautiously.
Propranolol: May increase propranolol and trifluoperazine levels. Monitor patient.
Warfarin: May decrease effect of oral anticoagulants. Monitor PT and INR.
Drug-herb. *St. John's wort:* May cause photosensitivity reactions. Advise patient to avoid excessive sunlight exposure.
Drug-lifestyle. *Alcohol use:* May increase CNS depression, particularly psychomotor skills. Strongly discourage alcohol use.
Sun exposure: May increase risk of photosensitivity reactions. Advise patient to avoid excessive sunlight exposure.

EFFECTS ON LAB TEST RESULTS

● May increase liver enzyme levels.
● May decrease WBC and granulocyte counts.

● May cause false-positive results for urinary porphyrin, urobilinogen, amylase, and 5-hydroxyindoleacetic acid tests and for urine pregnancy tests that use human chorionic gonadotropin.

CONTRAINDICATIONS & CAUTIONS

● Contraindicated in patients hypersensitive to phenothiazines and in those with CNS depression, coma, bone marrow suppression, or liver damage.
● Use cautiously in elderly or debilitated patients and in patients with CV disease (may decrease blood pressure), seizure disorder, glaucoma, or prostatic hyperplasia; also, use cautiously in those exposed to extreme heat.
● Use only in children who are hospitalized or under close supervision.

NURSING CONSIDERATIONS

● Watch for orthostatic hypotension. Keep patient supine for 1 hour after giving drug, and tell him to change positions slowly.
● Monitor patient for tardive dyskinesia, which may occur after prolonged use. It may not appear until months or years later and may disappear spontaneously or persist for life, despite ending drug.
● *Alert:* Watch for evidence of neuroleptic malignant syndrome (extrapyramidal effects, hyperthermia, autonomic disturbance), which is rare but deadly.
● Monitor periodic CBC and liver function tests, and ophthalmic tests (long-term use).
● Withhold dose and notify prescriber if jaundice, signs and symptoms of blood dyscrasia (fever, sore throat, infection, cellulitis, weakness), or persistent extrapyramidal reactions (longer than a few hours) develop, especially in children or pregnant women.
■ **Black Box Warning** Elderly patients with dementia-related psychosis treated with atypical or conventional antipsychotics are at increased risk for death. Antipsychotics aren't approved for the treatment of dementia-related psychosis. ■
● Don't withdraw drug abruptly unless severe adverse reactions occur.
● After abrupt withdrawal of long-term therapy, gastritis, nausea, vomiting, dizziness, tremor, feeling of warmth or cold, diaphoresis, tachycardia, headache, insomnia, anorexia, muscle rigidity, altered

---

Reactions may be *common,* uncommon, *life-threatening,* or COMMON AND LIFE-THREATENING.
Interaction may have a *rapid onset* or *delayed onset.*

mental status, or evidence of autonomic instability may occur.

● *Look alike–sound alike:* Don't confuse trifluoperazine with triflupromazine.

PATIENT TEACHING

● Warn patient to avoid activities that require alertness until effects of drug are known.

● Tell patient to avoid alcohol while taking drug.

● Tell patient to report signs of urine retention or constipation.

● Tell patient to use sunblock and to wear protective clothing outdoors.

● Advise patient to relieve dry mouth with sugarless gum or hard candy.

ziprasidone
zih-PRAZ-i-done

Geodon

Pharmacologic class:
benzisoxazole derivative
Pregnancy risk category C

AVAILABLE FORMS

Capsules: 20 mg, 40 mg, 60 mg, 80 mg
I.M. injection: 20 mg/ml single-dose vials (after reconstitution)

INDICATIONS & DOSAGES

➤ **Symptomatic treatment of schizophrenia**

Adults: Initially, 20 mg b.i.d. with food. Dosages are highly individualized. Adjust dosage, if necessary, no more frequently than every 2 days; to allow for lowest possible doses, the interval should be several weeks to assess symptom response. Effective dosage range is usually 20 to 80 mg b.i.d. Maximum dosage is 100 mg b.i.d.

➤ **Rapid control of acute agitation in schizophrenic patients**

Adults: 10 to 20 mg I.M. as needed, up to a maximum dose of 40 mg daily. Doses of 10 mg may be given every 2 hours; doses of 20 mg may be given every 4 hours.

➤ **Acute bipolar mania, including manic and mixed episodes, with or without psychotic features**

Adults: 40 mg P.O. b.i.d., with food, on day 1. Increase to 60 to 80 mg P.O. b.i.d.,

with food, on day 2; then adjust dosage based on patient response from 40 to 80 mg b.i.d., with food.

ADMINISTRATION

P.O.

● Always give drug with food for optimal effect.

I.M.

● To prepare I.M. ziprasidone, add 1.2 ml of sterile water for injection to the vial and shake vigorously until drug is completely dissolved.

● Don't mix injection with other medicinal products or solvents other than sterile water for injection.

● Inspect parenteral drug products for particulate matter and discoloration before administration.

● The effects of giving I.M. for more than 3 consecutive days are unknown. If long-term therapy of drug is necessary, switch to P.O. as soon as possible.

● Store injection at controlled room temperature, 59° to 86° F (15° to 30° C) in dry form, and protect from light. After reconstituting, it may be stored away from light for up to 24 hours at 59° to 86° F (15° to 30° C) or up to 7 days refrigerated, 36° to 46° F (2° to 8° C).

ACTION

May inhibit dopamine and serotonin-2 receptors, causing reduction in schizophrenia symptoms.

Route	Onset	Peak	Duration
P.O.	1–3 days	6–8 hr	12 hr
I.M.	Unknown	1 hr	Unknown

Half-life: 2¼ to 7 hours.

ADVERSE REACTIONS

CNS: *dizziness, headache, somnolence, suicide attempt,* akathisia, dizziness, extrapyramidal symptoms, hypertonia, asthenia, dystonia (P.O.), anxiety, insomnia, agitation, cogwheel rigidity, paresthesia, personality disorder, psychosis, speech disorder (I.M.).

CV: *bradycardia, QT interval prolongation,* orthostatic hypotension, tachycardia (P.O.), hypertension, vasodilation (I.M.).

EENT: rhinitis, abnormal vision (P.O.).

GI: *nausea,* constipation, dyspepsia, diarrhea, dry mouth, anorexia, abdominal pain, *rectal hemorrhage,* vomiting, dyspepsia, tooth disorder (I.M.).
GU: dysmenorrhea, priapism (I.M.).
Metabolic: hyperglycemia.
Musculoskeletal: myalgia (P.O.), back pain (I.M.).
Respiratory: cough (P.O.).
Skin: rash (P.O.), injection site pain, furunculosis, sweating (I.M.).
Other: flulike syndrome (I.M.).

INTERACTIONS
Drug-drug. *Antiarrhythmics (amiodarone, bretylium, disopyramide, dofetilide, procainamide, quinidine, sotalol), arsenic trioxide, cisapride, dolasetron, droperidol, levomethadyl, mefloquine, pentamidine, phenothiazines, pimozide, quinolones, tacrolimus:* May increase the risk of life-threatening arrhythmias. Use together is contraindicated.
Antihypertensives: May enhance hypotensive effects. Monitor blood pressure.
Carbamazepine: May decrease ziprasidone level. May need to increase ziprasidone dose to achieve desired effect.
Drugs that decrease potassium or magnesium such as diuretics: May increase risk of arrhythmias. Monitor potassium and magnesium levels if using these drugs together.
Itraconazole, ketoconazole: May increase ziprasidone level. May need to reduce ziprasidone dose to achieve desired effect.

EFFECTS ON LAB TEST RESULTS
None reported.

CONTRAINDICATIONS & CAUTIONS
• Contraindicated in patients hypersensitive to drug and in those with recent MI or uncompensated heart failure.
• Contraindicated in those with history of prolonged QT interval or congenital long QT interval syndrome and in those taking other drugs that prolong QT interval, such as dofetilide, sotalol, quinidine, other class IA and III antiarrhythmics, mesoridazine, thioridazine, chlorpromazine, droperidol, pimozide, sparfloxacin, gatifloxacin, moxifloxacin, halofantrine, mefloquine, pentamidine, arsenic trioxide, levomethadyl

acetate, dolasetron mesylate, probucol, and tacrolimus.
P.O.
• Contraindicated in patients with a history of QT interval prolongation or congenital QT syndrome and in those taking other drugs that prolong QT interval.
• Use cautiously in patients with history of seizures, bradycardia, hypokalemia, or hypomagnesemia; in those with acute diarrhea; and in those with conditions that may lower the seizure threshold (such as Alzheimer dementia).
• Use cautiously in patients at risk for aspiration pneumonia.
• Don't use drug in breast-feeding women.
I.M.
• Contraindicated in schizophrenic patients already taking P.O. ziprasidone.
• Use cautiously in elderly and renally or hepatically impaired patients.

NURSING CONSIDERATIONS
■ **Black Box Warning** In elderly patients with dementia-related psychosis, drug isn't indicated for use because of increased risk of death from CV events or infection. ■
• *Alert:* Hyperglycemia may occur. Monitor patients with diabetes regularly. Patients with risk factors for diabetes should undergo fasting blood glucose testing at baseline and periodically. Monitor all patients for symptoms of hyperglycemia, including excessive hunger or thirst, frequent urination, and weakness. Hyperglycemia may be reversible when drug is stopped.
• *Alert:* Monitor patient for symptoms of metabolic syndrome (significant weight gain and increased body mass index, hypertension, hyperglycemia, hypercholesterolemia, and hypertriglyceridemia).
P.O.
• Stop drug in patients with a QTc interval more than 500 msec.
• Dizziness, palpitations, or syncope may be symptoms of a life-threatening arrhythmia such as torsades de pointes. Provide CV evaluation and monitoring in patients who experience these symptoms.
• Don't give to patients with electrolyte disturbances, such as hypokalemia or hypomagnesemia, because these increase the risk of arrhythmia.

Reactions may be *common,* uncommon, *life-threatening,* or COMMON AND LIFE-THREATENING.
Interaction may have a *rapid onset* or *delayed onset.*

• Patient taking an antipsychotic may develop life-threatening neuroleptic malignant syndrome (hyperpyrexia, muscle rigidity, altered mental status, and autonomic instability) or tardive dyskinesia. Assess abnormal involuntary movement before starting therapy, at dosage changes, and periodically thereafter, to monitor patient for tardive dyskinesia.

• Monitor patient for abnormal body temperature regulation, especially if he is exercising strenuously, is exposed to extreme heat, is also receiving anticholinergics, or is subject to dehydration.

• Symptoms may not improve for 4 to 6 weeks.

PATIENT TEACHING

• Tell patient to take drug with food.

• Tell patient to immediately report to prescriber signs or symptoms of dizziness, fainting, irregular heartbeat, or relevant heart problems.

• Advise patient to report any recent episodes of diarrhea, abnormal movements, sudden fever, muscle rigidity, or change in mental status.

• Advise patient that symptoms may not improve for 4 to 6 weeks.

42
Anxiolytics

alprazolam
buspirone hydrochloride
chlordiazepoxide hydrochloride
clorazepate dipotassium
diazepam
doxepin hydrochloride
  (See Chapter 38, ANTIDEPRESSANTS.)
hydroxyzine hydrochloride
hydroxyzine pamoate
lorazepam
midazolam
  (See Chapter 48, SEDATIVE HYPNOTICS.)
oxazepam
prochlorperazine
  (See Chapter 60, ANTIEMETICS.)

SAFETY ALERT!

alprazolam
al-PRAH-zoe-lam

Apo-Alpraz†, Apo-Alpraz TS†,
Niravam, Novo-Alprazol†,
Nu-Alpraz†, Xanax✦, Xanax XR

Pharmacologic class:
benzodiazepine
Pregnancy risk category D
Controlled substance schedule IV

AVAILABLE FORMS
Oral solution: 1 mg/ml (concentrate)
Orally disintegrating tablets (ODTs):
0.25 mg, 0.5 mg, 1 mg, 2 mg
Tablets: 0.25 mg, 0.5 mg, 1 mg, 2 mg
Tablets (extended-release): 0.5 mg, 1 mg,
2 mg, 3 mg

INDICATIONS & DOSAGES
➤ **Anxiety**
Adults: Usual first dose, 0.25 to 0.5 mg
P.O. t.i.d. Maximum, 4 mg daily in divided
doses.
Elderly patients: Usual first dose, 0.25 mg
P.O. b.i.d. or t.i.d. Maximum, 4 mg daily
in divided doses.
➤ **Panic disorders**
Adults: 0.5 mg P.O. t.i.d., increased at
intervals of 3 to 4 days in increments of no

more than 1 mg. Maximum, 10 mg daily
in divided doses. If using extended-release
tablets, start with 0.5 to 1 mg P.O. once
daily. Increase by no more than 1 mg
every 3 to 4 days. Maximum daily dose
is 10 mg.
Adjust-a-dose: For debilitated patients or
those with advanced hepatic disease, usual
first dose is 0.25 mg P.O. b.i.d. or t.i.d.
Maximum, 4 mg daily in divided doses.

ADMINISTRATION
P.O.
● Don't break or crush extended-release
tablets.
● Mix oral solution with liquids or semisolid food, such as water, juices, carbonated
beverages, applesauce, and puddings. Use
only calibrated dropper provided with this
product.
● Use dry hands to remove ODTs from
bottle. Discard cotton from inside bottle.
● Discard unused portion if breaking
scored ODT.

ACTION
Unknown. Probably potentiates the effects
of GABA, depresses the CNS, and suppresses the spread of seizure activity.

Route	Onset	Peak	Duration
P.O.	Unknown	1–2 hr	Unknown
P.O. (extended-release)	Unknown	Unknown	Unknown

Half-life: Immediate-release, 12 to 15 hours;
extended-release, 11 to 16 hours.

ADVERSE REACTIONS
CNS: *insomnia, irritability, dizziness,
headache, anxiety, confusion, drowsiness,
light-headedness, sedation, somnolence,
difficulty speaking, impaired coordination,
memory impairment, fatigue, depression,*
suicide, mental impairment, ataxia, paresthesia, dyskinesia, hypoesthesia, lethargy,
vertigo, malaise, tremor, nervousness,
restlessness, agitation, nightmare,
syncope, akathisia, mania.
CV: palpitations, chest pain, hypotension.

Reactions may be *common,* uncommon, *life-threatening,* or COMMON AND LIFE-THREATENING.
Interaction may have a *rapid onset* or **delayed onset.**

EENT: sore throat, allergic rhinitis, blurred vision, nasal congestion.
GI: *diarrhea, dry mouth, constipation,* nausea, increased or decreased appetite, anorexia, vomiting, dyspepsia, abdominal pain.
GU: dysmenorrhea, sexual dysfunction, premenstrual syndrome, difficulty urinating.
Metabolic: increased or decreased weight.
Musculoskeletal: arthralgia, myalgia, arm or leg pain, back pain, muscle rigidity, muscle cramps, muscle twitch.
Respiratory: upper respiratory tract infection, dyspnea, hyperventilation.
Skin: pruritus, increased sweating, dermatitis.
Other: influenza, injury, emergence of anxiety between doses, dependence, feeling warm, increased or decreased libido.

INTERACTIONS
Drug-drug. *Anticonvulsants, antidepressants, antihistamines, barbiturates, benzodiazepines, general anesthetics, narcotics, phenothiazines:* May increase CNS depressant effects. Avoid using together.
Azole antifungals (including fluconazole, itraconazole, ketoconazole, miconazole): May increase and prolong alprazolam level, CNS depression, and psychomotor impairment. Avoid using together.
Carbamazepine, *propoxyphene:* May induce alprazolam metabolism and may reduce therapeutic effects. May need to increase dose.
Cimetidine, fluoxetine, fluvoxamine, hormonal contraceptives, nefazodone: May increase alprazolam level. Use cautiously together, and consider alprazolam dosage reduction.
Tricyclic antidepressants: May increase levels of these drugs. Monitor patient closely.
Drug-herb. *Kava, valerian root:* May increase sedation. Discourage use together.
St. John's wort: May decrease drug level. Discourage use together.
Drug-food. *Grapefruit juice:* May increase drug level. Discourage use together.
Drug-lifestyle. *Alcohol use:* May cause additive CNS effects. Discourage use together.
Smoking: May decrease effectiveness of drug. Monitor patient closely.

EFFECTS ON LAB TEST RESULTS
● May increase ALT and AST levels.

CONTRAINDICATIONS & CAUTIONS
● Contraindicated in patients hypersensitive to drug or other benzodiazepines and in those with acute angle-closure glaucoma.
● Use cautiously in patients with hepatic, renal, of pulmonary disease or history of substance abuse.

NURSING CONSIDERATIONS
● The optimum duration of therapy is unknown.
● *Alert:* Don't withdraw drug abruptly; withdrawal symptoms, including seizures, may occur. Abuse or addiction is possible.
● Monitor hepatic, renal, and hematopoietic function periodically in patients receiving repeated or prolonged therapy.
● *Look alike–sound alike:* Don't confuse alprazolam with alprostadil or lorazepam. Don't confuse Xanax with Zantac, Xopenex, or Tenex.

PATIENT TEACHING
● Warn patient to avoid hazardous activities that require alertness and good coordination until effects of drug are known.
● Tell patient to avoid use of alcohol while taking drug.
● Advise patient that smoking may decrease drug's effectiveness.
● Warn patient not to stop drug abruptly because withdrawal symptoms or seizures may occur.
● Tell patient to swallow extended-release tablets whole.
● Tell patient using ODT to remove it from bottle using dry hands and to immediately place it on his tongue where it will dissolve and can be swallowed with saliva.
● Tell patient taking half a scored ODT to discard the unused half.
● Advise patient to discard the cotton from the bottle of ODTs and keep it tightly sealed to prevent moisture from dissolving the tablets.
● Warn women to avoid use during pregnancy and breast-feeding.

buspirone hydrochloride
byoo-SPYE-rone

BuSpar✧, Bustab†

Pharmacologic class:
azaspirodecanedione derivative
Pregnancy risk category B

AVAILABLE FORMS
Tablets: 5 mg, 7.5 mg, 10 mg, 15 mg, 30 mg

INDICATIONS & DOSAGES
➤ **Anxiety disorders**
Adults: Initially, 7.5 mg P.O. b.i.d. Increase dosage by 5 mg daily at 2- to 3-day intervals. Usual maintenance dosage is 20 to 30 mg daily in divided doses. Don't exceed 60 mg daily.

ADMINISTRATION
P.O.
• Don't give drug with grapefruit juice.
• Give drug at the same times each day, and always with or always without food.

ACTION
May inhibit neuronal firing and reduce serotonin turnover in cortical, amygdaloid, and septohippocampal tissue.

Route	Onset	Peak	Duration
P.O.	Unknown	40–90 min	Unknown

Half-life: 2 to 3 hours.

ADVERSE REACTIONS
CNS: *dizziness, drowsiness, headache,* nervousness, insomnia, light-headedness, fatigue, numbness.
CV: tachycardia, nonspecific chest pain.
EENT: blurred vision.
GI: dry mouth, nausea, diarrhea, abdominal distress.

INTERACTIONS
Drug-drug. *Azole antifungals:* May inhibit first-pass metabolism of buspirone. Monitor patient closely for adverse effects; adjust dosage as needed.
CNS depressants: May increase CNS depression. Use together cautiously.

Drugs metabolized by CYP3A4 (erythromycin, nefazodone): May increase buspirone level. Monitor patient; decrease buspirone dosage and adjust carefully.
MAO inhibitors: May elevate blood pressure. Avoid using together.
Drug-food. *Grapefruit juice:* May increase drug level, increasing adverse effects. Give with liquid other than grapefruit juice.
Drug-lifestyle. *Alcohol use:* May increase CNS depression. Discourage use together.

EFFECTS ON LAB TEST RESULTS
None reported.

CONTRAINDICATIONS & CAUTIONS
• Contraindicated in patients hypersensitive to drug and within 14 days of MAO inhibitor therapy.
• Drug isn't recommended for patients with severe hepatic or renal impairment.

NURSING CONSIDERATIONS
• Monitor patient closely for adverse CNS reactions. Drug is less sedating than other anxiolytics, but CNS effects may be unpredictable.
• *Alert:* Before starting therapy, don't stop a previous benzodiazepine regimen abruptly because a withdrawal reaction may occur.
• Drug shows no potential for abuse and isn't classified as a controlled substance.
• *Look alike–sound alike:* Don't confuse buspirone with bupropion or risperidone.

PATIENT TEACHING
• Warn patient to avoid hazardous activities that require alertness and good coordination until effects of drug are known.
• Remind patient that drug effects may not be noticeable for several weeks.
• Warn patient not to abruptly stop a benzodiazepine because of risk of withdrawal symptoms.
• Tell patient to avoid use of alcohol during therapy.
• Advise patient to take consistently, that is, always with or always without food.

Reactions may be *common,* uncommon, *life-threatening,* or COMMON AND LIFE-THREATENING.
Interaction may have a *rapid onset* or *delayed onset.*

chlordiazepoxide hydrochloride
klor-dye-az-e-POX-ide

Librium

Pharmacologic class:
benzodiazepine
Pregnancy risk category D
Controlled substance schedule IV

AVAILABLE FORMS
Capsules: 5 mg, 10 mg, 25 mg
Powder for injection: 100-mg ampule

INDICATIONS & DOSAGES
➤ **Mild to moderate anxiety**
Adults: 5 to 10 mg P.O. t.i.d. or q.i.d.
Children older than age 6: 5 mg P.O. b.i.d. to q.i.d. Maximum, 10 mg P.O. b.i.d. or t.i.d.
➤ **Severe anxiety**
Adults: 20 to 25 mg P.O. t.i.d. or q.i.d.
Elderly patients: 5 mg P.O. b.i.d. to q.i.d.
Adjust-a-dose: For debilitated patients, 5 mg P.O. b.i.d. to q.i.d.
➤ **Withdrawal symptoms of acute alcoholism**
Adults: 50 to 100 mg P.O. Repeat in 2 to 4 hours, as needed. Maximum, 300 mg daily.
➤ **Preoperative apprehension and anxiety**
Adults: 5 to 10 mg P.O. t.i.d. or q.i.d. on day before surgery.

ADMINISTRATION
P.O.
● *Alert:* 5-mg and 25-mg capsules may look similar in color through the packaging. Verify contents and read label carefully.
I.V.
● Parenteral form isn't recommended for children younger than age 12.
● Make sure equipment and staff needed for emergency airway management are available. Monitor respirations every 5 to 15 minutes and before each I.V. dose.
● Keep powder refrigerated and away from light; mix just before use and discard remainder.
● Injectable form comes in two ampules— diluent and powdered drug. Read directions carefully.

● Don't give prepackaged diluent I.V. because air bubbles may form.
● Use 5 ml of normal saline solution or sterile water for injection as diluent for an ampule containing 100 mg of drug.
● Give over 1 minute.
● **Incompatibilities:** Other I.V. drugs.
I.M.
● For I.M. use, add 2 ml of diluent to powder and agitate gently until clear. Don't use the supplied diluent for I.V. use. Use immediately.
● I.M. form may be absorbed erratically.

ACTION
A benzodiazepine that may potentiate the effects of GABA, depress the CNS, and suppress the spread of seizure activity.

Route	Onset	Peak	Duration
P.O.	Unknown	½–4 hr	Unknown
I.V.	1–5 min	Unknown	15–60 min
I.M.	Unknown	Unknown	Unknown

Half-life: 5 to 30 hours.

ADVERSE REACTIONS
CNS: *drowsiness, lethargy,* ataxia, confusion, extrapyramidal reactions, minor changes in EEG patterns.
CV: edema.
GI: nausea, constipation.
GU: menstrual irregularities.
Hematologic: *agranulocytosis.*
Hepatic: jaundice.
Skin: *swelling and pain at injection site,* skin eruptions.
Other: altered libido.

INTERACTIONS
Drug-drug. *Cimetidine:* May decrease chlordiazepoxide clearance and increase risk of adverse reactions. Monitor patient carefully.
CNS depressants: May increase CNS depression. Use together cautiously.
Digoxin: May increase digoxin level and risk of toxicity. Monitor patient and digoxin level closely.
Disulfiram: May decrease clearance and increase half-life of chlordiazepoxide. Monitor patient for enhanced effects. Consider dosage adjustment.
Fluconazole, itraconazole, ketoconazole, miconazole: May increase and prolong

chlordiazepoxide levels, CNS depression, and psychomotor impairment. Avoid using together.
Levodopa: May decrease control of parkinsonian symptoms in patients with Parkinson disease. Use together cautiously.
Drug-herb. *Kava:* May increase sedation. Discourage use together.
Drug-lifestyle. *Alcohol use:* May cause additive CNS effects. Discourage use together.
Smoking: May decrease effectiveness of drug. Monitor patient closely.

EFFECTS ON LAB TEST RESULTS
• May increase liver function test values. May decrease granulocyte count.
• May cause a false-positive pregnancy test result. May alter urinary 17-ketosteroid (Zimmerman reaction), urine alkaloid (Frings thin-layer chromatography method), and urinary glucose determinations (with Chemstrip uG and Diastix).

CONTRAINDICATIONS & CAUTIONS
• Contraindicated in patients hypersensitive to drug and in pregnant women, especially in first trimester.
• Use cautiously in patients with mental depression, history of substance abuse, porphyria, or hepatic or renal disease.

NURSING CONSIDERATIONS
• In patients receiving repeated or prolonged therapy, monitor hepatic, renal, and hematopoietic function periodically.
• Watch for paradoxical reaction in psychiatric patients and hyperactive, aggressive children.
• *Alert:* Use of this drug may lead to abuse and addiction. Don't withdraw drug abruptly after long-term use because withdrawal symptoms may occur.
• *Look alike–sound alike:* Don't confuse Librium with Librax.

PATIENT TEACHING
• Warn patient to avoid hazardous activities that require alertness and coordination until effects of drug are known.
• Tell patient to avoid use of alcohol while taking drug.

• Notify patient that smoking may decrease drug's effectiveness.
• Warn patient drug may cause psychological and physical dependence. Tell patient not to increase dose or abruptly stop the drug because withdrawal symptoms may occur.
• Warn woman to avoid use during pregnancy.

SAFETY ALERT!

diazepam
dye-AZ-e-pam

Diastat*, Diastat Acudial, Diazemuls†, Diazepam Intensol*, Novo-Dipam†, Valium⬥, Vivol†

Pharmacologic class: benzodiazepine
Pregnancy risk category D
Controlled substance schedule IV

AVAILABLE FORMS
Injection: 5 mg/ml
Oral solution: 5 mg/5 ml, 5 mg/ml*
Rectal gel twin packs:* 2.5 mg (pediatric), 5 mg (pediatric), 10 mg, 15 mg (adult), 20 mg (adult)
Tablets: 2 mg, 5 mg, 10 mg

INDICATIONS & DOSAGES
➤ **Anxiety**
Adults: Depending on severity, 2 to 10 mg P.O. b.i.d. to q.i.d. Or, 2 to 10 mg I.M. or I.V. every 3 to 4 hours, as needed.
Children age 6 months and older: 1 to 2.5 mg P.O. t.i.d. or q.i.d., increase gradually, as needed and tolerated.
Elderly patients: Initially, 2 to 2.5 mg once daily or b.i.d.; increase gradually.
➤ **Acute alcohol withdrawal**
Adults: 10 mg P.O. t.i.d. or q.i.d. first 24 hours; reduce to 5 mg P.O. t.i.d. or q.i.d., as needed. Or, initially, 10 mg I.V. or I.M. Then, 5 to 10 mg I.V. or I.M. every 3 to 4 hours, as needed.
➤ **Before endoscopic procedures**
Adults: Adjust I.V. dose to desired sedative response (up to 20 mg). Or, 5 to 10 mg I.M. 30 minutes before procedure.

Reactions may be *common*, uncommon, *life-threatening*, or COMMON AND LIFE-THREATENING.
Interaction may have a *rapid onset* or *delayed onset*.

➤ **Muscle spasm**
Adults: 2 to 10 mg P.O. b.i.d. to q.i.d.
Or, 5 to 10 mg I.V. or I.M. initially;
then 5 to 10 mg I.V. or I.M. every 3 to
4 hours, as needed. For tetanus, larger
doses up to 20 mg every 2 to 8 hours
may be needed.
Children age 5 and older: 5 to 10 mg I.V.
or I.M. every 3 to 4 hours, as needed.
Children ages 1 month to 5 years: 1 to
2 mg I.V. or I.M. slowly; repeat every 3 to
4 hours, as needed.
➤ **Preoperative sedation**
Adults: 10 mg I.M. (preferred) or I.V.
before surgery.
➤ **Cardioversion**
Adults: 5 to 15 mg I.V. within 5 to 10 minutes before procedure.
➤ **Adjunct treatment for seizure
disorders**
Adults: 2 to 10 mg P.O. b.i.d. to q.i.d.
Children age 6 months and older: 1 to
2.5 mg P.O. t.i.d. or q.i.d. initially; increase
as needed and as tolerated.
➤ **Status epilepticus, severe recurrent
seizures**
Adults: 5 to 10 mg I.V. or I.M. initially.
Use I.M. route only if I.V. access is un-
available. Repeat every 10 to 15 minutes,
as needed, up to maximum dose of 30 mg.
Repeat every 2 to 4 hours, if needed.
Children age 5 and older: 1 mg I.V. every
2 to 5 minutes up to maximum of 10 mg.
Repeat every 2 to 4 hours, if needed.
Children ages 1 month to 5 years: 0.2 to
0.5 mg I.V. slowly every 2 to 5 minutes up
to maximum of 5 mg. Repeat every 2 to
4 hours, if needed.
Neonates: 0.3 to 0.75 mg/kg/dose I.V.
slowly every 15 to 30 minutes for two to
three doses.
➤ **Patients on stable regimens
of antiepileptic drugs who need
diazepam intermittently to control
bouts of increased seizure activity**
Adults and children age 12 and older:
0.2 mg/kg P.R., rounding up to the nearest
available dose form. A second dose may
be given 4 to 12 hours later.
Children ages 6 to 11: 0.3 mg/kg P.R.,
rounding up to the nearest available dose
form. A second dose may be given 4 to
12 hours later.
Children ages 2 to 5: 0.5 mg/kg P.R.,
rounding up to the nearest available dose

form. A second dose may be given 4 to
12 hours later.
Adjust-a-dose: For elderly and debilitated
patients, reduce dosage to decrease the
likelihood of ataxia and oversedation.

ADMINISTRATION
P.O.
● When using oral solution, dilute dose
just before giving.
I.V.
● I.V. route is the more reliable parenteral
route; I.M. route isn't recommended
because absorption is variable and injection is painful.
● Keep emergency resuscitation equipment
and oxygen at bedside.
● Avoid infusion sets or containers made
from polyvinyl chloride.
● If possible, inject directly into a large
vein. If not, inject slowly through infusion
tubing as near to the insertion site as possible. Give at no more than 5 mg/minute.
Watch closely for phlebitis at injection
site.
● Monitor respirations every 5 to 15 minutes and before each dose.
● Don't store parenteral solution in plastic
syringes.
● **Incompatibilities:** All other I.V. drugs,
most I.V. solutions.
I.M.
● Use the I.M. route if I.V. administration
is impossible.
Rectal
● Use Diastat rectal gel to treat no more
than five episodes per month and no more
than one episode every 5 days because
tolerance may develop.
● *Alert:* Only caregivers who can distinguish the distinct cluster of seizures or
events from the patient's ordinary seizure
activity, who have been instructed and
can give the treatment competently, who
understand which seizures may be treated
with Diastat, and who can monitor the
clinical response and recognize when
immediate professional medical evaluation
is needed should give Diastat rectal gel.

ACTION
A benzodiazepine that probably potentiates the effects of GABA, depresses the
CNS, and suppresses the spread of seizure
activity.

Route	Onset	Peak	Duration
P.O.	30 min	2 hr	20–80 hr
I.V.	1–5 min	1–5 min	15–60 min
I.M.	Unknown	2 hr	Unknown
P.R.	Unknown	90 min	Unknown

Half-life: About 1 to 12 days.

ADVERSE REACTIONS

CNS: *drowsiness,* dysarthria, slurred speech, tremor, transient amnesia, fatigue, ataxia, headache, insomnia, paradoxical anxiety, hallucinations, minor changes in EEG patterns, *pain.*
CV: *CV collapse, bradycardia,* hypotension.
EENT: diplopia, blurred vision, nystagmus.
GI: nausea, constipation, diarrhea with rectal form.
GU: incontinence, urine retention.
Hematologic: *neutropenia.*
Hepatic: jaundice.
Respiratory: *respiratory depression, apnea.*
Skin: rash, *phlebitis at injection site.*
Other: altered libido, physical or psychological dependence.

INTERACTIONS

Drug-drug. *Cimetidine, disulfiram, fluoxetine, fluvoxamine, hormonal contraceptives, isoniazid, metoprolol, propoxyphene, propranolol, valproic acid:* May decrease clearance of diazepam and increase risk of adverse effects. Monitor patient for excessive sedation and impaired psychomotor function.
CNS depressants: May increase CNS depression. Use together cautiously.
Digoxin: May increase digoxin level and risk of toxicity. Monitor patient and digoxin level closely.
Diltiazem: May increase CNS depression and prolong effects of diazepam. Reduce dose of diazepam.
Fluconazole, itraconazole, ketoconazole, miconazole: May increase and prolong diazepam level, CNS depression, and psychomotor impairment. Avoid using together.
Levodopa: May decrease levodopa effectiveness. Monitor patient.
Phenobarbital: May increase effects of both drugs. Use together cautiously.

Drug-herb. *Kava:* May increase sedation. Discourage use together.
Drug-lifestyle. *Alcohol use:* May cause additive CNS effects. Discourage use together.
Smoking: May decrease effectiveness of drug. Monitor patient closely.

EFFECTS ON LAB TEST RESULTS
● May increase liver function test values.
● May decrease neutrophil count.

CONTRAINDICATIONS & CAUTIONS
● Contraindicated in patients hypersensitive to drug or soy protein; in patients experiencing shock, coma, or acute alcohol intoxication (parenteral form); in pregnant women, especially in first trimester; and in infants younger than age 6 months (oral form).
● Diastat rectal gel is contraindicated in patients with acute angle-closure glaucoma.
● Use cautiously in patients with liver or renal impairment, depression, history of substance abuse, or chronic open-angle glaucoma. Use cautiously in elderly and debilitated patients.

NURSING CONSIDERATIONS
● Monitor periodic hepatic, renal, and hematopoietic function studies in patients receiving repeated or prolonged therapy.
● Monitor elderly patients for dizziness, ataxia, mental status changes. Patients are at an increased risk for falls.
● *Alert:* Use of drug may lead to abuse and addiction. Don't withdraw drug abruptly after long-term use; withdrawal symptoms may occur.
● *Look alike–sound alike:* Don't confuse diazepam with diazoxide or Ditropan. Don't confuse Valium with Valcyte.

PATIENT TEACHING
● Warn patient to avoid activities that require alertness and good coordination until effects of drug are known.
● Tell patient to avoid alcohol while taking drug.
● Notify patient that smoking may decrease drug's effectiveness.
● Warn patient not to abruptly stop drug because withdrawal symptoms may occur.

Reactions may be *common,* uncommon, *life-threatening,* or COMMON AND LIFE-THREATENING.
Interaction may have a *rapid onset* or *delayed onset.*

• Warn woman to avoid use during pregnancy.
• Instruct patient's caregiver on the proper use of Diastat rectal gel.

---

hydroxyzine hydrochloride
hye-DROX-i-zeen

Atarax†, Vistaril

hydroxyzine pamoate
Vistaril

Pharmacologic class: piperazine derivative
Pregnancy risk category NR

AVAILABLE FORMS
hydroxyzine hydrochloride
Capsules: 10 mg†, 25 mg†, 50 mg†
Injection: 25 mg/ml, 50 mg/ml
Syrup: 2 mg/ml†, 10 mg/5 ml
Tablets: 10 mg, 25 mg, 50 mg
hydroxyzine pamoate
Capsules: 25 mg, 50 mg
Oral suspension: 25 mg/5 ml

INDICATIONS & DOSAGES
➤ **Anxiety**
Adults: 50 to 100 mg P.O. q.i.d.
Children age 6 and older: 50 to 100 mg P.O. daily in divided doses.
Children younger than age 6: 50 mg P.O. daily in divided doses.
➤ **Preoperative and postoperative adjunctive therapy for sedation**
Adults: 25 to 100 mg I.M. or 50 to 100 mg P.O.
Children: 0.6 mg/kg P.O or I.M.
➤ **Pruritus**
Adults: 25 mg P.O. or I.M. t.i.d. or q.i.d.
Children age 6 and older: 50 to 100 mg P.O. daily in divided doses.
Children younger than age 6: 50 mg P.O. daily in divided doses.
➤ **Psychiatric and emotional emergencies, including acute alcoholism**
Adults: 50 to 100 mg I.M. every 4 to 6 hours, p.r.n.
➤ **Nausea and vomiting (excluding nausea and vomiting of pregnancy)**
Adults: 25 to 100 mg I.M.
Children: 1.1 mg/kg I.M.

➤ **Antepartum and postpartum adjunctive therapy**
Adults: 25 to 100 mg I.M.

ADMINISTRATION
P.O.
• Give drug without regard for meals.
• Shake suspension well before giving.
I.M.
• Parenteral form (hydroxyzine hydrochloride) is for I.M. use only, preferably by Z-track injection. Never give drug I.V. or subcutaneously.
• Aspirate I.M. injection carefully to prevent inadvertent I.V. injection. Inject deeply into a large muscle.

ACTION
Suppresses activity in certain essential regions of the subcortical area of the CNS.

Route	Onset	Peak	Duration
P.O.	15–30 min	2 hr	4–6 hr
I.M.	Unknown	Unknown	4–6 hr

Half-life: 3 hours.

ADVERSE REACTIONS
CNS: *drowsiness,* involuntary motor activity.
GI: *dry mouth,* constipation.
Skin: pain at I.M. injection site.
Other: hypersensitivity reactions.

INTERACTIONS
Drug-drug. *Anticholinergics:* May cause additive anticholinergic effects. Use together cautiously.
CNS depressants: May increase CNS depression. Use together cautiously; dosage adjustments may be needed.
Epinephrine: May inhibit and reverse vasopressor effect of epinephrine. Avoid using together.
Drug-lifestyle. *Alcohol use:* May increase CNS depression. Discourage use together.

EFFECTS ON LAB TEST RESULTS
• May cause false increase in urinary 17-hydroxycorticosteroid level.
• May cause false-negative skin allergen tests by reducing or inhibiting the cutaneous response to histamine.

CONTRAINDICATIONS & CAUTIONS
● Contraindicated in patients hypersensitive to drug, patients in early pregnancy, and breast-feeding women.

NURSING CONSIDERATIONS
● If patient takes other CNS drugs, watch for oversedation.
● Elderly patients may be more sensitive to adverse anticholinergic effects; monitor these patients for dizziness, excessive sedation, confusion, hypotension, and syncope.
● *Look alike–sound alike:* Don't confuse hydroxyzine with hydroxyurea, Hydrogesic, or hydralazine. Don't confuse Vistaril with Restoril.

PATIENT TEACHING
● Warn patient to avoid hazardous activities that require alertness and good coordination until effects of drug are known.
● Tell patient to avoid use of alcohol while taking drug.
● Advise patient to use sugarless hard candy or gum to relieve dry mouth.
● Warn woman of childbearing age to avoid use during pregnancy and breast-feeding.

SAFETY ALERT!

lorazepam
lor-AZ-e-pam

Ativan, Lorazepam Intensol, Novo-Lorazem†, Nu-Loraz†

Pharmacologic class: benzodiazepine
Pregnancy risk category D
Controlled substance schedule IV

AVAILABLE FORMS
Injection: 2 mg/ml, 4 mg/ml
Oral solution (concentrated): 2 mg/ml
Tablets: 0.5 mg, 1 mg, 2 mg

INDICATIONS & DOSAGES
➤ **Anxiety**
Adults: 2 to 6 mg P.O. daily in divided doses. Maximum, 10 mg daily.
Elderly patients: 1 to 2 mg P.O. daily in divided doses. Maximum, 10 mg daily.

➤ **Insomnia from anxiety**
Adults: 2 to 4 mg P.O. at bedtime.
➤ **Preoperative sedation**
Adults: 2 mg I.V. total or 0.044 mg/kg I.V., whichever is smaller. Larger doses up to 0.05 mg/kg I.V., to total of 4 mg, may be needed. Or, 0.05 mg/kg I.M. 2 hours before procedure. Total dose shouldn't exceed 4 mg.
➤ **Status epilepticus**
Adults: 4 mg I.V. If seizures continue or recur after 10 to 15 minutes; then, an additional 4-mg dose may be given. Drug may be given I.M. if I.V. access isn't available.
➤ **Nausea and vomiting caused by emetogenic cancer chemotherapy ◆**
Adults: 2.5 mg P.O. the evening before and just after starting chemotherapy. Or, 1.5 mg/m² (usually up to a maximum dose of 3 mg) I.V. (over 5 minutes) 45 minutes before starting chemotherapy.

ADMINISTRATION
P.O.
● Mix oral solution with liquid or semi-solid food, such as water, juices, carbonated beverages, applesauce, or pudding.
I.V.
● Keep emergency resuscitation equipment and oxygen available.
● Dilute with an equal volume of sterile water for injection, normal saline solution for injection, or D₅W. Give slowly at no more than 2 mg/minute.
● Monitor respirations every 5 to 15 minutes and before each I.V. dose.
● Contains benzyl alcohol. Avoid use in neonates.
● Refrigerate intact vials and protect from light.
● **Incompatibilities:** Aldesleukin, aztreonam, buprenorphine, caffeine citrate, floxacillin, foscarnet, idarubicin, imipenem-cilastatin sodium, omeprazole, ondansetron hydrochloride, sargramostim, sufentanil citrate, thiopental.
I.M.
● For status epilepticus, drug may be given I.M. if I.V. access isn't available.
● For I.M. use, inject deeply into a muscle. Don't dilute.
● Refrigerate parenteral form to prolong shelf life.

Reactions may be *common,* uncommon, *life-threatening,* or COMMON AND LIFE-THREATENING.
Interaction may have a *rapid onset* or *delayed onset.*

ACTION
May potentiate the effects of GABA, depress the CNS, and suppress the spread of seizure activity.

Route	Onset	Peak	Duration
P.O.	1 hr	2 hr	12–24 hr
I.V.	5 min	60–90 min	6–8 hr
I.M.	15–30 min	60–90 min	6–8 hr

Half-life: 10 to 20 hours.

ADVERSE REACTIONS
CNS: *drowsiness, sedation,* amnesia, insomnia, agitation, dizziness, weakness, unsteadiness, disorientation, depression, headache.
CV: hypotension.
EENT: visual disturbances, nasal congestion.
GI: abdominal discomfort, nausea, change in appetite.

INTERACTIONS
Drug-drug. *CNS depressants:* May increase CNS depression. Use together cautiously.
Digoxin: May increase digoxin level and risk of toxicity. Monitor patient and digoxin level closely.
Drug-herb. *Kava:* May increase sedation. Discourage use together.
Drug-lifestyle. *Alcohol use:* May cause additive CNS effects. Discourage use together.
Smoking: May decrease drug's effectiveness. Monitor patient closely.

EFFECTS ON LAB TEST RESULTS
● May increase liver function test values.

CONTRAINDICATIONS & CAUTIONS
● Contraindicated in patients hypersensitive to drug, other benzo-diazepines, or the vehicle used in parenteral dosage form; in patients with acute angle-closure glaucoma; and in pregnant women, especially in the first trimester.
● Use cautiously in patients with pulmonary, renal, or hepatic impairment, or history of substance abuse.
● Use cautiously in elderly, acutely ill, or debilitated patients.

NURSING CONSIDERATIONS
● Monitor hepatic, renal, and hemato-poietic function periodically in patients receiving repeated or prolonged therapy.
● *Alert:* Use of this drug may lead to abuse and addiction. Don't stop drug abruptly after long-term use because withdrawal symptoms may occur.
● *Look alike–sound alike:* Don't confuse lorazepam with alprazolam or clonazepam. Don't confuse Ativan with Atgam.

PATIENT TEACHING
● When used before surgery, drug causes substantial preoperative amnesia. Patient teaching requires extra care to ensure adequate recall. Provide written materials or inform a family member, if possible.
● Warn patient to avoid hazardous activities that require alertness or good coordination until effects of drug are known.
● Tell patient to avoid use of alcohol while taking drug.
● Notify patient that smoking may decrease drug's effectiveness.
● Warn patient not to stop drug abruptly because withdrawal symptoms may occur.
● Advise woman to avoid becoming pregnant while taking drug.

SAFETY ALERT!

oxazepam
ox-AZ-e-pam

Novoxapam†, Oxpam†, Serax

Pharmacologic class:
benzodiazepine
Pregnancy risk category D
Controlled substance schedule IV

AVAILABLE FORMS
Capsules: 10 mg, 15 mg, 30 mg

INDICATIONS & DOSAGES
➤ **Alcohol withdrawal, severe anxiety**
Adults: 15 to 30 mg P.O. t.i.d. or q.i.d.
➤ **Mild to moderate anxiety**
Adults: 10 to 15 mg P.O. t.i.d. or q.i.d.
Elderly patients: Initially, 10 mg t.i.d.; cautiously increase to 15 mg t.i.d. to q.i.d.

ADMINISTRATION
P.O.
• Give drug without regard for meals.
• *Alert:* Serax tablets may contain tartrazine.

ACTION
May stimulate GABA receptors in the ascending reticular activating system.

Route	Onset	Peak	Duration
P.O.	Unknown	3 hr	Unknown

Half-life: 5 to 13 hours.

ADVERSE REACTIONS
CNS: *drowsiness, lethargy,* dizziness, vertigo, headache, syncope, tremor, slurred speech, changes in EEG patterns.
CV: edema.
GI: nausea.
Hepatic: *hepatic dysfunction.*
Skin: rash.
Other: altered libido.

INTERACTIONS
Drug-drug. *CNS depressants:* May increase CNS depression. Use together cautiously.
Digoxin: May increase digoxin level and risk of toxicity. Monitor patient closely.
Drug-herb. *Kava:* May increase sedation. Discourage use together.
Drug-lifestyle. *Alcohol use:* May cause additive CNS effects. Discourage use together.

EFFECTS ON LAB TEST RESULTS
• May increase liver function test values.

CONTRAINDICATIONS & CAUTIONS
• Contraindicated in patients hypersensitive to drug; in pregnant women, especially in the first trimester; and in those with psychoses.
• Use cautiously in elderly patients and in those with history of substance abuse or in whom a decrease in blood pressure might lead to cardiac problems.

NURSING CONSIDERATIONS
• Monitor hepatic, renal, and hemato-poietic function periodically in patients receiving repeated or prolonged therapy.

• *Alert:* Use of this drug may lead to abuse and addiction. Don't stop drug abruptly because withdrawal symptoms may occur.
• *Look alike–sound alike:* Don't confuse oxazepam with oxaprozin.

PATIENT TEACHING
• Warn patient to avoid hazardous activities that require alertness or good coordination until effects of drug are known.
• Tell patient to avoid use of alcohol while taking drug.
• Notify patient that smoking may decrease drug's effectiveness.
• Warn patient not to stop drug abruptly because withdrawal symptoms may occur.
• Warn woman of childbearing age to avoid use during pregnancy.

atomoxetine hydrochloride
dexmethylphenidate
hydrochloride
dextroamphetamine sulfate
lisdexamfetamine dimesylate
methylphenidate hydrochloride

---

atomoxetine hydrochloride
at-oh-MOX-ah-teen

Strattera✑

Pharmacologic class: selective
norepinephrine reuptake inhibitor
Pregnancy risk category C

AVAILABLE FORMS
Capsules: 10 mg, 18 mg, 25 mg, 40 mg,
60 mg, 80 mg, 100 mg

INDICATIONS & DOSAGES
➤ **Attention deficit hyperactivity**
disorder (ADHD)
Adults, children, and adolescents who
weigh more than 70 kg (154 lb): Initially,
40 mg P.O. daily; increase after at least
3 days to a total of 80 mg/day P.O., as a
single dose in the morning or two evenly
divided doses in the morning and late
afternoon or early evening. After 2 to
4 weeks, increase total dose to a maximum of 100 mg, if needed.
Children who weigh 70 kg or less: Initially,
0.5 mg/kg P.O. daily; increase after a
minimum of 3 days to a target total daily
dose of 1.2 mg/kg P.O. as a single dose in
the morning or two evenly divided doses
in the morning and late afternoon or early
evening. Don't exceed 1.4 mg/kg or
100 mg daily, whichever is less.
Adjust-a-dose: In patients with moderate
hepatic impairment, reduce to 50% of the
normal dose; in those with severe hepatic
impairment, reduce to 25% of the normal
dose. Poor metabolizers of CYP2D6 may
require a reduced dose. In children who
weigh less than 70 kg, adjust dosage to
0.5 mg/kg daily and increase to 1.2 mg/kg
daily if symptoms don't improve after
4 weeks and if first dose is tolerated.
In children and adults who weigh more
than 70 kg, start at 40 mg daily and
increase to 80 mg daily if symptoms
don't improve after 4 weeks and if first
dose is tolerated.

ADMINISTRATION
P.O.
● Give drug without regard for meals.
● Capsules should be swallowed whole
and not opened.

ACTION
May be related to selective inhibition of
the presynaptic norepinephrine trans-
porter.

Route	Onset	Peak	Duration
P.O.	Rapid	1–2 hr	Unknown

Half-life: 21½ hours.

ADVERSE REACTIONS
CNS: *headache, insomnia,* dizziness,
somnolence, crying, irritability, mood
swings, pyrexia, fatigue, sedation, depression, tremor, early-morning awakening,
paresthesia, abnormal dreams, sleep
disorder.
CV: orthostatic hypotension, tachycardia,
hypertension, palpitations, hot flashes.
EENT: ear infection, rhinorrhea, sore
throat, nasal congestion, nasopharyngitis,
sinus congestion, mydriasis, sinusitis.
GI: *abdominal pain, constipation,* dyspepsia, *nausea, vomiting, decreased appetite,*
gastroenteritis, *dry mouth,* flatulence.
GU: urinary retention, urinary hesitation,
ejaculatory problems, difficulty in micturition, dysmenorrhea, erectile disturbance,
impotence, delayed menses, menstrual
disorder, prostatitis.
Metabolic: weight loss.
Musculoskeletal: arthralgia, myalgia.
Respiratory: *cough,* upper respiratory
tract infection.
Skin: *dermatitis, pruritus, increased*
sweating.
Other: influenza, decreased libido, rigors.

INTERACTIONS
Drug-drug. *Albuterol:* May increase CV effects. Use together cautiously.
MAO inhibitors: May cause hyperthermia, rigidity, myoclonus, autonomic instability with possible rapid fluctuations of vital signs, and mental status changes. Avoid use within 2 weeks of MAO inhibitor.
Pressor agents: May increase blood pressure. Use together cautiously.
Strong CYP2D6 inhibitors (paroxetine, fluoxetine, quinidine): May increase atomoxetine level. Reduce first dose.

EFFECTS ON LAB TEST RESULTS
None reported.

CONTRAINDICATIONS & CAUTIONS
• Contraindicated in patients hypersensitive to atomoxetine or to components of drug, in those who have taken an MAO inhibitor within the past 2 weeks, and in those with angle-closure glaucoma.
• Use cautiously in patients with hypertension, tachycardia, or CV or cerebrovascular disease, and in pregnant or breast-feeding women.
• Safety and efficacy haven't been established in patients younger than age 6.

NURSING CONSIDERATIONS
• Use drug as part of a total treatment program for ADHD, including psychological, educational, and social intervention.
■ **Black Box Warning** Monitor children and adolescents closely for worsening of condition, agitation, irritability, suicidal thinking or behaviors, and unusual changes in behavior, especially the first few months of therapy or when the dosage is increased or decreased. ■
• Patients taking drug for extended periods must be reevaluated periodically to determine drug's usefulness.
• Monitor growth during treatment. If growth or weight gain is unsatisfactory, consider interrupting therapy.
• *Alert:* Severe liver injury may occur and progress to liver failure. Notify prescriber of any sign of liver injury: yellowing of the skin or the sclera of the eyes, pruritus, dark urine, upper right-sided tenderness, or unexplained flulike syndrome.

• Monitor blood pressure and pulse at baseline, after each dose increase, and during treatment periodically.
• Monitor for urinary hesitancy or retention and sexual dysfunction.
• Patient can stop drug without tapering off.

PATIENT TEACHING
• *Alert:* Advise parents to call prescriber immediately about unusual behavior or suicidal thoughts.
• Tell pregnant women, women planning to become pregnant, and breast-feeding women to consult prescriber before taking atomoxetine.
• Tell patient to use caution when operating a vehicle or machinery until the effects of drug are known.

---

dexmethylphenidate hydrochloride
decks-meth-ill-FEN-i-date

Focalin, Focalin XR

Pharmacologic class:
methylphenidate derivative
Pregnancy risk category C
Controlled substance schedule II

AVAILABLE FORMS
Capsules (extended-release): 5 mg, 10 mg, 15 mg, 20 mg
Tablets: 2.5 mg, 5 mg, 10 mg

INDICATIONS & DOSAGES
➤ **Attention deficit hyperactivity disorder (ADHD)**
immediate-release tablets
Adults and children age 6 and older:
For patients who aren't now taking methylphenidate, initially, 2.5 mg P.O. b.i.d., given at least 4 hours apart. Increase weekly by 2.5 to 5 mg daily, up to a maximum of 20 mg daily in divided doses.
   For patients who are now taking methylphenidate, initially give half the current methylphenidate dosage, up to a maximum of 20 mg P.O. daily in divided doses.
extended-release capsules
Adults: For patients who aren't now taking dexmethylphenidate or methylphenidate, or who are on stimulants other than

---

Reactions may be *common*, uncommon, *life-threatening*, or COMMON AND LIFE-THREATENING.
Interaction may have a *rapid onset* or **delayed onset.**

methylphenidate, give 10 mg P.O. once daily in the morning. May adjust in weekly increments of 10 mg to a maximum dose of 20 mg daily.

For patients who are now taking methylphenidate, initially give half the total daily dose of methylphenidate. Patients who are now taking the immediate-release form of dexmethylphenidate may be switched to the same daily dose of extended-release form. Maximum daily dose is 20 mg.

Children ages 6 and older: For patients who aren't now taking dexmethyl-phenidate or methylphenidate, or who are on stimulants other than methylphenidate, give 5 mg P.O. once daily in the morning. May adjust in weekly increments of 5 mg to a maximum daily dose of 20 mg.

For patients who are now taking methylphenidate, initially give half the total daily dose of methylphenidate. Patients who are now taking the immediate-release form of dexmethylphenidate may be switched to the same daily dose of extended-release form. Maximum daily dose is 20 mg.

ADMINISTRATION
P.O.
● Capsules may be swallowed whole or the contents sprinkled on a small amount of applesauce and eaten immediately.
● Don't crush or divide the capsule or its contents.

ACTION
Blocks presynaptic reuptake of norepi-nephrine and dopamine and increases their release, increasing concentration in the synapse.

Route	Onset	Peak	Duration
P.O. (immediate-release)	Unknown	1–1½ hr	Unknown
P.O. (extended-release)	Unknown	1–4 hr; 4½–7 hr	Unknown

Half-life: 2 to 3 hours.

ADVERSE REACTIONS
CNS: *headache, anxiety, feeling jittery,* nervousness, insomnia, fever, dizziness.
CV: tachycardia.

EENT: throat pain.
GI: *anorexia, abdominal pain,* nausea, dyspepsia, dry mouth.
Musculoskeletal: twitching (motor or vocal tics).
Other: hypersensitivity reactions.

INTERACTIONS
Drug-drug. *Antacids, acid suppressants:* May alter the release of extended-release form. Avoid using together.
Anticoagulants, phenobarbital, phenytoin, primidone, tricyclic antidepressants: May inhibit metabolism of these drugs. May need to decrease dosage of these drugs; monitor drug levels.
Antihypertensives: May decrease effectiveness of these drugs. Use together cautiously; monitor blood pressure.
Clonidine, other centrally acting alpha agonists: May cause serious adverse effects. Use together cautiously.
MAO inhibitors: May increase risk of hypertensive crisis. Using together within 14 days of MAO inhibitor therapy is contraindicated.

EFFECTS ON LAB TEST RESULTS
None reported.

CONTRAINDICATIONS & CAUTIONS
● Contraindicated in patients hypersensitive to methylphenidate or other components.
● Contraindicated in patients with severe anxiety, tension, or agitation; glaucoma; or motor tics or a family history or diagnosis of Tourette syndrome, or within 14 days of MAO inhibitor therapy.
■ **Black Box Warning** Use cautiously in patients with a history of substance abuse. ■
● Use cautiously in patients with a psychiatric illness, bipolar disorder, depression, or family history of suicide; seizures, hypertension, hyperthyroidism, heart failure, or recent MI.
● Use in pregnant women only if the benefits outweigh the risks; drug may delay skeletal ossification, suppress weight gain, and impair organ development in the fetus.
● Use cautiously in breast-feeding women. It's unknown if drug appears in breast milk.
● Don't use in children or adolescents with structural cardiac abnormalities or other serious heart problems.

NURSING CONSIDERATIONS
• Diagnosis of ADHD must be based on complete history and evaluation of the patient by psychological and educational experts.
• Obtain a detailed patient history, including a family history for mental disorders, family suicide, ventricular arrhythmias, or sudden death.
• Refer patient for psychological, educational, and social support.
• Periodically reevaluate the long-term usefulness of the drug.
• Monitor CBC and differential and platelet counts during prolonged therapy.
• Don't use for severe depression or normal fatigue states.
• Stop treatment or reduce dosage if symptoms worsen or adverse reactions occur.
• Long-term stimulant use may temporarily suppress growth. Monitor children for growth and weight gain. If growth slows or weight gain is lower than expected, stop drug.
• Routinely monitor blood pressure and pulse.
• Monitor patient for signs of drug dependence or abuse.
• If seizures occur, stop drug.

PATIENT TEACHING
• Stress the importance of taking the correct dose of drug at the same time every day. Report accidental overdose immediately.
• *Alert:* Warn patient the misuse of amphetamines can have serious effects including sudden death.
• Advise patients unable to swallow capsules to empty the contents of the capsule onto a spoonful of applesauce and eat immediately.
• *Alert:* Tell patient not to cut, crush, or chew the contents of the extended-release beaded capsule.
• Advise parents to monitor child for medication abuse or sharing. Also inform parents to watch for increased aggression or hostility and to report worsening behavior.
• Advise parents to monitor child's height and weight and to tell the prescriber if they suspect growth is slowing.
• Caution patient to expect blurred vision or difficulty with accommodation and to exercise caution while performing activities that require a clear visual field. Advise patient to report blurred vision to the prescriber.

dextroamphetamine sulfate
dex-troe-am-FET-a-meen

Dexedrine*, Dexedrine Spansule, DextroStat, Liquadd

Pharmacologic class: amphetamine
Pregnancy risk category C
Controlled substance schedule II

AVAILABLE FORMS
Capsules (extended-release): 5 mg, 10 mg, 15 mg
Oral solution: 5 mg/5 ml
Tablets: 5 mg, 10 mg

INDICATIONS & DOSAGES
➤ **Narcolepsy**
Adults: 5 to 60 mg P.O. daily in divided doses.
Children ages 6 to 12: 5 mg P.O. daily. Increase by 5 mg at weekly intervals as needed.
Children age 12 and older: 10 mg P.O. daily. Increase by 10 mg at weekly intervals, as needed. Give first dose on awakening; additional doses (one or two) given at intervals of 4 to 6 hours.
➤ **Attention deficit hyperactivity disorder (ADHD)**
Children age 6 and older: 5 mg P.O. once daily or b.i.d. Increase by 5 mg at weekly intervals, as needed. It's rarely necessary to exceed 40 mg/day.
Children ages 3 to 5: 2.5 mg P.O. daily. Increase by 2.5 mg at weekly intervals, as needed.

ADMINISTRATION
P.O.
• Give drug 30 to 60 minutes before meals if used for weight reduction and at least 6 hours before bedtime to avoid sleep interference.
• Certain formulations may contain tartrazine.

ACTION
Unknown. Probably promotes nerve impulse transmission by releasing

stored dopamine and norepinephrine from nerve terminals in the brain. Main sites of activity appear to be the cerebral cortex and the reticular activating system.

Route	Onset	Peak	Duration
P.O.	30–60 min	2 hr	4 hr
P.O. (extended)	60 min	2 hr	8 hr

Half-life: 10 to 12 hours.

ADVERSE REACTIONS
CNS: *insomnia, nervousness, restlessness,* tremor, dizziness, headache, chills, over-stimulation, dysphoria, euphoria.
CV: *tachycardia, palpitations, arrhythmias,* hypertension.
GI: dry mouth, taste perversion, diarrhea, constipation, anorexia, other GI disturbances.
GU: impotence.
Metabolic: weight loss.
Skin: urticaria.
Other: increased libido.

INTERACTIONS
Drug-drug. *Acetazolamide, alkalizing drugs, antacids, sodium bicarbonate:* May increase renal reabsorption. Monitor patient for enhanced amphetamine effects.
Acidifying drugs, ammonium chloride, ascorbic acid: May decrease level and increase renal clearance of dextroamphetamine. Monitor patient for decreased amphetamine effects.
Adrenergic blockers: May inhibit adrenergic blocking effects. Avoid using together.
Chlorpromazine: May inhibit central stimulant effects of amphetamines. May use to treat amphetamine poisoning.
Insulin, oral antidiabetics: May decrease antidiabetic requirements. Monitor glucose level.
MAO inhibitors: May cause severe hypertension or hypertensive crisis. Avoid using within 14 days of MAO inhibitor therapy.
Meperidine: May potentiate analgesic effect. Use together cautiously.
Methenamine: May increase urinary excretion of amphetamines and reduce effectiveness. Monitor drug effects.

Norepinephrine: May enhance adrenergic effect of norepinephrine. Monitor patient.
Phenobarbital, phenytoin: May delay absorption of these drugs. Monitor patient closely.
Drug-food. *Caffeine:* May increase amphetamine and related amine effects. Urge caution.
Fruit juice: May decrease effectiveness of oral solution. Avoid giving together.

EFFECTS ON LAB TEST RESULTS
● May increase corticosteroid level.

CONTRAINDICATIONS & CAUTIONS
● Contraindicated in patients hypersensitive to or with idiosyncratic reactions to sympathomimetic amines and in those with hyperthyroidism, moderate to severe hypertension, symptomatic CV disease, glaucoma, advanced arteriosclerosis, or history of drug abuse.
● Contraindicated as first-line treatment for obesity or within 14 days of MAO inhibitor therapy.
● Use cautiously in agitated patients and patients with motor tics, phonic tics, or Tourette syndrome. Also use cautiously in patients whose underlying condition may be worsened by an increase in blood pressure or heart rate (preexisting hypertension, heart failure, recent MI); patients with a psychiatric illness, bipolar disorder, depression, or family history of suicide; those with a seizure disorder.
● Don't use in children or adolescents with structural cardiac abnormalities or other serious heart problems.

NURSING CONSIDERATIONS
● Obtain a detailed patient history, including a family history for mental disorders, family suicide, ventricular arrhythmias, or sudden death.
● Drug shouldn't be used to prevent fatigue.
● Obese patients should follow a weight-reduction program.
■ **Black Box Warning** Drug has a high abuse potential and may cause dependence. Monitor patient closely. ■
● *Alert:* Overdose may cause seizures.

- If tolerance to anorexigenic effect develops, stop drug and notify prescriber.
- Monitor for growth retardation in children.
- *Look alike–sound alike:* Don't confuse Dexedrine with dextran or Excedrin.

PATIENT TEACHING
- *Alert:* Warn patient the misuse of amphetamines can cause serious CV adverse events including sudden death.
- Tell patient to take drug 30 to 60 minutes before meals if used for weight reduction and at least 6 hours before bedtime to avoid sleep interference.
- Warn patient to avoid activities that require alertness, a clear visual field, or good coordination until CNS effects of drug are known.
- Tell patient he may get tired as drug effects wear off.
- Ask patient to report signs and symptoms of excessive stimulation.
- Inform parents that children may show increased aggression or hostility and to report worsening of behavior.
- Advise patient to consume caffeine-containing products cautiously.
- Tell patient not to drink fruit juice at same time as oral solution.
- Warn patient with a seizure disorder that drug may decrease seizure threshold. Instruct him to notify prescriber if seizures occur.

---

lisdexamfetamine dimesylate
lis-DEX-am-FET-a-meen

Vyvanse

Pharmacologic class: amphetamine
Pregnancy risk category C
Controlled substance schedule II

AVAILABLE FORMS
Capsules: 20 mg, 30 mg, 40 mg, 50 mg, 60 mg, 70 mg

INDICATIONS & DOSAGES
➤ **Attention deficit hyperactivity disorder (ADHD)**
Adults and children ages 6 to 12: Initially, 30 mg P.O. once daily in the morning.

Increase by 10 or 20 mg at weekly intervals to a maximum of 70 mg daily.

ADMINISTRATION
P.O.
- Capsules may be swallowed whole or the contents dissolved in a glass of water and taken immediately.
- Give drug in the morning to prevent insomnia.

ACTION
May increase the release of norepinephrine and dopamine into extraneural spaces by blocking their reuptake into the presynaptic neuron.

Route	Onset	Peak	Duration
P.O.	Rapid	1 hr	Unknown

Half-life: Less than 1 hour.

ADVERSE REACTIONS
CNS: *headache, insomnia, irritability,* aggressive or hostile behavior, agitation, delusional thinking, dizziness, fever, hallucinations, labile affect, restlessness, somnolence, tic, tremor.
CV: *ventricular hypertrophy,* increased blood pressure, increased heart rate.
EENT: abnormal vision, blurred vision.
GI: *abdominal pain, decreased appetite,* dry mouth, nausea, vomiting.
Metabolic: slow growth, weight loss.
Respiratory: dyspnea.
Skin: hyperhidrosis, rash.

INTERACTIONS
Drug-drug. *Adrenergic blockers:* May inhibit adrenergic blocking effects. Avoid using together.
Antihistamines: May inhibit sedative effects of antihistamines. Monitor patient.
Antihypertensives, veratrum alkaloids: May inhibit antihypertensive effects of these drugs. Avoid using together.
Chlorpromazine, haloperidol: May decrease effectiveness of amphetamines. Monitor patient closely.
Ethosuximide: May delay absorption of this drug. Monitor patient closely.
Lithium: May inhibit anorectic and CNS stimulant effects of amphetamine. Monitor patient closely.

Reactions may be *common*, uncommon, *life-threatening*, or COMMON AND LIFE-THREATENING.
Interaction may have a *rapid onset* or *delayed onset.*

Tricyclic antidepressants: May cause adverse CV effects. Avoid using together.
MAO inhibitors: May cause severe hypertension or hypertensive crisis. Avoid using within 14 days of MAO inhibitor therapy.
Meperidine: May increase the analgesic effect of meperidine. Use together cautiously.
Norepinephrine: May increase adrenergic effects of norepinephrine. Monitor patient closely.
Phenobarbital, phenytoin: May delay intestinal absorption of these drugs and enhance their anticonvulsant effects. Monitor patient closely.
Propoxyphene: May cause fatal seizures if overdose of propoxyphene taken. Don't use together.
Urine acidifiers (ammonium chloride, sodium acid phosphate), methenamine: May decrease serum level due to increased renal excretion of amphetamine. Monitor patient for decreased drug effects.
Drug-food. *Caffeine:* May increase CNS stimulation. Discourage use together.

EFFECTS ON LAB TEST RESULTS
● May increase corticosteroid level.
● May interfere with urinary steroid test.

CONTRAINDICATIONS & CAUTIONS
● Contraindicated in patients hypersensitive to sympathomimetic amines or in those with idiosyncratic reactions to them, in agitated patients, and in those with a history of drug abuse.
● Contraindicated in patients with advanced arteriosclerosis, hyperthyroidism, symptomatic CV disease, structural cardiac abnormalities, moderate to severe hypertension, or glaucoma.
● Contraindicated within 14 days of MAO inhibitor therapy.
● Use cautiously in patients with a history of arrhythmias, MI, stroke, or seizures.
● Use cautiously in patients with preexisting psychosis, bipolar disorder, or aggressive behavior; or Tourette syndrome.

NURSING CONSIDERATIONS
● Diagnosis of ADHD must be based on complete history and evaluation of the child with consultation of psychological, educational, and social resources.

● Give the lowest effective dose in the morning. Afternoon doses may cause insomnia.
■ **Black Box Warning** Monitor patient for signs of drug dependence or abuse. Misuse may cause sudden death. ■
● Abruptly stopping the drug can cause severe fatigue and depression.
● Monitor patient closely for adverse CV effects, new or worsening behavior (aggression, mania), vision problems, or seizures.
● Monitor blood pressure and pulse routinely.
● Effectiveness of this drug when taken longer than 4 weeks isn't known. Periodically interrupt therapy to determine whether continuation is necessary.
● Growth may be suppressed with long-term stimulant use. Monitor the child for growth and weight gain. Stop treatment if growth is suppressed or if weight gain is lower than expected.
● The drug may trigger Tourette syndrome. Monitor patient, especially at the start of therapy.

PATIENT TEACHING
● Tell patient or caregiver that drug should be taken in the morning to prevent insomnia.
● Advise patient to swallow capsule whole. If he's unable to do so, the contents may be dissolved in a glass of water and taken immediately. Once dissolved, don't store for later use.
● Tell patient or caregiver that abruptly stopping drug can cause severe fatigue, depression, or general withdrawal reaction.
● Caution patient to avoid activities that require alertness or good psychomotor coordination until CNS effects of drug are known.
● Warn patient with seizure disorder that drug may decrease seizure threshold. Urge him to notify his prescriber if a seizure occurs.
● Instruct patient or caregiver to report palpitations or visual disturbances.
● Tell patient or caregiver to report worsening aggression, hallucinations, delusions, or mania.
● Advise patient to avoid caffeine consumption while taking drug.

methylphenidate hydrochloride
meth-ill-FEN-i-date

Concerta◊, Metadate CD, Metadate ER, Methylin, Methylin ER, Ritalin◊, Ritalin LA, Ritalin-SR◊

methylphenidate transdermal system
Daytrana

Pharmacologic class: piperidine derivative
Pregnancy risk category NR; C (for Concerta, Daytrana, Metadate CD, Ritalin LA)
Controlled substance schedule II

AVAILABLE FORMS
Oral solution (Methylin): 5 mg/5 ml, 10 mg/5 ml
Tablets (chewable): 2.5 mg, 5 mg, 10 mg
Tablets (Ritalin, Methylin): 5 mg, 10 mg, 20 mg
Extended-release
Capsules (Metadate CD): 10 mg, 20 mg, 30 mg, 40 mg, 50 mg, 60 mg
Capsules (Ritalin LA): 10 mg, 20 mg, 30 mg, 40 mg
Tablets (Concerta): 18 mg, 27 mg, 36 mg, 54 mg
Tablets (Metadate ER, Methylin ER): 10 mg, 20 mg
Sustained-release
Tablets (Ritalin-SR): 20 mg
Transdermal system
Patch: 10 mg, 15 mg, 20 mg, 30 mg

INDICATIONS & DOSAGES
➤ **Attention deficit hyperactivity disorder (ADHD)**
Children age 6 and older: Initially, 5 mg P.O. b.i.d. immediate-release form before breakfast and lunch, increasing by 5 to 10 mg at weekly intervals, as needed, until an optimum daily dose of 2 mg/kg is reached, not to exceed 60 mg/day. To use Ritalin-SR, Metadate ER, and Methylin ER tablets in place of immediate-release methylphenidate tablets, calculate methylphenidate dosage in 8-hour intervals.
Concerta
Adolescents age 13 to 17 not currently taking methylphenidate, or for patients taking other stimulants: 18 mg P.O. extended-release Concerta once daily in the morning. Adjust dosage by 18 mg at weekly intervals to a maximum of 72 mg P.O. (not to exceed 2 mg/kg) once daily in the morning.
Children age 6 to 12 not currently taking methylphenidate or patients taking stimulants other than methylphenidate: 18 mg extended-release P.O. once daily every morning. Adjust dosage by 18 mg at weekly intervals to a maximum of 54 mg daily every morning.
Adolescents and children age 6 and older currently taking methylphenidate: If previous methylphenidate dosage was 5 mg b.i.d. or t.i.d. or 20 mg sustained-release, give 18 mg P.O. every morning. If previous dosage was 10 mg b.i.d. or t.i.d. or 40 mg sustained-release, give 36 mg P.O. every morning. If previous dosage was 15 mg b.i.d. or t.i.d. or 60 mg sustained-release, give 54 mg P.O. every morning. Maximum conversion daily dose is 54 mg. Once conversion is complete, adjust adolescents age 13 to 17 to maximum dose of 72 mg once daily (not to exceed 2 mg/kg).
Metadate CD
Children age 6 and older: Initially, 20 mg P.O. daily before breakfast, increasing by 10 to 20 mg at weekly intervals to a maximum of 60 mg daily.
Ritalin LA
Children age 6 and older: 20 mg P.O. once daily. Increase by 10 mg at weekly intervals to a maximum of 60 mg daily. If previous methylphenidate dosage was 10 mg b.i.d. or 20 mg sustained-release, give 20 mg P.O. once daily. If previous methylphenidate dosage was 15 mg b.i.d., give 30 mg P.O. once daily. If previous methylphenidate dosage was 20 mg b.i.d. or 40 mg sustained-release, give 40 mg P.O. once daily. If previous methylphenidate dosage was 30 mg b.i.d. or 60 mg sustained-release, give 60 mg P.O. once daily.
Daytrana
Children age 6 to 12: Initially, apply one 10-mg patch to clean, dry, nonirritated skin on the hip, alternating sites daily.

Apply 2 hours before desired effect and remove 9 hours later. Increase dose weekly as needed to a maximum of 30 mg daily. Base final dose and wear time on patient response.

➤ **Narcolepsy**
Adults: 10 mg P.O. b.i.d. or t.i.d. immediate-release, 30 to 45 minutes before meals. Dosage varies; average is 40 to 60 mg/day. To use Ritalin-SR, Metadate ER, or Methylin ER tablets in place of immediate-release methylphenidate tablets, calculate the dose of methylphenidate in 8-hour intervals.

ADMINISTRATION
P.O.
● Give chewable tablet with at least 8 oz (237 ml) of water.
● Give drug after meals to reduce appetite-suppressant effects; give last daily dose at least 6 hours before bedtime to prevent insomnia.
● Metadate CD or Ritalin LA may be swallowed whole, or the contents of the capsule may be sprinkled onto a small amount of cool applesauce and taken immediately.
Transdermal
● Avoid placing the patch on the waistline or where tight clothing may rub it off.

ACTION
Releases nerve terminal stores of norepinephrine, promoting nerve impulse transmission. At high doses, effects are mediated by dopamine.

Route	Onset	Peak	Duration
P.O. (Methylin, Ritalin)	Unknown	2 hr	Unknown
P.O. (Methylin ER, Ritalin-SR)	Unknown	5 hr	8 hr
P.O. (Metadate CD)	Unknown	1½ hr; 4½ hr	Unknown
P.O. (Ritalin LA)	Unknown	1–3 hr; 4–7 hr	Unknown
P.O. (Concerta)	Unknown	6–8 hr	Unknown
Transdermal	2 hr	Variable	14 hr

Half-life: Conventional, 3 to 6 hours; extended-release (Metadate ER, Methylin ER, Ritalin SR), 3 to 8 hours, (Concerta, Metadate CD, Ritalin LA) 8 to 12 hours; transdermal, 3 to 4 hours.

ADVERSE REACTIONS
CNS: *nervousness, headache, insomnia, seizures,* tics, dizziness, akathisia, dyskinesia, drowsiness, mood swings.
CV: *palpitations, tachycardia, arrhythmias,* hypertension.
EENT: pharyngitis, sinusitis.
GI: *nausea, abdominal pain, anorexia, decreased appetite, vomiting.*
Hematologic: *thrombocytopenia, thrombocytopenic purpura, leukopenia,* anemia.
Metabolic: weight loss.
Respiratory: cough, upper respiratory tract infection.
Skin: *exfoliative dermatitis,* **erythema multiforme,** rash, urticaria, application site irritation (redness, swelling, papules).
Other: *viral infection.*

INTERACTIONS
Drug-drug. *Anticonvulsants (such as phenobarbital, phenytoin, primidone), SSRIs, tricyclic antidepressants (imipramine, clomipramine, desipramine), warfarin:* May increase levels of these drugs. Monitor patient for adverse reactions and decrease dose of these drugs as needed. Monitor drug levels (or coagulation times if patient is also taking warfarin).
Centrally acting alpha₂ agonists, clonidine: May cause serious adverse events. Avoid using together.
Centrally acting antihypertensives: May decrease antihypertensive effect. Monitor blood pressure.
MAO inhibitors: May cause severe hypertension or hypertensive crisis. Avoid using within 14 days of MAO inhibitor therapy.
Drug-food. *Caffeine:* May increase amphetamine and related amine effects. Discourage use together.

EFFECTS ON LAB TEST RESULTS
● May decrease hemoglobin level and hematocrit.
● May decrease platelet and WBC counts.

CONTRAINDICATIONS & CAUTIONS
● Contraindicated in patients hypersensitive to drug and in those with glaucoma, motor tics, family history or diagnosis of Tourette syndrome, or history of marked anxiety, tension, or agitation. Also contraindicated within 14 days of MAO inhibitor

therapy. Avoid use in patients with structural cardiac abnormalities.

• Because it doesn't dissolve, Concerta isn't recommended in patients with a history of peritonitis or with severe GI narrowing (such as small bowel inflammatory disease, short-gut syndrome caused by adhesions or decreased transit time, cystic fibrosis, chronic intestinal pseudo-obstruction, or Meckel diverticulum).

• Use cautiously in patients with a history of emotional disorder, seizures, EEG abnormalities, or hypertension, and in patients whose underlying medical conditions might be compromised by increases in blood pressure or heart rate, such as those with preexisting hypertension, heart failure, recent MI, or hyperthyroidism.

■ **Black Box Warning** Use cautiously in patients who have a history of drug dependence or alcoholism. ■

NURSING CONSIDERATIONS

• Chewable tablets contain phenylalanine.
• Don't use drug to prevent fatigue or treat severe depression.
• Drug may trigger Tourette syndrome in children. Monitor patient, especially at start of therapy.
• Observe patient for signs of excessive stimulation. Monitor blood pressure.
• Check CBC, differential, and platelet counts with long-term use, particularly if patient shows signs or symptoms of hematologic toxicity (fever, sore throat, easy bruising).
• Monitor height and weight in children on long-term therapy. Drug may delay growth spurt, but children will attain normal height when drug is stopped.
• Monitor patient for tolerance or psychological dependence.
• *Look alike–sound alike:* Don't confuse Ritalin with Rifadin, or Ritalin SR with Ritalin LA.

PATIENT TEACHING

• Tell patient or caregiver to give last daily dose at least 6 hours before bedtime to prevent insomnia and after meals to reduce appetite-suppressant effects.
• Warn patient against chewing sustained-release tablets.
• Metadate CD or Ritalin LA may be swallowed whole, or the contents of the capsule may be sprinkled onto a small amount of cool applesauce and taken immediately.

• *Alert:* Warn patient to take chewable tablet with at least 8 oz (237 ml) of water. Not using enough water to swallow tablet may cause the tablet to swell and block the throat, causing choking.

• Caution patient to avoid activities that require alertness or good psychomotor coordination until CNS effects of drug are known.

• Warn patient with seizure disorder that drug may decrease seizure threshold. Urge him to notify prescriber if seizure occurs.

• Advise patient to avoid beverages containing caffeine while taking drug.

• Tell parent to apply patch immediately after opening; don't use if pouch seal is broken. Press firmly in place for about 30 seconds using the palm of your hand, being sure there is good contact with the skin, especially around the edges. Once applied correctly, the child may shower, bathe, or swim as usual.

• Inform parent if patch comes off, a new one may be applied on a different site, but the total wear time for that day should be 9 hours. Upon removal, fold patch in half so the sticky sides adhere to itself, then flush down toilet or dispose of in a lidded container.

• Tell parent, if the applied patch is missing, to ask the child when or how the patch came off. Teach child that patch shouldn't be shared or removed except by parent or health care provider.

• Encourage parent to use the application chart provided with patch carton to keep track of application and removal.

• Tell parent to remove patch sooner than 9 hours if the child has decreased evening appetite or has difficulty sleeping.

• Tell parent the effects of the patch lasts for several hours after its removal.

• Warn parent and patient to avoid exposing patch to direct external heat sources, such as heating pads, electric blankets, and heated water beds.

• Tell parent to notify prescriber if the child develops bumps, swelling, or blistering at the application site or is experiencing blurred vision or other serious side effects.

44

CNS stimulants

armodafinil
dextroamphetamine sulfate
(See Chapter 43, ATTENTION DEFICIT
HYPERACTIVITY DISORDER DRUGS.)
doxapram hydrochloride
methylphenidate hydrochloride
(See Chapter 43, ATTENTION DEFICIT
HYPERACTIVITY DISORDER DRUGS.)
modafinil
phentermine hydrochloride
**sibutramine hydrochloride
monohydrate**

---

armodafinil
are-moe-DAFF-ih-nihl

Nuvigil

Pharmacologic class: CNS
stimulant
Pregnancy risk category C
Controlled substance schedule IV

AVAILABLE FORMS
Tablets: 50 mg, 150 mg, 250 mg

INDICATIONS & DOSAGES
➤ **To improve wakefulness in
patients with excessive sleepiness
caused by narcolepsy, obstructive
sleep apnea-hypoapnea syndrome
(OAHS), or shift-work sleep
disorder**
Adults: 150 mg to 250 mg P.O. daily
in the morning. For OAHS, doses
exceeding 150 mg daily may not be
more effective. For shift-work disorder,
150 mg P.O. daily, 1 hour before start of
shift.
Adjust-a-dose: Reduce dosage in patients
with severe hepatic impairment, with or
without cirrhosis.

ADMINISTRATION
P.O.
• Give drug consistently with or without
food at same time each day. Food may
delay effect of drug.

ACTION
Unknown. May be similar to sympathomimetics, such as amphetamine and
methylphenidate. Also may inhibit
dopamine reuptake.

Route	Onset	Peak	Duration
P.O.	Unknown	2 hr	Unknown

Half-life: 15 hours.

ADVERSE REACTIONS
CNS: agitation, anxiety, depression,
dizziness, fatigue, *headache,* insomnia,
migraine, nervousness, pain, paresthesia,
pyrexia, tremor.
CV: increased blood pressure, increased
pulse, palpitations.
GI: abdominal pain, anorexia, constipation, diarrhea, dry mouth, dyspepsia, loose
stools, nausea, vomiting.
Respiratory: dyspnea.
Skin: contact dermatitis, hyperhidrosis,
rash, *Stevens-Johnson syndrome.*
Other: allergic reactions, flulike illness,
thirst.

INTERACTIONS
Drug-drug. *CNS stimulants (amphetamine,
methylphenidate):* May produce additive
effects. Use cautiously together.
*Drugs metabolized by CYP2C19
(diazepam, omeprazole, phenytoin, propranolol):* May increase levels of these
drugs. Monitor patient and reduce doses
as needed.
*Drugs metabolized by CYP3A (cyclo-
sporine, ethinyl estradiol, midazolam,
triazolam):* May decrease levels of these
drugs. Adjust doses as needed.
*Drugs that induce CYP3A (carbama-
zepine, phenobarbital, rifampin):* May
decrease armodafinil level. Check drug
level and adjust dose as needed.
*Drugs that inhibit CYP3A (erythromycin,
ketoconazole):* May increase armodafinil
level. Monitor patient carefully and
decrease dose as needed.
Drug-food. *Any food:* May delay onset of
action by several hours. Monitor effect

and give drug consistently with or without food, at the same time daily.

Drug-lifestyle. *Alcohol use:* May counteract armodafinil's effect. Discourage use together.

EFFECTS ON LAB TEST RESULTS
● May increase GGT and alkaline phosphatase levels.

CONTRAINDICATIONS & CAUTIONS
● Contraindicated in patients younger than age 17.
● Contraindicated in patients hypersensitive to modafinil, armodafinil, or their inactive ingredients.
● Contraindicated with left ventricular hypertrophy and with mitral valve prolapse developed with other CNS stimulants.
● Use cautiously in breast-feeding or elderly patients.
● Use in pregnant patient only when benefit to mother outweighs risk to fetus.
● Use cautiously in those with a history of drug abuse or dependence.
● Use cautiously in patients with a psychiatric illness; drug may increase the risk of mania, delusion, hallucinations, and suicidal ideation.
● Use cautiously in patients with cardiac disease, multiorgan hypersensitivity, or rash, including Stevens-Johnson syndrome and severe hepatic impairment.

NURSING CONSIDERATIONS
● Obtain a thorough medication history to avoid potentially dangerous drug interactions.
● Obtain a complete cardiac history. Monitor patient for increased blood pressure and pulse rate, ECG changes, chest pain, and arrhythmias.
● Monitor patient carefully for evidence of allergic reaction. If rash or other symptoms appear, stop drug immediately, notify prescriber, and monitor carefully.
● Assess patient for abnormal level of sleepiness. Don't allow patient to engage in dangerous activities, such as driving, until effect of medication is known.
● Patients receiving continuous positive airway pressure therapy for OAHS should continue its use regardless of armodafinil therapy.

PATIENT TEACHING
● **Alert:** Instruct patient to stop taking drug and notify prescriber if rash, hives, mouth sores, blister, peeling skin, trouble swallowing or breathing, or other symptoms of allergic reaction occur.
● Tell patient not to perform hazardous tasks, such as driving, if he feels excessive sleepiness or until effects of drug are known.
● Tell patient to notify prescriber of all drugs he takes to avoid potentially dangerous drug interactions.
● Tell patient to take drug at the same time, with or without food, every day.
● Advise patient that taking drug with food may delay its effects.
● Urge patient to notify prescriber right away if she becomes pregnant or plans to breast-feed.

doxapram hydrochloride
DOCKS-a-pram

Dopram

Pharmacologic class: analeptic
Pregnancy risk category B

AVAILABLE FORMS
Injection: 20 mg/ml (benzyl alcohol 0.9%)

INDICATIONS & DOSAGES
➤ **Postanesthesia respiratory stimulation**
Adults: 0.5 to 1 mg/kg as a single I.V. injection (not to exceed 1.5 mg/kg) or as multiple injections every 5 minutes, total not to exceed 2 mg/kg. Or, 250 mg in 250 ml of normal saline solution or D_5W infused at initial rate of 5 mg/minute I.V. until satisfactory response is achieved. Maintain at 1 to 3 mg/minute. Don't exceed total dose for infusion of 4 mg/kg.
➤ **Drug-induced CNS depression**
Adults: For injection, priming dose of 2 mg/kg I.V., repeated in 5 minutes and again every 1 to 2 hours until patient awakens (and if relapse occurs). Maximum daily dose is 3 g.

For infusion, priming dose of 2 mg/kg I.V., repeated in 5 minutes and again in 1 to 2 hours, if needed. If response occurs, give I.V. infusion (1 mg/ml) at 1 to 3 mg/minute

until patient awakens. Don't infuse for longer than 2 hours or give more than 3 g/day. May resume I.V. infusion after rest period of 30 minutes to 2 hours, if needed.

➤ **Chronic pulmonary disease related to acute hypercapnia**
Adults: 1 to 2 mg/minute by I.V. infusion using 2 mg/ml solution. Maximum, 3 mg/minute for up to 2 hours.

ADMINISTRATION
I.V.
- Drug is compatible with D_5W, $D_{10}W$, and normal saline solution.
- Give slowly; rapid infusion may cause hemolysis.
- Watch for irritation and infiltration; it can cause tissue damage and necrosis.
- **Incompatibilities:** Aminophylline, ascorbic acid, cefoperazone, cefotaxime, cefuroxime sodium, dexamethasone sodium phosphate, diazepam, digoxin, dobutamine, folic acid, furosemide, hydrocortisone sodium phosphate, hydrocortisone sodium succinate, ketamine, methylprednisolone sodium succinate, minocycline, sodium bicarbonate, thiopental, ticarcillin disodium.

ACTION
Not clearly defined. Directly stimulates the central respiratory centers in the medulla and may indirectly act on carotid, aortic, or other peripheral chemoreceptors.

Route	Onset	Peak	Duration
I.V.	20–40 sec	1–2 min	5–12 min

Half-life: 2½ to 4 hours.

ADVERSE REACTIONS
CNS: *headache, dizziness, seizures,* apprehension, disorientation, hyperactivity, bilateral Babinski's signs, paresthesia.
CV: *chest pain and tightness, variations in heart rate, hypertension, arrhythmias,* T-wave depression on ECG, flushing.
EENT: *laryngospasm,* sneezing.
GI: nausea, vomiting, diarrhea.
GU: urine retention, bladder stimulation with incontinence, albuminuria.
Musculoskeletal: muscle spasms.
Respiratory: *bronchospasm,* cough, dyspnea, rebound hypoventilation, hiccups.
Skin: pruritus, diaphoresis.

INTERACTIONS
Drug-drug. *General anesthetics:* May cause self-limiting arrhythmias. Avoid using doxapram within 10 minutes of an anesthetic that sensitizes the myocardium to catecholamines.
MAO inhibitors, sympathomimetics: May increase adverse CV effects. Use together cautiously.

EFFECTS ON LAB TEST RESULTS
- May increase BUN level. May decrease hemoglobin level and hematocrit.
- May decrease erythrocyte, RBC, and WBC counts.

CONTRAINDICATIONS & CAUTIONS
- Contraindicated in patients with seizure disorders; head injury; CV disorders; frank, uncompensated heart failure; severe hypertension; stroke; respiratory failure or incompetence secondary to neuromuscular disorders, muscle paresis, flail chest, obstructed airway, pulmonary embolism, pneumothorax, restrictive respiratory disease, acute bronchial asthma, or extreme dyspnea; or hypoxia unrelated to hypercapnia.
- Use cautiously in patients with bronchial asthma, severe tachycardia or arrhythmias, cerebral edema, increased intracranial pressure, hyperthyroidism, pheochromocytoma, or metabolic disorders.

NURSING CONSIDERATIONS
- Drug is used only in surgical or emergency department situations.
- Separate end of anesthetic treatment and start of this drug by at least 10 minutes.
- *Alert:* Establish an adequate airway before giving drug. Prevent patient from aspirating vomitus by placing him on his side.
- Monitor blood pressure, heart rate, deep tendon reflexes, and arterial blood gases before giving drug and every 30 minutes afterward.
- Monitor patient for evidence of overdose, such as hypertension, tachycardia, arrhythmias, skeletal muscle hyperactivity, and dyspnea. Hold drug and notify prescriber if patient needs mechanical ventilation or shows signs of increased arterial carbon dioxide or oxygen tension.

• **Look alike–sound alike:** Don't confuse doxapram with doxorubicin, doxepin, or doxazosin. Don't confuse Dopram with dopamine.

PATIENT TEACHING
• Inform family and patient about need for drug.
• Answer patient's questions and address his concerns.

---

modafinil
moe-DAFF-in-ill

Alertec†, Provigil

Pharmacologic class: analeptic
Pregnancy risk category C
Controlled substance schedule IV

AVAILABLE FORMS
Tablets: 100 mg, 200 mg

INDICATIONS & DOSAGES
➤ **To improve wakefulness in patients with excessive daytime sleepiness caused by narcolepsy, obstructive sleep apnea-hypoapnea syndrome, and shift-work sleep disorder**
Adults: 200 mg P.O. daily, as single dose in the morning. Patients with shift-work sleep disorder should take dose about 1 hour before the start of their shift.
Adjust-a-dose: In patients with severe hepatic impairment, give 100 mg P.O. daily, as single dose in the morning.

ADMINISTRATION
P.O.
• Give drug without regard for food; however, food may delay effect of drug.

ACTION
Unknown. Similar to action of sympathomimetics, including amphetamines, but drug is structurally distinct from amphetamines and doesn't alter release of dopamine or norepinephrine to produce CNS stimulation.

Route	Onset	Peak	Duration
P.O.	Unknown	2–4 hr	Unknown

Half-life: 15 hours.

ADVERSE REACTIONS
CNS: *headache, nervousness, dizziness, insomnia,* fever, depression, anxiety, cataplexy, paresthesia, dyskinesia, hypertonia, confusion, syncope, amnesia, emotional lability, ataxia, tremor, mania, hallucination, ***suicidal ideation.***
CV: ***arrhythmias,*** hypotension, hypertension, vasodilation, chest pain.
EENT: *rhinitis,* pharyngitis, epistaxis, amblyopia, abnormal vision.
GI: *nausea,* diarrhea, dry mouth, anorexia, vomiting, mouth ulcer, gingivitis, thirst.
GU: abnormal urine, urine retention, abnormal ejaculation, albuminuria.
Hematologic: eosinophilia.
Metabolic: hyperglycemia.
Musculoskeletal: joint disorder, neck pain, neck rigidity.
Respiratory: asthma, dyspnea, lung disorder.
Skin: sweating.
Other: herpes simplex, chills.

INTERACTIONS
Drug-drug. *Carbamazepine, phenobarbital, rifampin, and other inducers of CYP3A4:* May alter modafinil level. Monitor patient closely.
Cyclosporine, theophylline: May reduce levels of these drugs. Use together cautiously.
Diazepam, phenytoin, propranolol, other drugs metabolized by CYP2C19: May inhibit CYP2C19 and lead to higher levels of drugs metabolized by this enzyme. Use together cautiously; adjust dosage as needed.
Hormonal contraceptives: May reduce contraceptive effectiveness. Advise patient to use alternative or additional method of contraception during modafinil therapy and for 1 month after drug is stopped.
Itraconazole, ketoconazole, other inhibitors of CYP3A4: May alter modafinil level. Monitor patient closely.
Methylphenidate: May cause 1-hour delay in modafinil absorption. Separate dosage times.
Phenytoin, warfarin: May inhibit CYP2C9 and increase phenytoin and warfarin levels. Monitor patient closely for toxicity.
Tricyclic antidepressants (such as clomipramine, desipramine): May increase

---

Reactions may be *common,* uncommon, *life-threatening,* or COMMON AND LIFE-THREATENING.
Interaction may have a *rapid onset* or **delayed onset.**

tricyclic antidepressant level. Reduce dosage of these drugs.

EFFECTS ON LAB TEST RESULTS
• May increase glucose, GGT, and AST levels.
• May increase eosinophil count.

CONTRAINDICATIONS & CAUTIONS
• Contraindicated in patients hypersensitive to drug and in those with a history of left ventricular hypertrophy or ischemic ECG changes, chest pain, arrhythmias, or other evidence of mitral valve prolapse linked to CNS stimulant use.
• Use cautiously in patients with recent MI or unstable angina and in those with history of psychosis.
• Use cautiously and give reduced dosage to patients with severe hepatic impairment, with or without cirrhosis.
• Use cautiously in patients taking MAO inhibitors.
• Safety and efficacy in patients with severe renal impairment haven't been determined.

NURSING CONSIDERATIONS
• Monitor hypertensive patients closely.
• Although single daily 400-mg doses have been well tolerated, the larger dose is no more beneficial than the 200-mg dose.

PATIENT TEACHING
• *Alert:* Advise patient to stop drug and notify prescriber if rash, peeling skin, trouble swallowing or breathing, or other symptoms of allergic reaction occur. Rare cases of serious rash including Stevens-Johnson syndrome, toxic epidermal necrolysis, and drug rash with eosinophilia and hypersensitivity have been reported.
• Advise woman to notify prescriber about planned, suspected, or known pregnancy, or if she's breast-feeding.
• Caution patient that use of hormonal contraceptives (including depot or implantable contraceptives) together with modafinil tablets may reduce contraceptive effectiveness. Recommend an alternative method of contraception during modafinil therapy and for 1 month after drug is stopped.
• Instruct patient to confer with prescriber before taking prescription or OTC drugs to avoid drug interactions.

• Tell patient to avoid alcohol while taking drug.
• Warn patient to avoid activities that require alertness or good coordination until CNS effects of drug are known.

phentermine hydrochloride
FEN-ter-meen

Adipex-P

Pharmacologic class:
sympathomimetic amine
Pregnancy risk category NR
Controlled substance schedule IV

AVAILABLE FORMS
Capsules: 18.75 mg, 30 mg, 37.5 mg
Capsules (resin complex, sustained-release): 15 mg, 30 mg
Tablets: 8 mg, 30 mg, 37.5 mg

INDICATIONS & DOSAGES
➤ **Short-term adjunct in exogenous obesity**
Adults: 8 mg P.O. t.i.d. 30 minutes before meals. Or, 15 to 37.5 mg or 15 to 30 mg (as resin complex) P.O. daily as a single dose in the morning. Give Adipex-P before breakfast or 1 to 2 hours after breakfast.

ADMINISTRATION
P.O.
• Give sustained-release capsule whole, at least 10 hours before bedtime.
• Give last dose of immediate-release capsule or tablet at least 4 to 6 hours before bedtime.

ACTION
Unknown. Probably promotes nerve impulse transmission by releasing stored norepinephrine from nerve terminals in the brain, especially in the cerebral cortex and reticular activating system.

Route	Onset	Peak	Duration
P.O.	Unknown	Unknown	12–14 hr

Half-life: 19 to 24 hours.

ADVERSE REACTIONS
CNS: *insomnia,* overstimulation, headache, euphoria, dysphoria, dizziness.

CV: *palpitations, tachycardia,* increased blood pressure.
GI: dry mouth, dysgeusia, constipation, diarrhea, unpleasant taste, other GI disturbances.
GU: impotence.
Skin: urticaria.
Other: altered libido.

INTERACTIONS

Drug-drug. *Acetazolamide, antacids, sodium bicarbonate:* May increase renal reabsorption. Monitor patient for enhanced effects.
Ammonium chloride, ascorbic acid: May decrease level and increase renal excretion of phentermine. Monitor patient for decreased phentermine effects.
Insulin, oral antidiabetics: May alter antidiabetic requirements. Monitor glucose level.
MAO inhibitors: May cause severe hypertension or hypertensive crisis. Avoid using within 14 days of MAO inhibitor therapy.
Drug-food. *Caffeine:* May increase CNS stimulation. Discourage use together.

EFFECTS ON LAB TEST RESULTS
None reported.

CONTRAINDICATIONS & CAUTIONS
● Contraindicated in patients hypersensitive to sympathomimetic amines, in those with idiosyncratic reactions to them, in agitated patients, and in those with hyperthyroidism, moderate-to-severe hypertension, advanced arteriosclerosis, symptomatic CV disease, or glaucoma.
● Contraindicated within 14 days of MAO inhibitor therapy.
● Use cautiously in patients with mild hypertension.

NURSING CONSIDERATIONS
● Use drug with a weight-reduction program.
● Monitor patient for tolerance or dependence.
● *Look alike–sound alike:* Don't confuse phentermine with phentolamine.

PATIENT TEACHING
● Tell patient to take sustained-release drug at least 10 hours before bedtime or last dose of immediate-release drug at least 4 to 6 hours before bedtime to avoid sleep interference.
● Advise patient to avoid products that contain caffeine. Tell him to report evidence of excessive stimulation.
● Warn patient that fatigue may result as drug effects wear off and that he'll need more rest.
● Warn patient that drug may lose its effectiveness over time.
● Tell patient to take sustained-release capsule whole and not to chew, crush, or open it.

---

sibutramine hydrochloride monohydrate
sih-BUH-trah-meen

Meridia

Pharmacologic class: norepinephrine, serotonin, and dopamine reuptake inhibitor
Pregnancy risk category C
Controlled substance schedule IV

AVAILABLE FORMS
Capsules: 5 mg, 10 mg, 15 mg

INDICATIONS & DOSAGES
➤ **To manage obesity**
Adults: 10 mg P.O. given once daily. May increase to 15 mg P.O. daily after 4 weeks if weight loss is inadequate. Patients who don't tolerate 10 mg daily may receive 5 mg P.O. daily. Don't exceed 15 mg daily.

ADMINISTRATION
P.O.
● Give drug without regard for food.

ACTION
Inhibits reuptake of norepinephrine and, to a lesser extent, serotonin and dopamine.

Route	Onset	Peak	Duration
P.O.	Unknown	3–4 hr	Unknown

Half-life: About 15 hours.

ADVERSE REACTIONS
CNS: *headache, insomnia,* dizziness, nervousness, anxiety, depression, paresthesia,

---

Reactions may be *common,* uncommon, *life-threatening,* or COMMON AND LIFE-THREATENING.
Interaction may have a *rapid onset* or *delayed onset.*

somnolence, CNS stimulation, emotional lability, asthenia, migraine.

CV: tachycardia, vasodilation, hypertension, palpitations, chest pain, generalized edema.

EENT: *rhinitis, pharyngitis,* sinusitis, ear disorder, ear pain.

GI: *anorexia, constipation, dry mouth,* thirst, increased appetite, nausea, dyspepsia, gastritis, vomiting, taste perversion, abdominal pain, rectal disorder.

GU: dysmenorrhea, UTI, vaginal candidiasis, metrorrhagia.

Musculoskeletal: arthralgia, myalgia, tenosynovitis, joint disorder, neck or back pain.

Respiratory: increased cough, laryngitis.

Skin: rash, sweating, acne.

Other: herpes simplex, flulike syndrome, accidental injury, allergic reaction.

INTERACTIONS

Drug-drug. *CNS depressants:* May enhance CNS depression. Use together cautiously.

Dextromethorphan, dihydroergotamine, fentanyl, fluoxetine, fluvoxamine, lithium, MAO inhibitors, meperidine, paroxetine, pentazocine, sertraline, sumatriptan, tryptophan, venlafaxine: May cause hyperthermia, tachycardia, and loss of consciousness. Avoid using together.

Ephedrine, pseudoephedrine: May increase blood pressure or heart rate. Use together cautiously.

Drug-lifestyle. *Alcohol use:* May enhance CNS depression. Discourage use together.

EFFECTS ON LAB TEST RESULTS
• May increase ALT, AST, GGT, LDH, alkaline phosphatase, and bilirubin levels.

CONTRAINDICATIONS & CAUTIONS
• Contraindicated in patients hypersensitive to drug or its active ingredients, in those taking MAO inhibitors or other centrally acting appetite suppressants, and in those with anorexia nervosa.
• Contraindicated in patients with severe renal or hepatic dysfunction, history of hypertension, coronary artery disease, heart failure, arrhythmias, or stroke.
• Contraindicated in elderly patients.
• Use cautiously in patients with history of seizures or angle-closure glaucoma.

NURSING CONSIDERATIONS
• Measure blood pressure and pulse before starting therapy, with dosage changes, and at regular intervals during therapy.
• Use drug in obese patients with a body mass index of 30 or more (27 or more if patient has other risk factors, such as hypertension, diabetes, or dyslipidemia).
• Avoid using drug within 2 weeks of MAO inhibitor.
• **Alert:** Combining this drug with triptans, SSRIs, or SSNRIs may cause serotonin syndrome. Symptoms include restlessness, hallucinations, loss of coordination, fast heartbeat, rapid changes in blood pressure, increased body temperature, hyperreflexia, nausea, vomiting, and diarrhea. The syndrome is more likely to occur when starting or increasing the dose of the triptan, SSRI, or SSNRI.

PATIENT TEACHING
• Advise patient to report rash, hives, or other allergic reactions immediately.
• Instruct patient to notify prescriber before taking other prescription or OTC drugs.
• Advise patient to have blood pressure and pulse monitored at regular intervals. Stress importance of regular follow-up visits with prescriber.
• Advise patient to follow a reduced-calorie diet.
• Tell patient that weight loss can cause gallstones. Teach signs and symptoms, and tell patient to notify prescriber promptly if they occur.
• Tell patient to take drug daily in the morning to avoid sleep disturbances.

45

Nonopioid analgesics and antipyretics

acetaminophen
aspirin
diflunisal

acetaminophen
(APAP, paracetamol)
a-seet-a-MIN-a-fen

Abenol† ◇ , Acephen, ACET† ◇ ,
Aceta ◇ , Aspirin Free Anacin ◇ ,
Atasol† ◇ , FeverAll ◇ , Genapap ◇ ,
Genebs ◇ , Infantaire ◇ , Mapap ◇ ,
Maranox ◇ , Panadol ◇ , Silapap ◇ ,
St. Joseph Aspirin-Free Fever
Reducer for Children ◇ , Tylenol ◇ ,
UN-Aspirin ◇

Pharmacologic class:
para-aminophenol derivative
Pregnancy risk category B

AVAILABLE FORMS
Caplets: 160 mg ◇ , 500 mg ◇
Caplets (extended-release): 650 mg ◇
Capsules: 325 mg ◇ , 500 mg ◇
Elixir: 80 mg/2.5 ml, 80 mg/5 ml,
120 mg/5 ml, 160 mg/5 ml* ◇
Gelcaps: 500 mg ◇
Oral liquid: 160 mg/5 ml ◇ , 167 mg/5 ml,
500 mg/15 ml ◇
Oral solution: 48 mg/ml ◇ , 80 mg/
0.8 ml ◇ , 100 mg/ml ◇
Oral suspension: 80 mg/0.8 ml ◇ ,
160 mg/5 ml ◇
Oral syrup: 16 mg/ml ◇
Sprinkles: 80 mg/capsule ◇ , 160 mg/
capsule ◇
Suppositories: 80 mg ◇ , 120 mg ◇ ,
125 mg ◇ , 300 mg ◇ , 325 mg ◇ , 650 mg ◇
Tablets: 160 mg ◇ , 325 mg ◇ , 500 mg ◇ ,
650 mg ◇
Tablets (chewable): 80 mg ◇ , 160 mg
Tablets (dispersible): 80 mg ◇

INDICATIONS & DOSAGES
➤ **Mild pain or fever**
P.O.
Adults: 325 to 650 mg P.O. every 4 to
6 hours; or 1 g P.O. t.i.d. or q.i.d., as
needed. Or, two extended-release caplets
P.O. every 8 hours. Maximum, 4 g daily.
For long-term therapy, don't exceed 2.6 g
daily unless prescribed and monitored
closely by health care provider.
Children older than age 12: 650 mg P.O.
every 4 to 6 hours p.r.n.
Children age 12: 640 mg P.O. every 4 to
6 hours p.r.n.
Children age 11: 480 mg P.O. every 4 to
6 hours p.r.n.
Children ages 9 to 10: 400 mg P.O. every
4 to 6 hours p.r.n.
Children ages 6 to 8: 320 mg P.O. every
4 to 6 hours p.r.n.
Children ages 4 to 5: 240 mg P.O. every
4 to 6 hours p.r.n.
Children ages 2 to 3: 160 mg P.O. every
4 to 6 hours p.r.n.
Children ages 12 to 23 months: 120 mg
P.O. every 4 to 6 hours p.r.n.
Children ages 4 to 11 months: 80 mg P.O.
every 4 to 6 hours p.r.n.
Children up to age 3 months: 40 mg P.O.
every 4 to 6 hours p.r.n. Or, 10 to 15 mg/
kg/dose every 4 hours p.r.n. Don't exceed
five doses in 24 hours.
P.R.
Adults and children older than age 12:
650 mg P.R. every 4 to 6 hours p.r.n. Maximum, 4 g daily. For long-term therapy, don't
exceed 2.6 g daily unless prescribed and
monitored closely by health care provider.
Children ages 6 to 12: 325 mg P.R. every
4 to 6 hours p.r.n.
Children ages 3 to 6: 120 to 125 mg P.R.
every 4 to 6 hours p.r.n.
Children ages 1 to 3: 80 mg P.R. every
4 to 6 hours p.r.n.
Children ages 3 months to 11 months:
80 mg P.R. every 6 hours p.r.n.

ADMINISTRATION
P.O.
• Use liquid form for children and patients
who have difficulty swallowing.
• Give drug without regard for food.
• Dispersible tablet should be allowed to
dissolve in the mouth or chewed before
swallowing.

Reactions may be *common*, uncommon, *life-threatening*, or COMMON AND LIFE-THREATENING.
Interaction may have a *rapid onset* or **delayed onset**.

Rectal
• If suppository is too soft, refrigerate for 15 minutes or run under cold water in wrapper.

ACTION
Thought to produce analgesia by inhibiting prostaglandin and other substances that sensitize pain receptors. Drug may relieve fever through central action in the hypothalamic heat-regulating center.

Route	Onset	Peak	Duration
P.O., P.R.	Unknown	½–2 hr	3–4 hr

Half-life: 1 to 4 hours.

ADVERSE REACTIONS
Hematologic: hemolytic anemia, *leukopenia, neutropenia, pancytopenia.*
Hepatic: jaundice.
Metabolic: *hypoglycemia.*
Skin: rash, urticaria.

INTERACTIONS
Drug-drug. *Barbiturates, carbamazepine, hydantoins, rifampin, sulfinpyrazone:* High doses or long-term use of these drugs may reduce therapeutic effects and enhance hepatotoxic effects of acetaminophen. Avoid using together.
Lamotrigine: May decrease lamotrigine level. Monitor patient for therapeutic effects.
Warfarin: May increase hypoprothrombinemic effects with long-term use with high doses of acetaminophen. Monitor INR closely.
Zidovudine: May decrease zidovudine effect. Monitor patient closely.
Drug-herb. *Watercress:* May inhibit oxidative metabolism of acetaminophen. Discourage use together.
Drug-food. *Caffeine:* May enhance analgesic effects of acetaminophen. Products may combine caffeine and acetaminophen for therapeutic advantage.
Drug-lifestyle. *Alcohol use:* May increase risk of hepatic damage. Discourage use together.

EFFECTS ON LAB TEST RESULTS
• May decrease glucose and hemoglobin levels and hematocrit.

• May decrease neutrophil, WBC, RBC, and platelet counts.
• May cause false-positive test result for urinary 5-hydroxyindoleacetic acid. May falsely decrease glucose level in home monitoring systems.

CONTRAINDICATIONS & CAUTIONS
• Contraindicated in patients hypersensitive to drug.
• Use cautiously in patients with any type of liver disease and in patients with long-term alcohol use because therapeutic doses cause hepatotoxicity in these patients.

NURSING CONSIDERATIONS
• *Alert:* Many OTC and prescription products contain acetaminophen; be aware of this when calculating total daily dose.
• In children, don't exceed five doses in 24 hours.

PATIENT TEACHING
• Tell parents to consult prescriber before giving drug to children younger than age 2.
• Advise parents that drug is only for short-term use; urge them to consult prescriber if giving to children for longer than 5 days or adults for longer than 10 days.
• *Alert:* Advise patient or caregiver that many OTC products contain acetaminophen and should be counted when calculating total daily dose.
• Tell patient not to use for marked fever (temperature higher than 103.1° F [39.5° C]), fever persisting longer than 3 days, or recurrent fever unless directed by prescriber.
• *Alert:* Warn patient that high doses or unsupervised long-term use can cause liver damage. Excessive alcohol use may increase the risk of liver damage. Caution long-term alcoholics to limit drug to 2 g/day or less.
• Tell breast-feeding woman that drug appears in breast milk in low levels (less than 1% of dose). Drug may be used safely if therapy is short-term and doesn't exceed recommended doses.

aspirin
(acetylsalicylic acid, ASA)
ASS-pir-in

Aspergum◊, Bayer ◊, Ecotrin◊, Empirin◊, Halfprin, Heartline◊, Norwich ◊, Novasen†◊, St Joseph's◊, ZORprin◊

Pharmacologic class: salicylate
Pregnancy risk category D

AVAILABLE FORMS
Chewing gum: 227.5 mg ◊
Suppositories: 120 mg ◊, 200 mg ◊, 300 mg ◊, 600 mg ◊
Tablets: 325 mg ◊, 500 mg ◊
Tablets (chewable): 81 mg ◊
Tablets (controlled-release): 800 mg
Tablets (enteric-coated): 81 mg ◊, 162 mg ◊, 325 mg ◊, 500 mg ◊, 650 mg ◊
Tablets (extended-release): 650 mg ◊

INDICATIONS & DOSAGES
➤ **Rheumatoid arthritis, osteo-arthritis, or other polyarthritic or inflammatory conditions**
Adults: Initially, 2.4 to 3.6 g P.O. daily in divided doses. Maintenance dosage is 3.2 to 6 g P.O. daily in divided doses.
➤ **Juvenile rheumatoid arthritis**
Children who weigh more than 25 kg (55 lb): 2.4 to 3.6 g P.O. daily in divided doses.
Children who weigh 25 kg or less: 60 to 130 mg/kg P.O. in divided doses. Increase by 10 mg/kg daily at no more than weekly intervals. Maintenance dosages usually range from 80 to 100 mg/kg daily; up to 130 mg/kg daily.
➤ **Mild pain or fever**
Adults and children older than age 12: 324 to 650 mg P.O. or P.R. every 4 hours p.r.n.
Children ages 2 to 11: Give 10 to 15 mg/kg/dose P.O. or P.R. every 4 hours up to 80 mg/kg daily.
➤ **Suspected acute MI**
Adults: Initial dose of 160 mg to 325 mg P.O. as soon as MI is suspected. Continue maintenance dose of 160 mg to 325 mg P.O. daily for 30 days post infarction.

After 30 days, consider further therapy for prevention of MI.
➤ **To reduce risk of MI in patients with previous MI, unstable angina, and chronic stable angina pectoris**
Adults: 75 to 325 mg P.O. daily.
➤ **Kawasaki syndrome (mucocuta-neous lymph node syndrome)**
Children: 80 to 100 mg/kg P.O. daily, divided q.i.d. with immune globulin I.V. After the fever subsides, reduce dosage to 3 to 5 mg/kg once daily. Aspirin therapy usually continues for 6 to 8 weeks.
➤ **Acute rheumatic fever**
Adults: 5 to 8 g P.O. daily.
Children: 100 mg/kg daily P.O. for 2 weeks; then 75 mg/kg daily P.O. for 4 to 6 weeks.
➤ **To reduce risk of recurrent transient ischemic attacks and stroke or death in patients at risk**
Adults: 50 to 325 mg P.O. daily.
➤ **Acute ischemic stroke**
Adults: 160 to 325 mg P.O. daily, started within 48 hours of stroke onset and continued for up to 2 to 4 weeks.
➤ **Acute pericarditis after MI**
Adults: 160 to 325 mg P.O. daily. Higher doses (650 mg P.O. every 4 to 6 hours) may be needed.
➤ **CABG**
Adults: 325 mg P.O. daily starting 6 hours postprocedure.
➤ **PTCA**
Adults: Initial dose of 325 mg P.O. 2 hours presurgery and then 160 mg to 325 mg P.O. daily.
➤ **Carotid endarterectomy**
Adults: 80 mg P.O. daily to 650 mg P.O. twice daily starting presurgery.

ADMINISTRATION
P.O.
• For patient with swallowing difficulties, crush non–enteric-coated aspirin and dis-solve in soft food or liquid. Give liquid immediately after mixing because drug will break down rapidly.
• Give drug with food, milk, antacid, or large glass of water to reduce GI effects.
• Give sustained-release or enteric-coated forms whole; don't crush or break these tablets.
Rectal
• Refrigerate suppositories.

Reactions may be *common*, uncommon, *life-threatening*, or COMMON AND LIFE-THREATENING.
Interaction may have a *rapid onset* or **delayed onset.**

ACTION
Thought to produce analgesia and exert its anti-inflammatory effect by inhibiting prostaglandin and other substances that sensitize pain receptors. Drug may relieve fever through central action in the hypothalamic heat-regulating center. In low doses, drug also appears to interfere with clotting by keeping a platelet-aggregating substance from forming.

Route	Onset	Peak	Duration
P.O. (buffered)	5–30 min	1–2 hr	1–4 hr
P.O. (enteric-coated)	5–30 min	Variable	1–4 hr
P.O. (extended-release)	5–30 min	1–4 hr	1–4 hr
P.O. (solution)	5–30 min	15–40 min	1–4 hr
P.O. (tablet)	5–30 min	25–40 min	1–4 hr
P.R.	Unknown	3–4 hr	Unknown

Half-life: 15 to 20 minutes.

ADVERSE REACTIONS
EENT: *tinnitus, hearing loss.*
GI: *nausea, GI bleeding,* dyspepsia, GI distress, occult bleeding.
Hematologic: *prolonged bleeding time, leukopenia, thrombocytopenia.*
Hepatic: *hepatitis.*
Skin: *rash,* bruising, urticaria.
Other: *angioedema, Reye syndrome,* hypersensitivity reactions.

INTERACTIONS
Drug-drug. *ACE inhibitors:* May decrease antihypertensive effects. Monitor blood pressure closely.
Ammonium chloride and other urine acidifiers: May increase levels of aspirin products. Watch for aspirin toxicity.
Antacids in high doses and other urine alkalinizers: May decrease levels of aspirin products. Watch for decreased aspirin effect.
Anticoagulants: May increase risk of bleeding. Use with extreme caution if must be used together.
Beta blockers: May decrease antihypertensive effect. Avoid long-term aspirin use if patient is taking antihypertensives.

Corticosteroids: May enhance salicylate elimination and decrease drug level. Watch for decreased aspirin effect.
Heparin: May increase risk of bleeding. Monitor coagulation studies and patient closely if used together.
Ibuprofen, other NSAIDs: May negate the antiplatelet effect of low-dose aspirin therapy. Patients using immediate-release aspirin (not enteric-coated) should take ibuprofen at least 30 minutes after or more than 8 hours before aspirin. Occasional use of ibuprofen is unlikely to have a negative effect.
Methotrexate: May increase risk of methotrexate toxicity. Avoid using together.
Nizatidine: May increase risk of salicylate toxicity in patients receiving high doses of aspirin. Monitor patient closely.
Oral antidiabetics: May increase hypoglycemic effect. Monitor patient closely.
Probenecid, sulfinpyrazone: May decrease uricosuric effect. Avoid using together.
Valproic acid: May increase valproic acid level. Avoid using together.
Drug-herb. *Dong quai, feverfew, ginkgo, horse chestnut, kelpware, red clover:* May increase risk of bleeding. Monitor patient closely for increased effects. Discourage use together.
White willow: May increase risk of adverse effects. Discourage use together.
Drug-food. *Caffeine:* May increase drug absorption. Watch for increased effects.
Drug-lifestyle. *Alcohol use:* May increase risk of GI bleeding. Discourage use together.

EFFECTS ON LAB TEST RESULTS
● May increase liver function test values, blood urea nitrogen, creatinine, and potassium levels
● May decrease platelet and WBC counts.
● May falsely increase protein-bound iodine level.
● May interfere with urine glucose analysis with Diastix, Chemstrip uG, Clinitest, and Benedict solution; with urinary 5-hydroxyindoleacetic acid and vanillylmandelic acid tests; and with Gerhardt test for urine acetoacetic acid.

CONTRAINDICATIONS & CAUTIONS
● Contraindicated in patients hypersensitive to drug and in those with NSAID-induced

sensitivity reactions, G6PD deficiency, or bleeding disorders, such as hemophilia, von Willebrand disease, or telangiectasia.
• Use cautiously in patients with GI lesions, impaired renal function, hypoprothrombinemia, vitamin K deficiency, thrombocytopenia, thrombotic thrombocytopenic purpura, or severe hepatic impairment.
• *Alert:* Oral and rectal OTC products containing aspirin and nonaspirin salicylates shouldn't be given to children or teenagers who have or are recovering from chickenpox or flulike symptoms because of the risk of Reye syndrome.

NURSING CONSIDERATIONS
• For inflammatory conditions, rheumatic fever, and thrombosis, give aspirin on a schedule rather than as needed.
• Because enteric-coated and sustained-release tablets are slowly absorbed, they aren't suitable for rapid relief of acute pain, fever, or inflammation. They cause less GI bleeding and may be better suited for long-term therapy, such as for arthritis.
• For patients who can't tolerate oral drugs, ask prescriber about using aspirin rectal suppositories. Watch for rectal mucosal irritation or bleeding.
• Febrile, dehydrated children can develop toxicity rapidly.
• Monitor elderly patients closely because they may be more susceptible to aspirin's toxic effects.
• Monitor salicylate level. Therapeutic salicylate level for arthritis is 150 to 300 mcg/ml. Tinnitus may occur at levels above 200 mcg/ml, but this isn't a reliable indicator of toxicity, especially in very young patients and those older than age 60. With long-term therapy, severe toxic effects may occur with levels exceeding 400 mcg/ml.
• During prolonged therapy, assess hematocrit, hemoglobin level, PT, INR, and renal function periodically.
• Drug irreversibly inhibits platelet aggregation. Stop drug 5 to 7 days before elective surgery to allow time for production and release of new platelets.
• Monitor patient for hypersensitivity reactions, such as anaphylaxis and asthma.

• *Look alike–sound alike:* Don't confuse aspirin with Asendin or Afrin.

PATIENT TEACHING
• Tell patient who's allergic to tartrazine to avoid aspirin.
• Advise patient on a low-salt diet that 1 tablet of buffered aspirin contains 553 mg of sodium.
• Advise patient to take drug with food, milk, antacid, or large glass of water to reduce GI reactions.
• Tell patient not to crush or chew sustained-release or enteric-coated forms but to swallow them whole.
• Instruct patient to discard aspirin tablets that have a strong vinegar-like odor.
• Tell patient to consult prescriber if giving drug to children for longer than 5 days or adults for longer than 10 days.
• Advise patient receiving prolonged treatment with large doses of aspirin to watch for small, round, red pinprick spots, bleeding gums, and signs of GI bleeding, and to drink plenty of fluids. Encourage use of a soft-bristled toothbrush.
• Because of the many drug interactions with aspirin, warn patient taking prescription drugs to check with prescriber or pharmacist before taking aspirin or OTC products containing aspirin.
• Ibuprofen can interfere with the antiplatelet effect of low-dose aspirin therapy, negating its effect. Tell patient how to safely use ibuprofen in relation to aspirin therapy.
• Urge pregnant woman to avoid aspirin during last trimester of pregnancy unless specifically directed by prescriber.
• Drug is a leading cause of poisoning in children. Caution parents to keep drug out of reach of children. Encourage use of child-resistant containers.

diflunisal
dye-FLOO-ni-sal

Pharmacologic class: salicylate; NSAID
Pregnancy risk category C

AVAILABLE FORMS
Tablets: 250 mg, 500 mg

INDICATIONS & DOSAGES
➤ **Osteoarthritis, rheumatoid arthritis**
Adults: 500 to 1,000 mg P.O. daily in two divided doses, usually every 12 hours. Maximum, 1,500 mg daily.
Elderly patients: In patients older than age 65, one-half usual adult dosage.
➤ **Mild to moderate pain**
Adults: 1 g P.O., then 500 mg every 8 to 12 hours. A lower dosage of 500 mg P.O., then 250 mg every 8 to 12 hours may be appropriate.

ADMINISTRATION
P.O.
• Give tablets with water, milk, or meals.
• Give drug whole; don't crush or break tablets.

ACTION
Unknown. Probably related to inhibition of prostaglandin synthesis.

Route	Onset	Peak	Duration
P.O.	1 hr	2–3 hr	8–12 hr

Half-life: 8 to 12 hours.

ADVERSE REACTIONS
CNS: dizziness, fatigue, headache, insomnia, somnolence.
EENT: tinnitus.
GI: constipation, diarrhea, dyspepsia, flatulence, GI pain, nausea, stomatitis, vomiting.
GU: *interstitial nephritis,* hematuria, renal impairment.
Skin: *erythema multiforme, Stevens-Johnson syndrome,* pruritus, rash, sweating.

INTERACTIONS
Drug-drug. *Acetaminophen, hydrochlorothiazide, indomethacin:* May substantially increase levels of these drugs, increasing risk of toxicity. Avoid using together.
Antacids, aspirin: May decrease diflunisal level. Monitor patient for reduced therapeutic effect.
Anticoagulants, thrombolytics: May enhance effects of these drugs. Use together cautiously.

Cyclosporine: May enhance the nephrotoxicity of cyclosporine. Avoid using together.
Methotrexate: May enhance the toxicity of methotrexate. Avoid using together.
Sulindac: May decrease level of sulindac's metabolite. Monitor patient for reduced effect.

EFFECTS ON LAB TEST RESULTS
• May falsely elevate salicylate level.

CONTRAINDICATIONS & CAUTIONS
■ **Black Box Warning** Contraindicated for the treatment of perioperative pain after CABG surgery. ■
• Contraindicated in patients hypersensitive to drug and in those for whom acute asthmatic attacks, urticaria, or rhinitis are precipitated by aspirin or other NSAIDs.
• Use cautiously in patients with GI bleeding, history of peptic ulcer disease, renal impairment, compromised cardiac function, hypertension, or other conditions predisposing patient to fluid retention.

NURSING CONSIDERATIONS
■ **Black Box Warning** NSAIDs may increase the risk of serious thrombotic events, MI or stroke. The risk may be greater with longer use or in patients with CV disease or risk factors for CV disease. ■
■ **Black Box Warning** NSAIDs cause an increased risk of serious GI adverse reactions, including bleeding, ulceration, and perforation of the stomach or intestines, which can be fatal. Elderly patients are at greater risk. ■
• *Alert:* The Centers for Disease Control and Prevention recommend not giving salicylates to children and teenagers with chickenpox or flulike illness because of the link to Reye syndrome.

PATIENT TEACHING
• Advise patient to take with water, milk, or meals.
• Tell patient that tablets must be swallowed whole.
• Instruct patient to avoid aspirin or acetaminophen while using diflunisal.
• Inform breast-feeding woman that drug appears in breast milk; she should stop either breast-feeding or taking drug.

Nonsteroidal anti-inflammatories

celecoxib
diclofenac potassium
diclofenac sodium
etodolac
hydroxychloroquine sulfate
(See Chapter 8, ANTIMALARIALS.)
ibuprofen
indomethacin
indomethacin sodium trihydrate
ketoprofen
ketorolac tromethamine
meloxicam
nabumetone
naproxen
naproxen sodium
piroxicam
sulindac

celecoxib
sell-ah-COCKS-ib

Celebrex⬦

Pharmacologic class:
cyclooxygenase-2 (COX-2)
inhibitor
*Pregnancy risk category C;
D in 3rd trimester*

AVAILABLE FORMS
Capsules: 50 mg, 100 mg, 200 mg,
400 mg

INDICATIONS & DOSAGES
➤ **To relieve signs and symptoms
of osteoarthritis**
Adults: 200 mg P.O. daily as a single dose
or divided equally b.i.d.
➤ **To relieve signs and symptoms
of rheumatoid arthritis**
Adults: 100 to 200 mg P.O. b.i.d.
➤ **To relieve signs and symptoms
of ankylosing spondylitis**
Adults: 200 mg P.O. once daily or divided
b.i.d. If no response after 6 weeks, may
increase dose to 400 mg daily. If no
response after 6 more weeks, consider
other treatment.

➤ **To relieve signs and symptoms of
juvenile rheumatoid arthritis**
*Children age 2 and older who weigh 10 to
25 kg (22 to 55 lb):* 50 mg P.O. b.i.d.
*Children age 2 and older who weigh more
than 25 kg:* 100 mg P.O. b.i.d.
➤ **Adjunctive treatment for familial
adenomatous polyposis to reduce the
number of adenomatous colorectal
polyps**
Adults: 400 mg P.O. b.i.d. with food, for
up to 6 months.
Elderly patients: Start at lowest dosage.
➤ **Acute pain and primary
dysmenorrhea**
Adults: 400 mg P.O., initially, followed
by another 200-mg dose if needed.
On subsequent days, 200 mg P.O. b.i.d.
as needed.
Elderly patients: Start at lowest dosage.
Adjust-a-dose: For patients who weigh
less than 50 kg (110 lb), start at lowest
dosage. For patients with Child-Pugh class
B hepatic impairment, reduce dosage by
about 50%.

ADMINISTRATION
P.O.
● Drug can be given without regard to
meals, but food may decrease GI upset.

ACTION
Thought to inhibit prostaglandin synthesis, impeding COX-2, to produce anti-
inflammatory, analgesic, and antipyretic
effects.

Route	Onset	Peak	Duration
P.O.	Unknown	3 hr	Unknown

Half-life: 11 hours.

ADVERSE REACTIONS
CNS: *headache,* dizziness, insomnia.
CV: hypertension, peripheral edema.
EENT: pharyngitis, rhinitis, sinusitis.
GI: abdominal pain, diarrhea, dyspepsia,
flatulence, nausea.
Metabolic: hyperchloremia.
Musculoskeletal: back pain.

Reactions may be *common,* uncommon, *life-threatening,* or COMMON AND LIFE-THREATENING.
Interaction may have a *rapid onset* or ***delayed onset.***

Respiratory: upper respiratory tract infection.

Skin: *erythema multiforme, exfoliative dermatitis, Stevens-Johnson syndrome, toxic epidermal necrolysis,* rash.

Other: accidental injury.

INTERACTIONS

Drug-drug. *ACE inhibitors, angiotensin II antagonists:* May decrease antihypertensive effects. Monitor patient's blood pressure.

Antacids containing aluminum or magnesium: May decrease celecoxib level. Separate doses.

Aspirin: May increase risk of ulcers; low aspirin dosages can be used safely to reduce the risk of CV events. Monitor patient for signs and symptoms of GI bleeding.

Fluconazole: May increase celecoxib level. Reduce dosage of celecoxib to minimal effective dose.

Furosemide, thiazides: May reduce sodium excretion caused by diuretics, leading to sodium retention. Monitor patient for swelling and increased blood pressure.

Lithium: May increase lithium level. Monitor lithium level closely during treatment.

Warfarin: May increase PT and bleeding complications. Monitor PT and INR, and check for signs and symptoms of bleeding.

Drug-herb. *Dong quai, feverfew, garlic, ginger, horse chestnut, red clover:* May increase risk of bleeding. Discourage use together.

White willow: Herb and drug contain similar components. Discourage use together.

Drug-lifestyle. *Long-term alcohol use, smoking:* May cause GI irritation or bleeding. Check for signs and symptoms of bleeding.

EFFECTS ON LAB TEST RESULTS

● May increase ALT, AST, BUN, creatinine, and chloride levels.
● May decrease phosphate level.

CONTRAINDICATIONS & CAUTIONS

■ **Black Box Warning** Contraindicated for the treatment of perioperative pain after CABG surgery. ■

● Contraindicated in patients hypersensitive to drug, sulfonamides, aspirin, or other NSAIDs.

● Contraindicated in those with severe hepatic impairment.

● Avoid use in the third trimester of pregnancy and with any dose of a non-aspirin NSAID.

● Use cautiously in patients with history of ulcers or GI bleeding, advanced renal disease, dehydration, anemia, symptomatic liver disease, hypertension, edema, heart failure, or asthma, and in poor CYP2C9 metabolizers.

● Use cautiously in elderly or debilitated patients.

NURSING CONSIDERATIONS

● *Alert:* Patients allergic to or with a history of anaphylactic reactions to sulfonamides, aspirin, or other NSAIDs may be allergic to this drug.

■ **Black Box Warning** NSAIDs cause an increased risk of serious GI adverse events, including bleeding, ulceration, and perforation of the stomach or intestines, which can be fatal. Elderly patients are at greater risk. ■

● Patient with history of ulcers or GI bleeding is at higher risk for GI bleeding while taking NSAIDs such as celecoxib. Other risk factors for GI bleeding include treatment with corticosteroids or anticoagulants, longer duration of NSAID treatment, smoking, alcoholism, older age, and poor overall health.

■ **Black Box Warning** NSAIDs may increase the risk of serious thrombotic events, MI, or stroke. The risk may be greater with longer use or in patients with CV disease or risk factors for CV disease. ■

● Although drug may be used with low aspirin dosages, the combination may increase risk of GI bleeding.

● Watch for signs and symptoms of overt and occult bleeding.

● Drug can cause fluid retention; monitor patient with hypertension, edema, or heart failure.

● Assess patient for CV risk factors before therapy.

● Drug may be hepatotoxic; watch for signs and symptoms of liver toxicity.

● Before starting drug therapy, rehydrate dehydrated patient.

● Monitor patient's renal function; renal insufficiency is possible in patients with preexisting renal disease. Long-term

administration may cause renal papillary necrosis and other renal injury.
● *Look alike–sound alike:* Don't confuse Celebrex with Cerebyx or Celexa.

PATIENT TEACHING
● Tell patient to report history of allergic reactions to sulfonamides, aspirin, or other NSAIDs before therapy.
● Instruct patient to promptly report signs of GI bleeding, such as blood in vomit, urine, or stool; or black, tarry stools.
● *Alert:* Advise patient to immediately report rash, unexplained weight gain, or swelling.
● Tell woman to notify prescriber if she becomes pregnant or is planning to become pregnant during drug therapy.
● Instruct patient to take drug with food if stomach upset occurs.
● Tell patient that drug may harm the liver. Advise patient to stop therapy and notify prescriber immediately if he experiences signs and symptoms of liver toxicity, including nausea, fatigue, lethargy, itching, yellowing of skin or eyes, right upper quadrant tenderness, and flulike syndrome.
● Inform patient that it may take several days before he feels consistent pain relief.
● Advise patient that using OTC NSAIDs with celecoxib may increase the risk of GI toxicity.

---

diclofenac epolamine
dye-KLOE-fen-ak

Flector

diclofenac potassium
Apo-Diclo Rapide†, Cataflam, Novo-Difenac-K†, Voltaren Rapide†

diclofenac sodium
Apo-Diclo†, Novo-Difenac†, Nu-Diclo†, Voltaren, Voltaren-XR, Voltaren SR†

Pharmacologic class: NSAID
Pregnancy risk category B;
D in 3rd trimester

AVAILABLE FORMS
diclofenac epolamine
Transdermal patch: 1.3%

diclofenac potassium
Tablets: 50 mg
diclofenac sodium
Suppositories: 50 mg†, 100 mg†
Tablets (delayed-release): 25 mg, 50 mg, 75 mg
Tablets (extended-release): 100 mg

INDICATIONS & DOSAGES
➤ **Ankylosing spondylitis**
Adults: 25 mg delayed-release diclofenac sodium P.O. q.i.d.; may add another 25-mg dose at bedtime.
➤ **Osteoarthritis**
Adults: 50 mg P.O. b.i.d. or t.i.d., or 75 mg P.O. b.i.d. diclofenac potassium or delayed-release diclofenac sodium only. Or, 100 mg P.O. daily extended-release diclofenac sodium only.
➤ **Rheumatoid arthritis**
Adults: 50 mg P.O. t.i.d. or q.i.d., or 75 mg P.O. b.i.d. diclofenac potassium or delayed-release diclofenac sodium only. Or, 100 mg P.O. daily or b.i.d. extended-release diclofenac sodium only, or 50 to 100 mg diclofenac sodium P.R. at bedtime as substitute for last P.O. dose of the day. Don't exceed 150 mg daily.
➤ **Analgesia, primary dysmenorrhea**
Adults: 50 mg diclofenac potassium P.O. t.i.d. For some patients, the first dose on the 1st day may be 100 mg, followed by 50 mg for the second and third doses; maximum dose for 1st day is 200 mg. Don't exceed 150 mg daily after the 1st day.
✱*NEW INDICATION:* **Acute pain due to minor strains, sprains, and contusions**
Adults: 1 patch to the most painful area b.i.d.

ADMINISTRATION
P.O.
● Give drug with milk, meals, or antacids.
● Don't crush or break enteric-coated tablets.
Rectal
● If suppository is too soft, refrigerate briefly or hold wrapped suppository under cold running water.
Transdermal
● Do not apply to damaged or non-intact skin.

Reactions may be *common*, uncommon, *life-threatening*, or COMMON AND LIFE-THREATENING.
Interaction may have a *rapid onset* or *delayed onset.*

• Patch should not be worn while bathing or showering.

ACTION
May inhibit prostaglandin synthesis, to produce anti-inflammatory, analgesic, and antipyretic effects.

Route	Onset	Peak	Duration
P.O. (delayed-release)	30 min	2–3 hr	8 hr
P.O. (extended-release)	Unknown	5–6 hr	Unknown
P.O., P.R.	10 min	1 hr	8 hr
Transdermal	Unknown	10–20 hr	Unknown

Half-life: 1 to 2 hours; 12 hours for transdermal patch.

ADVERSE REACTIONS
CNS: *aseptic meningitis,* anxiety, depression, dizziness, drowsiness, headache, insomnia, irritability.
CV: *heart failure,* edema, fluid retention, hypertension.
EENT: *laryngeal edema,* blurred vision, epistaxis, eye pain, night blindness, reversible hearing loss, swelling of the lips and tongue, tinnitus.
GI: abdominal distention, abdominal pain or cramps, *bleeding,* constipation, diarrhea, flatulence, indigestion, melena, nausea, peptic ulceration, taste disorder, bloody diarrhea, appetite change, colitis.
GU: *nephrotic syndrome,* **acute renal failure,** fluid retention, interstitial nephritis, oliguria, papillary necrosis, proteinuria.
Hepatic: jaundice, *hepatitis, hepatotoxicity.*
Metabolic: *hypoglycemia,* hyperglycemia.
Musculoskeletal: back, leg or joint pain.
Respiratory: *asthma.*
Skin: *Stevens-Johnson syndrome,* allergic purpura, alopecia, bullous eruption, dermatitis, eczema, photosensitivity reactions, pruritus, rash, urticaria.
Other: *anaphylactoid reactions, anaphylaxis, angioedema.*

INTERACTIONS
Drug-drug. *Anticoagulants, including warfarin:* May cause bleeding. Monitor patient closely.
Aspirin: May decrease effectiveness of diclofenac and increase GI toxicity. Avoid using together.
Beta blockers: May decrease antihypertensive effects. Monitor patient closely.
Cyclosporine, digoxin, lithium, methotrexate: May reduce renal clearance of these drugs and increase risk of toxicity. Monitor patient closely.
Diuretics: May decrease effectiveness of diuretics. Avoid using together.
Insulin, oral antidiabetics: May alter requirements for antidiabetics. Monitor patient closely.
Potassium-sparing diuretics: May enhance retention and increase level of potassium. Monitor potassium level.
Drug-herb. *Dong quai, feverfew, garlic, ginger, horse chestnut, red clover:* May cause bleeding based on the known effects or components. Discourage use together.
White willow: Herb and drug contain similar components. Discourage use together.
Drug-lifestyle. *Sun exposure:* May cause photosensitivity reactions. Advise patient to avoid excessive sunlight exposure.

EFFECTS ON LAB TEST RESULTS
• May increase ALT, AST, bilirubin, BUN, and creatinine levels.
• May increase or decrease glucose level.

CONTRAINDICATIONS & CAUTIONS
■ **Black Box Warning** Contraindicated for the treatment of perioperative pain after CABG surgery. ■
• Contraindicated in patients hypersensitive to drug and in those with hepatic porphyria or history of asthma, urticaria, or other allergic reactions after taking aspirin or other NSAIDs.
• Avoid using during late pregnancy or breast-feeding.
• Use cautiously in patients with history of peptic ulcer disease, hepatic dysfunction, cardiac disease, hypertension, fluid retention, or impaired renal function.

NURSING CONSIDERATIONS
• Because NSAIDs impair the synthesis of renal prostaglandins, they can decrease renal blood flow and lead to reversible renal impairment, especially in patients with renal or heart failure or liver dysfunction, in elderly patients, and in those

taking diuretics. Monitor these patients closely.

• Liver function test values may increase during therapy. Monitor transaminase, especially ALT, levels periodically in patients undergoing long-term therapy. Make first transaminase measurement no later than 8 weeks after therapy begins.

■ **Black Box Warning** NSAIDs cause an increased risk of serious GI adverse events including bleeding, ulceration, and perforation of the stomach or intestines, which can be fatal. Elderly patients are at greater risk. ■

■ **Black Box Warning** NSAIDs may increase the risk of serious thrombotic events, MI, or stroke, which can be fatal. The risk may be greater with longer use or in patients with CV disease or risk factors for CV disease. ■

• Because of their antipyretic and anti-inflammatory actions, NSAIDs may mask the signs and symptoms of infection.

• *Look alike–sound alike:* Don't confuse diclofenac with Diflucan.

PATIENT TEACHING
• Tell patient to take drug with milk, meals, or antacids to minimize GI distress.
• Instruct patient not to crush, break, or chew enteric-coated tablets.
• Advise patient not to take this drug with any other diclofenac-containing products (such as Arthrotec).
• Teach patient signs and symptoms of GI bleeding, including blood in vomit, urine, or stool; coffee-ground vomit; and black, tarry stool. Tell him to notify prescriber immediately if any of these occurs.
• Teach patient the signs and symptoms of damage to the liver, including nausea, fatigue, lethargy, itching, yellowed skin or eyes, right upper quadrant tenderness, and flulike symptoms. Tell patient to contact prescriber immediately if these symptoms occur.
• Advise patient to avoid drinking alcohol or taking aspirin during drug therapy.
• Tell patient to wear sunscreen or protective clothing because drug may cause sensitivity to sunlight.
• Warn patient to avoid hazardous activities that require alertness until it is known whether the drug causes CNS symptoms.

• Tell pregnant woman to avoid use of drug during last trimester.
• Advise patient that use of OTC NSAIDs and diclofenac may increase the risk of GI toxicity.

---

etodolac
ee-toe-DOE-lak

Pharmacologic class: NSAID
Pregnancy risk category C;
D in 3rd trimester

AVAILABLE FORMS
Capsules: 200 mg, 300 mg
Tablets: 400 mg, 500 mg
Tablets (extended-release): 400 mg, 500 mg, 600 mg

INDICATIONS & DOSAGES
➤ **Acute pain**
Adults: 200 to 400 mg P.O. every 6 to 8 hours p.r.n., not to exceed 1,200 mg daily. In patients who weigh 60 kg (132 lb) or less, don't exceed total daily dose of 20 mg/kg.
➤ **Short- and long-term management of osteoarthritis and rheumatoid arthritis**
Adults: 600 to 1,000 mg P.O. daily, divided into two or three doses. Maximum daily dose is 1,200 mg. For extended-release tablets, 400 to 1,000 mg P.O. daily. Maximum daily dose is 1,200 mg.
➤ **Juvenile rheumatoid arthritis**
Children ages 6 to 16: 400 mg (extended-release) P.O. once daily if weight is 20 to 30 kg; 600 mg (extended-release) P.O. once daily if weight is 31 to 45 kg; 800 mg (extended-release) P.O. once daily if weight is 46 to 60 kg; or 1,000 mg P.O. once daily if weight exceeds 60 kg.

ADMINISTRATION
P.O.
• Give drug with milk or meals to minimize GI discomfort.

ACTION
Unknown. Produces anti-inflammatory, analgesic, and antipyretic effects, possibly by inhibiting prostaglandin synthesis.

Route	Onset	Peak	Duration
P.O.	30 min	1–2 hr	4–12 hr
P.O. (extended-release)	Unknown	3–12 hr	6–12 hr

Half-life: 7¼ hours.

ADVERSE REACTIONS

CNS: asthenia, malaise, dizziness, depression, drowsiness, nervousness, insomnia, syncope, fever.
CV: hypertension, *heart failure,* flushing, palpitations, edema, fluid retention.
EENT: blurred vision, tinnitus, photophobia.
GI: *dyspepsia,* flatulence, abdominal pain, diarrhea, nausea, constipation, gastritis, melena, vomiting, anorexia, *peptic ulceration with or without GI bleeding or perforation,* ulcerative stomatitis, thirst, dry mouth.
GU: dysuria, urinary frequency, *renal failure.*
Hematologic: anemia, *leukopenia,* hemolytic anemia.
Hepatic: *hepatitis.*
Metabolic: weight gain.
Respiratory: *asthma.*
Skin: pruritus, rash, cutaneous vasculitis, *Stevens-Johnson syndrome.*
Other: chills.

INTERACTIONS

Drug-drug. *Antacids:* May decrease etodolac's peak level. Watch for decreased effect of etodolac.
Aspirin: May decrease protein-binding of etodolac without altering its clearance. May increase GI toxicity. Avoid using together.
Beta blockers, diuretics: May blunt effects of these drugs. Monitor patient closely.
Cyclosporine: May increase risk of nephrotoxicity. Avoid using together.
Digoxin, lithium, methotrexate: May impair elimination of these drugs, increasing risk of toxicity. Monitor drug levels.
Phenylbutazone: May increase etodolac level. Avoid using together.
Phenytoin: May increase phenytoin level. Monitor patient for toxicity.
Warfarin: May decrease the protein binding of warfarin but doesn't change its clearance. Although no dosage adjustment is needed, monitor INR closely and watch for bleeding.
Drug-herb. *Dong quai, feverfew, garlic, ginger, horse chestnut, red clover:* May increase risk of bleeding. Discourage use together.
White willow: Herb and drug contain similar components. Discourage use together.
Drug-lifestyle. *Alcohol use:* May increase risk of adverse effects. Discourage use together.
Sun exposure: May cause photosensitivity reactions. Advise patient to avoid excessive sunlight exposure.

EFFECTS ON LAB TEST RESULTS

• May increase BUN and creatinine. May decrease uric acid and hemoglobin levels and hematocrit.
• May decrease WBC count.
• May cause a false-positive test result for urine bilirubin, possibly from phenolic metabolites and ketone bodies.

CONTRAINDICATIONS & CAUTIONS

■ **Black Box Warning** Contraindicated for the treatment of perioperative pain after CABG surgery. ■
• Contraindicated in patients hypersensitive to drug and in those with history of aspirin- or NSAID-induced asthma, rhinitis, urticaria, or other allergic reactions.
• Use cautiously in patients with history of renal or hepatic impairment, preexisting asthma, or GI bleeding, ulceration, and perforation.

NURSING CONSIDERATIONS

• Because NSAIDs impair the synthesis of renal prostaglandins, they can decrease renal blood flow and lead to reversible renal impairment, especially in patients with renal or heart failure or liver dysfunction, in elderly patients, and in those taking diuretics. Monitor these patients closely.
■ **Black Box Warning** NSAIDs cause an increased risk of serious GI adverse events including bleeding, ulceration, and perforation of the stomach or intestines, which can be fatal. Elderly patients are at greater risk. ■
■ **Black Box Warning** NSAIDs may increase the risk of serious thrombotic events, MI, or stroke, which can be fatal.

The risk may be greater with longer use or in patients with CV disease or risk factors for CV disease. ■

• *Look alike–sound alike:* Don't confuse Lodine with codeine, iodine, or Iopidine.

PATIENT TEACHING
• Tell patient to take drug with milk or meals to minimize GI discomfort.
• Teach patient signs and symptoms of GI bleeding, including blood in vomit, urine, or stool; coffee-ground vomit; and black, tarry stool. Tell him to notify prescriber immediately if any of these occurs.
• Advise patient to avoid consuming alcohol or aspirin while taking drug.
• Warn patient to avoid hazardous activities that require alertness until harmful CNS effects of drug are known.
• Teach patient signs and symptoms of liver damage, including nausea, fatigue, lethargy, itching, yellowed skin or eyes, right upper quadrant tenderness, and flulike symptoms. Tell him to contact prescriber immediately if any of these symptoms occurs.
• Advise patient to use a sunblock, wear protective clothing, and avoid prolonged exposure to sunlight because of possible sensitivity to sunlight.
• Tell pregnant woman to avoid use of drug during last trimester.
• Advise patient that use of OTC NSAIDs and etodolac may increase the risk of GI toxicity.

---

ibuprofen
eye-byoo-PROH-fen

Advil ◊ , Bayer Select Ibuprofen Pain Relief Formula, Children's Advil, Children's Motrin ◊ , Excedrin IB ◊ , Ibutab ◊ , Medipren ◊ , Motrin ◊ ✔, Novo-Profen† , PediaCare Fever ◊

Pharmacologic class: NSAID
Pregnancy risk category D in 3rd trimester

AVAILABLE FORMS
Capsules: 200 mg ◊
Oral drops: 40 mg/ml ◊
Oral suspension: 100 mg/5 ml ◊
Tablets: 100 mg, 200 mg, 400 mg, 600 mg, 800 mg ◊
Tablets (chewable): 50 mg ◊ , 100 mg ◊

INDICATIONS & DOSAGES
➤ **Rheumatoid arthritis, osteoarthritis, arthritis**
Adults: 300 to 800 mg P.O. t.i.d. or q.i.d. Maximum daily dose is 3.2 g.
➤ **Mild to moderate pain, dysmenorrhea**
Adults: 400 mg P.O. every 4 to 6 hours p.r.n.
➤ **Fever**
Adults: 200 to 400 mg P.O. every 4 to 6 hours, for no longer than 3 days. Maximum daily dose is 1.2 g.
Children ages 6 months to 12 years: If child's temperature is below 102.5° F (39.2° C), give 5 mg/kg P.O. every 6 to 8 hours. Treat higher temperatures with 10 mg/kg every 6 to 8 hours. Maximum daily dose is 40 mg/kg.
➤ **Juvenile arthritis**
Children: 30 to 40 mg/kg daily P.O. in three or four divided doses. Maximum daily dose is 50 mg/kg.

ADMINISTRATION
P.O.
• Give drug with milk or meals.

ACTION
May inhibit prostaglandin synthesis, to produce anti-inflammatory, analgesic, and antipyretic effects.

Route	Onset	Peak	Duration
P.O.	Variable	1–2 hr	4–6 hr

Half-life: 2 to 4 hours.

ADVERSE REACTIONS
CNS: *aseptic meningitis,* dizziness, headache, nervousness.
CV: edema, fluid retention, peripheral edema.
EENT: tinnitus.
GI: abdominal pain, bloating, constipation, decreased appetite, diarrhea, dyspepsia, epigastric distress, flatulence, GI fullness, heartburn, nausea, occult blood loss, peptic ulceration.

Reactions may be *common*, uncommon, *life-threatening*, or COMMON AND LIFE-THREATENING.
Interaction may have a *rapid onset* or *delayed onset.*

GU: *acute renal failure,* azotemia, cystitis, hematuria.
Hematologic: *agranulocytosis, aplastic anemia, leukopenia, neutropenia, pancytopenia, thrombocytopenia,* anemia, prolonged bleeding time.
Metabolic: *hyperkalemia, hypoglycemia.*
Respiratory: *bronchospasm.*
Skin: *Stevens-Johnson syndrome,* pruritus, rash, urticaria.

INTERACTIONS
Drug-drug. *Antihypertensives, furosemide, thiazide diuretics:* May decrease the effectiveness of diuretics or antihypertensives. Monitor patient closely.
Aspirin: May negate the antiplatelet effect of low-dose aspirin therapy. Advise patient on the appropriate spacing of doses.
Aspirin, corticosteroids: May cause adverse GI reactions. Avoid using together.
Bisphosphonates: May increase risk of gastric ulceration. Monitor patient for signs of gastric irritation or bleeding.
Cyclosporine: May increase nephrotoxicity of both drugs. Avoid using together.
Digoxin, lithium, oral anticoagulants: May increase levels or effects of these drugs. Monitor patient toxicity.
Methotrexate: May decrease methotrexate clearance and increases toxicity. Use together cautiously.
Drug-herb. *Dong quai, feverfew, garlic, ginger, ginkgo biloba, horse chestnut, red clover:* May increase risk of bleeding, based on the known effects of components. Discourage use together.
White willow: Herb and drug contain similar components. Discourage use together.
Drug-lifestyle. *Alcohol use:* May cause adverse GI reactions. Discourage use together.
Sun exposure: May cause photosensitivity reactions. Advise patient to avoid excessive sunlight exposure.

EFFECTS ON LAB TEST RESULTS
• May increase BUN, creatinine, ALT, AST, and potassium levels.
• May decrease glucose and hemoglobin levels and hematocrit.
• May decrease neutrophil, WBC, RBC, platelet, and granulocyte counts.

CONTRAINDICATIONS & CAUTIONS
• Contraindicated in patients hypersensitive to drug and in those with angioedema, syndrome of nasal polyps, or bronchospastic reaction to aspirin or other NSAIDs.
■ **Black Box Warning** Contraindicated for the treatment of perioperative pain after CABG surgery. ■
• Contraindicated in pregnant women.
• Use cautiously in patients with GI disorders, history of peptic ulcer disease, hepatic or renal disease, cardiac decompensation, hypertension, asthma, or intrinsic coagulation defects.

NURSING CONSIDERATIONS
• Check renal and hepatic function periodically in patients on long-term therapy. Stop drug if abnormalities occur and notify prescriber.
• Because of their antipyretic and anti-inflammatory actions, NSAIDs may mask signs and symptoms of infection.
• Blurred or diminished vision and changes in color vision may occur.
• Full anti-inflammatory effects may take 1 or 2 weeks to develop.
■ **Black Box Warning** NSAIDs cause an increased risk of serious GI adverse events including bleeding, ulceration, and perforation of the stomach or intestines, which can be fatal. Elderly patients are at greater risk. ■
■ **Black Box Warning** NSAIDs may increase the risk of serious thrombotic events, MI, or stroke, which can be fatal. The risk may be greater with longer use or in patients with CV disease or risk factors for CV disease. ■
• If patient consumes three or more alcoholic drinks per day, drug may cause stomach bleeding.

PATIENT TEACHING
• Tell patient to take with meals or milk to reduce adverse GI reactions.
• *Alert:* Drug is available OTC. Instruct patient not to exceed 1.2 g daily, not to give to children younger than age 12, and not to take for extended periods (longer than 3 days for fever or longer than 10 days for pain) without consulting prescriber.

- Tell patient that full therapeutic effect for arthritis may be delayed for 2 to 4 weeks. Although pain relief occurs at low dosage levels, inflammation doesn't improve at dosages less than 400 mg q.i.d.
- Caution patient that use with aspirin, alcohol, or corticosteroids may increase risk of GI adverse reactions.
- Teach patient to watch for and report to prescriber immediately signs and symptoms of GI bleeding, including blood in vomit, urine, or stool; coffee-ground vomit; and black, tarry stool.
- Tell patient to contact prescriber before using this drug if fluid intake hasn't been adequate or if fluids have been lost as a result of vomiting or diarrhea.
- Warn patient to avoid hazardous activities that require mental alertness until effects on CNS are known.
- Advise patient to wear sunscreen to avoid hypersensitivity to sunlight.

indomethacin
in-doe-METH-a-sin

Indocid†, Indocid SR†, Indocin, Indocin SR, Novo-Methacin†

indomethacin sodium trihydrate
Indocin I.V., Novo-Methacin†

Pharmacologic class: NSAID
Pregnancy risk category B;
D in 3rd trimester

AVAILABLE FORMS
indomethacin
Capsules: 25 mg, 50 mg
Capsules (sustained-release): 75 mg
Oral suspension: 25 mg/5 ml
indomethacin sodium trihydrate
Injection: 1-mg vials

INDICATIONS & DOSAGES
➤ **Moderate to severe rheumatoid arthritis or osteoarthritis, ankylosing spondylitis**
Adults: 25 mg P.O. b.i.d. or t.i.d. with food or antacids; increase daily dose by 25 or 50 mg every 7 days, up to 200 mg daily. Or, 75 mg sustained-release capsules

P.O. to start, in morning or at bedtime, followed by 75 mg sustained-release capsules b.i.d. if needed.
➤ **Acute gouty arthritis**
Adults: 50 mg P.O. t.i.d. Reduce dose as soon as possible; then stop therapy. Don't use sustained-release form.
➤ **Acute painful shoulders (bursitis or tendinitis)**
Adults: 75 to 150 mg P.O. daily in divided doses t.i.d. or q.i.d. for 7 to 14 days.
➤ **To close a hemodynamically significant patent ductus arteriosus in premature neonates**
Neonates older than age 7 days: 0.2 mg/kg I.V.; then two doses of 0.25 mg/kg at 12- to 24-hour intervals.
Neonates ages 2 to 7 days: 0.2 mg/kg I.V.; then two doses of 0.2 mg/kg at 12- to 24-hour intervals.
Neonates younger than age 48 hours: 0.2 mg/kg I.V.; then two doses of 0.1 mg/kg at 12- to 24-hour intervals.

ADMINISTRATION
P.O.
- Give drug with food, milk, or antacid.
I.V.
- Reconstitute powder for injection with sterile water or normal saline solution. For each 1-mg vial, add 1 or 2 ml of diluent for a solution containing 1 mg/ml or 0.5 mg/ml, respectively. Give over 20 to 30 minutes.
- Use only preservative-free sterile saline solution or sterile water to prepare. Never use diluents containing benzyl alcohol because it has been linked to toxicity in newborns.
- Because injection contains no preservatives, reconstitute drug immediately before use and discard unused solution.
- If anuria or marked oliguria is evident, withhold administration of second or third scheduled I.V. dose and notify prescriber.
- Watch carefully for bleeding and for reduced urine output.
- **Incompatibilities:** Amino acid injection, calcium gluconate, cimetidine, dextrose injection, dobutamine, dopamine, gentamicin, levofloxacin, solutions with pH less than 6, tobramycin sulfate, tolazoline.

Reactions may be *common*, uncommon, *life-threatening*, or COMMON AND LIFE-THREATENING.
Interaction may have a *rapid onset* or *delayed onset*.

Rectal
● If suppository is too soft, place in refrigerator for 15 minutes or run under cold water in wrapper.

ACTION
May inhibit prostaglandin synthesis, to produce anti-inflammatory, analgesic, and antipyretic effects.

Route	Onset	Peak	Duration
P.O.	30 min	1–4 hr	4–6 hr
I.V.	Immediate	Immediate	4–6 hr
P.R.	Unknown	Unknown	4–6 hr

Half-life: 4¼ hours.

ADVERSE REACTIONS
P.O. and P.R.
CNS: *headache,* confusion, dizziness, depression, drowsiness, fatigue, peripheral neuropathy, psychic disturbances, somnolence, syncope, vertigo.
CV: edema, hypertension.
EENT: hearing loss, tinnitus.
GI: *pancreatitis,* abdominal pain, anorexia, constipation, diarrhea, dyspepsia, *GI bleeding,* nausea, peptic ulceration.
GU: hematuria, renal insufficiency.
Hematologic: iron deficiency anemia.
Metabolic: *hyperkalemia.*
Skin: *Stevens-Johnson syndrome,* pruritus, urticaria.
Other: hypersensitivity reactions.
I.V.
GU: hematuria, interstitial nephritis, proteinuria.

INTERACTIONS
Drug-drug. *Aminoglycosides, cyclosporine, methotrexate:* May enhance toxicity of these drugs. Avoid using together.
Anticoagulants: May cause bleeding. Monitor patient closely.
Antihypertensives: May decrease antihypertensive effect. Monitor patient closely.
Antihypertensives, furosemide, thiazide diuretics: May impair response to both drugs. Avoid using together, if possible.
Aspirin: May decrease level of indomethacin. Avoid using together.
Aspirin, corticosteroids: May increase risk of GI toxicity. Avoid using together.

Bisphosphonates: May increase risk of gastric ulceration. Monitor patient for symptoms of gastric irritation or GI bleeding.
Diflunisal, probenecid: May decrease indomethacin excretion. Watch for increased indomethacin adverse reactions.
Digoxin: May prolong half-life of digoxin. Use together cautiously.
Dipyridamole: May enhance fluid retention. Avoid using together.
Lithium: May increase lithium level. Monitor patient for toxicity.
Penicillamine: May increase bioavailability of penicillamine. Monitor patient closely.
Phenytoin: May increase phenytoin level. Monitor patient closely.
Triamterene: May cause nephrotoxicity. Avoid using together.
Drug-herb. *Dong quai, feverfew, garlic, ginger, horse chestnut, red clover:* May cause bleeding. Discourage use together.
Senna: May inhibit diarrheal effects. Discourage use together.
White willow: Herb and drug contain similar components. Discourage use together.
Drug-lifestyle. *Alcohol use:* May cause GI toxicity. Discourage use together.

EFFECTS ON LAB TEST RESULTS
● May increase potassium level.
● May decrease hemoglobin level and hematocrit.
● May increase liver function test values.

CONTRAINDICATIONS & CAUTIONS
● Contraindicated in patients hypersensitive to drug and in those with a history of aspirin- or NSAID-induced asthma, rhinitis, or urticaria.
● Contraindicated in pregnant or breast-feeding women and in neonates with untreated infection, active bleeding, coagulation defects or thrombocytopenia, congenital heart disease needing patency of the ductus arteriosus, necrotizing enterocolitis, or significant renal impairment. Suppositories are contraindicated in patients with history of proctitis or recent rectal bleeding.
■ **Black Box Warning** Contraindicated for the treatment of perioperative pain after CABG surgery. ■
● Use cautiously in elderly patients, those with history of GI disease, and those with

epilepsy, parkinsonism, hepatic or renal disease, CV disease, infection, and mental illness or depression.

NURSING CONSIDERATIONS
● Because of the high risk of adverse effects from long-term use, drug shouldn't be used routinely as an analgesic or anti-pyretic.
● Sustained-release capsules shouldn't be used for acute gouty arthritis.
● If ductus arteriosus reopens, a second course of one to three doses may be given. If ineffective, surgery may be needed.
● Watch for bleeding in patients receiving anticoagulants, patients with coagulation defects, and neonates.
● Because NSAIDs impair synthesis of renal prostaglandins, they can decrease renal blood flow and lead to reversible renal impairment, especially in patients with renal failure, heart failure, or liver dysfunction; in elderly patients; and in those taking diuretics. Monitor these patients closely.
● Drug causes sodium retention; watch for weight gain (especially in elderly patients) and increased blood pressure in patients with hypertension.
● Monitor patient for rash and respiratory distress, which may indicate a hyper-sensitivity reaction.
● Because of their antipyretic and anti-inflammatory actions, NSAIDs may mask signs and symptoms of infection.
■ **Black Box Warning** NSAIDs cause an increased risk of serious GI adverse events including bleeding, ulceration, and per-foration of the stomach or intestines, which can be fatal. Elderly patients are at greater risk. ■
■ **Black Box Warning** NSAIDs may increase the risk of serious thrombotic events, MI, or stroke, which can be fatal. The risk may be greater with longer use or in patients with CV disease or risk factors for CV disease. ■
● Monitor patient on long-term oral therapy for toxicity by conducting regular eye examinations, hearing tests, CBCs, and kidney function tests.

PATIENT TEACHING
● Tell patient to take oral dose with food, milk, or antacid to prevent GI upset.

● Alert patient that using oral form with aspirin, alcohol, other NSAIDs, or corticosteroids may increase risk of adverse GI reactions.
● Teach patient signs and symptoms of GI bleeding, including blood in vomit, urine, or stool; coffee-ground vomit; and black, tarry stool. Tell him to notify prescriber immediately if any of these occurs.
● Tell patient to immediately report signs or symptoms of cardiac events, such as chest pain, shortness of breath, weakness, and slurred speech.
● Warn patient to avoid hazardous activities that require mental alertness until CNS effects are known.
● Tell patient to notify prescriber immedi-ately if visual or hearing changes occur.

ketoprofen
kee-toe-PROE-fen

Apo-Keto†

Pharmacologic class: NSAID
Pregnancy risk category B; D in 3rd trimester

AVAILABLE FORMS
Capsules: 25 mg, 50 mg, 75 mg
Capsules (extended-release): 100 mg, 150 mg, 200 mg
Suppositories: 50 mg†, 100 mg†
Tablets (enteric-coated): 50 mg†, 100 mg†
Tablets (extended-release): 200 mg†

INDICATIONS & DOSAGES
➤ **Rheumatoid arthritis, osteoarthritis**
Adults: 75 mg t.i.d. or 50 mg q.i.d., or 200 mg as an extended-release tablet once daily. Maximum dose is 300 mg daily, or 200 mg daily for extended-release capsules. Or, 50 or 100 mg P.R. b.i.d.; or one suppository at bedtime (with oral ketoprofen during the day).
Adults older than age 75: 75 to 150 mg P.O. daily. Adjust dose according to patient's response and tolerance.
➤ **Mild to moderate pain, dysmenorrhea**
Adults: 25 to 50 mg P.O. every 6 to 8 hours p.r.n. Maximum dose is 300 mg daily.

Reactions may be *common,* uncommon, *life-threatening,* or COMMON AND LIFE-THREATENING.
Interaction may have a *rapid onset* or *delayed onset.*

Adjust-a-dose: For elderly patients and those with impaired renal function, reduce first dose to between one-third and one-half normal first dose.

ADMINISTRATION
P.O.
● Give drug 30 minutes before or 2 hours after meals with a full glass of water. If adverse GI reactions occur, drug may be given with milk or meals.
● Don't crush delayed-release or extended-release tablets.
Rectal
● Rectal suppository replaces oral dose; don't use suppository in addition to tablets or capsules.

ACTION
Unknown. Produces anti-inflammatory, analgesic, and antipyretic effects, possibly by inhibiting prostaglandin synthesis.

Route	Onset	Peak	Duration
P.O. (extended-release)	2–3 hr	6–7 hr	Unknown
P.O., P.R.	1–2 hr	30–120 min	3–4 hr

Half-life: 2 to 5½ hours for extended-release forms.

ADVERSE REACTIONS
CNS: headache, dizziness, CNS excitation (which includes insomnia, nervousness, and dreams) or CNS depression (which includes somnolence and malaise).
CV: peripheral edema.
EENT: tinnitus, visual disturbances.
GI: *dyspepsia,* abdominal pain, anorexia, constipation, diarrhea, flatulence, nausea, stomatitis, peptic ulceration, vomiting.
GU: *nephrotoxicity.*
Hematologic: prolonged bleeding time.
Respiratory: dyspnea.
Skin: photosensitivity reactions, rash.

INTERACTIONS
Drug-drug. *Aspirin, corticosteroids:* May increase risk of adverse GI reactions. Avoid using together.
Aspirin, probenecid: May increase ketoprofen level. Avoid using together.
Cyclosporine: May increase nephrotoxicity. Avoid using together.

Hydrochlorothiazide, other diuretics: May decrease diuretic effectiveness. Monitor patient for lack of effect.
Lithium, methotrexate, phenytoin: May increase levels of these drugs, leading to toxicity. Monitor patient closely.
Warfarin: May increase risk of bleeding. Monitor patient closely.
Drug-herb. *Dong quai, feverfew, garlic, ginger, horse chestnut, red clover:* May cause bleeding based on the known effects of components. Discourage use together.
White willow: Herb and drug contain similar components. Discourage use together.
Drug-lifestyle. *Alcohol use:* May cause GI toxicity. Discourage use together.
Sun exposure: May cause photosensitivity reactions. Advise patient to avoid excessive sunlight exposure.

EFFECTS ON LAB TEST RESULTS
● May increase creatinine, BUN, ALT, and AST levels.
● May increase bleeding time.
● May increase or decrease iron test results.
● May falsely increase bilirubin level.

CONTRAINDICATIONS & CAUTIONS
● Contraindicated in patients hypersensitive to drug and in those with history of aspirin- or NSAID-induced asthma, urticaria, or other allergic reactions.
■ **Black Box Warning** Contraindicated for the treatment of perioperative pain after CABG surgery. ■
● Avoid use during last trimester of pregnancy.
● Drug isn't recommended for children or breast-feeding women.
● Use cautiously in patients with history of peptic ulcer disease, renal dysfunction, hypertension, heart failure, or fluid retention.

NURSING CONSIDERATIONS
● Don't use sustained-release form for patients in acute pain.
● Because NSAIDs impair synthesis of renal prostaglandins, they can decrease renal blood flow and lead to reversible renal impairment, especially in patients with renal or heart failure or liver dysfunction, in elderly patients, and in those taking diuretics. Monitor these patients closely.

• Check renal and hepatic function every 6 months or as indicated.
• Drug decreases platelet adhesion and aggregation, and can prolong bleeding time about 3 to 4 minutes from baseline.
■ **Black Box Warning** NSAIDs cause an increased risk of serious GI adverse events including bleeding, ulceration, and perforation of the stomach or intestines, which can be fatal. Elderly patients are at greater risk. ■
■ **Black Box Warning** NSAIDs may increase the risk of serious thrombotic events, MI, or stroke, which can be fatal. The risk may be greater with longer use or in patients with CV disease or risk factors for CV disease. ■
• NSAIDs may mask signs and symptoms of infection because of their antipyretic and anti-inflammatory actions.

PATIENT TEACHING
• *Alert:* Drug is available without prescription. Instruct patient not to exceed 75 mg daily.
• Tell patient to take drug 30 minutes before or 2 hours after meals with a full glass of water. If adverse GI reactions occur, patient may take drug with milk or meals.
• Tell patient not to crush delayed-release or extended-release tablets.
• Tell patient that full therapeutic effect may be delayed for 2 to 4 weeks.
• Teach patient signs and symptoms of GI bleeding, including blood in vomit, urine, or stool; coffee-ground vomit; and black, tarry stool. Tell him to notify prescriber immediately if any of these occurs.
• Alert patient that using with aspirin, alcohol, other NSAIDs, or corticosteroids may increase risk of adverse GI reactions.
• Warn patient to avoid hazardous activities that require mental alertness until CNS effects are known.
• Because of possibility of sensitivity to the sun, advise patient to use a sunblock, wear protective clothing, and avoid prolonged exposure to sunlight.
• Instruct patient to report problems with vision or hearing immediately.
• Tell patient to protect drug from direct light and excessive heat and humidity.

ketorolac tromethamine
KEE-toe-role-ak

Pharmacologic class: NSAID
*Pregnancy risk category C;
D in 3rd trimester*

AVAILABLE FORMS
Injection; 15 mg/ml in 1- and 2-ml vials and 1-ml Tubex syringes, 30 mg/ml in 1- and 2-ml single-dose vials, 1- and 2-ml Tubex syringes, and 10-ml multiple-dose vials
Tablets: 10 mg

INDICATIONS & DOSAGES
➤ **Short-term management of moderately severe, acute pain for single-dose treatment**
Adults younger than age 65: 60 mg I.M. or 30 mg I.V.
Children ages 2 to 16: 1 mg/kg I.M. (maximum dose 30 mg) or 0.5 mg/kg I.V. (maximum dose 15 mg).
Adults age 65 and older: 30 mg I.M. or 15 mg I.V.
Adjust-a-dose: For renally impaired patients or those who weigh less than 50 kg (110 lb), 30 mg I.M. or 15 mg I.V.
➤ **Short-term management of moderately severe, acute pain for multiple-dose treatment**
Adults younger than age 65: 30 mg I.M. or 30 mg I.V. every 6 hours for maximum of 5 days. Maximum daily dose is 120 mg.
Adults age 65 and older: 15 mg I.M. or I.V. every 6 hours for maximum of 5 days. Maximum daily dose is 60 mg.
Adjust-a-dose: For renally impaired patients or those who weigh less than 50 kg, 15 mg I.M. or I.V. every 6 hours. Maximum daily dose is 60 mg.
➤ **Short-term management of moderately severe, acute pain when switching from parenteral to oral administration (oral therapy is indicated only as continuation of parenterally given drug and should never be given without patient first having received parenteral therapy)**
Adults younger than age 65: 20 mg P.O. as single dose; then 10 mg P.O. every 4 to 6 hours for maximum of 5 days. Maximum daily dose is 40 mg.

Reactions may be *common*, uncommon, *life-threatening*, or COMMON AND LIFE-THREATENING.
Interaction may have a *rapid onset* or *delayed onset*.

Adults age 65 and older: 10 mg P.O. as single dose; then 10 mg P.O. every 4 to 6 hours for maximum of 5 days. Maximum daily dose is 40 mg.

Adjust-a-dose: For renally impaired patients or those who weigh less than 50 kg, give 10 mg P.O. as single dose; then 10 mg P.O. every 4 to 6 hours. Maximum daily dose is 40 mg.

ADMINISTRATION
P.O.
● Give drug with food if GI upset occurs.
I.V.
● Dilute with normal saline solution, D_5W, 5% dextrose and normal saline solution, Ringer's solution, lactated Ringer's solution, or Plasma-Lyte A.
● Give injection over at least 15 seconds.
● Protect from light.
● **Incompatibilities:** Azithromycin; fenoldopam mesylate; haloperidol lactate; nalbuphine; solutions that result in a relatively low pH, such as hydroxyzine, meperidine, morphine sulfate, and prochlorperazine; thiethylperazine.
I.M.
● When appropriate, give by deep I.M. injection.
● Patient may feel pain at injection site.
● Put pressure on site for 15 to 30 seconds after injection to minimize local effects.

ACTION
May inhibit prostaglandin synthesis, to produce anti-inflammatory, analgesic, and antipyretic effects.

Route	Onset	Peak	Duration
P.O.	30–60 min	30–60 min	6–8 hr
I.V.	Immediate	1–3 min	6–8 hr
I.M.	10 min	30–60 min	6–8 hr

Half-life: 4 to 6 hours.

ADVERSE REACTIONS
CNS: *headache,* dizziness, drowsiness, sedation.
CV: *arrhythmias,* edema, hypertension, palpitations.
GI: *dyspepsia, GI pain, nausea,* constipation, diarrhea, flatulence, peptic ulceration, stomatitis, vomiting.
GU: *renal failure.*

Hematologic: decreased platelet adhesion, prolonged bleeding time, purpura.
Skin: diaphoresis, pruritus, rash.
Other: pain at injection site.

INTERACTIONS
Drug-drug. *ACE inhibitors:* May cause renal impairment, particularly in volume-depleted patients. Avoid using together in volume-depleted patients.
Anticoagulants: May increase anti-coagulant levels in the blood. Use together with extreme caution and monitor patient closely.
Antihypertensives, diuretics: May decrease effectiveness. Monitor patient closely.
Lithium: May increase lithium level. Monitor patient closely.
Methotrexate: May decrease methotrexate clearance and increased toxicity. Avoid using together.
Probenecid: May increase level and toxicity of ketorolac. Avoid using together.
Salicylates: May increase the risk of serious ketorolac adverse effects. Avoid using together.
Drug-herb. *Dong quai, feverfew, garlic, ginger, horse chestnut, red clover:* May cause bleeding. Discourage use together.
White willow: Herb and drug contain similar components. Discourage use together.

EFFECTS ON LAB TEST RESULTS
● May increase ALT and AST levels.
● May increase bleeding time.

CONTRAINDICATIONS & CAUTIONS
■ **Black Box Warning** Contraindicated in patients hypersensitive to drug and in those with active peptic ulcer disease, recent GI bleeding or perforation, advanced renal impairment, cerebrovascular bleeding, hemorrhagic diathesis, or incomplete hemostasis, and those at risk for renal impairment from volume depletion or at risk for bleeding. ■
■ **Black Box Warning** Contraindicated in children younger than age 2 and in patients with history of peptic ulcer disease or GI bleeding, past allergic reactions to aspirin or other NSAIDs, and during labor and delivery or breast-feeding. ■
■ **Black Box Warning** Contraindicated as prophylactic analgesic before major surgery or intraoperatively when hemostasis

is critical; and in patients currently receiving aspirin, an NSAID, or probenecid. ■

■ **Black Box Warning** Contraindicated for treatment of perioperative pain in patients requiring coronary artery bypass graft surgery. ■

■ **Black Box Warning** Contraindicated in patients currently receiving aspirin or NSAIDs. ■

• Use cautiously in patients who are elderly or have hepatic or renal impairment or cardiac decompensation.

NURSING CONSIDERATIONS
• Correct hypovolemia before giving.

■ **Black Box Warning** Oral therapy is only indicated as a continuation of I.V./I.M. therapy. The maximum combined duration of parenteral and oral therapy is 5 days. ■

• In children age 2 and older, use as a single dose only.

• Don't give drug epidurally or intrathecally because of alcohol content.

• Carefully observe patients with coagulopathies and those taking anticoagulants. Drug inhibits platelet aggregation and can prolong bleeding time. This effect disappears within 48 hours of stopping drug and doesn't alter platelet count, INR, PTT, or PT.

■ **Black Box Warning** NSAIDs may increase the risk of serious thrombotic events, MI, or stroke, which can be fatal. The risk may be greater with longer use or in patients with CV disease or risk factors for CV disease. ■

■ **Black Box Warning** NSAIDs cause an increased risk of serious GI adverse events including bleeding, ulceration, and perforation of the stomach or intestines, which can be fatal. Elderly patients are at greater risk. ■

• NSAIDs may mask signs and symptoms of infection because of their antipyretic and anti-inflammatory actions.

• **Look alike–sound alike:** Don't confuse Toradol with Tegretol or Foradil.

PATIENT TEACHING
• Warn patient receiving drug I.M. that pain may occur at injection site.

• Teach patient signs and symptoms of GI bleeding, including blood in vomit, urine, or stool; coffee-ground vomit; and black, tarry stool. Tell him to notify prescriber immediately if any of these occurs.

• Tell patient not to take drug for more than 5 days in a row.

---

meloxicam
mel-OX-i-kam

Mobic

Pharmacologic class: NSAID
Pregnancy risk category C;
D in 3rd trimester

AVAILABLE FORMS
Oral suspension: 7.5 mg/5 ml
Tablets: 7.5 mg, 15 mg

INDICATIONS & DOSAGES
➤ **To relieve signs and symptoms of osteoarthritis or rheumatoid arthritis (RA)**
Adults: 7.5 mg P.O. once daily. May increase as needed to maximum dose of 15 mg daily.
➤ **To relieve signs and symptoms of pauciarticular or polyarticular course juvenile RA**
Children ages 2 to 17: 0.125 mg/kg P.O. once daily up to a maximum dose of 7.5 mg.

ADMINISTRATION
P.O.
• Give drug without regard for meals.
• The oral suspension may be substituted for the tablets, milligram for milligram. Shake liquid gently before use.

ACTION
May inhibit prostaglandin synthesis, to produce anti-inflammatory, analgesic, and antipyretic effects.

Route	Onset	Peak	Duration
P.O.	Unknown	4–5 hr	Unknown

Half-life: 15 to 20 hours.

ADVERSE REACTIONS
CNS: *seizures,* anxiety, confusion, depression, dizziness, fatigue, fever, headache, insomnia, malaise, nervous-

---

ness, paresthesia, somnolence, syncope, tremor, vertigo.

CV: *arrhythmias, heart failure, MI,* angina pectoris, edema, hypertension, hypotension, palpitations, tachycardia.

EENT: abnormal vision, conjunctivitis, pharyngitis, taste perversion, tinnitus.

GI: *hemorrhage, pancreatitis,* abdominal pain, colitis, constipation, diarrhea, dyspepsia, dry mouth, duodenal ulcer, esophagitis, flatulence, gastric ulcer, gastritis, gastroesophageal reflux, increased appetite, nausea, vomiting.

GU: *renal failure,* albuminuria, hematuria, urinary frequency, UTI.

Hematologic: *agranulocytosis, leukopenia, thrombocytopenia,* anemia, purpura.

Hepatic: *hepatitis, liver failure,* jaundice.

Metabolic: dehydration, weight increase or decrease.

Musculoskeletal: arthralgia, back pain.

Respiratory: *asthma, bronchospasm,* coughing, dyspnea, upper respiratory tract infection.

Skin: *erythema multiforme, exfoliative dermatitis, Stevens-Johnson syndrome, toxic epidermal necrolysis,* alopecia, bullous eruption, photosensitivity reactions, pruritus, rash, sweating, urticaria.

Other: *anaphylactoid reactions including shock, angioedema,* accidental injury, allergic reaction, flulike symptoms.

INTERACTIONS

Drug-drug. *ACE inhibitors:* May decrease antihypertensive effects. Monitor blood pressure.

Aspirin: May cause adverse effects. Avoid using together.

Furosemide, thiazide diuretics: May reduce sodium excretion caused by diuretics, leading to sodium retention. Monitor patient for edema and increased blood pressure.

Lithium: May increase lithium level. Monitor lithium level closely.

Methotrexate: May increase the toxicity of methotrexate. Use cautiously together.

Warfarin: May increase PT, INR, and risk of bleeding complications. Monitor PT and INR, and check for signs and symptoms of bleeding.

Drug-lifestyle. *Alcohol use:* May cause GI irritation and bleeding. Discourage use together.

Smoking: May cause GI irritation and bleeding. Discourage use together.

EFFECTS ON LAB TEST RESULTS

● May increase BUN, creatinine, ALT, AST, and bilirubin levels.

● May decrease hemoglobin level and hematocrit.

● May decrease WBC and platelet counts.

CONTRAINDICATIONS & CAUTIONS

● Contraindicated in patients hypersensitive to drug and in those who have experienced asthma, urticaria, or allergic reactions after taking aspirin or other NSAIDs.

■ **Black Box Warning** Contraindicated in perioperative pain following coronary artery bypass graft surgery. ■

● Avoid use late in pregnancy.

● Use with caution in patients with history of ulcers, GI bleeding, or asthma. Use cautiously in patients with dehydration, anemia, hepatic disease, renal disease, hypertension, fluid retention, heart failure, or asthma. Also use cautiously in elderly and debilitated patients because of increased risk of fatal GI bleeding.

NURSING CONSIDERATIONS

● *Alert:* Patients, including those hypersensitive to aspirin and other NSAIDs, may have allergic reactions to drug.

■ **Black Box Warning** NSAIDs may increase the risk of serious thrombotic events, MI, or stroke. The risk may be greater with longer use or in patients with CV disease or risk factors for CV disease. ■

■ **Black Box Warning** NSAIDs cause an increased risk of serious GI adverse events including bleeding, ulceration, and perforation of the stomach or intestines, which can be fatal. Elderly patients are at greater risk. ■

● Rehydrate dehydrated patients before starting drug. Patient with a history of ulcers or GI bleeding is at higher risk for GI bleeding while taking NSAIDs. Other risk factors for GI bleeding include treatment with corticosteroids or

anticoagulants, longer duration of NSAID treatment, smoking, alcoholism, older age, and poor overall health.
● Watch for signs and symptoms of overt and occult bleeding.
● NSAIDs can cause fluid retention; closely monitor patients who have hypertension, edema, or heart failure.
● Drug may be hepatotoxic. Watch for elevated ALT and AST levels. If signs and symptoms of liver disease develop, or if systemic signs and symptoms such as eosinophilia or rash occur, stop drug and call prescriber.
● Abdominal pain, vomiting, diarrhea, headache, and pyrexia may occur more frequently in children than in adults. Monitor children for these symptoms.
● Monitor hemoglobin level and hematocrit in patients on long-term therapy.

PATIENT TEACHING
● Tell patient to report history of allergic reactions to aspirin or other NSAIDs before starting therapy.
● Tell patient drug can be taken without regard to meals.
● Advise patient to report signs and symptoms of GI ulcers and bleeding, such as blood in vomit or stool, and black, tarry stools, and to contact prescriber if they occur.
● Instruct patient to report any skin rash, weight gain, or swelling.
● Advise patient to report warning signs of liver damage, such as nausea, fatigue, lethargy, itching, yellowed skin or eyes, right upper quadrant tenderness, and flulike symptoms.
● Warn patient with history of asthma that drug may trigger an asthmatic attack. Tell him to stop drug and contact prescriber if he has an attack.
● Tell woman of childbearing age to notify prescriber if she becomes pregnant or is planning to become pregnant while taking drug.
● Inform patient that it may take several days to achieve consistent pain relief.
● Advise patient that use of OTC NSAIDs with meloxicam may increase the risk of GI toxicity.

nabumetone
nah-BYOO-meh-tone

Pharmacologic class: NSAID
*Pregnancy risk category C;
D in 3rd trimester*

AVAILABLE FORMS
Tablets: 500 mg, 750 mg

INDICATIONS & DOSAGES
➤ **Rheumatoid arthritis, osteoarthritis**
Adults: Initially, 1,000 mg P.O. daily as a single dose or in divided doses b.i.d. Maximum, 2,000 mg daily.
Adjust-a-dose: For patients with moderate or severe renal insufficiency the maximum starting dose should not exceed 500 or 750 mg P.O. once daily. With careful monitoring, daily doses may be increased to a maximum of 1,500 mg.

ADMINISTRATION
P.O.
● Take drug with food, milk, or antacids to increase absorption.
● Limit alcohol intake to avoid risk of GI problems.

ACTION
Unknown. Produces anti-inflammatory, analgesic, and antipyretic effects, possibly by inhibiting prostaglandin synthesis.

Route	Onset	Peak	Duration
P.O.	Unknown	9–12 hr	Unknown

Half-life: About 24 hours.

ADVERSE REACTIONS
CNS: dizziness, fatigue, headache, insomnia, nervousness, somnolence.
CV: edema, vasculitis.
EENT: tinnitus.
GI: *abdominal pain, diarrhea, dyspepsia, bleeding,* anorexia, constipation, dry mouth, flatulence, gastritis, nausea, stomatitis, ulceration, vomiting.
GU: *renal failure.*
Respiratory: dyspnea, pneumonitis.
Skin: increased diaphoresis, pruritus, rash.

Reactions may be *common,* uncommon, *life-threatening,* or COMMON AND LIFE-THREATENING.
Interaction may have a *rapid onset* or *delayed onset.*

INTERACTIONS

Drug-drug. *Diuretics:* May decrease diuretic effectiveness. Monitor patient closely.

Warfarin, other highly protein-bound drugs: May cause adverse effects from displacement of drugs by nabumetone. Use together cautiously.

Drug-herb. *Dong quai, feverfew, garlic, ginger, horse chestnut, red clover:* May cause bleeding. Discourage use together.

White willow: Herb and drug contain similar components. Discourage use together.

Drug-food. *Any food:* May increase absorption. Advise patient to take drug with food.

Drug-lifestyle. *Alcohol use:* May increase risk of additive GI toxicity. Discourage use together.

EFFECTS ON LAB TEST RESULTS
None reported.

CONTRAINDICATIONS & CAUTIONS
● Contraindicated in patients with hypersensitivity reactions and history of aspirin- or NSAID-induced asthma, urticaria, or other allergic-type reactions.
● Contraindicated in children and in pregnant women during third trimester of pregnancy.
■ **Black Box Warning** Contraindicated for the treatment of perioperative pain after CABG surgery. ■
● Use cautiously in patients with renal or hepatic impairment; heart failure, hypertension, or other conditions that may predispose patient to fluid retention; or a history of peptic ulcer disease.

NURSING CONSIDERATIONS
● Because NSAIDs impair synthesis of renal prostaglandins, they can decrease renal blood flow and lead to reversible renal impairment, especially in patients with renal or heart failure or liver dysfunction, in elderly patients, and in those taking diuretics. Monitor these patients closely.
● During long-term therapy, periodically monitor renal and liver function, CBC, and hematocrit; assess patients for signs and symptoms of GI bleeding.
■ **Black Box Warning** NSAIDs cause an increased risk of serious GI adverse events including bleeding, ulceration, and perforation of the stomach or intestines, which can be fatal. Elderly patients are at greater risk. ■
■ **Black Box Warning** NSAIDs may increase the risk of serious thrombotic events, MI, or stroke, which can be fatal. The risk may be greater with longer use or in patients with CV disease or risk factors for CV disease. ■

PATIENT TEACHING
● Instruct patient to take drug with food, milk, or antacids. Drug is absorbed more rapidly when taken with food or milk.
● Advise patient to limit alcohol intake because using drug with alcohol increases the risk of GI problems.
● Teach patient signs and symptoms of GI bleeding, including blood in vomit, urine, or stool; coffee-ground vomit; and black, tarry stool. Tell him to notify prescriber immediately if any of these occurs.
● Warn patient against hazardous activities that require mental alertness until CNS effects are known.
● Advise patient that use of OTC NSAIDs in combination with nabumetone may increase the risk of GI toxicity.

---

naproxen
na-PROX-en

EC-Naprosyn, Naprosyn✐, Naxent†, Novo-Naprox†, Nu-Naprox†

naproxen sodium
Aleve◇, Anaprox, Anaprox DS, Apo-Napro-Na◇†, Naprelan, Novo-Naprox Sodium†

Pharmacologic class: NSAID
Pregnancy risk category B; D in 3rd trimester

AVAILABLE FORMS
naproxen
Oral suspension: 125 mg/5 ml
Tablets: 250 mg, 375 mg, 500 mg
Tablets (delayed-release): 375 mg, 500 mg

Tablets (extended-release): 750 mg, 1,000 mg

naproxen sodium
Tablets (controlled-release): 412.5 mg, 550 mg
Tablets (film-coated): 220 mg ◊ , 275 mg, 550 mg
Note: 275 mg of naproxen sodium contains 250 mg of naproxen.

INDICATIONS & DOSAGES
➤ **Rheumatoid arthritis, osteo-arthritis, ankylosing spondylitis, pain, dysmenorrhea, tendinitis, bursitis**
Adults: 250 to 500 mg naproxen b.i.d.; maximum, 1.5 g daily for a limited time. Or, 375 to 500 mg delayed-release EC-Naprosyn b.i.d. Or, 750 to 1,000 mg controlled-release Naprelan daily. Or, 275 to 550 mg naproxen sodium b.i.d.
➤ **Juvenile arthritis**
Children: 10 mg/kg P.O. in two divided doses.
➤ **Acute gout**
Adults: 750 mg naproxen P.O.; then 250 mg every 8 hours until attack sub-sides. Or, 825 mg naproxen sodium; then 275 mg every 8 hours until attack subsides.
➤ **Mild to moderate pain, primary dysmenorrhea**
Adults: 500 mg naproxen P.O.; then 250 mg every 6 to 8 hours up to 1.25 g daily. Or, 550 mg naproxen sodium; then 275 mg every 6 to 8 hours up to 1,375 mg daily. Or, 1,000 mg controlled-release Naprelan once daily. In patients older than age 65, don't exceed 400 mg daily.

ADMINISTRATION
P.O.
● Take drug with food or milk to minimize GI upset. Drink a full glass of water or other liquid with each dose.

ACTION
May inhibit prostaglandin synthesis to produce anti-inflammatory, analgesic, and antipyretic effects.

Route	Onset	Peak	Duration
P.O.	1 hr	2–4 hr	7 hr

Half-life: 10 to 20 hours.

ADVERSE REACTIONS
CNS: dizziness, drowsiness, headache, vertigo.
CV: edema, palpitations.
EENT: *tinnitus,* auditory disturbances, visual disturbances.
GI: abdominal pain, constipation, diarrhea, dyspepsia, epigastric pain, heartburn, nausea, occult blood loss, peptic ulcera-tion, stomatitis, thirst.
GU: *renal failure.*
Hematologic: ecchymoses, increased bleeding time.
Metabolic: *hyperkalemia.*
Respiratory: dyspnea.
Skin: diaphoresis, pruritus, purpura, rash, urticaria.

INTERACTIONS
Drug-drug. *ACE inhibitors:* May cause renal impairment. Use together cautiously.
Antihypertensives, diuretics: May decrease effect of these drugs. Monitor patient closely.
Aspirin, corticosteroids: May cause adverse GI reactions. Avoid using together.
Lithium: May increase lithium level. Observe patient for toxicity and monitor level. Adjustment of lithium dosage may be required.
Methotrexate: May cause toxicity. Monitor patient closely.
Oral anticoagulants, other sulfonylureas, highly protein-bound drugs: May cause toxicity. Monitor patient closely.
Probenecid: May decrease elimination of naproxen. Monitor patient for toxicity.
Drug-herb. *Dong quai, feverfew, garlic, ginger, ginkgo, horse chestnut, red clover:* May cause bleeding, based on the known effects of components. Discourage use together.
White willow: Herb and drug contain sim-ilar components. Discourage use together.
Drug-lifestyle. *Alcohol use:* May cause adverse GI reactions. Discourage use together.

EFFECTS ON LAB TEST RESULTS
● May increase BUN, creatinine, ALT, AST, and potassium levels.
● May increase bleeding time.
● May interfere with urinary 5-hydroxy-indoleacetic acid and 17-hydroxycortico-steroid determinations.

Reactions may be *common,* uncommon, *life-threatening,* or COMMON AND LIFE-THREATENING.
Interaction may have a *rapid onset* or *delayed onset.*

CONTRAINDICATIONS & CAUTIONS
• Contraindicated in patients hypersensitive to drug and in those with the syndrome of asthma, rhinitis, and nasal polyps.
■ **Black Box Warning** Naproxen (except controlled-release tablets) is contraindicated for the treatment of perioperative pain after CABG surgery. ■
• Patient should avoid drug during last trimester of pregnancy.
• Use cautiously in elderly patients and in patients with renal disease, CV disease, GI disorders, hepatic disease, or history of peptic ulcer disease.

NURSING CONSIDERATIONS
• Because NSAIDs impair synthesis of renal prostaglandins, they can decrease renal blood flow and lead to reversible renal impairment, especially in patients with renal failure, heart failure, or liver dysfunction; in elderly patients; and in those taking diuretics. Monitor these patients closely.
• Monitor CBC and renal and hepatic function every 4 to 6 months during long-term therapy.
■ **Black Box Warning** NSAIDs cause an increased risk of serious GI adverse events including bleeding, ulceration, and perforation of the stomach or intestines, which can be fatal. Elderly patients are at greater risk. ■
■ **Black Box Warning** NSAIDs may increase the risk of serious thrombotic events, MI, or stroke, which can be fatal. The risk may be greater with longer use or in patients with CV disease or risk factors for CV disease. ■
• Because of their antipyretic and anti-inflammatory actions, NSAIDs may mask signs and symptoms of infection.
• Drug may have a heart benefit, similar to aspirin, in preventing blood clotting.

PATIENT TEACHING
• **Alert:** Drug is available without prescription (naproxen sodium, 200 mg). Instruct patient not to take more than 600 mg in 24 hours. Dosage in patient older than age 65 shouldn't exceed 400 mg daily.
• Advise patient to take drug with food or milk to minimize GI upset. Tell him to drink a full glass of water or other liquid with each dose.

• Tell patient taking prescription doses for arthritis that full therapeutic effect may be delayed 2 to 4 weeks.
• Warn patient against taking naproxen and naproxen sodium at the same time.
• Teach patient signs and symptoms of GI bleeding, including blood in vomit, urine, or stool; coffee-ground vomit; and black, tarry stool. Tell him to notify prescriber immediately if any of these occurs.
• Caution patient that use with aspirin, alcohol, other NSAIDs, or corticosteroids may increase risk of adverse GI reactions.
• Warn patient against hazardous activities that require mental alertness until CNS effects are known.

piroxicam
peer-OX-i-kam

Feldene, Novo-Pirocam†, Nu-Pirox†

Pharmacologic class: NSAID
Pregnancy risk category B; D in 3rd trimester

AVAILABLE FORMS
Capsules: 10 mg, 20 mg

INDICATIONS & DOSAGES
➤ **Osteoarthritis, rheumatoid arthritis**
Adults: 20 mg P.O. daily. If desired, dose may be divided b.i.d.

ADMINISTRATION
P.O.
• Give drug with milk, antacids, or meals if adverse GI reactions occur.

ACTION
May inhibit prostaglandin synthesis, to produce anti-inflammatory, analgesic, and antipyretic effects.

Route	Onset	Peak	Duration
P.O.	1 hr	3–5 hr	48–72 hr

Half-life: 50 hours.

ADVERSE REACTIONS
CNS: *dizziness, headache,* drowsiness, somnolence, vertigo.

CV: peripheral edema.
EENT: auditory disturbances.
GI: *severe GI bleeding,* abdominal pain, anorexia, constipation, diarrhea, dyspepsia, epigastric distress, flatulence, heartburn, nausea, occult blood loss, peptic ulceration, stomatitis, vomiting.
GU: *nephrotoxicity.*
Hematologic: *agranulocytosis, leukopenia,* anemia, eosinophilia, prolonged bleeding time.
Metabolic: *hyperkalemia, hypoglycemia in diabetic patients.*
Skin: *pruritus, rash.*

INTERACTIONS
Drug-drug. *Antihypertensives, diuretics:* May decrease effects of these drugs. Avoid using together.
Aspirin, corticosteroids: May cause GI toxicity and may decrease level of piroxicam. Avoid using together.
Cyclosporine, methotrexate: May increase toxicity. Monitor patient closely.
Lithium: May increase lithium level. Monitor patient for toxicity.
Oral anticoagulants, other highly protein-bound drugs: May be toxic. Monitor patient closely.
Oral antidiabetics: May enhance antidiabetic effects. Monitor patient closely.
Ritonavir: May increase piroxicam level. Avoid using together.
Drug-herb. *Dong quai, feverfew, garlic, ginger, horse chestnut, red clover:* May cause bleeding. Discourage use together.
St. John's wort: May cause photosensitivity reaction. Advise patient to avoid excessive sunlight exposure.
White willow: Herb contains components similar to those of aspirin. Discourage use together.
Drug-lifestyle. *Alcohol use:* May cause GI toxicity and may decrease level of piroxicam. Discourage use together.
Sun exposure: May cause photosensitivity reaction. Advise patient to avoid excessive sunlight exposure.

EFFECTS ON LAB TEST RESULTS
● May increase BUN, creatinine, liver enzyme, and potassium levels.
● May decrease glucose and hemoglobin levels and hematocrit.

● May decrease WBC, granulocyte, and eosinophil counts.

CONTRAINDICATIONS & CAUTIONS
● Contraindicated in patients hypersensitive to drug and in those with bronchospasm or angioedema precipitated by aspirin or NSAIDs.
■ **Black Box Warning** Contraindicated for the treatment of perioperative pain after CABG surgery. ■
● Contraindicated in pregnant or breast-feeding patients.
● Use cautiously in elderly patients and in patients with GI disorders, history of renal or peptic ulcer disease, cardiac disease, hypertension, or conditions predisposing to fluid retention.

NURSING CONSIDERATIONS
● Because NSAIDs impair renal prostaglandin synthesis, they can decrease renal blood flow and lead to reversible renal impairment, especially in elderly patients, those taking diuretics, and those with renal failure, heart failure, or liver dysfunction. Monitor these patients closely.
● Check renal, hepatic, and auditory function and CBC periodically during prolonged therapy. Stop drug and notify prescriber if abnormalities occur.
■ **Black Box Warning** NSAIDs may increase the risk of serious thrombotic events, MI, or stroke, which can be fatal. The risk may be greater with longer use or in patients with CV disease or risk factors for CV disease. ■
■ **Black Box Warning** NSAIDs cause an increased risk of serious GI adverse events including bleeding, ulceration, and perforation of the stomach or intestines, which can be fatal. Elderly patients are at greater risk. ■
● NSAIDs may mask signs and symptoms of infection because of their antipyretic and anti-inflammatory actions.

PATIENT TEACHING
● Tell patient to take drug with milk, antacids, or meals if adverse GI reactions occur.
● Inform patient that full therapeutic effects may be delayed for 2 to 4 weeks.

Reactions may be *common,* uncommon, *life-threatening,* or COMMON AND LIFE-THREATENING.
Interaction may have a *rapid onset* or *delayed onset.*

• Teach patient signs and symptoms of GI bleeding, including blood in vomit, urine, or stool; coffee-ground vomit; and black, tarry stool. Tell him to notify prescriber immediately if any of these occurs.

• Warn patient against hazardous activities that require mental alertness until CNS effects are known.

• Because drug causes adverse skin reactions more often than other drugs in its class, advise patient to use a sunblock, wear protective clothing, and avoid prolonged exposure to sunlight. Sensitivity to the sun is the most common reaction.

• Advise patient that use of OTC NSAIDs in combination with piroxicam may increase the risk of GI toxicity.

buprenorphine hydrochloride
butorphanol tartrate
codeine phosphate
codeine sulfate
fentanyl citrate
fentanyl transdermal system
fentanyl transmucosal
hydromorphone hydrochloride
meperidine hydrochloride
methadone hydrochloride
morphine hydrochloride
morphine sulfate
nalbuphine hydrochloride
oxycodone hydrochloride
oxymorphone hydrochloride
pentazocine hydrochloride
pentazocine hydrochloride and
   naloxone hydrochloride
pentazocine lactate
propoxyphene hydrochloride
propoxyphene napsylate
tramadol hydrochloride

SAFETY ALERT!

buprenorphine hydrochloride
byoo-pre-NOR-feen

Buprenex, Subutex

Pharmacologic class: opioid
agonist-antagonist, opioid partial
agonist
Pregnancy risk category C
Controlled substance schedule III

AVAILABLE FORMS
Injection: 0.324 mg (equivalent to 0.3 mg
base/ml)
Sublingual tablets: 2 mg, 8 mg
(as base)

INDICATIONS & DOSAGES
➤ **Moderate to severe pain**
Adults and children age 13 and older:
0.3 mg I.M. or slow I.V. every 6 hours
p.r.n., or around the clock; repeat dose
(up to 0.3 mg), as needed, 30 to 60 minutes
after first dose.

Children ages 2 to 12: 2 to 6 mcg/kg I.M.
or I.V. every 4 to 6 hours.
Elderly patients: Reduce dose by
one-half.
Adjust-a-dose: In high-risk patients, such
as debilitated patients, reduce dose by
one-half.
➤ **Postoperative pain** ♦
Adults: 25 to 250 mcg/hour by continuous
I.V. infusion. Or, 60 mcg by epidural
administration in single doses, up to a
mean total dose of 180 mcg over 48 hours.
➤ **Adjunct to surgical anesthesia
with a local anesthetic** ♦
Adults: 0.3 mg by the epidural route.
➤ **Severe, chronic pain in terminally
ill patients** ♦
Adults: 0.15 to 0.3 mg by the epidural
route every 6 hours, up to a mean total
daily dose of 0.86 mg (range 0.15 to
7.2 mg).
➤ **Adjunct to surgical anesthesia
during circumcision** ♦
Children ages 9 months to 9 years:
3 mcg/kg I.M., followed by additional
3 mcg/kg doses postoperatively p.r.n.
➤ **Opioid dependence**
Adults: 12 to 16 mg S.L. as a single daily
dose.

ADMINISTRATION
I.V.
● When mixed in a 1:1 volume ratio, drug
is compatible with atropine sulfate,
diphenhydramine hydrochloride, droperidol, glycopyrrolate, haloperidol lactate,
hydroxyzine hydrochloride, promethazine
hydrochloride, scopolamine hydrochloride,
D_5W, 5% dextrose in normal saline solution, sodium chloride solution, lactated
Ringer's solution, and normal saline
solution injections.
● For direct injection, give slowly over
at least 2 minutes into a vein or through
tubing of a free-flowing, compatible I.V.
solution.
● **Incompatibilities:** Diazepam,
furosemide, lorazepam.
I.M.
● Give drug as deep I.M. injection.

Reactions may be *common*, uncommon, *life-threatening*, or COMMON AND LIFE-THREATENING.
Interaction may have a *rapid onset* or ***delayed onset.***

S.L.
● Place all the tablets of the dose under the tongue until dissolved; if uncomfortable, patient should take at least two at the same time.

ACTION
Unknown. Binds with opioid receptors in the CNS, altering perception of and emotional response to pain.

Route	Onset	Peak	Duration
I.V.	Immediate	2 min	6 hr
I.M.	15 min	1 hr	6 hr
S.L.	Unknown	Unknown	Unknown

Half-life: 1 to 7 hours.

ADVERSE REACTIONS
CNS: *dizziness, sedation, vertigo,* ***increased intracranial pressure,*** asthenia (tablets only), confusion, depression, dreaming, euphoria, fatigue, headache, insomnia (tablets only), nervousness, pain (tablets only), paresthesia, psychosis, slurred speech, weakness.
CV: ***bradycardia,*** cyanosis, flushing, hypertension, hypotension, tachycardia, Wenckebach block.
EENT: blurred vision, conjunctivitis, diplopia, miosis, rhinitis (tablets only), tinnitus, visual abnormalities.
GI: *nausea,* abdominal pain (tablets only), constipation, diarrhea (tablets only), dry mouth, vomiting.
GU: urine retention.
Respiratory: ***respiratory depression,*** dyspnea, hypoventilation.
Skin: diaphoresis, injection site reactions, pruritus, sweating (tablets only).
Other: back pain (tablets only), chills, infection (tablets only), withdrawal syndrome.

INTERACTIONS
Drug-drug. *CNS depressants, MAO inhibitors:* May cause additive effects. Use together cautiously.
CYP3A4 inducers (carbamazepine, phenobarbital, phenytoin, rifampin): May increase clearance of buprenorphine. Monitor patient for clinical effects of drug.
CYP3A4 inhibitors (erythromycin, indinavir, ketoconazole, ritonavir, saquinavir): May decrease clearance of buprenorphine.

Monitor patient for increased adverse effects.
Drug-lifestyle. *Alcohol use:* May cause additive effects. Discourage use together.

EFFECTS ON LAB TEST RESULTS
None reported.

CONTRAINDICATIONS & CAUTIONS
● Contraindicated in patients hypersensitive to drug.
● Use cautiously in elderly or debilitated patients; patients who are opioid dependent; in those undergoing biliary tract surgery; and in those with head injury, intracranial lesions, and increased intracranial pressure; severe respiratory, liver, or kidney impairment; CNS depression or coma; thyroid irregularities; adrenal insufficiency; and prostatic hypertrophy, urethral stricture, acute alcoholism, delirium tremens, or kyphoscoliosis.

NURSING CONSIDERATIONS
● Reassess patient's level of pain 15 and 30 minutes after parenteral administration.
● Buprenorphine 0.3 mg is equal to 10 mg of morphine and 75 mg of meperidine in analgesic potency. It has longer duration of action than morphine or meperidine.
● *Alert:* Naloxone won't completely reverse the respiratory depression caused by buprenorphine overdose; an overdose may require mechanical ventilation. Larger-than-usual doses of naloxone (more than 0.4 mg) and doxapram also may be indicated.
● Treat accidental skin exposure by removing exposed clothing and rinsing skin with water.
● Drug may cause constipation. Assess bowel function and need for stool softeners and stimulant laxatives.
● *Alert:* Drug's opioid antagonist properties may cause withdrawal syndrome in opioid-dependent patients.
● If dependence occurs, withdrawal symptoms may appear up to 14 days after drug is stopped.
● *Look alike–sound alike:* Don't confuse Buprenex with Bumex or bupropion.

PATIENT TEACHING
● Caution ambulatory patient about getting out of bed or walking.

• When drug is used after surgery, encourage patient to turn, cough, and breathe deeply to prevent breathing problems.

• Tell patient to place all the tablets of the dose under his tongue until dissolved; if this is uncomfortable, tell him to take at least two at the same time.

SAFETY ALERT!

butorphanol tartrate
byoo-TOR-fa-nole

Stadol

Pharmacologic class: opioid agonist-antagonist, opioid partial agonist
Pregnancy risk category C
Controlled substance schedule IV

AVAILABLE FORMS
Injection: 1 mg/ml, 2 mg/ml
Nasal spray: 10 mg/ml

INDICATIONS & DOSAGES
➤ **Moderate to severe pain**
Adults: 1 to 4 mg I.M. every 3 to 4 hours p.r.n., or around the clock. Not to exceed 4 mg per dose. Or, 0.5 to 2 mg I.V. every 3 to 4 hours p.r.n., or around the clock. Or, 1 mg by nasal spray every 3 to 4 hours (1 spray in one nostril); repeat in 60 to 90 minutes if pain relief is inadequate. For severe pain, 2 mg (1 spray in each nostril) every 3 to 4 hours.
Elderly patients: 1 mg I.M. or 0.5 mg I.V.; wait 6 hours before repeating dose. For nasal use, 1 mg (1 spray in one nostril). May give another 1 mg in 1.5 to 2 hours. Wait 6 hours before repeating sequence.
Adjust-a-dose: For patients with renal or hepatic impairment, increase dosage interval to 6 to 8 hours.
➤ **Labor for patients at full term and in early labor**
Adults: 1 or 2 mg I.V. or I.M.; repeat after 4 hours as needed.
➤ **Preoperative anesthesia or pre-anesthesia**
Adults: 2 mg I.M. 60 to 90 minutes before surgery.

➤ **Adjunct to balanced anesthesia**
Adults: 2 mg I.V. shortly before induction, or 0.5 to 1 mg I.V. in increments during anesthesia.
Elderly patients: One-half usual dose at twice the interval for I.V. use.

ADMINISTRATION
I.V.
• Compatible solutions include D_5W and normal saline solutions.
• Give by direct injection into a vein or into the tubing of a free-flowing I.V. solution.
• **Incompatibilities:** Dimenhydrinate, pentobarbital sodium.
I.M.
• Give drug I.M.; don't give sub-cutaneously.
Intranasal
• Watch for nasal congestion with nasal spray use.

ACTION
May bind with opioid receptors in the CNS, altering perception of and emotional response to pain.

Route	Onset	Peak	Duration
I.V.	1 min	4–5 min	2–4 hr
I.M.	10–30 min	30–60 min	3–4 hr
Nasal	15 min	1–2 hr	2½–5 hr

Half-life: About 2 to 9¼ hours.

ADVERSE REACTIONS
CNS: *dizziness, insomnia, somnolence,* **increased intracranial pressure,** anxiety, asthenia, confusion, euphoria, hallucinations, headache, lethargy, nervousness, paresthesia.
CV: flushing, hypotension, palpitations, vasodilation.
EENT: *nasal congestion,* blurred vision, tinnitus.
GI: *nausea, unpleasant taste, vomiting,* anorexia, constipation.
Respiratory: *respiratory depression.*
Skin: clamminess, excessive diaphoresis, hives, rash.
Other: sensation of heat.

INTERACTIONS
Drug-drug. *CNS depressants:* May cause additive effects. Use together cautiously.

Reactions may be *common,* uncommon, *life-threatening,* or COMMON AND LIFE-THREATENING.
Interaction may have a *rapid onset* or **delayed onset.**

Drug-lifestyle. *Alcohol use:* May cause additive effects. Discourage use together.

EFFECTS ON LAB TEST RESULTS
None reported.

CONTRAINDICATIONS & CAUTIONS
● Contraindicated in patients hypersensitive to drug or to preservative, benzethonium chloride, and in those with opioid addiction; may cause withdrawal syndrome.
● Use cautiously in patients with head injury, increased intracranial pressure, acute MI, ventricular dysfunction, coronary insufficiency, respiratory disease or depression, and renal or hepatic dysfunction.
● Use cautiously in patients who have recently received repeated doses of opioid analgesic.

NURSING CONSIDERATIONS
● Reassess patient's level of pain 15 and 30 minutes after administration.
● Respiratory depression apparently doesn't increase with larger dosage.
● Drug may cause constipation. Assess bowel function and need for stool softener and stimulant laxatives.
● Psychological and physical addiction may occur.
● Periodically monitor postoperative vital signs and bladder function. Because drug decreases both rate and depth of respirations, monitor arterial oxygen saturation to help assess respiratory depression.
● *Look alike–sound alike:* Don't confuse Stadol with sotalol.

PATIENT TEACHING
● Caution ambulatory patient about getting out of bed or walking. Warn outpatient to avoid driving and other hazardous activities that require mental alertness until it's clear how the drug affects the CNS.
● Teach patient how to take and store nasal spray.
● Instruct patient to avoid alcohol during therapy.

SAFETY ALERT!

codeine phosphate
koe-DEEN

codeine sulfate

Pharmacologic class: opioid
Pregnancy risk category C
Controlled substance schedule II

AVAILABLE FORMS
codeine phosphate
Injection: 15 mg/ml, 30 mg/ml, 60 mg/ml†
Oral solution: 15 mg/5 ml, 10 mg/ml†
codeine sulfate
Tablets: 15 mg, 30 mg, 60 mg

INDICATIONS & DOSAGES
➤ **Mild to moderate pain**
Adults: 15 to 60 mg P.O. or 15 to 60 mg (phosphate) subcutaneously, I.M., or I.V. every 4 to 6 hours p.r.n. Maximum daily dose is 360 mg.
Children older than age 1: 0.5 mg/kg P.O., subcutaneously, or I.M. every 4 to 6 hours p.r.n. Don't give I.V. in children.
➤ **Nonproductive cough**
Adults: 10 to 20 mg P.O. every 4 to 6 hours. Maximum daily dose is 120 mg.
Children ages 6 to 12: 5 to 10 mg P.O. every 4 to 6 hours. Maximum daily dose is 60 mg.
Children ages 2 to 5: 1 mg/kg P.O. daily in 4 equally divided doses every 4 to 6 hours.

ADMINISTRATION
P.O.
● Give drug with milk or meals to avoid GI upset.
I.V.
● Don't give discolored solution.
● Give drug by direct injection into a large vein. Give very slowly.
● **Incompatibilities:** Aminophylline, ammonium chloride, amobarbital, bromides, chlorothiazide, heparin, iodides, pentobarbital, phenobarbital, phenytoin, salts of heavy metals, sodium bicarbonate, sodium iodide, thiopental.
I.M.
● Document injection site.
Subcutaneous
● Assess injection site for local irritation, pain, and induration.

ACTION

May bind with opioid receptors in the CNS, altering perception of and emotional response to pain. Also suppresses the cough reflex by direct action on the cough center in the medulla.

Route	Onset	Peak	Duration
P.O.	30–45 min	1–2 hr	4–6 hr
I.V.	Immediate	Immediate	4–6 hr
I.M.	10–30 min	30–60 min	4–6 hr
Subcut.	10–30 min	Unknown	4–6 hr

Half-life: 2½ to 4 hours.

ADVERSE REACTIONS

CNS: *clouded sensorium, sedation,* dizziness, euphoria, light-headedness, physical dependence.
CV: *bradycardia,* flushing, hypotension.
GI: *constipation,* dry mouth, ileus, nausea, vomiting.
GU: urine retention.
Respiratory: *respiratory depression.*
Skin: *diaphoresis,* pruritus.

INTERACTIONS

Drug-drug. *CNS depressants, general anesthetics, hypnotics, MAO inhibitors, other opioid analgesics, sedatives, tranquilizers, tricyclic antidepressants:* May cause additive effects. Use together cautiously; monitor patient response.
Drug-lifestyle. *Alcohol use:* May cause additive effects. Discourage use together.

EFFECTS ON LAB TEST RESULTS

• May increase amylase and lipase levels.

CONTRAINDICATIONS & CAUTIONS

• Contraindicated in patients hypersensitive to drug.
• I.V. use contraindicated in children.
• Use cautiously in elderly or debilitated patients and in those with head injury, increased intracranial pressure, increased CSF pressure, hepatic or renal disease, hypothyroidism, Addison disease, acute alcoholism, seizures, severe CNS depression, bronchial asthma, COPD, respiratory depression, and shock.

• *Alert:* Breast-feeding mothers may put their infants at increased risk of morphine overdose if the mother is an ultra-rapid codeine metabolizer.

NURSING CONSIDERATIONS

• Reassess patient's level of pain at least 15 and 30 minutes after use.
• Codeine and aspirin or acetaminophen are commonly prescribed together to provide enhanced pain relief.
• For full analgesic effect, give drug before patient has intense pain.
• Drug is an antitussive and shouldn't be used when cough is a valuable diagnostic sign or is beneficial (as after thoracic surgery).
• Monitor cough type and frequency.
• Monitor respiratory and circulatory status.
• Opioids may cause constipation. Assess bowel function and need for stool softeners and stimulant laxatives.
• Codeine may delay gastric emptying, increase biliary tract pressure from contraction of the sphincter of Oddi, and interfere with hepatobiliary imaging studies.
• *Look alike–sound alike:* Don't confuse codeine with Cardene, Lodine, or Cordran.

PATIENT TEACHING

• Advise patient that GI distress caused by taking drug P.O. can be eased by taking drug with milk or meals.
• Instruct patient to ask for or to take drug before pain is intense.
• Caution ambulatory patient about getting out of bed or walking. Warn outpatient to avoid driving and other hazardous activities that require mental alertness until drug's effects on the CNS are known.
• Advise patient to avoid alcohol during therapy.
• Warn breast-feeding woman to watch for increased sleepiness, difficulty breast-feeding, or breathing, or limpness of infant. Tell her to immediately seek medical attention if this occurs.

Reactions may be *common,* uncommon, *life-threatening,* or COMMON AND LIFE-THREATENING.
Interaction may have a *rapid onset* or *delayed onset.*

fentanyl citrate
FEN-ta-nil

Sublimaze

fentanyl transdermal system
Duragesic

fentanyl transmucosal
Actiq, Fentora

Pharmacologic class: opioid agonist
Pregnancy risk category C
Controlled substance schedule II

AVAILABLE FORMS
Injection: 50 mcg/ml
Transdermal system: Patches that release 12.5 mcg, 25 mcg, 50 mcg, 75 mcg, or 100 mcg of drug per hour
Transmucosal: 100 mcg, 200 mcg; 400 mcg; 600 mcg; 800 mcg; 1,200 mcg; 1,600 mcg

INDICATIONS & DOSAGES
➤ **Adjunct to general anesthetic**
Adults: For low-dose therapy, 2 mcg/kg I.V. For moderate-dose therapy, 2 to 20 mcg/kg I.V.; then 25 to 100 mcg I.V. or I.M. p.r.n. For high-dose therapy, 20 to 50 mcg/kg I.V.; then 25 mcg to one-half initial loading dose I.V. p.r.n.
➤ **Adjunct to regional anesthesia**
Adults: 50 to 100 mcg I.M. or slowly I.V. over 1 to 2 minutes p.r.n.
➤ **To induce and maintain anesthesia**
Children ages 2 to 12: 2 to 3 mcg/kg I.V.
➤ **Postoperative pain, restlessness, tachypnea, and emergence delirium**
Adults: 50 to 100 mcg I.M. every 1 to 2 hours p.r.n.
➤ **Preoperative medication**
Adults: 50 to 100 mcg I.M. 30 to 60 minutes before surgery.
➤ **To manage persistent, moderate to severe chronic pain in opioid-tolerant patients who require around-the-clock opioid analgesics for an extended time**
Adults and children age 2 and older: When converting to Duragesic, base the first dose on the daily dose, potency, and characteristics of the current opioid therapy; the reliability of the relative potency estimates used to calculate the needed dose; the degree of opioid tolerance; and the patient's condition. Each patch may be worn for 72 hours, although some adult patients may need a patch to be applied every 48 hours during the first dosage period. May increase dose 3 days after the first dose, then every 6 days thereafter.
➤ **To manage breakthrough cancer pain in patients already receiving and tolerating an opioid**
Adults: 200 mcg Actiq initially; may give second dose 15 minutes after completing the first (30 minutes after first lozenge placed in mouth). Maximum dose is 2 lozenges per breakthrough episode. If several episodes of breakthrough pain requiring 2 lozenges occur, dose may be increased to the next available strength. After a successful dosage has been reached, patient should limit use to no more than 4 lozenges daily.
Or, initially 100 mcg Fentora between the upper cheek and gum. May repeat same dose once per breakthrough episode after at least 30 minutes. Adjust in 100-mcg increments. Doses above 400 mcg can be increased by 200 mcg. Generally, dosage should be increased when patient requires more than one dose per breakthrough episode. Once a successful maintenance dose has been established, reevaluate if patient experiences more than four breakthrough episodes per day.
➤ **Switching from Actiq to Fentora to manage breakthrough cancer pain in opioid-tolerant patients**
Adults: If current Actiq dose is 200 to 400 mcg, start with 100 mcg Fentora; if current Actiq dose is 600 to 800 mcg, use 200 mcg Fentora; if current Actiq dose is 1,200 to 1,600 mcg, use 400 mcg Fentora. Actiq and Fentora aren't bioequivalent.
Adjust-a-dose: For patients with renal or hepatic impairment, use lowest possible dose.

ADMINISTRATION
I.V.
● Only those trained to give I.V. anesthetics and manage adverse effects should give this form.

- Keep opioid antagonist (naloxone) and resuscitation equipment available.
- I.V. form often used with droperidol to produce neuroleptanalgesia.
- Inject slowly over 1 to 2 minutes.
- **Incompatibilities:** Azithromycin, fluorouracil, lidocaine, methohexital, pentobarbital sodium, phenytoin, thiopental.

I.M.
- Document administration site.

Transdermal
- Dosage equivalent charts are available to calculate the fentanyl transdermal dose based on the daily morphine intake; for example, for every 90 mg of oral morphine or 15 mg of I.M. morphine per 24 hours, 25 mcg/hour of transdermal fentanyl is needed.
- Clip hair at application site but don't use a razor, which may irritate skin. Wash area with clear water, if needed, but not with soaps, oils, lotions, alcohol, or other substances that may irritate skin or prevent adhesion. Dry area completely before application.
- Remove transdermal system from package just before applying, hold in place for 30 seconds, and be sure edges of patch stick to skin.
- Don't cut or otherwise alter transdermal patch before applying.
- Place transdermal patch on the upper back for a child or patient who's cognitively impaired to reduce the chance the patch will be removed and placed in the mouth.
- Heat from fever or heating pads, electric blankets, heat lamps, hot tubs, or water beds may increase transdermal delivery and cause toxicity.

Buccal
- Remove foil just before giving.
- For Actiq: Place tablet or lozenge between patient's cheek and gum and allow to dissolve over about 15 to 20 minutes; it must not be bitten, sucked, or chewed. Tablet or lozenge may be moved from one side to the other using the stick. Discard stick in the trash after use or, if any drug matrix remains on the stick, place under hot running tap water until dissolved. Or, place in child-resistant container provided and discard as for schedule II drugs.

- For Fentora: Place tablet between patient's cheek and gum and leave there until disintegrated, usually 14 to 25 minutes. Tablet shouldn't be sucked, chewed, or swallowed; this results in lower plasma concentrations. After 30 minutes, if remnants from tablet remain, they may be swallowed with a glass of water.

ACTION
Unknown. Binds with opioid receptors in the CNS, altering perception of and emotional response to pain.

Route	Onset	Peak	Duration
I.V.	1–2 min	3–5 min	30–60 min
I.M.	7–15 min	20–30 min	1–2 hr
Transdermal	12–24 hr	1–3 days	Variable
Transmucosal	5–15 min	20–30 min	Unknown

Half-life: 3½ hours after parenteral use; 5 to 15 hours after transmucosal use; 18 hours after transdermal use.

ADVERSE REACTIONS
CNS: *asthenia, clouded sensorium, confusion, euphoria, sedation, somnolence, seizures,* anxiety, depression, dizziness, hallucinations, headache, nervousness.
CV: *arrhythmias,* chest pain, hypertension, hypotension.
GI: *constipation,* abdominal pain, anorexia, diarrhea, dyspepsia, dry mouth, ileus, nausea, vomiting.
GU: urine retention.
Musculoskeletal: skeletal muscle rigidity (dose-related).
Respiratory: *apnea, hypoventilation, respiratory depression,* dyspnea.
Skin: *diaphoresis, pruritus,* erythema at application site (transdermal).
Other: physical dependence.

INTERACTIONS
Drug-drug. *Amiodarone:* May cause hypotension, bradycardia, and decreased cardiac output. Monitor patient closely.
CNS depressants, general anesthetics, hypnotics, MAO inhibitors, other opioid analgesics, sedatives, tricyclic antidepressants: May cause additive effects. Use together cautiously. Reduce dosages

---

Reactions may be *common*, uncommon, *life-threatening*, or COMMON AND LIFE-THREATENING.
Interaction may have a *rapid onset* or **delayed onset.**

of these drugs and reduce fentanyl dose by one-fourth to one-third.

CYP3A4 inducers (carbamazepine, phenytoin, rifampin): May decrease analgesic effects. Monitor patient for adequate pain relief.

Diazepam: May cause CV depression when given with high doses of fentanyl. Monitor patient closely.

Droperidol: May cause hypotension and decrease pulmonary arterial pressure. Use together cautiously.

Potent CYP3A4 inhibitors (clarithromycin, erythromycin, itraconazole, ketoconazole, nefazodone, nelfinavir, ritonavir, troleandomycin): May cause increased analgesia, CNS depression, and hypotensive effects. Monitor patient's respiratory status and vital signs.

Protease inhibitors: May increase fentanyl levels and adverse effects. Monitor patient closely for respiratory depression.

Drug-lifestyle. *Alcohol use:* May cause additive effects. Discourage use together.

EFFECTS ON LAB TEST RESULTS
• May increase amylase and lipase levels.

CONTRAINDICATIONS & CAUTIONS
• Contraindicated in patients intolerant to drug.

■ **Black Box Warning** Transdermal form contraindicated in patients hypersensitive to adhesives, those who are opioid-naive, those who need postoperative pain management, and those with acute, mild, or intermittent pain that can be managed with nonopioids. Don't use in patients with increased intracranial pressure, head injury, impaired consciousness, or coma. ■

■ **Black Box Warning** Transmucosal forms contraindicated in those who need acute or postoperative pain management. ■

• Fentora contraindicated in patients with mucositis more severe than grade 1.

• Use with caution in patients with brain tumors, COPD, decreased respiratory reserve, potentially compromised respirations, hepatic or renal disease, or cardiac bradyarrhythmias.

• Use with caution in elderly or debilitated patients.

NURSING CONSIDERATIONS
• For better analgesic effect, give drug before patient has intense pain.

• **Alert:** High doses can produce muscle rigidity, which can be reversed with neuromuscular blockers; however, patient must be artificially ventilated.

• Monitor circulatory and respiratory status and urinary function carefully. Drug may cause respiratory depression, hypotension, urine retention, nausea, vomiting, ileus, or altered level of consciousness, no matter how it's given.

• Periodically monitor postoperative vital signs and bladder function. Because drug decreases both rate and depth of respirations, monitoring of arterial oxygen saturation (SaO_2) may help assess respiratory depression. Immediately report respiratory rate below 12 breaths/minute, decreased respiratory volume, or decreased SaO_2.

• Drug may cause constipation. Assess bowel function and need for stool softeners and stimulant laxatives.

■ **Black Box Warning** Fentanyl is an opioid agonist and schedule II controlled substance with potential for abuse. Be alert for signs of misuse, abuse, or diversion. ■

Transdermal form

• **Alert:** Transdermal drug levels peak between 24 and 72 hours after initial application and dose increases. Monitor patients for life-threatening hypoventilation, especially during these times.

• Fentanyl patches should be used only in patients age 2 or older who are opioid-tolerant, who have chronic moderate to severe pain poorly controlled by other drugs, and who need a total daily opioid dose at least equivalent to the 25-mcg/hour fentanyl patch.

• When converting a patient from another opioid, determine the initial fentanyl dosage with great care; overestimating the dosage could be dangerous or fatal.

• Identify all daily drugs particularly CYP3A4 inhibitors, which may increase fentanyl levels.

• Monitor patients closely, and provide immediate care for evidence of overdose, such as slow or shallow breathing, a slow heartbeat, severe sleepiness, cold and

clammy skin, trouble walking and talking, and feeling faint, dizzy, or confused.

• Give patients detailed instructions for using fentanyl patches correctly and safely.

• Make dosage adjustments gradually in patient using the transdermal system. Reaching steady-state level of a new dosage may take up to 6 days; delay dosage adjustment until after at least two applications.

• Monitor patient who develops adverse reactions to the transdermal system for at least 12 hours after removal. Drug level drops gradually and may take as long as 17 hours to decline by 50%.

• Most patients experience good control of pain for 3 days while wearing the transdermal system, but a few may need a new application after 48 hours.

• Because the drug level rises for the first 24 hours after application, analgesic effect can't be evaluated on the first day. Make sure patient has adequate supplemental analgesic to prevent breakthrough pain.

• When reducing opioid therapy or switching to a different analgesic, withdraw the transdermal system gradually. Because the drug level drops gradually after removal, give half the equianalgesic dose of the new analgesic 12 to 18 hours after removal.

Transmucosal form

■ **Black Box Warning** Fentora and Actiq are used only to manage breakthrough cancer pain in patients who are already receiving and tolerating opioids. ■

■ **Black Box Warning** Fentora and Actiq aren't bioequivalent and can't be substituted on a microgram-per-microgram basis. ■

• *Look alike–sound alike:* Don't confuse fentanyl with alfentanil.

PATIENT TEACHING

• When drug is used for pain control, instruct patient to request drug before pain becomes intense.

• *Alert:* Inform family members only the patient should be activating the Ionsys system for pain control to decrease the risk of fatal respiratory depression.

• When drug is used after surgery, encourage patient to turn, cough, and breathe deeply to prevent lung problems.

• Instruct patient to avoid hazardous activities until CNS effects subside.

• Tell home care patient to avoid drinking alcohol or taking other CNS-type drugs because additive effects can occur.

• Advise patient not to stop drug abruptly.

• Teach patient about proper application of transdermal patch. Tell patient to clip hair at application site but not to use a razor, which may irritate skin. Wash area with clear water, if needed, but not with soaps, oils, lotions, alcohol, or other substances that may irritate skin or prevent adhesion. Dry area completely before application.

• Tell patient to remove transdermal system from package just before applying, hold in place for 30 seconds, and be sure the edges of patch stick to skin.

• *Alert:* Teach patient not to alter the transdermal patch (such as by cutting it) before applying.

• Advise parent or caregiver to place transdermal patch on the upper back for a child or a patient who's cognitively impaired, to reduce the chance the patch will be removed and placed in the mouth.

• Teach patient to dispose of the transdermal patch by folding it so the adhesive side adheres to itself and then flushing it down the toilet.

• Tell patient that, if another patch is needed after 48 to 72 hours, he should apply it to a different skin site.

• Tell patient that pain relief with the patch may not occur for several hours after the patch is applied. Oral, immediate-release opioids may be needed for initial pain relief.

• Inform patient that heat from fever or environment, such as from heating pads, electric blankets, heat lamps, hot tubs, or water beds, may increase transdermal delivery and cause toxicity requiring dosage adjustment. Instruct patient to notify prescriber if fever occurs or if he'll be spending time in a hot climate.

■ **Black Box Warning** Warn patient and patient's family that the amount of drug in 1 Actiq lozenge or Fentora tablet can be fatal to a child. Keep well secured and out of children's reach. ■

Reactions may be *common*, uncommon, *life-threatening*, or COMMON AND LIFE-THREATENING.
Interaction may have a *rapid onset* or **delayed onset.**

SAFETY ALERT!

hydromorphone hydrochloride (dihydromorphinone hydrochloride)
hye-droe-MOR-fone

Dilaudid, Dilaudid-HP

Pharmacologic class: opioid
Pregnancy risk category C
Controlled substance schedule II

AVAILABLE FORMS
Injection: 1 mg/ml, 2 mg/ml, 4 mg/ml, 10 mg/ml
Liquid: 5 mg/5 ml
Lyophilized powder for injection: 10 mg/ml
Suppositories: 3 mg†
Tablets: 2 mg, 3 mg, 4 mg, 8 mg

INDICATIONS & DOSAGES
➤ **Moderate to severe pain**
Adults: 2 to 4 mg P.O. every 4 to 6 hours p.r.n. Or, 1 to 4 mg I.M., subcutaneously, or I.V. (slowly over at least 2 to 5 minutes) every 4 to 6 hours p.r.n. Or, 3 mg P.R. suppository every 6 to 8 hours p.r.n. Or, 2.5 to 10 mg oral liquid every 3 to 6 hours p.r.n.

ADMINISTRATION
P.O.
● Give drug with food if GI upset occurs.
I.V.
● For infusion, drug may be mixed in D₅W, normal saline solution, dextrose 5% in normal saline solution, dextrose 5% in half-normal saline solution, or Ringer's or lactated Ringer's solutions.
● Give by direct injection over no less than 2 minutes.
● Respiratory depression and hypotension can occur. Give slowly, and monitor patient constantly. Keep resuscitation equipment available.
● **Incompatibilities:** Alkalies, ampho-tericin B cholesterol complex, ampicillin sodium, bromides, cefazolin, dexametha-sone, diazepam, gallium nitrate, haloperi-dol, heparin sodium, iodides, minocycline, phenobarbital sodium, phenytoin sodium, prochlorperazine edisylate, sargramostim, sodium bicarbonate, sodium phosphate, thiopental.

I.M.
● Document administration site.
Subcutaneous
● Rotate injection sites to avoid induration with subcutaneous injection.
Rectal
● Refrigerate suppositories.

ACTION
Unknown. Binds with opioid receptors in the CNS, altering perception of and emo-tional response to pain. Also suppresses the cough reflex by direct action on the cough center in the medulla.

Route	Onset	Peak	Duration
P.O.	15–30 min	30–60 min	4–5 hr
I.V.	10–15 min	15–30 min	2–3 hr
I.M.	15 min	30–60 min	4–5 hr
Subcut.	15 min	30–90 min	4 hr
P.R.	Unknown	Unknown	4 hr

Half-life: 2½ to 4 hours.

ADVERSE REACTIONS
CNS: sedation, somnolence, clouded sensorium, dizziness, euphoria, light-headedness.
CV: hypotension, flushing, *bradycardia.*
EENT: blurred vision, diplopia, nystagmus.
GI: nausea, vomiting, *constipation,* ileus, dry mouth.
GU: urine retention.
Respiratory: *respiratory depression, bronchospasm.*
Skin: diaphoresis, pruritus.
Other: induration with repeated sub-cutaneous injections, physical dependence.

INTERACTIONS
Drug-drug. *CNS depressants, general anesthetics, hypnotics, MAO inhibitors, other opioid analgesics, sedatives, tranquilizers, tricyclic antidepressants:* May cause additive effects. Use together with caution; reduce hydromorphone dose and monitor patient response.
Drug-lifestyle. *Alcohol use:* May cause additive effects. Discourage use together.

EFFECTS ON LAB TEST RESULTS
● May increase amylase and lipase levels.
● May interfere with hepatobiliary imaging studies because delayed gastric emptying

---

†Canada   ◇ OTC   ♦ Off-label use   🔗Photoguide   *Liquid contains alcohol.

and contraction of sphincter of Oddi may increase biliary tract pressure.

CONTRAINDICATIONS & CAUTIONS
• Contraindicated in patients hypersensitive to drug; in those with intracranial lesions that cause increased intracranial pressure; and in those with depressed ventilation, such as in status asthmaticus, COPD, cor pulmonale, emphysema, and kyphoscoliosis.
• Use with caution in elderly or debilitated patients and in those with hepatic or renal disease, hypothyroidism, Addison's disease, prostatic hyperplasia, or urethral stricture.

NURSING CONSIDERATIONS
• Reassess patient's level of pain at least 15 and 30 minutes after administration.
• For better analgesic effect, give drug on a regular schedule, before patient has intense pain.
■ **Black Box Warning** Dilaudid-HP, a highly concentrated form (10 mg/ml), may be given in smaller volumes to prevent the discomfort of large-volume I.M. or subcutaneous injections. Don't confuse Dilaudid-HP with standard parenteral formulations. Check dosage carefully. ■
• Monitor respiratory and circulatory status and bowel function.
• Keep opioid antagonist (naloxone) available.
• Drug may worsen or mask gallbladder pain.
• Drug is a commonly abused opioid.
• Drug may cause constipation. Assess bowel function and need for stool softeners and stimulant laxatives.
• *Alert:* Cough syrup may contain tartrazine.
• *Look alike–sound alike:* Don't confuse hydromorphone with morphine or oxymorphone or Dilaudid with Dilantin.

PATIENT TEACHING
• Instruct patient to request or take drug before pain becomes intense.
• Tell patient to store suppositories in refrigerator.
• Advise patient to take drug with food if GI upset occurs.

• When drug is used after surgery, encourage patient to turn, cough, and breathe deeply to avoid lung problems.
• Caution patient about getting out of bed or walking. Warn outpatient to avoid hazardous activities that require mental alertness until drug's CNS effects are known.
• Advise patient to avoid alcohol during therapy.

SAFETY ALERT!

meperidine hydrochloride (pethidine hydrochloride)
me-PER-i-deen

Demerol◆

Pharmacologic class: opioid
Pregnancy risk category B;
D if used for prolonged periods or in high doses at term
Controlled substance schedule II

AVAILABLE FORMS
Injection: 25 mg/ml, 50 mg/ml, 75 mg/ml, 100 mg/ml
Syrup: 50 mg/5 ml
Tablets: 50 mg, 100 mg

INDICATIONS & DOSAGES
➤ **Moderate to severe pain**
Adults: 50 to 150 mg P.O., I.M., or subcutaneously every 3 to 4 hours p.r.n.
Children: 1.1 to 1.8 mg/kg P.O., I.M., or subcutaneously every 3 to 4 hours. Maximum, 100 mg every 4 hours p.r.n.
Adjust-a-dose: Reduce meperidine doses by 25% to 50% when administered with phenothiazines and other tranquilizers because they potentiate the action of meperidine.
➤ **Preoperative analgesia**
Adults: 50 to 100 mg I.M. or subcutaneously 30 to 90 minutes before surgery.
Children: 1 to 2.2 mg/kg I.M. or subcutaneously up to the adult dose 30 to 90 minutes before surgery.
➤ **Adjunct to anesthesia**
Adults: Repeated slow I.V. injections of fractional doses (10 mg/ml). Or, continuous I.V. infusion of a more dilute solution (1 mg/ml) titrated to patient's needs.

Reactions may be *common*, uncommon, *life-threatening*, or COMMON AND LIFE-THREATENING.
Interaction may have a *rapid onset* or **delayed onset**.

➤ **Obstetric analgesia**
Adults: 50 to 100 mg I.M. or subcutaneously when pain becomes regular;
repeated at 1- to 3-hour intervals.

ADMINISTRATION
P.O.
• Syrup has local anesthetic effect. Give
with full glass of water.
I.V.
• Keep opioid antagonist (naloxone)
available.
• Give drug slowly by direct injection.
• Drug may also be given by slow continuous infusion. Drug is compatible with
most solutions, including D$_5$W, normal
saline solution, and Ringer's or lactated
Ringer's solutions.
• Protect from light and store at room
temperature.
• **Incompatibilities:** Acyclovir, allopurinol, aminophylline, amobarbital, amphotericin B, cefepime, cefoperazone,
doxorubicin liposomal, ephedrine,
furosemide, heparin, hydrocortisone
sodium succinate, idarubicin, imipenem
and cilastatin sodium, methylprednisolone
sodium succinate, morphine, pentobarbital,
phenobarbital sodium, phenytoin, sodium
bicarbonate, sodium iodide, thiopental.
I.M.
• Oral dose is less than half as effective as
parenteral dose. Give I.M. if possible.
When changing from parenteral to oral
route, increase dosage.
Subcutaneous
• Subcutaneous injection isn't recommended because it's very painful, but
it may be suitable for occasional use.
Monitor patient for pain at injection site,
local tissue irritation, and induration after
subcutaneous injection.

ACTION
Unknown. Binds with opioid receptors
in the CNS, altering perception of and
emotional response to pain.

Route	Onset	Peak	Duration
P.O.	15 min	60–90 min	2–4 hr
I.V.	1 min	5–7 min	2–4 hr
I.M., Subcut.	10–15 min	30–50 min	2–4 hr

Half-life: 2½ to 4 hours.

ADVERSE REACTIONS
CNS: *clouded sensorium, dizziness,
euphoria, light-headedness, sedation,
somnolence,* **seizures,** hallucinations,
headache, paradoxical anxiety, physical
dependence, syncope, tremor.
CV: **bradycardia, cardiac arrest, shock,**
hypotension, tachycardia.
GI: biliary tract spasms, constipation,
dry mouth, ileus, *nausea, vomiting.*
GU: urine retention.
Musculoskeletal: muscle twitching.
Respiratory: **respiratory arrest,
respiratory depression.**
Skin: *diaphoresis,* pruritus, urticaria.
Other: induration, local tissue irritation,
pain at injection site, phlebitis after I.V.
delivery.

INTERACTIONS
Drug-drug. *Aminophylline, barbiturates, heparin, methicillin, morphine
sulfate, phenytoin, sodium bicarbonate,
sulfonamides:* Incompatible when mixed
in same I.V. container. Avoid using
together.
Cimetidine: May increase respiratory
and CNS depression. Monitor patient
closely.
Chlorpromazine: May cause excessive
sedation and hypotension. Avoid using
together.
*CNS depressants, general anesthetics,
hypnotics, other opioid analgesics,
phenothiazines, sedatives, tricyclic antidepressants:* May cause respiratory
depression, hypotension, profound sedation, or coma. Use together with caution;
reduce meperidine dosage.
MAO inhibitors: May increase CNS
excitation or depression that can be severe
or fatal. Avoid using together.
Phenytoin: May decrease meperidine
level. Watch for decreased analgesia.
Protease inhibitors: May increase respiratory and CNS depression. Avoid using
together.
Ritonavir: May significantly increase level
and toxic effects of meperidine. Avoid use
together.
Drug-lifestyle. *Alcohol use:* May cause
additive effects. Discourage use together.

EFFECTS ON LAB TEST RESULTS
• May increase amylase and lipase levels.

CONTRAINDICATIONS & CAUTIONS
• Contraindicated in patients hypersensitive to drug and in those who have received MAO inhibitors within past 14 days.
• Avoid use in patients with end-stage renal disease.
• Use with caution in elderly or debilitated patients and in those with increased intracranial pressure, head injury, asthma and other respiratory conditions, supraventricular tachycardias, seizures, acute abdominal conditions, hepatic or renal disease, hypothyroidism, Addison's disease, urethral stricture, and prostatic hyperplasia.

NURSING CONSIDERATIONS
• In elderly patients or in those with renal dysfunction, active metabolite may accumulate, causing increased adverse CNS reactions.
• Drug may be used in some patients who are allergic to morphine.
• Reassess patient's level of pain at least 15 and 30 minutes after administration.
• Because drug toxicity frequently appears after several days of treatment, drug isn't recommended for treatment of chronic pain.
• In neonates exposed to drug during labor, monitor respirations. Have resuscitation equipment and naloxone available.
• Monitor respiratory and CV status carefully. Don't give if respirations are below 12 breaths/minute, if respiratory rate or depth is decreased, or if change in pupils is noted.
• If drug is stopped abruptly after long-term use, monitor patient for withdrawal symptoms.
• In postoperative patients, monitor bladder function.
• Monitor bowel function. Patient may need a stimulant laxative and stool softener.
• **Look alike–sound alike:** Don't confuse Demerol with Demulen.

PATIENT TEACHING
• Encourage postoperative patient to turn, cough, deep-breathe, and use an incentive spirometer to prevent lung problems.
• Caution ambulatory patient about getting out of bed or walking. Warn outpatient to avoid driving and other potentially hazardous activities that require mental alertness until drug's CNS effects are known.
• Advise patient to avoid alcohol during therapy.
• Caution patient that drug isn't intended for long-term use.

SAFETY ALERT!

methadone hydrochloride
METH-a-done

Dolophine, Methadose

Pharmacologic class: opioid agonist
Pregnancy risk category C
Controlled substance schedule II

AVAILABLE FORMS
Dispersible tablets (for methadone maintenance therapy): 40 mg
Injection: 10 mg/ml
Oral solution: 5 mg/5 ml, 10 mg/5 ml, 10 mg/ml (concentrate)
Tablets: 5 mg, 10 mg

INDICATIONS & DOSAGES
➤ **Severe pain**
Adults: 2.5 to 10 mg P.O., I.M., or subcutaneously every 3 to 4 hours p.r.n.
➤ **Severe chronic pain**
Adults: 5 to 20 mg P.O. every 6 to 8 hours p.r.n.
➤ **Opioid withdrawal syndrome**
Adults: 15 to 20 mg P.O. daily often suppresses withdrawal symptoms (highly individualized; some patients may require a higher dose). Maintenance dose is 20 to 120 mg P.O. daily. Dosage adjusted, as needed.

ADMINISTRATION
P.O.
• Oral liquid form legally required in maintenance programs. Completely dissolve tablets in ½ cup of orange juice or powdered citrus drink.
• Oral dose is half as potent as injected dose.
I.M.
• For parenteral use, I.M. injection is preferred. Rotate injection sites.

Reactions may be *common*, uncommon, *life-threatening*, or COMMON AND LIFE-THREATENING.
Interaction may have a *rapid onset* or *delayed onset.*

Subcutaneous
• Monitor patient for pain at injection site, tissue irritation, and induration after injection.

ACTION
Unknown. Binds with opioid receptors in the CNS, altering perception of and emotional response to pain.

Route	Onset	Peak	Duration
P.O.	30–60 min	90–120 min	4–6 hr
I.M., Subcut.	10–20 min	1–2 hr	4–5 hr

Half-life: 15 to 25 hours.

ADVERSE REACTIONS
CNS: *clouded sensorium,* hallucinations, *dizziness, light-headedness, sedation, somnolence, seizures,* agitation, choreic movements, euphoria, headache, insomnia, syncope.
CV: *arrhythmias, bradycardia, prolonged QT interval, cardiac arrest, shock, cardiomyopathy, heart failure,* flushing, phlebitis, edema, hypotension, palpitations.
EENT: visual disturbances.
GI: *nausea, vomiting,* abdominal pain, anorexia, biliary tract spasm, constipation, dry mouth, glossitis, ileus.
GU: urine retention.
Metabolic: hypokalemia, *hypomagnesia,* weight gain.
Respiratory: *respiratory arrest, respiratory depression, pulmonary edema.*
Skin: diaphoresis, pruritus, urticaria.
Other: decreased libido, induration, pain at injection site, physical dependence, tissue irritation.

INTERACTIONS
Drug-drug. *Ammonium chloride, other urine acidifiers, phenytoin:* May reduce methadone effect. Watch for decreased pain control.
CNS depressants, general anesthetics, hypnotics, MAO inhibitors, sedatives, tranquilizers, tricyclic antidepressants: May cause respiratory depression, hypotension, profound sedation, or coma. Use together with caution. Monitor patient response.
Nonnucleoside reverse transcriptase inhibitors (delavirdine, efavirenz,

nevirapine), protease inhibitors (lopinavir and ritonavir, nelfinavir, ritonavir), rifamycins: May increase methadone metabolism causing opioid withdrawal symptoms. Monitor patient and adjust dose as needed.
Protease inhibitors, cimetidine, fluvoxamine: May increase respiratory and CNS depression. Monitor patient closely.
Drug-lifestyle. *Alcohol use:* May cause additive effects. Discourage use together.

EFFECTS ON LAB TEST RESULTS
• May increase amylase level.

CONTRAINDICATIONS & CAUTIONS
• Contraindicated in patients hypersensitive to drug.
• Use with caution in elderly or debilitated patients and in those with acute abdominal conditions, severe hepatic or renal impairment, hypothyroidism, Addison's disease, prostatic hyperplasia, urethral stricture, head injury, increased intracranial pressure, asthma, and other respiratory conditions.
■ **Black Box Warning** Deaths have been reported during initiation of methadone therapy for opioid dependence. Exercise extreme caution when initiating treatment. ■

NURSING CONSIDERATIONS
■ **Black Box Warning** Respiratory depression, QT interval prolongation, and torsades de pointes have been observed during treatment. Be vigilant during treatment initiation and dose titration. ■
• Reassess patient's level of pain at least 15 and 30 minutes after parenteral administration and 30 minutes after oral administration.
■ **Black Box Warning** When used in opioid withdrawal syndrome, treatment products shall be dispensed only by opioid treatment programs. ■
• Because Diskets are available in 10-mg doses, they may not be appropriate for initial dosing in many patients.
• An around-the-clock regimen is needed to manage severe, chronic pain.
• Patient treated for opioid withdrawal syndrome usually needs an additional analgesic if pain control is needed.
• Monitor patient closely because drug has cumulative effect; marked sedation can occur after repeated doses.

• Monitor circulatory and respiratory status and bladder and bowel function. Patient may need a stool softener and stimulant laxative.

• *Alert:* Respiratory depressant effects may last longer than analgesic effects. Monitor patient's respiratory status closely.

• When used as an adjunct in the treatment of opioid addiction (maintenance), withdrawal is usually delayed and mild.

• *Alert:* Use caution when dosing. Confusion has occurred between ml and mg doses.

• *Look alike–sound alike:* Don't confuse methadone with methylphenidate (Metadate CD, Metadate ER), dexmethylphenidate, and Mephyton.

PATIENT TEACHING
• Caution ambulatory patient about getting out of bed or walking. Warn outpatient to avoid hazardous activities that require mental alertness until drug's CNS effects are known.

• Instruct patient to increase fluid and fiber in diet, if not contraindicated, to combat constipation.

• Advise patient to avoid alcohol during therapy.

■ **Black Box Warning** Caution patients not to use CNS depressants during initiation of treatment with methadone. ■

SAFETY ALERT!

morphine hydrochloride
MOR-feen

Doloral†, M.O.S†, M.O.S.-S.R†

morphine sulfate
Astramorph PF, Avinza, DepoDur, Duramorph PF, Infumorph, Kadian, M-Eslon†, Morphine H.P†, MS Contin, MSIR, Oramorph SR, RMS Uniserts, Roxanol, Statex†

Pharmacologic class: opioid
Pregnancy risk category C
Controlled substance schedule II

AVAILABLE FORMS
morphine hydrochloride
Oral solution: 1 mg/ml†, 5 mg/ml†, 10 mg/ml†, 20 mg/ml†, 50 mg/ml†
Suppositories: 10 mg†, 20 mg†, 30 mg†
Syrup: 1 mg/ml†*, 5 mg/ml†*, 10 mg/ml†*, 20 mg/ml†*, 50 mg/ml†*
Tablets: 10 mg†, 20 mg†, 40 mg†, 60 mg†
Tablets (extended-release): 30 mg†, 60 mg†
morphine sulfate
Capsules (extended-release beads): 30 mg, 60 mg, 90 mg, 120 mg
Capsules (extended-release pellets): 10 mg, 20 mg, 30 mg, 50 mg, 60 mg, 80 mg, 100 mg, 200 mg
Injection (with preservative): 0.5 mg/ml, 1 mg/ml, 2 mg/ml, 4 mg/ml, 5 mg/ml, 8 mg/ml, 10 mg/ml, 15 mg/ml, 25 mg/ml, 50 mg/ml
Injection (without preservative): 0.5 mg/ml, 1 mg/ml, 10 mg/ml, 15 mg/ml, 25 mg/ml
Oral solution: 10 mg/5 ml, 20 mg/5 ml, 20 mg/ml (concentrate), 100 mg/5 ml (concentrate)
Soluble tablets: 10 mg, 15 mg, 30 mg
Suppositories: 5 mg, 10 mg, 20 mg, 30 mg
Tablets: 15 mg, 30 mg
Tablets (extended-release): 15 mg, 30 mg, 60 mg, 100 mg, 200 mg

INDICATIONS & DOSAGES
➤ **Severe pain**
Adults: 5 to 20 mg subcutaneously or I.M. or 2.5 to 15 mg I.V. every 4 hours p.r.n. Or, 5 to 30 mg P.O. or 10 to 20 mg P.R. every 4 hours p.r.n.

   For continuous I.V. infusion, give loading dose of 15 mg I.V.; then continuous infusion of 0.8 to 10 mg/hour.

   For extended-release tablet, give 15 or 30 mg P.O., every 8 to 12 hours.

   For extended-release Kadian capsules used as a first opioid, give 20 mg P.O. every 12 hours or 40 mg P.O. once daily; increase conservatively in opioid-naive patients.

   For epidural injection, give 5 mg by epidural catheter; then, if pain isn't relieved adequately in 1 hour, give supplementary doses of 1 to 2 mg at intervals sufficient to assess effectiveness. Maximum total epidural dose shouldn't exceed 10 mg/ 24 hours.

   For intrathecal injection, a single dose of 0.2 to 1 mg may provide pain relief for 24 hours (only in the lumbar area). Don't repeat injections.

Reactions may be *common,* uncommon, *life-threatening,* or COMMON AND LIFE-THREATENING.
Interaction may have a *rapid onset* or *delayed onset.*

Nursing2010 Drug Handbook
Photoguide to tablets and capsules

This photoguide presents nearly 400 tablets and capsules, representing the most commonly prescribed generic and trade name drugs. These drugs, organized alphabetically by generic name, are shown in actual size and color with cross-references to drug information. Each product is labeled with its trade name and its strength.

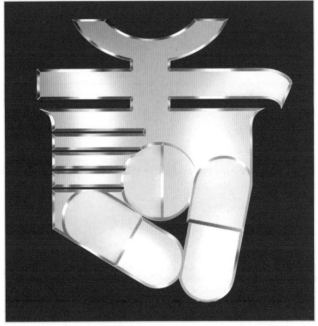

Adapted from Facts and Comparisons, St. Louis, Missouri.

For the list of companies permitting use of these photographs, see pages 1466–1467.

ACAMPROSATE CALCIUM

Campral
(page 1343)

333 mg

ACETAMINOPHEN AND HYDROCODONE BITARTRATE

Lortab
(page 1411)

2.5 mg/500 mg   5 mg/500 mg   7.5 mg/500 mg

Vicodin
(page 1409)

5 mg/500 mg

Vicodin ES
(page 1413)

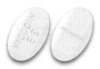

7.5 mg/750 mg

ACETAMINOPHEN WITH CODEINE

Tylenol with Codeine No. 3
(page 1412)

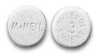

300 mg/30 mg

ALENDRONATE SODIUM

Fosamax
(page 784)

      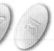

10 mg   40 mg   70 mg

ALFUZOSIN HYDROCHLORIDE

Uroxatral
(page 955)

10 mg

ALPRAZOLAM

Xanax
(page 682)

     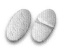

0.25 mg   0.5 mg   1 mg

2 mg

AMLODIPINE BESYLATE

Norvasc
(page 309)

2.5 mg   5 mg

ANASTROZOLE

Arimidex
(page 1182)

1 mg

ARIPIPRAZOLE

Abilify
(page 648)

10 mg   15 mg   30 mg

ATAZANAVIR SULFATE

Reyataz
(page 114)

 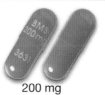

100 mg   200 mg

ATENOLOL

Tenormin
(page 356)

25 mg   50 mg   100 mg

ATOMOXETINE HYDROCHLORIDE

Strattera
(page 693)

10 mg   18 mg   25 mg

40 mg   60 mg

ATORVASTATIN CALCIUM

Lipitor
(page 406)

10 mg

20 mg

40 mg

80 mg

AZITHROMYCIN

Zithromax
(page 238)

250 mg

500 mg

600 mg

BENAZEPRIL HYDROCHLORIDE

Lotensin
(page 358)

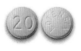

20 mg

40 mg

BUMETANIDE

Bumex
(page 426)

0.5 mg

1 mg

2 mg

BUSPIRONE HYDROCHLORIDE

BuSpar
(page 684)

5 mg

10 mg

15 mg

CARBIDOPA AND LEVODOPA

Sinemet
(page 635)

10 mg/100 mg   25 mg/250 mg

Sinemet CR
(page 635)

25 mg/100 mg

CARBIDOPA, LEVODOPA, AND ENTACAPONE

Stalevo
(page 637)

12.5 mg/50 mg/200 mg   25 mg/100 mg/200 mg

37.5 mg/150 mg/200 mg

CARISOPRODOL

Soma
(page 818)

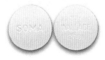

350 mg

CEFPROZIL

Cefzil
(page 197)

250 mg   500 mg

CELECOXIB

Celebrex
(page 716)

100 mg   200 mg

CIPROFLOXACIN

Cipro
(page 208)

  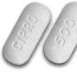 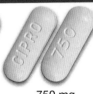

250 mg   500 mg   750 mg

CITALOPRAM HYDROBROMIDE

Celexa
(page 587)

20 mg   40 mg

CLARITHROMYCIN

Biaxin
(page 240)

250 mg   500 mg

Biaxin XL
(page 240)

500 mg

CLONAZEPAM

Klonopin
(page 555)

0.5 mg   1 mg   2 mg

CO-TRIMOXAZOLE

Bactrim DS
(page 272)

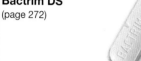

160 mg/800 mg

DARIFENACIN HYDROBROMIDE

Enablex
(page 966)

7.5 mg   15 mg

DESLORATADINE

Clarinex
(page 826)

5 mg

DIAZEPAM

Valium
(page 686)

2 mg   5 mg   10 mg

DILTIAZEM HYDROCHLORIDE

Cardizem
(page 310)

  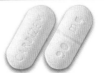

30 mg   90 mg

Cardizem CD
(page 310)

120 mg   180 mg   240 mg

300 mg   360 mg

Cardizem LA
(page 310)

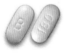

180 mg   240 mg   360 mg

DIVALPROEX SODIUM

Depakote
(page 578)

    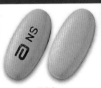

125 mg   250 mg   500 mg

Depakote Sprinkle
(page 578)

125 mg

DOXAZOSIN MESYLATE

Cardura
(page 367)

1 mg

2 mg

4 mg

8 mg

DULOXETINE HYDROCHLORIDE

Cymbalta
(page 596)

20 mg

30 mg

60 mg

ELETRIPTAN HYDROBROMIDE

Relpax
(page 618)

20 mg

40 mg

ENALAPRIL MALEATE

Vasotec
(page 368)

2.5 mg

5 mg

10 mg

20 mg

ERYTHROMYCIN BASE

Eryc
(page 242)

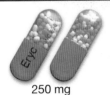

250 mg

Ery-Tab
(page 242)

333 mg

ESCITALOPRAM OXALATE

Lexapro
(page 598)

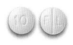

10 mg   20 mg

ESTRADIOL

Estrace
(page 990)

0.5 mg   1 mg   2 mg

ESTROGENS, CONJUGATED

Premarin
(page 996)

0.3 mg   0.45 mg   0.625 mg

0.9 mg   1.25 mg

ESZOPICLONE

Lunesta
(page 766)

1 mg   2 mg   3 mg

EZETIMIBE

Zetia
(page 410)

10 mg

FAMOTIDINE

Pepcid
(page 915)

20 mg   40 mg

FEXOFENADINE HYDROCHLORIDE

Allegra
(page 828)

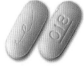

180 mg

FLUCONAZOLE

Diflucan
(page 87)

50 mg   100 mg   150 mg

200 mg

FLUOXETINE HYDROCHLORIDE

Prozac
(page 600)

10 mg   20 mg   40 mg

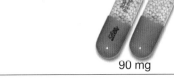

90 mg

Sarafem
(page 600)

10 mg   20 mg

FLUVASTATIN SODIUM

Lescol
(page 413)

20 mg   40 mg

FOSINOPRIL SODIUM

Monopril
(page 374)

10 mg   20 mg   40 mg

FROVATRIPTAN SUCCINATE

Frova
(page 619)

2.5 mg

FUROSEMIDE

Lasix
(page 429)

20 mg

40 mg

80 mg

GABAPENTIN

Neurontin
(page 559)

100 mg

300 mg

400 mg

GEMFIBROZIL

Lopid
(page 415)

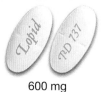
600 mg

GLIPIZIDE

Glucotrol
(page 1022)

5 mg   10 mg

Glucotrol XL
(page 1022)

2.5 mg   5 mg   10 mg

GLYBURIDE

DiaBeta
(page 1024)

1.25 mg   2.5 mg   5 mg

Micronase
(page 1024)

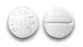

1.25 mg   2.5 mg   5 mg

IBUPROFEN

Motrin
(page 722)

400 mg   600 mg

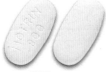

800 mg

INDINAVIR SULFATE

Crixivan
(page 131)

200 mg

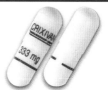

333 mg

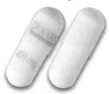

400 mg

LAMIVUDINE AND ZIDOVUDINE

Combivir
(page 1419)

150 mg/300 mg

LANSOPRAZOLE

Prevacid
(page 917)

15 mg

30 mg

LEVOFLOXACIN

Levaquin
(page 212)

250 mg

500 mg

LEVOTHYROXINE SODIUM

Levoxyl
(page 1090)

| 25 mcg | 50 mcg | 75 mcg |

| 88 mcg | 100 mcg | 112 mcg |

| 125 mcg | 137 mcg | 150 mcg |

| 175 mcg | 200 mcg | 300 mcg |

Synthroid
(page 1090)

| 25 mcg | 50 mcg | 75 mcg |

| 88 mcg | 100 mcg | 112 mcg |

  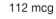

| 125 mcg | 150 mcg | 175 mcg |

 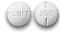

| 200 mcg | 300 mcg |

LISINOPRIL

Prinivil
(page 380)

    5 mg   10 mg   20 mg

40 mg

Zestril
(page 380)

   2.5 mg   5 mg   10 mg

 20 mg   40 mg

LOPINAVIR AND RITONAVIR

Kaletra
(page 135)

200 mg/50 mg

LOSARTAN POTASSIUM

Cozaar
(page 382)

25 mg   50 mg

LOVASTATIN

Mevacor
(page 416)

10 mg   20 mg   40 mg

LUBIPROSTONE

Amitiza
(page 941)

24 mcg

MEDROXYPROGESTERONE ACETATE

Provera
(page 1009)

2.5 mg   5 mg   10 mg

MEPERIDINE HYDROCHLORIDE

Demerol
(page 748)

50 mg   100 mg

METFORMIN HYDROCHLORIDE

Glucophage
(page 1025)

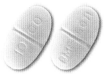

500 mg   850 mg

1,000 mg

Glucophage XR
(page 1025)

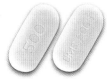

500 mg

METHYLPHENIDATE HYDROCHLORIDE

Concerta
(page 700)

18 mg   36 mg   54 mg

Ritalin
(page 700)

5 mg   10 mg   20 mg

Ritalin-SR
(page 700)

20 mg

METHYLPREDNISOLONE

Medrol
(page 1074)

4 mg   16 mg

METOPROLOL SUCCINATE

Toprol-XL
(page 385)

50 mg   100 mg   200 mg

MONTELUKAST SODIUM

Singulair
(page 875)

4 mg   5 mg   10 mg

NAPROXEN

Naprosyn
(page 733)

500 mg

NIFEDIPINE

Procardia XL
(page 317)

30 mg   60 mg   90 mg

NITROFURANTOIN

Macrobid
(page 302)

100 mg

NITROGLYCERIN

Nitrostat
(page 318)

0.4 mg

NORTRIPTYLINE HYDROCHLORIDE

Pamelor
(page 607)

10 mg   25 mg   50 mg

75 mg

OFLOXACIN

Floxin
(page 219)

          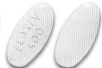

200 mg   300 mg   400 mg

OLMESARTAN MEDOXOMIL

Benicar
(page 391)

20 mg   40 mg

OMEPRAZOLE

Prilosec
(page 920)

10 mg   20 mg   40 mg

OXYCODONE HYDROCHLORIDE

OxyContin
(page 756)

10 mg   20 mg   40 mg

80 mg

PENTOXIFYLLINE

Trental
(page 470)

400 mg

PHENYTOIN SODIUM

Dilantin Kapseals
(page 570)

30 mg   100 mg

PRAVASTATIN SODIUM

Pravachol
(page 418)

10 mg   20 mg   40 mg

PROPRANOLOL HYDROCHLORIDE

Inderal
(page 321)

40 mg   60 mg   80 mg

Inderal LA
(page 321)

60 mg   80 mg   120 mg

160 mg

QUINAPRIL HYDROCHLORIDE

Accupril
(page 397)

5 mg   10 mg   20 mg

40 mg

RALOXIFENE HYDROCHLORIDE

Evista
(page 1394)

60 mg

RANITIDINE HYDROCHLORIDE

Zantac
(page 924)

150 mg   300 mg

RANOLAZINE

Ranexa
(page 323)

500 mg

RASAGILINE

Azilect
(page 640)

0.5 mg   1 mg

RISEDRONATE SODIUM

Actonel
(page 790)

5 mg   35 mg

RISPERIDONE

Risperdal
(page 671)

0.25 mg

0.5 mg

1 mg

2 mg

3 mg

4 mg

ROSIGLITAZONE MALEATE

Avandia
(page 1036)

2 mg

4 mg

8 mg

ROSUVASTATIN CALCIUM

Crestor
(page 420)

5 mg

10 mg

20 mg

40 mg

Nursing2010 Drug Handbook • C27

SERTRALINE HYDROCHLORIDE

Zoloft
(page 611)

50 mg

100 mg

SILDENAFIL CITRATE

Viagra
(page 960)

25 mg

50 mg

100 mg

SIMVASTATIN

Zocor
(page 422)

5 mg

10 mg

20 mg

40 mg

SITAGLIPTIN PHOSPHATE

Januvia
(page 1037)

100 mg

SORAFENIB

Nexavar
(page 1228)

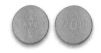

200 mg

SUCRALFATE

Carafate
(page 926)

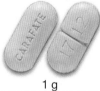

1 g

SUMATRIPTAN SUCCINATE

Imitrex
(page 624)

25 mg   50 mg

SUNITINIB MALATE

Sutent
(page 1229)

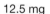

12.5 mg   25 mg   50 mg

TEMAZEPAM

Restoril
(page 773)

7.5 mg   15 mg   30 mg

TENOFOVIR DISOPROXIL FUMARATE

Viread
(page 149)

300 mg

TERAZOSIN HYDROCHLORIDE

Hytrin
(page 401)

1 mg   2 mg   5 mg

10 mg

TICLOPIDINE HYDROCHLORIDE

Ticlid
(page 531)

250 mg

TOLTERODINE TARTRATE

Detrol
(page 970)

1 mg   2 mg

TRAMADOL HYDROCHLORIDE AND ACETAMINOPHEN

Ultracet
(page 1407)

37.5 mg/325 mg

VALSARTAN

Diovan
(page 404)

40 mg

80 mg

160 mg

320 mg

VARDENAFIL HYDROCHLORIDE

Levitra
(page 964)

5 mg

10 mg

20 mg

VARENICLINE TARTRATE

Chantix
(page 1400)

0.5 mg

1 mg

VENLAFAXINE HYDROCHLORIDE

Effexor
(page 614)

25 mg

37.5 mg

50 mg

75 mg

100 mg

Effexor XR
(page 614)

75 mg

150 mg

VERAPAMIL HYDROCHLORIDE

Calan
(page 325)

40 mg

80 mg

120 mg

Isoptin SR
(page 325)

120 mg

180 mg

240 mg

Verelan
(page 325)

120 mg

180 mg

240 mg

WARFARIN SODIUM

Coumadin
(page 504)

1 mg

2 mg

2.5 mg

     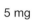

3 mg

4 mg

5 mg

6 mg

7.5 mg

10 mg

ZIDOVUDINE

Retrovir
(page 153)

 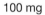

100 mg

300 mg

ZOLPIDEM TARTRATE

Ambien
(page 777)

5 mg

10 mg

30th Anniversary Edition

Nursing2010
DRUG
HANDBOOK®

30th Anniversary

MW00978196

midazolam HCl	morphine sulfate	nalbuphine HCl	pentazocine lactate	pentobarbital Na	perphenazine	phenobarbital Na	prochlorperazine edisylate	promazine HCl	promethazine HCl	ranitidine HCl	scopolamine HBr	secobarbital Na	sodium bicarbonate	thiethylperazine maleate	thiopental Na	
Y	P	Y	P	P*	Y		P	P	P	Y	P					atropine sulfate
Y	Y		Y	N	Y		Y		Y		Y			Y		butorphanol tartrate
Y	P		P	N	Y		P	P	P	N*	P				N	chlorpromazine HCl
Y	Y	Y	Y	N	Y		Y	Y	Y		Y	N				cimetidine HCl
																codeine phosphate
										Y						dexamethasone sodium phosphate
N	P	N	P	N	Y		N	N	N	Y	P		N		N	dimenhydrinate
Y	P	Y	P	N	Y		P	P	P	Y	P				N	diphenhydramine HCl
Y	P	Y	P	N	Y		P	P	P		P					droperidol
Y	P		P	N	Y		P	P	P	Y	P					fentanyl citrate
Y	Y	Y	N	N			Y	Y	Y	Y	Y	N	N		N	glycopyrrolate
N	N*		N		P(5)			N								heparin Na
Y			Y	Y		N	N*		Y	Y	Y			Y		hydromorphone HCl
Y	P	Y	P	N	Y		P	P	P	N	P					hydroxyzine HCl
Y	N		P	N	Y		P	P	P	Y	P					meperidine HCl
Y	P		P		P		P	P	P	Y	P		N			metoclopramide HCl
■	Y	Y		N	N		N	Y	Y	N	Y			Y		midazolam HCl
Y	■		P	N*	Y		P*	P	P*	Y	P				N	morphine sulfate
Y		■		N			Y		N*	Y	Y			Y		nalbuphine HCl
	P		■	N	Y		P	P*	P*	Y	P					pentazocine lactate
N	N*	N	N	■	N		N	N	N	N	P		Y		Y	pentobarbital Na
N	Y		Y	N	■		Y		Y	Y	Y			N		perphenazine
						■				N						phenobarbital Na
N	P*	Y	P	N	Y	N	■	P	P	Y	P				N	prochlorperazine edisylate
Y	P		P*	N			P	■	P		P					promazine HCl
Y	P*	N*	P*	N	Y		P	P	■	Y	P				N	promethazine HCl
N	Y	Y	Y	N	Y	N	Y		Y	■	Y			Y		ranitidine HCl
Y	P	Y	P	P	Y		P	P	P	Y	■				Y	scopolamine HBr
												■				secobarbital Na
				Y									■		N	sodium bicarbonate
Y		Y			N					Y				■		thiethylperazine maleate
	N			Y			N		N		Y		N		■	thiopental Na

Contents

Staff

Executive Publisher
Judith A. Schilling McCann, RN, MSN

Clinical Director
Joan M. Robinson, RN, MSN

Art Director
Elaine Kasmer

Clinical Project Manager
Lorraine Hallowell, RN, BSN, RVS

Electronic Project Manager
John Macalino

Clinical Editors
Lisa Morris Bonsall, RN, CRNP, MSN
Janet Rader Clark, RN, BSN
Kimberly A. Zalewski, RN, MSN

Editors
Karen C. Comerford
Diane Labus

Design Assistant
Kate Zulak

Associate Manufacturing Manager
Beth J. Welsh

Editorial Assistants
Karen J. Kirk, Jeri O'Shea, Linda K. Ruhf

Printed in China

NDH30-010509

ISSN 0273-320X
ISBN-13: 978-1-6054-7353-6

30th Anniversary Edition

Nursing2010

DRUG HANDBOOK®

30th Anniversary

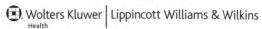

Wolters Kluwer | Lippincott Williams & Wilkins
Health

Philadelphia • Baltimore • New York • London
Buenos Aires • Hong Kong • Sydney • Tokyo

Children: 0.1 to 0.2 mg/kg subcutaneously or I.M. every 4 hours. Maximum single dose, 15 mg.

➤ **Moderate to severe pain requiring continuous, around-the-clock opioid**
Adults: Individualize dosage of Avinza. For patients with no tolerance to opioids, begin with 30 mg Avinza P.O. daily; adjust dosage by no more than 30 mg every 4 days. When converting from another oral morphine form, individualize the dosage schedule according to patient's schedule.

➤ **Single-dose, epidural extended pain relief after major surgery**
Adults: Inject 10 to 15 mg (maximum 20 mg) DepoDur via lumbar epidural administration before surgery or after clamping of umbilical cord during cesarean section. May be injected undiluted or may be diluted up to 5 ml total volume with preservative-free normal saline solution.

ADMINISTRATION
P.O.
• Oral solutions of various concentrations and an intensified oral solution (20 mg/ml) are available. Carefully note the strength given.
• Give morphine sulfate without regard to food.
• Oral capsules may be carefully opened and the entire contents poured into cool, soft foods, such as water, orange juice, applesauce, or pudding; patient should consume mixture immediately.
■ **Black Box Warning** Don't crush, break, or chew extended-release forms. ■
S.L.
• For S.L. use, measure oral solution with tuberculin syringe. Give dose a few drops at a time to allow maximal S.L. absorption and minimize swallowing.
I.V.
• For direct injection, dilute 2.5 to 15 mg in 4 or 5 ml of sterile water for injection and give slowly over 4 to 5 minutes.
• For continuous infusion, mix drug with D_5W to yield 0.1 to 1 mg/ml, and give by a continuous infusion device.
• In adults with severe, chronic pain, maintenance I.V. infusion is 0.8 to 80 mg/hour; sometimes higher doses are needed.
• Don't mix DepoDur with other drugs. Once DepoDur is given, don't give any

other drugs into epidural space for at least 48 hours. Don't use in-line filter during administration.
• Store DepoDur in refrigerator. Unopened vials can be stored at room temperature for up to 7 days. After drug is withdrawn from vial, it can be stored at room temperature for up to 4 hours before use.
• **Incompatibilities:** Aminophylline, amobarbital, cefepime, chlorothiazide, fluorouracil, haloperidol, heparin sodium, meperidine, pentobarbital, phenobarbital sodium, phenytoin sodium, prochlorperazine, promethazine hydrochloride, sodium bicarbonate, thiopental.
I.M.
• Document injection site.
• Store injection solution at room temperature and protect from light.
• Solution may darken with age. Don't use if injection is darker than pale yellow, discolored, or contains precipitate.
Subcutaneous
• Document injection site.
• Store injection solution at room temperature and protect from light.
• Solution may darken with age. Don't use if injection is darker than pale yellow, discolored, or contains precipitate.
Rectal
• Refrigeration of rectal suppository isn't needed.

ACTION
Unknown. Binds with opioid receptors in the CNS, altering perception of and emotional response to pain.

Route	Onset	Peak	Duration
P.O.	30 min	1–2 hr	4–12 hr
P.O. (extended-release)	1–2 hr	3–4 hr	12–24 hr
I.V.	5 min	20 min	4–5 hr
I.M.	10–30 min	30–60 min	4–5 hr
Subcut.	10–30 min	50–90 min	4–5 hr
P.R.	20–60 min	20–60 min	4–5 hr
Epidural	15–60 min	15–60 min	24 hr
Intrathecal	15–60 min	30–60 min	24 hr

Half-life: 2 to 3 hours.

ADVERSE REACTIONS

CNS: *dizziness, euphoria, light-headedness, nightmares, sedation, somnolence, **seizures**,* depression, hallucinations, nervousness, physical dependence, syncope.

CV: ***bradycardia, cardiac arrest, shock,*** hypertension, hypotension, tachycardia.

GI: *constipation, nausea, vomiting,* anorexia, biliary tract spasms, dry mouth, ileus.

GU: urine retention.

Hematologic: *thrombocytopenia.*

Respiratory: *apnea, respiratory arrest, respiratory depression.*

Skin: diaphoresis, edema, pruritus and skin flushing.

Other: decreased libido.

INTERACTIONS

Drug-drug. *Cimetidine:* May increase respiratory and CNS depression when given with morphine sulfate. Monitor patient closely.

CNS depressants, general anesthetics, hypnotics, MAO inhibitors, other opioid analgesics, sedatives, tranquilizers, tricyclic antidepressants: May cause respiratory depression, hypotension, profound sedation, or coma. Use together with caution, reduce morphine dose, and monitor patient response.

Drug-lifestyle. *Alcohol use:* May cause additive CNS effects. Warn patient to avoid alcohol.

EFFECTS ON LAB TEST RESULTS

● May increase amylase level. May decrease hemoglobin level (morphine sulfate).

● May decrease platelet count.

● May cause abnormal liver function test values (morphine sulfate).

CONTRAINDICATIONS & CAUTIONS

● Contraindicated in patients hypersensitive to drug and in those with conditions that would preclude I.V. administration of opioids (acute bronchial asthma or upper airway obstruction).

● Contraindicated in patients with GI obstruction.

● Use with caution in elderly or debilitated patients and in those with head injury, increased intracranial pressure, seizures, chronic pulmonary disease, prostatic hyperplasia, severe hepatic or renal disease, acute abdominal conditions, hypothyroidism, Addison's disease, and urethral stricture.

● Use with caution in patients with circulatory shock, biliary tract disease, CNS depression, toxic psychosis, acute alcoholism, delirium tremens, and seizure disorders.

NURSING CONSIDERATIONS

● Reassess patient's level of pain at least 15 and 30 minutes after giving parenterally and 30 minutes after giving orally.

● Keep opioid antagonist (naloxone) and resuscitation equipment available.

● Monitor circulatory, respiratory, bladder, and bowel functions carefully. Drug may cause respiratory depression, hypotension, urine retention, nausea, vomiting, ileus, or altered level of consciousness regardless of the route. If respirations drop below 12 breaths/minute, withhold dose and notify prescriber.

■ **Black Box Warning** Morphine has an abuse liability similar to other opioid analgesics and may be misused, abused, or diverted. ■

■ **Black Box Warning** Kadian capsules are not for use on an as-needed basis. ■

● Preservative-free preparations are available for epidural and intrathecal use.

■ **Black Box Warning** When the epidural or intrathecal route is used, observe patients in a fully equipped and staffed environment for at least 24 hours after the initial dose. ■

■ **Black Box Warning** Infumorph is not recommended for single-dose administration. ■

● When drug is given epidurally, monitor patient closely for respiratory depression up to 24 hours after the injection. Check respiratory rate and depth every 30 to 60 minutes for 24 hours. Watch for pruritus and skin flushing.

● Morphine is drug of choice in relieving MI pain; may cause transient decrease in blood pressure.

● An around-the-clock regimen best manages severe, chronic pain.

● Morphine may worsen or mask gallbladder pain.

Reactions may be *common*, uncommon, *life-threatening*, or COMMON AND LIFE-THREATENING.
Interaction may have a *rapid onset* or ***delayed onset.***

● Constipation is commonly severe with maintenance dose. Ensure that stool softener and/or stimulant laxative is ordered.
● Taper morphine sulfate therapy gradually when stopping therapy.
● *Look alike–sound alike:* Don't confuse morphine with hydromorphone or Avinza with Invanz.

PATIENT TEACHING
● When drug is used after surgery, encourage patient to turn, cough, deep-breathe, and use incentive spirometer to prevent lung problems.
● Caution ambulatory patient about getting out of bed or walking. Warn outpatient to avoid driving and other potentially hazardous activities that require mental alertness until drug's adverse CNS effects are known.
■ **Black Box Warning** Drinking alcohol or taking drugs containing alcohol while taking extended-release capsules may cause additive CNS effects. Warn patient to read labels on OTC drugs carefully and not to use alcohol in any form. ■
● Tell patient to swallow morphine sulfate whole or to open capsule and sprinkle beads or pellets on a small amount of applesauce immediately before taking.
● *Alert:* Warn patient not to crush, break, or chew extended-release forms.

SAFETY ALERT!

nalbuphine hydrochloride
NAL-byoo-feen

Pharmacologic class: opioid agonist-antagonist, opioid partial agonist
Pregnancy risk category B

AVAILABLE FORMS
Injection: 10 mg/ml, 20 mg/ml

INDICATIONS & DOSAGES
➤ **Moderate to severe pain**
Adults: For a patient of about 70 kg (154 lb), 10 to 20 mg subcutaneously, I.M., or I.V. every 3 to 6 hours p.r.n. Maximum, 160 mg daily.

➤ **Adjunct to balanced anesthesia**
Adults: 0.3 mg/kg to 3 mg/kg I.V. over 10 to 15 minutes; then maintenance doses of 0.25 to 0.50 mg/kg in single I.V. dose p.r.n.
Adjust-a-dose: In patients with renal or hepatic impairment, decrease dosage.

ADMINISTRATION
I.V.
● Inject slowly over at least 2 to 3 minutes into a vein or into an I.V. line containing a compatible, free-flowing I.V. solution, such as D_5W, normal saline solution, or lactated Ringer's solution.
● Respiratory depression can be reversed with naloxone. Keep resuscitation equipment available, particularly when giving I.V.
● **Incompatibilities:** Allopurinol, amphotericin B, cefepime, diazepam, docetaxel, ketorolac, methotrexate sodium, nafcillin, pentobarbital sodium, piperacillin and tazobactam sodium, promethazine, sargramostim, sodium bicarbonate, thiethylperazine.
I.M.
● Document injection site.
● Store vial in carton to protect from light.
Subcutaneous
● Document injection site.
● Store vial in carton to protect from light.

ACTION
Unknown. Binds with opioid receptors in the CNS, altering perception of and emotional response to pain.

Route	Onset	Peak	Duration
I.V.	2–3 min	30 min	3–6 hr
I.M.	15 min	1 hr	3–6 hr
Subcut.	15 min	Unknown	3–6 hr

Half-life: 5 hours.

ADVERSE REACTIONS
CNS: *dizziness, headache, sedation, vertigo,* confusion, crying, delusions, depression, euphoria, hallucinations, hostility, nervousness, restlessness, speech disorders, unusual dreams.
CV: *bradycardia,* hypertension, hypotension, tachycardia.
EENT: blurred vision, dry mouth.

GI: biliary tract spasms, constipation, cramps, dyspepsia, nausea, vomiting.
GU: urinary urgency.
Respiratory: *respiratory depression, asthma,* dyspnea, *pulmonary edema.*
Skin: burning, clamminess, diaphoresis, pruritus, urticaria.

INTERACTIONS
Drug-drug. *CNS depressants, general anesthetics, hypnotics, MAO inhibitors, sedatives, tranquilizers, tricyclic anti-depressants:* May cause respiratory depression, hypertension, profound seda-tion, or coma. Use together with caution, and monitor patient response.
Opioid analgesics: May decrease analgesic effect. Avoid using together.
Drug-lifestyle. *Alcohol use:* May cause additive effects. Discourage use together.

EFFECTS ON LAB TEST RESULTS
None reported.

CONTRAINDICATIONS & CAUTIONS
● Contraindicated in patients hypersensitive to drug.
● Use cautiously in patients with history of drug abuse and in those with emotional instability, head injury, increased intra-cranial pressure, impaired ventilation, MI accompanied by nausea and vomiting, upcoming biliary surgery, and hepatic or renal disease.
● *Alert:* Certain commercial preparations contain sodium metabisulfite.

NURSING CONSIDERATIONS
● Reassess patient's level of pain at least 15 and 30 minutes after parenteral administration.
● Drug acts as an opioid antagonist and may cause withdrawal syndrome. For patients who have received long-term opioids, give 25% of the usual dose initially. Watch for signs of withdrawal.
● *Alert:* Drug causes respiratory depres-sion, which at 10 mg is equal to respira-tory depression produced by 10 mg of morphine.
● Monitor circulatory and respiratory status and bladder and bowel function. If respirations are shallow or rate is below 12 breaths/minute, withhold dose and notify prescriber.

● Constipation is commonly severe with maintenance therapy. Make sure stool soft-ener or other stimulant laxative is ordered.
● Psychological and physical dependence may occur with prolonged use.
● *Look alike–sound alike:* Don't confuse Nubain with Navane.

PATIENT TEACHING
● Caution ambulatory patient about getting out of bed or walking. Warn outpatient to avoid driving and other hazardous activities that require mental alertness until drug's CNS effects are known.
● Teach patient how to manage trouble-some adverse effects such as constipation.

SAFETY ALERT!

oxycodone hydrochloride
ox-i-KOE-done

ETH-Oxydose, M-Oxy, OxyContin♦, OxyFAST, OxyIR, Roxicodone, Roxicodone Intensol, Supeudol†

Pharmacologic class: opioid
Pregnancy risk category B
Controlled substance schedule II

AVAILABLE FORMS
oxycodone hydrochloride
Capsules: 5 mg
Oral solution: 5 mg/5 ml, 20 mg/ml
Suppository: 10 mg†, 20 mg†
Tablets (immediate-release): 5 mg, 10 mg, 15 mg, 20 mg, 30 mg
Tablets (controlled-release): 10 mg, 20 mg, 40 mg, 60 mg, 80 mg

INDICATIONS & DOSAGES
➤ **Moderate to severe pain**
Adults: 5 mg immediate-release form P.O. every 6 hours. Or, one suppository P.R. three to four times daily p.r.n.
■ **Black Box Warning** Patients not currently receiving opioids, who need a continuous, around-the-clock analgesic for an extended period of time, give 10 mg controlled-release tablets P.O. every 12 hours. May increase dose every 1 to 2 days as needed. The 80-mg formulation is for opioid-tolerant patients only. ■

ADMINISTRATION
P.O.
- To minimize GI upset, give drug after meals or with milk.
- **Black Box Warning** Swallow extended-release tablets whole. ■
- **Black Box Warning** Reserve the 80-mg controlled-release tablets for opioid-tolerant patients who are taking daily doses of 160 mg or more. ■
- Patients taking the controlled-release form around-the-clock may need to take the immediate-release form for worsening of pain or prevention of incident pain.
Rectal
- Chill wrapped suppository in refrigerator for 30 minutes or under cold running water if too soft to administer.

ACTION
Unknown. Binds with opioid receptors in the CNS, altering perception of and emotional response to pain.

Route	Onset	Peak	Duration
P.O.	10–15 min	1 hr	3–6 hr
P.R.	Unknown	Unknown	Unknown

Half-life: 2 to 3 hours.

ADVERSE REACTIONS
CNS: clouded sensorium, dizziness, euphoria, light-headedness, physical dependence, sedation, somnolence.
CV: *bradycardia,* hypotension.
GI: *constipation, nausea, vomiting,* ileus.
GU: urine retention.
Respiratory: *respiratory depression.*
Skin: diaphoresis, pruritus.

INTERACTIONS
Drug-drug. *Anticoagulants:* Oxycodone hydrochloride products containing aspirin may increase anticoagulant effect. Monitor clotting times. Use together cautiously.
CNS depressants, general anesthetics, hypnotics, MAO inhibitors, other opioid analgesics, sedatives, tranquilizers, tricyclic antidepressants: May cause additive effects. Use together with caution. Reduce oxycodone dose and monitor patient response.
Drug-lifestyle. *Alcohol use:* May cause additive effects. Discourage use together.

EFFECTS ON LAB TEST RESULTS
- May increase amylase and lipase levels.

CONTRAINDICATIONS & CAUTIONS
- Contraindicated in patients hypersensitive to drug.
- Contraindicated in those suspected of having paralytic ileus.
- Use with caution in elderly and debilitated patients and in those with head injury, increased intracranial pressure, seizures, asthma, COPD, prostatic hyperplasia, severe hepatic or renal disease, acute abdominal conditions, urethral stricture, hypothyroidism, Addison's disease, and arrhythmias.

NURSING CONSIDERATIONS
- Reassess patient's level of pain at least 15 and 30 minutes after administration.
- For full analgesic effect, give drug before patient has intense pain.
- Single-drug oxycodone solution or tablets are especially useful for patients who shouldn't take aspirin or acetaminophen.
- Monitor circulatory and respiratory status. Withhold dose and notify prescriber if respirations are shallow or if respiratory rate falls below 12 breaths/minute.
- Monitor patient's bladder and bowel patterns. Patient may need a stimulant laxative because drug has a constipating effect.
- For patients who are taking more than 60 mg daily, stop drug gradually to prevent withdrawal symptoms.
- Drug isn't intended for as-needed use or for immediate postoperative pain. Drug is indicated only for postoperative use if patient was receiving it before surgery or if pain is expected to persist for an extended time.
- **Black Box Warning** Drug is potentially addictive and abused as much as morphine. Chewing, crushing, snorting, or injecting it can lead to overdose and death. ■

PATIENT TEACHING
- Instruct patient to take drug before pain is intense.
- Tell patient to take drug with milk or after eating.
- Tell patient to swallow extended-release tablets whole.

● Caution ambulatory patient about getting out of bed or walking. Warn outpatient to avoid driving and other hazardous activities that require mental alertness until drug's CNS effects are known.
● Advise patient to avoid alcohol use during therapy.
● Tell patient not to stop drug abruptly.

SAFETY ALERT!

oxymorphone hydrochloride
ox-i-MOR-fone

Opana, Opana ER

Pharmacologic class: opioid
Pregnancy risk category C;
D if used for prolonged periods or
high doses at term
Controlled substance schedule II

AVAILABLE FORMS
Injection: 1 mg/ml
Tablets: 5 mg, 10 mg
Tablets (extended-release [ER]): 5 mg, 7.5 mg, 10 mg, 15 mg, 20 mg, 30 mg, 40 mg

INDICATIONS & DOSAGES
➤ **Moderate to severe pain**
Adults: 1 to 1.5 mg I.M. or subcutaneously every 4 to 6 hours p.r.n. Or, 0.5 mg I.V. every 4 to 6 hours p.r.n. Or, in opioid-naive patients, 10 to 20 mg P.O. every 4 to 6 hours. If needed, begin dosing at 5 mg P.O. and adjust based on patient response.
➤ **Moderate to severe pain in patients requiring continuous, around-the-clock opioid treatment for an extended period of time**
Opioid-naive adults: Using ER form, give 5 mg P.O. every 12 hours. Increase 5 to 10 mg every 12 hours every 3 to 7 days as needed and tolerated. Patients taking Opana immediate-release tablets can be switched to Opana ER tablets by giving one-half the patient's total daily dose as Opana ER every 12 hours.
Adjust-a-dose: For patients with mild hepatic impairment or creatinine clearance less than 50 ml/minute, start with the lowest possible dose and slowly increase as tolerated.

➤ **Analgesia during labor**
Adults: 0.5 to 1 mg I.M.

ADMINISTRATION
P.O.
● Take tablets 1 hour before or 2 hours after a meal.
■ **Black Box Warning** Don't crush, break, chew, or dissolve ER tablets. ■
■ **Black Box Warning** ER tablets aren't for as-needed use. ■
I.V.
● Assess respiratory status before giving. Withhold dose and notify prescriber if respirations are shallow or rate falls below 12 breaths/minute.
● If necessary, dilute drug in normal saline solution.
● Give drug by direct I.V. injection.
● **Incompatibilities:** None reported.
I.M.
● Rotate administration sites and document.
● Assess respiratory status before giving. Withhold dose and notify prescriber if respirations are shallow or rate falls below 12 breaths/minute.
Subcutaneous
● Rotate administration sites and document.
● Assess respiratory status before giving. Withhold dose and notify prescriber if respirations are shallow or rate falls below 12 breaths/minute.

ACTION
May bind with opioid receptors in the CNS, altering perception of and emotional response to pain.

Route	Onset	Peak	Duration
P.O.	Varies	Varies	Varies
I.V.	5–10 min	15–30 min	3–4 hr
I.M.	10–15 min	30–90 min	3–6 hr
Subcut.	10–20 min	60–90 min	3–6 hr

Half-life: For parenteral, unknown. For ER tablets, 7 to 12 hours. For immediate-release tablets, 3 to 12 hours.

ADVERSE REACTIONS
CNS: *clouded sensorium, dizziness, euphoria, headache, sedation, somnolence,* **seizures,** dysphoria, light-headedness, hallucinations, physical dependence, restlessness.
CV: *hypotension,* **bradycardia.**

Reactions may be *common,* uncommon, *life-threatening,* or COMMON AND LIFE-THREATENING.
Interaction may have a *rapid onset* or **delayed onset.**

EENT: blurred vision, diplopia, miosis.
GI: *constipation, nausea, vomiting,* ileus.
GU: *urine retention.*
Respiratory: *respiratory depression.*
Skin: increased sweating, pruritus.

INTERACTIONS

Drug-drug. *Agonist or antagonist analgesics:* May reduce analgesic effect or precipitate withdrawal symptoms. Don't use together.
Anticholinergics: May increase risk of urine retention or severe constipation, leading to paralytic ileus. Monitor patient for abdominal pain or distention.
CNS depressants, general anesthetics, MAO inhibitors, phenothiazines, sedative hypnotics, tricyclic antidepressants: May cause additive effects. Use together with caution and reduce opioid dosage.
Drug-lifestyle. *Alcohol use:* May cause additive effects. Discourage use together.

EFFECTS ON LAB TEST RESULTS

• May increase amylase and lipase levels.

CONTRAINDICATIONS & CAUTIONS

• Contraindicated in patients hypersensitive to drug and in those with acute asthma attacks, severe respiratory depression, upper airway obstruction, paralytic ileus, or those with moderate to severe hepatic impairment.
• Contraindicated in patients with pulmonary edema caused by a respiratory irritant.
• Use with caution in elderly or debilitated patients and in those with head injury, increased intracranial pressure, seizures, asthma, COPD, acute abdominal conditions, biliary tract disease (including pancreatitis), acute alcoholism, delirium tremens, prostatic hyperplasia, renal or mild hepatic impairment, urethral stricture, respiratory depression, hypothyroidism, Addison disease, and arrhythmias.

NURSING CONSIDERATIONS

• Keep opioid antagonist (naloxone) and resuscitation equipment available.
• Use of this drug may worsen gallbladder pain.

• Drug isn't for mild pain. For better effect, give drug before patient has intense pain.
• Monitor CV and respiratory status. Withhold dose and notify prescriber if respirations decrease or rate is below 12 breaths/minute.
• Monitor bladder and bowel function. Patient may need a stimulant laxative.
■ **Black Box Warning** Drug has an abuse liability similar to other opioid analgesics. Consider this when concerned about an increased risk of misuse, abuse, or diversion. ■
• *Look alike–sound alike:* Don't confuse oxymorphone with oxymetholone or oxycodone, and don't confuse Numorphan with nalbuphine.

PATIENT TEACHING

• Instruct patient to ask for drug before pain is intense. Inform patient that ER tablets must be taken around-the-clock.
• When drug is used I.M. or I.V. after surgery, encourage patient to turn, cough, and deep-breathe and to use incentive spirometer to avoid lung problems.
• Caution ambulatory patient about getting out of bed or walking. Warn outpatient to avoid driving and other hazardous activities that require mental alertness until drug's CNS effects are known.
■ **Black Box Warning** Caution patient not to consume alcohol or take any prescription or OTC drug containing alcohol with oral form as this can lead to an overdose. ■
■ **Black Box Warning** Warn patient not to crush, break, chew, or dissolve ER tablets; doing so may lead to a fatal overdose. ■
• Tell patient to take tablets 1 hour before or 2 hours after a meal.
• Instruct patient to keep tablets in a child-resistant container in a safe place. Accidental ingestion by a child can result in death.

SAFETY ALERT!

pentazocine hydrochloride
pen-TAZ-oh-seen

Talwin†

pentazocine hydrochloride and naloxone hydrochloride
Talwin NX

pentazocine lactate
Talwin

Pharmacologic class: opioid agonist-antagonist, opioid partial agonist
Pregnancy risk category C
Controlled substance schedule IV

AVAILABLE FORMS
pentazocine hydrochloride
Tablets: 50 mg†
pentazocine hydrochloride and naloxone hydrochloride
Tablets: 50 mg pentazocine hydrochloride and 500 mcg naloxone hydrochloride
pentazocine lactate
Injection: 30 mg/ml

INDICATIONS & DOSAGES
➤ **Moderate to severe pain**
Adults: 50 to 100 mg P.O. every 3 to 4 hours p.r.n. Maximum oral dose is 600 mg/day. Or, 30 mg I.M., I.V., or subcutaneously every 3 to 4 hours p.r.n. Maximum parenteral dose is 360 mg/day. Single doses above 30 mg I.V. or 60 mg I.M. or subcutaneously aren't recommended.
➤ **Labor**
Adults: 30 mg I.M. as a single dose or 20 mg I.V. every 2 to 3 hours when contractions become regular for two to three doses.

ADMINISTRATION
P.O.
• Give drug with aspirin or acetaminophen for additive analgesic effect.
I.V.
• Give drug slowly by direct I.V. injection.
■ **Black Box Warning** Talwin NX, the oral form available in the United States,

contains the opioid antagonist naloxone, which discourages illicit I.V. use. ■
• **Incompatibilities:** Alkaline solutions, aminophylline, amobarbital, glycopyrrolate, heparin sodium, nafcillin sodium, pentobarbital sodium, phenobarbital sodium, sodium bicarbonate.
I.M.
• Rotate injection sites to minimize tissue irritation.
Subcutaneous
• Rotate injection sites to minimize tissue irritation. If possible, avoid giving subcutaneously.

ACTION
Unknown. Binds with opioid receptors in the CNS, altering perception of and emotional response to pain.

Route	Onset	Peak	Duration
P.O.	15–30 min	1–3 hr	2–3 hr
I.V.	2–3 min	15–30 min	2–3 hr
I.M., Subcut.	15–20 min	30–60 min	2–3 hr

Half-life: 2 to 3 hours.

ADVERSE REACTIONS
CNS: *dizziness, euphoria, lightheadedness, sedation,* confusion, drowsiness, hallucinations, headache, psychotomimetic effects, visual disturbances.
CV: *shock, circulatory depression,* hypertension, hypotension.
EENT: dry mouth.
GI: *nausea, vomiting,* constipation.
GU: urine retention.
Respiratory: *apnea, respiratory depression,* dyspnea.
Skin: diaphoresis, induration, nodules, sclerosis at injection site, pruritus, sloughing.
Other: *anaphylaxis,* hypersensitivity reactions, physical and psychological dependence.

INTERACTIONS
Drug-drug. *CNS depressants:* May cause additive effects. Use together cautiously.
Fluoxetine: May cause additive effects resulting in serotonin syndrome. Use together cautiously.

Reactions may be *common,* uncommon, *life-threatening,* or COMMON AND LIFE-THREATENING.
Interaction may have a *rapid onset* or *delayed onset.*

Opioid analgesics: May decrease analgesic effect. Avoid using together.

Drug-lifestyle. *Alcohol use:* May cause additive effects. Discourage use together.

Smoking: May increase requirements f or pentazocine. Monitor drug's effectiveness.

EFFECTS ON LAB TEST RESULTS
● May interfere with laboratory tests for urinary 17-hydroxycorticosteroids.

CONTRAINDICATIONS & CAUTIONS
● Contraindicated in patients hypersensitive to drug or its components and in children younger than age 12.
● Use cautiously in patients with hepatic or renal disease, acute MI, head injury, increased intracranial pressure, and respiratory depression.

NURSING CONSIDERATIONS
● Reassess patient's level of pain at least 15 and 30 minutes after parenteral administration and 30 minutes after oral administration.
● Drug may cause constipation. Assess bowel function and need for stool softeners and/or stimulant laxatives. Encourage fluids.
● Have naloxone readily available. Respiratory depression can be reversed with naloxone.
● Drug has opioid antagonist properties. May cause withdrawal syndrome in opioid-dependent patients.
● Psychological and physical dependence may occur with prolonged use.

PATIENT TEACHING
● Instruct patient to ask for drug before pain is intense.
● Caution ambulatory patient about getting out of bed or walking. Warn outpatient to avoid driving and other hazardous activities that require mental alertness until drug's CNS effects are known.
● Advise patient to avoid alcohol during therapy.
● Instruct patient or family to report skin rash, disorientation, or confusion to prescriber.

propoxyphene hydrochloride (dextropropoxyphene hydrochloride)
proe-POX-i-feen

Darvon, Darvon Pulvules, 642†

propoxyphene napsylate (dextropropoxyphene napsylate)
Darvon-N

Pharmacologic class: opioid
Pregnancy risk category C
Controlled substance schedule IV

AVAILABLE FORMS
propoxyphene hydrochloride
Capsules: 65 mg
propoxyphene napsylate
Tablets: 100 mg

INDICATIONS & DOSAGES
➤ **Mild to moderate pain**
Adults: 65 mg propoxyphene hydrochloride P.O. every 4 hours p.r.n. Maximum daily dose is 390 mg. Or, 100 mg propoxyphene napsylate P.O. every 4 hours p.r.n. Maximum daily dose is 600 mg.
Adjust-a-dose: For patients with hepatic or renal dysfunction, reduce dosage. Consider increasing dosing interval in elderly patients.

ADMINISTRATION
P.O.
● Give drug with food or milk to minimize GI upset.

ACTION
Unknown. Binds with opioid receptors in the CNS, altering perception of and emotional response to pain.

Route	Onset	Peak	Duration
P.O.	15–60 min	2–2½ hr	4–6 hr

Half-life: 6 to 12 hours.

ADVERSE REACTIONS
CNS: *dizziness, sedation,* euphoria, hallucinations, headache, light-headedness,

psychological and physical dependence, weakness.

GI: *nausea, vomiting,* abdominal pain, constipation.

Respiratory: *respiratory depression.*

INTERACTIONS

Drug-drug. *Carbamazepine:* May increase carbamazepine level. Monitor patient closely.

CNS depressants: May cause additive effects. Use together cautiously.

Tricyclic antidepressants (such as doxepin): May inhibit antidepressant metabolism. Monitor patient for toxicity.

Warfarin: May increase anticoagulant effect. Monitor PT and INR.

Drug-lifestyle. *Alcohol use:* May cause additive effects. Discourage use together.

Smoking: May increase metabolism of propoxyphene. Monitor patient closely.

EFFECTS ON LAB TEST RESULTS

• May alter liver function test values.

CONTRAINDICATIONS & CAUTIONS

• Contraindicated in patients hypersensitive to drug.

■ **Black Box Warning** Contraindicated in suicidal or addiction-prone patients. ■

• Use cautiously in patients with hepatic or renal disease, emotional instability, or history of drug or alcohol abuse.

■ **Black Box Warning** Use cautiously in patients taking tranquilizers or antidepressant drugs and patients who use alcohol in excess. ■

NURSING CONSIDERATIONS

• Reassess patient's pain level at least 30 minutes after giving drug.

• Propoxyphene hydrochloride 65 mg equals propoxyphene napsylate 100 mg.

• Drug may cause constipation. Assess bowel function and need for stool softeners and/or stimulant laxatives.

• Drug is considered a mild opioid analgesic, but pain relief is equivalent to that provided by aspirin. Drug is used with aspirin or acetaminophen to maximize analgesia. Patient may become tolerant and physically dependent on drug.

• Smokers may need increased dosage because smoking may induce liver

enzymes responsible for the metabolism of the drug, decreasing its effectiveness.

PATIENT TEACHING

• Advise patient to take drug with food or milk to minimize GI upset.

■ **Black Box Warning** Warn patient not to exceed recommended dosage. Respiratory depression, low blood pressure, profound sedation, coma, and death may result if used in excessive doses or with other CNS depressants. Advise patient to avoid alcohol or other CNS-type drugs when taking propoxyphene. ■

• Caution ambulatory patient about getting out of bed or walking. Warn outpatient to avoid driving and other hazardous activities that require mental alertness until drug's CNS effects are known.

---

tramadol hydrochloride
TRAM-uh-dohl

Ultram, Ultram ER

Pharmacologic class: synthetic, centrally active analgesic
Pregnancy risk category C

AVAILABLE FORMS

Tablets: 50 mg
Tablets (extended-release): 100 mg, 200 mg, 300 mg

INDICATIONS & DOSAGES

➤ **Moderate to moderately severe pain**

Adults age 17 and older: Initially, 25 mg P.O. in the morning. Adjust by 25 mg every 3 days to 100 mg/day (25 mg q.i.d.). Thereafter, adjust by 50 mg every 3 days to reach 200 mg/day (50 mg q.i.d.). Thereafter, give 50 to 100 mg P.O. every 4 to 6 hours p.r.n. Maximum, 400 mg daily.

Adults age 18 and older not taking tramadol immediate-release tablets: 100 mg P.O. once daily. Titrate by 100 mg every 5 days to relieve pain. Do not exceed 300 mg/day.

Elderly patients: For patients older than age 75, maximum is 300 mg daily in divided doses.

Reactions may be *common,* uncommon, *life-threatening,* or COMMON AND LIFE-THREATENING.
Interaction may have a *rapid onset* or **delayed onset.**

Adjust-a-dose: If creatinine clearance is less than 30 ml/minute, increase dose interval to every 12 hours; maximum is 200 mg daily. For patients with cirrhosis, give 50 mg every 12 hours.

ADMINISTRATION
P.O.
● Give drug without regard for meals.
● ER tablets must be swallowed whole; don't break or crush tablets.

ACTION
Unknown. Thought to bind to opioid receptors and inhibit reuptake of norepinephrine and serotonin.

Route	Onset	Peak	Duration
P.O.	Unknown	2 hr	Unknown
P.O. (ER)	Unknown	12 hr	Unknown

Half-life: 6 to 7 hours, ER 8 to 9 hours.

ADVERSE REACTIONS
CNS: *dizziness, headache, somnolence, vertigo, seizures,* anxiety, asthenia, CNS stimulation, confusion, coordination disturbance, euphoria, malaise, nervousness, sleep disorder.
CV: vasodilation.
EENT: visual disturbances.
GI: *constipation, nausea, vomiting,* abdominal pain, anorexia, diarrhea, dry mouth, dyspepsia, flatulence.
GU: menopausal symptoms, proteinuria, urinary frequency, urine retention.
Musculoskeletal: hypertonia.
Respiratory: *respiratory depression.*
Skin: diaphoresis, pruritus, rash.

INTERACTIONS
Drug-drug. *Carbamazepine:* May increase tramadol metabolism. Patients receiving long-term carbamazepine therapy up to 800 mg daily may need up to twice the recommended tramadol dose.
CNS depressants: May cause additive effects. Use together cautiously; tramadol dosage may need to be reduced.
Cyclobenzaprine, MAO inhibitors, neuroleptics, other opioids, tricyclic antidepressants: May increase risk of seizures. Monitor patient closely.
Quinidine: May increase level of tramadol. Monitor patient closely.

SSRIs: May increase risk of serotonin syndrome. Use cautiously and monitor patient for adverse effects.

EFFECTS ON LAB TEST RESULTS
● May increase liver enzyme level.
● May decrease creatinine and hemoglobin levels.

CONTRAINDICATIONS & CAUTIONS
● Contraindicated in patients hypersensitive to drug or other opioids, in breastfeeding women, and in those with acute intoxication from alcohol, hypnotics, centrally acting analgesics, opioids, or psychotropic drugs. Serious hypersensitivity reactions can occur, usually after the first dose. Patients with history of anaphylactic reaction to codeine and other opioids may be at increased risk.
● Use cautiously in patients at risk for seizures or respiratory depression; in patients with increased intracranial pressure or head injury, acute abdominal conditions, or renal or hepatic impairment; or in patients with physical dependence on opioids.

NURSING CONSIDERATIONS
● Reassess patient's level of pain at least 30 minutes after administration.
● Monitor CV and respiratory status. Withhold dose and notify prescriber if respirations are shallow or rate is below 12 breaths/minute.
● Monitor bowel and bladder function. Anticipate need for stimulant laxative.
● For better analgesic effect, give drug before onset of intense pain.
● Monitor patients at risk for seizures. Drug may reduce seizure threshold.
● In the case of an overdose, naloxone may also increase risk of seizures.
● Monitor patient for drug dependence. Drug can produce dependence similar to that of codeine or dextropropoxyphene and thus has potential for abuse.
● Withdrawal symptoms may occur if drug is stopped abruptly. Reduce dosage gradually.
● *Look alike–sound alike:* Don't confuse tramadol with trazodone or trandolapril.

PATIENT TEACHING

- Tell patient to take drug as prescribed and not to increase dose or dosage interval unless ordered by prescriber.
- Caution ambulatory patient to be careful when rising and walking. Warn outpatient to avoid driving and other potentially hazardous activities that require mental alertness until drug's CNS effects are known.
- Advise patient to check with prescriber before taking OTC drugs because drug interactions can occur.
- Warn patient not to stop the drug abruptly.

48

Sedative-hypnotics

chloral hydrate
diazepam
(See Chapter 42, ANXIOLYTICS.)
diphenhydramine hydrochloride
(See Chapter 55, ANTIHISTAMINES.)
eszopiclone
midazolam hydrochloride
phenobarbital sodium
(See Chapter 37, ANTICONVULSANTS.)
propofol
ramelteon
temazepam
triazolam
zaleplon
zolpidem tartrate

SAFETY ALERT!

chloral hydrate
KLOR-al HYE-drate

Aquachloral Supprettes, Somnote

Pharmacologic class: CNS
depressant
Pregnancy risk category C
Controlled substance schedule IV

AVAILABLE FORMS
Capsules: 500 mg
Suppositories: 325 mg, 500 mg, 650 mg
Syrup: 250 mg/5 ml, 500 mg/5 ml

INDICATIONS & DOSAGES
➤ **Sedation**
Adults: 250 mg P.O. or P.R. t.i.d. after
meals. Maximum single or daily dose is 2 g.
Children: 8 mg/kg P.O. t.i.d. Maximum
dosage is 500 mg t.i.d.
➤ **Insomnia**
Adults: 500 mg to 1 g P.O. or P.R. 15 to
30 minutes before bedtime. Maximum
daily dose is 2 g.
Children: 50 mg/kg P.O. or P.R. 15 to
30 minutes before bedtime. Maximum
single dose is 1 g.
➤ **Preoperatively to produce sedation
and relieve anxiety**
Adults: 500 mg to 1 g P.O. or P.R.
30 minutes before surgery.

➤ **Alcohol withdrawal**
Adults: 500 mg to 1 g P.R. every 6 hours
p.r.n.
➤ **Premedication for EEG**
Children: 20 to 25 mg/kg P.O. or P.R. up
to 500 mg/single dose. May give divided
doses.

ADMINISTRATION
P.O.
● Give drug after meals.
● Give capsule with full glass of water or
juice, and have patient swallow capsule
whole.
● To minimize unpleasant taste and stom-
ach irritation, dilute syrup or give with
liquid such as ½ glass water, fruit juice, or
ginger ale.
● Store capsules or liquid in dark container.
Rectal
● Refrigerate suppositories at least 2 hours
before intended use.
● Store suppositories in refrigerator.

ACTION
Unknown. Sedative effects may be caused
by drug's main metabolite,
trichloroethanol.

Route	Onset	Peak	Duration
P.O.	30 min	Unknown	4–8 hr
P.R.	Unknown	Unknown	4–8 hr

Half-life: 8 to 10 hours for trichloroethanol.

ADVERSE REACTIONS
CNS: drowsiness, nightmares, dizziness,
ataxia, paradoxical excitement, hangover,
somnolence, disorientation, delirium,
light-headedness, hallucinations, confusion,
somnambulism, vertigo, malaise, physical
and psychological dependence.
GI: *nausea, vomiting, diarrhea,*
flatulence.
Hematologic: eosinophilia, *leukopenia.*
Other: hypersensitivity reactions.

INTERACTIONS
Drug-drug. *CNS depressants including
opioid analgesics:* May cause excessive

CNS depression or vasodilation reaction.
Use together cautiously.
Furosemide I.V: May cause sweating,
flushes, variable blood pressure, nausea,
and uneasiness. Use together cautiously or
use a different hypnotic drug.
Oral anticoagulants: May increase risk of
bleeding. Monitor patient closely.
Phenytoin: May decrease phenytoin level.
Monitor patient closely.
Drug-lifestyle. *Alcohol use:* May react
synergistically, increasing CNS depression,
or, rarely, may produce a disulfiram-like
reaction. Strongly discourage alcohol use
with these drugs.

EFFECTS ON LAB TEST RESULTS
● May increase eosinophil count.
● May decrease WBC count.
● May cause false-positive results in urine
glucose tests that use cupric sulfate, such
as Benedict's reagent, and in phentolamine
tests.

CONTRAINDICATIONS & CAUTIONS
● Contraindicated in patients hypersensitive
to drug and in those with hepatic or renal
impairment.
● Oral administration is contraindicated in
patients with gastric disorders.
■ **Black Box Warning** Do not use when
less potentially dangerous agents would be
effective. ■
● Use with caution in patients with severe
cardiac disease.
● Use cautiously in patients with mental
depression, suicidal tendencies, or history
of drug abuse.
● Some products may contain tartrazine;
use cautiously in patients with aspirin
sensitivity.

NURSING CONSIDERATIONS
● *Alert:* Note two strengths of oral liquid
form. Double-check dose, especially when
giving to children. Fatal overdoses have
occurred.
● Take precautions to prevent hoarding or
overdosing by patients who are depressed,
suicidal, or drug dependent or who have
history of drug abuse.
● Long-term use isn't recommended;
drug loses its effectiveness in promoting
sleep after 14 days of continued use.
Long-term use may cause drug depen-

dence, and patient may experience
withdrawal symptoms if drug is
suddenly stopped.
● Monitor BUN level; large doses may
raise BUN level.
● Don't give drug for 48 hours before
fluorometric test.

PATIENT TEACHING
● Instruct patient to take capsule with a
full glass of water or juice and to swallow
capsule whole.
● Tell patient to avoid alcohol during drug
therapy.
● Caution patient to avoid performing
activities that require mental alertness or
physical coordination.
● Advise patient to store drug in dark
container and to store suppositories in
refrigerator.

SAFETY ALERT!

eszopiclone
ess-ZOP-ah-klone

Lunesta✦

Pharmacologic class:
pyrrolopyrazine derivative
Pregnancy risk category C
Controlled substance schedule IV

AVAILABLE FORMS
Tablets: 1 mg, 2 mg, 3 mg

INDICATIONS & DOSAGES
➤ **Insomnia**
Adults: 2 mg P.O. immediately
before bedtime. Increase to 3 mg as
needed.
*Elderly patients having trouble
falling asleep:* 1 mg P.O. immediately
before bedtime. Increase to 2 mg
as needed.
*Elderly patients having trouble staying
asleep:* 2 mg P.O. immediately before
bedtime.
Adjust-a-dose: In patients with
severe hepatic impairment, start with
1 mg P.O. In patients who also take
a potent CYP3A4 inhibitor, start with
1 mg and increase to 2 mg as
needed.

ADMINISTRATION
P.O.
- Avoid giving drug after a high-fat meal.
- Give drug immediately before bedtime because drug may cause dizziness or light-headedness.

ACTION
Probably interacts with GABA receptors at binding sites close or connected to benzodiazepine receptors.

Route	Onset	Peak	Duration
P.O.	Rapid	1 hr	Unknown

Half-life: 6 hours.

ADVERSE REACTIONS
CNS: abnormal dreams, anxiety, complex sleep-related behavior, confusion, decreased libido, depression, dizziness, hallucinations, *headache,* nervousness, pain, *somnolence,* neuralgia.
EENT: *unpleasant taste.*
GI: diarrhea, dry mouth, dyspepsia, nausea, vomiting.
GU: UTI.
Respiratory: *respiratory tract infection.*
Skin: pruritus, rash.
Other: *anaphylaxis, angioedema,* accidental injury, viral infection.

INTERACTIONS
Drug-drug. *CNS depressants:* May have additive CNS effects. Adjust dosage of either drug as needed.
CYP3A4 inhibitors (clarithromycin, itraconazole, ketoconazole, nefazodone, nelfinavir, ritonavir, troleandomycin): May decrease eszopiclone elimination, increasing the risk of toxicity. Use together cautiously.
Olanzapine: May impair cognitive function or memory. Use together cautiously.
Rifampicin: May decrease eszopiclone activity. Don't use together.
Drug-food. *High-fat meals:* May decrease drug absorption and effects. Discourage high-fat meals with or just before taking drug.
Drug-lifestyle. *Alcohol use:* May decrease psychomotor ability. Discourage use together.

EFFECTS ON LAB TEST RESULTS
None reported.

CONTRAINDICATIONS & CAUTIONS
- Use cautiously in patients with diseases or conditions that could affect metabolism or hemodynamic responses. Also use cautiously in patients with compromised respiratory function, severe hepatic impairment, or signs and symptoms of depression.

NURSING CONSIDERATIONS
- *Alert:* Anaphylaxis and angioedema may occur as early as the first dose; monitor the patient closely.
- Evaluate patient for physical and psychiatric disorders before treatment.
- Use the lowest effective dose.
- *Alert:* Give drug immediately before patient goes to bed or after patient has gone to bed and has trouble falling asleep.
- Use only for short periods (for example, 7 to 10 days). If patient still has trouble sleeping, check for other psychological disorders.
- Monitor patient for changes in behavior, including those that suggest depression or suicidal thinking.

PATIENT TEACHING
- *Alert:* Warn patient that drug may cause allergic reactions, facial swelling, and complex sleep-related behaviors, such as driving, eating, and making phone calls while asleep. Advise patient to report these adverse effects.
- Urge patient to take drug immediately before going to bed because drug may cause dizziness or light-headedness.
- Caution patient not to take drug unless he can get a full night's sleep.
- Advise patient to avoid taking drug after a high-fat meal.
- Tell patient to avoid activities that require mental alertness until the drug's effects are known.
- Advise patient to avoid alcohol while taking drug.
- Urge patient to immediately report changes in behavior and thinking.
- Warn patient not to stop drug abruptly or change dose without consulting the prescriber.
- Inform patient that tolerance or dependence may develop if drug is taken for a prolonged period.

midazolam hydrochloride
mid-AY-zoh-lam

Pharmacologic class:
benzodiazepine
Pregnancy risk category D
Controlled substance schedule IV

AVAILABLE FORMS
Injection: 1 mg/ml, 5 mg/ml
Syrup: 2 mg/ml

INDICATIONS & DOSAGES
➤ **Preoperative sedation (to induce sleepiness or drowsiness and relieve apprehension)**
Adults: 0.07 to 0.08 mg/kg I.M. about 1 hour before surgery.
➤ **Conscious sedation before short diagnostic or endoscopic procedures**
Adults younger than age 60: Initially, small dose not to exceed 2.5 mg I.V. given slowly; repeat in 2 minutes p.r.n., in small increments of first dose over at least 2 minutes to achieve desired effect. Total dose of up to 5 mg may be used. Additional doses to maintain desired level of sedation may be given by slow titration in increments of 25% of dose used to first reach the sedative end point.
Patients age 60 or older and debilitated patients: 0.5 to 1.5 mg I.V. over at least 2 minutes. Incremental doses shouldn't exceed 1 mg. A total dose of up to 3.5 mg is usually sufficient.
➤ **To induce sleepiness and amnesia and to relieve apprehension before anesthesia or before and during procedures**
P.O.
Children ages 6 to 16 who are cooperative: 0.25 to 0.5 mg/kg P.O. as a single dose, up to 20 mg.
Infants and children ages 6 months to 5 years or less cooperative, older children: 0.25 to 1 mg/kg P.O. as a single dose, up to 20 mg.
I.V.
Children ages 12 to 16: Initially, no more than 2.5 mg I.V. given slowly; repeat in 2 minutes, if needed, in small increments of first dose over at least 2 minutes to achieve desired effect. Total dose of up to 10 mg may be used. Additional doses to maintain desired level of sedation may be given by slow titration in increments of 25% of dose used to first reach the sedative end point.
Children ages 6 to 12: 0.025 to 0.05 mg/kg I.V. over 2 to 3 minutes. Additional doses may be given in small increments after 2 to 3 minutes. Total dose of up to 0.4 mg/kg, not to exceed 10 mg, may be used.
Children ages 6 months to 5 years: 0.05 to 0.1 mg/kg I.V. over 2 to 3 minutes. Additional doses may be given in small increments after 2 to 3 minutes. Total dose of up to 0.6 mg/kg, not to exceed 6 mg, may be used.
I.M.
Children: 0.1 to 0.15 mg/kg I.M. Use up to 0.5 mg/kg in more anxious patients.
Adjust-a-dose: For obese children, base dose on ideal body weight; high-risk or debilitated children and children receiving other sedatives need lower doses.
➤ **To induce general anesthesia**
Adults older than age 55: 0.3 mg/kg I.V. over 20 to 30 seconds if patient hasn't received premedication, or 0.2 mg/kg I.V. over 20 to 30 seconds if patient has received a sedative or opioid premedication. Additional increments of 25% of first dose may be needed to complete induction.
Adults younger than age 55: 0.3 to 0.35 mg/kg I.V. over 20 to 30 seconds if patient hasn't received premedication, or 0.25 mg/kg I.V. over 20 to 30 seconds if patient has received a sedative or opioid premedication. Additional increments of 25% of first dose may be needed to complete induction.
Adjust-a-dose: For debilitated patients, initially, 0.2 to 0.25 mg/kg. As little as 0.15 mg/kg may be needed.
➤ **As continuous infusion to sedate intubated patients in critical care unit**
Adults: Initially, 0.01 to 0.05 mg/kg may be given I.V. over several minutes, repeated at 10- to 15-minute intervals until adequate sedation is achieved. To maintain sedation, usual initial infusion rate is 0.02 to 0.1 mg/kg/hour. Higher loading dose or infusion rates may be needed in some patients. Use the lowest effective rate.

Children: Initially, 0.05 to 0.2 mg/kg may be given I.V. over 2 to 3 minutes or longer; then continuous infusion at rate of 0.06 to 0.12 mg/kg/hour. Increase or decrease infusion to maintain desired effect.
Neonates more than 32 weeks' gestational age: Initially, 0.06 mg/kg/hour. Adjust rate, as needed, using lowest possible rate.
Neonates less than 32 weeks' gestational age: Initially, 0.03 mg/kg/hour. Adjust rate, as needed, using lowest possible rate.

ADMINISTRATION
P.O.
● Give drug without regard for food, but don't give with grapefruit juice or grapefruit.
I.V.
● Drug may be mixed in the same syringe with morphine sulfate, meperidine, atropine, or scopolamine.
● When mixing infusion, use 5-mg/ml vial and dilute to 0.5 mg/ml with D₅W or normal saline solution.
■ **Black Box Warning** Give slowly over at least 2 minutes, and wait at least 2 minutes when titrating doses to produce therapeutic effect. ■
■ **Black Box Warning** Do not administer by rapid injection in the neonatal population. ■
● **Incompatibilities:** Albumin, amoxicillin sodium, amphotericin B, ampicillin sodium, bumetanide, butorphanol, ceftazidime, cefuroxime, clonidine, dexamethasone sodium phosphate, dimenhydrinate, dobutamine, foscarnet, fosphenytoin, furosemide, heparin sodium, hydrocortisone, imipenem-cilastatin sodium, lactated Ringer's injection, methotrexate sodium, nafcillin, omeprazole sodium, pentobarbital sodium, perphenazine, prochlorperazine edisylate, ranitidine hydrochloride, sodium bicarbonate, thiopental, some total parenteral nutrition formulations, trimethoprim-sulfamethoxazole.
I.M.
● Inject deeply into a large muscle.

ACTION
May potentiate the effects of GABA, depress the CNS, and suppress the spread of seizure activity.

Route	Onset	Peak	Duration
P.O.	10–20 min	45–60 min	2–6 hr
I.V.	90 sec–5 min	Rapid	2–6 hr
I.M.	15 min	15–60 min	2–6 hr

Half-life: 2 to 6 hours.

ADVERSE REACTIONS
CNS: *oversedation, drowsiness,* amnesia, headache, involuntary movements, nystagmus, paradoxical behavior or excitement.
CV: variations in blood pressure and pulse rate.
GI: *nausea,* vomiting.
Respiratory: APNEA, *decreased respiratory rate,* hiccups.
Other: *pain at injection site.*

INTERACTIONS
Drug-drug. *CNS depressants:* May cause apnea. Use together cautiously. Adjust dosage of midazolam if used with opiates or other CNS depressants.
Diltiazem: May increase CNS depression and prolonged effects of midazolam. Use lower dose of midazolam.
Erythromycin: May alter metabolism of midazolam. Use together cautiously.
Fluconazole, itraconazole, ketoconazole, miconazole: May increase and prolong midazolam level, CNS depression, and psychomotor impairment. Avoid using together.
Hormonal contraceptives: May prolong half-life of midazolam. Use together cautiously.
Rifampin: May decrease midazolam level. Monitor for midazolam effectiveness.
Theophylline: May antagonize sedative effect of midazolam. Use together cautiously.
Verapamil: May increase midazolam level. Monitor patient closely.
Drug-herb. *St. John's wort:* May decrease drug level. Discourage use together.
Drug-food. *Grapefruit juice:* May increase bioavailability of oral drug. Discourage use together.
Drug-lifestyle. *Alcohol use:* May cause additive CNS effects. Discourage use together.

EFFECTS ON LAB TEST RESULTS
None reported.

CONTRAINDICATIONS & CAUTIONS
• Contraindicated in patients hypersensitive to drug and in those with acute angle-closure glaucoma, shock, coma, or acute alcohol intoxication.
• Use cautiously in patients with uncompensated acute illness and in elderly or debilitated patients.

NURSING CONSIDERATIONS
■ **Black Box Warning** Have oxygen and resuscitation equipment available in case of severe respiratory depression. Excessive amounts and rapid infusion have been linked to respiratory arrest. Continuously monitor patient, including children taking syrup form, for life-threatening respiratory depression. ■
• Monitor blood pressure, heart rate and rhythm, respirations, airway integrity, and arterial oxygen saturation during procedure.

PATIENT TEACHING
• Because drug diminishes patient's recall of events around the time of surgery, provide written information, family member instructions, and follow-up contact.
• Warn patient to avoid hazardous activities that require alertness or good coordination until effects of drug are known.

SAFETY ALERT!

propofol
PRO-puh-fole

Diprivan

Pharmacologic class: phenol derivative
Pregnancy risk category B

AVAILABLE FORMS
Injection: 10 mg/ml in 20-ml ampules; 50-ml prefilled syringes; 50-ml and 100-ml infusion vials

INDICATIONS & DOSAGES
➤ **To induce anesthesia**
Adults younger than age 55 classified as American Society of Anesthesiologists (ASA) Physical Status (PS) category I or II: 2 to 2.5 mg/kg. Give in 40-mg boluses every 10 seconds until desired response is achieved.
Children ages 3 to 16 classified as ASA I or II: 2.5 to 3.5 mg/kg over 20 to 30 seconds.
Adjust-a-dose: In geriatric, debilitated, hypovolemic, or ASA PS III or IV patients, give half the usual induction dose, in 20-mg boluses, every 10 seconds. For cardiac anesthesia, give 20 mg (0.5 to 1.5 mg/kg) every 10 seconds until desired response is achieved. For neurosurgical patients, give 20 mg (1 to 2 mg/kg) every 10 seconds until desired response is achieved.
➤ **To maintain anesthesia**
Healthy adults younger than age 55: 0.1 to 0.2 mg/kg/minute (6 to 12 mg/kg/hour). Or, 20- to 50-mg intermittent boluses, p.r.n.
Healthy children ages 2 months to 16 years: 125 to 300 mcg/kg/minute (7.5 to 18 mg/kg/hour).
Adjust-a-dose: In geriatric, debilitated, hypovolemic, or ASA PS III or IV patients, give half the usual maintenance dose (0.05 to 0.1 mg/kg/minute or 3 to 6 mg/kg/hour). For cardiac anesthesia with secondary opioid, 100 to 150 mcg/kg/minute; low dose with primary opioid, 50 to 100 mcg/kg/minute. For neuro-surgical patients, 100 to 200 mcg/kg/minute (6 to 12 mg/kg/hour).
➤ **Monitored anesthesia care**
Healthy adults younger than age 55: Initially, 100 to 150 mcg/kg/minute (6 to 9 mg/kg/hour) for 3 to 5 minutes or a slow injection of 0.5 mg/kg over 3 to 5 minutes. For maintenance dose, give infusion of 25 to 75 mcg/kg/minute (1.5 to 4.5 mg/kg/hour), or incremental 10- or 20-mg boluses.
Adjust-a-dose: In geriatric, debilitated, or ASA PS III or IV patients, give 80% of usual adult maintenance dose. Don't use rapid bolus.
➤ **To sedate intubated intensive care unit (ICU) patients**
Adults: Initially, 5 mcg/kg/minute (0.3 mg/kg/hour) for 5 minutes. Increments of 5 to 10 mcg/kg/minute (0.3 to 0.6 mg/kg/hour) over 5 to 10 minutes may be used until desired sedation

is achieved. Maintenance rate, 5 to 50 mcg/kg/minute (0.3 to 3 mg/kg/hour).

ADMINISTRATION

I.V.
• Maintain aseptic technique when handling the solution. Drug can support the growth of microorganisms; don't use if solution might be contaminated.
• Protect drug from light. Shake well.
• Dilute only with D₅W. Don't dilute to less than 2 mg/ml.
• Don't use if emulsion shows evidence of separation.
• Don't infuse through a filter with a pore size smaller than 5 microns. Give via larger veins in arms to decrease injection site pain.
• Titrate drug daily to maintain minimum effective level. Allow 3 to 5 minutes between dosage adjustments to assess effects.
• Discard tubing and unused portions of drug after 12 hours.
• **Incompatibilities:** Other I.V. drugs, blood and plasma.

ACTION

Unknown. Rapid-acting I.V. sedative-hypnotic.

Route	Onset	Peak	Duration
I.V.	< 40 sec	Unknown	10–15 min

Half-life: Initial (distribution) phase, about 2 to 10 minutes; second (redistribution) phase, 21 to 70 minutes; terminal (elimination) phase, 1½ to 31 hours.

ADVERSE REACTIONS

CNS: dystonic or choreiform movement.
CV: *bradycardia,* hypotension, hypertension, decreased cardiac output.
Metabolic: hyperlipemia.
Respiratory: APNEA, *respiratory acidosis.*
Skin: rash.
Other: *burning or stinging at injection site.*

INTERACTIONS

Drug-drug. *Inhaled anesthetics (such as enflurane, halothane, isoflurane), opioids (alfentanil, fentanyl, meperidine, morphine), sedatives (such as barbiturates, benzodiazepines, chloral hydrate, droperidol):* May increase anesthetic and sedative effects and further decrease blood pressure and cardiac output. Monitor patient closely.
Drug-herb. *St. John's wort:* May prolong anesthetic effects. Advise patient to stop using herb 5 days before surgery.

EFFECTS ON LAB TEST RESULTS

• May increase lipid levels.

CONTRAINDICATIONS & CAUTIONS

• Contraindicated in patients hypersensitive to drug or its components (including egg lecithin, soybean oil, and glycerol), in pregnant women (because it may cause fetal depression), and in those unable to undergo general anesthesia or sedation.
• Use cautiously in patients who are hemodynamically unstable or who have seizures, disorders of lipid metabolism, or increased intracranial pressure.
• Because drug appears in breast milk, avoid using in breast-feeding women.

NURSING CONSIDERATIONS

• If drug is used for prolonged sedation in ICU, urine may turn green.
• For general anesthesia or monitored anesthesia care sedation, trained staff not involved in the surgical or diagnostic procedure should give drug. For ICU sedation, persons skilled in managing critically ill patients and trained in cardio-pulmonary resuscitation and airway management should give drug.
• Continuously monitor vital signs.
• *Alert:* The FDA issued an alert after receiving reports of chills, fever, and body aches in several clusters of patients shortly after patients received propofol for sedation or general anesthesia. Various lots of the drug were tested, but no toxins, bacteria, or other signs of contamination were found. The FDA advises all health care providers to carefully follow the handling and use sections of the prescribing information for this drug. They recommend that all patients be evaluated for possible reactions following use of the drug, and that anyone experiencing signs of acute febrile reactions be evaluated for possible bacterial sepsis. They ask that any adverse events following the use of propofol be reported to MedWatch.

- Monitor patient at risk for hyperlipidemia for elevated triglyceride levels.
- Drug contains 0.1 g of fat (1.1 kcal)/ml. Reduce other lipid products if given together.
- Drug contains ethylenediaminetetra-acetic acid (EDTA), a strong metal chelator. Consider supplemental zinc during prolonged therapy.
- When giving drug in the ICU, assess patient's CNS function daily to determine minimum dose needed.
- Stop drug gradually to prevent abrupt awakening and increased agitation.
- **Look alike–sound alike:** Don't confuse Diprivan with Ditropan or Dipivefrin.

PATIENT TEACHING
- Advise patient that performance of activities requiring mental alertness may be impaired for some time after drug use.

SAFETY ALERT!

ramelteon
rah-MELL-tee-on

Rozerem

Pharmacologic class: melatonin receptor agonist
Pregnancy risk category C

AVAILABLE FORMS
Tablets: 8 mg

INDICATIONS & DOSAGES
➤ **Insomnia characterized by trouble falling asleep**
Adults: 8 mg P.O. within 30 minutes of bedtime.

ADMINISTRATION
P.O.
- Don't give drug with or immediately after a high-fat meal.
- Give drug within 30 minutes of bedtime.

ACTION
Acts on receptors believed to maintain the circadian rhythm underlying the normal sleep-wake cycle.

Route	Onset	Peak	Duration
P.O.	Rapid	½-1½ hr	Unknown

Half-life: Parent compound, 1 to 2½ hours; metabolite M-II, 2 to 5 hours.

ADVERSE REACTIONS
CNS: complex sleep-related behaviors, depression, dizziness, fatigue, headache, somnolence, worsened insomnia.
GI: diarrhea, impaired taste, nausea.
Musculoskeletal: arthralgia, myalgia.
Respiratory: upper respiratory tract infection.
Other: *anaphylaxis, angioedema,* flulike symptoms.

INTERACTIONS
Drug-drug. *CNS depressants:* May cause excessive CNS depression. Use together cautiously.
Fluconazole (strong CYP2C9 inhibitor), ketoconazole (strong CYP3A4 inhibitor), weak CYP1A2 inhibitors: May increase ramelteon level. Use together cautiously.
Fluvoxamine (strong CYP1A2 inhibitor): May increase ramelteon level. Avoid use together.
Rifampin (strong CYP enzyme inducer): May decrease ramelteon level. Monitor patient for lack of effect.
Drug-food. *Food (especially high-fat meals):* May delay time to peak drug effect. Tell patient to take drug on an empty stomach.
Drug-lifestyle. *Alcohol use:* May cause excessive CNS depression. Discourage alcohol use.

EFFECTS ON LAB TEST RESULTS
- May increase prolactin level.
- May alter blood cortisol and testosterone levels.

CONTRAINDICATIONS & CAUTIONS
- Contraindicated in those hyper-sensitive to drug or its components. Don't use in patients taking fluvo-xamine or in those with severe hepatic impairment, severe sleep apnea, or severe COPD.
- Use cautiously in patients with depression or moderate hepatic impairment.

Reactions may be *common,* uncommon, *life-threatening,* or COMMON AND LIFE-THREATENING.
Interaction may have a *rapid onset* or **delayed onset.**

NURSING CONSIDERATIONS
● *Alert:* Anaphylaxis and angioedema may occur as early as the first dose. Monitor patient closely.
● Thoroughly evaluate the cause of insomnia before starting drug.
● Assess patient for behavioral or cognitive disorders.
● Drug doesn't cause physical dependence.

PATIENT TEACHING
● *Alert:* Warn patient that drug may cause allergic reactions, facial swelling, and complex sleep-related behaviors, such as driving, eating, and making phone calls while asleep. Advise patient to report these adverse effects.
● Instruct patient to take dose within 30 minutes of bedtime.
● Tell patient not to take drug with or after a heavy meal.
● Caution against performing activities that require mental alertness or physical coordination after taking drug.
● Caution patient to avoid alcohol while taking drug.
● Tell patient to consult prescriber if insomnia worsens or behavior changes.
● Urge woman to consult prescriber if menses stops, libido decreases, or galactorrhea or fertility problems develop.

SAFETY ALERT!

temazepam
te-MAZ-e-pam

Restoril*◆*

Pharmacologic class:
benzodiazepine
Pregnancy risk category X
Controlled substance schedule IV

AVAILABLE FORMS
Capsules: 7.5 mg, 15 mg, 22.5 mg, 30 mg

INDICATIONS & DOSAGES
➤ **Short-term treatment (7 to 10 days) of insomnia**
Adults: 15 to 30 mg P.O. at bedtime.
Elderly or debilitated patients: 15 mg P.O. at bedtime until individualized response is determined.

ADMINISTRATION
P.O.
● Give drug 15 to 30 minutes before bedtime.
● Give drug without regard for food.

ACTION
Probably acts on the limbic system, thalamus, and hypothalamus of the CNS to produce hypnotic effects.

Route	Onset	Peak	Duration
P.O.	Unknown	1–2 hr	3–18 hr

Half-life: 10 to 17 hours.

ADVERSE REACTIONS
CNS: complex sleep-related behaviors, drowsiness, dizziness, lethargy, disturbed coordination, daytime sedation, confusion, nightmares, vertigo, euphoria, weakness, headache, fatigue, nervousness, anxiety, depression, minor changes in EEG patterns (usually low-voltage fast activity).
EENT: blurred vision.
GI: diarrhea, nausea, dry mouth.
Other: *anaphylaxis, angioedema,* physical and psychological dependence.

INTERACTIONS
Drug-drug. *CNS depressants:* May increase CNS depression. Use together cautiously.
Drug-herb. *Calendula, hops, kava, lemon balm, passion flower, skullcap, valerian:* May enhance sedative effect of drug. Discourage use together.
Drug-lifestyle. *Alcohol use:* May cause additive CNS effects. Discourage use together.

EFFECTS ON LAB TEST RESULTS
● May increase liver function test values.

CONTRAINDICATIONS & CAUTIONS
● Contraindicated in pregnant patients and those hypersensitive to drug or other benzodiazepines.
● Use cautiously in patients with chronic pulmonary insufficiency, impaired hepatic or renal function, severe or latent depression, suicidal tendencies, and history of drug abuse.

NURSING CONSIDERATIONS

- **Alert:** Monitor patient closely. Anaphylaxis and angioedema may occur as early as the first dose.
- Assess mental status before starting therapy and reduce doses in elderly patients; these patients may be more sensitive to drug's adverse CNS effects.
- Take precautions to prevent hoarding by patients who are depressed, suicidal, or drug-dependent or who have history of drug abuse.
- **Look alike–sound alike:** Don't confuse Restoril with Vistaril.

PATIENT TEACHING

- **Alert:** Warn patient that drug may cause allergic reactions, facial swelling, and complex sleep-related behaviors, such as driving, eating, and making phone calls while asleep. Advise patient to report these adverse effects.
- Tell patient to avoid alcohol during therapy.
- Caution patient to avoid performing activities that require mental alertness or physical coordination.
- Warn patient not to stop drug abruptly if taken for 1 month or longer.
- Tell patient that onset of drug's effects may take as long as 2 to 2¼ hours.

SAFETY ALERT!

triazolam
trye-AY-zoe-lam

Apo-Triazo†, Halcion

Pharmacologic class:
benzodiazepine
Pregnancy risk category X
Controlled substance schedule IV

AVAILABLE FORMS
Tablets: 0.125 mg, 0.25 mg

INDICATIONS & DOSAGES
➤ **Short-term treatment (7 to 10 days) of insomnia**
Adults: 0.125 to 0.5 mg P.O. at bedtime. Reevaluate patient if drug is used for longer than 2 to 3 weeks.

Elderly or debilitated patients: 0.125 mg P.O. at bedtime; increase, as needed, to 0.25 mg P.O. at bedtime.

ADMINISTRATION
P.O.
- Give drug without regard for food, but avoid giving with grapefruit or grapefruit juice.

ACTION
Unknown. Probably acts on the limbic system, thalamus, and hypothalamus of the CNS to produce hypnotic effects.

Route	Onset	Peak	Duration
P.O.	Unknown	1–2 hr	1½–5½ hr

Half-life: 1½ to 5½ hours.

ADVERSE REACTIONS
CNS: complex sleep-related behaviors, drowsiness, amnesia, ataxia, depression, dizziness, headache, lack of coordination, mental confusion, nervousness, physical or psychological dependence, rebound insomnia.
GI: nausea, vomiting.
Other: *anaphylaxis, angioedema.*

INTERACTIONS
Drug-drug. *Cimetidine, erythromycin, fluoxetine, fluvoxamine, isoniazid, nefazodone, ranitidine:* May increase triazolam level. Avoid using with azole antifungals or nefazodone. Watch for increased sedation if used with other drugs.
CNS depressants: May cause excessive CNS depression. Use together cautiously.
Diltiazem: May increase CNS depression and prolonged effects of triazolam. Reduce triazolam dose.
Fluconazole, itraconazole, ketoconazole, miconazole: May increase and prolong drug level, CNS depression, and psychomotor impairment. Avoid using together.
Drug-herb. *Calendula, hops, kava, lemon balm, passion flower, skullcap, valerian:* May enhance sedative effect of drug. Discourage use together.
Drug-food. *Grapefruit:* May delay onset and increase drug effects. Discourage use together.

Reactions may be *common*, uncommon, *life-threatening*, or COMMON AND LIFE-THREATENING.
Interaction may have a *rapid onset* or **delayed onset.**

Drug-lifestyle. *Alcohol use:* May cause additive CNS effects. Discourage use together.
Smoking: May increase metabolism and clearance of drug. Advise patient who smokes to watch for decreased effectiveness of drug.

EFFECTS ON LAB TEST RESULTS
● May increase liver function test values.

CONTRAINDICATIONS & CAUTIONS
● Contraindicated in pregnant patients and those hypersensitive to benzodiazepines.
● Use cautiously in patients with impaired hepatic or renal function, chronic pulmonary insufficiency, sleep apnea, mental depression, suicidal tendencies, or history of drug abuse.
● Use cautiously in breast-feeding women.

NURSING CONSIDERATIONS
● *Alert:* Anaphylaxis and angioedema may occur as early as the first dose; monitor the patient closely.
● Assess mental status before starting therapy and reduce doses in elderly patients; these patients may be more sensitive to drug's adverse CNS effects.
● Monitor CBC, chemistry, and urinalysis.
● Take precautions to prevent hoarding or overdosing by patients who are depressed, suicidal, or drug-dependent or who have history of drug abuse.
● Minor changes in EEG patterns (usually low-voltage fast activity) may occur during and after therapy.
● *Look alike–sound alike:* Don't confuse Halcion with Haldol or halcinonide.

PATIENT TEACHING
● *Alert:* Warn patient that drug may cause allergic reactions, facial swelling, and complex sleep-related behaviors, such as driving, eating, and making phone calls while asleep. Advise patient to report these adverse effects.
● Warn patient not to take more than prescribed amount; overdose can occur at total daily dose of 2 mg (or four times highest recommended amount).
● Tell patient to avoid alcohol use while taking drug.
● Warn patient not to stop drug abruptly after taking for 2 weeks or longer.

● Caution patient to avoid performing activities that require mental alertness or physical coordination.
● Inform patient that drug doesn't tend to cause morning drowsiness.
● Tell patient that rebound insomnia may occur for 1 or 2 nights after stopping therapy.

SAFETY ALERT!

zaleplon
ZAL-ah-plon

Sonata

Pharmacologic class:
pyrazolopyrimidine
Pregnancy risk category C
Controlled substance schedule IV

AVAILABLE FORMS
Capsules: 5 mg, 10 mg

INDICATIONS & DOSAGES
➤ **Short-term treatment (7 to 10 days) of insomnia**
Adults: 10 mg P.O. daily at bedtime; may increase to 20 mg as needed. Low-weight adults may respond to 5-mg dose. Limit use to 7 to 10 days. Reevaluate patient if drug is used for more than 2 to 3 weeks.
Elderly patients: Initially, 5 mg P.O. daily at bedtime; doses of more than 10 mg aren't recommended.
Adjust-a-dose: For debilitated patients, initially, 5 mg P.O. daily at bedtime; doses of more than 10 mg aren't recommended. For patients with mild to moderate hepatic impairment or those also taking cimetidine, 5 mg P.O. daily at bedtime.

ADMINISTRATION
P.O.
● Don't give drug after a high-fat or heavy meal.

ACTION
A hypnotic with chemical structure unrelated to benzodiazepines that interacts with the GABA-benzodiazepine receptor complex in the CNS. Modulation of this complex is thought to be responsible for sedative, anxiolytic, muscle relaxant,

and anticonvulsant effects of benzodiazepines.

Route	Onset	Peak	Duration
P.O.	1 hr	1 hr	3–4 hr

Half-life: 1 hour.

ADVERSE REACTIONS
CNS: complex sleep-related behaviors,
headache, amnesia, anxiety, asthenia,
depersonalization, depression, difficulty
concentrating, dizziness, fever, hallucinations, hypertonia, hypesthesia, malaise,
migraine, nervousness, paresthesia,
somnolence, tremor, vertigo.
CV: chest pain, peripheral edema.
EENT: abnormal vision, conjunctivitis,
ear discomfort, epistaxis, eye discomfort,
hyperacusis, smell alteration.
GI: abdominal pain, anorexia, colitis,
constipation, dry mouth, dyspepsia,
nausea.
GU: dysmenorrhea.
Musculoskeletal: arthritis, back pain,
myalgia.
Respiratory: bronchitis.
Skin: photosensitivity reactions, pruritus,
rash.
Other: *anaphylaxis, angioedema.*

INTERACTIONS
Drug-drug. *Carbamazepine, phenobarbital, phenytoin, rifampin, other
CYP3A4 inducers:* May reduce
zaleplon bioavailability and peak
level by 80%. Consider using a different hypnotic.
Cimetidine: May increase zaleplon
bioavailability and peak level by 85%.
Use an initial zaleplon dose of 5 mg.
*CNS depressants (imipramine,
thioridazine):* May cause additive CNS
effects. Use together cautiously.
Drug-food. *High-fat foods, heavy meals:*
May prolong absorption, delaying peak
drug level by about 2 hours; may delay
sleep onset. Advise patient to avoid taking
with meals.
Drug-lifestyle. *Alcohol use:* May
increase CNS effects. Discourage use
together.

EFFECTS ON LAB TEST RESULTS
None reported.

CONTRAINDICATIONS & CAUTIONS
• Contraindicated in patients with severe
hepatic impairment.
• Use cautiously in elderly, depressed, or
debilitated patients, in breast-feeding
women, and in patients with compromised
respiratory function.

NURSING CONSIDERATIONS
• *Alert:* Monitor patient closely. Anaphylaxis and angioedema may occur as early
as the first dose.
• Because drug works rapidly, give
immediately before bedtime or after
patient has gone to bed and has had difficulty falling asleep.
• Closely monitor patients who have
compromised respiratory function caused
by illness or who are elderly or debilitated
because they are more sensitive to respiratory depression.
• Start treatment only after carefully evaluating patient because sleep disturbances
may be a symptom of an underlying
physical or psychiatric disorder.
• Adverse reactions are usually dose-
related. Consult prescriber about dose
reduction if adverse reactions occur.

PATIENT TEACHING
• *Alert:* Warn patient that drug may cause
allergic reactions, facial swelling, and
complex sleep-related behaviors, such as
driving, eating, and making phone calls
while asleep. Advise patient to report
these adverse effects.
• Advise patient that drug works
rapidly and should only be taken immediately before bedtime or after he has
gone to bed and has had trouble falling
asleep.
• Advise patient to take drug only if he will
be able to sleep for at least 4 undisturbed
hours.
• Caution patient that drowsiness, dizziness, light-headedness, and coordination
problems occur most often within 1 hour
after taking drug.
• Advise patient to avoid performing
activities that require mental alertness
until CNS adverse reactions are known.
• Advise patient to avoid alcohol use
while taking drug and to notify prescriber
before taking other prescription or OTC
drugs.

Reactions may be *common,* uncommon, *life-threatening,* or COMMON AND LIFE-THREATENING.
Interaction may have a *rapid onset* or *delayed onset.*

• Tell patient not to take drug after a high-fat or heavy meal.

• Advise patient to report sleep problems that continue despite use of drug.

• Notify patient that dependence can occur and that drug is recommended for short-term use only.

• Warn patient not to abruptly stop drug because of the risk of withdrawal symptoms, including unpleasant feelings, stomach and muscle cramps, vomiting, sweating, shakiness, and seizures.

• Notify patient that insomnia may recur for a few nights after stopping drug but should resolve on its own.

• Warn patient that drug may cause changes in behavior and thinking, including outgoing or aggressive behavior, loss of personal identity, confusion, strange behavior, agitation, hallucinations, worsening of depression, or suicidal thoughts. Tell patient to notify prescriber immediately if these symptoms occur.

SAFETY ALERT!

zolpidem tartrate
ZOL-pih-dem

Ambien✐, Ambien CR

Pharmacologic class:
imidazopyridine
Pregnancy risk category C
Controlled substance schedule IV

AVAILABLE FORMS
Tablets: 5 mg, 10 mg
Tablets (extended-release): 6.25 mg, 12.5 mg

INDICATIONS & DOSAGES
➤ **Short-term management of insomnia**
Adults: 10 mg immediate-release tablet, or 12.5 mg extended-release P.O. immediately before bedtime.
Elderly patients: 5 mg immediate-release tablet, or 6.25 mg extended-release P.O. immediately before bedtime. Maximum daily dose is 10 mg immediate-release or 6.25 mg extended-release.

Adjust-a-dose: For debilitated patients and those with hepatic insufficiency, 5 mg P.O. immediately before bedtime. Maximum daily dose is 10 mg immediate-release and 6.25 mg extended-release.

ADMINISTRATION
P.O.
• For rapid sleep onset, drug should be taken with or immediately after meals.
• For ODTs, the tablet is placed in the mouth, allowed to disintegrate, and then swallowed. Tablet may be taken with or without water. Don't crush, break, or split tablet.
• Don't crush, break, or divide extended-release tablets.

ACTION
Although drug interacts with one of three identified GABA-benzodiazepine receptor complexes, it isn't a benzodiazepine. It exhibits hypnotic activity and minimal muscle relaxant and anticonvulsant properties.

Route	Onset	Peak	Duration
P.O.	Rapid	30–120 min	Unknown

Half-life: 2½ hours.

ADVERSE REACTIONS
CNS: *headache,* amnesia, change in dreams, complex sleep-related behaviors, daytime drowsiness, depression, dizziness, hangover, lethargy, light-headedness, nervousness, sleep disorder.
CV: palpitations.
EENT: pharyngitis, sinusitis.
GI: abdominal pain, constipation, diarrhea, dry mouth, dyspepsia, nausea, vomiting.
Musculoskeletal: arthralgia, myalgia.
Skin: rash.
Other: *anaphylaxis, angioedema,* back or chest pain, flulike syndrome, hypersensitivity reactions.

INTERACTIONS
Drug-drug. *CNS depressants:* May cause excessive CNS depression. Use together cautiously.
Rifampin: May decrease effects of zolpidem. Avoid using together, if possible. Consider another hypnotic.

Drug-lifestyle. *Alcohol use:* May cause excessive CNS depression. Discourage use together.

EFFECTS ON LAB TEST RESULTS
None reported.

CONTRAINDICATIONS & CAUTIONS
• No known contraindications.
• Use cautiously in patients with compromised respiratory status.

NURSING CONSIDERATIONS
• *Alert:* Anaphylaxis and angioedema may occur as early as the first dose. Monitor patient closely.
• Use drug only for short-term management of insomnia, usually 7 to 10 days.
• Use the smallest effective dose in all patients.
• Take precautions to prevent hoarding by patients who are depressed, suicidal, or drug-dependent, or who have a history of drug abuse.
• *Look alike–sound alike:* Don't confuse Ambien with Amen.

PATIENT TEACHING
• *Alert:* Warn patient that drug may cause allergic reactions, facial swelling, and complex sleep-related behaviors, such as driving, eating, and making phone calls while asleep. Advise patient to report these adverse effects.
• For rapid sleep onset, instruct patient not to take drug with or immediately after meals.
• Instruct patient to take drug immediately before going to bed; onset of action is rapid.
• Tell patient to avoid alcohol use while taking drug.
• For ODTs, tell patient to place the tablet in the mouth, allow the tablet to disintegrate, and then tell the patient to swallow. The tablet may be taken with or without water. Tell the patient not to chew, break, or split the tablet.
• *Alert:* Tell patient not to crush, chew, or divide the extended-release tablets.
• Caution patient to avoid performing activities that require mental alertness or physical coordination during therapy.

Reactions may be *common*, uncommon, *life-threatening*, or COMMON AND LIFE-THREATENING.
Interaction may have a *rapid onset* or *delayed onset.*

49

Antigout drugs

allopurinol
allopurinol sodium
probenecid
sulfinpyrazone

---

allopurinol
al-oh-PURE-i-nole

Zyloprim

allopurinol sodium
Aloprim

Pharmacologic class: xanthine
oxidase inhibitor
Pregnancy risk category C

AVAILABLE FORMS
allopurinol
Tablets (scored): 100 mg, 300 mg
allopurinol sodium
Injection: 500 mg/30-ml vial

INDICATIONS & DOSAGES
➤ **Gout or hyperuricemia**
Adults: Mild gout, 200 to 300 mg P.O.
daily; severe gout with large tophi, 400 to
600 mg P.O. daily. Maximum 800 mg
daily. Dosage varies with severity of
disease; can be given as single dose or
divided, but doses greater than 300 mg
should be divided.
➤ **Hyperuricemia caused by
malignancies**
Adults and children older than age 10:
200 to 400 mg/m^2 daily I.V. as a single
infusion or in equally divided doses every
6, 8, or 12 hours. Maximum 600 mg daily.
Children age 10 and younger: Initially,
200 mg/m^2 daily I.V. as single infusion
or in equally divided doses every 6, 8, or
12 hours. Then titrate according to uric
acid levels. For children ages 6 to 10, give
300 mg P.O. daily or divided t.i.d.; for
children younger than age 6, give 150 mg
P.O. daily.
➤ **To prevent acute gout attacks**
Adults: 100 mg P.O. daily; increase at
weekly intervals by 100 mg without

exceeding maximum dose (800 mg) until
uric acid falls to 6 mg/dl or less.
➤ **To prevent uric acid nephropathy
during cancer chemotherapy**
Adults: 600 to 800 mg P.O. daily for 2 to
3 days, with high fluid intake.
➤ **Recurrent calcium oxalate calculi**
Adults: 200 to 300 mg P.O. daily in single
or divided doses.
Adjust-a-dose: If creatinine clearance
is 10 to 20 ml/minute, give 200 mg P.O.
or I.V. daily; if clearance is less than
10 ml/minute, give 100 mg P.O. or I.V.
daily; if clearance is less than 3 ml/minute,
give 100 mg P.O. or I.V. at extended
intervals.

ADMINISTRATION
P.O.
● Give drug with or immediately after
meals to minimize GI upset.
I.V.
● When possible, initiate therapy 24 to
48 hours before the start of chemotherapy
known to cause tumor lysis.
● Dissolve contents of each 30-ml vial
in 25 ml of sterile water for injection.
● Dilute solution to desired concentration
(no greater than 6 mg/ml) with normal
saline solution for injection or D$_5$W.
● Store solution at 68° to 77° F (20° to
25° C) and use within 10 hours. Don't
use solution if it contains particulates or
is discolored.
● **Incompatibilities:** Amikacin, amphotericin B, carmustine, cefotaxime,
chlorpromazine, cimetidine, clindamycin
phosphate, cytarabine, dacarbazine,
daunorubicin, diphenhydramine, doxorubicin, doxycycline hyclate, droperidol,
floxuridine, gentamicin, haloperidol
lactate, hydroxyzine, idarubicin, imipenem
and cilastatin sodium, mechlorethamine,
meperidine, methylprednisolone sodium
succinate, metoclopramide, minocycline,
nalbuphine, netilmicin, ondansetron,
prochlorperazine edisylate, promethazine,
sodium bicarbonate (or solutions containing sodium bicarbonate), streptozocin,
tobramycin sulfate, vinorelbine.

ACTION
Reduces uric acid production by inhibiting xanthine oxidase.

Route	Onset	Peak	Duration
P.O.	Unknown	30–120 hr	1–2 wk
I.V.	Unknown	30 min	Unknown

Half-life: Allopurinol, 1 to 2 hours; oxypurinol, about 15 hours.

ADVERSE REACTIONS
CNS: fever, drowsiness, headache, paresthesia, peripheral neuropathy, neuritis.
CV: hypersensitivity vasculitis, necrotizing angiitis.
EENT: epistaxis.
GI: nausea, vomiting, diarrhea, abdominal pain, gastritis, taste loss or perversion, dyspepsia.
GU: *renal failure,* uremia.
Hematologic: *agranulocytosis,* anemia, *aplastic anemia, thrombocytopenia, leukopenia,* leukocytosis, eosinophilia.
Hepatic: *hepatitis, hepatic necrosis,* hepatomegaly, cholestatic jaundice.
Musculoskeletal: arthralgia, myopathy.
Skin: *erythema multiforme,* rash, *toxic epidermal necrolysis,* exfoliative, urticarial, and purpuric lesions; severe furunculosis of nose; ichthyosis; alopecia.
Other: ecchymoses, chills.

INTERACTIONS
Drug-drug. *Amoxicillin, ampicillin:* May increase possibility of rash. Avoid using together.
Anticoagulants: May increase anti-coagulant effect. Dosage may need to be adjusted.
Antineoplastics: May increase potential for bone marrow suppression. Monitor patient carefully.
Azathioprine, mercaptopurine: May increase levels of these drugs. Concomitant administration of 300 to 600 mg of oral allopurinol per day requires dosage reduction to ⅓ to ¼ of usual dose of azathioprine or mercaptopurine. Make subsequent dosage adjustments based on thera-peutic response and appearance of toxic effects.

Chlorpropamide: May increase hypoglycemic effect. Avoid using together.
Ethacrynic acid, thiazide diuretics: May increase risk of allopurinol toxicity. Reduce allopurinol dosage, and monitor renal function closely.
Uricosurics: May have additive effect. May be used to therapeutic advantage.
Urine-acidifying drugs (ammonium chloride, ascorbic acid, potassium or sodium phosphate): May increase possibility of kidney stone formation. Monitor patient carefully.
Xanthines: May increase theophylline level. Adjust dosage of theophylline as needed.
Drug-lifestyle. *Alcohol use:* May increase uric acid level. Discourage use together.

EFFECTS ON LAB TEST RESULTS
● May increase alkaline phosphatase, ALT, and AST levels.
● May decrease hemoglobin level and hematocrit.
● May increase eosinophil count.
● May decrease granulocyte and platelet counts.
● May increase or decrease WBC count.

CONTRAINDICATIONS & CAUTIONS
● Contraindicated in patients hypersensitive to drug and in those with idiopathic hemochromatosis.

NURSING CONSIDERATIONS
● Monitor uric acid level to evaluate drug's effectiveness.
● Monitor fluid intake and output; daily urine output of at least 2 L and mainte-nance of neutral or slightly alkaline urine are desirable.
● Periodically monitor CBC and hepatic and renal function, especially at start of therapy.
● Optimal benefits may need 2 to 6 weeks of therapy. Because acute gout attacks may occur during this time, concurrent use of colchicine may be prescribed prophylactically.
● Don't restart drug in patients who have a severe reaction.
● *Look alike–sound alike:* Don't confuse Zyloprim with ZORprin.

Reactions may be *common,* uncommon, *life-threatening,* or COMMON AND LIFE-THREATENING.
Interaction may have a *rapid onset* or *delayed onset.*

PATIENT TEACHING
● To minimize GI adverse reactions, tell patient to take drug with or immediately after meals.
● Encourage patient to drink plenty of fluids while taking drug unless otherwise contraindicated.
● Drug may cause drowsiness; tell patient not to drive or perform hazardous tasks requiring mental alertness until CNS effects of drug are known.
● If patient is taking drug for recurrent calcium oxalate stones, advise him also to reduce his dietary intake of animal protein, sodium, refined sugars, oxalate-rich foods, and calcium.
● Tell patient to stop drug at first sign of rash, which may precede severe hypersensitivity or other adverse reactions. Rash is more common in patients taking diuretics and in those with renal disorders. Tell patient to report all adverse reactions.
● Advise patient to avoid alcohol during therapy.
● Teach patient importance of continuing drug even if asymptomatic.

---

probenecid
proe-BEN-e-sid

Pharmacologic class: sulfonamide derivative
Pregnancy risk category B

AVAILABLE FORMS
Tablets: 500 mg

INDICATIONS & DOSAGES
➤ **Adjunct to penicillin therapy**
Adults and children weighing more than 50 kg (110 lb): 500 mg P.O. q.i.d.
Children ages 2 to 14 or weighing 50 kg or less: Initially, 25 mg/kg P.O.; then 40 mg/kg/day in divided doses q.i.d.
➤ **Alternate therapy for uncomplicated gonorrhea**
Adults: Cefoxitin 2 g I.M. with probenecid 1 g P.O.
➤ **Hyperuricemia of gout, gouty arthritis**
Adults: 250 mg P.O. b.i.d. for first week; then 500 mg b.i.d., to maximum of 2 to 3 g daily. Review maintenance dose every

6 months and reduce by increments of 500 mg, if indicated.

ADMINISTRATION
P.O.
● To minimize GI distress, give drug with milk, food, or antacids. If unrelieved, consider reducing dosage.

ACTION
Blocks renal tubular reabsorption of uric acid, increasing excretion, and inhibits active renal tubular secretion of many weak organic acids, such as penicillins and cephalosporins.

Route	Onset	Peak	Duration
P.O.	Unknown	2–4 hr	Unknown

Half-life: 3 to 8 hours after 500-mg dose; 4 to 17 hours after larger doses.

ADVERSE REACTIONS
CNS: fever, *headache,* dizziness.
CV: flushing.
GI: anorexia, nausea, vomiting, sore gums.
GU: urinary frequency, renal colic, nephrotic syndrome, costovertebral pain.
Hematologic: *aplastic anemia,* hemolytic anemia, anemia.
Hepatic: *hepatic necrosis.*
Skin: dermatitis, pruritus.
Other: worsening of gout, hypersensitivity reactions including *anaphylaxis.*

INTERACTIONS
Drug-drug. *Acyclovir, cephalosporins, clofibrate, dapsone, ketamine, lorazepam, meclofenamate, penicillin, rifampin, sulfonamides, thiopental:* May increase levels of these drugs. Use together cautiously.
Allopurinol: May increase uric acid–lowering effects. May be used to therapeutic advantage.
Methotrexate: May impair excretion of methotrexate, causing increased level, effects, and toxicity of methotrexate. Monitor methotrexate level closely and adjust dosage accordingly.
Nitrofurantoin: May increase toxicity and reduce effectiveness of nitrofurantoin. Reduce probenecid dose.
NSAIDs: May increase NSAID toxicity. Avoid using together.

---

†Canada　　◇OTC　　◆ Off-label use　　✐Photoguide　　*Liquid contains alcohol.

Salicylates: May inhibit uricosuric effect of probenecid, causing urate retention. Avoid using together.
Sulfonylureas: May increase hypoglycemic effect. Monitor glucose level closely. Dosage may need to be adjusted.
Zidovudine: May increase zidovudine level and toxicity symptoms. Monitor patient.
Drug-lifestyle. *Alcohol use:* May increase urate level. Discourage use together.

EFFECTS ON LAB TEST RESULTS
● May decrease hemoglobin level and hematocrit.
● May falsely elevate theophylline level.

CONTRAINDICATIONS & CAUTIONS
● Contraindicated in patients hypersensitive to drug and in those with uric acid kidney stones or blood dyscrasias; also contraindicated in patients with an acute gout attack and in children younger than age 2.
● Use cautiously in patients with peptic ulcer or renal impairment.
● Use cautiously in patients with sulfa allergy because probenecid is a sulfonamide derivative.

NURSING CONSIDERATIONS
● Force fluids to maintain minimum daily output of 2 to 3 L. Alkalinize urine with sodium bicarbonate or potassium citrate. These measures prevent hematuria, renal colic, urate stone development, and costovertebral pain.
● Don't use to treat gout until acute attack subsides. Drug has no analgesic or anti-inflammatory effects and is of no value during acute gout attacks.
● Monitor BUN and renal function test results periodically in long-term therapy.
● Drug is suitable for long-term use; no cumulative effects or tolerance have been reported.
● Drug is ineffective in patients with glomerular filtration rate below 30 ml/minute.
● Drug may increase frequency, severity, and length of acute gout attacks during first 6 to 12 months of therapy. Appropriate therapy may be used preventively during first 3 to 6 months.
● *Look alike–sound alike:* Don't confuse probenecid with Procanbid.

PATIENT TEACHING
● Instruct patient with gout to take drug regularly to prevent recurrence.
● Tell patient to visit prescriber regularly so that uric acid can be monitored and dosage adjusted, if needed. Lifelong therapy may be needed in patients with hyperuricemia.
● Advise patient with gout to avoid all drugs that contain aspirin, which may precipitate gout. Acetaminophen may be used for pain.
● Instruct patient to drink at least 6 to 8 glasses of water per day.
● Urge patient with gout to avoid alcohol; it increases urate level.
● Tell patient with gout to limit intake of foods high in purine, such as anchovies, liver, sardines, kidneys, sweetbreads, peas, and lentils. Also tell him to identify and avoid other foods that may trigger gout attacks.
● Because drug may be prescribed with an antibiotic, instruct patient to take all medicine as prescribed.

sulfinpyrazone
sul-fin-PEER-a-zone

Pharmacologic class: pyrazolone derivative
Pregnancy risk category NR

AVAILABLE FORMS
Capsules: 200 mg
Tablets: 100 mg

INDICATIONS & DOSAGES
➤ **Intermittent or chronic gouty arthritis**
Adults: 200 to 400 mg P.O. daily, divided b.i.d. during the first week; then 400 mg P.O. daily divided b.i.d. Maximum dose is 800 mg daily.
➤ **To decrease the risk of sudden cardiac death 1 to 6 months after an MI ◆**
Adults: 300 mg P.O. q.i.d.

ADMINISTRATION
P.O.
● Give drug with food, milk, or antacids to reduce GI upset.

ACTION
Blocks renal tubular reabsorption of uric acid, increasing excretion, and inhibits platelet aggregation.

Route	Onset	Peak	Duration
P.O.	Unknown	1–2 hr	4–6 hr

Half-life: 3 hours.

ADVERSE REACTIONS
GI: *nausea, dyspepsia,* epigastric pain, reactivation of peptic ulcerations.
Hematologic: *leukopenia, agranulocytosis, thrombocytopenia, aplastic anemia,* anemia.
Respiratory: *bronchoconstriction in patients with aspirin-induced asthma.*
Skin: rash.

INTERACTIONS
Drug-drug. *Aspirin, niacin,* **salicylates:** May inhibit uricosuric effect of sulfinpyrazone. Avoid using together.
Cholestyramine: May bind and delay absorption of sulfinpyrazone. Give sulfinpyrazone 1 hour before or 4 to 6 hours after cholestyramine.
Oral anticoagulants: May increase anticoagulant effect and risk of bleeding. Use together cautiously.
Oral antidiabetics: May increase effects of these drugs. Monitor glucose level.
Probenecid: May inhibit renal excretion of sulfinpyrazone. Use together cautiously.
Theophylline, verapamil: May increase clearance of these drugs. Use together cautiously.
Drug-lifestyle. *Alcohol use:* May decrease effectiveness. Discourage use together.

EFFECTS ON LAB TEST RESULTS
• May increase BUN and creatinine levels.
• May decrease hemoglobin level and hematocrit.
• May decrease WBC, granulocyte, and platelet counts.

CONTRAINDICATIONS & CAUTIONS
• Contraindicated in patients hypersensitive to pyrazolones (including oxyphenbutazone and phenylbutazone) and in those with blood dyscrasias, active peptic ulcer, or symptoms of GI inflammation or ulceration.

• Use cautiously in patients with healed peptic ulcer and in pregnant women.

NURSING CONSIDERATIONS
• Monitor BUN, CBC, and renal function studies periodically during long-term use.
• Monitor fluid intake and output closely. Therapy, especially at start, may lead to renal colic and formation of uric acid stones until acid levels are normal (about 6 mg/dl).
• Force fluids to maintain minimum daily output of 2 to 3 L. Alkalinize urine with sodium bicarbonate or other drug.
• Drug has no anti-inflammatory or analgesic effects and is of no value during acute gout attacks.
• Drug may increase frequency, severity, and length of acute gout attacks during first 6 to 12 months of therapy. Appropriate therapy may be used preventively during first 3 to 6 months.
• Lifelong therapy may be needed in patients with hyperuricemia.

PATIENT TEACHING
• Instruct patient and family that drug must be taken regularly, even during acute exacerbations.
• Tell patient to take drug with food, milk, or antacids to reduce GI upset.
• Tell patient to visit prescriber regularly so blood levels can be monitored and dosage adjusted, if needed.
• Warn patient with gout not to take aspirin-containing drugs because these may precipitate gout. Acetaminophen may be used for pain.
• Tell patient with gout to avoid foods high in purine, such as anchovies, liver, sardines, kidneys, sweetbreads, peas, and lentils, and to identify and avoid any other foods that may trigger gout attacks.
• Instruct patient to drink at least 10 to 12 glasses of fluid daily.
• Advise patient to avoid alcohol during therapy.
• Instruct patient to report unusual bleeding, bruising, or flulike symptoms.

50

Antiresorptive drugs

alendronate sodium
calcitonin salmon
ibandronate sodium
pamidronate disodium
risedronate sodium
zoledronic acid

---

alendronate sodium
ah-LEN-dro-nate

Fosamax✦, Fosamax Plus D

Pharmacologic class:
bisphosphonate
Pregnancy risk category C

AVAILABLE FORMS
Tablets: 5 mg, 10 mg, 35 mg, 40 mg, 70 mg, 70 mg plus 2,800 international units vitamin D_3
Oral solution: 70 mg/75 ml

INDICATIONS & DOSAGES
➤ **Osteoporosis in postmenopausal women; to increase bone mass in men with osteoporosis**
Adults: 10 mg P.O. daily or 70-mg tablet or solution P.O. once weekly.
➤ **Paget disease of bone (osteitis deformans)**
Adults: 40 mg P.O. daily for 6 months.
➤ **To prevent osteoporosis in post-menopausal women**
Adults: 5 mg P.O. daily or 35-mg tablet P.O. once weekly.
➤ **Glucocorticoid-induced osteoporosis in patients receiving glucocorticoids in a daily dose equivalent to 7.5 mg or more of prednisone and who have low bone mineral density**
Adults: 5 mg P.O. daily. For postmenopausal women not receiving estrogen, recommended dose is 10 mg P.O. daily.

ADMINISTRATION
P.O.
• Give drug with 6 to 8 ounces of water at least 30 minutes before patient's first food or drink of the day to facilitate delivery to the stomach.
• Give at least 2 ounces of water after oral solution.
• Don't allow patient to lie down for 30 minutes after taking drug.

ACTION
Suppresses osteoclast activity on newly formed resorption surfaces, which reduces bone turnover. Bone formation exceeds resorption at remodeling sites, leading to progressive gains in bone mass.

Route	Onset	Peak	Duration
P.O.	Unknown	Unknown	Unknown

Half-life: More than 10 years.

ADVERSE REACTIONS
CNS: headache.
GI: abdominal pain, nausea, dyspepsia, constipation, diarrhea, flatulence, acid regurgitation, esophageal ulcer, vomiting, dysphagia, abdominal distention, gastritis, taste perversion.
Musculoskeletal: pain.

INTERACTIONS
Drug-drug. *Antacids, calcium supplements, many oral drugs:* May interfere with absorption of alendronate. Instruct patient to wait at least 30 minutes after taking alendronate before taking other drug orally.
Aspirin, NSAIDs: May increase risk of upper GI adverse reactions with drug doses greater than 10 mg daily. Monitor patient closely.
Ranitidine (I.V. form): May increase availability of alendronate. Reduce dosage as needed.
Drug-food. *Any food:* May decrease absorption of drug. Advise patient to take with full glass of water at least 30 minutes before food, beverages, or ingestion of other drugs.

Reactions may be *common*, uncommon, ***life-threatening***, or COMMON AND LIFE-THREATENING.
Interaction may have a *rapid onset* or **delayed onset**.

EFFECTS ON LAB TEST RESULTS
• May decrease calcium and phosphate levels.

CONTRAINDICATIONS & CAUTIONS
• Contraindicated in patients hypersensitive to drug and in those with hypocalcemia, severe renal insufficiency (CrCl less than 35 ml/min), or abnormalities of the esophagus that delay esophageal emptying.
• Use cautiously in patients with active upper GI problems (dysphagia, symptomatic esophageal diseases, gastritis, duodenitis, ulcers) or mild to moderate renal insufficiency.

NURSING CONSIDERATIONS
• Correct hypocalcemia and other disturbances of mineral metabolism (such as vitamin D deficiency) before therapy begins.
• When used to treat osteoporosis, disease may be confirmed by findings of low bone mass on diagnostic studies or by history of osteoporotic fracture.
• The recommended daily intake of vitamin D is 400 to 800 international units. Fosamax Plus D provides 400 international units daily when taken once weekly. Patients at risk for vitamin D deficiency, such as those who are chronically ill, who are nursing home bound, who have a GI malabsorption syndrome, or who are older than age 70, may require additional supplementation.
• In Paget disease, drug is indicated for patients with alkaline phosphatase level at least two times upper limit of normal, for those who are symptomatic, and for those at risk for future complications from the disease.
• Monitor patient's calcium and phosphate levels throughout therapy.
• Severe musculoskeletal pain has been associated with biophosphate use and may occur within days, months, or years of start of therapy. When drug is stopped, symptoms may resolve partially or completely.
• *Look alike–sound alike:* Don't confuse Fosamax with Flomax.

PATIENT TEACHING
• Stress importance of taking tablet only with 6 to 8 ounces of water at least 30 minutes before ingesting anything else, including food, beverages, and other drugs. Tell patient that waiting longer than 30 minutes improves absorption.
• Warn patient not to lie down for at least 30 minutes after taking drug to facilitate delivery to stomach and to reduce risk of esophageal irritation.
• Advise patient to report adverse effects immediately, especially chest pain or difficulty swallowing.
• Advise patient to take supplemental calcium and vitamin D if dietary intake is inadequate.
• Tell patient about benefits of weight-bearing exercises in increasing bone mass. If applicable, explain importance of reducing or eliminating cigarette smoking and alcohol use.

calcitonin salmon
kal-si-TOE-nin

Fortical, Miacalcin

Pharmacologic class: polypeptide hormone
Pregnancy risk category C

AVAILABLE FORMS
Injection: 200 units/ml in 2-ml ampules
Nasal spray: 200 units/activation

INDICATIONS & DOSAGES
➤ **Paget disease of bone (osteitis deformans)**
Adults: Initially, 100 units daily I.M. or subcutaneously. Maintenance dosage is 50 to 100 units daily I.M. or subcutaneously, every other day, or three times weekly.
➤ **Hypercalcemia**
Adults: 4 units/kg every 12 hours I.M. or subcutaneously. If response is inadequate after 1 or 2 days, increase dosage to 8 units/kg I.M. every 12 hours. If response remains unsatisfactory after 2 additional days, increase dosage to maximum of 8 units/kg I.M. every 6 hours.
➤ **Postmenopausal osteoporosis**
Adults: 200 units (one activation) daily intranasally, alternating nostrils daily. Or,

100 units I.M. or subcutaneously every other day. Patient should receive adequate vitamin D and calcium supplements (1.5 g calcium carbonate and 400 units of vitamin D) daily.

ADMINISTRATION
I.M.
● I.M. route is preferred if volume of dose exceeds 2 ml.
● Use freshly reconstituted solution within 2 hours.
● Give drug at bedtime, when possible, to minimize nausea and vomiting.
Intranasal
● Alternate nostrils daily.
● Give drug at bedtime, when possible, to minimize nausea and vomiting.
Subcutaneous
● Use freshly reconstituted solution within 2 hours.
● Give drug at bedtime, when possible, to minimize nausea and vomiting.
● Alternate injection sites.

ACTION
Decreases osteoclastic activity by inhibiting osteocytic osteolysis; decreases mineral release and matrix or collagen breakdown in bone.

Route	Onset	Peak	Duration
I.M., Subcut.	15 min	4 hr	8–24 hr
Intranasal	Rapid	30 min	1 hr

Half-life: 43 to 60 minutes.

ADVERSE REACTIONS
CNS: headache, weakness, dizziness, paresthesia.
CV: chest pressure, *facial flushing.*
EENT: eye pain, *nasal congestion, rhinitis.*
GI: *transient nausea,* unusual taste, diarrhea, anorexia, *vomiting,* epigastric discomfort, abdominal pain.
GU: *increased urinary frequency,* nocturia.
Respiratory: shortness of breath.
Skin: rash, pruritus of ear lobes, *inflammation at injection site.*
Other: hypersensitivity reactions, ***anaphylaxis,*** edema of feet, chills, tender palms and soles.

INTERACTIONS
Biphosphonates: Prior use of biphosphonates in patients with Paget disease may reduce the antiresorptive response to nasal spray. Monitor patient.

EFFECTS ON LAB TEST RESULTS
None reported.

CONTRAINDICATIONS & CAUTIONS
● Contraindicated in patients hypersensitive to drug.

NURSING CONSIDERATIONS
● Skin test is usually done in patients with suspected drug sensitivity before therapy.
● ***Alert:*** Systemic allergic reactions are possible because hormone is protein. Keep epinephrine nearby.
● ***Alert:*** Observe patient for signs of hypocalcemic tetany during therapy (muscle twitching, tetanic spasms, and seizures when hypocalcemia is severe).
● Monitor calcium level closely. Watch for symptoms of hypercalcemia relapse: bone pain, renal calculi, polyuria, anorexia, nausea, vomiting, thirst, constipation, lethargy, bradycardia, muscle hypotonicity, pathologic fracture, psychosis, and coma.
● Periodic examinations of urine sediment are recommended.
● Monitor periodic alkaline phosphatase and 24-hour urine hydroxyproline levels to evaluate drug effect.
● In Paget disease, maximum reductions of alkaline phosphatase and urinary hydroxyproline excretion may take 6 to 24 months of continuous treatment.
● In patients with good first response to drug who have a relapse, expect to evaluate antibody response to the hormone protein.
● If symptoms have been relieved after 6 months, treatment may be stopped until symptoms or radiologic signs recur.
● Refrigerate drug at 36° to 46° F (2° to 8° C).
● ***Look alike–sound alike:*** Don't confuse calcitonin with calcifediol or calcitriol.

PATIENT TEACHING
● When drug is given for postmenopausal osteoporosis, remind patient to take adequate calcium and vitamin D supplements.
● Show home care patient and family member how to give drug. Tell them to do

---

Reactions may be *common,* uncommon, ***life-threatening,*** or COMMON AND LIFE-THREATENING.
Interaction may have a *rapid onset* or ***delayed onset.***

so at bedtime if only one dose is needed daily. If nasal spray is prescribed, tell patient to alternate nostrils daily.
• Advise patient to notify prescriber if significant nasal irritation or evidence of an allergic response occurs.
• Inform patient that facial flushing and warmth occur in 20% to 30% of patients within minutes of injection and usually last about 1 hour.
• Tell patient that nausea and vomiting may occur at the onset of therapy.
• Tell patient to inform prescriber promptly if signs and symptoms of hypercalcemia occur. Inform patient that, if drug loses its hypocalcemic activity, other drugs or increased dosages won't help.

---

ibandronate sodium
eh-BAN-drow-nate

Boniva

Pharmacologic class:
bisphosphonate
Pregnancy risk category C

AVAILABLE FORMS
Injection: 3 mg/3-ml prefilled syringe
Tablets: 2.5 mg, 150 mg

INDICATIONS & DOSAGES
➤ **To treat or prevent postmenopausal osteoporosis**
Women: 2.5 mg P.O. daily or 150 mg P.O. once monthly, taken first thing in the morning, with a large glass of plain water, 1 hour before any food or other drugs. Or, for treatment, 3 mg I.V. bolus once every 3 months.

ADMINISTRATION
P.O.
• Give drug first thing in the morning 1 hour before eating or drinking and before any other drugs.
• Give drug with plain water only.
I.V.
• Prefilled syringes are for single use only.
• Give undiluted using needle provided with the syringe.
• Give by I.V. bolus over 15 to 30 seconds.
• Don't use if drug is discolored or contains particulate matter.

• Store at room temperature.
• **Incompatibilities:** Calcium-containing solutions and other I.V. drugs.

ACTION
Inhibits bone breakdown and removal to reduce bone loss and increase bone mass.

Route	Onset	Peak	Duration
P.O.	Unknown	½–2 hr	Unknown
I.V.	Rapid	Unknown	Unknown

Half-life: 1½ to 6½ days for the 150-mg dose.

ADVERSE REACTIONS
CNS: asthenia, dizziness, headache, insomnia, nerve root lesion, vertigo.
CV: hypertension.
EENT: nasopharyngitis, pharyngitis.
GI: *dyspepsia,* abdominal pain, constipation, diarrhea, gastritis, nausea, vomiting.
GU: UTI.
Musculoskeletal: *back pain,* arthralgia, arthritis, joint disorder, limb pain, localized osteoarthritis, muscle cramps, myalgia.
Respiratory: *bronchitis, upper respiratory tract infection,* pneumonia.
Skin: rash.
Other: allergic reaction, infection, influenza, tooth disorder.

INTERACTIONS
Drug-drug. *Aspirin, NSAIDs:* May increase GI irritation. Use together cautiously.
Products containing aluminum, calcium, magnesium, or iron: May decrease ibandronate absorption. Give oral ibandronate 1 hour before vitamins, minerals, or antacids.
Drug-food. *Food, milk, beverages (except water):* May decrease drug absorption. Give oral drug on an empty stomach with plain water.
Drug-lifestyle. *Alcohol use:* May decrease drug absorption and increase risk of esophageal irritation. Discourage use together.

EFFECTS ON LAB TEST RESULTS
• May increase cholesterol level.
• May decrease total alkaline phosphatase level. May interfere with bone-imaging agents.

CONTRAINDICATIONS & CAUTIONS
• Contraindicated in patients hypersensitive to drug and in those with uncorrected hypocalcemia. Oral form is contraindicated in those who can't stand or sit upright for 60 minutes.
• Don't give to patients with severe renal impairment.
• Use cautiously in patients with a history of GI disorders.

NURSING CONSIDERATIONS
• Correct hypocalcemia or other disturbances of bone and mineral metabolism before therapy.
• Make sure patient has adequate intake of calcium and vitamin D.
• Watch for signs or symptoms of esophageal irritation, including dysphagia, painful swallowing, retrosternal pain, and heartburn.
• Monitor patient for bone, joint, and muscle pain, which may be severe and incapacitating and may occur within days, months, or years of start of therapy. When drug is stopped, symptoms may resolve partially or completely.
• Watch for signs and symptoms of uveitis and scleritis.
• *Alert:* Drug may lead to osteonecrosis, mainly in the jaw. Dental surgery may worsen condition. Consider stopping drug if patient needs a dental procedure.
• Use during pregnancy only if benefit outweighs risk to fetus.
• Use cautiously in breast-feeding women.

PATIENT TEACHING
• Tell patient receiving I.V. form, if she misses a dose, reschedule the missed dose as soon as possible. Subsequent injections should be rescheduled once every 3 months from that dose. She shouldn't receive more than one dose in a 3-month time frame.
• Tell patient taking monthly dose to take it on same date each month and to wait at least 7 days between doses if she misses a scheduled dose.
• Tell patient taking daily dose not to take a missed dose later in the day. She should skip the missed dose and resume her normal schedule the next day.
• Instruct patient to take oral drug first thing in the morning 1 hour before eating or drinking and before any other drugs, including OTC drugs, such as calcium, antacids, and vitamins.
• Advise patient to swallow drug whole with a full glass of plain water while standing or sitting and to remain upright for at least 1 hour after taking drug.
• Caution patient to take only with plain water.
• Instruct patient not to chew or suck on the tablet.
• Advise patient to take calcium and vitamin D supplements as directed by prescriber.
• Tell patient to report any bone, joint, or muscle pain.
• Advise patient to stop drug and immediately report to prescriber signs and symptoms of esophageal irritation, such as dysphagia, painful swallowing, retrosternal pain, or heartburn.

pamidronate disodium
pah-MIH-dro-nate

Aredia

Pharmacologic class:
bisphosphonate
Pregnancy risk category D

AVAILABLE FORMS
Powder for injection: 30 mg/vial, 90 mg/vial
Solution for injection: 3 mg/ml, 6 mg/ml, 9 mg/ml, in 10-ml vials

INDICATIONS & DOSAGES
➤ **Moderate to severe hypercalcemia from cancer (with or without bone metastases)**
Adults: Dosage depends on severity of hypercalcemia. Correct calcium level for albumin. Corrected calcium (CCa) level is calculated using this formula:

$$\text{CCa (mg/dl)} = \text{serum calcium (mg/dl)} + 0.8(4 - \text{serum albumin (g/dl)})$$

Patients with CCa levels of 12 to 13.5 mg/dl may receive 60 to 90 mg by I.V. infusion as a single dose over 2 to 24 hours. Patients with CCa levels greater than 13.5 mg/dl may receive 90 mg by I.V. infusion over 2 to 24 hours. Allow at least 7 days before retreatment to permit full response to first dose.

➤ **Moderate to severe Paget disease**
Adults: 30 mg I.V. as a 4-hour infusion on 3 consecutive days for total dose of 90 mg. Repeat cycle as needed.

➤ **Osteolytic bone metastases of breast cancer with standard antineoplastic therapy**
Adults: 90 mg I.V. infusion over 2 hours every 3 to 4 weeks.

➤ **Osteolytic bone lesions of multiple myeloma**
Adults: 90 mg I.V. over 4 hours once monthly.

ADMINISTRATION
I.V.
- Reconstitute drug with 10 ml of sterile water for injection. After drug is completely dissolved, add to 250 ml (2-hour infusion), 500 ml (4-hour infusion), or 1,000 ml (up to 24-hour infusion) of half-normal or normal saline solution for injection or D₅W.
- Inspect solution for precipitate before use.
- Give drug only by I.V. infusion. Injecting a bolus may cause nephropathy.
- Infusions longer than 2 hours may reduce the risk of renal toxicity, particularly in patients with preexisting renal insufficiency.
- Solution is stable for 24 hours at room temperature.
- Store reconstituted drug at 36° to 46° F (2° to 8° C).
- **Incompatibilities:** Calcium-containing infusion solutions, such as Ringer's injection or lactated Ringer's solution.

ACTION
An antihypercalcemic that inhibits resorption of bone but apparently not bone formation. Adsorbs to hydroxyapatite crystals in bone and may directly block calcium phosphate dissolution and mature osteoclast formation.

Route	Onset	Peak	Duration
I.V.	Unknown	Unknown	Unknown

Half-life: Alpha, 1½ hours; beta, 27¼ hours.

ADVERSE REACTIONS
CNS: *seizures, fatigue,* somnolence, syncope, fever.
CV: *atrial fibrillation,* tachycardia, *hypertension, fluid overload.*
GI: *abdominal pain, anorexia, constipation, nausea, vomiting,* **GI hemorrhage.**
GU: renal dysfunction, *urinary tract infection,* **renal failure.**
Hematologic: *leukopenia, thrombocytopenia,* anemia.
Metabolic: hypophosphatemia, hypokalemia, *hypomagnesemia,* hypocalcemia.
Musculoskeletal: osteonecrosis of the jaw.
Skin: *infusion-site reaction, pain at infusion site.*

INTERACTIONS
None significant.

EFFECTS ON LAB TEST RESULTS
- May increase creatinine level.
- May decrease phosphate, potassium, magnesium, calcium, and hemoglobin levels.
- May decrease WBC and platelet counts.

CONTRAINDICATIONS & CAUTIONS
- Contraindicated in patients hypersensitive to drug or other bisphosphonates such as etidronate.
- Contraindicated in pregnancy.
- Use with caution, considering risks versus benefits, in patients with renal impairment.

NURSING CONSIDERATIONS
- Assess hydration before treatment. Use drug only after patient has been vigorously hydrated with normal saline solution. In patients with mild to moderate hypercalcemia, hydration alone may be sufficient.
- Because drug can cause electrolyte disturbances, carefully monitor electrolyte levels, especially calcium, phosphate, and magnesium. Short-term use of calcium may be needed in patients with severe hypocalcemia. Also monitor CBC and differential count, creatinine and hemoglobin levels, and hematocrit.
- Carefully monitor patients with anemia, leukopenia, or thrombocytopenia during first 2 weeks of therapy.

• Monitor patient's temperature. Patient may experience a slight elevation for 24 to 48 hours after therapy.
• *Alert:* Because renal dysfunction may lead to renal failure, single doses shouldn't exceed 90 mg.
• Monitor creatinine level before each treatment.
• In patients treated for bone metastases who have renal dysfunction, withhold dose until renal function returns to baseline. Treating bone metastases in patients with severe renal impairment isn't recommended. For other indications, determine whether the potential benefit outweighs the potential risk.
• Severe musculoskeletal pain has been associated with biophosphate use and may occur within days, months, or years of start of therapy. When drug is stopped, symptoms may resolve partially or completely.
• Bisphosphonates can interfere with bone-imaging agents.
• *Alert:* Patients should have a dental examination with appropriate preventive dentistry before taking drug, especially those with risk factors, including cancer, chemotherapy, corticosteroid therapy, and poor oral hygiene.
• Use cautiously in breast-feeding women; it's unknown if drug appears in breast milk.

PATIENT TEACHING
• Explain use and administration of drug to patient and family.
• Instruct patient to report adverse reactions promptly.
• Advise woman to alert her health care provider if she is pregnant or breast-feeding.

---

risedronate sodium
rah-SED-dro-nate

Actonel⌀

Pharmacologic class:
bisphosphonate
Pregnancy risk category C

AVAILABLE FORMS
Tablets: 5 mg, 30 mg, 35 mg, 75 mg, 150 mg

INDICATIONS & DOSAGES
➤ **To prevent and treat postmenopausal osteoporosis**
Women: 5-mg tablet P.O. once daily, or 35-mg tablet once weekly.
➤ **To prevent or treat post-menopausal osteoporosis when fewer dosing days are desirable**
Adults: 75 mg P.O. on 2 consecutive days for a total of 2 tablets each month. Or, one 150 mg tablet P.O. once each month.
➤ **To increase bone mass with osteoporosis**
Men: One 35-mg tablet P.O. once weekly.
➤ **Glucocorticoid-induced osteoporosis in patients taking 7.5 mg or more of prednisone or equivalent glucocorticoid daily**
Adults: 5 mg P.O. daily.
➤ **Paget disease**
Adults: 30 mg P.O. daily for 2 months. If relapse occurs or alkaline phosphatase level doesn't normalize, may repeat treatment course 2 months or more after completing first treatment course.
Adjust-a-dose: Don't use if creatinine clearance is less than 30 ml/minute.

ADMINISTRATION
P.O.
• Give drug at least 30 minutes before the first food or drink of the day, other than water. Give with 6 to 8 ounces of water while patient is sitting or standing.
• Warn patient against lying down for 30 minutes after taking drug.

ACTION
Reverses the loss of bone mineral density by reducing bone turnover and bone resorption. In patients with Paget disease, drug causes bone turnover to return to normal.

Route	Onset	Peak	Duration
P.O.	1 hr	Unknown	Unknown

Half-life: 1½ hours to 20 days.

ADVERSE REACTIONS
CNS: asthenia, *headache,* depression, dizziness, insomnia, anxiety, neuralgia, vertigo, hypertonia, paresthesia, *pain.*

Reactions may be *common,* uncommon, ***life-threatening,*** or COMMON AND LIFE-THREATENING.
Interaction may have a *rapid onset* or **delayed onset.**

CV: *hypertension,* CV disorder, angina pectoris, chest pain, peripheral edema.
EENT: pharyngitis, rhinitis, sinusitis, cataract, conjunctivitis, otitis media, amblyopia, tinnitus.
GI: *nausea, diarrhea, abdominal pain,* flatulence, gastritis, rectal disorder, constipation.
GU: *UTI,* cystitis.
Hematologic: ecchymosis, anemia
Musculoskeletal: *arthralgia,* neck pain, *back pain,* myalgia, bone pain, leg cramps, bursitis, tendon disorder.
Respiratory: dyspnea, pneumonia, bronchitis.
Skin: *rash,* pruritus, ***skin carcinoma.***
Other: *infection,* tooth disorder.

INTERACTIONS
Drug-drug. *Calcium supplements, antacids that contain calcium, magnesium, or aluminum:* May interfere with risedronate absorption. Advise patient to separate dosing times.
Drug-food. *Any food:* May interfere with absorption of drug. Advise patient to take drug at least 30 minutes before first food or drink of the day (other than water).

EFFECTS ON LAB TEST RESULTS
● May decrease calcium and phosphorus levels.

CONTRAINDICATIONS & CAUTIONS
● Contraindicated in patients hypersensitive to any component of the product, in hypocalcemic patients, in patients with creatinine clearance less than 30 ml/minute, and in those who can't stand or sit upright for 30 minutes after administration.
● Use cautiously in patients with upper GI disorders, such as dysphagia, esophagitis, and esophageal or gastric ulcers.

NURSING CONSIDERATIONS
● Risk factors for the development of osteoporosis include family history, previous fracture, smoking, a decrease in bone mineral density below the premenopausal mean, a thin body frame, White or Asian race, and early menopause.

● *Alert:* Drug may cause dysphagia, esophagitis, and esophageal or gastric ulcers. Monitor patient for symptoms of esophageal disease.
● Severe musculoskeletal pain has been associated with biophosphate use and may occur within days, months, or years of start of therapy. When drug is stopped, symptoms may resolve partially or completely.
● Give supplemental calcium and vitamin D if dietary intake is inadequate. Because calcium supplements and drugs containing calcium, aluminum, or magnesium may interfere with risedronate absorption, separate dosing times.
● Bisphosphonates can interfere with bone-imaging agents.

PATIENT TEACHING
● Explain that drug may reverse bone loss by stopping more bone loss and increasing bone strength.
● Caution patient about the importance of adhering to special dosing instructions.
● Tell patient not to chew or suck the tablet because doing so may irritate his mouth.
● Advise patient to contact prescriber immediately if he develops GI discomfort (such as difficulty or pain when swallowing, retrosternal pain, or severe heartburn).
● Advise patient to take calcium and vitamin D if dietary intake is inadequate, but to take them at a different time than risedronate.
● Advise patient to stop smoking and drinking alcohol, as appropriate. Also, advise patient to perform weightbearing exercise.
● Tell patient to store drug in a cool, dry place, at room temperature, and away from children.
● Urge patient to read the Patient Information Guide before starting therapy.
● Tell patient if he misses a dose of the 35-mg tablet, he should take 1 tablet on the morning after he remembers and return to taking 1 tablet once a week, as originally scheduled on his chosen day. Patient shouldn't take 2 tablets on the same day.

zoledronic acid
zoh-leh-DROH-nik

Reclast, Zometa

Pharmacologic class:
bisphosphonate
Pregnancy risk category D

AVAILABLE FORMS
*Injection as ready to infuse solution
(Reclast):* 5 mg/100 ml
Injection (Zometa): 4 mg/5-ml vial

INDICATIONS & DOSAGES
➤ **Hypercalcemia caused
by malignancy**
Adults: 4 mg (Zometa) by I.V. infusion
over at least 15 minutes. If albumin-
corrected calcium level doesn't return
to normal, may repeat 4 mg. Let at least
7 days pass before retreatment to allow a
full response to the first dose.
➤ **Multiple myeloma and bone
metastases of solid tumors in
conjunction with standard
antineoplastics**
Adults: 4 mg (Zometa) I.V. infused over
at least 15 minutes every 3 to 4 weeks.
Treatment duration depends on type of
cancer. Use for prostate cancer only after
it has progressed after treatment with at
least one course of hormonal therapy. Give
patients an oral calcium supplement of
500 mg and a multiple vitamin containing
400 international units of vitamin D daily.
Adjust-a-dose: For patients with creatinine clearance of 50 to 60 ml/minute, give
3.5 mg. If 40 to 49 ml/minute, give 3.3 mg.
If 30 to 39 ml/minute, give 3 mg. For
patients with normal baseline creatinine
level but an increase of 0.5 mg/dl and in
those with abnormal baseline creatinine
level who have an increase of 1 mg/dl,
withhold drug. Resume treatment only
when creatinine level has returned to
within 10% of baseline value. If creatinine
clearance is less than 30 ml/minute, don't
give drug.
➤ **Paget disease of bone
(osteitis deformans)**
Adults: 5 mg (Reclast) by I.V. infusion
over at least 15 minutes. Give through a
vented infusion line. May repeat if relapse

occurs. Patient also needs 1,500 mg
elemental calcium and 800 international
units vitamin D daily, especially during
the 2 weeks after dosing.
➤ **Treatment of osteoporosis in
postmenopausal women**
Adults: 5 mg (Reclast) by I.V. infusion
over no less than 15 minutes once a year.
✱*NEW INDICATION:* **To reduce the
incidence of fractures in postmenopausal women with osteoporosis and a recent low-trauma hip
fracture**
Adults: 5 mg (Reclast) by I.V. infusion
over no less than 15 minutes once a year.
Adjust-a-dose: Treatment with Reclast in
patients with severe renal impairment
(creatinine clearance less than
35 ml/minute) isn't recommended. Monitor
serum creatinine level before each dose.

ADMINISTRATION
I.V.
Zometa
● Reconstitute by adding 5 ml of sterile
water to each vial. Inspect solution to
make sure drug is dissolved completely
and there's no particulate matter or
discoloration.
● For patient with creatinine clearance
greater than 60 ml/minute, withdraw 5 ml
to obtain 4 mg of drug and mix in 100 ml
of normal saline solution or D₅W. For
patient with creatinine clearance of
60 ml/minute or less, withdraw 4.4 ml for
the 3.5-mg dose, 4.1 ml for the 3.3-mg
dose, or 3.8 ml for the 3-mg dose.
● Give as I.V. infusion over at least
15 minutes.
● If drug not used immediately after
reconstitution, refrigerate solution and
give within 24 hours.
Reclast
● Reclast is infused over not less than
15 minutes given at a constant infusion
rate. Give as a single I.V. solution through
a separate vented infusion line.
● If refrigerated, allow the refrigerated
solution to reach room temperature before
administration.
● After opening, solution is stable for
24 hours at 36° to 46° F (2° to 8° C).
● **Incompatibilities:** Solutions containing
calcium (such as lactated Ringer's solution)
or other I.V. drugs.

ACTION
Inhibits bone resorption, probably by inhibiting osteoclast activity and osteoclastic resorption of mineralized bone and cartilage. Decreases calcium release induced by the stimulatory factors produced by tumors.

Route	Onset	Peak	Duration
I.V. (Zometa)	Unknown	Unknown	7–28 days
I.V. (Reclast)	Unknown	Unknown	Unknown

Half-life: Alpha is 0.23 hours; beta is 1.75 hours for early distribution. Terminal half-life is 167 hours.

ADVERSE REACTIONS
CNS: *headache,* anxiety, somnolence, *insomnia,* confusion, agitation, *depression, paresthesia, hypoesthesia, fatigue, weakness, dizziness, fever.*
CV: *hypotension, hypertension,* atrial fibrillation, *leg edema.*
GI: *nausea, constipation, diarrhea, abdominal pain, vomiting, anorexia,* dysphagia, *increased appetite.*
GU: *increased creatinine level, urinary infection, candidiasis.*
Hematologic: anemia, *granulocytopenia, neutropenia, thrombocytopenia.*
Metabolic: *decreased calcium, phosphate, and, **magnesium** levels; dehydration; weight decrease.*
Musculoskeletal: *skeletal pain, arthralgia, myalgia, back pain,* osteonecrosis of the jaw.
Respiratory: *dyspnea, cough,* pleural effusion.
Skin: alopecia, dermatitis, rash.
Other: PROGRESSION OF CANCER, *rigors,* infection, influenza.

INTERACTIONS
Drug-drug. *Aminoglycosides, loop diuretics:* May have additive effects that lower calcium level. Use together cautiously, and monitor calcium level.
Nephrotoxic drugs, such as NSAIDs: Renal toxicity may be greater in patients with renal impairment. Use Reclast cautiously with other potentially nephrotoxic drugs. Monitor serum creatinine before each dose.

Thalidomide: May increase risk of renal dysfunction in patients with multiple myeloma. Use together cautiously.

EFFECTS ON LAB TEST RESULTS
● May increase creatinine level.
● May decrease calcium, phosphorus, magnesium, potassium, and hemoglobin levels and hematocrit.
● May decrease RBC, WBC, and platelet counts.

CONTRAINDICATIONS & CAUTIONS
● Contraindicated in patients hypersensitive to drug, other bisphosphonates, or any of its ingredients, in patients with hypercalcemia of malignancy whose creatinine level is more than 4.5 mg/dl, in patients with bone metastases and a creatinine level of more than 3 mg/dl, and in breast-feeding women.
● Reclast is contraindicated in patients with hypocalcemia. Patients must be adequately supplemented with calcium and vitamin D.
● Use cautiously in elderly patients and those with aspirin-sensitive asthma because other bisphosphonates have been linked to bronchoconstriction in aspirin-sensitive patients with asthma.

NURSING CONSIDERATIONS
● Reclast contains the same active ingredient found in Zometa, used for oncology indications. A patient being treated with Zometa shouldn't be treated with Reclast.
● Hydrate patient adequately before giving; urine output should be about 2 L daily.
● Each vial of Zometa contains 220 mg mannitol and 24 mg sodium citrate.
● **Alert:** Because of the risk of decreased renal function progressing to renal failure, don't exceed 4 mg as a single dose of Zometa and always infuse over at least 15 minutes.
● Monitor calcium, phosphate, magnesium, and creatinine levels carefully. Correct decreased calcium, phosphorus, and magnesium levels using I.V. calcium gluconate, potassium and sodium phosphate, and magnesium sulfate.
● Monitor renal function closely. Patients with renal impairment may be at a greater risk for adverse reactions.

• **Alert:** Patients, especially those who have cancer or poor oral hygiene or who are receiving chemotherapy or corticosteroids, should have a dental exam with appropriate preventive dentistry before therapy.
• Osteonecrosis of the jaw has been reported rarely in postmenopausal osteoporosis patients treated with bisphosphonates, including zoledronic acid. All patients should have a routine oral exam before treatment.
• Severe incapacitating bone, joint, and muscle pain may occur. Withhold future doses of Reclast if severe symptoms occur. When drug is stopped, symptoms may resolve partially or completely.

PATIENT TEACHING
• Review the use and administration of drug with patient and family.
• Instruct patient to report adverse effects promptly.
• Explain the importance of periodic laboratory tests to monitor therapy and renal function.
• If a woman becomes pregnant or is breast-feeding, advise her to alert prescriber.

Reactions may be *common*, uncommon, **_life-threatening_**, or **COMMON AND LIFE-THREATENING**.
Interaction may have a *rapid onset* or **_delayed onset_**.

51

Antirheumatics

abatacept
adalimumab
auranofin
aurothioglucose
gold sodium thiomalate
hydroxychloroquine sulfate
(See Chapter 8, ANTIMALARIALS.)
leflunomide

---

abatacept
uh-BAY-tuh-sept

Orencia

Pharmacologic class:
immunomodulator
Pregnancy risk category C

AVAILABLE FORMS
Lyophilized powder for injection:
250 mg single-use vial (25 mg/ml when
reconstituted)

INDICATIONS & DOSAGES
➤ **To reduce signs and symptoms
and structural damage and improve
physical function in patients with
moderate to severe rheumatoid
arthritis whose response to one or
more disease-modifying drugs has
been inadequate. Used alone or with
other disease-modifying drugs
(except tumor necrosis factor [TNF]
antagonists and anakinra)**
*Adults who weigh more than 100 kg
(220 lb):* 1 g I.V. over 30 minutes. Repeat
2 and 4 weeks after initial infusion and
then every 4 weeks thereafter.
*Adults who weigh 60 to 100 kg (132 to
220 lb):* 750 mg I.V. over 30 minutes.
Repeat 2 and 4 weeks after initial infusion
and then every 4 weeks thereafter.
Adults who weigh less than 60 kg: 500 mg
I.V. over 30 minutes. Repeat 2 and 4
weeks after initial infusion and then every
4 weeks thereafter.
✱*NEW INDICATION:* **As monotherapy
or with methotrexate to reduce signs
and symptoms of moderately to**
**severely active juvenile idiopathic
arthritis.**
*Children 6 to 17 years weighing less
than 75 kg (165 lb):* 10 mg/kg I.V. over
30 minutes. Repeat 2 and 4 weeks after
initial infusion and then every 4 weeks
thereafter.
*Children 6 to 17 years weighing 75 kg
(165 lb) or more:* Utilize adult dosing.

ADMINISTRATION
I.V.
● Reconstitute vial with 10 ml of sterile
water for injection, using only the silicone-
free disposable syringe provided, to yield
25 mg/ml.
● Gently swirl contents until completely
dissolved. Avoid vigorous shaking.
● Vent the vial with a needle to clear away
foam.
● The solution should be clear and colorless to pale yellow.
● Further dilute the solution to 100 ml
with normal saline solution. Infuse over
30 minutes using an infusion set and a
sterile, nonpyrogenic, low–protein-binding
filter.
● Store diluted solution at room temperature or refrigerate at 36° to 46° F (2° to
8° C). Complete infusion within 24 hours
of reconstituting.
● **Incompatibilities:** Don't infuse in the
same line with other I.V. drugs.

ACTION
Inhibits T-cell activation, decreases T-cell
proliferation, and inhibits production
of TNF-alpha, interferon-gamma, and
interleukin-2.

Route	Onset	Peak	Duration
I.V.	Unknown	Unknown	Unknown

Half-life: 13 days.

ADVERSE REACTIONS
CNS: *headache,* dizziness.
CV: hypertension.
EENT: *nasopharyngitis,* rhinitis, sinusitis.
GI: *nausea,* diverticulitis, dyspepsia.

GU: acute pyelonephritis, UTI.
Musculoskeletal: back pain, limb pain.
Respiratory: *upper respiratory tract infection,* bronchitis, cough, pneumonia.
Skin: cellulitis, rash.
Other: *infections, malignancies,* herpes simplex, influenza, infusion reactions.

INTERACTIONS
Drug-drug. *Anakinra, TNF antagonists:* May increase risk of infection. Don't use together.
Live-virus vaccines: May decrease effectiveness of vaccine. Avoid giving vaccines during or for 3 months after abatacept therapy.

EFFECTS ON LAB TEST RESULTS
None reported.

CONTRAINDICATIONS & CAUTIONS
• Contraindicated in patients hypersensitive to drug or its components.
• Don't use in patients taking a TNF antagonist or anakinra.
• Use cautiously in patients with active infection, history of chronic infections, scheduled elective surgery, or COPD.
• Patients who test positive for tuberculosis should be treated before receiving drug.

NURSING CONSIDERATIONS
• Make sure patient has been screened for tuberculosis before giving.
• Monitor patient, especially an older adult, carefully for infections and malignancies.
• If patient develops a severe infection, notify prescriber; therapy may need to be stopped.
• If patient has COPD, watch for worsening.
• Drug may cause serious adverse reactions in a breast-fed infant and may affect his developing immune system.
• Ensure the availability of appropriate supportive measures to treat possible hypersensitivity reactions.

PATIENT TEACHING
• Instruct patient to have tuberculosis screening before therapy.
• Tell patient to continue taking prescribed arthritis drugs. Caution against taking TNF antagonists, such as Enbrel, Remicade, and Humira, or anakinra.

• Tell patient to avoid exposure to infections.
• Tell patient to immediately report signs and symptoms of infection, swollen face or tongue, and difficulty breathing.
• Tell patient with COPD to report worsening signs and symptoms.
• Advise patient to avoid live-virus vaccines during and for 3 months after therapy.
• Advise woman to consult prescriber if she becomes pregnant or plans to breast-feed.
• Advise patient to contact prescriber before taking any other drugs or herbal supplements.
• Remind patient to contact prescriber before scheduling surgery.

adalimumab
ay-da-LIM-yoo-mab

Humira

Pharmacologic class: tumor necrosis factor (TNF)-alpha blocker
Pregnancy risk category B

AVAILABLE FORMS
Injection: 40 mg/0.8 ml as prefilled syringes or pens

INDICATIONS & DOSAGES
➤ **Rheumatoid arthritis (RA); psoriatic arthritis; ankylosing spondylitis**
Adults: 40 mg subcutaneously every other week. Patient may continue to take methotrexate, steroids, NSAIDs, salicylates, analgesics or other disease-modifying antirheumatic drugs (known as DMARDs) during therapy. Patients with RA who aren't also taking methotrexate may have the dose increased to 40 mg weekly, if needed.
➤ **Moderate to severe Crohn's disease when response to conventional therapy is inadequate or when response to infliximab is lost or patient can't tolerate the drug**
Adults: Initially, 160 mg subcutaneously on day 1 given as four 40-mg injections in 1 day or as two 40-mg injections per day

---

Reactions may be *common*, uncommon, *life-threatening*, or COMMON AND LIFE-THREATENING.
Interaction may have a *rapid onset* or **delayed onset**.

for 2 consecutive days; then 80 mg 2 weeks later (day 15), followed by a maintenance dose of 40 mg every other week starting at week 4 (day 29).

✳ *NEW INDICATION:* **To reduce the signs and symptoms of moderately to severely active polyarticular juvenile idiopathic arthritis.**

Children 4 to 17 years who weigh between 15 kg (33 lbs) and less than 30 kg (66 lbs): 20 mg subcutaneously every other week.

Children 4 to 17 years who weigh 30 kg (66 lbs) or more: 40 mg subcutaneously every other week.

✳ *NEW INDICATION:* **Moderate to severe chronic plaque psoriasis.**

Adults: 80 mg subcutaneously, followed by 40 mg subcutaneously every other week starting one week after the initial dose. Treatment beyond one year has not bee studied.

ADMINISTRATION
Subcutaneous
● Inject subcutaneously into abdomen or thigh.

ACTION
A recombinant human immunoglobulin G_1 monoclonal antibody that blocks human TNF-alpha. TNF-alpha participates in normal inflammatory and immune responses and in the inflammation and joint destruction of RA.

Route	Onset	Peak	Duration
Subcut.	Variable	Variable	Unknown

Half-life: 10 to 20 days.

ADVERSE REACTIONS
CNS: headache.
CV: *hemorrhage,* hypertension.
EENT: *sinusitis.*
GI: abdominal pain, nausea.
GU: hematuria, UTI.
Hematologic: *leukopenia, pancytopenia, thrombocytopenia.*
Metabolic: hypercholesterolemia, hyperlipidemia.
Musculoskeletal: back pain.
Respiratory: *upper respiratory tract infection,* bronchitis.
Skin: *rash.*

Other: *accidental injury, injection site reactions (erythema, itching, pain, swelling),* **anaphylaxis, malignancy,** allergic reactions, flulike syndrome.

INTERACTIONS
Drug-drug. *Anakinra:* May increase risk of serious infections and neutropenia. Don't use together.
Live-virus vaccines: No data are available on secondary transmission of infection from live-virus vaccines. Avoid using together.
Methotrexate: May decrease clearance of adalimumab. Dosage adjustment isn't necessary.

EFFECTS ON LAB TEST RESULTS
● May increase alkaline phosphatase and cholesterol levels.

CONTRAINDICATIONS & CAUTIONS
● Contraindicated in patients hypersensitive to drug or its components, in immunosuppressed patients, and those with an active chronic or localized infection.
● Use cautiously in patients with demyelinating disorders, a history of recurrent infection, those with underlying conditions that predispose them to infections, and those who have lived in areas where tuberculosis and histoplasmosis are endemic, and in the elderly.
● Use cautiously and monitor closely in heart failure patients.
● Don't give to pregnant women unless benefits outweigh risks. Because of the risk of serious adverse reactions, the patient should stop breast-feeding or stop using the drug.

NURSING CONSIDERATIONS
● Give first dose under supervision of prescriber.
■ **Black Box Warning** Patient should be evaluated, and treated if necessary for latent tuberculosis before starting adalimumab therapy. ■
■ **Black Box Warning** Serious infections and sepsis, including tuberculosis and invasive fungal infections, may occur. If patient develops new infection during treatment, monitor him closely and if infection becomes serious, stop drug. ■

- Drug may increase the risk of malignancy. Patients with highly active RA may be at an increased risk for lymphoma.
- If patient develops anaphylaxis, a severe infection, other serious allergic reaction, or evidence of a lupuslike syndrome, stop drug.
- Drug may cause reactivation of hepatitis B virus in chronic carriers.
- *Alert:* The needle cover contains latex and shouldn't be handled by those with latex sensitivity.

PATIENT TEACHING
- Tell patient to report evidence of tuberculosis or infection.
- Teach patient or caregiver how to give drug.
- *Alert:* Warn patient to seek immediate medical attention for symptoms of blood dyscrasias or infection, including fever, bruising, bleeding, and pallor.
- Tell patient to rotate injection sites and to avoid tender, bruised, red, or hard skin.
- Teach patient to dispose of used vials, needles, and syringes properly and not in the household trash or recyclables.
- Tell patient to refrigerate drug in its original container before use.

---

auranofin
or-RAIN-oh-fin

Ridaura

Pharmacologic class: gold compound
Pregnancy risk category C

AVAILABLE FORMS
Capsules: 3 mg

INDICATIONS & DOSAGES
➤ **Rheumatoid arthritis**
Adults: 3 mg b.i.d. or 6 mg once daily. After 6 months, may increase to 3 mg t.i.d. If response is inadequate after 3 months of 9 mg/day, stop use.

ADMINISTRATION
P.O.
- Give drug without regard for food.

ACTION
Probably acts by inhibiting sulfhydryl systems, which alters cellular metabolism. May also alter enzyme function and immune response and suppress phagocytic activity.

Route	Onset	Peak	Duration
P.O.	Unknown	2 hr	Unknown

Half-life: About 26 days.

ADVERSE REACTIONS
CNS: *seizures,* confusion, hallucinations.
EENT: conjunctivitis.
GI: *diarrhea, abdominal pain, nausea, stomatitis,* glossitis, anorexia, metallic taste, dyspepsia, flatulence, constipation, dysgeusia, ulcerative colitis.
GU: *acute renal failure,* proteinuria, hematuria, nephrotic syndrome, glomerulonephritis.
Hematologic: *thrombocytopenia, aplastic anemia, agranulocytosis, leukopenia,* eosinophilia, anemia.
Hepatic: jaundice.
Skin: *rash, pruritus, dermatitis,* exfoliative dermatitis, urticaria, erythema, alopecia.

INTERACTIONS
Drug-drug. *Phenytoin:* May increase phenytoin blood levels. Watch for toxicity.

EFFECTS ON LAB TEST RESULTS
- May increase alkaline phosphatase, ALT, and AST levels.
- May decrease hemoglobin level and hematocrit.
- May increase eosinophil count.
- May decrease granulocyte, platelet, and WBC counts.

CONTRAINDICATIONS & CAUTIONS
- Contraindicated in patients with history of severe gold toxicity or toxicity from previous exposure to other heavy metals and in those with necrotizing enterocolitis, pulmonary fibrosis, exfoliative dermatitis, bone marrow aplasia, or severe hemato-logic disorders.
- Contraindicated in patients with urticaria, eczema, colitis, severe debilitation, hemorrhagic conditions, or systemic lupus erythematosus and in patients who have recently received radiation therapy.

Reactions may be *common,* uncommon, *life-threatening,* or COMMON AND LIFE-THREATENING.
Interaction may have a *rapid onset* or **delayed onset.**

• Manufacturer recommends avoiding use during pregnancy.
• Use cautiously with other drugs that cause blood dyscrasias.
• Use cautiously in patients with rash, history of bone marrow depression, or renal, hepatic, or inflammatory bowel disease.

NURSING CONSIDERATIONS
■ **Black Box Warning** Monitor for signs of gold toxicity such as platelet count below 150,000/mm³, fall in hemoglobin granulocyte count less than 1,500/mm³, leukopenia (WBC count less than 4,000/mm³) or eosinophilia over 5%, proteinuria, hematuria, pruritis, rash, stomatitis, or persistent diarrhea. ■
• *Alert:* Monitor patient's urinalysis results monthly. If proteinuria or hematuria is detected, stop drug because it can cause nephrotic syndrome or glomerulonephritis, and notify prescriber.
• Monitor renal and liver function test results.
• Warn women of childbearing potential about risks of drug therapy during pregnancy.

PATIENT TEACHING
• Encourage patient to take drug as prescribed.
• Tell patient to continue other drug therapies if prescribed.
• Remind patient to see prescriber for monthly platelet counts.
• Suggest that patient have regular urinalysis.
• Tell patient to keep taking drug if mild diarrhea occurs but to immediately report blood in stool. Diarrhea is the most common adverse reaction.
• Advise patient to report rash or other skin problems and to stop drug until reaction subsides. Itching may precede dermatitis; consider itchy skin eruptions during drug therapy to be a reaction until proven otherwise.
• Inform patient that inflammation of the mouth may be preceded by a metallic taste; tell him to notify prescriber if this occurs. Promote careful oral hygiene during therapy.
• Advise patient to report unusual bleeding or bruising.

• Inform patient that beneficial effect may be delayed as long as 3 months. If response is inadequate and maximum dose has been reached, expect prescriber to stop drug.
• Warn patient not to give drug to others. Auranofin is prescribed only for selected patients with rheumatoid arthritis.

---

aurothioglucose
or-oh-thye-oh-GLUE-cose

Solganal

gold sodium thiomalate
Aurolate, Myochrysine

Pharmacologic class: gold compound
Pregnancy risk category C

AVAILABLE FORMS
aurothioglucose
Injection (suspension): 50 mg/ml in sesame oil in 10-ml vial
gold sodium thiomalate
Injection: 50 mg/ml with benzyl alcohol in 2-ml and 10-ml vials

INDICATIONS & DOSAGES
➤ **Rheumatoid arthritis**
aurothioglucose
Adults: Initially, 10 mg I.M., followed by 25 mg every week for second and third doses. Then, 50 mg every week to total dose of 800 mg to 1 g. If condition improves and no toxicity occurs, continue 25 to 50 mg every 3 to 4 weeks indefinitely.
Children ages 6 to 12: One-fourth usual adult dose. Don't exceed 25 mg per dose.
gold sodium thiomalate
Adults: Initially, 10 mg I.M., followed by 25 mg in 1 week. Then, 25 to 50 mg every week to total dose of 1 g. If condition improves and no toxicity occurs, give 25 to 50 mg every 2 weeks for 2 to 20 weeks; then, 25 to 50 mg every 3 to 4 weeks as maintenance therapy. If relapse occurs, resume injections at weekly intervals.
Children: Initially, a test dose of 10 mg I.M.; then, 1 mg/kg I.M. weekly, not to exceed 50 mg for a single injection. Follow adult spacing of doses.

ADMINISTRATION
I.M.
- Give drug I.M. only, preferably into gluteal muscle.
- Drug should be pale yellow; don't use if it darkens.
- When injecting gold sodium thiomalate, have patient lie down for 10 to 20 minutes to minimize hypotension.

ACTION
Probably acts by inhibiting sulfhydryl systems, which alters cellular metabolism. May also alter enzyme function and immune response and suppress phagocytic activity.

Route	Onset	Peak	Duration
I.M.	Unknown	3–6 hr	Unknown

Half-life: 3 to 27 days (single dose); 14 to 40 days (3rd dose); up to 168 days (11th dose).

ADVERSE REACTIONS
CNS: *seizures,* confusion, hallucinations.
CV: *bradycardia,* hypotension.
EENT: corneal gold deposition, corneal ulcers.
GI: *diarrhea, metallic taste, stomatitis,* anorexia, abdominal cramps, nausea, vomiting, ulcerative enterocolitis.
GU: *acute renal failure,* albuminuria, proteinuria, nephrotic syndrome, nephritis, acute tubular necrosis, hematuria.
Hematologic: *thrombocytopenia, aplastic anemia, agranulocytosis, leukopenia,* eosinophilia, anemia.
Hepatic: *hepatitis,* jaundice.
Skin: *rash, dermatitis,* erythema, exfoliative dermatitis, diaphoresis, photosensitivity reaction.
Other: *anaphylaxis, angioedema.*

INTERACTIONS
Drug-lifestyle. *Sun or ultraviolet light exposure:* May cause photosensitivity reaction. Advise patient to avoid excessive sunlight exposure.

EFFECTS ON LAB TEST RESULTS
- May increase alkaline phosphatase, ALT, and AST levels.
- May decrease hemoglobin level and hematocrit.
- May increase eosinophil count.
- May decrease granulocyte, platelet, and WBC counts.

CONTRAINDICATIONS & CAUTIONS
- Contraindicated in patients hypersensitive to drug and in those with history of severe toxicity from previous exposure to gold or other heavy metals.
- Contraindicated in those who have recently received radiation therapy and in those with hepatitis, exfoliative dermatitis, severe uncontrollable diabetes, renal disease, hepatic dysfunction, uncontrolled heart failure, systemic lupus erythematosus, colitis, Sjögren syndrome, urticaria, eczema, hemorrhagic conditions, or severe hematologic disorders.
- Use cautiously, if at all, in patients with rash, marked hypertension, compromised cerebral or CV circulation, or history of renal or hepatic disease, drug allergies, or blood dyscrasias.

NURSING CONSIDERATIONS
- Warn women about risks of gold therapy during pregnancy.
- **■ Black Box Warning** Give drug only under constant supervision of prescriber thoroughly familiar with drug's toxicities and benefits. **■**
- **■ Black Box Warning** Monitor for signs of gold toxicity including fall in hemoglobin, leukopenia < 4,000 wbc/mm³, proteinuria, hematuria, pruritis, rash, stomatitis, or persistent diarrhea. **■**
- Immerse aurothioglucose vial in warm water; shake vigorously before injecting.
- Analyze urine for protein and sediment changes before each injection.
- Watch for anaphylactoid reaction for 30 minutes after administration.
- *Alert:* Keep dimercaprol available to treat acute toxicity.
- Monitor CBC, including platelet count, before every second injection.
- If adverse reactions are mild, some rheumatologists resume gold therapy after 2 to 3 weeks' rest.
- Monitor platelet counts if patient develops purpura or ecchymoses.

PATIENT TEACHING
- Inform patient that increased joint pain may occur for 1 to 2 days after injection but usually subsides.
- Advise patient to report rash or skin problems immediately and to stop

drug until reaction subsides. Itching may precede skin inflammation; consider itchy skin eruptions during gold therapy to be a reaction until proven otherwise.
• Advise patient to report unusual bleeding or bruising.
• Instruct patient to report a metallic taste. Promote careful oral hygiene.
• Urge patient to avoid sunlight and artificial ultraviolet light, which may cause gray-blue skin pigmentation.
• Tell patient that benefits may not appear for 3 to 4 months.
• Stress need for follow-up care.

SAFETY ALERT!

leflunomide
leh-FLEW-no-mide

Arava

Pharmacologic class: pyrimidine synthesis inhibitor
Pregnancy risk category X

AVAILABLE FORMS
Tablets: 10 mg, 20 mg, 100 mg

INDICATIONS & DOSAGES
➤ **To reduce signs and symptoms of active rheumatoid arthritis; to slow structural damage as shown by erosions and joint space narrowing seen on X-ray; to improve physical function**
Adults: 100 mg P.O. every 24 hours for 3 days; then 20 mg (maximum daily dose) P.O. every 24 hours. Dose may be decreased to 10 mg daily if higher dose isn't well tolerated.
Adjust-a-dose: For confirmed ALT elevations between two and three times the upper limit of normal (ULN), reduce dose to 10 mg/day; if elevations persist despite dose reduction or if ALT elevations of greater than three times ULN are present, stop drug and give cholestyramine or charcoal.

ADMINISTRATION
P.O.
• Give drug without regard for food.

ACTION
An immunomodulatory drug that inhibits dihydroorotate dehydrogenase, an enzyme involved in pyrimidine synthesis, and that has antiproliferative activity and anti-inflammatory effects.

Route	Onset	Peak	Duration
P.O.	Unknown	6–12 hr	Unknown

Half-life: 15 to 18 days.

ADVERSE REACTIONS
CNS: anxiety, asthenia, depression, dizziness, fever, headache, insomnia, malaise, migraine, neuralgia, neuritis, pain, paresthesia, sleep disorder, vertigo.
CV: *hypertension,* angina pectoris, chest pain, palpitations, peripheral edema, tachycardia, varicose veins, vasculitis, vasodilation.
EENT: blurred vision, cataracts, conjunctivitis, epistaxis, eye disorder, pharyngitis, rhinitis, sinusitis.
GI: *diarrhea,* abdominal pain, anorexia, cholelithiasis, colitis, constipation, dry mouth, dyspepsia, enlarged salivary glands, esophagitis, flatulence, gastritis, gastroenteritis, gingivitis, melena, mouth ulcer, nausea, oral candidiasis, stomatitis, taste perversion, vomiting.
GU: albuminuria, cystitis, dysuria, hematuria, menstrual disorder, pelvic pain, prostate disorder, urinary frequency, UTI, vaginal candidiasis.
Hematologic: anemia.
Hepatic: *hepatotoxicity.*
Metabolic: *diabetes mellitus,* hyperglycemia, hyperlipidemia, hyperthyroidism, hypokalemia, weight loss.
Musculoskeletal: arthralgia, arthrosis, back pain, bone necrosis, bone pain, bursitis, joint disorder, leg cramps, muscle cramps, myalgia, neck pain, synovitis, tendon rupture, tenosynovitis.
Respiratory: *respiratory infection, asthma,* bronchitis, dyspnea, increased cough, lung disorder, pneumonia.
Skin: *alopecia, rash,* acne, contact dermatitis, dry skin, eczema, fungal dermatitis, hair discoloration, hematoma, maculopapular rash, nail disorder, pruritus, skin discoloration, skin disorder, skin nodule, skin ulcer, subcutaneous nodule.

Other: abscess, allergic reaction, cyst, ecchymoses, flulike syndrome, hernia, herpes simplex, herpes zoster, increased sweating, injury or accident, tooth disorder.

INTERACTIONS
Drug-drug. *Charcoal, cholestyramine:* May decrease leflunomide level. Sometimes used for this effect in overdose.
Methotrexate, other hepatotoxic drugs: May increase risk of hepatotoxicity. Monitor liver enzyme levels.
NSAIDs (diclofenac, ibuprofen): May increase NSAID level. Monitor patient.
Rifampin: May increase active leflunomide metabolite level. Use together cautiously.
Tolbutamide: May increase tolbutamide level. Monitor patient.

EFFECTS ON LAB TEST RESULTS
- May increase AST, ALT, glucose, lipid, and CK levels.
- May decrease potassium level.

CONTRAINDICATIONS & CAUTIONS
- Contraindicated in patients hypersensitive to drug or its components.
- ■ **Black Box Warning** Contraindicated in pregnant women and women of child-bearing potential who are not using reliable contraception. ■
- Drug isn't recommended for patients with significant hepatic impairment, evidence of infection with hepatitis B or C viruses, severe immunodeficiency, bone marrow dysplasia, or severe uncontrolled infections; in women who are breast-feeding; in patients younger than age 18; or in men attempting to father a child.
- Use cautiously in patients with renal insufficiency.

NURSING CONSIDERATIONS
- Vaccination with live vaccines isn't recommended. Consider the long half-life of drug when contemplating giving a live vaccine after stopping drug treatment.
- *Alert:* Men planning to father a child should stop drug therapy and follow recommended leflunomide removal protocol (cholestyramine 8 g, P.O. t.i.d. for 11 days). In addition to cholestyramine, verify drug levels are less than 0.02 mg/L by two separate tests at least 14 days apart. If

level is greater than 0.02 mg/L, consider additional cholestyramine treatment.
- Risk of malignancy, particularly lymphoproliferative disorders, is increased with use of some immunosuppressants, including leflunomide.
- *Alert:* Monitor ALT levels, platelet and WBC counts, and hemoglobin level or hematocrit at baseline and monthly for 6 months after starting therapy and every 6 to 8 weeks thereafter.
- *Alert:* Monitor AST, ALT, and serum albumin levels monthly if treatment includes methotrexate or other potential immunosuppressives.
- Stop drug and start cholestyramine or charcoal therapy if bone marrow suppression occurs.
- Watch for overlapping hematologic toxicity when switching to another antirheumatic.
- *Alert:* Rare cases of severe liver injury, including cases with fatal outcome, have occurred during leflunomide therapy. Most cases occur within 6 months of therapy and in a setting of multiple risk factors for hepatotoxicity (liver disease, other hepatotoxins).
- Carefully monitor patient after dose reduction. Because the active metabolite of leflunomide has a prolonged half-life, it may take several weeks for levels to decline.

PATIENT TEACHING
- Explain need for and frequency of required blood tests and monitoring.
- ■ **Black Box Warning** Instruct patient to use birth control during course of treatment and until it's been determined that drug is no longer active. ■
- Warn patient to immediately notify prescriber if signs or symptoms of pregnancy occur (such as late menstrual periods or breast tenderness).
- Advise woman to stop breast-feeding during therapy.
- Inform patient he may continue taking aspirin, other NSAIDs, and low-dose corticosteroids during treatment.
- Inform patient that it may take 4 weeks to begin to see improvement from therapy.

atracurium besylate
cisatracurium besylate
pancuronium bromide
succinylcholine chloride

SAFETY ALERT!

atracurium besylate
at-truh-KYOO-ree-um

Tracrium

Pharmacologic class: nondepolarizing neuromuscular blocker
Pregnancy risk category C

AVAILABLE FORMS
Injection: 10 mg/ml

INDICATIONS & DOSAGES
➤ **Adjunct to general anesthesia to**
facilitate endotracheal intubation
and relax skeletal muscles during
surgery or mechanical ventilation
Adults and children age 2 or older: 0.4 to
0.5 mg/kg by I.V. bolus. Give maintenance
dose of 0.08 to 0.1 mg/kg within 20 to
45 minutes during prolonged surgery.
Give maintenance doses every 15 to
25 minutes in patients receiving balanced
anesthesia. For prolonged procedures, use
a constant infusion at an initial rate of
9 to 10 mcg/kg/minute; then reduce to
5 to 9 mcg/kg/minute.
Children ages 1 month to 2 years: First
dose, 0.3 to 0.4 mg/kg I.V. for children
under halothane anesthesia. Frequent
maintenance doses may be needed.
Adjust-a-dose: In adults receiving enflurane or isoflurane at the same time, reduce
initial atracurium dose by 33% (0.25 to
0.35 mg/kg). In adults receiving atracurium
following succinylcholine, initial dose is
0.3 to 0.4 mg/kg.

ADMINISTRATION
I.V.
● Use drug only under direct supervision
by medical staff skilled in using neuromuscular blockers and maintaining patent

airway. Keep available emergency respiratory support (endotracheal equipment,
ventilator, oxygen, atropine, edrophonium,
neostigmine, and epinephrine).
● Give sedatives or general anesthetics
before neuromuscular blockers, which
don't reduce consciousness or alter pain
threshold.
● Drug usually is given by rapid I.V. bolus
injection but may be given by intermittent
infusion or continuous infusion.
● Don't give by I.M. injection.
● At concentrations of 0.2 mg/ml to
0.5 mg/ml, drug is compatible in D_5W,
normal saline solution for injection, or
dextrose 5% in normal saline solution for
injection for 24 hours (at room temperature
or refrigerated).
● Stable if undiluted for 6 weeks.
● Store in refrigerator. Don't freeze. Once
removed from refrigeration, use within
14 days, even if re-refrigerated.
● **Incompatibilities:** Alkaline solutions
(such as barbiturates), lactated Ringer's
solution.

ACTION
Prevents acetylcholine from binding to
receptors on motor end plate, thus
blocking neuromuscular transmission.

Route	Onset	Peak	Duration
I.V.	2 min	3–5 min	35–70 min

Half-life: 20 minutes.

ADVERSE REACTIONS
CV: *bradycardia,* hypotension,
tachycardia.
Respiratory: *prolonged, dose-related*
apnea, bronchospasm, laryngospasm,
wheezing, increased bronchial secretions,
dyspnea.
Skin: *skin flushing,* erythema, pruritus,
urticaria, rash.
Other: *anaphylaxis.*

INTERACTIONS
Drug-drug. *Amikacin, gentamicin,*
neomycin, streptomycin, tobramycin: May

increase the effects of nondepolarizing muscle relaxant including prolonged respiratory depression. Use together cautiously. May reduce nondepolarizing muscle relaxant dose.

Carbamazepine, phenytoin, theophylline: May reverse, or cause resistance to, neuromuscular blockade. May need to increase atracurium dose.

Clindamycin, general anesthetics (enflurane, halothane, isoflurane), kanamycin, polymyxin antibiotics (colistin, polymyxin B sulfate), procainamide, quinidine, quinine, thiazide and loop diuretics, trimethaphan, verapamil: May enhance neuromuscular blockade, increasing skeletal muscle relaxation and prolonging effect of atracurium. Use together cautiously during and after surgery.

Corticosteroids: May cause prolonged weakness. Monitor patient closely.

Edrophonium, neostigmine, pyridostigmine: May inhibit drug and reverse neuromuscular block. Monitor patient closely.

Lithium, magnesium salts, opioid analgesics: May enhance neuromuscular blockade, increasing skeletal muscle relaxation and possibly causing respiratory paralysis. Reduce atracurium dosage.

Succinylcholine: May cause quicker onset of atracurium; may increase depth of neuromuscular blockade. Monitor patient.

EFFECTS ON LAB TEST RESULTS
None reported.

CONTRAINDICATIONS & CAUTIONS
• Contraindicated in patients hypersensitive to drug.
• Use cautiously in elderly or debilitated patients and in those with CV disease; severe electrolyte disorder; bronchogenic carcinoma; hepatic, renal, or pulmonary impairment; neuromuscular disease; or myasthenia gravis.

NURSING CONSIDERATIONS
• Dosage depends on anesthetic used, individual needs, and response. Recommended dosages must be individually adjusted.
• Resistance may develop in burn patients; increase dosage if needed.
• Give analgesics for pain. Patient may have pain but may be unable to express it.

• Once spontaneous recovery starts, reverse atracurium-induced neuromuscular blockade with an anticholinesterase (such as neostigmine or edrophonium), usually given with an anticholinergic such as atropine. Complete reversal of neuromuscular blockade is usually achieved within 8 to 10 minutes after using an anticholinesterase.
• Monitor respirations and vital signs closely until patient has fully recovered from neuromuscular blockade, as indicated by tests of muscle strength (hand grip, head lift, and ability to cough).
• A nerve stimulator and train-of-four monitoring are recommended to confirm antagonism of neuromuscular blockade and recovery of muscle strength. Make sure spontaneous recovery is evident before attempting reversal with neostigmine.
• Prior use of succinylcholine doesn't prolong duration of action but quickens onset and may deepen neuromuscular blockade.
• Drug contains benzyl alcohol as a preservative.
• *Alert:* Careful dosage calculation is essential. Always verify dosage with another health care professional.

PATIENT TEACHING
• Explain all events and procedures to patient because he can still hear.

SAFETY ALERT!

cisatracurium besylate
sis-ah-trah-KYOO-ee-hum

Nimbex

Pharmacologic class:
nondepolarizing neuromuscular blocker
Pregnancy risk category B

AVAILABLE FORMS
Injection: 2 mg/ml, 10 mg/ml

INDICATIONS & DOSAGES
➤ **Adjunct to general anesthesia to facilitate endotracheal intubation and relax skeletal muscles during surgery**

Reactions may be *common*, uncommon, *life-threatening*, or COMMON AND LIFE-THREATENING.
Interaction may have a *rapid onset* or *delayed onset.*

Adults: First dose of 0.15 mg/kg I.V.; then maintenance dosages of 0.03 mg/kg I.V. every 40 to 50 minutes p.r.n. Or, first dose of 0.2 mg/kg I.V.; then maintenance dosages of 0.03 mg/kg I.V. every 50 to 60 minutes p.r.n. Or, after first dose, give a maintenance infusion at 3 mcg/kg/minute and reduce to 1 to 2 mcg/kg/minute as needed.

Children ages 2 to 12: 0.1 mg/kg I.V. over 5 to 10 seconds. After first dose, give a maintenance infusion of 3 mcg/kg/minute, then reduce to 1 to 2 mcg/kg/minute as needed.

Adjust-a-dose: During coronary artery bypass surgery with induced hypothermia, reduce infusion rate by 50%.

➤ **To maintain neuromuscular blockade during mechanical ventilation in intensive care unit (ICU)**
Adults: Principles for infusion in operating room apply to use in ICU. After first dose, give 3 mcg/minute by I.V. infusion. Range, 0.5 to 5 mcg/kg/minute.

Adjust-a-dose: In patients with neuromuscular disease, such as myasthenia gravis or Eaton-Lambert syndrome, don't exceed 0.02 mg/kg. Patients with burns may need increased amount.

ADMINISTRATION
I.V.
● Drug is colorless to slightly yellow or green-yellow. Inspect vials for particulates and discoloration before use. Don't use unclear solutions or those with visible particulates.
● The 20-ml vial is intended for use only in the ICU.
● Use only under direct supervision of medical staff skilled in using neuromuscular blockers and maintaining airway patency. Don't give drug unless resources for intubation, mechanical ventilation, and oxygen therapy are within reach.
● Keep refrigerated; don't freeze. Use drug within 21 days after removing from refrigeration.
● Use drug within 24 hours when diluted to a concentration of 0.1 mg/ml in D$_5$W, normal saline solution, or 5% dextrose and normal saline solution.
● **Incompatibilities:** Acyclovir, alkaline solutions with pH higher than 8.5, aminophylline, amphotericin B, amphotericin B

cholesteryl sulfate complex, ampicillin, ampicillin sodium and sulbactam sodium, cefazolin, cefoperazone, cefotaxime, cefoxitin, ceftazidime, ceftizoxime, cefuroxime, diazepam, furosemide, ganciclovir, heparin sodium, ketorolac, lactated Ringer's injection, methylprednisolone sodium succinate, piperacillin, piperacillin sodium and tazobactam sodium, propofol, sodium bicarbonate, sodium nitroprusside, thiopental sodium, ticarcillin disodium and clavulanate potassium, trimethoprim, and sulfamethoxazole.

ACTION
Binds to cholinergic receptors on the motor end plate, antagonizing acetylcholine and blocking neuromuscular transmission.

Route	Onset	Peak	Duration
I.V.	1–2 min	2–5 min	25–44 min

Half-life: 22 to 29 minutes; about 3 hours for laudanosine.

ADVERSE REACTIONS
CV: *bradycardia,* hypotension, flushing.
Respiratory: *bronchospasm, prolonged apnea.*
Skin: rash.

INTERACTIONS
Drug-drug. *Aminoglycosides, bacitracin, clindamycin, colistimethate sodium, colistin, lithium, local anesthetics, magnesium salts, polymyxins, procainamide, quinidine, quinine, tetracyclines:* May enhance neuromuscular blocking action of cisatracurium. Use together cautiously.
Carbamazepine, phenytoin: May decrease the effects of cisatracurium. May need to increase cisatracurium dose.
Enflurane or isoflurane given with nitrous oxide or oxygen: May prolong cisatracurium duration of action. Patient may need less frequent maintenance doses, lower maintenance doses, or reduced infusion rate of cisatracurium.
Succinylcholine: May shorten time to onset of maximal neuromuscular block. Monitor patient.

EFFECTS ON LAB TEST RESULTS
None reported.

CONTRAINDICATIONS & CAUTIONS
● Contraindicated in patients who are hypersensitive to drug, to other bisbenzylisoquinolinium drugs, or to benzyl alcohol (found in 10-ml vial).
● Use cautiously in pregnant or breast-feeding women.

NURSING CONSIDERATIONS
● Drug isn't recommended for rapid-sequence endotracheal intubation because of its intermediate onset.
● Dosage requirements vary widely among patients.
● *Alert:* Drug has no known effect on consciousness, pain threshold, or cerebration. To avoid patient distress, don't induce neuromuscular block before unconsciousness.
● Monitor neuromuscular function with nerve stimulator during drug administration. If stimulation doesn't elicit a response, stop infusion until response returns.
● To avoid inaccurate dosing, perform neuromuscular monitoring on a nonparetic arm or leg in patients with hemiparesis or paraparesis.
● Monitor acid-base balance and electrolyte levels. Abnormalities may potentiate or antagonize the action of cisatracurium.
● Monitor patient for malignant hyperthermia.
● Give analgesics, if indicated. Patient can feel pain but can't indicate its presence.
● *Alert:* Careful dosage calculation is essential. Always verify dosage with another health care professional.

PATIENT TEACHING
● Explain purpose of drug.
● Assure patient that monitoring will be continuous.
● Explain all procedures and events because patient can still hear.

pancuronium bromide
pan-kyoo-ROW-nee-uhm

Pharmacologic class:
nondepolarizing neuromuscular blocker
Pregnancy risk category C

AVAILABLE FORMS
Injection: 1 mg/ml, 2 mg/ml

INDICATIONS & DOSAGES
➤ **Adjunct to anesthesia to relax skeletal muscle, facilitate intubation, assist with mechanical ventilation**
Adults and children age 1 month and older: Initially, 0.04 to 0.1 mg/kg I.V.; then 0.01 mg/kg every 30 to 60 minutes.
Neonates: Individualize dosage.

ADMINISTRATION
I.V.
■ **Black Box Warning** This drug should be administered by adequately trained individuals familiar with its actions, characteristics, and hazards. ■
● Only staff skilled in airway management should use drug.
● Drug has no known effect on consciousness, pain threshold, or cerebration. To avoid patient distress, don't induce neuromuscular blockade before unconsciousness.
● Keep endotracheal equipment, ventilator, oxygen, atropine, edrophonium, epinephrine, and neostigmine immediately available.
● Store in refrigerator. Don't store in plastic containers or syringes, although plastic syringes may be used for administration.
● **Incompatibilities:** Alkaline solutions, barbiturates, diazepam, thiopental sodium.

ACTION
Prevents acetylcholine from binding to receptors on the motor end plate, blocking neuromuscular transmission.

Route	Onset	Peak	Duration
I.V.	30–45 sec	3–4½ min	35–65 min

Half-life: About 2 hours.

ADVERSE REACTIONS
CV: tachycardia, increased blood pressure.
EENT: excessive salivation.
Musculoskeletal: residual muscle weakness.
Respiratory: *prolonged respiratory insufficiency or apnea.*
Skin: transient rashes.
Other: allergic or idiosyncratic hypersensitivity reactions

INTERACTIONS
Drug-drug. *Aminoglycosides (amikacin, gentamicin, neomycin, streptomycin, tobramycin):* May increase the effects of nondepolarizing muscle relaxant, including prolonged respiratory depression. Use together only when necessary. Dose of nondepolarizing muscle relaxant may need to be reduced.
Azathioprine: May reverse neuromuscular blockade induced by pancuronium. Monitor patient.
Beta blockers, clindamycin, general anesthetics (such as enflurane, halothane, isoflurane), ketamine, lincomycin, magnesium sulfate, polymyxin antibiotics (colistin, polymyxin B sulfate), quinidine, quinine, verapamil: May enhance neuromuscular blockade, increasing skeletal muscle relaxation and prolonging effect of pancuronium. Use together cautiously during and after surgery.
Carbamazepine, phenytoin: May decrease effects of pancuronium. May need to increase pancuronium dose.
Diuretics: May cause electrolyte imbalance, or alter neuromuscular blockade. Monitor electrolytes before giving drug.
Lithium, opioid analgesics: May enhance neuromuscular blockade, increasing skeletal muscle relaxation and possibly causing respiratory paralysis. Use cautiously, and reduce dose of pancuronium.
Succinylcholine: May increase intensity and duration of neuromuscular blockade. Allow effects of succinylcholine to subside before giving pancuronium.
Theophylline: May produce a dose-dependent reversal of neuromuscular blocking effects. Monitor patient for clinical effect.
Tricyclic antidepressants (TCAs): May increase risk of ventricular arrhythmias in patients anesthetized with both halothane

and pancuronium. Monitor ECG closely in patients taking TCAs before surgery.

EFFECTS ON LAB TEST RESULTS
None reported.

CONTRAINDICATIONS & CAUTIONS
• Contraindicated in patients hypersensitive to bromides, those with tachycardia, and those for whom even a minor increase in heart rate is undesirable.
• Use cautiously in elderly or debilitated patients; in patients with renal, hepatic, or pulmonary impairment; and in those with respiratory depression, myasthenia gravis, myasthenic syndrome related to lung cancer, dehydration, thyroid disorders, CV disease, collagen diseases, porphyria, electrolyte disturbances, hyperthermia, and toxemic states. Also, use large doses cautiously in patients undergoing cesarean section.

NURSING CONSIDERATIONS
• Dosage depends on anesthetic used, individual needs, and response. Dosages are representative and must be adjusted.
• Allow succinylcholine effects to subside before giving this drug.
• Monitor baseline electrolyte determinations (electrolyte imbalance can potentiate neuromuscular effects) and vital signs, especially respirations and heart rate.
• Measure fluid intake and output; renal dysfunction may prolong duration of action because 25% of drug is excreted unchanged in the urine.
• A nerve stimulator and train-of-four monitoring are recommended to confirm antagonism of neuromuscular blockade and recovery of muscle strength. Make sure there's some evidence of spontaneous recovery before attempting pharmacologic reversal with neostigmine.
• Monitor respirations closely until patient recovers fully from neuromuscular blockade, as indicated by tests of muscle strength (hand grip, head lift, and ability to cough).
• After spontaneous recovery starts, neuromuscular blockade may be reversed with an anticholinesterase (such as neostigmine or edrophonium), which is usually given with an anticholinergic (such as atropine).

- Drug doesn't cause histamine release or hypotension, but it may raise heart rate and blood pressure.
- Give analgesics for pain.
- **Alert:** Careful dosage calculation is essential. Always verify dosage with another health care professional.

PATIENT TEACHING
- Explain all events and procedures to patient because he can still hear.

succinylcholine chloride (suxamethonium chloride)
SUK-seh-nil-KOH-leen

Anectine, Anectine Flo-Pack, Quelicin

Pharmacologic class: depolarizing neuromuscular blocker
Pregnancy risk category C

AVAILABLE FORMS
Injection: 20 mg/ml, 50 mg/ml, 100 mg/ml
Powder for infusion: 500-mg vial, 1-g vial

INDICATIONS & DOSAGES
➤ **Adjunct to anesthesia to relax skeletal muscles for surgery and orthopedic manipulations; to facilitate intubation and assist with mechanical ventilation; to lessen muscle contractions in pharmacologically or electrically induced seizures**
Adults: 0.6 mg/kg I.V. given over 10 to 30 seconds. Dosage range is 0.3 to 1.1 mg/kg. For longer response, give continuous infusion at 0.5 to 10 mg/minute, or give 0.04 to 0.07 mg/kg intermittently, as needed, to maintain relaxation. Or, 2.5 to 4 mg/kg I.M. Maximum I.M. dose is 150 mg.
Children: 1 to 2 mg/kg I.V. or 3 to 4 mg/kg I.M. Maximum I.M. dose is 150 mg.

ADMINISTRATION
I.V.
- Only staff skilled in airway management should use drug.
- Give test dose of 5 to 10 mg after patient has been anesthetized. If no respiratory

depression or transient depression for up to 5 minutes, then patient can metabolize drug, and it's OK to continue. Don't give if patient develops respiratory paralysis sufficient to need endotracheal intubation. (Recovery should occur within 30 to 60 minutes.)
- Use within 24 hours after reconstitution.
- Store injectable form in refrigerator. Store powder form at room temperature in tightly closed container.
- **Incompatibilities:** Alkaline solutions, barbiturates, nafcillin, sodium bicarbonate, solutions with pH above 4.5, thiopental sodium.
I.M.
- Inject deeply, preferably high into deltoid muscle.
- Store injectable form in refrigerator. Store powder form at room temperature in tightly closed container.

ACTION
Binds with a high affinity to cholinergic receptors, prolonging depolarization of the motor end plate and ultimately producing muscle paralysis.

Route	Onset	Peak	Duration
I.V.	30–60 sec	1–2 min	4–10 min
I.M.	2–3 min	Unknown	10–30 min

Half-life: Unknown.

ADVERSE REACTIONS
CV: *arrhythmias, bradycardia, cardiac arrest,* tachycardia, hypertension, hypotension, flushing.
EENT: increased intraocular pressure.
GI: excessive salivation.
Metabolic: *hyperkalemia.*
Musculoskeletal: *postoperative muscle pain,* muscle fasciculation, jaw rigidity.
Respiratory: *apnea, bronchoconstriction, prolonged respiratory depression.*
Skin: rash.
Other: allergic or idiosyncratic hypersensitivity reactions, *anaphylaxis, malignant hyperthermia, rhabdomyolysis with acute renal failure.*

INTERACTIONS
Drug-drug. *Aminoglycosides, anticholinesterases (such as echothiophate, edrophonium, neostigmine, physostigmine,*

Reactions may be *common*, uncommon, *life-threatening*, or COMMON AND LIFE-THREATENING.
Interaction may have a *rapid onset* or *delayed onset.*

pyridostigmine), aprotinin, general anesthetics (such as enflurane, halothane, isoflurane), glucocorticoids, hormonal contraceptives, lidocaine, lithium, magnesium, oxytocin, polymyxin antibiotics, (such as colistin, polymyxin B sulfate), procainamide, quinine: May enhance neuromuscular blockade, increasing skeletal muscle relaxation and potentiating effect. Use together cautiously during and after surgery.

Cardiac glycosides: May cause arrhythmias. Use together cautiously.

Cyclophosphamide, lithium, MAO inhibitors: May enhance neuromuscular blockade and prolong apnea. Use together cautiously.

Opioid analgesics: May enhance neuromuscular blockade, increasing skeletal muscle relaxation and possibly causing respiratory paralysis. Use together cautiously.

Parenteral magnesium sulfate: May enhance neuromuscular blockade, may increase skeletal muscle relaxation, and may cause respiratory paralysis. Use together cautiously, preferably at reduced doses.

Drug-herb. *Melatonin:* May potentiate blocking properties of drug. Ask patient about herbal remedy use, and recommend caution.

EFFECTS ON LAB TEST RESULTS
● May increase myoglobin and potassium levels.

CONTRAINDICATIONS & CAUTIONS
● Contraindicated in patients hypersensitive to drug and in those with abnormally low plasma pseudocholinesterase levels, angle-closure glaucoma, personal or family history of malignant hyperthermia, myopathies with elevated CK levels, acute major burns, multiple trauma, skeletal muscle denervation, upper motor neuron injury, or penetrating eye injuries.
● Drug may contain benzyl alcohol. Avoid use in neonates.
● Use cautiously in elderly or debilitated patients; in patients receiving quinidine or cardiac glycoside therapy; in patients with hepatic, renal, or pulmonary impairment; in those with respiratory depression, severe

burns or trauma, electrolyte imbalances, hyperkalemia, paraplegia, spinal CNS injury, stroke, degenerative or dystrophic neuromuscular disease, myasthenia gravis, myasthenic syndrome related to lung cancer, dehydration, thyroid disorders, collagen diseases, porphyria, fractures, muscle spasms, eye surgery, and pheochromocytoma. Also, use large doses cautiously in patients undergoing cesarean section.

NURSING CONSIDERATIONS
● Drug has no known effect on consciousness, pain threshold, or cerebration. To avoid patient distress, don't induce neuromuscular blockade before unconsciousness.
● Dosage depends on anesthetic used, individual needs, and response. Recommended dosages must be individually adjusted.
■ **Black Box Warning** Drug may cause acute rhabdomyolysis with hyperkalemia followed by ventricular arrhythmias, cardiac arrest, and death after administration to apparently healthy children who have undiagnosed skeletal muscle myopathy. Institute treatment for hyperkalemia when a healthy appearing infant or child develops cardiac arrest soon after administration of succinylcholine. ■
● Children may be less sensitive to drug than adults.
● Succinylcholine is the drug of choice for procedures less than 3 minutes and for orthopedic manipulations; use cautiously with fractures or dislocations.
● Monitor baseline electrolyte determinations and vital signs. Check respirations every 5 to 10 minutes during infusion.
● Monitor respirations closely until tests of muscle strength (hand grip, head lift, and ability to cough) indicate full recovery from neuromuscular blockade.
● *Alert:* Don't use reversing drugs. Unlike nondepolarizing drugs, neostigmine or edrophonium may worsen neuromuscular blockade.
● Repeated or continuous infusions aren't advisable; they may cause reduced response or prolonged muscle relaxation and apnea.

• Give analgesics for pain.
• Keep airway clear. Have emergency respiratory support equipment (endotracheal equipment, ventilator, oxygen, atropine, and epinephrine) immediately available.
• *Alert:* Careful dosage calculation is essential. Always verify dosage with another health care professional.

PATIENT TEACHING
• Explain all events and procedures to patient because he can still hear.
• Reassure patient that postoperative stiffness is normal and will soon subside.

53
Parathyroid-like drugs

calcitriol
cinacalcet hydrochloride
teriparatide

calcitriol
(1,25-dihydroxycholecalciferol)
kal-SIH-trye-ol

Calcijex, Rocaltrol

Pharmacologic class: vitamin D
analogue
Pregnancy risk category C

AVAILABLE FORMS
Capsules: 0.25 mcg, 0.5 mcg
Injection: 1 mcg/ml, 2 mcg/ml
Oral solution: 1 mcg/ml

INDICATIONS & DOSAGES
➤ **Hypocalcemia in patients under-**
going long-term dialysis
Adults: Initially, 0.25 mcg P.O. daily.
Increase by 0.25 mcg daily at 4- to 8-week
intervals. Maintenance P.O. dosage is
0.25 mcg every other day up to 1 mcg
daily. Or usual I.V. dosage is 1 to 2 mcg
I.V. three times weekly. Increase dose by
0.5 to 1 mcg at 2- to 4-week intervals.
➤ **Hypoparathyroidism, pseudo-**
hypoparathyroidism
Adults and children age 6 and older:
Initially, 0.25 mcg P.O. daily in the
morning. Dosage may be increased at 2- to
4-week intervals. Maintenance dosage is
0.25 to 2 mcg P.O. daily.
➤ **Hypoparathyroidism**
Children ages 1 to 5: Give 0.25 to
0.75 mcg P.O. daily.
➤ **To manage secondary hyper-**
parathyroidism and resulting
metabolic bone disease in predialysis
patients (with creatinine clearance
of 15 to 55 ml/minute)
Adults and children age 3 and older:
Initially, 0.25 mcg P.O. daily. Dosage may
be increased to 0.5 mcg/day if needed.
Children younger than age 3: Initially,
0.01 to 0.015 mcg/kg P.O. daily.

ADMINISTRATION
P.O.
● Give drug without regard for food.
● Don't give with magnesium-containing
antacids.
I.V.
● For hypocalcemia in patient undergoing
hemodialysis, give drug by rapid injection
through catheter at end of hemodialysis
session.
● **Incompatibilities:** None reported.

ACTION
Stimulates calcium absorption from the
GI tract and promotes movement of
calcium from bone to blood.

Route	Onset	Peak	Duration
P.O.	2–6 hr	3–6 hr	3–5 days
I.V.	Immediate	Unknown	3–5 days

Half-life: 3 to 6 hours.

ADVERSE REACTIONS
CNS: headache, somnolence, weakness,
irritability.
CV: hypertension, *arrhythmias.*
EENT: conjunctivitis, photophobia,
rhinorrhea, nephrocalcinosis.
GI: nausea, vomiting, constipation,
polydipsia, *pancreatitis,* metallic taste,
dry mouth, anorexia.
GU: polyuria, nocturia, nephrocalcinosis.
Metabolic: weight loss.
Musculoskeletal: bone and muscle pain.
Skin: pruritus.
Other: hyperthermia, decreased libido.

INTERACTIONS
Drug-drug. *Cardiac glycosides:* May
increase risk of arrhythmias. Use together
cautiously.
*Cholestyramine, colestipol, excessive use
of mineral oil:* May decrease absorption
of oral vitamin D analogues. Avoid using
together.
Corticosteroids: May counteract vitamin
D analogue effects. Avoid using together.
Magnesium-containing antacids: May
cause hypermagnesemia, especially in

patients with chronic renal failure. Avoid using together.

Phenytoin, phenobarbital: May inhibit calcitriol synthesis. Dose may need to be increased.

Thiazides: May cause hypercalcemia. Use together cautiously.

EFFECTS ON LAB TEST RESULTS
None reported.

CONTRAINDICATIONS & CAUTIONS
● Contraindicated in patients with hypercalcemia or vitamin D toxicity. Withhold all preparations containing vitamin D.
● Use cautiously in patients receiving cardiac glycosides and in those with sarcoidosis or hyperparathyroidism.

NURSING CONSIDERATIONS
● Effective therapy is dependent on adequate calcium intake.
● Monitor calcium level; this level times the phosphate level shouldn't exceed 70. During dose adjustment, determine calcium level twice weekly. If hypercalcemia occurs, stop drug and notify prescriber but resume after calcium level returns to normal. Patient should receive adequate daily intake of calcium. Observe for hypocalcemia, bone pain, and weakness before and during therapy.
● Monitor phosphorous level, especially in hypoparathyroid patients and dialysis patients.
● Reduce dose as parathyroid hormone levels decrease in response to therapy.
● The symptoms of vitamin D intoxication include headache, somnolence, weakness, irritability, hypertension, arrhythmias, conjunctivitis, photophobia, rhinorrhea, nausea, vomiting, constipation, polydipsia, pancreatitis, metallic taste, dry mouth, anorexia, nephrocalcinosis, polyuria, nocturia, weight loss, bone and muscle pain, pruritus, hyperthermia, and decreased libido.
● Protect drug from heat and light.
● *Look alike–sound alike:* Don't confuse calcitriol with calcifediol or calcitonin.

PATIENT TEACHING
● Tell patient to immediately report early symptoms of vitamin D intoxication:

weakness, nausea, vomiting, dry mouth, constipation, muscle or bone pain, or metallic taste.
● Instruct patient to adhere to diet and calcium supplementation and to avoid unapproved OTC drugs and antacids that contain magnesium.
● *Alert:* Tell patient that drug is the most potent form of vitamin D available and shouldn't be taken by anyone else.

---

cinacalcet hydrochloride
sin-ah-KAL-set

Sensipar

Pharmacologic class: calcimimetic
Pregnancy risk category C

AVAILABLE FORMS
Tablets: 30 mg, 60 mg, 90 mg

INDICATIONS & DOSAGES
➤ **Secondary hyperparathyroidism in patients with chronic kidney disease undergoing dialysis**
Adults: Initially, 30 mg P.O. once daily; adjust no more than every 2 to 4 weeks through sequential doses of 60 mg, 90 mg, 120 mg, and 180 mg P.O. once daily to reach target range of 150 to 300 picograms (pg)/ml for intact para-thyroid hormone (PTH).
➤ **Hypercalcemia in patients with parathyroid carcinoma**
Adults: Initially, 30 mg P.O. b.i.d.; adjust every 2 to 4 weeks through sequential doses of 30 mg, 60 mg, and 90 mg P.O. b.i.d., and 90 mg P.O. t.i.d. or q.i.d. daily if needed to normalize calcium level.

ADMINISTRATION
P.O.
● Don't break or crush tablets; give them whole, with food or shortly after a meal.

ACTION
Increases sensitivity of calcium-sensing receptor to extracellular calcium, letting calcium be absorbed despite decreased PTH.

Route	Onset	Peak	Duration
P.O.	Unknown	2–6 hr	Unknown

Half-life: Terminal half-life, 30 to 40 hours.

ADVERSE REACTIONS
CNS: *dizziness,* asthenia, *seizures.*
CV: chest pain, hypertension.
GI: *diarrhea, nausea, vomiting,* anorexia.
Metabolic: *hypocalcemia.*
Musculoskeletal: *myalgia.*
Other: access infection.

INTERACTIONS
Drug-drug. *Amitriptyline:* Amitriptyline and nortriptyline exposure increases by 20% in patients who are CYP2D6 extensive metabolizers. Avoid using together, if possible.
Drugs metabolized mainly by CYP2D6 with a narrow therapeutic index (such as flecainide, thioridazine, most tricyclic antidepressants, vinblastine): May strongly inhibit CYP2D6, decreasing metabolism and increasing levels of these drugs. Adjust dosage of other drugs, as needed.
Drugs that strongly inhibit CYP3A4 (such as erythromycin, itraconazole, ketoconazole): May increase cinacalcet level. Use together cautiously, monitoring PTH and calcium level closely and adjusting cinacalcet dosage, as needed.

EFFECTS ON LAB TEST RESULTS
● May decrease calcium, phosphorus, and testosterone levels.

CONTRAINDICATIONS & CAUTIONS
● Contraindicated in patients hypersensitive to drug or its components and in patients with calcium level less than 8.4 mg/dl.
● Use cautiously in patients with history of seizures and in those with moderate to severe hepatic impairment.

NURSING CONSIDERATIONS
● **Alert:** Monitor calcium level closely, especially if patient has a history of seizures, because decreased calcium level lowers seizure threshold.
● Patients with moderate to severe hepatic impairment may need dosage adjustment

based on PTH and calcium level. Monitor these patients closely.
● Give drug alone or with vitamin D sterols, phosphate binders, or both.
● Measure calcium level within 1 week after starting therapy or adjusting dosage. After maintenance dose is established, measure calcium level monthly for patients with chronic kidney disease receiving dialysis and every 2 months for those with parathyroid carcinoma.
● Watch carefully for evidence of hypocalcemia: paresthesias, myalgias, cramping, tetany, and seizures.
● If calcium level is 7.5 to 8.4 mg/dl or patient develops symptoms of hypocalcemia, give calcium-containing phosphate binders, vitamin D sterols, or both, to raise calcium level. If calcium level is below 7.5 mg/dl or hypocalcemia symptoms persist and the vitamin D dose can't be increased, withhold drug until calcium level reaches 8.0 mg/dl, hypocalcemia symptoms resolve, or both. Resume therapy with the next lowest dose.
● Measure intact PTH level 1 to 4 weeks after therapy starts or dosage changes. After the maintenance dose is established, monitor PTH level every 1 to 3 months. Levels in patients with chronic kidney disease receiving dialysis should be 150 to 300 pg/ml.
● Adynamic bone disease may develop if intact PTH levels are suppressed below 100 pg/ml. If this occurs, notify prescriber. The dosage of cinacalcet or vitamin D sterols may need to be reduced or stopped.
● **Alert:** Don't use drug in patients with chronic kidney disease who aren't receiving dialysis because they have an increased risk of hypocalcemia.

PATIENT TEACHING
● Tell patient not to divide tablets but to take them whole, with food or shortly after a meal.
● Advise patient to report to prescriber adverse reactions and signs of hypocalcemia, which include paresthesias, muscle weakness, muscle cramping, and muscle spasm.

teriparatide
(rDNA origin)
tehr-ih-PAHR-uh-tide

Forteo

Pharmacologic class: recombinant human parathyroid hormone (PTH)
Pregnancy risk category C

AVAILABLE FORMS
Injection: 750 mcg/3 ml in a prefilled pen

INDICATIONS & DOSAGES
➤ **Osteoporosis in postmenopausal women at high risk for fracture; primary or hypogonadal osteoporosis in men at high risk for fracture**
Adults: 20 mcg subcutaneously in thigh or abdominal wall once daily.

ADMINISTRATION
Subcutaneous
● Inspect solution before giving.
● Drug is a colorless, clear liquid.
● Don't use if solid particles are present or if the solution is cloudy or colored.
● Give while patient is in a sitting position to avoid orthostatic hypotension.
● Discard the pen after the 28-day use period, even if some unused solution still remains.

ACTION
Promotes new bone formation, skeletal bone mass, and bone strength by regulating calcium and phosphorus metabolism in bones and kidneys.

Route	Onset	Peak	Duration
Subcut.	Rapid	30 min	3 hr

Half-life: 1 hour.

ADVERSE REACTIONS
CNS: asthenia, depression, dizziness, headache, insomnia, *pain,* syncope, vertigo.
CV: angina pectoris, hypertension, orthostatic hypotension.
EENT: pharyngitis, rhinitis.
GI: constipation, diarrhea, dyspepsia, nausea, tooth disorder, vomiting.

Metabolic: hypercalcemia.
Musculoskeletal: *arthralgia,* leg cramps, neck pain.
Respiratory: dyspnea, increased cough, pneumonia.
Skin: rash, sweating.

INTERACTIONS
Drug-drug. *Calcium supplements:* May increase urinary calcium excretion. Dosage may need adjustment.
Digoxin: May predispose hypercalcemic patient to digitalis toxicity. Use together cautiously.

EFFECTS ON LAB TEST RESULTS
● May increase calcium and uric acid levels. May decrease phosphorus level.
● May increase urinary calcium and phosphorus excretion.

CONTRAINDICATIONS & CAUTIONS
● Contraindicated in patients hypersensitive to teriparatide or its components.
■ **Black Box Warning** Contraindicated in patients at increased risk for osteosarcoma, such as those with Paget disease or unexplained alkaline phosphatase elevations, children, and patients who have had skeletal radiation. ■
● Contraindicated in patients with bone metastases, a history of skeletal malignancies, hypercalcemia, or metabolic bone diseases other than osteoporosis; and in patients with hypercalcemia.
● Use cautiously in patients with active or recent urolithiasis or hepatic, renal, or cardiac disease, or hypotension.
● Don't use in nursing mothers.

NURSING CONSIDERATIONS
■ **Black Box Warning** Because of the risk of osteosarcoma, give drug only to patients for whom benefits outweigh risk. ■
● Treatment may last for up to 2 years.
● If patient may have urolithiasis or hypercalciuria, measure urinary calcium excretion before treatment.
● Monitor patient for orthostatic hypotension, which may occur within 4 hours of dosing.
● Monitor calcium level. If persistent hypercalcemia develops, stop drug and evaluate possible cause.

Reactions may be *common,* uncommon, *life-threatening,* or COMMON AND LIFE-THREATENING.
Interaction may have a *rapid onset* or **delayed onset.**

PATIENT TEACHING
- Instruct patient on proper use and disposal of prefilled pen.
- Tell patient not to share pen with others.
- Advise patient to remain in a sitting position while taking drug to prevent orthostatic hypotension.
- Advise patient to sit or lie down if drug causes a fast heart beat, light-headedness, or dizziness. Tell patient to report persistent or worsening symptoms.
- Urge patient to report persistent symptoms of hypercalcemia, which include nausea, vomiting, constipation, lethargy, and muscle weakness.

54
Skeletal muscle relaxants

baclofen
carisoprodol
cyclobenzaprine hydrochloride
dantrolene sodium
tizanidine hydrochloride

---

baclofen
BAK-loe-fen

Kemstro, Lioresal, Lioresal
Intrathecal

Pharmacologic class:
gamma-aminobutyric acid (GABA)
derivative
Pregnancy risk category C

AVAILABLE FORMS
Intrathecal injection: 50 mcg/ml,
500 mcg/ml, 2,000 mcg/ml
Tablets: 10 mg, 20 mg
Tablets (orally disintegrating): 10 mg,
20 mg

INDICATIONS & DOSAGES
➤ **Spasticity in multiple sclerosis;
spinal cord injury**
Adults: Initially, 5 mg P.O. t.i.d. for 3 days;
then 10 mg t.i.d. for 3 days, 15 mg t.i.d.
for 3 days, 20 mg t.i.d. for 3 days. Increase
daily dosage, based on response, to maximum of 80 mg.
Adjust-a-dose: For patients with psychiatric or brain disorders and for elderly
patients, increase dose gradually.
➤ **To manage severe spasticity in
patients who don't respond to or
can't tolerate oral baclofen therapy**
Adults: For screening phase, after test
dose to check responsiveness, give drug
via implantable infusion pump. Give test
dose of 1 ml of 50-mcg/ml dilution into
intrathecal space by barbotage over
1 minute or longer. Significantly decreased
severity or frequency of muscle spasm or
reduced muscle tone should appear within
4 to 8 hours. If response is inadequate,
give second test dose of 75 mcg/1.5 ml
24 hours after the first. If response is still

inadequate, give final test dose of
100 mcg/2 ml after 24 hours. Patients
unresponsive to the 100-mcg dose
shouldn't be considered candidates for
implantable pump.
Children: Initial test dose is the same as
that of adults (50 mcg); for very small
children, initial dose is 25 mcg.
For maintenance therapy: Adjust first dose
based on screening dose that elicited an
adequate response. Double this effective
dose and give over 24 hours. However, if
screening dose effectiveness was maintained for 12 hours or longer, don't double
the dose. After the first 24 hours, increase
dose slowly as needed and tolerated by
10% to 30% increments at 24-hour intervals in spasticity of spinal cord origin. In
children with spasticity of spinal cord origin and adults and children with spasticity
of cerebral origin, increase by 5% to 15%
increments at 24-hour intervals. During
prolonged maintenance therapy, increase
daily dose by 10% to 40% in spasticity of
spinal cord origin, or increase daily dose
by 5% to 15% in spasticity of cerebral
origin, if needed; if patient experiences
adverse effects, decrease dose by 10% to
20%. Maintenance dosages range from
12 mcg to 2,000 mcg daily, but experience
with dosages of more than 1,000 mcg
daily is limited. Most patients need
300 mcg to 800 mcg daily.
Adjust-a-dose: For patients with impaired
renal function, decrease oral and intrathecal doses.

ADMINISTRATION
P.O.
● Give drug with meals or milk to prevent
GI distress.
● Remove orally disintegrating tablet from
blister pack and immediately place on the
patient's tongue to dissolve; then have the
patient swallow with or without water.
Intrathecal
■ **Black Box Warning** Do not discontinue
abruptly. This can result in high fever,
altered mental status, exaggerated rebound
spasticity, and muscle rigidity, which in

Reactions may be *common*, uncommon, *life-threatening*, or COMMON AND LIFE-THREATENING.
Interaction may have a *rapid onset* or **delayed onset.**

rare cases, has led to rhabdomyolysis, multiple-organ-system failure, and death. ■

• Don't give intrathecal injection by I.V., I.M., subcutaneous, or epidural route.

• If patient suddenly requires a large intrathecal dose increase, check for a catheter complication, such as kinking or dislodgment.

• With long-term intrathecal use, about 5% of patients may develop tolerance to drug. In some cases, this may be treated by hospitalizing patient and slowly withdrawing drug over a 2-week period.

ACTION

Hyperpolarizes fibers to reduce impulse transmission. Appears to reduce transmission of impulses from the spinal cord to skeletal muscle, thus decreasing the frequency and amplitude of muscle spasms in patients with spinal cord lesions.

Route	Onset	Peak	Duration
P.O.	Unknown	2–3 hr	Unknown
P.O. (orally disintegrating)	Unknown	1½ hr	Unknown
Intrathecal	30 min–1 hr	4 hr	4–8 hr

Half-life: 2½ to 4 hours.

ADVERSE REACTIONS

CNS: *drowsiness,* high fever, *dizziness,* headache, *weakness,* fatigue, paresthesias, hypotonia, *confusion,* hallucinations, insomnia, dysarthria, **seizures with intrathecal use.**
CV: hypotension, hypertension.
EENT: blurred vision, nasal congestion, slurred speech.
GI: *nausea,* constipation, *vomiting.*
GU: urinary frequency.
Metabolic: hyperglycemia, weight gain.
Musculoskeletal: muscle rigidity or spasticity, **rhabdomyolysis,** muscle weakness.
Respiratory: dyspnea.
Skin: rash, pruritus, excessive sweating.
Other: *multiple organ-system failure.*

INTERACTIONS

Drug-drug. *CNS depressants:* May increase CNS depression. Avoid using together.

Drug-lifestyle. *Alcohol use:* May increase CNS depression. Discourage use together.

EFFECTS ON LAB TEST RESULTS

• May increase alkaline phosphatase, AST, CK, and glucose levels.

CONTRAINDICATIONS & CAUTIONS

• Contraindicated in patients hypersensitive to drug.
• Orally disintegrating tablets contraindicated in patients hypersensitive to aspartame or other components of the drug.
• Use cautiously in patients with impaired renal function or seizure disorder or when spasticity is used to maintain motor function.

NURSING CONSIDERATIONS

• *Alert:* Don't use oral drug to treat muscle spasm caused by rheumatic disorders, cerebral palsy, Parkinson disease, or stroke because drug's effectiveness for these indications hasn't been established.
• Watch for sensitivity reactions, such as fever, skin eruptions, and respiratory distress.
• Expect an increased risk of seizures in patients with seizure disorder.
• The amount of relief determines whether dosage (and drowsiness) can be reduced.
• Don't withdraw drug abruptly after long-term use unless severe adverse reactions demand it; doing so may precipitate seizures, hallucinations, or rebound spasticity.
• *Look alike–sound alike:* Don't confuse baclofen with Bactroban.

PATIENT TEACHING

• Instruct patient to take oral form with meals or milk.
• Tell patients with phenylketonuria that orally disintegrating tablets contain phenylalanine (3.9 mg/10 mg tablet and 7.9 mg/20 mg tablet).
• Instruct patient to remove orally disintegrating tablet from blister pack and immediately place on the tongue to dissolve; then swallow with or without water.
• Tell patient to avoid activities that require alertness until CNS effects of drug are known. Drowsiness usually is transient.

- Tell patient to avoid alcohol and OTC antihistamines while taking drug.
- Advise patient to follow prescriber's orders regarding rest and physical therapy.

---

carisoprodol
kar-eye-soe-PROE-dol

Soma♪

Pharmacologic class: carbamate derivative
Pregnancy risk category C

AVAILABLE FORMS
Tablets: 350 mg

INDICATIONS & DOSAGES
➤ **Adjunctive treatment for acute, painful musculoskeletal conditions**
Adults: 250 mg to 350 mg P.O. t.i.d. and at bedtime for a maximum of 2 to 3 weeks.

ADMINISTRATION
P.O.
- Give drug with food or milk if GI upset occurs.

ACTION
May modify central perception of pain without modifying pain reflexes. Muscle relaxant effects may be related to sedative properties.

Route	Onset	Peak	Duration
P.O.	½ hr	4 hr	4–6 hr

Half-life: 8 hours.

ADVERSE REACTIONS
CNS: *drowsiness, dizziness,* vertigo, ataxia, tremor, agitation, irritability, headache, depressive reactions, fever, insomnia, syncope.
CV: *orthostatic hypotension,* tachycardia, facial flushing.
GI: nausea, vomiting, epigastric distress, hiccups.
Respiratory: *asthmatic episodes,* hiccups.
Skin: *erythema multiforme,* pruritus, rash.
Other: *angioedema, anaphylaxis.*

INTERACTIONS
Drug-drug. *CNS depressants:* May increase CNS depression. Avoid using together.
Drug-lifestyle. *Alcohol use:* May increase CNS depression. Discourage use together.

EFFECTS ON LAB TEST RESULTS
- May increase eosinophil count.

CONTRAINDICATIONS & CAUTIONS
- Contraindicated in patients hypersensitive to related compounds (such as meprobamate) and in those with intermittent porphyria.
- Use cautiously in patients with impaired hepatic or renal function.
- Safety and effectiveness in children younger than age 16 haven't been established.

NURSING CONSIDERATIONS
- *Alert:* Watch for idiosyncratic reactions after first to fourth doses (weakness, ataxia, visual and speech difficulties, fever, skin eruptions, and mental changes) and for severe reactions, including bronchospasm, hypotension, and anaphylactic shock. After unusual reactions, withhold dose and notify prescriber immediately.
- Record amount of relief to help prescriber determine whether dosage can be reduced.
- Don't stop drug abruptly, which may cause mild withdrawal effects, such as insomnia, headache, nausea, or abdominal cramps.
- Drug may be habit forming.

PATIENT TEACHING
- Warn patient to avoid activities that require alertness until CNS effects of drug are known. Drowsiness is transient.
- Advise patient to avoid combining drug with alcohol or other CNS depressants.
- Tell patient to ask prescriber before using OTC cold or hay fever remedies.
- Instruct patient to follow prescriber's orders regarding rest and physical therapy.
- Advise patient to avoid sudden changes in posture if dizziness occurs.
- Tell patient to take drug with food or milk if GI upset occurs.

Reactions may be *common,* uncommon, *life-threatening,* or COMMON AND LIFE-THREATENING.
Interaction may have a *rapid onset* or **delayed onset.**

cyclobenzaprine hydrochloride

sye-kloe-BEN-za-preen

Amrix, Flexeril

Pharmacologic class: tricyclic antidepressant derivative
Pregnancy risk category B

AVAILABLE FORMS

Capsules (extended-release): 15 mg, 30 mg
Tablets: 5 mg, 7.5 mg, 10 mg

INDICATIONS & DOSAGES

➤ **Adjunct to rest and physical therapy to relieve muscle spasm from acute, painful musculoskeletal conditions**
Adults: 5 mg P.O. t.i.d. Based on response, dose may be increased to 10 mg t.i.d. Don't exceed 60 mg/day. Or, 15 to 30 mg extended-release capsule P.O. once daily. Use for longer than 2 or 3 weeks isn't recommended.
Adjust-a-dose: In elderly patients and in those with mild hepatic impairment, start with 5-mg conventional tablets and adjust slowly upward. Drug isn't recommended in patients with moderate to severe hepatic impairment. Don't use extended-release capsules in the elderly or those with impaired hepatic function.

ADMINISTRATION

P.O.
● Don't split the generic 10-mg tablets because of the high risk of inconsistent doses.
● Give extended-release capsules whole; don't crush or break.

ACTION

Unknown. Relieves skeletal muscle spasm of local origin without disrupting muscle function.

Route	Onset	Peak	Duration
P.O.	1 hr	4 hr	12–24 hr
P.O. (extended-release)	1.5 hr	7–8 hr	Unknown

Half-life: 1 to 3 days; 32 hours for extended-release capsules.

ADVERSE REACTIONS

CNS: *dizziness, drowsiness, **seizures,** headache,* tremor, insomnia, fatigue, asthenia, nervousness, confusion, paresthesia, depression, attention disturbances, dysarthria, ataxia, syncope.
CV: ***arrhythmias,*** palpitations, hypotension, tachycardia, vasodilation.
EENT: visual disturbances, blurred vision.
GI: *dry mouth,* dyspepsia, abnormal taste, constipation, nausea.
GU: urine retention, urinary frequency.
Skin: rash, urticaria, pruritus, sweating, acne.

INTERACTIONS

Drug-drug. *CNS depressants:* May increase CNS depression. Avoid using together.
Guanethidine: May block guanethidine's antihypertensive effect. Monitor patient's blood pressure.
MAO inhibitors: May cause hyperpyretic crisis, seizures, and death when MAO inhibitors are used with tricyclic antidepressants; may also occur with cyclobenzaprine. Avoid using within 2 weeks of MAO inhibitor therapy.
Naproxen: May increase drowsiness. Make patient aware of this interaction.
Tramadol: May increase risk of seizures. Use together cautiously.
Drug-lifestyle. *Alcohol use:* May increase CNS depression. Discourage use together.

EFFECTS ON LAB TEST RESULTS

None reported.

CONTRAINDICATIONS & CAUTIONS

● Contraindicated in patients hypersensitive to drug; in those with hyperthyroidism, heart block, arrhythmias, conduction disturbances, or heart failure; in those who have received MAO inhibitors within 14 days; and in those in the acute recovery phase of an MI.
● Use cautiously in elderly or debilitated patients and in those with a history of urine retention, acute angle-closure glaucoma, or increased intraocular pressure.
● Safety and effectiveness in children younger than age 15 haven't been established.

NURSING CONSIDERATIONS
• Drug may cause toxic reactions similar to those of tricyclic antidepressants. Observe same precautions as when giving tricyclic antidepressants.
• Monitor patient for nausea, headache, and malaise, which may occur if drug is stopped abruptly after long-term use.
• *Alert:* Notify prescriber immediately of signs and symptoms of overdose, including cardiac toxicity.
• *Look alike–sound alike:* Don't confuse Flexeril with Floxin.

PATIENT TEACHING
• Advise patient to report urinary hesitancy or urine retention. If constipation is a problem, suggest that patient increase fluid intake and use a stool softener.
• Warn patient to avoid activities that require alertness until CNS effects of drug are known.
• Warn patient not to combine with alcohol or other CNS depressants, including OTC cold or allergy remedies.
• Instruct patient not to split the generic 10-mg tablets because of the high risk of inconsistent doses.

---

dantrolene sodium
DAN-troe-leen

Dantrium, Dantrium Intravenous

Pharmacologic class: hydantoin derivative
Pregnancy risk category C

AVAILABLE FORMS
Capsules: 25 mg, 50 mg, 100 mg
Injection: 20 mg/vial

INDICATIONS & DOSAGES
➤ **Spasticity and sequelae from severe chronic disorders, such as multiple sclerosis, cerebral palsy, spinal cord injury, stroke**
Adults: 25 mg P.O. daily. Increase by 25-mg increments, up to 100 mg t.i.d. to q.i.d. Maintain each dosage level for 7 days to determine response. Maximum, 400 mg daily.
Children: Initially, 0.5 mg/kg P.O. daily for 7 days; then 0.5 mg/kg t.i.d. for 7 days,

1 mg/kg t.i.d. for 7 days, and finally, 2 mg/kg, t.i.d. for 7 days. May increase up to 3 mg/kg b.i.d. to q.i.d. if necessary. Maximum, 100 mg q.i.d.
➤ **To manage malignant hyperthermic crisis**
Adults and children: Initially, 1 mg/kg I.V. push. Repeat, as needed, up to cumulative dose of 10 mg/kg.
➤ **To prevent or attenuate malignant hyperthermic crisis in susceptible patients who need surgery**
Adults and children: 4 to 8 mg/kg P.O. daily in three or four divided doses for 1 or 2 days before procedure. Give final dose 3 or 4 hours before procedure. Or, 2.5 mg/kg I.V. about 1.25 hours before anesthesia; infuse over 1 hour.
➤ **To prevent recurrence of malignant hyperthermic crisis**
Adults: 4 to 8 mg/kg P.O. daily in four divided doses for up to 3 days after hyperthermic crisis.

ADMINISTRATION
P.O.
• Give drug with food or milk.
• Prepare oral suspension for single dose by dissolving capsule contents in juice or other liquid. For multiple doses, use acid vehicle and refrigerate. Use within several days.
I.V.
• Reconstitute drug by adding 60 ml of sterile water for injection and shaking vial until clear. Don't use a diluent that contains a bacteriostatic drug.
• Protect solution from light, and use within 6 hours.
• **Incompatibilities:** D_5W, normal saline solution, other I.V. drugs mixed in a syringe.

ACTION
Acts directly on skeletal muscle to decrease excitation and contraction coupling and reduce muscle strength by interfering with intracellular calcium movement.

Route	Onset	Peak	Duration
P.O.	Unknown	5 hr	Unknown
I.V.	Unknown	Unknown	3 hr after infusion

Half-life: P.O., 9 hours; I.V., 4 to 8 hours.

ADVERSE REACTIONS

CNS: *drowsiness, dizziness, malaise, fatigue, seizures,* headache, light-headedness, confusion, nervousness, insomnia, fever, depression.
CV: tachycardia, blood pressure changes, phlebitis, thrombophlebitis, heart failure.
EENT: excessive lacrimation, speech disturbance, diplopia, visual disturbances.
GI: anorexia, constipation, cramping, dysphagia, metallic taste, severe diarrhea, *GI bleeding,* vomiting.
GU: urinary frequency, hematuria, incontinence, nocturia, dysuria, crystal-luria, difficult erection, urine retention.
Hematologic: *leukopenia, thrombo-cytopenia, lymphocytic lymphoma,* anemia.
Hepatic: *hepatitis.*
Musculoskeletal: *muscle weakness,* myalgia, back pain.
Respiratory: pleural effusion with pericarditis, *pulmonary edema.*
Skin: eczematous eruption, pruritus, urticaria, abnormal hair growth, diaphoresis, photosensitivity.
Other: chills.

INTERACTIONS

Drug-drug. *Clofibrate, warfarin:* May decrease protein binding of dantrolene. Use together cautiously.
CNS depressants: May increase CNS depression. Avoid using together.
Estrogens: May increase risk of hepato-toxicity. Use together cautiously.
I.V. verapamil and other calcium channel blockers: May cause hyperkalemia, ventricular fibrillation, and myocardial depression. Stop verapamil before giving I.V. dantrolene.
Vecuronium: May increase neuromuscular blockade effect. Use together cautiously.
Drug-lifestyle. *Alcohol use:* May increase CNS depression. Discourage use together.
Sun exposure: May cause photosensitivity reactions. Advise patient to avoid excessive sunlight exposure.

EFFECTS ON LAB TEST RESULTS

● May increase ALT, AST, alkaline phosphatase, LDH, bilirubin, and BUN levels.

CONTRAINDICATIONS & CAUTIONS

● Contraindicated for spasms in rheumatic disorders and when spasticity is used to maintain motor function.
● Contraindicated in breast-feeding patients and patients with upper motor neuron disorders or active hepatic disease.
■ **Black Box Warning** Risk of hepatic injury is increased in women, patients older than age 35, and patients with hepatic disease (such as cirrhosis or hepatitis) or severely impaired cardiac or pulmonary function. ■

NURSING CONSIDERATIONS

● Start therapy as soon as malignant hyperthermia reaction is recognized.
■ **Black Box Warning** Liver damage may occur with long-term use. Use the lowest possible effective dose for each patient. If benefits don't occur within 45 days, stop therapy. ■
■ **Black Box Warning** Obtain liver func-tion test results at start of therapy. Monitor hepatic function, including AST and ALT, frequently. ■
● *Alert:* Watch for fever, jaundice, severe diarrhea, weakness, and sensitivity reac-tions, including skin eruptions. Withhold dose and notify prescriber.
● *Look alike–sound alike:* Don't confuse Dantrium with Daraprim.

PATIENT TEACHING

● Instruct patient to take drug with meals or milk in four divided doses.
● Tell patient to eat carefully to avoid choking. Some patients may have trouble swallowing during therapy.
● Warn patient to avoid driving and other hazardous activities until CNS effects of drug are known.
● Advise patient to avoid combining drug with alcohol or other CNS depressants.
● Advise patient to notify prescriber if skin or eyes turn yellow, skin itches, or fever develops.
● Tell patient to avoid photosensitivity reactions by using sunblock and wearing protective clothing, to report abdominal discomfort or GI problems immediately, and to follow prescriber's orders regarding rest and physical therapy.

tizanidine hydrochloride
tis-AN-i-deen

Zanaflex

Pharmacologic class: imidazoline
derivative, centrally acting alpha$_2$-
adrenergic agonist
Pregnancy risk category C

AVAILABLE FORMS
Capsules: 2 mg, 4 mg, 6 mg
Tablets: 2 mg, 4 mg

INDICATIONS & DOSAGES
➤ **Acute and intermittent management of increased muscle tone with spasticity**
Adults: Initially, 4 mg P.O. every 6 to
8 hours, as needed, to maximum of three
doses in 24 hours. Dosage can be
increased gradually in 2- to 4-mg increments, reaching optimum dose over 2 to
4 weeks. Maximum, 36 mg daily.
Adjust-a-dose: For patients with renal
insufficiency, reduce dosage. If higher
dosages are needed, increase individual
doses rather than frequency.

ADMINISTRATION
P.O.
● Give drug consistently with or without
food for same absorption rate and effect.

ACTION
Unknown. Acts as an alpha$_2$ agonist. May
reduce spasticity by increasing presynaptic inhibition of motor neurons at the level
of the spinal cord.

Route	Onset	Peak	Duration
P.O.	Unknown	1–2 hr	3–6 hr

Half-life: 2½ hours; metabolites, 20 to
40 hours.

ADVERSE REACTIONS
CNS: *somnolence, sedation, asthenia,
dizziness,* speech disorder, dyskinesia,
nervousness, hallucinations.
CV: *hypotension,* **bradycardia.**
EENT: amblyopia, pharyngitis, rhinitis.
GI: *dry mouth,* constipation, vomiting.
GU: *UTI,* urinary frequency.

Hepatic: hepatic injury.
Other: infection, flulike syndrome.

INTERACTIONS
Drug-drug. *Acetaminophen:* May delay
acetaminophen absorption time. Monitor
patient for clinical effect.
*Antihypertensives, other alpha agonists
such as clonidine:* May cause hypotension; monitor patient closely. Avoid using
together.
*Baclofen, benzodiazepines, other CNS
depressants:* May have additive CNS
depressant effects. Avoid using together.
*CYP1A2 inhibitors (amiodarone,
acyclovir, cimetidine, ciprofloxacin,
famotidine, fluoroquinolones, fluvoxamine,
mexiletine, propafenone, ticlodipine,
verapamil, zileuton):* May cause significant
increases in tizanidine levels. Use together
should be avoided; use of ciprofloxacin
or fluvoxamine with tizanidine is
contraindicated.
Oral contraceptives: May decrease
tizanidine clearance. Reduce tizanidine
dosage.
Drug-lifestyle. *Alcohol use:* May increase
CNS depression. Discourage use together.

EFFECTS ON LAB TEST RESULTS
● May increase AST and ALT levels.

CONTRAINDICATIONS & CAUTIONS
● Contraindicated in patients hypersensitive
to drug.
● Use of potent CYP1A2 inhibitors
ciprofloxacin and fluvoxamine with
tizanidine is contraindicated.
● Use cautiously in patients who are
taking antihypertensives, in those with
renal and hepatic impairment, in pregnant
or breast-feeding women, and in elderly
patients.
● Safety and effectiveness in children
haven't been established.

NURSING CONSIDERATIONS
● **Alert:** The capsules and tablets are
bioequivalent only if taken on an empty
stomach.
● Obtain liver function test results before
treatment; during treatment at 1, 3, and
6 months; and then periodically thereafter.
● **Alert:** Stop drug gradually, especially in
patients taking high doses for a prolonged

period. Decrease dose slowly to minimize the potential for rebound hypertension, tachycardia, and hypertonia.

● *Look alike–sound alike:* Don't confuse tizanidine with tiagabine; both have 4-mg starting doses.

PATIENT TEACHING

● Caution patient to avoid alcohol and activities that require alertness. Drug may cause drowsiness.

● Inform patient that dizziness upon standing quickly can be minimized by rising slowly and avoiding sudden position changes.

● Advise patient not to suddenly stop taking medication.

55
Antihistamines

cetirizine hydrochloride
chlorpheniramine maleate
desloratadine
diphenhydramine hydrochloride
fexofenadine hydrochloride
levocetirizine dihydrochloride
loratadine
promethazine hydrochloride

---

cetirizine hydrochloride
se-TEER-i-zeen

Zyrtec♦ ◊

Pharmacologic class: piperazine
derivative
Pregnancy risk category B

AVAILABLE FORMS
Oral solution: 5 mg/5 ml ◊
Tablets: 5 mg, 10 mg ◊
Tablets (chewable): 5 mg ◊, 10 mg ◊

INDICATIONS & DOSAGES
➤ **Seasonal allergic rhinitis**
Adults and children age 6 and older:
5 to 10 mg P.O. once daily.
Children ages 2 to 5: 2.5 mg P.O. once
daily. Maximum daily dose is 5 mg.
➤ **Perennial allergic rhinitis, chronic
urticaria**
Adults and children age 6 and older:
5 to 10 mg P.O. once daily.
Children ages 6 months to 5 years: 2.5 mg
P.O. once daily; in children ages 1 to 5,
increase to maximum of 5 mg daily.
Children ages 12 to 23 months should
receive the 5-mg dose as two divided doses.
Adjust-a-dose: In adults age 65 and older,
and adults and children age 6 and older
receiving hemodialysis, those with hepatic
impairment, and those with creatinine clearance less than 31 ml/minute, give 5 mg P.O.
daily. Don't use in children younger than
age 6 with renal or hepatic impairment.

ADMINISTRATION
P.O.
• Give drug without regard for food.

ACTION
A long-acting, nonsedating antihistamine
that selectively inhibits peripheral H_1
receptors.

Route	Onset	Peak	Duration
P.O.	Rapid	60 min	24 hr

Half-life: About 8 hours.

ADVERSE REACTIONS
CNS: *somnolence,* fatigue, dizziness,
headache.
EENT: pharyngitis.
GI: dry mouth, nausea, vomiting, abdomi-
nal distress.

INTERACTIONS
Drug-drug. *CNS depressants:* May cause
additive effect. Monitor patient closely
for excessive sedation or other adverse
effects.
Theophylline: May decrease cetirizine
clearance. Monitor patient closely.
Drug-lifestyle. *Alcohol use:* May
cause additive effects. Discourage
use together.

EFFECTS ON LAB TEST RESULTS
• May prevent, reduce, or mask positive
result in diagnostic skin test.

CONTRAINDICATIONS & CAUTIONS
• Contraindicated in patients hypersensitive
to drug or to hydroxyzine and in breast-
feeding women.
• Use cautiously in patients with renal or
hepatic impairment.

NURSING CONSIDERATIONS
• Stop drug 4 days before diagnostic skin
testing because antihistamines can
prevent, reduce, or mask positive skin test
response.
• *Look alike–sound alike:* Don't confuse
Zyrtec with Zyprexa or Zantac.

PATIENT TEACHING
• Warn patient not to perform hazardous
activities until CNS effects of drug are

Reactions may be *common,* uncommon, *life-threatening,* or COMMON AND LIFE-THREATENING.
Interaction may have a *rapid onset* or **delayed onset.**

known. Somnolence is a common adverse reaction.
• Advise patient not to use alcohol or other CNS depressants while taking drug.
• Inform patient that sugarless gum, hard candy, or ice chips may relieve dry mouth.

---

chlorpheniramine maleate
klor-fen-IR-a-meen

Aller-Chlor* ◊ , Allergy ◊ ,
Chlo-Amine ◊ , Chlor-Trimeton
Allergy 8 Hour ◊ , Chlor-Trimeton
Allergy 12 Hour ◊ , Efidac ◊

Pharmacologic class: alkylamine
Pregnancy risk category C

AVAILABLE FORMS
Capsules (sustained-release) ◊ : 8 mg, 12 mg
Syrup ◊ : 2 mg/5 ml*
Tablets ◊ : 4 mg
Tablets (chewable) ◊ : 2 mg
Tablets (extended-release) ◊ : 8 mg, 12 mg, 16 mg

INDICATIONS & DOSAGES
➤ **Allergic rhinitis**
Adults and children age 12 and older:
4 mg P.O. every 4 to 6 hours, not to exceed 24 mg daily. Or, 8 to 12 mg timed-release P.O. every 8 to 12 hours, not to exceed 24 mg daily. Or, 16 mg timed-release P.O. once daily.
Children ages 6 to 12 years: 2 mg P.O. every 4 to 6 hours, not to exceed 12 mg daily. Or, 8 mg timed-release P.O. at bedtime.
Children ages 2 to 5 years: 1 mg P.O. every 4 to 6 hours, not to exceed 6 mg daily.

ADMINISTRATION
P.O.
• Give extended-release tablets whole and not crushed or divided.

ACTION
Competes with histamine for H_1-receptor sites on effector cells. Drug prevents, but doesn't reverse, histamine-mediated responses.

Route	Onset	Peak	Duration
P.O.	15–60 min	2–6 hr	24 hr

Half-life: Adults with normal renal and hepatic function, 12 to 43 hours; children with normal renal and hepatic function, 9½ to 13 hours; chronic renal failure on hemodialysis, 11½ to 13¾ days.

ADVERSE REACTIONS
CNS: *drowsiness, stimulation,* sedation, excitability in children.
CV: hypotension, palpitations, weak pulse.
GI: *dry mouth,* epigastric distress.
GU: urine retention.
Respiratory: thick bronchial secretions.
Skin: rash, urticaria, pallor.

INTERACTIONS
Drug-drug. *CNS depressants:* May increase sedation. Use together cautiously.
MAO inhibitors: May increase anticholinergic effects. Avoid using together.
Drug-lifestyle. *Alcohol use:* May increase CNS depression. Discourage use together.

EFFECTS ON LAB TEST RESULTS
• May prevent, reduce, or mask positive result in diagnostic skin test.

CONTRAINDICATIONS & CAUTIONS
• Contraindicated in patients having acute asthmatic attacks and in those with angle-closure glaucoma, symptomatic prostatic hyperplasia, pyloroduodenal obstruction, or bladder neck obstruction.
• Contraindicated in breast-feeding women and in patients taking MAO inhibitors.
• Use cautiously in elderly patients and in those with increased intraocular pressure, hyperthyroidism, CV or renal disease, hypertension, bronchial asthma, urine retention, prostatic hyperplasia, and stenosing peptic ulcerations.

NURSING CONSIDERATIONS
• Stop drug 4 days before diagnostic skin testing because antihistamines can prevent, reduce, or mask positive skin test response.

PATIENT TEACHING
• Warn patient to avoid alcohol and hazardous activities that require alertness until CNS effects of drug are known.

---

†Canada   ◊ OTC   ◆ Off-label use   ⌀Photoguide   *Liquid contains alcohol.

• Inform patient that sugarless gum, hard candy, or ice chips may relieve dry mouth.
• Instruct patient to notify prescriber if tolerance develops because a different antihistamine may need to be prescribed.
• Advise patient that extended-release tablets should be swallowed whole and not crushed, chewed, or divided.

---

desloratadine
dess-lor-AT-a-deen

Clarinex✓, Clarinex RediTabs

Pharmacologic class: piperidine
Pregnancy risk category C

AVAILABLE FORMS
Syrup: 0.5 mg/ml, 2.5 mg/5 ml
Tablets: 5 mg
Tablets (orally disintegrating): 2.5 mg, 5 mg

INDICATIONS & DOSAGES
➤ **Seasonal allergic rhinitis (patients age 2 and older); perennial allergic rhinitis; chronic idiopathic urticaria**
Adults and children age 12 and older: 5 mg P.O. tablets or syrup once daily.
Children ages 6 to 11: 2.5 mg orally disintegrating tablet (ODT) or syrup P.O. once daily.
Children ages 12 months to 5 years: 1.25 mg P.O. once daily.
Infants ages 6 to 11 months: 1 mg P.O. once daily.
Adjust-a-dose: In adults with hepatic or renal impairment, start dosage at 5 mg P.O. every other day.

ADMINISTRATION
P.O.
• Give drug without regard for meals.
• Give ODTs with or without water.
• Store tablets at 36° to 86° F (2° to 30° C); store ODTs at 59° to 86° F (15° to 30° C).

ACTION
Long-acting tricyclic antihistamine with selective H_1-receptor histamine antagonist activity. It inhibits histamine release from human mast cells in vitro.

Drug doesn't cross the blood-brain barrier.

Route	Onset	Peak	Duration
P.O.	< 1 hr	3 hr	up to 24 hr
P.O. (orally disintegrating)	< 1 hr	2½–4 hr	up to 24 hr

Half-life: 27 hours.

ADVERSE REACTIONS
CNS: *headache,* somnolence, fatigue, dizziness.
EENT: pharyngitis, dry throat.
GI: nausea, dry mouth.
Musculoskeletal: myalgia.
Other: flulike symptoms.

INTERACTIONS
None reported.

EFFECTS ON LAB TEST RESULTS
• May prevent, reduce, or mask positive result in diagnostic skin test.

CONTRAINDICATIONS & CAUTIONS
• Contraindicated in breast-feeding women and in patients hypersensitive to drug, to any of its components, or to loratadine.
• Use cautiously in elderly patients because of the greater likelihood of decreased hepatic, renal, or cardiac function, and concomitant disease or other drug therapy.

NURSING CONSIDERATIONS
• Stop drug 4 days before diagnostic skin testing because antihistamines can prevent, reduce, or mask positive skin test response.

PATIENT TEACHING
• Advise patient not to exceed recommended dosage. Higher doses don't increase effectiveness and may cause somnolence.
• Tell patient that drug can be taken without regard to meals.
• Instruct patient to remove ODTs from blister pack and place on tongue immediately to dissolve.
• ODTs may be taken with or without water.
• Tell patient to report adverse effects.

Reactions may be *common,* uncommon, *life-threatening,* or COMMON AND LIFE-THREATENING.
Interaction may have a *rapid onset* or **delayed onset.**

diphenhydramine hydrochloride
dye-fen-HYE-drah-meen

AllerMax*◇, AllerMax Caplets◇, Altaryl Children's Allergy†◇, Banophen◇, Benadryl◇, Benadryl Allergy◇, Children's Pedia Care Nighttime Cough†◇, Diphen Cough◇, Diphenhist◇, Diphenhist Captabs◇, Dytan◇, Genahist◇, Hydramine Cough*◇, Siladryl*◇, Silphen*◇, Triaminic MultiSymptom*◇, Tusstat*◇

Pharmacologic class: ethanolamine
Pregnancy risk category B

AVAILABLE FORMS
Capsules: 25 mg◇, 50 mg◇
Elixir: 12.5 mg/5 ml*◇
Injection: 50 mg/ml
Strips (orally disintegrating): 12.5 mg*◇, 25 mg*◇
Syrup: 12.5 mg/5 ml*◇
Tablets: 25 mg◇, 50 mg◇
Tablets (chewable): 12.5 mg◇

INDICATIONS & DOSAGES
➤ **Rhinitis, allergy symptoms, motion sickness, Parkinson's disease**
Adults and children age 12 and older: 25 to 50 mg P.O. every 4 to 6 hours. Maximum, 300 mg P.O. daily. Or, 10 to 50 mg I.V. or deep I.M. Maximum I.V. or I.M. dosage, 400 mg daily.
Children ages 6 to 11: 12.5 to 25 mg P.O. every 4 to 6 hours. Maximum dose is 150 mg daily. Or, 5 mg/kg day divided into four doses P.O., deep I.M., or I.V. Maximum dose is 300 mg daily.
Children ages 2 to 5: 6.25 mg every 4 to 6 hours. Maximum dose is 37.5 mg daily. Or, 5 mg/kg day divided into four doses P.O., deep I.M., or I.V. Maximum dose is 300 mg daily.
➤ **Sedation**
Adults: 25 to 50 mg P.O. or deep I.M. as needed.
➤ **Nighttime sleep aid**
Adults: 25 to 50 mg P.O. at bedtime.
➤ **Nonproductive cough**
Adults and children age 12 and older: 25 mg (syrup) P.O. every 4 hours. Don't exceed 150 mg daily. Or, 25 to 50 mg (liquid) every 4 hours. Don't exceed 300 mg daily.
Children ages 6 to 11: 12.5 mg (syrup) P.O. every 4 hours. Don't exceed 75 mg daily. Or, 12.5 to 25 mg (liquid) every 4 hours. Don't exceed 150 mg daily.
Children ages 2 to 5: 6.25 mg (syrup) P.O. every 4 hours. Don't exceed 25 mg daily.
➤ **Antipsychotic-induced dystonia** ◆
Adults: 50 mg I.M. or I.V.

ADMINISTRATION
P.O.
• Give drug with food or milk to reduce GI distress.
I.V.
• Don't exceed 25 mg/minute.
• **Incompatibilities:** Allopurinol, amobarbital, amphotericin B, cefepime, dexamethasone, foscarnet, haloperidol lactate, pentobarbital, phenobarbital, phenytoin, thiopental.
I.M.
• Give I.M. injection deep into large muscle.
• Alternate injection sites to prevent irritation.

ACTION
Competes with histamine for H_1-receptor sites. Prevents, but doesn't reverse, histamine-mediated responses, particularly those of the bronchial tubes, GI tract, uterus, and blood vessels. Structurally related to local anesthetics, drug provides local anesthesia and suppresses cough reflex.

Route	Onset	Peak	Duration
P.O.	15 min	1–4 hr	6–8 hr
I.V.	Immediate	1–4 hr	6–8 hr
I.M.	Unknown	1–4 hr	6–8 hr

Half-life: 2.4 to 9.3 hours.

ADVERSE REACTIONS
CNS: *drowsiness, sedation, sleepiness, dizziness, incoordination, seizures,* confusion, insomnia, headache, vertigo, fatigue, restlessness, tremor, nervousness.
CV: palpitations, hypotension, tachycardia.
EENT: diplopia, blurred vision, nasal congestion, tinnitus.

GI: *dry mouth, nausea, epigastric distress,* vomiting, diarrhea, constipation, anorexia.
GU: dysuria, urine retention, urinary frequency.
Hematologic: *thrombocytopenia, agranulocytosis,* hemolytic anemia.
Respiratory: *thickening of bronchial secretions.*
Skin: urticaria, photosensitivity, rash.
Other: *anaphylactic shock.*

INTERACTIONS
Drug-drug. *CNS depressants:* May increase sedation. Use together cautiously.
MAO inhibitors: May increase anticholinergic effects. Avoid using together.
Other products that contain diphenhydramine (including topical therapy): May increase risk of adverse reactions. Avoid using together.
Drug-lifestyle. *Alcohol use:* May increase CNS depression. Discourage use together.
Sun exposure: May cause photosensitivity reactions. Advise patient to avoid extensive sunlight exposure.

EFFECTS ON LAB TEST RESULTS
● May decrease hemoglobin level and hematocrit.
● May decrease granulocyte and platelet counts.
● May prevent, reduce, or mask positive result in diagnostic skin test.

CONTRAINDICATIONS & CAUTIONS
● Contraindicated in patients hypersensitive to drug; newborns; premature neonates; breast-feeding women; patients with angle-closure glaucoma, stenosing peptic ulcer, symptomatic prostatic hyperplasia, bladder neck obstruction, or pyloroduodenal obstruction; and those having an acute asthmatic attack.
● Avoid use in patients taking MAO inhibitors.
● Use with caution in patients with prostatic hyperplasia, asthma, COPD, increased intraocular pressure, hyperthyroidism, CV disease, and hypertension.
● Children younger than age 12 should use drug only as directed by prescriber.

NURSING CONSIDERATIONS
● Stop drug 4 days before diagnostic skin testing.
● Injection form is for I.V. or I.M. administration only.
● Dizziness, excessive sedation, syncope, toxicity, paradoxical stimulation, and hypotension are more likely to occur in elderly patients.
● *Look alike–sound alike:* Don't confuse diphenhydramine with dimenhydrinate; don't confuse Benadryl with Bentyl or benazepril.

PATIENT TEACHING
● Warn patient not to take this drug with any other products that contain diphenhydramine (including topical therapy) because of increased adverse reactions.
● Instruct patient to take drug 30 minutes before travel to prevent motion sickness.
● Tell patient to take diphenhydramine with food or milk to reduce GI distress.
● Warn patient to avoid alcohol and hazardous activities that require alertness until CNS effects of drug are known.
● Inform patient that sugarless gum, hard candy, or ice chips may relieve dry mouth.
● Tell patient to notify prescriber if tolerance develops because a different antihistamine may need to be prescribed.
● Drug is in many OTC sleep and cold products. Advise patient to consult prescriber before using these products.
● Warn patient of possible photosensitivity reactions. Advise use of a sunblock.

fexofenadine hydrochloride
fecks-oh-FEN-a-deen

Allegra✒, Allegra ODT

Pharmacologic class: piperidine
Pregnancy risk category C

AVAILABLE FORMS
Capsules: 60 mg
Oral suspension: 30 mg/5 ml
Tablets: 30 mg, 60 mg, 180 mg
Tablets (orally disintegrating): 30 mg

INDICATIONS & DOSAGES
➤ **Seasonal allergic rhinitis**
Adults and children age 12 and older:
60 mg P.O. b.i.d. or 180 mg P.O. once daily.
Children ages 2 to 11: 30 mg P.O. b.i.d. either as a tablet or 5 ml oral suspension.
➤ **Chronic idiopathic urticaria**
Adults and children age 12 and older:
60 mg P.O. b.i.d. or 180 mg P.O. once daily.
Children ages 2 to 11: 30 mg P.O. b.i.d. either as a tablet or 5 ml oral suspension.
Children ages 6 months to younger than 2 years: 15 mg (2.5 ml) P.O. b.i.d.
Adjust-a-dose: For patients with impaired renal function or a need for dialysis, give adults and children age 12 and older 60 mg daily, children ages 2 to 11, 30 mg daily, and children ages 6 months to 2 years, 15 mg daily.

ADMINISTRATION
P.O.
• Don't give antacid within 2 hours of this drug.
• Give orally disintegrating tablets (ODTs) to patient with an empty stomach. Allow ODT to disintegrate on the patient's tongue; and it may be swallowed with or without water.
• Don't remove ODT from blister package until time of administration.

ACTION
A long-acting nonsedating antihistamine that selectively inhibits peripheral H_1 receptors.

Route	Onset	Peak	Duration
P.O.	Rapid	3 hr	14 hr

Half-life: 14½ hours.

ADVERSE REACTIONS
CNS: fatigue, drowsiness, headache.
GI: nausea, dyspepsia.
GU: dysmenorrhea.
Other: viral infection.

INTERACTIONS
Drug-drug. *Aluminum or magnesium antacids:* May decrease fexofenadine level. Separate dosage times.

Erythromycin, ketoconazole: May increase fexofenadine level. Monitor patient for side effects.
Drug-food. *Apple juice, grapefruit juice, orange juice:* May decrease drug effects. Patients should take drug with liquid other than these juices.
Drug-lifestyle. *Alcohol use:* May increase CNS depression. Discourage use together.

EFFECTS ON LAB TEST RESULTS
• May prevent, reduce, or mask positive result in diagnostic skin test.

CONTRAINDICATIONS & CAUTIONS
• Contraindicated in patients hypersensitive to drug or its components.
• Use cautiously in patients with impaired renal function.

NURSING CONSIDERATIONS
• Stop drug 4 days before patient undergoes diagnostic skin tests because drug can prevent, reduce, or mask positive skin test response.
• It's unknown if drug appears in breast milk; use caution when using drug in breast-feeding woman.

PATIENT TEACHING
• Instruct patient or parent not to exceed prescribed dosage and to use drug only when needed.
• Warn patient to avoid alcohol and hazardous activities that require alertness until CNS effects of drug are known. Explain that drug may cause drowsiness.
• Tell patient not to take antacids within 2 hours of this drug.
• Advise patient with dry mouth to try sugarless gum, hard candy, or ice chips.
• Tell parents to keep the oral suspension in a cool, dry place, tightly closed, and to shake well before using.
• Instruct patient to let ODT disintegrate on the tongue then swallow with or without water.
• Tell patient ODT should be taken on an empty stomach.
• Tell patient to keep ODT in original blister package until time of use.

levocetirizine dihydrochloride
LEE-voe-se-TIR-a-zeen

Xyzal

Pharmacologic class: H$_1$-receptor antagonist
Pregnancy risk category B

AVAILABLE FORMS
Oral solution: 2.5 mg/5 ml
Tablets: 5 mg

INDICATIONS & DOSAGES
➤ **Seasonal and perennial allergic rhinitis**
Adults and children age 12 and older:
5 mg P.O. once daily in the evening.
Children ages 6 to 11: 2.5 mg P.O. once daily in the evening.
➤ **Uncomplicated skin manifestations of chronic idiopathic urticaria**
Adults and children age 12 and older:
5 mg P.O. once daily in the evening.
Children ages 6 to 11: 2.5 mg P.O. once daily in the evening.
Adjust-a-dose: For patients ages 12 and older with creatinine clearance of 50 to 80 ml/minute, give 2.5 mg P.O. once daily; with creatinine clearance of 30 to 50 ml/minute, give 2.5 mg P.O. every other day; and with creatinine clearance 10 to 30 ml/minute, give 2.5 mg P.O. twice weekly (once every 3 to 4 days). Avoid use in patients with end-stage renal disease or those undergoing hemodialysis. Avoid use in children ages 6 to 11 with impaired renal function.

ADMINISTRATION
P.O.
● Give drug without regard for food.

ACTION
H$_1$-receptor inhibition creates antihistamine effect, relieving allergy symptoms.

Route	Onset	Peak	Duration
P.O.	Unknown	1 hr	24 hr

Half-life: 8 hours.

ADVERSE REACTIONS
CNS: fatigue, pyrexia, somnolence.

EENT: dry mouth, epistaxis, nasopharyngitis, pharyngitis.
Respiratory: cough.

INTERACTIONS
Drug-drug. *CNS depressants:* May have additive effects when taken together. Avoid using together.
Ritonavir: May increase serum concentration and increase half-life of levocetirizine. Use cautiously together.
Theophylline: May decrease the clearance of levocetirizine. Use cautiously together.
Drug-lifestyle. *Alcohol use:* May have additive effect when taken with levocetirizine. Discourage use together.

EFFECTS ON LAB TEST RESULTS
● May prevent, reduce, or mask positive result skin wheal in diagnostic skin test.

CONTRAINDICATIONS & CAUTIONS
● Contraindicated in patients hypersensitive to drug or to cetirizine.
● Contraindicated in patients with creatinine clearance less than 10 ml/minute or those undergoing hemodialysis.
● Contraindicated in patients age 6 to 11 with impaired renal function.

NURSING CONSIDERATIONS
● Monitor patient's renal function.
● Patient should avoid engaging in hazardous occupations requiring mental alertness and motor coordination, such as operating machinery or driving a motor vehicle.
● Drug is excreted in breast milk; avoid use in nursing mothers.
● Safety and effectiveness in patients younger than age 6 haven't been established.
● Use drug during pregnancy only if benefits to mother clearly outweigh risk to fetus.

PATIENT TEACHING
● Warn patient not to perform hazardous tasks or those requiring alertness and coordination until CNS effects are known.
● Advise patient to avoid use of alcohol and other CNS depressants while taking this drug.

Reactions may be *common*, uncommon, *life-threatening*, or COMMON AND LIFE-THREATENING.
Interaction may have a *rapid onset* or **delayed onset**.

• Advise patient not to take more than the recommended dose because of increased risk of somnolence at higher doses.

Route	Onset	Peak	Duration
P.O.	Rapid	1.3–2.5 hr	24 hr

Half-life: 8½ hours.

loratadine
lor-AT-a-deen

Alavert ◇ , Alavert Children's ◇ , Claritin ◇ , Claritin Hives Relief ◇ , Claritin 24-Hour Allergy ◇ , Claritin RediTabs ◇ , Claritin Syrup ◇ , Dimetapp Children's Non-Drowsy Allergy ◇ , Triaminic Allerchews ◇

Pharmacologic class: piperidine
Pregnancy risk category B

AVAILABLE FORMS
Syrup: 1 mg/ml ◇
Tablets: 10 mg ◇
Tablets (chewable): 5 mg ◇
Tablets (orally disintegrating): 5 mg ◇ , 10 mg ◇

INDICATIONS & DOSAGES
➤ **Allergic rhinitis**
Adults and children age 6 and older: 10 mg P.O. daily.
Children ages 2 to 5: 5 mg P.O. daily.
➤ **Chronic idiopathic urticaria ◆**
Adults and children age 6 and older: 10 mg P.O. daily.
Children ages 2 to 5: 5 mg P.O. daily.
Adjust-a-dose: In adults and children age 6 and older with hepatic impairment or GFR less than 30 ml/minute, give 10 mg every other day. In children ages 2 to 5 years with hepatic or renal impairment, give 5 mg every other day.

ADMINISTRATION
P.O.
• Give Claritin Reditabs on the tongue, where it disintegrates within a few seconds.
• Give drug with or without water.

ACTION
Blocks effects of histamine at H_1-receptor sites. Drug is a nonsedating antihistamine; its chemical structure prevents entry into the CNS.

ADVERSE REACTIONS
CNS: *headache,* drowsiness, fatigue, insomnia, nervousness.
GI: dry mouth.

INTERACTIONS
Drug-drug. *Cimetidine, ketoconazole, macrolide antibiotics (clarithromycin, erythromycin, troleandomycin):* May increase loratadine level. Monitor patient closely.
Drug-lifestyle. *Alcohol use:* May increase CNS depression. Discourage use together.

EFFECTS ON LAB TEST RESULTS
• May prevent, reduce, or mask positive result in diagnostic skin test.

CONTRAINDICATIONS & CAUTIONS
• Contraindicated in patients hypersensitive to drug.
• Use cautiously in patients with hepatic or renal impairment and in breast-feeding women.

NURSING CONSIDERATIONS
• Stop drug 4 days before patient undergoes diagnostic skin tests because drug can prevent, reduce, or mask positive skin test response.

PATIENT TEACHING
• Make sure patient understands to take drug once daily. If symptoms persist or worsen, tell him to contact prescriber.
• Tell patient taking Claritin Reditabs to use tablet immediately after opening individual blister.
• Advise patient taking Claritin Reditabs to place tablet on the tongue, where it disintegrates within a few seconds. It can be swallowed with or without water.
• Warn patient to avoid alcohol and hazardous activities that require alertness until CNS effects of drug are known.
• Tell patient that dry mouth can be relieved with sugarless gum, hard candy, or ice chips.

---

†Canada   ◇ OTC   ◆ Off-label use   ✐Photoguide   *Liquid contains alcohol.

promethazine hydrochloride
proe-METH-a-zeen

Phenadoz◆

Pharmacologic class:
phenothiazine
Pregnancy risk category C

AVAILABLE FORMS
Injection: 25 mg/ml, 50 mg/ml
Suppositories: 12.5 mg, 25 mg, 50 mg
Syrup: 6.25 mg/5 ml*
Tablets: 12.5 mg, 25 mg, 50 mg

INDICATIONS & DOSAGES
➤ **Motion sickness**
Adults: 25 mg P.O. or P.R. taken 30 minutes to 1 hour before departure. May repeat dose 8 to 12 hours later p.r.n.
Children older than age 2: 12.5 to 25 mg P.O. or P.R. 30 minutes to 1 hour before departure. May repeat dose 8 to 12 hours later p.r.n.
➤ **Nausea and vomiting**
Adults: 12.5 to 25 mg P.O., I.M., or P.R. every 4 to 6 hours p.r.n.
Children older than age 2: 12.5 to 25 mg P.O. or P.R. every 4 to 6 hours p.r.n. Or, 6.25 to 12.5 mg I.M. every 4 to 6 hours p.r.n.
➤ **Rhinitis, allergy symptoms**
Adults: 25 mg P.O. or P.R. at bedtime; or, 12.5 mg P.O. or P.R. t.i.d. and at bedtime.
Children older than age 2: 25 mg P.O. or P.R. at bedtime; or, 6.25 to 12.5 mg P.O. or P.R. t.i.d.
➤ **Nighttime sedation**
Adults: 25 to 50 mg P.O., I.V., I.M., or P.R. at bedtime.
Children older than age 2: 12.5 to 25 mg P.O., I.M., or P.R. at bedtime.
➤ **Adjunct to analgesics for routine preoperative or postoperative sedation**
Adults: 25 to 50 mg I.V., I.M., P.O. or P.R.
Children older than age 2: 0.5 to 1.1 mg/kg P.O., I.M., or P.R.

ADMINISTRATION
P.O.
• Reduce GI distress by giving drug with food or milk.

I.V.
• If solution is discolored or contains a precipitate, discard.
• Give injection through a free-flowing I.V. line.
• Don't give at a concentration above 25 mg/ml or a rate above 25 mg/minute.
• **Incompatibilities:** Aldesleukin, allopurinol, aminophylline, amphotericin B, cephalosporins, chloramphenicol sodium succinate, chloroquine phosphate, chlorothiazide, diatrizoate, dimenhydrinate, doxorubicin liposomal, foscarnet, furosemide, heparin sodium, hydrocortisone sodium succinate, iodipamide meglumine (52%), iothalamate, ketorolac, methohexital, morphine, nalbuphine, penicillin G potassium and sodium, pentobarbital sodium, phenobarbital sodium, phenytoin sodium, thiopental, vitamin B complex.
I.M.
• I.M. injection is the preferred parenteral route. Inject deep I.M. into large muscle mass. Rotate injection sites.
• Don't give subcutaneously or intra-arterially.
Rectal
• If suppository is too soft, place wrapped in refrigerator for 15 minutes or run under cold water.

ACTION
Phenothiazine derivative that competes with histamine for H_1-receptor sites on effector cells. Prevents, but doesn't reverse, histamine-mediated responses. At high doses, drug also has local anesthetic effects.

Route	Onset	Peak	Duration
P.O.	15–60 min	Unknown	< 12 hr
I.V.	3–5 min	Unknown	< 12 hr
I.M., P.R.	20 min	Unknown	< 12 hr

Half-life: Unknown.

ADVERSE REACTIONS
CNS: *drowsiness, sedation,* confusion, sleepiness, dizziness, disorientation, extrapyramidal symptoms.
CV: hypotension, hypertension.
EENT: *dry mouth,* blurred vision.
GI: nausea, vomiting.
GU: urine retention.

Reactions may be *common*, uncommon, **life-threatening**, or COMMON AND LIFE-THREATENING.
Interaction may have a *rapid onset* or **delayed onset**.

Hematologic: *leukopenia, agranulo-cytosis, thrombocytopenia.*
Metabolic: hyperglycemia.
Respiratory: *respiratory depression, apnea.*
Skin: photosensitivity, rash.

INTERACTIONS
Drug-drug. *Anticholinergics, tricyclic antidepressants:* May increase anticholinergic effects. Avoid using together.
CNS depressants: May increase sedation. Use together cautiously. If used together, reduce opiate dose by at least 25% to 50%, and reduce barbiturate dose by at least 50%.
Epinephrine: May block or reverse effects of epinephrine. Use other pressor drugs instead.
Levodopa: May decrease antiparkinsonian action of levodopa. Avoid using together.
Lithium: May reduce GI absorption or enhance renal elimination of lithium. Avoid using together.
MAO inhibitors: May increase extrapyramidal effects. Avoid using together.
Quinolones: May cause life-threatening arrhythmias. Avoid using together.
Drug-herb. *Yohimbe:* May increase risk of herb toxicity. Ask patient about use of herbal remedies, and recommend caution.
Drug-lifestyle. *Alcohol use:* May increase sedation. Discourage use together.
Sun exposure: May cause photosensitivity reactions. Advise patient to avoid extensive sunlight exposure and to use sunblock.

EFFECTS ON LAB TEST RESULTS
• May increase hemoglobin level and hematocrit.
• May decrease WBC, platelet, and granulocyte counts.
• May prevent, reduce, or mask positive result in diagnostic skin test. May cause false-positive or false-negative pregnancy test result. May interfere with blood grouping in the ABO system.

CONTRAINDICATIONS & CAUTIONS
• Contraindicated in patients hypersensitive to drug, those who have experienced adverse reactions to phenothiazines, breast-feeding women, comatose patients, and acutely ill or dehydrated children.

■ **Black Box Warning** Contraindicated in children younger than age 2 because of the potential for fatal respiratory depression. Use the lowest effective dose in children older than age 2 and avoid administering with drugs that can cause respiratory depression. ■
• Use cautiously in patients with asthma or pulmonary, hepatic, or CV disease and in those with intestinal obstruction, prostatic hyperplasia, bladder-neck obstruction, angle-closure glaucoma, seizure disorders, CNS depression, and stenosing or peptic ulcerations.

NURSING CONSIDERATIONS
• Monitor patient for neuroleptic malignant syndrome: altered mental status, autonomic instability, muscle rigidity, and hyperpyrexia.
• Stop drug 4 days before diagnostic skin testing because antihistamines can prevent, reduce, or mask positive skin test response.
• Drug is used as an adjunct to analgesics, usually to increase sedation; it has no analgesic activity.
• Drug may be mixed with meperidine in same syringe.
• In patients scheduled for a myelogram, stop drug 48 hours before procedure. Don't resume drug until 24 hours after procedure because of the risk of seizures.

PATIENT TEACHING
• Tell patient to take oral form with food or milk.
• When treating motion sickness, tell patient to take first dose 30 to 60 minutes before travel; dose may be repeated in 8 to 12 hours, if necessary. On succeeding days of travel, patient should take dose upon arising and with evening meal.
• Warn patient to avoid alcohol and hazardous activities that require alertness until CNS effects of drug are known.
• Inform patient that sugarless gum, hard candy, or ice chips may relieve dry mouth.
• Warn patient about possible photosensitivity reactions. Advise use of a sunblock.

56

Bronchodilators

albuterol sulfate
arformoterol tartrate
ephedrine sulfate
    (See Chapter 28, VASOPRESSORS.)
epinephrine
epinephrine hydrochloride
formoterol fumarate
ipratropium bromide
isoproterenol hydrochloride
levalbuterol hydrochloride
pirbuterol acetate
salmeterol xinafoate
terbutaline sulfate
theophylline
tiotropium bromide

albuterol sulfate
al-BYOO-ter-ole

AccuNeb, ProAir HFA, Proventil HFA, Ventolin HFA, VoSpire ER

Pharmacologic class: adrenergic
Pregnancy risk category C

AVAILABLE FORMS
Inhalation aerosol: 90 mcg/metered spray
Solution for inhalation: 0.083% (2.5 mg/3 ml), 0.5% (5 mg/ml), 0.042% (1.25 mg/3 ml), 0.021% (0.63 mg/3 ml)
Syrup: 2 mg/5 ml
Tablets: 2 mg, 4 mg
Tablets (extended-release): 4 mg, 8 mg

INDICATIONS & DOSAGES
➤ **To prevent or treat bronchospasm in patients with reversible obstructive airway disease**
Tablets (extended-release)
Adults and children age 12 and older:
4 to 8 mg P.O. every 12 hours. Maximum, 32 mg daily.
Children ages 6 to 11: 4 mg P.O. every 12 hours. Maximum, 24 mg daily.
Tablets
Adults and children age 12 and older:
2 to 4 mg P.O. t.i.d. or q.i.d. Maximum, 32 mg daily.

Children ages 6 to 11: 2 mg P.O. t.i.d. or q.i.d. Maximum, 24 mg daily.
Solution for inhalation
Adults and children age 12 and older:
2.5 mg t.i.d. or q.i.d. by nebulizer, given over 5 to 15 minutes. To prepare solution, use 0.5 ml of 0.5% solution diluted with 2.5 ml of normal saline solution. Or, use 3 ml of 0.083% solution.
Children ages 2 to 12 weighing more than 15 kg (33 lb): 2.5 mg by nebulizer given over 5 to 15 minutes t.i.d. or q.i.d., with subsequent doses adjusted to response. Don't exceed 2.5 mg t.i.d. or q.i.d.
Children ages 2 to 12 weighing 15 kg or less: 0.63 mg or 1.25 mg by nebulizer given over 5 to 15 minutes t.i.d. or q.i.d. with subsequent doses adjusted to response. Don't exceed 2.5 mg t.i.d. or q.i.d.
Syrup
Adults and children older than age 14:
2 to 4 mg (1 to 2 tsp) P.O. t.i.d. or q.i.d. Maximum, 32 mg daily.
Children ages 6 to 13: 2 mg (1 tsp) P.O. t.i.d. or q.i.d. Maximum, 24 mg daily.
Children ages 2 to 5: Initially, 0.1 mg/kg P.O. t.i.d. Starting dose shouldn't exceed 2 mg (1 tsp) t.i.d. Maximum, 12 mg daily.
Adjust-a-dose: For elderly patients and those sensitive to sympathomimetic amines, 2 mg P.O. t.i.d. or q.i.d. as oral tablets or syrup. Maximum, 32 mg daily.
Inhalation aerosol
Adults and children age 4 and older:
1 to 2 inhalations every 4 to 6 hours as needed. Regular use for maintenance therapy to control asthma symptoms isn't recommended.
➤ **To prevent exercise-induced bronchospasm**
Adults and children age 4 and older:
2 inhalations using the inhalation aerosol 15 minutes before exercise; up to 12 inhalations may be taken in 24 hours.

ADMINISTRATION
P.O.
• When switching patient from regular to extended-release tablets, remember that a regular 2-mg tablet every 6 hours is equiv-

alent to an extended-release 4-mg tablet every 12 hours.
• Give drug whole; don't break or crush extended-release tablets or mix them with food.
Inhalational
• If more than 1 inhalation is ordered, wait at least 2 minutes between inhalations.
• Use spacer device to improve drug delivery, if appropriate.
• Shake the inhaler before use.

ACTION

Relaxes bronchial, uterine, and vascular smooth muscle by stimulating beta$_2$ receptors.

Route	Onset	Peak	Duration
P.O.	15–30 min	2–3 hr	4–8 hr
P.O. (extended)	Unknown	6 hr	12 hr
Inhalation	5–15 min	30–120 min	2–6 hr

Half-life: About 4 hours.

ADVERSE REACTIONS

CNS: *tremor, nervousness, headache, hyperactivity,* insomnia, dizziness, weakness, CNS stimulation, malaise.
CV: *tachycardia, palpitations,* hypertension.
EENT: dry and irritated nose and throat with inhaled form, nasal congestion, epistaxis, hoarseness.
GI: *nausea, vomiting,* heartburn, anorexia, altered taste, increased appetite.
Metabolic: hypokalemia.
Musculoskeletal: muscle cramps.
Respiratory: *bronchospasm,* cough, wheezing, dyspnea, bronchitis, increased sputum.
Other: hypersensitivity reactions.

INTERACTIONS

Drug-drug. *CNS stimulants:* May increase CNS stimulation. Avoid using together.
Digoxin: May decrease digoxin level. Monitor digoxin level closely.
MAO inhibitors, tricyclic antidepressants: May increase adverse CV effects. Monitor patient closely.
Propranolol and other beta blockers: May cause mutual antagonism. Monitor patient carefully.

EFFECTS ON LAB TEST RESULTS
• May decrease potassium level.

CONTRAINDICATIONS & CAUTIONS
• Contraindicated in patients hypersensitive to drug or its ingredients.
• Use cautiously in patients with CV disorders (including coronary insufficiency and hypertension), hyperthyroidism, or diabetes mellitus and in those who are unusually responsive to adrenergics.
• Use extended-release tablets cautiously in patients with GI narrowing.

NURSING CONSIDERATIONS
• Drug may decrease sensitivity of spirometry used for diagnosis of asthma.
• Syrup contains no alcohol or sugar and may be taken by children as young as age 2.
• In children, syrup may rarely cause erythema multiforme or Stevens-Johnson syndrome.
• The HFA form uses the propellant hydrofluoroalkane (HFA) instead of chlorofluorocarbons.
• *Alert:* Patient may use tablets and aerosol together. Monitor these patients closely for signs and symptoms of toxicity.
• *Look alike–sound alike:* Don't confuse albuterol with atenolol or Albutein.

PATIENT TEACHING
• Warn patient about risk of paradoxical bronchospasm and to stop drug immediately if it occurs.
• Teach patient to perform oral inhalation correctly. Give the following instructions for using the MDI:
– Shake the inhaler.
– Clear nasal passages and throat.
– Breathe out, expelling as much air from lungs as possible.
– Place mouthpiece well into mouth, seal lips around mouthpiece, and inhale deeply as you release a dose from inhaler. Or, hold inhaler about 1 inch (two fingerwidths) from open mouth; inhale while dose is released.
– Hold breath for several seconds, remove mouthpiece, and exhale slowly.
• If prescriber orders more than 1 inhalation, tell patient to wait at least 2 minutes before repeating procedure.
• Tell patient that use of a spacer device may improve drug delivery to lungs.

• If patient is also using a corticosteroid inhaler, instruct him to use the bronchodilator first and then to wait about 5 minutes before using the corticosteroid. This lets the bronchodilator open the air passages for maximal effectiveness of the corticosteroid.

• Tell patient to remove canister and wash inhaler with warm, soapy water at least once a week.

• Advise patient to contact prescriber if using more than 4 inhalations per day for 2 or more days or more than one canister in 8 weeks.

• Advise patient not to chew or crush extended-release tablets or mix them with food.

---

arformoterol tartrate
arr-fohr-MOH-tur-ahl

Brovana

Pharmacologic class: long-acting selective beta₂ agonist
Pregnancy risk category C

AVAILABLE FORMS
Solution for inhalation: 15 mcg/2-ml vials

INDICATIONS & DOSAGES
➤ **Long-term maintenance treatment of bronchoconstriction in patients with COPD, including chronic bronchitis and emphysema**
Adults: 15 mcg, inhaled b.i.d. (morning and evening) via nebulizer. Maximum dose is 30 mcg daily.

ADMINISTRATION
Inhalational
• Use only the recommended nebulizer and compressor for treatment.
• Don't mix drugs with other drugs or solutions in the nebulizer.
• Store vials in the foil pouches in the refrigerator and use immediately after opening.

ACTION
Relaxes bronchial and cardiac smooth muscle by acting on beta₂-adrenergic receptors; stimulates the enzyme adenyl cyclase, which catalyzes the conversion from ATP to cAMP. This further relaxes bronchial smooth muscle and inhibits release of mediators (like histamine and leukotrienes) from mast cells.

Route	Onset	Peak	Duration
Inhalation	Rapid	30 min	Unknown

Half-life: 26 hours.

ADVERSE REACTIONS
CNS: *pain.*
CV: *chest pain, AV block,* atrial flutter, **heart failure, MI, prolonged QT interval, supraventricular tachycardia,** inverted T wave, peripheral edema.
EENT: sinusitis.
GI: diarrhea.
Metabolic: *hypoglycemia,* hypokalemia.
Musculoskeletal: back pain, leg cramps.
Respiratory: dyspnea, pulmonary or chest congestion, **bronchospasm.**
Skin: rash.
Other: hypersensitivity reaction, flu syndrome.

INTERACTIONS
Drug-drug. *Aminophylline, corticosteroids (such as dexamethasone, prednisone), theophylline:* May increase the risk of hypokalemia. Monitor patient's potassium level.
Beta blockers (such as metoprolol, atenolol): May decrease effectiveness of arformoterol and increase risk of bronchospasm. Avoid using together, if possible; otherwise, use with extreme caution.
Non–potassium-sparing diuretics (such as furosemide, hydrochlorothiazide): May increase the risk of hypokalemia and ECG changes. Use cautiously together and monitor patient's ECG and potassium level.
Other beta₂ adrenergics (such as albuterol, formoterol): May cause additive effects. Avoid using together.
QT interval-prolonging drugs (such as MAO inhibitors, tricyclic antidepressants): May increase risk of ventricular arrhythmias. Use cautiously together.

EFFECTS ON LAB TEST RESULTS
• May increase PSA levels. May decrease potassium levels. May increase or decrease glucose levels.

Reactions may be *common*, uncommon, *life-threatening*, or COMMON AND LIFE-THREATENING.
Interaction may have a *rapid onset* or *delayed onset.*

CONTRAINDICATIONS & CAUTIONS
• Contraindicated in patients hypersensitive to drug, formoterol, or any other components of this drug.
• Don't use in patients with acutely deteriorating COPD.
• Use cautiously in patients with seizure disorder; thyrotoxicosis; hepatic insufficiency; preexisting cardiovascular disease, including coronary insufficiency, arrhythmias and hypertension; or in those unresponsive to sympathomimetic amines.

NURSING CONSIDERATIONS
■ **Black Box Warning** Drug may increase the risk of asthma-related death. ■
• Drug is twice as potent as formoterol inhaler.
• *Alert:* Make sure patient has a rescue inhaler, such as albuterol, to treat an acute asthma attack or bronchospasm.
• *Alert:* Notify prescriber if patient experiences decreasing control of symptoms or begins using his short-acting beta$_2$ agonist more often.
• If paradoxical bronchospasm occurs, stop drug immediately.
• Monitor blood pressure, pulse, and ECG, as indicated.
• *Look alike–sound alike:* Don't confuse Brovana (arformoterol tartrate) with Boniva (ibandronate sodium).

PATIENT TEACHING
• Tell patient to store vials in the foil pouches in the refrigerator and use immediately after opening.
• Tell patient to use only the recommended nebulizer and compressor for treatment and not to mix drug with other inhaled drugs or solutions.
• *Alert:* Warn patient that drug is for maintenance treatment only and shouldn't be used to stop an asthma attack or bronchospasm. For emergency treatment, use a short-acting rescue inhaler such as albuterol.
• Educate patient using a short-acting bronchodilator on a scheduled basis, to stop scheduled use and use only for rescue therapy.
• *Alert:* Warn patient that serious adverse effects, including death, can occur at higher than recommended doses and not to take more inhalations than prescribed.

• Tell patient to stop drug immediately and obtain medical help if life-threatening bronchospasm, severe rash, or swelling in throat occurs.
• Inform patient that he may experience palpitations, chest pain, rapid heartbeat, tremors, or nervousness.
• Tell patient not to swallow the inhalation solution.
• Caution patient to notify prescriber if he notices a decrease in symptom control or more frequent use of his rescue inhaler.

SAFETY ALERT!

epinephrine (adrenaline)
ep-i-NEF-rin

Primatene Mist◊

epinephrine hydrochloride
Adrenalin Chloride, EpiPen, EpiPen Jr, microNefrin◊, Nephron◊

Pharmacologic class: adrenergic
Pregnancy risk category C

AVAILABLE FORMS
Aerosol inhaler: 220 mcg◊
Injection: 0.1 mg/ml (1:10,000), 0.5 mg/ml (1:2,000), 1 mg/ml (1:1,000) parenteral
Nebulizer inhaler: 1% (1:100)◊, 1.125%◊

INDICATIONS & DOSAGES
➤ **Bronchospasm, hypersensitivity reactions, anaphylaxis**
Adults: 0.1 to 0.5 ml of 1:1,000 solution I.M. or subcutaneously. Repeat every 10 to 15 minutes as needed. Or, 0.1 to 0.25 ml of 1:1,000 solution I.V. slowly over 5 to 10 minutes (1 to 2.5 ml of a commercially available 1:10,000 injection or of a 1:10,000 dilution prepared by diluting 1 ml of a commercially available 1:1,000 injection with 10 ml of water for injection or normal saline solution for injection). May repeat every 5 to 15 minutes as needed, or follow with a continuous I.V. infusion, starting at 1 mcg/minute and increasing to 4 mcg/minute, as needed.
Children: 0.01 ml/kg (10 mcg) of 1:1,000 solution subcutaneously; repeat

every 20 minutes to 4 hours, as needed. Maximum single dose shouldn't exceed 0.5 mg.

➤ **Hemostasis**
Adults: 1:50,000 to 1:1,000, sprayed or applied topically.

➤ **Acute asthma attacks**
Adults and children age 4 and older: One inhalation, repeated once if needed after at least 1 minute; don't give subsequent doses for at least 3 hours. Or, 1 to 3 deep inhalations using a hand-bulb nebulizer containing 1% (1:100) solution of epinephrine repeated every 3 hours, as needed.

➤ **To prolong local anesthetic effect**
Adults and children: With local anesthetics, may be used in concentrations of 1:500,000 to 1:50,000; most commonly, 1:200,000.

➤ **To restore cardiac rhythm in cardiac arrest**
Adults: 0.5 to 1 mg I.V., repeated every 3 to 5 minutes, if needed. A higher dose may be used if 1 mg fails: 3 to 5 mg (about 0.1 mg/kg); repeat every 3 to 5 minutes.
Children: 0.01 mg/kg (0.1 ml/kg of 1:10,000 injection) I.V. First endotracheal dose is 0.1 mg/kg (0.1 ml/kg of a 1:1,000 injection) diluted in 1 to 2 ml of half-normal or normal saline solution. Give subsequent I.V. or intratracheal doses 0.1 (0.1 ml/kg of a 1:1,000 injection), repeated every 3 to 5 minutes, if needed.

ADMINISTRATION
I.V.
● Keep solution in light-resistant container, and don't remove before use.
● Just before use, mix with D₅W, normal saline solution for injection, lactated Ringer's injection, or combinations of dextrose in saline solution.
● Monitor blood pressure, heart rate, and ECG when therapy starts and frequently thereafter.
● Discard solution if it's discolored or contains precipitate or after 24 hours.
● **Incompatibilities:** Aminophylline; ampicillin sodium; furosemide; hyaluronidase; Ionosol D-CM, PSL, and T solutions with D₅W; mephentermine; thiopental sodium. Compatible with most other I.V. solutions. Rapidly destroyed by alkalies or oxidizing drugs, including

halogens, nitrates, nitrites, permanganates, sodium bicarbonate, and salts of easily reducible metals, such as iron, copper, and zinc. Don't mix with alkaline solutions.
I.M.
● Avoid I.M. use of parenteral suspension into buttocks. Gas gangrene may occur because drug reduces oxygen tension of the tissues, encouraging growth of contaminating organisms.
● Massage site after I.M. injection to counteract vasoconstriction. Repeated local injection can cause necrosis at injection site.
Subcutaneous
● Don't refrigerate and protect from light.
● Preferred route. Don't inject too deeply and enter muscle.
Inhalational
● Teach patient to perform oral inhalation correctly. See "Patient teaching" for complete instructions.
● Epinephrine 1:100 will turn from pink to brown if exposed to air, light, heat, alkalies, and some metals. Don't use solution that's discolored or has a precipitate.

ACTION
Relaxes bronchial smooth muscle by stimulating beta₂ receptors and alpha and beta receptors in the sympathetic nervous system.

Route	Onset	Peak	Duration
I.V.	Immediate	5 min	Short
I.M.	Variable	Unknown	1–4 hr
Subcut.	5–15 min	30 min	1–4 hr
Inhalation	1–5 min	Unknown	1–3 hr

Half-life: Unknown.

ADVERSE REACTIONS
CNS: *drowsiness, headache, nervousness, tremor, **cerebral hemorrhage, stroke,*** vertigo, pain, disorientation, agitation, fear, dizziness, weakness.
CV: *palpitations, **ventricular fibrillation, shock,*** widened pulse pressure, hypertension, tachycardia, anginal pain, altered ECG (including a decreased T-wave amplitude).
GI: *nausea, vomiting.*
Respiratory: dyspnea.

Reactions may be *common,* uncommon, *life-threatening,* or COMMON AND LIFE-THREATENING.
Interaction may have a *rapid onset* or **delayed onset.**

Skin: urticaria, hemorrhage at injection site, pallor.
Other: tissue necrosis.

INTERACTIONS
Drug-drug. *Alpha blockers:* May cause hypotension from unopposed beta-adrenergic effects. Avoid using together.
Antihistamines, thyroid hormones: When given with sympathomimetics, may cause severe adverse cardiac effects. Avoid using together.
Cardiac glycosides, general anesthetics (halogenated hydrocarbons): May increase risk of ventricular arrhythmias. Monitor ECG closely.
Carteolol, nadolol, penbutolol, pindolol, propranolol, timolol: May cause hypertension followed by bradycardia. Stop beta blocker 3 days before starting epinephrine.
Doxapram, methylphenidate: May enhance CNS stimulation or pressor effects. Monitor patient closely.
Ergot alkaloids: May decrease vaso-constrictor activity. Monitor patient closely.
Guanadrel, guanethidine: May enhance pressor effects of epinephrine. Monitor patient closely.
Levodopa: May enhance risk of arrhythmias. Monitor ECG closely.
MAO inhibitors: May increase risk of hypertensive crisis. Monitor blood pressure closely.
Tricyclic antidepressants: May potentiate the pressor response and cause arrhythmias. Use together cautiously.

EFFECTS ON LAB TEST RESULTS
● May increase BUN, glucose, and lactic acid levels.

CONTRAINDICATIONS & CAUTIONS
● Contraindicated in patients with angle-closure glaucoma, shock (other than anaphylactic shock), organic brain damage, cardiac dilation, arrhythmias, coronary insufficiency, or cerebral arteriosclerosis.
● Contraindicated in patients receiving general anesthesia with halogenated hydrocarbons or cyclopropane and in patients in labor (may delay second stage).
● Commercial products containing sulfites contraindicated in patients with sulfite allergies, except when epinephrine is being used to treat serious allergic reactions or other emergency situations.
● Contraindicated for use in fingers, toes, ears, nose, or genitalia when used with local anesthetic.
● Use cautiously in patients with long-standing bronchial asthma or emphysema who have developed degenerative heart disease.
● Use cautiously in elderly patients and in those with hyperthyroidism, CV disease, hypertension, psychoneurosis, and diabetes.

NURSING CONSIDERATIONS
● In patients with Parkinson disease, drug increases rigidity and tremor.
● Drug interferes with tests for urinary catecholamines.
● One mg equals 1 ml of 1:1,000 solution or 10 ml of 1:10,000 solution.
● Epinephrine is drug of choice in emergency treatment of acute anaphylactic reactions.
● Observe patient closely for adverse reactions. Notify prescriber if adverse reactions develop; adjusting dosage or stopping drug may be necessary.
● If blood pressure increases sharply, give rapid-acting vasodilators, such as nitrates and alpha blockers, to counteract the marked pressor effect of large doses.
● Drug is rapidly destroyed by oxidizing products, such as iodine, chromates, nitrites, oxygen, and salts of easily reducible metals (such as iron).
● When treating patient with reactions caused by other drugs given I.M. or subcutaneously, inject this drug into the site where the other drug was given to minimize further absorption.
● ***Look alike–sound alike:*** Don't confuse epinephrine with ephedrine or norepinephrine.

PATIENT TEACHING
● Teach patient to perform oral inhalation correctly. Give the following instructions for using a metered-dose inhaler:
– Shake canister.
– Clear nasal passages and throat.
– Breathe out, expelling as much air from lungs as possible.
– Place mouthpiece well into mouth, and inhale deeply as you release dose from

inhaler. Or, hold inhaler about 1 inch (two fingerwidths) from open mouth, and inhale while releasing dose.
– Hold breath for several seconds, remove mouthpiece, and exhale slowly.
• If more than one inhalation is prescribed, advise patient to wait at least 2 minutes before repeating procedure.
• Tell patient that use of a spacer device may improve drug delivery to lungs.
• If patient is also using a corticosteroid inhaler, instruct him to use the broncho-dilator first and then to wait about 5 min-utes before using the corticosteroid. This lets the bronchodilator open the air passages for maximal effectiveness.
• Instruct patient to remove canister and wash inhaler with warm, soapy water at least once weekly.
• If patient has acute hypersensitivity reactions (such as to bee stings), you may need to teach him to self-inject drug.

---

formoterol fumarate
for-MOH-te-rol

Perforomist, Foradil Aerolizer

Pharmacologic class: selective beta$_2$-adrenergic agonist
Pregnancy risk category C

AVAILABLE FORMS
Capsules for inhalation: 12 mcg
Inhalation solution: 20 mcg/2-ml vial

INDICATIONS & DOSAGES
➤ **Maintenance treatment and pre-vention of bronchospasm in patients with reversible obstructive airway disease or nocturnal asthma, who usually require treatment with short-acting inhaled beta$_2$ agonists**
Adults and children age 5 and older: One 12-mcg capsule by inhalation via Aerolizer inhaler every 12 hours. Total daily dosage shouldn't exceed 1 capsule b.i.d. (24 mcg/day). If symptoms occur between doses, use a short-acting beta$_2$ agonist for immediate relief.
➤ **To prevent exercise-induced bronchospasm**
Adults and children age 5 and older: One 12-mcg capsule by inhalation via Aerolizer

inhaler at least 15 minutes before exercise p.r.n. Don't give additional doses within 12 hours of first dose.
➤ **Maintenance treatment of bronchoconstriction in patients with COPD (chronic bronchitis, emphysema)**
Adults: One 20-mcg/2 ml vial (Perforomist) by oral inhalation through a jet nebulizer every 12 hours. Maximum dose, 40 mcg/day. Or, one 12-mcg capsule (Foradil) by inhalation via Aerolizer inhaler every 12 hours; total daily dosage shouldn't exceed 24 mcg/day.

ADMINISTRATION
Inhalational
Foradil
• Give Foradil capsules only by oral inhalation and only with the Aerolizer inhaler. They aren't for oral ingestion. Patient shouldn't exhale into the device. Capsules should remain in the unopened blister until administration time and be removed immediately before use.
• Pierce Foradil capsules only once. In rare instances, the gelatin capsule may break into small pieces and get delivered to the mouth or throat upon inhalation. The Aerolizer contains a screen that should catch any broken pieces before they leave the device. To minimize the possibility of shattering the capsule, strictly follow storage and use instructions.

Perforomist
• Give Perforomist inhalational solution through a standard jet nebulizer connected to an air compressor.

ACTION
Long-acting selective beta$_2$ agonist that causes bronchodilation. It ultimately increases cAMP, leading to relaxation of bronchial smooth muscle and inhibition of mediator release from mast cells.

Route	Onset	Peak	Duration
Inhalation	15 min	1–3 hr	12 hr

Half-life: 7 hours for Perforomist.

ADVERSE REACTIONS
CNS: tremor, dizziness, insomnia, nervousness, headache, fatigue, malaise.

Reactions may be *common*, uncommon, *life-threatening*, or COMMON AND LIFE-THREATENING.
Interaction may have a *rapid onset* or **delayed onset.**

CV: *arrhythmias,* chest pain, angina, hypertension, hypotension, tachycardia, palpitations.
EENT: dry mouth, tonsillitis, dysphonia, nasopharyngitis.
GI: nausea, vomiting, diarrhea.
Metabolic: *metabolic acidosis,* hypokalemia, hyperglycemia.
Musculoskeletal: muscle cramps.
Respiratory: bronchitis, chest infection, dyspnea.
Skin: rash.
Other: viral infection.

INTERACTIONS
Drug-drug. *Adrenergics:* May potentiate sympathetic effects of formoterol. Use together cautiously.
Beta blockers: May antagonize effects of beta agonists, causing bronchospasm in asthmatic patients. Avoid use except when benefit outweighs risks. Use cardioselective beta blockers with caution to minimize risk of bronchospasm.
Diuretics, steroids, xanthine derivatives: May increase hypokalemic effect of formoterol. Use together cautiously.
MAO inhibitors, tricyclic antidepressants, other drugs that prolong QT interval: May increase risk of ventricular arrhythmias. Use together cautiously.
Non–potassium-sparing diuretics, such as loop or thiazide diuretics: May worsen ECG changes or hypokalemia. Use together cautiously, and monitor patient for toxicity.

EFFECTS ON LAB TEST RESULTS
• May increase glucose level. May decrease potassium level.

CONTRAINDICATIONS & CAUTIONS
• Contraindicated in patients hypersensitive to drug or its components.
• Use cautiously in patients with CV disease, especially coronary insufficiency, cardiac arrhythmias, and hypertension, and in those who are unusually responsive to sympathomimetic amines.
• Use cautiously in patients with diabetes mellitus because hyperglycemia and ketoacidosis have occurred rarely with the use of beta agonists.
• Use cautiously in patients with seizure disorders or thyrotoxicosis and in breast-feeding women.

• Use for asthma only as additional therapy for patients whose condition is not adequately controlled with other asthma-controller medications.

NURSING CONSIDERATIONS
• Drug isn't indicated for patients who can control asthma symptoms with just occasional use of inhaled, short-acting beta$_2$ agonists or for treatment of acute bronchospasm requiring immediate reversal with short-acting beta$_2$ agonists or in patients with rapidly deteriorating or significantly worsening asthma.
• Drug may be used along with short-acting beta agonists, inhaled corticosteroids, and theophylline therapy for asthma management.
• **Alert:** Drug isn't a substitute for short-acting beta$_2$ agonists for immediate relief of bronchospasm or as substitute for inhaled or oral corticosteroids.
• Patients using drug twice daily shouldn't take additional doses to prevent exercise-induced bronchospasm.
• For patients formerly using regularly scheduled short-acting beta$_2$ agonists, decrease use of the short-acting drug to an as-needed basis when starting long-acting formoterol.
■ **Black Box Warning** Drug may increase the risk of asthma-related death. ■
• **Alert:** As with all beta$_2$ agonists, drug may produce life-threatening paradoxical bronchospasm. If bronchospasm occurs, notify prescriber immediately.
• **Alert:** If patient develops tachycardia, hypertension, or other CV adverse effects, drug may need to be stopped.
• Watch for immediate hypersensitivity reactions, such as anaphylaxis, urticaria, angioedema, rash, and bronchospasm.
• **Look alike–sound alike:** Don't confuse Foradil with Toradol.

PATIENT TEACHING
• Tell patient not to increase the dosage or frequency of use without medical advice.
• Warn patient not to stop or reduce other medication taken for asthma.
• Advise patient that drug isn't to be used for acute asthmatic episodes. Prescriber should give a short-acting beta$_2$ agonist for this use.

• Advise patient to report worsening symptoms, treatment that becomes less effective, or increased use of short-acting beta agonists.

• Tell patient to report nausea, vomiting, shakiness, headache, fast or irregular heart beat, or sleeplessness.

• Tell patient using drug for exercise-induced bronchospasm to take it at least 15 minutes before exercise and to wait 12 hours before taking additional doses.

• Tell patient not to use the Foradil Aerolizer with a spacer device or to exhale or blow into the Aerolizer.

• Advise patient to avoid washing the Aerolizer and to always keep it dry. Each refill contains a new device to replace the old one.

• Tell patient to avoid exposing capsules to moisture and to handle them only with dry hands.

• Advise woman to notify prescriber if she becomes pregnant or is breast-feeding.

---

ipratropium bromide
ih-pra-TROE-pee-um

Atrovent, Atrovent HFA

Pharmacologic class:
anticholinergic
Pregnancy risk category B

AVAILABLE FORMS
Inhaler: 17 mcg/metered dose (Atrovent HFA)
Nasal spray: 0.03% (21 mcg/metered dose), 0.06% (42 mcg/metered dose)
Solution (for inhalation): 0.02% (500 mcg/vial)

INDICATIONS & DOSAGES
➤ **Bronchospasm in chronic bronchitis and emphysema**
Adults: Usually, 2 inhalations q.i.d.; patient may take additional inhalations as needed but shouldn't exceed 12 inhalations in 24 hours. Or, 250 to 500 mcg every 6 to 8 hours via oral nebulizer.
➤ **Rhinorrhea caused by allergic and nonallergic perennial rhinitis**
Adults and children age 6 and older: Two 0.03% nasal sprays (42 mcg) per nostril b.i.d. or t.i.d.

➤ **Rhinorrhea caused by the common cold**
Adults and children age 12 and older: Two 0.06% nasal sprays (84 mcg) per nostril t.i.d. or q.i.d.
Children ages 5 to 11: Two 0.06% nasal sprays (84 mcg) per nostril t.i.d.
➤ **Rhinorrhea caused by seasonal allergic rhinitis**
Adults and children age 5 and older: Two 0.06% nasal sprays (84 mcg) per nostril q.i.d.

ADMINISTRATION
Inhalational
• Shake canister before use, except for Atrovent HFA.
• If more than 1 inhalation is ordered, wait at least 2 minutes between inhalations.
• Use spacer device to improve drug delivery, if appropriate.
Intranasal
• Prime nasal spray before first use and after unused for more than 24 hours.
• Tilt patient's head backward after dose to allow drug to spread to back of nose.

ACTION
Inhibits vagally mediated reflexes by antagonizing acetylcholine at muscarinic receptors on bronchial smooth muscle.

Route	Onset	Peak	Duration
Inhalation	5–15 min	1–2 hr	3–6 hr

Half-life: About 2 hours.

ADVERSE REACTIONS
CNS: dizziness, pain, headache, nervousness.
CV: palpitations, hypertension, chest pain.
EENT: blurred vision, rhinitis, pharyngitis, sinusitis, epistaxis.
GI: nausea, GI distress, dry mouth.
Musculoskeletal: back pain.
Respiratory: *upper respiratory tract infection, bronchitis, bronchospasm,* cough, dyspnea, increased sputum.
Skin: rash.
Other: flulike symptoms, hypersensitivity reactions.

INTERACTIONS
Drug-drug. *Anticholinergics:* May increase anticholinergic effects. Avoid using together.

Reactions may be *common*, uncommon, *life-threatening*, or COMMON AND LIFE-THREATENING.
Interaction may have a *rapid onset* or *delayed onset.*

Drug-herb. *Jaborandi tree:* May decrease effect of drug. Advise patient to use cautiously.
Pill-bearing spurge: May decrease effect of drug. Advise patient to use cautiously.

EFFECTS ON LAB TEST RESULTS
None reported.

CONTRAINDICATIONS & CAUTIONS
• Contraindicated in patients hypersensitive to drug, atropine, or its derivatives.
• Use cautiously in patients with angle-closure glaucoma, prostatic hyperplasia, or bladder-neck obstruction.
• Safety and effectiveness of nebulization or inhaler in children younger than age 12 haven't been established.

NURSING CONSIDERATIONS
• If patient uses a face mask for a nebulizer, take care to prevent leakage around the mask because eye pain or temporary blurring of vision may occur.
• Safety and effectiveness of use beyond 4 days in patients with a common cold haven't been established.
• *Look alike–sound alike:* Don't confuse Atrovent with Alupent.

PATIENT TEACHING
• Warn patient that drug isn't effective for treating acute episodes of bronchospasm when rapid response is needed.
• Teach patient to perform oral inhalation correctly. Give the following instructions for using an MDI:
– Shake canister. The HFA form doesn't need to be shaken.
– Clear nasal passages and throat.
– Breathe out, expelling as much air from lungs as possible.
– Place mouthpiece well into mouth, and inhale deeply as you release dose from inhaler. (Patient should close his eyes.)
– Hold breath for several seconds, remove mouthpiece, and exhale slowly.
• Inform patient that use of a spacer device with MDI may improve drug delivery to lungs.
• Warn patient to avoid accidentally spraying drug into eyes. Temporary blurring of vision may result.

• If more than 1 inhalation is prescribed, tell patient to wait at least 2 minutes before repeating procedure.
• Instruct patient to remove canister and wash inhaler in warm, soapy water at least once weekly.
• If patient is also using a corticosteroid inhaler, instruct him to use ipratropium first and then to wait about 5 minutes before using the corticosteroid. This lets the bronchodilator open air passages for maximal effectiveness of the corticosteroid.
• Instruct patient to prime nasal spray by pumping seven times before first use and after unused for 1 week. Prime with two pumps after unused for 1 day.
• Instruct patient to sniff deeply after each spray and to breathe out through mouth. Tell him to tilt head backward to allow drug to spread to back of nose.

---

isoproterenol hydrochloride
eye-soe-proe-TER-e-nole

Isuprel

Pharmacologic class: nonselective beta-adrenergic agonist
Pregnancy risk category C

AVAILABLE FORMS
Injection: 200 mcg/ml in 1- and 5-ml ampules and 5- and 10-ml vials

INDICATIONS & DOSAGES
➤ **Bronchospasm during anesthesia**
Adults: Dilute 1 ml of a 1:5,000 solution with 10 ml of normal saline or D_5W. Give 0.01 to 0.02 mg I.V. and repeat as necessary. Or, give 1:50,000 solution undiluted using same dose.
➤ **Heart block, ventricular arrhythmias**
Adults: Initially, 0.02 to 0.06 mg I.V.; then 0.01 to 0.2 mg I.V. or 5 mcg/minute I.V. Or, initially, 0.2 mg I.M.; then 0.02 to 1 mg I.M., as needed.
Children: Initial I.V. infusion of 0.1 mcg/kg/minute. Adjust dosage based on patient's response. Usual dosage range is 0.1 to 1 mcg/kg/minute.
➤ **Shock**
Adults and children: 0.5 to 5 mcg/minute isoproterenol hydrochloride by continuous

I.V. infusion. Usual concentration is 1 mg or 5 ml in 500 ml D$_5$W. Titrate infusion rate according to heart rate, central venous pressure, blood pressure, and urine flow.
➤ **Postoperative cardiac patients with bradycardia ◆**
Children: I.V. infusion of 0.029 mcg/kg/minute.
➤ **As an aid in diagnosing the cause of mitral regurgitation ◆**
Adults: 4 mcg/minute I.V. infusion.
➤ **As an aid in diagnosing coronary artery disease or lesions ◆**
Adults: 1 to 3 mcg/minute I.V. infusion.

ADMINISTRATION
I.V.
● For infusion, dilute with most common I.V. solutions, but don't use with sodium bicarbonate injection; drug decomposes rapidly in alkaline solutions.
● Don't use solution if it's discolored or contains precipitate.
● Give by direct injection or I.V. infusion.
● For shock, closely monitor blood pressure, central venous pressure, ECG, arterial blood gas measurements, and urine output. Carefully titrate infusion rate according to these measurements. Use a continuous infusion pump to regulate flow rate.
● Store at room temperature. Protect from light.
● **Incompatibilities:** Alkalies, aminophylline, furosemide, metals, sodium bicarbonate.

ACTION
Relaxes bronchial smooth muscle by stimulating beta$_2$ receptors. As a cardiac stimulant, acts on beta$_1$ receptors in the heart.

Route	Onset	Peak	Duration
I.V.	Immediate	Unknown	< 60 min

Half-life: Unknown.

ADVERSE REACTIONS
CNS: headache, mild tremor, weakness, dizziness, nervousness, insomnia, anxiety.
CV: *palpitations, rapid rise and fall in blood pressure, tachycardia, angina,* **arrhythmias, cardiac arrest.**
GI: nausea, vomiting.

Metabolic: hyperglycemia.
Skin: diaphoresis.
Other: swelling of parotid glands with prolonged use.

INTERACTIONS
Drug-drug. *Epinephrine, other sympathomimetics:* May increase risk of arrhythmias. Use together cautiously. If used together, give at least 4 hours apart.
Halogenated general anesthetics or cyclopropane: May increase risk of arrhythmias. Avoid using together.
Propranolol, other beta blockers: May block bronchodilating effect of isoproterenol. Monitor patient carefully.

EFFECTS ON LAB TEST RESULTS
● May increase glucose level.

CONTRAINDICATIONS & CAUTIONS
● Contraindicated in patients with tachycardia or AV block caused by digoxin intoxication, arrhythmias other than those that may respond to drug, angina pectoris, or angle-closure glaucoma.
● Contraindicated when used with general anesthetics with halogenated drugs or cyclopropane.
● Use cautiously in elderly patients and in those with renal or CV disease, coronary insufficiency, diabetes, hyperthyroidism, or history of sensitivity to sympathomimetic amines.

NURSING CONSIDERATIONS
● Correct volume deficit before giving vasopressors.
● *Alert:* If heart rate exceeds 110 beats/minute during I.V. infusion, notify prescriber. Doses that increase the heart rate to more than 130 beats/minute may induce ventricular arrhythmias.
● Drug may cause a slight increase in systolic blood pressure and a slight to marked decrease in diastolic blood pressure.
● Monitor patient for adverse reactions.
● *Look alike–sound alike:* Don't confuse Isuprel with Isordil.

PATIENT TEACHING
● Tell patient to report chest pain, fluttering in chest, or other adverse reactions.

Reactions may be *common,* uncommon, *life-threatening,* or COMMON AND LIFE-THREATENING.
Interaction may have a *rapid onset* or **delayed onset.**

• Remind patient to report pain at the I.V. injection site.

---

levalbuterol hydrochloride
lev-al-BYOO-ter-ol

Xopenex

levalbuterol tartrate
Xopenex HFA

Pharmacologic class: beta$_2$ agonist
Pregnancy risk category C

AVAILABLE FORMS
Inhalation aerosol: 45 mcg per actuation
Solution for inhalation: 0.31 mg, 0.63 mg, or 1.25 mg in 3-ml vials; 1.25 mg/0.5-ml vials (concentrate)

INDICATIONS & DOSAGES
➤ **To prevent or treat bronchospasm in patients with reversible obstructive airway disease**
Adults and adolescents age 12 and older: 0.63 mg given t.i.d. every 6 to 8 hours, by oral inhalation via a nebulizer. Patients with more severe asthma who don't respond adequately to 0.63 mg t.i.d. may benefit from 1.25 mg t.i.d.
Children ages 6 to 11: 0.31 mg inhaled t.i.d. by nebulizer. Routine dosage shouldn't exceed 0.63 mg t.i.d.
Adults and children age 4 and older: 2 inhalations Xopenex HFA (90 mcg) every 4 to 6 hours. In some patients, 1 inhalation every 4 hours is sufficient.

ADMINISTRATION
Inhalational
• Keep unopened vial in foil pouch. After opened, vial must be used within 2 weeks and protected from light.
• Release four test sprays before first use of inhaler or after unused for more than 3 days.
• Shake canister well before use.
• Use a spacer device to improve inhalation, as appropriate.

ACTION
Relaxes bronchial smooth muscle by stimulating beta$_2$ receptors; also, inhibits release of mediators from mast cells in the airway.

Route	Onset	Peak	Duration
Inhalation	5–15 min	1 hr	3–4 hr

Half-life: 3¼ to 4 hours.

ADVERSE REACTIONS
CNS: dizziness, migraine, nervousness, pain, tremor, anxiety.
CV: tachycardia.
EENT: *rhinitis,* sinusitis, turbinate edema.
GI: dyspepsia.
Musculoskeletal: leg cramps.
Respiratory: increased cough.
Other: *viral infection,* flulike syndrome, accidental injury.

INTERACTIONS
Drug-drug. *Beta blockers:* May block pulmonary effect of the drug and cause severe bronchospasm. Avoid using together, if possible. If use together is unavoidable, consider a cardioselective beta blocker, but use cautiously.
Digoxin: May decrease digoxin level up to 22%. Monitor digoxin level.
Loop or thiazide diuretics: May cause ECG changes and hypokalemia. Use together cautiously.
MAO inhibitors, tricyclic antidepressants: May potentiate action of levalbuterol on the vascular system. Avoid using within 2 weeks of MAO inhibitor or tricyclic antidepressant therapy.
Other short-acting sympathomimetic aerosol bronchodilators, epinephrine: May increase adrenergic adverse effects. Use together cautiously.

EFFECTS ON LAB TEST RESULTS
None reported.

CONTRAINDICATIONS & CAUTIONS
• Contraindicated in patients hypersensitive to drug or to racemic albuterol.
• Use cautiously in patients with CV disorders (especially coronary insufficiency, hypertension, and arrhythmias), seizure disorders, hyperthyroidism, or diabetes mellitus, and in those who are unusually responsive to sympathomimetic amines.

NURSING CONSIDERATIONS
• *Alert:* As with other inhaled beta agonists, drug can produce paradoxical bronchospasm or life-threatening CV effects. If this

occurs, stop drug immediately and notify prescriber.
• Drug may worsen diabetes mellitus and ketoacidosis.
• Drug may temporarily decrease potassium level, but potassium supplementation is usually unnecessary.
• The compatibility of levalbuterol mixed with other drugs in a nebulizer hasn't been established.

PATIENT TEACHING
• Warn patient that he may experience worsened breathing. Tell him to stop drug and contact prescriber immediately if this occurs.
• Tell patient not to increase dosage without consulting prescriber.
• Urge patient to seek medical attention immediately if levalbuterol becomes less effective, if signs and symptoms become worse, or if he's using drug more frequently than usual.
• Tell patient that the effects of levalbuterol may last up to 8 hours.
• Tell patient not to double the next dose if he misses one. Tell him to take doses at least 6 hours apart.
• Advise patient to use other inhalations and antiasthmatics only as directed while taking levalbuterol.
• Inform patient that common adverse reactions include palpitations, rapid heart rate, headache, dizziness, tremor, and nervousness.
• Encourage woman to contact prescriber if she becomes pregnant or is breast-feeding.
• Tell patient to keep unopened vials in foil pouch. After the foil pouch is opened, vials must be used within 2 weeks. Inform patient that vials removed from the pouch, if not used immediately, should be protected from light and excessive heat and used within 1 week.
• Teach patient to use drug correctly when inhaling by nebulizer.
• Instruct patient to breathe as calmly, deeply, and evenly as possible until no more mist is formed in the nebulizer reservoir (5 to 15 minutes).
• Tell patient using the inhaler to release four test sprays into the air away from the face before the first use or if it hasn't been used for more than 3 days.

pirbuterol acetate
peer-BYOO-ter-ole

Maxair Autohaler

Pharmacologic class: beta$_2$ agonist
Pregnancy risk category C

AVAILABLE FORMS
Inhaler: 0.2 mg/metered dose

INDICATIONS & DOSAGES
➤ **To prevent and reverse broncho-spasm; asthma**
Adults and children age 12 and older:
1 or 2 inhalations (0.2 to 0.4 mg), repeated every 4 to 6 hours. Don't exceed 12 inhalations daily.

ADMINISTRATION
Inhalational
• If more than one inhalation is ordered, wait 1 minute between inhalations.
• Have patient hold his breath for 10 seconds after inhalation, then exhale slowly.
• Give corticosteroid inhaler 5 minutes after bronchodilator.

ACTION
Relaxes bronchial smooth muscle by stimulating beta$_2$ receptors.

Route	Onset	Peak	Duration
Inhalation	5 min	30–60 min	5 hr

Half-life: About 2 hours.

ADVERSE REACTIONS
CNS: tremor, nervousness, dizziness, insomnia, headache, vertigo.
CV: tachycardia, palpitations, chest tightness.
EENT: dry or irritated throat.
GI: nausea, vomiting, diarrhea, dry mouth.
Respiratory: cough.

INTERACTIONS
Drug-drug. *Beta blockers, propranolol:* May decrease bronchodilating effects. Avoid using together.
MAO inhibitors, tricyclic antidepressants: May potentiate action of beta

---

Reactions may be *common*, uncommon, *life-threatening*, or COMMON AND LIFE-THREATENING.
Interaction may have a *rapid onset* or **delayed onset**.

agonist on vascular system. Use together cautiously.

EFFECTS ON LAB TEST RESULTS
None reported.

CONTRAINDICATIONS & CAUTIONS
• Contraindicated in patients hypersensitive to drug.
• Use cautiously in patients unusually responsive to sympathomimetic amines and patients with CV disorders, hyperthyroidism, diabetes, and seizure disorders.

NURSING CONSIDERATIONS
• Monitor patient for increased pulse or blood pressure during therapy.
• Stop drug immediately and notify prescriber if paradoxical bronchospasm occurs.
• The likelihood of paradoxical bronchospasm is increased with the first use of a new canister.
• Notify prescriber of decreasing effectiveness of the drug.

PATIENT TEACHING
• Give the following instructions for using Autohaler:
– Remove mouthpiece cover by pulling down lip on back cover. Inspect mouthpiece for foreign objects. Locate "Up" arrows and air vents.
– Hold Autohaler upright so that arrows point up; raise lever until it snaps into place.
– Hold Autohaler around the middle, and shake gently several times.
– Continue to hold upright, and be careful not to block air vents at bottom. Exhale normally before use.
– Seal lips around mouthpiece. Inhale deeply through mouthpiece with steady, moderate force to trigger release of the drug. You'll hear a click and feel a soft puff when drug is released. Continue to take a full, deep breath.
– Take Autohaler away from mouth when done inhaling. Hold breath for 10 seconds; then exhale slowly.
– Continue to hold Autohaler upright while lowering lever. Lower lever after each puff. If additional puffs are ordered, wait 1 minute before repeating process to obtain the next puff.

• Have patient clean inhaler per manufacturer's instructions.
• If patient also uses a corticosteroid inhaler, tell him to use the bronchodilator first, and then wait about 5 minutes before using the corticosteroid. This allows the bronchodilator to open air passages for maximal effectiveness of the corticosteroid.
• Instruct patient to call prescriber if bronchospasm increases after using drug.
• Advise patient to seek medical attention if a previously effective dosage doesn't control symptoms; this may signal worsening of disease.

salmeterol xinafoate
sal-MEE-ter-ol

Serevent Diskus

Pharmacologic class: long-acting selective beta₂ agonist
Pregnancy risk category C

AVAILABLE FORMS
Inhalation powder: 50 mcg/blister

INDICATIONS & DOSAGES
➤ **Long-term maintenance of asthma; to prevent bronchospasm in patients with nocturnal asthma or reversible obstructive airway disease who need regular treatment with short-acting beta agonists**
Adults and children age 4 and older:
1 inhalation (50 mcg) every 12 hours, morning and evening.
➤ **To prevent exercise-induced bronchospasm**
Adults and children age 4 and older:
1 inhalation (50 mcg) at least 30 minutes before exercise. Additional doses shouldn't be taken for at least 12 hours.
➤ **COPD or emphysema**
Adults: 1 inhalation (50 mcg) b.i.d. in the morning and evening, about 12 hours apart.

ADMINISTRATION
Inhalational
• Give drug 30 to 60 minutes before exercise to prevent exercise-induced bronchospasm.
• Don't use a spacer device with this drug.

ACTION
Unclear. Selectively activates beta$_2$ receptors, which results in bronchodilation; also, blocks the release of allergic mediators from mast cells lining the respiratory tract.

Route	Onset	Peak	Duration
Inhalation	10–20 min	3 hr	12 hr

Half-life: 5½ hours; xinafoate salt, 11 days.

ADVERSE REACTIONS
CNS: headache, sinus headache, tremor, nervousness, giddiness, dizziness.
CV: *ventricular arrhythmias,* tachycardia, palpitations.
EENT: *nasopharyngitis,* pharyngitis, nasal cavity or sinus disorder.
GI: nausea, vomiting, diarrhea, heartburn.
Musculoskeletal: joint and back pain, myalgia.
Respiratory: *upper respiratory tract infection,* **bronchospasm,** cough, lower respiratory tract infection.
Other: hypersensitivity reactions.

INTERACTIONS
Drug-drug. *Beta agonists, other methylxanthines, theophylline:* May cause adverse cardiac effects with excessive use. Monitor patient.
MAO inhibitors: May cause risk of severe adverse CV effects. Avoid use within 14 days of MAO inhibitor therapy.
Tricyclic antidepressants: May cause risk of moderate to severe adverse CV effects. Use together with caution.

EFFECTS ON LAB TEST RESULTS
None reported.

CONTRAINDICATIONS & CAUTIONS
• Contraindicated in patients hypersensitive to drug or its ingredients.
• Use cautiously in patients unusually responsive to sympathomimetics and those with coronary insufficiency, arrhythmias, hypertension, other CV disorders, thyrotoxicosis, or seizure disorders.

NURSING CONSIDERATIONS
■ **Black Box Warning** Drug may increase the risk of asthma-related death. Only use salmeterol as additional therapy for patients whose condition is not adequately controlled on other medications or patients whose disease severity warrants initiation of treatment with 2 maintenance therapies. ■
• Drug isn't indicated for acute bronchospasm.
• *Alert:* Monitor patient for rash and urticaria, which may signal a hypersensitivity reaction.
• *Look alike–sound alike:* Don't confuse Serevent with Serentil.

PATIENT TEACHING
• Remind patient to take drug at about 12-hour intervals for optimal effect and to take drug even when feeling better.
• If patient is taking drug to prevent exercise-induced bronchospasm, tell him to take it 30 to 60 minutes before exercise.
• *Alert:* Tell patient drug shouldn't be used to treat acute bronchospasm. He must use a short-acting beta agonist, such as albuterol, to treat worsening symptoms.
• *Alert:* Rare serious asthma episodes or asthma-related deaths may occur in patients using salmeterol. Black patients may be at greater risk.
• Tell patient to contact prescriber if the short-acting agonist no longer provides sufficient relief or if he needs more than 4 inhalations daily. This may be a sign that the asthma symptoms are worsening. Tell him not to increase the dosage of salmeterol.
• If patient takes an inhaled corticosteroid, he should continue to use it regularly. Warn patient not to take other drugs without prescriber's consent.
• If patient takes the inhalation powder (in a multidose inhaler), instruct him not to exhale into the device. He should activate and use it only in a level, horizontal position.
• Tell patient not to use the dry-powder multidose inhaler with a spacer.
• Instruct patient never to wash the mouthpiece or any part of the dry-powder multidose inhaler; it must be kept dry.

Reactions may be *common,* uncommon, *life-threatening,* or COMMON AND LIFE-THREATENING.
Interaction may have a *rapid onset* or **delayed onset.**

terbutaline sulfate
ter-BYOO-ta-leen

Pharmacologic class: beta$_2$ agonist
Pregnancy risk category B

AVAILABLE FORMS
Injection: 1 mg/ml
Tablets: 2.5 mg, 5 mg

INDICATIONS & DOSAGES
➤ **Bronchospasm in patients with reversible obstructive airway disease**
Adults and children age 12 and older: 0.25 mg subcutaneously. Repeat in 15 to 30 minutes, p.r.n. Maximum, 0.5 mg in 4 hours. If patient fails to respond to second dose, consider other measures.
Adults and adolescents older than age 15: 2.5 to 5 mg P.O. t.i.d. every 6 hours while awake. Maximum, 15 mg daily.
Children ages 12 to 15: 2.5 mg P.O. t.i.d. every 6 hours while awake. Maximum, 7.5 mg daily.
➤ **Preterm labor**
Adults: 2.5 to 10 mcg/minute I.V. Increase dosage at 10 to 20 minute intervals until desired effects are achieved. Effective maximum recommended dosage ranges from 17.5 to 30 mcg/minute. Continue infusion for 12 hours after contractions cease. After I.V. therapy is complete oral therapy can be initiated at 2.5 to 10 mg P.O. every 4 to 6 hours.

ADMINISTRATION
P.O.
• Give drug without regard for food.
Subcutaneous
• Give subcutaneous injections into the side of the deltoid.
• Protect drug from light. Don't use if discolored.

ACTION
Relaxes bronchial smooth muscle by stimulating beta$_2$ receptors.

Route	Onset	Peak	Duration
P.O.	30 min	2–3 hr	4–8 hr
Subcut.	15 min	30 min	1½–4 hr

Half-life: Unknown.

ADVERSE REACTIONS
CNS: *nervousness, tremor, drowsiness, dizziness, headache,* weakness.
CV: *palpitations,* **arrhythmias,** tachycardia, flushing.
GI: *vomiting, nausea,* heartburn.
Metabolic: hypokalemia.
Respiratory: ***paradoxical bronchospasm with prolonged use,*** dyspnea.
Skin: diaphoresis.

INTERACTIONS
Drug-drug. *Cardiac glycosides, cyclopropane, halogenated inhaled anesthetics, levodopa:* May increase risk of arrhythmias. Monitor patient closely, and avoid using together with levodopa.
CNS stimulants: May increase CNS stimulation. Avoid using together.
MAO inhibitors: When given with sympathomimetics, may cause severe hypertension (hypertensive crisis). Avoid using together.
Propranolol, other beta blockers: May block bronchodilating effects of terbutaline. Avoid using together.

EFFECTS ON LAB TEST RESULTS
• May decrease potassium level.

CONTRAINDICATIONS & CAUTIONS
• Contraindicated in patients hypersensitive to drug or sympathomimetic amines.
• Use cautiously in patient with CV disorders, hyperthyroidism, diabetes, or seizure disorders.

NURSING CONSIDERATIONS
• Drug may reduce the sensitivity of spirometry for the diagnosis of bronchospasm.
• *Look alike–sound alike:* Don't confuse terbutaline with tolbutamide or terbinafine.

PATIENT TEACHING
• Make sure patient and caregivers understand why patient needs drug.
• Remind patient to separate oral doses by 6 hours.

theophylline
thee-OFF-i-lin

Immediate-release liquids
Elixophyllin*

Immediate-release tablets
Theolair

Timed-release tablets
Theochron, Uniphyl

Timed-release capsules
TheoCap, Theo-24

Pharmacologic class: xanthine
derivative
Pregnancy risk category C

AVAILABLE FORMS
Capsules (extended-release): 100 mg,
125 mg, 200 mg, 300 mg, 400 mg
D_5W injection: 200 mg in 50 ml or
100 ml; 400 mg in 100 ml, 250 ml,
500 ml, or 1,000 ml; 800 mg in 500 ml
or 1,000 ml
Elixir: 27 mg/5 ml*
Syrup: 80 mg/15 ml*
Tablets: 125 mg, 250 mg
Tablets (extended-release): 100 mg,
200 mg, 300 mg, 400 mg, 450 mg,
600 mg

INDICATIONS & DOSAGES
Extended-release preparations shouldn't
be used to treat acute bronchospasm.
➤ **Oral theophylline for acute
bronchospasm in patients not
currently receiving theophylline**
*Adults age 60 and younger, children ages
16 and older, and children ages 1 to
15 weighing 45 kg or more:* 5 mg/kg P.O.,
then 300 mg P.O. daily in divided doses
every 6 to 8 hours for 3 days. If tolerated,
increase to 400 mg P.O. daily in divided
doses every 6 to 8 hours. If necessary,
dosage may be increased after 3 days to
600 mg P.O. daily in divided doses every
6 to 8 hours.
*Children ages 1 to 15 weighing less
than 45 kg:* 5 mg/kg P.O., then 12 to
14 mg/kg (maximum 300 mg) P.O. daily
in divided doses every 4 to 6 hours for
3 days. If tolerated, increase to 16 mg/kg
(maximum 400 mg) P.O. daily in divided

doses every 4 to 6 hours. After 3 days,
if necessary, increase to 20 mg/kg
(maximum 600 mg) P.O. daily in divided
doses every 4 to 6 hours.
Adjust-a-dose: For children ages 1 to 15
with risk factors for reduced theophylline
clearance or for whom serum concentrations can't be monitored, give 5 mg/kg
P.O., then 12 to 14 mg/kg (maximum
300 mg) P.O. daily in divided doses every
4 to 6 hours for 3 days. If tolerated,
increase to 16 mg/kg (maximum 400 mg)
P.O. daily in divided doses every 4 to
6 hours. For children age 16 and older
and adults with risk factors for reduced
theophylline clearance or for whom
serum concentrations can't be monitored,
give 5 mg/kg P.O., then 300 mg P.O.
daily in divided doses every 6 to 8 hours
for 3 days. If tolerated, increase to 400 mg
P.O. daily in divided doses every 6 to
8 hours.
➤ **Parenteral theophylline for
patients not currently receiving
theophylline**
Loading dose: 4.6 mg/kg slowly; then
maintenance infusion.
*Nonsmoking adults younger than age
60 and children older than age 16:*
0.4 mg/kg/hour (maximum 900 mg daily).
Nonsmoking children ages 12 to 16:
0.5 mg/kg/hour (maximum 900 mg daily).
*Children ages 12 to 16 who smoke and
children ages 9 to 12:* 0.7 mg/kg/hour.
Children ages 1 to 9: 0.8 mg/kg/hour.
Infants ages 6 weeks to 1 year: Calculate
mg/kg/hour dosage as follows: 0.008 ×
(age in weeks) + 0.21.
Neonates older than 24 days: 1.5 mg/kg
every 12 hours to achieve target theophylline concentration of 7.5 mcg/ml.
Neonates 24 days old and younger:
1 mg/kg every 12 hours to achieve a
target theophylline concentration of
7.5 mcg/ml.
Adjust-a-dose: For adults older than
age 60, give 0.3 mg/kg/hour, up to a
maximum of 17 mg/hour. For adults with
heart failure, cor pulmonale, sepsis with
multiorgan failure, or shock, give
0.2 mg/kg/hour, up to a maximum infusion
rate of 17 mg/hour unless serum theophylline concentrations are monitored at
24-hour intervals. Maximum daily dose is
400 mg.

Reactions may be *common*, uncommon, ***life-threatening***, or COMMON AND LIFE-THREATENING.
Interaction may have a *rapid onset* or ***delayed onset.***

> **Chronic bronchospasm using
8- to 12-hour extended-release
preparations**
*Adults age 60 or younger, children age
16 and older, and children ages 6 to 15
weighing more than 45 kg:* 300 mg P.O.
daily in divided doses every 8 to
12 hours for 3 days. If tolerated, increase
to 400 mg P.O. in divided doses every
8 to 12 hours. After 3 more days, if necessary, increase dose to 600 mg P.O. daily in
divided doses every 8 to 12 hours.
*Children ages 6 to 15 weighing less
than 45 kg:* 12 to 14 mg/kg (maximum
300 mg) daily in divided doses every
8 to 12 hours for 3 days. If tolerated,
increase to 16 mg/kg (maximum 400 mg)
daily in divided doses every 8 to 12 hours.
After 3 more days, if necessary, increase
to 20 mg/kg (maximum 600 mg) daily in
divided doses every 8 to 12 hours.
Adjust-a-dose: For children ages 6 to 15
with risk factors for reduced theophylline
clearance or for whom serum concentrations can't be monitored, give 12 to
14 mg/kg (maximum 300 mg) daily in
divided doses for 3 days. If tolerated,
increase to a maximum of 16 mg/kg
(maximum 400 mg) P.O. daily in divided
doses every 8 to 12 hours. For children age
16 and older and adults age 60 or younger
or for whom serum concentrations can't
be monitored, give 300 mg P.O. daily in
divided doses every 8 to 12 hours. After
3 days, if necessary, increase to maximum
of 400 mg P.O. daily in divided doses
every 8 to 12 hours. For adults older than
age 60, the recommended maximum
daily dose is 400 mg P.O. per day in
divided doses every 8 to 12 hours unless
symptoms continue and peak serum
concentration is less than 10 mcg/ml.
Administer dosages greater than 400 mg
P.O. daily cautiously.

ADMINISTRATION
P.O.
• Each 0.5 mg/kg P.O. loading dose will
increase drug level by 1 mcg/ml.
• Give drug with full glass of water after
meals, if needed, to relieve GI symptoms,
although taking with food delays
absorption.
• Give drug around-the-clock, using
extended-release product at bedtime.

• Don't dissolve or crush extended-release
products. Small children unable to swallow
these can ingest (without chewing) the
contents of capsules sprinkled over soft
food.
I.V.
• Each 0.5 mg/kg I.V. loading dose will
increase drug level by 1 mcg/ml.
• Use commercially available infusion
solution, or mix in D$_5$W solution.
• Use infusion pump for continuous
infusion.
• **Incompatibilities:** Ascorbic acid,
ceftriaxone, cimetidine, hetastarch,
phenytoin.

ACTION
Inhibits phosphodiesterase, the enzyme
that degrades cAMP, resulting in relaxation
of smooth muscle of the bronchial airways
and pulmonary blood vessels.

Route	Onset	Peak	Duration
P.O.	15–60 min	1–2 hr	Unknown
P.O. (extended)	15–60 min	4–7 hr	Unknown
I.V.	15 min	15–30 min	Unknown

Half-life: Adults, 7 to 9 hours; smokers,
4 to 5 hours; children, 3 to 5 hours;
premature infants, 20 to 30 hours.

ADVERSE REACTIONS
CNS: *restlessness, dizziness, insomnia,
seizures,* headache, irritability, muscle
twitching.
CV: *palpitations, sinus tachycardia,
arrhythmias,* extrasystoles, flushing,
marked hypotension.
GI: *nausea, vomiting,* diarrhea, epigastric
pain.
Metabolic: urinary catecholamines.
Respiratory: *respiratory arrest,*
tachypnea.

INTERACTIONS
Drug-drug. *Adenosine:* May decrease
antiarrhythmic effect. Higher doses of
adenosine may be needed.
*Allopurinol, calcium channel blockers,
cimetidine, disulfiram, influenza virus
vaccine, interferon, macrolides (such as
erythromycin), methotrexate, mexiletine,
oral contraceptives, quinolones (such as
ciprofloxacin):* May decrease hepatic

clearance of theophylline; may increase theophylline level. Monitor levels closely and adjust theophylline dose.
Barbiturates, ketoconazole, nicotine, **phenytoin, rifamycins:** May enhance metabolism and decrease theophylline level; may increase phenytoin metabolism. Monitor patient for decreased therapeutic effect; monitor levels and adjust dosage.
Carbamazepine, isoniazid, loop diuretics: May increase or decrease theophylline level. Monitor theophylline level.
Carteolol, pindolol, propranolol, timolol: May act antagonistically, reducing the effects of one or both drugs; may reduce elimination of theophylline. Monitor theophylline level and patient closely.
Ephedrine, other sympathomimetics: May exhibit synergistic toxicity with these drugs, predisposing patient to arrhythmias. Monitor patient closely.
Lithium: May increase lithium excretion. Monitor patient closely.
Tetracyclines: May enhance the adverse effects of theophylline. Monitor patient closely.
Drug-herb. *Cacao tree:* May inhibit drug metabolism. Discourage use together.
Cayenne: May increase risk of drug toxicity. Advise patient to use together cautiously.
Ephedra: May increase risk of adverse reactions. Discourage use together.
Guarana: May cause additive CNS and CV effects. Discourage use together.
Ipriflavone: May increase risk of drug toxicity. Advise patient to use together cautiously.
St. John's wort: May decrease drug level. Discourage use together.
Drug-food. *Any food:* May cause accelerated drug release from extended-release products. Tell patient to take extended-release products on an empty stomach.
Caffeine: May decrease hepatic clearance of drug and increase drug level. Monitor patient for toxicity.
Drug-lifestyle. *Smoking:* May increase elimination of drug, increasing dosage requirements. Monitor drug response and level.

EFFECTS ON LAB TEST RESULTS
● May increase free fatty acid level and blood glucose.

● May falsely elevate theophylline level in the presence of acetaminophen, furosemide, phenylbutazone, probenecid, theobromine, caffeine, tea, chocolate, and cola, depending on assay used.

CONTRAINDICATIONS & CAUTIONS
● Contraindicated in patients hypersensitive to xanthine compounds (caffeine, theobromine) and in those with active peptic ulcer or poorly controlled seizure disorders.
● Use cautiously in young children, infants, neonates, elderly patients, and those with COPD, cardiac failure, cor pulmonale, renal or hepatic disease, peptic ulceration, hyperthyroidism, diabetes mellitus, glaucoma, severe hypoxemia, hypertension, compromised cardiac or circulatory function, angina, acute MI, or sulfite sensitivity.

NURSING CONSIDERATIONS
● Dosage may need to be increased in cigarette smokers and in habitual marijuana smokers because smoking causes drug to be metabolized faster.
● Monitor vital signs; measure and record fluid intake and output. Expect improved quality of pulse and respirations.
● Patients metabolize xanthines at different rates; dosage is determined by monitoring response, tolerance, pulmonary function, and drug level. Drug levels range from 10 to 20 mcg/ml; toxicity may occur at levels above 20 mcg/ml.
● *Alert:* Evidence of toxicity includes tachycardia, anorexia, nausea, vomiting, diarrhea, restlessness, irritability, and headache. If these signs occur, check drug level and adjust dosage, as indicated.
● *Look alike–sound alike:* Don't confuse extended-release form with regular-release form.
● *Look alike–sound alike:* Don't confuse Theolair with Thyrolar.

PATIENT TEACHING
● Supply instructions for home care and dosage schedule.
● Warn patient not to dissolve, crush, or chew extended-release products. Small children unable to swallow these can ingest (without chewing) the contents of capsules sprinkled over soft food.

Reactions may be *common,* uncommon, *life-threatening,* or COMMON AND LIFE-THREATENING.
Interaction may have a *rapid onset* or **delayed onset.**

• Tell patient to relieve GI symptoms by taking oral drug with full glass of water after meals, although food in stomach delays absorption.

• Warn patient to take drug regularly, only as directed. Patients tend to want to take extra "breathing pills."

• Inform elderly patient that dizziness is common at start of therapy.

• Urge patient to tell prescriber about any other drugs taken. OTC drugs or herbal remedies may contain ephedrine or theophylline salts; excessive CNS stimulation may result.

• If a smoker quits, tell him to inform prescriber. Dosage reduction may be needed to prevent toxicity.

---

tiotropium bromide
tye-oh-TROH-pee-um

Spiriva

Pharmacologic class:
anticholinergic
Pregnancy risk category C

AVAILABLE FORMS
Capsules for inhalation: 18 mcg

INDICATIONS & DOSAGES
➤ **Maintenance treatment of bronchospasm in COPD, including chronic bronchitis and emphysema**
Adults: 1 capsule (18 mcg) inhaled orally once daily using the HandiHaler inhalation device.

ADMINISTRATION
Inhalational
• Give capsules only by oral inhalation with the HandiHaler device.
• Open capsule blister immediately before use.
• Capsules aren't for oral ingestion.

ACTION
Competitive, reversible inhibition of muscarinic receptors leads to bronchodilation.

Route	Onset	Peak	Duration
Inhalation	30 min	3 hr	> 24 hr

Half-life: 5 to 6 days.

ADVERSE REACTIONS
CNS: depression, paresthesia.
CV: *angina pectoris,* chest pain, edema.
EENT: *sinusitis,* cataract, dysphonia, epistaxis, glaucoma, laryngitis, pharyngitis, rhinitis.
GI: *dry mouth,* abdominal pain, constipation, dyspepsia, gastroesophageal reflux, stomatitis, vomiting.
GU: UTI.
Metabolic: hypercholesterolemia, hyperglycemia.
Musculoskeletal: arthritis, leg pain, myalgia, skeletal pain.
Respiratory: *upper respiratory tract infection,* cough.
Skin: rash.
Other: *accidental injury,* allergic reaction, candidiasis, flulike syndrome, herpes zoster, infections.

INTERACTIONS
Drug-drug. *Anticholinergics:* May increase the risk of adverse reactions. Avoid using together.

EFFECTS ON LAB TEST RESULTS
• May increase cholesterol and glucose levels.

CONTRAINDICATIONS & CAUTIONS
• Contraindicated in patients hypersensitive to atropine, its derivatives, ipratropium, or any component of the product.
• Use cautiously in women who are pregnant or breast-feeding, patients with creatinine clearance of 50 ml/minute or less, or patients with angle-closure glaucoma, prostatic hyperplasia, or bladder neck obstruction.

NURSING CONSIDERATIONS
• *Alert:* Use drug for maintenance treatment of COPD, not for acute bronchospasm.
• Watch for evidence of hypersensitivity (especially angioedema) and paradoxical bronchospasm.
• *Look alike–sound alike:* Don't confuse Spiriva with Inspra.

PATIENT TEACHING
• Inform patient that drug is for maintenance treatment of COPD and not for immediate relief of breathing problems.

● **Alert:** Explain that capsules are for inhalation and shouldn't be swallowed.
● Provide full instructions for the Handi-Haler device.
● Tell patient not to get powder in his eyes.
● Review signs and symptoms of hypersensitivity (especially angioedema) and paradoxical bronchospasm. Tell patient to stop the drug and contact the prescriber if they occur.
● Advise patient to report eye pain, blurred vision, visual halos, colored images, or red eyes immediately.
● Tell patient to keep capsules in sealed blisters and to remove each capsule just before use. Caution against storing capsules in the HandiHaler device.
● Instruct patient to store capsules at 77° F (25° C) and not to expose them to extreme temperatures or moisture.

acetylcysteine
beclomethasone dipropionate
benzonatate
beractant
budesonide
calfactant
ciclesonide
codeine phosphate
(See Chapter 47, OPIOID ANALGESICS.)
codeine sulfate
(See Chapter 47, OPIOID ANALGESICS.)
dextromethorphan hydrobromide
diphenhydramine hydrochloride
(See Chapter 55, ANTIHISTAMINES.)
flunisolide
flunisolide hemihydrate
fluticasone furoate
fluticasone propionate
fluticasone propionate and
salmeterol inhalation powder
guaifenesin
hydromorphone hydrochloride
(See Chapter 47, OPIOID ANALGESICS.)
mometasone furoate
montelukast sodium
omalizumab
triamcinolone acetonide
zafirlukast

---

acetylcysteine
a-se-teel-SIS-tay-een

Acetadote

Pharmacologic class: L-cysteine
derivative
Pregnancy risk category B

AVAILABLE FORMS
Solution: 10%, 20%
I.V. injection: 200 mg/ml

INDICATIONS & DOSAGES
➤ **Adjunct therapy for abnormal
viscid or thickened mucous secretions in patients with pneumonia,
bronchitis, bronchiectasis, primary
amyloidosis of the lung, tuberculosis,
cystic fibrosis, emphysema, atelectasis, pulmonary complications of
thoracic surgery, or CV surgery**
Adults and children: 1 to 2 ml 10% or
20% solution by direct instillation into
trachea as often as every hour. Or, 1 to
10 ml of 20% solution or 2 to 20 ml of
10% solution by nebulization every 2 to
6 hours, p.r.n.
➤ **Acetaminophen toxicity**
Adults and children: Initially, 140 mg/kg
P.O.; then 70 mg/kg P.O. every 4 hours
for 17 doses (total). Or, a loading dose of
150 mg/kg I.V. over 60 minutes; then I.V.
maintenance dose of 50 mg/kg infused
over 4 hours, followed by 100 mg/kg
infused over 16 hours.
➤ **Prevention of contrast media
nephrotoxicity** ♦
Adults: 600 mg P.O. b.i.d. starting one day
before administration of contrast media
and continued through the day of administration for a total of 4 doses.

ADMINISTRATION
P.O.
● Dilute oral dose (used for acetaminophen
overdose) with cola, fruit juice, or water.
Dilute 20% solution to 5% (add 3 ml of
diluent to each milliliter of drug). If patient
vomits within 1 hour of receiving loading
or maintenance dose, repeat dose. Use
diluted solution within 1 hour.
● Drug smells strongly of sulfur. Mixing
oral form with juice or cola improves
its taste.
● Drug delivered through nasogastric tube
may be diluted with water.
● Store opened, undiluted oral solution in
the refrigerator for up to 96 hours.
I.V.
● Drug may turn from a colorless liquid
to a slight pink or purple color once the
stopper is punctured. This color change
doesn't affect the drug.
● Drug is hyperosmolar and is compatible
with D_5W, half-normal saline, and sterile
water for injection.
● Adjust total volume given for patients
who weigh less than 40 kg or who are
fluid restricted.

- For patients who weigh 40 kg (88 lb) or more, dilute loading dose in 200 ml of D₅W, second dose in 500 ml, and third dose in 1,000 ml.
- For patients who weigh 25 to 40 kg (55 to 88 lb), dilute loading dose in 100 ml, second dose in 250 ml, and third dose in 500 ml.
- For patients who weigh 20 kg (44 lb), dilute loading dose in 60 ml, second dose in 140 ml, and third dose in 280 ml.
- For patients who weigh 15 kg (33 lb), dilute loading dose in 45 ml, second dose in 105 ml, and third dose in 210 ml.
- For patients who weigh 10 kg (22 lb), dilute loading dose in 30 ml, second dose in 70 ml, and third dose in 140 ml.
- Reconstituted solution is stable for 24 hours at room temperature.
- Vials contain no preservatives; discard after opening.
- **Incompatibilities:** Incompatible with rubber and metals, especially iron, copper, and nickel.

Inhalational
- Use plastic, glass, stainless steel, or another nonreactive metal when giving by nebulization. Hand-bulb nebulizers aren't recommended because output is too small and particle size too large.
- **Incompatibilities:** Physically or chemically incompatible with inhaled tetracyclines, erythromycin lactobionate, amphotericin B, and ampicillin sodium. If given by aerosol inhalation, nebulize these drugs separately. Iodized oil, trypsin, and hydrogen peroxide are physically incompatible with acetylcysteine; don't add to nebulizer.

ACTION
Reduces the viscosity of pulmonary secretions by splitting disulfide linkages between mucoprotein molecular complexes. Also, restores liver stores of glutathione to treat acetaminophen toxicity.

Route	Onset	Peak	Duration
P.O., I.V., inhalation	Unknown	Unknown	Unknown

Half-life: 6¼ hours.

ADVERSE REACTIONS
CNS: abnormal thinking, fever, drowsiness, gait disturbances.

CV: chest tightness, flushing, hypertension, hypotension, tachycardia.
EENT: *rhinorrhea,* ear pain, eye pain, pharyngitis, throat tightness.
GI: *nausea, stomatitis, vomiting.*
Respiratory: *bronchospasm,* cough, dyspnea, rhonchi.
Skin: clamminess, diaphoresis, pruritus, rash, urticaria.
Other: *anaphylactoid reaction, angioedema,* chills.

INTERACTIONS
Drug-drug. *Activated charcoal:* May limit acetylcysteine's effectiveness. Avoid using activated charcoal before or with acetylcysteine.

EFFECTS ON LAB TEST RESULTS
None reported.

CONTRAINDICATIONS & CAUTIONS
- Contraindicated in patients hypersensitive to drug.
- Use cautiously in elderly or debilitated patients with severe respiratory insufficiency. Use I.V. form cautiously in patients with asthma or a history of bronchospasm.

NURSING CONSIDERATIONS
- Monitor cough type and frequency.
- *Alert:* Monitor patient for bronchospasm, especially if he has asthma.
- Ingestion of more than 150 mg/kg of acetaminophen may cause liver toxicity. Measure acetaminophen level 4 hours after ingestion to determine risk of liver toxicity.
- *Alert:* Drug is used for acetaminophen overdose within 24 hours of ingestion. Start drug immediately; don't wait for results of acetaminophen level. Give within 10 hours of acetaminophen ingestion to minimize hepatic injury.
- If you suspect acetaminophen overdose, obtain baseline AST, ALT, bilirubin, PT, BUN, creatinine, glucose, and electrolyte levels.
- *Alert:* Monitor patient receiving I.V. form for anaphylactoid reactions. If anaphylactoid reaction occurs, stop infusion and treat anaphylaxis. Once anaphylaxis treatment starts, restart infusion. If anaphylactoid symptoms return, stop drug. Contact the

---

Reactions may be *common,* uncommon, *life-threatening,* or COMMON AND LIFE-THREATENING.
Interaction may have a *rapid onset* or **delayed onset.**

Poison Control Center at (800) 222-1222 for more information.
- Facial erythema may occur within 30 to 60 minutes of start of I.V. infusion and usually resolves without stopping infusion.
- When acetaminophen level is below toxic level according to nomogram, stop therapy.
- *Look alike–sound alike:* Don't confuse acetylcysteine with acetylcholine.
- The vial stopper doesn't contain natural rubber latex, dry natural rubber, or blends of natural rubber.

PATIENT TEACHING
- Warn patient that drug may have a foul taste or smell that may be distressing.
- For maximum effect, instruct patient to cough to clear his airway before aerosol administration.

---

beclomethasone dipropionate
be-kloe-METH-a-sone

QVAR 40, QVAR 80

Pharmacologic class: glucocorticoid
Pregnancy risk category C

AVAILABLE FORMS
Oral inhalation aerosol: 40 mcg/metered spray, 80 mcg/metered spray

INDICATIONS & DOSAGES
➤ **Chronic asthma**
Adults and children age 12 and older: Starting dose, 40 to 80 mcg b.i.d. when previously used bronchodilators alone, or 40 to 160 mcg b.i.d. when previously used inhaled corticosteroids. Maximum, 320 mcg b.i.d.
Children ages 5 to 12: 40 mcg b.i.d., up to 80 mcg b.i.d.

ADMINISTRATION
Inhalational
- Prime the inhaler before first use by depressing canister twice into the air.
- Allow 1 minute to elapse between inhalations.

ACTION
May decrease inflammation by decreasing the number and activity of inflammatory cells, inhibiting bronchoconstrictor mechanisms producing direct smooth-muscle relaxation, and decreasing airway hyperresponsiveness.

Route	Onset	Peak	Duration
Inhalation	1–4 wk	Unknown	Unknown

Half-life: 2.8 hours.

ADVERSE REACTIONS
EENT: *hoarseness, throat irritation,* fungal infection of throat.
GI: *fungal infection of mouth,* dry mouth.
Respiratory: *bronchospasm,* cough, wheezing.
Other: *angioedema,* facial edema, hypersensitivity reactions, *adrenal insufficiency,* suppression of hypothalamic-pituitary-adrenal function.

INTERACTIONS
None significant.

EFFECTS ON LAB TEST RESULTS
None reported.

CONTRAINDICATIONS & CAUTIONS
- Contraindicated in patients hypersensitive to drug or its ingredients and in those with status asthmaticus, nonasthmatic bronchial diseases, or asthma controlled by broncho-dilators or other noncorticosteroids alone.
- Use cautiously, if at all, in patients with tuberculosis, fungal or bacterial infections, ocular herpes simplex, or systemic viral infections.
- Use cautiously in patients receiving systemic corticosteroid therapy.

NURSING CONSIDERATIONS
- Check mucous membranes frequently for signs and symptoms of fungal infection.
- During times of stress (trauma, surgery, or infection), systemic corticosteroids may be needed to prevent adrenal insufficiency in previously corticosteroid-dependent patients.
- Periodic measurement of growth and development may be needed during high-dose or prolonged therapy in children.
- *Alert:* Taper oral corticosteroid therapy slowly. Acute adrenal insufficiency and death may occur in patients with asthma who change abruptly from oral cortico-steroids to beclomethasone.

PATIENT TEACHING
• Tell patient to prime the inhaler before first use, or after 10 days of not using it, by depressing canister twice into the air.
• Inform patient that drug doesn't relieve acute asthma attacks.
• Tell patient who needs a bronchodilator to use it several minutes before beclomethasone.
• Instruct patient to carry or wear medical identification indicating his need for supplemental systemic corticosteroids during stress.
• Advise patient to allow 1 minute to elapse between inhalations of drug and to hold his breath for a few seconds to enhance drug action.
• Tell patient it may take up to 4 weeks to feel the full benefit of the drug.
• Tell patient to keep inhaler clean by wiping it weekly with a dry tissue or cloth; don't get it wet.
• Advise patient to prevent oral fungal infections by gargling or rinsing his mouth with water after each use. Caution him not to swallow the water.
• Tell patient to report evidence of corticosteroid withdrawal, including fatigue, weakness, arthralgia, orthostatic hypotension, and dyspnea.
• Instruct patient to store drug at 77° F (25° C). Advise patient to ensure delivery of proper dose by gently warming canister to room temperature before using.

---

benzonatate
ben-ZOE-na-tate

Tessalon

Pharmacologic class: local anesthetic
Pregnancy risk category C

AVAILABLE FORMS
Capsules: 100 mg, 200 mg

INDICATIONS & DOSAGES
➤ **Symptomatic relief of cough**
Adults and children older than age 10: 100 to 200 mg P.O. t.i.d.; up to 600 mg daily.

ADMINISTRATION
P.O.
• Protect drug from light and moisture.

ACTION
Chemical relative of tetracaine that suppresses the cough reflex by direct action on the cough center in the medulla and through an anesthetic action on stretch receptors of vagal afferent fibers in the respiratory passages, lungs, and pleura.

Route	Onset	Peak	Duration
P.O.	15–20 min	Unknown	3–8 hr

Half-life: Unknown.

ADVERSE REACTIONS
CNS: dizziness, headache, sedation.
EENT: nasal congestion, burning sensation in eyes.
GI: nausea, constipation, GI upset.
Other: chills, hypersensitivity reactions.

INTERACTIONS
None significant.

EFFECTS ON LAB TEST RESULTS
None reported.

CONTRAINDICATIONS & CAUTIONS
• Contraindicated in patients hypersensitive to drug or related compounds.
• Use cautiously in patients hypersensitive to PABA anesthetics (procaine, tetracaine) because cross-sensitivity reactions may occur.

NURSING CONSIDERATIONS
• Don't use drug when cough is a valuable diagnostic sign or is beneficial (such as after thoracic surgery).
• Monitor cough type and frequency.
• Use with percussion and chest vibration.

PATIENT TEACHING
• Warn patient not to chew capsules or dissolve in mouth, which produces either local anesthesia that may result in aspiration, or CNS stimulation that may cause restlessness, tremor, and seizures.
• Instruct patient to report adverse reactions.
• Instruct patient to protect drug from light and moisture.
• Tell patient to contact his prescriber if cough lasts longer than 1 week, recurs frequently, or is accompanied by high fever, rash, or severe headache.

Reactions may be *common*, uncommon, *life-threatening*, or COMMON AND LIFE-THREATENING.
Interaction may have a *rapid onset* or *delayed onset*.

beractant
(natural lung surfactant)
ber-AK-tant

Survanta

Pharmacologic class: bovine lung extract
Pregnancy risk category NR

AVAILABLE FORMS
Suspension for intratracheal instillation: 25 mg/ml

INDICATIONS & DOSAGES
➤ **To prevent respiratory distress syndrome (RDS), also known as hyaline membrane disease, in premature neonates weighing 1,250 g (2 lb, 12 ounces) or less at birth, or having symptoms consistent with surfactant deficiency**
Neonates: 4 ml/kg intratracheally. Divide each dose into four quarter-doses and give each quarter-dose with infant in a different position to ensure even distribution of drug; between quarter-doses, use a hand-held resuscitation bag at 60 breaths/minute and sufficient oxygen to prevent cyanosis. Give drug as soon as possible, preferably within 15 minutes of birth. Repeat in 6 hours if respiratory distress continues. Give no more than four doses in 48 hours.
➤ **Rescue treatment of RDS in premature infants**
Neonates: 4 ml/kg intratracheally; before giving, increase ventilator rate to 60 breaths/minute with an inspiratory time of 0.5 second and a fraction of inspired oxygen of 1. Divide each dose into four quarter-doses and give each quarter-dose with infant in a different position to ensure even distribution of drug; between quarter-doses, continue mechanical ventilation for at least 30 seconds or until stable. Give dose as soon as RDS is confirmed by X-ray, preferably within 8 hours of birth. Repeat in 6 hours if respiratory distress continues. Give no more than four doses in 48 hours.

ADMINISTRATION
Inhalational
• Refrigerate at 36° to 46° F (2° to 8° C). Warm before use by allowing drug to

stand at room temperature for at least 20 minutes or by holding in hand for at least 8 minutes. Don't use artificial warming methods. Unopened vials that have been warmed to room temperature may be returned to the refrigerator within 24 hours; however, warm and return drug to the refrigerator only once. Vials are for single use only; discard unused drug.
• Beractant doesn't need sonication or reconstitution before use. Inspect contents before giving; make sure color is off-white to light brown and that contents are uniform. If settling occurs, swirl vial gently; don't shake. Some foaming is normal.
• Use a 20G or larger needle to draw up drug; don't use a filter. Give drug using a #5 French end-hole catheter. Premeasure and shorten catheter before use. Fill catheter with beractant and discard excess drug so that only total dose to be given remains in the syringe. Insert catheter into neonate's endotracheal tube; make sure catheter tip protrudes just beyond end of tube above neonate's carina. Don't instill drug into a mainstream bronchus.
• Even distribution of drug is important. Give each dose in four quarter-doses, with each quarter-dose being given over 2 to 3 seconds and with the patient positioned differently after each use. Between giving quarter-doses, remove the catheter and ventilate the patient. Give the first quarter-dose with the patient's head and body inclined slightly downward, and the head turned to the right. Give the second quarter-dose with the head turned to the left. Then, incline the head and body slightly upward with the head turned to the right to give the third quarter-dose. Turn the head to the left for the fourth quarter-dose.

ACTION
Lowers alveolar surface tension during respiration and stabilizes alveoli against collapse. Drug contains neutral lipids, fatty acids, surfactant-related proteins, and phospholipids that mimic naturally occurring surfactant.

Route	Onset	Peak	Duration
Intra-tracheal	30–120 min	Unknown	2–3 days

Half-life: Unknown.

ADVERSE REACTIONS
CV: TRANSIENT BRADYCARDIA, hypotension, vasoconstriction.
Respiratory: *apnea, endotracheal tube reflux or blockage, decreased oxygen saturation, hypercapnia, hypocapnia.*
Skin: pallor.

INTERACTIONS
None significant.

EFFECTS ON LAB TEST RESULTS
None reported.

CONTRAINDICATIONS & CAUTIONS
• In infants who weigh less than 600 g at birth or more than 1,750 g at birth, use hasn't been studied.

NURSING CONSIDERATIONS
• Only staff experienced in treating clinically unstable premature neonates, including neonatal intubation and airway management, should give drug.
• Accurate weight determination is essential for proper measurement of dosage.
• Continuously monitor neonate before, during, and after giving beractant. The endotracheal tube may be suctioned before giving drug; allow neonate to stabilize before proceeding with administration.
• Immediately after giving, moist breath sounds and crackles can occur. Don't suction the neonate for 1 hour unless he has other signs or symptoms of airway obstruction.
• Continuous monitoring of ECG and transcutaneous oxygen saturation are essential; frequent arterial blood pressure monitoring and frequent arterial blood gas sampling are highly desirable.
• Transient bradycardia and oxygen desaturation are common after dosing.
• *Alert:* Drug can rapidly affect oxygenation and lung compliance. Peak ventilator inspiratory pressures may need to be adjusted if chest expansion improves substantially after drug administration. Notify prescriber and adjust immediately as directed because failing to do so may cause lung overdistention and fatal pulmonary air leakage.
• Review manufacturer's audiovisual materials that describe dosage and usage procedures.

• *Look alike–sound alike:* Don't confuse Survanta with Sufenta.

PATIENT TEACHING
• Inform parents of neonate's need for drug, and explain drug action and use.
• Encourage parents to ask questions, and address their concerns.

---

budesonide
byoo-DES-oh-nide

Pulmicort Flexhaler, Pulmicort Respules, Pulmicort Turbuhaler

Pharmacologic class: corticosteroid
Pregnancy risk category B

AVAILABLE FORMS
Dry powder inhaler: 200 mcg/dose
Inhalation suspension: 0.25 mg, 0.5 mg

INDICATIONS & DOSAGES
➤ **As a preventative in maintenance of asthma**
All patients: Use lowest effective dose after stabilizing asthma.
➤ **Turbuhaler**
Adults previously taking bronchodilator alone: Initially, inhaled dose of 200 to 400 mcg b.i.d. to maximum of 400 mcg b.i.d.
Adults previously taking inhaled corticosteroid: Initially, inhaled dose of 200 to 400 mcg b.i.d. to maximum of 800 mcg b.i.d.
Adults previously taking oral corticosteroid: Initially, inhaled dose of 400 to 800 mcg b.i.d. to maximum of 800 mcg b.i.d.
Children older than age 6 previously taking bronchodilator alone or inhaled corticosteroid: Initially, inhaled dose of 200 mcg b.i.d. to maximum of 400 mcg b.i.d.
Children older than age 6 previously taking oral corticosteroid: 400 mcg b.i.d., maximum.
➤ **Respules**
Children ages 1 to 8: 0.25 mg Respules via jet nebulizer with compressor once daily. Increase to 0.5 mg daily or 0.25 mg b.i.d. in child not receiving systemic or inhaled corticosteroid or 1 mg daily or 0.5 mg b.i.d. in child receiving oral corticosteroid.

Reactions may be *common,* uncommon, *life-threatening,* or COMMON AND LIFE-THREATENING.
Interaction may have a *rapid onset* or *delayed onset.*

➤ **Flexhaler**
Adults: Initially, inhaled dose of 360 mcg
b.i.d. to maximum 720 mcg b.i.d.
Children: Initially, inhaled dose of
180 mcg b.i.d. to maximum 360 mcg b.i.d.

ADMINISTRATION
Inhalational
● Give inhalation suspension at regular
intervals once a day or b.i.d., as directed.
● Give suspension with a jet nebulizer
connected to a compressor with
adequate airflow. Make sure that it's
equipped with a mouthpiece or suitable
face mask.
● When aluminum foil envelope has
been opened, the shelf-life of unused
ampules is 2 weeks when protected
from light.

ACTION
Exhibits potent glucocorticoid activity and
weak mineralocorticoid activity. Drug
inhibits mast cells, macrophages, and
mediators (such as leukotrienes) involved
in inflammation.

Route	Onset	Peak	Duration
Inhalation, powder	24 hr	1–2 wk	Unknown
Inhalation, Respules	2–8 days	4–6 wk	Unknown

Half-life: 2 to 3 hours.

ADVERSE REACTIONS
CNS: *headache,* asthenia, fever,
hypertonia, insomnia, pain, syncope.
EENT: *sinusitis, pharyngitis,* rhinitis,
voice alteration.
GI: abdominal pain, dry mouth, dyspepsia,
gastroenteritis, nausea, oral candidiasis,
taste perversion, vomiting.
Metabolic: weight gain.
Musculoskeletal: back pain, fractures,
myalgia.
Respiratory: *respiratory tract infection,*
bronchospasm, increased cough.
Skin: ecchymoses.
Other: flulike symptoms, hypersensitivity
reactions.

INTERACTIONS
Drug-drug. *Ketoconazole:* May inhibit
metabolism and increase level of
budesonide. Monitor patient.

EFFECTS ON LAB TEST RESULTS
None reported.

CONTRAINDICATIONS & CAUTIONS
● Contraindicated in patients hypersensitive
to drug and in those with status asthmaticus
or other acute asthma episodes.
● Use cautiously, if at all, in patients with
active or inactive tuberculosis, ocular
herpes simplex, or untreated systemic fungal, bacterial, viral, or parasitic infections.

NURSING CONSIDERATIONS
■ **Black Box Warning** When transferring
from systemic corticosteroid to this
drug, use caution and gradually decrease
corticosteroid dose to prevent adrenal
insufficiency. ■
● Drug doesn't remove the need for systemic
corticosteroid therapy in some situations.
● If bronchospasm occurs after use, stop
therapy and treat with a bronchodilator.
● Lung function may improve within
24 hours of starting therapy, but maximum
benefit may not be achieved for 1 to
2 weeks or longer.
● For Pulmicort Respules, lung function
improves in 2 to 8 days, but maximum
benefit may not be seen for 4 to 6 weeks.
● Watch for *Candida* infections of the
mouth or pharynx.
● *Alert:* Corticosteroids may increase risk
of developing serious or fatal infections in
patients exposed to viral illnesses, such as
chickenpox or measles.
● In rare cases, inhaled corticosteroids
have been linked to increased intraocular
pressure and cataract development. Stop
drug if local irritation occurs.

PATIENT TEACHING
● Tell patient that budesonide inhaler isn't
a bronchodilator and isn't intended to treat
acute episodes of asthma.
● Instruct patient to use the inhaler at
regular intervals because effectiveness
depends on twice-daily use on a regular
basis, by following these instructions:
– Keep Pulmicort Turbuhaler upright
(mouthpiece on top) during loading, to
provide the correct dose.
– Prime Turbuhaler when using it for the
first time. To prime, hold unit upright and
turn brown grip fully to the right, then fully
to the left until it clicks. Repeat priming.

– Load first dose by holding unit upright and turning brown grip to the right and then to the left until it clicks.

– Turn your head away from the inhaler and breathe out.

– During inhalation, Turbuhaler must be in the upright or horizontal position.

– Don't shake inhaler.

– Place mouthpiece between lips and to inhale forcefully and deeply.

– You may not taste the drug or sense it entering your lungs, but this doesn't mean it isn't effective.

– Don't exhale through the Turbuhaler. If more than one dose is required, repeat steps.

– Rinse your mouth with water and then spit out the water after each dose to decrease the risk of developing oral candidiasis.

– When 20 doses remain in the Turbuhaler, a red mark appears in the indicator window. When red mark reaches the bottom, the unit's empty.

– Don't use Turbuhaler with a spacer device and don't chew or bite the mouthpiece.

– Replace mouthpiece cover after use and always keep it clean and dry.

● Pulmicort Flexhaler must be primed before use. Refer to patient information guide for complete administration instructions.

● Tell patient that improvement in asthma control may be seen within 24 hours, although the maximum benefit may not appear for 1 to 2 weeks. If signs or symptoms worsen during this time, instruct patient to contact prescriber.

● Advise patient to avoid exposure to chickenpox or measles and to contact prescriber if exposure occurs.

■ **Black Box Warning** Instruct patient to carry or wear medical identification indicating need for supplementary corticosteroids during periods of stress or an asthma attack. ■

● Advise patient that unused Respules are good for 2 weeks after the foil envelope has been opened; however, unused Respules should be returned to the envelope to protect them from light.

● Tell patient to read and follow the patient information leaflet contained in the package.

calfactant
kal-FAK-tant

Infasurf

Pharmacologic class: bovine lung extract
Pregnancy risk category NR

AVAILABLE FORMS
Intratracheal suspension: 35 mg phospholipids and 0.65 mg proteins/ml; 6-ml vial

INDICATIONS & DOSAGES
➤ **To prevent respiratory distress syndrome (RDS) in premature infants younger than 29 weeks' gestational age at high risk for RDS; to treat infants younger than 72 hours of age, who develop RDS (confirmed by clinical and radiologic findings) and need an endotracheal tube (ETT)**
Neonates: 3 ml/kg of body weight at birth intratracheally, given in two aliquots of 1.5 ml/kg each, every 12 hours for a total of up to three doses.

ADMINISTRATION
Inhalational
● Suspension settles during storage. Gentle swirling or agitation of the vial is commonly needed for redispersion. Don't shake vial. Visible flecks in the suspension and foaming at the surface are normal.

● Withdraw dose into a syringe from single-use vial using a 20G or larger needle; avoid excessive foaming.

● Give through a side-port adapter into the ETT. Make sure two medical staff are present while giving dose. Give dose in two aliquots of 1.5 ml/kg each. Place infant on one side after first aliquot and other side after second aliquot. Give while ventilation is continued over 20 to 30 breaths for each aliquot, with small bursts timed only during the inspiratory cycles. Evaluate respiratory status and reposition infant between each aliquot.

● Enter each single-use vial only once; discard unused material.

• Unopened, unused vials that have warmed to room temperature can be rerefrigerated within 24 hours for future use. Avoid repeated warming to room temperature.
• Store drug at 36° to 46° F (2° to 8° C). It isn't necessary to warm drug before use.

ACTION
Modifies alveolar surface tension, which stabilizes the alveoli.

Route	Onset	Peak	Duration
Intra-tracheal	Unknown	Unknown	Unknown

Half-life: Unknown.

ADVERSE REACTIONS
CV: BRADYCARDIA.
Respiratory: AIRWAY OBSTRUCTION, APNEA, *cyanosis, hypoventilation.*
Other: *reflux of drug into ETT, dislodgment of ETT.*

INTERACTIONS
None significant.

EFFECTS ON LAB TEST RESULTS
None reported.

CONTRAINDICATIONS & CAUTIONS
• None known

NURSING CONSIDERATIONS
• Give drug under supervision of medical staff experienced in the acute care of neonates with respiratory failure who need intubation.
• *Alert:* Drug intended only for intra-tracheal use; to prevent RDS, give to infant as soon as possible after birth, preferably within 30 minutes.
• Monitor patient for reflux of drug into ETT, cyanosis, bradycardia, or airway obstruction during the procedure. If these occur, stop drug and take appropriate measures to stabilize infant. After infant is stable, resume drug with appropriate monitoring.
• After giving drug, carefully monitor infant so that oxygen therapy and ventilatory support can be modified in response to improvements in oxygenation and lung compliance.

PATIENT TEACHING
• Explain to parents the function of drug in preventing and treating RDS.
• Notify parents that, although infant may improve rapidly after treatment, he may continue to need intubation and mechanical ventilation.
• Notify parents of possible adverse effects of drug, including bradycardia, reflux into ETT, airway obstruction, cyanosis, dislodgment of ETT, and hypoventilation.
• Reassure parents that infant will be carefully monitored.

✱ NEW DRUG

ciclesonide
si-CLEH-son-ide

Alvesco

Pharmacologic class: corticosteroid
Pregnancy risk category C

AVAILABLE FORMS
Oral inhalation aerosol: 80 mcg, 160 mcg

INDICATIONS & DOSAGES
➤ **Preventative during asthma maintenance**
Adults and children age 12 and older who were previously taking broncho-dilators alone: Initially, inhaled dose of 80 mcg b.i.d. to maximum of 160 mcg b.i.d.
Adults and children age 12 and older who were previously taking inhaled cortico-steroids: Initially, 80 mcg b.i.d. to maximum of 320 mcg b.i.d.
Adults and children age 12 and older who were previously taking oral corticosteroids: 320 mcg b.i.d.

ACTION
May decrease inflammation by inhibiting macrophages, eosinophils, and mediators such as leukotrienes involved in the asthmatic response.

Route	Onset	Peak	Duration
Inhalation	Unknown	1 hour	Unknown

Half-life of drug and its active metabolite: Less than an hour and 6 to 7 hours, respectively.

ADVERSE REACTIONS
CNS: *headache,* back pain.
EENT: *nasopharyngitis,* sinusitis, pharyngolaryngeal pain, upper respiratory tract infection, nasal congestion.
Musculoskeletal: arthralgia, pain in the extremities.

INTERACTIONS
Drug-drug. *Ketoconazole, other inhibitors of cytochrome P450:* May increase ciclesonide level and adverse effects. Use together cautiously.
Drug-herb. None reported
Drug-food. None reported
Drug-lifestyle. None reported

EFFECTS ON LAB TEST RESULTS
None reported.

CONTRAINDICATIONS & CAUTIONS
● Contraindicated as primary treatment of status asthmaticus or other acute asthmatic episodes, and in patients hypersensitive to drug or its components.
   Use cautiously, if at all, in patients with active or quiescent respiratory tuberculo-sis infection; untreated systemic fungal, bacterial, viral, or parasitic infections; or ocular herpes simplex.

NURSING CONSIDERATIONS
● *Alert:* Don't use for acute bronchospasm.
● Assess patient for bone loss during long-term use.
● Watch for evidence of localized mouth infections, glaucoma, cataracts, and immunosuppression.
● Closely monitor children for growth suppression.
Pregnant patients
● Use drug only if benefits to mother justify risks to fetus. If a woman takes a corticosteroid during pregnancy, monitor neonate for hypoadrenalism.
Breast-feeding patients
● It's unknown if drug appears in breast milk; use cautiously in breast-feeding women.

Pediatric patients
● Safety and efficacy haven't been established in children younger than age 12.
Geriatric patients
● Use cautiously; elderly patients may be more sensitive to drug's effects.

PATIENT TEACHING
● Inform patient that drug isn't indicated for the relief of acute bronchospasm.
● Instruct patient to rinse his mouth with water and spit out after inhalation.
● Advise patient to use drug at regular intervals, as directed.
● Inform patient that therapeutic results may take several weeks.
● Warn patient to avoid exposure to chickenpox, measles, or other infections, and if exposed to consult prescriber immediately.
● Instruct patient to contact prescriber if symptoms don't improve after 4 weeks of treatment or if condition worsens.
● Advise parents of child receiving long-term therapy that child should have periodic growth measurements.

dextromethorphan hydrobromide
dex-troe-meth-OR-fan

Belminil DM † ◊ , Buckley's Cough Mixture, Creomulsion ◊ , Creo-Terpin* ◊ , Delsym ◊ , DexAlone ◊ , ElixSure Children's Cough, Hold DM ◊ , Koffex DM† ◊ , Robitussin ◊ , Robitussin Pediatric ◊ , Scot-Tussin ◊ , Simply Cough ◊ , Sucrets Cough ◊ , Theraflu Thin Strips* ◊ , Triaminic* ◊ , Trocal ◊ , Vicks Formula 44 ◊

Pharmacologic class: levorphanol derivative
Pregnancy risk category C

AVAILABLE FORMS
Gelcaps: 15 mg ◊ , 30 mg ◊
Liquid (extended-release): 30 mg/5 ml ◊
Lozenges: 5 mg ◊ , 7.5 mg ◊ , 10 mg ◊
Solution: 3.5 mg/5 ml, 5 mg/5 ml* ◊ , 7.5 mg/5 ml ◊ , 10 mg/5 ml* ◊ ,

12.5 mg/5ml ◊ , 15 mg/5 ml* ◊ ,
15 mg/15 ml* ◊
Strips (orally disintegrating): 7.5 mg* ◊ ,
15 mg* ◊

INDICATIONS & DOSAGES
➤ **Nonproductive cough**
Adults and children age 12 and older:
10 to 20 mg P.O. every 4 hours, or 30 mg
every 6 to 8 hours. Or, 60 mg extended-
release liquid b.i.d. Maximum, 120 mg
daily. Or, give lozenges, 5 to 15 mg,
every 1 to 4 hours, up to 120 mg/day.
Children ages 6 to 11: 5 to 10 mg P.O.
every 4 hours, or 15 mg every 6 to
8 hours. Or, 30 mg extended-release liquid
b.i.d. Maximum, 60 mg daily. Or, give
lozenges, 5 to 10 mg, every 1 to 4 hours,
up to 60 mg/day.
Children ages 2 to 5: 2.5 to 5 mg P.O. every
4 hours, or 7.5 mg every 6 to 8 hours. Or,
15 mg extended-release liquid b.i.d. Maximum, 30 mg daily.

ADMINISTRATION
P.O.
• Store at controlled room temperature
(59° to 86°F [15° to 30°C]).

ACTION
Suppresses the cough reflex by direct
action on the cough center in the medulla.

Route	Onset	Peak	Duration
P.O.	< 30 min	Unknown	3–6 hr

Half-life: About 11 hours.

ADVERSE REACTIONS
CNS: drowsiness, dizziness.
GI: nausea, vomiting, stomach pain.

INTERACTIONS
Drug-drug. *MAO inhibitors:* May
cause risk of hypotension, coma,
hyperpyrexia, and death. Avoid using
together.
Quinidine: May increase the risk of
dextromethorphan adverse effects.
Consider decreasing dextromethorphan
dose if needed.
Sibutramine: Serotonin syndrome may
occur. Avoid using together.
Drug-herb. *Parsley:* May promote or
produce serotonin syndrome. Discourage
use together.

EFFECTS ON LAB TEST RESULTS
None reported.

CONTRAINDICATIONS & CAUTIONS
• Contraindicated in patients currently
taking MAO inhibitors or within 2 weeks
of stopping MAO inhibitors.
• Use cautiously in atopic children, sedated
or debilitated patients, and patients
confined to the supine position.
• Use cautiously in patients sensitive to
aspirin or tartrazine dyes.
• *Alert:* Use of OTC cough products is not
recommended for neonates and children
under 2 years.

NURSING CONSIDERATIONS
• Don't use dextromethorphan when
cough is a valuable diagnostic sign or
is beneficial (such as after thoracic
surgery).
• Dextromethorphan 15 to 30 mg is
equivalent to codeine 8 to 15 mg as an
antitussive.
• Drug produces no analgesia or addiction
and little or no CNS depression.
• Use drug with chest percussion and
vibration.
• Monitor cough type and frequency.

PATIENT TEACHING
• Instruct patient to take drug exactly as
prescribed.
• Tell patient to report adverse reactions.
• Tell patient to contact his health care
provider if cough lasts longer than 1 week,
recurs frequently, or is accompanied by
high fever, rash, or severe headache.

---

flunisolide
floo-NISS-oh-lide

AeroBid, AeroBid-M, Nasarel,
Rhinalar†

flunisolide hemihydrate
AeroSpan HFA

Pharmacologic class: glucocorticoid
Pregnancy risk category C

AVAILABLE FORMS
flunisolide
Nasal solution: 25 mcg/metered spray

Oral inhalant: 250 mcg/metered spray
(at least 100 metered inhalations/container)
flunisolide hemihydrate
*Oral inhalant in a hydrofluoroalkane
(HFA) inhaler:* 80 mcg/metered dose

INDICATIONS & DOSAGES
➤ **Chronic asthma**
*Adults and adolescents older than
age 15:* 2 inhalations (500 mcg) with
chlorofluorocarbon (CFC) inhaler b.i.d.
Maximum, 8 inhalations (2,000 mcg)
daily.
Children ages 6 to 15: 2 inhalations
(500 mcg) with CFC inhaler b.i.d. Maximum, 1,000 mcg daily.
➤ **Chronic asthma**
Adults and children age 12 and older:
2 inhalations (160 mcg) with HFA
inhaler b.i.d. Don't exceed 320 mcg
twice daily.
Children ages 6 to 11: 1 inhalation
(80 mcg) with HFA inhaler b.i.d. Don't
exceed 160 mcg twice daily.
➤ **Seasonal or perennial rhinitis**
*Adults and adolescents older than
age 14:* 2 sprays (50 mcg) in each
nostril b.i.d. May be increased to
t.i.d., as needed. Maximum dose is
8 sprays in each nostril daily
(400 mcg).
Children ages 6 to 14: 1 spray
(25 mcg) in each nostril t.i.d. or
2 sprays (50 mcg) in each nostril b.i.d.
Maximum dose is 4 sprays in each
nostril daily (200 mcg).

ADMINISTRATION
Inhalational
• For best results, the canister should be
at room temperature before use.
• Allow 1 minute between doses.
Intranasal
• Before the first use, prime the
nasal spray by pushing down on the
pump 5 or 6 times until a fine mist
appears.

ACTION
A corticosteroid that may decrease
inflammation of asthma by inhibiting
macrophages, T-cells, eosinophils, and
mediators such as leukotrienes, while
reducing the number of mast cells within
the airway.

Route	Onset	Peak	Duration
Inhalation (nasal)	< 3 wk	Unknown	Unknown
Inhalation (oral)	1–4 wk	Unknown	Unknown

Half-life: 1.8 hours.

ADVERSE REACTIONS
CNS: *headache,* dizziness, fever,
irritability, nervousness.
CV: chest pain, edema, palpitations.
EENT: *nasal congestion, sore throat,*
altered taste, hoarseness, nasal burning or
stinging, nasal irritation, nasopharyngeal
fungal infections, throat irritation.
GI: *diarrhea, nausea, unpleasant taste,
upset stomach, vomiting,* abdominal pain,
decreased appetite, dry mouth.
Respiratory: *cold symptoms, upper
respiratory tract infection.*
Skin: pruritus, rash.
Other: *influenza.*

INTERACTIONS
None significant.

EFFECTS ON LAB TEST RESULTS
None reported.

CONTRAINDICATIONS & CAUTIONS
• Contraindicated in patients hypersensitive
to drug and in those with status asthmaticus
or respiratory tract infections.
• Drug isn't recommended in patients with
nonasthmatic bronchial diseases or with
asthma controlled by bronchodilator or
other noncorticosteroid alone.

NURSING CONSIDERATIONS
• All patients with asthma should
have routine tests of adrenal cortical
function, including measurement of
early morning resting cortisol levels
to establish a baseline in the event of
an emergency.
■ **Black Box Warning** There is an
increased risk of death due to adrenal
insufficiency in patients transferred from
systemically active corticosteriods to
flunisolide inhaler. Monitor patient
carefully ■
• *Alert:* Withdraw drug slowly in patients
who have received long-term oral corticosteroid therapy.

Reactions may be *common,* uncommon, *life-threatening,* or COMMON AND LIFE-THREATENING.
Interaction may have a *rapid onset* or **delayed onset.**

■ **Black Box Warning** After withdrawing systemic corticosteroids, patient may need supplemental systemic corticosteroids if stress (trauma, surgery, or infection) causes adrenal insufficiency. ■

● Store drug at room temperature.

● *Look alike–sound alike:* Don't confuse flunisolide with fluocinonide.

● Stop nasal spray after 3 weeks if symptoms don't improve.

PATIENT TEACHING
Oral inhalant

● Warn patient that drug doesn't relieve acute asthma attacks.

● *Alert:* Instruct patient to immediately contact prescriber if asthma episodes unresponsive to bronchodilators occur during treatment.

● Advise patient to ensure delivery of proper dose by gently warming the canister to room temperature before using. Some patients carry the canister in a pocket to keep it warm.

● Tell patient who also uses a broncho-dilator to use it several minutes before beginning flunisolide treatment.

● Instruct patient to begin inhaling immediately before activating the canister to get the full dose.

● Instruct patient to allow 1 minute to elapse before repeating inhalations and to hold his breath for a few seconds to enhance drug action.

● Teach patient to keep inhaler clean and unobstructed. If he's using a CFC inhaler, tell him to wash it with warm water and dry it thoroughly after use. The HFA inhaler doesn't need cleaning during normal use.

● Teach patient to check mucous membranes frequently for signs and symptoms of fungal infection.

● Advise patient to prevent oral fungal infections by gargling or rinsing mouth with water after each inhaler use. Caution him not to swallow the water.

● Warn patient to avoid exposure to chickenpox or measles. If exposed, contact prescriber immediately.

● Advise parents of a child receiving long-term therapy that the child should have periodic growth measurements and be checked for evidence of hypo-thalamic-pituitary-adrenal axis suppression.

Nasal spray

● Tell patient to prime the nasal inhaler (5 to 6 sprays) before first use and after long periods of no use.

● Advise patient to clear nasal passageways before use.

● Patient should follow manufacturer's instructions for use and cleaning. Tell him to discard open containers after 3 months.

● Advise patient that therapeutic results may take several weeks.

fluticasone furoate
FLOO-tih-ka-sone

Veramyst

fluticasone propionate
Flonase, Flovent Diskus†, Flovent HFA

Pharmacologic class: corticosteroid
Pregnancy risk category C

AVAILABLE FORMS
Nasal spray (furoate): 27.5 mcg/spray
Nasal spray (propionate): 50 mcg/metered spray
Oral inhalation aerosol: 44 mcg, 110 mcg, 220 mcg
Oral inhalation powder†: 50 mcg, 100 mcg, 250 mcg

INDICATIONS & DOSAGES
➤ **As preventative in maintenance of chronic asthma in patients requiring oral corticosteroid**
Flovent Diskus†
Adults and children age 12 and older: In patients previously taking bronchodilators alone, initially, inhaled dose of 100 mcg b.i.d. to maximum of 500 mcg b.i.d.
Adults and children age 12 and older previously taking inhaled corticosteroids: Initially, inhaled dose of 100 to 250 mcg b.i.d. to maximum of 500 mcg b.i.d.
Adults and children age 12 and older previously taking oral corticosteroids: Inhaled dose of 500 to 1,000 mcg b.i.d. Maximum dose, 1,000 mcg b.i.d.
Children ages 4 to 11: For patients previously on bronchodilators alone or on inhaled corticosteroids, initially, inhaled

dose of 50 mcg b.i.d. to maximum of
100 mcg b.i.d.

Flovent HFA

Adults and children age 12 and older:
In those previously taking bronchodilators
alone, initially, inhaled dose of 88 mcg
b.i.d. to maximum of 440 mcg b.i.d.

*Adults and children age 12 and older
previously taking inhaled corticosteroids:*
Initially, inhaled dose of 88 to 220 mcg
b.i.d. to maximum of 440 mcg b.i.d.

*Adults and children age 12 and older
previously taking oral corticosteroids:*
Initially, inhaled dose of 440 mcg b.i.d.
to maximum of 880 mcg b.i.d.

Children ages 4 to 11 years: 88 mcg
inhaled b.i.d. regardless of prior therapy.

➤ **Nasal symptoms of seasonal and
perennial allergic and nonallergic
rhinitis**

Flonase

Adults: Initially, 2 sprays (100 mcg) in
each nostril daily or 1 spray b.i.d. Once
symptoms are controlled, decrease to
1 spray in each nostril daily. Or, for
seasonal allergic rhinitis, 2 sprays in
each nostril once daily, as needed, for
symptom control.

Adolescents and children age 4 and older:
Initially, 1 spray (50 mcg) in each nostril
daily. If not responding, increase to
2 sprays in each nostril daily. Once symptoms are controlled, decrease to 1 spray
in each nostril daily. Maximum dose is
2 sprays in each nostril daily.

Veramyst

Adults and children age 12 and older:
110 mcg once daily administered as
2 sprays (27.5 mcg/spray) in each
nostril.

Children ages 2 to 11 years: 55 mcg
once daily administered as 1 spray
(27.5 mcg/spray) in each nostril.

ADMINISTRATION
Inhalational
● Prime and shake well before each use.
Intranasal
● Prime and shake well before use.

ACTION
Anti-inflammatory and vasoconstrictor
that may decrease inflammation by
inhibiting mast cells, macrophages, and
mediators such as leukotrienes.

Route	Onset	Peak	Duration
Inhalation (nasal)	12 hr	Several days	1–2 wk
Inhalation (oral)	24 hr	Several days	1–2 wk

Half-life: 3 hours.

ADVERSE REACTIONS
CNS: *headache,* dizziness, fever,
migraine, nervousness.
EENT: *pharyngitis,* blood in nasal mucus,
cataracts, conjunctivitis, dry eye, dysphonia, epistaxis, eye irritation, hoarseness,
laryngitis, nasal burning or irritation,
nasal discharge, rhinitis, sinusitis.
GI: *oral candidiasis,* abdominal discomfort, abdominal pain, diarrhea, mouth
irritation, nausea, viral gastroenteritis,
vomiting.
GU: UTI.
Hematologic: eosinophilia.
Metabolic: cushingoid features, growth
retardation in children, hyperglycemia,
weight gain.
Musculoskeletal: aches and pains,
disorder or symptoms of neck sprain or
strain, joint pain, muscular soreness,
osteoporosis.
Respiratory: *upper respiratory tract
infection,* **bronchospasm,** asthma
symptoms, bronchitis, chest congestion,
cough, dyspnea.
Skin: dermatitis, urticaria.
Other: *angioedema,* influenza, viral
infections.

INTERACTIONS
Drug-drug. *Ketoconazole and other
cytochrome P-450 3A4 inhibitors:* May
increase mean fluticasone level. Use
together cautiously.
Ritonavir: May cause systemic corticosteroid
effects, such as Cushing syndrome and adrenal suppression. Avoid using together.

EFFECTS ON LAB TEST RESULTS
● May cause an abnormal response
to the 6-hour cosyntropin stimulation
test in patients taking high doses of
fluticasone.

CONTRAINDICATIONS & CAUTIONS
● Contraindicated in patients hypersensitive
to ingredients in these preparations.

• Contraindicated as primary treatment of patients with status asthmaticus or other acute, intense episodes of asthma.

• Use cautiously in breast-feeding women.

NURSING CONSIDERATIONS

• Because of risk of systemic absorption of inhaled corticosteroids, observe patient carefully for evidence of systemic corticosteroid effects.

■ **Black Box Warning** Monitor patient, especially postoperatively, during periods of stress or severe asthma attack for evidence of inadequate adrenal response. ■

■ **Black Box Warning** During withdrawal from oral corticosteroids, some patients may experience signs and symptoms of systemically active corticosteroid withdrawal, such as joint or muscle pain, lassitude, and depression, despite maintenance or even improvement of respiratory function. Deaths due to adrenal insufficiency have occurred with transfer from active corticosteroids to fluticasone propionate inhaler. ■

• For patients starting therapy who are currently receiving oral corticosteroid therapy, reduce dose of prednisone to no more than 2.5 mg/day on a weekly basis, beginning after at least 1 week of therapy with fluticasone.

• *Alert:* As with other inhaled asthma drugs, bronchospasm may occur with an immediate increase in wheezing after a dose. If bronchospasm occurs after a dose of inhalation aerosol, treat immediately with a fast-acting inhaled bronchodilator.

PATIENT TEACHING

• Tell patient that drug isn't indicated for the relief of acute bronchospasm.

• For proper use of drug and to attain maximal improvement, tell patient to carefully follow the accompanying patient instructions.

• Advise patient to use drug at regular intervals, as directed.

• Instruct patient to contact prescriber if nasal spray doesn't improve condition after 4 days of treatment.

• Instruct patient to immediately contact prescriber if asthma episodes unresponsive

to bronchodilators occur during treatment with fluticasone. During such episodes, patient may need therapy with oral corticosteroids.

• Warn patient to avoid exposure to chickenpox or measles and, if exposed, to consult prescriber immediately.

• Tell patient to carry or wear medical identification indicating that he may need supplementary corticosteroids during stress or a severe asthma attack.

■ **Black Box Warning** During periods of stress or a severe asthma attack, instruct patient who has been withdrawn from systemic corticosteroids to resume prescribed oral corticosteroids immediately and to contact prescriber for further instruction. ■

• Tell patient to prime inhaler with 4 test sprays (away from his face) before first use, shaking well before each spray. Also, prime with 1 spray if inhaler has been dropped or not used for 1 week or longer.

• Advise patient to avoid spraying inhalation aerosol into eyes.

• Instruct patient to shake canister well before using inhalation aerosol.

• Instruct patient to rinse his mouth and spit water out after inhalation.

• Advise patient to store fluticasone powder in a dry place.

Flonase nasal spray

• Tell patient to prime the nasal inhaler before first use or after 1 week or longer of nonuse.

• Have patient clear nasal passages before use.

• Advise patient to follow manufacturer's recommendations for use and cleaning.

• Advise patient to use at regular intervals for full benefit.

• Tell patient to contact provider if signs or symptoms don't improve within 4 days or if signs or symptoms worsen.

• Tell patient that the correct amount of spray can't be guaranteed after 120 sprays, even though the bottle may not be completely empty.

fluticasone propionate and salmeterol inhalation powder
FLOO-tih-ka-sone and sal-MEE-ter-ol

Advair Diskus 100/50, Advair Diskus 250/50, Advair Diskus 500/50, Advair HFA 45/21, Advair HFA 115/21, Advair HFA 230/21

Pharmacologic class: corticosteroid, long-acting beta₂-adrenergic agonist
Pregnancy risk category C

AVAILABLE FORMS
Inhalation powder: 100 mcg fluticasone and 50 mcg salmeterol, 250 mcg fluticasone and 50 mcg salmeterol, 500 mcg fluticasone and 50 mcg salmeterol
Aerosol spray: 45 mcg fluticasone propionate and 21 mcg salmeterol, 115 mcg fluticasone propionate and 21 mcg salmeterol, 230 mcg fluticasone propionate and 21 mcg salmeterol

INDICATIONS & DOSAGES
➤ **Long-term maintenance of asthma**
Adults and children age 12 and older:
1 inhalation b.i.d., at least 12 hours apart of Advair Diskus; or 2 inhalations twice daily of Advair HFA. Starting doses are dependent on the patient's current asthma therapy.
Adults and children age 12 and older not currently taking an inhaled corticosteroid:
1 inhalation of fluticasone 100 mcg/salmeterol 50 mcg Diskus or fluticasone 250 mcg/salmeterol 50 mcg Diskus twice daily; or 2 inhalations of fluticasone 45 mcg/salmeterol 21 mcg HFA or fluticasone 115 mcg/salmeterol 21 mcg HFA twice daily.
Adults and children age 12 and older currently on and not adequately controlled by an inhaled corticosteroid: Consult the table above.
For patients already using an inhaled corticosteroid: Maximum inhalation of Advair Diskus is 500/50 b.i.d. and maximum dose of Advair HFA is 2 inhalations of fluticasone 230 mcg/salmeterol 21 mcg b.i.d.

➤ **Asthma in children who remain symptomatic while taking an inhaled corticosteroid**
Children ages 4 to 11: 1 inhalation (100 mg fluticasone and 50 mg salmeterol) b.i.d., morning and evening, about 12 hours apart.
➤ **Maintenance therapy for airflow obstruction in patients with COPD from chronic bronchitis; to reduce exacerbations of COPD in patients with a history of exacerbations**
Adults: 1 inhalation of Advair Diskus 250/50 only, b.i.d., about 12 hours apart.

ADMINISTRATION
Inhalational
• Prime Advair HFA before first use.
• After administration, have the patient rinse his mouth without swallowing.

ACTION
Fluticasone is a synthetic corticosteroid with potent anti-inflammatory activity.
　Salmeterol xinafoate, a long-acting beta agonist, relaxes bronchial smooth muscle and inhibits release of mediators.

Route	Onset	Peak	Duration
Inhalation (fluticasone)	Unknown	1–2 hr	Unknown
Inhalation (salmeterol)	Unknown	5 min	Unknown

Half-life: Fluticasone: 8 hours; salmeterol: 5½ hours.

ADVERSE REACTIONS
CNS: *headache,* compressed nerve syndromes, hypnagogic effects, sleep disorders, tremors, pain.
CV: palpitations.
EENT: *pharyngitis,* blood in nasal mucosa, congestion, conjunctivitis, dental discomfort and pain, eye redness, hoarseness or dysphonia, keratitis, nasal irritation, rhinorrhea, rhinitis, sinusitis, sneezing, viral eye infections.
GI: abdominal pain and discomfort, appendicitis, constipation, diarrhea, gastroenteritis, nausea, oral candidiasis, oral discomfort and pain, oral erythema and rashes, oral ulcerations, unusual taste, vomiting.
Musculoskeletal: arthralgia, articular rheumatism, bone and cartilage disorders,

---

Reactions may be *common,* uncommon, *life-threatening,* or COMMON AND LIFE-THREATENING.
Interaction may have a *rapid onset* or **delayed onset.**

Name of current corticosteroid	Dose of current corticosteroid	Recommended strength of Advair Diskus (1 inhalation b.i.d.)	Recommended strength of Advair HFA (2 inhalations b.i.d.)
Beclomethasone	≤ 160 mcg	100 mcg/50 mcg	45 mcg/21 mcg
dipropionate HFA	320 mcg	250 mcg/50 mcg	115 mcg/21 mcg
inhalation aerosol	640 mcg	500 mcg/50 mcg	230 mcg/21 mcg
Budesonide inhalation	≤ 400 mcg	100 mcg/50 mcg	45 mcg/21 mcg
aerosol/powder	800 to 1,200 mcg	250 mcg/50 mcg	115 mcg/21 mcg
	1,600 mcg	500 mcg/50 mcg	230 mcg/21 mcg
Flunisolide CFC	≤ 1,000 mcg	100 mcg/50 mcg	45 mcg/21 mcg
inhalation aerosol	1,250 to 2,000 mcg	250 mcg/50 mcg	115 mcg/21 mcg
Flunisolide HFA	≤ 320 mcg	100 mcg/50 mcg	45 mcg/21 mcg
inhalation aerosol	640 mcg	250 mcg/50 mcg	115 mcg/21 mcg
Fluticasone propionate	≤ 176 mcg	100 mcg/50 mcg	45 mcg/21 mcg
HFA inhalation aerosol	440 mcg	250 mcg/50 mcg	115 mcg/21 mcg
	660 to 880 mcg	500 mcg/50 mcg	230 mcg/21 mcg
Fluticasone propionate	≤ 200 mcg	100 mcg/50 mcg	45 mcg/21 mcg
inhalation powder	500 mcg	250 mcg/50 mcg	115 mcg/21 mcg
	1,000 mcg	500 mcg/50 mcg	230 mcg/21 mcg
Mometasone furoate	220 mcg	100 mcg/50 mcg	45 mcg/21 mcg
inhalation powder	440 mcg	250 mcg/50 mcg	115 mcg/21 mcg
	880 mcg	500 mcg/50 mcg	230 mcg/21 mcg
Triamcinolone acetonide	≤ 1,000 mcg	100 mcg/50 mcg	45 mcg/21 mcg
inhalation aerosol	1,100 to 1,600 mcg	250 mcg/50 mcg	115 mcg/21 mcg

muscle pain, muscle stiffness, rigidity, tightness.

Respiratory: *upper respiratory tract infection,* bronchitis, cough, lower respiratory tract infections, pneumonia.

Skin: disorders of sweat and sebum, infection, skin flakiness, sweating, urticaria.

Other: allergic reactions, chest symptoms, fluid retention, viral or bacterial infections.

INTERACTIONS

Drug-drug. *Beta blockers:* Blocked pulmonary effect of salmeterol may produce severe bronchospasm in patients with asthma. Avoid using together. If necessary, use a cardioselective beta blocker cautiously.

Ketoconazole, other inhibitors of cytochrome P-450: May increase fluticasone level and adverse effects. Use together cautiously.

Loop diuretics, thiazide diuretics: Potassium-wasting diuretics may cause or worsen ECG changes or hypokalemia. Use together cautiously.

MAO inhibitors, tricyclic antidepressants: May potentiate the action of salmeterol on the vascular system. Separate doses by 2 weeks.

EFFECTS ON LAB TEST RESULTS
• May increase liver enzyme levels.

CONTRAINDICATIONS & CAUTIONS
• Contraindicated in patients hypersensitive to drug or its components.

■ **Black Box Warning** When treating asthma use only for patients not adequately controlled on other asthma-controller medications. ■

• Contraindicated as primary treatment of status asthmaticus or other acute asthmatic episodes.

• Use cautiously, if at all, in patients with active or quiescent respiratory tuberculosis infection; untreated systemic fungal, bacterial, viral, or parasitic infection; or ocular herpes simplex.

• Use cautiously in patients with CV disorders, seizure disorders or thyrotoxicosis; in patients unusually responsive to sympathomimetic amines; and in patients with hepatic impairment.

NURSING CONSIDERATIONS

• *Alert:* Patient shouldn't be switched from systemic corticosteroids to Advair Diskus or Advair HFA because of hypothalamic-pituitary-adrenal axis suppression. Death from adrenal insufficiency can occur. Several months are required for recovery of hypothalamic-pituitary-adrenal function after withdrawal of systemic corticosteroids.

• Don't start therapy during rapidly deteriorating or potentially life-threatening episodes of asthma. Serious acute respiratory events, including fatality, can occur.

• The benefit of Advair 250/50 in treating patients with COPD for more than 6 months is unknown. If drug is used for longer than 6 months, periodically reevaluate patient to assess for benefits or risks of therapy.

• Monitor patient for urticaria, angioedema, rash, bronchospasm, or other signs of hypersensitivity.

• Don't use this drug to stop an asthma attack. Patients should carry an inhaled, short-acting beta₂ agonist (such as albuterol) for acute symptoms.

• If drug causes paradoxical bronchospasm, treat immediately with a short-acting inhaled bronchodilator (such as albuterol), and notify prescriber.

■ **Black Box Warning** Rare, serious asthma episodes or asthma-related deaths have occurred in patients taking salmeterol; black patients may be at a greater risk. ■

• Monitor patient for increased use of inhaled short-acting beta₂ agonist. The dose of Advair may need to be increased.

• Closely monitor children for growth suppression.

PATIENT TEACHING

• Instruct patient on proper use of the prescribed inhaler to provide effective treatment.

• Tell patient to avoid exhaling into the dry-powder multidose inhaler, to activate and use the dry-powder multidose inhaler in a level, horizontal position and not to use Advair Diskus with a spacer device.

• Instruct patient to keep the dry-powder multidose inhaler in a dry place, away from direct heat or sunlight, and to avoid washing the mouthpiece or other parts of the device. Patient should discard device 1 month after removal from the moisture-protective overwrap pouch or after every blister has been used, whichever comes first. He shouldn't attempt to take device apart.

• Instruct patient to rinse mouth after inhalation to prevent oral candidiasis.

• Inform patient that improvement may occur within 30 minutes after dose, but the full benefit may not occur for 1 week or more.

• Advise patient not to exceed recommended prescribing dose.

• Instruct patient not to relieve acute symptoms with Advair. Treat acute symptoms with an inhaled short-acting beta₂ agonist.

• Instruct patient to report decreasing effects or use of increasing doses of their short-acting inhaled beta₂ agonist.

• Tell patient to report palpitations, chest pain, rapid heart rate, tremor, or nervousness.

• Instruct patient to call immediately if exposed to chickenpox or measles.

---

guaifenesin
(glyceryl guaiacolate)
gwye-FEN-e-sin

Allfen Jr, Altarussin ◊ , Balminil† ◊ , Benylin E† ◊ , Diabetic Tussin ◊ , Ganidin NR, Guiatuss ◊ , Humibid ◊ , Liquibid, Mucinex ◊ , Mucinex Mini-Melts ◊ , Naldecon Senior EX ◊ , Organidin NR, Robitussin ◊ , Scot-Tussin Expectorant ◊ , Siltussin ◊

Pharmacologic class: propanediol derivative
Pregnancy risk category C

AVAILABLE FORMS

Capsules: 200 mg ◊
Granules: 50 mg ◊ , 100 mg ◊
Liquid: 100 mg/5 ml* ◊ , 200 mg/5 ml ◊
Syrup: 100 mg/5 ml ◊
Tablets: 100 mg ◊ , 200 mg ◊ , 400 mg
Tablets (extended-release): 600 mg ◊ , 1,200 mg ◊

Reactions may be *common*, uncommon, *life-threatening*, or COMMON AND LIFE-THREATENING.
Interaction may have a *rapid onset* or **delayed onset**.

INDICATIONS & DOSAGES
➤ **Expectorant**
Adults and children age 12 and older:
200 to 400 mg P.O. every 4 hours, or
600 to 1,200 mg extended-release
capsules or tablets every 12 hours.
Maximum, 2,400 mg daily.
Children ages 6 to 11: 100 to 200 mg P.O.
every 4 hours. Maximum, 1,200 mg daily.
Children ages 2 to 5: 50 to 100 mg P.O.
every 4 hours. Maximum, 600 mg daily.

ADMINISTRATION
P.O.
• Don't break or crush extended-release
products.
• Empty entire contents of granule packet
on the patient's tongue. Tell patient to
swallow without chewing for best taste.

ACTION
Increases production of respiratory tract
fluids to help liquefy and reduce the
viscosity of tenacious secretions.

Route	Onset	Peak	Duration
P.O.	Unknown	Unknown	Unknown

Half-life: Unknown.

ADVERSE REACTIONS
CNS: dizziness, headache.
GI: vomiting, nausea.
Skin: rash.

INTERACTIONS
None significant.

EFFECTS ON LAB TEST RESULTS
• May interfere with uric acid level determination and with 5-hydroxyindoleacetic
acid and vanillylmandelic tests.

CONTRAINDICATIONS & CAUTIONS
• Contraindicated in patients hypersensitive
to drug.

NURSING CONSIDERATIONS
• Some liquid formulations contain
alcohol.
• Drug is used to liquefy thick, tenacious
sputum. Evidence suggests that guaifenesin is effective as an expectorant, but no
evidence exists to support its role as an
antitussive.
• Monitor cough type and frequency.

• Stop use 48 hours before 5-hydroxy-
indoleacetic acid and vanillylmandelic tests.
• ***Look alike–sound alike:*** Don't confuse
guaifenesin with guanfacine.

PATIENT TEACHING
• Tell patient to contact his health care
provider if cough lasts longer than 1 week,
recurs frequently, or is accompanied by
high fever, rash, or severe headache.
• Inform patient that drug shouldn't be
used for chronic or persistent cough, such
as with smoking, asthma, chronic bronchitis, or emphysema.
• Advise patient to take each dose with
one glass of water; increasing fluid intake
may prove beneficial.
• Tell patient to empty entire contents of
granule packet onto the tongue and to
swallow without chewing for best taste.
• Encourage deep-breathing exercises.

---

mometasone furoate
moe-MEH-tah-zone

Asmanex Twisthaler

Pharmacologic class: glucocorticoid
Pregnancy risk category C

AVAILABLE FORMS
Inhalation powder: 110 mcg/inhalation,
220 mcg/inhalation

INDICATIONS & DOSAGES
➤ **Maintenance therapy for asthma;
asthma in patients who take an oral
corticosteroid**
*Adults and children age 12 and older
who previously used a bronchodilator or
inhaled corticosteroid:* Initially, 220 mcg
by oral inhalation every day in the
evening. Maximum, 440 mcg/day.
*Adults and children age 12 and older
who take an oral corticosteroid:* 440 mcg
b.i.d. by oral inhalation. Maximum,
880 mcg/day. Reduce oral corticosteroid
dosage by no more than 2.5 mg/day at
weekly intervals, beginning at least 1 week
after starting mometasone. After stopping
oral corticosteroid, reduce mometasone
dose to lowest effective amount.
Children 4 to 11 years: 110 mcg by oral
inhalation once daily in the evening.

ADMINISTRATION
Inhalational
• Have patient breathe deeply and rapidly during administration.
• Have patient rinse his mouth after administration.

ACTION
Unknown, although corticosteroids inhibit many cells and mediators involved in inflammation and the asthmatic response.

Route	Onset	Peak	Duration
Inhalation	Unknown	1–2½ hr	Unknown

Half-life: 5 hours.

ADVERSE REACTIONS
CNS: *headache,* depression, fatigue, insomnia, pain.
EENT: *allergic rhinitis, pharyngitis,* dry throat, dysphonia, earache, epistaxis, nasal irritation, sinus congestion, sinusitis.
GI: abdominal pain, anorexia, dyspepsia, flatulence, gastroenteritis, nausea, oral candidiasis, vomiting.
GU: dysmenorrhea, menstrual disorder, UTI.
Musculoskeletal: arthralgia, back pain, myalgia.
Respiratory: *upper respiratory tract infection,* respiratory disorder.
Other: accidental injury, flulike symptoms, infection.

INTERACTIONS
Drug-drug. *Ketoconazole:* May increase mometasone level. Use together cautiously.

EFFECTS ON LAB TEST RESULTS
None reported.

CONTRAINDICATIONS & CAUTIONS
• Contraindicated in patients hypersensitive to drug or its ingredients and in those with status asthmaticus or other acute forms of asthma or bronchospasm (as primary treatment).
• Use cautiously in patients at high risk for decreased bone mineral content (those with a family history of osteoporosis, prolonged immobilization, long-term use of drugs that reduce bone mass), patients switching from a systemic to an inhaled corticosteroid, and patients with active or dormant tuberculosis, untreated systemic infections, ocular herpes simplex, or immunosuppression.
• Use cautiously in breast-feeding women.

NURSING CONSIDERATIONS
• **Alert:** Don't use for acute bronchospasm.
• Wean patient slowly from a systemic corticosteroid after he switches to mometasone. Monitor lung function tests, beta-agonist use, and asthma symptoms.
• **Alert:** If patient is switching from an oral corticosteroid to an inhaled form, watch closely for evidence of adrenal insufficiency, such as fatigue, lethargy, weakness, nausea, vomiting, and hypotension.
• After an oral corticosteroid is withdrawn, hypothalamic-pituitary-adrenal (HPA) function may not recover for months. If patient has trauma, stress, infection, or surgery during this HPA recovery period, he is particularly vulnerable to adrenal insufficiency or adrenal crisis.
• Because an inhaled corticosteroid can be systemically absorbed, watch for cushingoid effects.
• Assess patient for bone loss during long-term use.
• Watch for evidence of localized mouth infections, glaucoma, and immunosuppression.
• Use drug only if benefits to mother justify risks to fetus. If a woman takes a corticosteroid during pregnancy, monitor neonate for hypoadrenalism.
• Monitor elderly patients for increased sensitivity to drug effects.

PATIENT TEACHING
• Instruct patient on proper use and routine care of the inhaler.
• Tell patient to use drug regularly and at the same time each day. If he uses it only once daily, tell him to do so in the evening.
• Caution patient not to use drug for immediate relief of an asthma attack or bronchospasm.
• Inform patient that maximal benefits might not occur for 1 to 2 weeks or longer after therapy starts; instruct him to notify his prescriber if his condition fails to improve or worsens.
• Tell patient that if he has bronchospasm after taking drug, he should immediately

---

Reactions may be *common,* uncommon, *life-threatening,* or COMMON AND LIFE-THREATENING.
Interaction may have a *rapid onset* or **delayed onset.**

use a fast-acting bronchodilator. Urge him to contact prescriber immediately if bronchospasm doesn't respond to the fast-acting bronchodilator.

• **Alert:** If patient has been weaned from an oral corticosteroid, urge him to contact prescriber immediately if an asthma attack occurs or if he is experiencing a period of stress. The oral corticosteroid may need to be resumed.

• Warn patient to avoid exposure to chickenpox or measles and to notify prescriber if such contact occurs.

• Long-term use of an inhaled corticosteroid may increase the risk of cataracts or glaucoma; tell patient to report vision changes.

• Advise patient to write the date on a new inhaler on the day he opens it and to discard the inhaler after 45 days or when the dose counter reads "00."

---

montelukast sodium
mon-tell-OO-kast

Singulair⌀

Pharmacologic class:
leukotriene-receptor antagonist
Pregnancy risk category B

AVAILABLE FORMS
Oral granules: 4-mg packet
Tablets (chewable): 4 mg, 5 mg
Tablets (film-coated): 10 mg

INDICATIONS & DOSAGES
➤ **Asthma, seasonal allergic rhinitis, perennial allergic rhinitis**
Adults and children age 15 and older:
10 mg P.O. once daily in evening.
Children ages 6 to 14: 5 mg chewable tablet P.O. once daily in evening.
Children ages 2 to 5: 4 mg chewable tablet or 1 packet of 4-mg oral granules P.O. once daily in the evening.
Children ages 12 to 23 months (asthma only): 1 packet of 4-mg oral granules P.O. once daily in the evening.
Children ages 6 to 23 months (perennial allergic rhinitis only): 1 packet of 4-mg oral granules P.O. once daily in the evening.

➤ **Prevention of exercise-induced bronchospasm**
Adults and children age 15 and older:
10 mg P.O. at least 2 hours before exercise. Patients already taking a daily dose shouldn't take an additional dose. Also, an additional dose shouldn't be taken within 24 hours of a previous dose.

ADMINISTRATION
P.O.
• Give oral granules directly in the mouth, dissolved in 5 ml of cold or room temperature baby formula or breast milk, or mixed with a spoonful of cold or room temperature soft foods (use only applesauce, carrots, rice, or ice cream).
• Give oral granules without regard for food.

ACTION
Reduces early and late-phase bronchoconstriction from antigen challenge.

Route	Onset	Peak	Duration
P.O. (chewable, granules)	Unknown	2–2½ hr	24 hr
P.O. (film-coated)	Unknown	3–4 hr	24 hr

Half-life: 2¾ to 5½ hours.

ADVERSE REACTIONS
CNS: *headache,* asthenia, dizziness, fatigue, fever.
EENT: dental pain, nasal congestion.
GI: abdominal pain, dyspepsia, infectious gastroenteritis.
GU: pyuria.
Hematologic: systemic eosinophilia.
Respiratory: cough.
Skin: rash.
Other: influenza, trauma.

INTERACTIONS
Drug-drug. *Phenobarbital, rifampin:* May decrease bioavailability of montelukast because of hepatic metabolism induction. Monitor patient for effectiveness.

EFFECTS ON LAB TEST RESULTS
• May increase ALT and AST levels.

CONTRAINDICATIONS & CAUTIONS
• Contraindicated in patients hypersensitive to drug or its ingredients.

• Use cautiously and with appropriate monitoring in patients whose dosages of systemic corticosteroids are reduced.

NURSING CONSIDERATIONS
• Assess patient's underlying condition, and monitor him for effectiveness.
• *Alert:* Don't abruptly substitute drug for inhaled or oral corticosteroids. Dose of inhaled corticosteroids may be reduced gradually.
• Drug isn't indicated for use in patients with acute asthmatic attacks, status asthmaticus, or as monotherapy for management of exercise-induced bronchospasm. Continue appropriate rescue drug for acute worsening.

PATIENT TEACHING
• Inform caregiver that the oral granules may be given directly into the child's mouth, dissolved in 1 teaspoon of cold or room-temperature baby formula or breast milk, or mixed in a spoonful of applesauce, carrots, rice, or ice cream.
• Tell caregiver not to open packet until ready to use and, after opening, to give the full dose within 15 minutes. Tell her that if she's mixing the drug with food, not to store excess for future use and to discard the unused portion.
• Advise patient to take drug daily, even if asymptomatic, and to contact his prescriber if asthma isn't well controlled.
• Warn patient not to reduce or stop taking other prescribed antiasthmatics without prescriber's approval.
• Advise patient to seek medical attention if short-acting inhaled bronchodilators are needed more often than usual during drug therapy.
• Warn patient that drug isn't beneficial in acute asthma attacks or in exercise-induced bronchospasm, and advise him to keep appropriate rescue drugs available.
• Advise patient with known aspirin sensitivity to continue to avoid using aspirin and NSAIDs during drug therapy.
• Advise patient with phenylketonuria that chewable tablet contains phenylalanine.

omalizumab
oh-mah-LIZ-uh-mab

Xolair

Pharmacologic class: DNA-derived humanized immunoglobulin monoclonal antibody
Pregnancy risk category B

AVAILABLE FORMS
Powder for injection: 150 mg in 5-ml vial

INDICATIONS & DOSAGES
➤ **Moderate to severe persistent asthma in patients with positive skin test or in vitro reactivity to a perennial aeroallergen and whose symptoms aren't adequately controlled by inhaled corticosteroids**
Adults and adolescents age 12 and older: 150 to 375 mg subcutaneously every 2 or 4 weeks. Dose and frequency vary with pretreatment immunoglobulin E (IgE) level (international units/ml) and patient weight. Divide doses larger than 150 mg among more than one injection site.

ADMINISTRATION
Subcutaneous
• Reconstitute with sterile water for injection only. Swirl gently, don't shake. Use 18 g needle to draw medication into syringe, then replace with a 25 g needle for administration.
• The lyophilized product takes 15 to 20 minutes to dissolve.
• The fully reconstituted product will appear clear or slightly opalescent and may have a few small bubbles or foam around the edge of the vial.
• Because the solution is slightly viscous, it may take 5 to 10 seconds to give.
• Use reconstituted solution within 4 hours if at room temperature or within 8 hours if refrigerated.

ACTION
Inhibits binding of IgE to high-affinity receptor, on surface of mast cells and basophils, which limits release of allergic response mediators.

Reactions may be *common*, uncommon, *life-threatening*, or COMMON AND LIFE-THREATENING.
Interaction may have a *rapid onset* or *delayed onset*.

Route	Onset	Peak	Duration
Subcut.	Unknown	7–8 days	Unknown

Half-life: About 26 days.

ADVERSE REACTIONS
CNS: *headache,* dizziness, fatigue, pain.
EENT: *pharyngitis, sinusitis,* earache.
Musculoskeletal: arm pain, arthralgia, fracture, leg pain.
Respiratory: *upper respiratory tract infection.*
Skin: *injection site reaction,* dermatitis, pruritus.
Other: *viral infections.*

INTERACTIONS
None reported.

EFFECTS ON LAB TEST RESULTS
• May increase IgE level.

CONTRAINDICATIONS & CAUTIONS
• Contraindicated in patients severely hypersensitive to drug.
• Safety and effectiveness haven't been established in children younger than age 12.
• Drug should be given only in a health care setting under direct medical supervision because of the risk of anaphylaxis.

NURSING CONSIDERATIONS
• **Alert:** Don't use this drug to treat acute bronchospasm or status asthmaticus.
• Don't abruptly stop systemic or inhaled corticosteroid when omalizumab therapy starts; taper the dose gradually and under supervision.
• Injection site reactions may occur, such as bruising, redness, warmth, burning, stinging, itching, hives, pain, induration, and inflammation. Most occur within 1 hour after the injection, last fewer than 8 days, and decrease in frequency with subsequent injections.
■ **Black Box Warning** Observe patient for at least 2 hours after the injection, and keep drugs available to respond to anaphylactic reactions. These reactions usually occur within 2 hours of subcutaneous injection; however, delayed reactions may occur up to 24 hours after administration. If the patient has a severe hypersensitivity reaction, stop treatment. ■

• Drug increases IgE level, so it can't be used to determine appropriate dosage during therapy or for 1 year after therapy ends.
• Patient medication guide must be given with each dose.

PATIENT TEACHING
• Tell patients not to stop or reduce the dosage of any other asthma drugs unless directed by the prescriber. Patient medication guide must be given with each dose.
• Explain that patient may not notice an immediate improvement in asthma after therapy starts.

---

triamcinolone acetonide
trye-am-SIN-oh-lone

Azmacort, Nasacort AQ

Pharmacologic class: glucocorticoid
Pregnancy risk category C

AVAILABLE FORMS
Inhalation aerosol: 100 mcg/metered spray
Nasal spray: 55 mcg/metered spray, 50 mcg/metered spray

INDICATIONS & DOSAGES
➤ **Persistent asthma**
Adults and children older than age 12:
2 inhalations t.i.d. to q.i.d. Maximum, 16 inhalations daily. In some patients, maintenance can be achieved when total daily dose is given b.i.d.
Children ages 6 to 12: 1 to 2 inhalations t.i.d. to q.i.d. Maximum, 12 inhalations daily.
➤ **Nasal treatment of symptoms of seasonal and perennial allergic rhinitis**
Adults and children older than age 12:
2 sprays Nasacort AQ in each nostril daily; may decrease to 1 spray per nostril daily. Adjust to minimum effective dosage.
Children ages 6 to 12: Initially, give 1 spray Nasacort AQ in each nostril daily. If no response occurs, increase to 2 sprays in each nostril daily. Adjust to minimum effective dosage.

ADMINISTRATION
Inhalational
• Shake well before using.
• Have patient rinse mouth after use.
Intranasal
• Have patient clear nasal passages before use.

ACTION
May decrease inflammation through inhibitory activities against cell types such as mast cells and macrophages and against mediators such as leukotrienes.

Route	Onset	Peak	Duration
Inhalation (nasal)	12–24 hr	Several days	1–2 wk
Inhalation (oral)	1–4 wk	Unknown	Unknown

Half-life: 18 to 36 hours; 5.4 hours (HFA).

ADVERSE REACTIONS
CNS: *headache.*
EENT: *pharyngitis, sneezing,* dry or irritated nose or throat, hoarseness, rhinitis.
GI: dry or irritated tongue or mouth, oral candidiasis.
Respiratory: cough, wheezing.
Other: facial edema, *adrenal insufficiency,* hypothalamic-pituitary-adrenal function suppression.

INTERACTIONS
None significant.

EFFECTS ON LAB TEST RESULTS
None reported.

CONTRAINDICATIONS & CAUTIONS
• Contraindicated in patients hypersensitive to drug or its ingredients and in those with status asthmaticus.
• Use with extreme caution, if at all, in patients with tuberculosis of the respiratory tract, ocular herpes simplex, or untreated fungal, bacterial, or systemic viral infections.
• Because of risk of severe adverse effects, don't use in breast-feeding women. It's unknown if drug appears in breast milk.

NURSING CONSIDERATIONS
• Unlike other corticosteroids, drug has a spacer built into the drug-delivery device.

• Use cautiously in patients receiving systemic corticosteroids.
• Most adverse reactions to corticosteroids are dose- or duration-dependent.
• Patients who have recently been switched from systemic corticosteroids to oral inhaled corticosteroids may need to resume systemic corticosteroid therapy during periods of stress or severe asthma attacks.
• Taper oral therapy slowly.
• Store drug between 59° and 86° F (15° and 30° C).
• For nasal spray, if symptoms don't improve after 2 to 3 weeks, reevaluate the patient.
• *Look alike–sound alike:* Don't confuse triamcinolone with Triaminicin.

PATIENT TEACHING
Inhalation aerosol
• Inform patient that inhaled cortico-steroids don't relieve emergency asthma attacks.
• Advise patient to warm canister to room temperature before using. Some patients carry canister in a pocket to keep it warm.
• If patient needs a bronchodilator, tell him to use it several minutes before triamcinolone. Tell patient to allow 1 minute to elapse before repeat inhalations and to hold his breath for a few seconds to enhance drug action.
• Teach patient to check mucous membranes frequently for evidence of fungal infection. Advise patient to avoid exposure to chickenpox or measles and to contact provider if exposure occurs.
• Tell patient to prevent oral fungal infections by gargling or rinsing mouth with water after each use of the inhaler. Remind him not to swallow the water.
• Tell patient to keep inhaler clean and unobstructed and to wash it with warm water and dry it thoroughly after use.
• Instruct patient to contact prescriber if response to therapy decreases; dosage may need adjustment. Tell him not to exceed recommended dosage on his own.
• Instruct patient to wear or carry medical identification indicating his need for supplemental systemic glucocorticoids during periods of stress.

Reactions may be *common,* uncommon, *life-threatening,* or COMMON AND LIFE-THREATENING.
Interaction may have a *rapid onset* or *delayed onset.*

Nasal spray
● Advise patient to use at regular intervals for full therapeutic effect.
● Advise patient to clear nasal passages before use.
● Have patient follow manufacturer's recommendations for use and cleaning.

zafirlukast
zah-FUR-luh-kast

Accolate

Pharmacologic class:
leukotriene-receptor antagonist
Pregnancy risk category B

AVAILABLE FORMS
Tablets: 10 mg, 20 mg

INDICATIONS & DOSAGES
➤ **Prevention and long-term treatment of asthma**
Adults and children age 12 and older: 20 mg P.O. b.i.d.
Children ages 5 to 11: 10 mg P.O. b.i.d.

ADMINISTRATION
P.O.
● Give drug 1 hour before or 2 hours after meals.

ACTION
Selectively competes for leukotriene-receptor sites, blocking inflammatory action.

Route	Onset	Peak	Duration
P.O.	Rapid	3 hr	Unknown

Half-life: 10 hours.

ADVERSE REACTIONS
CNS: *headache,* asthenia, dizziness, pain, fever.
GI: abdominal pain, diarrhea, dyspepsia, gastritis, nausea, vomiting.
Musculoskeletal: back pain, myalgia.
Other: accidental injury, infection.

INTERACTIONS
Drug-drug. *Aspirin:* May increase zafirlukast level. Monitor patient for adverse effects.

Erythromycin, theophylline: May decrease zafirlukast level. Monitor patient for decreased effectiveness.
Warfarin: May increase PT. Monitor PT and INR, and adjust anticoagulant dosage.
Drug-food. *Food:* May reduce rate and extent of drug absorption. Advise patient to take drug 1 hour before or 2 hours after a meal.

EFFECTS ON LAB TEST RESULTS
● May increase liver enzyme levels.

CONTRAINDICATIONS & CAUTIONS
● Contraindicated in patients hypersensitive to drug.
● Use cautiously in elderly patients and those with hepatic impairment.
● Use in pregnant women only if clearly needed. Don't use in breast-feeding women.

NURSING CONSIDERATIONS
● *Alert:* Reducing oral corticosteroid dose has been followed in rare cases by eosinophilia, vasculitic rash, worsening pulmonary symptoms, cardiac complications, or neuropathy, sometimes as Churg-Strauss syndrome.
● Drug isn't indicated to reverse bronchospasm in acute asthma attacks.

PATIENT TEACHING
● Tell patient that drug is used for long-term treatment of asthma and to keep taking it even if symptoms resolve.
● Advise patient to continue taking other antiasthmatics, as prescribed.
● Instruct patient to take drug 1 hour before or 2 hours after meals.

58

Antacids, adsorbents, and antiflatulents

aluminum hydroxide
calcium carbonate
magnesium hydroxide
(See Chapter 63, LAXATIVES.)
magnesium oxide
simethicone
sodium bicarbonate

---

aluminum hydroxide
a-LOO-mi-num

AlternaGEL ◊, Alu-Cap ◊,
Alu-Tab ◊, Amphojel ◊, Dialume ◊

Pharmacologic class: aluminum salt
Pregnancy risk category C

AVAILABLE FORMS
Capsules: 400 mg ◊, 500 mg ◊
Liquid: 600 mg/5 ml ◊
Oral suspension: 320 mg/5 ml ◊,
450 mg/5 ml ◊, 675 mg/5 ml ◊
Tablets: 500 mg ◊, 600 mg ◊

INDICATIONS & DOSAGES
➤ Acid indigestion
Adults: 500 to 1,500 mg P.O. three to six
times daily between meals and at bedtime.
Or, 5 to 10 ml of liquid formulation or
5 to 30 ml of oral suspension between
meals and at bedtime or as directed by
prescriber.

ADMINISTRATION
P.O.
• Shake suspension well.
• When giving through nasogastric tube,
make sure tube is placed correctly and is
patent; after instilling drug, flush tube
with water to ensure passage to stomach
and to clear tube.

ACTION
Reduces total acid load in GI tract,
elevates gastric pH to reduce pepsin
activity, strengthens gastric mucosal
barrier, and increases esophageal
sphincter tone.

Route	Onset	Peak	Duration
P.O.	Variable	Unknown	20–180 min

Half-life: Unknown.

ADVERSE REACTIONS
CNS: *encephalopathy.*
GI: *constipation,* **intestinal obstruction.**
Metabolic: hypophosphatemia.
Musculoskeletal: osteomalacia.

INTERACTIONS
Drug-drug. *Allopurinol, antibiotics
(tetracyclines), corticosteroids, diflunisal,
digoxin, ethambutol, H_2-receptor
antagonists, iron salts, isoniazid,
penicillamine, phenothiazines, thyroid
hormones, ticlopidine:* May decrease
effect of these drugs by impairing absorption. Separate doses by 1 to 2 hours.
*Ciprofloxacin, levofloxacin, lomefloxacin,
moxifloxacin, norfloxacin, ofloxacin:* May
decrease quinolone effect. Give antacid at
least 6 hours before or 2 hours after
quinolone.
Enteric-coated drugs: May be released
prematurely in stomach. Separate doses
by at least 1 hour.

EFFECTS ON LAB TEST RESULTS
• May increase gastrin level. May decrease
phosphate level.

CONTRAINDICATIONS & CAUTIONS
• No known contraindications.
• Use cautiously in patients with chronic
renal disease.

NURSING CONSIDERATIONS
• *Alert:* Monitor long-term, high-dose use
in patient on restricted sodium intake.
Each tablet, capsule, or 5 ml of suspension
may contain 2 or 3 mg of sodium. Refer to
manufacturer's label for specific sodium
content.
• Record amount and consistency of
stools. Manage constipation with laxatives
or stool softeners; alternate with
magnesium-containing antacids (if patient
doesn't have renal disease).

Reactions may be *common,* uncommon, *life-threatening,* or COMMON AND LIFE-THREATENING.
Interaction may have a *rapid onset* or **delayed onset.**

- Monitor phosphate level.
- Watch for evidence of hypophosphatemia (anorexia, malaise, and muscle weakness) with prolonged use; also can lead to resorption of calcium and bone demineralization.
- Aluminum hydroxide therapy may interfere with imaging techniques using sodium pertechnetate Tc-99m, and thus impair evaluation of Meckel's diverticulum. It also may interfere with reticuloendothelial imaging of liver, spleen, or bone marrow using technetium-99m sulfur colloid. It may antagonize effect of pentagastrin during gastric acid secretion tests.
- Because drug contains aluminum, it's used in patients with renal failure to help control hyperphosphatemia by binding with phosphate in the GI tract.

PATIENT TEACHING
- Instruct patient to shake suspension well and to follow with a small amount of milk or water to facilitate passage.
- Advise patient not to take aluminum hydroxide indiscriminately or to switch antacids without prescriber's advice.
- Urge patient to notify prescriber about signs and symptoms of GI bleeding, such as tarry stools or coffee-ground vomitus.
- Instruct pregnant patient to seek medical advice before taking drug.

---

calcium carbonate
KAL-see-um

Alka-Mints ◊, Amitone ◊, Calci-Chew ◊, Cal-Gest ◊, Caltrate, Chooz ◊, Dicarbosil ◊, Equilet ◊, Maalox Antacid Caplets ◊, Nephro-Calci ◊, Oscal, Rolaids Calcium Rich ◊, Surpass ◊, Trial ◊, Tums ◊, Tums E-X ◊, Tums Ultra ◊, Viactiv ◊

Pharmacologic class: calcium salt
Pregnancy risk category C

AVAILABLE FORMS
Calcium carbonate contains 40% calcium; 20 mEq calcium per gram.
Capsules: 1,250 mg ◊
Chewing gum: 300 mg ◊, 450 mg ◊, 500 mg/piece ◊

Lozenges: 600 mg ◊
Oral suspension: 1,250 mg/5 ml
Tablets: 500 mg ◊, 600 mg ◊, 650 mg ◊, 1,000 mg ◊, 1,250 mg ◊, 1,500 mg ◊
Tablets (chewable): 350 mg ◊, 400 mg ◊, 420 mg ◊, 500 mg ◊, 750 mg ◊, 850 mg ◊, 1,000 mg ◊, 1,177 mg ◊, 1,250 mg ◊

INDICATIONS & DOSAGES
➤ **Acid indigestion, calcium supplement**
Adults: 350 mg to 1.5 g P.O. or two pieces of chewing gum 1 hour after meals and at bedtime, as needed.

ADMINISTRATION
P.O.
- Shake suspension well before administration.

ACTION
Reduces total acid load in GI tract, elevates gastric pH to reduce pepsin activity, strengthens gastric mucosal barrier, and increases esophageal sphincter tone.

Route	Onset	Peak	Duration
P.O.	20 min	Unknown	20–180 min

Half-life: Unknown.

ADVERSE REACTIONS
CNS: headache, irritability, weakness.
GI: *nausea,* constipation, flatulence, rebound hyperacidity.

INTERACTIONS
Drug-drug. *Antibiotics (tetracyclines), hydantoins, iron salts, isoniazid, salicylates:* May decrease effect of these drugs because may impair absorption. Separate doses by 2 hours.
Ciprofloxacin, levofloxacin, lomefloxacin, moxifloxacin, norfloxacin, ofloxacin: May decrease quinolone effects. Give antacid at least 6 hours before or 2 hours after quinolone.
Enteric-coated drugs: May be released prematurely in stomach. Separate doses by at least 1 hour.
Drug-food. *Milk, other foods high in vitamin D:* May cause milk-alkali syndrome (headache, confusion, distaste for food, nausea, vomiting, hypercalcemia, hypercalciuria). Discourage use together.

EFFECTS ON LAB TEST RESULTS
• May decrease phosphate level.

CONTRAINDICATIONS & CAUTIONS
• Contraindicated in patients with ventricular fibrillation or hypercalcemia.
• Use cautiously, if at all, if patient takes a cardiac glycoside or has sarcoidosis or renal or cardiac disease.

NURSING CONSIDERATIONS
• Record amount and consistency of stools. Manage constipation with laxatives or stool softeners.
• Monitor calcium level, especially in patients with mild renal impairment.
• Watch for evidence of hypercalcemia (nausea, vomiting, headache, confusion, and anorexia).

PATIENT TEACHING
• Advise patient not to take calcium carbonate indiscriminately or to switch antacids without prescriber's advice.
• Tell patient who takes chewable tablets to chew thoroughly before swallowing and to follow with a glass of water.
• Tell patient who uses suspension form to shake well and take with a small amount of water to facilitate passage.
• Urge patient to notify prescriber about signs and symptoms of GI bleeding, such as tarry stools, or coffee-ground vomitus.

---

magnesium oxide
mag-NEE-see-um

Mag-Caps◊, Mag-Ox 400◊, Maox◊, Uro-Mag◊

Pharmacologic class: magnesium salt
Pregnancy risk category B

AVAILABLE FORMS
Capsules: 140 mg◊
Tablets: 400 mg◊, 420 mg◊, 500 mg

INDICATIONS & DOSAGES
➤ **Acid indigestion**
Adults: 140 mg P.O. with water or milk after meals and at bedtime.

➤ **Oral replacement therapy in mild hypomagnesemia**
Adults: 400 to 840 mg P.O. daily. Monitor magnesium level.

ADMINISTRATION
P.O.
• When used to treat acid indigestion, give with water or milk.

ACTION
Reduces total acid load in GI tract, elevates gastric pH to reduce pepsin activity, strengthens gastric mucosal barrier, and increases esophageal sphincter tone.

Route	Onset	Peak	Duration
P.O.	20 min	Unknown	20–180 min

Half-life: Unknown.

ADVERSE REACTIONS
GI: *diarrhea,* abdominal pain, nausea.
Metabolic: hypermagnesemia.

INTERACTIONS
Drug-drug. *Allopurinol, antibiotics, digoxin, iron salts, penicillamine, phenothiazines:* May decrease effects of these drugs because may impair absorption. Separate doses by 1 to 2 hours.
Enteric-coated drugs: May be released prematurely in stomach. Separate doses by at least 1 hour.

EFFECTS ON LAB TEST RESULTS
• May increase magnesium level.

CONTRAINDICATIONS & CAUTIONS
• Contraindicated in patients with severe renal disease.
• Use cautiously in patients with mild renal impairment.

NURSING CONSIDERATIONS
• *Alert:* Monitor magnesium level. With prolonged use and renal impairment, watch for evidence of hypermagnesemia (hypotension, nausea, vomiting, depressed reflexes, respiratory depression, and coma).
• If diarrhea occurs, use a different drug.

PATIENT TEACHING
• Advise patient not to take drug indiscriminately or to switch antacids without prescriber's advice.

Reactions may be *common*, uncommon, *life-threatening*, or COMMON AND LIFE-THREATENING.
Interaction may have a *rapid onset* or **delayed onset.**

● Urge patient to report signs of GI bleeding, such as tarry stools, or coffee-ground vomitus.

---

simethicone
sye-METH-ih-kone

Flatulex◇, Gas Relief◇, Gas-X◇, Gas-X Extra Strength◇, Gas-X Thin Strips◇, Genasyme◇, Infacol◇†, Mylanta Gas◇, Mylanta Gas Relief Extra Strength◇, Mylicon◇, Ovol†, Ovol Drops†, Pediacol◇†, Phazyme◇, Phazyme 95◇, Phazyme-125 ◇, Tums Gas Relief

Pharmacologic class:
polydimethylsiloxanes
Pregnancy risk category C

AVAILABLE FORMS
Capsules: 125 mg◇, 180 mg◇
Drops: 40 mg/0.6 ml◇
Strips (orally disintegrating): 62.5 mg◇
Tablets: 40 mg◇, 55 mg†◇, 60 mg◇, 80 mg◇, 95 mg◇, 125 mg◇
Tablets (chewable): 80 mg◇, 125 mg◇

INDICATIONS & DOSAGES
➤ **Flatulence, functional gastric bloating**
Adults and children older than age 12: 40 to 125 mg P.O. after each meal and at bedtime, up to 500 mg daily. For drops, 40 to 80 mg P.O. after each meal and at bedtime, up to 500 mg daily.
Children ages 2 to 12: 40 mg after meals and at bedtime, up to 240 mg daily.
Children younger than age 2: 20 mg after meals and at bedtime, up to 240 mg daily.

ADMINISTRATION
P.O.
● Shake drops well before giving.
● Fill the dropper to the ordered dosage level and then give slowly into the infant's mouth, toward the inner cheek.

● The dosage can also be mixed with 1 ounce of cool water, infant formula, or juice.

ACTION
Disperses or prevents formation of mucus-surrounded gas pockets in the GI tract.

Route	Onset	Peak	Duration
P.O.	Immediate	Immediate	Unknown

Half-life: Unknown.

ADVERSE REACTIONS
GI: belching, flatus.

INTERACTIONS
None significant.

EFFECTS ON LAB TEST RESULTS
None reported.

CONTRAINDICATIONS & CAUTIONS
● Contraindicated in patients hypersensitive to drug.
● For infant colic, safety is unknown.

NURSING CONSIDERATIONS
● Drug doesn't prevent gas formation.
● *Look alike–sound alike:* Don't confuse simethicone with cimetidine.

PATIENT TEACHING
● Tell patient to chew tablet before swallowing.
● Tell parent that drops may be mixed with 1 ounce of cool water, infant formula, or juice.
● Advise patient that changing positions often and walking will help pass flatus.

---

sodium bicarbonate
Arm & Hammer Baking Soda◇, Neut, Soda Mint◇

Pharmacologic class: alkalinizer
Pregnancy risk category C

AVAILABLE FORMS
Injection: 4% (2.4 mEq/5 ml), 4.2% (5 mEq/10 ml), 5% (297.5 mEq/500 ml), 7.5% (8.92 mEq/10 ml and 44.6 mEq/50 ml), 8.4% (10 mEq/10 ml and 50 mEq/50 ml)
Tablets◇: 325 mg, 650 mg

INDICATIONS & DOSAGES

➤ **Metabolic acidosis**

Adults and children: Dosage depends on blood carbon dioxide content, pH, and patient's condition; usually, 2 to 5 mEq/kg I.V. infused over 4- to 8-hour period. Or 7,800 mg to 15,600 mg (12 to 24 650-mg tablets) dissolved in 1 to 2 L of water and consumed over 1 hour.

➤ **Urinary alkalinization**

Adults: Initially, 3,900 mg P.O.; then 1,300 mg to 2,600 mg every 4 hours; dosage based on urine pH.

➤ **Antacid**

Adults: 300 mg to 2 g P.O. up to q.i.d. taken with glass of water.

➤ **Cardiac arrest**

Adults: 1 mEq/kg I.V. of 7.5% or 8.4% solution; then 0.5 mEq/kg I.V. every 10 minutes, depending on arterial blood gas (ABG) level. Base further dosages on results of ABG analysis.

Infants and children: 1 mEq/kg (1 ml/kg of 8.4% solution) I.V. slowly followed by 1 mEq/kg every 10 minutes of arrest. Don't give more than 8 mEq/kg I.V. total; a 4.2% solution may be preferred.

➤ **Prevention of contrast media nephrotoxicity ♦**

Adults: 154 mEq/L at 3 ml/kg/hour I.V. for 1 hour before contrast administration, followed by an infusion of 1 ml/kg/hour for 6 hours after the procedure.

ADMINISTRATION

P.O.

● Drug may contain 27% sodium.

I.V.

● Drug isn't routinely used in cardiac arrest because it may produce a paradoxical acidosis from carbon dioxide production. It shouldn't be routinely given during the early stages of resuscitation unless acidosis is clearly present.

● The 4% form is usually used for neutralizing I.V. drugs such as erythromycin. Consult pharmacist before use.

● Flush I.V. line thoroughly between medications.

● **Incompatibilities:** Alcohol 5% in dextrose 5%; allopurinol; amino acids; amiodarone; amobarbital; amphotericin B; ascorbic acid injection; atropine; bupivacaine; calcium salts; carbenicillin; carboplatin; carmustine; cefotaxime; chlorpro-

mazine; ciprofloxacin; cisatracurium; cisplatin; codeine; corticotropin; dextrose 5% in lactated Ringer's injection; diazepam; diltiazem; dobutamine; dopamine; doxapram; doxorubicin liposomal; doxycycline; epinephrine hydrochloride; fat emulsion 10%; fenoldopam; glycopyrrolate; hetastarch; hydromorphone; idarubicin; imipenem-cilastatin sodium; inamrinone; Ionosol B, D, or G with invert sugar 10%; isoproterenol; labetalol; lactated Ringer's injection; levorphanol; leucovorin calcium; lidocaine; magnesium sulfate; meperidine; meropenem; metaraminol; methylprednisolone sodium succinate; metoclopramide; midazolam; morphine sulfate; MVI-12 multivitamin; nafcillin; nalbuphine; nitrofurantoin; norepinephrine bitartrate; ondansetron; oxacillin; penicillin G potassium; pentazocine lactate; pentobarbital sodium; procaine; Ringer's injection; sargramostim; 1/6 M sodium lactate; streptomycin; succinylcholine; thiopental; ticarcillin disodium and clavulanate potassium; vancomycin; verapamil; vinca alkaloids; vitamin B complex with vitamin C. Drug inactivates catecholamines, such as norepinephrine, dobutamine, and dopamine, and it forms precipitate with calcium. Don't mix with these drugs, and flush line thoroughly.

ACTION

Restores buffering capacity of the body and neutralizes excess acid.

Route	Onset	Peak	Duration
P.O.	Unknown	Unknown	Unknown
I.V.	Immediate	Immediate	Unknown

Half-life: Unknown.

ADVERSE REACTIONS

CNS: tetany.

CV: edema.

GI: gastric distention, belching, flatulence.

Metabolic: hypokalemia, *metabolic alkalosis,* hypernatremia, hyperosmolarity with overdose.

Skin: pain and irritation at injection site.

INTERACTIONS

Drug-drug. *Anorexiants, flecainide, mecamylamine, methenamine, quinidine,*

sympathomimetics: May decrease renal
clearance of these drugs and increase risk
of toxicity. Monitor patient closely for
toxicity.
*Chlorpropamide, lithium, methotrexate,
salicylates, tetracycline:* May increase
urine alkalinization, increase renal clearance of these drugs, and decrease their
effect. Monitor patient closely for drug's
effect.
Enteric-coated drugs: May be released
prematurely in stomach. Avoid using
together.
Ketoconazole: May decrease ketoconazole
absorption. Separate use by at least
2 hours.

EFFECTS ON LAB TEST RESULTS
● May increase sodium and lactate levels.
● May decrease potassium level.

CONTRAINDICATIONS & CAUTIONS
● Contraindicated in patients with metabolic or respiratory alkalosis and in those
with hypocalcemia in which alkalosis may
produce tetany, hypertension, seizures, or
heart failure.
● Contraindicated in patients losing chloride because of vomiting or continuous GI
suction and in those receiving diuretics
that produce hypochloremic alkalosis.
Oral drug is contraindicated for acute
ingestion of strong mineral acids.
● Use with caution in patients with renal
insufficiency, heart failure, or other
edematous or sodium-retaining condition.

NURSING CONSIDERATIONS
● To avoid risk of alkalosis, obtain blood
pH, partial pressure of arterial oxygen,
partial pressure of arterial carbon dioxide,
and electrolyte levels. Tell prescriber
laboratory results.

PATIENT TEACHING
● Tell patient not to take drug with milk
because doing so may cause high levels
of calcium in the blood, abnormally high
alkalinity in tissues and fluids, or kidney
stones.

59

Antidiarrheals

bismuth subsalicylate
calcium polycarbophil
   (See Chapter 63, LAXATIVES.)
diphenoxylate hydrochloride and
   atropine sulfate
loperamide
octreotide acetate
rifaximin

bismuth subsalicylate
BIS-mith

Bismatrol◇, Bismatrol Extra
Strength◇, Children's
Kaopectate◇, Extra Strength
Kaopectate◇, Kaopectate◇,
Peptic Relief◇, Pepto-Bismol◇,
Pepto-Bismol Maximum Strength
Liquid◇, Pink Bismuth◇

Pharmacologic class: adsorbent
Pregnancy risk category NR

AVAILABLE FORMS
Caplets: 262 mg
Liquid: 87 mg/5 ml◇, 87.3 mg/5 ml◇,
175 mg/5 ml◇
Oral suspension: 262 mg/15 ml◇,
524 mg/15 ml◇, 130 mg/15 ml
Tablets (chewable): 262 mg◇

INDICATIONS & DOSAGES
➤ **Mild, nonspecific diarrhea**
Adults and children age 12 and older:
30 ml or 2 tablets P.O. every 30 minutes to
1 hour, up to maximum of eight doses and
for no longer than 2 days.
Children ages 9 to 11: 15 ml or 1 tablet
P.O. every 30 minutes to 1 hour, up to
maximum of eight doses and for no longer
than 2 days.
Children ages 6 to 8: 10 ml or ⅔ tablet
P.O. every 30 minutes to 1 hour, up to
maximum of eight doses and for no longer
than 2 days.
Children ages 3 to 5: 5 ml or ⅓ tablet
P.O. every 30 minutes to 1 hour, up to
maximum of eight doses and for no longer
than 2 days.

➤ **Traveler's diarrhea** ♦
Adults: 30 ml P.O. every 30 minutes for
8 doses.

ADMINISTRATION
P.O.
● Shake liquid well before administration.
● Have patient chew or dissolve tablets in
mouth.

ACTION
May have antisecretory, antimicrobial,
and anti-inflammatory effects against
bacterial and viral enteropathogens.

Route	Onset	Peak	Duration
P.O.	1 hr	Unknown	Unknown

Half-life: Unknown.

ADVERSE REACTIONS
GI: temporary darkening of tongue and
stools.
Other: salicylism with high doses.

INTERACTIONS
Drug-drug. *Aspirin, other salicylates:* May
cause salicylate toxicity. Monitor patient.
Oral anticoagulants, oral antidiabetics:
May increase effects of these drugs after
high doses of bismuth subsalicylate.
Monitor patient closely.
Tetracycline: May decrease tetracycline ab-
sorption. Separate doses by at least 2 hours.

EFFECTS ON LAB TEST RESULTS
None reported.

CONTRAINDICATIONS & CAUTIONS
● Contraindicated in patients hypersensitive
to salicylates.
● Use cautiously in patients taking aspirin.
Stop therapy if tinnitus occurs.
● Use cautiously in children and in patients
with bleeding disorders or salicylate
sensitivity.

NURSING CONSIDERATIONS
● Avoid use before GI radiologic procedures because drug is radiopaque and may
interfere with X-rays.

Reactions may be *common,* uncommon, *life-threatening,* or COMMON AND LIFE-THREATENING.
Interaction may have a *rapid onset* or **delayed onset.**

PATIENT TEACHING
● Advise patient that drug contains salicylate. Each tablet has 102 mg salicylate. Regular-strength liquid has 130 mg/15 ml. Extra-strength liquid has 230 mg/15 ml.
● Instruct patient to shake liquid before measuring dose and to chew tablets well before swallowing.
● Tell patient to call prescriber if diarrhea lasts longer than 2 days or is accompanied by high fever.
● Advise patient to drink plenty of clear fluids to help prevent dehydration, which may accompany diarrhea.
● Tell patient that tongue and stools may temporarily turn gray-black.
● Urge patient to consult with prescriber before giving drug to children or teenagers during or after recovery from the flu or chickenpox.
● Inform patient that all forms of drug are effective against traveler's diarrhea. Tablets and caplets may be more convenient to carry.

---

diphenoxylate hydrochloride and atropine sulfate
dye-fen-OKS-ul-ate and A-troe-peen

Lomotil*, Lonox

Pharmacologic class: opioid
Pregnancy risk category C
Controlled substance schedule V

AVAILABLE FORMS
Liquid: 2.5 mg/5 ml (with atropine sulfate 0.025 mg/5 ml)*
Tablets: 2.5 mg (with atropine sulfate 0.025 mg)

INDICATIONS & DOSAGES
➤ Acute, nonspecific diarrhea
Adults and children older than age 12: Initially, 5 mg P.O. q.i.d.; then adjust as needed. Maximum dosage 20 mg/day.
Children ages 2 to 12: 0.3 to 0.4 mg/kg liquid form P.O. daily in four divided doses. For maintenance, reduce dose when initial control of symptoms is achieved. Dosage may be reduced by

as much as 75%. Maximum dosage 20 mg/day.

ADMINISTRATION
P.O.
● Give drug without regard for food.

ACTION
Probably increases smooth muscle tone in GI tract, inhibits motility and propulsion, and diminishes secretions.

Route	Onset	Peak	Duration
P.O.	45–60 min	3 hr	3–4 hr

Half-life: Diphenoxylate, 2½ hours; its major metabolite, diphenoxylic acid, 4½ hours; atropine, 2½ hours.

ADVERSE REACTIONS
CNS: *dizziness, sedation,* confusion, depression, drowsiness, euphoria, headache, lethargy, malaise, numbness in limbs, restlessness.
CV: tachycardia.
EENT: blurred vision.
GI: *dry mouth, pancreatitis,* paralytic ileus, abdominal discomfort or distention, anorexia, fluid retention in bowel or megacolon, nausea, swollen gums, vomiting.
GU: urine retention.
Respiratory: *respiratory depression.*
Skin: dry skin, pruritus, rash.
Other: *anaphylaxis, angioedema,* possible physical dependence with long-term use.

INTERACTIONS
Drug-drug. *Barbiturates, CNS depressants, opioids, tranquilizers:* May enhance CNS depression. Monitor patient closely.
MAO inhibitors: May cause hypertensive crisis. Avoid using together.
Drug-lifestyle. *Alcohol use:* May enhance CNS depression. Discourage use together.

EFFECTS ON LAB TEST RESULTS
None reported.

CONTRAINDICATIONS & CAUTIONS
● Contraindicated in children younger than age 2 and in patients hypersensitive to

diphenoxylate or atropine, in those with obstructive jaundice, and with acute diarrhea resulting from poison, organisms that penetrate intestinal mucosa, or antibiotic-induced pseudomembranous enterocolitis.

• Use cautiously in children age 2 and older; in patients with hepatic disease, opioid dependence, or acute ulcerative colitis; and in pregnant women.

NURSING CONSIDERATIONS

• *Alert:* Monitor fluid and electrolyte balance. Correct fluid and electrolyte disturbances before starting drug. Dehydration, especially in young children, may increase risk of delayed toxicity. Fluid retention in bowel or megacolon may occur with drug use and may mask depletion of extracellular fluid and electrolytes, especially in young children treated for acute gastroenteritis.

• Stop therapy immediately and notify prescriber if abdominal distention or other signs or symptoms of toxic megacolon develop.

• Don't use for antibiotic-induced diarrhea.

• Drug is unlikely to be effective if no response occurs within 48 hours.

• Risk of physical dependence increases with high dosage and long-term use. Atropine sulfate helps discourage abuse.

• Monitor for signs of overdose, which may include restlessness, flushing, hyperthermia, and tachycardia, initially, followed by lethargy, coma, pinpoint pupils, hypotonicity, and respiratory depression.

• *Look alike–sound alike:* Don't confuse Lomotil with Lamictal.

PATIENT TEACHING

• Tell patient not to exceed recommended dosage.

• Warn patient not to use drug to treat acute diarrhea for longer than 2 days and to seek medical attention if diarrhea continues.

• Advise patient to avoid hazardous activities, such as driving, until CNS effects of drug are known.

loperamide
loe-PER-a-mide

Diar-aid Caplets◇, Imodium A-D◇, Imodium A-D EZ chews, K-pec II◇, Neo-Diaral◇

Pharmacologic class: piperidine derivative
Pregnancy risk category B

AVAILABLE FORMS
Chewable tablets: 2 mg◇
Tablets: 2 mg◇
Capsules: 2 mg
Oral liquid: 1 mg/5 ml◇, 1 mg/7.5 ml◇

INDICATIONS & DOSAGES
➤ **Acute, nonspecific diarrhea**
Adults and children older than age 12: Initially, give 4 mg P.O.; then 2 mg after each unformed stool. Maximum, 8 mg daily, unless otherwise directed.
Children ages 8 to 12: 2 mg P.O. t.i.d. on first day. Subsequent dosages of 5 ml or 0.1 mg/kg of body weight may be given after each unformed stool. Maximum, 6 mg daily.
Children ages 5 to younger than 8: 2 mg P.O. b.i.d. on first day. If diarrhea persists, contact prescriber. Maximum, 4 mg daily.
Children ages 2 to 5: 1 mg P.O. t.i.d. on first day. If diarrhea persists, contact prescriber.
➤ **Chronic diarrhea**
Adults: Initially, give 4 mg P.O.; then 2 mg after each unformed stool until diarrhea subsides. Adjust dosage to individual response.
➤ **Traveler's diarrhea ♦**
Adults: 4 mg P.O. followed by 2 mg after each unformed stool for a maximum of 16 mg/day.

ADMINISTRATION
P.O.
• Use the liquid formulation for children ages 2 to 5.

ACTION
Inhibits peristalsis.

Route	Onset	Peak	Duration
P.O.	Unknown	2½–5 hr	24 hr

Half-life: 9 to 14½ hours.

ADVERSE REACTIONS
CNS: dizziness, drowsiness, fatigue.
GI: *constipation,* abdominal pain, distention or discomfort, dry mouth, nausea, vomiting.
Skin: hypersensitivity reactions, rash.

INTERACTIONS
Drug-drug. *Saquinavir:* May increase loperamide levels and decrease saquinavir levels. Avoid using together.

EFFECTS ON LAB TEST RESULTS
None reported.

CONTRAINDICATIONS & CAUTIONS
• Contraindicated in patients hypersensitive to drug and in those who must avoid constipation.
• Contraindicated in patients with bloody diarrhea or diarrhea with fever greater than 101° F (38° C), in breast-feeding women, and in children younger than age 2.
• Use cautiously in patients with hepatic disease.

NURSING CONSIDERATIONS
• If symptoms don't improve within 48 hours, stop therapy and consider another drug.
• Drug produces antidiarrheal action similar to that of diphenoxylate but without as many adverse CNS effects.
• *Alert:* Monitor children closely for CNS effects; children may be more sensitive to these effects than adults.
• *Look alike–sound alike:* Don't confuse Imodium with Ionamin.

PATIENT TEACHING
• Advise patient not to exceed recommended dosage.
• Tell patient with acute diarrhea to stop drug and seek medical attention if no improvement occurs within 48 hours. In chronic diarrhea, tell patient to notify prescriber and to stop drug if no improvement occurs after taking 16 mg daily for at least 10 days.

• Advise patient with acute colitis to stop drug immediately and notify prescriber about abdominal distention.
• Warn patient to avoid activities that require mental alertness until CNS effects of drug are known.
• Tell patient to report nausea, abdominal pain, or abdominal discomfort.
• Advise patient to relieve dry mouth with ice chips or sugarless gum.

octreotide acetate
ok-TREE-oh-tide

Sandostatin, Sandostatin LAR

Pharmacologic class: synthetic octapeptide
Pregnancy risk category B

AVAILABLE FORMS
Injection ampules: 0.05 mg/ml, 0.1 mg/ml, 0.2 mg/ml, 0.5 mg/ml, 1 mg/ml
Injection (multidose vials): 0.2 mg/ml, 1 mg/ml
Injection (powder for suspension): 10 mg/5 ml, 20 mg/5 ml, 30 mg/5 ml

INDICATIONS & DOSAGES
➤ **Flushing and diarrhea from carcinoid tumors**
Adults: 0.1 to 0.6 mg daily subcutaneously in two to four divided doses for first 2 weeks of therapy. Usual daily dosage is 0.3 mg. Base subsequent dosage on individual response.
➤ **Watery diarrhea from vasoactive intestinal polypeptide-secreting tumors (VIPomas)**
Adults: 0.2 to 0.3 mg daily subcutaneously in two to four divided doses for first 2 weeks of therapy. Base subsequent dosage on individual response but usually shouldn't exceed 0.45 mg daily.
➤ **Acromegaly**
Adults: Initially, 50 mcg subcutaneously t.i.d.; then adjust based on somatomedin C levels every 2 weeks. If Sandostatin LAR is used, give 20 mg I.M. (intragluteally) at 4-week intervals.

➤ **Carcinoid crisis including hypotension** ◆
Adults: 50 to 500 mcg by rapid I.V. injection. Repeat dose as needed. Or, 50 mcg/hour I.V. infusion for 8 to 24 hours.
➤ **GI fistula** ◆
Adults: 50 to 200 mcg subcutaneously every 8 hours.
➤ **Variceal bleeding** ◆
Adults: 25 to 50 mcg/hour via continuous I.V. infusion, over 18 hours to 5 days.
➤ **AIDS-related diarrhea** ◆
Adults: 100 to 500 mcg subcutaneously t.i.d.
➤ **Short-bowel syndrome** ◆
Adults: I.V. infusion of 25 mcg/hour or 50 mcg subcutaneously b.i.d.
➤ **Diarrhea caused by chemotherapy or radiation therapy** ◆
Adults: 50 to 100 mcg subcutaneously t.i.d. for 1 to 3 days.
➤ **Pancreatic fistula** ◆
Adults: 50 to 200 mcg every 8 hours.

ADMINISTRATION
I.V.
● For emergency management of carcinoid crisis, give undiluted by rapid I.V. push.
● For other uses, dilute in 50 to 200 ml D$_5$W or normal saline solution and infuse over 15 to 30 minutes.
● Solution is stable for 24 hours.
● **Incompatibilities:** Total parenteral nutrition.
I.M.
● Don't use if particulates or discoloration are observed.
● Follow the mixing instructions included in the packaging and give immediately after mixing.
● Never give the injectable suspension by I.V. or subcutaneous routes.
Subcutaneous
● Don't use if particulates or discoloration are observed.

ACTION
Mimics action of naturally occurring somatostatin.

Route	Onset	Peak	Duration
I.V.	Rapid	30 min	< 12 hr
I.M.	Unknown	2–3 wk	Unknown
Subcut.	30 min	30 min	< 12 hr

Half-life: About 1½ hours, long-acting, unknown.

ADVERSE REACTIONS
CNS: dizziness, fatigue, headache, light-headedness.
CV: *arrhythmias, bradycardia,* conduction abnormalities, edema.
EENT: blurred vision.
GI: *abdominal pain or discomfort, diarrhea, gallbladder abnormalities, loose stools, nausea, pancreatitis,* constipation, fat malabsorption, flatulence, vomiting.
GU: pollakiuria, UTI.
Metabolic: *hypoglycemia,* hyperglycemia, hypothyroidism, suppressed secretion of growth hormone and gastroenterohepatic peptides (gastrin, vasoactive intestinal polypeptide, insulin, glucagon, secretin, motilin, and pancreatic polypeptide).
Musculoskeletal: backache, joint pain.
Skin: alopecia, erythema or pain at injection site, flushing, wheal.
Other: cold symptoms, flulike symptoms, pain or burning at subcutaneous injection site.

INTERACTIONS
Drug-drug. *Cyclosporine:* May decrease cyclosporine level. Monitor patient closely.

EFFECTS ON LAB TEST RESULTS
● May decrease vitamin B$_{12}$ level. May increase or decrease glucose level.
● May alter liver function test values.

CONTRAINDICATIONS & CAUTIONS
● Contraindicated in patients hypersensitive to drug or its components.

NURSING CONSIDERATIONS
● *Look alike–sound alike:* To avoid giving drug by the wrong route, don't confuse octreotide acetate injection with injectable depot suspension product.
● Monitor baseline thyroid function tests.
● Monitor IGF-I (somatomedin C) levels every 2 weeks. Dosage adjustments are based on this level.
● Periodically monitor laboratory tests, such as thyroid function, glucose, urine 5-hydroxyindoleacetic acid, plasma serotonin, and plasma substance P (for carcinoid tumors).
● Monitor patient regularly for gallbladder disease. Therapy may be related to the development of cholelithiasis because

of its effect on gallbladder motility or fat absorption.
• Monitor patient closely for signs and symptoms of glucose imbalance. Patients with type 1 diabetes mellitus and those receiving oral antidiabetics or oral diazoxide may need dosage adjustments during therapy. Monitor glucose level.
• Drug may alter fluid and electrolyte balance; other therapies may need adjusting.
• Half-life may be altered in patients with end-stage renal failure who are receiving dialysis.
• *Look alike–sound alike:* Don't confuse Sandostatin with Sandimmune or Sando-globulin.

PATIENT TEACHING
• Urge patient to report signs and symptoms of abdominal discomfort immediately.
• Stress importance of the need for periodic laboratory testing during octreotide therapy.

rifaximin
reh-FACKS-ah-men

Xifaxan

Pharmacologic class: rifamycin antibacterial
Pregnancy risk category C

AVAILABLE FORMS
Tablets: 200 mg

INDICATIONS & DOSAGES
➤ **Traveler's diarrhea from non-invasive strains of *Escherichia coli***
Adults and children age 12 and older: 200 mg P.O. t.i.d. for 3 days.
➤ **Hepatic encephalopathy**
Adults: 400 mg P.O. t.i.d. or every 8 hours.
➤ **Irritable bowel syndrome**
Adults: 400 mg P.O. b.i.d. or t.i.d. for 10 days.

ADMINISTRATION
P.O.
• Give drug without regard for food.

ACTION
Binds to the beta-subunit of bacterial DNA-dependent RNA polymerase, which inhibits bacterial RNA synthesis and kills *E. coli.*

Route	Onset	Peak	Duration
P.O.	Unknown	Unknown	Unknown

Half-life: Unknown.

ADVERSE REACTIONS
CNS: fever, headache.
GI: abdominal pain, constipation, defecation urgency, flatulence, nausea, rectal tenesmus, vomiting.

INTERACTIONS
None significant.

EFFECTS ON LAB TEST RESULTS
None reported.

CONTRAINDICATIONS & CAUTIONS
• Contraindicated in patients hypersensitive to rifaximin or any rifamycin antibacterial.

NURSING CONSIDERATIONS
• Don't use drug in patients whose illness may be caused by *Campylobacter jejuni, Shigella,* or *Salmonella.*
• *Alert:* Don't use drug in patients with blood in the stool, diarrhea with fever, or diarrhea from pathogens other than *E. coli.*
• Stop drug if diarrhea worsens or lasts longer than 24 to 48 hours. The patient may need a different antibiotic.
• Patients who have diarrhea after antibiotic therapy may have pseudomembranous colitis, which may range from mild to life-threatening.
• Monitor patient for overgrowth of nonsusceptible organisms.

PATIENT TEACHING
• Explain that drug may be taken with or without food.
• Tell patient to take all the prescribed drug, even if he feels better before the drug is finished.
• Advise patient to notify his prescriber if diarrhea worsens or lasts longer than 1 or 2 days after starting treatment. A different treatment may be needed.

● Tell patient to call the prescriber if he develops a fever or has blood in his stool.
● Explain that this drug is only for treating diarrhea caused by contaminated foods or beverages while traveling and not for any other type of infection.
● Caution patient not to share this drug with others.

aprepitant
chlorpromazine hydrochloride
(See Chapter 41, ANTIPSYCHOTICS.)
dimenhydrinate
dolasetron mesylate
dronabinol
fosaprepitant dimeglumine
granisetron
granisetron hydrochloride
meclizine hydrochloride
metoclopramide hydrochloride
ondansetron hydrochloride
palonosetron hydrochloride
perphenazine
(See Chapter 41, ANTIPSYCHOTICS.)
prochlorperazine
prochlorperazine edisylate
prochlorperazine maleate
promethazine hydrochloride
(See Chapter 55, ANTIHISTAMINES.)
scopolamine
scopolamine butylbromide
scopolamine hydrobromide
trimethobenzamide
    hydrochloride

---

aprepitant
ah-PRE-pit-ant

Emend

fosaprepitant dimeglumine
Emend

Pharmacologic class: substance P
and neurokinin-1 receptor
antagonist
Pregnancy risk category B

AVAILABLE FORMS
Capsules: 40 mg, 80 mg, 125 mg
Injection: 115 mg

INDICATIONS & DOSAGES
➤ **To prevent nausea and vomiting
after highly emetogenic chemotherapy (including cisplatin) and
moderately emetogenic chemotherapy, with a 5-HT$_3$ antagonist
and a corticosteroid**
Adults: On day 1 of chemotherapy, 125 mg
P.O. 1 hour before treatment, or 115 mg
by I.V. infusion over 15 minutes, given
30 minutes before treatment. On days 2
and 3, give 80 mg P.O. every morning.
➤ **To prevent postoperative nausea
and vomiting**
Adults: 40 mg P.O. within 3 hours before
induction of anesthesia.

ADMINISTRATION
P.O.
● Give drug without regard for food.
● Drug may be given with other antiemetics.
I.V.
● Reconstitute with 5 ml of normal saline
solution. Add the saline along the vial wall
to prevent foaming. Swirl gently and avoid
shaking.
● Add entire volume to infusion bag
containing 110 ml of saline. Total volume
will be 115 ml and final concentration is
1 mg/ml.
● Gently invert the bag 2 to 3 times.
● Administer over 15 minutes by I.V.
infusion.
● Final solution is stable for 24 hours at
ambient room temperature.
● **Incompatibilities:** Any solutions containing divalent cations (e.g. Ca^{2+}, Mg^{2+}),
including Ringer's lactate and Hartmann's
solution

ACTION
Inhibits emesis by selectively antagonizing substance P and neurokinin-1
receptors in the brain; appears to be
synergistic with 5-HT$_3$ antagonists and
corticosteroids.

Route	Onset	Peak	Duration
P.O.	Unknown	4 hr	Unknown

Half-life: 9 to 13 hours.

ADVERSE REACTIONS
CNS: *asthenia, fatigue,* dizziness, fever,
headache, insomnia.

CV: *bradycardia*, hypertension, hypotension.
EENT: mucous membrane disorder, tinnitus.
GI: *anorexia, constipation, diarrhea, nausea,* abdominal pain, epigastric pain, flatulence, gastritis, heartburn, vomiting.
GU: UTI.
Hematologic: *neutropenia,* anemia.
Respiratory: *hiccups.*
Skin: pruritus, infusion site pain, infusion site induration.
Other: dehydration.

INTERACTIONS
Drug-drug. *Alprazolam, midazolam, triazolam:* May increase levels of these drugs. Watch for CNS effects, such as increased sedation. Decrease benzodiazepine dose by 50%.
Carbamazepine, phenytoin, rifampin, other CYP3A4 inducers: May decrease aprepitant level. Watch for decreased antiemetic effect.
Clarithromycin, diltiazem, erythromycin, itraconazole, ketoconazole, nefazodone, nelfinavir, ritonavir, troleandomycin, other CYP3A4 inhibitors: May increase aprepitant level and risk of toxicity. Use together cautiously.
Dexamethasone, methylprednisolone: May increase levels of these drugs and risk of toxicity. Decrease P.O. corticosteroid dose by 50%; decrease I.V. methylprednisolone dose by 25%.
Diltiazem: May increase diltiazem level. Monitor heart rate and blood pressure. Avoid using together.
Docetaxel, etoposide, ifosfamide, imatinib, irinotecan, paclitaxel, vinorelbine, vinblastine, vincristine: May increase levels and risk of toxicity of these drugs. Use together cautiously.
Hormonal contraceptives: May decrease contraceptive effectiveness. Tell women to use additional birth control method during therapy.
Paroxetine: May decrease paroxetine and aprepitant effects. Monitor patient for effectiveness.
Phenytoin: May decrease phenytoin level. Monitor level carefully. Avoid using together. Increase phenytoin dose as needed during therapy.
Pimozide: May increase pimozide level. Avoid using together.
Tolbutamide: May decrease tolbutamide effects. Monitor glucose level.
Warfarin: May decrease warfarin effectiveness. Monitor INR carefully for 2 weeks after each aprepitant treatment.
Drug-herb. *St. John's wort:* May decrease antiemetic effects by inducing CYP3A4. Discourage use together.
Drug-food. *Grapefruit juice:* May increase drug level and risk of toxicity. Discourage use together.

EFFECTS ON LAB TEST RESULTS
● May increase alkaline phosphatase, AST, ALT, BUN, creatinine, glucose, and urine protein levels. May decrease sodium level.
● May increase RBC and WBC counts. May decrease neutrophil count.

CONTRAINDICATIONS & CAUTIONS
● Contraindicated in patients hypersensitive to fosaprepitant, aprepitant, or its components.
● Use cautiously in patients receiving chemotherapy drugs metabolized mainly via CYP3A4 and in those with severe hepatic disease.
● Use in pregnant women only when drug's benefits clearly outweigh its risks.
● Don't use in breast-feeding women; it's unknown if drug appears in breast milk.
● Safety and effectiveness haven't been established in children.

NURSING CONSIDERATIONS
● Avoid giving drug for more than 3 days per chemotherapy cycle.
● *Alert:* Fosaprepitant is given I.V. on day 1 only of a 3-day regimen.
● *Alert:* Before giving drug, screen patient carefully for possible drug and herb interactions.
● Don't give drug for existing nausea or vomiting.
● Expect to give drug with other antiemetics to treat breakthrough emesis.
● Monitor CBC, liver function test results, and creatinine level periodically during therapy.

Reactions may be *common,* uncommon, *life-threatening,* or COMMON AND LIFE-THREATENING.
Interaction may have a *rapid onset* or **delayed onset.**

PATIENT TEACHING
- If nausea or vomiting occurs, instruct patient to take breakthrough antiemetics rather than more aprepitant.
- Urge patient to report use of any other drugs or herbs.
- Caution patient against taking drug with grapefruit juice.
- Advise woman who takes a hormonal contraceptive to use an additional form of birth control.
- Tell patient who takes warfarin that PT and INR will be monitored closely for 2 weeks after therapy starts.

---

dimenhydrinate
dye-men-HYE-dri-nate

Calm-X◊, Children's Dramamine*◊, Dinate†◊, Dramamine*◊, Dramamine Liquid*◊, Dramanate, Dymenate, Gravol†, Gravol L/A†, Hydrate, Nauseatol†◊, Travel Tabs†, TripTone Caplets◊

Pharmacologic class: anticholinergic
Pregnancy risk category B

AVAILABLE FORMS
Injection: 50 mg/ml
Syrup: 12.5 mg/4 ml*◊, 12.5 mg/5 ml*◊, 15 mg/5 ml†◊, 15.62 mg/5 ml
Tablets: 50 mg◊
Tablets (chewable): 50 mg◊

INDICATIONS & DOSAGES
➤ **To prevent and treat motion sickness**
Adults and children age 12 and older: 50 to 100 mg P.O. every 4 to 6 hours; 50 mg I.M., as needed; or 50 mg I.V. diluted in 10 ml normal saline solution for injection, injected over 2 minutes. Maximum, 400 mg daily. For prevention, use drug 30 minutes before motion exposure.
Children ages 6 to 11: 25 to 50 mg P.O. every 6 to 8 hours, not to exceed 150 mg in 24 hours. Or, 1.25 mg/kg or 37.5 mg/m² I.M. or P.O. q.i.d. Maximum, 300 mg daily.

Children ages 2 to 5: 12.5 to 25 mg P.O. every 6 to 8 hours, not to exceed 75 mg in 24 hours. Or, 1.25 mg/kg or 37.5 mg/m² I.M. or P.O. q.i.d. Maximum, 300 mg daily.

ADMINISTRATION
P.O.
- May be given without regard for food.
- Give at least 30 minutes before activity or travel.
I.V.
- Dilute each milliliter (50 mg) of drug with 10 ml sterile water for injection, D_5W, or normal saline solution for injection.
- Give by direct injection over at least 2 minutes.
- Don't give if drug has particulate matter or discoloration.
- **Incompatibilities:** Aminophylline, ammonium chloride, amobarbital, butorphanol, chlorpromazine, glycopyrrolate, heparin, hydrocortisone sodium succinate, hydroxyzine hydrochloride, midazolam, pentobarbital sodium, phenobarbital sodium, phenytoin, prochlorperazine edisylate, promazine, promethazine hydrochloride, and thiopental.
I.M.
- Inspect drug for particulate matter or discoloration; don't give if present.

ACTION
May affect neural pathways originating in the labyrinth to inhibit nausea and vomiting.

Route	Onset	Peak	Duration
P.O.	15–30 min	Unknown	3–6 hr
I.V.	Immediate	Unknown	3–6 hr
I.M.	20–30 min	Unknown	3–6 hr

Half-life: Unknown.

ADVERSE REACTIONS
CNS: *drowsiness,* confusion, dizziness, excitation, headache, insomnia, lassitude, nervousness, tingling and weakness of hands, vertigo.
CV: hypotension, palpitations, tachycardia.
EENT: blurred vision, diplopia, dry respiratory passages, nasal congestion.
GI: anorexia, constipation, diarrhea, dry mouth, epigastric distress, nausea, vomiting.

GU: urine retention.
Respiratory: thickened bronchial secretions, wheezing.
Skin: photosensitivity reactions, rash, urticaria.
Other: *anaphylaxis,* tightness of chest.

INTERACTIONS
Drug-drug. *CNS depressants:* May cause additive CNS depression. Avoid using together.
Ototoxic drugs: Dimenhydrinate may mask symptoms of ototoxicity. Use together cautiously.
Tricyclic antidepressants, other anticholinergics: May increase anticholinergic activity. Monitor patient.
Drug-lifestyle. *Alcohol use:* May cause additive CNS depression. Discourage use together.

EFFECTS ON LAB TEST RESULTS
• May prevent, reduce, or mask diagnostic skin test response. May alter xanthine (caffeine, aminophylline) test results.

CONTRAINDICATIONS & CAUTIONS
• Contraindicated in patients hypersensitive to drug or its components.
• Use cautiously in elderly patients, patients receiving ototoxic drugs, and patients with seizures, acute angle-closure glaucoma, or enlarged prostate gland.

NURSING CONSIDERATIONS
• Elderly patients may be more susceptible to adverse CNS effects.
• Undiluted solution irritates veins and may cause sclerosis.
• Stop drug 4 days before diagnostic skin tests to prevent falsifying test response.
• Dramamine may contain tartrazine.
• *Alert:* Drug may mask symptoms of ototoxicity, brain tumor, or intestinal obstruction.
• *Look alike–sound alike:* Don't confuse dimenhydrinate with diphenhydramine.

PATIENT TEACHING
• Advise patient to avoid activities that require alertness until CNS effects of drug are known.
• Instruct patient to report adverse reactions promptly.

dolasetron mesylate
doe-LAZ-e-tron

Anzemet

Pharmacologic class: selective serotonin (5-HT$_3$) receptor antagonist
Pregnancy risk category B

AVAILABLE FORMS
Injection: 20 mg/ml as 12.5-mg/0.625-ml ampule or 100-mg/5-ml vial
Tablets: 50 mg, 100 mg

INDICATIONS & DOSAGES
➤ **To prevent nausea and vomiting from cancer chemotherapy**
Adults: 100 mg P.O. given as a single dose 1 hour before chemotherapy. Or, 1.8 mg/kg or a fixed dose of 100 mg as a single I.V. dose given 30 minutes before chemotherapy.
Children ages 2 to 16: 1.8 mg/kg P.O. given 1 hour before chemotherapy. Or, 1.8 mg/kg as a single I.V. dose given 30 minutes before chemotherapy. Injectable formulation can be mixed with apple juice and given P.O. Maximum dose is 100 mg.
➤ **To prevent postoperative nausea and vomiting**
Adults: 100 mg P.O. within 2 hours before surgery. Or, 12.5 mg as a single I.V. dose about 15 minutes before cessation of anesthesia or as soon as nausea or vomiting presents.
Children ages 2 to 16: 1.2 mg/kg P.O. given within 2 hours before surgery, to maximum of 100 mg. Or, 0.35 mg/kg, up to 12.5 mg given as a single I.V. dose about 15 minutes before stopping anesthesia or as soon as nausea or vomiting starts. I.V. form can be mixed with apple juice and given P.O.
➤ **Postoperative nausea and vomiting**
Adults: 12.5 mg as a single I.V. dose as soon as nausea or vomiting occurs.
Children ages 2 to 16: 0.35 mg/kg, to maximum dosage of 12.5 mg, given as a single I.V. dose as soon as nausea or vomiting occurs.

Reactions may be *common,* uncommon, *life-threatening,* or COMMON AND LIFE-THREATENING.
Interaction may have a *rapid onset* or *delayed onset.*

ADMINISTRATION
P.O.
• Mix injection for oral use in apple or apple-grape juice immediately before giving.
• Injection for oral use is stable in juice for 2 hours at room temperature.
I.V.
• Drug can be injected as rapidly as 100 mg over 30 seconds or diluted in 50 ml of compatible solution and infused over 15 minutes.
• **Incompatibilities:** Other I.V. drugs.

ACTION
Blocks the action of serotonin and prevents serotonin from stimulating the vomiting reflex.

Route	Onset	Peak	Duration
P.O.	Rapid	1 hr	8 hr
I.V.	Rapid	36 min	7 hr

Half-life: 8 hours.

ADVERSE REACTIONS
CNS: *headache,* dizziness, drowsiness, fatigue, fever.
CV: *arrhythmias,* ECG changes, edema, hypertension, hypotension, tachycardia.
GI: *diarrhea,* abdominal pain, anorexia, constipation, dyspepsia.
GU: hematuria, polyuria, urine retention.
Skin: pruritus, rash.
Other: chills, pain at injection site.

INTERACTIONS
Drug-drug. *Drugs that prolong ECG intervals such as antiarrhythmics:* May increase risk of arrhythmia. Monitor patient closely.
Drugs that inhibit CYP enzymes such as cimetidine: May increase level of hydrodolasetron, an active metabolite of dolasetron. Monitor patient for adverse effects.
Drugs that induce CYP enzymes such as rifampin: May decrease level of hydrodolasetron, an active metabolite of dolasetron. Monitor patient for decreased effectiveness of antiemetic.

EFFECTS ON LAB TEST RESULTS
• May increase ALT and AST levels.
• May increase PTT.

CONTRAINDICATIONS & CAUTIONS
• Contraindicated in patients hypersensitive to drug.
• *Alert:* Give with caution in patients who have or may develop prolonged cardiac conduction intervals, such as those with electrolyte abnormalities, history of arrhythmia, and cumulative high-dose anthracycline therapy.
• Drug isn't recommended for use in children younger than age 2. Use cautiously in breast-feeding women.

NURSING CONSIDERATIONS
• *Look alike–sound alike:* Don't confuse Anzemet with Aldomet or Avandamet.

PATIENT TEACHING
• Tell patient about possible adverse effects.
• Instruct patient to mix injection in juice for oral use immediately before giving.
• Tell patient to report nausea or vomiting.

---

dronabinol
(delta-9-tetrahydrocannabinol)
droe-NAB-i-nol

Marinol

Pharmacologic class: cannabinoid
Pregnancy risk category C
Controlled substance schedule III

AVAILABLE FORMS
Capsules: 2.5 mg, 5 mg, 10 mg

INDICATIONS & DOSAGES
➤ **Nausea and vomiting from cancer chemotherapy**
Adults: 5 mg/m^2 P.O. 1 to 3 hours before chemotherapy. Then, same dose every 2 to 4 hours after chemotherapy, for total of four to six doses daily. If needed, increase dosage in 2.5-mg/m^2 increments to maximum of 15 mg/m^2 per dose.
➤ **Anorexia and weight loss in patients with AIDS**
Adults: 2.5 mg P.O. b.i.d. before lunch and dinner. If patient can't tolerate it, decrease to 2.5 mg P.O. given as a single dose daily

in evening or at bedtime. May gradually increase to maximum of 20 mg daily given in divided doses.

ADMINISTRATION
P.O.
● Give 1 to 3 hours before chemotherapy.
● Store in cool environment, but protect from freezing.

ACTION
Unknown. A derivative of marijuana.

Route	Onset	Peak	Duration
P.O.	30–60 min	2–4 hr	4–6 hr

Half-life: 1 to 1½ days.

ADVERSE REACTIONS
CNS: *ataxia, dizziness, drowsiness, euphoria, paranoia,* amnesia, asthenia, confusion, depersonalization, hallucinations, headache, muddled thinking, somnolence.
CV: orthostatic hypotension, palpitations, tachycardia, vasodilation.
EENT: visual disturbances.
GI: *abdominal pain, dry mouth, nausea, vomiting,* diarrhea.

INTERACTIONS
Drug-drug. *CNS depressants, psychomimetic substances, sedatives:* May cause additive CNS depression. Avoid using together.
Drug-lifestyle. *Alcohol use:* May cause additive CNS depression. Discourage use together.

EFFECTS ON LAB TEST RESULTS
None reported.

CONTRAINDICATIONS & CAUTIONS
● Contraindicated in patients hypersensitive to sesame oil or cannabinoids.
● Use cautiously in the elderly, in pregnant or breast-feeding women, and in those with heart disease, psychiatric illness, or history of drug abuse.

NURSING CONSIDERATIONS
● Expect drug to be prescribed only for patients who haven't responded satisfactorily to other antiemetics.
● *Alert:* Drug is the principal active substance in *Cannabis sativa* (marijuana),

which can produce both physiologic and psychological dependence and has a high risk of abuse.
● CNS effects are intensified at higher dosages.
● Drug effects may persist for days after treatment ends.
● *Look alike–sound alike:* Don't confuse dronabinol with droperidol.

PATIENT TEACHING
● Tell patient that drug may induce unusual changes in mood or other adverse behavioral effects.
● Advise patient against performing activities that require alertness until CNS effects of drug are known.
● Warn caregivers to supervise patient during and immediately after treatment.
● Advise patient to take drug 1 to 3 hours before chemotherapy.

---

granisetron
Sancuso

granisetron hydrochloride
gran-IZ-e-tron

Kytril

Pharmacologic class: selective serotonin (5-HT$_3$) receptor antagonist
Pregnancy risk category B

AVAILABLE FORMS
Injection: 0.1 mg/ml in 1-ml single-use vials; 1 mg/ml in 1-ml, single-dose, preservative-free vials and 4-ml multidose vials containing benzyl alcohol
Oral solution: 1 mg/5 ml
Tablets: 1 mg
Transdermal patch: 3.1 mg per 24 hours

INDICATIONS & DOSAGES
➤ **To prevent nausea and vomiting from emetogenic cancer chemotherapy**
Adults and children age 2 and older: 10 mcg/kg I.V. undiluted and given by direct injection over 30 seconds, or diluted and infused over 5 minutes. Start giving at least 30 minutes before

chemotherapy. Or, for adults, 1 mg P.O. up to 1 hour before chemotherapy and repeated 12 hours later. Or, for adults, 2 mg P.O. daily given up to 1 hour before chemotherapy. Or, apply a single patch to the upper outer arm 24 to 48 hours before chemotherapy. Remove the patch a minimum of 24 hours after completion of chemotherapy or a maximum of 7 days.

➤ **To prevent nausea and vomiting from radiation, including total body irradiation and fractionated abdominal radiation**
Adults: 2 mg P.O. once daily within 1 hour of radiation.

➤ **Postoperative nausea and vomiting**
Adults: 1 mg I.V. undiluted and given over 30 seconds. For prevention, give before anesthesia induction or immediately before reversal.

ADMINISTRATION
P.O.
• Store bottle of oral solution in an upright position.
I.V.
• For direct injection, give drug undiluted over 30 seconds.
• For intermittent infusion, dilute with normal saline solution for injection or D_5W to a volume of 20 to 50 ml.
• Infuse over 5 minutes, starting within 30 minutes before chemotherapy and only on days chemotherapy is given.
• Diluted solutions are stable 24 hours at room temperature.
• Don't freeze vials.
• Once the multiuse vial is penetrated, use contents within 30 days.
• **Incompatibilities:** Other I.V. drugs.
Transdermal
• Apply patch to intact, healthy skin.
• Each patch is packed in a pouch and should be applied directly after the pouch has been opened.
• Do not cut the patch into pieces

ACTION
May block $5\text{-}HT_3$ in the CNS in the chemoreceptor trigger zone and in the peripheral nervous system on nerve terminals of the vagus nerve.

Route	Onset	Peak	Duration
P.O., I.V.	Unknown	Unknown	Unknown

Half-life: 5 to 9 hours.

ADVERSE REACTIONS
CNS: *asthenia, headache, fever,* agitation, anxiety, CNS stimulation, dizziness, insomnia, somnolence, *pain.*
CV: *bradycardia,* hypertension, hypotension.
GI: *constipation, nausea, vomiting,* abdominal pain, decreased appetite, diarrhea, dyspepsia, flatulence, taste disorder.
GU: oliguria, UTI.
Hematologic: *anemia, leukocytosis, leukopenia, thrombocytopenia.*
Respiratory: cough, increased sputum.
Skin: alopecia, rash, dermatitis.
Other: hypersensitivity reactions (*anaphylaxis,* urticaria, dyspnea, hypotension), infection.

INTERACTIONS
None known.

EFFECTS ON LAB TEST RESULTS
• May increase ALT and AST levels. May decrease hemoglobin level and hematocrit. May alter fluid and electrolyte levels with prolonged use.
• May decrease platelet and WBC counts.

CONTRAINDICATIONS & CAUTIONS
• Contraindicated in patients hypersensitive to drug.

NURSING CONSIDERATIONS
• Drug regimen is given only on days when chemotherapy is given. Treatment at other times isn't useful.

PATIENT TEACHING
• Stress importance of taking second dose of oral drug 12 hours after the first for maximum effectiveness.
• Tell patient to report adverse reactions immediately.

meclizine hydrochloride (meclozine hydrochloride)
MEK-li-zeen

Antivert, Antivert/25◇, Antivert/50, Bonamine†, Bonine◇, Dramamine Less Drowsy Formula

Pharmacologic class: anticholinergic
Pregnancy risk category B

AVAILABLE FORMS
Tablets: 12.5 mg, 25 mg◇, 50 mg
Tablets (chewable): 25 mg◇

INDICATIONS & DOSAGES
➤ **Vertigo**
Adults: 25 to 100 mg P.O. daily in divided doses. Dosage varies with response.
➤ **Motion sickness**
Adults and children age 12 and older: 25 to 50 mg P.O. 1 hour before travel; then daily for duration of trip.

ADMINISTRATION
P.O.
● Chewable tablets may be chewed or swallowed with water.

ACTION
Unknown. May affect neural pathways originating in the labyrinth to inhibit nausea and vomiting.

Route	Onset	Peak	Duration
P.O.	1 hr	Unknown	8–24 hr

Half-life: About 6 hours.

ADVERSE REACTIONS
CNS: *drowsiness,* auditory and visual hallucinations, excitation, nervousness, restlessness.
CV: hypotension, palpitations, tachycardia.
EENT: blurred vision, diplopia, dry nose and throat, tinnitus.
GI: anorexia, constipation, diarrhea, dry mouth, nausea, vomiting.
GU: urinary frequency, urine retention.
Skin: rash, urticaria.

INTERACTIONS
Drug-drug. *CNS depressants:* May increase drowsiness. Use together cautiously.

EFFECTS ON LAB TEST RESULTS
● May prevent, reduce, or mask diagnostic skin test response.

CONTRAINDICATIONS & CAUTIONS
● Contraindicated in patients hypersensitive to drug.
● Use cautiously in patients with asthma, glaucoma, or prostatic hyperplasia.

NURSING CONSIDERATIONS
● Stop drug 4 days before diagnostic skin tests to avoid interference with test response.
● Drug may mask signs and symptoms of ototoxicity, brain tumor, or intestinal obstruction.
● *Look alike–sound alike:* Don't confuse Antivert with Axert. Don't confuse Dramamine Less Drowsy with other Dramamine formulations.

PATIENT TEACHING
● Advise patient to avoid hazardous activities that require alertness until CNS effects of drug are known.
● Urge patient to report persistent or serious adverse reactions promptly.

---

metoclopramide hydrochloride
met-oh-KLOE-pra-mide

Apo-Metoclop†, Octamide PFS, Reglan, Reglan ODT

Pharmacologic class: dopamine antagonist
Pregnancy risk category B

AVAILABLE FORMS
Injection: 5 mg/ml
Syrup: 5 mg/5 ml
Tablets: 5 mg, 10 mg
Tablets (orally-disintegrating): 5 mg, 10 mg

Reactions may be *common,* uncommon, *life-threatening,* or COMMON AND LIFE-THREATENING.
Interaction may have a *rapid onset* or **delayed onset.**

INDICATIONS & DOSAGES

➤ **To prevent or reduce nausea and vomiting from emetogenic cancer chemotherapy**

Adults: 1 to 2 mg/kg I.V. 30 minutes before chemotherapy; repeat every 2 hours for two doses, then every 3 hours for three doses.

➤ **To prevent or reduce post-operative nausea and vomiting**

Adults: 10 to 20 mg I.M. near end of surgical procedure; repeat every 4 to 6 hours, as needed.

➤ **To facilitate small-bowel intubation, to aid in radiologic examinations**

Adults and children older than age 14: 10 mg or 2 ml I.V. as a single dose over 1 to 2 minutes.

Children ages 6 to 14: 2.5 to 5 mg or 0.5 to 1 ml I.V.

Children younger than age 6: 0.1 mg/kg I.V.

➤ **Delayed gastric emptying secondary to diabetic gastroparesis**

Adults: 10 mg P.O. 30 minutes before each meal and at bedtime for mild symptoms. Give by slow I.V. infusion over 1 to 2 minutes 30 minutes before each meal and at bedtime for up to 10 days for severe symptoms; then P.O. dose may be started and continued for 2 to 8 weeks.

➤ **Gastroesophageal reflux disease**

Adults: 10 to 15 mg P.O. q.i.d., as needed, 30 minutes before meals and at bedtime.

Adjust-a-dose: For patients with creatinine clearance below 40 ml/minute, decrease dosage by half.

➤ **To improve lactation ◆**

Adults: 30 to 45 mg P.O. daily.

ADMINISTRATION

P.O.
● Give drug before each meal and at bedtime.

I.V.
● Drug is compatible with D₅W, normal saline solution for injection, dextrose 5% in half-normal saline solution, Ringer's injection, and lactated Ringer's injection. Normal saline solution is the preferred diluent; drug is most stable in this solution.

● Give doses of 10 mg or less by direct injection over 1 to 2 minutes. Dilute doses larger than 10 mg in 50 ml of compatible diluent, and infuse over at least 15 minutes. Monitor blood pressure closely.

● No need to protect drug from light if infusion mixture is given within 24 hours. If protected from light and refrigerated, it's stable for 48 hours.

● **Incompatibilities:** Allopurinol, ampicillin, amphotericin B, calcium gluconate, cefepime, chloramphenicol sodium succinate, cisplatin, doxorubicin liposomal, erythromycin lactobionate, fluorouracil, furosemide, methotrexate sodium, penicillin G potassium, propofol, sodium bicarbonate.

I.M.
● Inspect for particulate matter and discoloration. If either is present, don't use.

ACTION

Stimulates motility of upper GI tract, increases lower esophageal sphincter tone, and blocks dopamine receptors at the chemoreceptor trigger zone.

Route	Onset	Peak	Duration
P.O.	30–60 min	1–2 hr	1–2 hr
I.V.	1–3 min	Unknown	1–2 hr
I.M.	10–15 min	Unknown	1–2 hr

Half-life: 4 to 6 hours.

ADVERSE REACTIONS

CNS: *anxiety, drowsiness, dystonic reactions, fatigue, lassitude, restlessness, neuroleptic malignant syndrome, seizures, suicide ideation,* akathisia, confusion, depression, dizziness, extrapyramidal symptoms, fever, hallucinations, headache, insomnia, tardive dyskinesia.

CV: *bradycardia, supraventricular tachycardia,* hypotension, transient hypertension.

GI: bowel disorders, diarrhea, nausea.

GU: incontinence, urinary frequency.

Hematologic: *agranulocytosis, neutropenia.*

Skin: rash, urticaria.

Other: loss of libido, prolactin secretion.

INTERACTIONS
Drug-drug. *Anticholinergics, opioid analgesics:* May antagonize GI motility effects of metoclopramide. Use together cautiously.
CNS depressants: May cause additive CNS effects. Avoid using together.
Levodopa: Levodopa and metoclopramide have opposite effects on dopamine receptors. Avoid using together.
MAO inhibitors: May increase release of catecholamines in patients with hypertension. Use together cautiously.
Phenothiazines: May increase risk of extrapyramidal effects. Monitor patient closely.
Drug-lifestyle. *Alcohol use:* May cause additive CNS effects. Discourage use together.

EFFECTS ON LAB TEST RESULTS
● May increase liver function tests, aldosterone and prolactin levels.
● May decrease neutrophil and granulocyte counts.

CONTRAINDICATIONS & CAUTIONS
● Contraindicated in patients hypersensitive to drug and in those with pheochromocytoma or seizure disorders.
● Contraindicated in patients for whom stimulation of GI motility might be dangerous (those with hemorrhage, obstruction, or perforation).
● Use cautiously in patients with history of depression, Parkinson disease, or hypertension.

NURSING CONSIDERATIONS
● Monitor bowel sounds.
● Safety and effectiveness of drug haven't been established for therapy lasting longer than 12 weeks.
● *Alert:* Use 25 mg diphenhydramine I.V. to counteract extrapyramidal adverse effects from high doses.

PATIENT TEACHING
● Tell patient to avoid activities that require alertness for 2 hours after doses.
● Urge patient to report persistent or serious adverse reactions promptly.
● Advise patient not to drink alcohol during therapy.

ondansetron

ondansetron hydrochloride
on-DAN-sah-tron

Zofran, Zofran ODT

Pharmacologic class: selective serotonin (5-HT$_3$) receptor antagonist
Pregnancy risk category B

AVAILABLE FORMS
Injection: 2 mg/ml
Oral solution: 4 mg/5 ml
Orally disintegrating tablets (ODTs): 4 mg, 8 mg
Premixed injection: 32 mg/50 ml
Tablets: 4 mg, 8 mg, 24 mg

INDICATIONS & DOSAGES
➤ **To prevent nausea and vomiting from emetogenic chemotherapy**
Adults and children age 12 and older: 8 mg P.O. 30 minutes before chemotherapy. Then, 8 mg P.O. 8 hours after first dose. Then, 8 mg every 12 hours for 1 to 2 days. Or, a single dose of 32 mg by I.V. infusion over 15 minutes beginning 30 minutes before chemotherapy. Or, three doses of 0.15 mg/kg I.V. For 3 dose regimen, give first dose 30 minutes before chemotherapy and subsequent doses 4 and 8 hours after first dose. Infuse drug over 15 minutes.
Children ages 4 to 11: 4 mg P.O. 30 minutes before chemotherapy. Then, 4 mg P.O. 4 and 8 hours after first dose. Then, 4 mg every 8 hours for 1 to 2 days.
Infants and children ages 6 months to 11 years: Three doses of 0.15 mg/kg I.V. Give first dose 30 minutes before chemotherapy; give subsequent doses 4 and 8 hours after first dose. Infuse drug over 15 minutes.
➤ **To prevent postoperative nausea and vomiting**
Adults: 4 mg undiluted solution for injection I.M. or I.V. over 2 to 5 minutes immediately before induction of anesthesia. Or, 16 mg P.O. 1 hour before induction of anesthesia.
Children ages 1 month to 12 years who weigh more than 40 kg (88 lb): 4 mg I.V. as a single dose.

Children ages 1 month to 12 years who weigh 40 kg or less: 0.1 mg/kg I.V. as a single dose.

➤ **To prevent nausea and vomiting from radiation therapy in patients receiving total body irradiation, single high-dose fraction to abdomen, or daily fractions to abdomen**

Adults: 8 mg P.O. t.i.d. For patients receiving total body irradiation, give 8 mg P.O. 1 to 2 hours before each fraction of radiation therapy each day. For patients receiving single high-dose fraction radiation therapy to the abdomen, give 8 mg P.O. 1 to 2 hours before therapy, then every 8 hours for 1 to 2 days after completion of therapy. For patients receiving daily fractionated radiation therapy, give 8 mg P.O. 1 to 2 hours before therapy, then every 8 hours for each day therapy is given.

Adjust-a-dose: For patients with severe hepatic impairment, total daily dose shouldn't exceed 8 mg.

ADMINISTRATION
P.O.
● Open blister of ODT just before use by peeling backing off. Don't push ODT through foil blister.
I.V.
● If precipitate is noted in vial, shake vigorously until dissolved.
● Dilute drug in 50 ml of D$_5$W injection or normal saline solution for injection.
● Drug is stable for up to 48 hours after dilution in D$_5$W, 5% dextrose in half-normal saline solution for injection, 5% dextrose in normal saline solution, and 3% sodium chloride solution for injection.
● Infuse over 15 minutes.
● **Incompatibilities:** Acyclovir sodium, allopurinol, aminophylline, amphotericin B, ampicillin sodium, ampicillin sodium and sulbactam sodium, cefepime, cefoperazone, dacarbazine with doxorubicin, dexamethasone sodium phosphate, droperidol, fluorouracil, furosemide, ganciclovir, lorazepam, meropenem, methylprednisolone sodium succinate, piperacillin sodium, sargramostim, sodium bicarbonate.
I.M.
● Document injection site.
● If precipitate is noted in vial, shake vigorously until dissolved.

ACTION
May block 5-HT$_3$ in the CNS in the chemoreceptor trigger zone and in the peripheral nervous system on nerve terminals of the vagus nerve.

Route	Onset	Peak	Duration
P.O.	Unknown	Unknown	Unknown
I.V.	Immediate	10 min	Unknown
I.M.	Unknown	41 min	Unknown

Half-life: 4 hours.

ADVERSE REACTIONS
CNS: *dizziness, fatigue, headache, malaise, sedation,* extrapyramidal syndrome, fever, *pain.*
CV: *arrhythmias,* chest pain.
GI: *constipation, diarrhea,* abdominal pain, decreased appetite, xerostomia.
GU: gynecologic disorders, urine retention.
Respiratory: hypoxia.
Skin: pruritus, rash.
Other: chills, injection site reaction.

INTERACTIONS
Drug-drug. *Drugs such as cimetidine that alter hepatic drug-metabolizing enzymes, phenobarbital, rifampin:* May change pharmacokinetics of ondansetron. No need to adjust dosage.
Drug-herb. *Horehound:* May enhance serotoninergic effects. Discourage use together.

EFFECTS ON LAB TEST RESULTS
● May increase ALT and AST levels.

CONTRAINDICATIONS & CAUTIONS
● Contraindicated in patients hypersensitive to drug.
● Use cautiously in patients with hepatic impairment.

NURSING CONSIDERATIONS
● Monitor liver function test results. Don't exceed 8 mg in patients with hepatic impairment.
● *Look alike–sound alike:* Don't confuse Zofran with Zosyn, Zantac, or Zoloft.

PATIENT TEACHING
● Instruct patient to immediately report difficulty breathing after drug administration.

• Tell patient receiving drug I.V. to report discomfort at insertion site.
• For patient taking ODTs, tell him to open blister just before use by peeling backing off and not by pushing through foil blister, and tell him that taking it with liquid isn't required.

---

palonosetron hydrochloride
pal-on-OS-e-tron

Aloxi

Pharmacologic class: selective serotonin (5-HT$_3$) receptor antagonist
Pregnancy risk category B

AVAILABLE FORMS
Capsules: 0.5 mg
Injection: 0.25 mg in 5-ml, single-use vial

INDICATIONS & DOSAGES
➤ **To prevent acute nausea and vomiting from moderately or highly emetogenic chemotherapy or delayed nausea and vomiting from moderately emetogenic chemotherapy**
Adults: 0.25 mg given I.V. over 30 seconds, 30 minutes before chemotherapy starts. Drug is given on the first day of each cycle, no more than every 7 days. Or, one 0.5 mg capsule P.O. 1 hour prior to the start of chemotherapy.
✳ *NEW INDICATION:* **To prevent postoperative nausea and vomiting for up to 24 hours following surgery**
Adults: 0.075 mg I.V. over 10 seconds immediately before anesthesia induction.

ADMINISTRATION
P.O.
• May be given without regard to food.
I.V.
• Flush with normal saline solution before and after injection.
• Give by rapid I.V. injection through a peripheral or central I.V. line.
• **Incompatibilities:** Other I.V. drugs.

ACTION
Antagonizes 5-HT$_3$ receptors in the GI tract and brain, which inhibits emesis caused by chemotherapy.

Route	Onset	Peak	Duration
I.V.	30 min	Unknown	5 days

Half-life: 40 hours.

ADVERSE REACTIONS
CNS: anxiety, dizziness, headache, weakness.
CV: *bradycardia, nonsustained ventricular tachycardia,* hypotension.
GI: constipation, diarrhea.
Metabolic: *hyperkalemia.*

INTERACTIONS
Drug-drug. *Antiarrhythmics or other drugs that prolong the QTc interval, diuretics that induce electrolyte abnormalities, high-dose anthracycline:* May increase risk of prolonged QTc interval. Use together cautiously.

EFFECTS ON LAB TEST RESULTS
• May increase potassium level.

CONTRAINDICATIONS & CAUTIONS
• Contraindicated in patents hypersensitive to palonosetron or its ingredients.
• Use cautiously in patients hypersensitive to other 5-HT$_3$ antagonists, in those taking drugs that affect cardiac conduction, and in those with cardiac conduction abnormalities, hypokalemia, or hypomagnesemia.
• Safety and efficacy in children haven't been established.

NURSING CONSIDERATIONS
• Before giving this drug, check patient's potassium level.
• Consider adding corticosteroids to the antiemetic regimen, particularly for patients receiving highly emetogenic chemotherapy.
• Make sure patient has additional antiemetics to take for breakthrough nausea or vomiting.
• If patient has cardiac conduction abnormalities, check the ECG before giving drug.

Reactions may be *common,* uncommon, *life-threatening,* or COMMON AND LIFE-THREATENING.
Interaction may have a *rapid onset* or **delayed onset.**

PATIENT TEACHING
● Advise patient to take a different antiemetic for breakthrough nausea or vomiting, at the first sign of nausea rather than waiting until symptoms are severe.
● Urge patient with a history of cardiac conduction abnormalities to report any changes in drug regimen such as adding or stopping an antiarrhythmic.

---

prochlorperazine
proe-klor-PER-a-zeen

Compro

prochlorperazine edisylate

prochlorperazine maleate
Nu-Prochlor†

Pharmacologic class: dopamine antagonist
Pregnancy risk category C

AVAILABLE FORMS
prochlorperazine
Suppository: 25 mg
prochlorperazine edisylate
Injection: 5 mg/ml
Suppository: 25 mg
prochlorperazine maleate
Tablets: 5 mg, 10 mg, 25 mg

INDICATIONS & DOSAGES
➤ **To control preoperative nausea**
Adults: 5 to 10 mg I.M. 1 to 2 hours before induction of anesthesia; repeat once in 30 minutes, if needed. Or, 5 to 10 mg I.V. 15 to 30 minutes before induction of anesthesia; repeat once, if needed.
➤ **Severe nausea and vomiting**
Adults: 5 to 10 mg P.O., t.i.d. or q.i.d.; 25 mg P.R., b.i.d.; or 5 to 10 mg I.M., repeated every 3 to 4 hours, as needed. Maximum I.M. dose is 40 mg daily. Or, 2.5 to 10 mg I.V. at no more than 5 mg/minute.
Children who weigh 18 to 39 kg (39 to 86 lb): 2.5 mg P.O. or P.R., t.i.d.; or 5 mg P.O. or P.R., b.i.d. Maximum, 15 mg daily. Or, 0.132 mg/kg by deep I.M. injection. Control is usually achieved with one dose.

Children who weigh 14 to 17 kg (30 to 38 lb): 2.5 mg P.O. or P.R., b.i.d. or t.i.d. Maximum, 10 mg daily. Or, 0.132 mg/kg by deep I.M. injection. Control is usually achieved with one dose.
Children who weigh 9 to 13 kg (20 to 29 lb): 2.5 mg P.O. or P.R. once daily or b.i.d. Maximum, 7.5 mg daily. Or, 0.132 mg/kg by deep I.M. injection. Control is usually achieved with one dose.
➤ **To manage symptoms of psychotic disorders**
Adults and children age 12 and older: 5 to 10 mg P.O., t.i.d. or q.i.d.
Children ages 2 to 12: 2.5 mg P.O. or P.R., b.i.d. or t.i.d. Don't exceed 10 mg on day 1. Increase dosage gradually to maximum, if needed. In children ages 2 to 5, maximum is 20 mg daily. In children ages 6 to 12, maximum is 25 mg daily.
➤ **To manage symptoms of severe psychosis**
Adults and children age 12 and older: 10 to 20 mg I.M., repeated in 2 to 4 hours, if needed. Rarely, patients may receive 10 to 20 mg every 4 to 6 hours. Start oral therapy after symptoms are controlled.
Children ages 2 to 12: 0.13 mg/kg I.M.
➤ **Nonpsychotic anxiety**
Adults: 5 to 10 mg P.O., t.i.d., or q.i.d. Or, 15 mg extended-release capsule once daily. Or, 10 mg extended-release capsule every 12 hours. Don't exceed 20 mg daily, and don't give for longer than 12 weeks.

ADMINISTRATION
P.O.
● Dilute oral solution with tomato juice, fruit juice, milk, coffee, carbonated beverage, tea, water, or soup. Or, mix with pudding.
● To prevent contact dermatitis, avoid getting concentrate solution on hands or clothing.
I.V.
● Add 20 mg of drug per liter of D_5W and normal saline solution, 15 to 30 minutes before induction of anesthesia.
● Infuse slowly; rate shouldn't exceed 5 mg/minute. Maximum parenteral dose is 40 mg daily.
● To prevent contact dermatitis, avoid getting injection solution on hands or clothing.

• **Incompatibilities:** Aldesleukin, allopurinol, amifostine, aminophylline, amphotericin B, ampicillin sodium, aztreonam, calcium gluconate, chloramphenicol sodium succinate, chlorothiazide, dexamethasone sodium phosphate, dimenhydrinate, etoposide, filgrastim, fludarabine, foscarnet, furosemide, gemcitabine, heparin sodium, hydrocortisone sodium succinate, hydromorphone, ketorolac, solutions containing methylparabens, midazolam hydrochloride, morphine, penicillin G potassium, penicillin G sodium, pentobarbital, phenobarbital sodium, phenytoin sodium, piperacillin sodium and tazobactam sodium, solutions containing propylparabens, thiopental, vitamin B complex with C.

I.M.
• For I.M. use, inject deeply into upper outer quadrant of gluteal region.
• Don't give by subcutaneous route or mix in syringe with another drug.
• To prevent contact dermatitis, avoid getting injection solution on hands or clothing.
• Store in light-resistant container. Slight yellowing doesn't affect potency; discard extremely discolored solutions.

Rectal
• Protect from light.

ACTION

Acts on the chemoreceptor trigger zone to inhibit nausea and vomiting; in larger doses, it partially depresses vomiting center.

Route	Onset	Peak	Duration
P.O.	30–40 min	Unknown	3–12 hr
P.O. (extended-release)	30–40 min	Unknown	10–12 hr
I.V.	Unknown	Unknown	Unknown
I.M.	10–20 min	Unknown	3–4 hr
P.R.	1 hr	Unknown	3–4 hr

Half-life: Unknown.

ADVERSE REACTIONS

CNS: *extrapyramidal reactions,* dizziness, EEG changes, pseudoparkinsonism, sedation.
CV: *orthostatic hypotension,* ECG changes, tachycardia.
EENT: *blurred vision, ocular changes.*

GI: *constipation, dry mouth,* increased appetite.
GU: *urine retention,* dark urine, inhibited ejaculation, menstrual irregularities.
Hematologic: *agranulocytosis, transient leukopenia.*
Hepatic: cholestatic jaundice.
Metabolic: weight gain.
Skin: *mild photosensitivity reactions,* allergic reactions, exfoliative dermatitis.
Other: gynecomastia, hyperprolactinemia.

INTERACTIONS

Drug-drug. *Antacids:* May inhibit absorption of oral phenothiazines. Separate antacid and phenothiazine doses by at least 2 hours.
Anticholinergics, including antidepressants and antiparkinsonians: May increase anticholinergic activity and may aggravate parkinsonian symptoms. Use together cautiously.
Barbiturates: May decrease phenothiazine effect. Monitor patient for decreased antiemetic effect.
Drug-herb. *Dong quai, St. John's wort:* May increase risk of photosensitivity. Advise patient to avoid excessive sun exposure.
Kava: May increase risk of dystonic reactions. Discourage use together.
Drug-lifestyle. *Alcohol use:* May increase CNS depression, particularly psychomotor skills. Strongly discourage use together.

EFFECTS ON LAB TEST RESULTS

• May decrease WBC and granulocyte counts.
• May cause false-positive results for urinary porphyrins, urobilinogen, amylase, and 5-hydroxyindoleacetic acid, and false-positive results in urine pregnancy tests using human chorionic gonadotropin. May cause abnormal liver function test results.

CONTRAINDICATIONS & CAUTIONS

• Contraindicated in patients hypersensitive to phenothiazines and in patients with CNS depression, including those in a coma.
• Contraindicated during pediatric surgery, when using spinal or epidural anesthetic or adrenergic blockers, and in children younger than age 2.

Reactions may be *common,* uncommon, *life-threatening,* or COMMON AND LIFE-THREATENING.
Interaction may have a *rapid onset* or *delayed onset.*

• Use cautiously in patients with impaired CV function, glaucoma, seizure disorders, and Parkinson disease; in those who have been exposed to extreme heat; and in children with acute illness.

NURSING CONSIDERATIONS
• Watch for orthostatic hypotension, especially when giving drug I.V.
• Monitor CBC and liver function studies during long-term therapy.
• **Alert:** Use drug only when vomiting can't be controlled by other measures or when only a few doses are needed. If more than four doses are needed in 24 hours, notify prescriber.

PATIENT TEACHING
• Teach patient what to use to dilute oral solution.
• Advise patient to wear protective clothing when exposed to sunlight.
• Tell patient to call prescriber if more than four doses are needed within 24 hours.

scopolamine (hyoscine)
skoe-POL-a-meen

Transderm-Scop, Scopace

scopolamine butylbromide (hyoscine butylbromide)
Buscopan†

scopolamine hydrobromide (hyoscine hydrobromide)
Scopolamine Hydrobromide Injection

Pharmacologic class: belladonna alkaloid, antimuscarinic
Pregnancy risk category C

AVAILABLE FORMS
scopolamine
Tablets: 0.4 mg
Transdermal patch: 1.5 mg/2.5 cm² (1 mg/72 hours)
scopolamine butylbromide
Injection: 20 mg/ml
Suppositories: 10 mg†
Tablets: 10 mg†

scopolamine hydrobromide
Injection: 0.3 mg, 0.4 mg, 0.86 mg and 1 mg/ml

INDICATIONS & DOSAGES
➤ **Spastic states and post-encephalitic parkinsonism**
Adults: 0.4 to 0.8 mg P.O.; adjust dosage and frequency to individual needs.
➤ **Delirium, preanesthetic sedation, and obstetric amnesia with analgesics**
Adults: 0.3 to 0.65 mg I.V., I.M., or subcutaneously 30 to 60 minutes before or with other agents at the time of anesthesia. Dilute solution with sterile water for injection before giving I.V.
Children: 0.006 mg/kg I.V., I. M., or subcutaneously 30 to 60 minutes before or with other agents at the time of anesthesia. Maximum dose, 0.3 mg. Dilute solution with sterile water for injection before giving I.V.
➤ **To prevent nausea and vomiting from motion sickness**
Adults: One Transderm-Scop, formulated to deliver 1 mg scopolamine over 3 days, applied to the skin behind the ear at least 4 hours before antiemetic is needed. Or, 0.3 to 0.65 mg hydrobromide I.V., I.M. or subcutaneously, t.i.d. or q.i.d., as needed. Or, 0.25 to 0.8 mg P.O. 1 hour before exposure to motion. Further doses of 0.25 to 0.8 mg may be given t.i.d., as needed.
Children: 6 mcg/kg or 200 mcg/m² hydrobromide I.V., I.M., or subcutaneously.

ADMINISTRATION
P.O.
• Give 30 to 60 minutes before a meal, but may be given with food if stomach upset occurs.
I.V.
• For direct injection, dilute with sterile water and inject at ordered rate through patent I.V. line. Intermittent and continuous infusions aren't recommended.
• Protect I.V. solutions from freezing and light, and store at room temperature.
• **Incompatibilities:** Alkalies, anticholinergics, methohexital.
I.M.
• Rotate injection sites and document.

- Only use clear solution.

Transdermal
- Keep in foil wrapper until ready to use.
- Wear gloves to apply or remove patch.
- Place patch behind ear, on clean, dry, hairless area.
- If patch is dislodged, replace with a new one.

Rectal
- If suppository is too soft to insert, refrigerate for 30 minutes or hold wrapped suppository under cold running water.

Subcutaneous
- Rotate injection sites and document.
- Only use clear solution.

ACTION

Inhibits muscarinic actions of acetylcholine on autonomic effectors innervated by postganglionic cholinergic neurons. May affect neural pathways originating in the inner ear to inhibit nausea and vomiting.

Route	Onset	Peak	Duration
P.O., I.M.	1 hr	1–2 hr	4–6 hr
I.V.	10 min	50–80 min	2 hr
Trans-dermal	4 hr	Unknown	72 hr
P.R., Subcut.	Unknown	Unknown	Unknown

Half-life: 8 hours.

ADVERSE REACTIONS

CNS: disorientation, restlessness, irritability, dizziness, drowsiness, headache, confusion, hallucinations, delirium, impaired memory.
CV: *paradoxical bradycardia,* palpitations, tachycardia, flushing.
EENT: dilated pupils, blurred vision, photophobia, increased intraocular pressure, difficulty swallowing.
GI: *constipation, dry mouth, epigastric distress, nausea, vomiting.*
GU: urinary hesitancy, urine retention.
Respiratory: bronchial plugging, depressed respirations.
Skin: rash, dryness, contact dermatitis with transdermal patch.
Other: heat intolerance.

INTERACTIONS

Drug-drug. *Amantadine, antihistamines, antiparkinsonians, disopyramide,* *glutethimide, meperidine, phenothiazines, procainamide, quinidine, tricyclic antidepressants:* May increase risk of adverse CNS reactions. Avoid using together.
Antacids: May decrease oral absorption of anticholinergics. Separate doses by 2 or 3 hours.
Atenolol: May increase pharmacologic effects of atenolol. Monitor patient for adverse effects.
CNS depressants: May increase risk of CNS depression. Monitor patient closely.
Digoxin: May increase digoxin level. Monitor patient for digoxin toxicity.
Ketoconazole: May interfere with ketoconazole absorption. Separate doses by 2 or 3 hours.
Drug-herb. *Jaborandi tree:* May decrease drug effects. Discourage use together.
Pill-bearing spurge: May decrease drug effects. Inform patient of this interaction.
Squaw vine: May decrease metabolic breakdown. Discourage use together.
Drug-lifestyle. *Alcohol use:* May increase risk of CNS depression. Discourage use together.

EFFECTS ON LAB TEST RESULTS
None reported.

CONTRAINDICATIONS & CAUTIONS

- Contraindicated in patients with angle-closure glaucoma, obstructive uropathy, obstructive disease of the GI tract, asthma, chronic pulmonary disease, myasthenia gravis, paralytic ileus, intestinal atony, unstable CV status in acute hemorrhage, tachycardia from cardiac insufficiency, or toxic megacolon.
- Contraindicated in patients hypersensitive to belladonna or barbiturates.
- Use cautiously in patients with autonomic neuropathy, hyperthyroidism, coronary artery disease, arrhythmias, heart failure, hypertension, hiatal hernia with reflux esophagitis, hepatic or renal disease, known or suspected GI infection, or ulcerative colitis.
- Use cautiously in children.
- Use cautiously in patients in hot or humid environments; drug can cause heatstroke.

Reactions may be *common,* uncommon, *life-threatening,* or COMMON AND LIFE-THREATENING.
Interaction may have a *rapid onset* or **delayed onset.**

NURSING CONSIDERATIONS
● Raise side rails as a precaution because some patients become temporarily excited or disoriented and some develop amnesia or become drowsy. Reorient patient, as needed.
● Tolerance may develop when therapy is prolonged.
● Atropine-like toxicity may cause dose-related adverse reactions. Individual tolerance varies greatly.
● *Alert:* Overdose may cause curare-like effects such as respiratory paralysis. Keep emergency equipment available.

PATIENT TEACHING
● Advise patient to apply patch the night before a planned trip. Transdermal method releases a controlled therapeutic amount of drug. Transderm-Scop is effective if applied 2 or 3 hours before experiencing motion but is more effective if applied 12 hours before.
● Instruct patient to remove one patch before applying another.
● Instruct patient to wash and dry hands thoroughly before and after applying the transdermal patch (on dry skin behind the ear) and before touching the eye because pupil may dilate. Tell patient to discard patch after removing it and to wash application site thoroughly.
● Tell patient that if patch becomes displaced, he should remove it and apply another patch on a fresh skin site behind the ear.
● Alert patient to possible withdrawal signs or symptoms (nausea, vomiting, headache, dizziness) when transdermal system is used for longer than 72 hours.
● Advise patient that eyes may be more sensitive to light while wearing patch. Advise patient to wear sunglasses for comfort.
● Warn patient to avoid activities that require alertness until CNS effects of drug are known.
● Instruct patient to ask pharmacist for brochure that comes with the transdermal product.
● Urge patient to report urinary hesitancy or urine retention.

trimethobenzamide hydrochloride
trye-meth-oh-BEN-za-mide

Tigan

Pharmacologic class: anticholinergic
Pregnancy risk category C

AVAILABLE FORMS
Capsules: 300 mg
Injection: 100 mg/ml

INDICATIONS & DOSAGES
➤ **Nausea and vomiting**
Adults: 300 mg P.O. t.i.d. or q.i.d.; or 200 mg I.M. When treating postoperative nausea and vomiting, repeat I.M. dose after 1 hour.

ADMINISTRATION
P.O.
● Adjust dosage according to indication, severity, and patient response.
I.M.
● For I.M. use, reduce pain and local irritation by injecting deep into upper outer quadrant of gluteal region.

ACTION
Probably acts on the chemoreceptor trigger zone to inhibit nausea and vomiting.

Route	Onset	Peak	Duration
P.O.	10–20 min	Unknown	3–4 hr
I.M.	15–35 min	Unknown	2–3 hr

Half-life: 7 to 9 hours.

ADVERSE REACTIONS
CNS: *drowsiness,* **coma, seizures,** depression, disorientation, dizziness with large doses, headache, parkinsonian-like symptoms.
CV: hypotension.
EENT: blurred vision.
GI: diarrhea.
Hepatic: jaundice.
Musculoskeletal: muscle cramps.
Other: hypersensitivity reactions.

INTERACTIONS

Drug-drug. *CNS depressants:* May cause additive CNS depression. Avoid using together.

Drug-lifestyle. *Alcohol use:* May cause additive CNS depression. Discourage use together.

EFFECTS ON LAB TEST RESULTS

None reported.

CONTRAINDICATIONS & CAUTIONS

• Contraindicated in patients hypersensitive to drug. Suppositories contraindicated in patients hypersensitive to benzocaine hydrochloride or similar local anesthetic. I.M. form is contraindicated in children.

• Use cautiously in children because drug may be linked to Reye syndrome.

NURSING CONSIDERATIONS

• Drug may mask signs and symptoms of toxic drug overdose, intestinal obstruction, brain tumor, or other conditions.

• Drug may cause pain, stinging, burning, redness, or swelling at I.M. injection site. Withhold drug if skin hypersensitivity reaction occurs.

• *Look alike–sound alike:* Don't confuse Tigan with Ticar.

PATIENT TEACHING

• Advise patient of possible drowsiness and dizziness; caution against performing hazardous activities requiring alertness until CNS effects of drug are known.

61

Antiulceratives and reflux drugs

cimetidine
cimetidine hydrochloride
esomeprazole magnesium
esomeprazole sodium
famotidine
lansoprazole
misoprostol
omeprazole
omeprazole magnesium
pantoprazole sodium
rabeprazole sodium
ranitidine hydrochloride
sucralfate

cimetidine
sye-MET-i-deen

Tagamet, Tagamet HB ◇

cimetidine hydrochloride
Tagamet

Pharmacologic class: H$_2$ receptor antagonist
Pregnancy risk category B

AVAILABLE FORMS
Injection: 300 mg/2 ml, 300 mg in 50 ml normal saline solution, 300 mg/2 ml ADD-Vantage vial
Oral liquid: 300 mg/5 ml*
Tablets: 200 mg ◇ , 300 mg, 400 mg, 800 mg

INDICATIONS & DOSAGES
➤ **To prevent upper GI bleeding in critically ill patients**
Adults: 50 mg/hour by continuous I.V. infusion for up to 7 days; 25 mg/hour to patients with creatinine clearance below 30 ml/minute.
➤ **Short-term treatment of duodenal ulcer; maintenance therapy**
Adults and children age 16 and older: 800 mg P.O. at bedtime. Or, 400 mg P.O. b.i.d. or 300 mg q.i.d. (with meals and at bedtime). Or, 200 mg t.i.d. with a 400-mg bedtime dose. Treatment lasts 4 to 6 weeks unless endoscopy shows healing. For

maintenance therapy, 400 mg at bedtime. For parenteral therapy, 300 mg diluted to 20 ml total volume with normal saline solution or other compatible I.V. solution by I.V. push over at least 5 minutes every 6 to 8 hours; or 300 mg diluted in 50 ml D$_5$W or other compatible I.V. solution by I.V. infusion over 15 to 20 minutes every 6 to 8 hours; or 300 mg I.M. every 6 to 8 hours (no dilution needed). To increase dosage, give 300-mg doses more frequently to maximum of 2,400 mg daily, as needed. Or, 900 mg/day (37.5 mg/hour) I.V. diluted in 100 to 1,000 ml of compatible solution by continuous I.V. infusion.
➤ **Active benign gastric ulceration**
Adults: 800 mg P.O. at bedtime or 300 mg P.O. q.i.d. (with meals and at bedtime) for up to 8 weeks.
➤ **Pathologic hypersecretory conditions, such as Zollinger-Ellison syndrome, systemic mastocytosis, and multiple endocrine adenomas**
Adults and children age 16 and older: 300 mg P.O. q.i.d. with meals and at bedtime; adjusted to patient needs. Maximum oral amount, 2,400 mg daily.
For parenteral therapy, 300 mg diluted to 20 ml with normal saline solution or other compatible I.V. solution by I.V. push over at least 5 minutes every 6 to 8 hours; or 300 mg diluted in 50 ml D$_5$W or other compatible I.V. solution by I.V. infusion over 15 to 20 minutes every 6 to 8 hours. Increase parenteral dosage by giving 300-mg doses more frequently to maximum of 2,400 mg daily, as needed.
➤ **Gastroesophageal reflux disease with erosive esophagitis**
Adults: 800 mg P.O. b.i.d. or 400 mg q.i.d. before meals and at bedtime for up to 12 weeks.
Adjust-a-dose: In patients with renal impairment, decrease dosage to 300 mg P.O. or I.V. every 12 hours, increasing frequency to every 8 hours with caution. A renally impaired patient who also has liver dysfunction may require even further dose reduction.

➤ Heartburn

Adults: 200 mg Tagamet HB P.O. with water as symptoms occur, or as directed, up to b.i.d. For prevention, 200 mg right before or up to 30 minutes before eating food or drinking beverages that cause heartburn. Maximum, 400 mg daily. Drug shouldn't be taken daily for longer than 2 weeks.

ADMINISTRATION

P.O.
● Give dose at end of hemodialysis.
I.V.
● Drug is commonly added to total parenteral nutrition solutions, with or without fat emulsions.
● Dilute I.V. solutions with normal saline solution, D_5W, dextrose 10% in water (and combinations of these), lactated Ringer's solution, or 5% sodium bicarbonate injection.
● For direct injection, give over 5 minutes. Rapid I.V. injection may result in arrhythmias and hypotension.
● For intermittent infusion, give drug over at least 30 minutes to minimize risk of adverse cardiac effects.
● For continuous infusion, if giving a total volume of 250 ml over 24 hours or less, use an infusion pump.
● Give dose at end of hemodialysis.
● **Incompatibilities:** Allopurinol, amphotericin B, barbiturates, cefazolin, cefepime, chlorpromazine, combination atropine sulfate and pentobarbital sodium, indomethacin sodium trihydrate, pentobarbital sodium, secobarbital, warfarin. Don't dilute with sterile water for injection.
I.M.
● I.M. injection may be given undiluted.
● Give dose at end of hemodialysis.

ACTION

Competitively inhibits action of histamine on the H_2 receptor sites of parietal cells, decreasing gastric acid secretion.

Route	Onset	Peak	Duration
P.O.	Unknown	45–90 min	4–5 hr
I.V.	Unknown	Immediate	Unknown
I.M.	Unknown	Unknown	Unknown

Half-life: 2 hours.

ADVERSE REACTIONS

CNS: confusion, dizziness, hallucinations, headache, peripheral neuropathy, somnolence.
GI: mild and transient diarrhea.
GU: impotence.
Musculoskeletal: arthralgia, muscle pain.
Other: mild gynecomastia if used longer than 1 month, hypersensitivity reactions.

INTERACTIONS

Drug-drug. *Antacids:* May interfere with cimetidine absorption. Separate doses by at least 1 hour, if possible.
Carmustine: May enhance the bone marrow suppression effects of carmustine. Avoid use together.
Digoxin, fluconazole, indomethacin, iron salts, ketoconazole, tetracycline: May decrease drug absorption. Separate doses by at least 2 hours.
Fosphenytoin, phenytoin, some benzodiazepines, theophylline, warfarin: May inhibit hepatic microsomal enzyme metabolism of these drugs. Monitor drug level.
I.V. lidocaine: May decrease clearance of lidocaine, increasing the risk of toxicity. Consider using a different H_2 antagonist, if possible. Monitor lidocaine level closely.
Metoprolol, propranolol, timolol: May increase the effects of beta-blocker. Consider another H_2 agonist or decrease the dose of beta-blocker.
Procainamide: May increase procainamide level. Avoid this combination, if possible. Monitor procainamide level closely and adjust the dose as necessary.
Drug-herb. *Guarana:* May increase caffeine level or prolong caffeine half-life. Monitor patient.
Pennyroyal: May change rate at which herb's toxic metabolites form. Monitor patient.
Yerba maté: May decrease clearance of herb's methylxanthines and cause toxicity. Discourage use together.
Drug-lifestyle. *Alcohol use:* May increase blood alcohol level. Discourage use together.
Smoking: May decrease drug's ability to inhibit nocturnal gastric secretion. Urge patient to quit smoking.

Reactions may be *common*, uncommon, *life-threatening*, or COMMON AND LIFE-THREATENING.
Interaction may have a *rapid onset* or **delayed onset.**

EFFECTS ON LAB TEST RESULTS
• May increase ALT, AST, and creatinine levels.
• May antagonize pentagastrin's effect during gastric acid secretion tests. May cause false-negative results in skin tests using allergen extracts. May impair interpretation of Hemoccult and Gastroccult test results on gastric content aspirate because of FD&C blue dye number 2 used in tablets.

CONTRAINDICATIONS & CAUTIONS
• Contraindicated in patients hypersensitive to drug.
• Use cautiously in elderly or debilitated patients because they may be more susceptible to drug-induced confusion.

NURSING CONSIDERATIONS
• Assess patient for abdominal pain. Note blood in emesis, stool, or gastric aspirate.
• Identify tablet strength when obtaining a drug history.
• Schedule dose at end of hemodialysis treatment because hemodialysis reduces drug levels. Adjust dosage for patients with renal impairment.
• Wait at least 15 minutes after giving tablet before drawing sample for Hemoccult or Gastroccult test, and follow test manufacturer's instructions closely.
• Treatment of gastric ulcer isn't as effective as treatment of duodenal ulcer.
• *Look alike–sound alike:* Don't confuse cimetidine with simethicone.

PATIENT TEACHING
• Remind patient taking drug once daily to take it at bedtime and to take multiple daily doses with meals.
• Instruct patient taking Tagamet HB not to exceed recommended dosage and not to take daily for longer than 14 days.
• Warn patient receiving drug I.M. that injection may be painful.
• Urge patient to avoid cigarette smoking because it may increase gastric acid secretion and worsen disease.
• Advise patient to report abdominal pain, blood in stools or emesis, black tarry stools, and coffee-ground emesis.

esomeprazole magnesium
ess-oh-ME-pray-zol

Nexium

esomeprazole sodium
Nexium I.V.

Pharmacologic class: proton pump inhibitor
Pregnancy risk category B

AVAILABLE FORMS
esomeprazole magnesium
Capsules (delayed-release): 20 mg, 40 mg
Powder for suspension (delayed-release): 10 mg, 20 mg, 40 mg
esomeprazole sodium
Powder for injection: 20 mg, 40 mg single-use vials

INDICATIONS & DOSAGES
➤ **Gastroesophageal reflux disease (GERD); to heal erosive esophagitis**
Adults: 20 or 40 mg P.O. daily for 4 to 8 weeks. Maintenance dose for healing erosive esophagitis is 20 mg P.O. for up to 6 months.
Children and adolescents age 12 to 17: For GERD only, 20 or 40 mg P.O. once daily for up to 8 weeks.
Children age 1 to 11: For GERD only, 10 mg P.O. once daily for up to 8 weeks.
➤ **Symptomatic GERD**
Adults: 20 mg P.O. daily for 4 weeks. If symptoms are unresolved, may continue treatment for 4 more weeks.
➤ **Short-term therapy (up to 10 days) of GERD in patients with a history of erosive esophagitis who are unable to take drug orally**
Adult: Reconstitute 20 or 40 mg with 5 ml of D$_5$W, normal saline solution, or lactated Ringer's injection and give by I.V. bolus over 3 minutes. Or, further dilute to a total volume of 50 ml and give I.V. over 10 to 30 minutes. Switch patient to oral therapy as soon as he can tolerate it.
➤ **To heal erosive esophagitis**
Children age 1 to 11 who weigh less than 20 kg (44 lb): 10 mg P.O. once daily for up to 8 weeks.

Children age 1 to 11 who weigh 20 kg or more: 10 or 20 mg P.O. once daily for up to 8 weeks.

➤ **To reduce the risk of gastric ulcers in patients receiving continuous NSAID therapy**
Adults: 20 or 40 mg P.O. once daily for up to 6 months.

➤ **Long-term treatment of patho-logical hypersecretory conditions, including Zollinger-Ellison syndrome**
Adults: 40 mg P.O. b.i.d. Adjust dosage based on patient response.

➤ **To eliminate *Helicobacter pylori***
Adults: 40 mg esomeprazole magnesium P.O. daily, 1,000 mg amoxicillin P.O. b.i.d., and 500 mg clarithromycin P.O. b.i.d., given together for 10 days to reduce duodenal ulcer recurrence.
Adjust-a-dose: For patient with severe hepatic failure, maximum daily dose is 20 mg.

ADMINISTRATION
P.O.
● Give drug at least 1 hour before meals. If patient has difficulty swallowing the capsule, contents of the capsule can be emptied and mixed with 1 tablespoon of applesauce and swallowed (without chewing the enteric-coated pellets).
● If giving capsule via nasogastric (NG) tube, open capsule and empty the granules into a 60-ml syringe. Mix with 50 ml of water. Replace the plunger and shake vigorously for 15 seconds. Flush NG tube with additional water after use. Don't give if pellets have dissolved or disintegrated.
● For oral suspension, mix contents of packet with 1 tablespoon of water, and then let it sit for 2 to 3 minutes to thicken. The suspension can then be stirred and drunk within 30 minutes.
● To give oral suspension via NG tube, add 15 ml of water to a syringe, then add contents of packet. Shake syringe and leave for 2 to 3 minutes to thicken. Shake syringe again and inject through NG or gastric tube within 30 minutes.
I.V.
● Flush I.V. line with D_5W, normal saline solution, or lactated Ringer's injection before and after administration.

● Use reconstituted solution within 12 hours.
● Use admixture diluted with D_5W within 6 hours.
● If diluted with normal saline solution or lactated Ringer's injection, use within 12 hours.
● Store reconstituted solution and admixture at room temperature.
● **Incompatibilities:** Other I.V. drugs.

ACTION
Reduces gastric acid secretion and decreases gastric acidity.

Route	Onset	Peak	Duration
P.O.	Unknown	1½ hr	13–17 hr
I.V.	Unknown	Unknown	Unknown

Half-life: 1 to 1½ hours.

ADVERSE REACTIONS
CNS: headache.
GI: abdominal pain, constipation, diarrhea, dry mouth, flatulence, nausea, vomiting.

INTERACTIONS
Drug-drug. *Amoxicillin, clarithromycin:* May increase levels of esomeprazole. Monitor patient for toxicity.
Diazepam: May decrease clearance of diazepam. Monitor patient for diazepam toxicity.
Drugs metabolized by CYP2C19: May alter clearance of esomeprazole, especially in elderly patients or patients with hepatic insufficiency. Monitor patient for toxicity.
Warfarin: May prolong PT and INR, causing abnormal bleeding. Monitor the patient and his PT and INR.
Drug-food. *Any food:* May reduce drug level. Advise patient to take drug 1 hour before food.

EFFECTS ON LAB TEST RESULTS
None reported.

CONTRAINDICATIONS & CAUTIONS
● Contraindicated in patients hyper-sensitive to drug or components of esomeprazole or omeprazole (a drug similar to this one).
● Use cautiously in patients with hepatic insufficiency and in pregnant or breast-

---

Reactions may be *common*, uncommon, *life-threatening*, or COMMON AND LIFE-THREATENING.
Interaction may have a *rapid onset* or *delayed onset*.

feeding women. It's unknown if this drug appears in breast milk, but omeprazole does.

• Use cautiously in patients receiving continuous NSAID therapy who are at increased risk for gastric ulcers (those age 60 and older and those with a history of gastric ulcers).

NURSING CONSIDERATIONS

• Antacids can be used while taking drug, unless otherwise directed by prescriber.
• Monitor patient for rash or signs and symptoms of hypersensitivity. Monitor GI symptoms for improvement or worsening. Monitor liver function tests, especially in patients with preexisting hepatic disease.
• **Alert:** Amoxicillin may trigger anaphylaxis in patients with a history of penicillin hypersensitivity.
• Long-term therapy may cause atrophic gastritis.
• **Look alike–sound alike:** Don't confuse Nexium with Nexavar.

PATIENT TEACHING

• Instruct patient to take drug exactly as prescribed.
• Tell patient to take drug at least 1 hour before a meal.
• Advise patient that antacids can be used while taking drug unless otherwise directed by prescriber.
• Warn patient not to chew or crush drug pellets because this inactivates the drug.
• If patient has difficulty swallowing capsule, tell him to mix contents of capsule with 1 tablespoon of soft applesauce and swallow immediately.
• Advise patient to store capsules at room temperature in a tight container.
• Tell patient to inform prescriber of worsening signs and symptoms or pain.
• Instruct patient to alert prescriber if rash or other signs and symptoms of allergy occur.

famotidine
fa-MOE-ti-deen

Pepcid✒, Pepcid AC ◊

Pharmacologic class: H$_2$ receptor antagonist
Pregnancy risk category B

AVAILABLE FORMS
Gelcaps: 10 mg ◊
Injection: 10 mg/ml
Powder for oral suspension: 40 mg/5 ml after reconstitution
Premixed injection: 20 mg/50 ml in normal saline solution
Tablets: 10 mg ◊ , 20 mg ◊ , 40 mg
Tablets (chewable): 10 mg ◊

INDICATIONS & DOSAGES
➤ **Short-term treatment for duodenal ulcer**
Adults: For acute therapy, 40 mg P.O. once daily at bedtime or 20 mg P.O. b.i.d. Healing usually occurs within 4 weeks. For maintenance therapy, 20 mg P.O. once daily at bedtime.
➤ **Short-term treatment for benign gastric ulcer**
Adults: 40 mg P.O. daily at bedtime for 8 weeks.
Children ages 1 to 16: 0.5 mg/kg/day P.O. at bedtime or divided b.i.d., up to 40 mg daily.
➤ **Pathologic hypersecretory conditions (such as Zollinger-Ellison syndrome)**
Adults: 20 mg P.O. every 6 hours, up to 160 mg every 6 hours.
➤ **Hospitalized patients who can't take oral drug or who have intractable ulcers or hypersecretory conditions**
Adults: 20 mg I.V. every 12 hours.
➤ **Gastroesophageal reflux disease (GERD)**
Adults: 20 mg P.O. b.i.d. for up to 6 weeks. For esophagitis caused by GERD, 20 to 40 mg b.i.d. for up to 12 weeks.
Children ages 1 to 16: 1 mg/kg/day P.O. divided twice daily up to 40 mg b.i.d.
➤ **To prevent or treat heartburn**
Adults: 10 mg Pepcid AC P.O. 1 hour before meals to prevent symptoms, or

10 mg Pepcid AC P.O. with water when symptoms occur. Maximum daily dose is 20 mg. Drug shouldn't be taken daily for longer than 2 weeks.
Adjust-a-dose: For patients with creatinine clearance below 50 ml/minute, give half the dose, or increase dosing interval to every 36 to 48 hours.

ADMINISTRATION
P.O.
● Reconstitute and shake oral suspension before use.
● Store reconstituted oral suspension below 86° F (30° C). Discard after 30 days.
I.V.
● Compatible solutions include sterile water for injection, normal saline solution for injection, D_5W or dextrose 10% in water for injection, 5% sodium bicarbonate injection, and lactated Ringer's injection. Drug also can be added to total parenteral nutrition solutions.
● For direct injection, dilute 2 ml (20 mg) with compatible solution to a total volume of either 5 or 10 ml.
● Inject over at least 2 minutes.
● For intermittent infusion, dilute 20 mg (2 ml) in 100-ml compatible solution. The premixed 50-ml solution doesn't need further dilution.
● Infuse over 15 to 30 minutes.
● After dilution, solution is stable 48 hours at 36° to 46° F (2° to 8° C).
● **Incompatibilities:** Amphotericin B cholesterol complex, azithromycin, cefepime, piperacillin with tazobactam.

ACTION
Competitively inhibits action of histamine on the H_2 at receptor sites of parietal cells, decreasing gastric acid secretion.

Route	Onset	Peak	Duration
P.O.	1 hr	1–3 hr	12 hr
I.V.	1 hr	1–4 hr	12 hr

Half-life: 2½ to 3½ hours.

ADVERSE REACTIONS
CNS: *headache,* dizziness, fever, malaise, paresthesia, vertigo.
CV: flushing, palpitations.

EENT: orbital edema, tinnitus.
GI: anorexia, constipation, diarrhea, dry mouth, taste perversion.
Musculoskeletal: bone and muscle pain.
Skin: acne, dry skin.
Other: transient irritation at I.V. site.

INTERACTIONS
None significant.

EFFECTS ON LAB TEST RESULTS
● May increase BUN, creatinine, and liver enzyme levels.
● May cause false-negative results in skin tests using allergen extracts. May antagonize pentagastrin in gastric acid secretion tests.

CONTRAINDICATIONS & CAUTIONS
● Contraindicated in patients hypersensitive to drug.

NURSING CONSIDERATIONS
● Assess patient for abdominal pain.
● Look for blood in emesis, stool, or gastric aspirate.

PATIENT TEACHING
● Instruct patient in proper use of OTC product, if appropriate.
● Warn patient with phenylketonuria that Pepcid AC chewable tablets contain phenylalanine.
● Tell patient to take prescription drug with a snack, if desired.
● Remind patient that prescription drug is most effective if taken at bedtime. Tell patient taking 20 mg twice daily to take one dose at bedtime.
● Advise patient to limit use of prescription drug to no longer than 8 weeks, unless ordered by prescriber, and OTC drug to no longer than 2 weeks.
● With prescriber's knowledge, let patient take antacids together, especially at beginning of therapy when pain is severe.
● Urge patient to avoid cigarette smoking because it may increase gastric acid secretion and worsen disease.
● Advise patient to report abdominal pain, blood in stools or vomit, black tarry stools, or coffee-ground emesis.

Reactions may be *common,* uncommon, *life-threatening,* or COMMON AND LIFE-THREATENING.
Interaction may have a *rapid onset* or *delayed onset.*

lansoprazole
lanz-AH-pray-zol

Prevacid✐, Prevacid I.V., Prevacid
SoluTab

Pharmacologic class: proton pump
inhibitor
Pregnancy risk category B

AVAILABLE FORMS
Capsules (delayed-release): 15 mg, 30 mg
Oral suspension (delayed-release):
15 mg/packet, 30 mg/packet
*Orally disintegrating tablet (ODT)
(delayed-release):* 15 mg, 30 mg
Powder for injection: 30-mg single-use vial

INDICATIONS & DOSAGES
➤ **Short-term treatment of active
duodenal ulcer**
Adults: 15 mg P.O. daily before eating for
4 weeks.
➤ **Maintenance of healed duodenal
ulcers**
Adults: 15 mg P.O. daily.
➤ **Short-term treatment of active
benign gastric ulcer**
Adults: 30 mg P.O. once daily for up to
8 weeks.
➤ **Short-term I.V. therapy for
erosive esophagitis when patient
can't take P.O. drug**
Adults: 30 mg I.V. daily over 30 minutes
for up to 7 days. As soon as patient can
take drug orally, switch to P.O. form and
continue for 6 to 8 weeks.
➤ **Short-term treatment of erosive
esophagitis**
Adults: 30 mg P.O. daily before eating for
up to 8 weeks. If healing doesn't occur,
8 more weeks of therapy may be given.
Maintenance dosage for healing is 15 mg
P.O. daily.
Children ages 12 to 17: 30 mg P.O. once
daily for up to 8 weeks.
*Children ages 1 to 11 who weigh more
than 30 kg (66 lb):* 30 mg P.O. once daily
for up to 12 weeks. Increase dosage up
to 30 mg b.i.d. in patients who remain
symptomatic after 2 weeks.
*Children ages 1 to 11 who weigh 30 kg
or less:* 15 mg P.O. once daily for up to
12 weeks. Increase dosage up to 30 mg

b.i.d. in patients who remain symptomatic
after 2 weeks.
➤ **Long-term treatment of pathologic hypersecretory conditions,
including Zollinger-Ellison syndrome**
Adults: Initially, 60 mg P.O. once daily.
Increase dosage, as needed. Give daily
amounts above 120 mg in evenly divided
doses.
➤ ***Helicobacter pylori* eradication
to reduce risk of duodenal ulcer
recurrence**
Adults: For patients receiving dual therapy,
30 mg P.O. lansoprazole with 1 g P.O.
amoxicillin, each given t.i.d. for 14 days.
For patients receiving triple therapy,
30 mg P.O. lansoprazole with 1 g P.O.
amoxicillin and 500 mg P.O. clarithromycin, all given b.i.d. for 10 to 14 days.
➤ **Short-term treatment of
symptomatic gastroesophageal
reflux disease**
Adults: 15 mg P.O. once daily for up to
8 weeks.
Children ages 12 to 17: 15 mg P.O. once
daily for up to 8 weeks.
*Children ages 1 to 11 who weigh more
than 30 kg (66 lb):* 30 mg P.O. once daily
for up to 12 weeks. Dosage can be
increased up to 30 mg b.i.d. in patients
who remain symptomatic after 2 weeks.
*Children ages 1 to 11 who weigh 30 kg
or less:* 15 mg P.O. once daily for up to
12 weeks. Dosage can be increased up
to 30 mg b.i.d. in patients who remain
symptomatic after 2 weeks.
➤ **NSAID-related ulcer in patients
who continue NSAID use**
Adults: 30 mg P.O. daily for 8 weeks.
➤ **To reduce risk of NSAID-related
ulcer in patients with history of
gastric ulcer who need NSAIDs**
Adults: 15 mg P.O. daily for up to
12 weeks.

ADMINISTRATION
P.O.
● Contents of capsule can be mixed with
40 ml of apple juice in a syringe and given
within 3 to 5 minutes via a nasogastric
(NG) tube. Flush with additional apple
juice to give entire dose and maintain
patency of the tube.
● To give ODTs using an oral syringe,
dissolve a 15-mg tablet in 4 ml water or a

30-mg tablet in 10 ml water and give within 15 minutes. Refill syringe with about 2 ml (15-mg tablet) or 5 ml (30-mg tablet) of water, shake gently, and give any remaining contents.
• To give ODTs through an NG tube 8 French or larger, dissolve a 15-mg tablet in 4 ml water or a 30-mg tablet in 10 ml water and give within 15 minutes. Refill syringe with about 5 ml of water, shake gently, and flush the NG tube.
• ODTs contain 2.5 mg phenylalanine/15-mg tablet and 5.1 mg phenylalanine/30-mg tablet.

I.V.
• Reconstitute with 5 ml sterile water for injection only.
• Mix gently until powder is dissolved.
• Further dilute with 50 ml normal saline solution, lactated Ringer's injection or D_5W.
• Flush the I.V. line with normal saline solution, lactated Ringer's injection, or D_5W before giving infusion.
• Infuse over 30 minutes using the 1.2 micron inline filter provided with drug.
• The inline filter will remove any precipitate that forms when reconstituted solution comes in contact with I.V. solutions.
• Solutions mixed with normal saline or lactated Ringer's injection are stable at room temperature for 24 hours. Solutions mixed with D_5W are stable for 12 hours.
• Protect from light.
• **Incompatibilities:** Other I.V. drugs.

ACTION
Inhibits proton pump activity by binding to hydrogen-potassium adenosine triphosphates, located at secretory surface of gastric parietal cells; to suppress gastric acid secretions.

Route	Onset	Peak	Duration
P.O.	1–3 hr	Unknown	24 hr
I.V.	Unknown	Unknown	24 hr

Half-life: Less than 2 hours.

ADVERSE REACTIONS
GI: abdominal pain, diarrhea, nausea.

INTERACTIONS
Drug-drug. *Ampicillin esters, digoxin, iron salts, ketoconazole:* May inhibit

absorption of these drugs. Monitor patient closely.
Atazanavir: May reduce GI absorption of atazanavir, reducing antiviral activity. Don't use together.
Clarithromycin: May increase lansoprazole levels and adverse effects. Monitor patient.
Sucralfate: May cause delayed lansoprazole absorption. Give lansoprazole at least 30 minutes before sucralfate.
Theophylline: May mildly increase theophylline clearance. Adjust theophylline dosage when lansoprazole is started or stopped. Use together cautiously.
Drug-herb. *Male fern:* May inactivate herb. Discourage use together.
St. John's wort: May increase risk of sun sensitivity. Advise patient to avoid excessive sunlight exposure.
Drug-food. *Food:* May decrease rate and extent of GI absorption. Advise patient to take before meals.

EFFECTS ON LAB TEST RESULTS
None reported.

CONTRAINDICATIONS & CAUTIONS
• Contraindicated in patients hypersensitive to drug.
• It's unknown if drug appears in breast milk. Breast-feeding women should either stop breast-feeding or stop drug.

NURSING CONSIDERATIONS
• Patients with severe liver disease may need dosage adjustment, but don't adjust dosage for elderly patients or those with renal insufficiency.
• Just because symptoms respond to therapy, gastric malignancy shouldn't be ruled out.
• **Alert:** Amoxicillin may trigger anaphylaxis in patients with a history of penicillin hypersensitivity.
• **Look alike–sound alike:** Don't confuse Prevacid with Pepcid, Prilosec, or Prevpac.

PATIENT TEACHING
• For best effect, instruct patient to take drug no more than 30 minutes before eating.
• Tell patient he may mix the capsule's contents with a small amount (about 2 ounces) of apple, cranberry, grape, orange, pineapple, prune, tomato, or

---
Reactions may be *common*, uncommon, **life-threatening**, or COMMON AND LIFE-THREATENING.
Interaction may have a *rapid onset* or **delayed onset.**

vegetable juice. The patient must drink the mixture within 30 minutes. To ensure complete delivery of the dose, the patient should fill the glass two or more times with juice and swallow the contents immediately.
• Contents of capsule can be mixed with 1 tablespoon of applesauce, Ensure, pudding, cottage cheese, yogurt, or strained pears and swallowed immediately. The granules shouldn't be chewed or crushed.
• For the oral suspension, instruct patient to empty packet contents into 30 ml of water, stir well, and drink immediately. Tell him not to crush or chew the granules and not to take with other liquids or food. If any material remains after drinking, tell him to add more water, stir, and drink immediately.
• Tell patient taking ODTs to allow tablet to dissolve on tongue until all particles can be swallowed.

---

misoprostol
mye-soe-PROST-ole

Cytotec

Pharmacologic class: prostaglandin E$_1$ analogue
Pregnancy risk category X

AVAILABLE FORMS
Tablets: 100 mcg, 200 mcg

INDICATIONS & DOSAGES
➤ **To prevent NSAID-induced gastric ulcer in elderly or debilitated patients at high risk for complications from gastric ulcer and in patients with history of NSAID-induced ulcer**
Adults: 200 mcg P.O. q.i.d. with food; if not tolerated, decrease to 100 mcg P.O. q.i.d. Give dosage for duration of NSAID therapy.

ADMINISTRATION
P.O.
• Give drug with food.
• Give last dose at bedtime.

ACTION
A synthetic prostaglandin E$_1$ analogue that replaces gastric prostaglandins depleted by NSAID therapy, decreases basal and stimulated gastric acid secretion, and increases gastric mucus and bicarbonate production.

Route	Onset	Peak	Duration
P.O.	30 min	60–90 min	3 hr

Half-life: 20 to 40 minutes.

ADVERSE REACTIONS
CNS: headache.
GI: *abdominal pain, diarrhea,* constipation, dyspepsia, flatulence, nausea, vomiting.
GU: cramps, dysmenorrhea, hypermenorrhea, menstrual disorders, postmenopausal vaginal bleeding, spotting.

INTERACTIONS
Drug-food. *Any food:* May decrease absorption rate of drug. However, manufacturer recommends that patient take drug with food.

EFFECTS ON LAB TEST RESULTS
None reported.

CONTRAINDICATIONS & CAUTIONS
• Contraindicated in those allergic to prostaglandins, pregnant women, or those who are breast-feeding.
• Use with caution in patients with inflammatory bowel disease.

NURSING CONSIDERATIONS
■ **Black Box Warning** Take special precautions to prevent use of drug during pregnancy. Uterine rupture is linked to certain risk factors, including later trimester pregnancies, higher doses of the drug, prior cesarean delivery or uterine surgery, or five or more previous pregnancies. Make sure woman understands dangers of drug to herself and her fetus and that she receives both oral and written warnings about these dangers. Also, make sure she can comply with effective contraception and that the result of a pregnancy test performed within 2 weeks of starting therapy is negative. ■
• Drug causes modest decrease in basal pepsin secretion.
• *Look alike–sound alike:* Don't confuse misoprostol with mifepristone.

PATIENT TEACHING

• Instruct patient not to share drug.

■ **Black Box Warning** Remind pregnant woman that drug may cause miscarriage, often with potentially life-threatening bleeding. ■

■ **Black Box Warning** Advise woman not to begin therapy until second or third day of next normal menstrual period. ■

• Advise patient to take drug as prescribed for duration of NSAID therapy.

• Tell patient that diarrhea usually occurs early in the course of therapy and is usually self-limiting. Taking drug with food helps minimize the diarrhea.

omeprazole
oh-ME-pray-zole

Losec†, Prilosec◊, Zegerid

omeprazole magnesium
Prilosec OTC◊

Pharmacologic class: proton pump inhibitor
Pregnancy risk category C

AVAILABLE FORMS

Capsules (delayed-release): 10 mg, 20 mg, 40 mg
Powder for oral suspension: 20 mg/packet, 40 mg/packet
Tablets (delayed-release): 20 mg ◊

INDICATIONS & DOSAGES

➤ **Symptomatic gastroesophageal reflux disease (GERD) without esophageal lesions**
Adults: 20 mg P.O., as delayed-release or oral suspension, daily for 4 weeks for patients who respond poorly to customary medical treatment, usually including an adequate course of H$_2$-receptor antagonists.
Children ages 2 to 16 weighing 20 kg (44 lb) or more: 20 mg P.O. daily.
Children ages 2 to 16 weighing less than 20 kg: 10 mg P.O. daily.
➤ **Erosive esophagitis and accompanying symptoms caused by GERD**
Adults: 20 mg P.O. daily for 4 to 8 weeks.

Children ages 2 to 16 weighing 20 kg or more: 20 mg P.O. daily.
Children ages 2 to 16 weighing less than 20 kg: 10 mg P.O. daily.
➤ **Maintenance of healing erosive esophagitis**
Adults: 20 mg P.O., as delayed-release or oral suspension, daily.
Children ages 2 to 16 weighing 20 kg or more: 20 mg P.O. daily.
Children ages 2 to 16 weighing less than 20 kg: 10 mg P.O. daily.
➤ **Pathologic hypersecretory conditions (such as Zollinger-Ellison syndrome)**
Adults: Initially, 60 mg P.O. daily; adjust dosage based on patient response. If daily dose exceeds 80 mg, give in divided doses. Doses up to 120 mg t.i.d. have been given. Continue therapy as long as clinically indicated.
➤ **Duodenal ulcer (short-term treatment)**
Adults: 20 mg P.O., as delayed-release or oral suspension, daily for 4 to 8 weeks.
➤ *Helicobacter pylori* **infection and duodenal ulcer disease, to eradicate** *H. pylori* **with clarithromycin (dual therapy)**
Adults: 40 mg P.O. every morning with clarithromycin 500 mg P.O. t.i.d. for 14 days. For patients with an ulcer at start of therapy, give another 14 days of omeprazole 20 mg P.O. once daily.
➤ *H. pylori* **infection and duodenal ulcer disease, to eradicate** *H. pylori* **with clarithromycin and amoxicillin (triple therapy)**
Adults: 20 mg P.O. with clarithromycin 500 mg P.O. and amoxicillin 1,000 mg P.O., each given b.i.d. for 10 days. For patients with an ulcer at start of therapy, give another 18 days of omeprazole 20 mg P.O. once daily.
➤ **Short-term treatment of active benign gastric ulcer**
Adults: 40 mg P.O. once daily for 4 to 8 weeks.
➤ **Frequent heartburn (2 or more days a week)**
Adults: 20 mg P.O. Prilosec OTC once daily before breakfast for 14 days.
May repeat the 14-day course every 4 months.

Reactions may be *common*, uncommon, *life-threatening*, or COMMON AND LIFE-THREATENING.
Interaction may have a *rapid onset* or **delayed onset.**

ADMINISTRATION

P.O.
- Don't open or crush tablets or capsules.
- Empty contents of Zegerid packet into a small cup containing 2 tablespoons of water. Stir contents and give to patient to drink immediately. Refill cup with water and repeat.
- Give drug 30 minutes before meals. Zegerid powder for oral suspension should be taken on an empty stomach at least 1 hour before a meal.

ACTION
Inhibits proton pump activity by binding to hydrogen-potassium adenosine triphosphatase, located at secretory surface of gastric parietal cells, to suppress gastric acid secretion.

Route	Onset	Peak	Duration
P.O.	1 hr	30 min–2 hr	< 3 days

Half-life: 30 to 60 minutes.

ADVERSE REACTIONS
CNS: asthenia, dizziness, headache.
GI: abdominal pain, constipation, diarrhea, flatulence, nausea, vomiting.
Musculoskeletal: back pain.
Respiratory: cough, upper respiratory tract infection.
Skin: rash.

INTERACTIONS
Drug-drug. *Ampicillin esters, iron derivatives, ketoconazole:* May cause poor bioavailability of these drugs because they need a low gastric pH for optimal absorption. Avoid using together.
Diazepam, fosphenytoin, phenytoin, warfarin: May decrease hepatic clearance, possibly leading to increased levels of these drugs. Monitor drug levels.
Drug-herb. *Ginkgo biloba:* May decrease therapeutic effects of drug. Discourage use together.
Male fern: May inactivate herb. Discourage use together.
Pennyroyal: May change rate at which herb's toxic metabolites form. Ask patient about the use of herb, and discourage use together.
St. John's wort: May increase risk of sun sensitivity. Advise patient to avoid excessive sunlight exposure.

EFFECTS ON LAB TEST RESULTS
None reported.

CONTRAINDICATIONS & CAUTIONS
- Contraindicated in patients hypersensitive to drug or its components.
- Zegerid is contraindicated in patients with metabolic alkalosis and hypocalcemia.
- Use cautiously in patients with Bartter syndrome, hypokalemia, and respiratory alkalosis.
- Long-term administration of bicarbonate with calcium or milk can cause milk-alkali syndrome.

NURSING CONSIDERATIONS
- Dosage adjustments may be necessary in Asians and patients with hepatic impairment.
- *Alert:* Amoxicillin may trigger anaphylaxis in patients with a history of penicillin hypersensitivity.
- Drug increases its own bioavailability with repeated doses. Drug is unstable in gastric acid; less drug is lost to hydrolysis because drug increases gastric pH.
- Zegerid contains 460 mg sodium per dose in the form of sodium bicarbonate.
- Gastrin level rises in most patients during the first 2 weeks of therapy.
- *Look alike–sound alike:* Don't confuse Prilosec with Prozac, Prilocaine, or Prinivil.

PATIENT TEACHING
- Tell patient to swallow tablets or capsules whole and not to open, crush, or chew them.
- Warn patients that Zegerid contains 460 mg sodium bicarbonate per dose. Those following a sodium-restricted diet should be cautious.
- Tell patient to empty contents of Zegerid packet into a small cup containing 2 tablespoons of water. Instruct him not to use other liquids or foods. Stir contents and drink immediately. Refill cup with water and drink.
- Instruct patient to take drug 30 minutes before meals. Zegerid powder for oral suspension should be taken on an empty stomach at least 1 hour before a meal.
- Caution patient to avoid hazardous activities if he gets dizzy.

• Advise patient that Prilosec OTC isn't intended to treat infrequent heartburn (one episode of heartburn a week or less), or for those who want immediate relief of heartburn.

• Inform patient that Prilosec OTC may take 1 to 4 days for full effect, although some patients may get complete relief of symptoms within 24 hours.

---

pantoprazole sodium
pan-TOE-pray-zol

Protonix, Protonix I.V.

Pharmacologic class: proton pump inhibitor
Pregnancy risk category B

AVAILABLE FORMS
Injection: 40 mg/vial
Suspension (delayed-release): 40 mg
Tablet (delayed-release): 20 mg, 40 mg

INDICATIONS & DOSAGES
➤ **Erosive esophagitis with gastro-esophageal reflux disease (GERD)**
Adults: 40 mg P.O. once daily for up to 8 weeks. For patients who haven't healed after 8 weeks of treatment, another 8-week course may be considered.
➤ **Short-term treatment of GERD in patients who can't take delayed-release tablets orally**
Adults: 40 mg I.V. daily for 7 to 10 days.
➤ **Short-term treatment of GERD linked to history of erosive esophagitis**
Adults: 40 mg I.V. once daily for 7 to 10 days. Switch to P.O. form as soon as patient is able to take orally.
➤ **Long-term maintenance of healing erosive esophagitis and reduction in relapse rates of daytime and night-time heartburn symptoms in patients with GERD**
Adults: 40 mg P.O. once daily.
➤ **Short-term treatment of patho-logic hypersecretion caused by Zollinger-Ellison syndrome or other neoplastic conditions**
Adults: Individualize dosage. Usual dose is 80 mg I.V. every 12 hours for no more than 6 days. For those needing a higher dose, 80 mg every 8 hours is expected to maintain acid output below 10 mEq/hour. Maximum daily dose is 240 mg/day.
➤ **Long-term treatment of pathologic hypersecretory conditions, including Zollinger-Ellison syndrome**
Adults: Individualize dosage. Usual start-ing dose is 40 mg P.O. b.i.d. Adjust dose to a maximum of 240 mg/day. Stop I.V. drug when P.O. drug is warranted.

ADMINISTRATION
P.O.
• Give drug without regard for food.
• Don't crush or split tablets.
• Give delayed-release suspension in apple sauce or apple juice 30 minutes prior to a meal.
• Do not split, chew, or crush granules for delayed-release oral suspension.
I.V.
• Safety and effectiveness of the I.V. form to start therapy for GERD are unknown.
• Reconstitute each vial with 10 ml of normal saline solution.
• Compatible diluents for infusion include normal saline solution, D_5W, or lactated Ringer's solution for injection.
• For patients with GERD, further dilute with 100 ml of diluent to yield 0.4 mg/ml.
• For patients with hypersecretion, combine two reconstituted vials and further dilute with 80 ml of diluent to a total volume of 100 ml, to yield 0.8 mg/ml.
• Infuse diluted solutions over 15 minutes at a rate of about 7 ml/minute.
• For a 2-minute infusion, give the recon-stituted vials (final yield of about 4 mg/ml) over at least 2 minutes.
• The reconstituted solution may be stored for up to 2 hours and the diluted solutions for up to 22 hours at room temperature.
• **Incompatibilities:** Midazolam, zinc-containing products or solutions. Don't give another infusion simultaneously through the same line.

ACTION
Inhibits proton pump activity by binding to hydrogen-potassium adenosine triphos-phatase, located at secretory surface of gastric parietal cells, to suppress gastric acid secretion.

Reactions may be *common*, uncommon, *life-threatening*, or COMMON AND LIFE-THREATENING.
Interaction may have a *rapid onset* or *delayed onset*.

Route	Onset	Peak	Duration
P.O.	Unknown	2½ hr	> 24 hr
I.V.	15–30 min	Unknown	24 hr

Half-life: 1 hour.

ADVERSE REACTIONS
CNS: anxiety, asthenia, dizziness, headache, insomnia, migraine, pain.
CV: chest pain.
EENT: pharyngitis, rhinitis, sinusitis.
GI: abdominal pain, constipation, diarrhea, dyspepsia, eructation, flatulence, gastroenteritis, GI disorder, nausea, rectal disorder, vomiting.
GU: urinary frequency, UTI.
Metabolic: hyperglycemia, hyperlipemia.
Musculoskeletal: arthralgia, back pain, hypertonia, neck pain.
Respiratory: bronchitis, dyspnea, increased cough, upper respiratory tract infection.
Skin: rash.
Other: flulike syndrome, infection.

INTERACTIONS
Drug-drug. *Ampicillin esters, iron salts, ketoconazole:* May decrease absorption of these drugs. Monitor patient closely and separate doses.
Drug-herb. *St. John's wort:* May increase risk of sunburn. Advise patient to avoid excessive sunlight exposure.
Drug-lifestyle. *Sunlight:* May increase risk of sunburn. Advise patient to avoid excessive sunlight exposure.

EFFECTS ON LAB TEST RESULTS
• May increase glucose and lipid levels.
• May increase liver function test result values.

CONTRAINDICATIONS & CAUTIONS
• Contraindicated in patients hypersensitive to any component of the formulation.

NURSING CONSIDERATIONS
• Symptomatic response to therapy doesn't preclude the presence of gastric malignancy.
• *Look alike–sound alike:* Don't confuse Protonix with Prilosec, Prozac, or Prevacid.

PATIENT TEACHING
• Instruct patient to take exactly as prescribed and at about the same time every day.
• Advise patient that drug can be taken without regard to meals.
• Tell patient to swallow tablet whole and not to crush, split, or chew it.
• Tell patient that antacids don't affect drug absorption.

rabeprazole sodium
rah-BEH-pray-zol

Aciphex

Pharmacologic class: proton pump inhibitor
Pregnancy risk category B

AVAILABLE FORMS
Tablets (delayed-release): 20 mg

INDICATIONS & DOSAGES
➤ **Healing of erosive or ulcerative gastroesophageal reflux disease (GERD)**
Adults: 20 mg P.O. daily for 4 to 8 weeks. Additional 8-week course may be considered, if needed.
➤ **Maintenance of healing of erosive or ulcerative GERD**
Adults: 20 mg P.O. daily.
➤ **Healing of duodenal ulcers**
Adults: 20 mg P.O. daily after morning meal for up to 4 weeks.
➤ **Pathologic hypersecretory conditions, including Zollinger-Ellison syndrome**
Adults: 60 mg P.O. daily; may be increased, as needed, to 100 mg P.O. daily or 60 mg P.O. b.i.d.
➤ **Symptomatic GERD, including daytime and nighttime heartburn**
Adults: 20 mg P.O. daily for 4 weeks. Additional 4-week course may be considered, if needed.
Children age 12 and older: 20 mg P.O. daily for up to 8 weeks.
➤ *Helicobacter pylori* **eradication, to reduce the risk of duodenal ulcer recurrence**
Adults: 20 mg P.O. b.i.d., combined with amoxicillin 1,000 mg P.O. b.i.d.

and clarithromycin 500 mg P.O. b.i.d., for 7 days.

ADMINISTRATION
P.O.
- Don't crush or split tablets.
- Give drug without regard for food.

ACTION
Blocks proton pump activity and gastric acid secretion by inhibiting gastric hydrogen-potassium adenosine triphosphatase (an enzyme) at secretory surface of gastric parietal cells.

Route	Onset	Peak	Duration
P.O.	< 1 hr	2–5 hr	> 24 hr

Half-life: 1 to 2 hours.

ADVERSE REACTIONS
CNS: headache.

INTERACTIONS
Drug-drug. *Clarithromycin:* May increase rabeprazole level. Monitor patient closely.
Cyclosporine: May inhibit cyclosporine metabolism. Use together cautiously.
Digoxin, ketoconazole, other gastric pH-dependent drugs: May decrease or increase drug absorption at increased pH values. Monitor patient closely.
Warfarin: May inhibit warfarin metabolism. Monitor PT and INR.

EFFECTS ON LAB TEST RESULTS
None reported.

CONTRAINDICATIONS & CAUTIONS
- Contraindicated in patients hypersensitive to drug, other benzimidazoles (lansoprazole, omeprazole), or components of these formulations.
- In *H. pylori* eradication, clarithromycin is contraindicated in pregnant women, patients hypersensitive to macrolides, and those taking pimozide; amoxicillin is contraindicated in patients hypersensitive to penicillin.
- Use cautiously in patients with severe hepatic impairment.

NURSING CONSIDERATIONS
- Consider additional courses of therapy if duodenal ulcer or GERD

isn't healed after first course of therapy.
- If *H. pylori* eradication is unsuccessful, do susceptibility testing. If patient is resistant to clarithromycin or susceptibility testing isn't possible, expect to start therapy using a different antimicrobial.
- *Alert:* Amoxicillin may trigger anaphylaxis in patients with a history of penicillin hypersensitivity.
- Symptomatic response to therapy doesn't preclude presence of gastric malignancy.
- *Alert:* Patients treated for *H. pylori* eradication have developed pseudomembranous colitis with nearly all antibiotics, including clarithromycin and amoxicillin. Monitor patient closely.

PATIENT TEACHING
- Explain importance of taking drug exactly as prescribed.
- Advise patient to swallow delayed-release tablet whole and not to crush, chew, or split.
- Inform patient that drug may be taken without regard to meals.

---

ranitidine hydrochloride
ra-NYE-te-deen

Nu-Ranit†, Zantac*✦, Zantac-C†, Zantac 75◇, Zantac 150◇, Zantac EFFERdose Tablets, Zantac 300

Pharmacologic class: H$_2$ receptor antagonist
Pregnancy risk category B

AVAILABLE FORMS
Granules (effervescent): 150 mg
Infusion: 1 mg/ml in 50-ml containers
Injection: 25 mg/ml
Syrup: 15 mg/ml*
Tablets: 75 mg◇, 150 mg◇, 300 mg
Tablets (effervescent): 25 mg, 150 mg

INDICATIONS & DOSAGES
➤ **Active duodenal and gastric ulcer**
Adults: 150 mg P.O. b.i.d. or 300 mg daily at bedtime. Or, 50 mg I.V. or I.M. every

---

Reactions may be *common*, uncommon, *life-threatening*, or COMMON AND LIFE-THREATENING.
Interaction may have a *rapid onset* or **delayed onset**.

6 to 8 hours. Maximum daily I.V. dose, 400 mg. Or, 150 mg by continuous infusion at 6.25 mg/hour over 24 hours.
Children ages 1 month to 16 years: For duodenal and gastric ulcers only, 2 to 4 mg/kg P.O. b.i.d., up to 300 mg/day.

➤ **Maintenance therapy for duodenal or gastric ulcer**
Adults: 150 mg P.O. at bedtime.
Children ages 1 month to 16 years: 2 to 4 mg/kg P.O. daily, up to 150 mg daily.

➤ **Pathologic hypersecretory conditions, such as Zollinger-Ellison syndrome (ZES)**
Adults: 150 mg P.O. b.i.d.; doses up to 6 g or more frequent intervals may be needed in patients with severe disease. Or, infuse continuously at 1 mg/kg/hour. After 4 hours, if patient remains symptomatic or gastric acid output is greater than 10 mEq/hour, increase dose in increments of 0.5 mg/kg/hour and recheck gastric acid output. Doses up to 2.5 mg/kg/hour and infusion rates up to 220 mg/hour have been used.

➤ **Gastroesophageal reflux disease**
Adults: 150 mg P.O. b.i.d.
Children ages 1 month to 16 years: 5 to 10 mg/kg P.O. daily given as two divided doses.

➤ **Erosive esophagitis**
Adults: 150 mg P.O. q.i.d. Maintenance dosage is 150 mg P.O. b.i.d.
Children ages 1 month to 16 years: 5 to 10 mg/kg P.O. daily given as two divided doses.

➤ **Heartburn**
Adults and children age 12 and older: 75 mg of Zantac 75 P.O. as symptoms occur, up to 150 mg daily, not to exceed 2 weeks of continuous treatment.

Adjust-a-dose: For patients with creatinine clearance below 50 ml/minute, 150 mg P.O. every 24 hours or 50 mg I.V. every 18 to 24 hours.

ADMINISTRATION
P.O.
• Give once-daily dose at bedtime.
• Dissolve 150-mg EFFERdose tablet in 6 to 8 ounces of water.
• Dissolve 25-mg EFFERdose tablet in at least 5 ml of water and give with a dosing cup, medicine dropper, or oral syringe.

I.V.
• To prepare I.V. injection, dilute 2 ml (50 mg) ranitidine with compatible I.V. solution to a total volume of 20 ml, and inject over at least 5 minutes. Compatible solutions include sterile water for injection, normal saline solution for injection, D_5W, or lactated Ringer's injection.
• To give drug by intermittent I.V. infusion, dilute 50 mg (2 ml) in 100 ml compatible solution and infuse at a rate of 5 to 7 ml/minute. The premixed solution is 50 ml and doesn't need further dilution. Infuse over 15 to 20 minutes.
• For continuous infusion to treat active duodenal or gastric ulcer, dilute 150 mg in 250 ml of D_5W. For hypersecretory conditions such as ZES, dilute with D_5W or other compatible solution to no more than 2.5 mg/ml.
• After dilution, solution is stable for 48 hours at room temperature.
• Store I.V. injection at 39° to 86° F (4° to 30° C). Store premixed containers at 36° to 77° F (2° to 25° C).
• **Incompatibilities:** Amphotericin B, atracurium, cefazolin, cefoxitin, ceftazidime, cefuroxime, chlorpromazine, clindamycin phosphate, diazepam, ethacrynate sodium, hetastarch, hydroxyzine, insulin, methotrimeprazine, midazolam, norepinephrine, pentobarbital sodium, phenobarbital, phytonadione.

ACTION
Competitively inhibits action of histamine on the H_2 at receptor sites of parietal cells, decreasing gastric acid secretion.

Route	Onset	Peak	Duration
P.O.	1 hr	1–3 hr	13 hr
I.V.	Unknown	Unknown	Unknown

Half-life: 2 to 3 hours.

ADVERSE REACTIONS
CNS: headache, malaise, vertigo.
EENT: blurred vision.
Hepatic: jaundice.
Other: *anaphylaxis, angioedema,* burning and itching at injection site.

INTERACTIONS
Drug-drug. *Antacids:* May interfere with ranitidine absorption. Stagger doses, if possible.
Diazepam: May decrease absorption of diazepam. Monitor patient closely.
Glipizide: May increase hypoglycemic effect. Adjust glipizide dosage, as directed.
Procainamide: May decrease renal clearance of procainamide. Monitor patient closely for toxicity.
Warfarin: May interfere with warfarin clearance. Monitor patient closely.

EFFECTS ON LAB TEST RESULTS
• May increase creatinine and ALT levels.
• May cause false-positive results in urine protein tests using Multistix.

CONTRAINDICATIONS & CAUTIONS
• Contraindicated in patients hypersensitive to drug and those with acute porphyria.
• Use cautiously in patients with hepatic dysfunction. Adjust dosage in patients with impaired renal function.

NURSING CONSIDERATIONS
• Assess patient for abdominal pain. Note presence of blood in emesis, stool, or gastric aspirate.
• Drug may be added to total parenteral nutrition solutions.
• *Look alike–sound alike:* Don't confuse ranitidine with rimantadine; don't confuse Zantac with Xanax or Zyrtec.

PATIENT TEACHING
• Instruct patient on proper use of OTC preparation, as indicated.
• Remind patient to take once-daily prescription drug at bedtime for best results.
• Instruct patient to take without regard to meals because absorption isn't affected by food.
• Tell patient taking 150-mg EFFERdose to dissolve drug in 6 to 8 ounces of water before taking.
• Tell parent to dissolve 25-mg EFFERdose tablet in at least 5 ml of water and give with a dosing cup, medicine dropper, or oral syringe.
• Urge patient to avoid cigarette smoking because this may increase gastric acid secretion and worsen disease.

• Advise patient to report abdominal pain, blood in stool or emesis, black, tarry stools, or coffee-ground emesis.
• Warn patients with phenylketonuria that EFFERdose granules and tablets contain aspartame.

---

sucralfate
soo-KRAL-fayt

Carafate✱

Pharmacologic class: gastrointestinal protectant
Pregnancy risk category B

AVAILABLE FORMS
Suspension: 1 g/10 ml
Tablets: 1 g

INDICATIONS & DOSAGES
➤ **Short-term (up to 8 weeks) treatment of duodenal ulcer**
Adults: 1 g P.O. q.i.d. 1 hour before meals and at bedtime.
➤ **Maintenance therapy for duodenal ulcer**
Adults: 1 g P.O. b.i.d.

ADMINISTRATION
P.O.
• Shake suspension well before pouring.
• Following administration, flush nasogastric tube with water to ensure passage into stomach.
• Give drug on an empty stomach 1 hour before or 2 hours after meals.

ACTION
Probably adheres to and protects surface of ulcer by forming a barrier.

Route	Onset	Peak	Duration
P.O.	Unknown	Unknown	6 hr

Half-life: 6 to 20 hours.

ADVERSE REACTIONS
CNS: dizziness, headache, sleepiness, vertigo.
GI: *constipation,* bezoar formation, diarrhea, dry mouth, flatulence, gastric discomfort, indigestion, nausea, vomiting.
Musculoskeletal: back pain.

Reactions may be *common,* uncommon, *life-threatening*, or COMMON AND LIFE-THREATENING.
Interaction may have a *rapid onset* or **delayed onset.**

Skin: pruritus, rash.

INTERACTIONS
Drug-drug. *Antacids:* May decrease binding of drug to gastroduodenal mucosa, impairing effectiveness. Separate doses by 30 minutes.

Cimetidine, digoxin, fosphenytoin, keto-conazole, phenytoin, quinidine, ranitidine, tetracycline, theophylline: May decrease absorption. Separate doses by at least 2 hours.

Ciprofloxacin, lomefloxacin, moxifloxacin, norfloxacin, ofloxacin: May decrease absorption of these drugs, reducing anti-infective response. If use together can't be avoided, give at least 6 hours apart.

EFFECTS ON LAB TEST RESULTS
None reported.

CONTRAINDICATIONS & CAUTIONS
• Use cautiously in patients with chronic renal failure.

NURSING CONSIDERATIONS
• Drug is minimally absorbed and causes few adverse reactions.
• Monitor patient for severe, persistent constipation.
• Drug is as effective as cimetidine in healing duodenal ulcer.
• Drug contains aluminum but isn't classified as an antacid. Monitor patient with renal insufficiency for aluminum toxicity.

PATIENT TEACHING
• Tell patient to take sucralfate on an empty stomach, 1 hour before each meal and at bedtime.
• Instruct patient to continue prescribed regimen to ensure complete healing. Pain and other ulcer signs and symptoms may subside within first few weeks of therapy.
• Urge patient to avoid cigarette smoking, which may increase gastric acid secretion and worsen disease.
• Antacids may be used while taking drug, but separate doses by 30 minutes.

62

Bowel disorder drugs

alosetron hydrochloride
atropine sulfate
(See Chapter 22, ANTIARRHYTHMICS.)
budesonide
dicyclomine hydrochloride
mesalamine
natalizumab
(See Chapter 88,
IMMUNOSUPPRESSANTS.)
octreotide acetate
(See Chapter 59, ANTIDIARRHEALS.)
olsalazine sodium
sulfasalazine

alosetron hydrochloride
ah-LOSS-e-tron

Lotronex✐

Pharmacologic class: selective
5-HT$_3$ receptor antagonist
Pregnancy risk category B

AVAILABLE FORMS
Tablets: 0.5 mg, 1 mg

INDICATIONS & DOSAGES
➤ **Severe diarrhea-predominant**
irritable bowel syndrome (IBS)
Women: 0.5 mg P.O. b.i.d. If, after 4 weeks,
drug is well tolerated but doesn't adequately control IBS symptoms, increase to
1 mg b.i.d. After 4 weeks at this dosage, if
symptoms aren't controlled, stop drug.

ADMINISTRATION
P.O.
● Give drug without regard for food.

ACTION
Selectively inhibits 5-HT$_3$ receptors in the
GI tract, which blocks neuronal depolarization, resulting in less visceral pain,
colonic transit, and GI secretions.

Route	Onset	Peak	Duration
P.O.	Unknown	1 hr	Variable

Half-life: 1½ hours.

ADVERSE REACTIONS
CNS: headache.
GI: CONSTIPATION, nausea, GI discomfort
and pain, abdominal discomfort and pain,
abdominal distention, hemorrhoids,
regurgitation, reflux, *ileus perforation,*
ischemic colitis, small bowel mesenteric
ischemia, impaction, obstruction.
Skin: rash.

INTERACTIONS
Drug-drug. *Hydralazine, isoniazid,*
and procainamide: May cause slower
metabolism of these drugs because of
N-acetyltransferase inhibition. Monitor
patient for toxicity.

EFFECTS ON LAB TEST RESULTS
● May increase ALT level.

CONTRAINDICATIONS & CAUTIONS
● Contraindicated in patients hypersensitive
to drug or any of its components, and in
those with a history of or current chronic
or severe constipation, sequelae from
constipation, intestinal obstruction, stricture, toxic megacolon, GI perforation,
GI adhesions, ischemic colitis, impaired
intestinal circulation, thrombophlebitis,
or hypercoagulable state.
● Contraindicated in patients with a history
of or current Crohn disease, ulcerative
colitis, or diverticulitis and in those who
are unable to understand or comply with
the Patient-Physician Agreement.
● Don't use drug if predominant symptom
is constipation.
● Use cautiously in patients with mild to
moderate liver impairment; contraindicated
in patients with severe liver impairment.
● Use cautiously in women who are
pregnant, breast-feeding, or planning to
become pregnant.
● Use in children younger than age
18 hasn't been studied.

NURSING CONSIDERATIONS
■ **Black Box Warning** Drug is only
appropriate for women who experience
symptoms for at least 6 months, have no

anatomic or biochemical GI tract abnormalities, and haven't responded to other therapies. ■
● Diarrhea-predominant IBS is considered severe if one or more of the following accompanies the diarrhea:
– frequent and severe abdominal pain or discomfort
– frequent bowel urgency or fecal incontinence
– disability or restriction of daily activities
■ **Black Box Warning** Patients taking drug have developed ischemic colitis and serious complications of constipation, resulting in death. If patient develops ischemic colitis (acute colitis, rectal bleeding, or sudden worsening of abdominal pain) while taking drug, stop therapy. If patient taking drug develops constipation, stop drug until symptoms subside. ■
■ **Black Box Warning** Only providers who are enrolled in the manufacturer's prescribing program should prescribe this drug. ■
● Drug is approved for use only in women with IBS. This drug isn't indicated for use in men.
● Elderly people may be at greater risk for complications of constipation.

PATIENT TEACHING
■ **Black Box Warning** Have patient sign a Patient-Physician Agreement before starting therapy. ■
● Urge patient to read the Medication Guide before starting drug and each time she refills the prescription.
● Tell patient that this drug won't cure but may alleviate some IBS symptoms.
● Inform patient that most women notice their symptoms improving after about 1 week of therapy, but some may take up to 4 weeks to get relief from abdominal pain, discomfort, and diarrhea. Let patient know that symptoms usually return within 1 week after stopping the drug.
● Advise patient that drug may be taken with or without food.
■ **Black Box Warning** If constipation or signs of ischemic colitis occur (rectal bleeding, bloody diarrhea, or worsened abdominal pain or cramping), tell patient to stop the drug and consult prescriber immediately. Therapy can be resumed

after the situation is discussed with prescriber and constipation resolves. ■
● Inform patient not to share drug with other people having similar symptoms. This drug hasn't been shown to be safe or effective for men.
● Tell woman to notify the prescriber immediately if she becomes pregnant.

budesonide
byoo-DES-oh-nide

Entocort EC

Pharmacologic class:
glucocorticoids
Pregnancy risk category B

AVAILABLE FORMS
Capsules: 3 mg

INDICATIONS & DOSAGES
➤ **Mild to moderate active Crohn's disease involving the ileum, ascending colon, or both**
Adults: 9 mg P.O. once daily in morning for up to 8 weeks. For recurrent episodes of active Crohn's disease, a repeat 8-week course may be given. Taper to 6 mg P.O. daily for 2 weeks before completely stopping.
➤ **To maintain remission in mild to moderate Crohn's disease that involves the ileum or ascending colon**
Adults: 6 mg P.O. daily for up to 3 months. If symptom control is maintained at 3 months, taper dose to stop therapy. Therapy for longer than 3 months doesn't have added benefit.
Adjust-a-dose: In patients with moderate to severe liver disease who have increased signs or symptoms of hypercorticism, reduce dose.

ADMINISTRATION
P.O.
● Give drug whole; don't break or crush capsule.

ACTION
Significant glucocorticoid effects caused by drug's high affinity for glucocorticoid receptors.

Route	Onset	Peak	Duration
P.O.	Unknown	½–10 hr	Unknown

Half-life: About 2 hours.

ADVERSE REACTIONS

CNS: *headache,* dizziness, asthenia, hyperkinesia, paresthesia, tremor, vertigo, fatigue, malaise, agitation, confusion, insomnia, nervousness, somnolence, pain.
CV: chest pain, hypertension, palpitations, tachycardia, flushing.
EENT: facial edema, ear infection, eye abnormality, abnormal vision, sinusitis.
GI: *nausea, diarrhea,* dyspepsia, abdominal pain, flatulence, vomiting, anal disorder, aggravated Crohn disease, enteritis, epigastric pain, fistula, glossitis, hemorrhoids, intestinal obstruction, tongue edema, tooth disorder, increased appetite.
GU: dysuria, micturition frequency, nocturia, intermenstrual bleeding, menstrual disorder, hematuria, pyuria.
Hematologic: leukocytosis, anemia.
Metabolic: *hypercorticism,* dependent edema, hypokalemia, increased weight.
Musculoskeletal: back pain, aggravated arthritis, cramps, arthralgia, myalgia.
Respiratory: *respiratory tract infection,* bronchitis, dyspnea.
Skin: *acne,* alopecia, dermatitis, eczema, skin disorder, increased sweating.
Other: flulike disorder, sleep disorder, candidiasis, viral infection.

INTERACTIONS

Drug-drug. *CYP inhibitors (erythromycin, indinavir, itraconazole, ketoconazole, ritonavir, saquinavir):* May increase effects of budesonide. If use together is unavoidable, reduce budesonide dosage.
Drug-food. *Grapefruit juice:* May increase drug effects. Discourage use together.

EFFECTS ON LAB TEST RESULTS

• May increase alkaline phosphatase and C-reactive protein levels. May decrease potassium and hemoglobin levels.
• May increase erythrocyte sedimentation rate and WBC count.

CONTRAINDICATIONS & CAUTIONS

• Contraindicated in patients hypersensitive to drug.
• Use cautiously in patients with tuberculosis, hypertension, diabetes mellitus, osteoporosis, peptic ulcer disease, glaucoma, or cataracts; those with a family history of diabetes or glaucoma; and those with any other condition in which glucocorticosteroids may have unwanted effects.
• Glucocorticoids appear in breast milk, and infants may have adverse reactions. Use cautiously in breast-feeding women only if benefits outweigh risks.

NURSING CONSIDERATIONS

• Reduced liver function affects elimination of this drug; systemic availability of drug may increase in patients with liver cirrhosis.
• Patients undergoing surgery or other stressful situations may need systemic glucocorticoid supplementation in addition to budesonide therapy.
• Carefully monitor patients transferred from systemic glucocorticoid therapy to budesonide for signs and symptoms of corticosteroid withdrawal. Watch for immunosuppression, especially in patients who haven't had diseases, such as chickenpox or measles; these can be fatal in patients who are immunosuppressed or receiving glucocorticoids.
• Replacement of systemic glucocorticoids with this drug may unmask allergies, such as eczema and rhinitis, which were previously controlled by systemic drug.
• Long-term use of drug may cause hypercorticism and adrenal suppression.

PATIENT TEACHING

• Tell patient to swallow capsules whole and not to chew or break them.
• Advise patient to avoid grapefruit juice while taking drug.
• Tell patient to notify prescriber immediately if he is exposed to or develops chickenpox or measles.
• Tell patient to keep container tightly closed.

Reactions may be *common,* uncommon, ***life-threatening,*** or COMMON AND LIFE-THREATENING.
Interaction may have a *rapid onset* or ***delayed onset.***

dicyclomine hydrochloride
dye-SYE-kloe-meen

Bentyl, Bentylol†, Di-Spaz, Formulex†

Pharmacologic class:
anticholinergic, antimuscarinic
Pregnancy risk category B

AVAILABLE FORMS
Capsules: 10 mg, 20 mg
Injection: 10 mg/ml
Syrup: 10 mg/5 ml
Tablets: 10 mg†, 20 mg

INDICATIONS & DOSAGES
➤ **Irritable bowel syndrome, other functional GI disorders**
Adults: Initially, 20 mg P.O. q.i.d., increased to 40 mg q.i.d. Or, 20 mg I.M. q.i.d.

ADMINISTRATION
P.O.
• Give drug 30 to 60 minutes before meals and at bedtime. Bedtime dose can be larger; give at least 2 hours after last meal of day.
I.M.
• *Alert:* Don't give subcutaneously or I.V.
• *Alert:* The dicyclomine labeling may be misleading. Injection concentration is 10 mg/ml. Carefully calculate appropriate amount of solution for administering correct dose.

ACTION
Inhibits action of acetylcholine on postganglionic, parasympathetic muscarinic receptors, decreasing GI motility. Drug possesses local anesthetic properties that may be partly responsible for spasmolysis.

Route	Onset	Peak	Duration
P.O., I.M.	Unknown	1–1½ hr	Unknown

Half-life: Initial, about 2 hours; secondary, 9 to 10 hours.

ADVERSE REACTIONS
CNS: *headache, dizziness,* fever, insomnia, light-headedness, drowsiness, nervousness, confusion, and excitement in elderly patients.
CV: *palpitations,* tachycardia.
EENT: *blurred vision,* increased intraocular pressure, mydriasis, photophobia.
GI: *constipation, dry mouth, thirst,* vomiting, *nausea,* abdominal distention, heartburn, paralytic ileus.
GU: *urinary hesitancy or retention,* impotence.
Skin: urticaria, decreased sweating or inability to sweat, local irritation.
Other: allergic reactions, heat prostration.

INTERACTIONS
Drug-drug. *Amantadine, antihistamines, antiparkinsonians, disopyramide, glutethimide, meperidine, phenothiazines, procainamide, quinidine, tricyclic antidepressants:* May have additive adverse effects. Avoid using together.
Antacids: May interfere with dicyclomine absorption. Give dicyclomine at least 1 hour before antacid.

EFFECTS ON LAB TEST RESULTS
None reported.

CONTRAINDICATIONS & CAUTIONS
• Contraindicated in patients hypersensitive to anticholinergics and in those with obstructive uropathy, obstructive disease of the GI tract, reflux esophagitis, severe ulcerative colitis, toxic megacolon, myasthenia gravis, unstable CV status in acute hemorrhage, tachycardia secondary to cardiac insufficiency or thyrotoxicosis, or glaucoma.
• Contraindicated in breast-feeding patients and in children younger than age 6 months.
• Use cautiously in patients with autonomic neuropathy, hyperthyroidism, coronary artery disease, arrhythmias, heart failure, hypertension, hiatal hernia, hepatic or renal disease, prostatic hyperplasia, known or suspected GI infection, and ulcerative colitis.
• Use cautiously in patients in hot or humid environments; drug can cause heatstroke.

NURSING CONSIDERATIONS
• Adjust dosage based on patient's needs and response. Dosages up to 40 mg P.O. q.i.d. have been used in adults, but safety

and effectiveness for longer than 2 weeks haven't been established.

• Dicyclomine is a synthetic tertiary derivative that may have atropine-like adverse reactions.

• *Alert:* Overdose may cause curarelike effects such as respiratory paralysis. Keep emergency equipment available.

• Monitor patient's vital signs and urine output carefully.

• *Look alike–sound alike:* Don't confuse dicyclomine with dyclonine or doxycycline; don't confuse Bentyl with Aventyl or Benadryl.

PATIENT TEACHING

• Tell patient when to take drug, and stress importance of doing so on time and at evenly spaced intervals.

• Advise patient to avoid driving and other hazardous activities if drowsiness, dizziness, or blurred vision occurs; to drink plenty of fluids to help prevent constipation; and to report rash or other skin eruption.

mesalamine
me-SAL-a-meen

Asacol, Canasa, Lialda, Pentasa, Rowasa

Pharmacologic class: salicylate
Pregnancy risk category B

AVAILABLE FORMS

Capsules (controlled-release): 250 mg, 500 mg
Rectal suspension: 4 g/60 ml
Suppositories: 1,000 mg
Tablets (delayed-release): 400 mg, 1.2 g

INDICATIONS & DOSAGES

➤ **Active mild to moderate distal ulcerative colitis, proctitis, or proctosigmoiditis**
Adults: Two 400-mg tablets (800 mg) P.O. t.i.d. for total dose of 2.4 g daily for 6 weeks. Or 1 g capsules P.O. q.i.d. for total dose of 4 g up to 8 weeks. Or 1,000 mg suppository P.R., retained in the rectum for 1 to 3 hours or longer, once daily at bedtime. Or 4 g retention enema once daily (preferably at bedtime).

➤ **Remission-induction of active, mild to moderate ulcerative colitis**
➤ **Lialda**
Adults: Two to four 1.2 g tablets (2.4 to 4.8 g) P.O. once daily with a meal for up to 8 weeks.
➤ **Asacol**
Adults: 1.6 g P.O. daily in divided doses for 6 months.
➤ **Pentasa**
Adults: Four 250-mg capsules or two 500-mg capsules (1 g) P.O. 4 times daily for a total dose of 4 g for up to 8 weeks.

ADMINISTRATION

P.O.
• Give Lialda with food.
• Don't crush or cut delayed-release or controlled-release forms.
• Intact or partially intact tablets may be seen in stool. Notify prescriber if this occurs repeatedly.
Rectal
• Patient should retain rectal dosage form overnight (for about 8 hours). Usual course of therapy for rectal form is 3 to 6 weeks.
• Shake suspension well before each use and remove sheath before inserting into rectum.

ACTION

An active metabolite of sulfasalazine, drug probably acts topically by inhibiting prostaglandin production in the colon.

Route	Onset	Peak	Duration
P.O., P.R.	Unknown	3–12 hr	Unknown

Half-life: About 5 to 10 hours.

ADVERSE REACTIONS

CNS: *headache,* dizziness, fever, fatigue, malaise, asthenia.
CV: chest pain.
EENT: *pharyngitis.*
GI: abdominal pain, cramps, discomfort, flatulence, diarrhea, rectal pain, bloating, nausea, *pancolitis,* vomiting, constipation, eructation.
GU: interstitial nephritis, nephropathy, *nephrotoxicity.*
Musculoskeletal: arthralgia, myalgia, back pain, hypertonia.

Reactions may be *common,* uncommon, *life-threatening*, or COMMON AND LIFE-THREATENING.
Interaction may have a *rapid onset* or *delayed onset.*

Respiratory: wheezing.
Skin: itching, rash, urticaria, hair loss.
Other: chills, acne.

INTERACTIONS
Drug-drug. *Lactulose:* May impair release of delayed- or extended-release products. Monitor patient closely.
Omeprazole: May increase absorption of mesalamine. Monitor patient closely.

EFFECTS ON LAB TEST RESULTS
● May increase BUN, creatinine, AST, ALT, alkaline phosphatase, LDH, amylase, and lipase levels.

CONTRAINDICATIONS & CAUTIONS
● Contraindicated in children and in patients allergic to mesalamine, sulfites (including sulfasalazine), any salicylates, or any component of the preparation.
● Use cautiously in renally impaired, elderly, pregnant, and breast-feeding patients.

NURSING CONSIDERATIONS
● Monitor periodic renal function studies in patients on long-term therapy.
● Because the mesalamine rectal suspension contains potassium metabisulfite, it may cause hypersensitivity reactions in patients sensitive to sulfites.
● Absorption of drug may be nephrotoxic.
● *Look alike–sound alike:* Don't confuse Asacol with Os-Cal.

PATIENT TEACHING
● Instruct patient to carefully follow instructions supplied with drug and to swallow tablets whole without crushing or chewing.
● Advise patient to stop drug if fever or rash occurs. Patient intolerant of sulfasalazine may also be hypersensitive to mesalamine.
● Tell patient to remove foil wrapper from suppositories before inserting into rectum.
● Teach patient about proper use of retention enema.
● Tell patient that enema solution may stain bedsheets and clothing. Patient should use protective underpads and linens.

olsalazine sodium
ol-SAL-uh-zeen

Dipentum

Pharmacologic class: salicylate
Pregnancy risk category C

AVAILABLE FORMS
Capsules: 250 mg

INDICATIONS & DOSAGES
➤ **Maintenance of remission of ulcerative colitis in patients intolerant of sulfasalazine**
Adults: 500 mg P.O. b.i.d. with meals.

ADMINISTRATION
P.O.
● Give drug with food.

ACTION
Unknown. After oral use, converts to 5-aminosalicylic acid (5-ASA or mesalamine) in the colon, where it has local anti-inflammatory effect.

Route	Onset	Peak	Duration
P.O.	Unknown	1 hr	Unknown

Half-life: About 1 hour.

ADVERSE REACTIONS
CNS: headache, depression, vertigo, dizziness, fatigue.
GI: *diarrhea,* nausea, *abdominal pain,* dyspepsia, bloating, anorexia.
Musculoskeletal: arthralgia.
Skin: rash, itching.

INTERACTIONS
Drug-drug. *Anticoagulants:* May prolong PT or INR. Monitor bleeding study results.
Drug-food. *Any food:* May decrease GI irritation. Advise patient to take drug with food.

EFFECTS ON LAB TEST RESULTS
● May increase ALT and AST levels.

CONTRAINDICATIONS & CAUTIONS
● Contraindicated in patients hypersensitive to salicylates.
● Use cautiously in patients with renal disease.

NURSING CONSIDERATIONS
- Regularly monitor BUN and creatinine levels and urinalysis in patients with renal disease.
- Absorption of drug or its metabolites may cause renal tubular damage.
- Diarrhea sometimes occurs during therapy. Although diarrhea appears to be dose-related, it's difficult to distinguish from worsening of disease symptoms.
- Similar drugs have caused worsening of disease.
- *Look alike–sound alike:* Don't confuse olsalazine with olanzapine.

PATIENT TEACHING
- Teach patient to take drug in evenly divided doses and with food to minimize adverse GI reactions.
- Instruct patient to report persistent or severe adverse reactions promptly.

---

sulfasalazine (salazosulfapyridine, sulphasalazine)
sul-fuh-SAL-uh-zeen

Azulfidine, Azulfidine EN-tabs, Salazopyrin†, Salazopyrin EN-Tabs†

Pharmacologic class: sulfonamide, salicylate
Pregnancy risk category B

AVAILABLE FORMS
Enteric-coated tablets: 500 mg
Oral suspension: 250 mg/5 ml
Tablets: 500 mg
Tablets (delayed-release): 500 mg

INDICATIONS & DOSAGES
➤ **Mild to moderate ulcerative colitis, adjunctive therapy in severe ulcerative colitis, Crohn disease**
Adults: Initially, 3 to 4 g P.O. daily in evenly divided doses; usual maintenance dose is 2 g P.O. daily in divided doses every 6 hours. Dosage may be started with 1 to 2 g, with gradual increase to minimize adverse effects.
Children 6 years and older: Initially, 40 to 60 mg/kg P.O. daily, divided into three to six doses; then 30 mg/kg daily in four doses. Dosage may be started at lower dose if GI intolerance occurs.
➤ **Rheumatoid arthritis in patients who have responded inadequately to salicylates or NSAIDs**
Adults (delayed-release tablets): 2 g P.O. daily in evenly divided doses. To reduce possible GI intolerance, start at 0.5 to 1 g daily.
➤ **Polyarticular-course juvenile rheumatoid arthritis in patients who have responded inadequately to salicylates or other NSAIDs**
Children age 6 and older (delayed-release tablets): 30 to 50 mg/kg P.O. daily in two divided doses. Maximum dose is 2 g daily. To reduce possible GI intolerance, start with one-quarter to one-third of planned maintenance dose and increase weekly until reaching maintenance dose at 1 month.

ADMINISTRATION
P.O.
- Give drug with food to decrease GI irritation.
- Don't cut or crush enteric-coated tablets.

ACTION
Unknown.

Route	Onset	Peak	Duration
P.O.	Unknown	3–12 hr	Unknown

Half-life: 6 to 8 hours.

ADVERSE REACTIONS
CNS: *seizures,* headache, depression, hallucinations.
GI: *nausea, vomiting, diarrhea,* abdominal pain, anorexia, stomatitis.
GU: *toxic nephrosis with oliguria and anuria,* crystalluria, hematuria, oligospermia, infertility.
Hematologic: *agranulocytosis, leukopenia, thrombocytopenia, aplastic anemia,* megaloblastic anemia, hemolytic anemia.
Hepatic: *hepatotoxicity,* jaundice.
Skin: *generalized skin eruption, erythema multiforme, Stevens-Johnson syndrome, epidermal necrolysis,* exfoliative dermatitis, photosensitivity reaction, urticaria, pruritus.

Reactions may be *common,* uncommon, *life-threatening*, or COMMON AND LIFE-THREATENING.
Interaction may have a *rapid onset* or **delayed onset.**

Other: *serum sickness, drug fever, anaphylaxis,* hypersensitivity reactions.

INTERACTIONS
Drug-drug. *Antibiotics:* May alter action of sulfasalazine by changing intestinal flora. Monitor patient closely.
Digoxin: May reduce absorption of digoxin. Monitor patient closely.
Folic acid: May decrease absorption. Monitor patient.
Iron: May decrease levels of sulfasalazine caused by iron chelation. Monitor patient closely.
Methotrexate: May displace methotrexate from protein-binding sites and decrease renal clearance. Monitor patient for hematologic toxicity and adverse GI events, especially nausea.
Oral anticoagulants: May increase anti-coagulant effect. Watch for bleeding.
Oral antidiabetics: May increase hypoglycemic effect. Monitor glucose levels.

EFFECTS ON LAB TEST RESULTS
● May increase ALT and AST levels. May decrease hemoglobin level.
● May decrease granulocyte, platelet, and WBC counts.

CONTRAINDICATIONS & CAUTIONS
● Contraindicated in patients hypersensitive to drug or its metabolites, in those with porphyria or intestinal and urinary obstruction, and in children younger than age 2.
● Use cautiously and in reduced doses in patients with impaired hepatic or renal function, severe allergy, bronchial asthma, or G6PD deficiency.

NURSING CONSIDERATIONS
● Therapeutic response in patients with rheumatoid arthritis may occur as soon as 4 weeks after starting therapy, but it may take up to 12 weeks in others.
● Drug may cause urine discoloration.
● *Alert:* Stop drug immediately and notify prescriber if patient shows signs and symptoms of hypersensitivity.
● *Look alike–sound alike:* Don't confuse sulfasalazine with sulfisoxazole, salsalate, or sulfadiazine.

PATIENT TEACHING
● Instruct patient to take drug after eating and to space doses evenly.
● Warn patient to avoid ultraviolet light.
● Advise patient that drug may produce an orange-yellow discoloration of skin and urine and may cause contact lenses to turn yellow.
● Instruct patient that if his skin or urine is discolored, to notify prescriber immediately.
● Tell patient to drink plenty of water and to swallow tablets whole without crushing or chewing.

63

Laxatives

bisacodyl
calcium polycarbophil
docusate calcium
docusate sodium
glycerin
lactulose
lubiprostone
magnesium citrate
magnesium hydroxide
magnesium sulfate
polyethylene glycol
polyethylene glycol and
**   electrolyte solution**
sodium phosphate monohydrate
**   and sodium phosphate dibasic**
**   anhydrous**
sodium phosphates

---

bisacodyl
bye-suh-KOH-dil

Alophen ◇ , Bisac-Evac ◇ ,
Bisa-Lax ◇ , Codulax† ◇ ,
Correctol ◇ , Doxidan, Dulcolax ◇ ,
Ex-Lax Ultra ◇ , Feen-a-Mint ◇ ,
Fleet Bisacodyl ◇ , Fleet Bisacodyl
Enema ◇ , Fleet Laxative ◇ ,
Modane ◇ , Soflax EX† ◇ ,
The Magic Bullet† ◇ , Woman's
Laxative† ◇

Pharmacologic class:
diphenylmethane derivative
Pregnancy risk category B

AVAILABLE FORMS
Enema: 0.33 mg/ml ◇
Suppositories: 10 mg ◇
Tablets (delayed release): 10 mg ◇
Tablets (enteric-coated): 5 mg ◇

INDICATIONS & DOSAGES
➤ **Chronic constipation; preparation for childbirth, surgery, or rectal or bowel examination**
Adults and children age 12 and older:
10 to 15 mg P.O. in evening or before breakfast. Or, 10 mg P.R. for evacuation before examination or surgery.
Children ages 6 to 11: 5 mg P.O. or P.R. at bedtime or before breakfast. Oral dose isn't recommended if child can't swallow tablet whole.

ADMINISTRATION
P.O.
● Don't give tablets within 1 hour after taking an antacid or milk.
● Don't crush or split tablets.
Rectal
● Insert suppository as high as possible into the rectum, and try to position suppository against the rectal wall. Avoid embedding within fecal material because doing so may delay onset of action.

ACTION
Unknown. Stimulant laxative that increases peristalsis, probably by direct effect on smooth muscle of the intestine, by irritating the muscle or stimulating the colonic intramural plexus. Drug also promotes fluid accumulation in colon and small intestine.

Route	Onset	Peak	Duration
P.O.	6–12 hr	Variable	Variable
P.R.	15–60 min	Variable	Variable

Half-life: Unknown.

ADVERSE REACTIONS
CNS: dizziness, faintness, muscle weakness with excessive use.
GI: *abdominal cramps, burning sensation in rectum with suppositories, nausea, vomiting,* diarrhea with high doses, laxative dependence with long-term or excessive use, protein-losing enteropathy with excessive use.
Metabolic: alkalosis, fluid and electrolyte imbalance, hypokalemia.
Musculoskeletal: tetany.

Reactions may be *common*, uncommon, *life-threatening*, or COMMON AND LIFE-THREATENING.
Interaction may have a *rapid onset* or **delayed onset**.

INTERACTIONS
Drug-drug. *Antacids:* May cause gastric irritation or dyspepsia from premature dissolution of enteric coating. Separate doses by at least 1 or 2 hours.
Drug-food. *Milk:* May cause gastric irritation or dyspepsia from premature dissolution of enteric coating. Don't use within 1 or 2 hours of drinking milk.

EFFECTS ON LAB TEST RESULTS
• May increase phosphate and sodium levels. May decrease calcium, magnesium, and potassium levels.

CONTRAINDICATIONS & CAUTIONS
• Contraindicated in patients hypersensitive to drug or its components and in those with rectal bleeding, gastroenteritis, intestinal obstruction, abdominal pain, nausea, vomiting, or other symptoms of appendicitis or acute surgical abdomen.

NURSING CONSIDERATIONS
• Give drug at times that don't interfere with scheduled activities or sleep. Soft, formed stools are usually produced 15 to 60 minutes after rectal use.
• Before giving for constipation, determine whether patient has adequate fluid intake, exercise, and diet.
• Tablets and suppositories are used together to clean the colon before and after surgery and before barium enema.

PATIENT TEACHING
• Advise patient to swallow enteric-coated tablet whole to avoid GI irritation. Instruct him not to take within 1 hour of milk or antacid.
• Tell patient that drug is for 1-week treatment only. (Stimulant laxatives are often abused.) Discourage excessive use.
• Advise patient to report adverse effects to prescriber.
• Teach patient about dietary sources of bulk, including bran and other cereals, fresh fruit, and vegetables.
• Tell patient to take drug with a full glass of water or juice.

calcium polycarbophil
KAL-see-um

Equalactin◊, Fiberall◊, FiberCon◊, Fiber-Lax◊, Konsyl Fiber◊, Phillips' Fibercaps◊

Pharmacologic class: hydrophilic drug
Pregnancy risk category A

AVAILABLE FORMS
Tablets: 500 mg◊, 625 mg◊
Tablets (chewable): 500 mg◊

INDICATIONS & DOSAGES
➤ **Constipation**
Adults and children older than age 12: 1 g P.O. once daily to q.i.d., p.r.n. Maximum, 4 g in 24 hours.
Children ages 7 to 12: 500 mg P.O. once daily to t.i.d., p.r.n. Maximum, 2 g in 24 hours.
➤ **Diarrhea from irritable bowel syndrome; acute, nonspecific diarrhea**
Adults and children older than age 12: 1 g P.O. once daily to q.i.d., p.r.n. Maximum, 4 g in 24 hours.
Children ages 7 to 12: 500 mg P.O. once daily to t.i.d., p.r.n. Maximum, 2 g in 24 hours.

ADMINISTRATION
P.O.
• Equalactin tablets should be chewed thoroughly before swallowing and followed by an 8-ounce glass of water with each dose.
• When drug is used as an antidiarrheal, don't give with glass of water.

ACTION
Absorbs water and expands to increase bulk and moisture content of stools. The increased bulk encourages peristalsis and bowel movement. As an antidiarrheal, drug absorbs free fecal water, thereby producing formed stools.

Route	Onset	Peak	Duration
P.O.	12–24 hr	3 days	Variable

Half-life: Unknown.

ADVERSE REACTIONS
GI: *intestinal obstruction,* abdominal fullness and increased flatus.
Other: laxative dependence with long-term or excessive use.

INTERACTIONS
Drug-drug. *Tetracyclines:* May impair tetracycline absorption. Avoid using together.

EFFECTS ON LAB TEST RESULTS
None reported.

CONTRAINDICATIONS & CAUTIONS
• Contraindicated in patients with signs or symptoms of GI obstruction or those with swallowing difficulty.

NURSING CONSIDERATIONS
• Before giving drug for constipation, determine whether patient has adequate fluid intake, exercise, and diet.
• In children younger than age 6, use must be directed by prescriber.
• *Alert:* Rectal bleeding or failure to respond to therapy may indicate need for surgery.

PATIENT TEACHING
• Full benefit of drug may take 1 to 3 days.
• Advise patient to chew Equalactin tablets thoroughly before swallowing and to drink an 8-ounce glass of water with each dose. When drug is used as an anti-diarrheal, tell patient not to drink the glass of water.
• Advise patient to seek medical attention if he experiences vomiting, chest pain, or difficulty breathing or swallowing after taking medication.
• Teach patient about dietary sources of fiber, including bran and other cereals, fresh fruit, and vegetables.
• For severe diarrhea, advise patient to repeat dose every 30 minutes, but not to exceed maximum daily dose. Tell patient not to use for longer than 2 days, unless directed by a prescriber.

docusate calcium (dioctyl calcium sulfosuccinate)
DOK-yoo-sayt

DC Softgels ◇ , Surfak ◇

docusate sodium (dioctyl sodium sulfosuccinate)
Colace ◇ , Diocto ◇ , Dioctyn, D.O.S ◇ , D-S-S ◇ , Dulcolax Stool Softener ◇ , Ex-Lax Stool Softener Caplets ◇ , Genasoft ◇ , Modane Soft ◇ , Phillips' Liqui-Gels ◇ , Regulax SS ◇ , Selax† ◇ , Silace ◇ , Soflax† ◇

Pharmacologic class: surfactant
Pregnancy risk category C

AVAILABLE FORMS
docusate calcium
Capsules: 240 mg ◇
docusate sodium
Capsules: 50 mg ◇ , 100 mg ◇ , 240 mg ◇ , 250 mg ◇
Enema concentrate: 18 g/100 ml (must be diluted)‡
Oral liquid: 150 mg/15 ml ◇
Oral solution: 10 mg/ml ◇ , 50 mg/ml ◇
Syrup: 20 mg/5 ml, 50 mg/15 ml ◇ , 60 mg/15 ml ◇
Tablets: 50 mg ◇ , 100 mg ◇

INDICATIONS & DOSAGES
➤ **Stool softener**
Adults and children older than age 12: 50 to 300 mg docusate calcium or sodium P.O. daily until bowel movements are normal. Or, give enema. Dilute 1:24 with sterile water before use, and give 100 to 150 ml retention enema, 300 to 500 ml evacuation enema, or 0.5 to 1.5 L flushing enema P.R.
Children ages 2 to 12: 50 to 150 mg docusate sodium P.O. daily.
Children younger than age 2: 25 mg docusate sodium P.O. daily.

ADMINISTRATION
P.O.
• Give liquid (not syrups) in milk, fruit juice, or infant formula to mask bitter taste.

• Store drug at 59° to 86° F (15° to 30° C), and protect liquid from light.
Rectal
• Follow instructions accompanying rectal suspension.

ACTION
Stool softener that reduces surface tension of interfacing liquid contents of the bowel. This detergent activity promotes incorporation of additional liquid into stools, thus forming a softer mass.

Route	Onset	Peak	Duration
P.O.	1–3 days	Unknown	Unknown
P.R.	Unknown	Unknown	Unknown

Half-life: Unknown.

ADVERSE REACTIONS
GI: bitter taste, mild abdominal cramping, diarrhea.
Other: laxative dependence with long-term or excessive use.

INTERACTIONS
Drug-drug. *Mineral oil:* May increase mineral oil absorption and cause toxicity and lipid pneumonia. Separate doses.

EFFECTS ON LAB TEST RESULTS
None reported.

CONTRAINDICATIONS & CAUTIONS
• Contraindicated in patients hypersensitive to drug and in those with intestinal obstruction or signs and symptoms of appendicitis, fecal impaction, or acute surgical abdomen, such as undiagnosed abdominal pain or vomiting.

NURSING CONSIDERATIONS
• Drug isn't used to treat existing constipation but prevents constipation from developing.
• Before giving drug, determine whether patient has adequate fluid intake, exercise, and diet.
• Drug is laxative of choice for patients who shouldn't strain during defecation, including patients recovering from MI or rectal surgery, those with rectal or anal disease that makes passage of

firm stools difficult, and those with postpartum constipation.

PATIENT TEACHING
• Teach patient about dietary sources of fiber, including bran and other cereals, fresh fruit, and vegetables.
• Instruct patient to use drug only occasionally and not for longer than 1 week without prescriber's knowledge.
• Tell patient to stop drug and notify prescriber if severe cramping occurs.
• Notify patient that it may take from 1 to 3 days to soften stools.

glycerin
GLI-ser-in

Fleet Babylax ◇ , Sani-Supp ◇

Pharmacologic class: trihydric alcohol
Pregnancy risk category NR

AVAILABLE FORMS
Enema (pediatric): 4 ml/applicator ◇
Suppositories: Adult, children, and infant sizes ◇

INDICATIONS & DOSAGES
➤ **Constipation**
Adults and children age 6 and older: 2 to 3 g as rectal suppository; or 5 to 15 ml as enema.
Children ages 2 to 6: 1 to 1.7 g as rectal suppository; or 2 to 5 ml as enema.

ADMINISTRATION
Rectal
• Give drug into the rectum as directed. The patient should retain the drug for at least 15 minutes.

ACTION
Draws water from the tissues into the feces, thus stimulating evacuation.

Route	Onset	Peak	Duration
P.R.	15–30 min	Unknown	Unknown

Half-life: Unknown.

ADVERSE REACTIONS
GI: *cramping pain,* hyperemia of rectal mucosa, rectal discomfort.

INTERACTIONS
None significant.

EFFECTS ON LAB TEST RESULTS
None reported.

CONTRAINDICATIONS & CAUTIONS
• Contraindicated in patients hypersensitive to drug and in those with intestinal obstruction or signs and symptoms of appendicitis, fecal impaction, or acute surgical abdomen, such as undiagnosed abdominal pain or vomiting.

NURSING CONSIDERATIONS
• Drug is used mainly to reestablish proper toilet habits in laxative-dependent patients.

PATIENT TEACHING
• Tell patient that drug must be retained for at least 15 minutes and that it usually acts within 1 hour. Entire suppository need not melt to be effective.
• Warn patient about adverse GI reactions.

---

lactulose
LAK-tyoo-lose

Cholac, Constilac, Constulose, Enulose, Kristalose

Pharmacologic class: disaccharide
Pregnancy risk category B

AVAILABLE FORMS
Packets: 10 g, 20 g
Syrup: 10 g/15 ml

INDICATIONS & DOSAGES
➤ **Constipation**
Adults: 10 to 20 g or 15 to 30 ml P.O. daily, increased to 60 ml/day, if needed.
➤ **To prevent and treat hepatic encephalopathy, including hepatic precoma and coma in patients with severe hepatic disease**
Adults: Initially, 20 to 30 g or 30 to 45 ml P.O. t.i.d. or q.i.d., until two or three soft stools are produced daily. Usual dose is 60 to 100 g daily in divided doses. Or, 200 g or 300 ml diluted with 700 ml of

water or normal saline solution and given as retention enema P.R. every 4 to 6 hours, as needed.

ADMINISTRATION
P.O.
• To minimize sweet taste, dilute with water or fruit juice or give with food.
Rectal
• Prepare enema (not commercially available) by adding 200 g (300 ml) to 700 ml of water or normal saline solution. The diluted solution is given as retention enema for 30 to 60 minutes. Use a rectal balloon.
• If enema isn't retained for at least 30 minutes, repeat dose.

ACTION
Produces an osmotic effect in colon; resulting distention promotes peristalsis. Also decreases ammonia, probably as a result of bacterial degradation, which lowers the pH of colon contents.

Route	Onset	Peak	Duration
P.O.	24–48 hr	Variable	Variable
P.R.	Unknown	Unknown	Unknown

Half-life: Unknown.

ADVERSE REACTIONS
GI: *abdominal cramps, belching, diarrhea, flatulence, gaseous distention,* nausea, vomiting.

INTERACTIONS
Drug-drug. *Antacids, antibiotics, oral neomycin:* May decrease lactulose effectiveness. Avoid using together.

EFFECTS ON LAB TEST RESULTS
None reported.

CONTRAINDICATIONS & CAUTIONS
• Contraindicated in patients on a low-galactose diet.
• Use cautiously in patients with diabetes mellitus.

NURSING CONSIDERATIONS
• Monitor sodium level for hypernatremia, especially when giving in higher doses to treat hepatic encephalopathy.

Reactions may be *common,* uncommon, *life-threatening,* or COMMON AND LIFE-THREATENING.
Interaction may have a *rapid onset* or *delayed onset.*

• Monitor mental status and potassium levels when giving to patients with hepatic encephalopathy.
• Replace fluid loss.
• *Look alike–sound alike:* Don't confuse lactulose with lactose.

PATIENT TEACHING
• Show home care patient how to mix and use drug.
• Inform patient about adverse reactions and tell him to notify prescriber if reactions become bothersome or if diarrhea occurs.
• Instruct patient not to take other laxatives during lactulose therapy.

---

lubiprostone
loo-bee-PRAHS-tohn

Amitiza &

Pharmacologic class: chloride channel activator
Pregnancy risk category C

AVAILABLE FORMS
Capsules: 8 mcg, 24 mcg

INDICATIONS & DOSAGES
➤ **Chronic idiopathic constipation**
Adults: 24 mcg P.O. b.i.d. with food.
✱*NEW INDICATION:* **Irritable bowel syndrome with constipation**
Women 18 years and older: 8 mcg P.O. b.i.d. with food and water.

ADMINISTRATION
P.O.
• Give drug with food.

ACTION
Increases intestinal fluid secretion by activating chloride channels, and increases intestinal motility.

Route	Onset	Peak	Duration
P.O.	Unknown	1 hr	Unknown

ADVERSE REACTIONS
CNS: *headache,* anxiety, depression, dizziness, fatigue, insomnia, pyrexia.
CV: chest pain, peripheral edema.

EENT: nasopharyngitis, pharyngolaryngeal pain, sinusitis.
GI: *diarrhea, nausea,* abdominal distension, abdominal pain or discomfort, constipation, dry mouth, dyspepsia, flatulence, gastroesophageal reflux disease, loose stools, stomach discomfort, viral gastroenteritis, vomiting.
GU: UTI.
Metabolic: weight gain.
Musculoskeletal: arthralgia, back pain, limb pain, muscle cramps.
Respiratory: bronchitis, cough, dyspnea, upper respiratory tract infection.
Other: influenza.

INTERACTIONS
None reported.

EFFECTS ON LAB TEST RESULTS
None reported.

CONTRAINDICATIONS & CAUTIONS
• Contraindicated in patients hypersensitive to drug or its components and in those with a history of mechanical GI obstruction.
• Use cautiously in women who are or may become pregnant.

NURSING CONSIDERATIONS
• Periodically assess patient's need for continued therapy.
• Monitor patient for diarrhea.
• Don't give drug to a patient with severe diarrhea.
• Safety and effectiveness in children haven't been established.

PATIENT TEACHING
• Tell patient to take drug with food.
• Explain to patient he may experience diarrhea; advise him not to take drug if he develops severe diarrhea.
• Advise patient about a proper diet and the need to drink plenty of fluids.

magnesium citrate
(citrate of magnesia)
Citro-Nesia ◇

magnesium hydroxide
(milk of magnesia)
Milk of Magnesia ◇, Milk of
Magnesia-Concentrated ◇,
Phillips' Milk of Magnesia ◇

magnesium sulfate ◇
(Epsom salts ◇)

Pharmacologic class: magnesium
salt
Pregnancy risk category B

AVAILABLE FORMS
magnesium citrate
Oral solution: About 168 mEq magnesium/
240 ml ◇
magnesium hydroxide
Chewable tablets: 300 mg, 600 mg
Oral suspension: 400 mg/5 ml,
800 mg/5 ml
magnesium sulfate
Granules: About 40 mEq magnesium/
5 g ◇

INDICATIONS & DOSAGES
➤ **Constipation, to evacuate bowel
before surgery**
Adults and children age 12 and older:
11 to 25 g magnesium citrate P.O. daily as
a single or divided dose. Or, 2.4 to 4.8 g
or 30 to 60 ml magnesium hydroxide P.O.
(2 to 4 tablespoons at bedtime or upon
arising, followed by 8 ounces of liquid)
daily as a single dose or divided. Or,
10 to 30 g magnesium sulfate P.O. daily
as a single or divided dose.
Children ages 6 to 11: 5.5 to 12.5 g
magnesium citrate P.O. daily as a single or
divided dose. Or, 1.2 to 2.4 g or 15 to 30 ml
magnesium hydroxide P.O. (1 to 2 tablespoons, followed by 8 ounces of liquid)
daily as a single or divided dose. Or,
5 to 10 g magnesium sulfate P.O. daily
as a single or divided dose. Don't use
dosage cup.
Children ages 2 to 5: 2.7 to 6.25 g
magnesium citrate P.O. daily as a single
or divided dose. Or, 0.4 to 1.2 g or 5 to
15 ml magnesium hydroxide P.O. (1 to

3 tsp, followed by 8 ounces of liquid)
daily as a single or divided dose. Or,
2.5 to 5 g magnesium sulfate P.O. daily
as a single or divided dose. Don't use
dosage cup.

ADMINISTRATION
P.O.
● Give drug at times that don't interfere
with scheduled activities or sleep.
Drug produces watery stools in 3 to
6 hours.
● Chill magnesium citrate before use to
improve its palatability.
● Shake suspension well; give with a large
amount of water when used as laxative.
When giving by nasogastric tube, make
sure tube is placed properly and is patent.
After instilling drug, flush tube with water
to ensure passage to stomach and maintain
tube patency.

ACTION
Saline laxative that produces an osmotic
effect in the small intestine by drawing
water into the intestinal lumen.

Route	Onset	Peak	Duration
P.O.	30 min–3 hr	Variable	Variable

Half-life: Unknown.

ADVERSE REACTIONS
GI: *abdominal cramping, diarrhea,
nausea.*
Metabolic: fluid and electrolyte disturbances with daily use.
Other: laxative dependence with long-term
or excessive use.

INTERACTIONS
Drug-drug. *Oral drugs:* May impair
absorption. Separate doses.

EFFECTS ON LAB TEST RESULTS
● May alter fluid and electrolyte levels
with prolonged use.

CONTRAINDICATIONS & CAUTIONS
● Contraindicated in pregnant patients
about to deliver and in patients with
myocardial damage, heart block, fecal
impaction, rectal fissures, intestinal
obstruction or perforation, renal disease,
or signs and symptoms of appendicitis or

Reactions may be *common,* uncommon, *life-threatening,* or COMMON AND LIFE-THREATENING.
Interaction may have a *rapid onset* or **delayed onset.**

acute surgical abdomen, such as abdominal pain, nausea, or vomiting.
● Use cautiously in patients with rectal bleeding.

NURSING CONSIDERATIONS
● Before giving drug for constipation, determine whether patient has adequate fluid intake, exercise, and diet.
● *Alert:* Monitor electrolyte levels during prolonged use. Magnesium may accumulate if patient has renal insufficiency.
● Drug is recommended for short-term use only.
● Magnesium sulfate is more potent than other saline laxatives.

PATIENT TEACHING
● Teach patient how to use drug.
● Teach patient about dietary sources of fiber, including bran and other cereals, fresh fruit, and vegetables.
● Warn patient that frequent or prolonged use as a laxative may cause dependence.

---

polyethylene glycol (PEG)
pol-ee-ETH-ih-leen

GlycoLax, MiraLax

Pharmacologic class: osmotic drug
Pregnancy risk category C

AVAILABLE FORMS
Powder: single-dose 17-g packets; 16-ounce (255-g), 24-ounce (527-g) containers

INDICATIONS & DOSAGES
➤ **Short-term treatment of occasional constipation**
Adults: 17 g (about 1 heaping tablespoon) powder P.O. daily.

ADMINISTRATION
P.O.
● Before giving, rule out bowel obstruction in patients who have nausea, vomiting, abdominal pain, or distention.
● Dissolve powder in 8 ounces (240 ml) of water, juice, soda, coffee, or tea.

ACTION
Causes water to be retained in stool.

Route	Onset	Peak	Duration
P.O.	48–96 hr	Unknown	Unknown

Half-life: Unknown.

ADVERSE REACTIONS
GI: abdominal bloating, cramping, diarrhea, excess stool frequency, flatulence, nausea.

INTERACTIONS
Drug-drug. *Drugs containing polyethylene glycol:* May cause urticaria. Monitor patient.

EFFECTS ON LAB TEST RESULTS
None reported.

CONTRAINDICATIONS & CAUTIONS
● Contraindicated in patients allergic to drug and those with known or suspected bowel obstruction.

NURSING CONSIDERATIONS
● It may take 2 to 4 days before a bowel movement occurs.
● Drug should be taken for 2 weeks or less to avoid risk of laxative dependence.
● Occasional use as directed doesn't affect absorption or secretion of glucose or electrolytes.
● Prolonged, frequent, or excessive use may cause electrolyte imbalance and laxative dependence.
● Drug may be more likely to cause diarrhea in older patients.

PATIENT TEACHING
● Explain that proper eating habits and lifestyle changes may produce more regular bowel movements. Tell patient to eat adequate amounts of dietary fiber, drink ample fluids, and get appropriate exercise.
● If patient uses bottled form of drug, urge him to measure each 17-g dose using the measuring cup provided in the package. If patient uses drug packets, each one contains 17 g.
● Instruct patient to dissolve dose in 8 ounces of water, juice, soda, coffee, or tea.
● Inform patient that it may take 2 to 4 days to produce a bowel movement.

- Warn patient that taking more than the recommended dose can cause dehydration and severe diarrhea.
- Tell patient that drug should be used for 2 weeks or less to avoid risk of laxative dependence.
- Urge patient to report unusual cramping, bloating, or diarrhea.

polyethylene glycol (PEG) and electrolyte solution
pol-ee-ETH-ih-leen

Colyte, Go-Evac, GoLYTELY, MoviPrep, NuLYTELY, TriLyte, OCL

Pharmacologic class: polyethylene glycol (PEG) nonabsorbable solution
Pregnancy risk category C

AVAILABLE FORMS
Powder for oral solution: 4L dose of solution contains PEG 3350 (17.6 mmol/L), sodium (125 mmol/L), sulfate (40 mmol/L; Colyte 80 mmol/L), chloride (35 mmol/L), bicarbonate (20 mmol/L), and potassium (10 mmol/L)
Oral solution: PEG 3350 (6 g), sodium sulfate decahydrate (1.29 g), sodium chloride (146 mg), potassium chloride (75 mg), sodium bicarbonate (168 mg), polysorbate-80 (30 mg) per 100 ml (OCL)

INDICATIONS & DOSAGES
➤ **Bowel preparation before GI examination**
Adults: 240 ml P.O. every 10 minutes until 4 L are consumed or until watery stool is clear. Typically, give 4 hours before examination, allowing 3 hours for drinking and 1 hour for bowel evacuation.

ADMINISTRATION
P.O.
- Use tap water to reconstitute powder. Shake vigorously to dissolve all powder. Refrigerate reconstituted solution, but use within 48 hours.
- *Alert:* Don't add flavoring or additional ingredients to the solution or give chilled solution. Hypothermia has been reported after ingesting large amounts of chilled solution.

- Give solution early in the morning if patient is scheduled for a midmorning examination. Oral solution induces diarrhea (onset 30 to 60 minutes) that rapidly cleans the bowel, usually within 4 hours.
- When using to prepare for barium enema, give solution the evening before the examination to avoid interfering with barium coating of the colonic mucosa.
- If given to semiconscious patient or to patient with impaired gag reflex, take care to prevent aspiration.
- Give drug at least 2 hours after solid food.

ACTION
PEG 3350, a nonabsorbable solution, acts as an osmotic. Sodium sulfate greatly reduces sodium absorption. The electrolyte level causes virtually no net absorption or secretion of ions.

Route	Onset	Peak	Duration
P.O.	1 hr	Variable	Variable

Half-life: None.

ADVERSE REACTIONS
EENT: rhinorrhea.
GI: *abdominal fullness, bloating, cramps, nausea, vomiting.*
Skin: allergic reaction, anal irritation, dermatitis, urticaria.

INTERACTIONS
Drug-drug. *Oral drugs:* May decrease absorption if given within 1 hour of starting therapy. Give at least 2 to 3 hours before starting therapy.

EFFECTS ON LAB TEST RESULTS
None reported.

CONTRAINDICATIONS & CAUTIONS
- Contraindicated in patients with GI obstruction or perforation, gastric retention, toxic colitis, or megacolon.

NURSING CONSIDERATIONS
- No major shifts in fluid or electrolyte balance have been reported.
- Patient preparation for barium enema may be less satisfactory with this solution

because it may interfere with the barium coating of the colonic mucosa using the double-contrast technique.

PATIENT TEACHING
• Tell patient to fast for 3 to 4 hours before taking solution, and thereafter to drink only clear fluids until examination is complete.
• Warn patient about adverse reactions.

sodium phosphate monohydrate and sodium phosphate dibasic anhydrous
OsmoPrep, Visicol

Pharmacologic class: osmotic laxative
Pregnancy risk category C

AVAILABLE FORMS
Tablets: 1.5 g sodium phosphate (1.102 g sodium phosphate monohydrate and 0.398 g sodium phosphate dibasic anhydrous)

INDICATIONS & DOSAGES
➤ **To cleanse the bowel before colonoscopy (Visicol)**
Adults age 18 and older: 40 tablets taken in the following manner: The evening before the procedure, 3 tablets P.O. with at least 8 ounces of clear liquid every 15 minutes, for a total of 20 tablets. The last dose will be only 2 tablets. The day of the procedure, 3 tablets P.O. with at least 8 ounces of clear liquid every 15 minutes, for a total of 20 tablets, starting 3 to 5 hours before the procedure. The last dose will be only 2 tablets.
➤ **To cleanse the bowel before colonoscopy (OsmoPrep)**
Adults age 18 and older: 32 tablets taken in the following manner: The evening before the procedure 4 tablets P.O. with 8 ounces of clear liquid every 15 minutes for a total of 20 tablets. 3 to 5 hours before the procedure take 4 tablets P.O. with at least 8 ounces of clear liquid every 15 minutes for a total of 12 tablets.

ADMINISTRATION
P.O.
• Give each dose with at least 8 ounces of clear liquid.

ACTION
Induces diarrhea by causing large amounts of water to be drawn into the colon, promoting rapid and effective evacuation.

Route	Onset	Peak	Duration
P.O.	Rapid	Varies	1–3 hr

Half-life: Unknown.

ADVERSE REACTIONS
CNS: dizziness, headache.
GI: abdominal bloating, abdominal pain, nausea, vomiting.

INTERACTIONS
Drug-drug. *Any drugs:* Reduces absorption of these drugs. Separate doses.

EFFECTS ON LAB TEST RESULTS
• May increase phosphorus level (typically normalizes 48 to 72 hours after giving drug). May decrease potassium and calcium levels.

CONTRAINDICATIONS & CAUTIONS
• Contraindicated in patients hypersensitive to sodium phosphate or any of its ingredients. Avoid giving drug to patients with heart failure, ascites, unstable angina, gastric retention, ileus, acute intestinal obstruction, pseudo-obstruction, severe chronic constipation, bowel perforation, acute colitis, toxic megacolon, or hypomotility syndrome (hypothyroidism, scleroderma).
• Use cautiously in patients with a history of electrolyte abnormalities, current electrolyte abnormalities, or impaired renal function. Also use cautiously in patients who take drugs that can induce electrolyte abnormalities or prolong the QT interval.
• Use cautiously in elderly patients because they may be more sensitive to drug effects.

NURSING CONSIDERATIONS
• Correct electrolyte imbalances before giving drug.

• As with other sodium phosphate cathartic preparations, this drug may induce colonic mucosal ulceration.
• Monitor patient for signs of dehydration.
• Don't repeat administration within 7 days.
• No enema or laxative is needed in addition to drug. Patients shouldn't take any additional purgatives, particularly those that contain sodium phosphate.
• *Alert:* Administration of other sodium phosphate products has caused death from significant fluid shifts, electrolyte abnormalities, and cardiac arrhythmias. Patients with electrolyte disturbances have an increased risk of prolonged QT interval. Use drug cautiously in patients who are taking other drugs known to prolong the QT interval.

PATIENT TEACHING
• Urge patient to drink at least 8 ounces of clear liquid with each dose. Inadequate fluid intake may lead to excessive fluid loss and hypovolemia.
• Tell patient to drink only clear liquids for at least 12 hours before starting the purgative regimen.
• Caution patient against taking an additional enema or laxative, particularly one that contains sodium phosphate.
• Tell patient that undigested or partially digested Visicol or OsmoPrep tablets and other drugs may appear in the stool.

sodium phosphates
Fleet Enema ◇, Fleet Phospho-soda ◇

Pharmacologic class: acid salt
Pregnancy risk category NR

AVAILABLE FORMS
Enema: 160 mg/ml sodium phosphate and 60 mg/ml sodium biphosphate ◇
Liquid: 2.4 g/5 ml sodium phosphate and 900 mg sodium biphosphate/5 ml ◇

INDICATIONS & DOSAGES
➤ **Constipation**
Adults and children age 12 and older: 20 to 45 ml solution mixed with 120 ml

cold water P.O. Or, 60 to 150 ml as an enema.
Children ages 10 to 11: 10 to 20 ml solution mixed with 120 ml cold water P.O.
Children ages 5 to 9: 5 to 10 ml solution mixed with 120 ml cold water P.O. Or, 30 to 60 ml as an enema.
Children ages 2 to 5: 60 ml P.R. as an enema.

ADMINISTRATION
P.O.
• Mix drug with cold water.
Rectal
• Follow instructions accompanying enema.

ACTION
Saline laxative that produces an osmotic effect in the small intestine by drawing water into the intestinal lumen.

Route	Onset	Peak	Duration
P.O.	30–180 min	Variable	Variable
P.R.	5–10 min	With effect	With effect

Half-life: Unknown.

ADVERSE REACTIONS
GI: *abdominal cramping.*
Metabolic: fluid and electrolyte disturbances, such as hypernatremia and hyperphosphatemia, with daily use.
Other: laxative dependence with long-term or excessive use.

INTERACTIONS
None significant.

EFFECTS ON LAB TEST RESULTS
• May increase sodium and phosphate levels. May decrease electrolyte level with prolonged use.

CONTRAINDICATIONS & CAUTIONS
• Contraindicated in patients on sodium-restricted diets and in patients with intestinal obstruction, intestinal perforation, edema, heart failure, megacolon, impaired renal function, or signs and symptoms of appendicitis or acute surgical abdomen, such as abdominal pain, nausea, or vomiting.
• Use cautiously in patients with large hemorrhoids or anal abrasions.

NURSING CONSIDERATIONS
• Before giving drug for constipation, determine whether patient has adequate fluid intake, exercise, and diet.
• *Alert:* Up to 10% of sodium content of drug may be absorbed.
• *Alert:* Severe electrolyte imbalances may occur if recommended dosage is exceeded.

PATIENT TEACHING
• Teach patient about dietary sources of fiber, including bran and other cereals, fresh fruit, and vegetables.
• Warn patient about adverse reactions, and stress importance of using drug only for short-term therapy.

64

Miscellaneous gastrointestinal tract drugs

cevimeline hydrochloride
hyoscyamine
L-hyoscyamine sulfate
pancreatin
pancrelipase
pilocarpine hydrochloride

---

cevimeline hydrochloride
seh-vih-MEH-leen

Evoxac

Pharmacologic class: cholinergic agonist
Pregnancy risk category C

AVAILABLE FORMS
Capsules: 30 mg

INDICATIONS & DOSAGES
➤ **Dry mouth in patients with Sjögren syndrome**
Adults: 30 mg P.O. t.i.d.

ADMINISTRATION
P.O.
- Give drug without regard for food.
- Encourage fluids.

ACTION
Stimulates the muscarinic receptors of the exocrine glands (salivary, sweat) and increases GI and urinary smooth muscle tone.

Route	Onset	Peak	Duration
P.O.	Unknown	1½–2 hr	Unknown

Half-life: 4 to 6 hours.

ADVERSE REACTIONS
CNS: *headache,* anxiety, depression, fever, dizziness, fatigue, hypoesthesia, insomnia, migraine, pain, tremor, vertigo.
CV: chest pain, palpitations, peripheral edema.
EENT: *rhinitis, sinusitis,* abnormal vision, conjunctivitis, earache, epistaxis, eye infection, eye pain, otitis media, pharyngitis, xerophthalmia, eye abnormality.
GI: *diarrhea, nausea,* abdominal pain, anorexia, constipation, dry mouth, eructation, excessive salivation, flatulence, gastroesophageal reflux, salivary gland enlargement and pain, salivary calculi, ulcerative stomatitis, vomiting, dyspepsia, increased amylase.
GU: cystitis, candidiasis, UTI, vaginitis.
Hematologic: anemia.
Musculoskeletal: arthralgia, back pain, hypertonia, hyporeflexia, leg cramps, myalgia, rigors, skeletal pain.
Respiratory: *upper respiratory tract infection,* bronchitis, pneumonia, coughing, hiccups.
Skin: *excessive sweating,* rash, pruritus, skin disorder, erythematous rash.
Other: fungal infections, flulike symptoms, injury, hot flushes, tooth disorder, toothache, postoperative pain, allergic reaction, infection, abscess.

INTERACTIONS
Drug-drug. *Antimuscarinics:* May cause antagonistic effects. Monitor patient for effectiveness.
Beta blockers: May cause conduction disturbances. Use together cautiously.
CYP inhibitors: May inhibit metabolism of cevimeline. Monitor patient closely.
Parasympathomimetics: May have additive effects. Use together cautiously.

EFFECTS ON LAB TEST RESULTS
- May increase amylase level. May decrease hemoglobin level.

CONTRAINDICATIONS & CAUTIONS
- Contraindicated in patients hypersensitive to drug and in those for whom miosis is undesirable (as in those who have acute iritis or angle-closure glaucoma).
- Contraindicated in patients with uncontrolled asthma.
- Use cautiously in patients with significant CV disease, controlled asthma, chronic bronchitis, or COPD and in those with a history of kidney stones or gallstones.

Reactions may be *common,* uncommon, ***life-threatening***, or COMMON AND LIFE-THREATENING.
Interaction may have a *rapid onset* or ***delayed onset.***

NURSING CONSIDERATIONS
• Monitor patients with a history of asthma, COPD, or chronic bronchitis for an increase in signs or symptoms, such as wheezing, increased sputum production, or cough.
• Monitor patients with a history of cardiac disease for changes in heart rate or increased frequency, severity, or duration of angina.
• Monitor elderly patients closely because they have an increased risk of impaired renal, hepatic, and cardiac function.

PATIENT TEACHING
• Advise patient not to interrupt or stop treatment without consulting prescriber.
• Tell patient that sweating is a common adverse effect. Urge adequate fluid intake to prevent dehydration.
• Inform patient that drug may cause visual disturbances that can impair driving ability, especially at night.

hyoscyamine
hye-AH-ska-meen

Cystospaz, Hyospaz

L-hyoscyamine sulfate
Anaspaz, Cystospaz, Cystospaz-M, IB-Stat, Levbid, Levsin*, Levsin Drops*, Levsin SL, Levsinex Timecaps, NuLev

Pharmacologic class: belladonna alkaloid, anticholinergic
Pregnancy risk category C

AVAILABLE FORMS
hyoscyamine
Tablets: 0.15 mg
L-hyoscyamine sulfate
Capsules (extended-release): 0.375 mg
Elixir: 0.125 mg/5 ml*
Injection: 0.5 mg/ml
Oral spray: 0.125 mg/ml*
Oral solution: 0.125 mg/ml*
Tablets: 0.125 mg, 0.15 mg
Tablets (extended-release): 0.375 mg
Tablets (orally disintegrating): 0.125 mg, 0.25 mg
Tablets (S.L.): 0.125 mg

INDICATIONS & DOSAGES
➤ **GI tract disorders caused by spasm; as adjunctive therapy for peptic ulcers, cystitis, renal colic; as drying agent to relieve symptoms of allergic rhinitis, parkinsonism**
Adults and children age 11 and older: 0.125 to 0.25 mg P.O. or S.L. t.i.d. or q.i.d. before meals and at bedtime. Or, 0.375 to 0.75 mg extended-release form P.O. every 12 hours. Or, 0.25 to 0.5 mg I.V., I.M., or subcutaneously every 4 hours, b.i.d. to q.i.d. Substitute oral drug when symptoms are controlled. Maximum, 1.5 mg daily.
Children ages 2 to 11: Individualize dosage according to weight. Don't exceed 0.75 mg in 24 hours.
Children younger than age 2: Individualize dosage according to weight. Maximum dose is based on weight.
➤ **To diminish secretions and block cardiac vagal reflexes preoperatively**
Adults and children older than age 2: 0.005 mg/kg I.V., I.M., or subcutaneously 30 to 60 minutes before anesthesia. Intra-operatively, adults may receive 0.125 mg I.V. as needed to reduce drug-induced bradycardia.
➤ **Diagnostic procedures**
Adults: 0.25 to 0.5 mg I.V., I.M., or subcutaneously 5 to 10 minutes before the procedure.
➤ **To block adverse muscarinic effects of anticholinesterase agents**
Adults: 0.3 to 0.6 mg I.V. for each 0.5 to 2 mg of neostigmine methylsulfate or physostigmine salicylate, or 10 to 20 mg of pyridostigmine bromide. Give hyoscyamine with or a few minutes before the anti-cholinesterase in a separate syringe.
➤ **Organophosphate pesticide toxicity**
Adults: Initially, 1 to 2 mg I.V. Additional 1 mg doses I.V. or I.M. every 3 to 10 minutes as needed; up to 25 mg may be needed in first 24 hours. Maintenance, 0.5 to 1 mg P.O. in intervals of several hours until symptoms are gone.

ADMINISTRATION
P.O.
• Give drug 30 minutes to 1 hour before meals and at bedtime. Bedtime dose can be larger; give at least 2 hours after last meal of day.

- Don't crush or split extended-release tablets.
- Hyoscyamine orally disintegrating tablets may be taken with or without water.

I.V.
- Use when P.O. and S.L. routes aren't possible or when rapid effect is needed.
- Injection contains sodium metabisulfite, which may cause allergic reaction in certain people.
- **Incompatibilities:** None reported.

I.M.
- Injection contains sodium metabisulfite, which may cause allergic reaction in certain people.

Subcutaneous
- Injection contains sodium metabisulfite, which may cause allergic reaction in certain people.

S.L.
- Hyoscyamine sublingual tablets are formulated for sublingual administration; however, they may be chewed or taken orally.

ACTION
Blocks acetylcholine action at muscarinic receptors, which decreases GI motility and inhibits gastric acid secretion.

Route	Onset	Peak	Duration
P.O.	20–30 min	½–1 hr	4–12 hr
P.O. (extended)	20–30 min	40–90 min	12 hr
I.V.	2–3 min	15–30 min	4 hr
I.M., Subcut.	Unknown	15–30 min	4–12 hr
S.L.	5–20 min	½–1 hr	4 hr

Half-life: Conventional tablets, 2 to 3½ hours; extended-release capsules or tablets, 5 to 6 or 9 hours, respectively; I.M., 12½ hours or longer. Prolonged in patients with renal dysfunction.

ADVERSE REACTIONS
CNS: *confusion or excitement in elderly patients,* fever, headache, insomnia, drowsiness, dizziness, nervousness, weakness, fever (especially in children).
CV: *palpitations,* tachycardia.
EENT: *blurred vision,* mydriasis, increased intraocular pressure, cycloplegia, photophobia.
GI: *constipation, dry mouth, paralytic ileus,* dysphagia, heartburn, loss of taste, nausea, vomiting.

GU: *urinary hesitancy, urine retention,* impotence.
Skin: urticaria, decreased or lack of sweating.
Other: hypersensitivity reactions.

INTERACTIONS
Drug-drug. *Amantadine, antihistamines, antiparkinsonians, disopyramide, glutethimide, MAO inhibitors, meperidine, phenothiazines, procainamide, quinidine, tricyclic antidepressants:* May have additive adverse effects. Avoid using together.
Antacids: May decrease absorption of oral anticholinergics. Separate doses by 2 or 3 hours.
Ketoconazole: May interfere with ketoconazole absorption. Separate doses by 2 or 3 hours.

EFFECTS ON LAB TEST RESULTS
None reported.

CONTRAINDICATIONS & CAUTIONS
- Contraindicated in patients hypersensitive to anticholinergics and in those with glaucoma, obstructive uropathy, obstructive disease of the GI tract, severe ulcerative colitis, myasthenia gravis, paralytic ileus, intestinal atony, unstable CV status in acute hemorrhage, tachycardia secondary to cardiac insufficiency of thyrotoxicosis, or toxic megacolon.
- Use cautiously in patients with autonomic neuropathy, hyperthyroidism, coronary artery disease, arrhythmias, heart failure, hypertension, hiatal hernia with reflux esophagitis, hepatic or renal disease, known or suspected GI infection, and ulcerative colitis.
- Use cautiously in patients in hot or humid environments; drug can cause heatstroke.
- Use cautiously in children and the elderly because they may be more susceptible to adverse effects.

NURSING CONSIDERATIONS
- **Alert:** Overdose may cause curare-like effects, such as respiratory paralysis. Keep emergency equipment available. Drug is dialyzable.
- Monitor patient's vital signs and urine output carefully.
- **Look alike–sound alike:** Don't confuse Anaspaz with Anaprox or Antispas.

Reactions may be *common,* uncommon, *life-threatening,* or COMMON AND LIFE-THREATENING.
Interaction may have a *rapid onset* or **delayed onset.**

PATIENT TEACHING
- Urge patient to take drug as prescribed.
- Caution patient not to crush or chew extended-release tablets.
- Advise patient to avoid driving and other hazardous activities if drowsiness, dizziness, or blurred vision occurs; to drink plenty of fluids to help prevent constipation; and to report rash or other skin eruption.
- Advise patient not to take any new drug or OTC preparation unless directed by prescriber.

pancreatin
PAN-kree-a-tin

Kutrase, Ku-Zyme

Pharmacologic class: pancreatic enzyme
Pregnancy risk category C

AVAILABLE FORMS
Kutrase
Capsules: 2,400 units lipase, 30,000 units protease, 30,000 units amylase
Ku-Zyme
Capsules: 1,200 units lipase, 15,000 units protease, 15,000 units amylase

INDICATIONS & DOSAGES
➤ **Exocrine pancreatic secretion insufficiency; digestive aid in diseases related to deficiency of pancreatic enzymes, such as cystic fibrosis**
Adults and children: Dosage varies with condition treated. Usual first dose is 8,000 to 24,000 units of lipase activity P.O. before or with each meal or snack. Total daily dose also may be given in divided doses every 1 to 2 hours throughout.

ADMINISTRATION
P.O.
- Give drug before or with meals and snacks.
- Don't crush enteric-coated forms. Capsules containing enteric-coated micro-spheres may be opened and sprinkled on a small quantity of cool, soft food. The food should be swallowed immediately, without chewing, and followed with a glass of water or juice.

ACTION
Replaces endogenous exocrine pancreatic enzymes and aids digestion of starches, fats, and proteins.

Route	Onset	Peak	Duration
P.O.	Unknown	Unknown	1–2 hr

Half-life: Unknown.

ADVERSE REACTIONS
GI: diarrhea with high doses, nausea.
Skin: perianal irritation.
Other: allergic reactions.

INTERACTIONS
Drug-drug. *Antacids:* May counteract pancreatin's beneficial effect. Avoid using together.
Oral iron supplement: May reduce oral iron supplement level. Separate doses.

EFFECTS ON LAB TEST RESULTS
- May increase uric acid level.

CONTRAINDICATIONS & CAUTIONS
- Contraindicated in patients hypersensitive to drug, pork protein, or pork enzymes and in those with acute pancreatitis or acute worsening of chronic pancreatitis.
- Use with caution in pregnant or breast-feeding women.

NURSING CONSIDERATIONS
- The different available products aren't interchangeable.
- To avoid indigestion, monitor patient's diet to ensure proper balance of fat, protein, and starch. Dosage varies according to degree of maldigestion and malabsorption, amount of fat in diet, and enzyme activity of individual preparations.
- Fewer bowel movements and improved stool consistency indicate effective therapy.
- Drug isn't effective in GI disorders unrelated to pancreatic enzyme deficiency.
- Enteric coating on some products may reduce available enzyme in upper portion of jejunum.

PATIENT TEACHING
- Instruct patient to take drug before or with meals and snacks.
- Tell patient not to crush or chew enteric-coated forms. Capsules containing enteric-coated microspheres may be opened and

sprinkled on a small quantity of cool, soft food. Stress importance of swallowing immediately, without chewing, and following with a glass of water or juice.

• Warn patient not to inhale powder form or powder from capsules; it may irritate skin or mucous membranes.

• Tell patient to store drug in airtight container at room temperature.

• Instruct patient not to change brands without consulting prescriber.

---

pancrelipase
pan-kre-LYE-pase

Creon 5, Creon 10, Creon 20, Ku-Zyme HP, Lipram 4500, Lipram-CR5, Lipram-CR10, Lipram-CR20, Lipram-PN10, Lipram-PN16, Lipram-PN20, Lipram-UL12, Lipram-UL18, Lipram-UL20, Pancrease, Pancrease MT4, Pancrease MT10, Pancrease MT16, Pancrease MT20, Pancrecarb MS4, Pancrecarb MS8, Panokase, Plaretase 8000, Ultrase, Ultrase MT12, Ultrase MT18, Ultrase MT20, Viokase, Viokase 8, Viokase 16, Viokase Powder, Viokase Tablets

Pharmacologic class: pancreatic enzyme
*Pregnancy risk category C;
B for Pancrease and Pancrease MT*

AVAILABLE FORMS
Creon 5, Lipram-CR5
Capsules (enteric-coated microspheres):
5,000 units lipase, 18,750 units protease, and 16,600 units amylase
Creon 10, Lipram-CR10
Capsules (enteric-coated microspheres):
10,000 units lipase, 37,500 units protease, and 33,200 units amylase
Creon 20, Lipram-CR20
Capsules (enteric-coated microspheres):
20,000 units lipase, 75,000 units protease, and 66,400 units amylase
Ku-Zyme HP, Panokase, Plaretase 8000, Viokase 8
Capsules or tablets: 8,000 units lipase, 30,000 units protease, and 30,000 units amylase

Lipram-PN10, Pancrease MT10
Capsules (enteric-coated contents):
10,000 units lipase, 30,000 units protease, and 30,000 units amylase
Lipram-PN16, Pancrease MT16
Capsules (enteric-coated contents):
16,000 units lipase, 48,000 units protease, and 48,000 units amylase
Lipram-PN20, Pancrease MT20
Capsules (enteric-coated contents):
20,000 units lipase, 44,000 units protease, and 56,000 units amylase
Lipram-UL12, Ultrase MT12
Capsules (enteric-coated contents):
12,000 units lipase, 39,000 units protease, and 39,000 units amylase
Lipram-UL18, Ultrase MT18
Capsules (enteric-coated contents):
18,000 units lipase, 58,500 units protease, and 58,500 units amylase
Lipram-UL20, Ultrase MT20
Capsules (enteric-coated contents):
20,000 units lipase, 65,000 units protease, and 65,000 units amylase
Pancrease, Lipram 4,500, Ultrase
Capsules (enteric-coated microspheres):
4,500 units lipase, 25,000 units protease, and 20,000 units amylase
Pancrease MT4
Capsules (enteric-coated microtablets):
4,000 units lipase, 12,000 units protease, and 12,000 units amylase
Pancrecarb MS4
Capsules (enteric-coated microspheres):
4,000 units lipase; 25,000 units protease; 25,000 units amylase
Pancrecarb MS8
Capsules (enteric-coated microspheres):
8,000 units lipase; 45,000 units protease; 40,000 units amylase
Viokase
Powder: 16,800 units lipase, 70,000 units protease, and 70,000 units amylase per 0.7 g powder
Viokase 16
Tablets: 16,000 units lipase, 60,000 units protease, and 60,000 units amylase

INDICATIONS & DOSAGES
➤ **Exocrine pancreatic secretion insufficiency; cystic fibrosis in adults and children; steatorrhea and other disorders of fat metabolism caused by insufficient pancreatic enzymes**

Reactions may be *common*, uncommon, *life-threatening*, or COMMON AND LIFE-THREATENING.
Interaction may have a *rapid onset* or **delayed onset.**

Adults and children older than age 12:
Adjust dosage to patient's response. Usual first dosage 4,000 to 33,000 units of lipase with each meal.
Children ages 7 to 12: 4,000 to 12,000 units of lipase activity with each meal or snack. More can be taken, if needed.
Children ages 1 to 6: 4,000 to 8,000 units of lipase with each meal and 4,000 units of lipase with each snack.
Children ages 6 months to 11 months: 2,000 units of lipase with each meal.

ADMINISTRATION
P.O.
• Give drug before or with meals and snacks.
• Don't crush enteric-coated forms. Capsules containing enteric-coated microspheres may be opened and sprinkled on a small quantity of cool, soft food. Have patient swallow immediately, without chewing, and follow dose with glass of water or juice.
• For infants, mix powder with applesauce and give with meals. Avoid contact with or inhalation of powder because it may be highly irritating. Older children may swallow capsules with food.

ACTION
Replaces endogenous exocrine pancreatic enzymes and aids digestion of starches, fats, and proteins.

Route	Onset	Peak	Duration
P.O.	Variable	Variable	Variable

Half-life: Unknown.

ADVERSE REACTIONS
GI: *nausea,* cramping, diarrhea with high doses.

INTERACTIONS
Drug-drug. *Antacids:* May destroy enteric coating and enhance degradation of pancrelipase. Avoid using together.
Oral iron supplement: May decrease iron response. Monitor patient for decreased effectiveness.

EFFECTS ON LAB TEST RESULTS
• May increase uric acid level.

CONTRAINDICATIONS & CAUTIONS
• Contraindicated in patients with severe hypersensitivity to pork and in those with

acute pancreatitis or acute worsening of chronic pancreatic diseases.

NURSING CONSIDERATIONS
• **Alert:** Use drug only for confirmed exocrine pancreatic insufficiency. It isn't effective in GI disorders unrelated to enzyme deficiency.
• Lipase activity is greater than with other pancreatic enzymes.
• Monitor patient's stools. Adequate replacement decreases number of bowel movements and improves stool consistency.
• Individual products aren't bioequivalent and shouldn't be interchanged without prescriber supervision.
• Dosage varies with degree of maldigestion and malabsorption, amount of fat in diet, and enzyme activity of individual preparations.
• Enteric coating on some products may reduce available enzyme in upper portion of jejunum.

PATIENT TEACHING
• Instruct patient to take drug before or with meals and snacks.
• Advise patient not to crush or chew enteric-coated forms. Capsules containing enteric-coated microspheres may be opened and sprinkled on a small quantity of cool, soft food. Stress importance of swallowing immediately, without chewing, and following with glass of water or juice.
• Warn patient not to inhale powder form or powder from capsules; it may irritate skin or mucous membranes.
• Tell patient to store drug in airtight container at room temperature.
• Instruct patient not to change brands without consulting prescriber.

pilocarpine hydrochloride
pye-loe-CAR-peen

Salagen

Pharmacologic class: cholinergic agonist
Pregnancy risk category C

AVAILABLE FORMS
Tablets: 5 mg, 7.5 mg

INDICATIONS & DOSAGES
➤ **Xerostomia from salivary gland hypofunction caused by radiotherapy for cancer of head and neck**
Adults: 5 mg P.O. t.i.d.; may increase to 10 mg P.O. t.i.d., as needed.
➤ **Dry mouth in patients with Sjögren syndrome**
Adults: 5 mg P.O. q.i.d.
Adjust-a-dose: For patients with moderate hepatic impairment, initial dose is 5 mg P.O. b.i.d. Adjust dose based on tolerance.
➤ **Keratoconjunctivitis sicca (dry eye syndrome)** ◆
Adult: 5 mg P.O. q.i.d. maximum of 30 mg/day.

ADMINISTRATION
P.O.
● Don't give drug with a high-fat meal.

ACTION
Cholinergic parasympathomimetic that increases secretion of salivary glands, eliminating dryness.

Route	Onset	Peak	Duration
P.O.	20 min	1 hr	3–5 hr

Half-life: 45 minutes to 1½ hours.

ADVERSE REACTIONS
CNS: *asthenia, dizziness, headache,* tremor.
CV: *flushing,* hypertension, tachycardia, edema.
EENT: *abnormal vision, rhinitis, sinusitis,* lacrimation, amblyopia, pharyngitis, voice alteration, conjunctivitis, epistaxis.
GI: *nausea,* dyspepsia, diarrhea, abdominal pain, vomiting, dysphagia, taste perversion.
GU: *urinary frequency.*
Musculoskeletal: myalgia.
Skin: *sweating,* rash, pruritus.
Other: *chills.*

INTERACTIONS
Drug-drug. *Beta blockers:* May increase risk of conduction disturbances. Use together cautiously.
Drugs with anticholinergic effects: May antagonize anticholinergic effects. Use together cautiously.

Drugs with parasympathomimetic effects: May result in additive pharmacologic effects. Monitor patient closely.
Drug-food. *High-fat meals:* May reduce drug absorption. Discourage patient from eating high-fat meals.

EFFECTS ON LAB TEST RESULTS
None reported.

CONTRAINDICATIONS & CAUTIONS
● Contraindicated in patients hypersensitive to pilocarpine, in breast-feeding women, in those with uncontrolled asthma, and in those for whom miosis is undesirable, as in acute iritis or angle-closure glaucoma.
● Use in severe hepatic insufficiency isn't recommended.
● Use cautiously in patients with CV disease, controlled asthma, chronic bronchitis, COPD, cholelithiasis, biliary tract disease, nephrolithiasis, cognitive or psychiatric disturbances, or in pregnant women.
● Safety and effectiveness of drug in children haven't been established.

NURSING CONSIDERATIONS
● Examine patient's fundus carefully before beginning therapy because retinal detachment may occur in patients with retinal disease.
● Monitor patient for signs and symptoms of toxicity: headache, visual disturbance, lacrimation, sweating, respiratory distress, GI spasm, nausea, vomiting, diarrhea, AV block, tachycardia, bradycardia, hypotension, hypertension, shock, mental confusion, arrhythmia, and tremors. Immediately notify prescriber of suspected toxicity.

PATIENT TEACHING
● Warn patient that driving ability may be impaired, especially at night, by drug-induced visual disturbances.
● Advise patient to drink plenty of fluids to prevent dehydration.
● Tell elderly patient with Sjögren syndrome that he may be especially prone to urinary frequency, diarrhea, and dizziness.
● Advise patient not to take drug with a high-fat meal.

65

Benign prostatic hyperplasia drugs

alfuzosin hydrochloride
dutasteride
finasteride
tamsulosin hydrochloride

alfuzosin hydrochloride
al-foo-ZOE-sin

Uroxatral🖊

Pharmacologic class: alpha₁ blocker
Pregnancy risk category B

AVAILABLE FORMS
Tablets (extended-release): 10 mg

INDICATIONS & DOSAGES
➤ **BPH**
Men: 10 mg P.O. immediately after same meal each day.

ADMINISTRATION
P.O.
● Give drug after same meal each day.
● Don't crush tablets.

ACTION
Selectively blocks alpha receptors in the prostate, which relaxes the smooth muscles in the bladder neck and prostate, improving urine flow and reducing symptoms of BPH.

Route	Onset	Peak	Duration
P.O.	Unknown	8 hr	Unknown

Half-life: 10 hours.

ADVERSE REACTIONS
CNS: dizziness, fatigue, headache, pain.
EENT: pharyngitis, sinusitis.
GI: abdominal pain, constipation, dyspepsia, nausea.
GU: impotence.
Respiratory: bronchitis, upper respiratory tract infection.

INTERACTIONS
Drug-drug. *Antihypertensives (diltiazem):* May cause hypotension. Monitor blood pressure and use together cautiously.
Atenolol: May cause hypotension and reduce heart rate. Monitor blood pressure and heart rate for these effects.
Cimetidine: May increase alfuzosin level. Use together cautiously.
Potent CYP3A4 inhibitors (itraconazole, ketoconazole, ritonavir): May inhibit hepatic metabolism of alfuzosin. Use together is contraindicated.

EFFECTS ON LAB TEST RESULTS
None reported.

CONTRAINDICATIONS & CAUTIONS
● Contraindicated in patients with Child-Pugh categories B and C and those hypersensitive to alfuzosin or its ingredients.
● Use cautiously in patients with severe renal insufficiency, congenital or acquired QT-interval prolongation, or symptomatic hypotension and hypotensive responses to other drugs.

NURSING CONSIDERATIONS
● Don't use drug to treat hypertension.
● Asymptomatic orthostatic hypotension may develop within a few hours.
● Symptoms of BPH and prostate cancer are similar; rule out prostate cancer before therapy.
● If angina pectoris develops or worsens, stop drug.
● Current or previous use of an alpha blocker may predispose the patient to intraoperative floppy iris syndrome during cataract surgery.

PATIENT TEACHING
● Tell patient to take drug just after the same meal each day.
● At start of therapy, warn patient about possible hypotension and explain that it may cause dizziness. Caution patient against performing hazardous

activities until he knows how the drug affects him.
- Tell patient to avoid situations in which he could be injured if he became light-headed or fainted.
- Warn patient not to crush or chew the tablets.
- Advise patient planning cataract surgery to alert his ophthalmologist about this drug and current or previous alpha blocker therapy.

---

dutasteride
doo-TAS-teh-ride

Avodart

Pharmacologic class: 5-alpha-reductase enzyme inhibitor
Pregnancy risk category X

AVAILABLE FORMS
Capsules: 0.5 mg

INDICATIONS & DOSAGES
➤ **To improve the symptoms of BPH, reduce the risk of acute urine retention, and reduce the need for BPH-related surgery**
Men: 0.5 mg P.O. once daily.
✱*NEW INDICATION: Symptomatic BPH*
Men: 0.5 mg P.O. once daily with tamsulosin 0.4 mg P.O. once daily.

ADMINISTRATION
P.O.
- Don't crush or break capsules.
- Give drug without regard for food.

ACTION
Inhibits conversion of testosterone to dihydrotestosterone, the androgen primarily responsible for the initial development and subsequent enlargement of the prostate gland.

Route	Onset	Peak	Duration
P.O.	Unknown	2–3 hr	Unknown

Half-life: About 5 weeks.

ADVERSE REACTIONS
GU: impotence, decreased libido, ejaculation disorder.
Other: gynecomastia.

INTERACTIONS
Drug-drug. *Cytochrome P-450 inhibitors (such as cimetidine, ciprofloxacin, diltiazem, ketoconazole, ritonavir, verapamil):* May increase dutasteride level. Use together cautiously.

EFFECTS ON LAB TEST RESULTS
- May lower prostate-specific antigen (PSA) level.

CONTRAINDICATIONS & CAUTIONS
- Contraindicated in women and children and in patients hypersensitive to dutasteride or its ingredients or to other 5-alpha-reductase inhibitors.
- Use cautiously in patients with hepatic disease and in those taking long-term potent cytochrome P-450 inhibitors.

NURSING CONSIDERATIONS
- Because drug may be absorbed through the skin, women who are or may become pregnant shouldn't handle the drug.
- If contact is made with leaking capsules, wash the contact area immediately with soap and water.
- Carefully monitor patients with a large residual urine volume or severely diminished urine flow, or both, for obstructive uropathy.
- Patients should wait at least 6 months after their last dose before donating blood.
- Establish a new baseline PSA level in men treated for 3 to 6 months and use it to assess potentially cancer-related changes in PSA level.
- To interpret PSA values in men treated for 6 months or more, double the PSA value for comparison with normal values in untreated men.
- Evaluate patients for prostate cancer prior to initiating therapy and periodically thereafter.

PATIENT TEACHING
- Tell patient to swallow the capsule whole.
- Inform patient that ejaculate volume may decrease but that sexual function should remain normal.
- Teach women who are pregnant or may become pregnant not to handle drug. A

Reactions may be *common*, uncommon, *life-threatening*, or COMMON AND LIFE-THREATENING.
Interaction may have a *rapid onset* or *delayed onset.*

male fetus exposed to drug by the mother's swallowing or absorbing the drug through her skin may be born with abnormal sex organs.
• **Alert:** Tell patient not to donate blood for at least 6 months after final dose.
• Tell patient he'll need periodic blood tests to monitor therapeutic effects.

finasteride
fin-AS-teh-ride

Propecia, Proscar

Pharmacologic class: steroid derivative
Pregnancy risk category X

AVAILABLE FORMS
Tablets: 1 mg, 5 mg

INDICATIONS & DOSAGES
➤ **Male pattern hair loss (andro-genetic alopecia) in men only**
Men: 1 mg P.O. Propecia daily.
➤ **To improve symptoms of BPH and reduce risk of acute urine retention and need for surgery, including transurethral resection of prostate and prostatectomy**
Men: 5 mg P.O. Proscar daily.
➤ **With doxazosin, to reduce the risk of BPH symptom progression (Proscar)**
Men: 5 mg P.O. daily.
➤ **Women with polycystic ovary syndrome hirsutism ♦**
Adults: 2.5 to 5 mg P.O. daily.

ADMINISTRATION
P.O.
• Give drug without regard for food.

ACTION
Inhibits conversion of testosterone to dihydrotestosterone (DHT), the androgen primarily responsible for the initial development and subsequent enlarge-ment of the prostate gland. In male pattern baldness, the scalp contains miniaturized hair follicles and increased DHT level; drug decreases scalp DHT level in such cases.

Route	Onset	Peak	Duration
P.O.	Unknown	1–2 hr	24 hr

Half-life: Unknown.

ADVERSE REACTIONS
GU: impotence, decreased volume of ejaculate, decreased libido.

INTERACTIONS
None significant.

EFFECTS ON LAB TEST RESULTS
• May decrease prostate-specific antigen (PSA) level.

CONTRAINDICATIONS & CAUTIONS
• Contraindicated in patients hypersensitive to drug or to other 5-alpha-reductase inhibitors, such as dutasteride. Although drug isn't used in women or children, manufacturer indicates pregnancy as a contraindication.
• Use cautiously in patients with liver dysfunction.

NURSING CONSIDERATIONS
• Before therapy, evaluate patient for conditions that mimic BPH, including hypotonic bladder, prostate cancer, infection, or stricture.
• Carefully monitor patients who have a large residual urine volume or severely diminished urine flow.
• Sustained increase in PSA level could indicate noncompliance with therapy.
• A minimum of 6 months of therapy may be needed for treatment of BPH.

PATIENT TEACHING
• Tell patient that drug may be taken with or without meals.
• Warn woman who is or may become pregnant not to handle crushed tablets because of risk of adverse effects on male fetus.
• Inform patient that signs of improve-ment may require at least 3 months of daily use when drug is used to treat hair loss or at least 6 months when taken for BPH.
• Reassure patient that drug may decrease volume of ejaculate without impairing normal sexual function.

tamsulosin hydrochloride
tam-soo-LOE-sin

Flomax

Pharmacologic class: alpha blocker
Pregnancy risk category B

AVAILABLE FORMS
Capsules: 0.4 mg

INDICATIONS & DOSAGES
➤ **BPH**
Adults: 0.4 mg P.O. once daily, given
30 minutes after same meal each day. If
no response after 2 to 4 weeks, increase
dosage to 0.8 mg P.O. once daily.

ADMINISTRATION
P.O.
● Don't crush or open capsules.
● Give drug 30 minutes after same meal
each day.

ACTION
Selectively blocks alpha receptors in the
prostate, leading to relaxation of smooth
muscles in the bladder neck and prostate,
improving urine flow and reducing symptoms of BPH.

Route	Onset	Peak	Duration
P.O.	Unknown	4–5 hr	9–15 hr

Half-life: 9 to 13 hours.

ADVERSE REACTIONS
CNS: *dizziness, headache,* asthenia,
insomnia, somnolence, syncope, vertigo.
CV: chest pain, orthostatic hypotension.
EENT: *rhinitis,* amblyopia, pharyngitis,
sinusitis.
GI: diarrhea, nausea.
GU: decreased libido, abnormal ejacula-
tion, priapism.
Musculoskeletal: back pain.
Respiratory: increased cough.
Other: *infection,* tooth disorder.

INTERACTIONS
Drug-drug. *Alpha blockers:* May interact
with tamsulosin. Avoid using together.
Cimetidine: May decrease tamsulosin
clearance. Use together cautiously.

EFFECTS ON LAB TEST RESULTS
None reported.

CONTRAINDICATIONS & CAUTIONS
● Contraindicated in patients hypersensitive
to drug or its components.

NURSING CONSIDERATIONS
● Monitor patient for decreases in blood
pressure.
● Symptoms of BPH and prostate cancer
are similar; rule out prostate cancer before
starting therapy.
● If treatment is interrupted for several
days or more, restart therapy at the 0.4 mg
P.O. once daily dose.
● *Look alike–sound alike:* Don't confuse
Flomax with Fosamax or Volmax.

PATIENT TEACHING
● Instruct patient not to crush, chew, or
open capsules.
● Tell patient to rise slowly from chair or
bed when starting therapy and to avoid
situations in which injury could occur as
a result of fainting. Advise him that drug
may cause sudden drop in blood pressure,
especially after first dose or when changing doses.
● Inform patient about the rare, but serious,
possibility of priapism.
● Instruct patient not to drive or perform
hazardous tasks for 12 hours after first
dose or changes in dose until response can
be monitored.
● Tell patient to take drug about 30 minutes
after same meal each day.
● Advise patient considering cataract
surgery to inform the ophthalmologist
that he is taking the drug. Floppy iris
syndrome may occur during surgery.

Reactions may be *common,* uncommon, *life-threatening,* or COMMON AND LIFE-THREATENING.
Interaction may have a *rapid onset* or ***delayed onset.***

66

Erectile dysfunction drugs

alprostadil
sildenafil citrate
tadalafil
vardenafil hydrochloride

---

alprostadil
al-PROSS-ta-dil

Caverject, Caverject Impulse,
Edex, Muse

Pharmacologic class: prostaglandin
Pregnancy risk category NR

AVAILABLE FORMS
Injection: 5 mcg/ml, 10 mcg/0.5 ml,
10 mcg/ml, 20 mcg/0.5 ml, 20 mcg/ml,
40 mcg/ml after reconstitution
Urogenital suppository: 125 mcg,
250 mcg, 500 mcg, 1,000 mcg

INDICATIONS & DOSAGES
➤ **Erectile dysfunction of vasculo-**
genic, psychogenic, or mixed causes
Injection
Men: Dosages are highly individualized;
initially, inject 2.5 mcg intracavernously.
If partial response occurs, give second
dose of 2.5 mcg; then increase in
increments of 5 to 10 mcg until patient
achieves erection suitable for intercourse and lasting no longer than
1 hour. If patient doesn't respond to
first dose, increase second dose to
7.5 mcg within 1 hour, and then
increase further in increments of 5 to
10 mcg until patient achieves suitable
erection. Patient must remain in
prescriber's office until complete
detumescence occurs. Don't
repeat procedure for at least 24 hours.
Urogenital suppository
Men: Initially, 125 to 250 mcg, under
supervision of prescriber. Adjust dosage
as needed until response is sufficient for
sexual intercourse. Maximum of two
administrations in 24 hours; maximum
dose is 1,000 mcg.

➤ **Erectile dysfunction of neurogenic**
cause (spinal cord injury)
Men: Dosages are highly individualized;
initially, inject 1.25 mcg intracavernously.
If partial response occurs, give second
dose of 1.25 mcg. Increase in increments
of 2.5 mcg, to dose of 5 mcg; then increase
in increments of 5 mcg until patient
achieves erection suitable for intercourse
and lasting no longer than 1 hour. If
patient doesn't respond to first dose, give
next higher dose within 1 hour. Patient
must remain in prescriber's office until
complete detumescence occurs. If there is
a response, don't repeat procedure for at
least 24 hours.

ADMINISTRATION
● For intracavernous injection, teach patient
to follow instructions on package insert.
● Store injection at or below room temperature (77° F [25° C]).
● Vial is designed for a single use. Discard
vial if injection solution is discolored or
contains precipitate.
● Don't shake injection contents of reconstituted vial.
● Store unopened urogenital suppositories
in refrigerator (36° to 46° F [2° to 8° C]).
● Have patient urinate before inserting
suppository because moisture makes it
easier to insert drug in penis and will help
dissolve it.

ACTION
Induces erection by relaxing trabecular
smooth muscle and dilating cavernosal
arteries. This leads to expansion of
lacunar spaces and entrapment of
blood by compressing venules against
the tunica albuginea, a process referred
to as the corporal veno-occlusive
mechanism.

Route	Onset	Peak	Duration
Intra-cavernous	5–20 min	5–20 min	1–6 hr
Urogenital	10 min	16 min	1 hr

Half-life: About 5 to 10 minutes.

ADVERSE REACTIONS

CNS: headache, dizziness.
CV: hypertension, hypotension.
EENT: sinusitis, nasal congestion.
GU: *penile pain, urethral burning,* prolonged erection, penile fibrosis, rash, or edema, prostatic disorder, pelvic pain, minor bleeding or spotting, testicular pain.
Musculoskeletal: back pain.
Respiratory: upper respiratory tract infection, cough, rhinitis.
Skin: injection site hematoma or ecchymosis.
Other: localized trauma or pain, flulike syndrome, accidental injury.

INTERACTIONS

Drug-drug. *Anticoagulants:* May increase risk of bleeding from intracavernosal injection site. Monitor patient closely.
Cyclosporine: May decrease cyclosporine level. Monitor cyclosporine level closely.
Vasoactive drugs: Safety and effectiveness haven't been studied. Avoid using together.

EFFECTS ON LAB TEST RESULTS

None reported.

CONTRAINDICATIONS & CAUTIONS

● Contraindicated in patients hypersensitive to drug, in those with conditions predisposing them to priapism (sickle cell anemia or trait, multiple myeloma, leukemia) or penile deformation (angulation, cavernosal fibrosis, Peyronie disease), in men with penile implants or for whom sexual activity is inadvisable or contraindicated, in women or children, and in sexual partners of pregnant women unless condoms are used.

NURSING CONSIDERATIONS

● Stop drug in patients who develop penile angulation, cavernosal fibrosis, or Peyronie disease.

PATIENT TEACHING

● Teach patient how to prepare and give drug before he begins treatment at home. Stress importance of reading and following patient instructions in each package insert. Tell him to store unopened suppositories in refrigerator (36° to 46° F [2° to 8° C]) and store

injection at or below room temperature (77° F [25° C]).
● Tell patient not to shake contents of reconstituted vial, and remind him that vial is designed for a single use. Tell him to discard vial if solution is discolored or contains precipitate.
● Instruct patient to urinate before inserting suppository because moisture makes it easier to insert drug in penis and will help dissolve it.
● Review administration and aseptic technique.
● Inform patient that he can expect an erection 5 to 20 minutes after administration, with a preferable duration of no more than 1 hour. If his erection lasts more than 6 hours, tell him to seek medical attention immediately.
● Remind patient to take drug as instructed (generally, no more than three times weekly, with at least 24 hours between each use). Warn him not to change dosage without consulting prescriber.
● Caution patient to use a condom if his sexual partner could be pregnant.
● Review possible adverse reactions. Tell patient to inspect his penis daily and to report redness, swelling, tenderness, curvature, excessive erection (priapism), unusual pain, nodules, or hard tissue.
● Urge patient not to reuse or share needles, syringes, or drug.
● Warn patient that drug doesn't protect against sexually transmitted diseases. Also, caution him that bleeding at injection site can increase risk of transmitting blood-borne diseases to his partner.
● Remind patient to keep regular follow-up appointments so prescriber can evaluate drug effectiveness and safety.

---

sildenafil citrate
sill-DEN-ah-fill

Revatio, Viagra♪

Pharmacologic class:
phosphodiesterase type-5 inhibitor
Pregnancy risk category B

AVAILABLE FORMS

Tablets: 20 mg, 25 mg, 50 mg, 100 mg

Reactions may be *common*, uncommon, *life-threatening*, or COMMON AND LIFE-THREATENING.
Interaction may have a *rapid onset* or **delayed onset**.

INDICATIONS & DOSAGES
➤ **Erectile dysfunction**
Adults younger than age 65: About 1 hour before sexual activity, 50 mg P.O., p.r.n. Dosage range is 25 to 100 mg based on effectiveness and tolerance. Maximum is one dose daily.
Elderly patients (age 65 and older): 25 mg P.O., as needed, about 1 hour before sexual activity. Dosage may be adjusted based on patient response. Maximum is one dose daily.
Adjust-a-dose: For adults with hepatic or severe renal impairment, 25 mg P.O. about 1 hour before sexual activity. Dosage may be adjusted based on patient response. Maximum is one dose daily.
➤ **Pulmonary arterial hypertension (Revatio only)**
Adults: 20 mg P.O. t.i.d. with doses taken 4 to 6 hours apart.

ADMINISTRATION
P.O.
● For most rapid absorption, give to patient on empty stomach.

ACTION
Increases effect of nitric oxide by inhibiting phosphodiesterase type 5 (PDE_5), which is responsible for degradation of cyclic guanosine monophosphate (cGMP) in the corpus cavernosum. When sexual stimulation causes local release of nitric oxide, inhibition of PDE_5 by sildenafil causes increased levels of cGMP in the corpus cavernosum, resulting in smooth muscle relaxation and inflow of blood to the corpus cavernosum.

Route	Onset	Peak	Duration
P.O.	15–30 min	30–120 min	4 hr

Half-life: 4 hours.

ADVERSE REACTIONS
CNS: *headache, seizures,* anxiety, dizziness, somnolence, vertigo.
CV: *MI, sudden cardiac death, ventricular arrhythmias, cerebrovascular hemorrhage, transient ischemic attack,* hypotension, flushing.
EENT: diplopia, temporary vision loss, decrease or loss of hearing, tinnitus, ocular redness or bloodshot appearance, increased

intraocular pressure, retinal vascular disease, retinal bleeding, vitreous detachment or traction, paramacular edema, photophobia, altered color perception, blurred vision, burning, swelling, pressure, nasal congestion.
GI: *dyspepsia,* diarrhea.
GU: hematuria, prolonged erection, priapism, UTI.
Musculoskeletal: arthralgia, back pain.
Respiratory: respiratory tract infection
Skin: rash.
Other: flulike syndrome.

INTERACTIONS
Drug-drug. *Beta blockers, loop and potassium-sparing diuretics:* May increase sildenafil metabolite level. Monitor patient.
Cytochrome P-450 inducers, rifampin: May reduce sildenafil level. Monitor effect.
Delavirdine, protease inhibitors: May increase sildenafil level, increasing risk of adverse events, including hypotension, visual changes, and priapism. Reduce initial sildenafil dose to 25 mg.
Hepatic isoenzyme inhibitors (such as cimetidine, erythromycin, itraconazole, ketoconazole): May reduce sildenafil clearance. Avoid using together.
Isosorbide, nitroglycerin: May cause severe hypotension. Use of nitrates in any form with sildenafil is contraindicated.
Drug-food. *High-fat meal:* May reduce absorption rate and peak level of drug. Advise patient to take drug on empty stomach.
Grapefruit: May increase drug level, while delaying absorption. Advise patient to avoid using together.

EFFECTS ON LAB TEST RESULTS
None reported.

CONTRAINDICATIONS & CAUTIONS
● Contraindicated in patients hypersensitive to drug or its components and in those taking organic nitrates.
● Use cautiously in patients age 65 and older; in patients with hepatic or severe renal impairment, retinitis pigmentosa, bleeding disorders, or active peptic ulcer disease; in those who have suffered an MI, a stroke, or life-threatening arrhythmia within last 6 months; in those with history of cardiac failure, coronary artery disease,

uncontrolled high or low blood pressure, or anatomic deformation of the penis (such as angulation, cavernosal fibrosis, or Peyronie disease); and in those with conditions that may predispose them to priapism (such as sickle cell anemia, multiple myeloma, or leukemia).

NURSING CONSIDERATIONS
• *Alert:* Drug increases risk of cardiac events. Systemic vasodilatory properties cause transient decreases in supine blood pressure and cardiac output (about 2 hours after ingestion). Patients with underlying CV disease are at increased risk for cardiac effects related to sexual activity.
• *Alert:* Serious CV events, including MI, sudden cardiac death, ventricular arrhythmias, cerebrovascular hemorrhage, transient ischemic attack, and hypertension, may occur with drug use. Most, but not all, of these incidents involve CV risk factors. Many events occur during or shortly after sexual activity; a few occur shortly after drug use without sexual activity, and others occur hours to days after drug use and sexual activity.
• Drug isn't indicated for use in neonates, children, or women.

PATIENT TEACHING
• Advise patient that drug shouldn't be used with nitrates under any circumstances.
• Advise patient of potential cardiac risk of sexual activity, especially in presence of CV risk factors. Instruct patient to notify prescriber and refrain from further activity if such symptoms as chest pain, dizziness, or nausea occur when starting sexual activity.
• Warn patient that erections lasting longer than 4 hours and priapism (painful erections lasting longer than 6 hours) may occur, and tell him to seek immediate medical attention. Penile tissue damage and permanent loss of potency may result if priapism isn't treated immediately.
• Inform patient that drug doesn't protect against sexually transmitted diseases; advise patient to use protective measures such as condoms.
• Tell patient receiving HIV medications that he's at increased risk for sildenafil adverse events, including low blood pressure, visual changes, and priapism,

and that he should promptly report such symptoms to his prescriber. Tell him not to exceed 25 mg of sildenafil in 48 hours.
• Instruct patient to take drug 30 minutes to 4 hours before sexual activity; maximum benefit can be expected less than 2 hours after ingestion.
• Advise patient that drug is most rapidly absorbed if taken on an empty stomach.
• Inform patient that impairment of color discrimination (blue, green) may occur and to avoid hazardous activities that rely on color discrimination.
• Instruct patient to notify prescriber of vision or hearing changes.
• Advise patient that drug is effective only in presence of sexual stimulation.
• Caution patient to take drug only as prescribed.

---

tadalafil
tah-DAL-ah-fill

Cialis

Pharmacologic class:
phosphodiesterase type-5 inhibitor
Pregnancy risk category B

AVAILABLE FORMS
Tablets (film-coated): 2.5 mg, 5 mg, 10 mg, 20 mg

INDICATIONS & DOSAGES
➤ **Erectile dysfunction**
Adults: 10 mg P.O. as a single dose, as needed, before sexual activity. Range is 5 to 20 mg, based on effectiveness and tolerance. Maximum is one dose daily. Or 2.5 mg P.O. once daily without regard to timing of sexual activity. May increase to 5 mg P.O. daily.
Adjust-a-dose: If creatinine clearance is 31 to 50 ml/minute, starting dosage is 5 mg once daily and maximum is 10 mg once every 48 hours. If clearance is 30 ml/minute or less, maximum is 5 mg once daily. Patients with Child-Pugh category A or B shouldn't exceed 10 mg daily. Patients taking potent cytochrome P-450 inhibitors (such as erythromycin, itraconazole, ketoconazole, and ritonavir) shouldn't exceed one 10-mg dose every 72 hours.

Reactions may be *common*, uncommon, *life-threatening*, or COMMON AND LIFE-THREATENING.
Interaction may have a *rapid onset* or **delayed onset**.

ADMINISTRATION
P.O.
● Give drug without regard for food.

ACTION
Increases cGMP levels, prolongs smooth muscle relaxation, and promotes blood flow into the corpus cavernosum.

Route	Onset	Peak	Duration
P.O.	Immediate	½–6 hr	Unknown

Half-life: 17½ hours.

ADVERSE REACTIONS
CNS: dizziness, *headache.*
CV: flushing.
EENT: decrease or loss of hearing, nasal congestion, tinnitus.
GI: *dyspepsia.*
Musculoskeletal: back pain, limb pain, myalgia.

INTERACTIONS
Drug-drug. *Alpha blockers (except 0.4 mg tamsulosin daily), nitrates:* May enhance hypotensive effects. Use together is contraindicated.
Potent cytochrome P-450 inhibitors (such as erythromycin, itraconazole, ketoconazole, ritonavir): May increase tadalafil level. Don't exceed a 10-mg dose every 72 hours.
Rifampin and other cytochrome P-450 inducers: May decrease tadalafil level. Monitor patient closely.
Drug-food. *Grapefruit:* May increase drug level. Discourage use together.
Drug-lifestyle. *Alcohol use:* May increase risk of headache, dizziness, orthostatic hypotension, and increased heart rate. Discourage use together.

EFFECTS ON LAB TEST RESULTS
None reported.

CONTRAINDICATIONS & CAUTIONS
● Contraindicated in patients hypersensitive to drug or its components and in those taking nitrates or alpha blockers (other than tamsulosin 0.4 mg once daily).
● Drug isn't recommended for patients with Child-Pugh category C, unstable angina, angina that occurs during sexual intercourse, New York Heart Association class II or greater heart failure within past 6 months, uncontrolled arrhythmias, hypotension (lower than 90/50 mm Hg), uncontrolled hypertension (higher than 170/100 mm Hg), stroke within past 6 months, or an MI within past 90 days.
● Drug isn't recommended for patients whose cardiac status makes sexual activity inadvisable or for those with hereditary degenerative retinal disorders.
● Use cautiously in patients taking potent cytochrome P-450 inhibitors (such as erythromycin, itraconazole, ketoconazole, and ritonavir) and in patients with bleeding disorders, significant peptic ulceration, or renal or hepatic impairment.
● Use cautiously in patients with conditions predisposing them to priapism (such as sickle cell anemia, multiple myeloma, and leukemia), anatomical penis abnormalities, or left ventricular outflow obstruction.
● Use cautiously in elderly patients, who may be more sensitive to drug effects.

NURSING CONSIDERATIONS
● *Alert:* Sexual activity may increase cardiac risk. Evaluate patient's cardiac risk before he starts taking drug.
● Before patient starts drug, assess him for underlying causes of erectile dysfunction.
● Transient decreases in supine blood pressure may occur.
● Prolonged erections and priapism may occur.

PATIENT TEACHING
● Warn patient that taking drug with nitrates could cause a serious drop in blood pressure, which increases the risk of heart attack or stroke.
● Tell patient to seek immediate medical attention if chest pain develops after taking the drug.
● Tell patient that drug doesn't protect against sexually transmitted diseases and that he should use protective measures.
● Urge patient to seek emergency medical care if his erection lasts more than 4 hours.
● Tell patient to take drug about 60 minutes before anticipated sexual activity. Explain that drug has no effect without sexual stimulation.
● Warn patient not to change dosage unless directed by prescriber.

• Caution patient against drinking large amounts of alcohol while taking drug.
• Instruct patient to notify prescriber of hearing changes.

---

vardenafil hydrochloride
var-DEN-ah-fill

Levitra◆

Pharmacologic class:
phosphodiesterase type-5 inhibitor
Pregnancy risk category B

AVAILABLE FORMS
Tablets (film-coated): 2.5 mg, 5 mg, 10 mg, 20 mg

INDICATIONS & DOSAGES
➤ **Erectile dysfunction**
Adults: 10 mg P.O. as a single dose, as needed, 1 hour before sexual activity. Dosage range is 5 to 20 mg, based on effectiveness and tolerance. Maximum, one dose daily.
Elderly patients age 65 and older: Initially 5 mg as a single dose, as needed, 1 hour before sexual activity.
Adjust-a-dose: For patients with Child-Pugh category B, first dose is 5 mg daily, as needed. Don't exceed 10 mg daily in patients with hepatic impairment.

ADMINISTRATION
P.O.
• Give drug without regard for food.

ACTION
Increases cGMP levels, prolongs smooth muscle relaxation, and promotes blood flow into the corpus cavernosum.

Route	Onset	Peak	Duration
P.O.	Immediate	30–120 min	Unknown

Half-life: 4 to 5 hours.

ADVERSE REACTIONS
CNS: *headache,* dizziness.
CV: *flushing.*
EENT: decrease or loss of hearing, tinnitus, rhinitis, sinusitis.
GI: dyspepsia, nausea.
Musculoskeletal: back pain.
Other: flulike syndrome.

INTERACTIONS
Drug-drug. *Alpha blockers, nitrates:* May enhance hypotensive effects. Avoid using together.
Antiarrhythmics of class IA (quinidine, procainamide) and class III (amiodarone, sotalol): May prolong QTc interval. Avoid using together.
Erythromycin, indinavir, itraconazole, ketoconazole, ritonavir: May increase vardenafil level. Reduce dose of vardenafil. If taken with ritonavir, reduce and extend dosage interval to once every 72 hours.
Drug-food. *High-fat meals:* May reduce peak level of drug. Discourage use with a high-fat meal.

EFFECTS ON LAB TEST RESULTS
• May increase CK level.

CONTRAINDICATIONS & CAUTIONS
• Contraindicated in patients hypersensitive to drug or its components and in those taking nitrates or alpha blockers.
• Contraindicated in patients with unstable angina, hypotension (systolic less than 90 mm Hg), uncontrolled hypertension (over 170/110 mm Hg), stroke, life-threatening arrhythmia, an MI within past 6 months, severe cardiac failure, Child-Pugh category C, end-stage renal disease requiring dialysis, congenital QTc-interval pro-longation, or hereditary degenerative retinal disorders.
• Use cautiously in patients with bleed-ing disorders or significant peptic ulceration.
• Use cautiously in those with anatomical penis abnormalities or conditions that predispose patient to priapism (such as sickle cell anemia, multiple myeloma, or leukemia).

NURSING CONSIDERATIONS
• **Alert:** Sexual activity may increase cardiac risk. Evaluate patient's cardiac risk before he starts taking drug.
• Before patient starts drug, assess for underlying causes of erectile dysfunction.
• Transient decreases in supine blood pressure may occur.
• Prolonged erections and priapism may occur.

Reactions may be *common,* uncommon, *life-threatening,* or COMMON AND LIFE-THREATENING.
Interaction may have a *rapid onset* or *delayed onset.*

PATIENT TEACHING
● Tell patient that drug doesn't protect against sexually transmitted diseases and that he should use protective measures.
● Advise patient that drug is absorbed most rapidly if taken on an empty stomach.
● Tell patient to notify prescriber about vision or hearing changes.
● Urge patient to seek immediate medical care if erection lasts more than 4 hours.
● Tell patient to take drug 60 minutes before anticipated sexual activity. Explain that drug has no effect without sexual stimulation.
● Warn patient not to change dosage unless directed by prescriber.

67
Incontinence drugs

darifenacin hydrobromide
flavoxate hydrochloride
oxybutynin chloride
solifenacin succinate
tolterodine tartrate
trospium chloride

---

darifenacin hydrobromide
da-ree-FEN-ah-sin

Enablex✏

Pharmacologic class:
antimuscarinic
Pregnancy risk category C

AVAILABLE FORMS
Tablets (extended-release): 7.5 mg, 15 mg

INDICATIONS & DOSAGES
➤ **Urge incontinence, urgency,**
and frequency from an overactive
bladder
Adults: Initially, 7.5 mg P.O. once daily.
After 2 weeks, may increase to 15 mg P.O.
once daily if needed.
Adjust-a-dose: If patient has a Child-Pugh
score of B or takes a potent CYP3A4 inhibitor, such as clarithromycin, itraconazole,
ketoconazole, nefazodone, nelfinavir, ritonavir, don't exceed 7.5 mg P.O. once daily.

ADMINISTRATION
P.O.
● Don't crush tablet; swallow whole.
● Give drug without regard for food.

ACTION
Relaxes smooth muscle of bladder by
antagonizing muscarinic receptors,
relieving symptoms of overactive bladder.

Route	Onset	Peak	Duration
P.O.	Unknown	7 hr	Unknown

Half-life: 13 to 19 hours.

ADVERSE REACTIONS
CNS: asthenia, dizziness, pain.
CV: hypertension, peripheral edema.

EENT: abnormal vision, dry eyes,
pharyngitis, rhinitis, sinusitis.
GI: *dry mouth, constipation,* abdominal
pain, diarrhea, dyspepsia, nausea, vomiting.
GU: urinary tract disorder, UTI,
vaginitis.
Metabolic: weight gain.
Musculoskeletal: arthralgia, back pain.
Respiratory: bronchitis.
Skin: dry skin, pruritus, rash.
Other: accidental injury, flulike syndrome.

INTERACTIONS
Drug-drug. *Anticholinergics:* May
increase anticholinergic effects, such as dry
mouth, blurred vision, and constipation.
Monitor patient closely.
Digoxin: May increase digoxin level.
Monitor digoxin level.
*Drugs metabolized by CYP2D6 (such as
flecainide, thioridazine, tricyclic antidepressants):* May increase levels of these
drugs. Use together cautiously.
Midazolam: May increase midazolam
level. Monitor patient carefully.
*Potent CYP3A4 inhibitors (such as
clarithromycin, itraconazole, ketoconazole,
nefazodone, nelfinavir, ritonavir):* May
increase darifenacin level. Maintain
dosage no higher than 7.5 mg P.O. daily.
Drug-lifestyle. *Hot weather:* May cause
heat prostration from decreased sweating.
Urge caution.

EFFECTS ON LAB TEST RESULTS
None reported.

CONTRAINDICATIONS & CAUTIONS
● Contraindicated in patients hypersensitive
to drug or its ingredients.
● Contraindicated in patients who have or
who are at risk for urine retention, gastric
retention, or uncontrolled narrow-angle
glaucoma.
● Avoid use in patients with a Child-Pugh
score of C.
● Use cautiously in patients with bladder
outflow or GI obstruction, ulcerative colitis,
myasthenia gravis, severe constipation,
controlled narrow-angle glaucoma,

Reactions may be *common,* uncommon, *life-threatening,* or COMMON AND LIFE-THREATENING.
Interaction may have a *rapid onset* or ***delayed onset.***

decreased GI motility, or a Child-Pugh score of B.

NURSING CONSIDERATIONS
● Assess bladder function, and monitor drug effects.
● If patient has bladder outlet obstruction, watch for urine retention.
● Assess patient for decreased gastric motility and constipation.
● Use during pregnancy only if maternal benefit outweighs fetal risk.
● It's unknown if drug appears in breast milk.

PATIENT TEACHING
● Tell patient to swallow tablet whole with plenty of liquid; caution against crushing or chewing tablet.
● Inform patient that drug may be taken with or without food.
● Tell patient to use caution, especially when performing hazardous tasks, until drug effects are known.
● Tell patient to report blurred vision, constipation, and urine retention.
● Discourage use of other drugs that may cause dry mouth, constipation, urine retention, or blurred vision.
● Tell patient that drug decreases sweating, and advise cautious use in hot environments and during strenuous activity.

---

flavoxate hydrochloride
fla-VOX-ate

Urispas

Pharmacologic class: flavone derivative
Pregnancy risk category B

AVAILABLE FORMS
Tablets: 100 mg

INDICATIONS & DOSAGES
➤ **Symptomatic relief of dysuria, urinary frequency and urgency, nocturia, incontinence, and suprapubic pain from urologic disorders**
Adults and children older than age 12: 100 to 200 mg P.O. t.i.d. to q.i.d. Reduce dosage when symptoms improve.

ADMINISTRATION
P.O.
● Give drug without regard for food.

ACTION
Produces a direct spasmolytic effect on urinary tract smooth muscles and provides local anesthesia and analgesia.

Route	Onset	Peak	Duration
P.O.	Unknown	2 hr	Unknown

Half-life: Unknown.

ADVERSE REACTIONS
CNS: *confusion,* nervousness, dizziness, headache, drowsiness, vertigo, fever.
CV: tachycardia, palpitations.
EENT: *blurred vision,* disturbed eye accommodation, increased ocular tension.
GI: dry mouth, nausea, vomiting.
GU: dysuria.
Hematologic: *leukopenia,* eosinophilia.
Skin: urticaria, dermatoses.

INTERACTIONS
Drug-lifestyle. *Exercise, hot weather:* May cause heatstroke. Advise patient to use with caution in hot weather.

EFFECTS ON LAB TEST RESULTS
● May increase eosinophil count. May decrease WBC count.

CONTRAINDICATIONS & CAUTIONS
● Contraindicated in patients with pyloric or duodenal obstruction, obstructive intestinal lesions or ileus, achalasia, GI hemorrhage, or obstructive uropathies of lower urinary tract.
● Safety and effectiveness of drug in children age 12 and younger are unknown.
● Use cautiously in patients who may have glaucoma and in pregnant or breast-feeding women.

NURSING CONSIDERATIONS
● Check patient history for other drug use before giving drugs with anticholinergic adverse reactions. Such reactions may be intensified by flavoxate.
● *Look alike–sound alike:* Don't confuse Urispas with Urised.

PATIENT TEACHING
• Warn patient to avoid hazardous activities, such as operating machinery or driving, until CNS effects of drug are known.
• Tell patient to contact prescriber if adverse reactions occur or if symptoms aren't diminished.
• Caution patient that using drug during very hot weather may cause fever or heatstroke because it suppresses diaphoresis.
• Tell patient drug may cause dry mouth or blurred vision.

oxybutynin chloride
ox-i-BYOO-ti-nin

Ditropan, Ditropan XL, Oxytrol

Pharmacologic class:
antimuscarinic
Pregnancy risk category B

AVAILABLE FORMS
Syrup: 5 mg/5 ml
Tablets: 5 mg
Tablets (extended-release): 5 mg, 10 mg, 15 mg
Transdermal patch: 36-mg patch delivering 3.9 mg/day

INDICATIONS & DOSAGES
➤ **Uninhibited or reflex neurogenic bladder**
Adults: 5 mg P.O. b.i.d. to t.i.d., to maximum of 5 mg q.i.d.
Children age 5 and older: 5 mg P.O. b.i.d., to maximum of 5 mg t.i.d.
➤ **Overactive bladder**
Adults: Initially, 5 mg P.O. Ditropan XL once daily. Dosage adjustments may be made weekly in 5-mg increments, as needed, to maximum of 30 mg P.O. daily. Or, apply one patch twice weekly to dry, intact skin on the abdomen, hip, or buttock.
➤ **Symptoms of detrusor overactivity associated with a neurological condition (e.g. spina bifida)**
Children age 6 and older: 5 mg P.O. Ditropan XL once daily. May increase in 5-mg increments, as needed, to maximum of 20 mg P.O. daily.

ADMINISTRATION
P.O.
• Don't crush extended-release tablets.
• Give extended-release tablets without regard for food.
Transdermal
• Apply to dry, intact skin on the abdomen, hip, or buttock.
• Avoid reapplication to the same site within 7 days.

ACTION
Relaxes smooth muscle of bladder by antagonizing muscarinic receptors, relieving symptoms of overactive bladder.

Route	Onset	Peak	Duration
P.O.	30–60 min	3–4 hr	6–10 hr
P.O. (extended-release)	Unknown	4–6 hr	24 hr
Trans-dermal	24–48 hr	Varies	96 hr

Half-life: For tablets or oral solution, 2 to 3 hours; for extended-release tablets, 12 to 13 hours; for patch, 7 to 8 hours.

ADVERSE REACTIONS
CNS: dizziness, insomnia, restlessness, hallucinations, asthenia, fever.
CV: *palpitations, tachycardia,* vasodilation.
EENT: mydriasis, cycloplegia, decreased lacrimation, amblyopia.
GI: *constipation, dry mouth,* nausea, vomiting, decreased GI motility.
GU: *urinary hesitancy, urine retention,* impotence.
Skin: rash, decreased diaphoresis.
Other: suppression of lactation.
Transdermal patch
CNS: fatigue, somnolence, headache.
CV: flushing.
EENT: abnormal vision.
GI: *dry mouth,* diarrhea, abdominal pain, nausea, flatulence.
GU: dysuria.
Musculoskeletal: back pain.
Skin: *pruritus,* erythema, vesicles, macules, rash, burning at injection site.

INTERACTIONS
Drug-drug. *Anticholinergics:* May increase anticholinergic effects. Use together cautiously.

Reactions may be *common,* uncommon, *life-threatening,* or COMMON AND LIFE-THREATENING.
Interaction may have a *rapid onset* or **delayed onset.**

Atenolol, digoxin: May increase levels of these drugs. Monitor drug levels closely.
CNS depressants: May increase CNS effects. Use together cautiously.
Haloperidol: May decrease haloperidol level. Monitor drug level closely.
Drug-lifestyle. *Alcohol use:* May increase CNS effects. Discourage use together.
Exercise, hot weather: May cause heatstroke. Advise patient to use with caution in hot weather.

EFFECTS ON LAB TEST RESULTS
None reported.

CONTRAINDICATIONS & CAUTIONS
● Contraindicated in patients hypersensitive to drug or its components and in those with myasthenia gravis, GI obstruction, untreated angle-closure glaucoma, megacolon, adynamic ileus, severe colitis, ulcerative colitis with megacolon, urine or gastric retention, or obstructive uropathy.
● Contraindicated in elderly or debilitated patients with intestinal atony and in hemorrhaging patients with unstable CV status.
● Use cautiously in elderly, pregnant, or breast-feeding patients and in those with autonomic neuropathy, reflux esophagitis, or hepatic or renal disease.
● Extended-release form is not recommended for children who can't swallow the tablet whole without chewing, dividing, or crushing, or children under 6 years.
● Use extended-release form cautiously in patients with bladder outflow obstruction, gastric obstruction, ulcerative colitis, intestinal atony, myasthenia gravis, or gastroesophageal reflux and in those taking drugs that worsen esophagitis (bisphosphonates).

NURSING CONSIDERATIONS
● Before giving drug, get confirmation of neurogenic bladder by cystometry and rule out partial intestinal obstruction in patients with diarrhea, especially those with colostomy or ileostomy.
● If patient has UTI, treat him with antibiotics.
● Drug may aggravate symptoms of hyperthyroidism, coronary artery disease, heart failure, arrhythmias, tachycardia, hypertension, or prostatic hyperplasia.

● Obtain periodic cystometry as directed to evaluate response to therapy.
● ***Look alike–sound alike:*** Don't confuse Ditropan with diazepam or Dithranol.

PATIENT TEACHING
● Warn patient to avoid hazardous activities, such as operating machinery or driving, until CNS effects of drug are known.
● Caution patient that using drug during very hot weather may cause fever or heatstroke because it suppresses sweating.
● Tell patient to swallow Ditropan XL whole and not to chew or crush it.
● Instruct patient to measure syrup with a teaspoon.
● Advise patient to store drug in tightly closed container at 59° to 86° F (15° to 30° C).
● Instruct patient using transdermal patch to change patch twice a week and to choose a new application site with each new patch to avoid the same site within 7 days. Warn patient to only wear one patch at a time. Tell patient to dispose of old patches carefully in the trash in a manner that prevents accidental application or ingestion by children and pets.
● Advise patient to avoid alcohol while taking drug.
● Tell patient that drug may cause dry mouth.

solifenacin succinate
sole-ah-FEN-ah-sin

VESIcare

Pharmacologic class: antimuscarinic
Pregnancy risk category C

AVAILABLE FORMS
Tablets (film-coated): 5 mg, 10 mg

INDICATIONS & DOSAGES
➤ **Overactive bladder with urinary urgency, frequency, and urge incontinence**
Adults: 5 mg P.O. once daily. May increase to 10 mg once daily if 5-mg dose is well tolerated.
Adjust-a-dose: If creatinine clearance is less than 30 ml/minute or the patient has

moderate liver impairment (Child-Pugh score B), or drug is taken concurrently with CYP3A4 inhibitors, maintain the dose at 5 mg.

ADMINISTRATION
P.O.
● Give drug without regard for food.
● Drug should be swallowed whole with liquid.

ACTION
Relaxes smooth muscle of bladder by antagonizing muscarinic receptors, relieving symptoms of overactive bladder.

Route	Onset	Peak	Duration
P.O.	Unknown	3–8 hr	Unknown

Half-life: 2 to 3 days.

ADVERSE REACTIONS
CNS: depression, dizziness, fatigue.
CV: hypertension, leg swelling.
EENT: blurred vision, dry eyes, pharyngitis.
GI: *constipation, dry mouth,* dyspepsia, nausea, upper abdominal pain, vomiting.
GU: urinary retention, UTI.
Respiratory: cough.
Other: influenza.

INTERACTIONS
Drug-drug. *Drugs that prolong the QT interval:* May increase the risk of serious cardiac arrhythmias. Monitor patient and ECG closely.
Potent CYP3A4 inhibitors (such as ketoconazole): May increase solifenacin levels. Don't exceed solifenacin dose of 5 mg daily when used together.

EFFECTS ON LAB TEST RESULTS
None reported.

CONTRAINDICATIONS & CAUTIONS
● Contraindicated in patients hypersensitive to drug or its components and in patients with urine or gastric retention or uncontrolled narrow-angle glaucoma. Don't use in patients with severe hepatic impairment (Child Pugh score C).
● Use cautiously in patients with a history of prolonged QT interval, those being treated for narrow-angle glaucoma, and those with bladder outflow obstruction,

decreased GI motility, renal insufficiency, or moderate liver impairment.

NURSING CONSIDERATIONS
● Assess bladder function, and monitor drug effects.
● If patient has bladder outlet obstruction, watch for urine retention.
● Monitor patient for decreased gastric motility and constipation.
● Safety and effectiveness are similar in older and younger adults, but levels and half-life may be increased in the elderly.

PATIENT TEACHING
● Explain that drug may cause blurred vision. Tell patient to use caution when performing hazardous activities or tasks that require clear vision until effects of the drug are known.
● Discourage use of other drugs that may cause dry mouth, constipation, urine retention, or blurred vision.
● Urge patient to notify prescriber about abdominal pain or constipation that lasts 3 days or longer.
● Tell patient that drug decreases the ability to sweat normally, and advise cautious use in hot environments or during strenuous activity.
● Tell patient to swallow tablet whole with liquid.
● Inform patient that drug may be taken with or without food.

---

tolterodine tartrate
toll-TEAR-oh-deen

Detrol✒, Detrol LA

Pharmacologic class:
antimuscarinic
Pregnancy risk category C

AVAILABLE FORMS
Capsules (extended-release): 2 mg, 4 mg
Tablets: 1 mg, 2 mg

INDICATIONS & DOSAGES
➤ **Overactive bladder in patients with symptoms of urinary frequency, urgency, or urge incontinence**
Adults: 2-mg tablet P.O. b.i.d. or 4-mg extended-release capsule P.O. daily. Dose

may be reduced to 1-mg tablet P.O. b.i.d. or 2-mg extended-release capsule P.O. daily, based on patient response and tolerance.

Adjust-a-dose: For patients with significantly reduced hepatic or renal function or those taking a potent CYP3A4 inhibitor, 1-mg tablet P.O. b.i.d. or 2-mg extended-release capsule P.O. daily.

ADMINISTRATION
P.O.
● Give extended-release capsules with liquid to be swallowed whole.

ACTION
Relaxes smooth muscle of bladder by antagonizing muscarinic receptors, relieving symptoms of overactive bladder.

Route	Onset	Peak	Duration
P.O.	Unknown	1–2 hr	Unknown
P.O. (extended-release)	Unknown	2–6 hr	Unknown

Half-life: 2 to 4 hours; about 8 hours with hepatic impairment.

ADVERSE REACTIONS
CNS: headache, fatigue, paresthesia, vertigo, dizziness, nervousness, somnolence.
CV: hypertension, chest pain.
EENT: abnormal vision, xerophthalmia, pharyngitis, rhinitis, sinusitis.
GI: *dry mouth,* abdominal pain, constipation, diarrhea, dyspepsia, flatulence, nausea, vomiting.
GU: dysuria, micturition frequency, urine retention, UTI.
Metabolic: weight gain.
Musculoskeletal: arthralgia, back pain.
Respiratory: bronchitis, coughing, upper respiratory tract infection.
Skin: pruritus, rash, erythema, dry skin.
Other: flulike syndrome, accidental injury, fungal infection, infection.

INTERACTIONS
Drug-drug. *Antifungals (itraconazole, ketoconazole, miconazole), CYP3A4 inhibitors (such as clarithromycin and erythromycin):* May increase tolterodine level. Don't give more than 1-mg tablet

b.i.d. or 2-mg extended-release capsule daily of tolterodine if used together.
Fluoxetine: May increase tolterodine level. Monitor patient. No dosage adjustment is needed.

EFFECTS ON LAB TEST RESULTS
None reported.

CONTRAINDICATIONS & CAUTIONS
● Contraindicated in patients hypersensitive to drug or its components and in those with uncontrolled angle-closure glaucoma or urine or gastric retention.
● Use cautiously in patients with significant bladder outflow obstruction, GI obstructive disorders (such as pyloric stenosis), controlled angle-closure glaucoma, and hepatic or renal impairment.

NURSING CONSIDERATIONS
● Assess baseline bladder function and monitor therapeutic effects.

PATIENT TEACHING
● Tell patient that sugarless gum, hard candy, or saliva substitute may help relieve dry mouth.
● Advise patient to avoid driving or other potentially hazardous activities until visual effects of drug are known.
● Advise women to stop breast-feeding during therapy.
● Instruct patient to immediately report signs of infection, urine retention, or GI problems.
● Tell patient taking extended-release form to swallow capsule whole and take with liquids.

trospium chloride
TROZ-pee-um

Sanctura, Sanctura XR

Pharmacologic class:
antimuscarinic
Pregnancy risk category C

AVAILABLE FORMS
Capsules (extended-release): 60 mg
Tablets: 20 mg

INDICATIONS & DOSAGES
➤ **Overactive bladder with symptoms of urinary urge incontinence, urgency, and frequency**
Adults younger than age 75: 20 mg P.O. b.i.d. taken on an empty stomach or at least 1 hour before a meal. Or 60 mg extended release capsule P.O. daily in morning.
Adults age 75 and older: Based on patient tolerance, reduce dose to 20 mg once daily.
Adjust-a-dose: If patient's creatinine clearance is less than 30 ml/minute, give 20 mg P.O. once daily at bedtime. Extended release form is not recommended if creatinine clearance is less than 30 ml/minute.

ADMINISTRATION
P.O.
• Give at least 1 hour before meals or on an empty stomach.
• Give extended release form with water on an empty stomach at least 1 hour before meal.

ACTION
Relaxes smooth muscle of bladder by antagonizing muscarinic receptors, relieving symptoms of overactive bladder.

Route	Onset	Peak	Duration
P.O.	Unknown	5–6 hr	Unknown

Half-life: About 20 hours.

ADVERSE REACTIONS
CNS: fatigue, headache.
EENT: dry eyes.
GI: *constipation, dry mouth,* abdominal pain, dyspepsia, flatulence.
GU: urine retention.

INTERACTIONS
Drug-drug. *Anticholinergics:* May increase dry mouth, constipation, or other adverse effects. Monitor patient.
Digoxin, metformin, morphine, procainamide, pancuronium, tenofovir, vancomycin: May alter elimination of these drugs or trospium, increasing levels. Monitor patient closely.
Drug-food. *High-fat foods:* May significantly decrease absorption. Give drug at least 1 hour before meals or on an empty stomach.

Drug-lifestyle. *Alcohol use:* May increase drowsiness. Discourage use together.

EFFECTS ON LAB TEST RESULTS
None reported.

CONTRAINDICATIONS & CAUTIONS
• Contraindicated in patients hypersensitive to the drug or any of its ingredients and in those with or at risk for urine retention, gastric retention, or uncontrolled narrow-angle glaucoma.
• Use cautiously in patients with significant bladder outflow obstruction, obstructive GI disorders, ulcerative colitis, intestinal atony, myasthenia gravis, renal insufficiency, moderate or severe hepatic impairment, or controlled narrow-angle glaucoma.

NURSING CONSIDERATIONS
• Assess patient to determine baseline bladder function, and monitor patient for therapeutic effects.
• If patient has bladder outflow obstruction, watch for evidence of urine retention.
• Monitor patient for decreased gastric motility and constipation.
• Elderly patients typically need a reduced dosage because they have an increased risk of anticholinergic effects.

PATIENT TEACHING
• Tell patient to take drug on an empty stomach or at least 1 hour before meals.
• Tell patient to take extended release form with water in the morning on an empty stomach, at least one hour before a meal.
• Discourage use of other drugs that may cause dry mouth, constipation, blurred vision, or urine retention.
• Tell patient that alcohol may increase drowsiness and fatigue. Urge him to avoid excessive alcohol consumption while taking trospium.
• Explain that drug may decrease sweating and increase the risk of heatstroke when used in hot environments or during strenuous activities.
• Urge patient to avoid activities that are hazardous or require mental alertness until he knows how the drug affects him.

Reactions may be *common*, uncommon, *life-threatening*, or COMMON AND LIFE-THREATENING.
Interaction may have a *rapid onset* or **delayed onset**.

68

Miscellaneous urinary tract drugs

bethanechol chloride
neostigmine bromide
neostigmine methylsulfate
phenazopyridine hydrochloride

---

bethanechol chloride
be-THAN-e-kole

Duvoid, Urecholine

Pharmacologic class: cholinergic agonist
Pregnancy risk category C

AVAILABLE FORMS
Tablets: 5 mg, 10 mg, 25 mg, 50 mg

INDICATIONS & DOSAGES
➤ **Acute postoperative and post-partum nonobstructive (functional) urine retention, neurogenic atony of urinary bladder with urine retention**
Adults: 10 to 50 mg P.O. t.i.d. to q.i.d. Determine minimum effective dose by giving 5 or 10 mg and repeating same amount at hourly intervals until satisfactory response or maximum of 50 mg has been given.

ADMINISTRATION
P.O.
• Give drug 1 hour before or 2 hours after meals because drug may cause nausea and vomiting if taken soon after eating.

ACTION
Directly stimulates muscarinic cholinergic receptors, mimicking acetylcholine action, increasing GI tract tone and peristalsis and contraction of the detrusor muscle of the urinary bladder.

Route	Onset	Peak	Duration
P.O.	30–90 min	1 hr	6 hr

Half-life: Unknown.

ADVERSE REACTIONS
CNS: headache, malaise.

CV: *bradycardia,* profound hypotension with reflexive tachycardia, flushing.
EENT: lacrimation, miosis.
GI: *abdominal cramps, diarrhea,* excessive salivation, nausea, belching, borborygmus.
GU: urinary urgency.
Respiratory: *bronchoconstriction,* increased bronchial secretions.
Skin: diaphoresis.

INTERACTIONS
Drug-drug. *Anticholinergics, atropine, belladonna alkaloids, procainamide, quinidine:* May reverse cholinergic effects. Observe patient for lack of drug effect.
Cholinesterase inhibitors (donepezil), cholinergic agonists: May cause additive effects or increase toxicity. Avoid using together.
Ganglionic blockers: May cause critical drop in blood pressure, usually preceded by severe abdominal pain. Avoid using together.

EFFECTS ON LAB TEST RESULTS
• May increase amylase, lipase, and liver enzyme levels.

CONTRAINDICATIONS & CAUTIONS
• Contraindicated in patients hypersensitive to drug or its components and in those with uncertain strength or integrity of bladder wall, mechanical obstruction of GI or urinary tract, hyperthyroidism, peptic ulceration, latent or active bronchial asthma, obstructive pulmonary disease, pronounced bradycardia or hypotension, vasomotor instability, cardiac or coronary artery disease, AV conduction defects, hypertension, seizure disorder, Parkinson disease, spastic GI disturbances, acute inflammatory lesions of the GI tract, peritonitis, or marked vagotonia.
• Use cautiously in pregnant or breast-feeding women.

NURSING CONSIDERATIONS
• Adverse effects are rare with P.O. use.
• Monitor vital signs frequently, especially respirations. Always have atropine injection

available, and be prepared to give 0.6 mg subcutaneously or by slow I.V. push. Provide respiratory support, if needed.
• Monitor patient for orthostatic hypotension.
• Watch for toxicity.
• Watch closely for adverse reactions that may indicate drug toxicity.

PATIENT TEACHING
• Tell patient to take drug on an empty stomach and at regular intervals.
• Inform patient that drug is usually effective 30 to 90 minutes after use.

---

neostigmine bromide
nee-oh-STIG-meen

Prostigmin

neostigmine methylsulfate
Prostigmin

Pharmacologic class:
cholinesterase inhibitor
Pregnancy risk category C

AVAILABLE FORMS
neostigmine bromide
Tablets: 15 mg
neostigmine methylsulfate
Injection: 0.25 mg/ml, 0.5 mg/ml, 1 mg/ml

INDICATIONS & DOSAGES
➤ **To control myasthenia gravis symptoms**
Adults: Initially, 15 mg P.O. t.i.d.; increase gradually, as needed. Range is 15 to 375 mg/day. Average dosage is 150 mg/day with intervals individualized. Or, 0.5 mg I.M. or subcutaneously; base subsequent parenteral doses on patient's response.
Children: 2 mg/kg/day P.O. divided every 3 to 4 hours.
➤ **To prevent and treat postoperative distention and urine retention**
Adults: For prevention, 0.25 mg I.M. or subcutaneously as soon as possible after surgery; then every 4 to 6 hours for 2 to 3 days. For treatment, 0.5 mg I.M. or subcutaneously. If urination hasn't occurred in 1 hour, catheterize. Continue 0.5-mg injections every 3 hours for at least 5 doses.

➤ **Antidote for nondepolarizing neuromuscular blockers**
Adults: 0.5 to 2 mg I.V. slowly. Repeat, as needed, to total of 5 mg. Before antidote dose, give 0.6 to 1.2 mg atropine sulfate I.V. if patient is bradycardic.

ADMINISTRATION
P.O.
• For myasthenia gravis, schedule doses before periods of fatigue. For example, if patient has difficulty swallowing, schedule dose 30 minutes before each meal.
• Give drug with food or milk to reduce adverse GI reactions.
I.V.
• Inspect visually for particulate matter and discoloration before administration.
• Give as slow I.V. injection.
• If patient's muscle weakness is severe, prescriber will determine if it's from drug toxicity or worsening myasthenia gravis. Test dose of edrophonium I.V. will aggravate drug-induced weakness but will temporarily relieve disease-induced weakness.
• **Incompatibilities:** None reported.
I.M.
• Inspect visually for particulate matter and discoloration before administration.
Subcutaneous
• Inspect visually for particulate matter and discoloration before administration.

ACTION
Inhibits acetylcholinesterase, blocking destruction of acetylcholine from the parasympathetic and somatic efferent nerves.

Route	Onset	Peak	Duration
P.O.	45–75 min	1–2 hr	2–4 hr
I.V.	4–8 min	1–2 hr	2–4 hr
I.M., Subcut.	20–30 min	1–2 hr	2–4 hr

Half-life: About 53 minutes.

ADVERSE REACTIONS
CNS: *seizures,* dizziness, headache, muscle weakness, loss of consciousness, drowsiness, syncope.

Reactions may be *common,* uncommon, *life-threatening,* or COMMON AND LIFE-THREATENING.
Interaction may have a *rapid onset* or **delayed onset.**

CV: *bradycardia, AV block, cardiac arrest,* hypotension, tachycardia, flushing, thrombophlebitis (I.V.).
EENT: blurred vision, lacrimation, miosis.
GI: *nausea, vomiting, diarrhea, abdominal cramps,* excessive salivation, flatulence, increased peristalsis.
GU: urinary frequency, incontinence, urinary urgency.
Musculoskeletal: *muscle cramps,* muscle weakness, muscle fasciculations, arthralgia.
Respiratory: *bronchospasm, respiratory depression, respiratory arrest, laryngospasm, paralysis of respiratory muscles, central respiratory paralysis,* dyspnea, increased secretions.
Skin: rash, urticaria, diaphoresis.
Other: *anaphylaxis,* hypersensitivity reactions.

INTERACTIONS
Drug-drug. *Aminoglycosides, anticholinergics, atropine, local and general anesthetics, magnesium sulfate, procainamide, quinidine:* May reverse cholinergic effects; watch for lack of drug effect. Stop all other cholinergics before giving this drug.
Corticosteroids: May antagonize the effects of cholinesterase inhibitors in myasthenia gravis. Monitor patient for severe muscle deterioration.
Other cholinesterase inhibitors: May cause cholinergic crisis; myasthenic weakness may mimic symptoms of cholinesterase inhibitor overdose in myasthenia gravis patients. Monitor patient.
Succinylcholine: May worsen blockade produced by succinylcholine when used to reverse the effects of nondepolarizing neuromuscular blockers in surgical patients. Monitor patient.

EFFECTS ON LAB TEST RESULTS
None reported.

CONTRAINDICATIONS & CAUTIONS
● Contraindicated in patients hypersensitive to cholinergics or bromides and in those with peritonitis or mechanical obstruction of the intestinal or urinary tract.
● Don't give if patient has received high concentrations of halothane or cyclopropane.

● Use cautiously in patients with bronchial asthma, bradycardia, seizure disorders, recent coronary occlusion, vagotonia, hyperthyroidism, arrhythmias, and peptic ulcer.

NURSING CONSIDERATIONS
● Dosage for the treatment of myasthenia gravis must be highly individualized, depending on response and tolerance of adverse effects. Therapy may be needed day and night.
● *Alert:* Monitor vital signs frequently, especially respirations. Keep atropine injection available, and provide respiratory support, as needed.
● *Look alike–sound alike:* Don't confuse neostigmine vials with etomidate vials, which look similar.
● Monitor and document patient's response after each dose. Ideal dosage is difficult to judge. Watch closely for improvement in strength, vision, and ptosis 45 to 60 minutes after each dose.
● When drug is used to prevent abdominal distention and GI distress, inserting a rectal tube may help passage of gas.
● When drug is given for postoperative abdominal distention and bladder atony, rule out mechanical obstruction before dose is given. If no response within 1 hour after first dose, catheterize patient.
● Patient may develop resistance to drug.
● Many patients with long-standing disease insist on self-administration. Provide bedside supply of tablets.

PATIENT TEACHING
● Tell patient to take drug with food or milk to reduce adverse GI reactions.
● When giving drug for myasthenia gravis, explain that it will relieve ptosis, double vision, chewing and swallowing problems, and trunk and limb weakness. Stress the importance of taking drug exactly as prescribed, including nighttime doses. Explain that patient may need to take drug for life.
● Teach patient how to observe and record variations in muscle strength.
● Advise patient to wear or carry medical identification.

phenazopyridine hydrochloride
fen-az-oh-PEER-i-deen

Azo-Gesic ◊, Azo-Standard ◊, Baridium ◊, Geridium, Phenazo†, Prodium ◊, Pyridiate, Pyridium, Urodine, Urogesic, UTI-Relief

Pharmacologic class: azo dye
Pregnancy risk category B

AVAILABLE FORMS
Tablets: 95 mg ◊, 97.2 mg, 100 mg, 200 mg

INDICATIONS & DOSAGES
➤ **Pain with urinary tract irritation or infection**
Adults: 200 mg P.O. t.i.d. after meals for 2 days.
Children ages 6 to 12: 12 mg/kg P.O. daily in three equally divided doses after meals for 2 days.

ADMINISTRATION
P.O.
• Give drug with meals to minimize GI distress.

ACTION
Unknown; exerts local anesthetic action on urinary mucosa.

Route	Onset	Peak	Duration
P.O.	Unknown	Unknown	Unknown

Half-life: Unknown.

ADVERSE REACTIONS
CNS: headache.
EENT: staining of contact lenses.
GI: nausea, GI disturbances.
Hematologic: hemolytic anemia, methemoglobinemia.
Skin: rash, pruritus.
Other: *anaphylactoid reactions.*

INTERACTIONS
None significant.

EFFECTS ON LAB TEST RESULTS
• May decrease hemoglobin level and hematocrit.

• May alter Diastix or Chemstrip uG results and interfere with urinary ketone tests (Acetest or Ketostix).

CONTRAINDICATIONS & CAUTIONS
• Contraindicated in patients hypersensitive to drug and in those with glomerulonephritis, severe hepatitis, uremia, renal insufficiency, or pyelonephritis during pregnancy.

NURSING CONSIDERATIONS
• When drug is used with an antibacterial, therapy shouldn't extend beyond 2 days.
• Patients with red blood cell G-6-PD deficiency may be predisposed to hemolysis.
• *Look alike–sound alike:* Don't confuse Pyridium with pyridoxine.

PATIENT TEACHING
• Advise patient that taking drug with meals may minimize GI distress.
• Caution patient to stop drug and notify prescriber immediately if skin or sclera becomes yellow-tinged, which may indicate drug accumulation from impaired renal excretion.
• Inform patient that drug colors urine red or orange and may stain fabrics and contact lenses.
• Tell diabetic patient to use Clinitest for accurate urine glucose test results. Also tell patient that drug may interfere with urinary ketone tests (Acetest or Ketostix).
• Advise patient to notify prescriber if urinary tract pain persists. Tell him that drug shouldn't be used for long-term treatment.

69

Androgens and anabolic steroids

fluoxymesterone
methyltestosterone
testosterone
testosterone cypionate
testosterone enanthate
testosterone propionate
testosterone transdermal

---

fluoxymesterone
flew-ox-ee-MESS-teh-rone

Pharmacologic class: androgen
Pregnancy risk category X
Controlled substance schedule III

AVAILABLE FORMS
Tablets: 10 mg

INDICATIONS & DOSAGES
➤ **Hypogonadism from testicular deficiency**
Adults: 5 to 20 mg P.O. daily.
➤ **Delayed puberty in boys**
Adolescents: Highly individualized; usually 2.5 to 10 mg daily for 4 to 6 months.
➤ **Palliation of breast cancer**
Women: 10 to 40 mg P.O. daily in divided doses. Treatment should be continued for 3 months or more. Individualize and use lowest effective dose.

ADMINISTRATION
P.O.
● Give as a single daily dose or in divided doses.

ACTION
Stimulates target tissues to develop normally in androgen-deficient men. May have some antiestrogen properties, making it useful in treating certain estrogen-dependent breast cancers.

Route	Onset	Peak	Duration
P.O.	Unknown	Unknown	9 hr

Half-life: 9¼ hours.

ADVERSE REACTIONS
CNS: headache, anxiety, depression, paresthesia, sleep apnea.
CV: edema.
GI: nausea.
GU: decreased ejaculatory volume, oligospermia, priapism, amenorrhea.
Hematologic: polycythemia, *suppression of clotting factors.*
Hepatic: reversible jaundice, *cholestatic hepatitis.*
Metabolic: hypercalcemia, hypernatremia, *hyperkalemia,* hyperphosphatemia.
Musculoskeletal: impaired bone maturation in boys with delayed puberty.
Skin: hypersensitivity reactions.
Other: *hypoestrogenic effects in women,* excessive hormonal effects in men, androgenic effects in women, altered libido, male pattern baldness.

INTERACTIONS
Drug-drug. *Hepatotoxic drugs:* May increase risk of hepatotoxicity. Monitor liver function closely.
Insulin, oral antidiabetics: May alter dosage requirements. Monitor glucose levels in diabetic patients.
Oral anticoagulants: May increase sensitivity to oral anticoagulants; may alter dosage requirements. Monitor INR.

EFFECTS ON LAB TEST RESULTS
● May increase calcium, lipid, liver enzyme, phosphate, potassium, and sodium levels. May decrease thyroxine-binding globulin and total T_4 levels.
● May increase RBC count and resin uptake of T_3 and T_4.
● May cause abnormal glucose tolerance test results.

CONTRAINDICATIONS & CAUTIONS
● Contraindicated in patients hypersensitive to drug; in men with breast cancer or known or suspected prostate cancer; in patients with cardiac, hepatic, or renal decompensation; and in pregnant or breast-feeding women.

• Use cautiously in prepubertal boys or patients with benign prostatic hyperplasia or aspirin sensitivity.

NURSING CONSIDERATIONS
• **Alert:** Don't use in women of childbearing age until pregnancy is ruled out.
• Monitor INR in patients taking oral anticoagulants because dosage may need adjustment.
• Unless contraindicated, use with high-calorie, high-protein diet. Give small, frequent meals.
• Watch for evidence of jaundice, and periodically evaluate hepatic function. If liver function test results are abnormal, notify prescriber because therapy should be stopped.
• Edema can be controlled with sodium restriction or diuretics. Monitor weight routinely.
• Monitor boys and men for evidence of excessive androgenic effects. In prepubertal boys, watch for premature epiphyseal closure, acne, priapism, growth of body and facial hair, and phallic enlargement. If postpubertal men, watch for testicular atrophy, oligospermia, decreased ejaculatory volume, impotence, gynecomastia, and epididymitis.
• The effect on bone maturation should be monitored by assessing bone age of wrist and hand every 6 months.
• Evaluate semen routinely every 3 to 4 months, especially in adolescent boys.
• **Alert:** Hypercalcemia symptoms may be difficult to distinguish from those caused by the condition being treated, unless anticipated and thought of as a symptom cluster. Hypercalcemia is particularly likely to occur in immobilized patients and in women with metastatic breast cancer, and may indicate bone metastases.
• **Alert:** Don't give drug to enhance patient's athletic performance or physique.
• Watch for signs and symptoms of hypoglycemia in diabetic patients. Check glucose levels. Dosage of antidiabetic may need adjustment.
• When given for breast cancer, subjective effects may not occur for about 1 month; objective effects on clinical symptoms may take 3 months.
• Hypoestrogenic effects in women include flushing, diaphoresis, vaginal bleeding, nervousness, emotional lability, menstrual irregularities, and vaginitis, including itching, dryness, and burning.

PATIENT TEACHING
• If GI upset occurs, tell patient to take drug with food or meals.
• Make sure patient understands importance of using an effective nonhormonal contraceptive during therapy.
• Advise woman to wear cotton underwear and to wash after intercourse to decrease risk of vaginitis.
• Tell woman of childbearing age to report menstrual irregularities and to stop drug until she can be examined.
• Instruct woman to stop drug immediately and notify prescriber if pregnancy is suspected.
• Explain to woman taking drug for palliation of breast cancer that virilization usually occurs. Give emotional support. Tell her to immediately report androgenic effects (acne, swelling, weight gain, increased hair growth, hoarseness, clitoral enlargement, deepening voice, decreased breast size, changes in libido, male pattern baldness, and oily skin or hair).
• Tell patient that stopping drug prevents further androgenic changes but probably won't reverse existing effects.
• Warn patient with diabetes to be alert for signs and symptoms of hypoglycemia and to notify prescriber if these occur.
• Tell patient to report sudden weight gain.

---

methyltestosterone
meth-ill-tes-TOSS-ter-own

Android, Metandren†, Testred, Virilon

Pharmacologic class: androgenic anabolic steroid hormone
Pregnancy risk category X
Controlled substance schedule III

AVAILABLE FORMS
Capsules: 10 mg
Tablets: 10 mg, 25 mg

INDICATIONS & DOSAGES
➤ **Breast cancer**
Women 1 to 5 years after menopause: 50 to 200 mg P.O. daily.

Reactions may be *common*, uncommon, **life-threatening**, or COMMON AND LIFE-THREATENING.
Interaction may have a *rapid onset* or **delayed onset**.

➤ **Hypogonadism**
Men: 10 to 50 mg P.O. daily.
➤ **Postpubertal cryptorchidism**
Men: 30 mg P.O. daily.

ADMINISTRATION
P.O.
● Give without regard for food.
● Have patient rinse mouth after tablet dissolves.

ACTION
Stimulates target tissues to develop normally in androgen-deficient men. May have some antiestrogen properties, making it useful in treating certain estrogen-dependent breast cancers.

Route	Onset	Peak	Duration
P.O.	Unknown	2 hr	Unknown

Half-life: Unknown.

ADVERSE REACTIONS
CNS: headache, anxiety, depression, paresthesia.
CV: edema.
GI: irritation of oral mucosa with buccal administration, nausea.
GU: oligospermia, decreased ejaculatory volume, priapism, amenorrhea.
Hematologic: *suppression of clotting factors,* polycythemia.
Hepatic: reversible jaundice, *cholestatic hepatitis.*
Metabolic: hypernatremia, *hyperkalemia,* hyperphosphatemia, hypercholesterolemia, hypercalcemia.
Musculoskeletal: muscle cramps or spasms.
Skin: hypersensitivity reactions, acne.
Other: androgenic effects in women, altered libido, *hypoestrogenic effects in women,* excessive hormonal effects in men, male pattern baldness.

INTERACTIONS
Drug-drug. *Cyclosporine:* May increase cyclosporine toxicity. Monitor cyclosporine levels.
Hepatotoxic drugs: May increase risk of hepatotoxicity. Monitor liver function closely.
Imipramine: May cause dramatic paranoid response. Monitor patient closely.
Insulin, oral antidiabetics: May decrease glucose level; may alter dosage requirements. Monitor glucose level in diabetic patients.
Oral anticoagulants: May increase sensitivity to oral anticoagulants; may alter dosage requirements. Monitor PT and INR.

EFFECTS ON LAB TEST RESULTS
● May increase sodium, potassium, phosphate, liver enzyme, lipid, and calcium levels. May decrease thyroxine-binding globulin and total T_4 levels.
● May increase RBC count and resin uptake of T_3 and T_4.

CONTRAINDICATIONS & CAUTIONS
● Contraindicated in pregnant or breast-feeding women and in men with breast or prostate cancer.
● Contraindicated in patients with cardiac, hepatic, or renal disease.
● Use cautiously in elderly patients; patients with cardiac, renal, or hepatic disease; and healthy males with delayed puberty.

NURSING CONSIDERATIONS
● Don't give to woman of childbearing age until pregnancy is ruled out.
● In children, obtain X-rays of wrist bones before therapy begins to establish bone maturation level. During treatment, bones may mature more rapidly than they grow in length. Periodically review X-rays to monitor bone maturation.
● Drug is typically used only for intermittent therapy. Because of potential hepatotoxicity, watch closely for jaundice.
● Promptly report evidence of virilization in women, such as deepening of the voice, increased hair growth, acne, or baldness.
● Watch for hypoestrogenic effects in women (flushing, diaphoresis, vaginal bleeding, nervousness, emotional lability, menstrual irregularities, and vaginitis, including itching, dryness, and burning).
● Watch for excessive hormonal effects in men. If patient is prepubertal, watch for premature epiphyseal closure, acne, priapism, growth of body and facial hair, and phallic enlargement. If he's postpubertal, watch for testicular atrophy, oligospermia, decreased ejaculatory volume, impotence, gynecomastia, and epididymitis.

• Unless contraindicated, use with high-calorie, high-protein diet. Give small, frequent meals.
• Periodically check cholesterol, calcium, and hemoglobin levels, hematocrit, and cardiac and liver function test results.
• Check weight regularly. Control edema with sodium restriction or diuretics.
• *Alert:* In breast cancer, therapeutic response usually occurs within 3 months. If disease appears to progress, stop drug.
• Report signs of hypercalcemia. In metastatic breast cancer, hypercalcemia may indicate progression of bone metastases.
• Evaluate semen every 3 to 4 months, especially in adolescent boys.
• *Alert:* Don't use to enhance athletic performance or physique.
• *Look alike–sound alike:* Testosterone and methyltestosterone aren't interchangeable. Don't confuse methyltestosterone with medroxyprogesterone.

PATIENT TEACHING
• Make sure patient understands importance of using effective contraception during therapy.
• Tell woman of childbearing age to report menstrual irregularities and to stop drug while awaiting examination.
• Instruct patient to stop drug immediately and notify prescriber if pregnancy is suspected.
• Tell patient to place buccal tablet in upper or lower buccal pouch between cheek and gum; tablet needs 30 to 60 minutes to dissolve. Tell patient not to eat, drink, chew, or smoke while buccal tablet is in place and not to swallow tablet.
• Instruct patient to change buccal tablet absorption site with each dose to minimize risk of irritation. Advise patient to rinse mouth after using buccal tablet.
• Tell woman to immediately report evidence of virilization, such as acne, swelling, weight gain, increased hair growth, hoarseness, clitoral enlargement, decreased breast size, deepening of voice, changes in libido, male pattern baldness, and oily skin or hair.
• Teach patient signs and symptoms of low glucose level (hypoglycemia) and method for checking glucose level; drug

enhances hypoglycemia. Instruct patient to report signs or symptoms of hypoglycemia immediately.
• Advise woman to wear cotton underwear and to wash after intercourse to decrease risk of vaginitis.

---

testosterone
Striant

testosterone cypionate
Depo-Testosterone

testosterone enanthate
Delatestryl

testosterone propionate

Pharmacologic class: androgen
Pregnancy risk category X
Controlled substance schedule III

AVAILABLE FORMS
testosterone
Blister packs (buccal; extended-release): 30 mg
Pellets (subcutaneous implant): 75 mg
testosterone cypionate
Injection (in oil): 100 mg/ml, 200 mg/ml
testosterone enanthate
Injection (in oil): 200 mg/ml
testosterone propionate
Injection (in oil): 25 mg/ml, 50 mg/ml, 100 mg/ml

INDICATIONS & DOSAGES
➤ **Hypogonadism**
Men: 10 to 25 mg propionate I.M. two to three times weekly; or 50 to 400 mg cypionate or enanthate I.M. every 2 to 4 weeks. Or, 150 to 450 mg (2 to 6 pellets) implanted subcutaneously every 3 to 6 months. Or, apply 1 buccal system (30 mg) to the gum region just above the incisor tooth on either side of the mouth, b.i.d., morning and evening about 12 hours apart. Alternate sides of the mouth with each application.
➤ **Delayed puberty**
Men and boys: 50 to 200 mg enanthate I.M. every 2 to 4 weeks for 4 to 6 months.
➤ **Metastatic breast cancer**
Women 1 to 5 years after menopause: 50 to 100 mg propionate I.M. three times

---

weekly; or 200 to 400 mg cypionate or enanthate I.M. every 2 to 4 weeks.

ADMINISTRATION
I.M.
● Store I.M. preparations at room temperature. If crystals appear, warm and shake bottle to disperse them.
● Inject deep into upper outer quadrant of gluteal muscle. Rotate injection sites; report soreness at site.
Subcutaneous
● In most men, the pellets are implanted in an area on the anterior abdominal wall.
Buccal
● The buccal system should be placed in the gum region just above the incisor tooth on either side of the mouth.
● Have the patient rotate sides of the mouth with each administration.
● Make sure the patient doesn't chew or swallow the buccal system.
● The buccal system should remain in place until the next dosing. Check placement after toothbrushing, mouthwash use, eating, and drinking.
● To remove the system, gently slide it downward from the gum toward the tooth.

ACTION
Stimulates target tissues to develop normally in androgen-deficient men. May have some antiestrogen properties, making it useful in treating certain estrogen-dependent breast cancers.

Route	Onset	Peak	Duration
I.M.	Unknown	10–100 min	Unknown
Subcut.	Unknown	Unknown	3–6 mo
Buccal	Unknown	10–12 hr	2–4 hr

Half-life: 10 to 100 minutes.

ADVERSE REACTIONS
CNS: headache, anxiety, depression, paresthesia, sleep apnea.
CV: edema.
GI: nausea, gum or mouth irritation, bitter taste, gum pain, tenderness, or edema, taste perversion (with buccal application).
GU: amenorrhea, oligospermia, decreased ejaculatory volume, priapism.
Hematologic: polycythemia, *suppression of clotting factors.*
Hepatic: reversible jaundice, *cholestatic hepatitis.*

Metabolic: hypernatremia, *hyperkalemia,* hypercalcemia, hyperphosphatemia, hypercholesterolemia.
Skin: pain, induration at injection site, local edema, acne.
Other: androgenic effects in women, gynecomastia, hypersensitivity reactions, hypoestrogenic effects in women, excessive hormonal effects in men, male pattern baldness.

INTERACTIONS
Drug-drug. *Corticosteroids:* May increase risk of edema. Use together cautiously, especially in patients with cardiac or hepatic disease.
Hepatotoxic drugs: May increase risk of hepatotoxicity. Monitor liver function closely.
Insulin, oral antidiabetics: May decrease glucose level; may alter dosage requirements. Monitor glucose level in diabetic patients.
Oral anticoagulants: May increase sensitivity; may alter dosage requirements. Monitor PT and INR; decrease anticoagulant dose if necessary.
Oxyphenbutazone: May increase oxyphenbutazone level. Monitor patient.

EFFECTS ON LAB TEST RESULTS
● May increase sodium, potassium, phosphate, cholesterol, liver enzyme, calcium, creatinine, and serum PSA levels. May decrease thyroxine-binding globulin, total T_4 levels, serum creatinine, and 17-ketosteroid levels.
● May increase RBC count and resin uptake of T_3 and T_4.
● May cause abnormal glucose tolerance test results.

CONTRAINDICATIONS & CAUTIONS
● Contraindicated in patients hypersensitive to drug and in those with hypercalcemia or cardiac, hepatic, or renal decompensation.
● Contraindicated in men with breast or prostate cancer and in pregnant or breast-feeding women.
● Use cautiously in elderly patients.

NURSING CONSIDERATIONS
● Unless contraindicated, use with high-calorie, high-protein diet. Give small, frequent meals to help avoid nausea.

- Don't give to woman of childbearing age until pregnancy is ruled out.
- Cypionate and enanthate are long-acting solutions.
- Monitor patient's liver function, PSA, cholesterol, and high-density lipoprotein periodically.
- Check hemoglobin and hematocrit levels periodically.
- In patients with metastatic breast cancer, hypercalcemia usually indicates progression of bone metastases. Report signs and symptoms of hypercalcemia.
- Report evidence of virilization in women. Androgenic effects include acne, edema, weight gain, increased hair growth, hoarseness, clitoral enlargement, decreased breast size, changes in libido, male pattern baldness, and oily skin or hair.
- Watch for hypoestrogenic effects in women (flushing; diaphoresis; vaginitis, including itching, drying, and burning; vaginal bleeding; menstrual irregularities).
- Watch for excessive hormonal effects in men and boys. In prepubertal boy, watch for premature epiphyseal closure, acne, priapism, growth of body and facial hair, and phallic enlargement. In postpubertal men, watch for testicular atrophy, oligospermia, decreased ejaculatory volume, impotence, gynecomastia, and epididymitis.
- Monitor patient's weight and blood pressure routinely.
- Monitor prepubertal boys by X-ray for rate of bone maturation.
- The treatment of hypogonadal men with testosterone esters may potentiate sleep apnea. Monitor patients with risk factors such as obesity or chronic lung diseases.
- **Alert:** Therapeutic response in breast cancer is usually apparent within 3 months. If disease progresses, stop drug.
- Androgens may alter results of laboratory studies during therapy and for 2 to 3 weeks after therapy ends.
- **Look alike–sound alike:** Don't confuse testosterone with testolactone.
- **Alert:** Testosterone salts aren't interchangeable.

PATIENT TEACHING
- Make sure patient understands importance of using an effective nonhormonal contraceptive during therapy.

- Instruct patient to stop drug immediately and notify prescriber if pregnancy is suspected.
- Review signs and symptoms of virilization with woman, and instruct her to notify prescriber if they occur.
- Advise woman to wear cotton underwear and to wash after intercourse to decrease risk of vaginitis.
- Instruct man to notify prescriber about priapism, reduced ejaculatory volume, or gynecomastia.
- Warn diabetic patient to be alert for hypoglycemia and to notify prescriber if it occurs.
- Instruct boys using testosterone for delayed puberty to have X-rays of hand and wrist obtained every 6 months during treatment.
- Tell patient to report sudden weight gain.
- Warn patient that drug shouldn't be used to enhance athletic performance.
- Instruct patient how to use the buccal system.
- Advise patient to avoid dislodging buccal system and ensure that the system is in place after toothbrushing, use of mouthwash, and eating or drinking.
- Tell men not to chew or swallow buccal system.

---

testosterone transdermal
Androderm, AndroGel, Testim

Pharmacologic class: androgen
Pregnancy risk category X
Controlled substance schedule III

AVAILABLE FORMS
1% gel: 25 mg, 50 mg per unit dose;
1.25 g per nonaerosol metered pump
Transdermal system: 2.5 mg/day, 5 mg/day

INDICATIONS & DOSAGES
➤ **Primary or hypogonadotropic hypogonadism**
Men: One or two Androderm patches applied to back, abdomen, arm, or thigh nightly for total dosage of 5 mg daily. Dose may be increased to 7.5 mg once daily or decreased to 2.5 mg once daily, depending upon a.m. serum testosterone levels. Or, initially, 50 mg of testosterone gel applied every morning to shoulders, upper arms, or abdomen. Don't apply

Testim to abdomen. Check testosterone level after about 2 weeks. If response is inadequate, may increase AndroGel to 75 mg daily. Then, adjust to 100 mg (either gel) if needed. Or, for AndroGel pump, 5 g (4 pumps) applied every morning to shoulders, upper arms, or abdomen. Check testosterone level after about 2 weeks. If response is inadequate, may increase to 7.5 g (6 pumps) daily or from 7.5 g to 10 g (8 pumps) daily.

ADMINISTRATION
Transdermal
● Wear gloves when handling patches. Fold used patches with adhesive sides together to discard.
● Apply patch nightly to clean, dry, intact skin of the shoulders, upper arms, or abdomen only and not to scrotum or bony prominences.
Topical
● Fully prime the AndroGel pump by pumping three times before first use. Discard that gel.
● Wear gloves to apply gel to clean, dry, intact skin of the shoulders, upper arms, or abdomen only and not to scrotum or bony prominences. Testim shouldn't be applied to the abdomen.
● Application in the morning is preferable.

ACTION
Releases testosterone, which stimulates target tissues to develop normally in androgen-deficient men.

Route	Onset	Peak	Duration
Trans-dermal, topical	Unknown	2–4 hr	2 hr after removal

Half-life: 10 to 100 minutes.

ADVERSE REACTIONS
CNS: *stroke,* asthenia, depression, headache.
GI: *GI bleeding.*
GU: prostatitis, prostate abnormalities, UTI.
Hepatic: *cholestatic hepatitis,* reversible jaundice.
Metabolic: hypernatremia, hyperkalemia, hypercalcemia, hyperphosphatemia, hypercholesterolemia.
Skin: *pruritus, blister under patch,* acne irritation, allergic contact dermatitis, burning.

Other: gynecomastia, breast tenderness, flulike syndrome.

INTERACTIONS
Drug-drug. *Corticosteroids:* May increase risk of edema. Use together cautiously, especially in patients with cardiac or hepatic disease.
Insulin: May alter insulin dosage requirements. Monitor glucose level.
Oral anticoagulants. May alter anticoagulant dosage requirements. Monitor PT and INR.
Oxyphenbutazone: May increase oxyphenbutazone level. Monitor patient.
Propranolol: May increase propranolol clearance. Monitor patient.

EFFECTS ON LAB TEST RESULTS
● May increase sodium, potassium, phosphate, cholesterol, liver enzyme, calcium, and creatinine levels and resin uptake of T_3 and T_4. May decrease total T_4 levels.
● May increase RBC count.

CONTRAINDICATIONS & CAUTIONS
● Contraindicated in patients hypersensitive to drug, in women, in men with known or suspected breast or prostate cancer, and in patients with CV, renal, or hepatic disease.
● Use cautiously in elderly men.

NURSING CONSIDERATIONS
● Periodically assess liver function test results, lipid profiles, hemoglobin level, hematocrit (with long-term use), and levels of prostatic acid phosphatase and prostate-specific antigen.
● Watch for excessive hormonal effects.

PATIENT TEACHING
● Tell patient to fully prime the AndroGel pump by pumping three times before first use and to discard that gel.
● Tell patient to apply gel or patch to clean, dry, intact skin of the shoulders, upper arms, or abdomen only and not to scrotum or bony prominences. Testim shouldn't be applied to the abdomen. Tell him that he can first pump gel into his hand.
● Tell patient using patch to apply it at night.
● Tell patient using gel to apply in the morning.
● Tell patient to wash his hands thoroughly with soap and water after applying.

- Instruct patient that patch must be changed every 24 hours.
- For best results, advise patient not to swim or shower for at least 5 hours after applying gel. Showering or swimming at least 1 hour after applying, if done infrequently, should have minimal effects on drug absorption.
- Tell patient that if the patch falls off, it may be reapplied. If patch falls off and can't be reapplied, and it has been worn at least 12 hours, a new patch may be applied at the next application time.
- Warn diabetic patient that drug may decrease glucose level and to be alert for hypoglycemia.
- Advise patient to report persistent erections, nausea, vomiting, changes in skin color, ankle swelling, or sudden weight gain to prescriber.
- Tell patient that drug may cause virilization in his female sexual partner, who should report acne or changes in body hair distribution.
- Tell patient that Androderm doesn't have to be removed during sexual intercourse or while showering.

Reactions may be *common*, uncommon, *life-threatening*, or COMMON AND LIFE-THREATENING.
Interaction may have a *rapid onset* or ***delayed onset***.

drospirenone and ethinyl estradiol
esterified estrogens
estradiol
estradiol and norethindrone
   acetate transdermal system
estradiol cypionate
estradiol gel
estradiol hemihydrate
estradiol valerate
estrogens, conjugated
estropipate
ethinyl estradiol and desogestrel
ethinyl estradiol and ethynodiol
   diacetate
ethinyl estradiol and levonorgestrel
ethinyl estradiol and norethindrone
ethinyl estradiol and
   norethindrone acetate
ethinyl estradiol and
   norgestimate
ethinyl estradiol and norgestrel
ethinyl estradiol, norethindrone
   acetate, and ferrous fumarate
etonogestrel and ethinyl estradiol
   vaginal ring
medroxyprogesterone acetate
mestranol and norethindrone
norelgestromin and ethinyl
   estradiol transdermal system
norethindrone
norethindrone acetate

---

drospirenone and ethinyl estradiol
droh-SPYE-re-none and ETH-i-nill

Yasmin, YAZ

Pharmacologic class: estrogenic and progestinic steroids
Pregnancy risk category X

AVAILABLE FORMS
Tablets: 3 mg drospirenone and 0.03 mg ethinyl estradiol as 21 yellow tablets and 7 white (inert) tablets (Yasmin); 3 mg drospirenone and 0.02 mg ethinyl estradiol as 24 light pink active tablets and 4 white (inert) tablets (YAZ).

INDICATIONS & DOSAGES
➤ **Contraception**
Women: 1 yellow Yasmin tablet P.O. daily for 21 days beginning on day 1 of menstrual cycle or first Sunday after onset of menstruation. Then 1 white inert tablet P.O. daily on days 22 through 28. Or 1 light pink YAZ tablet P.O. daily for 24 days beginning on day 1 of menstrual cycle or first Sunday after onset of menstruation. Then 1 white inert tablet P.O. daily on days 25 through 28. Begin next and all subsequent 28-day regimens on same day of week that first regimen began, following same schedule. Restart yellow or light pink tablets on next day after last white tablet.
➤ **Premenstrual dysphoric disorder**
Adults: 1 light pink YAZ tablet P.O. daily for 24 days beginning on day 1 of menstrual cycle or first Sunday after menstruation begins. Then 1 white inert tablet P.O. daily on days 25 through 28. Begin next and all subsequent 28-day regimens on same day of week that first regimen began, following same schedule. Restart light pink tablets on next day after last white tablet.

ADMINISTRATION
P.O.
● Give pill at same time each day.

ACTION
Reduces chance of conception by inhibiting ovulation, inhibiting sperm progression, and reducing chance of implantation.

Route	Onset	Peak	Duration
P.O.	Unknown	1–3 hr	Unknown

Half-life: drospirenone, 30 hours; ethinyl estradiol, 24 hours.

ADVERSE REACTIONS
CNS: *cerebral hemorrhage, cerebral thrombosis,* asthenia, depression, dizziness, emotional lability, headache, migraine, nervousness.

CV: *arterial thromboembolism, mesenteric thrombosis, MI,* hypertension, thrombophlebitis, fluid retention, edema.
EENT: cataracts, steepening of corneal curvature, intolerance to contact lenses, pharyngitis, retinal thrombosis, sinusitis.
GI: abdominal pain, abdominal cramping, bloating, changes in appetite, colitis, diarrhea, gastroenteritis, nausea, vomiting, gallbladder disease.
GU: amenorrhea, breakthrough bleeding, change in cervical erosion and secretion, change in menstrual flow, cystitis, cystitis-like syndrome, dysmenorrhea, impaired renal function, leukorrhea, menstrual disorder, premenstrual syndrome, spotting, temporary infertility after discontinuing treatment, UTI, vaginal candidiasis, vaginitis.
Hepatic: *Budd-Chiari syndrome, hepatic adenomas,* cholestatic jaundice, benign liver tumors.
Metabolic: reduced glucose tolerance, porphyria, weight change, *hyperkalemia.*
Musculoskeletal: back pain.
Respiratory: *pulmonary embolism,* bronchitis, upper respiratory tract infection.
Skin: *erythema multiforme,* acne, erythema nodosum, hemorrhagic eruption, hirsutism, loss of scalp hair, melasma, pruritus, rash.
Other: changes in libido, breast tenderness, *hemolytic-uremic syndrome.*

INTERACTIONS
Drug-drug. *ACE inhibitors, aldosterone antagonists, angiotensin II receptor antagonists, NSAIDs, potassium-sparing diuretics:* May increase risk of hyperkalemia. Monitor potassium level.
Acetaminophen: May increase level of contraceptive and decrease effectiveness of acetaminophen. Monitor patient for adverse effects. Adjust acetaminophen dose as needed.
Antibiotics, griseofulvin, penicillins, tetracycline: May decrease contraceptive effect. Advise patient to use additional method of birth control while taking the antibiotic.
Ascorbic acid, atorvastatin: May increase level of contraceptive. Monitor patient for adverse effects.
Carbamazepine, modafinil, oxcarbazepine, phenobarbital, phenytoin, protease inhibitors: May increase metabolism of ethinyl estradiol and decrease contraceptive effectiveness. Advise patient to use another method of birth control.
Clofibrate, morphine, salicylic acid, temazepam: May decrease levels and increase clearance of these drugs. Monitor patient for effectiveness.
Cyclosporine, prednisolone, theophylline: May increase levels of these drugs. Monitor patient for adverse effects and toxicity.
Phenylbutazone, rifampin: May decrease contraceptive effectiveness and increase menstrual irregularities. Advise patient to use another method of birth control.
Troleandomycin: May increase risk of intrahepatic cholestasis and decrease contraceptive effect. Advise patient to use an alternative method of birth control.
Drug-herb. *St. John's wort:* May decrease contraceptive effectiveness and increase breakthrough bleeding. Discourage use together, or advise use of additional method of birth control.
Drug-lifestyle. *Smoking:* May increase risk of CV adverse effects. Advise patient to avoid smoking.

EFFECTS ON LAB TEST RESULTS
• May increase corticoid; factor VII, VIII, IX, and X; prothrombin; thyroid-binding globulin; total circulating sex steroid; total thyroid hormone; triglyceride levels, amylase, GGT, iron-binding capacity, transferrin, prolactin, renin activity, and vitamin A. May decrease antithrombin III level, folate, albumin, zinc, and vitamin B_{12}.
• May increase norepinephrine-induced platelet aggregation. May decrease glucose tolerance and free T_3 resin uptake.

CONTRAINDICATIONS & CAUTIONS
• Contraindicated in women with hepatic dysfunction, tumor, or disease; renal or adrenal insufficiency; thrombophlebitis, thromboembolic disorders, or history of deep vein thrombosis or thromboembolic disorders; cerebrovascular or coronary artery disease; known or suspected breast cancer, endometrial cancer, or other estrogen-dependent neoplasia; abnormal genital bleeding; or cholestatic jaundice

of pregnancy or jaundice with other hormonal contraceptive use.

• Contraindicated in women who are or may be pregnant and in women age 65 or older.

• Use cautiously in patients with CV risk factors such as hypertension, hyperlipidemias, obesity, and diabetes.

• Use cautiously in patients with conditions aggravated by fluid retention.

NURSING CONSIDERATIONS

• *Alert:* The use of contraceptives causes increased risk of MI, thromboembolism, stroke, hepatic neoplasia, gallbladder disease, and hypertension. Risk increases in patients with hypertension, diabetes, hyperlipidemia, and obesity.

■ **Black Box Warning** Smoking increases the risk of serious CV adverse effects. The risk increases with age (especially age older than 35 years) and in patients who smoke 15 or more cigarettes daily. ■

• The relationship between the use of hormonal contraceptives and breast and cervical cancers is unclear. Encourage women to schedule a complete gynecologic examination at least yearly and to perform breast self-examinations monthly.

• In patients scheduled to have elective surgery that may increase the risk of thromboembolism, stop contraceptive use from at least 4 weeks before until 2 weeks after surgery. Also stop use during and after prolonged immobilization.

• Because of increased risk of thromboembolism in the postpartum period, don't start contraceptive earlier than 4 to 6 weeks after delivery.

• Stop use and evaluate patient if loss of vision, proptosis, diplopia, papilledema, or retinal vascular lesions occur. Recommend that contact lens wearers be evaluated by an ophthalmologist if visual changes or lens intolerance occurs.

• If patient misses two consecutive periods, she should obtain a negative pregnancy test result before continuing use of contraceptive.

• Immediately stop use if pregnancy is confirmed.

• Closely monitor patient with diabetes. Glucose intolerance may occur.

• Closely monitor patient with hypertension or a history of depression. Stop drug if these events occur.

• In patient at high risk for hyperkalemia and patient taking medications that may increase potassium, check potassium level during the first treatment cycle.

• Stop drug and evaluate patient if persistent, severe headaches occur or if migraines occur or are worsened.

• Evaluate patient for malignancy or pregnancy if she experiences breakthrough bleeding or spotting.

• Closely monitor patient with hyperlipidemias.

• Stop use if jaundice occurs.

• *Look alike–sound alike:* Don't confuse Yaz with Yasmin.

PATIENT TEACHING

• Advise patient to use additional method of birth control during the first 7 days of the first cycle of hormonal contraceptive.

• Inform patient that pills don't protect against sexually transmitted diseases such as HIV.

• Advise patient of the dangers of smoking while taking hormonal contraceptives. Suggest smokers choose a different form of birth control.

• Tell patient to schedule gynecologic examinations yearly and perform breast self-examination monthly.

• Inform patient that spotting, light bleeding, or stomach upset may occur during the first 1 to 3 packs of pills. Tell her to continue taking the pills and to notify her health care provider if these symptoms persist.

• Tell patient to take the pill at the same time each day.

• Tell patient to immediately report sharp chest pain; coughing of blood or sudden shortness of breath; calf pain; crushing chest pain or chest heaviness; sudden severe headache or vomiting; dizziness or fainting; visual or speech disturbances, weakness or numbness in an arm or leg; vision loss; breast lumps; severe stomach pain or tenderness; difficulty sleeping, lack of energy, fatigue, or change in mood; jaundice with fever, fatigue, loss of appetite, dark urine, or light-colored bowel movements.

• Tell patient to notify health care provider if she wears contact lenses and notices a change in vision or has trouble wearing the lenses.
• Tell patient that the risk of pregnancy increases with each active yellow or light pink tablet she forgets to take. Inform patient what to do if she misses pills.
• Tell patient to use an additional method of birth control and to notify health care provider if she isn't sure what to do about missed pills.
• Small amounts of hormonal contraceptives appear in breast milk. Yellow skin and eyes (jaundice) and breast enlargement may occur in breast-fed neonates.

esterified estrogens
ESS-tehr-eh-fide ESS-troe-jenz

Menest, Neo-Estrone†

Pharmacologic class: estrogen
Pregnancy risk category X

AVAILABLE FORMS
Tablets (film-coated): 0.3 mg, 0.625 mg, 1.25 mg, 2.5 mg

INDICATIONS & DOSAGES
➤ **Inoperable prostate cancer**
Men: 1.25 to 2.5 mg P.O. t.i.d.
➤ **Palliative treatment for metastatic breast cancer**
Men and postmenopausal women: 10 mg P.O. t.i.d. for 3 or more months.
➤ **Hypogonadism**
Women: 2.5 to 7.5 mg daily in divided doses in cycles of 20 days on, 10 days off.
➤ **Castration, primary ovarian failure**
Women: 1.25 mg daily in cycles of 3 weeks on, 1 week off. Adjust for symptoms. Can be given continuously.
➤ **Vasomotor menopausal symptoms**
Women: 1.25 mg P.O. daily in cycles of 3 weeks on, 1 week off. Dosage may be increased to 2.5 to 3.75 mg P.O. daily, if needed.
➤ **Atrophic vaginitis, kraurosis vulvae**
Women: 0.3 to 1.25 mg or more P.O. daily in cycles of 3 weeks on, 1 week off.

ADMINISTRATION
P.O.
• Use lowest effective dose needed for specific indication.

ACTION
Mimics the actions of endogenous estrogens; increases synthesis of DNA, RNA, and protein in responsive tissues; reduces release of follicle-stimulating and luteinizing hormones from pituitary gland.

Route	Onset	Peak	Duration
P.O.	Unknown	Unknown	Unknown

Half-life: Unknown.

ADVERSE REACTIONS
CNS: headache, dizziness, chorea, depression, *stroke, seizures.*
CV: thrombophlebitis, *thromboembolism,* hypertension, *edema, pulmonary embolism, MI.*
EENT: worsening myopia or astigmatism, intolerance of contact lenses.
GI: *nausea,* vomiting, abdominal cramps, bloating, anorexia, increased appetite, *pancreatitis,* increased risk of gallbladder disease.
GU: breakthrough bleeding, altered menstrual flow, dysmenorrhea, amenorrhea, *increased risk of endometrial cancer,* cervical erosion, altered cervical secretions, enlargement of uterine fibromas, vaginal candidiasis, testicular atrophy, impotence.
Hepatic: cholestatic jaundice, *hepatic adenoma.*
Metabolic: hypercalcemia, weight changes, hypertriglyceridemia.
Skin: melasma, rash, hirsutism or hair loss, erythema nodosum, dermatitis.
Other: *breast tenderness, enlargement, or secretion; gynecomastia; increased risk of breast cancer.*

INTERACTIONS
Drug-drug. *Carbamazepine, fosphenytoin, phenobarbital, phenytoin, rifampin:* May decrease effectiveness of estrogen therapy. Monitor patient closely.
Corticosteroids: May enhance effects. Monitor patient closely.
Cyclosporine: May increase risk of toxicity. Use together with caution, and monitor cyclosporine level frequently.

Reactions may be *common,* uncommon, *life-threatening,* or COMMON AND LIFE-THREATENING.
Interaction may have a *rapid onset* or *delayed onset.*

Dantrolene, hepatotoxic drugs: May increase risk of hepatotoxicity. Monitor liver function closely.

Oral anticoagulants: May decrease anticoagulant effects. Adjust dosage if needed. Monitor PT and INR.

Tamoxifen: May interfere with tamoxifen effectiveness. Avoid using together.

Drug-herb. *St. John's wort:* May decrease effects of drug. Discourage use together.

Drug-food. *Caffeine:* May increase caffeine level. Urge caution.

Grapefruit, grapefruit juice: May increase risk of adverse effects. Discourage use together.

Drug-lifestyle. *Smoking:* May increase risk of CV effects. If smoking continues, may need another form of therapy.

EFFECTS ON LAB TEST RESULTS
• May increase calcium, thyroid-binding globulin, serum triglyceride, serum phospholipid, and clotting factor VII, VIII, IX, and X levels.
• May increase norepinephrine-induced platelet aggregation and PT.
• May reduce metyrapone test results and cause impaired glucose tolerance.

CONTRAINDICATIONS & CAUTIONS
• Contraindicated in pregnant women, in patients hypersensitive to drug, and in patients with breast cancer (except metastatic disease), estrogen-dependent neoplasia, active thrombophlebitis, thromboembolic disorders, undiagnosed abnormal genital bleeding, or history of thromboembolic disease.
• Use cautiously in patients with history of hypertension, mental depression, cardiac or renal dysfunction, liver impairment, gallbladder disease, bone disease, migraine, seizures, or diabetes.

NURSING CONSIDERATIONS
• When used for vasomotor symptoms in menstruating women, cyclic administration is started on day 5 of bleeding.
• When given cyclically for short-term use, administration should be cyclic and attempts to discontinue or taper the medication should be made at 3 to 6 month intervals.
• Make sure patient has thorough physical examination before starting estrogen

therapy. Patients receiving long-term therapy should have annual examinations. Periodically monitor body weight, blood pressure, lipid levels, and hepatic function.
• Notify pathologist about patient's estrogen therapy when sending specimens to laboratory for evaluation.
• **Alert:** Because of risk of thromboembolism, stop therapy at least 1 month before procedures that cause prolonged immobilization or increased risk of thromboembolism, such as knee or hip surgery.
■ **Black Box Warning** Estrogens have been reported to increase the risk of endometrial carcinoma. ■
■ **Black Box Warning** Estrogens should not be used during pregnancy. ■
• Glucose tolerance may be impaired. Monitor glucose level closely in patients with diabetes.

PATIENT TEACHING
• Tell patient to read package insert describing estrogen's adverse effects; also, give patient verbal explanation.
• Emphasize importance of regular physical examinations. Postmenopausal women who use estrogen replacement for longer than 5 years to treat menopausal symptoms may be at increased risk for endometrial cancer. This risk is reduced by using cyclic rather than continuous therapy and the lowest possible estrogen dosage. Adding progestins to the regimen decreases risk of endometrial hyperplasia, but it's unknown whether progestins affect risk of endometrial cancer.
• **Alert:** Warn patient to immediately report abdominal pain; pain, numbness, or stiffness in legs or buttocks; pressure or pain in chest or shortness of breath; severe headaches; visual disturbances, such as blind spots, flashing lights, or blurriness; vaginal bleeding or discharge; breast lumps; swelling of hands or feet; yellow skin or sclera; dark urine; or light-colored stools.
• Tell diabetic patient to report elevated glucose level so that antidiabetic dosage can be adjusted.
• Explain to woman receiving cyclic therapy for postmenopausal symptoms

that she may experience withdrawal bleeding during week off drug. Tell her to report unusual vaginal bleeding.

• Teach woman to perform routine breast self-examination.

• Advise woman of childbearing age to consult prescriber before taking drug and to advise prescriber immediately if she becomes pregnant.

• Teach patient methods to decrease risk of blood clots.

• Encourage patient to stop smoking or reduce number of cigarettes smoked because of the risk of CV complications.

---

estradiol (oestradiol)
ess-tra-DYE-ole

Alora, Climara, Estrace✲, Estrace Vaginal Cream, Estraderm, Estring Vaginal Ring, Evamist, Gynodiol, Menostar, Vivelle, Vivelle-Dot

estradiol acetate
Femring, Femtrace

estradiol cypionate
Depo-Estradiol

estradiol gel
Divigel, Elestrin, EstroGel

estradiol hemihydrate
Estrasorb, Vagifem

estradiol valerate (oestradiol valerate)
Delestrogen

Pharmacologic class: estrogen
Pregnancy risk category X

AVAILABLE FORMS
estradiol
Spray, topical solution: 1.53 mg
Tablets (micronized): 0.5 mg, 1 mg, 1.5 mg, 2 mg
Transdermal: 0.014 mg/24 hours, 0.025 mg/24 hours, 0.0375 mg/24 hours, 0.05 mg/24 hours, 0.06 mg/24 hours, 0.075 mg/24 hours, 0.1 mg/24 hours
Vaginal cream (in nonliquefying base): 0.1 mg/g

estradiol acetate
Tablets: 0.45 mg, 0.9 mg, 1.8 mg
Vaginal ring: 0.05 mg/24 hours; 0.1 mg/24 hours
estradiol cypionate
Injection (in oil): 5 mg/ml
estradiol gel
Transdermal gel: 0.06% (1.25 g/metered dose), 0.1% (in 0.25-, 0.5-, and 1-g single-dose packets)
estradiol hemihydrate
Topical emulsion: 0.25%
Vaginal tablets: 25 mcg
estradiol valerate
Injection (in oil): 10 mg/ml, 20 mg/ml, 40 mg/ml

INDICATIONS & DOSAGES
➤ **Vasomotor menopausal symptoms, female hypogonadism, female castration, primary ovarian failure**
Women: 0.5 to 2 mg P.O. estradiol daily in cycles of 21 days on and 7 days off or cycles of 5 days on and 2 days off. Or, for vasomotor symptoms, 1 to 5 mg cypionate I.M. once every 3 to 4 weeks; for female hypogonadism, 1.5 to 2 mg cypionate I.M. once every month.
Transdermal patch
Women: Apply patch according to manufacturer's instructions. Alora, Estraderm, Vivelle, and Vivelle-Dot are applied twice weekly. Climara and Menostar are applied once a week. Apply to clean, dry area of the trunk. Adjust dose, if necessary, after the first 2 or 3 weeks of therapy; then every 3 to 6 months as needed. Rotate application sites weekly with an interval of at least 1 week between particular sites used. Adjust dosage as needed.
➤ **Postmenopausal urogenital symptoms**
Women: One ring inserted into the upper third of the vagina. Ring is kept in place for 3 months.
➤ **Vulvar and vaginal atrophy**
Women: 0.05 mg/24 hours Estraderm applied twice weekly in a cyclic regimen. Or, 0.05 mg/24 hours Climara applied weekly in a cyclic regimen. Or, 2 to 4 g vaginal applications of cream daily for 1 to 2 weeks. When vaginal mucosa is restored, maintenance dose is 1 g one to three times weekly in a cyclic regimen. If

---

using Vagifem for atrophic vaginitis, give 1 tablet vaginally once daily for 2 weeks. Maintenance dose is 1 tablet inserted vaginally twice weekly. Or, 10 to 20 mg valerate I.M. every 4 weeks as needed. Or, 1 to 5 mg estradiol cypionate I.M. once every 3 to 4 weeks.

➤ **Moderate to severe vasomotor symptoms, as well as vulval and vaginal atrophy associated with menopause**
Women: 1.25 g EstroGel applied once daily to skin in a thin layer from wrist to shoulder of one upper extremity.

➤ **Palliative treatment of advanced, inoperable breast cancer**
Men and postmenopausal women: 10 mg P.O. estradiol t.i.d. for 3 months.

➤ **Palliative treatment of advanced, inoperable prostate cancer**
Men: 30 mg valerate I.M. every 1 to 2 weeks, or 1 to 2 mg P.O. estradiol t.i.d.

➤ **To prevent postmenopausal osteoporosis**
Women: Place a 6.5-cm² (0.025 mg/24 hours) Climara patch once weekly on clean, dry skin of lower abdomen or upper quadrant of buttock. Or, place a 3.25-cm² (0.014 mg/24 hours) Menostar patch once weekly to clean, dry area of the lower abdomen. Or, place a 0.5 mg/24 hours Estraderm patch twice weekly in a cyclic regimen in women with an intact uterus. In women with a hysterectomy, apply one Estraderm patch twice weekly in a continuous regimen. For each system, press firmly in place for about 10 seconds; ensure complete contact, especially around edges. Or, 0.025-mg/24 hours Vivelle, Vivelle-Dot, or Alora system applied to a clean, dry area of the trunk twice weekly. Or, 0.5 mg P.O. daily for 21 days, followed by 7 days without drug.

➤ **Moderate to severe vasomotor symptoms from menopause**
Women: Apply contents of two 1.74-g foil pouches (total 3.48 g) of Estrasorb daily. Or, Divigel 0.1% at dose of 0.25, 0.5, or 1 g/day. Start with Divigel 0.25 g daily and adjust dose based on individual patient response. Or, 1 pump per day of Elestrin applied to the upper arm. Or, Evamist 1 spray per day initially; may adjust dose based on clinical response.

ADMINISTRATION
P.O.
● Give drug without regard for food. If stomach upset occurs, give with food.
● Don't give drug with grapefruit juice.
● Store at controlled room temperature.
I.M.
● To give I.M. injection, make sure drug is well dispersed by rolling vial between palms. Inject deep into large muscle. Rotate injection sites to prevent muscle atrophy. Never give drug I.V.
Transdermal
● Open each pouch of Estrasorb individually and use contents of one pouch for each leg. Rub emulsion into thigh and calf for 3 minutes until thoroughly absorbed; rub emulsion remaining on hands onto the buttocks. Allow areas to dry before covering with clothing. Wash hands with soap and water to remove excess drug.
● Apply Elestrin once daily to the upper arm.
● Apply EstroGel over the entire area of one arm.
● Apply Evamist each morning to adjacent, non-overlapping areas on the inner surface of the forearm, starting near the elbow. Allow to dry for 2 minutes and do not wash the site for 30 minutes.
● Apply Divigel once daily on skin of either right or left upper thigh. Application surface area should be about 5 by 7 inches (about the size of two palm prints). Apply entire contents of a unit dose packet each day. To avoid potential skin irritation, apply Divigel to right or left upper thigh on alternating days. Don't apply Divigel on face, breasts, or irritated skin, or in or around the vagina. After application, allow gel to dry before dressing. Don't wash application site within 1 hour after applying Divigel. Avoid contact of gel with eyes. Wash hands after application.
● Apply transdermal patch to clean, hairless, intact skin on abdomen or buttock. Don't apply to breasts, waistline, or other areas where clothing can loosen patch. When applying, ensure thorough contact between patch and skin, especially around edges, and hold in place for about 10 seconds. Apply patch immediately after opening and removing protective cover. Rotate application sites.

Vaginal
• Using the applicator, insert Vagifem as far into vagina as it can comfortably go, without using force.

ACTION
Increases synthesis of DNA, RNA, and protein in responsive tissues; reduces release of follicle-stimulating and luteinizing hormones from the pituitary gland.

Route	Onset	Peak	Duration
P.O., I.M., vaginal	Unknown	Unknown	Unknown
Trans-dermal (Esclim)	Unknown	27–30 hr	Unknown
Trans-dermal (Estrasorb)	Immediate	Unknown	Unknown
Trans-dermal gel (EstroGel)	Immediate	1 hr	24–36 hr

Half-life: Unknown.

ADVERSE REACTIONS
CNS: *stroke, headache,* dizziness, chorea, depression, *seizures,* insomnia (Vagifem).
CV: thrombophlebitis, *thromboembolism,* hypertension, *edema, pulmonary embolism (PE), MI.*
EENT: worsening myopia or astigmatism, intolerance of contact lenses, sinusitis (Vagifem).
GI: *nausea,* vomiting, abdominal cramps, bloating, increased appetite, *pancreatitis,* anorexia, gallbladder disease, dyspepsia (Vagifem).
GU: breakthrough bleeding, altered menstrual flow, dysmenorrhea, amenorrhea, *increased risk of endometrial cancer,* cervical erosion, abnormal Pap smear, altered cervical secretions, enlargement of uterine fibromas, vaginal candidiasis in women, testicular atrophy, impotence in men, genital pruritus, hematuria, vaginal discomfort, vaginitis (Vagifem).
Hepatic: cholestatic jaundice, *hepatic adenoma.*
Metabolic: weight changes, hypothyroidism, hypercalcemia (in patients with breast cancer and bone metastases).
Respiratory: *upper respiratory tract infection,* allergy, bronchitis (Vagifem).

Skin: melasma, urticaria, erythema nodosum, dermatitis, hair loss, pruritus.
Other: *gynecomastia, increased risk of breast cancer,* hot flashes, pain (Vagifem), *breast tenderness, enlargement, or secretion,* flulike syndrome.

INTERACTIONS
Drug-drug. *Carbamazepine, fosphenytoin, phenobarbital, phenytoin, rifampin:* May decrease effectiveness of estrogen therapy. Monitor patient closely.
Corticosteroids: May enhance effects of corticosteroids. Monitor patient closely.
Cyclosporine: May increase risk of toxicity. Use together with caution, and monitor cyclosporine level frequently.
Dantrolene, other hepatotoxic drugs: May increase risk of hepatotoxicity. Monitor liver function closely.
Oral anticoagulants: May decrease anticoagulant effect. Dosage adjustments may be needed. Monitor PT and INR.
Tamoxifen: May interfere with tamoxifen effectiveness. Avoid using together.
Drug-herb. *Black cohosh:* May increase drug's adverse effects. Discourage use together.
Saw palmetto: May negate drug's effects. Discourage use together.
St. John's wort: May decrease effects of drug. Discourage use together.
Drug-food. *Caffeine:* May increase caffeine level. Advise patient to avoid or minimize use of caffeine.
Grapefruit juice: May elevate drug level. Tell patient to take drug with liquid other than grapefruit juice.
Drug-lifestyle. *Smoking:* May increase risk of adverse CV effects. If smoking continues, may need another therapy.
Sunscreen use: May increase absorption of Estrasorb. Tell patient to separate application times.

EFFECTS ON LAB TEST RESULTS
• May increase clotting factor VII, VIII, IX, and X; total T_4; thyroid-binding globulin; liver function test; and triglyceride levels.
• May increase norepinephrine-induced platelet aggregation and PT.
• May decrease metyrapone test results.

Reactions may be *common,* uncommon, *life-threatening,* or COMMON AND LIFE-THREATENING.
Interaction may have a *rapid onset* or *delayed onset.*

CONTRAINDICATIONS & CAUTIONS

• Contraindicated in pregnant patients and patients with thrombophlebitis or thrombo-embolic disorders, estrogen-dependent neoplasia, breast or reproductive organ cancer (except for palliative treatment), undiagnosed abnormal genital bleeding, or history of thrombophlebitis or thrombo-embolic disorders linked to previous estrogen use (except for palliative treatment of breast and prostate cancer).

• Contraindicated in patients with liver dysfunction or disease.

• Use cautiously in patients with cerebrovascular or coronary artery disease, asthma, bone disease, migraine, seizures, or cardiac or renal dysfunction.

• Use cautiously in women who have a strong family history (grandmother, mother, sister) of breast cancer, breast nodules, fibrocystic breasts, or abnormal mammogram findings.

• **Alert:** Postmenopausal women ages 50 to 79 who are taking estrogen and progestin have an increased risk of MI, stroke, invasive breast cancer, PE, and thrombosis. Postmenopausal women age 65 or older also have an increased risk of dementia.

NURSING CONSIDERATIONS

• Ensure that patient has physical examination before starting therapy. Patients receiving long-term therapy should have yearly examinations. Monitor lipid levels, blood pressure, body weight, and hepatic function.

• Ask patient about allergies, especially to foods and plants. Estradiol is available as an aqueous solution or as a solution in peanut oil; estradiol cypionate, as a solution in cottonseed oil; estradiol valerate, as a solution in castor oil or sesame oil.

■ **Black Box Warning** Estrogen increases the risk of endometrial cancer. Use adequate diagnostic measures, including endometrial sampling when indicated, to rule out malignancy in all cases of undiagnosed persistent or recurring abnormal vaginal bleeding. ■

■ **Black Box Warning** Do not use estrogens with or without progestins to prevent cardiovascular disease or dementia. ■

• When estrogen is prescribed for a postmenopausal woman with a uterus, also initiate a progestin to reduce the risk of endometrial cancer.

• **Alert:** EstroGel contains alcohol. Avoid fire, flame, or smoking until area dries in 2 to 5 minutes.

• In women also taking oral estrogen, treatment with the Estraderm transdermal patch can begin 1 week after withdrawal of oral therapy, or sooner if menopausal symptoms appear before the end of the week.

• Transdermal systems may be used continually rather than cyclically. Other alternative regimens are 1 to 5 mg cypionate I.M. every 3 to 4 weeks and 10 to 20 mg (valerate) I.M. every 4 weeks, as needed.

• Instruct patients using Vagifem who have severely atrophic vaginal mucosa to be careful when inserting the applicator. After gynecologic surgery, tell patient to use any vaginal applicator cautiously and only if clearly indicated.

• The prescriber should assess the patient's need to continue estradiol therapy. Make attempts to stop or taper at 3- to 6-month intervals.

• Because of risk of thromboembolism, stop therapy at least 1 month before high-risk procedures or those that cause prolonged immobilization, such as knee or hip surgery.

• Glucose tolerance may be impaired. Monitor glucose level closely in patients with diabetes.

• Notify pathologist about estrogen therapy when sending specimens to laboratory for evaluation.

• Estrace 2 mg micronized tablets contain tartrazine.

PATIENT TEACHING

• Tell patient to read package insert describing estrogen's adverse effects and give verbal explanation.

• Emphasize importance of regular physical examinations. Postmenopausal women who use estrogen replacement for longer than 5 years may be at increased risk for endometrial cancer. Risk is reduced by using cyclic rather than continuous therapy and the lowest possible dosages of estrogen. Adding progestins to the regimen decreases risk of endometrial hyperplasia; however, it isn't known whether progestins affect risk of

endometrial cancer. No increased risk of breast cancer has been reported.
- Teach woman how to use cream. She should wash vaginal area with soap and water before applying and insert cream high into the vagina (about two-thirds the length of the applicator). She should take drug at bedtime, or lie flat for 30 minutes after instillation to minimize drug loss.
- Tell patient using topical emulsion not to apply it with sunscreen.
- Tell patient to use transdermal system correctly, to rotate sites, to avoid breasts and waistline, and to reapply patch if it falls off.
- Teach patient using transdermal gel (EstroGel) to apply in a thin layer on one arm and allow to dry before smoking, getting near flames, dressing, or touching the arm. Recommend bathing before application to maintain full dosage.
- Tell patient that estradiol gel should never be applied directly to the breast.
- Tell patient to insert Vagifem by the applicator as far into vagina as it can comfortably go, without using force.
- **Alert:** Warn patient to immediately report abdominal pain, pressure or pain in chest, shortness of breath, severe headaches, visual disturbances, vaginal bleeding or discharge, breast lumps, swelling of hands or feet, yellow skin or sclera, dark urine, light-colored stools, and pain, numbness, or stiffness in legs or buttocks.
- Explain to patient receiving cyclic therapy for postmenopausal symptoms that withdrawal bleeding may occur during week off drug. Tell her to report unusual vaginal bleeding.
- Tell diabetic patient to report elevated glucose level so that antidiabetic dosage can be adjusted.
- Teach woman how to perform routine breast self-examination.
- Teach patient methods to decrease risk of blood clots.
- Advise woman not to become pregnant during estrogen therapy.
- Advise woman of childbearing age to consult prescriber before taking drug and to advise prescriber immediately if she becomes pregnant.
- Encourage patient to stop or reduce smoking because of the risk of CV complications.

estradiol and norethindrone acetate transdermal system
ess-tra-DYE-ole and nor-ETH-in-drone

CombiPatch

Pharmacologic class: estrogen and progestin
Pregnancy risk category X

AVAILABLE FORMS
Transdermal: 9-cm² system releasing 0.05 mg estradiol and 0.14 mg norethindrone acetate daily; 16-cm² system releasing 0.05 mg estradiol and 0.25 mg norethindrone acetate daily

INDICATIONS & DOSAGES
➤ **Moderate to severe vasomotor symptoms from menopause; vulval and vaginal atrophy; hypoestrogenemia from hypogonadism, castration, or primary ovarian failure in women with intact uterus**
Continuous combined regimen
Women: Wear 9-cm² patch continuously on lower abdomen. Replace system twice weekly during 28-day cycle. May increase to 16-cm² patch.
Continuous sequential regimen
Women: For use in sequential regimen with an estradiol transdermal system (such as Alora, Esclim, Estraderm, Vivelle), wear 0.05-mg estradiol transdermal patch for first 14 days of 28-day cycle; replace system twice weekly. Wear 9-cm² patch system on lower abdomen for rest of 28-day cycle; replace system twice weekly. May increase to 16-cm² patch as needed.

ADMINISTRATION
Transdermal
- Apply patch system to a smooth (fold-free), clean, dry, nonirritated area of skin on lower abdomen, avoiding the waistline. Rotate application sites, with an interval of at least 1 week between applications to same site.
- Don't apply patch on or near breasts.
- Avoid applying to areas that may get prolonged sun exposure.
- Reapply patch, if needed, to another area of lower abdomen. If patch fails to adhere, replace with a new one.

ACTION
A matrix transdermal system in which estradiol and norethindrone are released continuously. Estrogen replacement therapy can reduce menopausal symptoms and release of follicle-stimulating and luteinizing hormones in postmenopausal women.

Route	Onset	Peak	Duration
Trans-dermal	12–24 hr	Unknown	3–4 days

Half-life: 6 to 20 hours (estradiol); 5 to 14 hours (norethindrone).

ADVERSE REACTIONS
CNS: *asthenia,* **stroke,** depression, insomnia, nervousness, dizziness, *head-ache, pain.*
CV: **thromboembolism,** thrombophlebitis, hypertension, *edema,* **pulmonary embolism, MI.**
EENT: pharyngitis, *rhinitis, sinusitis,* retinal vascular thrombosis, intolerance to contact lenses.
GI: *abdominal pain, diarrhea,* dyspepsia, changes in appetite, flatulence, *nausea,* constipation, gallbladder disease.
GU: *dysmenorrhea, leukorrhea, men-strual disorder,* suspicious Papanicolaou smears, *vaginitis,* menorrhagia, **vaginal hemorrhage.**
Hepatic: cholestatic jaundice.
Metabolic: weight changes, hyper-calcemia, hypertriglyceridemia.
Musculoskeletal: arthralgia, *back pain.*
Respiratory: *respiratory disorder,* bronchitis.
Skin: application site reactions, acne, melasma, chloasma.
Other: *accidental injury, flulike syndrome, breast pain,* tooth disorder, peripheral edema, breast enlargement, infection, changes in libido.

INTERACTIONS
Drug-drug. *Carbamazepine, fosphenytoin, phenobarbital, phenytoin, rifampin:* May decrease estrogen therapy effectiveness. Monitor patient closely.
Corticosteroids: May enhance effects of corticosteroids. Monitor patient closely.
Cyclosporine: May increase risk of toxicity. Use together with caution; monitor cyclo-sporine level frequently.

Dantrolene, hepatotoxic drugs: May increase risk of hepatotoxicity. Monitor liver function closely.
Oral anticoagulants: May decrease effect of anticoagulant. May need to adjust dose. Monitor PT and INR.
Tamoxifen: May interfere with tamoxifen effectiveness. Avoid using together.
Drug-herb. *Black cohosh:* May increase adverse effects of drug. Discourage use together.
Saw palmetto: May cause antiestrogenic effects. Discourage use together.
St. John's wort: May decrease effects of drug. Discourage use together.
Drug-food. *Caffeine:* May increase caffeine level. Advise patient to avoid caffeine.
Grapefruit juice: May elevate estrogen level. Advise patient to take with liquid other than grapefruit juice.
Drug-lifestyle. *Smoking:* May increase risk of adverse CV effects. If smoking continues, may need alternative therapy.

EFFECTS ON LAB TEST RESULTS
● May increase T_3 and T_4, HDL, and triglyceride levels. May decrease LDL levels.
● May increase fibrinogen activity and platelet count. May decrease T_3 resin uptake. May alter activated PTT, INR, and platelet aggregation times.
● May reduce metyrapone test values. May alter glucose tolerance test results.

CONTRAINDICATIONS & CAUTIONS
● Contraindicated in women hypersensitive to estrogen, progestin, or any component of the patch; in pregnant patients; and in patients with known or suspected breast cancer, known or suspected estrogen-dependent neoplasia, undiagnosed abnor-mal genital bleeding, active thrombo-phlebitis, thromboembolic disorders, or stroke.
● Use cautiously in breast-feeding women and in patients with impaired liver function, asthma, epilepsy, migraine, or cardiac or renal dysfunction.

NURSING CONSIDERATIONS
■ **Black Box Warning** Do not use estrogens, with or without progestins,

to prevent cardiovascular disease or dementia. ■

■ **Black Box Warning** Postmenopausal women treated for 5 years have an increased risk of MI, stroke, invasive breast cancer, pulmonary emboli and deep vein thrombosis. ■

• Women not receiving continuous estrogen or combined estrogen and progestin therapy may start therapy at any time.

• Women receiving continuous hormone replacement therapy should complete the current cycle before starting therapy. Women commonly have withdrawal bleeding at completion of cycle; first day of withdrawal bleeding is appropriate time to start therapy.

• Store patches in refrigerator before dispensing. Patient may then store patches at room temperature for up to 6 months, or the expiration date, whichever comes first.

• Reevaluate therapy at 3- to 6-month intervals.

• A combined estrogen and progestin regimen is indicated for a woman with an intact uterus. Progestins taken with estrogen significantly reduce, but don't eliminate, risk of endometrial cancer linked to use of estrogen alone.

• Because of risk of thromboembolism stop therapy at least 4 to 6 weeks before surgery associated with an increased risk of thromboembolism, or during periods of prolonged immobilization.

• Blood pressure increases have been linked to estrogen use. Monitor patient's blood pressure regularly.

• Treatment of postmenopausal symptoms usually starts during menopause stage when vasomotor symptoms occur.

• Monitor glucose level closely in patients with diabetes.

• **Alert:** Don't interchange CombiPatch with other estrogen patches. Verify therapy before application.

PATIENT TEACHING

• Teach woman how to apply patch properly. She should wear only one patch at any time during therapy. Tell her to apply patch immediately after opening protective cover.

• Tell patient an oil-based cream or lotion may help remove adhesive from the skin

after patch has been removed and the area allowed to dry for 15 minutes.

• Advise woman not to use patch if she's pregnant or plans to become pregnant.

• Urge woman of childbearing age to consult prescriber before applying patch and to advise prescriber immediately if she becomes pregnant.

• Instruct patient that the continuous combined regimen may lead to irregular bleeding, particularly in the first 6 months, but that it usually decreases with time, and often stops completely.

• Tell patient that, for the continuous sequential regimen, monthly withdrawal bleeding is common.

• Advise patient to alert prescriber and remove patch at first sign of clotting disorders (thrombophlebitis, cerebrovascular disorders, and pulmonary embolism).

• Instruct patient to stop using patch and call prescriber about any loss of vision, sudden onset of protrusion of the eyeball (proptosis), double vision, or migraine.

• Encourage patient to stop or reduce smoking because of the risk of CV complications.

• Tell patient to perform monthly self breast exams and to have annual gynecologic and breast examinations by a health care provider.

• Advise patient not to store patches where extreme temperatures can occur.

estrogens, conjugated (estrogenic substances, conjugated; oestrogens, conjugated)
ESS-troe-jenz

C.E.S†, Cenestin, Enjuvia, Premarin◆, Premarin Intravenous

Pharmacologic class: estrogen
Pregnancy risk category X

AVAILABLE FORMS
Injection: 25 mg/5 ml
Tablets: 0.3 mg, 0.45 mg, 0.625 mg, 0.9 mg, 1.25 mg
Vaginal cream: 0.625 mg/g

Reactions may be *common,* uncommon, *life-threatening,* or COMMON AND LIFE-THREATENING.
Interaction may have a *rapid onset* or **delayed onset.**

INDICATIONS & DOSAGES
➤ **Abnormal uterine bleeding (hormonal imbalance)**
Adults: 25 mg I.V. or I.M. Repeat dose in 6 to 12 hours, if necessary.
➤ **Vulvar or vaginal atrophy**
Adults: 0.5 to 2 g cream intravaginally once daily in cycles of 3 weeks on, 1 week off.
➤ **Castration and primary ovarian failure**
Adults: Initially, 1.25 mg Premarin P.O. daily in cycles of 3 weeks on, 1 week off. Adjust dose as needed.
➤ **Female hypogonadism**
Adults: 0.3 to 0.625 mg Premarin P.O. daily, given cyclically 3 weeks on, 1 week off.
➤ **Moderate to severe vasomotor symptoms with or without moderate to severe symptoms of vulvar and vaginal atrophy associated with menopause**
Adults: Initially, 0.3 mg Premarin or Enjuvia P.O. daily. Premarin may also be given cyclically 25 days on, 5 days off. Adjust dosage based on patient response.
➤ **Moderate to severe vasomotor symptoms from menopause**
Adults: 0.45 to 1.25 mg Cenestin P.O. daily. Adjust dose based on patient response.
➤ **Moderate to severe symptoms of vulvar and vaginal atrophy from menopause**
Adults: 0.3 mg Cenestin P.O. daily.
➤ **To prevent osteoporosis**
Adults: 0.3 mg Premarin P.O. daily, or cyclically, 25 days on, 5 days off. Adjust dose based on response of bone mineral density testing.
➤ **Palliative treatment of inoperable prostatic cancer**
Adults: 1.25 to 2.5 mg Premarin P.O. t.i.d.
➤ **Palliative treatment of breast cancer**
Adults: 10 mg Premarin P.O. t.i.d. for at least 3 months.

ADMINISTRATION
P.O.
● Give drug at same time each day.
I.V.
● Refrigerate before reconstituting.
● Reconstitute only with diluent provided. Agitate gently after adding diluent.

● Drug is compatible with normal saline, dextrose, or invert sugar solutions.
● Use reconstituted solution within a few hours, if possible. Reconstituted solution is stable under refrigeration for 60 days. Don't use if solution darkens or precipitates.
● Give direct injection slowly to avoid flushing reaction.
● **Incompatibilities:** Acidic solutions, ascorbic acid, protein hydrolysate.
I.M.
● Reconstitute only with diluent provided. Agitate gently after adding diluent.
● Inject deep into large muscle. Rotate injection sites to prevent muscle atrophy.
Vaginal
● Wash the vaginal area with soap and water, insert about two-thirds the length of the applicator into the vagina, and release drug. Give drug at bedtime or when the patient will lie flat for 30 minutes after use to minimize drug loss.

ACTION
Increases synthesis of DNA, RNA, and protein in responsive tissues. Also reduces release of follicle-stimulating and luteinizing hormones from the pituitary gland.

Route	Onset	Peak	Duration
P.O., I.V., I.M., vaginal	Unknown	Unknown	Unknown

Half-life: Unknown.

ADVERSE REACTIONS
CNS: headache, dizziness, chorea, depression, *stroke, seizures.*
CV: flushing with rapid I.V. administration, thrombophlebitis, *thromboembolism,* hypertension, *edema, pulmonary embolism, MI.*
EENT: worsening myopia or astigmatism, intolerance of contact lenses.
GI: *nausea,* vomiting, abdominal cramps, bloating, anorexia, increased appetite, *pancreatitis,* gallbladder disease.
GU: breakthrough bleeding, altered menstrual flow, dysmenorrhea, amenorrhea, *increased risk of endometrial cancer,* cervical erosion, altered cervical secretions, enlargement of uterine fibromas,

vaginal candidiasis, testicular atrophy, impotence.

Hepatic: cholestatic jaundice, *hepatic adenoma.*

Metabolic: weight changes, hypercalcemia, hypertriglyceridemia.

Skin: melasma, chloasma, urticaria, hirsutism or hair loss, erythema nodosum, dermatitis.

Other: *breast tenderness, enlargement, or secretion, gynecomastia, **increased risk of breast cancer,*** changes in libido.

INTERACTIONS

Drug-drug. *Carbamazepine, fosphenytoin, phenobarbital, phenytoin, rifampin:* May decrease effectiveness of estrogen therapy. Monitor patient closely.
Corticosteroids: May enhance corticosteroid effects. Monitor patient closely.
Cyclosporine: May increase risk of toxicity. Use together with caution, and monitor cyclosporine level frequently.
Dantrolene, other hepatotoxic drugs: May increase risk of hepatotoxicity. Monitor liver function closely.
Oral anticoagulants: May decrease anticoagulant effects. May need to adjust dosage. Monitor PT and INR.
Tamoxifen: May interfere with tamoxifen effectiveness. Avoid using together.
Drug-herb. *Black cohosh:* May increase adverse effects of drug. Discourage use together.
Red clover: May interfere with hormonal therapies. Discourage use together.
Saw palmetto: May have antiestrogenic effects. Discourage use together.
St. John's wort: May decrease effects of drug. Discourage use together.
Drug-food. *Caffeine:* May increase caffeine level. Advise caution.
Grapefruit juice: May increase concentration of estrogen. Avoid using together.
Drug-lifestyle. *Smoking:* May increase risk of adverse CV effects. If smoking continues, recommend nonhormonal contraception.

EFFECTS ON LAB TEST RESULTS

• May increase clotting factor VII, VIII, IX, and X; total T_4; phospholipid; thyroid-binding globulin; and triglyceride levels.
• May increase norepinephrine-induced platelet aggregation and PT.

• May cause a false-positive metyrapone test result.

CONTRAINDICATIONS & CAUTIONS

■ **Black Box Warning** Contraindicated in pregnant patients. ■
• Contraindicated in patients with thrombophlebitis, thromboembolic disorders, estrogen-dependent neoplasia, breast or reproductive cancer (except for palliative treatment), or undiagnosed abnormal genital bleeding.
• Use cautiously in patients with cerebrovascular or coronary artery disease, asthma, bone disease, migraine, seizures, or cardiac, hepatic, or renal dysfunction.
• Use cautiously in women who have a strong family history (mother, grandmother, sister) of breast or genital tract cancer, breast nodules, fibrocystic breasts, or abnormal mammogram findings.

NURSING CONSIDERATIONS

• Make sure patient has thorough physical exam before starting therapy, and patients receiving long-term therapy should have yearly exams. Periodically monitor lipid levels, blood pressure, body weight, and hepatic function.
• Rapid treatment of dysfunctional uterine bleeding or reduction of surgical bleeding usually requires delivery by I.V. or I.M. route.
■ **Black Box Warning** Don't use to prevent CV disease. In postmenopausal women receiving therapy for more than 5 years, drugs may increase risks of MI, stroke, invasive breast cancer, pulmonary emboli, and deep vein thrombosis. Use the lowest effective doses for the shortest time, considering the benefits and risks. ■
■ **Black Box Warning** In postmenopausal women receiving therapy for more than 5 years, drug may increase risk of endometrial cancer. Cyclic therapy and the lowest possible dose reduces risk. Adding progestins decreases risk of endometrial hyperplasia, but it's unknown whether they affect risk of endometrial cancer. ■
■ **Black Box Warning** In postmenopausal women 65 years of age or older during 4 years of treatment with conjugated estrogens plus medroxyprogesterone acetate, drug may increase the risk of dementia. ■

Reactions may be *common,* uncommon, *life-threatening,* or COMMON AND LIFE-THREATENING.
Interaction may have a *rapid onset* or **delayed onset.**

• When used solely for the treatment of vulval and vaginal atrophy, consider topical products.

• Notify pathologist about estrogen therapy when sending specimens to laboratory for evaluation.

• Because of thromboembolism risk, stop therapy at least 1 month before procedures that prolong immobilization or raise the risk of thromboembolism, such as knee or hip surgery.

• Glucose tolerance may be impaired. Monitor glucose level closely in patients with diabetes.

• Re-evaluate need for therapy at 3 to 6 month intervals.

• *Look alike–sound alike:* Don't confuse Premarin with Primaxin, Provera, or Remeron.

PATIENT TEACHING
• Tell patient to read package insert describing estrogen's adverse effects and to explain them back to you.

• Emphasize importance of regular physical exams.

• Teach woman how to use vaginal cream. Tell patient to wash the vaginal area with soap and water, insert about two-thirds the length of the applicator into the vagina, and release drug. Tell her to use drug at bedtime or to lie flat for 30 minutes after use to minimize drug loss.

• Explain to patient that cyclic therapy for postmenopausal symptoms may cause withdrawal bleeding during week off drug. Tell her to report unusual vaginal bleeding.

• *Alert:* Warn patient to immediately report abdominal pain; pain, numbness, or stiffness in legs or buttocks; pressure or pain in chest; shortness of breath; severe headaches; visual disturbances, such as blind spots, flashing lights, or blurriness; vaginal bleeding or discharge; breast lumps; swelling of hands or feet; yellow skin or sclera; dark urine; and light-colored stools.

• Tell diabetic patient to report elevated glucose level so that antidiabetic dosage can be adjusted.

• Teach woman how to perform routine breast self-examination.

• Advise woman not to become pregnant during estrogen therapy.

• Advise woman of childbearing age to consult prescriber before taking drug and to advise prescriber immediately if she becomes pregnant.

• Encourage patient to stop smoking or reduce number of cigarettes smoked because of the risk of CV complications.

• Tell patient using drug for osteoporosis prevention to ensure adequate intake of calcium and vitamin D.

• Inform patient that vaginal cream has been reported to weaken latex condoms and to use an alternative method of birth control.

estropipate (piperazine estrone sulfate)
ess-troe-PIH-pate

Ogen, Ortho-Est

Pharmacologic class: estrogen
Pregnancy risk category X

AVAILABLE FORMS
Tablets: 0.75 mg, 1.5 mg, 3 mg, 6 mg
Vaginal cream: 1.5 mg/g

INDICATIONS & DOSAGES
➤ **Vulval and vaginal atrophy**
Women: 0.75 to 6 mg P.O. daily, 3 weeks on and 1 week off; or 2 to 4 g vaginal cream daily.

➤ **Primary ovarian failure, female castration, female hypogonadism**
Women: 1.5 to 9 mg P.O. daily for first 3 weeks; then a rest period of 8 to 10 days. If bleeding doesn't occur by end of rest period, cycle is repeated.

➤ **Vasomotor menopausal symptoms**
Women: 0.75 to 6 mg P.O. daily in cyclic method, 3 weeks on and 1 week off. Can be given continuously.

➤ **To prevent osteoporosis**
Women: 0.75 mg P.O. daily for 25 consecutive days of a 31-day cycle, followed by 6 days without drug. Repeat regimen as indicated.

ADMINISTRATION
P.O.
• Give drug with meals to minimize GI upset.

Vaginal

• Wash vaginal area with soap and water and then insert vaginal cream high into vagina (about two-thirds the length of applicator). Use drug at bedtime or when patient is able to lie flat for 30 minutes after application to minimize drug loss.

ACTION

Increases synthesis of DNA, RNA, and proteins in responsive tissues; reduces follicle-stimulating and luteinizing hormones.

Route	Onset	Peak	Duration
P.O., vaginal	Unknown	Unknown	Unknown

Half-life: Unknown.

ADVERSE REACTIONS

CNS: depression, headache, dizziness, migraine, *seizures, stroke.*
CV: *edema,* thrombophlebitis, hypertension, *pulmonary embolism (PE), MI, thromboembolism.*
EENT: steepening of corneal curvature, intolerance to contact lenses.
GI: nausea, vomiting, gallbladder disease, abdominal cramps, bloating.
GU: increased size of uterine fibromas, *endometrial cancer,* vaginal candidiasis, cystitis-like syndrome, dysmenorrhea, amenorrhea, breakthrough bleeding, condition resembling premenstrual syndrome.
Hepatic: cholestatic jaundice, *hepatic adenoma.*
Metabolic: weight changes, hypercalcemia, hypertriglyceridemia.
Skin: hemorrhagic eruption, erythema nodosum, *erythema multiforme,* hirsutism or hair loss, melasma.
Other: breast engorgement or enlargement, *breast cancer,* breast tenderness, changes in libido.

INTERACTIONS

Drug-drug. *Carbamazepine, fosphenytoin, phenobarbital, phenytoin, rifampin:* May decrease estrogen effect. Monitor patient closely.
Corticosteroids: May enhance corticosteroid effect. Monitor patient closely.

Cyclosporine: May increase risk of toxicity. Use together with caution; frequently monitor cyclosporine level.
Dantrolene, other hepatotoxic drugs: May increase risk of hepatotoxicity. Monitor liver function closely.
Oral anticoagulants: May decrease anticoagulant effect. Dosage adjustments may be needed. Monitor PT and INR.
Tamoxifen: May interfere with tamoxifen effect. Avoid using together.
Drug-herb. *Black cohosh:* May increase adverse effects of estrogen. Discourage use together.
Red clover: May interfere with hormonal therapies. Discourage use together.
Saw palmetto: May have antiestrogenic effect. Discourage use together.
St. John's wort: May decrease estrogen effect. Discourage use together.
Drug-food. *Caffeine:* May increase caffeine level. Advise caution.
Drug-lifestyle. *Smoking:* May increase risk of adverse CV effects. If smoking continues, may need alternative therapy.

EFFECTS ON LAB TEST RESULTS

• May increase clotting factor VII, VIII, IX, and X; total T_4; phospholipid; thyroid-binding globulin; and triglyceride levels.
• May increase norepinephrine-induced platelet aggregation and PT.
• May reduce metyrapone test results.

CONTRAINDICATIONS & CAUTIONS

■ **Black Box Warning** Contraindicated during pregnancy or during the immediate postpartum period. ■
• Contraindicated in patients with active thrombophlebitis; thromboembolic disorders; estrogen-dependent neoplasia; undiagnosed genital bleeding; and breast, reproductive organ, or genital cancer.
• Use cautiously in patients with cerebrovascular or coronary artery disease; asthma; mental depression; bone disease; migraine; seizures; or cardiac, hepatic, or renal dysfunction.
• Use cautiously in women who have a family history (mother, grandmother,

---

Reactions may be *common,* uncommon, *life-threatening,* or COMMON AND LIFE-THREATENING.
Interaction may have a *rapid onset* or *delayed onset.*

sister) of breast or genital tract cancer, breast nodules, fibrocystic breasts, or abnormal mammogram findings.

NURSING CONSIDERATIONS
● Make sure patient has thorough physical examination before starting estrogen therapy. Patients receiving long-term therapy should have examinations yearly. Periodically monitor lipid levels, blood pressure, body weight, and hepatic function.

■ **Black Box Warning** Estrogens and progestins shouldn't be used to prevent CV disease. The Women's Health Initiative study reported increased risks of MI, stroke, invasive breast cancer, PE, and deep vein thrombosis in postmenopausal women during 5 years of combination therapy. Because of these risks, estrogens and progestins should be prescribed at the lowest effective doses and for the shortest duration consistent with treatment goals and risks for the individual woman. ■

■ **Black Box Warning** Estrogens may increase the risk of endometrial cancer in postmenopausal women. ■

● When used to treat hypogonadism, duration of therapy needed to produce withdrawal bleeding depends on patient's endometrial response to drug. If satisfactory withdrawal bleeding doesn't occur, an oral progestin is added to the regimen. Explain to patient that, despite return of withdrawal bleeding, pregnancy can't occur because she doesn't ovulate.

● Estropipate-estrone equivalents are:

0.75 mg estropipate = 0.625 mg estrone

1.5 mg estropipate = 1.25 mg estrone

3 mg estropipate = 2.5 mg estrone

6 mg estropipate = 5 mg estrone

● Because of risk of thromboembolism, stop therapy at least 1 month before procedures that prolong immobilization or raise the risk of thromboembolism, such as knee or hip surgery.

● Glucose tolerance may be impaired. Monitor glucose level closely in patients with diabetes.

PATIENT TEACHING
● Tell patient to read package insert describing estrogen's adverse effects; also, explain effects verbally.
● Teach woman how to use vaginal cream. Patient should wash the vaginal area with soap and water and then insert vaginal cream high into the vagina (about two-thirds the length of the applicator). Tell her to use drug at bedtime or to lie flat for 30 minutes after application to minimize drug loss.
● Tell diabetic patient to report elevated glucose level to prescriber.
● Stress importance of regular physical examinations. Postmenopausal women who use estrogen replacement for longer than 5 years may have increased risk of endometrial cancer. Using cyclic therapy and lowest possible estrogen dosage reduces risk. Adding progestins to regimen decreases risk of endometrial hyperplasia; however, it isn't known whether progestins affect risk of endometrial cancer.
● *Alert:* Warn patient to immediately report abdominal pain; pain, stiffness, or numbness in legs or buttocks; pressure or pain in chest; shortness of breath; severe headaches; visual disturbances, such as blind spots or flashing lights; vaginal bleeding or discharge; breast lumps; swelling of hands or feet; yellow skin or sclera; dark urine; and light-colored stools.
● Teach woman how to perform routine breast self-examination.
● Advise woman not to become pregnant while on estrogen therapy.
● Encourage patient to stop or reduce smoking because of the risk of CV complications.
● Advise woman of childbearing age to consult prescriber before taking drug and to tell prescriber immediately if she becomes pregnant.
● Teach patient at risk for osteoporosis about the importance of adequate calcium and vitamin D intake.

ethinyl estradiol and desogestrel
ETH-i-nill and DAY-so-jest-rul

monophasic
Apri, Desogen, Ortho-Cept

biphasic
Kariva, Mircette

triphasic
Cyclessa, Velivet

ethinyl estradiol and ethynodiol diacetate
monophasic
Demulen 1/35, Demulen 1/50, Zovia 1/35E, Zovia 1/50E

ethinyl estradiol and levonorgestrel
monophasic
Aviane, Lessina, Levlen, Levlite, Levora-28, Lybrel, Nordette-28, Portia-28, Seasonale

biphasic
Seasonique

triphasic
Enpresse, Tri-Levlen, Triphasil, Trivora-28

ethinyl estradiol and norethindrone
monophasic
Brevicon, Modicon, Necon 1/35, Necon 0.5/35, Norethin 1/35E, Norinyl 1 + 35, Nortrel 0.5/35, Nortrel 1/35, Ortho-Novum 1/35, Ovcon-35, Ovcon-50

biphasic
Necon 10/11, Ortho-Novum 10/11

triphasic

Necon 7/7/7, Ortho-Novum 7/7/7, Tri-Norinyl

ethinyl estradiol and norethindrone acetate
monophasic
Junel 21 Day 1/20, Junel 21 Day 1.5/30, Junel Fe 1/20, Loestrin 21 1.5/30, Loestrin 21 1/20, Microgestin 1.5/30, Microgestin 1/20

ethinyl estradiol and norgestimate
monophasic
MonoNessa, Ortho-Cyclen, Sprintec

triphasic
Ortho Tri-Cyclen, Ortho Tri-Cyclen Lo, Tri-Sprintec

ethinyl estradiol and norgestrel
monophasic
Cryselle, Lo/Ovral, Low-Ogestrel, Ogestrel

ethinyl estradiol, norethindrone acetate, and ferrous fumarate
monophasic
Femcon Fe, Loestrin 24 Fe, Loestrin Fe 1/20, Loestrin Fe 1.5/30, Microgestin Fe 1/20, Microgestin Fe 1.5/30

triphasic
Estrostep Fe

mestranol and norethindrone
monophasic
Necon 1/50, Norinyl 1 + 50, Ortho-Novum 1/50-28

Pharmacologic class: estrogenic and progestinic steroids
Pregnancy risk category X

AVAILABLE FORMS
monophasic hormonal contraceptives
ethinyl estradiol and desogestrel
Tablets: ethinyl estradiol 30 mcg and desogestrel 0.15 mg (Apri, Desogen, Ortho-Cept)

ethinyl estradiol and ethynodiol diacetate
Tablets: ethinyl estradiol 35 mcg and ethynodiol diacetate 1 mg (Demulen 1/35, Zovia 1/35E); ethinyl estradiol 50 mcg and ethynodiol diacetate 1 mg (Demulen 1/50, Zovia 1/50E)
ethinyl estradiol and levonorgestrel
Tablets: ethinyl estradiol 20 mcg and levonorgestrel 0.1 mg (Aviane, Lessina); ethinyl estradiol 20 mcg and levonorgestrel 0.9 mg (Lybrel); ethinyl estradiol 30 mcg and levonorgestrel 0.15 mg (Levlen, Levlite, Levora, Nordette-28, Portia, Seasonale); ethinyl estradiol 30 mcg and 0.15 mg levonorgestrel (84 tablets), and 10 mcg ethinyl estradiol (7 tablets) (Seasonique)
ethinyl estradiol and norethindrone
Tablets: ethinyl estradiol 35 mcg and norethindrone 0.4 mg (Ovcon-35); ethinyl estradiol 35 mcg and norethindrone 0.5 mg (Brevicon, Modicon, Necon 0.5/35, Nortel 0.5/35-28); ethinyl estradiol 35 mcg and norethindrone 1 mg (N.E.E. 1/35, Nelova 1/35E, Norethin 1/35E, Norinyl 1+35, Nortel 1/35-21, Ortho-Novum 1/35); ethinyl estradiol 50 mcg and norethindrone 1 mg (Ovcon-50)
ethinyl estradiol and norethindrone acetate
Tablets: ethinyl estradiol 20 mcg and norethindrone acetate 1 mg (Junel 21 day 1/20, Loestrin 1/20, Microgestin 1/20); ethinyl estradiol 30 mcg and norethindrone acetate 1.5 mg (Junel 21 day 1.5/30, Loestrin 1.5/30, Microgestin 1/35)
ethinyl estradiol and norgestimate
Tablets: ethinyl estradiol 35 mcg and norgestimate 0.25 mg (MonoNessa, Ortho-Cyclen, Sprintec)
ethinyl estradiol and norgestrel
Tablets: ethinyl estradiol 30 mcg and norgestrel 0.3 mg (Cryselle, Lo/Ovral, Lo-Ogestrel); ethinyl estradiol 50 mcg and norgestrel 0.5 mg (Ogestrel)
ethinyl estradiol, norethindrone acetate, and ferrous fumarate
Tablets: ethinyl estradiol 20 mcg, norethindrone acetate 1 mg, and ferrous fumarate 75 mg (Loestrin Fe 1/20, Loestrin 24 Fe, Microgesin Fe 1/20); ethinyl estradiol 30 mcg, norethindrone

acetate 1.5 mg, and ferrous fumarate 75 mg (Loestrin Fe 1.5/30, Microgesin Fe 1.5/30)
Chewable tablets: norethindrone 0.4 mg/ethinyl estradiol 35 mcg; inactive tablets contain ferrous fumarate 75 mg
mestranol and norethindrone
Tablets: mestranol 50 mcg and norethindrone 1 mg (Necon 1/50, Norinyl 1 + 50, Ortho-Novum 1/50)
biphasic hormonal contraceptives
ethinyl estradiol and desogestrel
Tablets: ethinyl estradiol 20 mcg and desogestrel 0.15 mg (21 days), then inert tablets (2 days), then ethinyl estradiol 10 mcg (5 days) (Kariva, Mircette)
ethinyl estradiol and levonorgestrel
Tablets: ethinyl estradiol 50 mcg and levonorgestrel 0.25 mg (Preven Emergency Contraceptive Kit)
ethinyl estradiol and norethindrone
Tablets: ethinyl estradiol 35 mcg and norethindrone 0.5 mg (10 days); ethinyl estradiol 35 mcg and norethindrone 1 mg (11 days) (Necon 10/11-21, Necon 10/11-28, Ortho-Novum 10/11)
triphasic hormonal contraceptives
ethinyl estradiol and desogestrel
Tablets: 0.1 mg desogestrel with 25 mcg ethinyl estradiol (7 tablets); 0.125 mg desogestrel with 25 mcg ethinyl estradiol (7 tablets); 0.15 mg desogestrel with 25 mcg ethinyl estradiol (7 tablets) (Cyclessa, Velivet)
ethinyl estradiol and levonorgestrel
Tablets: ethinyl estradiol 30 mcg and levonorgestrel 0.05 mg (6 days); ethinyl estradiol 40 mcg and levonorgestrel 0.075 mg (5 days); ethinyl estradiol 30 mcg and levonorgestrel 0.125 mg (10 days) (Enpresse, Tri-Levlen, Triphasil, Trivora-28)
ethinyl estradiol and norethindrone
Tablets: ethinyl estradiol 35 mcg and norethindrone 0.5 mg (7 days); ethinyl estradiol 35 mcg and norethindrone 1 mg (9 days); ethinyl estradiol 35 mcg and norethindrone 0.5 mg (5 days) (Tri-Norinyl); ethinyl estradiol 35 mcg and norethindrone 0.5 mg (7 days); ethinyl estradiol 35 mcg and norethindrone 0.75 mg (7 days); ethinyl estradiol 35 mcg and norethindrone 1 mg (7 days) (Necon 7/7/7, Ortho-Novum 7/7/7)

ethinyl estradiol and norgestimate

Tablets: ethinyl estradiol 25 mcg and norgestimate 0.18 mg (7 days); ethinyl estradiol 25 mcg and norgestimate 0.215 mg (7 days); ethinyl estradiol 25 mcg and norgestimate 0.25 mg (7 days) (Ortho Tri-Cyclen Lo); ethinyl estradiol 35 mcg and norgestimate 0.18 mg (7 days); ethinyl estradiol 35 mcg and norgestimate 0.215 mg (7 days); ethinyl estradiol 35 mcg and norgestimate 0.25 mg (7 days) (Ortho Tri-Cyclen, TriSprintec)

ethinyl estradiol, norethindrone acetate, and ferrous fumarate

Tablets: ethinyl estradiol 20 mcg and norethindrone acetate 1 mg (5 days); ethinyl estradiol 30 mcg and norethindrone acetate 1 mg (7 days); ethinyl estradiol 35 mcg and norethindrone acetate 1 mg (9 days); and 75-mg ferrous fumarate tablets (7 days) (Estrostep Fe)

INDICATIONS & DOSAGES

➤ **Contraception**

Monophasic hormonal contraceptives

Women: 1 tablet P.O. daily beginning on first day of menstrual cycle or first Sunday after menstrual cycle begins. With 20- and 21-tablet package, new cycle begins 7 days after last tablet taken. With 28-tablet package, dosage is 1 tablet daily without interruption; extra tablets taken on days 22 to 28 are placebos or contain iron. Or, for Seasonale, 1 pink tablet P.O. daily beginning on first Sunday after menstrual cycle begins, for 84 consecutive days, followed by 7 days of white (inert) tablets. Or, for Lybrel, 1 tablet P.O. daily beginning on the first day of menstrual cycle. When changing from 21-day or 28-day combination oral contraceptive, begin on first day of withdrawal bleeding, at the latest 7 days after last active tablet. When changing from progestin-only pill begin the next day. When changing from implant contraceptive, begin the day of implant removal. When changing from injection contraceptive, begin the day when next injection is due.

Biphasic hormonal contraceptives

Women: 1 color tablet P.O. daily for 10 days; then next color tablet for 11 days. With 21-tablet packages, new cycle begins 7 days after last tablet taken. With 28-tablet packages, dosage is 1 tablet daily without interruption. Or, for Seasonique, 1 light blue-green tablet P.O. once daily for 84 consecutive days followed by 1 yellow tablet for 7 consecutive days; then repeat cycle.

Triphasic hormonal contraceptives

Women: 1 tablet P.O. daily in the sequence specified by the brand. With 21-tablet packages, new dosing cycle begins 7 days after last tablet taken. With 28-tablet packages, dosage is 1 tablet daily without interruption.

➤ **Moderate acne vulgaris in women age 15 and older who have no known contraindications to hormonal contraceptive therapy, who want oral contraception for at least 6 months, who have reached menarche, and who are unresponsive to topical antiacne drugs**

Women age 15 and older: 1 tablet Ortho Tri-Cyclen or Estrostep P.O. daily (21 tablets contain active ingredients and 7 are inert).

ADMINISTRATION

P.O.

● Give drug at the same time each day; give at night to reduce nausea and headaches.

● Chewable tablet may be swallowed whole or chewed and followed with a full glass of liquid.

ACTION

Inhibit ovulation and may prevent transport of the ovum (if ovulation should occur) through the fallopian tubes.

Estrogen suppresses follicle-stimulating hormone, blocking follicular development and ovulation.

Progestin suppresses luteinizing hormone so that ovulation can't occur even if the follicle develops; it also thickens cervical mucus, interfering with sperm migration, and prevents implantation of the fertilized ovum.

Route	Onset	Peak	Duration
P.O.	Unknown	2 hours (ethinyl estradiol) 0.5 to 4 hr (varies by progestin)	Unknown

Half-life: 6 to 20 hours (ethinyl estradiol); 5 to 45 hours (varies by progestin).

ADVERSE REACTIONS

CNS: *headache, dizziness,* depression, lethargy, migraine, *stroke, cerebral hemorrhage.*
CV: *thromboembolism,* hypertension, edema, *pulmonary embolism, MI.*
EENT: worsening myopia or astigmatism, intolerance of contact lenses, exophthalmos, diplopia.
GI: *nausea, vomiting, abdominal cramps,* bloating, anorexia, changes in appetite, gallbladder disease, *pancreatitis.*
GU: *breakthrough bleeding, spotting,* granulomatous colitis, dysmenorrhea, amenorrhea, cervical erosion or abnormal secretions, enlargement of uterine fibromas, vaginal candidiasis.
Hepatic: cholestatic jaundice, *liver tumors, gallbladder disease.*
Metabolic: weight change, additive insulin resistance in diabetics.
Skin: rash, acne, *erythema multiforme,* melasma, hirsutism.
Other: breast tenderness, enlargement, or secretion, *anaphylaxis, hemolytic uremic syndrome.*

INTERACTIONS

Drug-drug. *Anti-infectives (chloramphenicol, fluconazole, griseofulvin, neomycin, nitrofurantoin, penicillins, sulfonamides, tetracyclines):* May decrease contraceptive effect. Advise patient to use another method of contraception.
Atorvastatin: May increase norethindrone and ethinyl estradiol levels. Monitor patient for adverse effects.
Benzodiazepines: May decrease or increase benzodiazepine levels. Adjust dosage, if necessary.
Beta blockers: May increase beta blocker level. Dosage adjustment may be necessary.
Carbamazepine, fosphenytoin, phenobarbital, phenytoin, rifampin: May decrease estrogen effect. Use together cautiously.
Corticosteroids: May enhance corticosteroid effect. Monitor patient closely.
Insulin, sulfonylureas: Glucose intolerance may decrease antidiabetic effects. Monitor these effects.
Nonnucleoside reverse transcriptase inhibitors, protease inhibitors: May decrease hormonal contraceptive effect. Avoid using together, if possible.

Oral anticoagulants: May decrease anticoagulant effect. Dosage adjustments may be needed. Monitor PT and INR.
Tamoxifen: May inhibit tamoxifen effect. Avoid using together.
Drug-herb. *Black cohosh:* May increase adverse effects of estrogen. Discourage use together.
Red clover: May interfere with drug. Discourage use together.
Saw palmetto: May have antiestrogenic effect. Discourage use together.
St. John's wort: May decrease drug effect because of increased hepatic metabolism. Discourage use together, or advise patient to use an additional method of contraception.
Drug-food. *Caffeine:* May increase caffeine level. Urge caution.
Grapefruit juice: May increase estrogen level. Advise patient to take with liquid other than grapefruit juice.
Drug-lifestyle. *Smoking:* May increase risk of adverse CV effects. If smoking continues, may need alternative therapy.

EFFECTS ON LAB TEST RESULTS

• May increase clotting factor II, VII, VIII, IX, X, and XII; fibrinogen; phospholipid; plasminogen; thyroid-binding globulin; total T_4; and triglyceride levels.
• May increase norepinephrine-induced platelet aggregation and PT.
• May reduce metyrapone test results. May cause false-positive result in nitro-blue tetrazolium test.

CONTRAINDICATIONS & CAUTIONS

• Contraindicated in patients with thromboembolic disorders, cerebrovascular or coronary artery disease, diplopia or ocular lesions arising from ophthalmic vascular disease, classic migraine, MI, known or suspected breast cancer, known or suspected estrogen-dependent neoplasia, benign or malignant liver tumors, active liver disease or history of cholestatic jaundice with pregnancy or previous use of hormonal contraceptives, and undiagnosed abnormal vaginal bleeding.
• Contraindicated in women who are or may be pregnant or breast-feeding.
• Use cautiously in patients with hyperlipidemia, hypertension, migraines, seizure disorders, asthma, or cardiac,

renal, or hepatic insufficiency, bleeding irregularities, gallbladder disease, ocular disease, diabetes, and emotional disorders.

NURSING CONSIDERATIONS

■ **Black Box Warning** Cigarette smoking increases the risk of serious cardiovascular side effects from oral contraceptives. This risk increases with age and with heavy smoking (at least 15 cigarettes daily) and is quite marked in women older than 35 years. Women who use oral contraceptives should not smoke. ■

• Triphasic hormonal contraceptives may cause fewer adverse reactions, such as breakthrough bleeding and spotting.
• The Centers for Disease Control and Prevention reports that use of hormonal contraceptives may decrease risk of ovarian and endometrial cancers and doesn't seem to increase risk of breast cancer. However, the FDA reports that hormonal contraceptives may be linked to an increase in cervical cancer.
• Monitor lipid levels, blood pressure, body weight, and hepatic function.
• *Alert:* Many hormonal contraceptives share similar names. Make sure to check the hormone strength for verification.
• Estrogens and progestins may alter glucose tolerance, thus changing dosage requirements for antidiabetics. Monitor glucose level.
• Stop hormonal contraceptives for a few weeks before adrenal function tests.
• Stop hormonal contraceptive and notify prescriber if patient develops granulomatous colitis.
• Stop drug at least 1 week before surgery to decrease risk of thromboembolism. Tell patient to use an alternative method of birth control.
• Women who are nonlactating mothers or those who have had second-trimester abortion must wait 28 days before starting oral contraception.
• In case of first-trimester abortion, patient may start Lybrel immediately without additional contraceptive method.

PATIENT TEACHING

• Tell patient to take tablets at same time each day; nighttime doses may reduce nausea and headaches.

• Advise patient to use additional method of birth control, such as condom or diaphragm with spermicide, for first week of first cycle.
• Tell patient that missing doses in midcycle greatly increases likelihood of pregnancy.
• Tell patient that missing a dose may cause spotting or light bleeding.
• Tell patient that hormonal contraceptives don't protect against HIV or other sexually transmitted diseases.
• Tell patient using Seasonale that there will be four planned menses per year, but spotting or bleeding between menses may occur.
• If 1 pill is missed, tell patient to take it as soon as possible (2 pills if remembered on the next day) and then to continue regular schedule. Advise an additional method of contraception for remainder of cycle. If 2 consecutive pills are missed, tell patient to take 2 pills a day for next 2 days and then resume regular schedule. Advise an additional method of contraception for the next 7 days or preferably for the remainder of cycle. If 2 consecutive pills are missed in the 3rd or 4th week or if patient misses 3 consecutive pills, tell patient to contact prescriber for instructions.
• Warn patient of common adverse effects, such as headache, nausea, dizziness, breast tenderness, spotting, and breakthrough bleeding, which usually diminish after 3 to 6 months.
• Instruct patient to weigh herself at least twice a week and to report any sudden weight gain or swelling to prescriber.
• Warn patient to avoid exposure to ultraviolet light or prolonged exposure to sunlight.
• *Alert:* Warn patient to immediately report abdominal pain; numbness, stiffness, or pain in legs or buttocks; pressure or pain in chest; shortness of breath; severe headache; visual disturbances, such as blind spots, blurriness, or flashing lights; undiagnosed vaginal bleeding or discharge; two consecutive missed menstrual periods; lumps in the breast; swelling of hands or feet; or severe pain in the abdomen (tumor rupture in liver).
• Advise patient of increased risks created by simultaneous use of cigarettes and hormonal contraceptives.

Reactions may be *common,* uncommon, *life-threatening,* or COMMON AND LIFE-THREATENING.
Interaction may have a *rapid onset* or **delayed onset.**

• If one menstrual period is missed and tablets have been taken on schedule, tell patient to continue taking them. If two consecutive menstrual periods are missed, tell patient to stop drug and have pregnancy test. Progestins may cause birth defects if taken early in pregnancy.

• Tell patient to chew chewable tablet and follow with a full glass of liquid or swallow whole.

• Advise patient not to take same drug for longer than 12 months without consulting prescriber. Stress importance of Papanicolaou tests and annual gynecologic examinations.

• Advise patient to check with prescriber about how soon pregnancy may be attempted after hormonal therapy is stopped. Many prescribers recommend that women not become pregnant within 2 months after stopping drug.

• Warn patient of possible delay in achieving pregnancy when drug is stopped.

• Teach woman how to perform routine breast self-examination.

• Teach patient methods to decrease risk of thromboembolism.

• Advise patient taking hormonal contraceptives to use additional form of birth control during concurrent treatment with certain antibiotics.

• Advise patient that hormonal contraceptives may change the fit of contact lenses.

---

etonogestrel and ethinyl estradiol vaginal ring
e-toe-noe-JES-trel and ETH-i-nill

NuvaRing

Pharmacologic class: estrogenic and progestinic steroids
Pregnancy risk category X

AVAILABLE FORMS
Vaginal ring: Delivers 0.12 mg etonogestrel and 0.015 mg ethinyl estradiol daily

INDICATIONS & DOSAGES
➤ **Contraception**
Women: Insert one ring into the vagina and leave in place for 3 weeks. Insert new ring 1 week after the previous ring is removed.

ADMINISTRATION
Vaginal
• In women who did not use hormonal contraception during the previous month, therapy should be initiated on the first day of the menstrual cycle. A woman using a combination oral contraceptive may switch to NuvaRing on any day, but at the latest on the day following the usual hormone-free interval.

• Leave ring in place continuously for a full 3 weeks to maintain effect. It's then removed for 1 week. During this time, withdrawal bleeding occurs (usually starting 2 or 3 days after removal). Insert a new ring inserted 1 week after removal of the previous one, regardless of whether patient is still menstruating.

ACTION
Suppresses gonadotropins, which inhibits ovulation, increases the viscosity of cervical mucus (decreasing the ability of sperm to enter the uterus), and alters the endometrial lining (reducing potential for implantation).

Route	Onset	Peak	Duration
Vaginal	Immediate	Unknown	Unknown

Half-life: ethinyl estradiol, 45 hours; etonogestrel, 29 hours.

ADVERSE REACTIONS
CNS: *headache,* emotional lability, *cerebral thrombosis, cerebral hemorrhage.*
CV: hypertension, *thromboembolic events, MI.*
EENT: *sinusitis,* changes in corneal curvature, intolerance to contact lenses.
GI: *nausea.*
GU: *vaginitis, leukorrhea,* device-related events (for example, foreign body sensation, coital difficulties, device expulsion), vaginal discomfort, breakthrough bleeding.
Hematologic: *coagulation abnormalities.*
Hepatic: *hepatic adenomas,* benign liver tumors, cholestatic jaundice.
Metabolic: weight gain.
Respiratory: *upper respiratory tract infection.*
Skin: melasma.

INTERACTIONS

Drug-drug. *Acetaminophen:* May decrease acetaminophen level and increase ethinyl estradiol level. Monitor patient for effects.

Ampicillin, barbiturates, carbamazepine, felbamate, griseofulvin, oxcarbazepine, phenylbutazone, phenytoin, rifampin, tetracyclines, topiramate: May decrease contraceptive effect and increase risk of pregnancy, breakthrough bleeding, or both. Tell patient to use an additional form of contraception while taking these drugs.

Ascorbic acid, atorvastatin, itraconazole: May increase ethinyl estradiol level. Monitor patient for adverse effects.

Clofibric acid, morphine, salicylic acid, temazepam: May increase clearance of these drugs. Monitor patient for effectiveness.

Cyclosporine, prednisolone, theophylline: May increase levels of these drugs. Monitor levels if appropriate and adjust dosage.

HIV protease inhibitors: May affect contraceptive effect. Refer to the specific protease inhibitor drug literature. May need to use a backup method of contraception.

Miconazole (oil-based vaginal capsule): May increase serum concentrations of etonogestrel and ethinyl estradiol. Monitor patient for adverse effects.

Drug-herb. *St. John's wort:* May reduce drug effectiveness and increase the risk of breakthrough bleeding and pregnancy. Discourage use together.

Drug-lifestyle. *Smoking:* May increase risk of serious CV adverse effects, especially in those older than age 35 who smoke 15 or more cigarettes daily. Urge patient to avoid smoking.

EFFECTS ON LAB TEST RESULTS

● May increase clotting factor VII, VIII, IX, and X; prothrombin; thyroid-binding globulin (leading to increased circulating total thyroid hormone levels); sex hormone–binding globulin (and other binding proteins); and triglyceride levels. May decrease antithrombin III and folate levels.

● May increase norepinephrine-induced platelet aggregation. May decrease T_3 resin uptake.

CONTRAINDICATIONS & CAUTIONS

● Contraindicated in patients hypersensitive to any component of drug, patients who are or may be pregnant, patients older than age 35 who smoke 15 or more cigarettes daily, and patients with thrombophlebitis, thromboembolic disorder, history of deep vein thrombophlebitis, cerebral vascular or coronary artery disease (current or previous), valvular heart disease with complications, severe hypertension, diabetes with vascular complications, headache with focal neurologic symptoms, major surgery with prolonged immobilization, known or suspected cancer of the endometrium or breast, estrogen-dependent neoplasia, abnormal undiagnosed genital bleeding, jaundice related to pregnancy or previous use of hormonal contraceptive, active liver disease, or benign or malignant hepatic tumors.

● Use cautiously in patients with hypertension, hyperlipidemias, obesity, or diabetes.

● Use cautiously in patients with conditions that could be aggravated by fluid retention, and in patients with a history of depression.

NURSING CONSIDERATIONS

● *Alert:* Drug may increase the risk of MI, thromboembolism, stroke, hepatic neoplasia, and gallbladder disease.

■ **Black Box Warning** Cigarette smoking increases the risk of serious adverse cardiac effects. The risk increases with age and in patients who smoke 15 or more cigarettes daily. ■

● Stop drug at least 4 weeks before and for 2 weeks after procedures that may increase the risk of thromboembolism, and during and after prolonged immobilization.

● Stop drug and notify prescriber if patient develops unexplained partial or complete loss of vision, proptosis, diplopia, papilledema, retinal vascular lesions, migraines, depression, or jaundice.

● Monitor blood pressure closely if patient has hypertension or renal disease.

Reactions may be *common*, uncommon, *life-threatening*, or COMMON AND LIFE-THREATENING.
Interaction may have a *rapid onset* or **delayed onset**.

• Rule out pregnancy if woman hasn't adhered to the prescribed regimen and a period is missed, if prescribed regimen has been adhered to and two periods are missed, or if the patient has retained the ring for longer than 4 weeks.

PATIENT TEACHING
• Stress importance of having regular annual physical examinations to check for adverse effects or developing contraindications.
• Tell patient that drug doesn't protect against HIV and other sexually transmitted diseases.
• Advise patient not to smoke while using contraceptive.
• Tell patient to use backup method until ring has been used continuously for 7 days. Tell patient not to use diaphragm if backup method of birth control is needed.
• Tell patient who wears contact lenses to contact an ophthalmologist if vision or lens tolerance changes.
• Advise patient to follow manufacturer's instructions for use if switching from different form of hormonal contraceptive.
• Tell patient to insert ring into vagina (using fingers) and keep it in place continuously for 3 weeks to maintain effect, saving foil package for later disposal. Explain that it is then removed for 1 full week and that, during this time, withdrawal bleeding occurs (usually starting 2 or 3 days after removal). Tell patient to insert new ring 1 week after removing previous one, regardless of menstrual bleeding. Tell patient to reseal ring in the package after removing it from vagina.
• Advise patient that, if the ring is removed or expelled (such as while removing a tampon, straining, or moving bowels), it should be washed with cool to lukewarm (not hot) water and reinserted immediately. Stress that contraceptive effect may be compromised if the ring stays out for longer than 3 hours and that she should use a backup method of contraception until the newly reinserted ring is used continuously for 7 days.

medroxyprogesterone acetate
me-DROX-ee-proe-JESS-te-rone

Depo-Provera, Depo-subQ Provera 104, Provera☙

Pharmacologic class: progestin
Pregnancy risk category X

AVAILABLE FORMS
Tablets: 2.5 mg, 5 mg, 10 mg
Injection (suspension): 104 mg/0.65 ml, 150 mg/ml, 400 mg/ml

INDICATIONS & DOSAGES
➤ **Abnormal uterine bleeding caused by hormonal imbalance**
Women: 5 to 10 mg P.O. daily for 5 to 10 days beginning on day 16 of menstrual cycle. If patient also has received estrogen, give 10 mg P.O. daily for 10 days beginning on day 16 or 21 of cycle.
➤ **Secondary amenorrhea**
Women: 5 to 10 mg P.O. daily for 5 to 10 days. Start at any time during menstrual cycle (usually during latter half of cycle).
➤ **Endometrial or renal cancer**
Adults: 400 to 1,000 mg I.M. weekly. Dosage may be decreased to 400 mg/month when disease has stabilized.
➤ **Contraception**
Women: 150 mg (Depo-Provera) I.M. once every 3 months. Or, 104 mg Depo-subQ Provera subcutaneously once every 3 months.
➤ **Endometriosis**
Adults: 104 mg Depo-subQ Provera subcutaneously once every 3 months. Therapy for longer than 2 years isn't recommended.

ADMINISTRATION
P.O.
• Give drug with food if GI upset occurs.
I.M.
• Shake vigorously before use.
• Give by deep I.M. injection in the gluteal or deltoid muscle.
• I.M. injection may be painful. Monitor sites for evidence of sterile abscess.
Rotate injection sites to prevent muscle atrophy.

Subcutaneous
● Shake vigorously before use.
● Give subcutaneous injection into the anterior thigh or abdomen.

ACTION
Suppresses ovulation, possibly by inhibiting pituitary gonadotropin secretion, thus preventing follicular maturation and causing endometrial thinning.

Route	Onset	Peak	Duration
P.O.	Rapid	2 to 4 hr	3 to 5 days
I.M.	Slow	24 hr	3 to 4 mo
Subcut.	Unknown	Unknown	Unknown

Half-life: 2¼ to 9 hours P.O., 50 days I.M., 40 days subcutaneous.

ADVERSE REACTIONS
CNS: depression, *stroke,* pain, dizziness.
CV: thrombophlebitis, *pulmonary embolism,* edema, *thromboembolism,* syncope.
EENT: exophthalmos, diplopia.
GI: *bloating, abdominal pain.*
GU: *breakthrough bleeding,* dysmenorrhea, *amenorrhea,* cervical erosion, abnormal secretions.
Hepatic: cholestatic jaundice.
Metabolic: weight changes.
Musculoskeletal: loss of bone mineral density.
Skin: rash, induration, sterile abscesses, acne, pruritus, melasma, alopecia, hirsutism.
Other: breast tenderness, enlargement, or secretion, hot flashes.

INTERACTIONS
Drug-drug. *Aminoglutethimide, carbamazepine, fosphenytoin, phenobarbital, phenytoin, rifampin:* May decrease progestin effects. Monitor patient for diminished therapeutic response. Tell patient to use a nonhormonal contraceptive during therapy with these drugs.
Anticonvulsants, corticosteroids: These drugs can also reduce bone mass. Monitor patient.
Drug-food. *Caffeine:* May increase caffeine level. Advise caution.
Drug-lifestyle. *Smoking:* May increase risk of adverse CV effects. If smoking continues, may need alternative therapy.

EFFECTS ON LAB TEST RESULTS
● May increase liver function test values, coagulation tests, and prothrombin factors VII, VIII, IX, and X.
● May reduce metyrapone test results. May cause abnormal thyroid function test results.

CONTRAINDICATIONS & CAUTIONS
● Contraindicated in patients hypersensitive to drug and in those with active thromboembolic disorders or history of thromboembolic disorders, cerebrovascular disease, apoplexy, breast cancer, undiagnosed abnormal vaginal bleeding, missed abortion, or hepatic dysfunction; also contraindicated during pregnancy. Tablets are contraindicated in patients with liver dysfunction or known or suspected malignant disease of genital organs.
● Use cautiously in patients with diabetes, seizures, migraine, cardiac or renal disease, asthma, or depression.

NURSING CONSIDERATIONS
● Drug shouldn't be used as test for pregnancy; it may cause birth defects and masculinization of female fetus.
● Depo-Provera and Depo-subQ Provera may cause a significant loss of bone mineral density.
● Monitor patient for pain, swelling, warmth, or redness in calves; sudden, severe headaches; visual disturbances; numbness in extremities; signs of depression; signs of liver dysfunction (abdominal pain, dark urine, jaundice).

PATIENT TEACHING
● According to FDA regulations, patient must read package insert explaining possible adverse effects of progestins before receiving first dose. Also, give patient verbal explanation.
■ **Black Box Warning** Teach patient that this product does not protect against HIV or other sexually-transmitted diseases. ■
● Advise patient to take medication with food if GI upset occurs.
● *Alert:* Tell patient to report unusual symptoms immediately and to stop drug and notify prescriber about visual disturbances or migraine.

Reactions may be *common,* uncommon, *life-threatening,* or COMMON AND LIFE-THREATENING.
Interaction may have a *rapid onset* or *delayed onset.*

• Teach woman how to perform routine breast self-examination.

• Advise patient to immediately report to prescriber any breast abnormalities, vaginal bleeding, swelling, yellowed skin or eyes, dark urine, clay-colored stools, shortness of breath, chest pain, or pregnancy.

• Advise patient that injection must be given every 3 months to maintain adequate contraceptive effects.

• Tell patient that because this is a long-acting method of birth control, it may take some time for fertility to return after the last injection.

• Tell woman to immediately report to prescriber a suspected pregnancy.

• Advise patient that amenorrhea is possible with prolonged use.

• Encourage adequate intake of calcium and vitamin D.

---

norelgestromin and ethinyl estradiol transdermal system
nor-el-JES-troe-min and ETH-i-nill

Ortho Evra

Pharmacologic class: estrogenic and progestogenic steroids
Pregnancy risk category X

AVAILABLE FORMS
Transdermal patch: norelgestromin 6 mg and ethinyl estradiol 0.75 mg per patch, delivering 150 mcg norelgestromin and 20 mcg ethinyl estradiol daily

INDICATIONS & DOSAGES
➤ Contraception
Women: Apply 1 patch weekly for 3 weeks. Apply each new patch on the same day of the week. Week 4 is patch free. On the day after week 4 ends, apply a new patch to start a new 4-week cycle. The patch-free interval between cycles should never be longer than 7 days.

ADMINISTRATION
Transdermal
• Apply patch to a clean, dry area of the skin on the buttocks, abdomen, upper outer arm, or upper torso. Don't apply to

the breasts or to skin that is red, irritated, or cut.

ACTION
Combination hormonal contraceptives act by suppressing gonadotropins. The primary mechanism of this action is ovulation inhibition. However, changes in cervical mucus increase the difficulty of sperm entry into the uterus, and changes in the endometrium decrease the likelihood of implantation.

Route	Onset	Peak	Duration
Trans-dermal	Rapid	2 days	Unknown

Half-life: ethinyl estradiol, 6 to 45 hours; norelgestromin, 28 hours.

ADVERSE REACTIONS
CNS: *headache,* emotional lability.
CV: ***thromboembolic events, MI,*** hypertension, edema, ***cerebral hemorrhage.***
EENT: contact lens intolerance, changes in corneal curvature.
GI: *nausea, abdominal pain,* vomiting, gallbladder disease, cholestatic jaundice.
GU: *menstrual cramps,* changes in menstrual flow, vaginal candidiasis.
Hepatic: ***hepatic adenomas,*** benign liver tumors.
Metabolic: weight changes.
Respiratory: *upper respiratory tract infection.*
Skin: *application site reaction,* melasma.
Other: *breast tenderness, enlargement, or secretion.*

INTERACTIONS
Drug-drug. *Acetaminophen, clofibric acid, morphine, salicylic acid, temazepam:* May decrease levels or increase clearance of these drugs. Monitor patient for lack of effect.
Ampicillin, barbiturates, carbamazepine, felbamate, griseofulvin, oxcarbazepine, phenylbutazone, phenytoin, rifampin, tetracyclines, topiramate: May reduce contraceptive effectiveness, resulting in unintended pregnancy or breakthrough bleeding. Encourage backup method of contraception if used together.
Anticoagulants: May increase or decrease effect of anticoagulant. Monitor patient and lab values.

Ascorbic acid, atorvastatin, itraconazole, ketoconazole: May increase hormone levels. Use together cautiously.
Cyclosporine, prednisolone, theophylline: May increase levels of these drugs. Monitor patient for adverse reactions.
HIV protease inhibitors: May affect contraceptive effectiveness and safety. Use together cautiously.
Drug-herb. *St. John's wort:* May reduce effectiveness of drug and cause breakthrough bleeding. Discourage use together.
Drug-lifestyle. *Smoking:* May increase risk of CV adverse effects, related to age and smoking 15 or more cigarettes daily. Urge patient not to smoke.

EFFECTS ON LAB TEST RESULTS
• May increase circulating total thyroid hormone, triglyceride, other binding protein, sex hormone–binding globulin, total circulating endogenous sex steroid, corticoid, and factor VII, VIII, IX, and X levels. May decrease antithrombin III and folate levels.
• May decrease free T_3 resin uptake and glucose tolerance.

CONTRAINDICATIONS & CAUTIONS
• Contraindicated in patients hypersensitive to any component of this drug and in those with past history of deep vein thrombosis or related disorder; current or past history of cerebrovascular or coronary artery disease; past or current known or suspected breast cancer, endometrial cancer, or other known or suspected estrogen-dependent neoplasia; or hepatic adenoma or cancer; and in those who are or may be pregnant.
• Contraindicated in patients with thrombophlebitis, thromboembolic disorders, valvular heart disease with complications, severe hypertension, diabetes with vascular involvement, headaches with focal neurologic symptoms, major surgery with prolonged immobilization, undiagnosed abnormal genital bleeding, cholestatic jaundice of pregnancy or jaundice with previous hormonal contraceptive use, or acute or chronic hepatocellular disease with abnormal liver function.

• Use cautiously in patients with CV disease risk factors, with conditions that might be aggravated by fluid retention, or with a history of depression.

NURSING CONSIDERATIONS
• *Alert:* Patients taking combination hormonal contraceptives may be at increased risk for thrombophlebitis, venous thrombosis with or without embolism, pulmonary embolism, MI, cerebral hemorrhage, cerebral thrombosis, hypertension, gallbladder disease, hepatic adenomas, benign liver tumors, mesenteric thrombosis, and retinal thrombosis.
• Increased risk of MI occurs primarily in smokers and women with hypertension, hypercholesterolemia, morbid obesity, and diabetes.
• Encourage women with a history of hypertension or renal disease to use a different contraceptive. If this drug is used, monitor blood pressure closely and stop use if hypertension occurs.
• Drug may be less effective in women who weigh 90 kg (198 lb) or more.
■ **Black Box Warning** Cigarette smoking increases the risk of serious adverse cardiac effects. The risk increases with age especially in women over 35, and in those who smoke 15 or more cigarettes daily. ■
• The risk of thromboembolic disease increases if therapy is used postpartum or postabortion.
• Birth control patch users may be at higher risk for developing serious blood clots versus birth control pill users.
• Rule out pregnancy if withdrawal bleeding fails to occur for two consecutive cycles.
• If skin becomes irritated, the patch may be removed and a new patch applied at a different site.
• Stop drug and notify prescriber at least 4 weeks before and for 2 weeks after an elective surgery that increases the risk of thromboembolism, and during and after prolonged immobilization. Teach the patient about alternative methods of contraception during this time.
• Stop drug and notify prescriber if patient has headaches, vision loss, proptosis, diplopia, papilledema, retinal vascular lesions, jaundice, or depression.

Reactions may be *common*, uncommon, *life-threatening*, or COMMON AND LIFE-THREATENING. Interaction may have a *rapid onset* or *delayed onset.*

PATIENT TEACHING

- Emphasize the importance of having regular annual physical examinations to check for adverse effects or developing contraindications.
- Tell patient that drug doesn't protect against HIV and other sexually transmitted diseases.
- Advise woman to apply patch on the first day of menstrual cycle or the first Sunday of menstrual cycle.
- Advise patient to use a backup method of contraception for the first 7 days.
- Tell patient switching from estrogen-progestin oral contraceptives to apply first patch on the first day of withdrawal bleeding. If no bleeding within 5 days of last hormonally active pill, advise patient to obtain a pregnancy test.
- Advise patient to immediately apply a new patch once the used patch is removed, on the same day of the week every 7 days for 3 weeks. Week 4 is patch free. Bleeding is expected to occur during this time.
- Tell patient to apply each patch to a clean, dry area of the skin on the buttocks, abdomen, upper outer arm, or upper torso. Tell patient not to apply to the breasts or to skin that's red, irritated, or cut.
- Tell patient to carefully fold the used patch in half so that it sticks to itself, before discarding.
- Tell woman to immediately stop use if pregnancy is confirmed.
- Tell patient who wears contact lenses to report visual changes or changes in lens tolerance.
- Advise patient not to smoke while using the patch.
- Tell patient that if a patch becomes detached for less than one day, to reapply it or replace it immediately and continue the schedule. If the patch is detached for more than one day, a new cycle should be started and back-up contraception should be used for the first week.
- Stress that if woman isn't sure what to do about mistakes with patch use, she should use a backup method of birth control and contact her health care provider.

norethindrone
nor-ETH-in-drone

Camila, Errin, Micronor, Nor-QD

norethindrone acetate
Aygestin

Pharmacologic class: progestin
Pregnancy risk category X

AVAILABLE FORMS
norethindrone
Tablets: 0.35 mg
norethindrone acetate
Tablets: 5 mg

INDICATIONS & DOSAGES
➤ **Amenorrhea, abnormal uterine bleeding**
Women: 2.5 to 10 mg norethindrone acetate P.O. daily for 5 to 10 days, beginning in the assumed latter half of the menstrual cycle.
➤ **Endometriosis**
Women: 5 mg norethindrone acetate P.O. daily for 14 days; then increased by 2.5 mg daily every 2 weeks, up to 15 mg daily. Therapy may continue for 6 to 9 months or until breakthrough bleeding warrants temporary termination.
➤ **Contraception**
Women: Initially, 0.35 mg norethindrone P.O. on first day of menstruation; then 0.35 mg daily.

ADMINISTRATION
P.O.
- Give drug at same time every day, continuously, with no interruption between pill packs.

ACTION
Suppresses ovulation, possibly by inhibiting pituitary gonadotropin secretion, and forms thick cervical mucus.

Route	Onset	Peak	Duration
P.O.	Unknown	Unknown	Unknown

Half-life: 5 to 14 hours.

ADVERSE REACTIONS

CNS: depression, *stroke.*
CV: thrombophlebitis, *pulmonary embolism,* edema, *thromboembolism.*
EENT: exophthalmos, diplopia.
GI: *bloating, abdominal pain or cramping.*
GU: *breakthrough bleeding,* dysmenorrhea, *amenorrhea,* cervical erosion, abnormal secretions.
Hepatic: cholestatic jaundice.
Metabolic: weight changes.
Skin: melasma, rash, acne, pruritus, alopecia, hirsutism, hemorrhagic skin eruptions.
Other: breast tenderness, enlargement, or secretion; premenstrual-like syndrome.

INTERACTIONS

Drug-drug. *Barbiturates, carbamazepine, fosphenytoin, phenytoin, rifampin:*
May decrease progestin effects. Monitor patient for diminished therapeutic response.
Drug-food. *Caffeine:* May increase caffeine level. Urge caution.
Drug-lifestyle. *Smoking:* May increase risk of adverse CV effects. If smoking continues, may need alternative therapy.

EFFECTS ON LAB TEST RESULTS

• May increase liver function test values. May alter coagulation factors and thyroid function tests.
• May decrease metyrapone test results.

CONTRAINDICATIONS & CAUTIONS

• Contraindicated in pregnant women, patients hypersensitive to drug, and patients with breast cancer, undiagnosed abnormal vaginal bleeding, severe hepatic disease, missed abortion, or current or previous thromboembolic disorders.
• Use cautiously in patients with diabetes, seizures, migraines, cardiac or renal disease, asthma, and depression.

NURSING CONSIDERATIONS

• If switching from combined oral contraceptives to progestin-only pills (POPs), take the first POP the day after the last active combined pill.
• If switching from POPs to combined pills, take the first active combined pill on the first day of menstruation, even if the POP pack isn't finished.

• *Alert:* Norethindrone acetate is twice as potent as norethindrone. Norethindrone acetate shouldn't be used for contraception.
• Patients with menstrual disorders usually need preliminary estrogen treatment.
• Watch patient closely for signs of edema.
• Monitor blood pressure.
• *Look alike–sound alike:* Don't confuse Micronor with Micro-K or Micronase.

PATIENT TEACHING

• According to FDA regulations, patient must read package insert explaining possible adverse effects before receiving first dose. Also, give patient verbal explanation.
• Tell patient to take drug at the same time every day when used as a contraceptive. If she's more than 3 hours late taking the pill or if she has missed a pill, she should take the pill as soon as she remembers, and then continue the normal schedule. Also tell her to use a backup method of contraception for the next 48 hours.
• *Alert:* Tell patient to report unusual symptoms immediately and to stop drug and notify prescriber about visual disturbances or migraine, or pain or numbness in her arms or legs.
• Teach woman how to perform routine breast self-examination.
• Tell woman to report suspected pregnancy to prescriber.
• Encourage patient to stop or reduce smoking because of the risk of CV complications.
• Tell patient with diabetes that glucose levels may be affected and to closely monitor her levels.
• Tell patient that drug does not protect against HIV or other sexually transmitted diseases.
• Tell patient that if she vomits soon after taking a pill to use a back-up method of birth control for 48 hours.

Reactions may be *common,* uncommon, *life-threatening,* or COMMON AND LIFE-THREATENING.
Interaction may have a *rapid onset* or **delayed onset.**

71

Fertility drugs

cetrorelix acetate
clomiphene citrate
menotropins

cetrorelix acetate
set-ROH-re-lix

Cetrotide

Pharmacologic class: gonadotropin-releasing hormone (GnRH) antagonist
Pregnancy risk category X

AVAILABLE FORMS
Powder for injection: 0.25 mg, 3 mg

INDICATIONS & DOSAGES
➤ **To inhibit premature luteinizing hormone (LH) surges in women undergoing controlled ovarian stimulation**
Women: 3 mg subcutaneously once during early to middle follicular phase, given when estradiol level indicates an appropriate stimulation response, usually on stimulation day 7 (range, days 5 to 9). If human chorionic gonadotropin (hCG) hasn't been given within 4 days after injection, give drug 0.25 mg subcutaneously once daily until the day of hCG administration. Or, give 0.25-mg multiple-dose regimen subcutaneously on stimulation day 5 (morning or evening) or day 6 (morning), and continue once daily until the day of hCG administration.

ADMINISTRATION
Subcutaneous
• Store 3-mg form at room temperature (77° F [25° C]) and 0.25-mg form in refrigerator (36° to 46° F [2° to 8° C]).
• Follow proper administration technique, as follows. Wash hands thoroughly with soap and water. Flip off plastic cover of vial and wipe top with an alcohol swab. Attach needle with yellow mark to prefilled syringe. Push needle through rubber stopper of vial and slowly inject liquid into vial. Leave syringe in place and gently swirl (don't shake) vial until solution is clear and without residue. Draw liquid

from vial into syringe. If necessary, invert vial and pull needle back as far as needed to withdraw entire contents of vial. Detach needle with yellow mark from syringe and replace it with needle with gray mark. Invert syringe and push plunger until all air bubbles are gone.
• Choose an injection site on lower abdomen, around the navel. If giving a multiple-dose (0.25-mg) regimen, choose a different site each day to minimize local irritation. Clean site with alcohol swab and gently pinch a skinfold surrounding injection site. Insert needle completely into skin at about a 45-degree angle and, after needle has been inserted completely, release grasp of skin. Gently pull back plunger of syringe to check for correct positioning of needle. If no blood appears, inject entire solution.

ACTION
Competes with natural GnRH for binding to membrane receptors on pituitary cells, which controls the release of LH and follicle-stimulating hormone.

Route	Onset	Peak	Duration
Subcut.	1–2 hr	1–2 hr	> 4 days

Half-life: 62.8 hours (single 3-mg dose); 5 hours (single 0.25-mg dose); 20.6 hours (multiple 0.25-mg doses).

ADVERSE REACTIONS
CNS: headache.
GI: nausea.
GU: *ovarian hyperstimulation syndrome.*

INTERACTIONS
None reported.

EFFECTS ON LAB TEST RESULTS
• May increase alkaline phosphatase, ALT, AST, and GGT levels.

CONTRAINDICATIONS & CAUTIONS
• Contraindicated in patients hypersensitive to drug, extrinsic peptide hormones, mannitol, GnRH, or GnRH analogues.
• Contraindicated in patients with severe renal impairment.

• Contraindicated in pregnant and breast-feeding women, and in patients age 65 or older.

NURSING CONSIDERATIONS
• **Alert:** Carefully monitor for hypersensitivity reaction after the first injection.
• Rule out pregnancy before starting treatment.
• Prescriber should be experienced in fertility treatment.
• Adjust dose according to patient response.
• When ultrasound shows enough follicles of adequate size, give hCG to induce ovulation and maturation of oocytes.
• To reduce the risk of ovarian hyperstimulation syndrome, don't give hCG if ovaries show an excessive response to treatment.

PATIENT TEACHING
• Instruct patient to store 3-mg form at room temperature (77° F [25° C]) and 0.25-mg form in refrigerator (36° to 46° F [2° to 8° C]). Tell patient to keep this product away from children.
• Tell patient to report any adverse effects that become bothersome.
• Teach patient the importance of following the regimen exactly as prescribed to achieve best results.
• If blood appears when patient pulls back on plunger, tell her to withdraw needle and gently press an alcohol swab onto injection site. Explain that she'll need to discard syringe and drug vial and repeat procedure using a new pack.
• Urge patient to use a syringe and needle only once and then to dispose of them properly, in a medical waste container, if available.

clomiphene citrate
KLOE-mi-feen

Clomid, Milophene, Serophene

Pharmacologic class:
chlorotrianisene derivative
Pregnancy risk category X

AVAILABLE FORMS
Tablets: 50 mg

INDICATIONS & DOSAGES
➤ **To induce ovulation**
Women: 50 mg P.O. daily for 5 days, starting on day 5 of menstrual cycle (first day of menstrual flow is day 1) if bleeding occurs, or at any time if patient hasn't had recent uterine bleeding. If ovulation doesn't occur, may increase dose to 100 mg P.O. daily for 5 days as soon as 30 days after previous course. Repeat until conception occurs or until three courses of therapy are completed.

ADMINISTRATION
P.O.
• Protect drug from heat, light, and excessive humidity.
• Give drug without regard for food.

ACTION
Appears to stimulate release of follicle-stimulating hormone, luteinizing hormone, and pituitary gonadotropins, resulting in maturation of the ovarian follicle, ovulation, and development of the corpus luteum.

Route	Onset	Peak	Duration
P.O.	Unknown	Unknown	Unknown

Half-life: 5 days.

ADVERSE REACTIONS
CNS: headache, restlessness, insomnia, dizziness, light-headedness, depression, fatigue.
EENT: blurred vision, diplopia, scotoma, photophobia.
GI: nausea, vomiting, bloating, distention.
GU: *ovarian enlargement,* urinary frequency and polyuria, abnormal uterine bleeding, ovarian cyst that regresses spontaneously when drug is stopped.
Metabolic: weight gain.
Skin: reversible alopecia, urticaria, rash, dermatitis.
Other: *hot flashes, breast discomfort.*

INTERACTIONS
None significant.

EFFECTS ON LAB TEST RESULTS
None reported.

Reactions may be *common,* uncommon, *life-threatening,* or COMMON AND LIFE-THREATENING.
Interaction may have a *rapid onset* or **delayed onset.**

CONTRAINDICATIONS & CAUTIONS
● Contraindicated in pregnant women and in those with undiagnosed abnormal genital bleeding, ovarian cyst not related to polycystic ovarian syndrome, hepatic disease or dysfunction, uncontrolled thyroid or adrenal dysfunction, or organic intracranial lesion (such as a pituitary tumor).

NURSING CONSIDERATIONS
● Monitor patient closely because of potentially serious adverse reactions.
● Long-term cyclic therapy isn't recommended.
● **Look alike–sound alike:** Don't confuse clomiphene with clomipramine or clonidine. Don't confuse Serophene with Sarafem.

PATIENT TEACHING
● Tell patient about the risk of multiple births, which increases with higher doses.
● Teach patient to take and chart basal body temperature to ascertain if ovulation has occurred.
● Reinforce importance of compliance with drug regimen.
● Reassure patient that ovulation typically occurs after first course of therapy. If pregnancy doesn't occur, therapy may be repeated twice.
● Advise patient to stop drug and contact prescriber immediately if pregnancy is suspected because drug may have teratogenic effect.
● **Alert:** Advise patient to stop drug and contact prescriber immediately if abdominal symptoms or pain occur; these symptoms may indicate ovarian enlargement or ovarian cyst. Also, tell patient to immediately notify prescriber if signs and symptoms of impending visual toxicity occur, such as blurred vision, double vision, vision defect in one part of the eye (scotoma), or sensitivity to the sun.
● Warn patient to avoid hazardous activities, such as driving or operating machinery, until CNS effects are known. Drug may cause dizziness and visual disturbances.

menotropins
men-oh-TROE-pins

Menopur, Repronex

Pharmacologic class: gonadotropin
Pregnancy risk category X

AVAILABLE FORMS
Injection: 75 international units of luteinizing hormone (LH) and 75 international units of follicle-stimulating hormone (FSH) activity per ampule; 150 international units of LH and 150 international units of FSH activity per ampule

INDICATIONS & DOSAGES
➤ **Assisted reproductive technologies**
Adults: Initially, 225 units subcutaneously (Menopur, Repronex) or I.M. (Repronex only) for patients who have received gonadotropin-releasing hormone (GnRH) agonist or antagonist pituitary suppression. Adjust dose based on ultrasound and estradiol levels not more frequently than every 2 days and not to exceed 75 to 150 units Repronex or 150 units Menopur per adjustment. Maximum daily dose is 450 units. Use for maximum of 12 days (Repronex) or 20 days (Menopur). Then, 5,000 to 10,000 units of human chorionic gonadotropin (hCG) after adequate follicular development.
➤ **Infertility with oligo-anovulation (Repronex)**
Adults: Initially, 150 units subcutaneously or I.M. daily for 5 days in patients who have received GnRH agonist or antagonist pituitary suppression. Adjust based on response; 75 to 150 units per adjustment and not more frequently than every 2 days. Maximum daily dose is 450 units; don't use for more than 12 days. If patient response is adequate, 5,000 to 10,000 units of hCG. Hold hCG if estradiol level is greater than 2,000 picograms/ml.

ADMINISTRATION
I.M.
● Refrigerate powder or store at room temperature.
● Reconstitute with 1 to 2 ml of sterile normal saline solution for injection. Do

not shake; gently swirl until the solution is clear. Use immediately.
• Rotate injection sites.
• Only Repronex should be given I.M.
Subcutaneous
• Refrigerate powder or store at room temperature.
• Reconstitute with 1 to 2 ml of sterile normal saline solution for injection. Do not shake; gently swirl until the solution is clear. Use immediately.
• Use alternating sides of the lower abdomen for subcutaneous administration. Rotate injection sites.

ACTION
In women who haven't had primary ovarian failure, drug mimics FSH in inducing follicular growth and LH in aiding follicular maturation.

Route	Onset	Peak	Duration
I.M., Subcut.	9–12 days	12–18 hr	Unknown

Half-life: Menopur, 11 to 13 hours; Repronex, 54 to 60 hours.

ADVERSE REACTIONS
CNS: *stroke, headache,* migraine, malaise, fever, dizziness.
CV: tachycardia, venous thrombophlebitis, *arterial occlusion, pulmonary embolism.*
GI: *nausea,* vomiting, diarrhea, *abdominal cramps,* bloating.
GU: *ovarian enlargement with pain and abdominal distention,* multiple births, *ovarian hyperstimulation syndrome,* ovarian cysts, *ectopic pregnancy,* menstrual disorder.
Musculoskeletal: aches, back pain, joint pains.
Respiratory: *acute respiratory distress syndrome, pulmonary infarction,* atelectasis, dyspnea, tachypnea.
Skin: rash.
Other: *gynecomastia, anaphylaxis,* hypersensitivity reactions, injection site reaction, chills.

INTERACTIONS
None significant.

EFFECTS ON LAB TEST RESULTS
None reported.

CONTRAINDICATIONS & CAUTIONS
• Contraindicated in patients hypersensitive to drug and in those with primary ovarian failure, uncontrolled thyroid or adrenal dysfunction, pituitary tumor, abnormal uterine bleeding, uterine fibromas, ovarian cysts or enlargement not due to polycystic ovarian syndrome, sex hormone–dependent tumor of the reproductive tract (Menopur only), or any cause of infertility other than anovulation (Repronex only).
• Contraindicated in pregnant women.

NURSING CONSIDERATIONS
• Prescriber should be experienced in fertility treatment.
• Monitor woman closely to ensure adequate ovarian stimulation without hyperstimulation.
• *Alert:* Watch for ovarian hyperstimulation syndrome, which may rapidly progress to a life-threatening condition, characterized by dramatic increase in vascular permeability, which causes rapid accumulation of fluid in the peritoneal cavity, thorax, and pericardium. Signs and symptoms are hypovolemia, hemoconcentration, electrolyte imbalance, ascites, hemoperitoneum, pleural effusion, hydrothorax, and thromboembolism. Condition is common and severe if woman becomes pregnant.

PATIENT TEACHING
• Tell woman about possibility of multiple births (which occur about 20% of the time).
• In women being treated for infertility, encourage daily intercourse from day before hCG is given until ovulation occurs.
• Instruct patient to immediately report severe abdominal pain, bloating, swelling of hands or feet, nausea, vomiting, diarrhea, substantial weight gain, or dyspnea.

Reactions may be *common,* uncommon, *life-threatening,* or COMMON AND LIFE-THREATENING.
Interaction may have a *rapid onset* or **delayed onset.**

acarbose
glimepiride
glipizide
glyburide
metformin hydrochloride
miglitol
nateglinide
pioglitazone hydrochloride
pramlintide acetate
repaglinide
rosiglitazone maleate
sitagliptin phosphate

SAFETY ALERT!

acarbose
a-KAR-boz

Precose

Pharmacologic class: alpha-
glucosidase inhibitor
Pregnancy risk category B

AVAILABLE FORMS
Tablets: 25 mg, 50 mg, 100 mg

INDICATIONS & DOSAGES
➤ **Adjunct to diet and exercise
or with a sulfonylurea, metformin or insulin, to lower glucose
level in patients with type 2
diabetes**
Adults: Individualized. Initially, 25 mg
P.O. t.i.d. with first bite of each main meal.
Adjust dosage every 4 to 8 weeks, based
on 1-hour postprandial glucose level and
tolerance. Maintenance dosage is 50 to
100 mg P.O. t.i.d.
Adjust-a-dose: For patients who weigh
less than 60 kg (132 lb), don't exceed
50 mg P.O. t.i.d. For patients who weigh
more than 60 kg, don't exceed 100 mg
P.O. t.i.d.

ADMINISTRATION
P.O.
● Give dose with first bite of each main
meal.

ACTION
Delays digestion of carbohydrates, resulting in a smaller increase in glucose level
after meals.

Route	Onset	Peak	Duration
P.O.	Unknown	1 hr	2–4 hr

Half-life: 2 hours.

ADVERSE REACTIONS
GI: *abdominal pain, diarrhea, flatulence.*

INTERACTIONS
Drug-drug. *Calcium channel blockers,
corticosteroids, estrogens, fosphenytoin,
hormonal contraceptives, isoniazid,
nicotinic acid, phenothiazine, phenytoin,
sympathomimetics, thiazides and other
diuretics, thyroid products:* May cause
hyperglycemia when used together or
hypoglycemia when withdrawn. Monitor
glucose level.
*Digestive enzyme preparations containing
carbohydrate-splitting enzymes (such as
amylase, pancreatin), intestinal adsorbents
(such as activated charcoal):* May reduce
effect of acarbose. Avoid using together.
Digoxin: May reduce digoxin level.
Monitor digoxin level.

EFFECTS ON LAB TEST RESULTS
● May increase ALT and AST levels.
May decrease calcium, vitamin B_6, and
hemoglobin levels and hematocrit.

CONTRAINDICATIONS & CAUTIONS
● Contraindicated in patients hypersensitive
to drug and in those with diabetic ketoacidosis, cirrhosis, inflammatory bowel
disease, colonic ulceration, renal impairment, partial intestinal obstruction, predisposition to intestinal obstruction,
chronic intestinal disease with marked
disorder of digestion or absorption, or
conditions that may deteriorate because
of increased intestinal gas formation.
● Contraindicated in pregnant or breast-
feeding women and those with creatinine
level greater than 2 mg/dl.

• Use cautiously in patients receiving a sulfonylurea or insulin.
• Safety and effectiveness of drug haven't been established in children.

NURSING CONSIDERATIONS
• Closely monitor patients receiving a sulfonylurea or insulin; drug may increase risk of hypoglycemia. If hypoglycemia occurs, give oral glucose (dextrose). Severe hypoglycemia may require I.V. glucose infusion or glucagon administration. Because dosage adjustments may be needed to prevent further hypoglycemia, report hypoglycemia and treatment required to prescriber.
• Insulin therapy may be needed during increased stress (infection, fever, surgery, or trauma). Monitor patient closely for hyperglycemia.
• Monitor patient's 1-hour postprandial glucose level to determine therapeutic effectiveness of drug and to identify appropriate dose. Report hyperglycemia to prescriber. Thereafter, measure glycosylated hemoglobin level every 3 months.
• Monitor transaminase level every 3 months in first year of therapy and periodically thereafter in patients receiving more than 50 mg t.i.d. Report abnormalities; dosage adjustment or drug withdrawal may be needed.

PATIENT TEACHING
• Tell patient to take drug daily with first bite of each of three main meals.
• Explain that therapy relieves symptoms but doesn't cure disease.
• Stress importance of adhering to therapeutic regimen, specific diet, weight reduction, exercise, and hygiene programs. Show patient how to monitor glucose level and to recognize and treat hyperglycemia.
• Teach patient taking a sulfonylurea how to recognize hypoglycemia. Advise treating symptoms with a form of dextrose rather than with a product containing table sugar.
• Urge patient to wear or carry medical identification at all times.
• Advise patient that adverse reactions usually occur in the first few weeks of therapy and diminish over time.

SAFETY ALERT!

glimepiride
glye-MEH-per-ide

Amaryl

Pharmacologic class: sulfonylurea
Pregnancy risk category C

AVAILABLE FORMS
Tablets: 1 mg, 2 mg, 4 mg

INDICATIONS & DOSAGES
➤ **Adjunct to diet and exercise to lower glucose level in patients with type 2 diabetes whose hyperglycemia can't be managed by diet and exercise alone**
Adults: Initially, 1 or 2 mg P.O. once daily; usual maintenance dose is 1 to 4 mg P.O. once daily. After reaching 2 mg, dosage is increased in increments not exceeding 2 mg every 1 to 2 weeks, based on patient's glucose level response. Maximum dose is 8 mg daily.
➤ **Adjunct to diet and exercise in conjunction with insulin or metformin therapy in patients with type 2 diabetes whose hyperglycemia can't be managed with the maximum dosage of glimepiride alone**
Adults: 8 mg P.O. once daily; used with low-dose insulin. Increase insulin dosage weekly, if needed, based on patient's glucose level response. If patients do not respond adequately to maximum dose of glimepiride, addition of metformin may be considered.
Adjust-a-dose: For patients with renal or hepatic impairment, initially, 1 mg P.O. once daily then adjust to appropriate dosage, if needed.

ADMINISTRATION
P.O.
• Give drug with first meal of the day.

ACTION
Lowers glucose level, possibly by stimulating release of insulin from functioning pancreatic beta cells, and may lead to increased sensitivity of peripheral tissues to insulin.

Reactions may be *common*, uncommon, *life-threatening*, or COMMON AND LIFE-THREATENING.
Interaction may have a *rapid onset* or ***delayed onset***.

Route	Onset	Peak	Duration
P.O.	1 hr	2–3 hr	> 24 hr

Half-life: 9 hours.

ADVERSE REACTIONS
CNS: dizziness, asthenia, headache.
EENT: changes in accommodation.
GI: nausea.
Hematologic: *leukopenia,* hemolytic anemia, *agranulocytosis, thrombocytopenia, aplastic anemia, pancytopenia.*
Hepatic: cholestatic jaundice.
Metabolic: *hypoglycemia,* dilutional hyponatremia.
Skin: pruritus, erythema, urticaria, morbilliform or maculopapular eruptions, photosensitivity reactions.

INTERACTIONS
Drug-drug. *Beta blockers:* May mask symptoms of hypoglycemia. Monitor glucose level.
Drugs that tend to produce hyperglycemia (such as corticosteroids, estrogens, fosphenytoin, hormonal contraceptives, isoniazid, nicotinic acid, other diuretics, phenothiazines, phenytoin, thyroid products): May lead to loss of glucose control. Adjust dosage.
Insulin: May increase risk of hypoglycemia. Use together cautiously.
NSAIDs, other drugs that are highly protein-bound (such as beta blockers, chloramphenicol, coumarin, MAO inhibitors, probenecid, sulfonamides): May increase hypoglycemic action of sulfonylureas such as glimepiride. Monitor glucose level carefully.
Rifamycins, thiazide diuretics: May increase risk of hyperglycemia. Monitor glucose level.
Salicylates: May increase hypoglycemic effects of sulfonylurea. Monitor glucose level.
Drug-herb. *Burdock, dandelion, eucalyptus, marshmallow:* May increase drug effects. Discourage use together.
Drug-lifestyle. *Alcohol use:* May alter glycemic control, most commonly causing hypoglycemia. May also cause disulfiram-like reaction. Discourage use together.

EFFECTS ON LAB TEST RESULTS
• May increase alkaline phosphatase, AST, BUN, and creatinine levels. May decrease glucose, hemoglobin, and sodium levels.
• May decrease granulocyte, platelet, RBC, and WBC counts.

CONTRAINDICATIONS & CAUTIONS
• Contraindicated in patients hypersensitive to drug and in those with diabetic ketoacidosis, which should be treated with insulin.
• Contraindicated in pregnant women or elderly patients and as sole therapy for type 1 diabetes.
• Contraindicated in breast-feeding women because it may cause hypoglycemia in breast-fed infants.
• Use cautiously in debilitated or malnourished patients and in those with adrenal, pituitary, hepatic, or renal insufficiency; these patients are more susceptible to the hypoglycemic action of glucose-lowering drugs.
• Use cautiously in patients allergic to sulfonamides.
• In children, safety and effectiveness haven't been established.

NURSING CONSIDERATIONS
• Glimepiride and insulin may be used together in patients who lose glucose control after first responding to therapy.
• Monitor fasting glucose level periodically to determine therapeutic response. Also monitor glycosylated hemoglobin level, usually every 3 to 6 months, to precisely assess long-term glycemic control.
• Use of oral hypoglycemics may carry higher risk of CV mortality than use of diet alone or of diet and insulin therapy.
• When changing patient from other sulfonylureas to glimepiride, a transition period isn't needed. Monitor patient carefully for 1 to 2 weeks when changing from longer half-life sulfonylureas, such as chlorpropamide.
• *Look alike–sound alike:* Don't confuse glimepiride with glyburide or glipizide. Don't confuse Amaryl with Altace.

PATIENT TEACHING
• Tell patient to take drug with first meal of the day.

• Make sure patient understands that therapy relieves symptoms but doesn't cure the disease. He should also understand potential risks and advantages of taking drug and of other treatment methods.

• Stress importance of adhering to diet, weight reduction, exercise, and personal hygiene programs. Explain to patient and family how and when to monitor glucose level, and teach recognition of and intervention for signs and symptoms of high and low glucose levels.

• Advise patient to wear or carry medical identification at all times.

• Advise woman to consult prescriber before planning pregnancy. Insulin may be needed during pregnancy and breastfeeding.

• Advise patient to consult prescriber before taking any OTC products.

• Teach patient to carry candy or other simple sugars to treat mild episodes of low glucose level. Patient experiencing severe episode may need hospital treatment.

• Advise patient to avoid alcohol, which lowers glucose level.

SAFETY ALERT!

glipizide
GLIP-i-zide

Glucotrol◆, Glucotrol XL◆

Pharmacologic class: sulfonylurea
Pregnancy risk category C

AVAILABLE FORMS
Tablets (extended-release): 2.5 mg, 5 mg, 10 mg
Tablets (immediate-release): 5 mg, 10 mg

INDICATIONS & DOSAGES
➤ **Adjunct to diet to lower glucose level in patients with type 2 (non–insulin-dependent) diabetes**
Immediate-release tablets
Patients older than age 65: First dose is 2.5 mg P.O. daily.
Adults: Initially, 5 mg P.O. daily 30 minutes before breakfast. Maximum once-daily dose is 15 mg. Divide doses of

more than 15 mg. Maximum daily dose is 40 mg.
Extended-release tablets
Adults: Initially, 5 mg P.O. with breakfast daily. Increase by 5 mg every 3 months, depending on level of glycemic control. Maximum daily dose is 20 mg.
Adjust-a-dose: For patients with liver disease, first dose is 2.5 mg P.O. daily.
➤ **To replace insulin therapy**
Adults: If insulin dosage is more than 20 units daily, start patient at usual dosage in addition to 50% of insulin. If insulin dosage is less than or equal to 20 units daily, insulin may be stopped when glipizide starts.

ADMINISTRATION
P.O.
• Give immediate-release tablet about 30 minutes before meals.
• Don't split or crush extended-release tablets.

ACTION
Unknown. Probably stimulates insulin release from pancreatic beta cells, reduces glucose output by the liver, and increases peripheral sensitivity to insulin.

Route	Onset	Peak	Duration
P.O. (immediate-release)	15–30 min	1–3 hr	24 hr
P.O. (extended-release)	2–3 hr	6–12 hr	24 hr

Half-life: 2 to 4 hours.

ADVERSE REACTIONS
CNS: dizziness, drowsiness, headache, syncope, *asthenia.*
GI: nausea, dyspepsia, flatulence, constipation, diarrhea.
GU: polyuria.
Hematologic: *leukopenia,* hemolytic anemia, *agranulocytosis, thrombocytopenia, aplastic anemia.*
Hepatic: cholestatic jaundice.
Metabolic: *hypoglycemia.*
Musculoskeletal: arthralgia, leg cramps.
Respiratory: rhinitis.
Skin: rash, pruritus, photosensitivity reactions.

Reactions may be *common,* uncommon, *life-threatening,* or COMMON AND LIFE-THREATENING.
Interaction may have a *rapid onset* or *delayed onset.*

INTERACTIONS
Drug-drug. *Amantadine, anabolic steroids, antifungals, chloramphenicol, clofibrate, guanethidine, MAO inhibitors, NSAIDs, probenecid, salicylates, sulfonamides:* May increase hypoglycemic activity. Monitor glucose level.
Beta blockers: May prolong hypoglycemic effect and mask symptoms of hypoglycemia. Use together cautiously.
Corticosteroids, glucagon, phenytoin, rifamycins, thiazide diuretics: May decrease hypoglycemic response. Monitor glucose level.
Oral anticoagulants: May increase hypoglycemic activity or enhance anticoagulant effect. Monitor glucose level, PT, and INR.
Drug-herb. *Burdock, dandelion, eucalyptus, marshmallow:* May increase drug effects. Discourage use together.
Drug-lifestyle. *Alcohol use:* May alter glycemic control, most commonly causing hypoglycemia. May cause disulfiram-like reaction. Discourage use together.

EFFECTS ON LAB TEST RESULTS
• May increase alkaline phosphatase, AST, LDH, BUN, cholesterol, and creatinine levels. May decrease glucose and hemoglobin levels.
• May decrease granulocyte, platelet, and WBC counts.

CONTRAINDICATIONS & CAUTIONS
• Contraindicated in patients hypersensitive to drug and in those with diabetic ketoacidosis with or without coma.
• Contraindicated in pregnant or breast-feeding women and as sole therapy in type 1 diabetes.
• Use cautiously in patients with severe GI narrowing, renal or hepatic disease, in those allergic to sulfonamides, and in debilitated, malnourished, or elderly patients.

NURSING CONSIDERATIONS
• Some patients may achieve effective control on a once-daily regimen, whereas others respond better with divided dosing.
• Patient may switch from immediate-release dose to extended-release tablets at the nearest equivalent total daily dose.
• Glipizide is a second-generation sulfonylurea. The frequency of adverse reactions appears to be lower than with first-generation drugs such as chlorpropamide.
• During periods of increased stress, patient may need insulin therapy. Monitor patient closely for hyperglycemia in these situations.
• Patient switching from insulin therapy to an oral antidiabetic should check glucose level at least three times a day before meals. Patient may need hospitalization during transition.
• **Look alike–sound alike:** Don't confuse glipizide with glyburide or glimepiride.

PATIENT TEACHING
• Instruct patient about disease and importance of following therapeutic regimen, adhering to diet, losing weight, getting exercise, following personal hygiene programs, and avoiding infection. Explain how and when to monitor glucose level, and teach recognition of episodes of low and high glucose levels.
• Tell patient to carry candy or other simple sugars to treat mild low-glucose episodes. Patient experiencing severe episode may need hospital treatment.
• Instruct patient not to change drug dosage without prescriber's consent and to report abnormal blood or urine glucose test results.
• Tell patient not to take other drugs, including OTC drugs, without first checking with prescriber.
• Advise patient to wear or carry medical identification at all times.
• Advise woman planning pregnancy to first consult prescriber. Insulin may be needed during pregnancy and breast-feeding.
• Advise patient to avoid alcohol, which lowers glucose level.
• Tell patient that he may occasionally notice something in his stool that looks like a tablet.

SAFETY ALERT!

glyburide (glibenclamide)
GLYE-byoor-ide

DiaBeta✲, Euglucon†, Gen Glybe†, Glynase PresTab, Micronase✲

Pharmacologic class: sulfonylurea
Pregnancy risk category B (Glynase, Micronase); C (DiaBeta)

AVAILABLE FORMS
Tablets: 1.25 mg, 2.5 mg, 5 mg
Tablets (micronized): 1.5 mg, 3 mg, 4.5 mg, 6 mg

INDICATIONS & DOSAGES
➤ **Adjunct to diet to lower glucose level in patients with type 2 (non–insulin-dependent) diabetes**
Nonmicronized form
Adults: Initially, 2.5 to 5 mg P.O. once daily with breakfast or first main meal. Adjust to maintenance dose at no more than 2.5-mg increments at weekly intervals. Usual daily maintenance dose is 1.25 to 20 mg, in single dose or divided doses. Maximum daily dose is 20 mg P.O.
Micronized form
Adults: Initially, 1.5 to 3 mg daily with breakfast or first main meal. Adjust to maintenance dose at no more than 1.5-mg increments at weekly intervals. Usual daily maintenance dose is 0.75 to 12 mg. Dosages exceeding 6 mg daily may have better response with b.i.d. dosing. Maximum dose is 12 mg P.O. daily.
Adjust-a-dose: For patients who are more sensitive to antidiabetics and for those with adrenal or pituitary insufficiency, start with 1.25 mg daily. When using micronized tablets, patients who are more sensitive to antidiabetics should start with 0.75 mg daily.
➤ **To replace insulin therapy**
Adults: If insulin dosage is less than 40 units/day, patient may be switched directly to glyburide when insulin is stopped. If insulin dose is less than 20 units/day, initial dose is 2.5 to 5 mg (1.5 to 3 mg micronized) P.O. daily. If insulin dose is 20 to 40 units/day, initial

dose is 5 mg (3 mg micronized) P.O. daily. If insulin dosage is 40 or more units/day, initially, 5 mg (3 mg micronized) P.O. once daily in addition to 50% of insulin dose.

ADMINISTRATION
P.O.
● Give drug with breakfast or first main meal.

ACTION
Unknown. Probably stimulates insulin release from pancreatic beta cells, reduces glucose output by the liver, and increases peripheral sensitivity to insulin.

Route	Onset	Peak	Duration
P.O. (micronized)	1 hr	1 hr	12–24 hr
P.O. (non-micronized)	2–4 hr	2–4 hr	16–24 hr

Half-life: 10 hours.

ADVERSE REACTIONS
EENT: changes in accommodation or blurred vision.
GI: nausea, epigastric fullness, heartburn.
Hematologic: *leukopenia,* hemolytic anemia, *agranulocytosis, thrombo-cytopenia, aplastic anemia.*
Hepatic: cholestatic jaundice, *hepatitis.*
Metabolic: *hypoglycemia,* hyponatremia.
Musculoskeletal: arthralgia, myalgia.
Skin: rash, pruritus, other allergic reactions.
Other: *angioedema.*

INTERACTIONS
Drug-drug. *Anabolic steroids, chloramphenicol, clofibrate, fluoroquinolones, guanethidine, MAO inhibitors, miconazole, NSAIDs, probenecid, phenylbutazone,* **salicylates,** *sulfonamides:* May increase hypoglycemic activity. Monitor glucose level.
Beta blockers: May prolong hypoglycemic effect and mask symptoms of hypoglycemia. Use together cautiously.
Carbamazepine, corticosteroids, glucagon, **rifamycins, thiazide diuretics:** May decrease hypoglycemic response. Monitor glucose level.

Reactions may be *common,* uncommon, *life-threatening,* or COMMON AND LIFE-THREATENING.
Interaction may have a *rapid onset* or **delayed onset.**

Oral anticoagulants: May increase hypo-glycemic activity or enhance anticoagulant effect. Monitor glucose level, PT, and INR.

Drug-herb. *Burdock, dandelion, eucalyptus, marshmallow:* May increase hypoglycemic effect. Discourage use together.

Drug-lifestyle. *Alcohol use:* May alter glycemic control, most commonly causing hypoglycemia. May cause disulfiram-like reaction. Discourage use together.

EFFECTS ON LAB TEST RESULTS
● May increase alkaline phosphatase, AST, ALT, bilirubin, BUN, and cholesterol levels. May decrease glucose, sodium, and hemoglobin levels.
● May decrease granulocyte, platelet, and WBC counts.

CONTRAINDICATIONS & CAUTIONS
● Contraindicated in patients hypersensitive to drug and in those with diabetic ketoacidosis with or without coma.
● Contraindicated as sole therapy for type 1 diabetes and in pregnant or breast-feeding women.
● Use cautiously in patients with hepatic or renal impairment; in debilitated, malnourished, or elderly patients; and in patients allergic to sulfonamides.

NURSING CONSIDERATIONS
● *Alert:* Micronized glyburide (Glynase PresTab) contains drug in a smaller particle size and isn't bioequivalent to regular glyburide tablets. In patients who have been taking Micronase or DiaBeta, adjust dosage.
● Although most patients may take drug once daily, those taking more than 10 mg daily may achieve better results with twice-daily dosage.
● Drug is a second-generation sulfonylurea. Adverse effects are less common with second-generation drugs than with first-generation drugs such as chlorpropamide.
● During periods of increased stress, such as infection, fever, surgery, or trauma, patient may need insulin therapy. Monitor patient closely for hyperglycemia in these situations.
● Patient switching from insulin therapy to an oral antidiabetic should check glucose

level at least three times a day before meals. Patient may need hospitalization during transition.
● *Look alike–sound alike:* Don't confuse glyburide with glimepiride or glipizide.

PATIENT TEACHING
● Teach patient about diabetes and the importance of following therapeutic regimen, adhering to specific diet, losing weight, getting exercise, following personal hygiene programs, and avoiding infection. Explain how and when to monitor glucose level, and teach recognition of and intervention for low and high glucose levels.
● Tell patient not to change drug dosage without prescriber's consent and to report abnormal blood or urine glucose test results.
● Teach patient to carry candy or other simple sugars for mild low-glucose level. Patient experiencing severe episode may need hospital treatment.
● Advise patient not to take other drugs, including OTC drugs, without first checking with prescriber.
● Advise patient to wear or carry medical identification at all times.
● *Alert:* Instruct patient to report episodes of low glucose to prescriber immediately; a severely low glucose level is sometimes fatal in patients receiving as little as 2.5 to 5 mg daily.
● Advise patient to avoid alcohol, which may lower glucose level.

SAFETY ALERT!

metformin hydrochloride
met-FORE-min

Fortamet, Glucophage⬦, Glucophage XR⬦, Glumetza, Riomet

Pharmacologic class: biguanide
Pregnancy risk category B

AVAILABLE FORMS
Oral solution: 500 mg/5 ml
Tablets: 500 mg, 850 mg, 1,000 mg
Tablets (extended-release): 500 mg, 750 mg, 1,000 mg

INDICATIONS & DOSAGES

➤ **Adjunct to diet to lower glucose level in patients with type 2 (non–insulin-dependent) diabetes**

Adults: If using regular-release tablets or oral solution, initially 500 mg P.O. b.i.d. given with morning and evening meals, or 850 mg P.O. once daily given with morning meal. When 500-mg dose of regular-release form is used, may increase dosage by 500 mg weekly to maximum dose of 2,500 mg P.O. daily in divided doses. When 850-mg dose of regular-release form is used, may increase dosage by 850 mg every other week to maximum dose of 2,550 mg P.O. daily in divided doses. If using extended-release formulation, start therapy at 500 mg (1,000 mg for Glumetza and Fortamet) P.O. once daily with the evening meal. May increase dose weekly in increments of 500 mg daily, up to a maximum dose of 2,000 mg once daily (2,500 mg for Fortamet). If higher doses are required, consider a trial of 1,000 mg b.i.d. or using the regular-release formulation up to its maximum dose.

Children ages 10 to 16: 500 mg P.O. b.i.d. using the regular-release formulation only. Increase dosage in increments of 500 mg weekly up to a maximum of 2,000 mg daily in divided doses.

Elderly patients: Dosage should be conservative because of potential decrease in renal function.

Adjust-a-dose: For debilitated patients, dosage should be conservative because of potential decrease in renal function.

➤ **Adjunct to diet and exercise in type 2 diabetes as monotherapy or with a sulfonylurea or insulin (Fortamet)**

Adults age 17 and older: Initially, 500 mg P.O. with evening meal for patients on insulin therapy. Increase dosage based on glucose level in increments of 500 mg weekly to a maximum of 2,500 mg daily. Decrease insulin dose by 10% to 25% when fasting blood glucose level is less than 120 mg/dl.

If patient has not responded to four weeks of maximum dose Fortamet monotherapy, consider the gradual addition of an oral sulfonylurea.

Elderly patients: Use conservative initial and maintenance dosage because of potential decrease in renal function. Adjust dosage carefully. Don't adjust to maximum dosage.

➤ **Adjunct to diet and exercise in type 2 diabetes as monotherapy or with a sulfonylurea or insulin (Glumetza)**

Adults: Initially, 500 mg P.O. once daily in the evening with food for patients on insulin therapy. Increase as needed in weekly increments of 500 mg, to a maximum of 2,000 mg daily. If glycemic control not attained at this dose, give 1,000 mg b.i.d. Decrease insulin dose by 10% to 25% when fasting glucose level is less than 120 mg/dl.

If patient has not responded to four weeks of maximum dose Glumetza monotherapy, consider the gradual addition of an oral sulfonylurea.

Adjust-a-dose: For malnourished or debilitated patients, don't adjust to maximum dosage.

ADMINISTRATION
P.O.
● Give drug with meals. Maximum doses may be better tolerated if total dose is divided into t.i.d. dosing and given with meals (immediate-release tablets only.)
● Don't cut or crush extended-release tablets.

ACTION
Decreases hepatic glucose production and intestinal absorption of glucose and improves insulin sensitivity (increases peripheral glucose uptake and use).

Route	Onset	Peak	Duration
P.O. (conventional)	Unknown	2–4 hr	Unknown
P.O. (extended-release)	Unknown	4–8 hr	Unknown
P.O. (solution)	Unknown	2½ hr	Unknown

Half-life: About 6 hours.

ADVERSE REACTIONS
CNS: asthenia, headache.
GI: *diarrhea, nausea, vomiting,* abdominal bloating, *flatulence,* anorexia, taste perversion.

Hematologic: megaloblastic anemia.
Metabolic: *lactic acidosis,* HYPO-
GLYCEMIA.
Other: accidental injury, *infection.*

INTERACTIONS
Drug-drug. *Beta-blockers:* Hypoglycemia
may be difficult to recognize in patients
using beta-blockers. Monitor patient and
blood glucose.
*Calcium channel blockers, corticosteroids,
estrogens, fosphenytoin, hormonal contraceptives, isoniazid, nicotinic acid, phenothiazines, phenytoin, sympathomimetics,
thiazide and other diuretics, thyroid drugs:*
May produce hyperglycemia. Monitor
patient's glycemic control. Metformin
dosage may need to be increased.
*Cationic drugs (such as amiloride, cimeti-
dine, digoxin, morphine, procainamide,
quinidine, quinine, ranitidine, triamterene,
trimethoprim, vancomycin):* May compete
for common renal tubular transport
systems, which may increase metformin
level. Monitor glucose level.
Nifedipine: May increase metformin level.
Monitor patient closely. Metformin
dosage may need to be decreased.
Radiologic contrast dye: May cause acute
renal failure. Withhold metformin at the
time of or prior to the procedure and
48 hours after the procedure. Restart drug
only after renal function is evaluated and
found to be normal.
Drug-herb. *Guar gum:* May decrease
hypoglycemic effect. Discourage use
together.
Drug-lifestyle. *Alcohol use:* May increase
drug effects. Discourage use together.

EFFECTS ON LAB TEST RESULTS
• May decrease vitamin B_{12} and hemoglobin levels.

CONTRAINDICATIONS & CAUTIONS
• Contraindicated in patients hypersensitive
to drug and in those with hepatic disease or
metabolic acidosis.
• Contraindicated in patients with renal
disease and in those with a serum creatinine greater than or equal to 1.5 mg/dl
(males) or greater than or equal to
1.4 mg/dl (females).
• Contraindicated in patients with acute
heart failure requiring pharmacologic

intervention and in patients with conditions predisposing to renal dysfunction,
CV collapse, MI, hypoxia, and septicemia. Temporarily withhold from
patients having radiologic studies involving use of contrast media containing
iodine.
■ **Black Box Warning** Contraindicated
in patients older than age 80, unless
creatinine clearance indicates normal
renal function. ■
• Use caution when giving drug to elderly,
debilitated, or malnourished patients and
to those with adrenal or pituitary insufficiency because of increased risk of
hypoglycemia.

NURSING CONSIDERATIONS
• Before therapy begins and at least
annually thereafter, assess patient's
renal function. If renal impairment is
detected, a different antidiabetic may be
indicated.
• When switching patients from chlorpropamide to metformin, take care during
the first 2 weeks of metformin therapy
because the prolonged retention of chlorpropamide increases the risk of hypoglycemia during this time.
• Monitor patient's glucose level regularly
to evaluate effectiveness of therapy. Notify
prescriber if glucose level increases
despite therapy.
• If patient hasn't responded to 4 weeks of
therapy with maximum dosage, an oral
sulfonylurea can be added while keeping
metformin at maximum dosage. If patient
still doesn't respond after several months
of therapy with both drugs at maximum
dosage, prescriber may stop both and start
insulin therapy.
• Monitor patient closely during times of
increased stress, such as infection, fever,
surgery, or trauma. Insulin therapy may be
needed in these situations.
■ **Black Box Warning** Risk of drug-
induced lactic acidosis is very low; however, when it occurs, it is fatal in approximately 50% of cases. Reported cases have
occurred primarily in diabetic patients
with significant renal insufficiency; in those
with other medical or surgical problems;
and in those with other drug regimens.
Risk increases with degree of renal
impairment and patient age. Suspect

lactic acidosis in any diabetic patient with metabolic acidosis lacking evidence of ketoacidosis. ■

■ **Black Box Warning** Stop drug immediately and notify prescriber if patient develops a condition related to hypoxemia or dehydration because of risk of lactic acidosis. ■

● Stop drug temporarily for surgical procedures (except minor procedures that don't restrict intake of food and fluids) and for patients undergoing radiologic studies involving use of contrast media containing iodine. Don't restart drug until patient's oral intake has resumed and renal function has been deemed normal by prescriber and at least 48 hours after contrast media.

● Monitor patient's hematologic status for evidence of megaloblastic anemia. Patients with inadequate vitamin B_{12} or calcium intake or absorption appear to be predisposed to developing subnormal vitamin B_{12} level. These patients should have routine vitamin B_{12} level determinations every 2 to 3 years.

● *Look alike–sound alike:* Don't confuse Glucophage with Glucovance or Glucotrol.

PATIENT TEACHING

● Instruct patient about nature of diabetes and importance of following therapeutic regimen, adhering to specific diet, losing weight, getting exercise, following personal hygiene programs, and avoiding infection. Explain how and when to monitor glucose level. Teach evidence of low and high glucose levels. Explain emergency measures.

■ **Black Box Warning** Instruct patient to stop drug and immediately notify prescriber about unexplained hyperventilation, muscle pain, malaise, dizziness, light-headedness, unusual sleepiness, unexplained stomach pain, feeling of coldness, slow or irregular heart rate, or other nonspecific symptoms of early lactic acidosis. ■

● Warn patient not to consume excessive alcohol while taking drug.

● Tell patient not to change drug dosage without prescriber's consent. Encourage patient to report abnormal glucose level test results.

● *Alert:* Advise patient not to cut, crush, or chew extended-release tablets; instead, he should swallow them whole.

● Tell patient that inactive ingredients may be eliminated in the stool as a soft mass resembling the original tablet.

● Advise patient not to take other drugs, including OTC drugs, without first checking with prescriber.

● Instruct patient to carry medical identification at all times.

● Tell patient that adverse effects of diarrhea, nausea, and upset stomach generally subside over time.

SAFETY ALERT!

miglitol
MIG-lah-tall

Glyset

Pharmacologic class:
alpha-glucosidase inhibitor
Pregnancy risk category B

AVAILABLE FORMS
Tablets: 25 mg, 50 mg, 100 mg

INDICATIONS & DOSAGES
➤ **Adjunct to diet in patients with type 2 diabetes, alone or with a sulfonylurea**
Adults: 25 mg P.O. t.i.d. May start with 25 mg P.O. daily and increase gradually to t.i.d. to minimize GI upset; dosage may be increased after 4 to 8 weeks to 50 mg P.O. t.i.d. Dosage may then be further increased after 3 months, based on glycosylated hemoglobin level, to maximum of 100 mg P.O. t.i.d.

ADMINISTRATION
P.O.
● Give drug t.i.d. with first bite of each main meal.

ACTION
Lowers glucose level by inhibiting the alpha-glucosidases in the small intestine, which convert carbohydrates to glucose. Inhibiting these enzymes delays the digestion of carbohydrates after a meal, resulting in a smaller increase in postprandial glucose level.

Reactions may be *common*, uncommon, *life-threatening*, or COMMON AND LIFE-THREATENING.
Interaction may have a *rapid onset* or *delayed onset.*

Route	Onset	Peak	Duration
P.O.	Unknown	2–3 hr	Unknown

Half-life: About 2 hours.

ADVERSE REACTIONS
GI: *abdominal pain, diarrhea, flatulence.*
Skin: rash.

INTERACTIONS
Drug-drug. *Digoxin, propranolol,
ranitidine:* May decrease bioavailability
of these drugs. Watch for loss of effect of
these drugs and adjust dosage.
*Intestinal absorbents (such as charcoal),
digestive enzyme preparations (such as
amylase, pancreatin):* May reduce effect
of miglitol. Avoid using together.

EFFECTS ON LAB TEST RESULTS
• May decrease iron level.

CONTRAINDICATIONS & CAUTIONS
• Contraindicated in patients hypersensitive
to drug or its components and in those
with diabetic ketoacidosis, inflammatory
bowel disease, colonic ulceration, partial
intestinal obstruction, chronic intestinal
diseases with marked disorders of digestion
or absorption, or conditions that may
deteriorate because of increased gas
formation in the intestine.
• Contraindicated in those predisposed to
intestinal obstruction and in those with
creatinine level greater than 2 mg/dl.
• Use cautiously in patients also receiving
insulin or a sulfonylurea because drug
may increase hypoglycemic potential of
these drugs.

NURSING CONSIDERATIONS
• In patients also taking insulin or a
sulfonylurea, dosage adjustment of these
drugs may be needed. Monitor patient for
hypoglycemia.
• Diabetes management should include
diet control, an exercise program, and
regular testing of urine and glucose
level.
• Monitor glucose level regularly, especially during situations of increased stress,
such as infection, fever, surgery, or trauma.
• Monitor glycosylated hemoglobin level
every 3 months to evaluate long-term
glycemic control.

• Treat mild to moderate hypoglycemia
with a ready form of sugar, such as glucose
tablets or gel. Severe hypoglycemia may
necessitate I.V. glucose or glucagon.
• Monitor patient for adverse GI effects.

PATIENT TEACHING
• Stress importance of adhering to diet,
weight reduction, and exercise instructions.
Urge patient to have glucose and glycosylated hemoglobin levels tested regularly.
• Inform patient that drug treatment
relieves symptoms but doesn't cure
diabetes.
• Teach patient how to recognize high and
low glucose levels.
• Instruct patient to have a source of
glucose readily available to treat
hypoglycemia.
• Advise patient to seek medical advice
promptly during periods of stress, such
as fever, trauma, infection, or surgery,
because dosage may have to be adjusted.
• Instruct patient to take drug three times
daily with first bite of each main meal.
• Show patient how and when to monitor
glucose level.
• Advise patient that sucrose (table sugar,
cane sugar) or fruit juices shouldn't be
used to treat low-glucose reactions with
this drug. Oral glucose (dextrose) or
glucagon is necessary to increase glucose.
• Advise patient that adverse GI effects
are most common during first few weeks
of therapy and should improve over time.
• Urge patient to carry medical identification at all times.

nateglinide
nah-TEG-lah-nyde

Starlix

Pharmacologic class: meglitinide
derivative
Pregnancy risk category C

AVAILABLE FORMS
Tablets: 60 mg, 120 mg

INDICATIONS & DOSAGES
➤ **Type 2 diabetes, as monotherapy,
or with metformin or a thiazolidinedione**

Adults: 120 mg P.O. t.i.d. taken 1 to 30 minutes before meals. Patients near goal HbA$_{1c}$ when treatment is started may receive 60 mg P.O. t.i.d.

ADMINISTRATION
P.O.
● Give drug 1 to 30 minutes before a meal.

ACTION
Lowers glucose level by stimulating insulin secretion from pancreatic beta cells.

Route	Onset	Peak	Duration
P.O.	20 min	1 hr	4 hr

Half-life: About 1½ hours.

ADVERSE REACTIONS
CNS: dizziness.
GI: diarrhea.
Metabolic: *hypoglycemia.*
Musculoskeletal: back pain, arthropathy.
Respiratory: *upper respiratory tract infection,* bronchitis, coughing.
Other: flulike symptoms, accidental trauma.

INTERACTIONS
Drug-drug. *Corticosteroids, rifamycins, sympathomimetics, thiazides, thyroid products:* May reduce hypoglycemic action of nateglinide. Monitor glucose level closely. *MAO inhibitors, nonselective beta blockers, NSAIDs, salicylates:* May increase hypoglycemic action of nateglinide. Monitor glucose level closely.

EFFECTS ON LAB TEST RESULTS
● May increase uric acid level. May decrease glucose level.

CONTRAINDICATIONS & CAUTIONS
● Contraindicated in patients hypersensitive to drug, in those with type 1 diabetes or diabetic ketoacidosis, and in pregnant or breast-feeding patients.
● Use cautiously in patients with moderate to severe liver dysfunction or adrenal or pituitary insufficiency, and in elderly and malnourished patients.

NURSING CONSIDERATIONS
● Don't use with or as a substitute for glyburide or other oral antidiabetics;

may use with metformin or a thiazolidinedione.
● Monitor glucose level regularly to evaluate drug's effectiveness.
● Observe patient for signs and symptoms of hypoglycemia. To minimize risk of hypoglycemia, make sure that patient has a meal immediately after dose. If hypoglycemia occurs and patient remains conscious, give him an oral form of glucose. If he's unconscious, treat with I.V. glucose.
● Risk of hypoglycemia increases with strenuous exercise, alcohol ingestion, or insufficient caloric intake.
● Symptoms of hypoglycemia may be masked in patients with autonomic neuropathy and in those who use beta blockers.
● Insulin therapy may be needed for glycemic control in patients with fever, infection, or trauma and in those undergoing surgery.
● Monitor glucose level closely when other drugs are started or stopped, to detect possible drug interactions.
● Periodically monitor HbA$_{1c}$ level.
● Drug's effectiveness may decrease over time.
● No special dosage adjustments are usually necessary in elderly patients, but some elderly patients may have greater sensitivity to glucose-lowering effect.

PATIENT TEACHING
● Tell patient to take drug 1 to 30 minutes before a meal.
● Advise patient to skip the scheduled dose if he skips a meal to reduce risk of hypoglycemia.
● Instruct patient on risk of hypoglycemia, its signs and symptoms (sweating, rapid pulse, trembling, confusion, headache, irritability, and nausea), and ways to treat these symptoms by eating or drinking something containing sugar.
● Teach patient how to monitor and log glucose levels to evaluate diabetes control.
● Advise patient to notify prescriber for persistent low or high glucose level.
● Instruct patient to adhere to prescribed diet and exercise regimen.
● Explain possible long-term complications of diabetes and importance of regular preventive therapy.

Reactions may be *common,* uncommon, *life-threatening,* or COMMON AND LIFE-THREATENING.
Interaction may have a *rapid onset* or **delayed onset.**

● Encourage patient to wear a medical identification bracelet.

pioglitazone hydrochloride
pie-oh-GLIT-ah-zohn

Actos

Pharmacologic class:
thiazolidinedione
Pregnancy risk category C

AVAILABLE FORMS
Tablets: 15 mg, 30 mg, 45 mg

INDICATIONS & DOSAGES
➤ **Type 2 diabetes, alone or with a sulfonylurea, metformin, or insulin**
Adults: Initially, 15 or 30 mg P.O. once daily. Maximum daily dose, if used alone or in combination therapy, is 45 mg.
Adjust-a-dose: For patients taking pioglitazone with insulin, reduce insulin by 10% to 25% if patient reports hypoglycemia or if glucose level is less than 100 mg/dl.

ADMINISTRATION
P.O.
● Give drug without regard for meals.

ACTION
Lowers glucose level by decreasing insulin resistance and hepatic glucose production. Improves sensitivity of insulin in muscle and adipose tissue.

Route	Onset	Peak	Duration
P.O.	Unknown	≤ 2 hr	Unknown

Half-life: 3 to 7 hours.

ADVERSE REACTIONS
CNS: headache.
CV: *edema, heart failure.*
EENT: sinusitis, pharyngitis.
Hematologic: anemia.
Metabolic: *hypoglycemia with combination therapy, aggravated diabetes,* weight gain.
Musculoskeletal: myalgia, fractures.

Respiratory: upper respiratory tract infection.
Other: tooth disorder.

INTERACTIONS
Drug-drug. *Atorvastatin:* May decrease atorvastatin and pioglitazone levels. Monitor patient and glucose level.
Hormonal contraceptives: May decrease level of hormonal contraceptives, reducing contraceptive effectiveness. Advise patient taking drug and hormonal contraceptives to consider additional birth control measures.
Ketoconazole: May inhibit pioglitazone metabolism. Monitor glucose level more frequently.
Drug-herb. *Burdock, dandelion, eucalyptus, marshmallow:* May increase hypoglycemic effects. Discourage use together.
Drug-lifestyle. *Alcohol use:* May alter glycemic control and increase risk of hypoglycemia. Discourage use together.

EFFECTS ON LAB TEST RESULTS
● May increase ALT, HDL, LDL, and total cholesterol levels. May decrease glucose, triglyceride, hematocrit, and hemoglobin levels.

CONTRAINDICATIONS & CAUTIONS
■ **Black Box Warning** Contraindicated in patients with symptomatic heart failure and in those with New York Heart Association (NYHA) Class III or IV heart failure. ■
● Contraindicated in patients hypersensitive to drug or its components and in those with type 1 diabetes, diabetic ketoacidosis, active liver disease, ALT level greater than two and a half times the upper limit of normal, and in those who experienced jaundice while taking troglitazone.
■ **Black Box Warning** Use cautiously in patients with edema or heart failure or patients at risk for heart failure. ■

NURSING CONSIDERATIONS
● *Alert:* Measure liver enzyme levels at start of therapy, every 2 months for first year of therapy, and periodically thereafter. Obtain liver function test results in patients who develop signs and symptoms of liver dysfunction, such as nausea, vomiting, abdominal pain, fatigue, anorexia, and dark urine. Stop drug if patient develops jaundice or if liver function test results

show ALT level greater than three times the upper limit of normal.

■ **Black Box Warning** Drug can cause fluid retention, leading to or worsening heart failure. Observe patients carefully for signs and symptoms of heart failure (including excessive, rapid weight gain, dyspnea, and/or edema). If these signs and symptoms develop, the heart failure should be managed according to the current standards of care. Also, stopping or reducing dose of pioglitazone must be considered. ■

• Hemoglobin level and hematocrit may drop, usually during first 4 to 12 weeks of therapy.

• Management of type 2 diabetes should include diet control. Because caloric restrictions, weight loss, and exercise help improve insulin sensitivity and help make drug therapy effective, these measures are essential for proper diabetes management.

• Watch for hypoglycemia, especially in patients receiving combination therapy. Dosage adjustments of these drugs may be needed.

• Monitor glucose level regularly, especially during situations of increased stress, such as infection, fever, surgery, and trauma.

• Safety and efficacy of drug in children haven't been evaluated.

• Use during pregnancy only if the benefit justifies risk to fetus; insulin is the preferred antidiabetic during pregnancy.

• Macular edema has been reported in some patients. Persons with diabetes should have regular eye exams by an ophthalmologist.

• Risk of fractures (forearm, hand, wrist, foot, ankle, fibula, and tibia) in female patients receiving long-term treatment is increased. Give only if risk outweighs benefits.

• *Look alike–sound alike:* Don't confuse pioglitazone with rosiglitazone.

PATIENT TEACHING

• Instruct patient to adhere to dietary instructions and to have glucose and glycosylated hemoglobin levels tested regularly.

• Teach patient taking pioglitazone with insulin or oral antidiabetics the signs and symptoms of hypoglycemia.

• Advise patient to notify prescriber during periods of stress, such as fever, trauma, infection, or surgery, because dosage may need adjustment.

• Instruct patient how and when to monitor glucose level.

• Notify patient that blood tests of liver function will be performed before therapy starts, every 2 months for the first year, and periodically thereafter.

• Tell patient to report unexplained nausea, vomiting, abdominal pain, fatigue, anorexia, and dark urine immediately because these symptoms may indicate liver problems.

• Warn patient to contact his health care provider if he has signs or symptoms of heart failure (unusually rapid increase in weight or swelling, shortness of breath).

• Advise anovulatory, premenopausal women with insulin resistance that therapy may cause resumption of ovulation; recommend using contraception.

• Tell patient to have regular eye exams and to report any visual changes immediately.

SAFETY ALERT!

pramlintide acetate
PRAM-lin-tyde

Symlin

Pharmacologic class: human amylin analogue
Pregnancy risk category C

AVAILABLE FORMS
Injection: 0.6 mg/ml in 5-ml vials, 1 mg/ml in 1.5-ml and 2.7-ml multidose pen injectors

INDICATIONS & DOSAGES
➤ **Adjunct to insulin in patients with type 1 diabetes**
Adults: Initially, 15 mcg subcutaneously before meals of more than 250 calories or 30 g of carbohydrates. Reduce preprandial rapid-acting or short-acting insulin dose, including fixed-mix insulin such as 70/30, by 50%. Increase pramlintide dose by 15-mcg increments every 3 days if no nausea occurs, to a maintenance dose

Reactions may be *common,* uncommon, *life-threatening,* or COMMON AND LIFE-THREATENING.
Interaction may have a *rapid onset* or **delayed onset**.

of 30 to 60 mcg. Adjust insulin dose as needed.

Adjust-a-dose: If significant nausea at 45 or 60 mcg persists, decrease to 30 mcg. If nausea persists at 30 mcg, consider stopping.

➤ **Adjunct to insulin in patients with type 2 diabetes, with or without a sulfonylurea or metformin**
Adults: Initially, 60 mcg subcutaneously immediately before major meals. Reduce preprandial rapid-acting or short-acting insulin dose, including fixed-mix insulin, by 50%. Increase pramlintide dose to 120 mcg if no significant nausea occurs for 3 to 7 days. Adjust insulin dose as needed.

Adjust-a-dose: If significant nausea persists at 120 mcg, decrease to 60 mcg.

ADMINISTRATION
Subcutaneous
• Before starting drug, review patient's HbA$_{1c}$ level, recent blood glucose monitoring data, hypoglycemic episodes, current insulin regimen, and body weight.
• To give drug, use a U-100 insulin syringe, preferably a 0.3-ml size.
• Give each dose subcutaneously into abdomen or thigh. Rotate injection sites, and use site separate from insulin site used at same time.
• Don't mix drug with any type of insulin; give drug as separate injection.
• Drug concentration in pen injector is higher than in vials. Don't transfer drug to syringe for administration.
• Refrigerate pen injectors and unopened and opened vials. Contents of opened vials should be used within 28 days and those of unopened vials before expiration date.

ACTION
Slows rate at which food leaves the stomach, reducing the initial postprandial increase in glucose level. Decreases hyperglycemia by reducing postprandial glucagon level and reduces total caloric intake by reducing appetite.

Route	Onset	Peak	Duration
Subcut.	Unknown	19–21 min	Unknown

Half-life: About 48 minutes each (parent drug and active metabolite).

ADVERSE REACTIONS
CNS: dizziness, fatigue, *headache.*
EENT: pharyngitis.
GI: abdominal pain, *anorexia, nausea, vomiting.*
Metabolic: *hypoglycemia.*
Musculoskeletal: arthralgia.
Respiratory: cough.
Skin: injection site reaction.
Other; allergic reaction, *accidental injury.*

INTERACTIONS
Drug-drug. *ACE inhibitors, disopyramide, fibrates, fluoxetine, MAO inhibitors, oral antidiabetics, pentoxifylline, propoxyphene, salicylates, sulfonamide antibiotics:* May increase risk of hypoglycemia. Monitor glucose level closely.
Alpha glucosidase inhibitors (such as acarbose), anticholinergics (such as atropine, tricyclic antidepressants, benztropine): May alter GI motility and slow intestinal absorption. Avoid using together.
Beta blockers, clonidine, guanethidine, reserpine: May mask signs of hypoglycemia. Monitor glucose level closely.
Oral drugs dependent on rapid onset of action (such as analgesics): May delay absorption because of slowed gastric emptying. If rapid effect is needed, give oral drug 1 hour before or 2 hours after pramlintide.

EFFECTS ON LAB TEST RESULTS
None reported.

CONTRAINDICATIONS & CAUTIONS
• Contraindicated in patients hypersensitive to drug or its components, including metacresol, and in patients with gastroparesis or hypoglycemia unawareness.
• Don't use in patients noncompliant with current insulin and glucose monitoring regimen, patients with a glycosylated hemoglobin (HbA$_{1c}$) level greater than 9%, patients with severe hypoglycemia during the previous 6 months, and patients who take drugs that stimulate GI motility.
• Use cautiously in pregnant or breast-feeding women and in elderly patients.

NURSING CONSIDERATIONS
■ **Black Box Warning** Drug may increase the risk of insulin-induced severe hypo-

glycemia, particularly in patients with type 1 diabetes. The risk of severe hypoglycemia is highest within the first 3 hours after an injection. ■

• Symptoms of hypoglycemia may be masked in patients with a long history of diabetes, diabetic nerve disease, or intensified diabetes control.

• Notify prescriber of severe nausea and vomiting. A reduced dose may be needed.

• If patient has persistent nausea or recurrent, unexplained hypoglycemia that requires medical assistance, stop drug.

• If patient doesn't comply with glucose monitoring or drug dosage adjustments, stop drug.

PATIENT TEACHING

• Teach patient how to take drug exactly as prescribed, at mealtimes. Explain that it doesn't replace daily insulin but may lower the amount of insulin needed.

• Explain that a meal is considered more than 250 calories or 30 g of carbohydrates.

• Caution patient not to mix drug with insulin; instruct him to give the injections at separate sites.

• Instruct patient not to change doses of pramlintide or insulin without consulting prescriber.

• Instruct patient not to transfer drug from pen injector to syringe. Drug in pen injector is a higher concentration than in vial.

• Tell patient to refrain from driving, operating heavy machinery, or performing other risky activities where he could hurt himself or others, until it's known how drug affects his glucose level.

• Caution patient about possibility of severe hypoglycemia, particularly within 3 hours after injection.

• Teach patient and family members the signs and symptoms of hypoglycemia, including hunger, headache, sweating, tremor, irritability, and difficulty concentrating.

• Instruct patient and family members what to do if patient develops hypoglycemia.

• Tell patient to report to prescriber severe nausea and vomiting.

• Advise women of childbearing age to tell the prescriber if they are, could be, or are planning to become pregnant.

• Teach patient how to handle unplanned situations, such as illness or stress, low or forgotten insulin dose, accidental use of too much insulin or drug, not enough food, or missed meals.

• Tell patient to refrigerate pen injectors and unopened and opened vials. Contents of opened vials should be used within 28 days and those of unopened vials before expiration date.

SAFETY ALERT!

repaglinide
re-PAG-lah-nyde

Prandin

Pharmacologic class: meglitinide
Pregnancy risk category C

AVAILABLE FORMS
Tablets: 0.5 mg, 1 mg, 2 mg

INDICATIONS & DOSAGES
➤ **Type 2 diabetes alone or with metformin or a thiazolidinedione**
Adults: For patients not previously treated or whose HbA_{1c} is below 8%, starting dose is 0.5 mg P.O. taken about 15 minutes before each meal. For patients previously treated with glucose-lowering drugs and whose HbA_{1c} is 8% or more, first dose is 1 to 2 mg P.O. with each meal. Recommended dosage range is 0.5 to 4 mg with meals b.i.d., t.i.d., or q.i.d. Maximum daily dose is 16 mg.

Determine dosage by glucose response. May double dosage up to 4 mg with each meal until satisfactory glucose response is achieved. At least 1 week should elapse between dosage adjustments to assess response to each dose.

Metformin or a thiazolidinedione may be added if repaglinide monotherapy is inadequate; no repaglinide dosage adjustment is necessary.
Adjust-a-dose: In patients with severe renal impairment, starting dose is 0.5 mg P.O. with meals.

ADMINISTRATION
P.O.
• Give drug before meals, usually 15 minutes before start of meal; however, time can vary from immediately preceding meal to up to 30 minutes before meal.

ACTION
Stimulates insulin release from beta cells in the pancreas by closing ATP-dependent potassium channels in beta cell membranes, which causes calcium channels to open. Increased calcium influx induces insulin secretion; the overall effect is to lower glucose level.

Route	Onset	Peak	Duration
P.O.	30 min	1 hr	Unknown

Half-life: 1 hour.

ADVERSE REACTIONS
CNS: *headache,* paresthesia.
CV: angina.
EENT: rhinitis, sinusitis.
GI: constipation, diarrhea, dyspepsia, nausea, vomiting.
GU: UTI.
Metabolic: HYPOGLYCEMIA, hyperglycemia.
Musculoskeletal: arthralgia, back pain.
Respiratory: bronchitis, *upper respiratory tract infection.*
Other: tooth disorder.

INTERACTIONS
Drug-drug. *Barbiturates, carbamazepine, rifampin:* May increase repaglinide metabolism. Monitor glucose level.
Beta blockers, chloramphenicol, coumarin derivatives, MAO inhibitors, NSAIDs, other drugs that are highly protein bound, probenecid, salicylates, sulfonamides: May increase hypoglycemic action of repaglinide. Monitor glucose level.
Calcium channel blockers, corticosteroids, estrogens, fosphenytoin, hormonal contraceptives, isoniazid, nicotinic acid, phenothiazines, phenytoin, sympathomimetics, thiazides and other diuretics, thyroid products: May produce hyperglycemia, resulting in a loss of glycemic control. Monitor glucose level.
Clarithromycin: May increase repaglinide levels. Adjust repaglinide dosage.
Erythromycin, itraconazole, ketoconazole, miconazole, similar inhibitors of CYP3A4: May inhibit repaglinide metabolism. Monitor glucose level.
Gemfibrozil: May increase repaglinide levels. Avoid using together, if possible.

Monitor glucose level and adjust repaglinide dosage, if indicated.
Drug-herb. *Burdock, dandelion, eucalyptus, marshmallow:* May increase hypoglycemic effects. Discourage use together.
Drug-food. *Grapefruit juice:* May inhibit metabolism of drug. Discourage use together.
Drug-lifestyle. *Alcohol use:* May alter glycemic control, most commonly causing hypoglycemia. Discourage use together.

EFFECTS ON LAB TEST RESULTS
● May increase or decrease glucose level.

CONTRAINDICATIONS & CAUTIONS
● Contraindicated in patients hypersensitive to drug or its inactive ingredients and in those with type 1 diabetes or diabetic ketoacidosis.
● Use cautiously in elderly, debilitated, or malnourished patients and in those with hepatic, adrenal, or pituitary insufficiency.

NURSING CONSIDERATIONS
● Increase dosage carefully in patients with impaired renal function or renal failure requiring dialysis.
● Metformin may be added if repaglinide alone is inadequate.
● Drug may increase CV mortality compared with diet alone or diet plus insulin.
● Monitor patient for loss of glycemic control, especially during stress, such as fever, trauma, infection, or surgery.
● Hypoglycemia may be difficult to recognize in elderly patients and in patients taking beta blockers.
● When switching to a different oral hypoglycemic, begin new drug on day after last dose of repaglinide.
● **Look alike–sound alike:** Don't confuse Prandin with Avandia.

PATIENT TEACHING
● Stress importance of diet and exercise with drug therapy.
● Discuss symptoms of hypoglycemia with patient and family.
● Encourage patient to keep regular appointments and have his HbA_{1c} level checked every 3 months to determine long-term glucose control.
● Tell patient to take drug before meals, usually 15 minutes before start of meal;

however, time can vary from immediately preceding meal to up to 30 minutes before meal.
● Tell patient that, if a meal is skipped or added, he should skip dose or add an extra dose of drug for that meal, respectively.
● Instruct patient to monitor glucose level carefully and tell him what to do when he's ill, undergoing surgery, or under added stress.
● Advise woman planning pregnancy to first consult prescriber. Insulin may be needed during pregnancy and breast-feeding.
● Teach patient to carry candy or other simple sugars to treat mild hypoglycemia episodes. Patient experiencing severe episode may need emergency treatment.
● Advise patient to avoid alcohol, which lowers glucose level.

SAFETY ALERT!

rosiglitazone maleate
roh-zee-GLIT-ah-zohn

Avandia✣

Pharmacologic class:
thiazolidinedione
Pregnancy risk category C

AVAILABLE FORMS
Tablets: 2 mg, 4 mg, 8 mg

INDICATIONS & DOSAGES
➤ Type 2 diabetes, alone or with a sulfonylurea, metformin, or insulin
Adults: Initially, 4 mg P.O. daily in the morning or in divided doses b.i.d. (morning and evening). Increase to 8 mg P.O. daily or in divided doses b.i.d. if fasting glucose level doesn't improve after 12 weeks of treatment.
Adjust-a-dose: For patients stabilized on insulin, continue the insulin dose when rosiglitazone therapy starts. Don't use rosiglitazone doses greater than 4 mg daily with insulin. Decrease insulin dose by 10% to 25% if patient reports hypoglycemia or if fasting glucose level falls to below 100 mg/dl. Adjust based on glucose-lowering response.

ADMINISTRATION
P.O.
● *Alert:* Check liver enzyme levels before therapy starts. Don't use drug in patients with increased baseline liver enzyme levels.
● Give drug without regard for food.

ACTION
Lowers glucose level by improving insulin sensitivity.

Route	Onset	Peak	Duration
P.O.	Unknown	1 hr	Unknown

Half-life: 3 to 4 hours.

ADVERSE REACTIONS
CNS: headache, fatigue.
CV: edema, *worsening heart failure.*
EENT: sinusitis.
GI: diarrhea.
Hematologic: anemia.
Metabolic: hyperglycemia, weight gain.
Musculoskeletal: back pain, fractures.
Respiratory: upper respiratory tract infection.
Other: accidental injury.

INTERACTIONS
Drug-drug. *Gemfibrozil, ketoconazole:* May increase rosiglitazone levels, increasing hypoglycemic effects and other adverse reactions. Monitor glucose; dosage adjustment may be necessary.
Insulin: May increase incidence of edema. Monitor patient.
Rifampin: May decrease rosiglitazone levels. Monitor glucose; dosage adjustment may be necessary.

EFFECTS ON LAB TEST RESULTS
● May increase glucose, HDL, LDL, total cholesterol, and ALT levels. May decrease hemoglobin level and hematocrit.

CONTRAINDICATIONS & CAUTIONS
● Contraindicated in patients hypersensitive to drug or its components.
■ **Black Box Warning** Contraindicated in patients with symptomatic heart failure or those with established New York Heart Association Class III or IV heart failure. ■
● Contraindicated in patients with active liver disease, increased baseline liver

---

Reactions may be *common,* uncommon, *life-threatening,* or COMMON AND LIFE-THREATENING.
Interaction may have a *rapid onset* or **delayed onset.**

enzyme levels (ALT level greater than two and a half times upper limit of normal), type 1 diabetes, or diabetic ketoacidosis and in those who experienced jaundice while taking troglitazone.
● Use cautiously in patient with underlying heart disease or those at high risk for MI. Monitor patient closely.
● Use cautiously in patients with edema or heart failure.

NURSING CONSIDERATIONS
● *Alert:* Monitor liver enzyme levels every 2 months for first 12 months and periodically thereafter. If ALT level becomes elevated, recheck as soon as possible. Stop drug if levels remain elevated.
■ **Black Box Warning** Drug can cause fluid retention leading to or worsening heart failure. Monitor patients for signs and symptoms of heart failure. Notify prescriber if any deterioration in cardiac status occurs. ■
● Management of type 2 diabetes should include diet control. Because caloric restriction, weight loss, and exercise help improve insulin sensitivity and effectiveness of drug therapy, these measures are essential to proper diabetes treatment.
● Check glucose and glycosylated hemoglobin levels periodically to monitor therapeutic response to drug.
● Hemoglobin level and hematocrit may drop during therapy, usually during first 4 to 8 weeks. Increases in total cholesterol, low-density lipoprotein, and high-density lipoprotein levels and decreases in free fatty acid level also may occur.
● For patients inadequately controlled with a maximum dose of a sulfonylurea or metformin, add rosiglitazone to, rather than substitute it for, a sulfonylurea or metformin.
● Drug may increase the incidence of bone fractures (most common in the arm, hand, and foot) in women.
● *Look alike–sound alike:* Don't confuse rosiglitazone with pioglitazone; or Avandia with Prandin.

PATIENT TEACHING
● Advise patient that drug can be taken with or without food.
● Notify patient that blood will be tested to check liver function before therapy

starts, every 2 months for first 12 months, and then periodically thereafter.
● Tell patient to immediately notify prescriber about unexplained signs and symptoms, such as nausea, vomiting, abdominal pain, fatigue, anorexia, or dark urine; these may indicate liver problems.
● Warn patient to contact his health care provider about signs or symptoms of heart failure (unusually rapid increase in weight or swelling, shortness of breath).
● *Alert:* Warn patients with underlying heart disease or those at high risk for an MI that they're at an increased risk for an MI while on rosiglitazone. Patient should notify his health care provider of any change in cardiac condition.
● Recommend use of contraceptives to premenopausal, anovulatory women with insulin resistance because ovulation may resume with therapy.
● Advise patient that management of diabetes includes diet control, calorie restriction, weight loss, and exercise, and that these measures improve effectiveness of drug therapy.
● Instruct patient to monitor glucose level carefully and tell him what to do when he's ill, undergoing surgery, or under added stress.

sitagliptin phosphate
sit-ah-GLIP-ten

Januvia◈

Pharmacologic class: Dipeptidyl peptidase-4 (DPP-4) enzyme inhibitor
Pregnancy risk category B

AVAILABLE FORMS
Tablets: 25 mg, 50 mg, 100 mg

INDICATIONS & DOSAGES
➤ **To improve glycemic control in type 2 diabetes, alone or with metformin or a thiazolidinedione**
Adults: 100 mg P.O. once daily.
Adjust-a-dose: For patients with creatinine clearance of 30 to 50 ml/minute, give 50 mg once daily; for patients with clearance less than 30 ml/minute or end-

stage renal disease with hemodialysis or peritoneal dialysis, give 25 mg once daily. Give without regard to timing of dialysis session.

ADMINISTRATION
P.O.
• Give drug without regard for food.

ACTION
Inhibits DPP-4, an enzyme that rapidly inactivates incretin hormones, which play a part in the body's regulation of glucose. By increasing and prolonging active incretin levels, the drug helps to increase insulin release and decrease circulating glucose.

Route	Onset	Peak	Duration
P.O.	Rapid	1–4 hr	Unknown

Half-life: 12.4 hours.

ADVERSE REACTIONS
CNS: headache.
EENT: nasopharyngitis.
GI: abdominal pain, nausea, diarrhea.
Metabolic: *hypoglycemia.*
Respiratory: upper respiratory tract infection.
Skin: exfoliative skin conditions, *(Stevens-Johnson syndrome).*
Other: *angioedema, anaphylaxis,* hypersensitivity reaction.

INTERACTIONS
None significant.

EFFECTS ON LAB TEST RESULTS
• May increase creatinine level.
• May increase WBC count.

CONTRAINDICATIONS & CAUTIONS
• Contraindicated in patients with type 1 diabetes or diabetic ketoacidosis.
• Contraindicated in patients with a history of hypersensitivity to sitagliptin.
• Use cautiously in patients with moderate to severe renal insufficiency and in those taking other antidiabetics.

NURSING CONSIDERATIONS
• In elderly patients and those at risk for renal insufficiency, periodically assess renal function.

• Monitor glycosylated hemoglobin level periodically to assess long-term glycemic control.
• Management of type 2 diabetes should include diet control. Because caloric restrictions, weight loss, and exercise help improve insulin sensitivity and help make drug therapy effective, these measures are essential for proper diabetes management.
• Watch for hypoglycemia, especially in patients receiving combination therapy.
• Safety and effectiveness of drug in children haven't been evaluated.

PATIENT TEACHING
• Tell patient that drug isn't a substitute for diet and exercise and that it's important to follow a prescribed dietary and physical activity routine and to monitor his glucose levels.
• Inform patient and family members of the signs and symptoms of hyperglycemia and hypoglycemia and the steps to take if these symptoms occur.
• Provide patient with information on complications associated with diabetes and ways to assess for them.
• Tell patient to notify prescriber during periods of stress, such as fever, infection, or surgery; dosage may need adjustment.
• Tell patient drug may be taken without regard for food.

Reactions may be *common,* uncommon, *life-threatening,* or COMMON AND LIFE-THREATENING.
Interaction may have a *rapid onset* or **delayed onset.**

carboprost tromethamine
dinoprostone
methylergonovine maleate
oxytocin, synthetic injection

Route	Onset	Peak	Duration
I.M.	Unknown	15–60 min	24 hr

Half-life: Unknown.

---

carboprost tromethamine
KAR-boe-prost

Hemabate

Pharmacologic class:
prostaglandin
Pregnancy risk category C

AVAILABLE FORMS
Injection: 250 mcg/ml

INDICATIONS & DOSAGES
➤ **To terminate pregnancy between weeks 13 and 20 of gestation**
Adults: Initially, 250 mcg deep I.M. Give subsequent doses of 250 mcg at intervals of 1½ to 3½ hours, depend-ing on uterine response. Dosage may be increased in increments to 500 mcg if contractility is inadequate after several 250-mcg doses. Total dose shouldn't exceed 12 mg or continuous administration for more than 2 days.
➤ **Postpartum hemorrhage from uterine atony not managed by conventional methods**
Adults: 250 mcg by deep I.M. injection. Repeat doses every 15 to 90 minutes as needed. Maximum total dose is 2 mg.

ADMINISTRATION
I.M.
● Only trained personnel in a hospital setting should give drug.
● Give deep in the muscle using a tuberculin syringe.

ACTION
Produces strong, prompt contractions of uterine smooth muscle, possibly mediated by calcium and cAMP.

ADVERSE REACTIONS
CNS: *fever,* headache, anxiety, paresthesia, syncope, weakness.
CV: *arrhythmias,* chest pain, flushing.
EENT: blurred vision, eye pain.
GI: *vomiting, diarrhea, nausea.*
GU: *uterine rupture,* endometritis, uterine or vaginal pain.
Musculoskeletal: backache, leg cramps.
Respiratory: coughing, wheezing.
Skin: rash, diaphoresis.
Other: breast tenderness, chills, hot flashes.

INTERACTIONS
Drug-drug. *Other oxytocics:* May increase action. Avoid using together.

EFFECTS ON LAB TEST RESULTS
None reported.

CONTRAINDICATIONS & CAUTIONS
● Contraindicated in patients hypersensitive to drug and in those with acute pelvic inflammatory disease or active cardiac, pulmonary, renal, or hepatic disease.
● Use cautiously in patients with history of asthma, hypotension, hypertension, anemia, jaundice, or diabetes; and those with seizure disorders, previous uterine surgery, or CV, adrenal, renal, or hepatic disease.

NURSING CONSIDERATIONS
● Unlike other prostaglandin abortifacients, drug is given by I.M. injection. Injectable form avoids risk of expelling vaginal suppositories if patient has profuse vaginal bleeding.
● Pretreating and giving with antiemetics and antidiarrheals decreases the risk of common GI effects.

PATIENT TEACHING
- Explain use and administration of drug to patient and family.
- Instruct patient to report adverse reactions promptly.

---

dinoprostone
dye-noe-PROST-ohn

Cervidil, Prepidil, Prostin E2

Pharmacologic class: prostaglandin
Pregnancy risk category C

AVAILABLE FORMS
Endocervical gel: 0.5 mg/application (2.5-ml syringe)
Vaginal insert: 10 mg
Vaginal suppositories: 20 mg

INDICATIONS & DOSAGES
■ **Black Box Warning** Strictly adhere to recommended dosages. ■
➤ **To terminate second-trimester pregnancy; to evacuate uterine contents in missed abortion, intrauterine fetal death up to 28 weeks' gestation, or benign hydatidiform mole**
Women: Insert 20-mg suppository high into posterior vaginal fornix; repeat every 3 to 5 hours until abortion is complete, for a maximum of 2 days.
➤ **To ripen an unfavorable cervix in pregnant woman at or near term**
Women: Apply 0.5 mg endocervical gel intravaginally; if cervix remains unfavorable after 6 hours, repeat dose. Don't exceed 1.5 mg (three applications) within 24 hours. Or, place 10-mg vaginal insert transversely in posterior vaginal fornix immediately after removing insert from foil. Take insert out when active labor begins or after 12 hours have passed, whichever occurs first.

ADMINISTRATION
Vaginal
- For cervical ripening, have patient lie on her back; use a speculum to examine cervix. Use catheter provided with drug to insert gel into cervical canal just below level of the internal os.

- Bring gel to room temperature just before giving. Don't force warming with water bath, microwave, or other external heat source.
- When giving gel form, don't try to give small amount of drug remaining in catheter.
- Patient should lie down for 15 to 30 minutes after using gel.
- Bring vaginal suppository to room temperature just before giving. Patient should lie down for 10 minutes following vaginal suppository insertion.
- When using the vaginal insert, a small amount of water-soluble jelly may be used to aid insertion. There's no need to warm the vaginal insert before insertion.
- Patient should lie down for 2 hours after using vaginal insert. Remove insert at onset of active labor or 12 hours after insertion.

ACTION
Produces strong, prompt contractions of uterine smooth muscle, possibly mediated by calcium and cAMP. Also has a local cervical effect in initiating softening, effacement, and dilation.

Route	Onset	Peak	Duration
Vaginal (gel)	15–30 min	Unknown	Unknown
Vaginal (insert)	Unknown	Unknown	Unknown
Vaginal (suppository)	10 min	Unknown	2–6 hr

Half-life: 2½ to 5 minutes.

ADVERSE REACTIONS
CNS: *fever, headache, dizziness,* anxiety, paresthesia, weakness, syncope.
CV: *arrhythmias,* chest pain.
EENT: blurred vision, eye pain.
GI: *nausea, vomiting, diarrhea.*
GU: vaginal pain, vaginitis, endometritis, *uterine hyperstimulation, uterine rupture.*
Musculoskeletal: *nocturnal leg cramps,* backache, muscle cramps.
Respiratory: coughing, dyspnea.
Skin: rash, diaphoresis.
Other: *shivering, chills,* breast tenderness, hot flashes, *fetal heart rate*

Reactions may be *common,* uncommon, *life-threatening,* or COMMON AND LIFE-THREATENING.
Interaction may have a *rapid onset* or **delayed onset.**

abnormality, premature rupture of membranes, fetal depression, fetal acidosis.

INTERACTIONS

Drug-drug. *Other oxytocics:* May increase action. Avoid using together.
Drug-lifestyle. *Alcohol use:* May inhibit effectiveness of drug with high doses. Discourage use together.

EFFECTS ON LAB TEST RESULTS

None reported.

CONTRAINDICATIONS & CAUTIONS

● Gel form contraindicated in patients hypersensitive to prostaglandins or constituents of gel; in those for whom prolonged uterine contractions are undesirable; in those with placenta previa or unexplained vaginal bleeding during pregnancy; and in those for whom vaginal delivery isn't indicated (because of vasa previa or active genital herpes).
● Suppository form contraindicated in patients hypersensitive to drug, in those with acute pelvic inflammatory disease, and in those with active cardiac, pulmonary, renal, or hepatic disease.
● Insert form contraindicated in patients hypersensitive to drug and in those with evidence of fetal distress when delivery isn't imminent, with unexplained vaginal bleeding during pregnancy, or with evidence of marked fetal cephalopelvic disproportion; also contraindicated when oxytocics are contraindicated, when prolonged uterine contraction may be detrimental to fetal safety or uterine integrity, when membranes have ruptured, when patient is already receiving an oxytocic, and when patient is multipara with six or more previous term pregnancies.
● Use gel form cautiously in patients with asthma or history of asthma, renal or hepatic dysfunction, ruptured membranes, glaucoma, or increased intraocular pressure.
● Use suppository form cautiously in patients with asthma, seizure disorders, anemia, diabetes, hypertension or hypotension, jaundice, scarred uterus, cervicitis, acute vaginitis, or CV, renal, or hepatic disease.

NURSING CONSIDERATIONS

■ **Black Box Warning** Give drug only in a hospital where critical care and surgical facilities are available. ■
● Treat drug-induced fever with water sponging and increased fluid intake, not with aspirin.
● Check vaginal discharge regularly.
● Abortion should be complete within 30 hours when suppository form is used.

PATIENT TEACHING

● Explain use and administration of drug to patient and family.
● Instruct patient to report adverse reactions promptly.

---

methylergonovine maleate
meth-ill-er-goe-NOE-veen

Methergine

Pharmacologic class: ergot alkaloid
Pregnancy risk category C

AVAILABLE FORMS

Injection: 0.2 mg/ml in 1-ml ampules
Tablets: 0.2 mg

INDICATIONS & DOSAGES

➤ **To prevent and treat postpartum hemorrhage caused by uterine atony or subinvolution**
Adults: 0.2 mg I.M. every 2 to 4 hours to a maximum of five doses. For excessive uterine bleeding or other emergencies, 0.2 mg I.V. over 1 minute while monitoring blood pressure and uterine contractions. After first I.M. or I.V. dose, 0.2 mg P.O. every 6 to 8 hours for 2 to 7 days. Decrease dosage if severe cramping occurs.

ADMINISTRATION

P.O.
● Store tablets in tightly closed, light-resistant container. Discard if discolored.
I.V.
● Don't routinely use this form because of risk of severe hypertension and stroke.
● Dilute to 5 ml with normal saline solution, as needed.
● Give slowly over at least 1 minute while carefully monitoring blood pressure.

• Store solution below 46° F (8° C). Daily stock may be kept at room temperature for 60 to 90 days.
• **Incompatibilities:** None reported.
I.M.
• Store in refrigerator and protect from light.
• Drug may be given after delivery of the anterior shoulder, after delivery of the placenta, or during the puerperium.

ACTION
Increases motor activity of the uterus by direct stimulation of the smooth muscle, shortening the third stage of labor, and reducing blood loss.

Route	Onset	Peak	Duration
P.O.	5–10 min	30 min	3 hr
I.V.	Immediate	Unknown	45 min
I.M.	2–5 min	Unknown	3 hr

Half-life: 1½ to 12¾ hours.

ADVERSE REACTIONS
CNS: *seizures, stroke with I.V. use,* dizziness, headache, hallucinations.
CV: hypertension, transient chest pain, palpitations, hypotension, thrombophlebitis.
EENT: tinnitus, nasal congestion.
GI: *nausea, vomiting,* diarrhea, foul taste.
GU: hematuria.
Musculoskeletal: leg cramps.
Respiratory: dyspnea.
Skin: diaphoresis.

INTERACTIONS
Drug-drug. *Dopamine, ergot alkaloids, I.V. oxytocin, regional anesthetics, vasoconstrictors:* May cause excessive vasoconstriction. Use together cautiously.
Clarithromycin, delavirdine, erythromycin, indinavir, itraconazole, ketoconazole, nelfinavir, ritonavir, telithromycin, troleandomycin, voriconazole: May cause vasospasm, leading to ischemia. Avoid using together.
Clotrimazole, fluconazole, fluoxetine, fluvoxamine, nefazodone, saquinavir, zileuton: May increase risk of vasospasm. Use together cautiously.

EFFECTS ON LAB TEST RESULTS
• May decrease prolactin level.

CONTRAINDICATIONS & CAUTIONS
• Contraindicated in pregnant patients, in patients sensitive to ergot preparations, and in patients with hypertension or toxemia.
• Use cautiously in patients with sepsis, obliterative vascular disease, or hepatic or renal disease.
• Use cautiously during last stage of labor.

NURSING CONSIDERATIONS
• Monitor and record blood pressure, pulse rate, and uterine response; report sudden change in vital signs, frequent periods of uterine relaxation, and character and amount of vaginal bleeding.
• Monitor contractions, which may begin immediately. Contractions may continue for up to 45 minutes after I.V. use or for 3 hours or more after P.O. or I.M. use.
• *Look alike–sound alike:* Don't confuse Methergine with terbutaline.

PATIENT TEACHING
• Explain use of drug to patient and family.
• Instruct patient to report adverse reactions promptly.

oxytocin, synthetic injection
ox-i-TOE-sin

Pitocin

Pharmacologic class: exogenous hormone
Pregnancy risk category NR

AVAILABLE FORMS
Injection: 10 units/ml in 1-ml ampule, 1-ml, 3-ml, and 10-ml vials, or syringe

INDICATIONS & DOSAGES
➤ **To induce or stimulate labor**
Adults: Initially, 10 units in 1,000 ml of D_5W injection, lactated Ringer's, or normal saline solution I.V. infused at 0.5 to 2 milliunits/minute. Increase rate by 1 to 2 milliunits/minute at 30- to 60-minute intervals until normal contraction pattern is established. Decrease rate when labor is firmly established. Rates exceeding 9 to 10 milliunits/minute are rarely required.

➤ **To reduce postpartum bleeding after expulsion of placenta**
Adults: 10 to 40 units in 1,000 ml of D₅W injection, lactated Ringer's, or normal saline solution I.V. infused at rate needed to control bleeding, which is usually 20 to 40 milliunits/minute. Also, 10 units may be given I.M. after delivery of placenta.

➤ **Incomplete or inevitable abortion**
Adults: 10 units I.V. in 500 ml of normal saline solution, lactated Ringer's, or dextrose 5% in normal saline solution. Infuse at 10 to 20 milliunits (20 to 40 drops)/minute. Don't exceed 30 units in 12 hours.

ADMINISTRATION
I.V.
● Never give drug simultaneously by more than one route.
● To induce or stimulate labor, dilute drug by adding 10 units to 1 L of normal saline, lactated Ringer's, or D₅W solution.
● To produce intense uterine contractions and reduce postpartum bleeding, dilute drug by adding 10 units to 500 ml of normal saline, lactated Ringer's, or D₅W solution.
● Don't give bolus injection; use an infusion pump. Give drug only by piggyback infusion so that it may be stopped without interrupting I.V. line.
● **Incompatibilities:** Fibrinolysin (human), norepinephrine bitartrate, Normosol-M with dextrose 5%, plasmin, prochlorperazine, sodium bisulfite, warfarin sodium.
I.M.
● Drug isn't recommended for routine I.M. use, but 10 units may be given I.M. after delivery of placenta to control postpartum uterine bleeding.
● Never give drug simultaneously by more than one route.

ACTION
Causes potent and selective stimulation of uterine and mammary gland smooth muscle.

Route	Onset	Peak	Duration
I.V.	Immediate	Unknown	1 hr
I.M.	3–5 min	Unknown	2–3 hr

Half-life: 3 to 5 minutes.

ADVERSE REACTIONS
Maternal
CNS: *subarachnoid hemorrhage, seizures, coma.*
CV: *arrhythmias,* hypertension, increased heart rate, systemic venous return, and cardiac output.
GI: nausea, vomiting.
GU: *abruptio placentae,* tetanic uterine contractions, *postpartum hemorrhage, uterine rupture,* impaired uterine blood flow, pelvic hematoma, increased uterine motility.
Hematologic: *afibrinogenemia, possibly related to postpartum bleeding.*
Other: *anaphylaxis, death from oxytocin-induced water intoxication,* hypersensitivity reactions.
Fetal
CNS: *infant brain damage.*
CV: *bradycardia, arrhythmias,* PVCs.
EENT: neonatal retinal hemorrhage.
Hepatic: neonatal jaundice.
Respiratory: *anoxia, asphyxia.*
Other: *low Apgar scores at 5 minutes.*

INTERACTIONS
Drug-drug. *Cyclopropane anesthetics:* May cause less pronounced bradycardia and hypotension. Use together cautiously.
Thiopental anesthetics: May delay induction. Use together cautiously.
Vasoconstrictors: May cause severe hypertension if oxytocin is given within 3 to 4 hours of vasoconstrictor in patient receiving caudal block anesthetic. Avoid using together.

EFFECTS ON LAB TEST RESULTS
None reported.

CONTRAINDICATIONS & CAUTIONS
● Contraindicated in patients hypersensitive to drug.
● Contraindicated when vaginal delivery isn't advised (placenta previa, vasa previa, invasive cervical carcinoma, genital herpes), when cephalopelvic disproportion is present, or when delivery requires conversion, as in transverse lie.
● Contraindicated in fetal distress when delivery isn't imminent, in prematurity, in other obstetric emergencies, and in patients with severe toxemia or hypertonic uterine patterns.

• Use cautiously during first and second stages of labor because cervical laceration, uterine rupture, and maternal and fetal death have been reported.
• Use cautiously, if at all, in patients with invasive cervical cancer and in those with previous cervical or uterine surgery (including cesarean section), grand multi-parity, uterine sepsis, traumatic delivery, or overdistended uterus.

NURSING CONSIDERATIONS
■ **Black Box Warning** Drug is only indicated for the medical, rather than the elective, induction of labor. ■
• Drug is used to induce or reinforce labor only when pelvis is known to be adequate, when vaginal delivery is indicated, when fetal maturity is assured, and when fetal position is favorable. Use drug only in hospital where critical care facilities and prescriber are immediately available.
• Monitor fluid intake and output. Anti-diuretic effect may lead to fluid overload, seizures, and coma from water intoxication.
• Monitor and record uterine contractions, heart rate, blood pressure, intrauterine pressure, fetal heart rate, and character of blood loss every 15 minutes.
• Have 20% magnesium sulfate solution available to relax the myometrium.
• If contractions occur less than 2 minutes apart, exceed 50 mm, or last 90 seconds or longer, stop infusion, turn patient on her side, and notify prescriber.
• Drug doesn't cause fetal abnormalities when used as indicated.
• *Look alike–sound alike:* Don't confuse Pitocin with Pitressin.

PATIENT TEACHING
• Explain use and administration of drug to patient and family.
• Instruct patient to report adverse reactions promptly.

Reactions may be *common*, uncommon, *life-threatening*, or COMMON AND LIFE-THREATENING.
Interaction may have a *rapid onset* or **delayed onset.**

exenatide
glucagon
insulin (lispro)
insulin (regular)
insulin aspart (rDNA origin)
    injection
insulin aspart (rDNA origin)
    protamine suspension and
    insulin aspart (rDNA origin)
    injection
insulin detemir (rDNA origin)
    injection
insulin glargine (rDNA origin)
    injection
insulin glulisine (rDNA origin)
    injection
insulin lispro protamine and
    insulin lispro
isophane insulin suspension (NPH)
isophane insulin suspension and
    insulin injection combinations

SAFETY ALERT!

exenatide
eks-EHN-uh-tyde

Byetta

Pharmacologic class: incretin
mimetic
Pregnancy risk category C

AVAILABLE FORMS
Injection: 5 mcg/dose in 1.2-ml prefilled
pen (60 doses); 10 mcg/dose in 2.4-ml
prefilled pen (60 doses)

INDICATIONS & DOSAGES
➤ **Adjunctive therapy to improve
glycemic control in patients with
type 2 diabetes who take metformin,
a sulfonylurea, a thiazolidinedione,
a combination of metformin and a
sulfonylurea, or a combination of
metformin and a thiazolidinedione,
but who haven't achieved glycemic
control**
Adults: 5 mcg subcutaneously b.i.d. within
60 minutes before morning and evening
meals. If needed, increase to 10 mcg b.i.d.
after 1 month.

ADMINISTRATION
Subcutaneously
• Drug comes in two strengths; check
cartridge carefully before use.
• Give as a subcutaneous injection in the
thigh, abdomen, or upper arm.
• Before first use, store drug in refrigerator at 36° to 46° F (2° to 8° C). After first
use, drug can be kept at temperature up to
77° F (25° C). Don't freeze, and don't use
drug if it has been frozen. Protect drug
from light. Discard pen 30 days after first
use, even if some drug remains.

ACTION
Reduces fasting and postprandial glucose
levels in type 2 diabetes by stimulating
insulin production in response to elevated glucose levels, inhibiting glucagon
release after meals, and slowing gastric
emptying.

Route	Onset	Peak	Duration
Subcut.	Unknown	2 hr	Unknown

Half-life: 2½ hours.

ADVERSE REACTIONS
CNS: dizziness, headache, jittery feeling,
weakness.
GI: anorexia, *diarrhea,* dyspepsia, *nausea,
pancreatitis, vomiting.*
Metabolic: *hypoglycemia.*
Skin: excessive sweating, pruritus, urticaria,
rash.
Other: hypersensitivity reactions, injection
site reaction, *angioedema, anaphylaxis.*

INTERACTIONS
Drug-drug. *Acetaminophen:* May
decrease acetaminophen concentration.
Give acetaminophen 1 hour before
exenatide injection.
Digoxin, lisinopril, lovastatin: May
decrease concentrations of these drugs.
Monitor patient.
Drugs that are rapidly absorbed: May
slow gastric emptying and reduce

absorption of some oral drugs. Separate administration by 1 hour.
Oral drugs that need to maintain a threshold concentration to maintain effectiveness (antibiotics, hormonal contraceptives): May reduce rate and extent of absorption of these drugs. Give these drugs at least 1 hour before giving exenatide.
Sulfonylureas: May increase the risk of hypoglycemia. Reduce sulfonylurea dose as needed, and monitor patient closely.

EFFECTS ON LAB TEST RESULTS
None reported.

CONTRAINDICATIONS & CAUTIONS
• Contraindicated in patients hypersensitive to drug or its components.
• Don't use in patients with type 1 diabetes or diabetic ketoacidosis.
• Don't use in patients with end-stage renal disease, creatinine clearance less than 30 ml/minute, or severe GI disease (including gastroparesis).
• Use cautiously in pregnant or breast-feeding women.

NURSING CONSIDERATIONS
• Assess GI function before and during treatment.
• Monitor glucose level regularly and glycosylated hemoglobin level periodically.
• *Alert:* Stop drug if pancreatitis is suspected. Initiate appropriate treatment and monitor patient carefully. Byetta should not be readministered.
• *Look alike–sound alike:* Don't confuse exenatide with ezetimibe.

PATIENT TEACHING
• Explain the risks of drug.
• Review proper use and storage of dosage pen, particularly the one-time setup for each new pen.
• Inform patient that prefilled pen doesn't include a needle; explain which needle length and gauge is appropriate.
• Instruct patient to inject drug in the thigh, abdomen, or upper arm within 60 minutes before morning and evening meals. Caution against injecting drug after a meal.
• Advise patient that drug may decrease appetite, food intake, and body weight, and that these changes don't warrant a change in dosage.

• Advise patient to seek immediate medical care if unexplained, persistent, severe abdominal pain, with or without vomiting, occurs.
• Review steps for managing hypoglycemia, especially if patient takes a sulfonylurea.
• Stress importance of proper storage (refrigerated), infection prevention, and timing of exenatide dose in relation to other oral drugs.
• Tell patient that if a dose is missed, resume treatment as prescribed with the next scheduled dose.

glucagon
GLOO-ka-gon

GlucaGen Diagnostic Kit, GlucaGen HypoKit, Glucagon Emergency Kit

Pharmacologic class: antihypoglycemic
Pregnancy risk category B

AVAILABLE FORMS
Powder for injection: 1-mg (1-unit) vial

INDICATIONS & DOSAGES
➤ **Hypoglycemia**
Glucagon
Adults and children who weigh more than 20 kg (44 lb) or older than 6 to 8 years: 1 mg (1 unit) I.V., I.M., or subcutaneously.
Children who weigh 20 kg or less: 0.5 mg (0.5 units) or 20 to 30 mcg/kg I.V., I.M., or subcutaneously; maximum dose 1 mg. May repeat in 15 minutes, if needed. I.V. glucose must be given if patient fails to respond.
GlucaGen
Adults and children (more than 25 kg or older than 6 to 8 years and weight is unknown): 1 ml I.V., I.M., or subcutaneously.
Children (less than 25 kg or younger than 6 to 8 years and weight is unknown): 0.5 ml I.V., I.M., or subcutaneously.
➤ **Diagnostic aid for radiologic examination**
Adults: 0.25 to 2 mg I.V. or 1 to 2 mg I.M. before radiologic examination.

ADMINISTRATION
I.V.
- Reconstitute drug in 1-unit vial with 1 ml of diluent.
- Use only diluent supplied by manufacturer when preparing doses of 2 mg or less. For larger doses, dilute with sterile water for injection.
- Unstable hypoglycemic diabetic patients may not respond to glucagon; give dextrose I.V. instead.
- Store at room temperature before reconstituting. Avoid freezing and protect from light. After reconstitution, use immediately.
- **Incompatibilities:** Sodium chloride solution, solutions with pH 3 to 9.5.
I.M.
- Store at room temperature before reconstituting. Avoid freezing and protect from light. After reconstitution, use immediately.
Subcutaneously
- Store at room temperature before reconstituting. Avoid freezing and protect from light. After reconstitution, use immediately.

ACTION
Raises glucose level by promoting catalytic depolymerization of hepatic glycogen to glucose. Relaxes the smooth muscle of the stomach, duodenum, small bowel, and colon.

Route	Onset	Peak	Duration
I.V. (hypo-glycemia)	Immediate	30 min	60–90 min
I.V. (gastric relaxation)	1 min	30 min	9–25 min
I.M.	4–10 min	13 min	12–32 min
Subcut.	4–10 min	20 min	12–32 min

Half-life: 8 to 18 minutes.

ADVERSE REACTIONS
CV: hypotension.
GI: nausea, vomiting.
Respiratory: *bronchospasm, respiratory distress.*
Other: hypersensitivity reactions.

INTERACTIONS
Drug-drug. *Anticoagulants:* May enhance anticoagulant effect. Monitor prothrombin activity, and watch for signs of bleeding.

EFFECTS ON LAB TEST RESULTS
- May decrease potassium level.

CONTRAINDICATIONS & CAUTIONS
- Contraindicated in patients hypersensitive to drug and in those with pheochromocytoma.
- Use cautiously in patients with history of insulinoma or pheochromocytoma.

NURSING CONSIDERATIONS
- For hypoglycemia, use drug only in emergency situations.
- Monitor glucose level before, during, and after administration.
- *Alert:* Arouse patient from coma as quickly as possible, and give additional carbohydrates orally to prevent secondary hypoglycemic reactions.

PATIENT TEACHING
- Instruct patient and caregivers how to give glucagon and recognize a low glucose episode.
- Explain importance of calling prescriber immediately in emergencies.
- Teach patient and caregivers how to prevent hypoglycemia.

SAFETY ALERT!

insulin aspart (rDNA origin) injection
IN-su-lin AS-part

NovoLog, NovoRapid†

insulin aspart (rDNA origin) protamine suspension and insulin aspart (rDNA origin) injection
NovoLog Mix 70/30, NovoLog Mix 50/50

Pharmacologic class: human insulin analog
Pregnancy risk category B

AVAILABLE FORMS
PenFill cartridges: 3 ml (100 units/ml)
Prefilled syringes: 3 ml (100 units/ml)

Vial: 10 ml, containing 100 units of insulin aspart per ml (U-100)

INDICATIONS & DOSAGES
➤ Control of hyperglycemia in patients with diabetes
NovoLog
Adults and children age 2 and older:
Dosage is highly individualized. Typical daily insulin requirement is 0.5 to 1 unit/kg/day, divided in a meal-related treatment regimen. About 50% to 70% of dose is provided with NovoLog and the remainder by an intermediate- or long-acting insulin. Give 5 to 10 minutes before start of meal by subcutaneous injection in the abdominal wall, thigh, or upper arm.
External insulin infusion pumps (adults and children age 4 and older): initially, based on the total daily insulin dose of the previous regimen. Usually 50% of the total dose is given as meal-related boluses, and the remainder as basal infusion. Adjust dose if needed.

NovoLog Mix 70/30
Adults: Dosage is individualized based on the needs of the patient. Doses are usually given twice daily within 15 minutes of meals.

NovoLog Mix 50/50
Adults: Dosage is individualized based on the needs of the patient. Doses may be administered up to three times daily within 15 minutes of meal initiation.

ADMINISTRATION
Subcutaneous
● Inspect insulin vials before use. NovoLog is a clear, colorless solution. It should not contain particulate matter or be cloudy, viscous, or discolored. NovoLog Mix 70/30 and NovoLog Mix 50/50 should be uniformly white and cloudy and should not contain particulate matter or be discolored.
● Give NovoLog 5 to 10 minutes before start of meal. Give NovoLog Mix 70/30 and NovoLog Mix 50/50 up to 15 minutes before start of meal. Because of its rapid onset of action and short duration of action, patients also may need longer-acting insulins to prevent hyperglycemia.

● Let insulin warm to room temperature before giving to minimize discomfort. Give by subcutaneous injection into the abdominal wall, thigh, or upper arm. Rotate sites to minimize lipodystrophies.
● When giving and mixing NovoLog with NPH human insulin, draw up NovoLog into syringe first and give immediately after dose is drawn up.
● Store drug between 36° and 46° F (2° and 8° C). Don't freeze. Don't expose vials to excessive heat or sunlight. Opened vials of NovoLog Mix 70/30 and opened vials and cartridges of NovoLog are stable at room temperature for 28 days. Unopened cartridges of NovoLog Mix 50/50 are stable at room temperature for 14 days; if refrigerated, they are stable until the expiration date. Punctured cartridges of NovoLog Mix 70/30 and NovoLog Mix 50/50 may be stored at room temperature up to 14 days; don't refrigerate punctured cartridges.
Subcutaneous
External insulin pump
● Don't dilute or mix insulin aspart with any other insulin when using an external insulin pump.
● Insulin aspart is recommended for use with Disetronic H-TRON plus V100 with Disetronic 3.15 plastic cartridges and Classic or Tender infusion sets, Polyfin or Sof-set infusion sets, and MiniMed Models 505, 506, and 507 with MiniMed 3-ml syringes.
● Replace infusion sets, insulin aspart in the reservoir, and choose a new infusion site every 48 hours or less to avoid insulin degradation and infusion set malfunction.
● Discard insulin exposed to temperatures higher than 98.6° F (37° C). The temperature of the insulin may exceed ambient temperature when the pump housing, cover, tubing, or sport case is exposed to sunlight or radiant heat.
I.V.
● NovoLog may also be given as an I.V. infusion with close medical monitoring of glucose and potassium levels. Using a polypropylene bag, dilute insulin aspart to a concentration of 0.05 to 1 unit/ml in normal saline solution, D_5W, or 10% dextrose injection with 40 mEq/L of potassium chloride.
● *Alert:* Don't give 70/30 or 50/50 form I.V.

Reactions may be *common*, uncommon, *life-threatening*, or COMMON AND LIFE-THREATENING.
Interaction may have a *rapid onset* or **delayed onset**.

ACTION
Regulates glucose metabolism. It has the same glucose-lowering effect as regular human insulin, but its effect is more rapid and of shorter duration.

Route	Onset	Peak	Duration
I.V.	Immediate	Unknown	3–5 hr
Subcut.	15 min	1–3 hr	3–5 hr
Subcut. (70/30)	Rapid	1–4 hr	≤ 24 hr

Half-life: 81 minutes.

ADVERSE REACTIONS
Metabolic: *hypoglycemia,* hypokalemia.
Skin: injection site reactions, lipodystrophy, pruritus, rash.
Other: *allergic reactions.*

INTERACTIONS
Drug-drug. *ACE inhibitors, disopyramide, fibrates, fluoxetine, oral antidiabetics, propoxyphene, salicylates, somatostatin analogue (octreotide), sulfonamide antibiotics:* May enhance the glucose-lowering effect of insulin and may potentiate hypoglycemia. Monitor glucose level, and watch for signs and symptoms of hypoglycemia. May need insulin dose adjustment.
Beta blockers, clonidine: May increase or decrease the glucose-lowering effect of insulin and cause hypoglycemia or hyperglycemia. May reduce or mask symptoms of hypoglycemia. Monitor glucose level.
Corticosteroids, danazol, diuretics, estrogens, isoniazid, niacin, phenothiazine derivatives, progestins (as in hormonal contraceptives), somatropin, sympathomimetics (epinephrine, salbutamol, terbutaline), thyroid hormones: May decrease the glucose-lowering effect of insulin and cause hyperglycemia. Monitor glucose level. May require insulin dose adjustment.
Crystalline zinc preparations: May be incompatible with NovoLog. Don't mix together.
Guanethidine, reserpine: May reduce or mask symptoms of hypoglycemia. Monitor glucose level.
Lithium salts, pentamidine: May increase or decrease glucose-lowering effect of insulin and may cause hypoglycemia or hyperglycemia. Pentamidine may cause hypoglycemia, sometimes

followed by hyperglycemia. Monitor glucose level.
MAO inhibitors: May increase insulin's effects. Monitor patient and glucose level closely.
Drug-herb. *Burdock, dandelion, eucalyptus, marshmallow:* May increase drug's effects. Discourage use together.
Drug-lifestyle. *Alcohol use:* May increase or decrease drug effect, causing hypoglycemia or hyperglycemia. Advise patient to monitor glucose level.
Exercise: May alter the need for drug, requiring dose adjustment. Advise patient to report changes in physical activity.
Marijuana use: May increase glucose level. Inform patient of this interaction.
Smoking: May increase glucose level and decrease response to insulin. Monitor glucose level.

EFFECTS ON LAB TEST RESULTS
● May increase alkaline phosphatase level. May decrease glucose and potassium levels.

CONTRAINDICATIONS & CAUTIONS
● Contraindicated during episodes of hypoglycemia and in patients hypersensitive to NovoLog or one of its components.
● Use cautiously in patients susceptible to hypoglycemia and hypokalemia, such as those who have autonomic neuropathy or are fasting, taking potassium-lowering drugs, or taking drugs sensitive to potassium level.

NURSING CONSIDERATIONS
● The time course of NovoLog action may vary among people or at different times in the same person and depends on the site of injection, blood supply, temperature, and physical activity.
● Adjustments in the dose of NovoLog or of any insulin may be needed with changes in physical activity or meal routine. Insulin requirements also may be altered during emotional disturbances, illness, or other stresses.
● Adjust dose regularly, according to patient's glucose measurements. Monitor glucose level regularly.
● *Look alike–sound alike:* Don't confuse NovoLog Mix 70/30 with Novolin 70/30.

• Periodically monitor glycosylated hemoglobin level.

• Assess patient for rash (including pruritus) over whole body, shortness of breath, wheezing, hypotension, rapid pulse, or sweating, which may signify a generalized allergy to insulin. Severe cases, including anaphylactic reactions, may be life-threatening.

• Patients with renal dysfunction and hepatic impairment may need close glucose monitoring and dose adjustments of NovoLog.

• Observe injection sites for reactions, such as redness, swelling, itching, or burning. These reactions should resolve within a few days to a few weeks.

• Assess patient and notify prescriber for signs and symptoms of hypoglycemia (sweating, shaking, trembling, confusion, headache, irritability, hunger, rapid pulse, nausea) and hyperglycemia (drowsiness, fruity breath odor, frequent urination, thirst).

• Symptoms of hypoglycemia may occur in patients with diabetes, regardless of glucose value.

• Patients with long duration of diabetes, diabetic nerve disease, or intensified diabetes control may have different or less-pronounced early warning symptoms of hypoglycemia; severe hypoglycemia may occur in such patients with virtually no warning.

For external pump use with NovoLog

• Monitor patient with an external insulin pump for erythematous, pruritic, or thickened skin at injection site.

• *Alert:* Pump or infusion set malfunctions or insulin degradation can lead to hyperglycemia and ketosis in a short time because there's a subcutaneous depot of fast-acting insulin.

• Teach patient how to properly use the external insulin pump.

PATIENT TEACHING

• Tell patient not to stop insulin therapy without medical approval.

• Advise patient of the warning signs of low glucose level (shaking, sweating, moodiness, irritability, confusion, or agitation). Tell patient to carry sugar (candy, sugar packets) to counteract low glucose level.

• Instruct patient to roll the cartridge or pen between his palms 10 times before inserting the NovoLog Penfill cartridge into a compatible delivery device or using the NovoLog FlexPen. Then, to turn the device upside down so the glass ball inside the cartridge or pen travels the length of the cartridge and to repeat this rolling and turning technique at least 10 times until the suspension is uniformly white and cloudy.

• Teach patient proper insulin injection technique and importance of timing dose to meals and adhering to meal plans.

• Tell patient to report swelling, redness, and itching at injection site, and instruct patient on the importance of rotating injection sites to avoid lipodystrophies.

• Instruct patient on correct use of injection pen, if indicated.

• Instruct patient to use the same brand of insulin, especially if mixing insulin. Changing brands of insulin may necessitate dosage changes.

• Tell patient not to dilute or mix insulin aspart with any other insulin when using an external insulin pump.

• Instruct patient to monitor glucose level regularly.

• Advise patient to avoid vigorous exercise immediately after insulin injection, especially of the area where injection was given; it causes increased absorption and increased risk of low glucose level.

• Advise patient to store insulin at 36° to 46° F (2° to 8° C), and avoid freezing or excessive heat or sunlight.

• Advise woman to notify prescriber about planned, suspected, or known pregnancy.

• Urge patient to carry medical identification at all times.

• Instruct patient about the importance of diet and exercise. Explain long-term complications of diabetes and the importance of yearly eye and foot examinations.

Reactions may be *common*, uncommon, *life-threatening*, or COMMON AND LIFE-THREATENING. Interaction may have a *rapid onset* or **delayed onset**.

insulin detemir (rDNA origin) injection
IN-su-lin DEH-teh-meer

Levemir

Pharmacologic class: insulin analog
Pregnancy risk category C

AVAILABLE FORMS
Injection: 100 units/ml in 10-ml vials,
3-ml cartridges (PenFill), 3-ml prefilled
syringes (InnoLet, FlexPen)

INDICATIONS & DOSAGES
➤ **Hyperglycemia in patients with
diabetes mellitus who need basal
(long-acting) insulin**
Adults and children age 6 and older: Base
dosage on patient response and glucose
level. In insulin-naive patients with type 2
diabetes, start with 0.1 to 0.2 units/kg
subcutaneously once daily in the evening
or 10 units once or twice daily based on
glucose level. Patients with type 1 or
2 diabetes already receiving basal-bolus
treatment or basal insulin may switch to
this drug on a unit-for-unit basis, adjusted
to glycemic target.

ADMINISTRATION
Subcutaneous
● *Alert:* Don't give I.V. or I.M.
● *Alert:* Don't mix or dilute with other
insulins.
● Give by subcutaneous injection in the
thigh, abdominal wall, or upper arm.
Rotate injection sites within the same
region.
● Store unused insulin detemir between
36° and 46° F (2° and 8° C). Don't freeze.
Don't use insulin detemir if it has been
frozen.
● After initial use, store vials in
a refrigerator, never in a freezer.
If refrigeration isn't possible, keep
in-use vial unrefrigerated at room
temperature, below 86° F (30° C),
for up to 42 days. Keep vial as cool
as possible, away from direct heat
and light.
● After initial use, a cartridge or prefilled
syringe may be used for up to 42 days if

kept at room temperature, below 86° F
(30° C). Don't store in-use cartridges and
prefilled syringes in a refrigerator or with
the needle in place. Keep all cartridges
and prefilled syringes away from direct
heat and sunlight. Unopened cartridges
and prefilled syringes can be used until
the expiration date printed on the label
if they're stored in a refrigerator. Keep
unused cartridges and prefilled syringes
in the carton so they'll stay clean and
protected from light.

ACTION
Regulates glucose metabolism by binding
to insulin receptors, facilitating cellular
uptake of glucose into muscle and fat, and
inhibiting release of glucose from liver.

Route	Onset	Peak	Duration
Subcut.	Unknown	6–8 hr	6–23 hr

Half-life: 5 to 7 hours.

ADVERSE REACTIONS
CV: edema.
Metabolic: HYPOGLYCEMIA, sodium
retention, *weight gain.*
Skin: injection site reactions, lipodystro-
phy, pruritus, rash.
Other: *allergic reactions.*

INTERACTIONS
Drug-drug. *ACE inhibitors, antidiabetic
drugs, disopyramide, fibrates, fluoxetine,*
MAO inhibitors, *octreotide, propoxyphene,
salicylates, sulfonamides:* May increase
the glucose-lowering effect of insulin and
risk of hypoglycemia. Monitor glucose
level carefully.
*Beta blockers, clonidine, guanethidine,
reserpine:* May decrease or conceal signs
of hypoglycemia. Avoid using together, if
possible.
Clonidine, lithium salts: May increase
or decrease glucose-lowering effect of
insulin. Monitor glucose level carefully.
*Corticosteroids, danazol, diuretics,
estrogens, isoniazid, phenothiazines,
progestogens, somatropin, sympathomimetics, thyroid hormones:* May decrease
glucose-lowering effect of insulin. Monitor
glucose level carefully.
Other insulins: May alter the action of one
or both insulins if mixed together. Don't
mix or dilute insulin detemir with other

insulins.
Pentamidine: May cause initial hypoglycemia followed by hyperglycemia. Use together cautiously.
Drug-lifestyle. *Alcohol use:* May increase or decrease effect of drug. Discourage use together.

EFFECTS ON LAB TEST RESULTS
• May decrease glucose level.

CONTRAINDICATIONS & CAUTIONS
• Contraindicated in patients hypersensitive to drug or its components. Don't give drug with an insulin infusion pump.
• Use cautiously in patients with hepatic or renal impairment; they may need dosage adjustment.

NURSING CONSIDERATIONS
• Monitor glucose level routinely in all patients receiving insulin.
• Measure patient's glycosylated hemoglobin level periodically.
• Watch for hyperglycemia, especially if patient's diet or exercise pattern changes.
• Assess patient for signs and symptoms of hypoglycemia. Insulin doses may need adjustment.
• Early warning symptoms of hypoglycemia may be less pronounced in patients who take beta blockers and those with longstanding diabetes, diabetic nerve disease, or intensified diabetes control. Monitor glucose level closely in these patients because severe hypoglycemia could develop before symptoms do.
• Insulin requirements may be altered during illness, emotional disturbance, or stress, or if patient changes his usual meal plan or exercise level.
• Starting dosage, increments of change, and maintenance dosage should be conservative in elderly patients as hypoglycemia may be harder to recognize.

PATIENT TEACHING
• Teach diabetes management, including glucose monitoring, injection techniques, and continuous rotation of injection sites.
• *Alert:* Urge patient not to mix with any other insulin or solution.
• Instruct patient to use only solution that's clear and colorless, with no visible particles.

• Tell patient to recognize and report signs and symptoms of hyperglycemia, such as nausea, vomiting, drowsiness, flushed dry skin, dry mouth, increased urination, thirst, and loss of appetite.
• Urge patient to check glucose level often to achieve control and avoid hyperglycemia and hypoglycemia.
• Teach patient to recognize and report signs and symptoms of hypoglycemia, such as sweating, dizziness, lightheadedness, headache, drowsiness, and irritability.
• Advise patient to carry a quick source of simple sugar, such as hard candy or glucose tablets, in case of hypoglycemia.
• Caution patient not to stop insulin abruptly or change the amount or type of insulin used without consulting prescriber.
• Advise patient to avoid alcohol because it lowers the glucose level.
• Caution woman to consult prescriber before trying to become pregnant.
• Tell patient to store unused vials, cartridges, and prefilled syringes in the refrigerator at 36° to 46° F (2° to 8° C).
• After initial use, vials may be refrigerated or stored at room temperature, below 86° F (30° C), away from direct heat and light, for up to 42 days. Cartridges or prefilled syringes may be stored at room temperature, below 86° F (30° C). Tell patient not to store or refrigerate insulin with a needle in place.
• Caution against freezing drug and against using drug that has been frozen.

SAFETY ALERT!

insulin glargine (rDNA origin) injection
IN-su-lin GLAR-gene

Lantus

Pharmacologic class: pancreatic hormone
Pregnancy risk category C

AVAILABLE FORMS
Injection: 100 units/ml in 10-ml vials, 3-ml cartridge (OptiClik), 3-ml disposable insulin device (SoloStar)

Reactions may be *common,* uncommon, *life-threatening,* or COMMON AND LIFE-THREATENING.
Interaction may have a *rapid onset* or **delayed onset.**

INDICATIONS & DOSAGES
➤ **To manage type 1 (insulin-dependent) diabetes in patients who need basal (long-acting) insulin to control hyperglycemia**
Adults and children age 6 and older:
Individualize dosage, and give subcutaneously once daily at the same time each day.
➤ **To manage type 2 (non-insulin-dependent) diabetes in patients who need basal (long-acting) insulin to control hyperglycemia**
Adults: Individualize dosage, and give subcutaneously once daily at the same time each day. If patient is insulin-naive, start with 10 units subcutaneously daily. Adjust dose to patient response.

ADMINISTRATION
Subcutaneous
● *Alert:* Don't give I.V.
● *Alert:* Don't mix or dilute with other insulins or solutions.
● Rotate injection sites with each dose.
● Store unopened insulin vials and 3-ml cartridge system in the refrigerator; opened vials may be stored at 86° F (30° C) or less and away from direct heat. Discard opened vials or cartridge system after 28 days whether refrigerated or not. Don't freeze or refrigerate the open, in-use cartridge system if inserted in OptiClik.

ACTION
Reduces glucose level by stimulating peripheral glucose uptake, especially by skeletal muscle and fat, and by inhibiting hepatic glucose production.

Route	Onset	Peak	Duration
Subcut.	1 hr	None	24 hr

Half-life: Unknown.

ADVERSE REACTIONS
Metabolic: *hypoglycemia.*
Skin: lipodystrophy, pruritus, rash.
Other: allergic reactions, pain at injection site.

INTERACTIONS
Drug-drug. *ACE inhibitors, disopyramide, fibrates, fluoxetine,* **MAO inhibitors,** *octreotide, oral antidiabetics, propoxyphene, salicylates, sulfonamide antibiotics:* May cause hypoglycemia and increase insulin effect. Monitor glucose level. May need to adjust dosage of insulin glargine.
Beta blockers, clonidine: May mask signs of hypoglycemia and may either increase or reduce insulin's glucose-lowering effect. Avoid using together, if possible. If used together, monitor glucose level carefully.
Corticosteroids, danazol, diuretics, estrogens, isoniazid, phenothiazines (such as prochlorperazine, promethazine hydrochloride), progestins (such as hormonal contraceptives), somatropin, sympathomimetics (such as albuterol, epinephrine, terbutaline), thyroid hormones: May reduce the glucose-lowering effect of insulin. Monitor glucose level. May need to adjust dosage of insulin glargine.
Guanethidine, reserpine: May mask the signs of hypoglycemia. Avoid using together, if possible. Monitor glucose level carefully.
Lithium: May either increase or decrease the glucose-lowering effect of insulin. Monitor glucose level. May require dosage adjustments of insulin glargine.
Pentamidine: May cause hypoglycemia, which may be followed by hyperglycemia. Avoid using together, if possible.
Drug-herb. *Burdock, dandelion, eucalyptus, marshmallow:* May increase hypoglycemic effects. Discourage use together.
Licorice root: May increase dosage requirements of insulin. Discourage use together.
Drug-lifestyle. *Alcohol use, emotional stress:* May increase or decrease the glucose-lowering effect of insulin. Advise patient to self-monitor glucose level.

EFFECTS ON LAB TEST RESULTS
● May decrease glucose level.

CONTRAINDICATIONS & CAUTIONS
● Contraindicated during hypoglycemic episodes and in patients hypersensitive to drug or its components.
● Use cautiously in patients with renal or hepatic impairment.

NURSING CONSIDERATIONS
● Because of prolonged duration, this isn't the insulin of choice for diabetic ketoacidosis.

• The rate of absorption, onset, and duration of action may be affected by exercise and other variables, such as illness and emotional stress.

• As with any insulin therapy, lipodystrophy may occur at the injection site and delay insulin absorption. Reduce this risk by rotating the injection site with each injection.

• Hypoglycemia is the most common adverse effect of insulin. Early symptoms may be different or less pronounced in patients with long duration of diabetes, diabetic nerve disease, or intensified diabetes control. Monitor glucose level closely in these patients because severe hypoglycemia may result before the patient develops symptoms.

• *Look alike–sound alike:* Don't confuse Lente with Lantus.

PATIENT TEACHING

• Teach proper glucose monitoring, injection techniques, and diabetes management.

• Tell patient to take dose once daily at the same time each day.

• *Alert:* Educate diabetic patients about signs and symptoms of low glucose level, such as fatigue, weakness, confusion, headache, pallor, and profuse sweating.

• Urge patient to wear or carry medical identification at all times.

• Advise patient to treat mild hypoglycemia with oral glucose tablets. Encourage patient to always carry glucose tablets in case of a low-glucose episode.

• Educate patients on the importance of maintaining prescribed diet, and explain that adjustments in drug dosage, meal patterns, and exercise may be needed to regulate glucose.

• *Alert:* Advise patient not to dilute or mix any other insulin or solution with insulin glargine. If the solution is cloudy, urge patient to discard the vial. Use solution only if it's clear and colorless.

• *Alert:* Make any change of insulin cautiously and only under medical supervision. Changes in insulin type, strength, manufacturer, type (such as regular, NPH, or insulin analogues), species (animal, human), or method of manufacturer (rDNA versus animal source insulin) may require a change in dosage. Oral

antidiabetic treatment taken at the same time may need to be adjusted.

• Tell patient to consult prescriber before using OTC medications.

• Inform patient to avoid alcohol, which lowers glucose level.

• Advise patient to avoid vigorous exercise immediately after insulin injection, especially of the area where injection was given; it causes increased absorption and increased risk of low glucose.

• Advise woman planning pregnancy to first consult prescriber.

• Advise patient that if OptiClik device malfunctions, drug may be drawn from the cartridge system into a U-100 syringe and injected.

• Advise patient on proper drug storage: store unopened insulin vials and 3-ml cartridge system in the refrigerator, opened vials may be stored at 86° F (30° C) or less and away from direct heat, discard opened vials or cartridge system after 28 days whether refrigerated or not, and don't freeze or refrigerate the open, in-use cartridge system if inserted in OptiClik.

SAFETY ALERT!

insulin glulisine (rDNA origin) injection
IN-su-lin GLUE-lih-seen

Apidra

Pharmacologic class: human insulin analog
Pregnancy risk category C

AVAILABLE FORMS
Injection: 100 units/ml in 10-ml vial or 3-ml cartridge (OptiClik)

INDICATIONS & DOSAGES
➤ **Diabetes mellitus**
Adults and children age 4 and older: Individualize dosage. Give by subcutaneous injection within 15 minutes before a meal. If regimen also includes a longer-acting insulin or basal insulin analogue, give within 20 minutes after meal starts. Or, give drug as continuous subcutaneous infusion using an external

infusion pump. Or, drug may be given I.V. under strict medical supervision with close monitoring of blood glucose and potassium levels.

ADMINISTRATION
Subcutaneous
● **Alert:** Drug has a more rapid onset and shorter duration of action than regular human insulin. Give within 15 minutes before or within 20 minutes after the start of a meal.
● Don't mix drug in a syringe with any other insulin except NPH.
● When used in an external subcutaneous infusion pump, don't mix drug with any other insulin or diluent.
● Store unopened vials in the refrigerator and opened vials in the refrigerator or below 77° F (25° C). Use opened vials within 28 days. Infusion bags are stable at room temperature for 48 hours. Protect from direct heat and light.
I.V.
● Use at a concentration of insulin glulisine 1 unit/ml in infusion systems with the infusion fluid, sterile 0.9% sodium chloride solution, using polyvinyl chloride (PVC) Viaflex infusion bags and PVC tubing (Clearlink system Continu-Flo solution set) with a dedicated infusion line. The use of other bags and tubing hasn't been studied.

ACTION
Lowers glucose level by increasing peripheral glucose uptake and decreasing hepatic glucose production. When drug is given by subcutaneous injection, onset of action is more rapid and duration of action shorter than those of regular human insulin.

Route	Onset	Peak	Duration
I.V.	Immediate	Unknown	Unknown
Subcut.	15 min	55 min	Unknown

Half-life: 13 minutes (I.V.), 42 minutes (Subcut.)

ADVERSE REACTIONS
Metabolic: *hypoglycemia.*
Skin: *injection site reactions,* lipodystrophy, pruritus, rash.
Other: allergic reactions, *anaphylaxis,* insulin antibody production.

INTERACTIONS
Drug-drug. *ACE inhibitors, disopyramide, fibrates, fluoxetine,* **MAO inhibitors,** *oral antidiabetics, pentoxifylline, propoxyphene, salicylates, sulfonamide antibiotics:* May increase glucose-lowering effects. Monitor glucose level, and watch for evidence of hypoglycemia.
Beta blockers, clonidine, lithium, pentamidine: May cause unpredictable response to insulin. Use together cautiously; monitor patient closely.
Clozapine, corticosteroids, danazol, diazoxide, diuretics, estrogens, glucagons, isoniazid, olanzapine, phenothiazines, progestogens, protease inhibitors, somatropin, sympathomimetics (such as epinephrine, albuterol, and terbutaline), thyroid hormone: May decrease glucose-lowering effects. Monitor glucose level carefully.
Drug-lifestyle. *Alcohol:* May potentiate or reduce insulin effects, resulting in either hypoglycemia or hyperglycemia. Discourage alcohol use.

EFFECTS ON LAB TEST RESULTS
● May decrease glucose level.

CONTRAINDICATIONS & CAUTIONS
● Contraindicated during periods of hypoglycemia and in patients hypersensitive to insulin glulisine or one of its ingredients.
● Use cautiously in patients with impaired renal or hepatic function and in pregnant or breast-feeding women.

NURSING CONSIDERATIONS
● Use with a longer-acting or basal insulin analogue.
● Changes in insulin strength, manufacturer, type, or species may cause a need for dosage adjustment.
● Changes in physical activity or usual meal plan may cause a need for dosage adjustment.
● Insulin requirements may be altered during illness, emotional disturbances, or stress.
● Early warning signs of hypoglycemia may be different or less pronounced in patients who take beta blockers, who have had an oral antidiabetic added to the

regimen, or who have long-term diabetes or diabetic nerve disease.
• Monitor patient for lipodystrophy at injection site; it may delay insulin absorption.
• Redness, swelling, or itching may occur at injection site.

PATIENT TEACHING
• Tell patient to take drug within 15 minutes before starting a meal to 20 minutes after starting a meal, depending on regimen.
• Teach patient how to give subcutaneous insulin injections.
• Tell patient not to mix insulin glulisine in a syringe with any insulin other than NPH.
• If patient is mixing insulin glulisine with NPH, tell patient to use U-100 syringes, to draw insulin glulisine into the syringe first, followed by NPH insulin, and to inject the mixture immediately.
• Instruct patient to rotate injection sites to avoid injection-site reactions.
• If patient is using an external infusion pump, teach proper use of the device. Tell patient not to mix insulin glulisine with any other insulin or diluents. Instruct patient to change the infusion set, reservoir with insulin, and infusion site at least every 48 hours.
• Teach patient the signs and symptoms of hypoglycemia (sweating, rapid pulse, trembling, confusion, headache, irritability, and nausea). Advise the patient to treat these symptoms by eating or drinking something containing sugar.
• Instruct the patient to contact a health care provider for possible dosage adjustments if hypoglycemia occurs frequently.
• Show patient how to monitor and log glucose levels to evaluate diabetes control.
• Explain the possible long-term complications of diabetes and the importance of regular preventive therapy. Urge patient to follow prescribed diet and exercise regimen. To further reduce the risk of heart disease, encourage patient to stop smoking and lose weight.
• Instruct patient to carry medical identification showing that he has diabetes.
• Tell patient to store unopened vials in the refrigerator and opened vials in the refrigerator or below 77° F (25° C). Opened vials should be used within 28 days. Protect from direct heat and light.

SAFETY ALERT!

insulin (regular)
IN-su-lin

Humulin R ◇ , Humulin R Regular U-500 (concentrated), Novolin R ◇ , Novolin R PenFill ◇ , Novolin R Prefilled ◇

insulin (lispro)
Humalog

insulin lispro protamine and insulin lispro
Humalog Mix 75/25, Humalog Mix 50/50

isophane insulin suspension (NPH)
Humulin N ◇ , Novolin N ◇ , Novolin N PenFill ◇ , Novolin N Prefilled ◇

isophane insulin suspension and insulin injection combinations
Humulin 50/50 ◇ , Humulin 70/30 ◇ , Novolin 70/30 ◇ , Novolin 70/30 PenFill ◇ , Novolin 70/30 Prefilled ◇

Pharmacologic class: pancreatic hormone
Pregnancy risk category B

AVAILABLE FORMS
Available without a prescription
insulin (regular)
Injection (human): 100 units/ml (Humulin R, Novolin R, Novolin R PenFill, Novolin R Prefilled)
isophane insulin suspension (NPH)
Injection (human): 100 units/ml (Humulin N, Novolin N, Novolin N PenFill, Novolin N Prefilled)
isophane insulin suspension and insulin injection combinations
Injection (human): 100 units/ml (Humulin 50/50, Humulin 70/30, Novolin 70/30, Novolin 70/30 PenFill, Novolin 70/30 Prefilled)
Available by prescription only
insulin (regular)
Injection (human): 500 units/ml (Humulin R Regular U-500 [concentrated])

Reactions may be *common,* uncommon, *life-threatening,* or COMMON AND LIFE-THREATENING.
Interaction may have a *rapid onset* or **delayed onset.**

insulin (lispro)
Injection (human): 100 units/ml (Humalog)
insulin lispro protamine and insulin
lispro
Injection (human): 100 units/ml (Humalog
Mix 75/25, Humalog Mix 50/50)

INDICATIONS & DOSAGES
➤ **Moderate to severe diabetic
ketoacidosis or hyperosmolar
hyperglycemia**
regular insulin
Adults older than age 20: Loading dose of
0.15 units/kg I.V. by direct injection, followed by 0.1 unit/kg/hour as a continuous
infusion. If glucose level doesn't fall by
50 mg/dl in the first hour, double the
insulin infusion rate every hour until
glucose level decreases steadily by 50 to
75 mg/dl. Decrease rate of insulin infusion
to 0.05 to 0.1 unit/kg/hour when glucose
level reaches 250 to 300 mg/dl. Start infusion of D_5W in half-normal saline solution
separately from the insulin infusion when
glucose level is 150 to 200 mg/dl in
patients with diabetic ketoacidosis or 250
to 300 mg/dl in those with hyperosmolar
hyperglycemia. Give dose of insulin subcutaneously 1 to 2 hours before stopping
insulin infusion (intermediate-acting
insulin is recommended).
Adults and children age 20 and younger:
Loading dose isn't recommended. Begin
therapy at 0.1 unit/kg/hour I.V. infusion.
After condition improves, decrease rate of
insulin infusion to 0.05 unit/kg/hour. Start
infusion of D_5W in half-normal saline
solution separately from the insulin
infusion when glucose level is 250 mg/dl.
➤ **Mild diabetic ketoacidosis**
regular insulin
Adults older than age 20: Loading dose
of 0.4 to 0.6 unit/kg divided in two
equal parts, with half the dose given
by direct I.V. injection and half given
I.M. or subcutaneously. Subsequent
doses can be based on 0.1 unit/kg/hour
I.M. or subcutaneously.
➤ **Newly diagnosed diabetes**
regular insulin
Adults older than age 20: Individualize
therapy. Initially, 0.5 to 1 unit/kg/day
subcutaneously as part of a regimen with
short-acting and long-acting insulin
therapy.

Adults and children age 20 and younger:
Individualize therapy. Initially, 0.1 to
0.25 unit/kg subcutaneously every 6 to
8 hours for 24 hours; then adjust
accordingly.
➤ **Control of hyperglycemia with
Humalog and longer-acting insulin
in patients with type 1 diabetes**
Adults: Dosage varies among patients and
must be determined by prescriber familiar
with patient's metabolic needs, eating
habits, and other lifestyle variables. Inject
subcutaneously within 15 minutes before
or after a meal.
➤ **Control of hyperglycemia with
Humalog and sulfonylureas in
patients with type 2 diabetes**
Adults and children older than age 3:
Dosage varies among patients and must
be determined by prescriber familiar with
patient's metabolic needs, eating habits,
and other lifestyle variables. Inject subcutaneously within 15 minutes before or
after a meal.
➤ **Hyperkalemia** ◆
Adults: 50 ml of dextrose 50% given over
5 minutes, followed by 5 to 10 units of
regular insulin by I.V. push.

ADMINISTRATION
I.V.
● Give only regular insulin I.V.
● Inject directly into vein or into a port
close to I.V. access site. Intermittent infusion isn't recommended.
● For continuous infusion, dilute drug
in normal saline solution and give at
prescribed rate.
● **Incompatibilities:** Aminophylline,
amobarbital, chlorothiazide, cytarabine,
digoxin, diltiazem, dobutamine, dopamine,
levofloxacin, methylprednisolone sodium
succinate, nafcillin, norepinephrine,
pentobarbital sodium, phenobarbital
sodium, phenytoin sodium, ranitidine,
sodium bicarbonate, thiopental.
Subcutaneous
● Injection dosage is expressed in USP
units. Use only the syringes calibrated
for that concentration of insulin.
● To mix insulin suspension, swirl
vial gently or rotate between palms or
between palm and thigh. Don't shake
vigorously, to avoid bubbling and air in
syringe.

- Regular insulin may be mixed with NPH insulin in any proportion. When mixing regular insulin with NPH, always draw up regular insulin into syringe first.
- Switching from separate injections to a prepared mixture may alter patient response. When NPH is mixed with regular insulin in the same syringe, give immediately to avoid loss of potency.
- Lispro insulin may be mixed with Humulin N; give within 15 minutes before a meal to prevent a hypoglycemic reaction.
- Don't use insulin that changes color or becomes clumped or granular in appearance.
- Check expiration date on vial before using contents.
- Drug is usually given subcutaneously. To give, pinch a fold of skin with fingers at least 3 inches (7.6 cm) apart and insert needle at a 45- to 90-degree angle.
- Press, don't rub, site after injection. Rotate injection sites to avoid overuse of one area. Diabetic patients may achieve better control if injection site is rotated within same anatomic region.
- Store injectable insulin in cool area. Refrigeration is desirable. Don't freeze.

ACTION

Increases glucose transport across muscle and fat cell membranes to reduce glucose level. Helps convert glucose to glycogen; triggers amino acid uptake and conversion to protein in muscle cells; stimulates triglyceride formation and inhibits release of free fatty acids from adipose tissue; and stimulates lipoprotein lipase activity, which converts circulating lipoproteins to fatty acids.

Route	Onset	Peak	Duration
I.V. (regular)	Immediate	Unknown	Unknown
Subcut. (rapid)	½–1½ hr	2–3 hr	5–7 hr
Subcut. (intermediate)	1–2½ hr	4–15 hr	24 hr
Subcut. (long-acting)	4–8 hr	10–30 hr	36 hr

Half-life: About 9 minutes after I.V. use.

ADVERSE REACTIONS

EENT: blurred vision.
GI: *dry mouth.*
Metabolic: *hypoglycemia,* hyperglycemia, *hypomagnesemia,* hypokalemia.
Skin: rash, urticaria, pruritus, swelling, redness, stinging, warmth at injection site.
Respiratory: *increased cough, respiratory tract infection,* dyspnea, reduced pulmonary function.
Other: *lipoatrophy, lipohypertrophy, anaphylaxis,* hypersensitivity reactions.

INTERACTIONS

Drug-drug. *ACE inhibitors, anabolic steroids, antidiabetics, calcium, chloroquine, clonidine, disopyramide, fibrates, fluoxetine, guanethidine, lithium, MAO inhibitors, mebendazole, octreotide, pentamidine, propoxyphene, pyridoxine, salicylates, sulfinpyrazone, sulfonamides, tetracyclines:* May enhance hypoglycemic effects of insulin. Monitor glucose level.
Acetazolamide, adrenocorticosteroids, albuterol, antiretrovirals, asparaginase, calcitonin, cyclophosphamide, danazol, diazoxide, diltiazem, diuretics, dobutamine, epinephrine, estrogens, ethacrynic acid, hormonal contraceptives containing estrogen, isoniazid, lithium, morphine, niacin, nicotine, phenothiazines, phenytoin, progestogens, somatropin, terbutaline, thyroid hormones: May diminish insulin response. Monitor glucose level.
Bronchodilators and other inhaled drugs: May alter the absorption of inhaled insulin. Consistently time doses of other inhaled drugs with inhaled insulin, and monitor glucose level closely.
Carteolol, nadolol, pindolol, propranolol, timolol: May mask symptoms of hypoglycemia as a result of beta blockade (such as tachycardia). May delay recovery from hypoglycemic episodes. Use together cautiously in patients with diabetes.
Rosiglitazone: May cause fluid retention that may lead to or worsen heart failure. Monitor patient closely.
Drug-herb. *Basil, bay, bee pollen, burdock, ginseng, glucomannan, horehound, marshmallow, myrrh, sage:* May affect glycemic control. Discourage use together, and monitor glucose level carefully.

Reactions may be *common*, uncommon, *life-threatening*, or COMMON AND LIFE-THREATENING.
Interaction may have a *rapid onset* or *delayed onset.*

Drug-food. *Unregulated diet:* May cause hyperglycemia or hypoglycemia. Urge caution and monitor patient's diet.

Drug-lifestyle. *Alcohol use:* May cause hypoglycemic effect. Discourage use together.

Marijuana use: May increase glucose level. Inform patient of this interaction.

Smoking: May increase glucose level and decrease response to drug. Monitor glucose level.

EFFECTS ON LAB TEST RESULTS
● May decrease glucose, magnesium, and potassium levels.

CONTRAINDICATIONS & CAUTIONS
● Contraindicated in patients with history of systemic allergic reaction to pork when porcine-derived products are used or hypersensitivity to any component of preparation.
● Contraindicated during episodes of hypoglycemia.

NURSING CONSIDERATIONS
● *Alert:* Regular insulin is for patients with circulatory collapse, diabetic ketoacidosis, or hyperkalemia. Don't use Humulin R (concentrated) U-500 I.V. Don't use intermediate- or long-acting insulins for coma or other emergencies requiring rapid drug action. Also, ketosis-prone type 1, severely ill, and newly diagnosed diabetic patients with very high glucose levels may need hospitalization and I.V. treatment with regular fast-acting insulin.
● *Alert:* Some patients may develop insulin resistance and need large insulin doses to control symptoms of diabetes. U-500 insulin is available as Humulin R (concentrated) U-500 for such patients. Give pharmacy sufficient notice when requesting refill prescription. Never store U-500 insulin in same area with other insulin preparations because of the risk of severe overdose if accidentally given to the wrong patient.
● Monitor patient for hyperglycemia (rebound, or Somogyi, effect).

PATIENT TEACHING
● Make sure patient knows that drug relieves symptoms but doesn't cure disease.
● Instruct patient about the disease and importance of following therapeutic

regimen, adhering to specific diet, losing weight, getting exercise, following personal hygiene program, and avoiding infection. Emphasize importance of timing injections with eating and of not skipping meals.
● Stress that accuracy of measurement is important, especially with concentrated regular insulin. A magnifying sleeve or dose magnifier may improve accuracy. Show patient and caregivers how to measure and give insulin.
● Advise patient not to change order in which insulins are mixed or model or brand of insulin, syringe, or needle. Be sure patient knows when mixing two insulins to always draw the regular into the syringe first.
● Teach patient that glucose level and urine ketone tests provide essential guides to dosage and success of therapy. It's important for patient to recognize symptoms of high and low glucose levels. Insulin-induced low glucose level is hazardous and may cause brain damage if prolonged; most adverse effects are temporary. Instruct patient on insulin peak times and their importance.
● Instruct patient on proper use of equipment for monitoring glucose level.
● Advise patient not to smoke within 30 minutes after insulin injection because smoking decreases amount of insulin absorbed subcutaneously.
● Advise patient to avoid vigorous exercise immediately after insulin injection, especially of the area where injection was given, because it increases absorption and risk of low glucose episodes.
● Teach patient to avoid alcohol because it lowers glucose level.
● Advise patient to wear or carry medical identification at all times, to carry ample insulin and syringes on trips, to keep carbohydrates (lump of sugar or candy) on hand for emergencies, and to note time zone changes for dosage schedule when traveling.
● Advise woman planning pregnancy to first consult prescriber.
● Advise patient to store injectable insulin at 36° to 46° F (2° to 8° C). Tell him not to freeze or expose vials to excessive heat or sunlight.

desmopressin acetate
somatropin
vasopressin

---

desmopressin acetate
des-moe-PRESS-in

DDAVP, Minirin, Stimate

Pharmacologic class: posterior
pituitary hormone
Pregnancy risk category B

AVAILABLE FORMS
Injection: 4 mcg/ml
Nasal solution: 0.1 mg/ml, 1.5 mg/ml
Tablets: 0.1 mg, 0.2 mg

INDICATIONS & DOSAGES
➤ **Nonnephrogenic diabetes**
insipidus, temporary polyuria,
and polydipsia related to pituitary
trauma
Adults and children older than age 12:
0.1 to 0.4 ml intranasally daily in one
to three doses. Most adults need 0.2 ml
daily in two divided doses. Or, give
0.5 to 1 ml (2 to 4 mg) I.V. or subcutaneously daily, usually in two divided
doses. Or, give 0.05 mg P.O. b.i.d.;
adjust dosage to patient response. If
patient previously received the drug
intranasally, begin oral therapy 12 hours
after last intranasal dose.
Children ages 3 months to 12 years:
0.05 to 0.3 ml intranasally daily in one
or two doses.
➤ **Hemophilia A and von Willebrand**
disease
Adults and children: 0.3 mcg/kg diluted
in normal saline solution and infused I.V.
over 15 to 30 minutes. Repeat dose, if
needed, as indicated by laboratory response
and patient's condition. If used preoperatively, give 30 minutes prior to the scheduled procedure. Or, 300 mcg (one spray
in each nostril) of solution containing
1.5 mcg/ml. Dose of 150 mcg (one spray
of solution containing 1.5 mg/ml into a

single nostril) may be adequate for patients
weighing less than 50 kg (110 lb). Give
drug 2 hours before surgery.
➤ **Primary nocturnal enuresis**
Children age 6 and older: Initially, 0.2 mg
P.O. at bedtime, and adjust dose up to
0.6 mg to achieve desired response.

ADMINISTRATION
P.O.
• Discontinue in patient with acute illness
that may result in fluid or electrolyte
imbalance.
• Store at controlled room temperature.
I.V.
• Don't give injection to patients with
hemophilia A with factor VIII of up
to 5% or with severe von Willebrand
disease.
• For adults and children who weigh more
than 10 kg (22 lb), dilute with 50 ml
sterile physiologic saline solution. For
children who weigh 10 kg or less, 10 ml
of diluent is recommended.
• Inspect drug for particulates and
discoloration before infusing.
• Monitor blood pressure and pulse during
infusion.
• The comparable antidiuretic dose
of the injection is about ¹⁄₁₀ of the
intranasal dose.
• **Incompatibilities:** None reported.
Intranasal
• Ensure nasal passages are intact, clean,
and free of obstruction before giving
intranasally.
• Nasal spray pump delivers only doses
of 10 mcg DDAVP or 150 mcg Stimate.
If doses other than those are required,
use the nasal tube delivery system or
injection.
Subcutaneous
• Teach patient to rotate injection sites to
prevent tissue damage.

ACTION
Increases the permeability of renal
tubular epithelium to adenosine monophosphate and water, enabling the
epithelium to promote reabsorption of

water and produce a concentrated urine. Also increases factor VIII activity by releasing endogenous factor VIII from plasma storage sites.

Route	Onset	Peak	Duration
P.O.	1 hr	1–1½ hr	8–12 hr
I.V.	15–30 min	1½–2 hr	4–12 hr
Intranasal	1 hr	1–5 hr	8–12 hr
Subcut.	Unknown	Unknown	Unknown

Half-life: Fast phase, about 8 minutes; slow phase, 114 hours.

ADVERSE REACTIONS
CNS: headache, *seizures.*
CV: flushing, slight rise in blood pressure.
EENT: rhinitis, epistaxis, sore throat.
GI: nausea, abdominal cramps.
GU: vulval pain.
Metabolic: hyponatremia.
Respiratory: cough.
Skin: local erythema, swelling, or burning after injection.

INTERACTIONS
Drug-drug. *Carbamazepine, chlorpropamide:* May increase ADH; may increase desmopressin effect. Avoid using together.
Clofibrate: May enhance and prolong effects of desmopressin. Monitor patient closely.
Demeclocycline, epinephrine, heparin, lithium: May increase risk of adverse effects. Monitor patient closely.
Pressor agents: May enhance pressor effects with large doses of desmopressin. Monitor patient closely.
Drug-lifestyle. *Alcohol use:* May increase risk of adverse effects. Discourage use together.

EFFECTS ON LAB TEST RESULTS
• May decrease sodium level.

CONTRAINDICATIONS & CAUTIONS
• Contraindicated in patients hypersensitive to drug and in those with type IIB von Willebrand disease.
• Use cautiously in patients with coronary artery insufficiency, hypertensive CV disease, and conditions linked to fluid and electrolyte imbalances, such as cystic fibrosis, because these patients are susceptible to hyponatremia.
• Use cautiously in patients at risk for water intoxication with hyponatremia.
• Use cautiously in breast-feeding women; it's unknown if drug appears in breast milk.

NURSING CONSIDERATIONS
• Morning and evening doses are adjusted separately for adequate diurnal rhythm of water turnover.
• Intranasal use can cause changes in the nasal mucosa, resulting in erratic, unreliable absorption. Report worsening condition to prescriber, who may recommend injectable DDAVP.
• Restrict fluid intake to reduce risk of water intoxication and sodium depletion, especially in children or elderly patients.
• **Alert:** Overdose may cause oxytocic or vasopressor activity. Withhold drug and notify prescriber. If fluid retention is excessive, give furosemide.
• **Look alike–sound alike:** Don't confuse desmopressin with vasopressin.

PATIENT TEACHING
• Some patients may have trouble measuring and inhaling drug into nostrils. Teach patient and caregivers correct administration method.
• Instruct patient to clear nasal passages before giving drug.
• Instruct patient to press down four times to prime pump. Tell him to discard the bottle after 25 (150 mcg/spray) or 50 doses (10 mcg/spray), depending on the strength, because the amount left may be less than desired dose.
• Advise patient to report nasal congestion, allergic rhinitis, or upper respiratory tract infection to prescriber; dosage adjustment may be needed.
• Teach patient using subcutaneous drug to rotate injection sites to prevent tissue damage.
• Warn patient to drink only enough water to satisfy thirst.
• Inform patient with hemophilia A or von Willebrand disease that taking desmopressin may prevent hazards of using blood products.
• Advise patient to carry medical identification indicating use of drug.

somatropin
soe-ma-TROE-pin

Accretropin, Genotropin, Genotropin Miniquick, Humatrope, Norditropin, Nutropin, Nutropin AQ, Omnitrope, Saizen, Serostim, Serostim LQ, Tev-Tropin, Zorbtive

Pharmacologic class: anterior pituitary hormone
Pregnancy risk category C; B (Serostim)

AVAILABLE FORMS
Accretropin injection: 5 mg/ml
Genotropin injection: 1.5 mg (about 4.5 international units/vial), 5.8 mg (about 17.4 international units/vial), 13.8 mg (about 41.4 international units/vial)
Genotropin Miniquick injection: 0.2 mg/vial, 0.4 mg/vial, 0.6 mg/vial, 0.8 mg/vial, 1 mg/vial, 1.2 mg/vial, 1.4 mg/vial, 1.6 mg/vial, 1.8 mg/vial, 2 mg/vial
Humatrope injection: 2 mg (about 6 international units/vial)†, 5 mg (about 15 international units/vial), 6 mg (18 international units/cartridge), 12 mg (36 international units/cartridge), 24 mg (72 international units/cartridge)
Norditropin injection: 5 mg/1.5 ml cartridges, 10 mg/1.5 ml cartridges, 15 mg/1.5 ml cartridges
Nutropin injection: 5 mg (about 15 international units/vial), 10 mg (about 30 international units/vial)
Nutropin AQ injection: 10 mg (about 30 international units/vial)
Omnitrope injection: 1.5 mg (about 4.5 international units/vial), 5.8 mg/vial, 5 mg/1.5 ml injection cartridge, 10 mg/1.5 ml injection cartridge
Saizen injection: 5 mg (about 15 international units/vial)
Serostim injection: 4 mg (about 12 international units/vial), 5 mg (about 15 international units/vial), 6 mg (about 18 international units/vial)
Serostim LQ injection: 6 mg (about 18 international units) per 0.5 ml
Tev-Tropin injection: 5 mg (15 international units/vial)
Zorbtive injection: 8.8 mg (approximately 26.4 international units/vial)

INDICATIONS & DOSAGES
➤ **Long-term treatment of growth failure in children with inadequate secretion of endogenous growth hormone (GH)**
Children: 0.18 mg/kg Humatrope I.M. or subcutaneously weekly, divided equally and given on 3 alternate days, six times weekly or once daily. Or, 0.3 mg/kg Nutropin or Nutropin AQ subcutaneously weekly in daily divided doses; in pubertal patients, a weekly dosage of 0.7 mg/kg (Nutropin or Nutropin AQ) in daily divided doses may be used. Or, 0.06 mg/kg Saizen I.M. or subcutaneously three times weekly. Or, 0.024 to 0.034 mg/kg Norditropin subcutaneously six to seven times weekly. Or, 0.48 mg/kg Genotropin subcutaneously weekly, divided into six or seven doses. Or, up to 0.1 mg/kg Tev-Tropin subcutaneously three times weekly. Or, 0.18 mg/kg to 0.3 mg/kg Accretropin subcutaneously every week, divided into equal daily doses given six to seven times per week.
➤ **Growth failure from chronic renal insufficiency up to time of renal transplantation**
Children: Up to 0.35 mg/kg/week Nutropin or Nutropin AQ subcutaneously divided into daily doses.
➤ **Long-term treatment of short stature from Turner syndrome**
Children: Up to 0.375 mg/kg/week Humatrope, Nutropin, or Nutropin AQ subcutaneously divided into equal doses given three to seven times weekly. Or, up to 0.067 mg/kg/day Norditropin subcutaneously. Or, 0.36 mg/kg Accretropin subcutaneously per week, divided into equal daily doses given six or seven times each week.
➤ **Short stature in children with Noonan syndrome**
Children: Up to 0.066 mg/kg/day Norditropin subcutaneously.
➤ **Long-term treatment of growth failure in children with Prader-Willi syndrome diagnosed by genetic testing**
Children: 0.24 mg/kg Genotropin subcutaneously weekly, divided into six to seven doses.

Reactions may be *common*, uncommon, *life-threatening*, or COMMON AND LIFE-THREATENING.
Interaction may have a *rapid onset* or **delayed onset**.

➤**Replacement of endogenous GH in adult patients with GH deficiency**

Adults: Initially, not more than 0.006 mg/kg Humatrope, Nutropin, or Nutropin AQ subcutaneously daily. May be increased to maximum of 0.0125 mg/kg Humatrope daily.

Nutropin or Nutropin AQ dosages may be increased to maximum of 0.025 mg/kg daily in patients younger than age 35 or 0.0125 mg/kg daily in patients older than age 35. Or, starting dosages not exceeding 0.04 mg/kg Genotropin subcutaneously weekly, divided into six to seven doses, may be increased at 4- to 8-week intervals to a maximum dose of 0.08 mg/kg subcutaneously weekly, divided into six to seven doses.

➤**Replacement of endogenous GH in adult patients with GH deficiency**

Adults: Initially, not more than 0.005 mg/kg Saizen daily. May increase after 4 weeks to a maximum dose of 0.01 mg/kg daily based on patient tolerance and clinical response.

➤**AIDS wasting or cachexia**

Adults and children who weigh more than 55 kg (121 lb): 6 mg Serostim or Serostim LQ subcutaneously at bedtime.

Adults and children who weigh 45 to 55 kg (99 to 121 lb): 5 mg Serostim or Serostim LQ subcutaneously at bedtime.

Adults and children who weigh 35 to 45 kg (77 to 99 lb): 4 mg Serostim or Serostim LQ subcutaneously at bedtime.

Adults and children who weigh less than 35 kg: 0.1 mg/kg/day Serostim or Serostim LQ subcutaneously at bedtime.

➤**Long-term treatment of growth failure in children born small for gestational age (SGA) who don't catch up by age 2**

Children: 0.48 mg/kg Genotropin subcutaneously weekly, divided into six to seven doses.

➤**Idiopathic short stature**

Children: Up to 0.37 mg/kg Humatrope subcutaneously weekly, divided into six to seven equal doses.

➤**Short bowel syndrome**

Adults: 0.1 mg/kg/day subcutaneously daily for 4 weeks.

ADMINISTRATION
I.M.

● To prepare solution, inject supplied diluent into vial containing drug by aiming stream of liquid against wall of glass vial. Then swirl vial gently until contents are completely dissolved. Don't shake vial.

● After reconstitution, make sure solution is clear. Don't inject solution if it's cloudy or contains particles.

● For patients on hemodialysis, give drug before bedtime or 3 to 4 hours after dialysis. For long-term cycling peritoneal dialysis, give drug in the morning after completion of dialysis. For long-term ambulatory peritoneal dialysis, give drug in the evening at the time of the overnight exchange.

● Store reconstituted drug in refrigerator; use within 14 days.

● If patient develops sensitivity to diluent, reconstitute drug with sterile water for injection. When drug is reconstituted in this way, use only one reconstituted dose per vial, refrigerate solution if it isn't used immediately after reconstitution, use reconstituted dose within 24 hours, and discard unused portion.

● *Alert:* When administering to newborn, reconstitute with sterile water for injection.
Subcutaneous

● To prepare solution, inject supplied diluent into vial containing drug by aiming stream of liquid against wall of glass vial. Then swirl vial gently until contents are completely dissolved. Don't shake vial.

● After reconstitution, make sure solution is clear. Don't inject solution if it's cloudy or contains particles.

● For patients on hemodialysis, give drug before bedtime or 3 to 4 hours after dialysis. For long-term cycling peritoneal dialysis, give drug in the morning after completion of dialysis. For long-term ambulatory peritoneal dialysis, give drug in the evening at the time of the overnight exchange.

● Store reconstituted drug in refrigerator; use within 14 days.

● If patient develops sensitivity to diluent, reconstitute drug with sterile water for injection. When drug is reconstituted in this way, use only one reconstituted dose

per vial, refrigerate solution if it isn't used immediately after reconstitution, use reconstituted dose within 24 hours, and discard unused portion.
• *Alert:* When administering to newborn, reconstitute with sterile water for injection.

ACTION
Purified GH of recombinant DNA origin that stimulates skeletal, linear, muscle, and organ growth.

Route	Onset	Peak	Duration
I.M., Subcut.	Unknown	3–5 hr	12–48 hr

Half-life: 20 to 30 minutes.

ADVERSE REACTIONS
CNS: headache, weakness.
CV: mild, transient edema.
Hematologic: *leukemia.*
Metabolic: mild hyperglycemia, hypothyroidism.
Musculoskeletal: localized muscle pain.
Skin: injection site pain.
Other: antibodies to GH.

INTERACTIONS
Drug-drug. *Corticotropin, corticosteroids:* Long-term use may inhibit growth response to GH. Monitor patient for lack of effect.

EFFECTS ON LAB TEST RESULTS
• May increase glucose, inorganic phosphorus, alkaline phosphatase, and parathyroid hormone levels.

CONTRAINDICATIONS & CAUTIONS
• Contraindicated in patients with closed epiphyses, active malignancy, or an active underlying intracranial lesion.
• For patients hypersensitive to either metacresol or glycerin, don't use supplied diluent to reconstitute Humatrope.
• Contraindicated (Genotropin only) in patients with Prader-Willi syndrome who are severely obese or have severe respiratory impairment.
• Don't begin therapy in patients with acute critical illness due to complications following open heart or abdominal surgery, trauma, or acute respiratory failure.

• Use cautiously in children with hypothyroidism and in those with GH deficiency caused by intracranial lesion.
• Use cautiously in patients with diabetes.

NURSING CONSIDERATIONS
• Frequently examine children with hypothyroidism and those whose GH deficiency is caused by an intracranial lesion for progression or recurrence of underlying disease.
• *Alert:* In patients with Prader-Willi syndrome who are morbidly obese and in those with a history of respiratory impairment, sleep apnea, or unidentified respiratory infection, therapy may be life-threatening. Assess patients with Prader-Willi syndrome for sleep apnea and upper airway obstruction before treatment. Interrupt treatment if signs of upper airway obstruction occur.
• Monitor patient with Prader-Willi syndrome for signs of respiratory infection.
• Monitor child's height regularly. Regular checkups, including monitoring of blood and radiologic studies, are also needed.
• Monitor patient's glucose level regularly because GH may induce a state of insulin resistance.
• Excessive glucocorticoid therapy inhibits somatropin's growth-promoting effect. Patients with coexisting corticotropin deficiency should have their glucocorticoid replacement dosage carefully adjusted to avoid growth inhibition.
• Watch for slipped capital femoral epiphysis or progression of scoliosis in patients with rapid growth.
• Monitor results of periodic thyroid function tests for hypothyroidism; condition may need thyroid hormone treatment. Laboratory measurements of thyroid hormone may change.
• Patient should have ophthalmic exams to monitor for intracranial hypertension before therapy (to establish baseline) and periodically thereafter.
• *Look alike–sound alike:* Don't confuse somatropin with somatrem or sumatriptan.
• Only adults with GH deficiency alone or together with multiple hormone deficiencies from pituitary or hypothalamic disease, surgery, radiation, or trauma or those who were GH deficient as children and

Reactions may be *common,* uncommon, *life-threatening,* or COMMON AND LIFE-THREATENING.
Interaction may have a *rapid onset* or **delayed onset.**

have been confirmed GH deficient as
adults can take Saizen.

PATIENT TEACHING
• Inform parents that child with endocrine
disorders (including GH deficiency)
may have an increased risk of slipped
capital epiphyses. Tell parents to notify
prescriber if they notice their child
limping.
• Instruct patients with diabetes to monitor
glucose level closely and report changes to
prescriber.
• Stress importance of close follow-up
care.

---

vasopressin (ADH)
vay-soe-PRESS-in

Pitressin

Pharmacologic class: posterior
pituitary hormone
Pregnancy risk category C

AVAILABLE FORMS
Injection: 20 units/ml

INDICATIONS & DOSAGES
➤ **Nonnephrogenic, nonpsychogenic
diabetes insipidus**
Adults: 5 to 10 units I.M. or subcutaneously b.i.d. to q.i.d., p.r.n. Or,
intranasally (aqueous solution used
as spray or applied to cotton balls) in
individualized dosages, based on
response.
Children: 2.5 to 10 units I.M. or subcutaneously b.i.d. to q.i.d., p.r.n. Or,
intranasally (aqueous solution used as
spray or applied to cotton balls) in
individualized doses.
➤ **To prevent and treat abdominal
distention**
Adults: Initially, 5 units I.M.; give
subsequent injections every 3 to
4 hours, increasing to 10 units, if
needed. Children may receive reduced
dosages. Or, for adults, aqueous vasopressin 5 to 15 units subcutaneously at
2 hours before and again at 30 minutes
before abdominal radiography or kidney
biopsy.

➤ **Abdominal roentgenography**
Adults: 2 injections of 10 units each I.M.
or subcutaneously, given 2 hours and
½ hour before films are exposed.
➤ **GI bleeding ◆**
Adults: Initially, 0.2 to 0.4 units/minute
I.V.; increase to 0.9 units/minute as
needed. For intra-arterial infusion, 0.1 to
0.5 units/minute.
➤ **Pulseless cardiac arrest ◆**
Adults: One dose of 40 units I.V. or intra-
osseously may replace either the first or
second epinephrine dose.
➤ **Septic shock and vasodilatory
shock ◆**
Adults: 0.01 to 0.04 units/minute by I.V.
infusion.

ADMINISTRATION
I.V.
• For I.V. or intra-arterial infusion, dilute
aqueous vasopressin in normal saline
solution or D_5W to a concentration of
0.1 to 1 unit/ml.
I.M.
• Warm the vial in your hands, and mix
until the hormone is distributed throughout
the solution before administration.
• Rotate injection sites to prevent tissue
damage.
Subcutaneous
• Warm vial in hands, and mix until the
hormone is distributed throughout the
solution before administration.
• Rotate injection sites to prevent tissue
damage.
Intranasal
• Give drug intranasally on cotton pledgets,
by nasal spray, or by dropper. Determine
dosage and interval between treatments
for each patient.

ACTION
Increases permeability of the renal tubular
epithelium to adenosine monophosphate
and water; the epithelium promotes
reabsorption of water and produces a
concentrated urine.

Route	Onset	Peak	Duration
I.V.	Unknown	Unknown	Unknown
I.M., Subcut., intranasal	Unknown	Unknown	2–8 hr

Half-life: 10 to 20 minutes.

ADVERSE REACTIONS
CNS: tremor, headache, vertigo.
CV: vasoconstriction, *arrhythmias,*
cardiac arrest, myocardial ischemia,
circumoral pallor, *decreased cardiac*
output, angina in patients with vascular
disease.
GI: abdominal cramps, nausea, vomiting,
flatulence.
GU: uterine cramps.
Respiratory: *bronchoconstriction.*
Skin: diaphoresis, cutaneous gangrene,
urticaria.
Other: *anaphylaxis,* water intoxication.

INTERACTIONS
Drug-drug. *Carbamazepine, chlorpro-*
pamide, clofibrate, fludrocortisone,
tricyclic antidepressant, urea: May
increase antidiuretic response. Use
together cautiously.
Demeclocycline, heparin, lithium, norepi-
nephrine: May reduce antidiuretic activity.
Use together cautiously.
Ganglionic blocking agents: May increase
sensitivity to pressor effects. Monitor
patient and blood pressure.
Drug-lifestyle. *Alcohol use:* May reduce
antidiuretic activity. Discourage use
together.

EFFECTS ON LAB TEST RESULTS
None reported.

CONTRAINDICATIONS & CAUTIONS
● Contraindicated in patients allergic to
vasopressin or any of its components and
in those with chronic nephritis and nitrogen retention.
● Use cautiously in children; elderly
patients; pregnant women; patients with
preoperative or postoperative polyuria;
and those with seizure disorders,
migraines, asthma, CV disease, heart
failure, renal disease, goiter with cardiac
complications, arteriosclerosis, or fluid
overload.

NURSING CONSIDERATIONS
● Monitor patient for hypersensitivity
reactions, including urticaria, angioedema,
bronchoconstriction, and anaphylaxis.
● Synthetic desmopressin is sometimes
preferred because of its longer duration of
action and less frequent adverse reactions.

Desmopressin also is available commercially as a nasal solution.
● Drug may be used for transient polyuria
from ADH deficiency in neurosurgery or
head injury.
● Use minimum effective dose to reduce
adverse reactions.
● Give with 1 or 2 glasses of water to
reduce adverse reactions and improve
therapeutic response.
● Monitor urine specific gravity and fluid
intake and output to aid evaluation of drug
effectiveness.
● Monitor ECG and fluid or electrolyte
status at periodic intervals.
● To prevent possible seizures, coma, and
death, observe patient closely for early
evidence of water intoxication, including
drowsiness, listlessness, headache,
confusion, and weight gain.
● Water intoxication may be treated with
water restriction and temporary withdrawal
of drug until polyuria occurs. Severe water
intoxication may require osmotic diuresis
with mannitol, hypertonic dextrose, or
urea, alone or with furosemide.
● Monitor blood pressure of patient taking
vasopressin twice daily. Watch for excessively elevated blood pressure or lack of
response to drug, which may be indicated
by hypotension. Also, monitor weight
daily.
● *Look alike–sound alike:* Don't confuse
vasopressin with desmopressin.

PATIENT TEACHING
● Instruct patient to rotate injection sites to
prevent tissue damage.
● Tell patient to report adverse reactions,
drowsiness, listlessness, and headache to
prescriber promptly.
● Tell patient to avoid alcohol and OTC
drugs unless approved by prescriber.
● Tell patient to restrict water intake.
However, such side effects as skin blanching, abdominal cramps, and nausea may
be reduced by drinking 1 to 2 glasses of
water at the time of administration.

Reactions may be *common,* uncommon, *life-threatening,* or COMMON AND LIFE-THREATENING.
Interaction may have a *rapid onset* or *delayed onset.*

dexamethasone
dexamethasone sodium
   phosphate
fludrocortisone acetate
hydrocortisone
hydrocortisone acetate
hydrocortisone cypionate
hydrocortisone sodium
   succinate
methylprednisolone
methylprednisolone acetate
methylprednisolone sodium
   succinate
prednisolone
prednisolone sodium phosphate
prednisone
triamcinolone acetonide
triamcinolone hexacetonide

---

dexamethasone
dex-a-METH-a-sone

Dexamethasone Intensol*, Dexpak
Taperpak

dexamethasone sodium
phosphate

Pharmacologic class: glucocorticoid
Pregnancy risk category C

AVAILABLE FORMS
dexamethasone
Elixir: 0.5 mg/5 ml*
Oral solution: 0.5 mg/5 ml,
0.5 mg/0.5 ml*
Tablets: 0.25 mg, 0.5 mg, 0.75 mg, 1 mg,
1.5 mg, 2 mg, 4 mg, 6 mg
dexamethasone sodium phosphate
Injection: 4 mg/ml, 10 mg/ml

INDICATIONS & DOSAGES
➤ **Cerebral edema**
Adults: Initially, 10 mg phosphate I.V.;
then 4 mg I.M. every 6 hours until
symptoms subside (usually 2 to 4 days);
then taper over 5 to 7 days. Oral therapy
(1 to 3 mg t.i.d.) should replace I.M.
dosing as soon as possible.

➤ **Palliative management of
recurrent or inoperable brain
tumors**
Adults: 2 mg b.i.d. to t.i.d. for maintenance therapy.
➤ **Inflammatory conditions,
neoplasias**
Adults: 0.75 to 9 mg/day P.O. or 0.5 to
9 mg/day phosphate I.M., depending on
size and location of affected area.
➤ **Acute, self-limited allergic disorders, acute exacerbations of
chronic allergic disorders**
Adults: On day one, give 4 or 8 mg
I.M. (using 4 mg/ml preparation). On
days two and three, give four 0.75 mg
tablets P.O. in two divided doses. On
day four, give two 0.75 mg tablets P.O.
in two divided doses. On days five
and six, give one 0.75 mg tablet P.O.
A follow-up visit should take place on
day eight.
➤ **Shock**
Adults: 20 mg phosphate as single first
dose; then 3 mg/kg/24 hours via continuous I.V. infusion. Or, 2 to 6 mg/kg
phosphate I.V. as single dose. Or, 40 mg
phosphate I.V. every 2 to 6 hours, as
needed, continued only until patient is
stabilized (usually not longer than 48 to
72 hours).
➤ **Dexamethasone suppression test
for Cushing's syndrome**
Adults: Determine baseline 24-hour urine
levels of 17-hydroxycorticosteroids; then,
give 0.5 mg P.O. every 6 hours for 48
hours. Repeat 24-hour urine collection to
determine 17-hydroxycorticosteroid
excretion during second 24 hours of
dexamethasone administration. Or, 1 mg
P.O. as single dose at 11:00 p.m. with
determination of plasma cortisol at 8 a.m.
the next morning.
➤ **Adrenocortical insufficiency**
Children: 0.02 to 3 mg/kg or 0.6 to
9 mg/m² P.O. daily, in four divided
doses.
➤ **Tuberculosis meningitis**
Adults: 8 to 12 mg phosphate I.M. daily;
taper over 6 to 8 weeks.

➤**Adjunctive treatment in bacterial meningitis** ◆
Adults, children, infants: 0.15 mg/kg phosphate I.V. q.i.d. for the first 2 to 4 days of anti-infective therapy.

ADMINISTRATION
P.O.
● Give oral dose with food when possible. Patient may need measures to prevent GI irritation.
I.V.
● For direct injection, inject undiluted over at least 1 minute.
● For intermittent or continuous infusion, dilute solution according to manufacturer's instructions and give over prescribed duration.
● During continuous infusion, change solution every 24 hours.
● **Incompatibilities:** Ciprofloxacin, daunorubicin, diphenhydramine, doxapram, doxorubicin, glycopyrrolate, idarubicin, midazolam, vancomycin.
I.M.
● Give I.M. injection deep into gluteal muscle. Rotate injection sites to prevent muscle atrophy. Avoid subcutaneous injection because atrophy and sterile abscesses may occur.

ACTION
Unclear. Decreases inflammation, mainly by stabilizing leukocyte lysosomal membranes; suppresses immune response; stimulates bone marrow; and influences protein, fat, and carbohydrate metabolism.

Route	Onset	Peak	Duration
P.O.	1–2 hr	1–2 hr	2½ days
I.V.	1 hr	1 hr	Variable
I.M.	1 hr	1 hr	6 days

Half-life: About 1 to 2 days.

ADVERSE REACTIONS
CNS: *euphoria, insomnia,* psychotic behavior, *pseudotumor cerebri,* vertigo, headache, paresthesia, *seizures,* depression.
CV: *heart failure,* hypertension, edema, *arrhythmias,* thrombophlebitis, *thrombo-embolism.*
EENT: cataracts, glaucoma.

GI: *peptic ulceration,* GI irritation, increased appetite, *pancreatitis,* nausea, vomiting.
GU: menstrual irregularities, increased urine glucose and calcium levels.
Metabolic: hypokalemia, hyperglycemia, carbohydrate intolerance, hypercholes-terolemia, hypocalcemia, sodium retention.
Musculoskeletal: growth suppression in children, muscle weakness, osteoporosis, tendon rupture, myopathy.
Skin: hirsutism, delayed wound healing, acne, various skin eruptions, atrophy at I.M. injection site.
Other: cushingoid state, susceptibility to infections, acute adrenal insufficiency after increased stress or abrupt withdrawal after long-term therapy, *angioedema.*
After abrupt withdrawal: rebound inflammation, fatigue, weakness, arthralgia, fever, dizziness, lethargy, fainting, orthostatic hypotension, dyspnea, anorexia, *hypoglycemia. After prolonged use, sudden withdrawal may be fatal.*

INTERACTIONS
Drug-drug. *Aminoglutethimide:* May cause loss of dexamethasone-induced adrenal suppression. Use together cautiously.
Antidiabetics, including insulin: May decrease response. May need dosage adjustment.
Aspirin, indomethacin, other NSAIDs: May increase risk of GI distress and bleeding. Use together cautiously.
Barbiturates, carbamazepine, phenytoin, rifampin: May decrease corticosteroid effect. Increase corticosteroid dosage.
Cardiac glycosides: May increase risk of arrhythmia resulting from hypokalemia. May need dosage adjustment.
Cyclosporine: May increase toxicity. Monitor patient closely.
Ephedrine: May cause decreased half-life and increased clearance of dexametha-sone. Monitor patient.
Oral anticoagulants: May alter dosage requirements. Monitor PT and INR closely.
Potassium-depleting drugs such as thiazide diuretics: May enhance potassium-wasting effects of dexamethasone. Monitor potassium level.

Reactions may be *common,* uncommon, *life-threatening,* or COMMON AND LIFE-THREATENING.
Interaction may have a *rapid onset* or *delayed onset.*

Salicylates: May decrease salicylate level. Monitor patient for lack of salicylate effectiveness.

Skin-test antigens: May decrease response. Postpone skin testing until therapy is completed.

Toxoids, vaccines: May decrease antibody response and may increase risk of neurologic complications. Avoid using together.

Drug-lifestyle. *Alcohol use:* May increase risk of gastric irritation and GI ulceration. Discourage use together.

EFFECTS ON LAB TEST RESULTS
● May increase cholesterol and glucose levels.
● May decrease calcium, potassium, T_3, and T_4 levels. May decrease ^{131}I uptake and protein-bound iodine levels in thyroid function tests. May cause false-negative results in nitroblue tetrazolium test for systemic bacterial infections. May alter reactions to skin tests.

CONTRAINDICATIONS & CAUTIONS
● Contraindicated in patients hypersensitive to drug or its ingredients, in those with systemic fungal infections, and in those receiving immunosuppressive doses together with live virus vaccines. I.M. administration is contraindicated in patients with idiopathic thrombocytopenic purpura.
● Use with caution in patient with recent MI.
● Use cautiously in patients with GI ulcer, renal disease, hypertension, osteoporosis, diabetes mellitus, hypothyroidism, cirrhosis, diverticulitis, nonspecific ulcerative colitis, recent intestinal anastomoses, thromboembolic disorders, seizures, myasthenia gravis, heart failure, tuberculosis, active hepatitis, ocular herpes simplex, emotional instability, or psychotic tendencies and in women who are breast-feeding.
● Because some forms contain sulfite preservatives, also use cautiously in patients sensitive to sulfites.

NURSING CONSIDERATIONS
● Most adverse reactions to corticosteroids are dose- or duration-dependent.
● For better results and less toxicity, give once-daily dose in morning.

● Always adjust to lowest effective dose.
● Monitor patient's weight, blood pressure, and electrolyte levels.
● Monitor patient for cushingoid effects, including moon face, buffalo hump, central obesity, thinning hair, hypertension, and increased susceptibility to infection.
● Watch for depression or psychotic episodes, especially in high-dose therapy.
● Diabetic patient may need increased insulin; monitor glucose levels.
● Drug may mask or worsen infections, including latent amebiasis.
● Elderly patients may be more susceptible to osteoporosis with long-term use.
● Inspect patient's skin for petechiae.
● Gradually reduce dosage after long-term therapy.
● ***Look alike–sound alike:*** Don't confuse dexamethasone with desoximetasone.

PATIENT TEACHING
● Tell patient not to stop drug abruptly or without prescriber's consent.
● Instruct patient to take drug with food or milk.
● Teach patient signs and symptoms of early adrenal insufficiency: fatigue, muscle weakness, joint pain, fever, anorexia, nausea, shortness of breath, dizziness, and fainting.
● Instruct patient to carry medical identification indicating his need for supplemental systemic glucocorticoids during stress, especially when dosage is decreased. This card should contain prescriber's name and name and dosage of drug.
● Warn patient on long-term therapy about cushingoid effects (moon face, buffalo hump) and the need to notify prescriber about sudden weight gain or swelling.
● Warn patient about easy bruising.
● Advise patient receiving long-term therapy to consider exercise or physical therapy. Tell him to ask prescriber about vitamin D or calcium supplement.
● Instruct patient receiving long-term therapy to have periodic eye examinations.
● Advise patient to avoid exposure to infections (such as measles and chickenpox) and to notify prescriber if such exposure occurs.
● Tell patient to avoid alcohol.

fluordocortisone acetate
floo-droe-KOR-ti-sone

Pharmacologic class:
mineralocorticoid
Pregnancy risk category C

AVAILABLE FORMS
Tablets: 0.1 mg

INDICATIONS & DOSAGES
➤ **Salt-losing adrenogenital syndrome**
Adults: 0.1 to 0.2 mg P.O. daily.
➤ **Addison disease (adrenocortical insufficiency)**
Adults: 0.1 mg P.O. daily. Usual dosage range is 0.1 mg three times weekly to 0.2 mg daily. Decrease dosage to 0.05 mg daily if transient hypertension develops as a result of drug therapy.
➤ **Postural hypotension ♦**
Adults: 0.1 to 0.4 mg P.O. daily in patients with diabetes; 0.05 to 0.2 mg daily in patients with postural hypotension as a result of levodopa therapy.

ADMINISTRATION
P.O.
• Continually monitor patients for signs that dosage adjustment is needed, such as remissions or exacerbations of the disease, and stress (surgery, infection, trauma).
• Store at room temperature and avoid excessive heat.

ACTION
Increases sodium resorption and potassium and hydrogen secretion at the distal convoluted tubules of nephrons.

Route	Onset	Peak	Duration
P.O.	Variable	2 hr	1–2 days

Half-life: 18 to 36 hours.

ADVERSE REACTIONS
CNS: *convulsions, increased intracranial pressure with papilledema (pseudotumor cerebri),* vertigo, headache, severe mental disturbances.
CV: *heart failure,* hypertension, cardiac hypertrophy, edema, syncope.
EENT: cataracts, glaucoma, increased intraocular pressure, exophthalmos.
GI: *peptic ulcer with possible perforation and hemorrhage, pancreatitis,* abdominal distension, ulcerative esophagitis.
Hematologic: bruising.
Metabolic: *sodium and water retention,* hypokalemia, hyperglycemia.
Musculoskeletal: muscle weakness.
Skin: diaphoresis, urticaria, allergic rash, impaired wound healing, acne.
Other: *anaphylaxis,* insomnia.

INTERACTIONS
Drug-drug. *Anabolic steroids, estrogen:* May increase fludrocortisone levels. Monitor patient for adverse effects and increased edema.
Barbiturates, carbamazepine, fosphenytoin, phenytoin, rifampin: May increase clearance of fludrocortisone acetate. Monitor patient for possible diminished effect of corticosteroid. Corticosteroid dosage may need to be increased.
Digoxin: May increase the risk of digoxin toxicity associated with hypokalemia. Monitor potassium and digoxin levels.
Potassium-depleting drugs such as amphotericin B, thiazide diuretics: May enhance potassium-wasting effects of fludrocortisone. Monitor potassium level. Use potassium supplements as needed.
Salicylates: May decrease salicylate effectiveness. Coadministration also may increase the ulcerogenic effects of each. Monitor patient for decreased effect and for ulcers.
Drug-food. *Sodium-containing drugs or foods:* May increase blood pressure. Advise patient of need for sodium intake adjustment.

EFFECTS ON LAB TEST RESULTS
• May decrease potassium level.
• May affect the nitroblue tetrazolium test for bacterial infection and produce false-negative results.

CONTRAINDICATIONS & CAUTIONS
• Contraindicated in patients hypersensitive to drug and in those with systemic fungal infections.

• Use cautiously in patients with hypothyroidism, recent MI, cirrhosis, ocular
herpes simplex, emotional instability,
psychotic tendencies, diverticulitis,
fresh intestinal anastamoses, active or
latent peptic ulcer, renal insufficiency,
hypertension, osteoporosis, myasthenia
gravis, active hepatitis, active tuberculosis, or nonspecific ulcerative colitis.
Also use cautiously in breast-feeding
women.
• Patients shouldn't be vaccinated against
smallpox while taking drug.

NURSING CONSIDERATIONS
• Drug is used with cortisone or hydrocortisone in adrenal insufficiency.
• Perform glucose tolerance tests only if
needed because addisonian patients tend
to develop severe hypoglycemia within
3 hours of the test.
• *Alert:* Monitor patient's blood
pressure and electrolyte levels. If
hypertension occurs, notify prescriber
and expect dosage to be decreased
by 50%.
• Weigh patient daily; notify prescriber
about sudden weight gain.
• Unless contraindicated, give low-
sodium diet that's high in potassium
and protein. Potassium supplements
may be needed.
• Drug may cause adverse effects similar
to those of glucocorticoids.
• *Look alike–sound alike:* Don't confuse
Florinef with Fiorinal.

PATIENT TEACHING
• Tell patient to notify prescriber if low
blood pressure, weakness, cramping, or
palpitations worsen, or if changes in
mental status occur.
• Warn patient that mild swelling is
common.
• Caution patient to avoid exposure to
infections (such as chickenpox or measles)
and to notify prescriber if such exposure
occurs.

hydrocortisone
hye-droe-KOR-ti-sone

Cortef, Cortenema

hydrocortisone acetate
Anucort-HC, Anusol-HC,
Cortifoam, Proctocort

hydrocortisone cypionate
Cortef

hydrocortisone sodium succinate
A-Hydrocort, Solu-Cortef

Pharmacologic class: glucocorticoid
Pregnancy risk category C

AVAILABLE FORMS
hydrocortisone
Enema: 100 mg/60 ml
Tablets: 5 mg, 10 mg, 20 mg
hydrocortisone acetate
Injection: 25 mg/ml, 50 mg/ml
suspension
Rectal aerosol foam: 10% aerosol foam
(provides 90 mg/application)
Rectal suppository: 25 mg, 30 mg
hydrocortisone cypionate
Oral suspension: 2 mg/ml
hydrocortisone sodium succinate
Injection: 100-mg vial, 250-mg vial,
500-mg vial, 1,000-mg vial

INDICATIONS & DOSAGES
➤ **Severe inflammation, adrenal
insufficiency**
Adults: 10 to 320 mg P.O. daily in three or
four divided doses. Or, initially, 100 to
500 mg succinate I.M. or I.V.; repeat every
2 to 10 hours as needed. Or, 5 to 75 mg
acetate into joints or soft tissue repeated at
3 to 5 days for bursae and 1 to 4 weeks for
joints. Dosage varies with size of joint.
Local anesthetics commonly are injected
with dose.
➤ **Shock**
Adults: Initially, 50 mg/kg succinate I.V.,
repeated in 4 hours. Repeat dosage every
24 hours as needed. Or, 0.5 to 2 g every
2 to 6 hours, continued until patient is
stabilized (usually not longer than 48 to
72 hours).

Children: Succinate (I.M. or I.V.) 0.16 to 1 mg/kg or 6 to 30 mg/m² given once or twice daily.

➤ **Adjunct treatment for ulcerative colitis and proctitis**

Adults: 1 enema (100 mg) P.R. nightly for 21 days. Or, 1 applicatorful (90-mg foam) P.R. daily or b.i.d. for 14 to 21 days. Or, 25 mg rectal suppository b.i.d. for 2 weeks. For severe proctitis, 25 mg P.R. t.i.d. or 50 mg b.i.d.

ADMINISTRATION
P.O.
• Give drug with milk or food when possible. Patient may need another drug to prevent GI irritation.
I.V.
• Don't use acetate or suspension form for I.V. route.
• Reconstitute hydrocortisone sodium succinate with bacteriostatic water or bacteriostatic saline solution before adding to I.V. solutions. For direct injection, inject over 30 seconds to 10 minutes. For infusion, dilute with D₅W, normal saline solution, or dextrose 5% in normal saline solution to 1 mg/ml or less.
• **Incompatibilities:** Amobarbital, ampicillin sodium, bleomycin, ciprofloxacin, colistimethate, cytarabine, dacarbazine, diazepam, dimenhydrinate, ephedrine, ergotamine, furosemide, heparin sodium, hydralazine, idarubicin, Ionosol B with invert sugar 10%, kanamycin, methylprednisolone sodium succinate, midazolam, nafcillin, pentobarbital sodium, phenobarbital sodium, phenytoin, prochlorperazine edisylate, promethazine hydrochloride, sargramostim, vancomycin, vitamin B complex with C.
I.M.
• Inject deep into gluteal muscle. Rotate injection sites to prevent muscle atrophy. Avoid subcutaneous injection because atrophy and sterile abscesses may occur.
• Injectable forms aren't used for alternate-day therapy.
Rectal
• Have the patient lie on his left side during administration and for 30 minutes afterward to allow fluid to distribute throughout the left colon. Have patient try to retain the enema for at least 1 hour but preferably all night.

ACTION
Not clearly defined. Decreases inflammation, mainly by stabilizing leukocyte lysosomal membranes; suppresses immune response; stimulates bone marrow; and influences protein, fat, and carbohydrate metabolism.

Route	Onset	Peak	Duration
P.O., I.V., I.M., P.R.	Variable	Variable	Variable

Half-life: 8 to 12 hours.

ADVERSE REACTIONS
CNS: *euphoria, insomnia,* psychotic behavior, ***pseudotumor cerebri,*** vertigo, headache, paresthesia, *seizures.*
CV: *heart failure,* hypertension, edema, *arrhythmias,* thrombophlebitis, ***thromboembolism.***
EENT: cataracts, glaucoma.
GI: *peptic ulceration,* GI irritation, increased appetite, *pancreatitis,* nausea, vomiting.
GU: menstrual irregularities, increased urine calcium levels.
Hematologic: easy bruising.
Metabolic: hypokalemia, hyperglycemia, carbohydrate intolerance, hypercholesterolemia, hypocalcemia.
Musculoskeletal: growth suppression in children, muscle weakness, osteoporosis, tendon rupture.
Skin: hirsutism, delayed wound healing, acne, skin eruptions.
Other: cushingoid state, susceptibility to infections, ***acute adrenal insufficiency after increased stress or abrupt withdrawal after long-term therapy.***
After abrupt withdrawal: rebound inflammation, fatigue, weakness, arthralgia, fever, dizziness, lethargy, depression, fainting, orthostatic hypotension, dyspnea, anorexia, *hypoglycemia. After prolonged use, sudden withdrawal may be fatal.*

INTERACTIONS
Drug-drug. *Aspirin, indomethacin, other NSAIDs:* May increase risk of GI distress and bleeding. Use together cautiously. *Barbiturates, carbamazepine, fosphenytoin, phenytoin, rifampin:* May decrease corticosteroid effect. Increase corticosteroid dosage.

Reactions may be *common,* uncommon, *life-threatening,* or COMMON AND LIFE-THREATENING.
Interaction may have a *rapid onset* or **delayed onset.**

Cyclosporine: May increase toxicity. Monitor patient closely.

Live attenuated virus vaccines, other toxoids and vaccines: May decrease antibody response and increase risk of neurologic complications. Avoid using together.

Oral anticoagulants: May alter dosage requirements. Monitor PT and INR closely.

Potassium-depleting drugs such as thiazide diuretics: May enhance potassium-wasting effects of hydrocortisone. Monitor potassium level.

Skin-test antigens: May decrease response. Postpone skin testing until after therapy.

Drug-herb. *Echinacea:* May increase immune-stimulating effects. Discourage use together.

Ginseng: May increase immune-modulating response. Discourage use together.

EFFECTS ON LAB TEST RESULTS

● May increase glucose and cholesterol levels. May decrease T_3, T_4, potassium, and calcium levels.

● May cause decreased ^{131}I uptake and protein-bound iodine levels in thyroid function tests. May cause false-negative results in nitroblue tetrazolium test for systemic bacterial infections. May alter reactions to skin tests.

CONTRAINDICATIONS & CAUTIONS

● Contraindicated in patients hypersensitive to drug or its ingredients, in those with systemic fungal infections, in those receiving immunosuppressive doses together with live virus vaccines, and in premature infants (succinate).

● Use with caution in patient with recent MI.

● Use cautiously in patients with GI ulcer, renal disease, hypertension, osteoporosis, diabetes mellitus, hypothyroidism, cirrhosis, diverticulitis, nonspecific ulcerative colitis, active hepatitis, recent intestinal anastomoses, thromboembolic disorders, seizures, myasthenia gravis, heart failure, tuberculosis, ocular herpes simplex, emotional instability, and psychotic tendencies or in women who are breast-feeding.

NURSING CONSIDERATIONS

● Determine whether patient is sensitive to other corticosteroids.

● Most adverse reactions to corticosteroids are dose- or duration-dependent.

● For better results and less toxicity, give a once-daily dose in morning.

● *Alert:* Salts aren't interchangeable.

● *Alert:* Only hydrocortisone sodium succinate can be given I.V.

● Enema may produce same systemic effects as other forms of hydrocortisone. If enema therapy must exceed 21 days, taper off by giving every other night for 2 to 3 weeks.

● High-dose therapy usually isn't continued beyond 48 hours.

● Always adjust to lowest effective dose.

● Monitor patient's weight, blood pressure, and electrolyte level.

● Monitor patient for cushingoid effects, including moon face, buffalo hump, central obesity, thinning hair, hypertension, and increased susceptibility to infection.

● Unless contraindicated, give a low-sodium diet that's high in potassium and protein. Give potassium supplements.

● Drug may mask or worsen infections, including latent amebiasis.

● Stress (fever, trauma, surgery, and emotional problems) may increase adrenal insufficiency. Increase dosage.

● Watch for depression or psychotic episodes, especially during high-dose therapy.

● Inspect patient's skin for petechiae.

● Diabetic patient may need increased insulin; monitor glucose level.

● Periodic measurement of growth and development may be needed during high-dose or prolonged therapy in children.

● Elderly patients may be more susceptible to osteoporosis with prolonged use.

● Gradually reduce dosage after long-term therapy.

● *Look alike–sound alike:* Don't confuse Solu-Cortef with Solu-Medrol (methyl-prednisolone sodium succinate), or hydrocortisone with hydroxychloroquine.

PATIENT TEACHING

● Tell patient not to stop drug abruptly or without prescriber's consent.

● Instruct patient to take oral form of drug with milk or food.

• Warn patient on long-term therapy about cushingoid effects (moon face, buffalo hump) and the need to notify prescriber about sudden weight gain or swelling.

• Teach patient signs and symptoms of early adrenal insufficiency: fatigue, muscle weakness, joint pain, fever, anorexia, nausea, shortness of breath, dizziness, and fainting.

• Instruct patient to carry a card with his prescriber's name and name and dosage of drug, indicating his need for supplemental systemic glucocorticoids during stress.

• Warn patient about easy bruising.

• Urge patient receiving long-term therapy to consider exercise or physical therapy. Also, tell him to ask prescriber about vitamin D or calcium supplement.

• Advise patient receiving long-term therapy to have periodic eye examinations.

• Caution patient to avoid exposure to infections (such as chickenpox or measles) and to notify prescriber if such exposure occurs.

---

methylprednisolone
meth-ill-pred-NISS-oh-lone

Medrol✧, Medrol Dosepak, Meprolone Unipak

methylprednisolone acetate
Depo-Medrol

methylprednisolone sodium succinate
A-Methapred, Solu-Medrol

Pharmacologic class: glucocorticoid
Pregnancy risk category C

AVAILABLE FORMS
methylprednisolone
Tablets: 2 mg, 4 mg, 8 mg, 16 mg, 24 mg, 32 mg
methylprednisolone acetate
Injection (suspension): 20 mg/ml, 40 mg/ml, 80 mg/ml
methylprednisolone sodium succinate
Injection: 40-mg vial, 125-mg vial, 500-mg vial, 1,000-mg vial, 2,000-mg vial

INDICATIONS & DOSAGES
➤ **Severe inflammation or immuno-suppression**
Adults: 2 to 60 mg base P.O. usually in four divided doses. Or, initially, 24 mg (six 4-mg tablets) on the first day; taper by 4 mg per day until 21 tablets have been given. Or, 10 to 80 mg acetate I.M. daily, or 10 to 250 mg succinate I.M. or I.V. up to six times daily. Or, 4 to 40 mg acetate into smaller joints or 20 to 80 mg acetate into larger joints. Intralesional use is usually 20 to 60 mg acetate. Repeat intralesional and intra-articular injections every 1 to 5 weeks.
Children: 0.117 to 1.66 mg/kg or 3.3 to 50 mg/m^2 P.O. daily in three or four divided doses. Or, 0.03 to 0.2 mg/kg or 1 to 6.25 mg/m^2 succinate I.M. once daily or b.i.d.
➤ **Congenital adrenogenital syndrome**
Children: 40 mg acetate I.M. every 2 weeks.
➤ **Shock**
Adults: 100 to 250 mg succinate I.V. every 2 to 6 hours. Or, 30 mg/kg I.V. initially; repeat every 4 to 6 hours as needed. Give over 3 to 15 minutes. Continue therapy for 2 to 3 days or until patient is stable.

ADMINISTRATION
P.O.
• Give drug with milk or food when possible. Critically ill patients may need to take drug with an antacid or H$_2$-receptor antagonist.
I.V.
• Use only methylprednisolone sodium succinate, never the acetate form.
• Reconstitute according to manufacturer's directions using supplied diluent, or use bacteriostatic water for injection with benzyl alcohol.
• Compatible solutions include D$_5$W, normal saline solution, and dextrose 5% in normal saline solution.
• For direct injection, inject diluted drug into vein or free-flowing compatible I.V. solution over at least 1 minute.
• For intermittent or continuous infusion, dilute solution according to manufacturer's instructions and give over prescribed duration. If used for

---

continuous infusion, change solution every 24 hours.
• For shock, give massive doses over at least 10 minutes to prevent arrhythmias and circulatory collapse.
• Discard reconstituted solution after 48 hours.
• **Incompatibilities:** Allopurinol, aminophylline, calcium gluconate, ciprofloxacin, cytarabine, diltiazem, docetaxel, doxapram, etoposide, filgrastim, gemcitabine, glycopyrrolate, nafcillin, ondansetron, paclitaxel, penicillin G sodium, potassium chloride, propofol, sargramostim, vinorelbine, vitamin B complex with C.

I.M.
• Give injection deeply into gluteal muscle. Avoid subcutaneous injection because atrophy and sterile abscesses may occur.
• Dermal atrophy may occur with large doses of acetate form. Use several small injections rather than a single large dose, and rotate injection sites.

ACTION
Not clearly defined. Decreases inflammation, mainly by stabilizing leukocyte lysosomal membranes; suppresses immune response; stimulates bone marrow; and influences protein, fat, and carbohydrate metabolism.

Route	Onset	Peak	Duration
P.O.	Rapid	2–3 hr	30–36 hr
I.V.	Rapid	Immediate	1 wk
I.M.	6–48 hr	4–8 days	4–8 days
Intra-articular	Rapid	7 days	1–5 wk

Half-life: 18 to 36 hours.

ADVERSE REACTIONS
CNS: *euphoria, insomnia,* psychotic behavior, *pseudotumor cerebri,* vertigo, headache, paresthesia, *seizures.*
CV: *arrhythmias, heart failure,* hypertension, edema, thrombophlebitis, *thromboembolism, cardiac arrest, circulatory collapse after rapid use of large I.V. dose.*
EENT: cataracts, glaucoma.
GI: *peptic ulceration,* GI irritation, increased appetite, *pancreatitis,* nausea, vomiting.
GU: menstrual irregularities.

Metabolic: hypokalemia, hyperglycemia, carbohydrate intolerance, hypercholesterolemia, hypocalcemia.
Musculoskeletal: growth suppression in children, muscle weakness, osteoporosis.
Skin: hirsutism, delayed wound healing, acne, various skin eruptions.
Other: cushingoid state, susceptibility to infections, *acute adrenal insufficiency after increased stress or abrupt withdrawal after long-term therapy.* **After abrupt withdrawal (may be fatal after prolonged use):** rebound inflammation, fatigue, weakness, arthralgia, fever, dizziness, lethargy, depression, fainting, orthostatic hypotension, dyspnea, anorexia, *hypoglycemia.*

INTERACTIONS
Drug-drug. *Aspirin, indomethacin, other NSAIDs:* May increase risk of GI distress and bleeding. Use together cautiously.
Barbiturates, carbamazepine, phenytoin, rifampin: May decrease corticosteroid effect. Increase corticosteroid dosage.
Cyclosporine: May increase toxicity. Monitor patient closely.
Ketoconazole and macrolide antibiotics: May decrease methylprednisolone clearance. Decreased dose may be required.
Oral anticoagulants: May alter dosage requirements. Monitor PT and INR closely.
Potassium-depleting drugs such as thiazide diuretics: May enhance potassium-wasting effects of methylprednisolone. Monitor potassium level.
Salicylates: May decrease salicylate levels. Monitor patient for lack of salicylate effectiveness.
Skin-test antigens: May decrease response. Postpone skin testing until after therapy.
Toxoids, vaccines: May decrease antibody response and may increase risk of neurologic complications. Avoid using together.
Drug-herb. *Echinacea:* May increase immune-stimulating effects. Discourage use together.
Ginseng: May increase immune-regulating response. Discourage use together.

EFFECTS ON LAB TEST RESULTS
• May increase glucose and cholesterol levels and urine calcium levels. May

decrease T_3, T_4, potassium, and calcium levels.

• May decrease ^{131}I uptake and protein-bound iodine levels in thyroid function tests. May cause false-negative results in nitroblue tetrazolium test for systemic bacterial infections. May alter reactions to skin tests.

CONTRAINDICATIONS & CAUTIONS

• Contraindicated in patients hypersensitive to drug or its ingredients, in those with systemic fungal infections, in premature infants (acetate and succinate), and in patients receiving immunosuppressive doses together with live virus vaccines.

• Use cautiously in patients with GI ulceration or renal disease, hypertension, osteoporosis, diabetes mellitus, hypothyroidism, cirrhosis, diverticulitis, nonspecific ulcerative colitis, recent intestinal anastomoses, thromboembolic disorders, seizures, active hepatitis, myasthenia gravis, heart failure, tuberculosis, ocular herpes simplex, emotional instability, and psychotic tendencies or in breast-feeding women.

NURSING CONSIDERATIONS

• Medrol may contain tartrazine. Watch for allergic reaction to tartrazine in patients with sensitivity to aspirin.

• Drug may be used for alternate-day therapy.

• Most adverse reactions to corticosteroids are dose- or duration-dependent. For better results and less toxicity, give a once-daily dose in the morning.

• *Alert:* Different salts aren't interchangeable.

• *Alert:* Don't give Solu-Medrol intrathecally because severe adverse reactions may occur.

• If immediate onset of action is needed, don't use acetate form.

• Always adjust to lowest effective dose.

• Monitor patient's weight, blood pressure, electrolyte level, and sleep patterns. Euphoria may initially interfere with sleep, but patients typically adjust to therapy in 1 to 3 weeks.

• Monitor patient for cushingoid effects, including moon face, buffalo hump, central obesity, thinning hair, hypertension, and increased susceptibility to infection.

• Measure growth and development periodically in children during high-dose or prolonged treatment.

• Drug may mask or worsen infections, including latent amebiasis.

• Watch for depression or psychotic episodes, especially in high-dose therapy.

• Diabetic patient may need increased insulin; monitor glucose level.

• Watch for an enhanced response to drug in patients with hypothyroidism or cirrhosis.

• Unless contraindicated, give low-sodium diet that's high in potassium and protein. Give potassium supplements as needed.

• Elderly patients may be more susceptible to osteoporosis with prolonged use.

• Taper off dosage after long-term therapy.

• *Look alike–sound alike:* Don't confuse Solu-Medrol with Solu-Cortef or methylprednisolone with medroxyprogesterone.

PATIENT TEACHING

• Tell patient not to stop drug abruptly or without prescriber's consent.

• Instruct patient to take oral form of drug with milk or food.

• Teach patient signs and symptoms of early adrenal insufficiency: fatigue, muscle weakness, joint pain, fever, anorexia, nausea, shortness of breath, dizziness, and fainting.

• Instruct patient to carry or wear medical identification indicating his need for supplemental systemic glucocorticoids during stress. This card should contain prescriber's name, name of drug, and dosage taken.

• Warn patient on long-term therapy about cushingoid effects (moon face, buffalo hump) and the need to notify prescriber about sudden weight gain or swelling.

• Advise patient receiving long-term therapy to consider exercise or physical therapy. Also, tell patient to ask prescriber about vitamin D or calcium supplement.

• Instruct patient to avoid exposure to infections (such as chickenpox or measles) and to contact prescriber if such exposure occurs.

Reactions may be *common,* uncommon, *life-threatening,* or COMMON AND LIFE-THREATENING.
Interaction may have a *rapid onset* or *delayed onset.*

prednisolone
pred-NISS-oh-lone

Prelone

prednisolone acetate
Flo-Pred

prednisolone sodium phosphate
Orapred, Orapred ODT, Pediapred

Pharmacologic class:
glucocorticoid, mineralocorticoid
Pregnancy risk category C

AVAILABLE FORMS
prednisolone
Syrup: 5 mg/5 ml, 15 mg/5 ml*
Tablets: 5 mg
prednisolone acetate
Oral suspension: 15 mg/5 ml
prednisolone sodium phosphate
Oral solution: 5 mg/5 ml, 15 mg/5 ml
Orally disintegrating tablets (ODTs):
10 mg, 15 mg, 30 mg

INDICATIONS & DOSAGES
➤ **Severe inflammation, immuno-suppression**
prednisolone
Adults: 2.5 to 15 mg P.O. b.i.d., t.i.d., or q.i.d.
Children: Initially, 0.14 to 2 mg/kg/day P.O. or 4 to 60 mg/m²/day, divided q.i.d.
prednisolone acetate, prednisolone sodium phosphate
Adults: 5 to 60 mg P.O. daily in divided doses b.i.d., t.i.d., or q.i.d.
Children: Initially, 0.14 to 2 mg/kg daily, or 4 to 60 mg/m² or P.O. daily, divided t.i.d. or q.i.d.
➤ **Uncontrolled asthma in those taking inhaled corticosteroids and long-acting bronchodilators**
Children: 1 to 2 mg/kg/day prednisolone sodium phosphate or prednisolone acetate P.O. in single or divided doses. Continue short course (or "burst" therapy) until child achieves a peak expiratory flow rate of 80% of his personal best, or until symptoms resolve. This usually requires 3 to 10 days of treatment but can take longer. Tapering

the dose after improvement doesn't necessarily prevent relapse.
➤ **Acute exacerbations of multiple sclerosis**
Adults and children: 200 mg/day prednisolone sodium phosphate or prednisolone acetate P.O. as single or divided dose for 7 days; then 80 mg every other day for 1 month.
➤ **Nephrotic syndrome**
Children: 60 mg/m² daily prednisolone sodium phosphate or prednisolone acetate P.O., divided t.i.d. for 4 weeks, followed by 4 weeks of single-dose alternate-day therapy at 40 mg/m²/day.

ADMINISTRATION
P.O.
● Give drug with food to reduce GI irritation. Patient may need another drug to prevent GI irritation.
● Don't cut or crush ODTs.

ACTION
Not clearly defined. Decreases inflammation, mainly by stabilizing leukocyte lysosomal membranes; suppresses immune response; stimulates bone marrow; and influences protein, fat, and carbohydrate metabolism.

Route	Onset	Peak	Duration
P.O.	Rapid	1–2 hr	3–36 hr

ADVERSE REACTIONS
CNS: *euphoria, insomnia, **pseudotumor cerebri, seizures,*** psychotic behavior, vertigo, headache, paresthesia.
CV: ***arrhythmias, heart failure, thromboembolism,*** hypertension, edema, thrombophlebitis.
EENT: cataracts, glaucoma.
GI: *peptic ulceration, **pancreatitis,*** GI irritation, increased appetite, nausea, vomiting.
GU: menstrual irregularities, increased urine calcium levels.
Metabolic: hypokalemia, hyperglycemia, carbohydrate intolerance, hypercholesterolemia, hypocalcemia.
Musculoskeletal: growth suppression in children, muscle weakness, osteoporosis.
Skin: hirsutism, delayed wound healing, acne, various skin eruptions.

Other: *acute adrenal insufficiency,* susceptibility to infections, cushingoid state, after increased stress or abrupt withdrawal after long-term therapy.

After abrupt withdrawal: rebound inflammation, fatigue, weakness, arthralgia, fever, dizziness, lethargy, depression, fainting, orthostatic hypotension, dyspnea, anorexia, *hypoglycemia. After prolonged use, sudden withdrawal may be fatal.*

INTERACTIONS
Drug-drug. *Aspirin, indomethacin, other NSAIDs:* May increase risk of GI distress and bleeding. Use together cautiously.
Barbiturates, carbamazepine, fosphenytoin, phenytoin, rifampin: May decrease corticosteroid effect. Increase corticosteroid dosage.
Cyclosporine: May increase toxicity and risk of seizures. Monitor patient closely.
Drugs that deplete potassium, such as thiazide diuretics and amphotericin B: May enhance potassium-wasting effects of prednisolone. Monitor potassium level.
Oral anticoagulants: May alter dosage requirements. Monitor PT and INR closely.
Salicylates: May decrease salicylate level. Monitor patient for lack of salicylate effectiveness.
Skin-test antigens: May decrease response. Postpone skin testing until therapy is completed.
Toxoids, vaccines: May decrease antibody response and may increase risk of neurologic complications. Avoid using together.

EFFECTS ON LAB TEST RESULTS
• May increase glucose and cholesterol levels. May decrease T_3, T_4, potassium, and calcium levels.
• May decrease ^{131}I uptake and protein-bound iodine levels in thyroid function tests. May alter skin-test results. May cause false-negative results in nitroblue tetrazolium test for systemic bacterial infections.

CONTRAINDICATIONS & CAUTIONS
• Contraindicated in patients hypersensitive to drug or its ingredients, in those with systemic fungal infections, and in those receiving immunosuppressive doses together with live-virus vaccines.
• Use with caution in patients with recent MI.
• Use cautiously in patients with GI ulcer, renal disease, hypertension, osteoporosis, diabetes mellitus, hypothyroidism, cirrhosis, active hepatitis, diverticulitis, nonspecific ulcerative colitis, recent intestinal anastomoses, thromboembolic disorders, seizures, myasthenia gravis, heart failure, tuberculosis, ocular herpes simplex, emotional instability, and psychotic tendencies or in breast-feeding women.

NURSING CONSIDERATIONS
• Determine whether patient is sensitive to other corticosteroids.
• Always adjust to lowest effective dose.
• Drug may be used for alternate-day therapy.
• Most adverse reactions to corticosteroids are dose- or duration-dependent.
• Monitor patient's weight, blood pressure, and electrolyte level.
• Monitor patient for cushingoid effects, including moon face, buffalo hump, central obesity, thinning hair, hypertension, and increased susceptibility to infection.
• Watch for depression or psychotic episodes, especially during high-dose therapy.
• Diabetic patient may need increased insulin; monitor glucose level.
• Give patient low-sodium diet that's high in potassium and protein. Give potassium supplements as needed.
• Drug may mask or worsen infections, including latent amebiasis.
• Elderly patients may be more susceptible to osteoporosis with long-term use.
• Gradually reduce dosage after long-term therapy.
• *Look alike–sound alike:* Don't confuse prednisolone with prednisone.

PATIENT TEACHING
• Tell patient not to stop drug abruptly or without prescriber's consent.
• Instruct patient to take oral form of drug with food or milk.

Reactions may be *common*, uncommon, *life-threatening*, or COMMON AND LIFE-THREATENING.
Interaction may have a *rapid onset* or *delayed onset.*

• Teach patient signs and symptoms of early adrenal insufficiency: fatigue, muscle weakness, joint pain, fever, anorexia, nausea, shortness of breath, dizziness, and fainting.

• Instruct patient to carry medical identification that includes prescriber's name and name and dosage of drug and indicates his need for supplemental systemic glucocorticoids during stress.

• Warn patient on long-term therapy about cushingoid effects and the need to notify prescriber about sudden weight gain or swelling.

• Tell patient to report slow healing.

• Advise patient receiving long-term therapy to consider exercise or physical therapy. Also, tell him to ask prescriber about vitamin D or calcium supplement.

• Instruct patient to avoid exposure to infections and to notify prescriber if exposure occurs.

• Tell patient to avoid immunizations while taking drug.

• *Alert:* Tell patient not to cut, crush, or chew ODTs.

• Instruct patient not to remove the ODT from the blister pack until he's ready to take it. The tablet can be swallowed whole or allowed to dissolve on the tongue with or without water.

• Tell patient to store Orapred in the refrigerator at 36° to 46° F (2° to 8° C).

prednisone
PRED-ni-sone

Prednisone Intensol*, Sterapred, Sterapred DS, Winpred†

Pharmacologic class:
adrenocorticoid
Pregnancy risk category C

AVAILABLE FORMS
Oral solution: 5 mg/5 ml*, 5 mg/ml (concentrate)*
Tablet: 1 mg, 2.5 mg, 5 mg, 10 mg, 20 mg, 50 mg

INDICATIONS & DOSAGES
➤ **Severe inflammation, immuno-suppression**
Adults: 5 to 60 mg P.O. daily in single dose or as two to four divided doses. Maintenance dose given once daily or every other day. Dosage must be individualized.
Children: 0.14 to 2 mg/kg or 4 to 60 mg/m² daily P.O. in four divided doses.
➤ **Contact dermatitis; poison ivy**
Adults: Initially, 30 mg (six 5-mg tablets); taper by 5 mg daily until 21 tablets have been given.
➤ **Acute exacerbations of multiple sclerosis**
Adults: 200 mg P.O. daily for 7 days; then 80 mg P.O. every other day for 1 month.
➤ **Advanced pulmonary tuberculosis**
Adults: 40 to 60 mg P.O. daily; taper over 4 to 8 weeks.
➤ **Tuberculosis meningitis**
Adults: 1 mg/kg P.O. daily for 30 days; taper over several weeks.
➤ **Adjunctive treatment in *Pneumocystis carinii* pneumonia in patients with AIDS ◆**
Adults and children age 13 and older: 40 mg P.O. b.i.d. for 5 days; then 40 mg P.O. daily for 5 days; then 20 mg P.O. daily for 11 days or until completion of anti-infective therapy.

ADMINISTRATION
P.O.
• Unless contraindicated, give drug with food to reduce GI irritation. Patient may need another drug to prevent GI irritation.
• Solution may be diluted in juice or other flavored diluent or semisolid food such as applesauce before using.

ACTION
Not clearly defined. Decreases inflammation, mainly by stabilizing leukocyte lysosomal membranes; suppresses immune response; stimulates bone marrow; and influences protein, fat, and carbohydrate metabolism.

Route	Onset	Peak	Duration
P.O.	Variable	Variable	Variable

Half-life: 18 to 36 hours.

ADVERSE REACTIONS

CNS: *euphoria, insomnia,* psychotic behavior, ***pseudotumor cerebri,*** vertigo, headache, paresthesia, ***seizures.***

CV: ***heart failure,*** hypertension, edema, ***arrhythmias,*** thrombophlebitis, ***thromboembolism.***

EENT: cataracts, glaucoma.

GI: *peptic ulceration,* ***pancreatitis,*** GI irritation, increased appetite, nausea, vomiting.

GU: menstrual irregularities, increased urine calcium level.

Metabolic: hypokalemia, hyperglycemia, carbohydrate intolerance, hypercholesterolemia, hypocalcemia.

Musculoskeletal: growth suppression in children, muscle weakness, osteoporosis.

Skin: hirsutism, delayed wound healing, acne, various skin eruptions.

Other: cushingoid state, susceptibility to infections, ***acute adrenal insufficiency,*** after increased stress or abrupt withdrawal after long-term therapy.

After abrupt withdrawal: rebound inflammation, fatigue, weakness, arthralgia, fever, dizziness, lethargy, depression, fainting, orthostatic hypotension, dyspnea, anorexia, *hypoglycemia. After prolonged use, sudden withdrawal may be fatal.*

INTERACTIONS

Drug-drug. *Aspirin, indomethacin, other NSAIDs:* May increase risk of GI distress and bleeding. Use together cautiously.

Barbiturates, carbamazepine, fosphenytoin, phenobarbital, phenytoin, rifampin: May decrease corticosteroid effect. Increase corticosteroid dosage.

Cyclosporine: May increase toxicity and cause seizures. Monitor patient closely.

Oral anticoagulants: May alter dosage requirements. Monitor PT and INR closely.

Potassium-depleting drugs, such as thiazide diuretics and amphotericin B: May enhance potassium-wasting effects of prednisone. Monitor potassium level.

Salicylates: May decrease salicylate level. Monitor patient for lack of salicylate effectiveness.

Skin-test antigens: May decrease response. Postpone skin testing until therapy is completed.

Toxoids, vaccines: May decrease antibody response and may increase risk of neurologic complications. Avoid using together.

Troleandomcyin, ketoconazole: May inhibit the metabolism of corticosteroids and decrease their clearance. Titrate the dose of corticosteroid to avoid toxicity.

EFFECTS ON LAB TEST RESULTS

- May increase glucose and cholesterol levels. May decrease T_3, T_4, potassium, and calcium levels.
- May decrease ^{131}I uptake and protein-bound iodine values in thyroid function tests. May cause false-negative results in nitroblue tetrazolium test for systemic bacterial infections. May alter reactions to skin tests.

CONTRAINDICATIONS & CAUTIONS

- Contraindicated in patients hypersensitive to drug or its ingredients, in those with systemic fungal infections, and in those receiving immunosuppressive doses together with live-virus vaccines.
- Use cautiously in patients with recent MI, GI ulcer, renal disease, hypertension, osteoporosis, diabetes mellitus, hypothyroidism, cirrhosis, active hepatitis, diverticulitis, nonspecific ulcerative colitis, recent intestinal anastomoses, thromboembolic disorders, seizures, myasthenia gravis, heart failure, tuberculosis, ocular herpes simplex, emotional instability, and psychotic tendencies or in breast-feeding women.

NURSING CONSIDERATIONS

- Determine whether patient is sensitive to other corticosteroids.
- Drug may be used for alternate-day therapy.
- Always adjust to lowest effective dose.
- Most adverse reactions to corticosteroids are dose- or duration-dependent.
- For better results and less toxicity, give a once-daily dose in the morning.
- Drug may be used in conjunction with mineralocorticoids when needed.

Reactions may be *common,* uncommon, *life-threatening,* or COMMON AND LIFE-THREATENING.
Interaction may have a *rapid onset* or ***delayed onset.***

- Monitor patient's blood pressure, sleep patterns, and potassium level.
- Weigh patient daily; report sudden weight gain to prescriber.
- Monitor patient for cushingoid effects, including moon face, buffalo hump, central obesity, thinning hair, hypertension, and increased susceptibility to infection.
- Watch for depression or psychotic episodes, especially during high-dose therapy.
- Diabetic patient may need increased insulin; monitor glucose level.
- Elderly patients may be more susceptible to osteoporosis with long-term use.
- Drug may mask or worsen infections, including latent amebiasis.
- Unless contraindicated, give low-sodium diet that's high in potassium and protein. Give potassium supplements as needed.
- Gradually reduce dosage after long-term therapy.
- *Look alike–sound alike:* Don't confuse prednisone with prednisolone or primidone.

PATIENT TEACHING
- Tell patient not to stop drug abruptly or without prescriber's consent.
- Instruct patient to take drug with food or milk.
- Teach patient signs and symptoms of early adrenal insufficiency: fatigue, muscle weakness, joint pain, fever, anorexia, nausea, shortness of breath, dizziness, and fainting.
- Instruct patient to carry or wear medical identification indicating his need for supplemental systemic glucocorticoids during stress. It should include prescriber's name and name and dosage of drug.
- Warn patient on long-term therapy about cushingoid effects (moon face, buffalo hump) and the need to notify prescriber about sudden weight gain or swelling.
- Advise patient receiving long-term therapy to consider exercise or physical therapy. Also, tell patient to ask prescriber about vitamin D or calcium supplement.
- Tell patient to report slow healing.
- Advise patient receiving long-term therapy to have periodic eye examinations.
- Instruct patient to avoid exposure to infections and to contact prescriber if exposure occurs.

triamcinolone acetonide
trye-am-SIN-oh-lone

Kenalog-10, Kenalog-40, Trivaris

triamcinolone hexacetonide
Aristospan Intra-articular,
Aristospan Intralesional

Pharmacologic class: glucocorticoid
Pregnancy risk category C

AVAILABLE FORMS
triamcinolone acetonide
Injection (suspension): 10 mg/ml, 40 mg/ml
Injection (gel suspension): 80 mg/ml
triamcinolone hexacetonide
Injection (suspension): 5 mg/ml (intralesional); 20 mg/ml (intra-articular)

INDICATIONS & DOSAGES
➤ **Severe inflammation, immuno-suppression**
Adults: 60 mg acetonide I.M., then 20 to 100 mg I.M. acetonide as needed every 6 weeks, if possible. Or, 1 mg acetonide into lesions. Or, initially, 2.5 to 15 mg acetonide into joints (depending on joint size) or soft tissue; then may increase to 40 mg for larger areas. For Trivaris, doses up to 10 mg (smaller areas) and up to 40 mg (larger areas) have usually been sufficient. A local anesthetic is commonly injected with triamcinolone into the joint. For hexacetonide, up to 0.5 mg (of 5 mg/ml suspension) intralesional or sublesional injection per square inch of affected skin. Additional injections based on patient's response. Or, 2 to 20 mg (using the 20 mg/ml suspension) via intra-articular injection. Repeat every 3 to 4 weeks.
Children older than age 12: Initially, 60 mg acetonide I.M.; repeat with additional I.M. doses of 20 to 100 mg, as needed, at 6 week intervals, if possible.
Children ages 6 to 12: 0.03 to 0.2 mg/kg acetonide, or 1 to 6.25 mg/m^2 I.M. 1- to 7-day intervals.

ADMINISTRATION
I.M.
- Give deep into gluteal muscle. Rotate injection sites to prevent muscle atrophy.

● Don't use 10 mg/ml strength for this route.

Intra-articular
● Strict aseptic technique is mandatory.
● Prior use of a local anesthetic may be desirable.
● Each syringe of Trivaris should only be used for a single treatment.

Intralesional
● Strict aseptic technique is mandatory.
● Inject directly into the lesion intra-dermally or subcutaneously.
● It is preferable to use a tuberculin syringe and small-bore needle (not smaller than 24 gauge)

ACTION

Not clearly defined. Decreases inflammation, mainly by stabilizing leukocyte lysosomal membranes; suppresses immune response; stimulates bone marrow; and influences protein, fat, and carbohydrate metabolism.

Route	Onset	Peak	Duration
I.M., intra-articular, intralesional	Variable	Variable	Variable

Half-life: 18 to 36 hours.

ADVERSE REACTIONS

CNS: *euphoria, insomnia,* **pseudotumor cerebri, seizures,** headache, paresthesia, psychotic behavior, vertigo.
CV: **arrhythmias, heart failure, thrombo-embolism,** hypertension, edema, thrombophlebitis.
EENT: cataracts, glaucoma.
GI: **pancreatitis,** *peptic ulceration,* GI irritation, increased appetite, nausea, vomiting.
GU: menstrual irregularities, increased urine calcium level.
Metabolic: hypokalemia, hyperglycemia and carbohydrate intolerance, hypercholesterolemia, hypokalemia, hypocalcemia.
Musculoskeletal: growth suppression in children, muscle weakness, osteoporosis.
Skin: hirsutism, delayed wound healing, acne, various skin eruptions.
Other: **acute adrenal insufficiency,** cushingoid state, susceptibility to infections after increased stress or abrupt withdrawal after long-term therapy.

After abrupt withdrawal: *After prolonged use, sudden withdrawal may be fatal;* rebound inflammation, fatigue, weakness, arthralgia, fever, dizziness, lethargy, depression, fainting, orthostatic hypotension, dyspnea, anorexia, **hypoglycemia.**

INTERACTIONS

Drug-drug. *Antidiabetics:* May increase blood glucose level. Adjust dosage of antidiabetics as needed.
Aspirin, indomethacin, other NSAIDs: May increase risk of GI distress and bleeding. Use together cautiously.
Barbiturates, carbamazepine, fosphenytoin, phenytoin, rifampin: May decrease corticosteroid effect. Increase corticosteroid dosage.
Cyclosporine: May increase toxicity and seizures. Monitor patient closely.
Ketoconazole, macrolide antibiotics: May decrease metabolism or clearance of triamcinolone, respectively. Decrease triamcinolone dose or dosing interval if needed.
Oral anticoagulants: May alter dosage requirements. Monitor PT and INR closely.
Potassium-depleting drugs, such as thiazide diuretics and amphotericin B: May enhance potassium-wasting effects of triamcinolone. Monitor potassium level.
Salicylates: May decrease salicylate level. Monitor patient for lack of salicylate effectiveness.
Skin-test antigens: May decrease response. Postpone skin testing until after therapy.
Toxoids, vaccines: May decrease antibody response and increase risk of neurologic complications. Avoid using together.

EFFECTS ON LAB TEST RESULTS

● May increase glucose and cholesterol levels. May decrease potassium and calcium levels.
● May decrease ^{131}I uptake and protein-bound iodine values in thyroid function tests. May alter reactions to skin tests.
● May cause false-negative results in nitroblue tetrazolium test for systemic bacterial infections.

Reactions may be *common,* uncommon, *life-threatening,* or COMMON AND LIFE-THREATENING.
Interaction may have a *rapid onset* or **delayed onset.**

CONTRAINDICATIONS & CAUTIONS

• Contraindicated in patients hypersensitive to drug or its ingredients, in those with systemic fungal infections, and in those receiving immunosuppressive doses together with live-virus vaccines.
• Use cautiously in patients with recent MI, GI ulcer, renal disease, hypertension, osteoporosis, diabetes mellitus, hypothyroidism, cirrhosis, diverticulitis, nonspecific ulcerative colitis, recent intestinal anastomoses, thromboembolic disorders, seizures, myasthenia gravis, active hepatitis, lactation, heart failure, tuberculosis, ocular herpes simplex, emotional instability, or psychotic tendencies.

NURSING CONSIDERATIONS

• Determine whether patient is sensitive to other corticosteroids.
• Drug isn't used for alternate-day therapy.
• Always adjust to lowest effective dose.
• Most adverse reactions to corticosteroids are dose- or duration-dependent.
• Monitor patient's weight, blood pressure, and electrolyte level.
• Monitor patient for cushingoid effects, such as moon face, buffalo hump, central obesity, thinning hair, hypertension, and increased susceptibility to infection.
• Watch for allergic reaction to tartrazine in patients sensitive to aspirin.
• Watch for depression or psychotic episodes, especially during high-dose therapy.
• Diabetic patient may need increased insulin dosage; monitor glucose level.
• Drug may mask or worsen infections, including latent amebiasis.
• Elderly patients may be more susceptible to osteoporosis with long-term use.
• Unless contraindicated, give low-sodium diet that's high in potassium and protein. Give potassium supplements as needed.
• Gradually reduce dosage after long-term therapy. Drug may affect patient's sleep.
• *Look alike–sound alike:* Don't confuse triamcinolone with Triaminic.

PATIENT TEACHING

• Tell patient not to stop drug abruptly or without prescriber's consent.
• Teach patient signs and symptoms of early adrenal insufficiency: fatigue, muscle weakness, joint pain, fever, anorexia, nausea, shortness of breath, dizziness, and fainting.
• Instruct patient to carry medical identification that includes prescriber's name and drug's name and dosage and indicates his need for supplemental systemic glucocorticoids during stress.
• Warn patient on long-term therapy about cushingoid effects (moon face, buffalo hump) and the need to notify prescriber about sudden weight gain and swelling.
• Tell patient to report slow healing.
• Advise patient receiving long-term therapy to consider exercise or physical therapy. Also, tell patient to ask prescriber about vitamin D or calcium supplement.
• Instruct patient to avoid exposure to infections and to notify prescriber if exposure occurs.

77

Thyroid hormone antagonists

methimazole
potassium iodide
propylthiouracil
radioactive iodine

methimazole
meth-IM-a-zole

Tapazole

Pharmacologic class: thyroid
hormone antagonist
Pregnancy risk category D

AVAILABLE FORMS
Tablets: 5 mg, 10 mg, 15 mg, 20 mg

INDICATIONS & DOSAGES
➤ **Hyperthyroidism**
Adults: If mild, 15 mg P.O. daily. If
moderately severe, 30 to 40 mg daily. If
severe, 60 mg daily. Daily amount is
divided into three equal doses and given
at 8-hour intervals. Maintenance dosage
is 5 to 30 mg daily.
Children: 0.4 mg/kg P.O. in three divided
doses daily. Maintenance dosage is
0.2 mg/kg in divided doses daily.

ADMINISTRATION
P.O.
● Give drug with meals to minimize
adverse GI effects.

ACTION
Inhibits synthesis of thyroid hormones.

Route	Onset	Peak	Duration
P.O.	Rapid	30–60 min	Unknown

Half-life: 5 to 13 hours.

ADVERSE REACTIONS
CNS: headache, drowsiness, vertigo,
paresthesia, neuritis, neuropathies, CNS
stimulation, depression, fever.
CV: edema.
GI: diarrhea, nausea, vomiting, salivary gland
enlargement, loss of taste, epigastric distress.
GU: nephritis.

Hematologic: *agranulocytosis, leukopenia,
thrombocytopenia, aplastic anemia.*
Hepatic: jaundice, hepatic dysfunction,
hepatitis.
Metabolic: hypothyroidism.
Musculoskeletal: arthralgia, myalgia.
Skin: rash, urticaria, discoloration, pruritus,
erythema nodosum, exfoliative dermatitis,
lupuslike syndrome, abnormal hair loss.
Other: lymphadenopathy.

INTERACTIONS
Drug-drug. *Aminophylline, theophylline:*
May decrease clearance of these drugs.
Dosage may need to be adjusted.
Beta blockers: Beta-blocker clearance
may be enhanced by hyperthyroidism.
Dosage of beta blocker may need to be
reduced when patient becomes euthyroid.
Cardiac glycosides: May increase cardiac
glycoside level. Cardiac glycoside dosage
may need to be reduced.
Potassium iodide: May decrease response
to drug. Methimazole dosage may need to
be increased.
Warfarin: May alter dosage requirements.
Monitor PT, PTT, and INR.

EFFECTS ON LAB TEST RESULTS
● May decrease hemoglobin level.
● May decrease granulocyte, WBC, and
platelet counts.
● May alter thyroid uptake of ^{123}I or ^{131}I.

CONTRAINDICATIONS & CAUTIONS
● Contraindicated in patients hypersensitive
to drug and in breast-feeding women.
● Use cautiously in pregnant patients.

NURSING CONSIDERATIONS
● Pregnant women may need less drug as
pregnancy progresses. Monitor thyroid
function studies closely. Thyroid hormone
may be added to regimen. Drug may be
stopped during last few weeks of pregnancy.
● Monitor CBC periodically to detect
impending leukopenia, thrombocytopenia,
and agranulocytosis; also monitor hepatic
function. Stop drug if liver abnormality
occurs.

Reactions may be *common,* uncommon, *life-threatening,* or COMMON AND LIFE-THREATENING.
Interaction may have a *rapid onset* or *delayed onset.*

• *Alert:* Doses higher than 30 mg daily increase risk of agranulocytosis.
• *Alert:* Patients older than age 40 may have an increased risk of drug-induced agranulocytosis.
• Watch for evidence of hypothyroidism (mental depression, cold intolerance, and hard, nonpitting edema); notify prescriber because patient may need dosage adjustment.
• *Alert:* Stop drug and notify prescriber if severe rash or enlarged cervical lymph nodes develop.
• *Look alike–sound alike:* Don't confuse methimazole with mebendazole, methazolamide, metolazone, or metronidazole.

PATIENT TEACHING
• Tell patient to take drug with meals to reduce adverse GI reactions.
• Warn patient to report fever, sore throat, mouth sores, skin eruptions, anorexia, itching, right upper quadrant pain, or yellow skin or eyes.
• Tell patient to ask prescriber about using iodized salt and eating shellfish because the iodine in these foods may make the drug less effective.
• Warn patient that drug may cause drowsiness; advise patient to use caution when operating machinery or a vehicle.
• Instruct patient to store drug in light-resistant container.
• Teach patient to watch for evidence of hypothyroidism (unexplained weight gain, fatigue, cold intolerance) and to notify prescriber if it arises.
• Tell woman not to use drug while breast-feeding.

---

potassium iodide
po-TASS-ee-um

Iosat ◇, Pima, saturated solution (SSKI), strong iodine solution (Lugol's solution), ThyroSafe ◇, ThyroShield ◇

Pharmacologic class: salt of stable iodine
Pregnancy risk category D

AVAILABLE FORMS
Oral solution (Lugol's solution): iodine 5% and potassium iodide 10%

Oral solution (SSKI): 1 g/ml
Oral solution (ThyroShield): 65 mg/ml
Syrup (Pima): 325 mg/5 ml
Tablets: 65 mg, 130 mg

INDICATIONS & DOSAGES
➤ **To prepare for thyroidectomy**
Adults and children: 2 to 6 drops strong iodine solution P.O. t.i.d.; or 1 to 5 drops SSKI in water P.O. t.i.d. after meals for 10 days before surgery.
➤ **Thyrotoxic crisis**
Adults and children: 500 mg P.O. every 4 hours (about 10 drops of SSKI); or 1 ml of strong iodine solution t.i.d. Give at least 1 hour after the first dose of propylthiouracil or methimazole.
➤ **Radiation protectant for thyroid gland (strong iodine solution)**
Adults and children age 1 and older: 130 mg P.O. daily for 10 days unless directed otherwise by public health authorities. Start no later than 3 to 4 hours after exposure. Avoid repeat dosing, if possible, in pregnant or breast-feeding women.
Infants up to age 1: 65 mg P.O. daily for 10 days unless directed otherwise by public health authorities. Start no later than 3 to 4 hours after exposure.
➤ **Radiation protectant for thyroid gland (ThyroShield)**
Adults and children ages 12 to 18 weighing at least 68 kg (150 lb): 130 mg (2 ml) P.O. every 24 hours for 10 days unless directed otherwise by public health authorities. Start no later than 3 to 4 hours after exposure. Avoid repeat dosing in pregnant or breast-feeding women.
Children ages 3 to 12 or children ages 12 to 18 weighing less than 68 kg (150 lb): 65 mg (1 ml) P.O. every 24 hours for 10 days unless directed otherwise by public health authorities. Start no later than 3 to 4 hours after exposure.
Children ages 1 month to 3 years: 32.5 mg (0.5 ml) P.O. every 24 hours for 10 days unless directed otherwise by public health authorities. Start no later than 3 to 4 hours after exposure.
Neonates from birth to 1 month: 16.25 mg (0.25 ml) P.O. every 24 hours for 10 days unless directed otherwise by public health authorities. Start no later than 3 to 4 hours after exposure. Avoid repeat dosing, if possible.

➤ Expectorant
Adults: 5 to 10 ml (325 mg to 650 mg) Pima P.O. t.i.d. Or, 300 to 600 mg SSKI P.O. t.i.d. to q.i.d.
Children: 2.5 to 5 ml (162.5 mg to 325 mg) Pima P.O. t.i.d.

ADMINISTRATION
P.O.
• Dilute oral solution in water, milk, or fruit juice, and give after meals to prevent gastric irritation, hydrate patient, and mask salty taste.
• Give iodides through straw to avoid tooth discoloration.
• Store in light-resistant container.

ACTION
Inhibits thyroid hormone formation, limits iodide transport into the thyroid gland, and blocks thyroid hormone release.

Route	Onset	Peak	Duration
P.O.	< 24 hr	10–15 days	Unknown

Half-life: Unknown.

ADVERSE REACTIONS
CNS: fever.
EENT: periorbital edema.
GI: nausea, vomiting, diarrhea, inflammation of salivary glands, burning mouth and throat, sore teeth and gums, *metallic taste.*
Metabolic: *potassium toxicity.*
Skin: acneiform rash.
Other: hypersensitivity reactions (including ***angioedema***).

INTERACTIONS
Drug-drug. *ACE inhibitors, potassium-sparing diuretics:* May cause hyperkalemia. Avoid using together.
Antithyroid drugs: May increase hypothyroid or goitrogenic effects. Monitor patient closely.
Lithium carbonate: May cause hypothyroidism. Use together cautiously.
Drug-food. *Iodized salt, shellfish:* May alter drug's effectiveness. Urge caution.

EFFECTS ON LAB TEST RESULTS
• May increase potassium level.
• May alter thyroid function test results.

CONTRAINDICATIONS & CAUTIONS
• Contraindicated in patients with tuberculosis, acute bronchitis, iodide hypersensitivity, or hyperkalemia. Some formulations contain sulfites, which may cause allergic reactions in hypersensitive patients.
• Use cautiously in patients with hypocomplementemic vasculitis, goiter, or autoimmune thyroid disease.

NURSING CONSIDERATIONS
• The FDA doesn't recommend prophylaxis with potassium iodide for a radiation emergency in adults over age 40 unless a large internal radiation dose is anticipated.
• For thyrotoxicosis, first iodine dose is given at least 1 hour after first dose of propylthiouracil and methimazole.
• ***Alert:*** Earliest signs of delayed hypersensitivity reactions caused by iodides are irritation and swollen eyelids.
• Signs of an iodide hypersensitivity reaction include angioedema, cutaneous and mucosal hemorrhage, fever, arthralgia, lymph node enlargement, and eosinophilia.
• Monitor patient for iodism, which can cause metallic taste, burning in mouth and throat, sore teeth and gums, increased salivation, coryza, sneezing, eye irritation with swelling of eyelids, severe headache, productive cough, GI irritation, diarrhea, rash, or soreness of the pharynx, larynx, and tonsils.

PATIENT TEACHING
• Show patient how to mask salty taste of oral solution. Tell him to take all forms of drug after meals.
• ***Alert:*** Warn patient that sudden withdrawal may precipitate thyroid crisis.
• ***Alert:*** Teach patient signs and symptoms of potassium toxicity, including confusion, irregular heart beat, numbness, tingling, pain or weakness of hands or feet, and tiredness.
• Tell patient to ask prescriber about using iodized salt and eating shellfish. These foods contain iodine and may alter drug's effectiveness.
• Tell patient not to increase the amount of potassium through diet.
• Tell patient to stop drug and notify prescriber if epigastric pain, rash, metallic taste, nausea, or vomiting occurs.

Reactions may be *common*, uncommon, *life-threatening*, or COMMON AND LIFE-THREATENING.
Interaction may have a *rapid onset* or *delayed onset*.

propylthiouracil (PTU)

proe-pill-thye-oh-YOOR-a-sill

Propyl-Thyracil†

Pharmacologic class: thyroid hormone antagonist
Pregnancy risk category D

Route	Onset	Peak	Duration
P.O.	Unknown	60–90 min	Unknown

Half-life: 1 to 2 hours.

AVAILABLE FORMS
Tablets: 50 mg, 100 mg†

INDICATIONS & DOSAGES
➤ **Hyperthyroidism**
Adults: 300 to 450 mg P.O. daily in divided doses. Patients with severe hyperthyroidism or very large goiters may need initial doses of 600 to 1,200 mg daily. Continue until patient is euthyroid; then start maintenance dose of 100 mg to 150 mg P.O. daily.
Children older than age 10: Initially, 150 to 300 mg or 150 mg/m² P.O. daily in divided doses. Continue until patient is euthyroid. Individualize maintenance dose.
Children ages 6 to 10: Initially, 50 to 150 mg P.O. daily in divided doses every 8 hours. Continue until patient is euthyroid. Individualize maintenance dose.
Neonates: 5 to 10 mg/kg P.O. daily in divided doses t.i.d.
➤ **Thyrotoxic crisis**
Adults: 200 mg P.O. every 4 to 6 hours on first day; after symptoms are fully controlled, gradually reduce dosage to usual maintenance levels.

ADMINISTRATION
P.O.
• Give in three equally divided doses about 8 hours apart.
• Give drug with meals to reduce adverse GI reactions.
• Store drug in light-resistant container.

ACTION
Inhibits oxidation of iodine in thyroid gland, blocking ability of iodine to combine with tyrosine to form T_4, and may prevent coupling of monoiodotyrosine and diiodotyrosine to form T_4 and T_3.

ADVERSE REACTIONS
CNS: headache, drowsiness, vertigo, paresthesia, neuritis, neuropathies, CNS stimulation, depression, fever.
CV: vasculitis.
EENT: visual disturbances, loss of taste.
GI: diarrhea, *nausea, vomiting,* epigastric distress, salivary gland enlargement.
GU: nephritis.
Hematologic: *agranulocytosis, leukopenia, thrombocytopenia, aplastic anemia.*
Hepatic: jaundice, *hepatotoxicity.*
Metabolic: dose-related hypothyroidism.
Musculoskeletal: arthralgia, myalgia.
Skin: rash, urticaria, skin discoloration, pruritus, erythema nodosum, exfoliative dermatitis, lupuslike syndrome.
Other: lymphadenopathy.

INTERACTIONS
Drug-drug. *Aminophylline, oxtriphylline, theophylline:* May decrease clearance of these drugs. Dosage may need to be adjusted.
Cardiac glycosides: May increase glycoside level. Dosage may need to be reduced.
Potassium iodide: May decrease response to drug. Dosage of antithyroid drug may need to be increased.
Warfarin: May increase anticoagulation. Monitor PT and INR.
Drug-food. *Iodized salt, shellfish:* May alter drug's effectiveness. Urge caution.

EFFECTS ON LAB TEST RESULTS
• May decrease hemoglobin level.
• May decrease granulocyte, WBC, and platelet counts and liothyronine uptake.

CONTRAINDICATIONS & CAUTIONS
• Contraindicated in patients hypersensitive to drug and in breast-feeding women.
• Use cautiously in pregnant patients.

NURSING CONSIDERATIONS
• Pregnant women may need less drug as pregnancy progresses. Monitor thyroid function studies closely. Thyroid hormone may be added to regimen. Drug may

be stopped during last few weeks of pregnancy.

• **Alert:** Patients older than age 40 may have an increased risk of agranulocytosis.

• Watch for hypothyroidism (mental depression, cold intolerance, and hard, nonpitting edema); adjust dosage.

• Monitor CBC periodically to detect impending leukopenia, thrombocytopenia, and agranulocytosis.

• **Alert:** Stop drug and notify prescriber if severe rash develops or cervical lymph nodes enlarge.

• Monitor hepatic function. Stop drug if transaminase levels are greater than three times the upper limit of normal.

• **Look alike–sound alike:** Don't confuse propylthiouracil with Purinethol.

PATIENT TEACHING

• Instruct patient to take drug with meals.

• Warn patient to report fever, sore throat, mouth sores, and skin eruptions.

• Tell patient to report unusual bleeding or bruising.

• Tell patient to ask prescriber about using iodized salt and eating shellfish. These foods contain iodine and may alter effectiveness of drug.

• Teach patient to watch for signs and symptoms of hypothyroidism (unexplained weight gain, fatigue, cold intolerance) and to notify prescriber if they occur.

SAFETY ALERT!

radioactive iodine (sodium iodide, I¹³¹)
Hicon, Sodium Iodide, I¹³¹
Therapeutic

Pharmacologic class: thyroid hormone antagonist
Pregnancy risk category X

AVAILABLE FORMS

All radioactivity concentrations are determined at time of calibration.

Sodium Iodide ¹³¹I Therapeutic
Capsules: Radioactivity range 0.75 to 100 mCi/capsule
Oral solution: Radioactivity range 3.5 to 150 mCi/vial
Concentrated oral solution: 1,000 mCi/ml

INDICATIONS & DOSAGES

➤ **Hyperthyroidism**
Adults: Usual dosage is 4 to 10 mCi P.O. Dosage is based on estimated weight of thyroid gland and thyroid uptake. Repeat treatment after 6 weeks, based on T₄ level.

➤ **Thyroid cancer**
Adults: Initially, 50 to 100 mCi P.O., with subsequent doses of 100 to 150 mCi. Dosage is based on estimated malignant thyroid tissue and metastatic tissue as determined by total body scan. Repeat treatment according to clinical status.

ADMINISTRATION

P.O.

• Institute full radiation precautions. Have patient use proper disposal methods when coughing and expectorating. After dose for hyperthyroidism, patient's urine and saliva are slightly radioactive for 24 hours; vomitus is highly radioactive for 6 to 8 hours.

• After dose for thyroid cancer, patient's urine, saliva, and perspiration are radioactive for 3 days. Isolate patient and observe these precautions: Don't allow pregnant personnel to care for patient; provide disposable eating utensils and linens; instruct patient to save urine in lead container for 24 to 48 hours; limit contact with patient to 30 minutes per shift per person on day 1, and increase time, as needed, to 1 hour on day 2 and longer on day 3.

ACTION

Limits thyroid hormone secretion by destroying thyroid tissue. Affinity of thyroid tissue for radioactive iodine facilitates uptake of drug by cancerous thyroid tissue that has metastasized to other sites in the body.

Route	Onset	Peak	Duration
P.O.	Unknown	60–90 min	Unknown

Half-life: Unknown.

ADVERSE REACTIONS

CV: chest pain, tachycardia.
EENT: *fullness in neck,* pain on swallowing, sore throat.
GI: nausea, vomiting.

Reactions may be *common*, uncommon, *life-threatening*, or COMMON AND LIFE-THREATENING.
Interaction may have a *rapid onset* or **delayed onset.**

Hematologic: anemia, blood dyscrasia, *leukopenia, thrombocytopenia.*
Metabolic: hypothyroidism, radiation-induced thyroiditis.
Respiratory: cough.
Skin: rash, pruritus, urticaria, temporary thinning of hair.
Other: radiation sickness, allergic-type reactions.

INTERACTIONS
Drug-drug. *Lithium carbonate:* May cause hypothyroidism. Use together cautiously.
These drugs may interfere with the action of ^{131}I and should be withheld for the specified time before the ^{131}I dose is given:
Adrenocorticoids: 1 week.
Benzodiazepines: 1 month.
Cholecystographic drugs: 6 to 9 months.
Contrast media that contain iodine: 1 to 2 months.
Products containing iodine, including topical drugs, and vitamins: 2 weeks.
Salicylates: 1 to 2 weeks.
Also, the uptake of radioiodide will be affected by the use of thyroid and antithyroid drugs.

EFFECTS ON LAB TEST RESULTS
• May decrease hemoglobin, T_4, and thyroid-stimulating hormone levels. May increase or decrease protein-bound iodine level.
• May decrease platelet and WBC counts. May alter ^{131}I thyroid uptake.

CONTRAINDICATIONS & CAUTIONS
• Contraindicated in women who are or may become pregnant or are breast-feeding.
• Contraindicated in a patient who is vomiting or has diarrhea.

NURSING CONSIDERATIONS
• All antithyroid drugs and thyroid preparations must be stopped 1 week before ^{131}I dose. If this isn't possible, patient may receive thyroid-stimulating hormone for 3 days before ^{131}I dose.
• Measure the dose by a radioactivity calibration system immediately before administration.
• Sodium iodide ^{131}I is not typically used for treatment of hyperthyroidism in patients younger than age 30.

• When treating women of childbearing age, give dose during menstruation or within 7 days afterward.
• After therapy for hyperthyroidism, patient shouldn't resume antithyroid drugs but should continue propranolol or other drugs used to treat symptoms of hyperthyroidism until onset of full ^{131}I effect (usually 6 weeks).
• Monitor thyroid function by T_4 and thyroid-stimulating hormone levels.

PATIENT TEACHING
• Tell patient to fast overnight before therapy and to drink as much fluid as possible for 48 hours afterward.
• Instruct patient about appropriate radiation exposure precautions to use after receiving drug.
• Warn patient who's discharged fewer than 7 days after ^{131}I dose for thyroid cancer to avoid close contact with small children and not to sleep in same room with another person for 7 days after treatment.
• Teach patient the signs and symptoms of hypothyroidism (unexplained weight gain, fatigue, cold intolerance) and instruct him to notify prescriber if they occur.

78

Thyroid hormones

levothyroxine sodium
liothyronine sodium
liotrix

---

levothyroxine sodium
(T_4 L-thyroxine sodium)
lee-voe-thye-ROX-een

Eltroxin†, Euthyrox†, Levo-T, Levothroid, Levoxyl✿, Synthroid✿, Unithroid Direct

Pharmacologic class: thyroid hormone
Pregnancy risk category A

AVAILABLE FORMS
Tablets: 25 mcg, 50 mcg, 75 mcg, 88 mcg, 100 mcg, 112 mcg, 125 mcg, 137 mcg, 150 mcg, 175 mcg, 200 mcg, 300 mcg

INDICATIONS & DOSAGES
➤ **Thyroid hormone replacement**
Adults: For patients younger than age 50 or those older than age 50 who have been recently treated for hyperthyroidism, or have been hypothyroid for a short time, give 1.7 mcg/kg P.O. once daily. Monitor thyroid-stimulating hormone (TSH) levels every 6 to 8 weeks, making dosage adjustments in 12.5- to 25-mcg increments until patient is euthyroid and TSH level normalizes.
Adults: For patients age 50 or older or those younger than age 50 with underlying cardiac disease, give 25 to 50 mcg P.O. daily. Adjust dose every 6 to 8 weeks, if needed, until patient is euthyroid and TSH level normalizes.
Children older than age 12: More than 150 mcg or 2 to 3 mcg/kg P.O. daily.
Children ages 6 to 12: 100 to 150 mcg or 4 to 5 mcg/kg P.O. daily.
Children ages 1 to 5: 75 to 100 mcg or 5 to 6 mcg/kg P.O. daily.
Children ages 6 months to 1 year: 50 to 75 mcg or 6 to 8 mcg/kg P.O. daily.
Children ages 3 to 6 months: 25 to 50 mcg or 8 to 10 mcg/kg P.O. daily.

Infants and neonates birth to 3 months: 10 to 15 mcg/kg P.O. daily. In neonates at risk for cardiac failure, use a lower initial dose (such as 25 mcg daily), and increase every 4 to 6 weeks as needed.
Elderly patients with underlying cardiovascular disease: 12.5 to 25 mcg P.O. daily; increase by 12.5 to 25 mcg every 4 to 6 weeks, depending on response.
➤ **Severe, long-standing hypo-thyroidism**
Adults: 12.5 to 25 mcg P.O. daily. Increase in increments of 25 mcg every 2 to 4 weeks as needed.
Children: 25 mcg P.O. daily. Increase in increments of 25 mcg every 2 to 4 weeks as needed.

ADMINISTRATION
P.O.
● Synthroid may contain tartrazine.
● Give drug at same time each day on an empty stomach, preferably ½ to 1 hour before breakfast.
● Give levoxyl with a full glass of water to prevent choking, gagging, and difficulty swallowing.
● If necessary, crush tablet and suspend it in small amount of formula (except soy formula, which may decrease the absorption), breast milk, or water, and give by spoon or dropper. Crushed tablet can also be sprinkled over food, except foods containing large amounts of soybean, fiber, or iron.

ACTION
Not completely defined. Stimulates metabolism of all body tissues by accelerating rate of cellular oxidation.

Route	Onset	Peak	Duration
P.O.	24 hr	Unknown	Unknown

Half-life: 3 to 4 days in hyperthyroidism; 9 to 10 days in hypothyroidism.

ADVERSE REACTIONS
CNS: *nervousness, insomnia, tremor,* headache, fever.

Reactions may be *common,* uncommon, *life-threatening,* or COMMON AND LIFE-THREATENING.
Interaction may have a *rapid onset* or **delayed onset.**

Thyroid hormones 1091

CV: *tachycardia, palpitations, **arrhythmias**, angina pectoris, **cardiac arrest.***
GI: diarrhea, vomiting.
GU: menstrual irregularities.
Metabolic: weight loss.
Musculoskeletal: decreased bone density.
Skin: allergic skin reactions, diaphoresis.
Other: heat intolerance.

INTERACTIONS

Drug-drug. *Amiodarone, iodide (including iodine-containing radiographic contrast agents), lithium:* May reduce thyroid hormone secretion. Monitor thyroid function studies if used together.
Antacids, calcium carbonate, cholestyramine, colestipol, ferrous sulfate, sucralfate: May impair levothyroxine absorption. Separate doses by 4 to 5 hours.
Beta blockers: May reduce beta-blocker effects. Monitor patient.
Carbamazepine, hydantoins, phenobarbital, rifampin: May increase hepatic metabolism, resulting in hypothyroidism. Monitor patient.
Digoxin: May decrease glycoside effects. Monitor patient for clinical effect.
Estrogens: May decrease thyroid levels. Monitor levels after 12 weeks of therapy and adjust levothyroxine dose as needed.
Fosphenytoin, phenytoin: May release free thyroid hormone. Monitor patient for tachycardia.
Insulin, oral antidiabetics: May alter glucose level. Monitor glucose level. Dosage adjustments may be needed.
Ketamine: May produce marked hypertension and tachycardia. Use together cautiously.
Sympathomimetics such as epinephrine: May increase risk of coronary insufficiency. Monitor patient closely.
Selective serotonin reuptake inhibitors: May increase levothyroxine requirements. Adjust dosage as needed.
Theophylline: May decrease theophylline clearance in hypothyroidism; clearance may return to normal when euthyroid state is achieved. Monitor theophylline level.
Tricyclic antidepressants, tetracyclic antidepressants: May increase therapeutic effects and toxicity of both drugs. Monitor patient closely.
Warfarin: May increase anticoagulant effects. Monitor patient for bleeding and check PT and INR closely. Warfarin dosage adjustment may be needed.
Drug-herb. *Horseradish:* May cause abnormal thyroid function. Discourage use in patients undergoing thyroid function tests.
Lemon balm: May have antithyroid effects; may inhibit TSH. Discourage use together.
Drug-food. *Cottonseed meal, dietary fiber, soybean flour, walnuts.* May decrease absorption of drug. Dosage adjustments may be needed.

EFFECTS ON LAB TEST RESULTS
• May decrease thyroid function test results. May alter results of liothyronine, protein-bound iodine, and radioactive ^{131}I uptake studies.

CONTRAINDICATIONS & CAUTIONS
• Contraindicated in patients hypersensitive to drug and in those with acute MI uncomplicated by hypothyroidism, untreated subclinical or overt thyrotoxicosis, or uncorrected adrenal insufficiency.
• Use cautiously in elderly patients and in those with angina pectoris, hypertension, other CV disorders, renal insufficiency, or ischemia.
• Use cautiously in patients with diabetes mellitus, diabetes insipidus, or myxedema and during rapid replacement in those with arteriosclerosis.

NURSING CONSIDERATIONS
• Patients with diabetes mellitus may need increased antidiabetic doses when starting thyroid hormone replacement.
• Watch for angina, coronary occlusion, or stroke in patients with arteriosclerosis who are receiving rapid replacement.
• In patients with coronary artery disease who must receive thyroid hormone, observe carefully for possible coronary insufficiency.
• Patients with adult hypothyroidism are unusually sensitive to thyroid hormone. Start at lowest dosage, and adjust to higher dosages according to patient's symptoms and laboratory data until euthyroid state is reached.
• When changing from levothyroxine to liothyronine, stop levothyroxine and begin

†Canada ◇OTC ♦Off-label use ✔Photoguide *Liquid contains alcohol.

liothyronine. Increase dosage in small increments after residual effects of levo-thyroxine have disappeared. When changing from liothyronine to levothyroxine, start levothyroxine several days before withdrawing liothyronine to avoid relapse. Drugs aren't interchangeable.

• Long-term therapy causes bone loss in premenopausal and postmenopausal women. Consider a basal bone density measurement, and monitor patient closely for osteoporosis.

• Patients taking levothyroxine who need to have ^{131}I uptake studies performed must stop drug 4 weeks before test.

• Patients taking anticoagulants may need their dosage modified and require careful monitoring of coagulation status.

• Dosage may need to be increased in pregnant patients.

• Drug shouldn't be used for infertility (unless associated with hypothyroidism).

■ **Black Box Warning** Drug should not be used for the treatment of obesity or for weight loss. ■

• *Look alike–sound alike:* Don't confuse levothyroxine with liothyronine or liotrix or Lamictal.

PATIENT TEACHING
• Teach patient the importance of compliance. Tell him to take drug at same time each day, preferably ½ to 1 hour before breakfast, to maintain constant hormone levels and help prevent insomnia.

• Make sure patient understands that replacement therapy is usually for life. The drug should never be stopped unless directed by prescriber.

• Warn patient (especially elderly patient) to notify prescriber immediately about chest pain, palpitations, sweating, nervousness, shortness of breath, or other signals of overdose or aggravated CV disease.

• Tell caregiver of infant or child who can't swallow tablets to crush tablet and suspend in small amount of formula (except soy formula, which may decrease the absorption), breast milk, or water, and give by spoon or dropper. Crushed tablet can be sprinkled over food, except foods containing large amounts of soybean, fiber, or iron.

• Tell patient using Levoxyl to take pill with plenty of water to avoid choking,

gagging, or getting the pill stuck in his throat.

• Advise patient who has achieved stable response not to change brands.

• Tell patient to report unusual bleeding and bruising.

• Advise patient not to take OTC or other prescription drugs without first consulting prescriber.

• Advise patient to report pregnancy to prescriber because dosage may need adjustment.

• Advise patient to protect tablets from light and moisture.

---

liothyronine sodium (T₃)
lye-oh-THYE-roe-neen

Cytomel, Triostat

Pharmacologic class: thyroid hormone
Pregnancy risk category A

AVAILABLE FORMS
Injection: 10 mcg/ml in 1-ml vials*
Tablets: 5 mcg, 25 mcg, 50 mcg

INDICATIONS & DOSAGES
➤ **Congenital hypothyroidism**
Children: 5 mcg P.O. daily; increase by 5 mcg every 3 to 4 days until desired response is achieved.
➤ **Myxedema**
Adults: Initially, 5 mcg P.O. daily; increase by 5 to 10 mcg every 1 to 2 weeks until daily dose reaches 25 mcg. Then increase by 5 to 25 mcg daily every 1 to 2 weeks. Maintenance dosage is 50 to 100 mcg daily.
➤ **Myxedema coma, premyxedema coma**
Adults: Initially, 10 to 20 mcg I.V. for patients with CV disease; 25 to 50 mcg I.V. for patients who don't have CV disease. Adjust dosage based on patient's condition and response. Switch patient to oral therapy as soon as possible.
➤ **Simple (nontoxic) goiter**
Adults: Initially, 5 mcg P.O. daily; may increase by 5 to 10 mcg daily every 1 to 2 weeks, until daily dose reaches 25 mcg. Then increase by 12.5 to 25 mcg daily

---

Reactions may be *common*, uncommon, *life-threatening*, or COMMON AND LIFE-THREATENING.
Interaction may have a *rapid onset* or **delayed onset**.

every 1 to 2 weeks. Usual maintenance dosage is 75 mcg daily.
Patients older than age 65 and children: 5 mcg daily; increase by 5 mcg daily every 1 to 2 weeks.
➤ **Thyroid hormone replacement**
Adults: Initially, 25 mcg P.O. daily; increase by 12.5 to 25 mcg every 1 to 2 weeks until satisfactory response occurs. Usual maintenance dosage is 25 to 75 mcg daily.
➤ **T₃ suppression test to differentiate hyperthyroidism from euthyroidism**
Adults: 75 to 100 mcg P.O. daily for 7 days.

ADMINISTRATION
P.O.
● When switching from I.V. therapy, discontinue I.V. dose, begin P.O. at a low dose, and increase gradually according to patient response.
● Give drug at same time each day, preferably before breakfast.
I.V.
● **Alert:** Don't give I.M. or subcutaneously.
● Give repeat doses 4 to 12 hours apart.
● To store, refrigerate vials.
● When switching to P.O. levothyroxine from I.V. liothyronine, decrease I.V. dose gradually.
● **Incompatibilities:** None reported.

ACTION
Unclear. Enhances oxygen consumption by most tissues of the body; increases the basal metabolic rate and the metabolism of carbohydrates, lipids, and proteins.

Route	Onset	Peak	Duration
P.O.	Unknown	2–3 days	3 days
I.V.	Unknown	Unknown	Unknown

Half-life: Less than or equal to 2½ days.

ADVERSE REACTIONS
CNS: *nervousness, insomnia, tremor,* headache, fever.
CV: *tachycardia, arrhythmias,* angina, *cardiac decompensation and collapse, MI.*
GI: diarrhea, vomiting.
GU: menstrual irregularities.
Metabolic: weight loss.
Musculoskeletal: accelerated bone maturation in infants and children.
Skin: skin reactions, diaphoresis.
Other: heat intolerance.

INTERACTIONS
Drug-drug. *Beta blockers:* May reduce beta-blocker effect. Monitor patient for clinical effect.
Aluminum and magnesium antacids, cholestyramine, colestipol, sucralfate: May impair liothyronine absorption. Separate doses by 4 to 5 hours.
Digoxin: May decrease glycoside effect. Monitor patient for clinical effect.
Insulin, oral antidiabetics: First thyroid replacement therapy may increase insulin or oral hypoglycemic requirements. Monitor glucose level. Dosage adjustments may be needed.
Ketamine: May cause hypertension and tachycardia. Use with caution and be prepared to treat hypertension.
Sympathomimetics such as epinephrine: May increase risk of coronary insufficiency. Monitor patient closely.
Theophylline: May decrease theophylline clearance in hypothyroidism; clearance may return to normal when euthyroid state is achieved. Monitor theophylline level.
Tricyclic antidepressants: May enhance both drugs. May cause transient cardiac arrhythmias. Monitor patient.
Warfarin: May increase warfarin effect. Monitor patient for bleeding and check PT and INR closely. Warfarin dosage adjustment may be needed.
Drug-herb. *Lemon balm:* May have antithyroid effects; may inhibit thyroid-stimulating hormone. Discourage use together.
Drug-food. *Cottonseed meal, dietary fiber, soybean flour, walnuts:* May decrease absorption of drug. Advise patient that dosage adjustments may be needed.

EFFECTS ON LAB TEST RESULTS
● May decrease thyroid function test results. May alter results of liothyronine, protein-bound iodine, and radioactive ¹³¹I uptake studies.

CONTRAINDICATIONS & CAUTIONS
● Contraindicated in patients hypersensitive to drug and in those with acute MI uncomplicated by hypothyroidism, untreated thyrotoxicosis, or uncorrected adrenal insufficiency. Also contraindicated with artificial rewarming of patients.

- Use cautiously in elderly patients and in those with angina pectoris, hypertension, other CV disorders, renal insufficiency, or ischemia.
- Use cautiously in patients with diabetes mellitus, diabetes insipidus, or myxedema and during rapid replacement in those with arteriosclerosis.

NURSING CONSIDERATIONS

- Watch for angina, coronary occlusion, or stroke in patients with arteriosclerosis who are receiving rapid replacement. In patients with coronary artery disease who must receive thyroid hormones, watch for possible coronary insufficiency.
- *Alert:* Drug may be used when a rapid-onset or a rapidly reversible drug is desirable, or in patients with impaired peripheral conversion of levothyroxine to liothyronine.
- Long-term therapy causes bone loss in premenopausal and postmenopausal women. Consider a basal bone density measurement, and monitor patient closely for osteoporosis.
- Thyroid hormone replacement requirements are about 25% lower in patients older than age 60 than in young adults.
- Monitor pulse and blood pressure.
- When changing from levothyroxine to this drug, stop levothyroxine and start this drug at a low dosage. Increase dosage in small increments after residual effects of levothyroxine have disappeared. When changing from this drug to levothyroxine, start levothyroxine several days before stopping this drug to avoid relapse.
- Patients who need ^{131}I uptake studies done must stop drug 7 to 10 days before test.
- In pregnant patients, dosage may need to be increased.
- *Look alike–sound alike:* Don't confuse levothyroxine with liothyronine or liotrix. Don't confuse Cytomel with Cytotec.

PATIENT TEACHING

- Teach patient importance of compliance. Tell him to take thyroid hormones at same time each day, preferably before breakfast, to maintain constant hormone levels and help prevent insomnia.
- Make sure patient understands that replacement therapy is usually for life.

Drug should never be stopped unless directed by prescriber.
- Advise patient who has achieved a stable response not to change brands.
- Warn patient (especially elderly patient) to notify prescriber at once about chest pain, palpitations, sweating, nervousness, or other signals of overdose or aggravated CV disease.
- Tell patient to report unusual bleeding and bruising.
- For diabetic patients, advise them to monitor glucose level closely.
- Tell patient not to take OTC or other prescription medications without first consulting his prescriber.
- Advise woman to report pregnancy to prescriber because dosage may need adjustment.

liotrix

LYE-oh-trix

Thyrolar

Pharmacologic class: thyroid hormone
Pregnancy risk category A

AVAILABLE FORMS

Tablets: Levothyroxine sodium 12.5 mcg and liothyronine sodium 3.1 mcg (Thyrolar-¼); levothyroxine sodium 25 mcg and liothyronine sodium 6.25 mcg (Thyrolar-½); levothyroxine sodium 50 mcg and liothyronine sodium 12.5 mcg (Thyrolar-1); levothyroxine sodium 100 mcg and liothyronine sodium 25 mcg (Thyrolar-2); levothyroxine sodium 150 mcg and liothyronine sodium 37.5 mcg (Thyrolar-3)

INDICATIONS & DOSAGES

Dosages are expressed in thyroid equivalents and must be individualized to approximate the deficit in patient's thyroid secretion.
➤ **Hypothyroidism**
Adults: Initially, a single daily dose of Thyrolar-½. Adjust dosage by 1 tablet of Thyrolar-¼ at 2- to 3-week intervals. Maintenance dose is 1 tablet of Thyrolar-1 or Thyrolar-2 daily. Readjust dose within the first 4 weeks of therapy after proper

clinical and laboratory evaluations of T_4 and TSH.

Adjust-a-dose: For elderly patients and patients with long-standing myxedema with cardiovascular impairment, initial dose is 1 tablet of Thyrolar-¼ daily. Reduce dose if angina occurs.

➤ **Congenital hypothyroidism**

Children older than age 12: More than 18.75/75 (T_3/T_4) mcg P.O. daily.

Children ages 6 to 12: 12.5/50 (T_3/T_4) to 18.75/75 mcg (T_3/T_4) P.O. daily.

Children ages 1 to 5: 9.35/37.5 (T_3/T_4) to 12.5/50 (T_3/T_4) mcg P.O. daily.

Children ages 6 to 12 months: 6.25/25 (T_3/T_4) to 9.35/37.5 (T_3/T_4) mcg P.O. daily.

Newborns and infants birth to 6 months: 3.1/12.5 (T_3/T_4) to 6.25/25 (T_3/T_4) mcg P.O. daily.

ADMINISTRATION
P.O.
● Give drug at same time each day, preferably before breakfast.

ACTION

Not clearly defined. Stimulates metabolism of all body tissues by accelerating the rate of cellular oxidation and provides both T_3 and T_4 to the tissues.

Route	Onset	Peak	Duration
P.O.	Unknown	Unknown	Unknown

Half-life: Unknown.

ADVERSE REACTIONS

CNS: *nervousness, insomnia, tremor,* headache.
CV: *tachycardia,* **arrhythmias,** angina pectoris, **cardiac decompensation and collapse.**
GI: diarrhea, vomiting.
GU: menstrual irregularities.
Metabolic: weight loss.
Musculoskeletal: accelerated rate of bone maturation in infants and children.
Skin: allergic skin reactions, diaphoresis.
Other: heat intolerance.

INTERACTIONS

Drug-drug. *Beta blockers:* May reduce beta-blocker effect. Monitor patient for clinical effect.

Cholestyramine, colestipol: May impair liotrix absorption. Separate doses by 4 to 5 hours.
Digoxin: May decrease glycoside effect. Monitor patient for clinical effect.
Estrogens: May decrease thyroid levels. Monitor levels after 12 weeks of therapy and adjust liotrix dose as needed.
Fosphenytoin, phenytoin: May release free thyroid hormone. Monitor patient for tachycardia.
Insulin, oral antidiabetics: May alter glucose level. Monitor glucose level. Dosage adjustments may be needed.
Sympathomimetics such as epinephrine: May increase risk of coronary insufficiency. Monitor patient closely.
Theophylline: May decrease theophylline clearance in hypothyroidism; clearance may return to normal when euthyroid state is achieved. Monitor theophylline level.
Warfarin: May increase anticoagulant effects. Monitor patient for bleeding and check PT and INR closely. Warfarin dosage adjustment may be needed.
Drug-herb. *Lemon balm:* May have antithyroid effects; may inhibit thyroid-stimulating hormone. Discourage use together.

EFFECTS ON LAB TEST RESULTS
● May decrease thyroid function test results. May alter results of liothyronine, protein-bound iodine, and radioactive ^{131}I uptake studies.

CONTRAINDICATIONS & CAUTIONS
● Contraindicated in patients hypersensitive to drug and in those with acute MI uncomplicated by hypothyroidism, untreated thyrotoxicosis, or uncorrected adrenal insufficiency.
● Use cautiously in elderly patients and in those with angina pectoris, hypertension, other CV disorders, renal insufficiency, or ischemia.
● Use cautiously in patients with diabetes mellitus, diabetes insipidus, or myxedema and during rapid replacement in those with arteriosclerosis.

NURSING CONSIDERATIONS
● Watch for angina, coronary occlusion, or stroke in patients with arteriosclerosis who are receiving rapid replacement.

- In patients with coronary artery disease who must receive thyroid hormones, monitor patient for possible coronary insufficiency. Also watch carefully during surgery because arrhythmias may arise.
- Thyroid hormone replacement requirements are about 25% lower in patients older than age 60 than in young adults.
- Dosage may need to be increased in pregnant patients.
- Monitor pulse and blood pressure.
- Long-term therapy causes bone loss in premenopausal and postmenopausal women. Consider a basal bone density measurement and monitor patient closely for osteoporosis.
- Patients taking liotrix must stop drug 7 to 10 days before undergoing ^{131}I uptake studies.
- **■ Black Box Warning** Don't use drug to treat obesity. ■
- *Look alike–sound alike:* Don't confuse Thyrolar with thyroid or Synthroid; don't confuse liotrix with levothyroxine or liothyronine.

PATIENT TEACHING

- Teach patient importance of compliance. He should take thyroid hormones at same time each day, preferably before breakfast, to maintain constant hormone levels and help prevent insomnia.
- Tell patient that drug should never be stopped unless directed by prescriber.
- Warn patient (especially elderly patient) to notify prescriber immediately about chest pain, palpitations, sweating, nervousness, or other signs of overdose or aggravated CV disease.
- Tell patient to report unusual bleeding and bruising.
- Advise patient not to take other drugs (OTC or prescription) without first consulting his prescriber.
- Advise patient to report pregnancy to prescriber because dosage may need adjustment.

79

Topical anti-inflammatories

betamethasone dipropionate
betamethasone valerate
clobetasol propionate
desoximetasone
diclofenac epolamine
diclofenac sodium
fluocinolone acetonide
fluocinonide
fluticasone propionate
hydrocortisone
hydrocortisone acetate
hydrocortisone butyrate
hydrocortisone probutate
hydrocortisone valerate
triamcinolone acetonide

---

betamethasone dipropionate
bay-ta-METH-a-sone

Diprolene, Diprolene AF

betamethasone valerate
Beta-Val, Dermabet, Luxiq, Valnar

Pharmacologic class: corticosteroid
Pregnancy risk category C

AVAILABLE FORMS
betamethasone dipropionate
Aerosol: 0.1%
Cream: 0.05%
Gel: 0.05%
Lotion: 0.05%
Ointment: 0.05%
betamethasone valerate
Cream: 0.05%, 0.1%
Foam: 0.12%
Lotion: 0.1%
Ointment: 0.1%

INDICATIONS & DOSAGES
➤ **Inflammation and pruritus from corticosteroid-responsive dermatoses**
Adults and children older than age 12:
Clean area; apply cream, ointment, lotion, aerosol spray, or gel sparingly. Give dipropionate products once daily to b.i.d.; give valerate 0.1% solution b.i.d., or valerate 0.1% cream or ointment once daily to t.i.d. Maximum dosage of augmented betamethasone dipropionate 0.05% ointment, cream, gel, or lotion is 45 g, 50 g, 45 g, or 50 ml per week, respectively. Therapy with augmented formulations shouldn't exceed 2 weeks.
➤ **Inflammation and pruritus from corticosteroid-responsive dermatoses of scalp (valerate only)**
Adults: Gently massage small amounts of foam into affected scalp areas b.i.d., morning and evening, until control is achieved. If no improvement is seen in 2 weeks, reassess diagnosis.

ADMINISTRATION
Topical
• Gently wash skin before applying. To prevent skin damage, rub in gently, leaving a thin coat. When treating hairy sites, part hair and apply directly to lesions.
• Decrease dosing frequency to once daily following clinical improvement.
• Avoid applying near eyes or mucous membranes or in ear canal, groin area, or armpit.
• Don't dispense foam directly into warm hands because foam will begin to melt upon contact.
• For patients with eczematous dermatitis whose skin may be irritated by adhesive material, hold dressing in place with gauze, elastic bandages, stockings, or stockinette.
• *Alert:* Don't use occlusive dressings.
• Continue drug for a few days after lesions clear.

ACTION
Unclear. Is diffused across cell membranes to form complexes with receptors. Has anti-inflammatory, antipruritic, vasoconstrictive, and antiproliferative activity. Considered a medium-potency to very-high-potency drug (depending on product), according to vasoconstrictive properties.

Route	Onset	Peak	Duration
Topical	Unknown	Unknown	Unknown

Half-life: Unknown.

ADVERSE REACTIONS
GU: glycosuria with dipropionate.
Metabolic: hyperglycemia.
Skin: burning, pruritus, irritation, dryness, erythema, folliculitis, striae, acneiform eruptions, perioral dermatitis, hypopigmentation, hypertrichosis, allergic contact dermatitis, secondary infection, maceration, atrophy, miliaria with occlusive dressings.
Other: *hypothalamic-pituitary-adrenal axis suppression,* Cushing syndrome.

INTERACTIONS
None significant.

EFFECTS ON LAB TEST RESULTS
• May increase glucose level.

CONTRAINDICATIONS & CAUTIONS
• Contraindicated in patients hypersensitive to corticosteroids.
• Don't use as monotherapy in primary bacterial infections (impetigo, paronychia, erysipelas, cellulitis, angular cheilitis), rosacea, perioral dermatitis, or acne.
• Don't use augmented betamethasone dipropionate 0.05% ointment, betamethasone dipropionate 0.05% gel, cream, and ointment; betamethasone valerate 0.1% ointment on the face, groin, or axilla.
• Use cautiously in pregnant or breast-feeding women.

NURSING CONSIDERATIONS
• Drug isn't for ophthalmic use.
• Because of alcohol content of vehicle, gel products may cause mild, transient stinging, especially when used on or near excoriated skin.
• If antifungal or antibiotic combined with corticosteroid fails to provide prompt improvement, stop corticosteroid until infection is controlled.
• Systemic absorption is likely with prolonged or extensive body surface treatment. Watch for symptoms.
• Avoid using plastic pants or tight-fitting diapers on treated areas in young children. Children may absorb larger amounts of

drug and be more susceptible to systemic toxicity.
• **Alert:** Diprolene and Diprolene AF may not be replaced with generics because other products have different potencies.

PATIENT TEACHING
• Teach patient how to apply drug.
• Emphasize that drug is for external use only.
• Tell patient to wash hands after application.
• Tell patient to stop drug and report signs of systemic absorption, skin irritation or ulceration, hypersensitivity, or infection.
• Instruct patient not to use occlusive dressings.
• Discuss personal hygiene measures to reduce chance of infection.

clobetasol propionate
kloe-BAY-ta-sol

Clobex, Cormax, Embeline, Embeline E, Olux, Olux-E, Temovate, Temovate Emollient

Pharmacologic class: corticosteroid
Pregnancy risk category C

AVAILABLE FORMS
Cream: 0.05%
Foam: 0.05%
Gel: 0.05%
Lotion: 0.05%
Ointment: 0.05%
Scalp application: 0.05%*
Shampoo: 0.05%
Solution: 0.05%

INDICATIONS & DOSAGES
➤ **Inflammation and pruritus from corticosteroid-responsive dermatoses; short-term topical treatment of mild to moderate plaque-type psoriasis of nonscalp regions, excluding the face and intertriginous areas**
Adults: Apply thin layer of Clobex lotion to affected skin areas b.i.d., morning and evening, for maximum of 14 days. For lesions of moderate to severe plaque psoriasis that haven't improved sufficiently, continue treatment for up to

2 more weeks, as long as 10% or less of the body surface area is affected. Total dose shouldn't exceed 50 g (50 ml) of lotion weekly.

➤ **Inflammation and pruritus from corticosteroid-responsive dermatoses; short-term topical treatment of mild to moderate plaque-type psoriasis of nonscalp regions, excluding the face and intertriginous areas**
Adults and children age 12 and older: Apply thin layer to affected skin areas b.i.d., morning and evening, for maximum of 14 days. Total dose shouldn't exceed 50 g of foam, cream, or ointment or 50 ml of lotion or solution weekly.

➤ **Inflammation and pruritus of moderate to severe corticosteroid-responsive dermatoses of the scalp**
Adults: Apply to the affected scalp area b.i.d., morning and evening. Gently massage into affected scalp area until the foam disappears. Repeat until entire affected scalp area is treated. Limit treatment to 14 days, with no more than 50 g of foam weekly.

➤ **Moderate to severe scalp psoriasis**
Adults: Apply Clobex shampoo to affected areas of dry scalp in thin film once daily. Leave in place for 15 minutes before lathering and rinsing. Limit treatment to 4 consecutive weeks.

ADMINISTRATION
Topical
● Gently wash skin before applying. To prevent skin damage, rub medication in gently and completely. When treating hairy sites, part hair and apply directly to lesions.
● Avoid applying near eyes or mucous membranes or in ear canal.
● *Alert:* Don't use occlusive dressings or bandages. Don't cover or wrap treated areas unless directed by prescriber.

ACTION
Unclear. Diffuses across cell membranes to form complexes with receptors, showing anti-inflammatory, antipruritic, vasoconstrictive, and antiproliferative activity. Considered a very-high-potency to high-potency drug, according to vasoconstrictive properties.

Route	Onset	Peak	Duration
Topical	Unknown	Unknown	Unknown

Half-life: Unknown.

ADVERSE REACTIONS
GU: glycosuria.
Metabolic: hyperglycemia.
Skin: burning, pruritus, irritation, dryness, erythema, folliculitis, perioral dermatitis, allergic contact dermatitis, hypopigmentation, hypertrichosis, acneiform eruptions, skin atrophy, telangiectasia.
Other: *hypothalamic-pituitary-adrenal axis suppression,* Cushing syndrome, finger numbness.

INTERACTIONS
None significant.

EFFECTS ON LAB TEST RESULTS
● May increase glucose level.

CONTRAINDICATIONS & CAUTIONS
● Contraindicated in patients hypersensitive to corticosteroids and in those with primary scalp infections.
● Don't use as monotherapy for primary bacterial infections (impetigo, paronychia, erysipelas, cellulitis, angular cheilitis, erythrasma), rosacea, perioral dermatitis, or acne.
● Don't use very high-potency or high-potency agents on the face, groin, or axilla areas.
● Drug isn't for ophthalmic use.
● Use cautiously in children and in pregnant or breast-feeding women.

NURSING CONSIDERATIONS
● If antifungal or antibiotic combined with corticosteroid fails to provide prompt improvement, stop corticosteroid until infection is controlled.
● Stop drug and notify prescriber if skin infection, striae, or atrophy occurs.
● Hypothalamic-pituitary-adrenal axis suppression occurs at doses as low as 2 g daily.

PATIENT TEACHING
● Teach patient how to apply drug and to avoid contact with eyes.
● Tell patient to wash hands after application.

• Tell patient to stop drug and report signs of systemic absorption, skin irritation or ulceration, hypersensitivity, or infection.
• Warn patient to use drug for no longer than 14 consecutive days.
• Tell patient using the foam to invert can and dispense a small amount of Olux foam (up to a golfball–size dollop) into the cap of the can, onto a saucer or other cool surface, or directly on the lesion, taking care to avoid contact with the eyes. Dispensing directly onto hands isn't recommended because the foam will melt immediately upon contact with warm skin. Tell him to move hair away from affected area of scalp so that foam can be applied to each affected area.
• Tell patient using foam that contents are flammable and under pressure, so he should avoid smoking during and immediately after application and keep can away from flames. Also tell him not to puncture or incinerate container.

---

desoximetasone
dess-OX-ee-MET-ah-sone

Topicort, Topicort LP

Pharmacologic class: corticosteroid
Pregnancy risk category C

AVAILABLE FORMS
Cream: 0.05%, 0.25%
Gel: 0.05%
Ointment: 0.25%

INDICATIONS & DOSAGES
➤ **Inflammation from corticosteroid-responsive dermatoses**
Adults and children: Clean area; apply a thin film and rub in gently b.i.d.

ADMINISTRATION
Topical
• Gently wash skin before applying. To prevent skin damage, rub in gently, leaving thin coat. When treating hairy sites, part hair and apply directly to lesions.
• Avoid applying near eyes, mucous membranes, or in ear canal.
• ***Alert:*** Do not bandage, cover, or wrap the treated skin area unless ordered.

• Stop drug and notify prescriber if skin infection, striae, or atrophy occur.
• Continue drug for a few days after lesions clear.

ACTION
Unclear. Diffuses across cell membranes to form complexes with receptors, showing anti-inflammatory, antipruritic, vasoconstrictive, and antiproliferative activity. Considered a high-potency drug (0.25% cream and ointment, 0.05% gel) or medium-potency drug (0.05% cream) according to vasoconstrictive properties.

Route	Onset	Peak	Duration
Topical	Unknown	Unknown	Unknown

Half-life: Unknown.

ADVERSE REACTIONS
GU: glycosuria.
Metabolic: hyperglycemia.
Skin: burning, pruritus, irritation, dryness, erythema, folliculitis, hypertrichosis, acneiform eruptions, perioral dermatitis, hypopigmentation, allergic contact dermatitis, *maceration, secondary infection, atrophy, striae, miliaria with occlusive dressings.*
Other: *hypothalamic-pituitary-adrenal axis suppression,* Cushing syndrome.

INTERACTIONS
None significant.

EFFECTS ON LAB TEST RESULTS
• May increase glucose level.

CONTRAINDICATIONS & CAUTIONS
• Contraindicated in patients hypersensitive to drug or its components.
• Don't use as monotherapy in primary bacterial infections (impetigo, paronychia, erysipelas, cellulitis, angular cheilitis), treatment of rosacea, perioral dermatitis, or acne.
• Don't use very-high-potency or high-potency agents on the face, groin, or axillae.
• Drug isn't for ophthalmic use.
• Use cautiously in children and pregnant or breast-feeding women.

Reactions may be *common,* uncommon, *life-threatening,* or COMMON AND LIFE-THREATENING.
Interaction may have a *rapid onset* or **delayed onset.**

NURSING CONSIDERATIONS

- If fever develops and occlusive dressing is in place, notify prescriber and remove occlusive dressing.
- If antifungal or antibiotic combined with corticosteroid fails to provide prompt improvement, stop corticosteroid until infection is controlled.
- Systemic absorption is likely with use of occlusive dressings, prolonged treatment, or extensive body surface treatment. Watch for symptoms of HPA axis suppression, Cushing syndrome, hyperglycemia, and glucosuria.
- Avoid using plastic pants or tight-fitting diapers on treated areas in young children. Children may absorb larger amounts of drug and be more susceptible to systemic toxicity.
- Gel contains alcohol and may cause burning or irritation in open lesions.
- *Look alike–sound alike:* Don't confuse desoximetasone with dexamethasone.

PATIENT TEACHING

- Teach patient how to apply drug.
- Tell patient this drug is for external use only and to avoid contact with the eyes.
- If an occlusive dressing is ordered, advise patient to leave it in place for no longer than 12 hours each day and not to use the dressing on infected or weeping lesions.
- Tell patient to stop drug and report signs of systemic absorption, skin irritation or ulceration, hypersensitivity, or infection.

---

diclofenac epolamine
dye-KLOE-fen-ak

Flector

diclofenac sodium
Solaraze, Voltaren

Pharmacologic class: NSAID
Pregnancy risk category B

AVAILABLE FORMS
Topical gel: 1%, 3%
Topical patch: 1.3%

INDICATIONS & DOSAGES

➤ **Actinic keratosis (Solaraze only)**
Adults: Apply gently to lesion b.i.d. for 60 to 90 days.

➤ **Osteoarthritis (Voltaren only)**
Adults: Apply 4 q of gel to affected foot, knee, or ankle q.i.d. Maximum dose of 16 g to any single joint of the lower extremities . Or apply 2 g of gel to affected hand, elbow, or wrist q.i.d. Maximum dose of 8 g to any single joint of the upper extremities. Total dose shouldn't exceed 32 g daily for all affected joints.

ADMINISTRATION
Topical

- Don't apply to open wounds or broken skin.
- Avoid contact with eyes.
- Use enough gel to cover the lesion; for example, use 0.5 g of gel on a 5- × 5-cm lesion.
- Don't apply Flector Patch to nonintact or damaged skin, including from exudative dermatitis, eczema, infected lesions, burns, or wounds.
- Measure gel using supplied dosing cards in package.
- Wear gloves to gently massage Voltaren into skin of entire joint.

ACTION
Unknown. May produce anti-inflammatory and analgesic effects by ability to inhibit prostaglandin synthesis.

Route	Onset	Peak	Duration
Topical	Unknown	4–12 hr	Unknown

Half-life: 1 to 3 hours; 12 hours for patch.

ADVERSE REACTIONS
CNS: *paresthesia,* headache, pain, asthenia, migraine, hypokinesia.
CV: chest pain, hypertension.
EENT: sinusitis, pharyngitis, rhinitis, conjunctivitis, eye pain.
GI: diarrhea, dyspepsia, abdominal pain.
GU: hematuria, renal impairment.
Hepatic: liver impairment.
Metabolic: hypercholesterolemia, hyperglycemia.
Musculoskeletal: arthralgia, arthrosis, back pain, myalgia, neck pain.

Respiratory: *asthma,* dyspnea, pneumonia.
Skin: *reaction at application site, contact dermatitis, dry skin, exfoliation, localized pain, pruritus, rash,* localized edema, acne, alopecia, photosensitivity reactions, skin ulcer.
Other: *anaphylaxis, flulike syndrome,* infection, allergic reaction.

INTERACTIONS
Drug-drug. *Oral NSAIDs:* May increase drug effects. Minimize use together.
Drug-lifestyle. *Sun exposure:* May increase risk of photosensitivity reactions. Advise patient to avoid excessive sun exposure.

EFFECTS ON LAB TEST RESULTS
● May increase ALT, AST, cholesterol, creatinine, glucose, and phosphokinase levels.

CONTRAINDICATIONS & CAUTIONS
● Contraindicated in patients hypersensitive to diclofenac, benzyl alcohol, polyethylene glycol monomethyl ether 350, or hyaluronic acid.
■ **Black Box Warning** Contraindicated for perioperative pain for coronary artery bypass graft surgery. ■
● Avoid use during late pregnancy.
● Use cautiously in patients with the aspirin triad; these patients are usually asthmatics who develop rhinitis, with or without nasal polyps, after taking aspirin or other NSAIDs.
● Use cautiously in patients with active GI bleeding or ulceration and in those with severe renal or hepatic impairment.
● Use cautiously in breast-feeding women; it's unknown if drug appears in breast milk. Patient should either stop breast-feeding or stop treatment, taking into account importance of drug to mother.

NURSING CONSIDERATIONS
■ **Black Box Warning** NSAIDs may increase the risk of serious CV thrombotic events. The risk may increase with duration of use. Patients with CV disease or risk factors for CV disease may be at greater risk. ■
■ **Black Box Warning** NSAIDs increase the risk of serious GI adverse reactions

including bleeding, ulceration, and perforation of the stomach or intestines, which can be fatal. These reactions can occur at any time and without warning. Elderly patients are at greater risk. ■
● Safety and effectiveness of sunscreens, cosmetics, or other topical medications used with drug are unknown.
● Complete healing or optimal therapeutic effect may not be seen until 30 days after therapy is complete.
● Reevaluate lesions that don't respond to therapy.
● Because of the risk of premature closure of the ductus arteriosus, avoid drug in late pregnancy.

PATIENT TEACHING
● Inform patient about risk of skin reactions (rash, itchiness, pain, irritation) at the application site. Urge patient to seek medical attention if adverse reactions persist or worsen.
● Encourage patient to minimize sun exposure during therapy. Explain that sunscreen may be helpful but that the safety of using sunscreen with drug is unknown.
● Caution patient not to apply gel to open wounds or broken skin.
● Instruct patient to avoid contact with eyes.
● Instruct patient not to apply other topical drugs or cosmetics to affected area while using drug, unless directed.
● Advise patient to use only on intact skin unless otherwise directed.
● Inform patient that if Flector Patch begins to peel off, the edges may be taped down. Instruct patient not to wear Flector Patch during bathing or showering. Bathing should take place in between scheduled patch removal and application.
● Tell patient to wash his hands after applying gel unless the hands are the treated area; then don't wash for at least one hour after application.
● Instruct patient not to cover area with clothing for at least 10 minutes after applying gel and to wait at least one hour before showering or bathing.
● Tell woman to notify prescriber if she's pregnant or breast-feeding.

Reactions may be *common,* uncommon, *life-threatening,* or COMMON AND LIFE-THREATENING.
Interaction may have a *rapid onset* or *delayed onset.*

fluocinolone acetonide
floo-oh-SIN-oh-lone

Derma-Smoothe/FS,
FS Shampoo, Synalar

Pharmacologic class: corticosteroid
Pregnancy risk category C

AVAILABLE FORMS
Cream: 0.01%, 0.025%
Oil: 0.01%
Ointment: 0.025%
Shampoo: 0.01%
Topical solution: 0.01%

INDICATIONS & DOSAGES
➤ **Inflammation from corticosteroid-responsive dermatoses**
Adults and children: Clean area; apply product sparingly t.i.d. to q.i.d.
➤ **Atopic dermatitis**
Adults: Apply thin film of topical oil t.i.d.
Children 3 months and older: Apply thin film of topical oil b.i.d. for maximum of 4 weeks. Avoid face and diaper area.
➤ **Scalp psoriasis**
Adults: Wet or dampen hair and scalp thoroughly. Apply a thin film of topical oil and massage into scalp. Cover with supplied shower cap overnight or for a minimum of 4 hours before washing thoroughly with regular shampoo and then rinsing thoroughly with water.
➤ **Seborrheic dermatitis of the scalp**
Adults: Apply no more than 30 ml of 0.01% shampoo to the scalp once daily, lather, and rinse thoroughly with water after 5 minutes.

ADMINISTRATION
Topical
● Gently wash skin before applying. To prevent skin damage, rub in gently, leaving a thin coat. When treating hairy sites, part hair and apply directly to lesions.
● Avoid application near eyes or mucous membranes; in armpits, groin, or rectal area; or in ear canal if eardrum is perforated.
● Do not use occlusive dressing unless ordered.

● For patients with eczematous dermatitis whose skin may be irritated by adhesive material, hold dressing in place with gauze, elastic bandages, stockings, or stockinette.
● Change dressing as prescribed. Stop drug and notify prescriber if skin infection, striae, or atrophy occur.
● Shake shampoo well prior to use.

ACTION
Unclear. Is diffused across cell membranes to form complexes with receptors. Shows anti-inflammatory, antipruritic, vasoconstrictive, and antiproliferative activity. Considered a medium-potency to low-potency drug, according to vasoconstrictive properties.

Route	Onset	Peak	Duration
Topical	Unknown	Unknown	Unknown

Half-life: Unknown.

ADVERSE REACTIONS
GU: glycosuria.
Metabolic: hyperglycemia.
Skin: burning, pruritus, irritation, dryness, erythema, folliculitis, hypertrichosis, hypopigmentation, acneiform eruptions, perioral dermatitis, allergic contact dermatitis, *maceration, secondary infection, atrophy, striae, miliaria with occlusive dressings.*
Other: *hypothalamic-pituitary-adrenal axis suppression,* Cushing syndrome.

INTERACTIONS
None significant.

EFFECTS ON LAB TEST RESULTS
● May increase glucose level.

CONTRAINDICATIONS & CAUTIONS
● Contraindicated in patients hypersensitive to drug or its components.
● Don't use as monotherapy in primary bacterial infections (impetigo, paronychia, erysipelas, cellulitis, angular cheilitis), treatment of rosacea, perioral dermatitis, or acne.
● Drug isn't for ophthalmic use.
● Use cautiously in pregnant or breast-feeding women.

NURSING CONSIDERATIONS
• If an occlusive dressing has been applied and a fever develops, notify prescriber and remove dressing.
• If antifungal or antibiotic combined with corticosteroid fails to provide prompt improvement, stop corticosteroid until infection is controlled.
• Systemic absorption is likely with use of occlusive dressings, prolonged treatment, or extensive body surface treatment. Watch for symptoms, such as hyperglycemia, glycosuria, hypothalamic-pituitary-adrenal axis suppression, or Cushing syndrome.
• Avoid using plastic pants or tight-fitting diapers on treated areas in young children. Children may absorb larger amounts of drug and be more susceptible to systemic toxicity.
• **Alert:** Body oil and scalp oil formulations contain peanut oil.
• **Look alike–sound alike:** Don't confuse fluocinolone with fluocinonide or fluticasone.

PATIENT TEACHING
• Teach patient or family how to apply drug using gloves or sterile applicator.
• Tell patient to wash hands after application.
• If an occlusive dressing is used, advise patient to leave it in place for no longer than 12 hours each day and not to use dressing on infected or weeping lesions.
• Tell patient to stop using solution and notify prescriber if he develops signs of systemic absorption, skin irritation or ulceration, hypersensitivity, or infection.
• Advise patient using the shampoo not to bandage, cover, or wrap the treated scalp area unless directed.

---

fluocinonide
floo-oh-SIN-oh-nide

Lidex, Lidex-E, Vanos

Pharmacologic class: corticosteroid
Pregnancy risk category C

AVAILABLE FORMS
Cream: 0.05%, 0.1%
Gel: 0.05%

Ointment: 0.05%
Topical solution: 0.05%

INDICATIONS & DOSAGES
➤ **Inflammation from corticosteroid-responsive dermatoses**
Adults and children: Clean area; apply cream, gel, ointment, or topical solution sparingly b.i.d. to q.i.d. In children, use lowest dosage that promotes healing. If using Vanos 0.1% cream in adults and children age 12 and older, apply a thin layer once or twice daily for up to 2 weeks. Don't use more than 60 g/week.

ADMINISTRATION
Topical
• Gently wash skin before applying. To prevent skin damage, rub in gently, leaving a thin coat. When treating hairy sites, part hair and apply directly to lesion.
• Avoid applying near eyes or mucous membranes or in ear canal.
• Occlusive dressings may be used in severe or resistant dermatoses.
• For patients with eczematous dermatitis whose skin may be irritated by adhesive material, hold dressing in place with gauze, elastic bandages, stockings, or stockinette.
• Change dressing as prescribed. Stop drug and notify prescriber if skin infection, striae, or atrophy occur.
• Continue treatment for a few days after lesions clear.

ACTION
Unclear. Diffuses across cell membranes to form complexes with cytoplasmic receptors, showing anti-inflammatory, antipruritic, vasoconstrictive, and anti-proliferative activity. Considered a high-potency drug, according to vasoconstrictive properties.

Route	Onset	Peak	Duration
Topical	Unknown	Unknown	Unknown

Half-life: Unknown.

ADVERSE REACTIONS
GU: glycosuria.
Metabolic: hyperglycemia.
Skin: burning, pruritus, irritation, dryness, erythema, folliculitis, hypertrichosis, hypopigmentation, acneiform eruptions,

---

Reactions may be *common*, uncommon, *life-threatening*, or COMMON AND LIFE-THREATENING.
Interaction may have a *rapid onset* or **delayed onset**.

perioral dermatitis, allergic contact dermatitis, *maceration, secondary infection, atrophy, striae, miliaria with occlusive dressings.*
Other: *hypothalamic-pituitary-adrenal axis suppression,* Cushing syndrome.

INTERACTIONS
None significant.

EFFECTS ON LAB TEST RESULTS
• May increase glucose level.

CONTRAINDICATIONS & CAUTIONS
• Contraindicated in patients hypersensitive to drug or its components.
• Don't use as monotherapy in primary bacterial infections (impetigo, paronychia, erysipelas, cellulitis, angular cheilitis), treatment of rosacea, perioral dermatitis, or acne.
• Don't use very-high-potency or high-potency agents on the face, groin, or armpits.
• Drug isn't for ophthalmic use.
• Use cautiously in pregnant or breast-feeding women.

NURSING CONSIDERATIONS
• If an occlusive dressing has been applied and a fever develops, notify prescriber and remove dressing.
• If antifungal or antibiotic combined with corticosteroid fails to provide prompt improvement, stop corticosteroid until infection is controlled.
• Systemic absorption is likely with use of occlusive dressings, prolonged treatment, or extensive body surface treatment. Watch for such symptoms as hyperglycemia, glycosuria, and hypothalamic-pituitary-adrenal axis suppression.
• Avoid using plastic pants or tight-fitting diapers on treated areas in young children. Children may absorb larger amounts of drug and be more susceptible to systemic toxicity.
• *Look alike–sound alike:* Don't confuse fluocinonide with fluocinolone or fluticasone.

PATIENT TEACHING
• Teach patient and family how to apply drug using careful hand washing and gloves or sterile applicator.

• If an occlusive dressing is ordered, advise patient to leave it in place no more than 12 hours each day and not to use the dressing on infected or weeping lesions.
• Tell patient to stop drug and report signs of systemic absorption, skin irritation or ulceration, hypersensitivity, or infection.

fluticasone propionate
FLOO-ti-ka-sone

Cutivate

Pharmacologic class: corticosteroid
Pregnancy risk category C

AVAILABLE FORMS
Cream: 0.05%
Lotion: 0.05%
Ointment: 0.005%

INDICATIONS & DOSAGES
➤ **Inflammation and pruritus from dermatoses responsive to corticosteroids**
Adults: Apply sparingly to affected area b.i.d.; rub in gently and completely.
Children age 3 months and older: Apply a thin film of cream (0.05%) to affected areas b.i.d. Rub in gently. Don't use for longer than 4 weeks. If using lotion (0.05%) in adults and children 1 year and older, apply once daily.
➤ **Inflammation and pruritus from atopic dermatitis**
Children age 3 months and older: Apply thin film (0.05%) to affected areas once daily or b.i.d. Rub in gently. Don't use for longer than 4 weeks.

ADMINISTRATION
Topical
• Don't use drug with an occlusive dressing or in diaper area.

ACTION
Unclear. Is diffused across cell membranes to form complexes with cytoplasmic receptors. Shows anti-inflammatory, antipruritic, vasoconstrictive, and anti-proliferative activity. Considered a medium-potency drug, according to vasoconstrictive properties.

Route	Onset	Peak	Duration
Topical	Rapid	Unknown	10 hr

Half-life: Unknown.

ADVERSE REACTIONS
CNS: light-headedness.
GU: glycosuria.
Metabolic: hyperglycemia.
Skin: urticaria, burning, hypertrichosis, pruritus, irritation, erythema, hives, dryness.
Other: *hypothalamic-pituitary-adrenal axis suppression,* Cushing syndrome.

INTERACTIONS
None significant.

EFFECTS ON LAB TEST RESULTS
● May increase glucose level.

CONTRAINDICATIONS & CAUTIONS
● Contraindicated in patients hypersensitive to drug or its components.
● Don't use as monotherapy in primary bacterial, viral, fungal, herpetic, or tubercular skin infections; for treatment of rosacea, perioral dermatitis, or acne.
● Drug isn't for ophthalmic use.
● Use cautiously in pregnant or breast-feeding women.

NURSING CONSIDERATIONS
● Don't mix drug with other bases or vehicles because doing so may affect potency.
● If adverse reactions occur, prescriber may order less potent drug.
● Stop drug if local irritation or systemic infection, absorption, or hypersensitivity occurs.
● Absorption of corticosteroid is increased when drug is applied to inflamed or damaged skin, eyelids, or scrotal area; it's lowest when applied to intact normal skin, palms of hands, or soles of feet.
● *Look alike–sound alike:* Don't confuse fluticasone with fluconazole.

PATIENT TEACHING
● Teach patient or family member how to apply drug using gloves, sterile applicator, or after careful hand washing.
● Tell patient to wash hands after application.

● Tell patient to avoid prolonged use and contact with eyes. Warn him not to apply to face, in skin creases, or around eyes, genitals, underarms, or rectum.
● Instruct patient to notify prescriber if condition persists or worsens or if burning or irritation develops.

---

hydrocortisone
hye-droe-KOR-ti-sone

Ala-Cort, Ala-Scalp, Anusol-HC, Cetacort, Cortizone-5◇, Cortizone-10◇, Cortizone-10 Quickshot◇, Dermolate◇, Hi-Cor 2.5, Hycort, HydroSkin, HydroTex, Hytone, LactiCare-HC, Maximum Strength Cortaid Faststick, Procort◇, Scalpicin◇, Synacort, Tegrin-HC◇, Texacort, T/Scalp

hydrocortisone acetate
Anusol HC◇, Cortaid◇, Cortef Feminine Itch◇, Corticaine◇, Gynecort◇, Lanacort-5◇, Lanacort 10◇, ProctoCream-HC, ProctoFoam-HC, Tucks, U-cort

hydrocortisone butyrate
Locoid, Locoid Lipocream

hydrocortisone probutate
Pandel

hydrocortisone valerate
Westcort

Pharmacologic class: corticosteroid
Pregnancy risk category C

AVAILABLE FORMS
hydrocortisone
Cream: 0.5%◇, 1%◇, 2.5%
Gel: 1%, 2%
Lotion: 0.25%, 0.5%◇, 1%◇, 1%, 2%, 2.5%
Ointment: 0.5%◇, 1%◇, 2.5%
Rectal cream: 1%◇
Rectal ointment: 1%
Spray: 1%◇
Stick roll-on: 1%
Topical solution: 1%, 2.5%

Reactions may be *common,* uncommon, *life-threatening,* or COMMON AND LIFE-THREATENING.
Interaction may have a *rapid onset* or **delayed onset.**

hydrocortisone acetate
Cream: 0.5%◊, 1%◊, 1%, 2%, 2.5%
Lotion: 0.5%
Ointment: 0.5%◊, 1%◊
Rectal foam: 90 mg per application
Suppositories: 25 mg, 30 mg
hydrocortisone butyrate
Cream: 0.1%
Ointment: 0.1%
Solution: 0.1%
hydrocortisone probutate
Cream: 0.1%
hydrocortisone valerate
Cream: 0.2%
Ointment: 0.2%

INDICATIONS & DOSAGES
➤ **Inflammation and pruritus from corticosteroid-responsive dermatoses, adjunctive topical management of seborrheic dermatitis of scalp**
Adults and children: Clean area; apply cream, gel, lotion, ointment, or topical solution sparingly daily to q.i.d. Spray aerosol onto affected area daily to q.i.d. until acute phase is controlled; then reduce dosage to one to three times weekly as needed. Give children lowest dose that provides positive results.
➤ **Inflammation from proctitis**
Adults: 1 applicatorful of rectal foam P.R. daily or b.i.d. for 2 to 3 weeks; then every other day as needed. Give enema once nightly for 21 days or until patient improves; may use every other night for 2 to 3 months. Insert suppository b.i.d. for 2 weeks.

ADMINISTRATION
Topical
● Gently wash skin before applying. To prevent skin damage, rub in gently, leaving a thin coat. When treating hairy sites, part hair and apply directly to lesions.
● Check individual products for frequency of administration.
● Avoid applying near eyes or mucous membranes or in ear canal; may be safely used on face, groin, armpits, and under breasts.
● Change dressing as prescribed. Stop drug and tell prescriber if skin infection, striae, or atrophy occurs.
● When using aerosol near the face, cover patient's eyes and warn against inhaling

spray. Aerosol contains alcohol and may cause irritation or burning when used on open lesions. Don't spray longer than 3 seconds or from closer than 6 inches (15 cm) to avoid freezing tissues. If spray is applied to dry scalp after shampooing, drug doesn't need to be massaged into scalp.
● Continue treatment for a few days after lesions clear.
Rectal
● Insert suppositories blunt end first after removing foil wrapper.

ACTION
Unclear. Diffuses across cell membranes to form complexes with cytoplasmic receptors, showing anti-inflammatory, antipruritic, vasoconstrictive, and anti-proliferative activity. Considered a low-potency (hydrocortisone, hydrocortisone acetate) and a medium-potency (hydrocortisone butyrate, hydrocortisone probutate, hydrocortisone valerate) drug, according to vasoconstrictive properties.

Route	Onset	Peak	Duration
Topical, P.R.	Unknown	Unknown	Unknown

Half-life: Unknown.

ADVERSE REACTIONS
Topical
GU: glycosuria.
Metabolic: hyperglycemia.
Skin: burning, pruritus, irritation, dryness, erythema, folliculitis, hypertrichosis, hypopigmentation, acneiform eruptions, allergic contact dermatitis, *atrophy, maceration, secondary infection, striae, miliaria with occlusive dressings.*
Other: *hypothalamic-pituitary-adrenal axis suppression,* Cushing syndrome.
Rectal
CNS: *seizures, increased intracranial pressure,* vertigo, headache.
CV: hypertension.
EENT: cataracts, glaucoma.
GI: peptic ulcer, *pancreatitis,* abdominal distention.
GU: menstrual irregularities.
Metabolic: fluid or electrolyte disturbances, decreased carbohydrate tolerance.

Musculoskeletal: muscle weakness, osteoporosis, necrosis and fractures in bone.
Skin: impaired wound healing, fragile skin, petechiae, erythema, sweating.

INTERACTIONS
None significant.

EFFECTS ON LAB TEST RESULTS
• May increase glucose level.

CONTRAINDICATIONS & CAUTIONS
• Contraindicated in patients hypersensitive to drug or its components.
• Don't use as monotherapy in primary bacterial infections (impetigo, paronychia, erysipelas, cellulitis, angular cheilitis), treatment of rosacea, perioral dermatitis, or acne.
• Drug isn't for ophthalmic use.
• Use cautiously in pregnant or breast-feeding women.

NURSING CONSIDERATIONS
• If an occlusive dressing is applied and a fever develops, notify prescriber and remove dressing.
• If antifungal or antibiotic combined with corticosteroid fails to provide prompt improvement, stop corticosteroid until infection is controlled.
• Systemic absorption is likely with use of occlusive dressings, prolonged treatment, or extensive body surface treatment. Watch for symptoms, such as hyperglycemia, glycosuria, and hypothalamic-pituitary-adrenal axis suppression.
• Avoid using plastic pants or tight-fitting diapers on treated areas in young children. Children may absorb larger amounts of drug and be more susceptible to systemic toxicity.
• Monitor patient for fluid or electrolyte disturbances (sodium and fluid retention, potassium loss, hypokalemic alkalosis, negative nitrogen balance from catabolism of protein).
• Drug may suppress skin reaction testing.
• **Look alike–sound alike:** Don't confuse hydrocortisone with hydroxychloroquine.

PATIENT TEACHING
• Teach patient or family member how to apply drug.

• Tell patient to wash hands after application.
• If an occlusive dressing is ordered, advise patient to leave it in place for no longer than 12 hours each day and not to use the dressing on infected or weeping lesions.
• Tell patient to stop drug and report signs of systemic absorption, skin irritation or ulceration, hypersensitivity, infection, or lack of improvement.
• Instruct patient to insert suppositories blunt end first after removing foil wrapper.
• For perianal application, instruct patient to place small amount of drug on a tissue and gently rub in.
• Tell patient to disassemble applicator or aerosol cap and clean with warm water after each use.
• Tell patient to stop using this product if condition worsens or if symptoms persist for more than 7 days.

---

triamcinolone acetonide
trye-am-SIN-oh-lone

Kenalog, Triacet, Triderm

Pharmacologic class: corticosteroid
Pregnancy risk category C

AVAILABLE FORMS
Aerosol: 0.2 mg/2-second spray
Cream: 0.025%, 0.1%, 0.5%
Lotion: 0.025%, 0.1%
Ointment: 0.025%, 0.1%, 0.5%
Paste: 0.1%

INDICATIONS & DOSAGES
➤ **Inflammation and pruritus from corticosteroid-responsive dermatoses**
Adults and children: Clean area; apply aerosol, cream, lotion, or ointment sparingly b.i.d. to q.i.d. Rub in lightly.
➤ **Inflammation from oral lesions**
Adults and children: Apply paste at bedtime and, if needed, b.i.d. or t.i.d., preferably after meals. Apply small amount without rubbing; press to lesion in mouth until thin film develops.

Reactions may be *common*, uncommon, *life-threatening*, or COMMON AND LIFE-THREATENING.
Interaction may have a *rapid onset* or **delayed onset**.

ADMINISTRATION
Topical
● Gently wash skin before applying.
To avoid skin damage, rub in gently,
leaving a thin coat. When treating hairy
sites, part hair and apply directly to
lesions.
● Don't apply near eyes or in ear canal.
● When using aerosol near the face,
cover patient's eyes and warn against
inhaling spray. Aerosol contains alcohol
and may cause irritation or burning
when used on open lesions. Don't spray
longer than 3 seconds or from closer
than 6 inches (15 cm) to avoid freezing
tissues.
● Occlusive dressings may be used in
severe or resistant dermatoses.

ACTION
Unclear. Diffuses across cell membranes
to form complexes with cytoplasmic
receptors, showing anti-inflammatory,
antipruritic, vasoconstrictive, and anti-
proliferative activity. Considered a
medium-potency (0.025% and 0.1% cream,
ointment, lotion) and high-potency
(0.5% cream, ointment) drug, according
to vasoconstrictive properties.

Route	Onset	Peak	Duration
Topical	Several hr	Unknown	> 1 wk

Half-life: Unknown.

ADVERSE REACTIONS
CV: syncope.
GI: peptic ulcer.
GU: glycosuria.
Metabolic: hyperglycemia.
Skin: burning, pruritus, irritation, dryness,
erythema, folliculitis, hypertrichosis,
hypopigmentation, acneiform eruptions,
perioral dermatitis, allergic contact dermatitis, *maceration, secondary infection,
atrophy, striae, miliaria with occlusive
dressings.*
Other: *hypothalamic-pituitary-adrenal
axis suppression,* Cushing syndrome.

INTERACTIONS
None significant.

EFFECTS ON LAB TEST RESULTS
● May increase glucose level.

CONTRAINDICATIONS & CAUTIONS
● Contraindicated in patients hypersensitive
to drug or its components.
● Contraindicated in the presence of
fungal, viral, or bacterial infections of the
mouth or throat (paste).
● Don't use as monotherapy in primary
bacterial infections (impetigo, paronychia,
erysipelas, cellulitis, angular cheilitis),
treatment of rosacea, perioral dermatitis,
or acne.
● Don't use very-high-potency or high-
potency agents on the face, groin, or axilla
areas.
● Drug isn't for ophthalmic use.
● Use cautiously in pregnant or breast-
feeding women.

NURSING CONSIDERATIONS
● Stop drug and tell prescriber if skin
infection, striae, or atrophy occur.
● If antifungal or antibiotic combined with
corticosteroid fails to provide prompt
improvement, stop corticosteroid until
infection is controlled.
● Systemic absorption is likely with the use
of occlusive dressings, prolonged treatment, or extensive body surface treatment.
Watch for symptoms, such as hyperglycemia, glycosuria, and hypothalamic-
pituitary-adrenal axis suppression.
● Avoid using plastic pants or tight-fitting
diapers on treated areas in young children.
Children may absorb larger amounts of
drug and be more susceptible to systemic
toxicity.

PATIENT TEACHING
● Teach patient or family member how to
apply drug.
● If an occlusive dressing is ordered,
advise patient to leave it in place for no
longer than 12 hours each day and not to
use the dressing on infected or weeping
lesions.
● Tell patient to stop drug and report signs
of systemic absorption, skin irritation or
ulceration, hypersensitivity, infection, or
lack of improvement.

80

Alkylating drugs

bendamustine hydrochloride
busulfan
carboplatin
carmustine
chlorambucil
cisplatin
cyclophosphamide
dacarbazine
ifosfamide
lomustine
mechlorethamine hydrochloride
melphalan
melphalan hydrochloride
oxaliplatin
thiotepa

✱ NEW DRUG

bendamustine hydrochloride
ben-dah-MOO-steen
hy-dro-CHLOR-ide

Treanda

Pharmacologic class:
mechlorethamine derivative
Pregnancy risk category D

AVAILABLE FORMS
Lyophilized powder for injection: 100 mg
in single-use vials

INDICATIONS & DOSAGES
➤ **Chronic lymphocytic leukemia
(CLL)**
Adults: 100 mg/m² I.V. over 30 minutes on
days 1 and 2 of a 28-day cycle, given up to
6 cycles.
Adjust-a-dose: For patients with grade 4
hematologic toxicity or clinically significant grade 2, 3, or 4 nonhematologic
toxicity, delay treatment. Resume treatment when nonhematologic toxicity has
improved to grade 1 or absolute neutrophil
count is 1×10^9/L or higher and platelet
count is 75×10^9/L or higher. In those with
grade 3 or greater hematologic toxicity,
give 50 mg/m² on days 1 and 2 of each
cycle; if grade 3 or greater toxicity recurs,
reduce dose to 25 mg/m² on days 1 and 2

of each cycle. In patients with clinically
significant grade 3 nonhematologic toxicity
or greater, give 50 mg/m² on days 1 and 2
of each cycle. Increase dose in subsequent
cycles, as tolerated.

ADMINISTRATION
I.V.
● Preparation and administration of
parenteral form of drug may be mutagenic,
teratogenic, or carcinogenic to staff.
Follow institutional policy to reduce
risks.
● Reconstitute powder using sterile water
for injection. Add 20 ml to a 100-mg vial.
Drug should dissolve within 5 minutes.
Inspect vial for particulate matter and
discoloration; discard if present.
● Reconstituted solutions must be further
diluted within 30 minutes using 500 ml of
normal saline solution. Discard cloudy or
discolored solution (solution should be
clear and colorless to slightly yellow).
● Reconstituted solution is stable for
24 hours when refrigerated, or 3 hours
at room temperature.
● **Incompatibilities:** Compatibility with
solutions other than normal saline and
sterile water for injection hasn't been
established.

ACTION
Mechlorethamine splits into electrophilic
alkyl groups, which covalently bond
with electron-rich nucleophilic moieties,
causing cell death.

PHARMACOKINETICS
Absorption: Given I.V.
Distribution: About 95% protein-bound
in plasma.
Metabolism: Primarily through hydro-
lysis to metabolites with low cytotoxic
activity.
Excretion: About 90% excreted in feces.

Route	Onset	Peak	Duration
I.V.	Rapid	30 minutes	Unknown

Half-life: About 3½ hours.

Reactions may be *common*, uncommon, *life-threatening*, or COMMON AND LIFE-THREATENING.
Interaction may have a *rapid onset* or **delayed onset.**

ADVERSE REACTIONS
CNS: *pyrexia, fatigue, asthenia,* chills.
EENT: nasopharyngitis.
GI: *nausea, vomiting, diarrhea.*
Hematologic: NEUTROPENIA, THROMBO-
CYTOPENIA, anemia, LEUKOPENIA,
lymphopenia.
Metabolic: *weight loss, hyperuricemia,*
tumor lysis syndrome.
Respiratory: cough.
Skin: *rash,* pruritus.
Other: *hypersensitivity,* infection, herpes
simplex, ***infusion reactions.***

INTERACTIONS
Drug-drug. *CYP1A2 inducers (omepra-*
zole): May decrease drug levels. Use
together cautiously.
CYP1A2 inhibitors (fluvoxamine,
ciprofloxacin): May increase drug levels.
Use together cautiously.
Drug-lifestyle. *Smoking:* May decrease
drug levels. Discourage smoking.

EFFECTS ON LAB TEST RESULTS
• May increase uric acid, bilirubin, AST,
ALT, and creatinine levels.
• May decrease neutrophil, platelet, RBC,
leukocyte, hemoglobin, and lymphocyte
counts.

CONTRAINDICATIONS & CAUTIONS
• Contraindicated in patients hypersensitive to the drug, bendamustine
or mannitol.
• Use cautiously in patients with mild
to moderate renal impairment or mild
hepatic impairment. Avoid use in
patients with creatinine clearance
less than 40 ml/minute. Avoid use in
those with moderate to severe hepatic
impairment.

NURSING CONSIDERATIONS
• Give through a separate I.V. line using
an infusion pump.
• Routinely monitor BUN, creatinine and
uric acid levels, liver function studies, and
complete blood count.
• Monitor closely for signs of allergic
reaction, including chills, rash, and
pruritus.
• Administer antipyretics, corticosteroids, and antihistamines, as
prescribed.

• Monitor for signs of infection (fever,
chills, malaise).
• Monitor fluid intake and output
closely, and maintain adequate
hydration.
• Allopurinol may be necessary during
the first 2 weeks of treatment to combat
elevated uric acid levels associated with
tumor lysis syndrome.
Pregnant patients
• Risk to fetus must be weighed against
potential benefit to mother.
Breast-feeding patients
• It isn't known if drug appears in
breast milk. However, because of the
risk of serious adverse reactions,
mutagenicity, and carcinogenicity
in infants, breast-feeding isn't
recommended.
Pediatric patients
• Safety and efficacy haven't been
established.
Geriatric patients
• Response rate was lower in elderly
patients as compared to younger
patients.

PATIENT TEACHING
• Advise patient to avoid exposure to
people with infections.
• Instruct patient to watch for signs and
symptoms of infection (fever, sore throat,
malaise) or bleeding.
• Advise patient to report any signs
of allergic reaction immediately
(rash, facial swelling, or difficulty
breathing) during or soon after
infusion.
• Caution women of childbearing
age to avoid pregnancy throughout
treatment and for 3 months after
therapy.
• Advise male patients to use reliable
contraception during treatment and for
3 months after therapy.
• Advise women to stop breast-feeding
during therapy because of toxicity risk to
infant.
• Tell patient that drug may cause
tiredness and to avoid driving or
operating dangerous tools or
machinery until the effects of drug
are known.
• Advise patient to report nausea, vomiting,
or diarrhea.

busulfan
byoo-SUL-fan

Busulfex, Myleran

Pharmacologic class: alkyl sulfonate
Pregnancy risk category D

AVAILABLE FORMS
Injection: 6 mg/ml
Tablets: 2 mg

INDICATIONS & DOSAGES
➤ **Chronic myelocytic (granulocytic) leukemia**
Adults: 4 to 8 mg P.O. daily until WBC count falls to 15,000/mm³; stop drug until WBC count rises to 50,000/mm³, and then resume dosage as before. Or, 4 to 8 mg P.O. daily until WBC count falls to 10,000 to 20,000/mm³; then reduce daily dose, as needed, to maintain WBC count at this level. Dosage is highly variable; range is 2 mg weekly to 4 mg daily.
Children: 0.06 to 0.12 mg/kg daily or 1.8 to 4.6 mg/m² P.O.; adjust dosage to maintain WBC count at 20,000/mm³ but never below 10,000/mm³.
➤ **Allogeneic hematopoietic stem cell transplantation in patients with chronic myelogenous leukemia**
Adults: 0.8 mg/kg I.V. every 6 hours for 4 days (a total of 16 doses). Give cyclophosphamide 60 mg/kg I.V. over 1 hour daily for 2 days beginning 6 hours after the 16th dose of busulfan injection.
Children who weigh more than 12 kg (26.5 lb): 0.8 mg/kg I.V. with cyclophosphamide.
Children who weigh 12 kg or less: 1.1 mg/kg I.V. with cyclophosphamide.

ADMINISTRATION
P.O.
● Give drug on an empty stomach to minimize nausea and vomiting.
I.V.
● Give antiemetic before first dose of busulfan injection and then on a fixed schedule during therapy; give phenytoin to prevent seizures.

● Follow facility policy when preparing and handling drug. Label as a hazardous drug.
● Dilute drug in either D_5W or normal saline solution to at least 0.5 mg/ml.
● Use the 5-micron nylon filter to withdraw the calculated volume from the ampule. Then use a new needle to inject the drug into the I.V. bag or syringe.
● Invert several times to ensure mixing.
● Use a central venous access device.
● Flush access device with 5 ml of D_5W or normal saline solution before and after each infusion.
● Infuse over 2 hours through a central venous access device using a controlled-infusion device.
● Solutions are stable 8 hours at room temperature or 12 hours when diluted in normal saline solution and refrigerated. Infusions must be completed within these times.
● **Incompatibilities:** Don't mix or give with other I.V. solutions of unknown compatibility.

ACTION
Unknown. Thought to cross-link strands of cellular DNA and interfere with RNA transcription, causing an imbalance of growth that leads to cell death. Not specific to cell cycle.

Route	Onset	Peak	Duration
P.O.	1–2 wk	Unknown	Unknown
I.V.	Unknown	Unknown	Unknown

Half-life: About 2½ hours.

ADVERSE REACTIONS
CNS: *fever, headache, asthenia, pain, insomnia, anxiety, dizziness, depression,* delirium, agitation, ***encephalopathy, confusion,*** hallucination, lethargy, somnolence, ***seizures.***
CV: *edema, chest pain, tachycardia, hypertension, hypotension, **thrombosis,** vasodilation, **heart rhythm abnormalities,*** cardiomegaly, ***heart failure, pericardial effusion,*** tachycardia.
EENT: *rhinitis, epistaxis, pharyngitis, sinusitis, ear disorder, cataracts, corneal thinning, lens changes.*
GI: *nausea, stomatitis, vomiting, anorexia, diarrhea, abdominal pain and enlarge-*

ment, dyspepsia, constipation, dry mouth, rectal disorder, pancreatitis.
GU: dysuria, *oliguria,* hematuria, hemorrhagic cystitis.
Hematologic: GRANULOCYTOPENIA, THROMBOCYTOPENIA, LEUKOPENIA, *anemia,* APLASTIC ANEMIA.
Hepatic: *jaundice,* hepatomegaly, *hyperbilirubinemia, **hepatic veno-occlusive disease.***
Metabolic: *hypomagnesemia, hyperglycemia, hypokalemia, hypocalcemia, hypervolemia, weight gain, hypophosphatemia,* hyponatremia.
Musculoskeletal: *back pain, myalgia, arthralgia.*
Respiratory: *lung disorder, cough, dyspnea, **irreversible pulmonary fibrosis, alveolar hemorrhage, asthma,** atelectasis,* pleural effusion hypoxia, hemoptysis.
Skin: *inflammation at injection site, rash, pruritus, alopecia,* exfoliative dermatitis, erythema nodosum, acne, skin discoloration, *hyperpigmentation.*
Other: Addison-like wasting syndrome, *chills, allergic reaction, **infection,** hiccup.*

INTERACTIONS
Drug-drug. *Acetaminophen, itraconazole:* May decrease busulfan clearance. Use together cautiously.
Anticoagulants, aspirin: May increase risk of bleeding. Avoid using together.
Cyclophosphamide: May increase risk of cardiac tamponade in patients with thalassemia. Monitor patient.
Metronidazole: May increase busulfan toxicity. Avoid using together.
Myelosuppressives: May increase myelosuppression. Monitor patient.
Other cytotoxic agents causing pulmonary injury: May cause additive pulmonary toxicity. Avoid using together.
Phenytoin: May decrease busulfan level. Monitor busulfan level.
Thioguanine: May cause hepatotoxicity, esophageal varices, or portal hypertension. Use together cautiously.

EFFECTS ON LAB TEST RESULTS
• May increase alkaline phosphatase, ALT, bilirubin, BUN, creatinine, and glucose levels. May decrease calcium, hemoglobin, magnesium, phosphorus, potassium, and sodium levels.

• May decrease WBC and platelet counts.

CONTRAINDICATIONS & CAUTIONS
• Contraindicated in patients with chronic myelogenous leukemia resistant to drug and in those with chronic lymphocytic or acute leukemia or in the blastic crisis of chronic myelogenous leukemia.
• Use cautiously in patients recently given other myelosuppressives or radiation treatment and in those with depressed neutrophil or platelet count.
• Use cautiously in patients with history of head trauma or seizures and in those receiving other drugs that lower the seizure threshold because high-dose therapy has been linked to seizures.

NURSING CONSIDERATIONS
■ **Black Box Warning** Do not use busulfan unless a diagnosis of CML has been adequately established. ■
■ **Black Box Warning** Reduce or discontinue the dosage if unusual depression of bone marrow function occurs. ■
■ **Black Box Warning** Malignant tumors and acute leukemias have been reported in patients who have received busulfan therapy. ■
• Therapeutic effects are commonly accompanied by toxicity.
• To prevent bleeding, avoid all I.M. injections when platelet count is less than 50,000/mm³.
• Monitor patient response (increased appetite and sense of well-being, decreased total WBC count, reduced size of spleen), which usually begins in 1 to 2 weeks.
• Monitor for jaundice and liver function abnormalities in patients receiving high-dose busulfan.
• Anticipate possible blood transfusion during treatment because of cumulative anemia. Patients may receive injections of RBC colony-stimulating factor to promote RBC production and decrease the need for blood transfusions.
• *Alert:* Pulmonary fibrosis may occur as late as 8 months to 10 years after therapy. (Average length of therapy is 4 years.)

PATIENT TEACHING
• Advise patient to watch for signs of infection (fever, sore throat, fatigue) and

bleeding (easy bruising, nosebleeds, bleeding gums, tarry stools). Tell patient to take temperature daily.

• Instruct patient to report signs and symptoms of toxicity so dosage can be adjusted. Persistent cough and progressive labored breathing with liquid in the lungs, suggestive of pneumonia, may be caused by drug toxicity.

• Advise patient to report signs of sudden weakness, anorexia, melanoderma, nausea and vomiting, unusual fatigue, and weight loss.

• Instruct patient to avoid OTC products containing aspirin and NSAIDs.

• Inform patient that drug may cause skin darkening.

• Advise woman of childbearing age to avoid becoming pregnant during therapy. Recommend that she consult prescriber before becoming pregnant.

• Advise patient not to breast-feed during therapy because of risk of toxicity to infant.

• Instruct patient to take drug on empty stomach to decrease nausea and vomiting.

• Because of risk of impotence and sterility, advise men who want to father a child about sperm banking before therapy.

SAFETY ALERT!

carboplatin
KAR-bo-pla-tin

Paraplatin

Pharmacologic class: platinum coordination compound
Pregnancy risk category D

AVAILABLE FORMS
Aqueous solution for injection: 50 mg/5 ml, 150 mg/15 ml, 450 mg/45 ml
Lyophilized powder for injection: 50-mg, 150-mg, 450-mg vials

INDICATIONS & DOSAGES
➤ **Advanced ovarian cancer**
Adults: 360 mg/m^2 I.V. on day 1 every 4 weeks. Or, 300 mg/m^2 on day 1 every 4 weeks for six cycles when used with

other chemotherapy drugs. Doses shouldn't be repeated until platelet count exceeds 100,000/mm^3 and neutrophil count exceeds 2,000/mm^3. Subsequent doses are based on blood counts: If platelets are greater than 100,000/mm^3 and neutrophils are greater than 2,000/mm^3, give 125% of dose. If platelets are 50,000/mm^3 to 100,000/mm^3 and neutrophils are 500/mm^3 to 2,000/mm^3, keep same dose. If platelets are less than 50,000/mm^3 and neutrophils are less than 500/mm^3, give 75% of dose.

Adjust-a-dose: If creatinine clearance is 41 to 59 ml/minute, first dose is 250 mg/m^2. If creatinine clearance is 16 to 40 ml/minute, first dose is 200 mg/m^2. Drug isn't recommended for patients with creatinine clearance of 15 ml/minute or less.

ADMINISTRATION
I.V.
■ **Black Box Warning** Anaphylaxis may occur within minutes of administration. Keep epinephrine, corticosteroids, and antihistamines available when giving carboplatin. ■

• Preparing and giving parenteral form of drug may be mutagenic, teratogenic, or carcinogenic. Follow facility policy to reduce risks.

• Don't use aluminum needles or I.V. administration sets because drug may precipitate or lose potency.

• For premixed aqueous solution of 10 mg/ml, dilute for infusion with normal saline solution or D$_5$W to a concentration as low as 0.5 mg/ml.

• For vials of lyophilized powder, reconstitute with sterile water for injection, D$_5$W, or normal saline. For 50-mg vial, use 5 ml solution; for 150-mg vial, use 15 ml solution; for 450-mg vial, use 45 ml solution to yield a concentration of 10 mg/ml.

• Give drug by continuous or intermittent infusion over at least 15 minutes.

• Store unopened vials at room temperature. Protect from light.

• Once reconstituted and diluted as directed, drug is stable at room temperature for 8 hours.

• Because drug contains no preservatives, discard after 8 hours.

Reactions may be *common*, uncommon, *life-threatening*, or COMMON AND LIFE-THREATENING.
Interaction may have a *rapid onset* or **delayed onset**.

• **Incompatibilities:** Amphotericin B cholesteryl sulfate complex, fluorouracil, mesna, sodium bicarbonate.

ACTION
May cross-link strands of cellular DNA and interfere with RNA transcription, causing an imbalance of growth that leads to cell death. Not specific to cell cycle.

Route	Onset	Peak	Duration
I.V.	Unknown	Unknown	Unknown

Half-life: 5 hours.

ADVERSE REACTIONS
CNS: dizziness, confusion, *stroke,* peripheral neuropathy, CENTRAL NEUROTOXICITY.
CV: *heart failure, embolism.*
EENT: ototoxicity.
GI: *abdominal pain,* constipation, diarrhea, *nausea, vomiting,* mucositis, change in taste, stomatitis.
Hematologic: THROMBOCYTOPENIA, *leukopenia,* NEUTROPENIA, anemia, BONE MARROW SUPPRESSION, *bleeding.*
Skin: alopecia.
Other: hypersensitivity reactions.

INTERACTIONS
Drug-drug. *Aspirin, NSAIDs:* May increase risk of bleeding. Avoid using together.
Bone marrow suppressants, including radiation therapy: May increase hematologic toxicity. Monitor CBC with differential closely.
Nephrotoxic drugs, especially aminoglycosides and amphotericin B: May enhance nephrotoxicity of carboplatin. Use together cautiously.

EFFECTS ON LAB TEST RESULTS
• May increase alkaline phosphatase, AST, BUN, and creatinine levels. May decrease electrolyte and hemoglobin levels and hematocrit.
• May decrease neutrophil, platelet, RBC, and WBC counts.

CONTRAINDICATIONS & CAUTIONS
• Contraindicated in patients with severe bone marrow suppression or bleeding or with history of hypersensitivity to cisplatin,

platinum-containing compounds, or mannitol.

NURSING CONSIDERATIONS
■ **Black Box Warning** Carboplatin should be administered under the supervision of a physician experienced in the use of chemotherapeutic agents. ■
• Determine electrolyte, creatinine, and BUN levels; CBC; platelet count; and creatinine clearance before first infusion and before each course of treatment.
• Monitor CBC and platelet count frequently during therapy and, when indicated, until recovery. Lowest WBC and platelet counts usually occur by day 21. Levels usually return to baseline by day 28. Don't repeat unless platelet count exceeds 100,000/mm³.
■ **Black Box Warning** Bone marrow suppression is dose related and may be severe, resulting in infection or bleeding. ■
■ **Black Box Warning** Vomiting is another frequent drug-related side effect. ■
• Bone marrow suppression may be more severe in patients with creatinine clearance below 60 ml/minute; adjust dosage.
• *Alert:* Carefully check ordered dose against laboratory test results. Only one increase in dosage is recommended. Subsequent doses shouldn't exceed 125% of starting dose.
• Therapeutic effects are commonly accompanied by toxicity.
• Drug has less nephrotoxicity and neurotoxicity than cisplatin, but it causes more severe myelosuppression.
• To prevent bleeding, avoid all I.M. injections when platelet count is below 50,000/mm³.
• Monitor vital signs during infusion.
• Give antiemetic to reduce nausea and vomiting.
■ **Black Box Warning** Anticipate blood transfusions during treatment because of cumulative anemia. Patient may receive injections of RBC colony-stimulating factor to promote cell production. ■
• Patients older than age 65 are at greater risk for neurotoxicity.
• *Look alike–sound alike:* Don't confuse carboplatin with cisplatin.

PATIENT TEACHING
• Advise patient of most common adverse reactions: nausea, vomiting, bone marrow suppression, anemia, and reduction in blood platelets.
• Advise patient to watch for signs of infection (fever, sore throat, fatigue) and bleeding (easy bruising, nosebleeds, bleeding gums, tarry stools). Tell patient to take temperature daily.
• Instruct patient to avoid OTC products containing aspirin and NSAIDs.
• Advise women to stop breast-feeding during therapy because of risk of toxicity to infant.
• Because of risk of impotence, sterility, and menstruation cessation, counsel both men and women of childbearing age before starting therapy. Also recommend that women consult prescriber before becoming pregnant.

carmustine (BCNU)
kar-MUS-teen

BiCNU, Gliadel Wafer

Pharmacologic class: nitrosourea
Pregnancy risk category D

AVAILABLE FORMS
Injection: 100-mg vial (lyophilized), with a 3-ml vial of absolute alcohol supplied as a diluent
Wafer: 7.7 mg, for intracavitary use

INDICATIONS & DOSAGES
➤ **Brain tumor, Hodgkin lymphoma, malignant lymphoma, multiple myeloma**
Adults: 150 to 200 mg/m^2 I.V. by slow infusion every 6 weeks; may be divided into daily injections of 75 to 100 mg/m^2 on 2 successive days; repeat dose every 6 weeks if platelet count is greater than 100,000/mm^3 and WBC count is greater than 4,000/mm^3.
Adjust-a-dose: Dosage is reduced by 30% when WBC nadir is 2,000 to 2,999/mm^3 and platelet nadir is 25,000 to 74,999/mm^3. Dosage is reduced by 50% when WBC nadir is less than 2,000/mm^3 and platelet nadir is less than 25,000/mm^3.
➤ **Adjunct to surgery to prolong survival in patients with recurrent glioblastoma multiforme for whom surgical resection is indicated**
Adults: 8 wafers placed in the resection cavity if size and shape of cavity allow. If 8 wafers can't be accommodated, use maximum number of wafers allowed. Or, 150 to 200 mg/m^2 I.V. by slow infusion as single dose, repeated every 6 to 8 weeks.
➤ **Adjunct to surgery and radiation in patients with newly diagnosed high-grade malignant glioma**
Adults: 8 wafers placed in the resection cavity if size and shape of cavity allow. If 8 wafers can't be accommodated, use maximum number of wafers allowed.

ADMINISTRATION
I.V.
• Preparing and giving parenteral form of drug may be mutagenic, teratogenic, or carcinogenic. Follow facility policy to reduce risks. Wear gloves when handling any form of drug.
• Prepare drug only in glass containers. Solution is unstable in plastic I.V. bags.
• If powder liquefies or appears oily, discard because decomposition has occurred.
• To reconstitute, dissolve 100 mg of drug in 3 ml of absolute alcohol provided by manufacturer.
• Dilute solution with 27 ml of sterile water for injection. Resulting solution contains 3.3 mg of carmustine/ml in 10% alcohol.
• For infusion, dilute in normal saline solution or D$_5$W.
• Don't mix with other drugs during administration.
• Give at least 250 ml over 1 to 2 hours.
• To reduce pain on infusion, dilute further or slow infusion rate.
• Solution may be stored in refrigerator for 24 hours or at room temperature for 8 hours. It may decompose at temperatures above 80° F (27° C). Protect from light.
• **Incompatibilities:** Sodium bicarbonate.

Reactions may be *common,* uncommon, *life-threatening,* or COMMON AND LIFE-THREATENING.
Interaction may have a *rapid onset* or **delayed onset.**

Topical
● Unopened foil pouches of wafer may be kept at room temperature for a maximum of 6 hours.
● Wafers broken in half may be used; however, discard wafers broken into more than two pieces.

ACTION

Inhibits enzymatic reactions involved with DNA synthesis, cross-links strands of cellular DNA, and interferes with RNA transcription, causing an imbalance of growth that leads to cell death. Not specific to cell cycle.

Route	Onset	Peak	Duration
I.V. intra-cavitary	Unknown	Unknown	Unknown

Half-life: 15 to 30 minutes.

ADVERSE REACTIONS

CNS: ataxia, *brain edema, seizures.*
EENT: visual disturbances.
GI: *nausea, vomiting,* anorexia, diarrhea, dysphagia, *GI hemorrhage.*
GU: *nephrotoxicity,* renal impairment.
Hematologic: *cumulative bone marrow suppression, leukopenia, thrombocytopenia, acute leukemia or bone marrow dysplasia,* anemia, *hemorrhage.*
Hepatic: *hepatotoxicity.*
Metabolic: hyperglycemia, *hypokalemia,* hyponatremia.
Respiratory: *pulmonary fibrosis.*
Other: *intense pain at infusion site from venous spasm.*

INTERACTIONS

Drug-drug. *Cimetidine:* May increase carmustine's bone marrow toxicity. Avoid using together.
Digoxin, phenytoin: May decrease levels of these drugs. Monitor patient.
Myelosuppressives: May increase myelosuppression. Monitor patient.

EFFECTS ON LAB TEST RESULTS

● May increase alkaline phosphatase, AST, bilirubin, hemoglobin, and urine urea levels.
● May decrease platelet and WBC counts.

CONTRAINDICATIONS & CAUTIONS

● Contraindicated in patients hypersensitive to drug.

NURSING CONSIDERATIONS

■ **Black Box Warning** Carmustine for injection should be administered under the supervision of a physician experienced in the use of cancer chemotherapeutic agents. ■
■ **Black Box Warning** Bone marrow suppression, notably thrombocytopenia and leukopenia is the most common and severe of the toxic effects. ■
■ **Black Box Warning** Pulmonary toxicity appears to be dose related. Patients receiving greater than 1,400 mg/m^2 cumulative dose are at higher risk. Pulmonary toxicity can occur years after treatment and can result in death, particularly in patients treated in childhood. ■
● Obtain pulmonary function tests before and during therapy.
■ **Black Box Warning** Bone marrow suppression is delayed with carmustine. Blood counts should be monitored weekly for at least 6 weeks after a dose and drug shouldn't be given more often than every 6 weeks. ■
● Give antiemetic before drug to reduce nausea.
● If drug touches skin, wash off thoroughly. Avoid contact with skin because drug will stain skin brown.
● Perform liver, renal function, and pulmonary function tests periodically.
● Monitor CBC with differential. The absolute neutrophil count may be used to better calculate the patient's immunosuppressive state.
● Monitor uric acid level. To prevent hyperuricemia with resulting uric acid nephropathy, allopurinol may be used with adequate hydration.
● Therapeutic levels are commonly toxic.
● Acute leukemia or bone marrow dysplasia may occur after long-term use.
● To prevent bleeding, avoid using I.M. when platelet count is less than 50,000/mm^3.
● Anticipate blood transfusions during treatment because of cumulative anemia. Patient may receive injections of RBC colony-stimulating factor to promote cell production.

PATIENT TEACHING
• Advise patient about common adverse reactions to drug.
• Tell patient to watch for signs and symptoms of infection (fever, sore throat, fatigue) and bleeding (easy bruising, nosebleeds, bleeding gums, tarry stools). Tell him to take temperature daily.
• Instruct patient to avoid OTC products containing aspirin and NSAIDs.
• Advise women to stop breast-feeding during therapy because of possible risk of toxicity to infant.
• Caution woman of childbearing age to avoid becoming pregnant during therapy. Recommend that she consult prescriber before becoming pregnant.

SAFETY ALERT!

chlorambucil
klor-AM-byoo-sill

Leukeran

Pharmacologic class: nitrogen mustard
Pregnancy risk category D

AVAILABLE FORMS
Tablets: 2 mg

INDICATIONS & DOSAGES
➤ **Chronic lymphocytic leukemia; malignant lymphomas, including lymphosarcoma, giant follicular lymphoma, and Hodgkin lymphoma**
Adults: 0.1 to 0.2 mg/kg P.O. daily for 3 to 6 weeks, then adjust for maintenance (usually 4 to 10 mg daily).
Adjust-a-dose: Reduce first dose if given within 4 weeks after a full course of radiation therapy or myelosuppressive drugs, or if pretreatment leukocyte or platelet counts are depressed from bone marrow disease.

ADMINISTRATION
P.O.
• For initial therapy and short courses of therapy, give entire daily dose at one time.

ACTION
Cross-links strands of cellular DNA and interferes with RNA transcription, causing an imbalance of growth that leads to cell death. Not specific to cell cycle.

Route	Onset	Peak	Duration
P.O.	Unknown	1 hr	Unknown

Half-life: 2 hours for parent compound; 2½ hours for phenylacetic acid metabolite.

ADVERSE REACTIONS
CNS: *seizures,* tremor.
GI: *nausea, vomiting, stomatitis, diarrhea.*
Hematologic: *neutropenia, bone marrow suppression, thrombocytopenia,* anemia, *myelosuppression.*
Skin: rash.
Other: *allergic reaction.*

INTERACTIONS
None reported.

EFFECTS ON LAB TEST RESULTS
• May increase alkaline phosphatase, AST, and blood and urine uric acid levels. May decrease hemoglobin level. May decrease granulocyte, neutrophil, platelet, RBC, and WBC counts.

CONTRAINDICATIONS & CAUTIONS
• Contraindicated in patients with hypersensitivity or resistance to previous therapy. Patients hypersensitive to other alkylating drugs may also be hypersensitive to this drug.
• Use cautiously in patients with history of head trauma or seizures and in patients receiving other drugs that lower the seizure threshold.
• Use cautiously within 4 weeks of a full course of radiation or chemotherapy.

NURSING CONSIDERATIONS
■ **Black Box Warning** Chlorambucil can severely suppress bone marrow function. It is a carcinogen in humans and is probably mutagenic and teratogenic in humans. It also produces human infertility. ■
• Monitor CBC with differential.
• Monitor patient for neutropenia, which may not appear until after the 3rd week of treatment. The absolute neutrophil count (ANC) may continue to decrease for up to 10 days after treatment ends.

Reactions may be *common,* uncommon, *life-threatening,* or COMMON AND LIFE-THREATENING.
Interaction may have a *rapid onset* or *delayed onset.*

• Use the ANC to calculate the patient's immunosuppression.

• Monitor uric acid level. To prevent hyperuricemia with resulting uric acid nephropathy, allopurinol may be used with adequate hydration.

• If WBC count falls below 2,000/mm^3 or granulocyte count falls below 1,000/mm^3, follow institutional policy for infection control in immunocompromised patients. Patients may receive injections of WBC colony-stimulating factor to increase WBC count recovery.

• Therapeutic effects are frequently accompanied by toxicity.

• To prevent bleeding, avoid all I.M. injections when platelet count is below 50,000/mm^3.

• Anticipate blood transfusions during treatment because of cumulative anemia. Patient may receive injections of RBC colony-stimulating factor to promote RBC production and decrease need for blood transfusions.

PATIENT TEACHING

• Advise patient to watch for signs of infection (fever, sore throat, fatigue) and bleeding (easy bruising, nosebleeds, bleeding gums, tarry stools). Tell patient to take temperature daily.

• Instruct patient to avoid OTC products containing aspirin and NSAIDs.

• Advise women to stop breast-feeding during therapy because of risk of toxicity to infant.

• Advise women of childbearing age to avoid becoming pregnant during therapy and to notify prescriber immediately if pregnancy is suspected.

SAFETY ALERT!

---

cisplatin (CDDP)
SIS-pla-tin

Platinol, Platinol AQ

Pharmacologic class: platinum coordination complex
Pregnancy risk category D

AVAILABLE FORMS
Injection: 1 mg/ml

INDICATIONS & DOSAGES
➤ **Adjunctive therapy in metastatic testicular cancer**
Adults: 20 mg/m^2 I.V. daily for 5 days. Repeat every 3 weeks for three or four cycles.
➤ **Adjunctive therapy in metastatic ovarian cancer**
Adults: 100 mg/m^2 I.V.; repeat every 4 weeks. Or, 75 to 100 mg/m^2 I.V. once every 4 weeks with cyclophosphamide.
➤ **Advanced bladder cancer**
Adults: 50 to 70 mg/m^2 I.V. every 3 to 4 weeks. Give 50 mg/m^2 every 4 weeks in patients who have received other antineoplastics or radiation therapy.

ADMINISTRATION
I.V.
• Preparing and giving parenteral form of drug may be mutagenic, teratogenic, or carcinogenic. Follow facility policy to reduce risks.

• Hydrate patient with normal saline solution for 8 to 12 hours before giving drug. Maintain urine output of at least 100 ml/hour for 4 consecutive hours before therapy and for 24 hours after therapy.

• Reconstitute powder using sterile water for injection. Add 10 ml to 10-mg vial or 50 ml to 50-mg vial to make a solution containing 1 mg/ml.

• Infusions are most stable in solutions containing chloride (such as normal or half-normal saline solution and 0.22% sodium chloride). Don't use D$_5$W alone.

• Further dilute with dextrose 5% in 0.3% sodium chloride injection or dextrose 5% in half-normal saline solution for injection with 37.5 g mannitol added.

• Administer over 6 to 8 hours.

• Solutions are stable for 20 hours at room temperature. Don't refrigerate.

• **Incompatibilities:** Aluminum administration sets, amifostine, amphotericin B cholesteryl sulfate complex, cefepime, D$_5$W, etoposide with mannitol and potassium chloride, fluorouracil, mesna, 0.1% sodium chloride solution, paclitaxel, piperacillin sodium with tazobactam sodium, sodium bicarbonate, sodium bisulfate, sodium thiosulfate, solutions with a chloride content less than 2%, thiotepa.

ACTION

May cross-link strands of cellular DNA and interfere with RNA transcription, causing an imbalance of growth that leads to cell death. Not specific to cell cycle.

Route	Onset	Peak	Duration
I.V.	Unknown	Unknown	Several days

Half-life: Initial phase, 25 to 79 minutes; terminal phase, 58 to 78 hours.

ADVERSE REACTIONS

CNS: *peripheral neuritis,* **seizures.**
EENT: *tinnitus, hearing loss.*
GI: anorexia, diarrhea, loss of taste, *nausea, vomiting.*
GU: PROLONGED RENAL TOXICITY WITH REPEATED COURSES OF THERAPY.
Hematologic: MYELOSUPPRESSION, *leukopenia, thrombocytopenia,* anemia.
Metabolic: *hypomagnesemia, hypokalemia, hypocalcemia.*
Other: *anaphylactoid reaction.*

INTERACTIONS

Drug-drug. *Aminoglycosides:* May increase nephrotoxicity. Carefully monitor renal function study results.
Aminoglycosides, bumetanide, ethacrynic acid, furosemide, torsemide: May increase ototoxicity. Avoid using together, if possible.
Aspirin, NSAIDs: May increase risk of bleeding. Avoid using together.
Fosphenytoin, phenytoin: May decrease phenytoin and fosphenytoin levels. Monitor levels.
Myelosuppressives: May increase myelosuppression. Monitor patient.

EFFECTS ON LAB TEST RESULTS

• May increase uric acid level. May decrease calcium, hemoglobin, magnesium, phosphate, potassium, and sodium levels.
• May decrease platelet and WBC counts.

CONTRAINDICATIONS & CAUTIONS

• Contraindicated in patients hypersensitive to drug or other platinum-containing compounds and in those with severe renal disease, hearing impairment, or myelosuppression.
• Use cautiously in patients previously treated with radiation or cytotoxic drugs

and in those with peripheral neuropathies; also use cautiously with other ototoxic and nephrotoxic drugs.

NURSING CONSIDERATIONS

■ **Black Box Warning** Drug should be administered under the supervision of a physician experienced in the use of cancer chemotherapeutic agents. ■
• Monitor CBC, electrolyte levels (especially potassium and magnesium), platelet count, and renal function studies before initial and subsequent doses.
■ **Black Box Warning** Ototoxicity may be more pronounced in children and is manifested by tinnitus or loss of high frequency hearing and occasionally, deafness. ■
• To detect hearing loss, obtain audiometry tests before initial and subsequent doses.
• Prehydration and mannitol diuresis may significantly reduce renal toxicity and ototoxicity.
• Therapeutic effects are frequently accompanied by toxicity.
• Patients may experience vomiting 3 to 5 days after treatment, requiring prolonged antiemetic treatment. Some prescribers combine metoclopramide with dexamethasone and antihistamines, or ondansetron or granisetron with dexamethasone to control vomiting. Monitor intake and output. Continue I.V. hydration until patient can tolerate adequate oral intake.
■ **Black Box Warning** Renal toxicity is cumulative; don't give next dose until renal function returns to normal. ■
• Don't repeat dose unless platelet count exceeds 100,000/mm³, WBC count exceeds 4,000/mm³, creatinine level is below 1.5 mg/dl, creatinine clearance is 50 ml/minute or more, and BUN level is below 25 mg/dl.
■ **Black Box Warning** Be careful to avoid overdose. Doses greater than 100 mg/m² per cycle every 3 to 4 weeks are rare. Confirm that dose is total dose per cycle, not daily dose. ■
• To prevent bleeding, avoid all I.M. injections when platelet count is less than 50,000/mm³.
• Anticipate need for blood transfusions during treatment because of cumulative anemia.

Reactions may be *common,* uncommon, *life-threatening,* or COMMON AND LIFE-THREATENING.
Interaction may have a *rapid onset* or *delayed onset.*

■ **Black Box Warning** Immediately give epinephrine, corticosteroids, or antihistamines for anaphylactoid reactions. ■

● Safety of drug in children hasn't been established.

● *Look alike–sound alike:* Don't confuse cisplatin with carboplatin; they aren't interchangeable.

PATIENT TEACHING
● Advise patient to watch for signs and symptoms of infection (fever, sore throat, fatigue) and bleeding (easy bruising, nosebleeds, bleeding gums, tarry stools). Tell patient to take temperature daily.
● Tell patient to immediately report ringing in the ears or numbness in hands or feet.
● Instruct patient to avoid OTC products containing aspirin.
● Advise women to stop breast-feeding during therapy because of risk of toxicity to infant.
● Advise women of childbearing age to consult prescriber before becoming pregnant.

SAFETY ALERT!

cyclophosphamide
sye-kloe-FOSS-fa-mide

Lyophilized Cytoxan, Procytox†

Pharmacologic class: nitrogen mustard
Pregnancy risk category D

AVAILABLE FORMS
Injection: 100-mg, 200-mg, 500-mg, 1-g, 2-g vials
Tablets: 25 mg, 50 mg

INDICATIONS & DOSAGES
➤ **Breast or ovarian cancer, Hodgkin lymphoma, chronic lymphocytic leukemia, chronic myelocytic leukemia, acute lymphoblastic leukemia, acute myelocytic and monocytic leukemia, neuroblastoma, retinoblastoma, malignant lymphoma, multiple myeloma, mycosis fungoides, sarcoma**
Adults and children: Initially for induction, 40 to 50 mg/kg I.V. in divided doses over 2 to 5 days. Or, 10 to 15 mg/kg I.V. every 7 to 10 days, 3 to 5 mg/kg I.V. twice weekly, or 1 to 5 mg/kg P.O. daily, based on patient tolerance.

Adjust subsequent doses according to evidence of antitumor activity or leukopenia.
➤ **Minimal-change nephrotic syndrome**
Children: 2.5 to 3 mg/kg P.O. daily for 60 to 90 days.

ADMINISTRATION
P.O.
● Don't give drug at bedtime; infrequent urination during the night may increase possibility of cystitis.
I.V.
● Preparing and giving parenteral form of drug may be mutagenic, teratogenic, or carcinogenic. Follow facility policy to reduce risks.
● Reconstitute powder using sterile water for injection or bacteriostatic water for injection containing only parabens.
● Add 5 ml to 100-mg vial, 10 ml to 200-mg vial, 25 ml to 500-mg vial, 50 ml to 1-g vial, or 100 ml to 2-g vial to produce a solution containing 20 mg/ml. Shake vigorously to dissolve. If powder doesn't dissolve completely, let vial stand for a few minutes.
● Check reconstituted solution for small particles. Filter solution, if needed.
● Give by direct I.V. injection or infusion.
● For infusion, further dilute with D_5W, dextrose 5% in normal saline solution for injection, dextrose 5% in Ringer's injection, lactated Ringer's injection, sodium lactate injection, or half-normal saline solution for injection.
● Reconstituted solution is stable 6 days if refrigerated or 24 hours at room temperature. Use stored solutions cautiously because drug contains no preservatives.
● **Incompatibilities:** Amphotericin B cholesteryl sulfate complex.

ACTION
Cross-links strands of cellular DNA and interferes with RNA transcription, causing an imbalance of growth that leads to cell death. Not specific to cell cycle.

Route	Onset	Peak	Duration
P.O.	Unknown	Unknown	Unknown
I.V.	Unknown	2–3 hr	Unknown

Half-life: 3 to 12 hours.

ADVERSE REACTIONS
CV: *cardiotoxicity with very high doses and with doxorubicin.*
GI: *nausea and vomiting,* anorexia, stomatitis.
GU: HEMORRHAGIC CYSTITIS, impaired fertility.
Hematologic: *leukopenia, thrombocytopenia,* anemia.
Hepatic: *hepatotoxicity.*
Metabolic: hyperuricemia, SIADH.
Respiratory: *pulmonary fibrosis with high doses.*
Skin: *alopecia.*
Other: *secondary malignant disease, anaphylaxis,* hypersensitivity reactions.

INTERACTIONS
Drug-drug. *Allopurinol, myelosuppressives:* May increase myelosuppression. Monitor patient for toxicity.
Anticoagulants: May increase anticoagulant effect. Monitor patient for bleeding.
Aspirin, NSAIDs: May increase risk of bleeding. Avoid using together.
Barbiturates: May enhance cyclophosphamide toxicity. Monitor patient closely.
Cardiotoxic drugs: May increase adverse cardiac effects. Monitor patient for toxicity.
Chloramphenicol, corticosteroids: May reduce activity of cyclophosphamide. Use together cautiously.
Ciprofloxacin: May decrease antimicrobial effect. Monitor patient for effect.
Digoxin: May decrease digoxin level. Monitor level closely.
Quinolones: May decrease the antimicrobial effects of quinolones. Monitor patient.
Succinylcholine: May prolong neuromuscular blockade. Avoid using together.
Thiazide diuretics: May prolong antineoplastic-induced leukopenia. Monitor patient closely.

EFFECTS ON LAB TEST RESULTS
• May increase uric acid level. May decrease hemoglobin and pseudocholinesterase levels.

• May decrease platelet, RBC, and WBC counts.
• May suppress positive reaction to *Candida,* mumps, *Trichophyton,* and tuberculin skin test results. May cause a false-positive Papanicolaou test result.

CONTRAINDICATIONS & CAUTIONS
• Contraindicated in patients hypersensitive to drug and in those with severe bone marrow suppression.
• Use cautiously in patients with leukopenia, thrombocytopenia, malignant cell infiltration of bone marrow, or hepatic or renal disease and in those who have recently undergone radiation therapy or chemotherapy.

NURSING CONSIDERATIONS
• If cystitis occurs, stop drug and notify prescriber. Cystitis can occur months after therapy ends. Mesna may be given to reduce frequency and severity of bladder toxicity. Test urine for blood.
• Adequately hydrate patients before and after dose to decrease risk of cystitis.
• Use caution to ensure correct dose to decrease risk of cardiac toxicity.
• Monitor CBC and renal and liver function test results.
• Monitor patient closely for leukopenia (nadir between days 8 and 15, recovery in 17 to 28 days).
• Monitor uric acid level. To prevent hyperuricemia with resulting uric acid nephropathy, allopurinol may be used with adequate hydration.
• To prevent bleeding, avoid all I.M. injections when platelet count is less than 50,000/mm³.
• Anticipate blood transfusions because of cumulative anemia. Patients may receive injections of RBC colony-stimulating factor to promote RBC production and decrease need for blood transfusions.
• Therapeutic effects are often accompanied by toxicity.
• In boys, using drug for nephrotic syndrome for more than 60 days increases the incidence of oligospermia and azoospermia. Use for more than 90 days increases the risk of sterility.
• Drug may be used to treat nononcologic disorders, such as lupus, nephritis, and rheumatoid arthritis.

Reactions may be *common*, uncommon, *life-threatening*, or COMMON AND LIFE-THREATENING.
Interaction may have a *rapid onset* or **delayed onset.**

PATIENT TEACHING
• Warn patient that hair loss is likely to occur but is reversible.
• Advise patient to watch for signs and symptoms of infection (fever, sore throat, fatigue) and bleeding (easy bruising, nosebleeds, bleeding gums, tarry stools). Tell patient to take temperature daily.
• Instruct patient to avoid OTC products that contain aspirin.
• To minimize risk of hemorrhagic cystitis, encourage patient to urinate every 1 to 2 hours while awake and to drink at least 3 L of fluid daily.
• If patient is taking tablets, tell him not to take it at bedtime because infrequent urination increases risk of cystitis.
• Advise both men and women to practice contraception during therapy and for 4 months afterward; drug may cause birth defects.
• Advise women to stop breast-feeding during therapy because of risk of toxicity to infant.
• Drug can cause irreversible sterility in both men and women. Before therapy, counsel patients who are considering parenthood. Also recommend that women consult prescriber before becoming pregnant.

SAFETY ALERT!

dacarbazine (DTIC)
da-KAR-ba-zeen

DTIC-Dome

Pharmacologic class: triazene
Pregnancy risk category C

AVAILABLE FORMS
Injection: 100-mg, 200-mg, 500-mg vials

INDICATIONS & DOSAGES
➤ **Metastatic malignant melanoma**
Adults: 2 to 4.5 mg/kg I.V. daily for 10 days; repeat every 4 weeks as tolerated. Or, 250 mg/m² I.V. daily for 5 days; repeat every 3 weeks.
➤ **Hodgkin lymphoma**
Adults: 150 mg/m² I.V. daily (with other drugs) for 5 days; repeat every 4 weeks.

Or, 375 mg/m² on first day of combination regimen; repeat every 15 days.

ADMINISTRATION
I.V.
• Preparing and giving parenteral drug may be mutagenic, teratogenic, or carcinogenic. Follow facility policy to reduce risks.
• Reconstitute drug using sterile water for injection. Add 9.9 ml to 100-mg vial or 19.7 ml to 200-mg vial to yield a concentration of 10 mg/ml.
• For infusion, dilute with up to 250 ml of normal saline solution or D_5W.
• Infuse over at least 15 to 30 minutes.
• To decrease pain at insertion site, dilute drug further or decrease infusion rate.
• Watch for irritation and infiltration during infusion; extravasation can cause severe pain, tissue damage, and necrosis. If solution infiltrates, stop immediately, apply ice to area for 24 to 48 hours, and notify prescriber.
• Reconstituted solutions in the vial are stable 8 hours at room temperature and with normal lighting conditions, or up to 3 days if refrigerated.
• Solution should be colorless to clear yellow. If solution turns pink, it has decomposed. Discard it.
• Diluted solutions are stable 8 hours at room temperature and with normal lighting, or up to 24 hours if refrigerated.
• **Incompatibilities:** Allopurinol sodium, cefepime, hydrocortisone sodium succinate, piperacillin with tazobactam.

ACTION
May cross-link strands of cellular DNA and interfere with RNA and protein synthesis. Not specific to cell cycle.

Route	Onset	Peak	Duration
I.V.	Unknown	Unknown	Unknown

Half-life: Initial phase, 19 minutes; terminal phase, 5 hours.

ADVERSE REACTIONS
GI: *anorexia, severe nausea and vomiting,* stomatitis.
Hematologic: *leukopenia, thrombocytopenia.*
Skin: alopecia.

Other: *anaphylaxis,* severe pain with infiltration or a too-concentrated solution, tissue damage.

INTERACTIONS
Drug-lifestyle. *Sun exposure:* May cause photosensitivity reaction, especially during first 2 days of therapy. Advise patient to avoid excessive sunlight exposure.

EFFECTS ON LAB TEST RESULTS
• May increase BUN and liver enzyme levels.
• May decrease platelet, RBC, and WBC counts.

CONTRAINDICATIONS & CAUTIONS
• Contraindicated in patients hypersensitive to drug.
■ **Black Box Warning** Use cautiously because drug may be carcinogenic and teratogenic. ■
• Use cautiously in patients with impaired bone marrow function and those with severe renal or hepatic dysfunction.

NURSING CONSIDERATIONS
■ **Black Box Warning** Dacarbazine should be administered under the super-vision of a physician experienced in the use of cancer chemotherapeutic agents. ■
• Give antiemetics before giving this drug. Nausea and vomiting may subside after several doses.
• To prevent bleeding, avoid all I.M. injections when platelet count is below 50,000/mm^3.
■ **Black Box Warning** Hemopoietic depression is the most common toxicity. ■
• Anticipate need for blood transfusions to combat anemia. Patient may receive injections of RBC colony-stimulating factors to promote RBC production and decrease need for blood transfusions.
• Therapeutic effects commonly occur with toxicity. Monitor CBC and platelet count.
■ **Black Box Warning** Hepatic necrosis may occur. Monitor liver function tests. ■
• For Hodgkin lymphoma, drug is usually given with bleomycin, vinblastine, and doxorubicin.
■ **Black Box Warning** The physician must carefully weigh the possibility of therapeutic benefit against the risk of toxicity for each patient. ■
• *Look alike–sound alike:* Don't confuse dacarbazine with procarbazine.

PATIENT TEACHING
• Tell patient to watch for evidence of infection (fever, sore throat, fatigue) and bleeding (easy bruising, nosebleeds, bleeding gums, tarry stools). Tell him to take temperature daily.
• Tell patient to avoid people with upper respiratory tract infections.
• Instruct patient to avoid OTC products that contain aspirin or NSAIDs.
• Advise patient to avoid sunlight and sunlamps for first 2 days after treatment.
• Reassure patient that fever, malaise, and muscle pain, beginning 7 days after treatment ends and possibly lasting 7 to 21 days, may be treated with mild fever reducers such as acetaminophen.
• Tell patient that restricting food intake for 4 to 6 hours before dose may help to decrease adverse GI effects.
• Reassure patient that hair loss is reversible.
• Advise woman to avoid pregnancy and breast-feeding during therapy.

SAFETY ALERT!

ifosfamide
eye-FOSS-fa-mide

Ifex

Pharmacologic class: nitrogen mustard
Pregnancy risk category D

AVAILABLE FORMS
Powder for injection: 1 g, 3 g

INDICATIONS & DOSAGES
➤ **Testicular cancer**
Adults: 1.2 g/m^2 daily I.V. for 5 consecutive days. Repeat treatment every 3 weeks or after patient recovers from hematologic toxicity. Don't repeat doses until WBC count exceeds 4,000/mm^3 and platelet count exceeds 100,000/mm^3.

Reactions may be *common,* uncommon, *life-threatening,* or COMMON AND LIFE-THREATENING.
Interaction may have a *rapid onset* or **delayed onset.**

ADMINISTRATION
I.V.
● Preparing and giving drug may be mutagenic, teratogenic, or carcinogenic. Follow facility policy to reduce risks.
● Give a protective drug such as mesna to prevent hemorrhagic cystitis. Ifosfamide and mesna are physically compatible and may be mixed in the same I.V. solution.
● Obtain urinalysis before each dose. If microscopic hematuria occurs, notify prescriber. Adjust dosage of mesna, if needed. Adequate fluid intake (2 L daily, either P.O. or I.V.) is essential before, and 72 hours after, therapy.
● Reconstitute each gram of drug with 20 ml of diluent to yield a solution of 50 mg/ml. Use sterile water for injection or bacteriostatic water for injection. Solutions may then be further diluted with sterile water, dextrose 2.5% or 5% in water, half-normal or normal saline solution for injection, dextrose 5% and normal saline solution for injection, or lactated Ringer's injection.
● Infuse each dose over at least 30 minutes.
● Reconstituted solution is stable for 1 week at room temperature or 6 weeks if refrigerated. However, use solution within 6 hours if drug was reconstituted with sterile water without a preservative (such as benzyl alcohol or parabens).
● **Incompatibilities:** Cefepime, mesna with epirubicin, methotrexate sodium.

ACTION
Cross-links strands of cellular DNA and interferes with RNA transcription, causing an imbalance of growth that leads to cell death. Not specific to cell cycle.

Route	Onset	Peak	Duration
I.V.	Unknown	Unknown	Unknown

Half-life: About 14 hours.

ADVERSE REACTIONS
CNS: *somnolence, confusion,* hallucinations, depressive psychosis, fever.
GI: *nausea, vomiting.*
GU: *hemorrhagic cystitis, hematuria.*
Hematologic: *leukopenia, thrombocytopenia, myelosuppression.*
Skin: *alopecia.*
Other: infection, phlebitis.

INTERACTIONS
Drug-drug. *Anticoagulants, aspirin, NSAIDs:* May increase risk of bleeding. Avoid using together.
Barbiturates, chloral hydrate, fosphenytoin, phenytoin: May increase ifosfamide toxicity. Monitor patient closely.
Corticosteroids: May inhibit hepatic enzymes, reducing ifosfamide's effect. Monitor patient for increased ifosfamide toxicity if corticosteroid dosage is suddenly reduced or stopped.
Cyclophosphamide: May increase risk of cardiac tamponade in patients with thalassemia. Monitor patient closely.
Myelosuppressives: May enhance hematologic toxicity. Dosage adjustment may be needed.

EFFECTS ON LAB TEST RESULTS
● May increase liver enzyme levels.
● May decrease WBC and platelet counts.

CONTRAINDICATIONS & CAUTIONS
● Contraindicated in patients hypersensitive to drug and in those with severe bone marrow suppression.
● Use cautiously in patients with renal impairment or compromised bone marrow reserve as indicated by leukopenia, granulocytopenia, extensive bone marrow metastases, previous radiation therapy, or previous therapy with cytotoxic drugs.

NURSING CONSIDERATIONS
■ **Black Box Warning** Drug should be administered under the supervision of a physician experienced in the use of cancer chemotherapeutic agents. ■
■ **Black Box Warning** Urotoxic side effects, especially hemorrhagic cystitis, and CNS toxicities, such as confusion and coma, may require cessation of ifosfamide therapy. ■
■ **Black Box Warning** Severe myelosuppression has been reported. ■
● Give antiemetic before drug, to reduce nausea.
● Ensure that patient is adequately hydrated during therapy.
● Don't give drug at bedtime; infrequent urination during the night may increase possibility of cystitis. If cystitis develops, stop drug and notify prescriber.

- Bladder irrigation with normal saline solution may be done to treat cystitis.
- Monitor CBC and renal and liver function tests.
- To prevent bleeding, avoid all I.M. injections when platelet count is less than 50,000/mm³.
- Anticipate blood transfusions because of cumulative anemia. Patients may receive injections of RBC colony-stimulating factor to promote RBC production and decrease need for blood transfusions.
- Assess patient for mental status changes; dosage may have to be decreased.
- *Look alike–sound alike:* Don't confuse ifosfamide with cyclophosphamide.

PATIENT TEACHING
- Remind patient to urinate frequently to minimize contact of drug and its metabolites with the lining of the bladder.
- Advise patient to watch for signs and symptoms of infection (fever, sore throat, fatigue) and bleeding (easy bruising, nosebleeds, bleeding gums, tarry stools). Tell patient to take temperature daily.
- Instruct patient to avoid OTC products that contain aspirin.
- Advise women to stop breast-feeding during therapy because of possible risk of toxicity to infant.
- Caution woman of childbearing age to avoid becoming pregnant during therapy. Recommend that she consult prescriber before becoming pregnant.

SAFETY ALERT!

lomustine (CCNU)
loe-MUS-teen

CeeNU

Pharmacologic class: nitrosourea
Pregnancy risk category D

AVAILABLE FORMS
Capsules: 10-mg, 40-mg, 100-mg dose pack (two 10-mg, two 40-mg, two 100-mg capsules)

INDICATIONS & DOSAGES
➤ **Brain tumor, Hodgkin lymphoma**
Adults and children: 100 to 130 mg/m² P.O. as single dose every 6 weeks. Repeat doses shouldn't be given until WBC count exceeds 4,000/mm³ and platelet count is greater than 100,000/mm³.
Adjust-a-dose: Reduce dosage according to degree of bone marrow suppression or when used with other myelosuppressive drugs. Reduce dosage by 30% for WBC count nadir 2,000 to 2,999/mm³ and platelet count nadir 25,000 to 74,999/mm³; by 50% for WBC count nadir less than 2,000/mm³ and platelet count nadir less than 25,000/mm³.

ADMINISTRATION
P.O.
- Give antiemetic before drug to reduce nausea.
- Give 2 to 4 hours after meals; drug will be more completely absorbed if taken when stomach is empty.
- Store capsules at room temperature. Avoid exposure to moisture, and protect from temperatures greater than 104° F (40° C).

ACTION
Cross-links strands of cellular DNA and interferes with RNA transcription, causing an imbalance of growth that leads to cell death. Not specific to cell cycle.

Route	Onset	Peak	Duration
P.O.	Unknown	Unknown	Unknown

Half-life: 1 to 2 days.

ADVERSE REACTIONS
CNS: disorientation, lethargy, ataxia.
GI: *nausea, vomiting,* stomatitis.
GU: *nephrotoxicity,* progressive azotemia, *renal failure,* amenorrhea, azoospermia.
Hematologic: anemia, LEUKOPENIA, THROMBOCYTOPENIA, BONE MARROW SUPPRESSION.
Hepatic: *hepatotoxicity.*
Skin: alopecia.
Other: *secondary malignant disease.*

Reactions may be *common*, uncommon, *life-threatening*, or COMMON AND LIFE-THREATENING.
Interaction may have a *rapid onset* or *delayed onset.*

INTERACTIONS
Drug-drug. *Anticoagulants, aspirin, NSAIDs:* May increase risk of bleeding. Avoid using together.
Myelosuppressives: May increase myelosuppression. Monitor patient.

EFFECTS ON LAB TEST RESULTS
• May increase urine urea level. May decrease hemoglobin level.
• May decrease WBC, RBC, and platelet counts.

CONTRAINDICATIONS & CAUTIONS
• Contraindicated in patients hypersensitive to drug.
• Use cautiously in patients with decreased platelet, WBC, or RBC counts and in those receiving other myelosuppressives.

NURSING CONSIDERATIONS
■ **Black Box Warning** Monitor CBC weekly. Usually not given more often than every 6 weeks; bone marrow toxicity is cumulative and delayed, usually occurring 4 to 6 weeks after drug administration. ■
• Periodically monitor liver function test results.
• To prevent bleeding, avoid all I.M. injections when platelet count is less than 50,000/mm³.
• Anticipate blood transfusions because of cumulative anemia. Patients may receive RBC colony-stimulating factor to promote RBC production and decrease need for blood transfusions.
• Therapeutic effects come with toxicity.
■ **Black Box Warning** Bone marrow suppression, notably thrombocytopenia and leukopenia is the most common and severe of the toxic effects of the drug. ■

PATIENT TEACHING
• Advise patient to take capsules on an empty stomach, if possible.
• Advise patient to watch for signs and symptoms of infection (fever, sore throat, fatigue) and bleeding (easy bruising, nosebleeds, bleeding gums, tarry stools). Tell patient to take temperature daily.
• *Alert:* Tell patients that to give the proper dose of lomustine, two or more different types and colors of capsules may be dispensed.

• Instruct patient to avoid OTC products that contain aspirin or NSAIDs.
• Advise women to stop breast-feeding during therapy because of possible risk of toxicity to infant.
• Caution woman of childbearing age to avoid becoming pregnant during therapy. Recommend that she consult prescriber before becoming pregnant.

SAFETY ALERT!

mechlorethamine hydrochloride (nitrogen mustard)
me-klor-ETH-a-meen

Mustargen

Pharmacologic class: nitrogen mustard
Pregnancy risk category D

AVAILABLE FORMS
Powder for injection: 10-mg vials

INDICATIONS & DOSAGES
Dosage is based on patient response and degree of toxicity.
➤ **Hodgkin lymphoma**
Adults and children: 6 mg/m² daily on days 1 and 8 of 28-day cycle in combination with other antineoplastics, such as mechlorethamine-vincristine-procarbazine-prednisone (MOPP) regimen. Repeat dosage for six cycles.
Adjust-a-dose: Subsequent doses reduced by 50% in MOPP regimen when WBC count is 3,000 to 3,999/mm³ and by 75% when WBC count is 1,000 to 2,999/mm³ or platelet count is 50,000 to 100,000/mm³.
➤ **Polycythemia vera, chronic lymphocytic leukemia, chronic myelocytic leukemia, bronchogenic cancer, mycosis fungoides**
Adults and children: 0.4 mg/kg as single dose or in divided doses of 0.1 to 0.2 mg/kg daily.
➤ **Malignant effusions (pericardial, peritoneal, pleural)**
Adults: Consult specialized references. Usual dose 0.2 to 0.4 mg/kg.

ADMINISTRATION
I.V.
■ **Black Box Warning** Drug is highly toxic. Avoid inhaling dust or vapors. Also avoid contact with skin or mucous membranes. Use personal protection equipment, clean drug equipment, and neutralize unused drug according to manufacturer's instructions. ■
• Reconstitute drug using 10 ml of sterile water for injection or normal saline solution for injection. Resulting solution contains 1 mg/ml of drug. Give by direct injection into a vein or into tubing of a free-flowing I.V. solution.
• Prepare immediately before infusion. Solution is very unstable. Visually inspect before using to make sure solution is colorless. Use within 15 minutes, and discard unused solution.
• Dispose of equipment used in preparation and administration of mechlorethamine properly and according to institutional policy. Neutralize unused solution with an equal volume of 5% sodium bicarbonate and 5% sodium thiosulfate for 45 minutes.
■ **Black Box Warning** Drug is a potent vesicant. If extravasation occurs, apply cold compresses for 6 to 12 hours, and infiltrate area with isotonic sodium thiosulfate. ■
• **Incompatibilities:** Allopurinol, cefepime, D_5W, methohexital, normal saline solution.
Topical
• When given intracavitarily for sclerosing effect, dilute, using up to 100 ml of normal saline solution for injection. Turn patient from side to side every 5 to 10 minutes for 1 hour to distribute drug.

ACTION
Cross-links strands of cellular DNA and interferes with RNA transcription, causing an imbalance of growth that leads to cell death. Not specific to cell cycle.

Route	Onset	Peak	Duration
I.V., topical	Few sec– few min	Unknown	Unknown

Half-life: Unknown.

ADVERSE REACTIONS
CNS: weakness, vertigo, neurotoxicity.
CV: *thrombophlebitis.*
EENT: tinnitus, deafness with high doses.

GI: *nausea, vomiting, anorexia,* diarrhea, metallic taste.
GU: menstrual irregularities, impaired spermatogenesis.
Hematologic: *agranulocytosis, thrombo-cytopenia, lymphocytopenia,* mild anemia beginning in 2 to 3 weeks.
Hepatic: jaundice.
Metabolic: hyperuricemia.
Skin: *alopecia,* rash, sloughing, severe skin irritation with extravasation or contact.
Other: *anaphylaxis, secondary malignant disease,* precipitation of herpes zoster.

INTERACTIONS
Drug-drug. *Anticoagulants, aspirin, NSAIDs:* May increase risk of bleeding. Avoid using together.
Myelosuppressives: May increase myelo-suppression. Monitor patient.

EFFECTS ON LAB TEST RESULTS
• May increase urine urea level. May decrease hemoglobin level.
• May decrease granulocyte, lymphocyte, RBC, and platelet counts.

CONTRAINDICATIONS & CAUTIONS
• Contraindicated in patients hypersensitive to drug and in those with infectious diseases.
• Use cautiously in patients with severe anemia or depressed neutrophil or platelet count and in those who have recently undergone radiation therapy or chemotherapy.

NURSING CONSIDERATIONS
■ **Black Box Warning** Administer only under the supervision of a physician experienced in the use of cancer chemo-therapeutic agents. ■
• Monitor uric acid level. To prevent hyperuricemia with resulting uric acid or nephropathy, make sure patient is adequately hydrated. Alkalinizing the urine and using allopurinol may also be helpful.
• Therapeutic effects are commonly accompanied by toxicity.
• Neurotoxicity increases with dosage and patient age.
• To prevent bleeding, avoid all I.M. injections when platelet count is less than 50,000/mm³.

Reactions may be *common,* uncommon, *life-threatening,* or COMMON AND LIFE-THREATENING.
Interaction may have a *rapid onset* or *delayed onset.*

• Monitor patient closely for bone marrow suppression (nadir of myelosuppression occurring between days 4 and 10 and lasting 10 to 21 days).

• Give blood transfusions for cumulative anemia. Patients may receive RBC colony-stimulating factor to promote RBC cell production and decrease need for blood transfusions.

PATIENT TEACHING

• Advise patient to report any pain or burning at site of injection during or after administration.

• Advise patient to watch for signs and symptoms of infection (fever, sore throat, fatigue) and bleeding (easy bruising, nosebleeds, bleeding gums, tarry stools). Tell patient to take temperature daily.

• Tell patient that severe nausea and vomiting can occur.

• Instruct patient to avoid OTC products that contain aspirin or NSAIDs.

• Advise women to stop breast-feeding during therapy because of risk of toxicity to infant.

• Advise women of childbearing age to consult prescriber before becoming pregnant.

• Tell patient about the risk of sterility.

SAFETY ALERT!

melphalan (L-PAM, phenylalanine mustard)
MEL-fa-lan

Alkeran

melphalan hydrochloride
Alkeran

Pharmacologic class: nitrogen mustard
Pregnancy risk category D

AVAILABLE FORMS
Lyophilized powder for injection: 50 mg
Tablets (scored): 2 mg

INDICATIONS & DOSAGES
➤ **Multiple myeloma**
Adults: Initially, 6 mg P.O. daily for 2 to 3 weeks; then stop drug for up to 4 weeks or until WBC and platelet counts stop dropping and begin to rise again; maintenance dose is 2 mg daily. Or, 10 mg/day for 7 to 10 days, followed by 2 mg/day when WBC is greater than 4,000 cells/mcL and platelet count is greater than 100,00 cells, mcL; dosage is adjusted to between 1 and 3 mg/day depending on hematologic response. Or, 0.15 mg/kg P.O. daily for 7 days followed by a rest period of at least 14 days; maintenance dose is 0.05 mg/kg/day or less. Or 0.25 mg/kg/day for 4 days (or 0.2 mg/kg/day for 5 days); repeat every 4 to 6 weeks.

Or, give I.V. to patients who can't tolerate oral therapy, 16 mg/m^2 given by infusion over 15 to 20 minutes at 2-week intervals for four doses. After patient has recovered from toxicity, give drug at 4-week intervals.

Adjust-a-dose: For patients with renal insufficiency, reduce dosage by up to 50%.
➤ **Nonresectable advanced ovarian cancer**
Adults: 0.2 mg/kg P.O. daily for 5 days. Repeat every 4 to 6 weeks, depending on bone marrow recovery.

ADMINISTRATION
P.O.
• Give drug when patient has an empty stomach; food decreases drug absorption.
I.V.
• Preparing and giving this form may be mutagenic, teratogenic, or carcinogenic. Follow facility policy to reduce risks.
• Because drug isn't stable in solution, reconstitute immediately before giving with the 10 ml of sterile diluent supplied by manufacturer. Shake vigorously until solution is clear. The resulting solution will contain 5 mg/ml of melphalan. Immediately dilute required dose in normal saline solution for injection to no more than 0.45 mg/ml. Give infusion over 15 to 20 minutes.
• Monitor infusion carefully. Extravasation causes painful inflammation.
• Reconstituted product begins to degrade within 30 minutes. After final dilution, nearly 1% of drug degrades every 10 minutes. Administration must be finished within 60 minutes of reconstitution.

• Don't refrigerate reconstituted product because precipitate will form.
• **Incompatibilities:** Amphotericin B, chlorpromazine, D_5W, lactated Ringer's injection. Compatibility with normal saline injection depends on the concentration; don't prepare solutions with a concentration exceeding 0.45 mg/ml.

ACTION
Cross-links strands of cellular DNA and interferes with RNA transcription, causing an imbalance of growth that leads to cell death. Not specific to cell cycle.

Route	Onset	Peak	Duration
P.O., I.V.	Unknown	Unknown	Unknown

Half-life: 2 hours.

ADVERSE REACTIONS
CV: hypotension, tachycardia, edema.
GI: nausea, vomiting, diarrhea, oral ulceration, stomatitis.
Hematologic: *thrombocytopenia, leukopenia, bone marrow suppression,* hemolytic anemia.
Hepatic: *hepatotoxicity.*
Metabolic: hyperuricemia.
Respiratory: *pneumonitis, pulmonary fibrosis,* dyspnea, *bronchospasm.*
Skin: pruritus, alopecia, urticaria, ulceration at injection site.
Other: *anaphylaxis,* hypersensitivity reactions.

INTERACTIONS
Drug-drug (I.V. melphalan only).
Anticoagulants, aspirin, NSAIDs: May increase risk of bleeding. Avoid using together.
Carmustine: May decrease threshold for pulmonary toxicity. Use together cautiously.
Cimetidine: May decrease melphalan level. Monitor patient closely.
Cisplatin: May increase renal impairment, decreasing melphalan clearance. Monitor patient closely.
Cyclosporine: May cause severe renal impairment. Monitor renal function closely.
Interferon alfa: May increase melphalan elimination. Monitor patient closely.
Myelosuppressives: May increase myelosuppression. Monitor patient.

Vaccines: May decrease effectiveness of killed-virus vaccines and increase risk of toxicity from live-virus vaccines. Postpone routine immunization for at least 3 months after last dose of melphalan.
Drug-food. *Any food:* May decrease oral drug absorption. Advise patient to take drug on an empty stomach.

EFFECTS ON LAB TEST RESULTS
• May increase urine urea level. May decrease hemoglobin level.
• May decrease RBC, WBC, and platelet counts.
• May cause a false-positive direct Coombs' test.

CONTRAINDICATIONS & CAUTIONS
• Contraindicated in patients hypersensitive to drug and in those with disease resistant to drug. Patients hypersensitive to chlorambucil may have cross-sensitivity to this drug.
• Contraindicated in patients with severe leukopenia, thrombocytopenia, or anemia and in those with chronic lymphocytic leukemia.
• Use cautiously in patients receiving radiation and chemotherapy.
■ **Black Box Warning** Drug produces chromosomal changes in vitro and in vivo, and should be considered mutagenic. ■

NURSING CONSIDERATIONS
■ **Black Box Warning** Administer drug only under the supervision of a physician experienced in the use of cancer chemotherapeutic agents. ■
■ **Black Box Warning** Severe bone marrow suppression with resulting bleeding or infection may occur. ■
■ **Black Box Warning** Drug is leukemogenic and potentially mutagenic. ■
• Dosage may need to be reduced in patients with renal impairment.
• Monitor uric acid level and CBC.
• To prevent bleeding, avoid all I.M. injections when platelet count is less than 50,000/mm³.
• Give blood transfusions for cumulative anemia. Patients may receive RBC colony-stimulating factor to promote RBC production and decrease need for blood transfusions.

• Anaphylaxis may occur. Keep antihistamines and steroids readily available to give if needed.

• **Look alike–sound alike:** Don't confuse melphalan with Mephyton.

PATIENT TEACHING

• Advise patient to take tablets on empty stomach.

• Advise patient to report pain or redness at I.V. site.

• Advise patient to watch for signs and symptoms of infection (fever, sore throat, fatigue) and bleeding (easy bruising, nosebleeds, bleeding gums, tarry stools). Tell patient to take temperature daily.

• Instruct patient to avoid OTC products that contain aspirin or NSAIDs.

• Advise women to stop breast-feeding during therapy because of risk of toxicity to infant.

• Advise women of childbearing age to consult prescriber before becoming pregnant.

SAFETY ALERT!

oxaliplatin
ox-ah-li-PLA-tin

Eloxatin

Pharmacologic class: platinum coordination complex
Pregnancy risk category D

AVAILABLE FORMS

Solution for injection: 5 mg/ml in 50-, 100-mg or 200 mg single-use vials

INDICATIONS & DOSAGES

➤ **First-line treatment of advanced colorectal cancer with 5-fluorouracil and leucovorin (5-FU/LV)**
Adults: On day 1, give 85 mg/m² oxaliplatin I.V. in 250 to 500 ml D_5W and leucovorin 200 mg/m² I.V. in D_5W simultaneously over 120 minutes, in separate bags using a Y-line, followed by 5-FU 400 mg/m² I.V. bolus over 2 to 4 minutes, followed by 600 mg/m² 5-FU I.V. infusion in 500 ml D_5W over 22 hours.

On day 2, give 200 mg/m² leucovorin I.V. infusion over 120 minutes, followed by 400 mg/m² 5-FU I.V. bolus over 2 to 4 minutes, followed by 600 mg/m² 5-FU I.V. infusion in 500 ml D_5W over 22 hours.

Repeat cycle every 2 weeks.
Adjust-a-dose: In patients with unresolved and persistent grade 2 neurosensory events, reduce oxaliplatin to 65 mg/m². In those with persistent grade 3 neurosensory events, consider stopping drug. In patients recovering from grade 3 or 4 GI or hematologic events, reduce dose to 65 mg/m² and reduce dose of 5-FU by 20%.

➤ **With 5-FU/LV for the adjuvant treatment of stage III colon cancer in patients who have had complete resection of the primary tumor**
Adults: On day 1, give oxaliplatin, 85 mg/m² I.V. in 250 to 500 ml D_5W and 200 mg/m² leucovorin I.V. infusion in D_5W, both over 120 minutes at the same time, in separate bags, using a Y-line. Follow with 5-FU 400 mg/m² I.V. bolus over 2 to 4 minutes, then 600 mg/m² 5-FU in 500 ml D_5W as a 22-hour continuous infusion.

On day 2, give leucovorin, 200 mg/m² I.V. infused over 120 minutes, followed by 5-FU 400 mg/m² as an I.V. bolus over 2 to 4 minutes, then 600 mg/m² 5-FU in 500 ml D_5W as a 22-hour infusion.

Repeat cycle every 2 weeks for a total of 6 months. Premedicate with antiemetics, with or without dexamethasone.
Adjust-a-dose: For patients with persistent grade 2 neurotoxicity, consider an oxaliplatin dose reduction to 75 mg/m². For patients who recovered from grade 4 neutropenia, grade 3 or 4 thrombocytopenia, or a grade 3 or 4 GI event, reduce oxaliplatin to 75 mg/m² and 5-FU to a 300 mg/m² bolus and 500 mg/m² 22-hour infusion. Delay dose until neutrophils are 1.5×10^9/L or more and platelets are 75×10^9/L or more.

ADMINISTRATION
I.V.
• Preparing and giving drug may be mutagenic, teratogenic, or carcinogenic. Follow facility policy to reduce risks.

• Reconstitute powder using sterile water for injection or D_5W. Add 10 ml to a 50-mg vial or 20 ml to a 100-mg vial, for a yield of 5 mg/ml. Never reconstitute with sodium chloride solution or other solution containing chloride.

• Reconstituted solutions must be further diluted in an infusion solution of 250 to 500 ml of D_5W.

• Inspect bag for particulate matter and discoloration before giving, and discard if present.

• Don't use needles or I.V. administration sets that contain aluminum because it displaces the platinum, causing it to lose potency and form a black precipitate.

• Give oxaliplatin and leucovorin over 2 hours at the same time in separate bags, using a Y-line. Extend the infusion time to 6 hours to decrease acute toxicities.

• Store unopened vials at room temperature. Reconstituted solutions are stable if refrigerated (36° to 46° F [2° to 8° C]) for up to 24 hours. After final dilution, solutions are stable for 6 hours at room temperature and up to 24 hours under refrigeration.

• **Incompatibilities:** Alkaline solutions or drugs such as 5-FU. Flush infusion line with D_5W before giving any other drugs simultaneously.

ACTION

Probably inhibits cell replication and transcription by forming platinum complexes that cross-link with DNA molecules. Not specific to cell cycle.

Route	Onset	Peak	Duration
I.V.	Unknown	Unknown	Unknown

Half-life: Unknown.

ADVERSE REACTIONS

CNS: *pain, peripheral neuropathy, fatigue, headache, dizziness, insomnia, fever.*
CV: chest pain, ***thromboembolism,*** *edema, flushing, peripheral edema.*
EENT: *rhinitis,* pharyngolaryngeal dysesthesias, pharyngitis, epistaxis, abnormal lacrimation.
GI: *nausea, vomiting, diarrhea, stomatitis, abdominal pain, anorexia, constipation, dyspepsia, taste perversion,* gastroesophageal reflux, flatulence, mucositis.

GU: dysuria, hematuria.
Hematologic: FEBRILE NEUTROPENIA, *anemia,* LEUKOPENIA, THROMBOCYTOPENIA.
Hepatic: veno-occlusive disease.
Metabolic: hypokalemia, dehydration.
Musculoskeletal: *back pain, arthralgia.*
Respiratory: *dyspnea, cough, upper respiratory tract infection,* hiccups, ***pulmonary toxicity.***
Skin: *injection site reaction,* rash, alopecia.
Other: ***anaphylaxis,*** *hand-foot syndrome, allergic reaction,* rigors.

INTERACTIONS

Drug-drug. *Nephrotoxic drugs (such as gentamicin):* May decrease elimination of nephrotoxic drugs and increase gentamicin levels. Monitor patient for signs and symptoms of toxicity.

EFFECTS ON LAB TEST RESULTS

• May increase creatinine, bilirubin, AST, and ALT levels. May decrease potassium and hemoglobin levels.

• May decrease neutrophil, WBC, and platelet counts.

CONTRAINDICATIONS & CAUTIONS

• Contraindicated in patients allergic to drug or other platinum-containing compounds and in pregnant or breast-feeding patients.

• Use cautiously in patients with renal impairment or peripheral sensory neuropathy.

NURSING CONSIDERATIONS

■ **Black Box Warning** Administer drug under the supervision of a physician experienced in the use of cancer chemotherapeutic agents. ■

• Drug doesn't require patient prehydration.

• Give antiemetic with or without dexamethasone before drug to reduce nausea.

• Drug clearance is reduced in patients with renal impairment. Dosage adjustment for patients with renal impairment hasn't been established.

• Monitor CBC, platelet count, and liver and kidney function before each chemotherapy cycle.

Reactions may be *common,* uncommon, ***life-threatening,*** or COMMON AND LIFE-THREATENING.
Interaction may have a *rapid onset* or ***delayed onset.***

■ **Black Box Warning** Monitor patient for hypersensitivity reactions, which may occur within minutes of administration. Keep epinephrine, corticosteroids, and antihistamines available. ■

● Monitor patient for injection site reaction; extravasation may occur.

● Monitor patient for neuropathy and pulmonary toxicity. Peripheral neuropathy may be acute or persistent. Acute neuropathy is reversible; it occurs within 2 days of dosing and resolves within 14 days. Persistent peripheral neuropathy occurs more than 14 days after dosing and causes paresthesias, dysesthesias, hypoesthesias, and other neurologic impairment that can interfere with daily activities (such as walking or swallowing).

● Avoid ice and cold exposure during infusion of drug because cold temperatures can worsen acute neurologic symptoms. Cover patient with a blanket during infusion.

● Diarrhea, dehydration, hypokalemia, and fatigue may occur more frequently in elderly patients.

PATIENT TEACHING

● Inform patient of potential adverse reactions.

● Tell patient to avoid exposure to cold or cold objects (such as cold drinks or ice cubes), which can bring on or worsen acute symptoms of peripheral neuropathy. Advise patient to drink warm drinks, wear warm clothing, and cover any exposed skin (hands, face, and head). Have patient warm the air going into his lungs by wearing a scarf or ski mask. Have him wear gloves when touching cold objects (such as frozen foods, door knobs, or mailboxes).

● Tell patient to contact prescriber immediately if he has trouble breathing or experiences signs and symptoms of an allergic reaction, such as rash, hives, swelling of lips or tongue, or sudden cough.

● Tell patient to contact prescriber if fever, signs and symptoms of an infection, persistent vomiting, diarrhea, or signs and symptoms of dehydration (thirst, dry mouth, light-headedness, and decreased urination) occur.

thiotepa (TESPA, triethylenethiophosphoramide, TSPA)
thye-oh-TEE-pa

Pharmacologic class: alkylating drug
Pregnancy risk category D

AVAILABLE FORMS
Injection: 15- and 30-mg vials

INDICATIONS & DOSAGES
➤ **Breast and ovarian cancers, lymphoma, Hodgkin lymphoma**
Adults and children older than age 12: 0.3 to 0.4 mg/kg I.V. every 1 to 4 weeks or 0.2 mg/kg for 4 to 5 days at intervals of 2 to 4 weeks.
➤ **Bladder tumor**
Adults and children older than age 12: 30 to 60 mg in 30 to 60 ml of normal saline solution instilled in bladder for 2 hours once weekly for 4 weeks.
➤ **Neoplastic effusions**
Adults and children older than age 12: 0.6 to 0.8 mg/kg intracavitarily every 1 to 4 weeks.

ADMINISTRATION
I.V.
● Preparing and giving drug may be mutagenic, teratogenic, or carcinogenic. Follow facility policy to reduce risks.
● Reconstitute with 1.5 ml of sterile water for injection in 15-mg vial or 3 ml in 30-mg vial to yield 10 mg/ml. Don't reconstitute with other solutions.
● Further dilute with normal saline solution for injection. If larger volume is desired, further dilute with sodium chloride solution, D_5W, dextrose 5% in normal saline solution for injection, Ringer's injection, or lactated Ringer's injection.
● If solution appears grossly opaque or has a precipitate, discard it. Make sure solutions are clear to slightly opaque. To eliminate haze, filter solutions through a 0.22-micron filter before use.
● If pain occurs at insertion site, dilute drug further or use a local anesthetic to reduce pain. Make sure drug doesn't infiltrate.

- Use solutions within 8 hours.
- Refrigerate and protect dry powder from direct sunlight to avoid possible drug breakdown.
- **Incompatibilities:** Cisplatin, filgrastim, minocycline, vinorelbine.

Intravesical
- Preparing and giving drug may be mutagenic, teratogenic, or carcinogenic. Follow facility policy to reduce risks.
- For bladder instillation, dehydrate patient 8 to 10 hours before therapy. Instill drug into bladder by catheter; ask patient to retain solution for 2 hours. If discomfort is too great with 60 ml, reduce volume to 30 ml. Reposition patient every 15 minutes for maximum area contact.

Intracavitary
- Preparing and giving drug may be mutagenic, teratogenic, or carcinogenic. Follow facility policy to reduce risks.
- For intracavitary instillation, drug may be given through the same tubing used to remove the fluid from the cavity involved.

ACTION
Cross-links strands of cellular DNA and interferes with RNA transcription, causing an imbalance of growth that leads to cell death. Not specific to cell cycle.

Route	Onset	Peak	Duration
I.V., topical	Unknown	Unknown	Unknown

Half-life: 2¼ hours.

ADVERSE REACTIONS
CNS: headache, dizziness, fatigue, weakness, fever.
EENT: blurred vision, conjunctivitis.
GI: *nausea, vomiting,* abdominal pain, anorexia, stomatitis.
GU: amenorrhea, decreased spermatogenesis, dysuria, increased urine levels of uric acid, urine retention, hemorrhagic cystitis (with intravesical administration).
Hematologic: *leukopenia, thrombocytopenia, neutropenia,* anemia.
Metabolic: hyperuricemia.
Respiratory: *laryngeal edema.*
Skin: dermatitis, alopecia, pain at injection site, urticaria, rash.
Other: hypersensitivity reactions, *including anaphylaxis.*

INTERACTIONS
Drug-drug. *Anticoagulants, aspirin, NSAIDs:* May increase risk of bleeding. Avoid using together.
Myelosuppressives: May increase myelosuppression. Monitor patient.
Neuromuscular blockers: May prolong muscular paralysis. Monitor patient.
Other alkylating drugs, irradiation therapy: May intensify toxicity rather than enhance therapeutic response. Avoid using together.

EFFECTS ON LAB TEST RESULTS
- May increase uric acid level. May decrease pseudocholinesterase and hemoglobin levels.
- May decrease lymphocyte, platelet, WBC, RBC, and neutrophil counts.

CONTRAINDICATIONS & CAUTIONS
- Contraindicated in patients hypersensitive to drug, in breast-feeding patients, and in those with severe bone marrow, hepatic, or renal dysfunction.
- Use in pregnant women only when benefits to mother outweigh risk of teratogenicity.
- Use cautiously in patients with mild bone marrow suppression and renal or hepatic dysfunction.

NURSING CONSIDERATIONS
- Monitor CBC weekly for at least 3 weeks after last dose.
- If patient's WBC count drops below 3,000/mm³ or if platelet count falls below 150,000/mm³, stop drug and notify prescriber. If WBC count falls below 2,000/mm³ or granulocyte count falls below 1,000/mm³, follow institutional policy for infection control in immunocompromised patients.
- Monitor uric acid level. To prevent hyperuricemia with resulting uric acid nephropathy, give allopurinol along with adequate hydration.
- Therapeutic effects are commonly accompanied by toxicity.
- To prevent bleeding, avoid all I.M. injections when platelet count is below 50,000/mm³.
- Give blood transfusions for cumulative anemia. Inject RBC colony-stimulating

factor to promote RBC production and
decrease need for transfusions.

PATIENT TEACHING
● Advise patient to watch for signs and
symptoms of infection (fever, sore throat,
fatigue) and bleeding (easy bruising,
nosebleeds, bleeding gums, tarry stools).
Tell patient to take temperature daily.
Tell patient to report even mild infections.
● Instruct patient to avoid OTC products
containing aspirin or NSAIDs.
● Advise woman to stop breast-feeding
during therapy because of risk of toxicity
to infant.
● Caution woman of childbearing age
to consult prescriber before becoming
pregnant.

81

Antibiotic antineoplastics

bleomycin sulfate
daunorubicin citrate liposomal
daunorubicin hydrochloride
doxorubicin hydrochloride
doxorubicin hydrochloride liposomal
epirubicin hydrochloride
idarubicin hydrochloride
mitomycin

SAFETY ALERT!

bleomycin sulfate
blee-oh-MYE-sin

Blenoxane

Pharmacologic class: cytotoxic
glycopeptide antibiotic
Pregnancy risk category D

AVAILABLE FORMS
Injection: 15-unit vials, 30-unit vials

INDICATIONS & DOSAGES
➤ **Squamous cell carcinoma (head,
neck, skin, penis, cervix, and vulva),
non-Hodgkin lymphoma, testicular
carcinoma**
Adults: 2 units or less of bleomycin for
injection for the first two doses. If no acute
reaction occurs, then 10 to 20 units/m^2
I.V., I.M., or subcutaneously once or twice
weekly to total of 400 units.
➤ **Hodgkin lymphoma**
Adults: 2 units or less of bleomycin for
injection for the first two doses. If no acute
reaction occurs, then 10 to 20 units/m^2 I.V.,
I.M., or subcutaneously one or two times
weekly. After 50% response, maintenance
dose is 1 unit I.V. or I.M. daily or 5 units
I.V. or I.M. weekly. Total cumulative dose
is 400 units.
➤ **Malignant pleural effusion**
Adults: 60 units given as single-dose bolus
intrapleural injection.

ADMINISTRATION
I.V.
● Preparing and giving parenteral form of
drug may be mutagenic, teratogenic, and

carcinogenic. Follow facility policy to
reduce risks.
● Drug may adsorb to plastic I.V. bags. For
prolonged infusions, use glass containers.
● Reconstitute drug with 5 or 10 ml of
normal saline solution for injection to
equal 3 units/ml solution.
● Use reconstituted solution within 24 hours.
● Refrigerate unopened vials containing
dry powder.
● **Incompatibilities:** Amino acids; aminophylline; ascorbic acid injection; cefazolin;
diazepam; drugs containing sulfhydryl
groups; fluids containing dextrose;
furosemide; hydrocortisone; methotrexate;
mitomycin; nafcillin; penicillin G;
riboflavin; solutions containing divalent
and trivalent cations, especially calcium
salts and copper; terbutaline sulfate.
I.M.
● Dilute 15 unit-vial in 1 to 5 ml or 30 unit-
vial in 2 to 10 ml of sterile water for injection, bacteriostatic water for injection, or
normal saline solution for injection.
● Monitor injection site for irritation.
Subcutaneous
● Dilute 15 unit-vial in 1 to 5 ml or
30 unit-vial in 2 to 10 ml of sterile water
for injection, bacteriostatic water for injection, or normal saline solution for injection.
● Monitor injection site for irritation.

ACTION
May inhibit DNA synthesis and cause scis-
sion of single- and double-stranded DNA;
also inhibits RNA and protein synthesis.

Route	Onset	Peak	Duration
I.V. Subcut.	Unknown	Unknown	Unknown
I.M.	Unknown	30–60 min	Unknown

Half-life: 2 hours.

ADVERSE REACTIONS
CNS: fever.
GI: *stomatitis, anorexia, nausea, vomiting,*
diarrhea.
Metabolic: weight loss, hyperuricemia.
Respiratory: PNEUMONITIS, *pulmonary
fibrosis.*

Reactions may be *common*, uncommon, *life-threatening*, or COMMON AND LIFE-THREATENING.
Interaction may have a *rapid onset* or *delayed onset*.

Skin: *erythema, hyperpigmentation, acne, rash, striae, skin tenderness, pruritus, reversible alopecia,* hyperkeratosis, nail changes.
Other: *chills, anaphylactoid reactions.*

INTERACTIONS
Drug-drug. *Anesthesia:* May increase oxygen requirements. Monitor patient closely.
Cardiac glycosides: May decrease digoxin level. Monitor digoxin level closely.
Fosphenytoin, phenytoin: May decrease phenytoin and fosphenytoin levels. Monitor drug levels closely.

EFFECTS ON LAB TEST RESULTS
● May increase uric acid level.

CONTRAINDICATIONS & CAUTIONS
● Contraindicated in patients hypersensitive to drug.
● Use cautiously in patients with renal or pulmonary impairment.

NURSING CONSIDERATIONS
■ **Black Box Warning** Drug should be administered under the supervision of a physician experienced in the use of cancer chemotherapeutic agents. ■
● Obtain pulmonary function tests. If tests show a marked decline, stop drug.
■ **Black Box Warning** Fatal pulmonary fibrosis may occur, especially when cumulative dose exceeds 400 units. ■
■ **Black Box Warning** Monitor lymphoma patient for idiosyncratic reaction (hypotension, confusion, fever, and wheezing) after receiving drug. ■
● *Alert:* Adverse pulmonary reactions are more common in patients older than age 70. Also, in patients receiving radiation therapy, patients with lung disease, and patients who need oxygen therapy, pulmonary toxic adverse effects may be increased.
● Monitor chest X-ray and listen to lungs regularly.
● Obtain pulmonary function tests and chest X-rays before each course of therapy.
● Watch for fever, which may be treated with antipyretics. Fever usually occurs within 3 to 6 hours of administration.
● *Alert:* Watch for hypersensitivity reactions, which may be delayed for several hours, especially in patients with

lymphoma. (Give test dose of 1 to 2 units before first two doses in these patients. If no reaction occurs, follow regular dosage schedule.)
● For intrapleural use, dilute 60 units of drug in 50 to 100 ml normal saline solution for injection; give drug through a thoracotomy tube.
● If patient's condition requires sclerosis, instill drug when chest tube drainage is 100 to 300 ml/24 hours, ideally, drainage should be less than 100 ml. After instillation, clamp thoracotomy tube and move patient from his back to his left then right side for the next 4 hours. Remove clamp and reestablish suction. Amount of time chest tube is left in place after sclerosis depends on patient's condition.
● Don't use adhesive dressings.

PATIENT TEACHING
● Warn patient that hair loss may occur but is usually reversible.
● Tell patient to report adverse reactions promptly and to take infection-control and bleeding precautions.
● For patient who's to receive anesthesia, tell him to inform anesthesiologist that he has taken this drug. High oxygen levels inhaled during surgery may enhance pulmonary toxicity of drug.

SAFETY ALERT!

---

daunorubicin citrate liposomal
daw-nah-ROO-buh-sin

DaunoXome

Pharmacologic class: anthracycline glycoside antibiotic
Pregnancy risk category D

AVAILABLE FORMS
Injection: 2 mg/ml (equivalent to 50 mg daunorubicin base)

INDICATIONS & DOSAGES
➤ **First-line cytotoxic therapy for advanced HIV-related Kaposi sarcoma**
Adults: 40 mg/m² I.V. over 60 minutes once every 2 weeks. Continue treatment until progressive disease becomes evident or

until other complications of HIV infection preclude continuation of therapy.

Adjust-a-dose: For patients with impaired hepatic and renal function, if bilirubin level is 1.2 to 3 mg/dl, give three-fourths normal dose; if bilirubin or creatinine level exceeds 3 mg/dl, give one-half normal dose.

ADMINISTRATION

I.V.
● Preparing and giving drug may be mutagenic, teratogenic, or carcinogenic. Follow facility policy to reduce risks.
● To dilute, withdraw calculated volume of drug from vial and transfer into an equal amount of D_5W. Recommended concentration after dilution is 1 mg/ml.
● Use immediately after dilution.
● Don't use an in-line filter.
● Give over 60 minutes.
■ **Black Box Warning** Back pain, flushing, and chest tightness may develop during first 5 minutes of infusion. These symptoms subside after infusion stops and usually don't recur when drug is infused more slowly. ■
● Monitor I.V. site closely; watch for irritation and infiltration, which can cause tissue damage and necrosis. If it occurs, stop infusion, apply ice, and notify prescriber.
● If needed, drug may be refrigerated at 36° to 46° F (2° to 8° C) for up to 6 hours.
● **Incompatibilities:** Bacteriostatic agents, other I.V. drugs, saline and other solutions.

ACTION

Maximizes selectivity of daunorubicin for solid tumors in situ. After penetrating tumor, drug is released over time to exert antineoplastic activity by inhibiting DNA synthesis and DNA-dependent RNA synthesis.

Route	Onset	Peak	Duration
I.V.	Unknown	Unknown	Unknown

Half-life: 4½ hours.

ADVERSE REACTIONS

CNS: *headache, neuropathy,* depression, dizziness, insomnia, amnesia, anxiety, ataxia, confusion, *seizures,* hallucination, tremor, hypertonia, *meningitis, fatigue,* malaise, emotional lability, abnormal gait, hyperkinesia, somnolence, abnormal thinking, *fever.*

CV: chest pain, hypertension, palpitations, *arrhythmias, pericardial effusion, cardiac arrest,* angina pectoris, *pulmonary hypertension,* flushing, edema, tachycardia, *MI.*
EENT: *rhinitis,* stomatitis, sinusitis, abnormal vision, conjunctivitis, tinnitus, eye pain, deafness, earache.
GI: taste disturbances, dry mouth, gingival bleeding, *nausea, diarrhea, abdominal pain, vomiting, anorexia,* constipation, *GI hemorrhage,* gastritis, dysphagia, stomatitis, increased appetite, melena, hemorrhoids, tenesmus.
GU: dysuria, nocturia, polyuria.
Hematologic: NEUTROPENIA, THROMBO-CYTOPENIA.
Hepatic: hepatomegaly.
Metabolic: dehydration.
Musculoskeletal: *rigors, back pain,* arthralgia, myalgia.
Respiratory: *cough, dyspnea,* hemoptysis, hiccups, pulmonary infiltration, increased sputum.
Skin: alopecia, pruritus, *increased sweating,* dry skin, seborrhea, folliculitis, injection site inflammation.
Other: splenomegaly, lymphadenopathy, tooth caries, allergic reactions, flulike symptoms.

INTERACTIONS
None significant.

EFFECTS ON LAB TEST RESULTS
● May decrease neutrophil and platelet counts.

CONTRAINDICATIONS & CAUTIONS
● Contraindicated in patients who have experienced severe hypersensitivity reaction to drug or its components.
● Use cautiously in patients with myelo-suppression, cardiac disease, previous radiotherapy encompassing the heart, previous anthracycline use (doxorubicin cumulative dose is 300 mg/m² or above), or hepatic or renal dysfunction.

NURSING CONSIDERATIONS
● Drug causes less nausea, vomiting, alopecia, neutropenia, thrombocytopenia, and potentially less cardiotoxicity than conventional daunorubicin.
■ **Black Box Warning** Give only under supervision of prescriber specializing in chemotherapy. ■

Reactions may be *common,* uncommon, *life-threatening,* or COMMON AND LIFE-THREATENING.
Interaction may have a *rapid onset* or **delayed onset.**

■ **Black Box Warning** Monitor cardiac function regularly. Assess patient before giving each dose because of risk of cardiac toxicity and heart failure. Cardiac monitoring is especially advised in patients who have received prior anthracyclines, have pre-existing cardiac disease, or have had prior radiotherapy encompassing the heart. ■

● Determine left ventricular ejection fraction at total cumulative doses of 320 mg/m^2 and every 160 mg/m^2 thereafter. Total cumulative doses generally shouldn't exceed 550 mg/m^2.

■ **Black Box Warning** Provide careful hematologic monitoring because severe myelosuppression may occur. Repeat blood counts and evaluate before giving each dose. If absolute granulocyte count is below 750/mm^3, withhold drug. ■

● Monitor patient closely for signs and symptoms of opportunistic infection, especially because patients with HIV infection are immunocompromised.

■ **Black Box Warning** Reduce dosage in patients with impaired hepatic function. ■

● *Look alike–sound alike:* Don't confuse daunorubicin citrate liposomal with daunorubicin hydrochloride.

PATIENT TEACHING

● Inform patient that hair loss may occur but that it's usually reversible.

● Instruct patient to call prescriber if sore throat, fever, or other signs or symptoms of infection occur. Tell patient to avoid exposure to people with infections.

● Advise woman to report suspected or confirmed pregnancy during therapy.

● Tell patient to report back pain, flushing, or chest tightness during infusion.

SAFETY ALERT!

daunorubicin hydrochloride
daw-nah-ROO-buh-sin

Cerubidine

Pharmacologic class: anthracycline glycoside antibiotic
Pregnancy risk category D

AVAILABLE FORMS
Injection: 20-mg and 50-mg vials

INDICATIONS & DOSAGES
Dosages vary. Check treatment protocol with prescriber.

➤ **To induce remission in acute nonlymphocytic (myelogenous, monocytic, erythroid) leukemia**
Adults age 60 and older: In combination, 30 mg/m^2 per day I.V. on days 1, 2, and 3 of first course and on days 1 and 2 of subsequent courses with cytarabine infusions.
Adults younger than age 60: In combination, 45 mg/m^2 per day I.V. on days 1, 2, and 3 of first course and on days 1 and 2 of subsequent courses with cytarabine infusions.

➤ **To induce remission in acute lymphocytic leukemia (with combination therapy)**
Adults: 45 mg/m^2 per day I.V. on days 1, 2, and 3 of first course.
Children age 2 and older: 25 mg/m^2 I.V. on day 1 every week for up to 6 weeks, if needed.
Children younger than age 2 or with body surface area less than 0.5 m^2: Dose based on body weight, not surface area.
Adjust-a-dose: For patients with impaired hepatic and renal function, reduce dosage as follows: If bilirubin level is 1.2 to 3 mg/dl, give three-fourths normal dose; if bilirubin or creatinine level exceeds 3 mg/dl, give half normal dose.

ADMINISTRATION
I.V.
● Preparing and giving parenteral drug may be mutagenic, teratogenic, or carcinogenic. Follow facility policy to reduce risks.
● Reconstitute with 4 ml sterile water for injection to yield 5 mg/ml.
● Withdraw desired dose into syringe containing 10 to 15 ml of normal saline solution for injection.
● Inject as a slow I.V. push over 2 to 3 minutes into tubing of a free-flowing I.V. solution of D$_5$W or normal saline solution for injection.
■ **Black Box Warning** Give drug into a rapidly infusing I.V. infusion. Do not give I.M. or subcutaneously. Severe local tissue necrosis will result from extravasation. ■
● If extravasation occurs, stop infusion immediately, apply ice to area for 24 to 48 hours, and notify prescriber. Because

drug is a vesicant, extravasation could cause severe tissue necrosis.
• If possible, use within 8 hours of preparation. Reconstituted solution is stable 24 hours at room temperature, 48 hours if refrigerated.
• **Incompatibilities:** Other I.V. drugs. If mixed with dexamethasone or heparin, drug may precipitate; don't mix together.

ACTION
May interfere with DNA-dependent RNA synthesis by intercalation.

Route	Onset	Peak	Duration
I.V.	Unknown	Unknown	Unknown

Half-life: Initial, 45 minutes; terminal, 18½ hours.

ADVERSE REACTIONS
CNS: fever.
CV: IRREVERSIBLE CARDIOMYOPATHY, ECG changes.
GI: *nausea, vomiting,* diarrhea, abdominal pain, mucositis.
Hematologic: *bone marrow suppression.*
Metabolic: hyperuricemia.
Skin: *reversible alopecia, severe cellulitis and tissue sloughing with drug extravasation,* rash, darkening or redness of previously irradiated areas, contact dermatitis urticaria.

INTERACTIONS
Drug-drug. *Doxorubicin:* May cause additive cardiotoxicity. Monitor patient for toxicity.
Hepatotoxic drugs: May increase risk of additive hepatotoxicity. Monitor hepatic function closely.
Myelosuppressive drugs: May increase risk of myelosuppression. Monitor patient closely.

EFFECTS ON LAB TEST RESULTS
• May increase alkaline phosphatase, AST, bilirubin, and uric acid levels. May decrease hemoglobin level and hematocrit.
• May decrease platelet and WBC counts.

CONTRAINDICATIONS & CAUTIONS
• Contraindicated in patients hypersensitive to the drug.
• Use cautiously in patients with myelosuppression or impaired cardiac, renal, or hepatic function.

NURSING CONSIDERATIONS
■ **Black Box Warning** Only physicians experienced in leukemia chemotherapy should administer drug. Adequate laboratory and supportive resources must be available. ■
• Take preventive measures (including adequate hydration) before starting treatment. Hyperuricemia may result from rapid lysis of leukemic cells. Allopurinol may be ordered.
■ **Black Box Warning** Myocardial toxicity may occur when total cumulative dosage exceeds 400 to 550 mg/m^2 in adults, 300 mg/m^2 in children older than 2 years, or 10 mg/kg in children younger than 2 years. This may occur during therapy to several months to years after therapy. ■
• Perform cardiac function studies, including ECG and ejection fraction, before treatment and then periodically throughout therapy.
• *Alert:* Cumulative adult dosage is limited to 400 to 550 mg/m^2 (450 mg/m^2 when patient is also receiving or has received cyclophosphamide or radiation therapy to cardiac area).
■ **Black Box Warning** Reduce dosage in patients with renal or hepatic impairment. ■
• Monitor CBC and hepatic function tests; monitor ECG every month during therapy.
• *Alert:* If signs of heart failure, cardiomyopathy, or arrhythmia develop, stop drug immediately and notify prescriber.
• Watch for nausea and vomiting, which may last 24 to 48 hours.
■ **Black Box Warning** Severe myelosuppression occurs when used in therapeutic doses; this may lead to infection or hemorrhage. ■
• Blood transfusions may be needed to combat anemia. Patient may receive injected RBC colony-stimulating factor to promote RBC production and to decrease need for blood transfusions.
• **Look alike–sound alike:** Reddish color of drug is similar to that of doxorubicin; don't confuse the two.
• Lowest blood counts occur 10 to 14 days after dose.

Reactions may be *common,* uncommon, *life-threatening,* or COMMON AND LIFE-THREATENING.
Interaction may have a *rapid onset* or **delayed onset.**

● *Look alike–sound alike:* Don't confuse daunorubicin hydrochloride with daunorubicin citrate liposomal.

PATIENT TEACHING
● Advise patient to report any pain or burning at site of injection during or after administration.
● Advise patient to watch for signs and symptoms of infection (fever, sore throat, fatigue) and bleeding (easy bruising, nosebleeds, bleeding gums, tarry stools) and to take temperature daily.
● Inform patient that red urine for 1 to 2 days is normal and doesn't indicate the presence of blood in urine.
● Advise patient that hair loss may occur but that it's usually reversible.
● Caution woman of childbearing age to avoid becoming pregnant during therapy. Recommend that she consult prescriber before becoming pregnant.

SAFETY ALERT!

doxorubicin hydrochloride
dox-oh-ROO-bi-sin

Pharmacologic class: anthracycline glycoside antibiotic
Pregnancy risk category D

AVAILABLE FORMS
Injection (preservative-free): 2 mg/ml
Powder for injection: 10-mg, 20-mg, 50-mg, 100-mg, 150-mg vials

INDICATIONS & DOSAGES
➤ **Bladder, breast, lung, ovarian, stomach, and thyroid cancers; non-Hodgkin lymphoma; Hodgkin lymphoma; acute lymphoblastic and myeloblastic leukemia; Wilms tumor; neuroblastoma; lymphoma; soft tissue and bone sarcomas**
Adults: 60 to 75 mg/m² I.V. as single dose every 3 weeks; or when used in combination with other chemotherapy drugs, 40 to 60 mg/m² I.V. every 21 to 28 days.
Elderly patients: May need reduced dosages.
Adjust-a-dose: Reduce dosage for patients with myelosuppression or impaired cardiac or liver function. Be prepared to

decrease dosage if bilirubin level rises: Give 50% of dose when bilirubin level is 1.2 to 3 mg/100 ml; 25% when it's 3.1 to 5 mg/100 ml.

ADMINISTRATION
I.V.
● Preparing and giving parenteral drug may be mutagenic, teratogenic, or carcinogenic. Follow facility policy to reduce risks.
● If drug leaks or spills, inactivate with 5% sodium hypochlorite solution (household bleach).
● Reconstitute with preservative-free normal saline solution for injection to yield 2 mg/ml; add 5 ml to 10-mg vial, 10 ml to 20-mg vial, or 25 ml to 50-mg vial. Shake vial to dissolve drug.
● Don't place I.V. catheter over joints or in limbs with poor venous or lymphatic drainage.
● Give by direct injection over at least 3 minutes into the tubing of a free-flowing I.V. solution containing D₅W or normal saline solution for injection.
● If vein streaking occurs, slow administration rate. If welts appear, stop drug and notify prescriber.
● Some protocols give doxorubicin as a prolonged infusion, which requires central venous access.
■ **Black Box Warning** If extravasation occurs, stop infusion immediately and notify prescriber. Monitor area closely because extravasation may be progressive. Apply ice to the site for 15 minutes 4 times daily for 3 days. Drug is a strong vesicant and may cause tissue necrosis. Early consultation with a plastic surgeon may be advisable. ■
● Refrigerated, reconstituted solution is stable 15 days; at room temperature, it's stable 7 days.
● **Incompatibilities:** Allopurinol, aluminum, aminophylline, bacteriostatic diluents, cefepime, dexamethasone sodium phosphate, diazepam, fluorouracil, furosemide, ganciclovir, heparin sodium, hydrocortisone sodium succinate, piperacillin with tazobactam.

ACTION
May interfere with DNA-dependent RNA synthesis by intercalation.

Route	Onset	Peak	Duration
I.V.	Unknown	Unknown	Unknown

Half-life: Initial, 30 minutes; terminal, 16½ hours.

ADVERSE REACTIONS

CV: cardiac depression, *arrhythmias, acute left ventricular failure, irreversible cardiomyopathy.*
EENT: conjunctivitis.
GI: *nausea, vomiting,* diarrhea, *stomatitis,* esophagitis, anorexia.
GU: transient red urine.
Hematologic: *leukopenia, thrombocytopenia,* MYELOSUPPRESSION.
Metabolic: hyperuricemia.
Skin: *severe cellulitis and tissue sloughing with drug extravasation,* urticaria, facial flushing, *complete alopecia within 3 to 4 weeks,* hyperpigmentation of nail beds and dermal creases, radiation recall effect.
Other: chills, *anaphylaxis.*

INTERACTIONS

Drug-drug. *Aminophylline, cephalothin, dexamethasone, fluorouracil, heparin, hydrocortisone:* May form a precipitate. Don't mix together.
Calcium channel blockers: May increase cardiotoxic effects. Monitor patient's ECG closely.
Cyclosporine: May increase doxorubicin concentration. Monitor patient for toxicity.
Digoxin: May decrease digoxin level. Monitor digoxin level closely.
Fosphenytoin, phenytoin: May decrease level of phenytoin or fosphenytoin. Monitor drug level.
Paclitaxel: May decrease doxorubicin clearance. Monitor patient for toxicity.
Phenobarbital: May increase doxorubicin clearance. Monitor patient closely.
Progesterone: May enhance neutropenia and thrombocytopenia. Monitor patient and laboratory values closely.
Streptozocin: May increase and prolong doxorubicin level. Doxorubicin dosage may have to be adjusted.

EFFECTS ON LAB TEST RESULTS

• May increase uric acid level.
• May decrease platelet and WBC counts.

CONTRAINDICATIONS & CAUTIONS

• Contraindicated in patients with a history of sensitivity reactions to drug or its components.
• Contraindicated in patients with marked myelosuppression induced by previous treatment with other antitumor drugs or radiotherapy and in those who have received a lifetime cumulative dose of 550 mg/m² of doxorubicin or daunorubicin.

NURSING CONSIDERATIONS

■ **Black Box Warning** Drug should be administered under the supervision of a physician experienced with cancer chemotherapeutic agents. ■
• Perform cardiac function studies, including ECG and ejection fraction, before treatment and then periodically throughout therapy. Dexrazoxane may be given within 30 minutes of doxorubicin if the accumulated dose of doxorubicin has reached 300 mg/m².
• Take preventive measures, including adequate hydration of the patient, before starting treatment. Rapid lysis of leukemic cells may cause hyperuricemia. Allopurinol may be ordered.
• Premedicate with antiemetic to reduce nausea.
• If skin or mucosal contact occurs, immediately wash with soap and water.
■ **Black Box Warning** Never give drug I.M. or subcutaneously. ■
■ **Black Box Warning** Reduce dosage in patients with hepatic impairment. ■
■ **Black Box Warning** Severe myelosuppression may occur. ■
• Monitor CBC with differential and hepatic function tests; monitor ECG monthly during therapy. If WBC count falls below 2,000/mm³ or granulocyte count falls below 1,000/mm³, follow institutional policy for infection control in immunocompromised patients.
• Monitor ECG for changes, such as sinus tachycardia, T-wave flattening, ST-segment depression, and voltage reduction.
• Leukopenia may occur during days 10 to 15, with recovery by day 21.
• If tachycardia develops, stop drug or slow rate of infusion, and notify prescriber.
■ **Black Box Warning** Myocardial toxicity may occur during therapy or months to years after termination of therapy. ■

Reactions may be *common,* uncommon, *life-threatening,* or COMMON AND LIFE-THREATENING.
Interaction may have a *rapid onset* or **delayed onset.**

• *Alert:* If signs of heart failure develop, stop drug and notify prescriber. Heart failure can often be prevented by limiting cumulative dose to 550 mg/m^2 (400 mg/m^2 when patient is also receiving or has received cyclophosphamide or radiation therapy to cardiac area).

• *Look alike–sound alike:* Reddish color of drug is similar to that of daunorubicin; don't confuse the two drugs.

• Esophagitis is common in patients who also have received radiation therapy.

• *Alert:* If patient has previously received radiation therapy, he's susceptible to radiation recall effect.

• *Look alike–sound alike:* Don't confuse doxorubicin with doxorubicin liposomal.

PATIENT TEACHING

• Advise patient to report any pain or burning at site of injection during or after administration.

• Advise patient to watch for signs and symptoms of infection (fever, sore throat, fatigue) and bleeding (easy bruising, nosebleeds, bleeding gums, tarry stools) and to take temperature daily.

• Advise patient that orange to red urine for 1 to 2 days is normal and doesn't indicate presence of blood.

• Inform patient that hair loss may occur but that it's usually reversible. Hair may regrow 2 to 5 months after drug is stopped.

SAFETY ALERT!

doxorubicin hydrochloride liposomal
dox-oh-ROO-bi-sin

Doxil

Pharmacologic class: anthracycline glycoside antibiotic
Pregnancy risk category D

AVAILABLE FORMS
Injection: 20 mg/10 ml, 50 mg/30 ml

INDICATIONS & DOSAGES
➤ **Metastatic ovarian carcinoma refractory to both paclitaxel- and platinum-based chemotherapy regimens**

Women: 50 mg/m^2 I.V. initially at 1 mg/minute once every 4 weeks for minimum of four courses. Continue as long as condition doesn't progress, patient shows no evidence of cardiotoxicity, and patient continues to tolerate treatment. If no infusion-related adverse reactions develop, increase infusion rate to complete administration over 1 hour.

➤ **AIDS-related Kaposi sarcoma refractory to previous combination chemotherapy and in patients intolerant of such therapy**
Adults: 20 mg/m^2 I.V. over 30 minutes once every 3 weeks. Continue as long as patient responds satisfactorily and tolerates treatment.

Adjust-a-dose: For patients with impaired hepatic function, reduce dosage as follows: If bilirubin level is 1.2 to 3 mg/dl, give half normal dose; if bilirubin level is more than 3 mg/dl, give one-fourth normal dose. Dose modifications may be needed for stomatitis, myelosuppression, and hand-foot syndrome, based on toxicity grade.

✴ *NEW INDICATION*
➤ **Multiple myeloma**
Adults: 30 mg/m^2 I.V. on day 4 following bortezomib which is given at 1.3 mg/m^2 bolus on days 1, 4, 8, and 11, every 3 weeks. Treatment may continue for up to 8 cycles, until disease progression or occurrence of unacceptable toxicity.

ADMINISTRATION
I.V.
• Follow procedures for proper handling and disposal of antineoplastics.

• Dilute appropriate dose (maximum, 90 mg) in 250 ml D$_5$W using aseptic technique.

• Carefully check label on I.V. bag before giving drug. Accidentally substituting doxorubicin hydrochloride liposomal for conventional doxorubicin hydrochloride may cause severe adverse reactions. The two products can't be substituted on a milligram-per-milligram basis.

• Don't use an in-line filter.

• Infuse over 30 to 60 minutes, depending on dose. Monitor patient carefully during infusion.

■ **Black Box Warning** Acute infusion-related reactions include flushing, shortness of breath, facial swelling, headache, chills,

back pain, tightness in chest or throat, and hypotension. They may resolve when infusion rate is slowed, or over several hours to a day when infusion is stopped. ■
• If extravasation occurs, stop infusion immediately. Apply ice at the site for about 30 minutes to help alleviate local reaction. Restart infusion in another vein.
• Refrigerate diluted solution at 36° to 46° F (2° to 8° C) and give within 24 hours.
• **Incompatibilities:** Other I.V. drugs.

ACTION

Consists of doxorubicin hydrochloride encapsulated in liposomes. Action may involve drug's ability to bind DNA and inhibit nucleic acid synthesis.

Route	Onset	Peak	Duration
I.V.	Unknown	Unknown	Unknown

Half-life: 5 hours in first phase; 55 hours in second phase with doses of 10 to 20 mg/m^2.

ADVERSE REACTIONS

CNS: *asthenia,* paresthesia, headache, somnolence, dizziness, depression, insomnia, anxiety, malaise, emotional lability, fatigue, fever.
CV: chest pain, hypotension, tachycardia, peripheral edema, ***cardiomyopathy, heart failure, arrhythmias,*** pericardial effusion.
EENT: pharyngitis, rhinitis, conjunctivitis, retinitis, optic neuritis.
GI: *nausea, vomiting, constipation, anorexia, diarrhea,* abdominal pain, dyspepsia, oral candidiasis, enlarged abdomen, esophagitis, dysphagia, *stomatitis,* taste perversion, glossitis.
GU: albuminuria.
Hematologic: LEUKOPENIA, NEUTROPENIA, THROMBOCYTOPENIA, *anemia.*
Hepatic: hyperbilirubinemia.
Metabolic: dehydration, weight loss, hypocalcemia, hyperglycemia.
Musculoskeletal: myalgia, back pain.
Respiratory: dyspnea, increased cough, pneumonia.
Skin: *rash, alopecia,* dry skin, pruritus, skin discoloration, skin disorder, exfoliative dermatitis, sweating, *palmar-plantar erythrodysesthesia.*
Other: allergic reaction, chills, *herpes zoster,* infection, infusion-related reactions.

INTERACTIONS

None reported. However, drug may interact with drugs that interact with conventional form of doxorubicin hydrochloride.

EFFECTS ON LAB TEST RESULTS

• May increase bilirubin and glucose levels. May decrease calcium and hemoglobin levels.
• May increase PT and INR. May decrease neutrophil, platelet, and WBC counts.

CONTRAINDICATIONS & CAUTIONS

• Contraindicated in patients hypersensitive to conventional formulation of doxorubicin hydrochloride or any component in the liposomal form.
• Contraindicated in patients with marked myelosuppression and those who have received a lifetime cumulative dose of 550 mg/m^2 (400 mg/m^2 in patients who have received radiotherapy to the mediastinal area or therapy with other cardiotoxic drugs such as cyclophosphamide).
• Use cautiously in patients who have received other anthracyclines.

NURSING CONSIDERATIONS

• Consider previous or current therapy with related compounds such as daunorubicin when calculating total dose of drug to be given. Heart failure and cardiomyopathy may occur after stopping therapy.
■ **Black Box Warning** Cumulative dose over 550 mg/m^2 increases risk of cardiotoxicity. ■
• Give drug to patient with history of CV disease only when benefit outweighs risk to patient.
• Don't give I.M. or subcutaneously.
• *Alert:* Monitor patient for signs and symptoms of palmar-plantar erythrodysesthesia, hematologic toxicity, or stomatitis. These adverse reactions may be managed with dosage delays and adjustments.
■ **Black Box Warning** Evaluate patient's hepatic function before therapy, and adjust dosage accordingly. ■
■ **Black Box Warning** Drug exhibits pharmacokinetic properties different from those of conventional doxorubicin hydrochloride and shouldn't be substituted on a milligram-by-milligram basis. ■

Reactions may be *common,* uncommon, ***life-threatening,*** or COMMON AND LIFE-THREATENING.
Interaction may have a *rapid onset* or ***delayed onset.***

• Drug may increase toxicity of other antineoplastics.

• Closely monitor cardiac function by endomyocardial biopsy, echocardiography, or gated radionuclide scans. If results indicate possible cardiac injury, the benefit of continued therapy must be weighed against the risk of myocardial injury.

■ **Black Box Warning** Severe myelo-suppression may occur. ■

• Monitor CBC, including platelets, before each dose and frequently throughout therapy. Leukopenia is usually transient. Persistent severe myelosuppression may result in superinfection or hemorrhage. Patient may need granulocyte colony-stimulating factor (or granulocyte-macrophage colony-stimulating factor) to support blood counts.

PATIENT TEACHING

• Tell patient to notify prescriber if he experiences signs and symptoms of hand-foot syndrome (such as tingling or burning, redness, flaking, bothersome swelling, small blisters, or small sores on palms of hands or soles of feet).

• To reduce the risk of hand-foot syndrome, advise the patient to follow these guidelines at least 1 day before and for 3 to 5 days after treatment:

– Avoid direct sunlight and use sunblock SPF 15 or higher on all exposed skin.

– Wear loose clothing and comfortable, well-ventilated, low-heeled shoes.

– Avoid contact with hot water and take cool, short showers or baths.

– Don't put pressure on your skin. (Avoid kneeling, leaning on your elbows, wearing tight jewelry or undergarments, and chopping hard foods.)

• Advise patient to report signs and symptoms of mouth inflammation (such as painful redness, swelling, or sores in mouth).

• Warn patient to avoid exposure to people with infections. Tell patient to report temperature of 100.5° F (38° C) or higher.

• Tell patient to report nausea, vomiting, tiredness, weakness, rash, or mild hair loss.

• Advise woman of childbearing age to avoid pregnancy during therapy.

SAFETY ALERT!

epirubicin hydrochloride
ep-uh-ROO-bi-sin

Ellence

Pharmacologic class: anthracycline glycoside antibiotic
Pregnancy risk category D

AVAILABLE FORMS
Injection: 2 mg/ml
Powder for injection: 50 mg, 200 mg

INDICATIONS & DOSAGES
➤ **Adjuvant therapy in patients with evidence of axillary node tumor involvement after resection of primary breast cancer**
Adults: 100 to 120 mg/m² I.V. infusion over 3 to 5 minutes through a free-flowing I.V. solution on day 1 of each cycle, or divided equally in two doses on days 1 and 8 of each cycle; cycle repeated every 3 to 4 weeks for six cycles; used with regimens containing cyclophosphamide and fluorouracil.

Dosage modification after first cycle is based on toxicity. For patients with platelet count nadir below 50,000/mm³, absolute neutrophil count (ANC) below 250/mm³, neutropenic fever, or grade 3 or 4 nonhematologic toxicity, reduce day 1 dose in subsequent cycles to 75% of day 1 dose given in current cycle. Delay day 1 therapy in subsequent cycles until platelet count is at least 100,000/mm³, ANC is at least 1,500/mm³, and non-hematologic toxicities recover to grade 1.

For patients receiving divided doses (days 1 and 8), day 8 dose should be 75% of day 1 dose if platelet count is 75,000 to 100,000/mm³ and ANC is 1,000 to 1,499/mm³. If day 8 platelet count is below 75,000/mm³, ANC is below 1,000/mm³, or grade 3 or 4 non-hematologic toxicity has occurred, omit day 8 dose.

Adjust-a-dose: For patients with bone marrow dysfunction (heavily pretreated patients, patients with bone marrow depression, or those with neoplastic bone marrow infiltration), start at lower doses of 75 to 90 mg/m².

■ **Black Box Warning** For patients with hepatic dysfunction, if bilirubin is 1.2 to 3 mg/dl or AST is two to four times upper limit of normal, give half recommended starting dose. If bilirubin level is above 3 mg/dl or AST is more than four times upper limit of normal, give one-fourth recommended starting dose. ■

For patients with severe renal dysfunction (creatinine level over 5 mg/dl), consider lower doses.

ADMINISTRATION
I.V.
● Wear protective clothing (goggles, gown, disposable gloves) when handling drug, which is a vesicant.
■ **Black Box Warning** Never give drug I.M. or subcutaneously. Always give I.V. through free-flowing normal saline solution or D_5W. ■
● Avoid veins over joints or in limbs with compromised venous or lymphatic drainage.
● Avoid repeated injection into the same vein.
● Give drug over 3 to 5 minutes.
● Facial flushing and erythematous streaking along vein may indicate overly rapid delivery.
● If burning or stinging occurs, stop infusion immediately and restart in another vein.
● After vial has been penetrated, discard unused solution after 24 hours.
● **Incompatibilities:** Fluorouracil, heparin, ifosfamide with mesna, other I.V. drugs.

ACTION
May form a complex with DNA by getting between nucleotide base pairs, inhibiting DNA, RNA, and protein synthesis; DNA cleavage occurs, resulting in cyticidal activity. Drug may also interfere with replication and transcription of DNA and may generate cytotoxic free radicals.

Route	Onset	Peak	Duration
I.V.	Unknown	Unknown	Unknown

Half-life: 31 to 35 hours.

ADVERSE REACTIONS
CNS: *lethargy,* fever.
CV: *cardiomyopathy, heart failure,* hot flashes.
EENT: *conjunctivitis, keratitis.*

GI: *nausea, vomiting, diarrhea,* anorexia, *mucositis.*
GU: *amenorrhea,* red urine.
Hematologic: LEUKOPENIA, NEUTRO-PENIA, *febrile neutropenia,* anemia, THROMBOCYTOPENIA.
Skin: *alopecia,* rash, itch, skin changes, local toxicity.
Other: *infection.*

INTERACTIONS
Drug-drug. *Calcium channel blockers, other cardioactive compounds:* May increase risk of heart failure. Monitor cardiac function closely.
Cimetidine: May increase epirubicin level by 50%. Avoid using together.
Cytotoxic drugs: May cause additive toxicities (especially hematologic and GI). Monitor patient closely.

EFFECTS ON LAB TEST RESULTS
● May decrease hemoglobin level.
● May decrease neutrophil, platelet, and WBC counts.

CONTRAINDICATIONS & CAUTIONS
● Contraindicated in patients hypersensitive to drug, other anthracyclines, or anthracenediones, and in patients with baseline neutrophil counts below 1,500/mm³, severe myocardial insufficiency, recent MI, serious arrhythmias, or severe hepatic dysfunction.
● Contraindicated in patients who have had previous treatment with anthracyclines to total cumulative doses.
● Use cautiously in patients with active or dormant cardiac disease, previous or current radiotherapy to mediastinal and pericardial areas, or previous therapy with other anthracyclines or anthracenediones.
● Use cautiously in patients receiving other cardiotoxic drugs.

NURSING CONSIDERATIONS
■ **Black Box Warning** Give drug under supervision of prescriber experienced in cancer chemotherapy. ■
● Don't handle drug if you are pregnant.
● For patients taking 120 mg/m², give prophylactic co-trimoxazole or fluoroquinolones.
● Give antiemetic before drug to reduce nausea and vomiting.

Reactions may be *common,* uncommon, *life-threatening,* or COMMON AND LIFE-THREATENING.
Interaction may have a *rapid onset* or *delayed onset.*

• Before therapy, obtain total bilirubin, AST, and creatinine levels; CBC including ANC; and left ventricular ejection fraction (LVEF).
• Monitor LVEF regularly during therapy. Stop drug at first sign of impaired cardiac function. Early signs of cardiac toxicity include sinus tachycardia, ECG abnormalities, tachyarrhythmias, bradycardia, AV block, and bundle-branch block.

■ **Black Box Warning** Delayed cardiac toxicity may occur 2 to 3 months after treatment ends; indications include reduced LVEF and signs and symptoms of heart failure (tachycardia, dyspnea, pulmonary edema, dependent edema, hepatomegaly, ascites, pleural effusion, and gallop rhythm). Delayed cardiac toxicity depends on cumulative dose of epirubicin. Don't exceed cumulative dose of 900 mg/m^2. ■

■ **Black Box Warning** Severe myelosuppression may occur. ■

• Obtain total and differential WBC, CBC, platelet counts, and liver function tests before and during each cycle of therapy.
• WBC nadir is usually reached 10 to 14 days after drug administration, and returns to normal by day 21.
• Monitor uric acid, potassium, calcium phosphate, and creatinine levels immediately after initial chemotherapy administration in patients susceptible to tumor lysis syndrome. Hydration, urine alkalinization, and prophylaxis with allopurinol may prevent hyperuricemia and minimize potential complications of tumor lysis syndrome.
• Drug may enhance the effects of radiation therapy or cause an inflammatory cell reaction at irradiation site. Monitor patient closely.

■ **Black Box Warning** Secondary AML has been reported in patients with breast cancer treated with anthracyclines including epirubicin. ■

PATIENT TEACHING
• Advise patient to report any pain or burning at site of injection during or after administration.
• Advise patient to report nausea, vomiting, mouth inflammation, dehydration, fever, evidence of infection, or symptoms of heart failure (rapid heart beat, labored breathing, swelling).
• Tell patient that urine will be reddish pink for 1 to 2 days after treatment.

• Inform patient of risk of heart damage and treatment-related leukemia with use of drug.
• Advise men to use effective contraception during treatment.
• Advise women that irreversible, premature menopause may occur.
• Tell patient that hair usually regrows within 2 to 3 months after therapy stops.

SAFETY ALERT!

idarubicin hydrochloride
eye-duh-ROO-bi-sin

Idamycin PFS

Pharmacologic class: semisynthetic anthracycline
Pregnancy risk category D

AVAILABLE FORMS
Injection: 1 mg/ml in 5-, 10- and 20-ml single-dose vials

INDICATIONS & DOSAGES
Dosages vary. Check treatment protocol with prescriber.
➤ **Acute myeloid leukemia, including French-American-British classifications M1 through M7, with other approved antileukemic drugs**
Adults: 12 mg/m^2 daily for 3 days by slow I.V. injection (over 10 to 15 minutes) with 100 mg/m^2 daily of cytarabine for 7 days by continuous I.V. infusion. Or, the cytarabine may be given 25-mg/m^2 bolus; then 200 mg/m^2 daily for 5 days by continuous infusion. A second course may be given, if needed.
Adjust-a-dose: If patient experiences severe mucositis, delay therapy until recovery is complete and reduce dosage by 25%.

■ **Black Box Warning** Reduce dosage in patients with hepatic or renal impairment. Don't give idarubicin if bilirubin level exceeds 5 mg/dl. ■

ADMINISTRATION
I.V.
• Preparing and giving parenteral drug may be mutagenic, teratogenic, or carcinogenic. Follow facility policy to reduce risks.

● Reconstitute to final concentration of 1 mg/ml using normal saline solution for injection without preservatives. Add 5 ml to 5-mg vial, 10 ml to 10-mg vial, or 20 ml to 20-mg vial. Don't use bacteriostatic saline solution. Vial is under negative pressure.

■ **Black Box Warning** Give drug over 10 to 15 minutes into a free-flowing I.V. infusion of normal saline or D_5W solution running into a large vein. Do not give I.M. or subcutaneously. ■

■ **Black Box Warning** Drug is a vesicant; tissue necrosis may result. ■

● If extravasation occurs, stop infusion immediately and notify prescriber. Treat with intermittent ice packs for ½ hour immediately and then for ½ hour q.i.d. for 4 days.

● Reconstituted solutions are stable for 72 hours at 59° to 86° F (15° to 30° C); 7 days if refrigerated and protected from light. Label unused solutions with chemotherapy hazard label.

● **Incompatibilities:** Acyclovir sodium, alkaline solutions, allopurinol, ampicillin sodium with sulbactam, cefazolin, cefepime, ceftazidime, clindamycin phosphate, dexamethasone sodium phosphate, etoposide, furosemide, gentamicin, heparin, hydrocortisone sodium succinate, lorazepam, meperidine, methotrexate sodium, piperacillin sodium with tazobactam, sodium bicarbonate, teniposide, vancomycin, vincristine.

ACTION

Unknown. Probably inhibits nucleic acid synthesis and interacts with the enzyme topoisomerase II. Drug is highly lipophilic, which increases rate of cellular uptake.

Route	Onset	Peak	Duration
I.V.	Unknown	Few min	Unknown

Half-life: 20 to 22 hours.

ADVERSE REACTIONS

CNS: *headache, changed mental status,* peripheral neuropathy, **seizures,** *fever.*
CV: HEMORRHAGE, *heart failure, MI,* **myocardial insufficiency, arrhythmias, myocardial toxicity,** atrial fibrillation, chest pain, asymptomatic decline in left ventricular ejection fraction.

GI: *nausea, vomiting, cramps, diarrhea, mucositis.*
GU: renal dysfunction, red urine.
Hematologic: myelosuppression.
Hepatic: changes in hepatic function.
Metabolic: hyperuricemia.
Skin: *alopecia, rash, urticaria, bullous erythrodermatous rash on palms and soles,* urticaria, erythema at previously irradiated sites, tissue necrosis if extravasation occurs.
Other: INFECTION, hypersensitivity reactions.

INTERACTIONS

Drug-drug. *Alkaline solutions, heparin:* These combinations are incompatible. Don't mix idarubicin with other drugs unless specific compatibility data are known.

EFFECTS ON LAB TEST RESULTS

● May increase uric acid level. May decrease hemoglobin level.
● May decrease WBC, neutrophil, and platelet counts.

CONTRAINDICATIONS & CAUTIONS

● Use cautiously in patients with bone marrow suppression induced by previous drug therapy or radiotherapy, impaired hepatic or renal function, previous treatment with anthracyclines or cardiotoxic drugs, or a cardiac condition.

NURSING CONSIDERATIONS

■ **Black Box Warning** Drug should be given only under the supervision of a physician experienced in the use of cancer chemotherapeutic agents. ■

■ **Black Box Warning** Cardiotoxicity is the dose-limiting toxicity of drug. It is more common in those who have received prior anthracyclines or who have preexisting cardiac disease. ■

● Cardiovascular side effects occur with greater frequency in older patients.
● Make sure patient is adequately hydrated before treatment. Hyperuricemia may result from rapid lysis of leukemic cells. Allopurinol may be ordered.
● Assess patient for systemic infection and ensure that it's controlled before therapy begins.
● Give antiemetics to prevent or treat nausea and vomiting.

Reactions may be *common*, uncommon, *life-threatening*, or COMMON AND LIFE-THREATENING.
Interaction may have a *rapid onset* or *delayed onset.*

- Monitor hepatic and renal function tests and CBC frequently.
- To prevent bleeding, avoid all I.M. injections when platelet count is below 50,000/mm³.
- ■ **Black Box Warning** Severe myelosuppression may occur. ■
- Anticipate need for blood transfusions for anemia. Patient may receive injections of RBC colony-stimulating factor to promote RBC production and decrease need for blood transfusions.
- Notify prescriber if signs or symptoms of heart failure occur.
- *Look alike–sound alike:* Don't confuse idarubicin with daunorubicin or doxorubicin.

PATIENT TEACHING
- Teach patient to recognize signs and symptoms of leakage of drug into surrounding tissue, and tell him to report them if they occur.
- Warn patient to watch for signs and symptoms of infection (fever, sore throat, fatigue) and bleeding (easy bruising, nosebleeds, bleeding gums, tarry stools).
- Advise patient that red urine for several days is normal and doesn't indicate presence of blood.
- Caution woman of childbearing age to avoid becoming pregnant during therapy. Recommend that she consult prescriber before becoming pregnant.

SAFETY ALERT!

mitomycin (mitomycin-C)
mye-toe-MYE-sin

Mutamycin

Pharmacologic class: antineoplastic antibiotic
Pregnancy risk category D

AVAILABLE FORMS
Powder for injection: 5-, 20-, 40-mg vials

INDICATIONS & DOSAGES
Dosage and indications vary. Check treatment protocol with prescriber.
➤ **Disseminated adenocarcinoma of stomach or pancreas**

Adults: 20 mg/m² as an I.V. single dose. Repeat cycle at 15 mg/m² after 6 to 8 weeks when WBC and platelet counts have returned to normal.
Adjust-a-dose: For patients with myelosuppression, if leukocytes are 2,000 to 2,999/mm³ and platelets are 25,000 to 74,999/mm³, give 70% of initial dose. If leukocytes are less than 2,000/mm³ and platelets are less than 25,000/mm³, give 50% of initial dose.

ADMINISTRATION
I.V.
- Preparing and giving drug may be mutagenic, teratogenic, or carcinogenic. Follow institutional policy to reduce risks.
- Using sterile water for injection, reconstitute drug in 5-mg vials with 10 ml, 20-mg vials with 40 ml, and 40-mg vials with 80 ml.
- Give drug into the side arm of a free-flowing I.V.
- When reconstituted with sterile water, solution is stable for 14 days under refrigeration and 7 days at room temperature. When diluted, drug is stable in D₅W for no more than 4 hours, normal saline solution for no more than 48 hours, sodium lactate for no more than 24 hours.
- The combination of mitomycin (5 to 15 mg) and heparin (1,000 to 10,000 units) in 30 ml normal saline solution is stable for 72 hours at room temperature.
- Stop infusion immediately and notify prescriber if extravasation occurs because of potential for severe ulceration and necrosis.
- **Incompatibilities:** Aztreonam, bleomycin, cefepime, etoposide, filgrastim, gemcitabine, piperacillin sodium-tazobactam sodium, sargramostim, topotecan, vinorelbine.

ACTION
Similar to an alkylating drug, cross-linking strands of DNA and causing an imbalance of cell growth, leading to cell death.

Route	Onset	Peak	Duration
I.V.	Unknown	Unknown	Unknown

Half-life: About 50 minutes.

ADVERSE REACTIONS
CNS: headache, neurologic abnormalities, confusion, drowsiness, fatigue, *fever,* pain.
EENT: blurred vision.
GI: mucositis, *nausea, vomiting, anorexia, diarrhea, stomatitis.*
GU: *renal toxicity, hemolytic uremic syndrome.*
Hematologic: THROMBOCYTOPENIA, LEUKOPENIA, *microangiopathic hemolytic anemia.*
Respiratory: *interstitial pneumonitis, pulmonary edema,* dyspnea, nonproductive cough, *acute respiratory distress syndrome.*
Skin: cellulitis, induration, desquamation, pruritus, *pain at injection site, reversible alopecia,* purple bands on nails, rash, sloughing with extravasation.
Other: *septicemia,* ulceration.

INTERACTIONS
Drug-drug. *Vinca alkaloids:* May cause acute respiratory distress when given together. Monitor patient closely.

EFFECTS ON LAB TEST RESULTS
• May increase BUN and creatinine levels. May decrease hemoglobin level.
• May decrease WBC and platelet counts.

CONTRAINDICATIONS & CAUTIONS
• Contraindicated in patients hypersensitive to drug and in those with thrombocytopenia, coagulation disorders, or an increased bleeding tendency from other causes.

NURSING CONSIDERATIONS
■ **Black Box Warning** Administer drug under the supervision of a physician experienced with cancer chemotherapeutic agents. ■
• Never give drug I.M. or subcutaneously.
■ **Black Box Warning** Bone marrow suppression is the most common and severe toxic effect. ■
• Continue CBC and blood studies at least 8 weeks after therapy stops. Leukopenia and thrombocytopenia are cumulative. If WBC count falls below 2,000/mm^3 or granulocyte count falls below 1,000/mm^3, follow institutional policy for infection control in immunocompromised patients.
• To prevent bleeding, avoid all I.M. injections when platelet count is less than 100,000/mm^3.

• Anticipate need for blood transfusions to combat anemia. Patients may receive injections of RBC colony-stimulating factor to promote RBC production and to decrease need for blood transfusions.
• Monitor patient for dyspnea with nonproductive cough; chest X-ray may show infiltrates.
• Monitor renal function tests.
• Leukopenia may occur up to 8 weeks after therapy and may be cumulative with successive doses.
■ **Black Box Warning** Hemolytic uremic syndrome is characterized by microangiopathic hemolytic anemia, thrombocytopenia, and renal failure. ■

PATIENT TEACHING
• Advise patient to report any pain or burning at site of injection during or after administration.
• Warn patient to watch for signs and symptoms of infection (fever, sore throat, fatigue) and bleeding (easy bruising, nosebleeds, bleeding gums, tarry stools). Tell patient to take temperature daily.
• Inform patient that hair loss may occur but that it's usually reversible.

Reactions may be *common,* uncommon, *life-threatening,* or COMMON AND LIFE-THREATENING.
Interaction may have a *rapid onset* or *delayed onset.*

82

Antimetabolites

capecitabine
cytarabine
fludarabine phosphate
fluorouracil
gemcitabine hydrochloride
hydroxyurea
mercaptopurine
methotrexate
methotrexate sodium
pemetrexed

SAFETY ALERT!

capecitabine
kap-ah-SEAT-ah-been

Xeloda

Pharmacologic class: pyrimidine
analog
Pregnancy risk category D

AVAILABLE FORMS
Tablets: 150 mg, 500 mg

INDICATIONS & DOSAGES
➤ **With docetaxel or alone, meta-static breast cancer resistant to both paclitaxel and an anthracycline-containing chemotherapy regimen or resistant to paclitaxel in patients for whom further anthracycline therapy isn't indicated; first-line treatment of metastatic colorectal cancer when fluoropyrimidine therapy alone is preferred; Duke stage C colon cancer after complete resection of primary tumor when fluoropyrimidine alone is preferred**
Adults: 2,500 mg/m² daily P.O., in two divided doses, about 12 hours apart and after a meal, for 2 weeks, followed by a 1-week rest period; repeat every 3 weeks. Adjuvant treatment in patients with Duke C colon cancer is recommended for a total of 6 months.

Adjust-a-dose: Follow National Cancer Institute of Canada (NCIC) common toxicity criteria when adjusting dosage.

Toxicity criteria relate to degrees of severity of diarrhea, nausea, vomiting, stomatitis, and hand-and-foot syndrome. Refer to drug package insert for specific toxicity definitions. NCIC grade 1: Maintain dose level. NCIC grade 2: At first appearance, stop treatment until resolved to grade 0 to 1; then restart at 100% of starting dose for next cycle. At second appearance, stop treatment until resolved to grade 0 to 1 and use 75% of starting dose for next cycle. At third appearance, stop treatment until resolved to grade 0 to 1 and use 50% of starting dose for next cycle. At fourth appearance, stop treatment permanently. NCIC grade 3: At first appearance, stop treatment until resolved to grade 0 to 1 and use 75% of starting dose for next cycle. At second appearance, stop treatment until resolved to grade 0 to 1 and use 50% of starting dose for next cycle. At third appearance, stop treatment permanently. NCIC grade 4: At first appearance, stop treatment permanently or until resolved to grade 0 to 1, and use 50% of starting dose for next cycle. Reduce starting dose for patients with creatinine clearance 30 to 50 ml/minute to 75% of the starting dose.

ADMINISTRATION
P.O.
● Give drug with water within 30 minutes after breakfast and dinner.

ACTION
Converted to active 5-fluorouracil (5-FU), which causes cellular injury by interfering with DNA synthesis to inhibit cell division and with RNA processing and protein synthesis.

Route	Onset	Peak	Duration
P.O.	Unknown	90–120 min	Unknown

Half-life: About 45 minutes.

ADVERSE REACTIONS
CNS: dizziness, *fatigue,* headache, insomnia, *paresthesia, pyrexia, fever,* lethargy, *peripheral neuropathy.*

CV: edema, chest pain, **venous thrombosis.**
EENT: *eye irritation,* epistaxis, *increased lacrimation,* rhinorrhea.
GI: *diarrhea, nausea, vomiting, stomatitis, abdominal pain, constipation, anorexia, dyspepsia,* taste perversion.
Hematologic: NEUTROPENIA, **thrombocytopenia,** anemia, **lymphopenia.**
Metabolic: dehydration.
Musculoskeletal: myalgia, limb pain, *back pain.*
Respiratory: *dyspnea.*
Skin: *hand-foot syndrome, dermatitis,* nail disorder, alopecia, *rash.*

INTERACTIONS
Drug-drug. *Antacids containing aluminum hydroxide and magnesium hydroxide:* May increase exposure to capecitabine and its metabolites. Monitor patient.
Leucovorin: May increase cytotoxic effects of 5-FU with enhanced toxicity. Monitor patient carefully.
Phenytoin: May increase toxicity or phenytoin effect. Monitor phenytoin level.
■ **Black Box Warning** *Warfarin:* May decrease clearance of warfarin and increase risk of bleeding. Monitor PT and INR. ■

EFFECTS ON LAB TEST RESULTS
• May increase bilirubin level. May decrease hemoglobin level.
• May decrease neutrophil, platelet, and WBC counts.

CONTRAINDICATIONS & CAUTIONS
• Contraindicated in patients hypersensitive to 5-FU, patients with known dihydropyrimidine dehydrogenase deficiency, and in those with severe renal impairment.
• Use cautiously in elderly patients and those with history of coronary artery disease, mild to moderate hepatic dysfunction from liver metastases, hyperbilirubinemia, and renal insufficiency. Also, use cautiously in patients also taking warfarin.

NURSING CONSIDERATIONS
• Patients older than age 80 may have a greater risk of adverse GI effects.
• Assess patient for severe diarrhea, and notify prescriber if it occurs. Give fluid and electrolyte replacement if patient becomes dehydrated. Drug may need to be immediately interrupted until diarrhea resolves or becomes less intense.
• Monitor patient for hand-foot syndrome (numbness, paresthesia, painless or painful swelling, erythema, desquamation, blistering, and severe pain of hands or feet), hyperbilirubinemia, and severe nausea. Drug therapy must be immediately adjusted. Hand-foot syndrome is staged from 1 to 4; drug may be stopped if severe or recurrent episodes occur.
• Hyperbilirubinemia may require stopping drug.
■ **Black Box Warning** Frequently monitor the INR and PT of patients also taking capecitabine and oral coumarin-derivative anticoagulant therapy; adjust anticoagulant dose accordingly. ■
• **Alert:** Monitor patient carefully for toxicity, which may be managed by symptomatic treatment, dose interruptions, and dosage adjustments.

PATIENT TEACHING
• Tell patient how to take drug. Drug is usually taken for 14 days, followed by 7-day rest period (no drug), as a 21-day cycle. Prescriber determines number of treatment cycles.
• Instruct patient to take drug with water within 30 minutes after breakfast and dinner.
• If a combination of tablets is prescribed, teach patient importance of correctly identifying the tablets to avoid possible dosing error.
• For missed doses, instruct patient not to take the missed dose and not to double the next one. Instead, he should continue with regular dosing schedule and check with prescriber.
• Instruct patient to inform prescriber if he's taking folic acid.
• Inform patient and caregiver about expected adverse effects of drug, especially nausea, vomiting, diarrhea, and hand-foot syndrome (pain, swelling, or redness of hands or feet). Tell him that patient-specific dose adaptations during therapy are expected and needed.
• **Alert:** Instruct patient to stop taking drug and contact prescriber immediately if he develops diarrhea (more than four bowel movements daily or diarrhea at night), vomiting (two to five episodes in 24 hours),

---

Reactions may be *common,* uncommon, *life-threatening,* or COMMON AND LIFE-THREATENING.
Interaction may have a *rapid onset* or **delayed onset.**

nausea, appetite loss or decrease in amount of food eaten each day, stomatitis (pain, redness, swelling or sores in mouth), hand-foot syndrome, temperature of 100.5° F (38° C) or higher, or other evidence of infection.

• Tell patient that most adverse effects improve within 2 to 3 days after stopping drug. If patient doesn't improve, tell him to contact prescriber.

• Advise woman of childbearing age to avoid becoming pregnant during therapy.

• Advise breast-feeding woman to stop breast-feeding during therapy.

SAFETY ALERT!

cytarabine (ara-C, cytosine arabinoside)
sye-TARE-a-been

Cytosar†, Cytosar-U, DepoCyt, Tarabine PFS

Pharmacologic class: pyrimidine analog
Pregnancy risk category D

AVAILABLE FORMS
Injection: 20 mg/ml, 100 mg/ml
Liposomal injection: 10 mg/ml
Powder for injection: 100-mg, 500-mg, 1-g, 2-g vials

INDICATIONS & DOSAGES
➤ **Acute nonlymphocytic leukemia**
Adults and children: 100 mg/m² I.V. daily by continuous I.V. infusion or in two divided doses by rapid I.V. injection or I.V. infusion for 5 to 10 days in a course of therapy or daily until remission is attained.
➤ **Acute lymphocytic leukemia**
Consult literature for current recommendations.
➤ **Meningeal leukemia**
Adults and children: Varies from 5 to 75 mg/m² intrathecally. Frequency varies from once daily for 4 days to once every 2 to 7 days. The most frequently used dose is 30 mg/m² every 4 days until CSF fluid is normal; then one additional dose.
➤ **Lymphomatous meningitis**
Adults: For induction, give 50 mg liposomal injection intrathecally every

14 days for two doses (weeks 1 and 3); then, for consolidation therapy, give 50 mg liposomal injection intrathecally every 14 days for three doses (weeks 5, 7, and 9) followed by one additional dose at week 13. Maintenance dose, 50 mg liposomal injection intrathecally every 28 days for four doses (weeks 17, 21, 25, and 29).
Adjust-a-dose: For patients with neurotoxicity, reduce dose to 25 mg. If neurotoxicity persists, stop therapy.

ADMINISTRATION
I.V.
• Preparing and giving parenteral drug may be mutagenic, teratogenic, or carcinogenic. Follow facility policy to reduce risks.
• To reduce nausea, give antiemetic before drug. Nausea and vomiting are more likely with large doses given by I.V. push. Dizziness may occur with rapid infusion.
• Except for neonates or intrathecal use, reconstitute drug using the provided diluent, which is bacteriostatic water for injection containing benzyl alcohol.
• Reconstitute 100-mg vial with 5 ml of diluent, 500-mg or 1 g vials with 10 ml of diluent or 2 g vial with 20 ml of diluent.
• Discard cloudy reconstituted solution.
• For I.V. infusion, further dilute using normal saline solution for injection or D₅W.
• Reconstituted solution is stable for 48 hours.
• **Incompatibilities:** Allopurinol sodium, amphotericin B cholesteryl sulfate complex, fluorouracil, ganciclovir sodium, heparin sodium, hydrocortisone sodium succinate, insulin, methylprednisolone sodium succinate, nafcillin, oxacillin, penicillin.
I.M.
• Preparing and giving parenteral drug may be mutagenic, teratogenic, or carcinogenic. Follow facility policy to reduce risks.
Subcutaneous
• Preparing and giving parenteral drug may be mutagenic, teratogenic, or carcinogenic. Follow facility policy to reduce risks.

Intrathecal
■ **Black Box Warning** Give with dexamethasone to help decrease the symptoms of chemical arachnoiditis, which may be life-threatening. ■

• For intrathecal administration, use preservative-free normal saline solution. Use immediately after reconstitution. Discard unused drug.
• Withdraw intrathecal cytarabine liposome injection from the vial immediately before administration. It is a single-use vial, doesn't contain any preservative, and should be used within 4 hours of withdrawal from the vial. Discard unused portions of each vial properly.
• Don't use in-line filters when giving intrathecal cytarabine liposome injection.
• After drug administration by lumbar puncture, instruct patient to lie flat for 1 hour.
• Patients should be observed by the physician for immediate toxic reactions.
• Refrigerate liposomal form at 36° to 46° F (2° to 8° C).

ACTION
Inhibits DNA synthesis.

Route	Onset	Peak	Duration
I.V., I.M., intrathecal	Unknown	Unknown	Unknown
Subcut.	Unknown	20–60 min	Unknown

Half-life: Initial, 8 minutes; terminal, 1 to 3 hours; in CSF, 2 hours.

ADVERSE REACTIONS
CNS: *neurotoxicity,* malaise, dizziness, headache, cerebellar syndrome, *fever.*
CV: *thrombophlebitis,* edema.
EENT: conjunctivitis.
GI: *nausea, vomiting, diarrhea, anorexia, anal ulceration,* abdominal pain, oral ulcers in 5 to 10 days, projectile vomiting, **bowel necrosis with high doses given by rapid I.V.**
GU: urine retention, renal dysfunction.
Hematologic: *leukopenia,* anemia, reticulocytopenia, **thrombocytopenia,** *megaloblastosis.*
Hepatic: *hepatotoxicity,* jaundice.
Metabolic: hyperuricemia.
Musculoskeletal: myalgia, bone pain.
Respiratory: *pulmonary edema,* shortness of breath, pulmonary hypersensitivity.

Skin: *rash,* pruritus, alopecia, freckling.
Other: flulike syndrome, infection, ***anaphylaxis.***

INTERACTIONS
Drug-drug. *Digoxin, except oral liquid and liquid-filled capsules:* May decrease oral digoxin absorption. Monitor digoxin level closely.
Flucytosine: May decrease flucytosine activity. Avoid using together.
Gentamicin: May decrease activity against *Klebsiella pneumoniae.* Avoid using together.

EFFECTS ON LAB TEST RESULTS
• May increase bilirubin, phosphorus, potassium, and uric acid levels. May decrease hemoglobin level.
• May increase megaloblast count. May decrease platelet, RBC, reticulocyte, and WBC counts.

CONTRAINDICATIONS & CAUTIONS
• Contraindicated in patients hypersensitive to drug and active meningeal infection (liposomal altarabine).
• Use cautiously in patients with hepatic or renal compromise, gout, or myelosuppression.

NURSING CONSIDERATIONS
■ **Black Box Warning** Cytarabine should administered by physicians experienced in cancer chemotherapy. For induction therapy, patients should be treated in a facility with laboratory and supportive resources sufficient to monitor drug tolerance and protect and maintain a patient compromised by drug toxicity. The physician must judge possible benefit to the patient against known toxic effects of cytarabine. ■
• Monitor fluid intake and output carefully. Maintain high fluid intake and give allopurinol to reduce urate nephropathy in leukemia-induction therapy. Monitor uric acid level.
• Monitor hepatic and renal function studies and CBC.
• Therapy may be modified or stopped if granulocyte count is below 1,000/mm³ or platelet count is below 50,000/mm³.
• Corticosteroid eyedrops help prevent drug-induced conjunctivitis.

Reactions may be *common,* uncommon, *life-threatening,* or COMMON AND LIFE-THREATENING.
Interaction may have a *rapid onset* or **delayed onset.**

• Provide diligent mouth care to help prevent stomatitis.

• *Alert:* Assess patient receiving high doses for neurotoxicity, which may first appear as nystagmus but can progress to ataxia and cerebellar dysfunction.

• To prevent bleeding, avoid all I.M. injections when platelet count is below 50,000/mm³.

• Anticipate blood transfusions because of cumulative anemia. Patient may receive RBC colony-stimulating factors to promote RBC production and decrease need for blood transfusions.

■ **Black Box Warning** Monitor patient for toxic effects, including bone marrow suppression, nausea, vomiting, diarrhea, oral ulceration and hepatic dysfunction. ■

• In leukopenia, initial WBC count nadir occurs 7 to 9 days after drug is stopped. A second, more severe nadir occurs 15 to 24 days after drug is stopped. In thrombocytopenia, platelet count nadir occurs on days 12 to 15.

• *Alert:* A cytarabine syndrome has been described and is characterized by fever, myalgia, bone pain, occasionally chest pain, maculopapular rash, conjunctivitis, and malaise. It usually occurs 6 to 12 hours following drug administration. Corticosteroids have been shown to be beneficial in the treatment or prevention of this syndrome.

• *Look alike–sound alike:* Do not confuse conventional cytarabine with liposomal cytarabine.

PATIENT TEACHING
• Instruct patient to watch for signs and symptoms of infection (fever, sore throat, fatigue) and bleeding (easy bruising, nosebleeds, bleeding gums, tarry stools). Tell patient to take temperature daily.

• Advise patient to report visual changes, blurred vision, or eye pain to prescriber.

• Advise breast-feeding woman to stop breast-feeding during therapy because of risk of toxicity to infant.

• Caution woman of childbearing age to consult prescriber before becoming pregnant because drug may harm fetus.

fludarabine phosphate
floo-DAR-a-been

Fludara

Pharmacologic class: purine analog
Pregnancy risk category D

AVAILABLE FORMS
Liquid for injection: 50 mg/2 ml
Powder for injection: 50 mg

INDICATIONS & DOSAGES
➤ **B-cell chronic lymphocytic leukemia in patients with no or inadequate response to at least one standard alkylating drug regimen**
Adults: 25 mg/m² I.V. daily over 30 minutes for 5 consecutive days. Repeat cycle every 28 days.
Adjust-a-dose: In patients with creatinine clearance of 30 to 70 ml/minute, decrease dose by 20%. Don't use drug in patients with clearance less than 30 ml/minute.

ADMINISTRATION
I.V.
• Preparing and giving parenteral drug may be mutagenic, teratogenic, or carcinogenic. Follow facility policy to reduce risks.

• To prepare, add 2 ml of sterile water for injection to the vial. If using powder for injection, dissolution should occur within 15 seconds.

• Each milliliter contains 25 mg of drug.

• Dilute further in 100 or 125 ml of D_5W or normal saline solution for injection.

• Use within 8 hours of reconstitution.

• Store drug in refrigerator at 36° to 46° F (2° to 8° C).

• **Incompatibilities:** Acyclovir sodium, amphotericin B, chlorpromazine, daunorubicin, ganciclovir, hydroxyzine hydrochloride, prochlorperazine edisylate.

ACTION
Unknown. After conversion to its active metabolite, drug interferes with DNA synthesis by inhibiting DNA polymerase alpha, ribonucleotide reductase, and DNA primase.

Route	Onset	Peak	Duration
I.V.	Unknown	Unknown	Unknown

Half-life: About 10 hours.

ADVERSE REACTIONS

CNS: *fatigue, malaise, weakness, paresthesia,* peripheral neuropathy, **stroke,** headache, sleep disorder, depression, cerebellar syndrome, **transient ischemic attack,** agitation, *confusion, fever,* **coma,** *pain.*

CV: *edema,* angina, phlebitis, **arrhythmias, heart failure, MI,** supraventricular tachycardia, **deep vein thrombosis, aneurysm, hemorrhage.**

EENT: *visual disturbances,* hearing loss, delayed blindness, sinusitis, pharyngitis, epistaxis.

GI: *nausea, vomiting, diarrhea,* constipation, *anorexia,* stomatitis, **GI bleeding,** esophagitis, mucositis.

GU: dysuria, *UTI,* urinary hesitancy, proteinuria, hematuria, **renal failure.**

Hematologic: hemolytic anemia, MYELOSUPPRESSION.

Hepatic: *liver failure,* cholelithiasis.

Metabolic: hypocalcemia, hyperkalemia, hyperglycemia, dehydration, hyperuricemia, hyperphosphatemia.

Musculoskeletal: *myalgia.*

Respiratory: *cough, pneumonia, dyspnea, upper respiratory tract infection,* allergic pneumonia, hemoptysis, hypoxia, bronchitis.

Skin: *rash,* pruritus, alopecia, seborrhea, diaphoresis.

Other: *chills,* **tumor lysis syndrome,** INFECTION, **anaphylaxis.**

INTERACTIONS

Drug-drug. *Cytarabine:* May decrease metabolism of subsequently given fludarabine and inhibition of fludarabine activity. Monitor patient closely.

Myelosuppressives: May increase toxicity. Avoid using together, if possible.

■ **Black Box Warning** *Pentostatin:* May increase risk of pulmonary toxicity, which can be fatal. Avoid using together. ■

EFFECTS ON LAB TEST RESULTS

● May increase glucose, phosphate, potassium, and uric acid levels.

● May decrease calcium and hemoglobin levels. May decrease platelet, RBC, and WBC counts.

CONTRAINDICATIONS & CAUTIONS

● Contraindicated in patients hypersensitive to drug or its components and in those with creatinine clearance less than 30 ml/minute.

● Use cautiously in patients with renal insufficiency.

NURSING CONSIDERATIONS

■ **Black Box Warning** Administer under the supervision of a physician experienced in the use of antineoplastic therapy. ■

● *Alert:* Monitor patient closely and expect modified dosage based on toxicity. Most toxic effects are dose dependent. Advanced age, renal insufficiency, and bone marrow impairment may predispose patients to increased or excessive toxicity.

■ **Black Box Warning** Careful hematologic monitoring is needed, especially of neutrophil and platelet counts. Bone marrow suppression can be severe. ■

■ **Black Box Warning** Monitor patient for development of hemolytic anemia. ■

● Severe and fatal neurotoxicity may occur.

● To prevent bleeding, avoid all I.M. injections when platelet count is below 50,000/mm^3.

● Give blood transfusions because of cumulative anemia. Patient may receive RBC colony-stimulating factors to promote RBC production and decrease need for blood transfusions.

● Hyperuricemia, hypocalcemia, hyperkalemia, and renal failure may result from rapid lysis of tumor cells. Take preventative measures against tumor lysis syndrome, such as I.V. hydration, alkalinization of urine, and treatment with allopurinol as appropriate.

● *Look alike–sound alike:* Don't confuse fludarabine with floxuridine, fluorouracil, or flucytosine.

PATIENT TEACHING

● Instruct patient to watch for signs and symptoms of infection (fever, sore throat, fatigue) and bleeding (easy bruising, nosebleeds, bleeding gums, tarry stools). Tell patient to take temperature daily.

Reactions may be *common,* uncommon, *life-threatening,* or COMMON AND LIFE-THREATENING.
Interaction may have a *rapid onset* or **delayed onset.**

- Advise woman to consult prescriber before becoming pregnant.
- Caution woman to stop breast-feeding during therapy because of risk of toxicity to infant.

fluorouracil (5-fluorouracil, 5-FU)
flure-oh-YOOR-a-sill

Carac, Efudex, Fluoroplex

Pharmacologic class: pyrimidine analog
Pregnancy risk category D (injection); X (topical form)

AVAILABLE FORMS
Cream: 0.5%, 1%, 5%
Injection: 50 mg/ml
Topical solution: 2%, 5%

INDICATIONS & DOSAGES
➤ **Colon, rectal, breast, stomach, and pancreatic cancers**
Adults: Initially, 12 mg/kg I.V. daily for 4 days (daily dose shouldn't exceed 800 mg); if no toxicity, give 6 mg/kg on days 6, 8, 10, and 12; then give a single weekly maintenance dose of 10 to 15 mg/kg I.V. begun after toxicity (if any) from first course has subsided. (Recommended dosages are based on actual body weight unless patient is obese or retaining fluid.).
➤ **Palliative treatment of advanced colorectal cancer**
Adults: 425 mg/m^2 I.V. daily for 5 consecutive days. Give with 20 mg/m^2 of leucovorin I.V. Repeat at 4-week intervals for two additional courses; then repeat at 4- to 5-week intervals, if tolerated.
➤ **Early breast cancer**
Adults: 600 mg/m^2 I.V. on days 1 and 8 of each cycle, combined with cyclo-phosphamide 100 mg/m^2 on days 1 through 14 of each cycle and methotrexate 40 mg/m^2 on days 1 and 8 of each cycle. Repeat monthly for 6 to 12 months, allowing for a 2-week rest period between cycles. In adults older than age 60, first

fluorouracil dose is 400 mg/m^2 and methotrexate dose is 30 mg/m^2.
➤ **Multiple actinic (solar) keratoses**
Adults: Apply Carac cream once daily for up to 4 weeks. Or, apply Efudex or Fluoroplex cream or topical solution b.i.d. for 2 to 6 weeks.
➤ **Superficial basal cell carcinoma**
Adults: Apply 5% Efudex cream or topical solution b.i.d. usually for 3 to 6 weeks; maximum, 12 weeks.

ADMINISTRATION
I.V.
- Preparing and giving parenteral drug may be mutagenic, teratogenic, or carcinogenic. Follow facility policy to reduce risks.
- To reduce nausea, give antiemetic before fluorouracil.
- Don't use cloudy solution. If crystals form, redissolve by warming.
- Drug may be given by direct injection without dilution.
- For infusion, dilute drug with D$_5$W, sterile water for injection, or normal saline solution for injection.
- For continuous infusion, use plastic I.V. containers. Solution is more stable in plastic than in glass bottles.
- Don't refrigerate. Protect drug from sunlight.
- Discard unused portion of vial after 1 hour.
- **Incompatibilities:** Aldesleukin, amphotericin B cholesterol complex, carboplatin, cisplatin, cytarabine, diazepam, doxorubicin, droperidol, epirubicin, fentanyl citrate, filgrastim, gallium nitrate, leucovorin calcium, metoclopramide, morphine sulfate, ondansetron, topotecan, vinorelbine tartrate.
Topical
- Apply topical form cautiously near patient's eyes, nose, and mouth.
- Avoid occlusive dressings with topical form because they increase risk of inflammatory reactions in adjacent normal skin.
- Apply topical form with nonmetal applicator or suitable gloves. Wash hands immediately after handling topical form.
- The 1% topical strength is used on patient's face. Higher strengths, such as 5%, are used for thicker skinned areas or resistant lesions, such as superficial basal cell carcinoma.

ACTION

May interfere with DNA and RNA synthesis, leading to a thymine deficiency that provokes unbalanced growth and death of the cell.

Route	Onset	Peak	Duration
I.V., topical	Unknown	Unknown	Unknown

Half-life: 20 minutes.

ADVERSE REACTIONS

CNS: acute cerebellar syndrome, confusion, disorientation, euphoria, ataxia, headache, *weakness, malaise.*
CV: *myocardial ischemia,* angina, thrombophlebitis.
EENT: epistaxis, photophobia, lacrimation, lacrimal duct stenosis, nystagmus, visual changes, eye irritation.
GI: *stomatitis, GI ulcer, nausea, vomiting, diarrhea, anorexia, GI bleeding.*
Hematologic: *leukopenia, thrombocytopenia, agranulocytosis, anemia.*
Skin: *dermatitis, erythema, scaling, pruritus,* nail changes, pigmented palmar creases, erythematous contact dermatitis, desquamative rash of hands and feet, hand-foot syndrome with long-term use, photosensitivity reactions, *reversible alopecia, pain, burning,* soreness, suppuration, *swelling, dryness, erosion* with topical use.
Other: *anaphylaxis.*

INTERACTIONS

Drug-drug. *Leucovorin calcium:* May increase cytotoxicity and toxicity of fluorouracil. Monitor patient closely.
Drug-lifestyle. *Sun exposure:* May cause photosensitivity reactions. Advise patient to avoid excessive sunlight exposure.

EFFECTS ON LAB TEST RESULTS

• May increase alkaline phosphatase, AST, ALT, bilirubin, 5-hydroxyindoleacetic acid (in urine), and LDH levels. May decrease hemoglobin and plasma albumin levels.
• May decrease granulocyte, platelet, RBC, and WBC counts.

CONTRAINDICATIONS & CAUTIONS

• Contraindicated in patients hypersensitive to drug and in those with bone marrow suppression (WBC counts of 5,000/mm^3 or less or platelet counts of 100,000/mm^3 or less) or potentially serious infections.
• Contraindicated in patients in a poor nutritional state and those who have had major surgery within previous month.
• Topical formulations contraindicated in pregnant women.
• Use cautiously in patients who have received high-dose pelvic radiation or alkylating drugs and in those with impaired hepatic or renal function or widespread neoplastic infiltration of bone marrow.

NURSING CONSIDERATIONS

■ **Black Box Warning** Drug should be administered under the supervision of a physician experienced in cancer chemotherapy. ■
■ **Black Box Warning** Patient should be hospitalized at least during the initial course of therapy. ■
• Ingestion and systemic absorption of topical form may cause leukopenia, thrombocytopenia, stomatitis, diarrhea, or GI ulceration, bleeding, and hemorrhage. Application to large ulcerated areas may cause systemic toxicity.
• Watch for stomatitis or diarrhea (signs of toxicity). Consider using topical oral anesthetic to soothe lesions. Stop drug and notify prescriber if diarrhea occurs.
• Encourage diligent oral hygiene to prevent superinfection of denuded mucosa.
• Monitor WBC and platelet counts. WBC counts with differential are recommended before each dose. Watch for ecchymoses, petechiae, easy bruising, and anemia.
• Monitor fluid intake and output, CBC, and renal and hepatic function tests.
• Long-term use may cause erythematous, desquamative rash of the hands and feet, which may be treated with pyridoxine 50 to 150 mg P.O. daily for 5 to 7 days.
• Dermatologic adverse effects are reversible when drug is stopped.
• To prevent bleeding, avoid I.M. injections when platelet count is below 50,000/mm^3.
• Anticipate blood transfusions because of cumulative anemia. Patient may receive injections of RBC colony-stimulating factors to promote RBC production and decrease need for blood transfusions.
• *Alert:* Toxicity may be delayed for 1 to 3 weeks.

Reactions may be *common,* uncommon, *life-threatening,* or COMMON AND LIFE-THREATENING.
Interaction may have a *rapid onset* or *delayed onset.*

• The WBC count nadir occurs 9 to 14 days after first dose; the platelet count nadir occurs in 7 to 14 days.

• *Look alike–sound alike:* Drug may be ordered as "5-fluorouracil" or "5-FU." The numeral "5" is part of the drug name and shouldn't be confused with dosage units.

• *Look alike–sound alike:* Don't confuse fluorouracil with floxuridine, fludarabine, or flucytosine.

PATIENT TEACHING
• Warn patient that hair loss may occur but is reversible.

• Caution patient to avoid prolonged exposure to sunlight or ultraviolet light when topical form is used.

• Tell patient to use highly protective sunblock to avoid inflammatory skin irritation.

• Warn patient that topically treated area may be unsightly during therapy and for several weeks afterward. Complete healing may take 1 or 2 months.

• Caution woman of childbearing age to consult prescriber before becoming pregnant.

• Advise woman to stop breast-feeding during therapy because of risk of toxicity to infant.

SAFETY ALERT!

gemcitabine hydrochloride
jem-SITE-ah-been

Gemzar

Pharmacologic class: pyrimidine analog
Pregnancy risk category D

AVAILABLE FORMS
Powder for injection: 200-mg, 1-g vials

INDICATIONS & DOSAGES
➤ **Locally advanced or metastatic adenocarcinoma of pancreas**
Adults: 1,000 mg/m² I.V. over 30 minutes once weekly for up to 7 weeks, unless toxicity occurs. Monitor CBC with differential and platelet count before giving each dose.

Adjust-a-dose: If bone marrow suppression is detected, adjust therapy. If absolute granulocyte count (AGC) is 1,000/mm³ or more and platelet count is 100,000/mm³ or more, give full dose. If AGC is 500 to 999/mm³ or platelet count is 50,000 to 99,999/mm³, give 75% of dose. If AGC is below 500/mm³ or platelet count is below 50,000/mm³, withhold dose. Course of 7 weeks is followed by 1 week of rest. Subsequent dosage cycles consist of one infusion weekly for 3 of 4 consecutive weeks. Dosage adjustments for subsequent cycles are based on AGC and platelet count nadirs and degree of nonhematologic toxicity.

➤ **With cisplatin, first-line treatment of inoperable, locally advanced, or metastatic non–small-cell lung cancer**
Adults: For 4-week schedule, 1,000 mg/m² I.V. over 30 minutes on days 1, 8, and 15 of each 28-day cycle. 100 mg/m² cisplatin on day 1 after gemcitabine infusion.

For 3-week schedule, 1,250 mg/m² I.V. over 30 minutes on days 1 and 8 of each 21-day cycle. 100 mg/m² cisplatin on day 1 after gemcitabine infusion.

➤ **With carboplatin, for treatment of advanced ovarian cancer that relapsed at least 6 months after platinum-based therapy**
Adults: 1,000 mg/m²I.V. over 30 minutes on days 1 and 8 of each 21-day cycle. Give carboplatin AUC 4 I.V. on day 1 after gemcitabine. Check CBC with differential and platelet count before each dose. The AGC should be 1,500/mm³ or higher and platelet count 100,000/mm³ or higher before each cycle.

Adjust-a-dose: Base adjustment on AGC and platelet count results on day 8 of cycle. If AGC is 1,000 to 1,499/mm³, give 50% of dose. If AGC is below 1,000/mm³or platelet count is below 75,000/mm³, hold dose. Adjustments for subsequent cycles based on observed toxicities.

➤ **With paclitaxel, first-line therapy for metastatic breast cancer after failure of other adjuvant chemotherapy with an anthracycline**
Adults: 1,250 mg/m² I.V. over 30 minutes on days 1 and 8 of each 21-day cycle,

with 175 mg/m^2 paclitaxel I.V. as a 3-hour infusion given before gemcitabine dose on day 1 of the cycle. Adjust dosage based on total AGC and platelet counts taken on day 8 of the cycle.

Adjust-a-dose: If AGC is 1,000 to 1,199/mm^3 or platelet count is 50,000 to 75,000/mm^3, give 75% of dose. If AGC is 700 to 999/mm^3 and platelet count is 50,000/mm^3 or above, give 50% of dose. If AGC is below 700/mm^3 or platelet count is below 50,000/mm^3, withhold dose.

ADMINISTRATION
I.V.
• Preparing and giving parenteral drug may be mutagenic, teratogenic, or carcinogenic. Follow facility policy to reduce risks.
• To prepare solution, add 5 ml of unpreserved normal saline solution for injection to 200-mg vial or 25 ml to 1-g vial. Shake to dissolve.
• Resulting concentration is 40 mg/ml; reconstitution at higher concentrations isn't recommended.
• If needed, dilute to as little as 0.1 mg/ml by adding normal saline solution for injection.
• Make sure solution is clear to light straw-colored and free of particles.
• Don't extend infusion time beyond 60 minutes or give drug more often than once weekly; doing so may increase toxicity.
• Drug is stable 24 hours at room temperature.
• Don't refrigerate reconstituted drug because it may crystallize.
• **Incompatibilities:** Acyclovir, amphotericin B, cefoperazone, cefotaxime, furosemide, ganciclovir, imipenem and cilastatin, irinotecan, methotrexate, methylprednisolone, mitomycin, piperacillin, piperacillin and tazobactam sodium, prochlorperazine, sodium succinate.

ACTION
Cytotoxic and specific to cell cycle; inhibits DNA synthesis and blocks progression of cells.

Route	Onset	Peak	Duration
I.V.	Unknown	Unknown	Unknown

Half-life: About 2 to 19½ hours.

ADVERSE REACTIONS
CNS: *somnolence, paresthesia, pain, fever.*
CV: *edema, peripheral edema.*
GI: *stomatitis, nausea, vomiting, constipation, diarrhea.*
GU: *proteinuria, hematuria.*
Hematologic: anemia, **leukopenia, neutropenia, thrombocytopenia.**
Hepatic: **hepatotoxicity.**
Respiratory: *dyspnea,* **bronchospasm, pneumonitis.**
Skin: *alopecia, rash,* pain at injection site.
Other: *flulike syndrome, infection.*

INTERACTIONS
Warfarin: May increase the anticoagulant effect of warfarin. Monitor patient and INR.

EFFECTS ON LAB TEST RESULTS
• May increase ALT, AST, BUN, and creatinine levels. May decrease hemoglobin level.
• May decrease neutrophil, platelet, and WBC counts.

CONTRAINDICATIONS & CAUTIONS
• Contraindicated in patients hypersensitive to drug and in pregnant or breast-feeding women.
• Use cautiously in patients with renal or hepatic impairment.
• In children, safety and effectiveness haven't been determined.

NURSING CONSIDERATIONS
• Monitor patient closely. Expect dosage modification according to toxicity and degree of myelosuppression. Age, gender, and presence of renal impairment may predispose patient to toxicity.
• Carefully monitor hematologic values, especially of neutrophil and platelet counts.
• Obtain baseline and periodic renal and hepatic laboratory tests.

PATIENT TEACHING
• Advise patient to watch for evidence of infection (fever, sore throat, fatigue) and bleeding (easy bruising, nosebleeds, bleeding gums, tarry stools). Tell patient to take temperature daily.
• Advise patient to promptly report flulike symptoms or breathing problems.

Reactions may be *common,* uncommon, *life-threatening,* or COMMON AND LIFE-THREATENING.
ᵗnteraction may have a *rapid onset* or **delayed onset.**

• Tell patient that adverse effects may continue after treatment ends.
• Caution woman to avoid pregnancy or breast-feeding during therapy.

hydroxyurea
hye-drox-ee-yoor-EE-a

Droxia, Hydrea

Pharmacologic class:
antimetabolite
Pregnancy risk category D

AVAILABLE FORMS
Capsules: 200 mg, 300 mg, 400 mg, 500 mg

INDICATIONS & DOSAGES
➤ **Melanoma; resistant chronic myelocytic leukemia; recurrent, metastatic, or inoperable ovarian cancer; head and neck cancers**
Adults: 80 mg/kg Hydrea P.O. as single dose every 3 days; or 20 to 30 mg/kg P.O. as single daily dose.
➤ **To reduce frequency of painful crises and need for blood transfusions in adult patients with sickle cell anemia with recurrent moderate to severe painful crises**
Adults: 15 mg/kg Droxia P.O. once daily. If blood counts are in acceptable range, dose may be increased by 5 mg/kg daily every 12 weeks until maximum tolerated dose or 35 mg/kg daily has been reached. If blood counts are considered toxic, withhold drug until counts recover. Resume treatment after reducing dose by 2.5 mg/kg daily. Every 12 weeks, drug may then be adjusted up or down in 2.5-mg/kg daily increments until patient is at a stable, nontoxic dose for 24 weeks.

ADMINISTRATION
P.O.
• Wear gloves when handling drug or its container, and wash hands before and after contact with bottle or capsule. If powder from capsule is spilled, wipe up immediately with a damp towel. Dispose of towel in a closed container such as a plastic bag.

ACTION
May inhibit DNA synthesis.

Route	Onset	Peak	Duration
P.O.	Unknown	2 hr	24 hr

Half-life: 3 to 4 hours.

ADVERSE REACTIONS
CNS: *seizures,* hallucinations, headache, dizziness, disorientation, malaise, fever.
GI: *anorexia, nausea, vomiting, diarrhea,* stomatitis, constipation.
Hematologic: *leukopenia, thrombocytopenia, anemia, megaloblastosis, bone marrow suppression.*
Metabolic: hyperuricemia, weight gain.
Skin: rash, itching, alopecia, cutaneous vasculitic toxicities (including vasculitic ulcerations and gangrene).
Other: chills.

INTERACTIONS
Drug-drug. *Cytotoxic drugs, radiation therapy:* May enhance toxicity of hydroxyurea. Use together cautiously.
Interferon: May increase the risk of cutaneous vasculitic toxicities, including vasculitic ulcerations and gangrene. Stop drug.

EFFECTS ON LAB TEST RESULTS
• May increase BUN, creatinine, hepatic enzyme, and uric acid levels. May decrease hemoglobin level.
• May decrease WBC, RBC, and platelet counts.

CONTRAINDICATIONS & CAUTIONS
• Contraindicated in patients hypersensitive to drug and in those with WBC count less than 2,500/mm^3, platelet count less than 100,000/mm^3, or severe anemia.
• Use cautiously in patients with renal dysfunction and in the elderly.

NURSING CONSIDERATIONS
• Routinely measure BUN, uric acid, liver enzyme, and creatinine levels; monitor blood counts every 2 weeks.
• Acceptable blood counts during dosage adjustment are neutrophil count of 2,500/mm^3 or more, platelet count of 95,000/mm^3 or more, hemoglobin level more than 5.3 g/dl, and reticulocyte count

(if hemoglobin level is below 9 g/dl) at least 95,000/mm³. Toxic levels are neutrophil count less than 2,000/mm³, platelet count less than 80,000/mm³, hemoglobin level less than 4.5 g/dl, and reticulocyte count (if hemoglobin level is below 9 g/dl) less than 80,000/mm³.

• Hydroxyurea may dramatically lower WBC count in 24 to 48 hours.

• *Alert:* Patients who have received or are currently receiving interferon may be at a greater risk for developing cutaneous vasculitic toxicities. Monitor closely.

• Monitor fluid intake and output; keep patient hydrated.

• Allopurinol is used to treat or prevent tumor lysis syndrome.

• To prevent bleeding, avoid all I.M. injections when platelet count is less than 50,000/mm³.

• Give blood transfusions for cumulative anemia. Patient may receive injections of RBC colony-stimulating factors to promote RBC production and decrease need for blood transfusions.

• Dosage change may be needed after chemotherapy or radiation therapy.

• Auditory and visual hallucinations and hematologic toxicity increase when renal function decreases.

• Drug crosses blood-brain barrier.

• Radiation therapy may increase risk or severity of GI distress or stomatitis.

PATIENT TEACHING

• Tell patient and caregiver to wear gloves when handling drug or its container and to wash their hands before and after contact with the bottle or capsule. If powder from capsule is spilled, wipe up immediately with a damp towel and dispose of the towel in a closed container such as a plastic bag.

• Tell patient who can't swallow capsules that he may empty contents into water, drink immediately, and rinse mouth with water afterward. Inform patient that some inert material may not dissolve.

• Advise patient to watch for signs and symptoms of infection (fever, sore throat, fatigue) and bleeding (easy bruising, nosebleeds, bleeding gums, tarry stools). He also should take his temperature daily.

• Caution woman of childbearing age to consult prescriber before becoming pregnant.

mercaptopurine (6-mercaptopurine, 6-MP)
mer-kap-toe-PYOOR-een

Purinethol

Pharmacologic class: purine analogue
Pregnancy risk category D

AVAILABLE FORMS
Tablets (scored): 50 mg

INDICATIONS & DOSAGES
➤ **Acute lymphoblastic leukemia**
Adults and children: 2.5 mg/kg P.O. once daily (rounded to nearest 25 mg). May increase to 5 mg/kg daily after 4 weeks if no improvement.

   After remission is attained, usual maintenance dose for adults and children is 1.5 to 2.5 mg/kg once daily.

ADMINISTRATION
P.O.
• Give total daily dosage at one time, calculated to the nearest multiple of 25 mg.

• If giving allopurinol concurrently, reduce dosage of mercaptopurine to one-third to one-fourth of the usual dose.

ACTION
Inhibits RNA and DNA synthesis.

Route	Onset	Peak	Duration
P.O.	Unknown	Unknown	Unknown

Half-life: Unknown.

ADVERSE REACTIONS
GI: nausea, vomiting, anorexia, painful oral ulcers, diarrhea, *pancreatitis,* GI ulceration.
Hematologic: *leukopenia, thrombo-cytopenia, anemia.*
Hepatic: *jaundice, hepatotoxicity.*
Metabolic: hyperuricemia.
Skin: rash, hyperpigmentation.

INTERACTIONS
Drug-drug. *Allopurinol:* Slows inactivation of mercaptopurine. Decrease mercaptopurine to 25% or 33% of normal dose.

Reactions may be *common,* uncommon, *life-threatening,* or COMMON AND LIFE-THREATENING.
Interaction may have a *rapid onset* or **delayed onset.**

Azathioprine: Increased risk of severe myelosuppression. Avoid giving together.
Co-trimoxazole: May enhance bone marrow suppression. Monitor CBC with differential carefully.
Hepatotoxic drugs: May enhance hepatotoxicity of mercaptopurine. Monitor patient for hepatotoxicity.
Nondepolarizing neuromuscular blockers: May antagonize muscle relaxant effect. Notify anesthesiologist that patient is receiving mercaptopurine.
Warfarin: May decrease or increase anticoagulant effect. Monitor PT and INR.

EFFECTS ON LAB TEST RESULTS
● May increase uric acid, transaminase, alkaline phosphatase, and bilirubin levels. May decrease hemoglobin level.
● May decrease WBC, RBC, and platelet counts.

CONTRAINDICATIONS & CAUTIONS
● Contraindicated in patients resistant or hypersensitive to drug.

NURSING CONSIDERATIONS
■ **Black Box Warning** A diagnosis of acute lymphatic leukemia must be established before starting therapy. The supervising physician must be knowledgeable in assessing response to chemotherapy. ■
● Consider modifying dosage after chemotherapy or radiation therapy in patients who have depressed neutrophil or platelet counts or impaired hepatic or renal function.
● *Alert:* Drug may be ordered as "6-mercaptopurine" or as "6-MP." The numeral 6 is part of drug name and doesn't refer to dosage.
● Monitor CBC and transaminase, alkaline phosphatase, and bilirubin levels weekly during induction and monthly during maintenance.
● Leukopenia, thrombocytopenia, or anemia may persist for several days after drug is stopped.
● Watch for signs of bleeding and infection.
● Monitor fluid intake and output. Encourage 3 L fluid intake daily.
● *Alert:* Watch for jaundice, clay-colored stools, and frothy, dark urine. Hepatic dysfunction is reversible when drug is stopped. If right-sided abdominal tenderness occurs, stop drug and notify prescriber.

● Monitor uric acid level. Use allopurinol cautiously.
● To prevent bleeding, avoid all I.M. injections when platelet count is below 100,000/mm³.
● Anticipate need for blood transfusions because of cumulative anemia. Patient may receive injections of RBC colony-stimulating factors to promote RBC production and decrease need for blood transfusions.
● GI adverse reactions are less common in children than in adults.
● *Look alike–sound alike:* Don't confuse Purinethol and propylthiouracil (PTU). Both are available in 50 mg strengths.

PATIENT TEACHING
● Instruct patient to watch for signs and symptoms of infection (fever, sore throat, fatigue) and bleeding (easy bruising, nosebleeds, bleeding gums, tarry stools). Tell patient to take temperature daily.
● Caution woman of childbearing age to consult prescriber before becoming pregnant.
● Advise woman to stop breast-feeding during therapy because of risk of toxicity to infant.

SAFETY ALERT!

**methotrexate
(amethopterin, MTX)**
meth-oh-TREX-ate

methotrexate sodium
Methotrexate LPF, Rheumatrex, Trexall

Pharmacologic class: folic acid antagonist
Pregnancy risk category X

AVAILABLE FORMS
Injection: 25 mg/ml in 2-ml, 4-ml, 8-ml, 10-ml, 20-ml, and 40-ml preservative-free single-use vials; 25 mg/ml in 2-ml and 10-ml vials containing benzyl alcohol
Lyophilized powder: 1,000-mg vials, preservative-free; 2.5-mg/ml, 25-mg/ml vials
Tablets (scored): 5 mg, 7.5 mg, 10 mg, 15 mg

INDICATIONS & DOSAGES
➤ **Trophoblastic tumors (chorio-carcinoma, hydatidiform mole)**
Adults: 15 to 30 mg P.O. or I.M. daily for 5 days. Repeat after 1 or more weeks, based on response or toxicity. Number of courses is three to maximum of five.

➤ **Acute lymphocytic leukemia**
Adults and children: 3.3 mg/m² daily P.O., I.V., or I.M. with 40 to 60 mg/m² prednisone daily for 4 to 6 weeks or until remission occurs; then 30 mg/m² P.O. or I.M. weekly in two divided doses or 2.5 mg/kg I.V. every 14 days.

➤ **Meningeal leukemia**
Adults and children: 12 mg/m² or less (maximum 15 mg) intrathecally every 2 to 5 days until CSF is normal; then one additional dose. Or, for children, use dosages based on age.
Children age 3 and older: 12 mg intra-thecally every 2 to 5 days.
Children ages 2 to 3: 10 mg intrathecally every 2 to 5 days.
Children ages 1 to 2: 8 mg intrathecally every 2 to 5 days.
Children younger than age 1: 6 mg intrathecally every 2 to 5 days.

➤ **Burkitt lymphoma (stage I, II, or III)**
Adults: 10 to 25 mg P.O. daily for 4 to 8 days, with 1-week rest intervals.

➤ **Lymphosarcoma (stage III)**
Adults: 0.625 to 2.5 mg/kg daily P.O., I.M., or I.V.

➤ **Osteosarcoma**
Adults: Initially, 12 g/m² I.V. as 4-hour infusion. Give subsequent doses 15 g/m² I.V. as 4-hour I.V. infusion at postoperative weeks 4, 5, 6, 7, 11, 12, 15, 16, 29, 30, 44, and 45. Give with leucovorin, 15 mg P.O. every 6 hours for 10 doses, beginning 24 hours after start of methotrexate infusion.

➤ **Breast cancer**
Adults: 40 mg/m² I.V. on days 1 and 8 of each cycle, combined with cyclophos-phamide and fluorouracil.
Adjust-a-dose: In patients older than age 60, give 30 mg/m².

➤ **Mycosis fungoides**
Adults: 2.5 to 10 mg P.O. daily; or 5 to 50 mg I.M. weekly; or 15 to 37.5 mg I.M. twice weekly.

➤ **Psoriasis**
Adults: 10 to 25 mg P.O., I.M., or I.V. as single weekly dose; or 2.5 to 5 mg P.O. every 12 hours for three doses weekly. Dosage shouldn't exceed 30 mg per week.

➤ **Rheumatoid arthritis**
Adults: Initially, 7.5 mg P.O. weekly, either in single dose or divided as 2.5 mg P.O. every 12 hours for three doses once weekly. Dosage may be gradually increased to maximum of 20 mg weekly.

➤ **Poly-articular course JRA**
Children and adolescents age 2 to 16: 10 mg/m² P.O., or I.M. once weekly. Or, 20 to 30 mg/m²/week I.M. or subcutaneously.

➤ **Head and neck carcinomas**
Adults: 40 to 60 mg/m² I.V. weekly. Response to therapy is limited to 4 months.

ADMINISTRATION
P.O.
● Give drug when patient has an empty stomach.
● Tablets may contain lactose. If needed, give with OTC lactose enzyme supplement.
I.V.
● Preparing and giving parenteral drug may be mutagenic, teratogenic, or carcinogenic. Follow facility policy to reduce risks.
● Dilution of drug depends on product, and infusion guidelines vary, depending on dose.
● Reconstitute 20-mg vial to a con-centration no greater than 25 mg/ml. Reconstitute 1-g vial to a concentration of 50 mg/ml.
● If giving infusion, dilute total dose in D₅W.
● Reconstitute solutions without preserva-tives with normal saline solution or D₅W immediately before use, and discard unused drug.
● **Incompatibilities:** Bleomycin, chlor-promazine, droperidol, gemcitabine, idarubicin, ifosfamide, midazolam, nalbuphine, promethazine, propofol.
I.M.
● Preparing and giving parenteral drug may be mutagenic, teratogenic, or carcinogenic. Follow facility policy to reduce risks.
Intrathecal
● Preparing and giving parenteral drug may be mutagenic, teratogenic, or

---

Reactions may be *common*, uncommon, *life-threatening*, or COMMON AND LIFE-THREATENING.
Interaction may have a *rapid onset* or **delayed onset**.

carcinogenic. Follow facility policy to reduce risks.

■ **Black Box Warning** Use preservative-free form for intrathecal administration. ■

ACTION

Reversibly binds to dihydrofolate reductase, blocking reduction of folic acid to tetrahydrofolate, a cofactor necessary for purine, protein, and DNA synthesis.

Route	Onset	Peak	Duration
P.O.	Unknown	1–2 hr	Unknown
I.V.	Immediate	Immediate	Unknown
I.M.	Unknown	30 min–1 hr	Unknown
Intrathecal	Unknown	Unknown	Unknown

Half-life: For doses below 30 mg/m², about 3 to 10 hours; for doses of 30 mg/m² and above, 8 to 15 hours.

ADVERSE REACTIONS

CNS: *arachnoiditis within hours of intrathecal use, leukoencephalopathy, seizures,* subacute neurotoxicity possibly beginning a few weeks later, demyelination, malaise, fatigue, dizziness, headache, aphasia, hemiparesis, fever, drowsiness.

EENT: pharyngitis, blurred vision.

GI: gingivitis, *stomatitis, diarrhea,* abdominal distress, anorexia, GI ulceration and *bleeding,* enteritis, *nausea, vomiting.*

GU: nephropathy, *tubular necrosis, renal failure,* hematuria, menstrual dysfunction, defective spermatogenesis, infertility, abortion, cystitis.

Hematologic: *anemia, leukopenia, thrombocytopenia.*

Hepatic: *acute toxicity, chronic toxicity,* including cirrhosis and *hepatic fibrosis.*

Metabolic: *diabetes,* hyperuricemia.

Musculoskeletal: arthralgia, myalgia, osteoporosis in children on long-term therapy.

Respiratory: *pulmonary fibrosis, pulmonary interstitial infiltrates,* pneumonitis, dry, nonproductive cough.

Skin: *urticaria,* pruritus, hyperpigmentation, erythematous rashes, ecchymoses, rash, photosensitivity reactions, alopecia, acne, psoriatic lesions aggravated by exposure to sun.

Other: chills, reduced resistance to infection, *septicemia, sudden death.*

INTERACTIONS

Drug-drug. *Acitretin:* May increase the risk of hepatitis. Avoid using together.

Acyclovir: Use with intrathecal methotrexate may cause neurologic abnormalities. Monitor patient closely.

Digoxin: May decrease digoxin level. Monitor digoxin level closely.

Folic acid derivatives: Antagonizes methotrexate effect. Avoid using together, except for leucovorin rescue with high-dose methotrexate therapy.

Fosphenytoin, phenytoin: May decrease phenytoin and fosphenytoin levels. Monitor drug levels closely.

Hepatotoxic drugs: May increase risk of hepatotoxicity. Monitor patient closely.

NSAIDs, phenylbutazone, salicylates: May increase methotrexate toxicity. Avoid using together.

Oral antibiotics: May decrease absorption of methotrexate. Monitor patient closely.

Penicillins, sulfonamides, trimethoprim: May increase methotrexate level. Monitor patient for methotrexate toxicity.

Probenecid: May impair excretion of methotrexate, causing increased level, effect, and toxicity of methotrexate. Monitor methotrexate level closely and adjust dosage accordingly.

Procarbazine: May increase risk of nephrotoxicity. Monitor patient closely.

Theophylline: May increase theophylline level. Monitor theophylline level closely.

Thiopurines: May increase thiopurine level. Monitor patient closely.

Vaccines: May make immunizations ineffective; may cause risk of disseminated infection with live-virus vaccines. Postpone immunization, if possible.

Drug-food. *Any food:* May delay absorption and reduce peak level of methotrexate. Instruct patient to take drug on an empty stomach.

Drug-lifestyle. *Alcohol use:* May increase hepatotoxicity. Discourage use together.

Sun exposure: May cause photosensitivity reactions. Advise patient to avoid excessive sunlight exposure.

■ **Black Box Warning** Methotrexate given with radiotherapy may increase the risk of soft tissue necrosis and osteonecrosis. ■

EFFECTS ON LAB TEST RESULTS
• May increase uric acid level. May decrease hemoglobin level.
• May decrease WBC, RBC, and platelet counts.
• May alter results of laboratory assay for folate, which interferes with detection of folic acid deficiency.

CONTRAINDICATIONS & CAUTIONS
• Contraindicated in patients hypersensitive to drug and in those with psoriasis or rheumatoid arthritis who also have alcoholism, alcoholic liver, chronic liver disease, immunodeficiency syndromes, or blood dyscrasias.
■ **Black Box Warning** Contraindicated in pregnancy and do not use in women of childbearing potential unless benefits outweigh risks. ■
• Contraindicated in breast-feeding women.
■ **Black Box Warning** Use cautiously and at modified dosage in patients with impaired hepatic or renal function, bone marrow suppression, aplasia, leukopenia, thrombocytopenia, or anemia. ■
• Use cautiously in very young, elderly, or debilitated patients and in those with infection, peptic ulceration, or ulcerative colitis.

NURSING CONSIDERATIONS
■ **Black Box Warning** Methotrexate-induced lung disease is a potentially dangerous lesion that may occur at any time during therapy. It isn't always fully reversible. Pulmonary symptoms (especially a dry, nonproductive cough) may require interruption of treatment and careful investigation. ■
■ **Black Box Warning** Diarrhea and ulcerative stomatitis require interruption of therapy; hemorrhagic enteritis and death from intestinal perforation may occur. ■
■ **Black Box Warning** Malignant lymphomas may occur in patients receiving low-dose methotrexate. ■
■ **Black Box Warning** Methotrexate may induce tumor lysis syndrome in patients with rapidly growing tumors. ■
■ **Black Box Warning** Severe, occasionally fatal skin reactions have been reported following single or multiple doses of methotrexate. Reactions have occurred within days of methotrexate administra-

tion. Recovery has been reported with discontinuation of therapy. ■
■ **Black Box Warning** Potentially fatal opportunistic infections, especially Pneumocystis carinii pneumonia, may occur with methotrexate therapy. ■
■ **Black Box Warning** The high-dose regimens for osteosarcoma require meticulous care. ■
• *Alert:* Drug may be given daily or once weekly, depending on the disease. To avoid administration errors, know your patient's dosing schedule.
• Monitor pulmonary function tests periodically and fluid intake and output daily. Encourage fluid intake of 2 to 3 L daily.
• Monitor uric acid level.
• Drug distributes readily into pleural effusions and other third-space compartments, such as ascites, leading to prolonged systemic level and risk of toxicity. Use drug cautiously in these patients.
• *Alert:* Alkalinize urine by giving sodium bicarbonate tablets or fluids to prevent precipitation of drug, especially at high doses. Maintain urine pH above 7. If BUN level is 20 to 30 mg/dl or creatinine level is 1.2 to 2 mg/dl, reduce dosage. If BUN level exceeds 30 mg/dl or creatinine level is higher than 2 mg/dl, stop drug and notify prescriber.
■ **Black Box Warning** Watch for increases in AST, ALT, and alkaline phosphatase levels, which may signal hepatic dysfunction. Periodic liver biopsies are recommended for psoriatic patients who are under long-term treatment. ■
• Watch for signs and symptoms of bleeding (especially GI) and infection.
• To prevent bleeding, avoid all I.M. injections when platelet count is below 50,000/mm³.
• Give blood transfusions for cumulative anemia. Patient may receive injections of RBC colony-stimulating factors to promote RBC production and decrease need for blood transfusions.
• Leucovorin rescue is needed with doses of more than 100 mg and starts 24 hours after therapy starts. Leucovorin is continued until methotrexate level falls below 5×10^{-8} M. Consult specialized references for specific recommendations for leucovorin dosage. Monitor methotrexate level and adjust leucovorin dose.

Reactions may be *common*, uncommon, *life-threatening*, or COMMON AND LIFE-THREATENING.
Interaction may have a *rapid onset* or **delayed onset.**

• The WBC and platelet count nadirs usually occur on day 7.

PATIENT TEACHING
• Advise patient to watch for signs and symptoms of infection (fever, sore throat, fatigue) and bleeding (easy bruising, nosebleeds, bleeding gums, tarry stools). Tell patient to take temperature daily.

■ **Black Box Warning** Fully inform patient of the risks involved with methotrexate therapy. ■

• Teach and encourage diligent mouth care to reduce risk of superinfection in the mouth.
• Instruct patient how to take leucovorin. Stress the importance of taking as prescribed until instructed by prescriber to stop.
• Tell patient to use highly protective sunblock when exposed to sunlight.
• Warn both men and women to avoid conception during and for at least 12 weeks after therapy because of risk of abortion, birth defects, or fetal death.
• Advise woman to stop breast-feeding during therapy.

SAFETY ALERT!

pemetrexed
peh-meh-TREX-ed

Alimta

Pharmacologic class: folate antagonist
Pregnancy risk category D

AVAILABLE FORMS
Injection: 500 mg in single-use vials

INDICATIONS & DOSAGES
➤ **Malignant pleural mesothelioma or non-small cell (non-squamous) lung cancer with cisplatin, in patients whose disease is unresectable or who aren't candidates for surgery**
Adults: 500 mg/m² I.V. over 10 minutes on day 1 of each 21-day cycle. Starting 30 minutes after pemetrexed infusion ends, give cisplatin 75 mg/m² I.V. over 2 hours.

➤ **Locally advanced or metastatic non–small-cell lung cancer after chemotherapy**
Adults: 500 mg/m² I.V. over 10 minutes on day 1 of each 21-day cycle.
Adjust-a-dose: In patients who develop toxic reactions, adjust dosage according to the table.

Toxic reaction	Dosage change
– Grade 3 (severe or undesirable) or grade 4 (life-threatening or disabling) diarrhea – Diarrhea that warrants hospitalization – Any grade 3 toxicity (except mucositis and increased transaminase levels) – Any grade 4 toxicity (except mucositis) – Platelet count ≥ 50,000/mm³ and absolute neutrophil count < 500/mm³	Give 75% of previous pemetrexed and cisplatin doses.
Platelet count < 50,000/mm³	Give 50% of previous pemetrexed and cisplatin doses.
Grade 3 or 4 mucositis	Give 50% of previous pemetrexed dose and 100% of previous cisplatin dose.
Grade 2 (moderate) neurotoxicity	Give 100% of previous pemetrexed dose and 50% of previous cisplatin dose.
– Grade 3 or 4 neurotoxicity – Any grade 3 or 4 toxicity (except increased transaminase levels) present after two dose reductions	Stop therapy.

ADMINISTRATION
I.V.
• Reconstitute 500-mg vial with 20 ml of preservative-free normal saline solution to yield 25 mg/ml.
• Swirl vial gently until powder is completely dissolved. Solution should be clear and colorless to yellow or yellow-green.
• Calculate appropriate dose, and further dilute with 100 ml normal saline solution.

- Give over 10 minutes.
- Reconstituted solution and dilution are stable for 24 hours refrigerated or at room temperature.
- **Incompatibilities:** Calcium-containing diluents including Ringer's or lactated Ringer's for injection; other drugs or diluents.

ACTION
Disturbs cell replication by inhibiting several folate-dependent enzymes involved in nucleotide synthesis. When given with other antineoplastics, drug inhibits growth of mesothelioma cell lines.

Route	Onset	Peak	Duration
I.V.	Unknown	Unknown	Unknown

Half-life: 3½ hours.

ADVERSE REACTIONS
CNS: *depression, fatigue, fever, neuropathy.*
CV: **cardiac ischemia,** *chest pain, edema,* **emboli,** thrombosis.
EENT: *pharyngitis.*
GI: *anorexia, constipation, diarrhea, nausea, stomatitis, vomiting,* esophagitis, painful, difficult swallowing.
GU: **renal failure.**
Hematologic: *anemia,* LEUKOPENIA, NEUTROPENIA, THROMBOCYTOPENIA.
Metabolic: dehydration.
Musculoskeletal: arthralgia, *myalgia.*
Respiratory: *dyspnea.*
Skin: *alopecia, rash.*
Other: allergic reaction, *infection.*

INTERACTIONS
Drug-drug. *Nephrotoxic drugs, probenecid:* May delay pemetrexed clearance. Monitor patient.
NSAIDs: May decrease pemetrexed clearance in patients with mild to moderate renal insufficiency. For NSAIDs with short half-lives, avoid use for 2 days before, during, and 2 days after pemetrexed therapy. For NSAIDs with long half-lives, avoid use for 5 days before, during, and 2 days after pemetrexed therapy.

EFFECTS ON LAB TEST RESULTS
- May increase ALT, AST, and creatinine levels. May decrease hemoglobin level and hematocrit.

- May decrease absolute neutrophil, platelet, and WBC counts.

CONTRAINDICATIONS & CAUTIONS
- Contraindicated in patients with a history of severe hypersensitivity reaction to drug or its ingredients. Don't use in patients with creatinine clearance less than 45 ml/minute.

NURSING CONSIDERATIONS
- Patient shouldn't start a new cycle of treatment unless absolute neutrophil count is 1,500 cells/mm³ or more, platelet count is 100,000 cells/mm³ or more, and creatinine clearance is 45 ml/minute or more.
- Patients with pleural effusion and ascites may need to have effusion drained before therapy.
- Monitor renal function, CBC, platelet count, hemoglobin level, hematocrit, and liver function test values.
- Assess patient for neurotoxicity, mucositis, and diarrhea. Severe symptoms may warrant dosage adjustment.
- **Alert:** To reduce the occurrence and severity of cutaneous reactions, give a corticosteroid, such as dexamethasone 4 mg P.O. b.i.d., the day before, the day of, and the day after giving this drug.
- **Alert:** To reduce toxicity, patient should take 350 to 1,000 mcg of folic acid daily, 5 days before therapy until 21 days after therapy.
- **Alert:** Give vitamin B_{12} 1,000 mcg I.M. once during the week before the first dose and every three cycles thereafter. After the first cycle, vitamin injections may be given on the first day of the cycle.

PATIENT TEACHING
- Inform patient that he may receive corticosteroids and vitamins before pemetrexed to help minimize its adverse effects.
- Tell patient to avoid NSAIDs for several days before, during, and after treatment.
- Urge patient to report adverse effects, especially fever, sore throat, infection, diarrhea, fatigue, and limb pain.
- It's unknown if drug appears in breast milk. Advise patient to stop breast-feeding during treatment.

Reactions may be *common,* uncommon, *life-threatening,* or COMMON AND LIFE-THREATENING.
Interaction may have a *rapid onset* or **delayed onset.**

83

Antimitotic drugs

docetaxel
paclitaxel
paclitaxel protein-bound particles
vinblastine sulfate
vincristine sulfate
vinorelbine tartrate

SAFETY ALERT!

docetaxel
dohs-eh-TAX-ell

Taxotere

Pharmacologic class: taxoid
Pregnancy risk category D

AVAILABLE FORMS
Injection: 20 mg, 80 mg, in single-dose vials

INDICATIONS & DOSAGES
➤ **Locally advanced or metastatic breast cancer after failure of previous chemotherapy**
Adults: 60 to 100 mg/m^2 I.V. over 1 hour every 3 weeks.
Adjust-a-dose: In patients receiving 100 mg/m^2 who experience febrile neutropenia, neutrophil count of less than 500/mm^3 for longer than 1 week, severe or cumulative cutaneous reactions, or severe peripheral neuropathy, reduce subsequent dose by 25%, to 75 mg/m^2. In patients who continue to experience reactions with decreased dose, either decrease it further to 55 mg/m^2 or stop drug.
➤ **Adjuvant postsurgery treatment of operable, node-positive breast cancer**
Adults: 75 mg/m^2 I.V. as a 1-hour infusion given 1 hour after doxorubicin 50 mg/m^2 and cyclophosphamide 500 mg/m^2 every 3 weeks for six cycles.
Adjust-a-dose: Patients who experience febrile neutropenia should receive granulocyte colony-stimulating factor (G-CSF) in all subsequent cycles. If febrile neutropenia doesn't resolve, continue G-CSF

and reduce docetaxel dose to 60 mg/m^2. For patients who experience severe or cumulative cutaneous reactions or moderate neurosensory signs and symptoms, reduce dose to 60 mg/m^2. If these reactions persist at the reduced dosage, stop treatment.
➤ **Locally advanced or metastatic non–small-cell lung cancer after failure of previous cisplatin-based chemotherapy**
Adults: 75 mg/m^2 I.V. over 1 hour every 3 weeks.
Adjust-a-dose: In patients who experience febrile neutropenia, neutrophil count of less than 500/mm^3 for longer than 1 week, severe or cumulative cutaneous reactions, or severe peripheral neuropathy, withhold drug until toxicity resolves; then restart at 55 mg/m^2. In patients in whom grade 3 peripheral neuropathy or above develops, stop drug.
➤ **With cisplatin, unresectable, locally advanced, or metastatic non–small-cell lung cancer not previously treated with chemotherapy**
Adults: 75 mg/m^2 docetaxel I.V. over 1 hour, immediately followed by cisplatin 75 mg/m^2 I.V. over 30 to 60 minutes every 3 weeks.
Adjust-a-dose: In patients whose lowest platelet count during the previous course of therapy was less than 25,000/mm^3, and those with febrile neutropenia or serious nonhematologic toxicities, decrease docetaxel dosage to 65 mg/m^2. For patients who require a further dosage reduction, a dosage of 50 mg/m^2 is recommended. For cisplatin dosage adjustments, see manufacturers' prescribing information.
➤ **Androgen-independent metastatic prostate cancer, with prednisone**
Adults: 75 mg/m^2 I.V., as a 1-hour infusion every 3 weeks, given with 5 mg prednisone P.O. b.i.d. continuously. Premedicate with dexamethasone 8 mg P.O. at 12 hours, 3 hours, and 1 hour before docetaxel infusion.
Adjust-a-dose: In patients who experience febrile neutropenia, neutrophil count less

than 500/mm³ for more than 1 week, severe or cumulative cutaneous reactions, or moderate neurosensory signs or symptoms, reduce subsequent dose to 60 mg/m². In patients who continue to experience reactions with the decreased dose, stop treatment.

➤ **Advanced gastric adeno-carcinoma, in combination with cisplatin and fluorouracil (5-FU)**

Adults: Premedicate with antiemetics and hydration per cisplatin recommendations. Give 75 mg/m² docetaxel I.V. over 1 hour, followed by cisplatin 75 mg/m² I.V. over 1 to 3 hours both on day 1 only, then, fluorouracil 750 mg/m² I.V. daily as a 24-hour continuous infusion for 5 days beginning at the end of cisplatin infusion. Repeat cycle every 3 weeks.

Adjust-a-dose: Patients who experience febrile neutropenia should receive G-CSF in subsequent cycles. If episode recurs, reduce dose to 60 mg/m². If subsequent episodes of complicated neutropenia occur, reduce dose to 45 mg/m². In patients who experience grade 4 thrombo-cytopenia, reduce dosage to 60 mg/m². Don't retreat until neutrophils are greater than 1,500/mm³ and platelets are greater than 100,000/mm³. Stop treatment if toxicity persists.

For patients who experience diarrhea, adjust dosage as follows: for first episode of grade 3 diarrhea, reduce 5-FU dose by 20%; for second episode, reduce docetaxel dose by 20%; for first episode of grade 4 diarrhea, reduce docetaxel and 5-FU doses by 20%; for second episode, stop drug. For patients who experience stomatitis, adjust dosage as follows: For first episode of grade 3, reduce 5-FU dose by 20%; second episode, stop 5-FU in subsequent cycles; third episode, reduce docetaxel dose by 20%. For first episode of grade 4, stop 5-FU in subsequent cycles; second episode, reduce docetaxel dose by 20%. For patients who experience liver dysfunction, reduce docetaxel dose by 20%. If AST or ALT is greater than five times upper limit of normal (ULN) or alkaline phosphatase is greater than five times ULN, stop treatment.

➤ **Induction treatment of inoperable locally advanced squamous cell cancer of the head and neck (SCCHN), with cisplatin and 5-FU**

Adults: 75 mg/m² I.V. infusion over 1 hour, followed by cisplatin 75 mg/m² I.V. infusion over 1 hour, on day 1, followed by 5-FU 750 mg/m² daily as a continuous I.V. infusion for 5 days. Repeat this regimen every 3 weeks for four cycles. After chemotherapy, patients should receive radiotherapy. Premedicate with antiemetics and appropriate hydration before and after giving cisplatin.

Adjust-a-dose: Use the same dosage adjustment schedule as for advanced gastric adenocarcinoma.

➤ **Induction treatment for locally advanced SCCHN with cisplatin and 5-FU before chemoradiotherapy**

Adults: 75 mg/m² I.V. infusion over 1 hour, followed by cisplatin 100 mg/m² I.V. infusion over 30 minutes to 3 hours on day 1, followed by 5-FU 1,000 mg/m² daily as a continuous I.V. infusion from day 1 to day 4. Repeat this regimen every 3 weeks for three cycles. After chemotherapy, patients should receive chemoradiotherapy. Premedicate with antiemetics and oral corticosteroids.

Adjust-a-dose: Use the same dosage adjustment schedule as for advanced gastric adenocarcinoma.

ADMINISTRATION
I.V.

● Wear gloves to prepare and give drug. If solution contacts skin, wash immediately and thoroughly with soap and water. If solution contacts mucous membranes, flush thoroughly with water.

● Dilute using supplied diluent. Let drug and diluent stand at room temperature for 5 minutes before mixing. After adding all the diluent to drug vial, gently rotate vial for about 45 seconds. Let solution stand for a few minutes so foam dissipates. All foam need not dissipate before preparing infusion solution.

● Prepare infusion solution by withdrawing needed amount of premixed solution from vial and injecting it into 250 ml normal saline solution or D₅W to yield 0.3 to 0.74 mg/ml. Doses of more than 200 mg need a larger volume to stay below 0.74 mg/ml of drug. Mix infusion thoroughly by manual rotation.

Reactions may be *common*, uncommon, *life-threatening*, or COMMON AND LIFE-THREATENING.
Interaction may have a *rapid onset* or **delayed onset.**

• Prepare and store infusion solution in bottles (glass or polypropylene) or plastic bags, and give through polyethylene-lined administration sets.
• Contact between undiluted concentrate and polyvinyl chloride equipment or devices isn't recommended.
• If solution isn't clear or if it contains precipitate, discard.
• The first dilution is stable for 8 hours Use infusion solution within 4 hours.
• Infuse over 1 hour.
• Store unopened vials between 2° and 25° (36° and 77° F).
• Mark all waste materials with CHEMO-THERAPY HAZARD labels.
• **Incompatibilities:** None reported.

ACTION

Promotes formation and stabilization of nonfunctional microtubules. This prevents mitosis and leads to cell death.

Route	Onset	Peak	Duration
I.V.	Rapid	Unknown	Unknown

Half-life: Alpha phase, 4 minutes; beta phase, 36 minutes; terminal phase, 11 hours.

ADVERSE REACTIONS

CNS: *asthenia,* paresthesia, peripheral neuropathy.
CV: *fluid retention, peripheral edema, arrhythmias,* chest tightness, flushing, hypotension.
EENT: altered hearing, tearing.
GI: *anorexia, diarrhea, dysphagia, esophagitis, nausea, stomatitis, vomiting.*
Hematologic: FEBRILE NEUTROPENIA, LEUKOPENIA, MYELOSUPPRESSION, NEUTROPENIA, THROMBOCYTOPENIA, *anemia.*
Hepatic: *hepatotoxicity.*
Musculoskeletal: *myalgia,* arthralgia, back pain.
Respiratory: dyspnea, *pulmonary edema.*
Skin: *alopecia,* desquamation, skin eruptions, nail pigmentation alterations, nail pain, rash, reaction at injection site.
Other: *infection,* chills, drug fever, hypersensitivity reactions.

INTERACTIONS

Drug-drug. *Compounds that induce, inhibit, or are metabolized by CYP3A4,*

such as cyclosporine, erythromycin, ketoconazole, troleandomycin: May modify metabolism of docetaxel. Use together cautiously.
Ketoconazole or other CYP3A4 inhibitors:
May increase docetaxel level and toxicity, including neutropenia. Monitor patient closely.

EFFECTS ON LAB TEST RESULTS

• May increase alkaline phosphatase, ALT, AST, and bilirubin levels. May decrease hemoglobin level.
• May decrease platelet and WBC counts.

CONTRAINDICATIONS & CAUTIONS

• Contraindicated in patients severely hypersensitive to drug or to other forms containing polysorbate 80 and in those with neutrophil count below 1,500/mm³.
■ **Black Box Warning** Patients with severe hepatic impairment shouldn't receive this drug. Don't give drug to patients with bilirubin levels exceeding ULN, or those with ALT or AST levels above 1½ times ULN and alkaline phosphatase levels above 2½ times ULN. ■
• Safety and effectiveness in children haven't been established.

NURSING CONSIDERATIONS

■ **Black Box Warning** Drug should be administered only under the supervision of a physician experienced with anti-neoplastics. ■
• Give oral corticosteroid such as dexamethasone 16 mg P.O. (8 mg b.i.d.) daily for 3 days, starting 1 day before docetaxel administration, to reduce risk or severity of fluid retention and hypersensitivity reactions.
■ **Black Box Warning** Don't give drug to patients with baseline neutrophil count less than 1,500/mm³. ■
• Bone marrow toxicity is the most frequent and dose-limiting toxicity. Frequent blood count monitoring is needed during therapy.
■ **Black Box Warning** Monitor patient closely for hypersensitivity reactions, especially during first and second infusions. ■
■ **Black Box Warning** Fluid retention is dose related and may be severe. Monitor patient closely. ■

• **Alert:** When indicated, cisplatin dose should follow dose of docetaxel.
• **Look alike–sound alike:** Don't confuse Taxotere with Taxol.

PATIENT TEACHING
• Caution woman of childbearing age to avoid pregnancy or breast-feeding during therapy.
• Advise patient to report any pain or burning at injection site during or after administration.
• Warn patient that hair loss occurs in almost 80% of patients and reverses when treatment stops.
• Tell patient to promptly report sore throat, fever, or unusual bruising or bleeding, as well as signs and symptoms of fluid retention, such as swelling or shortness of breath.

SAFETY ALERT!

paclitaxel
pak-leh-TAX-ell

Onxol, Taxol

Pharmacologic class: taxoid
Pregnancy risk category D

AVAILABLE FORMS
Injection: 6 mg/ml in 5-, 16.7-, 25-, 50-ml vials

INDICATIONS & DOSAGES
➤ **Second-line treatment of AIDS-related Kaposi sarcoma**
Adults: 135 mg/m² Taxol I.V. over 3 hours every 3 weeks, or 100 mg/m² I.V. over 3 hours every 2 weeks.
Adjust-a-dose: Don't give drug if baseline or subsequent neutrophil counts are less than 1,000/mm³. Reduce subsequent doses of Taxol by 20% for patients who experience severe neutropenia (neutrophil count 500/mm³ for 1 week or longer). Patient also may need reduction in dexamethasone premedication dose (10 mg P.O. instead of 20 mg P.O.) and start of a hematopoietic growth factor.
➤ **First-line and subsequent therapy for advanced ovarian cancer**

Adults (previously untreated): 175 mg/m² over 3 hours every 3 weeks, followed by cisplatin 75 mg/m²; or, 135 mg/m² over 24 hours, followed by cisplatin 75 mg/m², every 3 weeks.
Adults (previously treated): 135 or 175 mg/m² I.V. over 3 hours every 3 weeks.
➤ **Breast cancer after failure of combination chemotherapy for metastatic disease or relapse within 6 months of adjuvant chemotherapy (previous therapy should have included an anthracycline unless contraindicated); adjuvant therapy for node-positive breast cancer given sequentially to standard doxorubicin-containing combination chemotherapy**
Adults: 175 mg/m² I.V. over 3 hours every 3 weeks.
➤ **First treatment of advanced non–small-cell lung cancer for patients who aren't candidates for curative surgery or radiation**
Adults: 135 mg/m² I.V. Taxol infusion over 24 hours, followed by cisplatin 75 mg/m². Repeat cycle every 3 weeks.
Adjust-a-dose: Subsequent courses shouldn't be repeated until neutrophil count is at least 1,500/mm³ and platelet count is at least 100,000/mm³. Reduce subsequent doses of Taxol by 20% for patients who experience severe neutropenia (neutrophil count less than 500/mm³ for a week or longer) or severe peripheral neuropathy. For patients with hepatic impairment, adjust doses for the first courses of therapy as follows: For 24-hour infusion of Taxol if transaminase levels are less than two times the upper limit of normal (ULN) and bilirubin levels are 1.5 mg/dl or less, give 135 mg/m². If transaminase levels are two to less than 10 times ULN and bilirubin levels are 1.5 mg/dl or less, give 100 mg/m². If transaminase levels are less than 10 times ULN and bilirubin levels are 1.6 to 7.5 mg/dl, give 50 mg/m². If transaminase levels are 10 times ULN or more, or bilirubin levels are more than 7.5 mg/dl, don't use drug. For 3-hour infusion of Taxol, if transaminase levels are less than 10 times ULN and bilirubin levels are 1.25 times ULN or less, give 175 mg/m². If transaminase levels are less

than 10 times ULN and bilirubin levels are 1.26 to 2 times ULN, give 135 mg/m². If transaminase levels are less than 10 times ULN and bilirubin levels are 2.01 to 5 times ULN, give 90 mg/m². If transaminase levels are 10 times ULN or more or bilirubin levels are more than five times ULN, don't use drug. For subsequent courses, base dosage adjustment on individual tolerance.

ADMINISTRATION
I.V.
● Preparing and giving drug may be mutagenic, teratogenic, or carcinogenic. Follow institutional policy to reduce risks. Mark all waste materials with CHEMOTHERAPY HAZARD labels.
● Prepare and store infusion solutions in glass containers. Undiluted concentrate shouldn't contact polyvinyl chloride I.V. bags or tubing.
● Dilute concentrate before infusion. Compatible solutions include normal saline solution for injection, D_5W, 5% dextrose in normal saline solution for injection, and 5% dextrose in Ringer's lactate injection. Dilute to yield 0.3 to 1.2 mg/ml. Diluted solutions are stable for 24 hours at room temperature. Prepared solution may appear hazy.
● Give through polyethylene-lined administration sets, and use an in-line 0.22-micron filter.
● Watch for irritation and infiltration; extravasation can cause tissue damage and necrosis.
● Closely monitor patient and vital signs during infusion, especially during the first hour.
● Store diluted solution in glass or polypropylene bottles, or use polypropylene or polyolefin bags.
● **Incompatibilities:** Amphotericin B, chlorpromazine, cisplatin, doxorubicin liposomal, hydroxyzine hydrochloride, methylprednisolone sodium succinate, mitoxantrone.

ACTION
Prevents depolymerization of cellular microtubules, inhibiting normal reorganization of microtubule network needed for mitosis and other vital cellular functions.

Route	Onset	Peak	Duration
I.V.	Unknown	Unknown	Unknown

Half-life: After 6- to 12-hour infusion, distribution and elimination half-lives average about 30 minutes and 6 hours, respectively. For 3-hour infusion, distribution and elimination half-lives average about 30 minutes and 2½ hours, respectively.

ADVERSE REACTIONS
CNS: *peripheral neuropathy, asthenia.*
CV: **bradycardia,** *hypotension, abnormal ECG.*
GI: *nausea, vomiting, diarrhea, mucositis.*
Hematologic: NEUTROPENIA, LEUKOPENIA, THROMBOCYTOPENIA, *anemia,* BLEEDING.
Musculoskeletal: *myalgia, arthralgia.*
Skin: *alopecia, cellulitis and phlebitis at injection site.*
Other: hypersensitivity reactions, **anaphylaxis,** *infections.*

INTERACTIONS
Drug-drug. *Carbamazepine, phenobarbital:* May increase metabolism and may decrease paclitaxel levels. Use together cautiously.
Cisplatin: May cause additive myelosuppressive effects. Give paclitaxel before cisplatin.
Doxorubicin, cyclosporine, felodipine, ketoconazole: May increase plasma levels of doxorubicin and its active metabolite, doxorubicinol. Use together cautiously.
Drugs that inhibit cytochrome P-450, such as cyclosporine, dexamethasone, diazepam, etoposide, **ketoconazole,** *quinidine, retinoic acid, teniposide, testosterone, verapamil, vincristine:* May increase paclitaxel level. Monitor patient for toxicity.

EFFECTS ON LAB TEST RESULTS
● May increase alkaline phosphatase, AST, and triglyceride levels. May decrease hemoglobin level.
● May decrease neutrophil, WBC, and platelet counts.

CONTRAINDICATIONS & CAUTIONS
● Contraindicated in patients hypersensitive to drug or polyoxyethylated castor oil (also known as Cremophor EL, a vehicle used in drug solution).

---

†Canada   ◇OTC   ◆Off-label use   ✐Photoguide   *Liquid contains alcohol.

■ **Black Box Warning** Contraindicated those with baseline neutrophil counts below 1,500/mm³ and platelet counts below 100,000/mm³, or AIDS-related Kaposi sarcoma with baseline neutrophil counts below 1,000/mm³. ■

● Use cautiously in patients with hepatic impairment.

NURSING CONSIDERATIONS
■ **Black Box Warning** Administer drug under the supervision of a physician experienced with cancer chemotherapeutic agents. ■

● Patient may experience peripheral neuropathies, which may be cumulative and dose related. Patients with severe symptoms may need dosage reduction.

■ **Black Box Warning** To reduce risk or severity of hypersensitivity, patients must receive pretreatment with corticosteroids, such as dexamethasone, and antihistamines. Both H₁-receptor antagonists, such as diphenhydramine, and H₂-receptor antagonists, such as cimetidine or ranitidine, may be used. ■

■ **Black Box Warning** Monitor blood counts often during therapy. Bone marrow toxicity is the most common and dose-limiting toxicity. Packed RBC or platelet transfusions may be needed in severe cases. Institute bleeding precautions, as indicated. ■

● RBC colony-stimulating factors may promote RBC production and decrease need for blood transfusions.

● Avoid all I.M. injections when platelet count is below 50,000/mm³.

● If patient develops significant cardiac conduction abnormalities, use indicated therapy and continuous cardiac monitoring during therapy and subsequent infusions.

● **Alert:** When indicated, cisplatin dose should follow dose of paclitaxel.

● **Look alike–sound alike:** Don't confuse paclitaxel with paroxetine; don't confuse Taxol with Paxil or Taxotere.

PATIENT TEACHING
● Advise patient to report any pain or burning at site of injection during or after administration.

● Urge patient to watch for fever, sore throat, and fatigue and for easy bruising,

nosebleeds, bleeding gums, or tarry stools. Tell patient to take temperature daily.

● Teach patient symptoms of peripheral neuropathy, such as a tingling or burning sensation or numbness in limbs, and to report these symptoms immediately.

● Warn patient that reversible hair loss will probably occur.

● Caution woman of childbearing age to avoid becoming pregnant during therapy. Recommend that she consult prescriber before becoming pregnant.

SAFETY ALERT!

paclitaxel protein-bound particles
pak-leh-TAX-ell

Abraxane

Pharmacologic class: taxoid
Pregnancy risk category D

AVAILABLE FORMS
Lyophilized powder for injection: 100 mg in single-use vials

INDICATIONS & DOSAGES
➤ **Metastatic breast cancer after failure of combination chemotherapy or relapse within 6 months of adjuvant chemotherapy (previous therapy should have included an anthracycline unless clinically contraindicated at the time)**
Adults: 260 mg/m² I.V. over 30 minutes every 3 weeks.

Adjust-a-dose: For patients with severe sensory neuropathy or a neutrophil count less than 500/mm³ for a week or longer, reduce dose to 220 mg/m². For recurring severe sensory neuropathy or severe neutropenia, reduce dose to 180 mg/m². For grade 3 (severe) sensory neuropathy, stop drug until condition improves to a grade 1 or 2 (mild to moderate); then restart at a reduced dose for the rest of treatment.

ADMINISTRATION
I.V.
● Because of drug's cytotoxicity, handle it cautiously and wear gloves. If drug contacts skin, wash area thoroughly with

soap and water. If drug contacts mucous membranes, flush them thoroughly with water.
• Reconstitute the vial with 20 ml of normal saline solution to yield 5 mg/ml of drug. Direct the stream slowly, over at least 1 minute, onto the inside wall of the vial to avoid foaming. Let the vial sit for 5 minutes to ensure proper wetting of the powder. Gently swirl or turn the vial for at least 2 minutes until completely dissolved. If foaming occurs, let the solution stand for 15 minutes for the foam to subside. If particles are visible, gently invert the vial again to ensure complete resuspension. The solution should appear milky and uniform. Inject the correct dose into an empty polyvinyl chloride–type I.V. bag and use immediately.
• Give drug over 30 minutes.
• The suspension for infusion, when prepared in an infusion bag, is stable at room temperature and normal lighting for up to 8 hours.
• Store unopened vials at room temperature in the original package. Store reconstituted vials at 36° to 46° F (2° to 8° C) for up to 8 hours, protected from light.
• **Incompatibilities:** None known.

ACTION
Prevents depolymerization of cellular microtubules, inhibiting reorganization of the microtubule network and disrupting mitosis and other vital cell functions.

Route	Onset	Peak	Duration
I.V.	Unknown	Unknown	Unknown

Half-life: 27 hours.

ADVERSE REACTIONS
CNS: *asthenia, sensory neuropathy.*
CV: *abnormal ECG, edema,* **cardiac arrest,** chest pain, **supraventricular tachycardia, thromboembolism, thrombosis,** hypertension, hypotension.
EENT: *visual disturbances.*
GI: *diarrhea, nausea, oral candidiasis, vomiting,* intestinal obstruction, **ischemic colitis, pancreatitis, perforation,** mucositis.
Hematologic: *anemia,* **NEUTROPENIA, thrombocytopenia, bleeding.**
Hepatic: **hepatic encephalopathy, hepatic necrosis.**

Musculoskeletal: *arthralgia, myalgia.*
Respiratory: **pulmonary embolism,** *cough, dyspnea, pneumonia, respiratory tract infection.*
Skin: *alopecia,* injection site reactions.
Other: *infections,* hypersensitivity reactions.

INTERACTIONS
Drug-drug. *Cytochrome P-450 inhibitors:* May decrease paclitaxel metabolism. Use together cautiously.

EFFECTS ON LAB TEST RESULTS
• May increase alkaline phosphatase, AST, bilirubin, creatinine, and GGT levels. May decrease hemoglobin level.
• May decrease neutrophil and platelet counts.

CONTRAINDICATIONS & CAUTIONS
■ **Black Box Warning** Contraindicated in patients with baseline neutrophil counts of under 1,500/mm³. ■
• Don't retreat until neutrophil counts recover to more than 1,500/mm³and platelet count recovers to more than 100,000/mm³.
• In patients with creatinine level over 2 mg/dl or bilirubin level over 1.5 mg/dl, use hasn't been studied.

NURSING CONSIDERATIONS
■ **Black Box Warning** Give only under supervision of practitioner experienced in using chemotherapy in a facility that can manage complications of therapy. ■
■ **Black Box Warning** Don't substitute Abraxane for other forms of paclitaxel. ■
• Because drug contains human albumin, a remote risk exists of transmitting viruses and Creutzfeldt-Jakob disease.
• Assess patient for symptoms of sensory neuropathy and severe neutropenia.
• Monitor liver and kidney function test results.
• Monitor infusion site closely.

PATIENT TEACHING
• Warn patient that alopecia commonly occurs but is reversible after therapy.
• Teach patient to recognize signs of neuropathy, such as tingling, burning, and numbness in arms and legs.

- Tell patient to report fever or other signs of infection, severe abdominal pain, or severe diarrhea.
- Advise patient to contact prescriber if nausea and vomiting persist or interfere with adequate nutrition. Reassure patient that an antiemetic can be prescribed.
- Explain that many patients experience weakness and fatigue, so it's important to rest. Tiredness, paleness, and shortness of breath may result from low blood counts, and patient may need a transfusion.
- To reduce or prevent mouth sores, remind patient to perform proper oral hygiene.
- Tell women to avoid becoming pregnant or breast-feeding and men to avoid fathering a child during therapy.

vinblastine sulfate (VLB)
vin-BLAS-teen

Pharmacologic class: vinca alkaloid
Pregnancy risk category D

AVAILABLE FORMS
Injection: 10-mg vials (lyophilized powder), 1 mg/ml in 10-ml and 25-ml vials

INDICATIONS & DOSAGES
➤ **Breast or testicular cancer, Hodgkin and malignant lymphoma, choriocarcinoma, lymphosarcoma, mycosis fungoides, Kaposi sarcoma, histiocytosis**
Adults: 3.7 mg/m^2 I.V. weekly. May increase to maximum dose of 18.5 mg/m^2 I.V. weekly based on response. Don't repeat dose if WBC count is below 4,000/mm^3. Increase dosage at weekly intervals in increments of 1.8 mg/m^2 until desired therapeutic response is obtained, leukocyte count decreases to 3,000/mm^3, or maximum weekly dose of 18.5 mg/m^2 is reached.
Children: First dose is 2.5 mg/m^2 I.V. weekly. Increase dosage by 1.25 mg/m^2 weekly until WBC count is below 3,000/mm^3 or tumor response is seen. Maximum dose is 12.5 mg/m^2 I.V. weekly.
Adjust-a-dose: For patients with direct bilirubin over 3 mg/dl, reduce dose by 50%. For patients with recent exposure to radiation therapy or chemotherapy, single doses usually don't exceed 5.5 mg/m^2. Once a dose is determined to produce a WBC count below 3,000/mm^3, give maintenance doses of one increment less than this amount at weekly intervals.

ADMINISTRATION
I.V.
- Preparing and giving drug may be mutagenic, teratogenic, or carcinogenic. Follow institutional policy to reduce risks.
- Reconstitute drug in 10-mg vial with 10 ml of bacteriostatic saline solution for injection. This yields 1 mg/ml. Don't use other diluents. Protect solution from light.
- Inject drug directly into tubing of running I.V. line over 1 minute.
- ■ **Black Box Warning** Make sure catheter is properly positioned in vein. Drug is a vesicant; if extravasation occurs, stop infusion immediately and notify prescriber. The manufacturer recommends that moderate heat be applied to area of leakage. Local injection of hyaluronidase may help disperse drug. Moderate heat may be applied on and off every 2 hours for 24 hours. ■
- Drug reconstituted with diluent containing preservatives is stable for 28 days if refrigerated. Immediately discard any unused portion of solution reconstituted with diluent that doesn't contain preservatives.
- **Incompatibilities:** Cefepime, doxorubicin, furosemide, heparin.

ACTION
Arrests mitosis in metaphase, blocking cell division.

Route	Onset	Peak	Duration
I.V.	Unknown	Unknown	Unknown

Half-life: Initial phase, 3 minutes; second phase, 1½ hours; terminal phase, 25 hours.

ADVERSE REACTIONS
CNS: *numbness, paresthesia, peripheral neuropathy and neuritis,* **seizures, stroke,** depression, headache.
CV: *MI,* hypertension.
EENT: pharyngitis.
GI: *anorexia, constipation, ileus, nausea, stomatitis, vomiting,* abdominal pain, bleeding ulcer, diarrhea.

Hematologic: *anemia, leukopenia, thrombocytopenia.*
Metabolic: *weight loss,* hyperuricemia.
Musculoskeletal: *loss of deep tendon reflexes, muscle pain and weakness,* jaw pain.
Respiratory: *acute bronchospasm,* shortness of breath.
Skin: *irritation, phlebitis,* cellulitis, reversible alopecia, vesiculation and necrosis with extravasation.
Other: SIADH.

INTERACTIONS
Drug-drug. *Azole antifungals, erythromycin, other drugs that inhibit cytochrome P-450 pathway:* May increase toxicity of vinblastine. Monitor patient closely for toxicity.
Mitomycin: May increase risk of bronchospasm and shortness of breath. Monitor patient's respiratory status.
Ototoxic drugs, such as platinum-containing antineoplastics: May cause temporary or permanent hearing impairment. Monitor hearing function.
Phenytoin: May decrease plasma phenytoin level. Monitor phenytoin level closely.

EFFECTS ON LAB TEST RESULTS
• May increase uric acid and bilirubin levels. May decrease hemoglobin level.
• May decrease WBC and platelet counts.

CONTRAINDICATIONS & CAUTIONS
• Contraindicated in patients with severe leukopenia or bacterial infection or in patients hypersensitive to the drug.
• Use cautiously in patients with hepatic dysfunction.

NURSING CONSIDERATIONS
■ **Black Box Warning** Drug is fatal if given intrathecally; it's for I.V. use only. ■
• To reduce nausea, give antiemetic before drug.
• Don't give drug into a limb with compromised circulation.
• *Alert:* After giving drug, check for development of life-threatening acute bronchospasm. If this occurs, notify prescriber immediately. Reaction is most likely to occur in patients who are also receiving mitomycin.

• Monitor patient for stomatitis. If stomatitis occurs, stop drug and notify prescriber.
• Assess bowel activity. Give laxatives as indicated. Stool softeners may be used prophylactically.
• Don't repeat dosage more frequently than every 7 days or severe leukopenia will occur. Nadir occurs on days 4 to 10 and lasts another 7 to 14 days.
• Assess patient for numbness and tingling in hands and feet. Assess gait for early evidence of footdrop.
• Drug is less neurotoxic than vincristine.
• Stop drugs known to cause urine retention for first few days after therapy, particularly in elderly patients.
• *Look alike–sound alike:* Don't confuse vinblastine with vincristine or vinorelbine.

PATIENT TEACHING
• Tell patient to report evidence of infection (fever, sore throat, fatigue) and bleeding (easy bruising, nosebleeds, bleeding gums, tarry stools). Tell patient to take temperature daily.
• Urge patient to report pain, swelling, burning, or any unusual feeling at injection site during infusion.
• Warn patient that hair loss may occur but that it's usually temporary.
• Caution woman to avoid pregnancy during therapy.
• Tell patient that pain may occur in jaw and in the organ with the tumor.

SAFETY ALERT!

vincristine sulfate (VCR)
vin-KRIS-teen

Pharmacologic class: vinca alkaloid
Pregnancy risk category D

AVAILABLE FORMS
Injection: 1 mg/ml in 1-ml, 2-ml, 5-ml multidose vials; 1 mg/ml in 1-ml, 2-ml, 5-ml preservative-free vials

INDICATIONS & DOSAGES
➤ **Acute lymphoblastic and other leukemias, Hodgkin lymphoma, malignant lymphoma, neuro-**

blastoma, rhabdomyosarcoma, Wilms tumor
Adults: 1.4 mg/m² I.V. weekly. Maximum weekly dose is 2 mg.
Children who weigh more than 10 kg (22 lb): Give 1.5 to 2 mg/m² I.V. weekly.
Children who weigh 10 kg and less or with body surface area less than 1 m²: Initially, 0.05 mg/kg I.V. weekly.
Adjust-a-dose: For patients with direct bilirubin over 3 mg/dl, reduce dose by 50%.

ADMINISTRATION
I.V.
• Preparing and giving drug may be mutagenic, teratogenic, or carcinogenic. Follow institutional policy to reduce risks.
• Inject directly into tube of running I.V. line of normal saline or dextrose in water only, slowly over 1 minute.
■ **Black Box Warning** Make sure catheter is positioned correctly in vein. Drug is a vesicant; if it extravasates, stop infusion immediately and notify prescriber. Apply heat on and off every 2 hours for 24 hours. ■
• If protocol requires a continuous infusion, use a central line.
• All vials contain 1 mg/ml solution; refrigerate them.
• **Incompatibilities:** Cefepime, furosemide, idarubicin, sodium bicarbonate.

ACTION
Arrests mitosis in metaphase, blocking cell division.

Route	Onset	Peak	Duration
I.V.	Unknown	Unknown	Unknown

Half-life: Initial phase, 4 minutes; second phase, 2¼ hours; terminal phase, 3½ days.

ADVERSE REACTIONS
CNS: *loss of deep tendon reflexes, pares-thesia, peripheral neuropathy, **coma, seizures,*** ataxia, cranial nerve palsies, fever, headache, sensory loss.
CV: hypertension, hypotension.
EENT: blindness, diplopia, hoarseness, optic and extraocular neuropathy, photo-phobia, ptosis, visual disturbances, vocal cord paralysis.

GI: *constipation, cramps, nausea, stomatitis, vomiting, **intestinal necrosis,*** anorexia, diarrhea, dysphagia, ileus that mimics surgical paralytic ileus.
GU: dysuria, polyuria, SIADH, urine retention.
Hematologic: ***leukopenia, thrombo-cytopenia,*** anemia.
Metabolic: hyponatremia, weight loss.
Musculoskeletal: *cramps, jaw pain, muscle weakness.*
Respiratory: ***acute bronchospasm,*** dyspnea.
Skin: *phlebitis,* cellulitis at injection site, rash, reversible alopecia, severe local reaction following extravasation.

INTERACTIONS
Drug-drug. *Asparaginase:* May decrease hepatic clearance of vincristine. Use together also may result in additive neuro-toxicity. Monitor patient for toxicity.
Digoxin: May decrease digoxin's effects. Monitor digoxin level.
Mitomycin: May increase frequency of bronchospasm and acute pulmonary reactions. Monitor patient's respiratory status.
Ototoxic drugs: May potentiate loss of hearing. Use together with caution.
Phenytoin: May reduce phenytoin level. Monitor phenytoin level closely.

EFFECTS ON LAB TEST RESULTS
• May decrease sodium and hemoglobin levels. May increase uric acid level.
• May decrease WBC and platelet counts.

CONTRAINDICATIONS & CAUTIONS
• Contraindicated in patients hyper-sensitive to drug and in those with demyelinating form of Charcot-Marie-Tooth syndrome.
• Don't give to patients who are receiving radiation therapy through ports that include the liver.
• Use cautiously in patients with hepatic dysfunction, neuromuscular disease, or infection.

NURSING CONSIDERATIONS
• Don't use the 5-mg vials for single doses.
• ***Alert:*** Patient also taking mitomycin has a higher risk of life-threatening bronchospasm. Monitor him after dose,

---

Reactions may be *common*, uncommon, ***life-threatening***, or COMMON AND LIFE-THREATENING.
Interaction may have a *rapid onset* or ***delayed onset.***

and notify prescriber immediately if it occurs.
- Watch for hyperuricemia, especially in patients with leukemia or lymphoma. Maintain hydration and give allopurinol to prevent uric acid nephropathy. Watch for toxicity.
- If SIADH develops, fluid restriction may be needed. Monitor fluid intake and output.
- Because of risk of neurotoxicity, don't give drug more often than once weekly. Children are more resistant to neurotoxicity than adults. Neurotoxicity is dose related and usually reversible.
- Elderly patients and those with underlying neurologic disease may be more susceptible to neurotoxic effects.
- Monitor patient for Achilles tendon reflex depression, numbness, tingling, footdrop or wristdrop, difficulty walking, ataxia, and slapping gait. Monitor his ability to walk on heels. Support him while walking.
- Monitor bowel function. Give stool softener, laxative, or water before giving dose. Constipation may be an early sign of neurotoxicity.
- Stop drugs known to cause urine retention, particularly in elderly patients, for first few days after therapy.
- **■ Black Box Warning** Drug is fatal if given intrathecally; it's for I.V. use only. ■
- *Look alike–sound alike:* Don't confuse vincristine with vinblastine or vinorelbine.

PATIENT TEACHING
- Advise patient to report any pain or burning at site of injection during or after administration.
- Tell patient to report evidence of infection (fever, sore throat, fatigue) and bleeding (easy bruising, nosebleeds, bleeding gums, tarry stools). Tell patient to take temperature daily.
- Warn patient that hair loss may occur, but explain that it's usually temporary.
- Caution woman to avoid becoming pregnant during therapy and to consult prescriber before becoming pregnant.

SAFETY ALERT!

vinorelbine tartrate
vin-oh-REL-been

Navelbine

Pharmacologic class: semisynthetic vinca alkaloid
Pregnancy risk category D

AVAILABLE FORMS
Injection: 10 mg/ml, 50 mg/5 ml

INDICATIONS & DOSAGES
➤ **Alone or as adjunct therapy with cisplatin for first-line treatment of ambulatory patients with nonresectable advanced non–small-cell lung cancer (NSCLC); alone or with cisplatin in stage IV of NSCLC; with cisplatin in stage III of NSCLC**
Adults: 30 mg/m^2 I.V. weekly. In combination treatment, 25 mg/m^2 I.V. weekly with cisplatin given every 4 weeks at a dose of 100 mg/m^2. Or, 30 mg/m^2 I.V. weekly in combination with cisplatin, given on days 1 and 29, then every 6 weeks at a dose of 120 mg/m^2.
Adjust-a-dose: If granulocyte count is 1,000/mm^3 to 1,499/mm^3, give 50% of dose. If less than 1,000/mm^3, dose is withheld. If total bilirubin is 2.1 to 3 mg/dl, reduce dose by 50%; if more than 3 mg/dl, give 25% of dose.

ADMINISTRATION
I.V.
- Drug may be a contact irritant; handle and give with care. Wear gloves. Avoid inhaling vapors and allowing contact with skin or mucous membranes, especially those of the eyes. In case of contact, wash with generous amounts of water for at least 15 minutes.
- Dilute drug before use to 1.5 to 3 mg/ml with D$_5$W or normal saline solution in a syringe. Or, dilute to 0.5 to 2 mg/ml in an I.V. bag.
- Give drug I.V. over 6 to 10 minutes into side port of a free-flowing I.V. line that is closest to I.V. bag; then flush with 75 to 125 ml or more of D$_5$W or normal saline solution.

• Monitor site for irritation and infiltration because drug can cause localized tissue damage, necrosis, and thrombophlebitis.

■ **Black Box Warning** Make sure catheter is properly positioned in vein. If extravasation occurs, stop drug immediately and inject remaining dose into a different vein; notify prescriber. ■

• Drug may be stored for up to 24 hours at room temperature.

• **Incompatibilities:** Acyclovir, allopurinol, aminophylline, amphotericin B, ampicillin sodium, cefazolin, ceftriaxone, cefuroxime, fluorouracil, furosemide, ganciclovir, methylprednisolone, mitomycin, piperacillin, sodium bicarbonate, thiotepa, trimethoprim-sulfamethoxazole.

ACTION
Exerts its primary antineoplastic effect by disrupting microtubule assembly, which in turn disrupts spindle formation and prevents mitosis.

Route	Onset	Peak	Duration
I.V.	Unknown	Unknown	Unknown

Half-life: About 27 to 43½ hours.

ADVERSE REACTIONS
CNS: *asthenia, fatigue, peripheral neuropathy.*
CV: chest pain.
GI: *anorexia, constipation, diarrhea, nausea, stomatitis, vomiting.*
Hematologic: *anemia,* **agranulocytosis, bone marrow suppression, granulocytopenia, thrombocytopenia,** LEUKOPENIA.
Hepatic: hyperbilirubinemia.
Musculoskeletal: arthralgia, jaw pain, loss of deep tendon reflexes, myalgia.
Respiratory: dyspnea, shortness of breath.
Skin: *alopecia, injection pain or reaction,* rash.

INTERACTIONS
Drug-drug. *Cisplatin:* May increase risk of bone marrow suppression when used with cisplatin. Monitor hematologic status closely.
Cytochrome P-450 inhibitors: May decrease metabolism of vinorelbine. Watch for increased adverse effects.
Mitomycin: May cause pulmonary reactions. Monitor respiratory status closely.

Paclitaxel: May increase risk of neuropathy. Monitor patient closely.

EFFECTS ON LAB TEST RESULTS
• May increase bilirubin level. May decrease hemoglobin level.
• May increase liver function test values. May decrease granulocyte, WBC, and platelet counts.

CONTRAINDICATIONS & CAUTIONS
• Contraindicated in patients with pretreatment granulocyte count below 1,000/mm³ and in patients hypersensitive to the drug.
• Use with caution in patients whose bone marrow may have been compromised by previous exposure to radiation therapy or chemotherapy or whose bone marrow is still recovering from chemotherapy.
• Use with caution in patients with hepatic impairment.
• Safety and effectiveness in children haven't been established.

NURSING CONSIDERATIONS
■ **Black Box Warning** Check patient's granulocyte count before giving; make sure count is 1,000/mm³ or higher before giving drug. ■

• If count is lower, withhold drug and notify prescriber. Granulocyte count nadir occurs between days 7 and 10.

■ **Black Box Warning** Drug is fatal if given intrathecally; it's for I.V. use only. ■

• Adjust dosage by hematologic toxicity or hepatic insufficiency, whichever results in the lower dosage. If granulocyte count falls below 1,500/mm³ but is greater than 1,000/mm³, reduce dosage by 50%. If three consecutive doses are skipped because of agranulocytosis, don't resume therapy.

• In patients with hepatic impairment, monitor liver enzyme levels.
• Patient may receive injections of WBC colony-stimulating factors to promote cell growth and decrease risk of infection.
• **Alert:** Monitor deep tendon reflexes; loss may represent cumulative toxicity.
• Monitor patient closely for hypersensitivity.
• As a guide to the effects of therapy, monitor patient's peripheral blood count and bone marrow.

Reactions may be *common*, uncommon, *life-threatening*, or COMMON AND LIFE-THREATENING.
Interaction may have a *rapid onset* or **delayed onset.**

• *Look alike–sound alike:* Don't confuse vinorelbine with vinblastine or vincristine.

PATIENT TEACHING
• Advise patient to report any pain or burning at site of injection.
• Instruct patient not to take other drugs, including OTC preparations, until approved by prescriber.
• Tell patient to report evidence of infection (fever, sore throat, fatigue) and bleeding (easy bruising, nosebleeds, bleeding gums, tarry stools). Tell him to take temperature daily.
• Advise patient to report increased shortness of breath, cough, abdominal pain, or constipation.
• Caution woman to avoid becoming pregnant during therapy.

84

Antineoplastics that alter hormone balance

anastrozole
estramustine phosphate sodium
exemestane
flutamide
fulvestrant
goserelin acetate
letrozole
leuprolide acetate
megestrol acetate
tamoxifen citrate
toremifene citrate

SAFETY ALERT!

anastrozole
an-AHS-troh-zol

Arimidex☙

Pharmacologic class: aromatase inhibitor
Pregnancy risk category D

AVAILABLE FORMS
Tablets: 1 mg

INDICATIONS & DOSAGES
➤ **First-line treatment of post-menopausal women with hormone receptor–positive or hormone receptor–unknown locally advanced or metastatic breast cancer; advanced breast cancer in postmenopausal women with disease progression after tamoxifen therapy; adjunctive treatment of postmenopausal women with hormone receptor–positive early breast cancer**
Adults: 1 mg P.O. daily.

ADMINISTRATION
P.O.
● Give drug without regard for meals.

ACTION
A selective nonsteroidal aromatase inhibitor that significantly lowers estradiol levels, which inhibits breast cancer cell growth in postmenopausal women.

Route	Onset	Peak	Duration
P.O.	< 24 hr	Unknown	< 7 days

Half-life: 50 hours.

ADVERSE REACTIONS
CNS: headache, asthenia, pain, dizziness, *depression,* paresthesia.
CV: *hot flashes,* **thromboembolic disease,** chest pain, edema, peripheral edema, hypertension.
EENT: *pharyngitis,* cataracts.
GI: *nausea,* vomiting, diarrhea, constipation, abdominal pain, anorexia, dry mouth, dyspepsia.
GU: vaginal dryness, pelvic pain.
Metabolic: weight gain, increased appetite.
Musculoskeletal: bone pain, *back pain, arthritis, arthralgia.*
Respiratory: dyspnea, increased cough.
Skin: *rash,* sweating.

INTERACTIONS
None significant.

EFFECTS ON LAB TEST RESULTS
● May increase liver enzyme levels.

CONTRAINDICATIONS & CAUTIONS
● Don't use in women who are or may be pregnant.
● Use cautiously in breast-feeding women.

NURSING CONSIDERATIONS
● Give drug under supervision of a prescriber experienced in use of antineoplastics.
● Patients with hormone receptor–negative disease and patients who didn't respond to previous tamoxifen therapy rarely respond to anastrozole.
● For patients with advanced breast cancer, continue anastrozole until tumor progresses.

Reactions may be *common*, uncommon, *life-threatening*, or COMMON AND LIFE-THREATENING.
Interaction may have a *rapid onset* or **delayed onset.**

PATIENT TEACHING
- Instruct patient to report adverse reactions, especially difficulty breathing or chest pain.
- Tell patient to take medication at the same time each day.
- Stress need for follow-up care.
- Counsel woman about risks of pregnancy during therapy.

SAFETY ALERT!

estramustine phosphate sodium
ESS-truh-muss-TEEN

Emcyt

Pharmacologic class: estrogen and nitrogen mustard
Pregnancy risk category X

AVAILABLE FORMS
Capsules: 140 mg

INDICATIONS & DOSAGES
➤ **Palliative treatment of metastatic or progressive prostate cancer**
Adults: 10 to 16 mg/kg daily P.O. in three or four divided doses. Usual dose is 14 mg/kg daily. Continue therapy for up to 3 months and, if successful, maintain as long as patient responds.

ADMINISTRATION
P.O.
- Give drug 1 hour before or 2 hours after meals.
- Don't give drug within 2 hours of dairy products.
- Store capsules in refrigerator.

ACTION
Unknown. Uptake into prostate cancer cells is facilitated by the estrogen component. Once intracellular, it may have weak alkylating activity.

Route	Onset	Peak	Duration
P.O.	Unknown	Unknown	Unknown

Half-life: Terminal, 20 hours.

ADVERSE REACTIONS
CNS: lethargy, insomnia, headache, anxiety, *stroke,* emotional lability.
CV: *MI, edema,* chest pain, thrombophlebitis, *heart failure,* flushing, *thrombosis.*
GI: *nausea,* vomiting, *diarrhea,* anorexia, flatulence, *GI bleeding,* thirst, *GI upset.*
Hematologic: *leukopenia, thrombocytopenia.*
Musculoskeletal: leg cramps.
Respiratory: *pulmonary embolism, dyspnea.*
Skin: rash, pruritus, dry skin, thinning of hair.
Other: *breast tenderness, painful gynecomastia.*

INTERACTIONS
Drug-drug. *Calcium-containing drugs such as antacids:* May impair absorption of estramustine. Avoid using together.
Drug-food. *Milk products and calcium-rich foods:* May impair absorption of drug. Discourage use together.

EFFECTS ON LAB TEST RESULTS
- May increase ALT, AST, ceruloplasmin, cortisol, LDH, phospholipid, prolactin, and triglyceride levels. May decrease folate, phosphate, pregnanediol, and pyroxidine levels.
- May increase PT. May decrease glucose tolerance and platelet and WBC counts.

CONTRAINDICATIONS & CAUTIONS
- Contraindicated in patients hypersensitive to estradiol or nitrogen mustard and in those with active thrombophlebitis or thromboembolic disorders, except when actual tumor mass is cause of thromboembolic phenomenon.
- Use cautiously in patients with history of thrombophlebitis, thromboembolic disorders, or cerebrovascular or coronary artery disease.
- Use cautiously in patients with impaired liver function.

NURSING CONSIDERATIONS
- Monitor weight regularly in patients with history of thrombophlebitis, thromboembolic disorders, or cerebrovascular or

coronary artery disease. Drug may worsen peripheral edema or heart failure.
• Monitor liver function periodically throughout therapy in patients with impaired liver function.
• Each 140-mg capsule contains 12.5 mg of sodium.
• Drug may increase blood pressure and decrease glucose level. Monitor periodically throughout therapy.
• Drug may be effective in patients who don't respond to estrogen therapy alone.
• Patient may continue therapy as long as response is favorable. Some patients have taken drug for more than 3 years.
• Drug may increase norepinephrine-induced platelet aggregation and decrease response to the metyrapone test.

PATIENT TEACHING
• Tell patient to take drug on an empty stomach (1 hour before or 2 hours after meals) and to avoid taking within 2 hours of dairy products.
• Because drug may harm fetus, advise contraception use during therapy.
• Instruct patient to store capsules in refrigerator.

SAFETY ALERT!

exemestane
ecks-eh-MES-tayn

Aromasin

Pharmacologic class: aromatase inhibitor
Pregnancy risk category D

AVAILABLE FORMS
Tablets: 25 mg

INDICATIONS & DOSAGES
➤ **Advanced breast cancer in postmenopausal women whose disease has progressed after treatment with tamoxifen**
Adults: 25 mg P.O. once daily after food.

ADMINISTRATION
P.O.
• Give drug after a meal.

ACTION
A highly protein-bound, irreversible, steroidal aromatase inactivator that reduces circulating estrogen levels, which decreases cell growth in estrogen-dependent breast cancer.

Route	Onset	Peak	Duration
P.O.	Unknown	1 hr	24 hr

Half-life: About 24 hours.

ADVERSE REACTIONS
CNS: *fatigue, insomnia, pain, depression,* anxiety, dizziness, headache, paresthesia, generalized weakness, asthenia, confusion, hypoesthesia, fever.
CV: *hot flashes,* hypertension, edema, chest pain.
EENT: sinusitis, rhinitis, pharyngitis.
GI: *nausea,* vomiting, abdominal pain, anorexia, constipation, diarrhea, increased appetite, dyspepsia.
GU: UTI.
Hematologic: *lymphopenia.*
Musculoskeletal: *arthralgia,* pathologic fractures, arthritis, back pain, skeletal pain.
Respiratory: *dyspnea,* bronchitis, cough, upper respiratory tract infection.
Skin: *increased sweating, alopecia,* itching, dermatitis, rash.
Other: infection, flulike syndrome, lymphedema.

INTERACTIONS
Drug-drug. *Drugs containing estrogen:* May interfere with exemestane's action. Avoid using together.
Potent CYP3A4 inducers, such as phenytoin and rifampicin: May increase the metabolism of exemestane, decreasing level. Increase exemestane dosage to 50 mg daily.
Drug-herb. *St. John's wort:* May decrease effectiveness of drug. Discourage use together.

EFFECTS ON LAB TEST RESULTS
• May increase bilirubin, alkaline phosphatase, and creatinine levels.

CONTRAINDICATIONS & CAUTIONS
• Contraindicated in patients hypersensitive to drug or its components.

Reactions may be *common,* uncommon, *life-threatening,* or COMMON AND LIFE-THREATENING.
Interaction may have a *rapid onset* or **delayed onset.**

NURSING CONSIDERATIONS
● Use drug only in postmenopausal women. Pregnancy must be ruled out before starting drug therapy.
● Patients with advanced disease should continue treatment until tumor progression is apparent.
● Patients with early-stage breast cancer who have taken tamoxifen for 2 to 3 years should take this drug to complete a 5-year course, unless cancer recurs or is found in the other breast.

PATIENT TEACHING
● Tell patient to take drug after a meal.
● Stress the importance of maintaining healthy bones by staying active, eating foods containing calcium and vitamin D, minimizing alcohol consumption, and quitting smoking.
● Advise patient to report adverse effects, especially fever or swelling of arms or legs.

SAFETY ALERT!

flutamide
FLOO-ta-mide

Euflex†

Pharmacologic class: nonsteroidal antiandrogen
Pregnancy risk category D

AVAILABLE FORMS
Capsules: 125 mg, 250 mg†

INDICATIONS & DOSAGES
➤ **Metastatic locally confined prostate cancer (stages B₂, C, D₂), combined with luteinizing hormone–releasing hormone analogues such as leuprolide acetate or goserelin**
Adults: 250 mg P.O. every 8 hours.
➤ **Hirsutism in women ♦**
Women: 125 to 500 mg P.O. daily.

ADMINISTRATION
P.O.
● Give drug with a full glass of water.
● Give drug without regard for food.

ACTION
Inhibits androgen uptake or prevents binding of androgens in nucleus of cells in target tissues.

Route	Onset	Peak	Duration
P.O.	Unknown	2 hr	Unknown

Half-life: For steady-state metabolite, about 6½ hours.

ADVERSE REACTIONS
CNS: drowsiness, confusion, depression, anxiety, nervousness, paresthesia.
CV: peripheral edema, hypertension, *hot flashes.*
GI: *diarrhea, nausea, vomiting,* anorexia.
GU: *impotence,* urine discoloration.
Hematologic: anemia, *leukopenia, thrombocytopenia,* hemolytic anemia.
Hepatic: *hepatic encephalopathy, liver failure.*
Skin: rash, photosensitivity reactions.
Other: *loss of libido,* gynecomastia.

INTERACTIONS
Drug-drug. *Warfarin:* May increase PT. Monitor PT and INR.
Drug-lifestyle. *Sun exposure:* May cause photosensitivity reactions. Advise patient to avoid excessive sunlight exposure.

EFFECTS ON LAB TEST RESULTS
● May increase BUN, creatinine, hemoglobin, and liver enzyme levels.
● May decrease platelet and WBC counts.
● May alter pituitary-gonadal system tests during therapy and for 12 weeks after.

CONTRAINDICATIONS & CAUTIONS
● Contraindicated in patients hypersensitive to drug and in those with severe liver dysfunction.

NURSING CONSIDERATIONS
■ **Black Box Warning** Obtain liver function test at the start of therapy and at the first signs and symptoms suggesting of liver dysfunction (nausea, vomiting, anorexia, fatigue). ■
● Monitor CBC periodically.
● Flutamide must be taken continuously with drug used for medical castration (such as leuprolide) to allow full therapeutic benefit. Leuprolide suppresses testos-

terone production, whereas flutamide inhibits testosterone action at cellular level; together, they can impair growth of androgen-responsive tumors.

PATIENT TEACHING
• Advise patient not to stop drug without consulting prescriber.
• Tell patient to take drug with a full glass of water.
• Tell patient drug may be taken without food, but if stomach irritation occurs, to take with food.
• Instruct patient to report adverse reactions promptly, especially dark yellow or brown urine, vomiting, or yellowing of the eyes or skin.

SAFETY ALERT!

fulvestrant
full-VES-trant

Faslodex

Pharmacologic class: estrogen antagonist
Pregnancy risk category D

AVAILABLE FORMS
Injection: 50 mg/ml in 2.5-ml and 5-ml prefilled syringes

INDICATIONS & DOSAGES
➤ **Hormone receptor–positive metastatic breast cancer with disease progression after antiestrogen therapy**
Postmenopausal women: 250 mg (one 5-ml syringe or two 2.5-ml syringes) by slow I.M. injection into buttocks once monthly.

ADMINISTRATION
I.M.
• Expel gas bubble from syringe before giving.
• When using the 2.5-ml syringes, both must be given to obtain full dose.
• Give slowly into buttocks.

ACTION
Competitively binds estrogen receptors and downregulates estrogen-receptor

protein in human breast cancer cells. It's effective in treating estrogen receptor–positive breast tumors.

Route	Onset	Peak	Duration
I.M.	Unknown	7 days	1 mo

Half-life: About 40 days.

ADVERSE REACTIONS
CNS: *asthenia, headache, pain,* dizziness, insomnia, fever, paresthesia, depression, anxiety.
CV: *hot flashes,* chest pain, peripheral edema.
EENT: *pharyngitis.*
GI: *nausea, vomiting, constipation, abdominal pain, diarrhea,* anorexia.
GU: UTI.
Hematologic: anemia.
Musculoskeletal: *bone pain, back pain, pelvic pain,* arthritis.
Respiratory: *dyspnea, cough.*
Skin: *injection site pain,* rash, sweating.
Other: accidental injury, flulike syndrome.

INTERACTIONS
None reported.

EFFECTS ON LAB TEST RESULTS
• May decrease hemoglobin level and hematocrit.

CONTRAINDICATIONS & CAUTIONS
• Contraindicated in pregnant women and in patients allergic to drug or any of its components.
• Use cautiously in patients with moderate or severe hepatic impairment.

NURSING CONSIDERATIONS
• Because drug is given I.M., don't use in patients with bleeding diatheses or thrombocytopenia, or in those taking anticoagulants.
• Make sure woman isn't pregnant before starting drug.

PATIENT TEACHING
• Caution woman to avoid pregnancy and to report suspected pregnancy immediately.
• Inform patient of the most common side effects, including pain at injection site, headache, GI symptoms, back pain, hot flashes, and sore throat.

Reactions may be *common,* uncommon, *life-threatening,* or COMMON AND LIFE-THREATENING.
Interaction may have a *rapid onset* or *delayed onset.*

goserelin acetate
GOE-se-rel-in

Zoladex

Pharmacologic class: gonadotropin-releasing hormone analogue
Pregnancy risk category X *(endometriosis and endometrial thinning); D (breast cancer)*

AVAILABLE FORMS
Implants: 3.6 mg, 10.8 mg

INDICATIONS & DOSAGES
➤ **Endometriosis, including pain relief and lesion reduction**
Women: 3.6 mg subcutaneously every 28 days into the anterior abdominal wall below the navel. Maximum length of therapy is 6 months.
➤ **Endometrial thinning before endometrial ablation**
Women: 3.6 mg subcutaneously into the anterior abdominal wall below the navel. Give one or two implants, 4 weeks apart.
➤ **Palliative treatment of advanced breast cancer in premenopausal and perimenopausal women**
Women: 3.6 mg subcutaneously every 28 days into the anterior abdominal wall below the navel.
➤ **Palliative treatment of advanced prostate cancer**
Men: 3.6 mg subcutaneously every 28 days or 10.8 mg subcutaneously every 12 weeks into the anterior abdominal wall below the navel.

ADMINISTRATION
Subcutaneous
• Implant comes in a preloaded syringe. If package is damaged, don't use the syringe. Make sure drug is visible in the translucent chamber of the syringe.
• Give drug into the anterior abdominal wall below the navel using aseptic technique.
• After cleaning area with an alcohol swab and injecting a local anesthetic, stretch patient's skin with one hand while grasping barrel of syringe with the other.

• Insert needle into the subcutaneous fat; then change direction of needle so that it parallels the abdominal wall. Push needle in until hub touches patient's skin; withdraw about 1 cm (this creates a gap for drug to be injected) before depressing plunger completely.
• To avoid need for a new syringe and injection site, don't aspirate after inserting needle. If needle penetrates a blood vessel, blood will appear in the syringe chamber. Withdraw needle, and inject elsewhere with a new syringe.
• Never give by I.V. injection.

ACTION
A luteinizing hormone–releasing hormone (LH-RH) analogue that acts on the pituitary gland to decrease the release of follicle-stimulating hormone and LH, dramatically lowering sex hormone levels (estrogen in women and testosterone in men).

Route	Onset	Peak	Duration
Subcut.	Rapid	30–60 min	Throughout therapy

Half-life: About 4½ hours.

ADVERSE REACTIONS
CNS: lethargy, *pain,* dizziness, *insomnia,* anxiety, *depression, headache,* chills, *emotional lability, stroke, asthenia.*
CV: edema, *heart failure, arrhythmias, peripheral edema,* hypertension, *MI,* peripheral vascular disorder, chest pain, *hot flashes.*
GI: nausea, vomiting, diarrhea, constipation, ulcer, anorexia, abdominal pain.
GU: *sexual dysfunction, impotence, lower urinary tract symptoms,* renal insufficiency, urinary obstruction, *vaginitis,* UTI, *amenorrhea.*
Hematologic: anemia.
Metabolic: hypercalcemia, hyperglycemia, weight increase, gout.
Musculoskeletal: back pain, osteoporosis.
Respiratory: COPD, upper respiratory tract infection.
Skin: rash, *diaphoresis, acne, seborrhea,* hirsutism.
Other: *changes in breast size, changes in libido, infection,* breast swelling, pain, and tenderness.

INTERACTIONS
None significant.

EFFECTS ON LAB TEST RESULTS
• May increase calcium and glucose levels. May decrease hemoglobin level.

CONTRAINDICATIONS & CAUTIONS
• Contraindicated in patients hypersensitive to LH-RH, LH-RH agonist analogues, or goserelin acetate.
• Contraindicated in pregnant or breast-feeding women and in patients with obstructive uropathy or vertebral metastases.
• The 10.8-mg implant is contraindicated in women because of insufficient data supporting reliable suppression of estradiol.
• Because drug may cause bone density loss in women, use cautiously in patients with risk factors for osteoporosis, such as family history of osteoporosis, chronic alcohol or tobacco abuse, or use of drugs such as corticosteroids or anticonvulsants that affect bone density.

NURSING CONSIDERATIONS
• Before giving to women, rule out pregnancy.
• When drug is used for prostate cancer, LH-RH analogues such as goserelin may initially worsen symptoms because drug first increases testosterone level. Some patients may temporarily have increased bone pain. Rarely, disease may get worse (spinal cord compression or ureteral obstruction), although the relationship to therapy is uncertain.
• When drug is used for endometrial thinning, if one implant is given, surgery should be performed 4 weeks later; if two implants are given, surgery should be performed 2 to 4 weeks after patient receives second implant.

PATIENT TEACHING
• Advise patient to return every 28 days for a new implant. A delay of a couple of days is permissible.
• Tell patient that pain may worsen for first 30 days of treatment.
• Tell woman to use a nonhormonal form of contraception during treatment. Caution patient about significant risks to fetus.

• Urge woman to call prescriber if menstruation persists or if breakthrough bleeding occurs. Menstruation should stop during treatment.
• Inform woman that a delayed return of menstruation may occur after therapy ends. Persistent lack of menstruation is rare.

SAFETY ALERT!

letrozole
LE-tro-zol

Femara

Pharmacologic class: aromatase inhibitor
Pregnancy risk category D

AVAILABLE FORMS
Tablets: 2.5 mg

INDICATIONS & DOSAGES
➤ **Metastatic breast cancer with disease progression after antiestrogen therapy (such as tamoxifen)**
Postmenopausal women: 2.5 mg P.O. as single daily dose.
➤ **First-line treatment of hormone receptor–positive or hormone receptor–unknown, locally advanced, or metastatic breast cancer**
Postmenopausal women: 2.5 mg P.O. once daily until tumor progression is evident.
➤ **Adjuvant treatment of hormone-sensitive early breast cancer**
Postmenopausal women: 2.5 mg P.O. daily.
➤ **Extended adjuvant treatment of early breast cancer following 5 years of adjuvant tamoxifen therapy**
Postmenopausal women: 2.5 mg P.O. once daily for 5 years.

ADMINISTRATION
P.O.
• Give drug without regard for meals.

ACTION
Inhibits conversion of androgens to estrogens, which decreases tumor mass or delays progression of tumor growth in some women.

Route	Onset	Peak	Duration
P.O.	Unknown	2 days	Unknown

Half-life: About 2 days.

ADVERSE REACTIONS
CNS: headache, somnolence, dizziness, fatigue, mood changes.
CV: *hot flashes,* **MI, thromboembolism,** chest pain, edema, hypertension.
GI: *nausea,* vomiting, constipation, diarrhea, abdominal pain, anorexia.
Metabolic: hypercholesterolemia, weight gain.
Musculoskeletal: *bone pain, limb pain, back pain, arthralgia.*
Respiratory: dyspnea, cough.
Skin: rash, pruritus.
Other: viral infections, breast pain, alopecia, diaphoresis.

INTERACTIONS
Drug-drug. *Tamoxifen:* May reduce plasma letrozole levels. Give letrozole immediately after tamoxifen course is completed.

EFFECTS ON LAB TEST RESULTS
• May increase cholesterol level.

CONTRAINDICATIONS & CAUTIONS
• Contraindicated in patients hypersensitive to drug or its components.
• Use cautiously in patients with severe liver impairment; dosage adjustment isn't needed in those with mild to moderate liver dysfunction.

NURSING CONSIDERATIONS
• Dosage adjustment isn't needed in patients with creatinine clearance of 10 ml/minute or more.
• ***Look alike–sound alike:*** Don't confuse Femara with FemHRT.

PATIENT TEACHING
• Instruct patient to take drug exactly as prescribed.
• Tell patient to take drug with a small glass of water, with or without food.
• Inform patient about potential adverse effects.
• Advise patient to use caution performing tasks that require alertness, coordination, or dexterity, such as driving, until effects are known.

SAFETY ALERT!

leuprolide acetate
loo-PROE-lide

Eligard, Lupron, Lupron Depot, Lupron Depot-Ped, Lupron Depot–3 Month, Lupron Depot–4 Month, Viadur

Pharmacologic class: gonadotropin-releasing hormone analogue
Pregnancy risk category X

AVAILABLE FORMS
Depot injection: 3.75 mg, 7.5 mg, 11.25 mg, 15 mg, 22.5 mg, 30 mg, 45 mg
Injection: 5 mg/ml in 2.8-ml multiple-dose vials
Implant: 65 mg

INDICATIONS & DOSAGES
➤ **Advanced prostate cancer**
Adults: 1 mg subcutaneously daily. Or, 7.5 mg I.M. depot injection monthly. Or, 7.5 mg subcutaneous Eligard once monthly. Or, 22.5 mg I.M. depot injection every 3 months. Or, 22.5 mg subcutaneous Eligard every 3 months. Or, 30 mg I.M. depot injection every 4 months. Or, 30 mg subcutaneous Eligard every 4 months. Or, 45 mg subcutaneous Eligard every 6 months. Or, 72-mg Viadur implant inserted subcutaneously every 12 months.
➤ **Endometriosis**
Adults: 3.75 mg I.M. depot injection as single injection once monthly for up to 6 months. Or, 11.25 mg I.M. every 3 months for up to 6 months.
➤ **Central precocious puberty**
Children: Initially, 0.3 mg/kg (minimum 7.5 mg) I.M. depot injection as single injection every 4 weeks. May increase in increments of 3.75 mg every 4 weeks, if needed. Stop drug before girl reaches age 11 or boy reaches age 12.
➤ **Anemia related to uterine fibroids (with iron therapy)**
Adults: 3.75 mg I.M. depot injection once monthly for up to 3 consecutive months.

---

†Canada   ◇ OTC   ♦ Off-label use   ✐Photoguide   *Liquid contains alcohol.

Or 11.25 mg I.M. depot injection for 1 dose.

ADMINISTRATION
• Products have specific mixing and administration instructions. Read manufacturer's directions closely.
I.M.
• Never give by I.V. injection.
• Give depot injections under medical supervision.
• Use supplied diluent to reconstitute drug (extra diluent is provided; discard remainder).
• Inject into vial; shake well. Suspension will appear milky. Use immediately.
• Draw 1 ml into a syringe with a 22G needle.
• When preparing Lupron Depot–3 Month 22.5 mg, use a 23G or larger needle. Withdraw 1.5 ml from ampule for the 3-month form.
• When using prefilled dual-chamber syringes, prepare for injection according to manufacturer's instructions.
• Gently shake syringe to form a uniform milky suspension. If particles adhere to stopper, tap syringe against your finger.
• Remove needle guard and advance plunger to expel air from syringe. Inject entire contents I.M. as with a normal injection.
Subcutaneous
• For the two-syringe mixing system, connect the syringes and inject the liquid contents according to manufacturer's instructions.
• Mix product by pushing contents back and forth between syringes for about 45 seconds; shaking the syringes won't mix the contents enough.
• Attach the needle provided in the kit and inject subcutaneously.
• Suspension settles very quickly. Remix if settling occurs. Must be given within 30 minutes.
• Never give by I.V. injection.

ACTION
Stimulates and then inhibits release of follicle-stimulating hormone and luteinizing hormone, which suppresses testosterone and estrogen levels.

Route	Onset	Peak	Duration
I.M., Subcut.	Variable	1–2 mo	60–90 days
Implant	Unknown	4 hr	12 mo

Half-life: Unknown.

ADVERSE REACTIONS
CNS: *dizziness, depression, headache, pain,* insomnia, paresthesia, *asthenia.*
CV: *arrhythmias,* angina, *MI, peripheral edema, ECG changes,* hypotension, hypertension, murmur, *hot flashes.*
GI: *nausea, vomiting,* anorexia, constipation.
GU: *impotence, vaginitis,* urinary frequency, hematuria, UTI, *amenorrhea.*
Hematologic: anemia.
Metabolic: *weight gain or loss.*
Musculoskeletal: transient bone pain during first week of treatment, joint disorder, myalgia, neuromuscular disorder, bone loss.
Respiratory: dyspnea, sinus congestion, *pulmonary fibrosis.*
Skin: reactions at injection site, dermatitis, acne.
Other: gynecomastia, androgen-like effects.

INTERACTIONS
None significant.

EFFECTS ON LAB TEST RESULTS
• May increase albumin, alkaline phosphatase, bilirubin, BUN, calcium, creatinine, glucose, LDH, phosphorus, and uric acid levels. May decrease hemoglobin level.
• May alter results of pituitary-gonadal system tests during therapy and for 12 weeks after.

CONTRAINDICATIONS & CAUTIONS
• Contraindicated in patients hypersensitive to drug or other gonadotropin-releasing hormone analogues, in women with undiagnosed vaginal bleeding, and in pregnant or breast-feeding women.
• The 30- and 45-mg depot injections and the Viadur implant are contraindicated in women and children.
• Use cautiously in patients hypersensitive to benzyl alcohol.

Reactions may be *common,* uncommon, *life-threatening,* or COMMON AND LIFE-THREATENING.
Interaction may have a *rapid onset* or *delayed onset.*

NURSING CONSIDERATIONS
● A fractional dose of drug formulated to give every 3, 4, or 6 months isn't equivalent to same dose of once-a-month formulation.
● After starting treatment for central precocious puberty, monitor patient response every 1 to 2 months with a gonadotropin-releasing hormone stimulation test and sex corticosteroid level determinations. Measure bone age for advancement every 6 to 12 months.
● *Alert:* During first few weeks of treatment for prostate cancer, signs and symptoms of disease may temporarily worsen or additional signs and symptoms may occur (tumor flare).

PATIENT TEACHING
● Before starting child on treatment for central precocious puberty, make sure parents understand importance of continuous therapy.
● Carefully instruct patient who will give himself subcutaneous injection about the proper technique and advise him to use only the syringes provided by manufacturer.
● Advise patient that, if another syringe must be substituted, a low-dose insulin syringe (U-100, 0.5 ml) may be an appropriate choice but that needle gauge should be no smaller than 22G (except when using Lupron Depot–3 Month 22.5 mg).
● Instruct patient to store leuprolide acetate powder (depot) and diluent at room temperature, to refrigerate unopened vials of leuprolide acetate injection, and to protect leuprolide acetate injection from heat and light.
● Inform patient with history of undesirable effects from other endocrine therapies that leuprolide is easier to tolerate.
● Reassure patient that adverse effects disappear after about 1 week. Explain that symptoms of prostate cancer or central precocious puberty may worsen at first.
● Advise patient to keep implant insertion site clean and dry for 24 hours after procedure and to avoid heavy physical activity until site has healed. Local insertion site reactions such as bruising, burning, itching, and pain may resolve within 2 weeks.
● Advise woman of childbearing age to use a nonhormonal form of contraception during treatment.

megestrol acetate
me-JESS-trole

Megace, Megace ES, Megace OS†

Pharmacologic class: progestin
Pregnancy risk category D (tablets);
X (oral suspension)

AVAILABLE FORMS
Oral suspension: 40 mg/ml
Oral suspension (concentrated): 125 mg/ml
Tablets: 20 mg, 40 mg

INDICATIONS & DOSAGES
➤ **Breast cancer**
Adults: 40 mg P.O. q.i.d.
➤ **Endometrial cancer**
Adults: 40 to 320 mg P.O. daily in divided doses.
➤ **Anorexia, cachexia, or unexplained significant weight loss in patients with AIDS**
Adults: 800 mg P.O. (20 ml regular oral suspension) or 625 mg P.O. (5 ml concentrated oral suspension) once daily.

ADMINISTRATION
P.O.
● Give drug without regard for meals.
● Shake suspension well before pouring.

ACTION
Inhibits hormone-dependent tumor growth by inhibiting pituitary and adrenal steroidogenesis. Drug may also have direct cytotoxicity; its appetite-stimulating mechanism is unknown.

Route	Onset	Peak	Duration
P.O.	Unknown	1–5 hr	Unknown

Half-life: About 10 days.

ADVERSE REACTIONS
CV: thrombophlebitis, *heart failure,* hypertension, *thromboembolism.*
GI: nausea, vomiting, *diarrhea,* flatulence, constipation, dry mouth, increased appetite.
GU: breakthrough menstrual bleeding, impotence, vaginal bleeding or discharge, UTI.

Metabolic: hyperglycemia, *weight gain.*
Musculoskeletal: carpal tunnel syndrome.
Respiratory: *pulmonary embolism,* dyspnea.
Skin: alopecia, rash.
Other: gynecomastia, tumor flare.

INTERACTIONS
None significant.

EFFECTS ON LAB TEST RESULTS
• May increase glucose level.

CONTRAINDICATIONS & CAUTIONS
• Contraindicated in patients hypersensitive to drug.
• Contraindicated in known or suspected pregnancy.
• Use cautiously in patients with history of thrombophlebitis or thromboembolism.

NURSING CONSIDERATIONS
• May increase glucose level in diabetic patients.
• Drug isn't intended for prophylactic use to avoid weight loss. Start treatment with megestrol acetate oral suspension only after treatable causes of weight loss are sought and addressed.
• Drug is relatively nontoxic with a low risk of adverse effects.
• Two months is an adequate trial period in patients with cancer.

PATIENT TEACHING
• Inform patient that therapeutic response isn't immediate. Drug must be taken for at least 2 months to determine effectiveness.
• Tell patient drug may be taken without regard to food.
• *Alert:* Tell patient that the ES oral suspension is more concentrated than the regular oral suspension, so a smaller amount is needed.
• Advise woman to stop breast-feeding during therapy because of risk of toxicity to infant.
• Advise woman of childbearing age to use an effective form of contraception while receiving drug.

tamoxifen citrate
ta-MOX-i-fen

APO-Tamox†, Nolvadex-D†, Tamofen†

Pharmacologic class: nonsteroidal antiestrogen
Pregnancy risk category D

AVAILABLE FORMS
Tablets: 10 mg, 20 mg

INDICATIONS & DOSAGES
➤ **Advanced breast cancer in women and men**
Adults: 20 mg to 40 mg P.O. daily; divide doses of more than 20 mg per day b.i.d.
➤ **Adjunct treatment of breast cancer**
Women: 20 mg to 40 mg P.O. daily for 5 years; divide doses of more than 20 mg per day b.i.d.
➤ **To reduce breast cancer occurrence**
High-risk women: 20 mg P.O. daily for 5 years.
➤ **Ductal carcinoma in situ (DCIS) after breast surgery and radiation**
Adults: 20 mg P.O. daily for 5 years.

ADMINISTRATION
P.O.
• Give drug without regard to food.

ACTION
Unknown. Drug is selective estrogen-receptor modulator.

Route	Onset	Peak	Duration
P.O.	1 mo–Several mo	Unknown	Several wk

Half-life: Distribution phase, 7 to 14 hours; terminal phase, more than 7 days.

ADVERSE REACTIONS
CNS: *stroke,* confusion, weakness, sleepiness, headache.
CV: *fluid retention, hot flashes, thromboembolism.*
EENT: corneal changes, cataracts, retinopathy.

Reactions may be *common,* uncommon, *life-threatening,* or COMMON AND LIFE-THREATENING.
Interaction may have a *rapid onset* or **delayed onset.**

GI: *nausea, vomiting, diarrhea.*
GU: *amenorrhea, irregular menses, vaginal discharge, **endometrial cancer, uterine sarcoma,** vaginal bleeding.*
Hematologic: ***leukopenia, thrombo-cytopenia.***
Hepatic: ***hepatic necrosis,*** fatty liver, cholestasis.
Metabolic: *hypercalcemia, weight gain or loss.*
Musculoskeletal: brief worsening of pain from osseous metastases.
Respiratory: ***pulmonary embolism (PE).***
Skin: *skin changes,* rash.
Other: temporary bone or tumor pain, alopecia.

INTERACTIONS

Drug-drug. *Bromocriptine:* May elevate tamoxifen level. Monitor patient closely.
Coumarin-type anticoagulants: May significantly increase anticoagulant effect. Monitor patient, PT, and INR closely.
CYP3A4 inducers (such as rifampin): May increase tamoxifen metabolism and may lower drug levels. Monitor patient for clinical effects.
Cytotoxic drugs: May increase risk of thromboembolic events. Monitor patient.

EFFECTS ON LAB TEST RESULTS

● May increase BUN, calcium, T_4, and liver enzyme levels.
● May decrease WBC and platelet counts.

CONTRAINDICATIONS & CAUTIONS

● Contraindicated in patients hypersensitive to drug.
● Contraindicated as therapy to reduce risk of breast cancer in high-risk women who also need anticoagulants or in women with history of deep vein thrombosis or PE.
● Use cautiously in patients with leukopenia or thrombocytopenia.

NURSING CONSIDERATIONS

● Monitor lipid levels during long-term therapy in patients with hyperlipidemia.
● Monitor calcium level. At start of therapy, drug may compound hypercalcemia related to bone metastases.
● Women should have baseline and periodic gynecologic examinations because of a slight increased risk of endometrial cancer.

● Monitor CBC closely in patients with leukopenia or thrombocytopenia.
● Rule out pregnancy before therapy.
● Patient may initially experience worsening symptoms.
● Adverse reactions are usually minor and well tolerated.
● In postmenopausal women, karyopyknotic index of vaginal smears and various degrees of estrogen effect of Papanicolaou smears may vary.
■ **Black Box Warning** Women who are at high risk for breast cancer or who have DCIS and are taking drug to reduce risk may experience life-threatening endometrial cancer, uterine sarcoma, stroke, or PE. The benefits of drug outweigh its risks in women already diagnosed with breast cancer. ■

PATIENT TEACHING

● Reassure patient that acute worsening of bone pain during therapy usually indicates drug will produce good response. Give analgesics to relieve pain.
● Strongly encourage woman who is taking or has taken drug to have regular gynecologic exams because drug may increase risk of uterine cancer.
● Encourage woman to have annual mammograms and breast exams.
● Advise patient to use a barrier form of contraception because short-term therapy induces ovulation in premenopausal women.
● Instruct patient to report vaginal bleeding or changes in menstrual cycle.
● Caution woman to avoid becoming pregnant during therapy and first 2 months after stopping drug. Advise her to consult prescriber before becoming pregnant.
● Advise patient that breast cancer risk assessment tools are available and that she should discuss her concerns with her prescriber.
● Tell patient to report symptoms of stroke, such as headache, vision changes, confusion, difficulty speaking or walking, and weakness of face, arm, or leg, especially on one side of the body.
● Tell patients to report symptoms of PE, such as chest pain, difficulty breathing, rapid breathing, sweating, and fainting.

toremifene citrate
tore-EM-ah-feen

Fareston

Pharmacologic class: nonsteroidal antiestrogen
Pregnancy risk category D

AVAILABLE FORMS
Tablets: 60 mg

INDICATIONS & DOSAGES
➤ **Metastatic breast cancer in post-menopausal women with estrogen receptor–positive or estrogen receptor–unknown tumors**
Adults: 60 mg P.O. once daily. Continue until disease progresses.

ADMINISTRATION
P.O.
● Give drug without regard for meals.

ACTION
A nonsteroidal triphenylethylene with antiestrogenic effect; competes with estrogen for binding sites in the tumor, which blocks the tumor's growth-stimulating effects of endogenous estrogen.

Route	Onset	Peak	Duration
P.O.	Unknown	3 hr	Unknown

Half-life: About 5 days.

ADVERSE REACTIONS
CNS: dizziness, fatigue, depression.
CV: edema, ***thromboembolism, heart failure, MI, pulmonary embolism,*** hot flashes.
EENT: visual disturbances, glaucoma, dry eyes, *cataracts.*
GI: *nausea,* vomiting.
GU: *vaginal discharge,* vaginal bleeding.
Hepatic: *hepatotoxicity.*
Metabolic: hypercalcemia.
Skin: *sweating.*

INTERACTIONS
Drug-drug. *Calcium-elevating drugs such as hydrochlorothiazide:* May increase risk of hypercalcemia. Monitor calcium level closely.

Coumarin-like anticoagulants such as warfarin: May prolong PT and INR. Monitor PT and INR closely.
CYP3A4 enzyme inducers such as carbamazepine, phenobarbital, and phenytoin: May increase toremifene metabolism rate. Monitor patient closely.
CYP3A4-6 enzyme inhibitors such as erythromycin, and ketoconazole: May increase toremifene metabolism rate. Monitor patient closely.

EFFECTS ON LAB TEST RESULTS
● May increase calcium and liver enzyme levels.

CONTRAINDICATIONS & CAUTIONS
● Contraindicated in patients hypersensitive to drug and in those with history of thromboembolic disease.

NURSING CONSIDERATIONS
● Obtain periodic CBC, calcium levels, and liver function tests.
● Monitor calcium level closely during first weeks of treatment in patients with bone metastases because of increased risk of hypercalcemia.

PATIENT TEACHING
● Instruct patient to take drug exactly as prescribed.
● Advise patient that doses may be taken without regard for meals.
● Warn patient not to stop therapy without consulting prescriber.
● Inform patient about vaginal bleeding and other adverse effects; tell her to notify prescriber if bleeding occurs.
● Warn patient that disease flare-up may occur during first weeks of therapy. Reassure her that this doesn't indicate treatment failure.
● Advise patient to report leg or chest pain, severe headache, visual changes, or shortness of breath.
● Counsel woman about risks of becoming pregnant during therapy.

Reactions may be *common*, uncommon, *life-threatening*, or COMMON AND LIFE-THREATENING.
Interaction may have a *rapid onset* or *delayed onset.*

85

Miscellaneous antineoplastics

asparaginase
azacitidine
bevacizumab
bortezomib
cetuximab
dasatinib
erlotinib
etoposide
etoposide phosphate
imatinib mesylate
irinotecan hydrochloride
ixabepilone
lapatinib
mitoxantrone hydrochloride
nelarabine
nilotinib
panitumumab
pegaspargase
procarbazine hydrochloride
rituximab
sorafenib
sunitinib malate
temsirolimus
teniposide
topotecan hydrochloride
trastuzumab

SAFETY ALERT!

asparaginase
a-SPARE-a-gi-nase

Elspar, Kidrolase†

Pharmacologic class: Escherichia coli–derived enzyme
Pregnancy risk category C

AVAILABLE FORMS
Injection: 10,000-international unit vial

INDICATIONS & DOSAGES
➤ **Acute lymphocytic leukemia with other drugs**
Adults and children: 1,000 international units/kg I.V. daily for 10 days beginning on day 22 of regimen, injected over 30 minutes. Or, 6,000 international units/m² I.M. at intervals specified in protocol.

➤ **Sole induction drug for acute lymphocytic leukemia**
Adults and children: 200 international units/kg I.V. daily for 28 days.

ADMINISTRATION
I.V.
• Preparing and giving parenteral form of drug may be mutagenic, teratogenic, or carcinogenic. Follow facility policy to reduce risks.
• Reconstitute drug with 5 ml of sterile water for injection or saline solution for injection.
• To avoid foaming, don't shake vial vigorously.
• Use only clear solution.
• Use of a 5-micron filter during infusion removes gelatinous fiberlike particles that occasionally form without reducing drug potency.
• Give injection over 30 minutes through a running infusion of normal saline solution or D_5W.
• Refrigerate unopened dry powder. Reconstituted solution is stable for 8 hours if refrigerated.
• If drug touches skin or mucous membranes, wash with a generous amount of water for at least 15 minutes.
• **Incompatibilities:** None reported.
I.M.
• For I.M. injection, reconstitute with 2 ml normal saline solution to the 10,000–international unit vial. Refrigerate and use within 8 hours.
• Don't give more than 2 ml I.M. at one injection site.
• Don't use cloudy solutions.
• If drug touches skin or mucous membranes, wash with a generous amount of water for at least 15 minutes.

ACTION
Leads to death of leukemic cells by destroying the essential amino acid asparagine, which is needed for protein synthesis in acute lymphocytic leukemia.

Route	Onset	Peak	Duration
I.V.	Immediate	Immediate	23–33 days
I.M.	Unknown	14–24 hr	23–33 days

Half-life: 8 to 30 hours.

ADVERSE REACTIONS
CNS: agitation, confusion, drowsiness, depression, fatigue, fever, hallucinations, headache, lethargy, somnolence.
GI: HEMORRHAGIC PANCREATITIS, *anorexia, nausea, vomiting,* cramps, stomatitis.
GU: *azotemia,* **renal failure,** glycosuria, polyuria, uric acid nephropathy.
Hematologic: *anemia,* **DIC, hypofibrinogenemia, leukopenia,** depression of clotting factor synthesis.
Hepatic: *hepatotoxicity.*
Metabolic: *hyperglycemia,* hyperammonemia, hyperuricemia, hypocalcemia, weight loss.
Skin: *rash, urticaria.*
Other: ANAPHYLAXIS, chills, hypersensitivity reactions.

INTERACTIONS
Drug-drug. *Methotrexate:* May decrease methotrexate effectiveness. Avoid using together, or give asparaginase after methotrexate.
Prednisone: May cause hyperglycemia. Monitor glucose level.
Vincristine: May increase neuropathy. Give asparaginase after vincristine, and monitor patient closely.

EFFECTS ON LAB TEST RESULTS
• May increase alkaline phosphatase, ammonia, AST, ALT, bilirubin, BUN, glucose, and uric acid levels. May decrease calcium, cholesterol, hemoglobin, and serum albumin levels.
• May decrease thyroid function test values and WBC count.

CONTRAINDICATIONS & CAUTIONS
• Contraindicated in patients hypersensitive to drug (unless desensitized) and in those with pancreatitis or history of pancreatitis.
• Use cautiously in patients with hepatic dysfunction.

NURSING CONSIDERATIONS
■ **Black Box Warning** Drug should be given in a hospital setting only under the supervision of an experienced physician who is prepared to treat anaphylaxis. ■
• Monitor blood and urine glucose levels before and during therapy. Watch for signs and symptoms of hyperglycemia.
• Start allopurinol before therapy begins to help prevent uric acid nephropathy.
• *Alert:* Risk of hypersensitivity increases with repeated doses. Give 2 international units I.D. before first dose and when 1 week or more has elapsed between doses. Observe site for at least 1 hour for erythema or a wheal, which indicates a positive skin test.
• *Alert:* Patient with negative skin test may still develop an allergic reaction; desensitization may be needed before first treatment dose and with retreatment. Give 1 international unit I.V. If no reaction occurs, double dose every 10 minutes until total daily dose is given.
• Drug shouldn't be used alone to induce remission unless combination therapy is inappropriate. Drug isn't recommended for maintenance therapy.
• Keep epinephrine, diphenhydramine, and I.V. corticosteroids available for treating anaphylaxis.
• Monitor CBC and bone marrow function tests.
• Obtain amylase and lipase levels to check pancreatic status. If levels are elevated, stop asparaginase.
• Increase patient's fluid intake to help prevent tumor lysis, which can result in uric acid nephropathy.
• Drug may affect clotting factor synthesis and cause hypofibrinogenemia, leading to thrombosis or, more commonly, severe bleeding. Monitor patient and bleeding studies closely.
• Because of vomiting, give fluids parenterally for 24 hours or until oral fluids are tolerated.
• Patient may become hypersensitive to drug derived from cultures of *Escherichia coli.* Erwinia asparaginase, which is derived from cultures of *E. carotovora,* may be used in these patients without causing cross-sensitivity.

Reactions may be *common,* uncommon, *life-threatening,* or COMMON AND LIFE-THREATENING.
Interaction may have a *rapid onset* or **delayed onset.**

- Drug toxicity is more likely to occur in adults than in children.
- There are several protocols for use of this drug.

PATIENT TEACHING
- Tell patient to watch for signs of infection (fever, sore throat, fatigue) and bleeding (easy bruising, nosebleeds, bleeding gums, tarry stools). Tell patient to take temperature daily.
- Stress importance of maintaining adequate fluid intake to help prevent hyperuricemia. If adverse GI reactions prevent patient from drinking fluids, tell him to notify prescriber.
- Urge patient to immediately report severe headache, stomach pain with nausea or vomiting, or inability to move a limb.
- Advise patient to report signs of a hypersensitivity reaction, including rash, itching, chills, dizziness, chest tightness, or difficulty breathing.

SAFETY ALERT!

azacitidine
az-uh-SIT-uh-deen

Vidaza

Pharmacologic class: pyrimidine nucleoside analog
Pregnancy risk category D

AVAILABLE FORMS
Powder for injection: 100-mg vials

INDICATIONS & DOSAGES
➤ **Myelodysplastic syndrome, including refractory anemia, refractory anemia with ringed sideroblasts (if patient has neutropenia or thrombocytopenia, or needs transfusions), refractory anemia with excess blasts, refractory anemia with excess blasts in transformation, or chronic myelomonocytic leukemia**
Adults: Initially, 75 mg/m² subcutaneously or I.V. daily for 7 days; repeat cycle every 4 weeks. May increase to 100 mg/m² if no response after two treatment cycles and

nausea and vomiting are the only toxic reactions. Four to six treatment cycles are recommended.
Adjust-a-dose: If bicarbonate level is less than 20 mEq/L, reduce next dose by 50%. If BUN or creatinine levels rise during treatment, delay the next cycle until they are normal; then give 50% of previous dose.

For patients with baseline WBC greater than or equal to 3×10^9/L, absolute neutrophil count (ANC) greater than or equal to 1.5×10^9/L, and platelets greater than or equal to 75×10^9/L, adjust the dose based on nadir counts as follows: If ANC is less than 0.5×10^9/L and platelets are less than 25×10^9/L, give 50% of dose. If ANC is 0.5 to 1.5×10^9/L and platelets are 25 to 50×10^9/L, give 67% of dose. Adjust further dosages during therapy based on hematologic or renal toxicities.

ADMINISTRATION
I.V.
- Reconstitute drug with 10 ml of sterile water for injection.
- Vigorously shake or roll the vial until powder is dissolved. The resulting solution will be 10 mg/ml.
- Use only clear solution.
- Withdraw proper dose and mix in a total volume of 50 to 100 ml of normal saline solution or lactated Ringer's solution.
- Give the infusion over 10 to 40 minutes. Infusion must be completed within 1 hour of reconstitution.
- **Incompatibilities:** Dextrose 5%, hespan, bicarbonate.
Subcutaneous
- Dilute using aseptic and hazardous substances techniques.
- Reconstitute with 4 ml sterile water for injection. Invert vial two to three times and gently rotate until a uniform suspension forms. The resulting cloudy suspension will be 25 mg/ml.
- Draw up suspension into syringes for injection (no more than 4 ml per syringe).
- Just before giving drug, resuspend drug by inverting the syringe two to three times and gently rolling between palms for 30 seconds. Divide doses greater than

4 ml into two syringes and inject into two separate sites.

● Give new injections at least 1 inch from previous site, and never into tender, bruised, red, or hardened skin.

● Reconstituted drug is stable 1 hour at room temperature and 8 hours refrigerated (36° to 46° F [2° to 8° C]). After refrigeration, suspension may be allowed to warm for 30 minutes at room temperature.

ACTION

Causes hypomethylation of DNA and is toxic to abnormal hematopoietic cells in bone marrow. Hypomethylation may restore normal function to genes needed for proliferation and differentiation. Drug has little effect on nonproliferating cells.

Route	Onset	Peak	Duration
I.V.	Unknown	Unknown	Unknown
Subcut.	Unknown	30 min	Unknown

Half-life: About 40 minutes after subcutaneous injection; unknown after I.V.

ADVERSE REACTIONS

CNS: *anxiety, depression, dizziness, fatigue, headache, insomnia, malaise, pain, weakness,* hypoesthesia, lethargy, syncope.

CV: *cardiac murmur, chest pain, edema,* hypotension, peripheral swelling, tachycardia.

EENT: *epistaxis, nasopharyngitis, pharyngitis, rhinorrhea,* nasal congestion, postnasal drip, sinusitis.

GI: *abdominal pain and tenderness, anorexia, constipation, decreased appetite, diarrhea, nausea, vomiting,* abdominal distention, dyspepsia, dysphagia, gingival bleeding, hemorrhoids, loose stools, mouth hemorrhage, oral mucosal petechiae, stomatitis, tongue ulceration.

GU: *dysuria,* UTI.

Hematologic: *anemia,* FEBRILE NEUTROPENIA, LEUKOPENIA, NEUTROPENIA, THROMBOCYTOPENIA, hematoma, postprocedural hemorrhage.

Metabolic: *decreased weight.*

Musculoskeletal: *arthralgia, back pain, limb pain, myalgia,* muscle cramps.

Respiratory: *atelectasis, cough, crackles, dyspnea, rales, rhonchi, pneumonia, upper respiratory tract infection,* pleural effusion, wheezing.

Skin: *bruising, contusion, ecchymosis, erythema, increased sweating, injection site reaction, pain, pallor, petechiae, pitting edema, rash, skin lesion,* cellulitis, dry skin, granuloma, night sweats, pigmentation, pruritus at injection site, skin nodules, swelling at injection site, urticaria.

Other: *pyrexia, rigors,* herpes simplex, lymphadenopathy.

INTERACTIONS

None reported.

EFFECTS ON LAB TEST RESULTS

● May increase BUN and creatinine levels. May decrease bicarbonate and potassium levels.

● May decrease neutrophil, platelet, and WBC counts.

CONTRAINDICATIONS & CAUTIONS

● Contraindicated in patients hypersensitive to azacitidine or mannitol and in patients with advanced malignant hepatic tumors.

● Use cautiously in patients with hepatic and renal disease.

NURSING CONSIDERATIONS

● Check liver function test results and creatinine level before therapy starts.

● Obtain CBC before each cycle or more often.

● Monitor renal function closely in elderly patients and in renally impaired patients receiving drug because renal impairment may increase toxicity.

● Store unreconstituted vials at room temperature (59° to 86° F [15° to 30° C]).

PATIENT TEACHING

● Inform patient that blood counts may decrease with febrile neutropenia, thrombocytopenia, and anemia.

● Advise men and women to use birth control during therapy.

Reactions may be *common,* uncommon, *life-threatening,* or COMMON AND LIFE-THREATENING.
Interaction may have a *rapid onset* or *delayed onset.*

bevacizumab
beh-vah-SIZZ-yoo-mab

Avastin

Pharmacologic class: monoclonal
antibody
Pregnancy risk category C

AVAILABLE FORMS
Solution: 25 mg/ml in 4-ml and 16-ml vials

INDICATIONS & DOSAGES
➤ **First- or second-line treatment,
with fluorouracil-based chemotherapy, for metastatic colon or
rectal cancer**
Adults: If used with bolus irinotecan,
fluorouracil, and leucovorin (IFL) regimen,
give 5 mg/kg I.V. every 14 days. If used
with oxaliplatin, fluorouracil, and leucovorin (known as FOLFOX 4) regimen, give
10 mg/kg I.V. every 14 days. Infusion rate
varies by patient tolerance and number of
infusions.
➤ **With carboplatin and paclitaxel
as first-line treatment of unresectable, locally advanced, recurrent,
or metastatic nonsquamous,
non–small cell lung cancer**
Adults: 15 mg/kg I.V. infusion once every
3 weeks.
✻*NEW INDICATION:* **With paclitaxel, for
metastatic HER2-negative breast
cancer in patients who have not
received chemotherapy.**
Adults: 10 mg/kg I.V. every 14 days.

ADMINISTRATION
I.V.
● Don't freeze or shake vials.
● Dilute drug using aseptic technique.
Withdraw proper dose and mix in a total
volume of 100 ml normal saline solution
in an I.V. bag.
● Don't give by I.V. push or bolus.
● Give the first infusion over 90 minutes
and, if tolerated, the second infusion over
60 minutes. Later infusions can be given
over 30 minutes if previous infusions were
tolerated.
● Discard unused portion; drug is
preservative-free.

● Drug is stable 8 hours if refrigerated at
36° to 46° F (2° to 8° C) and protected
from light.
● **Incompatibilities:** Dextrose solutions.

ACTION
A recombinant humanized vascular
endothelial growth factor (VEGF)
inhibitor. Because VEGF promotes angiogenesis to tumors, it may contribute to
metastatic tumor growth.

Route	Onset	Peak	Duration
I.V.	Unknown	Unknown	Unknown

Half-life: About 20 days.

ADVERSE REACTIONS
CNS: *asthenia, dizziness, headache,*
abnormal gait, confusion, pain, syncope.
CV: INTRA-ABDOMINAL THROMBOSIS,
*hypertension, **thromboembolism, deep vein
thrombosis,** heart failure, hypotension.*
EENT: *epistaxis,* excess lacrimation,
gum bleeding, taste disorder, voice
alteration.
GI: *anorexia, constipation, diarrhea,
dyspepsia, flatulence, stomatitis, vomiting,
GI hemorrhage,* abdominal pain, colitis,
dry mouth, nausea.
GU: *vaginal hemorrhage,* proteinuria,
urinary urgency.
Hematologic: *leukopenia, neutropenia,
thrombocytopenia.*
Metabolic: *hypokalemia, weight loss,*
bilirubinemia.
Musculoskeletal: *myalgia.*
Respiratory: HEMOPTYSIS, *dyspnea,
upper respiratory tract infection.*
Skin: *alopecia, dermatitis, discoloration,
dry skin, exfoliative dermatitis,* nail
disorder, skin ulcer.
Other: decreased wound healing, hypersensitivity.

INTERACTIONS
Drug-drug. *Irinotecan:* May increase
level of irinotecan metabolite. Monitor
patient.

EFFECTS ON LAB TEST RESULTS
● May increase bilirubin and urine protein
levels. May decrease potassium level.
● May decrease neutrophil, platelet, and
WBC counts.

CONTRAINDICATIONS & CAUTIONS
• Contraindicated in patients with recent hemoptysis or within 28 days after major surgery.
• Use cautiously in patients hypersensitive to drug or its components, in those who need surgery, are taking anticoagulants, or have significant CV disease.

NURSING CONSIDERATIONS
• *Alert:* Reversible posterior leuko-encephalopathy syndrome (RPLS)-associated symptoms (hypertension, headache, visual disturbances, altered mental function, and seizures) may occur 16 hours to 1 year after starting the drug. Monitor patient closely. If syndrome occurs, stop drug and provide supportive care.
• RPLS can be confirmed only by MRI.
• Hypersensitivity reactions can occur during infusion. Monitor the patient closely.
• In patients who develop nephrotic syndrome, severe hypertension, hypertensive crisis, serious hemorrhage, GI perforation, or wound dehiscence that needs intervention, stop drug.
• Before elective surgery, stop drug, considering drug's half-life is about 20 days. Don't resume therapy until incision is fully healed.
• *Alert:* Drug may increase risk of serious arterial thromboembolic events including MI, TIAs, stroke, and angina. Those patients at highest risk are age 65 or older, have a history of arterial thromboembolism, and have taken the drug before. If patient has an arterial thrombotic event, permanently stop drug.
■ **Black Box Warning** Drug may cause fatal GI perforation. Monitor patient closely. ■
■ **Black Box Warning** Bevacizumab can result in life-threatening wound dehiscence. Permanently discontinue bevacizumab therapy in patients who experience wound dehiscence that requires medical intervention. ■
■ **Black Box Warning** Fatal pulmonary hemorrhage can occur in patients with non-small cell lung cancer treated with chemotherapy and bevacizumab. ■
• Monitor urinalysis for worsening proteinuria. Patients with 2+ or greater urine

dipstick test should undergo 24-hour urine collection.
• Monitor patient's blood pressure every 2 to 3 weeks.
• It's unknown whether drug appears in breast milk. Women shouldn't breast-feed during therapy and for about 3 weeks after therapy ends.
• Adverse reactions occur more often in older patients.

PATIENT TEACHING
• Inform patient about potential adverse reactions.
• Tell patient to report adverse reactions immediately, especially abdominal pain, constipation, and vomiting.
• Advise patient that blood pressure and urinalysis will be monitored during treatment.
• Caution woman of childbearing age to avoid pregnancy during treatment.
• Urge patient to alert other health care providers about treatment and to avoid elective surgery during treatment.

SAFETY ALERT!

bortezomib
bore-TEZ-uh-mib

Velcade

Pharmacologic class: proteosome inhibitor
Pregnancy risk category D

AVAILABLE FORMS
Powder for injection: 3.5 mg

INDICATIONS & DOSAGES
✳ *NEW INDICATION:* **Previously untreated multiple myeloma**
Adults: 1.3 mg/m^2 I.V. over 3 to 5 seconds in combination with oral melphalan and oral prednisone for nine 6-week treatment cycles. In cycles 1–4, bortezomib is given twice weekly (days 1, 4, 8, 11, 22, 25, 29, and 32). In cycles 5–9, bortezomib is given once weekly (days 1, 8, 22, and 29). Separate consecutive doses of drug by at least 72 hours. Prior to initiating any cycle, platelet count should be 70 × 10^9/L or greater, ANC should be 1 × 10^9/L or

---

Reactions may be *common*, uncommon, *life-threatening*, or COMMON AND LIFE-THREATENING.
Interaction may have a *rapid onset* or **delayed onset**.

greater, and non-hematology toxicities should have resolved to Grade 1 or baseline.

Adjust-a-dose: If prolonged grade 4 neutropenia or thrombocytopenia, or thrombocytopenia with bleeding in previous cycle, consider reducing dose by 25% for next cycle. If platelet count less than or equal to 30 × 10⁹/L or ANC 0.75 × 10⁹/L or less on a day other than day 1, withhold dose. If several doses in consecutive cycles are withheld due to toxicity, reduce dose by 1 dose level (from 1.3 mg/m² to 1 mg/m², or from 1 mg/m² to 0.7 mg/m²). For grade 3 non-hematological toxicities, withhold drug until symptoms are grade 1 or baseline, then restart with one dose level reduction. If patient has neuropathic pain, peripheral neuropathy, or both, see table.

➤ **Multiple myeloma or mantle cell lymphoma that still progresses after at least one therapy**

Adults: 1.3 mg/m² by I.V. bolus twice weekly for 2 weeks (days 1, 4, 8, and 11), followed by a 10-day rest period (days 12 through 21). This 3-week period is a treatment cycle. For therapy longer than 8 cycles, may adjust dosage schedule to once weekly for 4 weeks on days 1, 8, 15, and 22, followed by a rest period on days 23 through 35. Separate consecutive doses of drug by at least 72 hours.

Adjust-a-dose: If grade 3 nonhematologic or grade 4 hematologic toxicity (excluding neuropathy) develops, withhold drug. When toxicity has resolved, restart at a 25% reduced dose. If patient has neuropathic pain, peripheral neuropathy, or both, see table.

Severity of neuropathy	Dosage
Grade 1 (paresthesias, loss of reflexes, or both) without pain or loss of function	No change.
Grade 1 with pain or grade 2 (function altered but not activities of daily living)	Reduce to 1 mg/m².
Grade 2 with pain or grade 3 (interference with activities of daily living)	Hold drug until toxicity resolves; then start at 0.7 mg/m² once weekly.
Grade 4 (permanent sensory loss that interferes with function)	Stop drug.

ADMINISTRATION
I.V.
● Use caution and aseptic technique when preparing and handling drug. Wear gloves and protective clothing to prevent skin contact.
● Reconstitute with 3.5 ml of normal saline solution and give by I.V. bolus.
● Reconstituted drug may be stored up to 3 hours in a syringe at 59° to 86° F (15° to 30° C), but total storage time must not exceed 8 hours.
● Store unopened vial at a controlled room temperature, in original packaging, protected from light.
● **Incompatibilities:** None reported.

ACTION
Disrupts intracellular homeostatic mechanisms by inhibiting the 26S proteosome, which regulates intracellular levels of certain proteins, causing cells to die.

Route	Onset	Peak	Duration
I.V.	Unknown	Unknown	Unknown

Half-life: 9 to 15 hours.

ADVERSE REACTIONS
CNS: *anxiety, asthenia, dizziness, dysesthesia, fever, headache, insomnia, paresthesia, peripheral neuropathy, rigors.*
CV: *edema, hypotension.*
EENT: *blurred vision.*
GI: *abdominal pain, constipation, decreased appetite, diarrhea, dysgeusia, dyspepsia, nausea, vomiting.*
Hematologic: NEUTROPENIA, THROMBOCYTOPENIA, *anemia.*
Musculoskeletal: *arthralgia, back pain, bone pain, limb pain, muscle cramps, myalgia.*
Respiratory: *cough, dyspnea, pneumonia, upper respiratory tract infection.*
Skin: *pruritus, rash.*
Other: *dehydration, herpes zoster, pyrexia.*

INTERACTIONS
Drug-drug. *Antihypertensives:* May cause hypotension. Monitor patient's blood pressure closely.
Drugs linked to peripheral neuropathy, such as amiodarone, antivirals, isoniazid, nitrofurantoin, statins: May worsen neuropathy. Use together cautiously.

Inhibitors or inducers of CYP3A4: May increase risk of toxicity or may reduce drug's effects. Monitor patient closely.
Oral antidiabetics: May cause hypoglycemia or hyperglycemia. Monitor glucose level closely.

EFFECTS ON LAB TEST RESULTS
● May decrease hemoglobin level.
● May decrease neutrophil and platelet counts.

CONTRAINDICATIONS & CAUTIONS
● Contraindicated in patients hypersensitive to bortezomib, boron, or mannitol.
● Use cautiously in patients with hepatic or renal impairment or with a history of syncope or in those who are dehydrated or receiving other drugs known to cause hypotension.
● Safety and effectiveness haven't been established for pregnant women or children.

NURSING CONSIDERATIONS
● Monitor for evidence of neuropathy, such as a burning sensation, hyperesthesia, hypoesthesia, paresthesia, discomfort, or neuropathic pain.
● Watch carefully for adverse effects, especially in the elderly.
● Be sure patient has an order for an antiemetic, antidiarrheal, or both to treat drug-induced nausea, vomiting, or diarrhea.
● Provide fluid and electrolyte replacement to prevent dehydration.
● To manage orthostatic hypotension, adjust antihypertensive dosage, maintain hydration status, and give mineralocorticoids.
● *Alert:* Because thrombocytopenia is common, monitor patient's CBC and platelet counts carefully during treatment, especially on day 11.

PATIENT TEACHING
● Tell patient to notify prescriber about new or worsening peripheral neuropathy.
● Urge women to use effective contraception and not to breast-feed during treatment.
● Teach patient how to avoid dehydration, and stress the need to tell prescriber about dizziness, light-headedness, or fainting spells.

● Tell patient to use caution when driving or performing other hazardous activities because drug may cause fatigue, dizziness, faintness, light-headedness, and doubled or blurred vision.

SAFETY ALERT!

cetuximab
seh-TUX-eh-mab

Erbitux

Pharmacologic class: monoclonal antibody
Pregnancy risk category C

AVAILABLE FORMS
Injection: 2 mg/ml in 50-ml vial

INDICATIONS & DOSAGES
➤ **Squamous cell carcinoma of the head and neck**
Adults: A loading dose of 400 mg/m^2 I.V. over 2 hours (maximum rate, 5 ml/minute) followed by weekly maintenance dose of 250 mg/m^2 I.V. over 1 hour. If used with radiation therapy, begin drug 1 week before radiation course and continue for the duration (6 or 7 weeks). If used as monotherapy for recurrent or metastatic disease after failure of platinum-based therapy, continue until disease progresses or unacceptable toxicity occurs.
➤ **Epidermal growth factor–expressing metastatic colorectal cancer, alone in patients intolerant of irinotecan-based and oxaliplatin-based chemotherapy or with irinotecan in patients refractory to irinotecan-based chemotherapy**
Adults: Loading dose, 400 mg/m^2 I.V. over 2 hours (maximum, 5 ml/minute), alone or with irinotecan. Maintenance dosage, 250 mg/m^2 I.V. weekly over 1 hour (maximum, 5 ml/minute).
Adjust-a-dose: If patient develops a grade 1 or 2 infusion reaction, permanently reduce infusion rate by 50%. If patient develops a grade 3 or 4 infusion reaction, stop drug immediately and permanently. If patient develops a severe acneiform rash, follow these guidelines:

Reactions may be *common,* uncommon, *life-threatening,* or COMMON AND LIFE-THREATENING.
Interaction may have a *rapid onset* or *delayed onset.*

• After first occurrence, delay infusion
1 to 2 weeks. If patient improves, continue
at 250 mg/m². If patient doesn't improve,
stop drug.
• After second occurrence, delay infusion
1 to 2 weeks. If patient improves, reduce
dose to 200 mg/m². If patient doesn't
improve, stop drug.
• After third occurrence, delay infusion
1 to 2 weeks. If patient improves, reduce
dose to 150 mg/m². If patient doesn't
improve, stop drug.
• After fourth occurrence, stop drug.

ADMINISTRATION
I.V.
• Solution should be clear and colorless
and may contain a small amount of
particulates.
• Don't shake or dilute.
• Drug can be given by infusion pump
or syringe pump, piggybacked into the
patient's infusion line. Don't give drug
by I.V. push or bolus.
• Give drug through a low–protein-binding
0.22-micrometer in-line filter.
• Flush line with normal saline solution at
the end of the infusion.
• Store vials at 36° to 46° F (2° to 8° C).
Don't freeze.
• Solution in infusion container is stable
up to 12 hours at 36° to 46° F (2° to 8° C)
and up to 8 hours at 68° to 77° F
(20° to 25° C).
• **Incompatibilities:** Don't dilute with
other solutions.

ACTION
An epidermal growth factor receptor
(EGFR) antagonist that binds to the
EGFR on normal and tumor cells,
inhibiting epidermal growth factor from
binding, which interrupts cell growth,
induces cell death, and decreases growth
factor production.

Route	Onset	Peak	Duration
I.V.	Unknown	Unknown	Unknown

Half-life: 4¾ days.

ADVERSE REACTIONS
CNS: *asthenia, depression, fever,
headache, insomnia, pain.*
CV: *edema, **cardiopulmonary arrest.***

EENT: *conjunctivitis.*
GI: *abdominal pain, anorexia, constipation, diarrhea, dyspepsia, dysphagia,
mucositis, nausea, stomatitis, vomiting,
xerostomia.*
GU: ***acute renal failure.***
Hematologic: *anemia,* LEUKOPENIA.
Metabolic: *dehydration,* HYPOMAGNESIA,
weight loss.
Musculoskeletal: *back pain.*
Respiratory: *cough, dyspnea, **pulmonary
embolus.***
Skin: *alopecia, maculopapular rash, nail
disorder, pruritus, radiation dermatitis,
acneiform rash.*
Other: ***anaphylactoid reaction,*** *chills,
infection,* infusion reaction, **sepsis.**

INTERACTIONS
Drug-lifestyle. *Sun exposure:* May worsen
skin reactions. Advise patient to avoid
excessive sun exposure.

EFFECTS ON LAB TEST RESULTS
• May decrease magnesium, calcium, and
potassium levels.

CONTRAINDICATIONS & CAUTIONS
• Use cautiously in patients hypersensitive
to drug, its components, or murine
proteins. If used with radiation, use
cautiously in patients with a history of
coronary artery disease, arrhythmias,
and heart failure.

NURSING CONSIDERATIONS
• Premedicate with 50 mg I.V. diphenhydramine.
■ **Black Box Warning** Severe infusion
reactions, including acute airway obstruction, urticaria, and hypotension, may
occur, usually with the first infusion.
If a severe infusion reaction occurs, stop
drug immediately and give symptomatic
treatment. ■
• Keep epinephrine, corticosteroids, I.V.
antihistamines, bronchodilators, and
oxygen available for severe infusion
reactions.
• Manage mild to moderate infusion
reactions by decreasing infusion rate and
premedicating with an antihistamine for
subsequent infusions.
• Monitor patient for infusion reactions
for 1 hour after infusion ends.

• Assess patient for acute onset or worsening of pulmonary symptoms. If interstitial lung disease is confirmed, stop drug.
• Monitor patient for skin toxicity, which starts most often during first 2 weeks of therapy. Treat with topical and oral antibiotics.
■ **Black Box Warning** In patients also receiving radiation therapy, closely monitor electrolytes, especially magnesium, potassium, and calcium, during and after therapy. Cardiopulmonary arrest has occurred. ■
• It's unknown if drug appears in breast milk. Women shouldn't breast-feed until 60 days after last dose.

PATIENT TEACHING
• Tell patient to promptly report adverse reactions.
• Inform patient that skin reactions may occur, typically during the first 2 weeks of treatment.
• Advise patient to avoid prolonged or unprotected sun exposure during treatment.

dasatinib
duh-SAH-tin-nib

Sprycel

Pharmacologic class: protein-tyrosine kinase inhibitor
Pregnancy risk category D

AVAILABLE FORMS
Tablets: 20 mg, 50 mg, 70 mg, 100 mg

INDICATIONS & DOSAGES
➤ **Accelerated, myeloid, or lymphoid blast-phase chronic myeloid leukemia (CML) with resistance or intolerance to earlier treatment, including imatinib; Philadelphia chromosome–positive acute lymphoblastic leukemia with resistance or tolerance to prior therapy**
Adults: 70 mg P.O. b.i.d., in the morning and evening. If patient tolerates this dose but fails to respond to treatment, increase to 100 mg b.i.d. Continue until disease progresses or intolerable adverse effects occur.

Adjust-a-dose: If patient has hematologic toxicity, consider reducing dose or interrupting or stopping therapy.
If patient has severe, nonhematologic toxicity, hold dose until condition resolves; then resume at previous or reduced dose.
➤ **Chronic-phase CML resistant or intolerant to previous therapy including imatinib**
Adults: 100 mg P.O. daily. May increase to 140 mg daily.

ADMINISTRATION
P.O.
• Give drug without regard for food.
• *Alert:* Don't crush or cut tablets. If tablet is crushed or broken, wear chemotherapy gloves to dispose of it. Pregnant women shouldn't handle broken tablets.

ACTION
Reduces leukemic cell growth by inhibiting a tyrosine kinase enzyme. As a result, bone marrow can resume production of normal RBCs, WBCs, and platelets.

Route	Onset	Peak	Duration
P.O.	Unknown	½–6 hr	Unknown

Half-life: 3 to 5 hours.

ADVERSE REACTIONS
CNS: *asthenia, chills, dizziness, fatigue, headache, neuropathy,* **bleeding,** *pyrexia,* **seizures,** anxiety, confusion, depression, insomnia, somnolence, syncope, tremor, vertigo, affect lability.
CV: ARRHYTHMIAS, *chest pain, edema,* **cardiac dysfunction, heart failure,** hypertension, hypotension, pericardial effusion, cardiomegaly, flushing, palpitations, MI.
EENT: *mucositis, stomatitis,* conjunctivitis, dry eyes, dysgeusia, tinnitus.
GI: *abdominal distention and pain, anorexia, constipation, diarrhea, nausea, vomiting,* **bleeding,** anal fissure, colitis, dyspepsia, dysphagia, gastritis.
GU: *renal failure,* urinary frequency.
Hematologic: *anemia,* **febrile neutropenia, pancytopenia, thrombocytopenia.**

Reactions may be *common,* uncommon, *life-threatening,* or COMMON AND LIFE-THREATENING.
Interaction may have a *rapid onset* or **delayed onset.**

Metabolic: *weight loss or gain,* hyperuricemia, appetite changes.
Musculoskeletal: *arthralgia, myalgia, pain,* inflammation, muscle stiffness, weakness.
Respiratory: *cough, dyspnea, upper respiratory tract infection, pleural effusion, pneumonia,* asthma, ***pulmonary edema, pulmonary hypertension,*** lung infiltrates, pneumonitis.
Skin: *pruritus, rash,* acne, alopecia, dry skin, nail or pigment disorders, sweating, dermatitis, photosensitivity reactions, urticaria.
Other: *infection,* ***tumor lysis syndrome,*** ascites, gynecomastia, herpes infection.

INTERACTIONS
Drug-drug. *Antacids:* May decrease dasatinib absorption. Give antacid 2 hours before or 2 hours after dasatinib.
CYP3A4 inducers (carbamazepine, dexamethasone, phenobarbital, phenytoin, rifampicin): May decrease dasatinib level. Avoid using together, or increase dasatinib dose in 20-mg increments.
CYP3A4 inhibitors (atazanavir, clarithromycin, erythromycin, indinavir, itraconazole, ketoconazole, nefazodone, nelfinavir, ritonavir, saquinavir, telithromycin): May increase dasatinib level and toxicity. Avoid using together; if unavoidable, monitor patient closely and consider decreasing dasatinib dose to 20 to 40 mg daily.
CYP3A4 substrates (cyclosporine, ergot alkaloids, fentanyl, pimozide, quinidine, sirolimus, tacrolimus): May alter levels of these drugs. Use cautiously together, and monitor patient.
H$_2$-blockers, proton pump inhibitors: May decrease dasatinib level because of gastric acid suppression. Avoid using together. Consider antacids as an alternative.
Simvastatin: May increase simvastatin level. Monitor patient.
Drug-herb. *St. John's wort:* May decrease drug level. Discourage use together.
Drug-food. *Grapefruit juice:* May increase dasatinib level. Avoid use together.

EFFECTS ON LAB TEST RESULTS
● May increase uric acid, bilirubin, creatinine, AST, ALT, CK, and troponin levels.
May decrease phosphate and calcium levels.
● May decrease RBC, platelet, and neutrophil counts.

CONTRAINDICATIONS & CAUTIONS
● Use cautiously in patients receiving antiarrhythmics, antiplatelets, or anticoagulants; patients receiving cumulative high-dose anthracycline therapy; patients with a prolonged QT interval or risk of prolonged QT interval (those with hypokalemia, hypomagnesemia, or current use of drugs that prolong the QT interval); patients with liver impairment; and patients who are lactose intolerant.

NURSING CONSIDERATIONS
● Monitor CBC weekly for the first 2 months of treatment, then monthly thereafter, or as indicated.
● Correct electrolyte imbalances, especially of potassium and magnesium, before treatment.
● Monitor for heart failure.
● Drug contains lactose.
● Drug may cause fetal harm. Don't use in pregnant women. If used, mother should be warned of potential harm.
● Drug affects older and younger adults similarly, although older adults may be more sensitive to drug's effects.
● It's unknown if drug appears in breast milk; mothers shouldn't breast-feed during treatment.

PATIENT TEACHING
● Tell patient to take the tablets at about the same time every day.
● Caution patient not to crush or cut the tablets.
● Warn women of childbearing age to use reliable contraception during treatment. Men who take drug should use condoms to avoid impregnating their partners.
● Tell patient to report weight gain, swelling, and shortness of breath.
● Advise patient to notify prescriber immediately about easy or unusual bruising.

SAFETY ALERT!

erlotinib
ur-LOE-tih-nib

Tarceva

Pharmacologic class: epidermal growth factor receptor inhibitor
Pregnancy risk category D

AVAILABLE FORMS
Tablets: 25 mg, 100 mg, 150 mg

INDICATIONS & DOSAGES
➤ **With gemcitabine, first-line treatment of locally advanced, unresectable, or metastatic pancreatic cancer**
Adults: 100 mg P.O. once daily taken at least 1 hour before or 2 hours after meals. Continue until disease progresses or intolerable toxicity occurs.
➤ **Locally advanced or metastatic non–small cell lung cancer after failure of at least one chemotherapy regimen**
Adults: 150 mg P.O. once daily taken at least 1 hour before or 2 hours after meals. Continue until disease progresses or intolerable toxicity occurs.
Adjust-a-dose: In patients with severe skin reactions or severe diarrhea refractory to loperamide, reduce dose in 50-mg decrements or stop therapy.

ADMINISTRATION
P.O.
● Give drug 1 hour before or 2 hours after a meal.

ACTION
Probably inhibits tyrosine kinase activity in epidermal growth factor receptors, which are expressed on the surface of normal and cancer cells. Is particularly selective for human epidermal growth factor receptor 1.

Route	Onset	Peak	Duration
P.O.	Unknown	4 hr	Unknown

Half-life: About 36 hours.

ADVERSE REACTIONS
CNS: *fatigue.*

EENT: *conjunctivitis, keratoconjunctivitis sicca.*
GI: *abdominal pain, anorexia, diarrhea, nausea, stomatitis, vomiting.*
Respiratory: *cough, dyspnea, **pulmonary toxicity.***
Skin: *dry skin, pruritus, rash.*
Other: *infection.*

INTERACTIONS
Drug-drug. *Anticoagulants, such as warfarin:* May increase risk of bleeding. Monitor PT and INR.
CYP3A4 inducers, such as carbamazepine, phenobarbital, phenytoin, rifabutin, rifampin: May increase erlotinib metabolism. Increase erlotinib dosage, as needed.
Strong CYP3A4 inhibitors, such as atazanavir, clarithromycin, indinavir, itraconazole, ketoconazole, nefazodone, nelfinavir, ritonavir, saquinavir, telithromycin, troleandomycin, voriconazole: May decrease erlotinib metabolism. Use together cautiously, and consider reducing erlotinib dosage.
Drug-herb. *St. John's wort:* May increase drug metabolism. Drug dosage may need to be increased. Discourage use together.

EFFECTS ON LAB TEST RESULTS
● May increase ALT, AST, and bilirubin levels.
● May increase INR and PT.

CONTRAINDICATIONS & CAUTIONS
● Use cautiously in patients with pulmonary disease or liver impairment. Also use cautiously in patients who have received or are receiving chemotherapy because it may worsen adverse pulmonary effects.

NURSING CONSIDERATIONS
● Monitor liver function tests periodically during therapy. Notify prescriber of abnormal findings.
● *Alert:* Closely monitor patients with baseline hepatic impairment, particularly those with total bilirubin level greater than 3 times the upper limit of normal. If liver function changes are severe, dose interruption or discontinuation should be considered.
● *Alert:* Rarely, serious interstitial lung disease may occur. If patient develops

---

Reactions may be *common*, uncommon, *life-threatening*, or COMMON AND LIFE-THREATENING.
Interaction may have a *rapid onset* or **delayed onset.**

dyspnea, cough, and fever, notify prescriber. Therapy may need to be interrupted or stopped.
• Monitor patient for severe diarrhea, and give loperamide if needed.
• Women shouldn't breast-feed while taking this drug.
• Drug has been used to treat squamous cell head and neck cancer.

PATIENT TEACHING
• *Alert:* Tell patient to immediately report new or worsened cough, shortness of breath, eye irritation, or severe or persistent diarrhea, nausea, anorexia, or vomiting.
• Instruct patient to take drug 1 hour before or 2 hours after food.
• Advise women to avoid pregnancy while taking this drug and for 2 weeks after treatment ends. Drug can harm fetus.
• Explain the likelihood of serious interactions with other drugs and herbal supplements and the need to tell prescriber about any change in drugs and supplements taken.

SAFETY ALERT!

etoposide (VP-16-213)
e-toe-POE-side

VePesid

etoposide phosphate
Etopophos

Pharmacologic class: podophyllotoxin derivative
Pregnancy risk category D

AVAILABLE FORMS
etoposide
Capsules: 50 mg
Injection: 20 mg/ml in 5-, 12.5-, and 25-ml vials
etoposide phosphate
Injection: 119.3-mg vials equivalent to 100 mg etoposide

INDICATIONS & DOSAGES
➤ **Testicular cancer**
Adults: 50 to 100 mg/m² daily I.V. on 5 consecutive days every 3 to 4 weeks.

Or, 100 mg/m² daily I.V. on days 1, 3, and 5 every 3 to 4 weeks for three or four courses of therapy.
➤ **Small cell carcinoma of the lung**
Adults: 35 mg/m² daily I.V. for 4 days. Or, 50 mg/m² daily I.V. for 5 days. P.O. dose is two times I.V. dose, rounded to nearest 50 mg.
Adjust-a-dose: For patients with creatinine clearance of 15 to 50 ml/minute, reduce dose by 25%.

ADMINISTRATION
P.O.
• Give drug without regard for food.
• Don't give drug with grapefruit juice.
I.V.
• Preparing and giving parenteral drug may be mutagenic, teratogenic, or carcinogenic. Follow facility policy to reduce risks.
• For etoposide infusion, dilute to 0.2 or 0.4 mg/ml in either D₅W or normal saline solution. Higher concentrations may crystallize.
• Give etoposide by slow infusion over at least 30 minutes to prevent severe hypotension.
• For etoposide phosphate, give without further dilution or dilute to as low as 0.1 mg/ml in either D₅W or normal saline solution.
• Give etoposide phosphate over 5 to 210 minutes.
• Check blood pressure every 15 minutes during infusion. Hypotension may occur if infusion is too rapid. If systolic pressure falls below 90 mm Hg, stop infusion and notify prescriber.
• Etoposide diluted to 0.2 mg/ml is stable 96 hours at room temperature in plastic or glass, unprotected from light; at 0.4 mg/ml, it's stable 24 hours under same conditions. Diluted etoposide phosphate solution is stable for same times at room temperature or 24 hours refrigerated.
• **Incompatibilities:** Cefepime hydrochloride, filgrastim, gallium nitrate, idarubicin.

ACTION
Inhibits topoisomerase II enzyme, causing inability to repair DNA strand breaks, which leads to cell death. Cell cycle specific to G₂ portion of cell cycle.

Route	Onset	Peak	Duration
P.O., I.V.	Unknown	Unknown	Unknown

Half-life: Initial phase, ½ to 2 hours; terminal phase, 5¼ hours.

ADVERSE REACTIONS
CNS: peripheral neuropathy.
CV: hypotension.
GI: *anorexia, diarrhea, nausea, vomiting,* abdominal pain, stomatitis, *mucositis.*
Hematologic: LEUKOPENIA, NEUTRO-PENIA, THROMBOCYTOPENIA, anemia, *myelosuppression.*
Hepatic: *hepatotoxicity.*
Skin: *reversible alopecia,* rash.
Other: *anaphylaxis,* hypersensitivity reactions.

INTERACTIONS
Drug-drug. *Cyclosporine:* May increase etoposide level and toxicity. Monitor CBC and adjust etoposide dose.
Phosphatase inhibitors: May decrease etoposide effectiveness. Monitor drug effects.
Warfarin: May further prolong PT. Monitor PT and INR closely.
Drug-food. *Grapefruit juice:* May reduce etoposide concentrations. Avoid using together.

EFFECTS ON LAB TEST RESULTS
• May decrease hemoglobin level.
• May decrease neutrophil, platelet, RBC, and WBC counts.

CONTRAINDICATIONS & CAUTIONS
• Contraindicated in patients hypersensitive to drug.
• Use cautiously in patients who have had cytotoxic or radiation therapy and in those with hepatic impairment.

NURSING CONSIDERATIONS
■ **Black Box Warning** Give drug under the supervision of a physician experienced in the use of cancer chemotherapy. ■
• Obtain baseline blood pressure before starting therapy.
• Anticipate need for antiemetics.
• Have diphenhydramine, hydrocortisone, epinephrine, and emergency equipment available to establish an airway in case anaphylaxis occurs.

• Store capsules in refrigerator.
■ **Black Box Warning** Monitor CBC. Watch for evidence of bone marrow suppression. ■
• Observe patient's mouth for signs of ulceration.
• To prevent bleeding, avoid all I.M. injections when platelet count is below 50,000/mm³.
• Anticipate need for RBC colony-stimulating factors or blood transfusions.
• Etoposide phosphate dose is expressed as etoposide equivalents; 119.3 mg of etoposide phosphate is equivalent to 100 mg of etoposide.

PATIENT TEACHING
• Tell patient to watch for signs and symptoms of infection (fever, sore throat, fatigue) and bleeding (easy bruising, nosebleeds, bleeding gums, tarry stools). Tell patient to take temperature daily.
• Inform patient of need for frequent blood pressure readings during I.V. administration.
• Caution woman of childbearing age to avoid pregnancy and breast-feeding during therapy.

SAFETY ALERT!

imatinib mesylate
eh-MAT-eh-nib

Gleevec

Pharmacologic class: protein-tyrosine kinase inhibitor
Pregnancy risk category D

AVAILABLE FORMS
Tablets: 100 mg, 400 mg

INDICATIONS & DOSAGES
➤ **Relapsed or refractory Philadelphia chromosome–positive (Ph+) ALL**
Adults: 600 mg P.O. daily.
➤ **Aggressive systemic mastocytosis (ASM) without the D816V c-Kit mutation or with c-Kit mutational status unknown**
Adults: 400 mg P.O. daily.

Reactions may be *common,* uncommon, *life-threatening,* or COMMON AND LIFE-THREATENING.
Interaction may have a *rapid onset* or **delayed onset.**

Adjust-a-dose: For patients with ASM associated with eosinophilia, a clonal hematologic disease related to the fusion kinase FIP1L1-PDGFRα, initial dose is 100 mg/day. Increase dose from 100 mg to 400 mg/day if no adverse drug reactions and if insufficient response to therapy.

➤ **Hypereosinophilic syndrome (HES) or chronic eosinophilic leukemia (CEL), or both**
Adults: 400 mg P.O. daily.
Adjust-a-dose: In HES/CEL patients with demonstrated FIP1L1-PDGFRα, fusion kinase, initial dose is 100 mg/day. Increase dose from 100 mg to 400 mg/day if no adverse drug reactions and if insufficient response to therapy.

➤ **Myelodysplastic (MDS) or myelo-proliferative (MPD) disease with PDGFR gene rearrangements**
Adults: 400 mg P.O. daily.

➤ **Unresectable, recurrent, or metastatic dermatofibrosarcoma protuberans (DFSP)**
Adults: 800 mg P.O. daily.

➤ **Chronic myeloid leukemia (CML) in blast crisis, in accelerated phase, or in chronic phase after failure of alfa interferon therapy; newly diagnosed Philadelphia chromosome–positive (Ph+) chronic phase CML**
Adults: For chronic-phase CML, 400 mg P.O. daily as single dose with a meal and large glass of water. For accelerated-phase CML or blast crisis, 600 mg P.O. daily as single dose with a meal and large glass of water. Continue treatment as long as patient continues to benefit. May increase daily dose to 600 mg P.O. in chronic phase or to 800 mg P.O. (400 mg P.O. b.i.d.) in accelerated phase or blast crisis.
Children age 2 and older: For newly diagnosed Ph+ chronic-phase CML only, give 340 mg/m² daily P.O. Don't exceed 600 mg.

➤ **Kit (CD117)-positive unresectable or metastatic malignant GI stromal tumors (GIST)**
Adults: 400 mg P.O. daily or b.i.d.

➤ **Ph+ chronic phase CML in patients whose disease has recurred after stem cell transplant or who are resistant to alfa interferon therapy**

Children age 2 and older: 260 mg/m² daily P.O. as a single dose or divided into two doses. Have patient take with meal and large glass of water. May increase dosage to 340 mg/m² daily.
Adjust-a-dose: Withhold treatment or reduce dosage based on bilirubin or liver transaminase levels, severity of fluid retention, or hematologic toxicities. See manufacturer's package insert for details on dosage adjustment.

ADMINISTRATION
P.O.
● For daily dosing of 800 mg and above, use the 400-mg tablet to reduce exposure to iron.
● For patients unable to swallow tablets, disperse the tablets in water or apple juice (50 ml for 100-mg tablet or 200 ml for 400-mg tablet). Stir and have patient drink immediately.

ACTION
Inhibits the abnormal tyrosine kinase created by the Philadelphia chromosome abnormality in CML; it inhibits tumor growth of murine myeloid cells and leukemia lines from CML patients in blast crisis.

Route	Onset	Peak	Duration
P.O.	Unknown	2–4 hr	Unknown

Half-life: Within 7 days.

ADVERSE REACTIONS
CNS: CEREBRAL HEMORRHAGE, *fatigue, headache, pyrexia, weakness, depression, dizziness, insomnia.*
CV: *edema.*
EENT: *epistaxis,* nasopharyngitis.
GI: GI HEMORRHAGE, *abdominal pain, anorexia, constipation, diarrhea, dyspepsia, nausea, vomiting.*
Hematologic: HEMORRHAGE, NEUTRO-PENIA, THROMBOCYTOPENIA, *anemia.*
Metabolic: *hypokalemia,* weight increase.
Musculoskeletal: *arthralgia, myalgia, muscle cramps, musculoskeletal pain.*
Respiratory: *cough, dyspnea, pneumonia.*
Skin: *petechiae, rash,* pruritus.
Other: *night sweats.*

INTERACTIONS
Drug-drug. *Acetaminophen:* May increase risk of hepatic toxicity. Monitor patient closely.
CYP3A4 inducers (carbamazepine, dexamethasone, phenobarbital, phenytoin, rifampin): May increase metabolism and decrease imatinib level. Use together cautiously.
CYP3A4 inhibitors (clarithromycin, erythromycin, itraconazole, ketoconazole): May decrease metabolism and increase imatinib level. Monitor patient for toxicity.
Dihydropyridine-calcium channel blockers, certain HMG-CoA reductase inhibitors (simvastatin), cyclosporine, pimozide, triazolo-benzodiazepines: May increase levels of these drugs. Monitor patient for toxicity, and obtain drug levels, if appropriate.
Levothyroxine: May increase levothyroxine clearance, causing increased thyroid stimulating hormone levels and symptoms of hypothyroidism. Monitor thyroid function.
Warfarin: May alter metabolism of warfarin. Avoid using together; use standard heparin or a low–molecular-weight heparin.
Drug-herb. *St. John's wort:* May decrease drug effects. Discourage use together.

EFFECTS ON LAB TEST RESULTS
• May increase creatinine, bilirubin, alkaline phosphatase, AST, and ALT levels. May decrease potassium and hemoglobin levels.
• May decrease neutrophil and platelet counts.

CONTRAINDICATIONS & CAUTIONS
• Contraindicated in patients hypersensitive to drug or its components.
• Use cautiously in elderly patients and in those with hepatic impairment.
• Severe congestive heart failure and left ventricular dysfunction have occurred in patients taking imatinib. Use cautiously in patients with cardiac disease or risk factors for cardiac failure.
• Safety and effectiveness in children younger than age 2 haven't been established.

NURSING CONSIDERATIONS
• Monitor patient closely for possibly severe fluid retention. Elderly patients may have an increased risk of edema.

• Monitor weight daily. Report unexpected, rapid weight gain.
• Monitor CBC weekly for first month; every other week for second month and periodically thereafter.
• Monitor liver function tests carefully because hepatotoxicity (occasionally severe) may occur; decrease dosage as needed.
• May increase dose if no severe adverse reactions or severe non–leukemia-related neutropenia or thrombocytopenia in the following circumstances: disease progression, failure to achieve a satisfactory hematologic response after at least 3 months of treatment, or loss of a previously achieved hematologic response.
• In patients with HES and cardiac involvement, cases of cardiogenic shock/ left ventricular dysfunction have been associated with the initiation of imatinib therapy. The condition is reversible with administration of systemic steroids, circulatory support measures, and by temporarily withholding imatinib. Monitor echocardiogram and serum troponin in patients with HES/CEL and in patients with MDS/MPD or ASM associated with high eosinophil levels.
• Grade 3/4 hemorrhage has been reported in patients with newly diagnosed CML and with GIST. GI tumor sites may be the source of GI bleeds in GIST.
• Gastrointestinal perforations, some fatal, have been reported.

PATIENT TEACHING
• Tell patient to take drug with food and a large glass of water.
• Advise patient unable to swallow tablets to mix them in water or apple juice (50 ml for 100-mg tablet or 200 ml for 400-mg tablet). Tell him to stir and drink immediately.
• Advise patient to report to prescriber any adverse effects, such as fluid retention.
• Advise patient to obtain periodic liver and kidney function tests and blood work to determine blood counts.
• Tell patient to avoid or limit the use of acetaminophen in OTC or prescription products because of potential toxic effects on the liver.

irinotecan hydrochloride
eh-rin-OH-te-kan

Camptosar

Pharmacologic class: DNA
topoisomerase inhibitor
Pregnancy risk category D

AVAILABLE FORMS
Injection: 20 mg/ml in 2- and 5-ml vials

INDICATIONS & DOSAGES
➤ **Metastatic carcinoma of the colon
or rectum that has recurred or
progressed after fluorouracil (5-FU)
therapy**
Adults: Initially, 125 mg/m² by I.V. infusion over 90 minutes on days 1, 8, 15,
and 22; then 2-week rest period. Thereafter, additional courses of treatment
may be repeated every 6 weeks with
4 weeks on and 2 weeks off. Subsequent
doses may be adjusted to low of
50 mg/m² or maximum of 150 mg/m²
in 25- to 50-mg/m² increments based on
patient's tolerance. Or, 350 mg/m² by
I.V. infusion over 90 minutes once every
3 weeks. Additional courses may continue indefinitely in patients who respond
favorably and in those whose disease
remains stable, provided intolerable
toxicity doesn't occur.
Adjust-a-dose: Consider reducing starting dose in patients age 65 and older,
in those who have received pelvic or
abdominal radiation, or in those who
have a performance status of 2 or increased bilirubin level. Give 300 mg/m²
by I.V. infusion over 90 minutes once
every 3 weeks. Or, give 100 mg/m² by
I.V. infusion over 90 minutes once
weekly.
➤ **First-line therapy for metastatic
colorectal cancer with 5-fluorouracil
(5-FU) and leucovorin**
Regimen 1
Adults: 125 mg/m² I.V. over 90 minutes
on days 1, 8, 15, and 22; then leucovorin
20 mg/m² I.V. bolus on days 1, 8, 15, and
22 and 5-FU 500 mg/m² I.V. bolus on
days 1, 8, 15, and 22. Courses are repeated
every 6 weeks.

Regimen 2
Adults: 180 mg/m² I.V. over 90 minutes
on days 1, 15, and 29; then leucovorin
200 mg/m² I.V. over 2 hours on days 1, 2,
15, 16, 29, and 30; then 5-FU 400 mg/m²
I.V. bolus on days 1, 2, 15, 16, 29, and 30
and 5-FU 600 mg/m² I.V. infusion over
22 hours on days 1, 2, 15, 16, 29, and 30.
Adjust-a-dose: See manufacturer's package
insert for details on dosage adjustment.

ADMINISTRATION
I.V.
● Drug packaged in plastic blister to protect against inadvertent breakage and
leakage. Inspect vial for damage and signs
of leakage before removing blister.
● Wear gloves while handling and preparing infusion solutions. If drug contacts
skin, wash thoroughly with soap and water.
If drug contacts mucous membranes, flush
thoroughly with water.
● Dilute drug in D₅W injection (preferred)
or normal saline solution for injection
before infusion to yield 0.12 to 2.8 mg/ml.
● Solution is stable for up to 24 hours at
77° F (25° C) in ambient fluorescent lighting. Solutions diluted in D₅W, stored at
36° to 46° F (2° to 8° C), and protected
from light are stable for 48 hours. However, because microbial contamination
may occur during dilution, use admixture
within 24 hours if refrigerated or 6 hours
if kept at room temperature. Refrigerating
admixtures using normal saline solution
isn't recommended because of low and
sporadic risk of visible particulate. Don't
freeze admixture because drug may
precipitate.
● Premedicate patient with antiemetic
drugs on day of treatment starting at least
30 minutes before giving irinotecan.
● Watch for irritation and infiltration;
extravasation can cause tissue damage and
necrosis. If extravasation occurs, flush site
with sterile water and apply ice. Notify
prescriber.
● Store vial at 59° to 86° F (15° to 30° C).
Protect from light.
● **Incompatibilities:** Other I.V. drugs.

ACTION
Interacts with topoisomerase I, inducing
reversible single-strand DNA breaks.
Drug binds to the topoisomerase I–DNA

complex and prevents relegation of these single-strand breaks.

Route	Onset	Peak	Duration
I.V.	Unknown	1 hr	Unknown

Half-life: About 6 to 12 hours.

ADVERSE REACTIONS
CNS: *asthenia, dizziness, fever, headache, insomnia, pain,* akathisia.
CV: *edema, vasodilation,* orthostatic hypotension.
EENT: *rhinitis.*
GI: DIARRHEA, *abdominal cramping, pain, and enlargement, anorexia, constipation, dyspepsia, flatulence, nausea, stomatitis, vomiting.*
Hematologic: *anemia, **leukopenia, neutropenia, thrombocytopenia.***
Metabolic: *dehydration, weight loss.*
Musculoskeletal: *back pain.*
Respiratory: *dyspnea, increased cough.*
Skin: *alopecia, rash, sweating.*
Other: *chills, infection.*

INTERACTIONS
Drug-drug. *CYP3A4 enzyme-inducing anticonvulsants (phenytoin, phenobarbital, or carbamazepine), rifampin, rifabutin:* May significantly decrease irinotecan levels. For patients requiring anticonvulsant treatment, consider substituting non–enzyme-inducing anticonvulsants at least 2 weeks before start of irinotecan therapy.
Dexamethasone: May increase risk of irinotecan-induced lymphocytopenia. Monitor patient closely.
Diuretics: May increase risk of dehydration and electrolyte imbalance. Consider stopping diuretic during active periods of nausea and vomiting.
Ketoconazole: May increase irinotecan levels leading to drug toxicity. Stop ketoconazole at least 1 week before starting irinotecan therapy. Ketoconazole is contraindicated during irinotecan therapy.
Laxatives: May increase risk of diarrhea. Avoid using together.
Neuromuscular-blocking agents: May prolong the neuromuscular-blocking effects of succinylcholine, and the neuromuscular blockade of nondepolarizing drugs may be antagonized. Monitor patient for

prolonged effects of succinylcholine if given together.
Prochlorperazine: May increase risk of akathisia. Monitor patient closely.
Other antineoplastics: May cause additive adverse effects, such as myelosuppression and diarrhea. Monitor patient closely.
Drug-herb. *St. John's wort:* May decrease drug levels by about 40%. Use together is contraindicated.

EFFECTS ON LAB TEST RESULTS
• May increase alkaline phosphatase, AST, and bilirubin levels. May decrease hemoglobin level.
• May decrease WBC and neutrophil counts.

CONTRAINDICATIONS & CAUTIONS
• Contraindicated in patients hypersensitive to drug.
• Safety and effectiveness of drug in children haven't been established.
• Use cautiously in elderly patients.

NURSING CONSIDERATIONS
■ **Black Box Warning** Administer drug under the supervision of a physician experienced with cancer chemotherapy. ■
■ **Black Box Warning** Drug may cause severe myelosuppression. ■
• Pelvic or abdominal irradiation may increase risk of severe myelosuppression. Avoid use of drug in patients undergoing irradiation.
■ **Black Box Warning** Drug can cause severe diarrhea. Treat diarrhea occurring within 24 hours of drug administration with 0.25 to 1 mg atropine I.V., unless contraindicated. ■
■ **Black Box Warning** Treat late diarrhea (more than 24 hours after irinotecan administration) promptly with loperamide. Monitor patient for dehydration, electrolyte imbalance, or sepsis, and treat appropriately. ■
• Delay subsequent doses until normal bowel function returns for at least 24 hours without antidiarrheal. If grade 2, 3, or 4 late diarrhea occurs, decrease subsequent doses within the current cycle.
• To decrease risk of dehydration, withhold diuretic during treatment and periods of active vomiting or diarrhea.

Reactions may be *common,* uncommon, *life-threatening,* or COMMON AND LIFE-THREATENING.
Interaction may have a *rapid onset* or ***delayed onset.***

• If neutropenic fever occurs or if absolute neutrophil count drops below 500/mm³, temporarily stop therapy. Reduce dosage, especially if WBC count is below 2,000/mm³, neutrophil count is below 1,000/mm³, hemoglobin level is below 8 g/dl, or platelet count is below 100,000/mm³.

• A colony-stimulating factor may be helpful in patients with significant neutropenia.

• Monitor WBC count with differential, hemoglobin level, and platelet count before each dose.

• **Look alike–sound alike:** Don't confuse irinotecan with topotecan.

PATIENT TEACHING
• Inform patient about risk of diarrhea and methods to treat it; tell him to avoid laxatives.

• Instruct patient to contact prescriber if any of the following occur: diarrhea for the first time during treatment; black or bloody stools; symptoms of dehydration such as light-headedness, dizziness, or faintness; inability to drink fluids due to nausea or vomiting; inability to control diarrhea within 24 hours; or fever or infection.

• Warn patient that hair loss may occur.

• Caution women to avoid pregnancy or breast-feeding during therapy.

ixabepilone
ecks-ah-BEH-pill-own

Ixempra

Pharmacologic class: microtubule inhibitor
Pregnancy risk category D

AVAILABLE FORMS
Injection: 15 mg, 45 mg vials

INDICATIONS & DOSAGES
➤ **With capecitabine for metastatic or locally advanced breast cancer, after failure of anthracycline and a taxane; or alone for metastatic or locally advanced breast cancer, after**

failure of anthracycline, taxanes, and capecitabine
Adults: 40 mg/m² I.V. over 3 hours every 3 weeks. Doses for patients with body surface area (BSA) greater than 2.2 m² should be calculated based on 2.2 m². Premedicate with an H_1 antagonist, such as diphenhydramine 50 mg P.O. and an H_2 antagonist such as ranitidine 150 to 300 mg 1 hour before ixabepilone infusion.

Adjust-a-dose: If toxicities occur, refer to package insert for adjustments for monotherapy and combination therapy.

In patients with hepatic impairment receiving combination therapy who have an AST or ALT up to 2.5 × ULN or bilirubin up to 1 × ULN, the standard dose may be given. Treatment is contraindicated with higher AST, ALT, or bilirubin levels. Patients with moderate hepatic impairment receiving monotherapy should be started at 20 mg/m². The dosage in subsequent cycles may be increased to 30 mg/m² if tolerated. Use in patients with AST or ALT greater than 10 × ULN or bilirubin greater than 2 × ULN isn't recommended. Refer to package insert for additional guidance.

ADMINISTRATION
I.V.
• Protect drug from light.

• Keep refrigerated. Let stand at room temperature for 30 minutes before administration.

• The white precipitate in diluent will clear at room temperature.

• Drug may be a contact irritant; handle and give with care. Wear gloves and avoid inhaling vapors.

• Reconstitute drug before use, using supplied diluent, to a concentration of 15 mg/8 ml or 45 mg/23.5 ml. Gently swirl and invert vial.

• Before giving drug, further dilute with lactated Ringer's solution supplied in di(2-ethylhexyl) phthalate (DEHP)–free bags. Final concentration should yield 0.2 mg/ml to 0.6 mg/ml.

• Infuse within 6 hours of preparation.

• Administer through a 0.2- to 1.2-micron in-line filter, using a DEHP-free administration set.

• **Incompatibilities:** Unknown. Don't give with other I.V. drugs.

ACTION
Causes cell death by inhibiting cell division.

Route	Onset	Peak	Duration
I.V.	Rapid	3 hr	3 wk

Half-life: 52 hours.

ADVERSE REACTIONS
CNS: insomnia, *peripheral neuropathy, headache, fatigue, asthenia,* dizziness, fever, pain.
CV: *edema,* chest pain, **supraventricular arrhythmias.**
EENT: increased lacrimation
GI: *anorexia, taste disorder, nausea, vomiting, stomatitis, mucositis, diarrhea, constipation, abdominal pain,* gastroesophageal reflux disease.
Hematologic: FEBRILE NEUTROPENIA, LEUKOPENIA, anemia, THROMBOCYTOPENIA.
Hepatic: *acute hepatic failure,* jaundice.
Metabolic: dehydration, weight loss.
Musculoskeletal: *myalgia, arthralgia, skeletal pain.*
Respiratory: upper respiratory tract infection, dyspnea, cough.
Skin: *alopecia, rash, nail disorder, palmer-plantar erythrodysesthesia disorder,* pruritus, exfoliation, *hyperpigmentation.*
Other: hypersensitivity reactions, hot flush.

INTERACTIONS
Drug-drug. *CYP3A4 inducers (such as dexamethasone, phenytoin, carbamazepine, rifampin, rifampicin, rifabutin, or phenobarbital):* May decrease ixabepilone level, causing treatment failure. Avoid using together.
CYP3A4 inhibitors (such as ketoconazole, itraconazole, clarithromycin, atazanavir, nefazodone, saquinavir, telithromycin, ritonavir, amprenavir, indinavir, nelfinavir, delavirdine, or voriconazole): May increase ixabepilone level. Avoid using together. If use together is necessary, decrease ixabepilone dose according to manufacturer's instructions.
Drug-herb. *St. John's wort:* May decrease drug level. Discourage use together.
Drug-food. *Grapefruit juice:* May increase drug level. Discourage use together.

EFFECTS ON LAB TEST RESULTS
• May increase bilirubin, AST, and ALT levels.
• May decrease neutrophil, WBC, RBC, and platelet counts.

CONTRAINDICATIONS & CAUTIONS
• Contraindicated in patients hypersensitive to drug or its components.
• Contraindicated in patients with neutrophil counts less than 1,500 cells/mm³ or platelet count less than 100,000 cells/mm³.
■ **Black Box Warning** Contraindicated in patients with AST or ALT > 2.5 × ULN or bilirubin > 1 × ULN in combination with capecitabine. ■
• Use cautiously in patients with cardiac disease.

NURSING CONSIDERATIONS
• Monitor baseline and periodic CBC and liver enzymes and adjust dose as needed.
• Premedicate with H₁ and H₂ antagonists 1 hour before infusion to avoid hypersensitivity reaction. If patient experiences a hypersensitivity reaction, also premedicate with corticosteroids.
• Monitor cardiac function. Discontinue drug in those who develop cardiac ischemia or impaired cardiac function.
• In patients with CNS changes, be aware that drug contains dehydrated alcohol.
• Monitor for signs of peripheral neuropathy, hypersensitivity reactions or infections.
• Peripheral neuropathy is generally reversible and should be managed by dose adjustment and delays.
• Drug may cause fetal harm. Tell patient to avoid becoming pregnant.
• Because of drug's potential risk, breastfeeding should be stopped or drug should be stopped.
• Elderly patients have a greater risk of grade 3 or 4 adverse effects when used with capecitabine.

PATIENT TEACHING
• Tell patient to report numbness or tingling of hands or feet.
• Advise patient to call prescriber for fever above 100.5° F or signs of infections such as chills, cough, or pain or burning on urination.

Reactions may be *common*, uncommon, *life-threatening*, or COMMON AND LIFE-THREATENING.
Interaction may have a *rapid onset* or **delayed onset**.

• Advise patient to call prescriber for skin rash, itching, flushing, swelling, difficulty breathing, or chest tightness.
• Tell patient that he will need periodic blood testing during treatment.
• Tell patient not to drink grapefruit juice while taking drug.
• *Alert:* Advise patient that ixabepilone contains alcohol. Avoid dangerous activities such as driving or operating machinery if dizzy or drowsy.
• Caution woman of childbearing age to avoid pregnancy and breast-feeding during therapy.

lapatinib
lah-PAH-tih-nihb

Tykerb

Pharmacologic class: kinase inhibitor
Pregnancy risk category D

AVAILABLE FORMS
Tablets: 250 mg

INDICATIONS & DOSAGES
➤ **Advanced or metastatic breast cancer with capecitabine when tumors overexpress HER2 and patient has had prior therapy, including an anthracycline, a taxane, and trastuzumab**
Adults: 1,250 mg (5 tablets) P.O. once daily as a single dose on days 1 through 21, with 2,000 mg/m²/day capecitabine given P.O. in two doses 12 hours apart on days 1 to 14. Repeat 21-day cycle.
Adjust-a-dose: In patients with decreased left ventricular ejection fraction (LVEF) that is grade 2 or higher by NCI Common Terminology Criteria for Adverse Events (NCI CTCAE), or LVEF that drops below the institution's lower limit of normal due to treatment, stop drug. After 2 weeks if patient has recovered normal LVEF and is asymptomatic, resume at reduced dose of 1,000 mg/day and monitor LVEF. In patients with severe hepatic impairment (Child Pugh class C), reduce dose to 750 mg/day. In patients with grade 2 or higher toxicity by NCI CTCAE, withhold drug. Resume normal dose of 1,250 mg/day

if initial episode of toxicity improves to grade 1 or lower. If toxicity recurs, resume at 1,000 mg/day.

ADMINISTRATION
P.O.
• Give drug once daily; don't divide doses.
• Give drug 1 hour before or 1 hour after a meal.
• Give capecitabine with or within 30 minutes after food.

ACTION
Inhibits ErbB-driven tumor cell growth; additive effects may be seen when given together with capecitabine.

Route	Onset	Peak	Duration
P.O.	Up to 1½ hr	4 hr	Unknown

Half-life: 14¼ hours; after repeated dosing, 24 hours.

ADVERSE REACTIONS
CNS: *insomnia.*
CV: *decreased LVEF, prolonged QT interval.*
EENT: *mucosal inflammation.*
GI: *diarrhea, nausea, vomiting, stomatitis, dyspepsia.*
Hematologic: *anemia,* NEUTROPENIA, THROMBOCYTOPENIA.
Musculoskeletal: *arm or leg pain, back pain.*
Respiratory: DYSPNEA.
Skin: *palmar-plantar erythrodysesthesia, rash, dry skin.*

INTERACTIONS
Drug-drug. *Antiarrhythmics, other drugs that prolong QT interval, cumulative high-dose anthracycline therapy:* May prolong QTc interval. Avoid using together.
CYP2C8 inhibitors, P-glycoprotein substrates: May increase lapatinib level. Avoid using together.
Strong CYP3A4 inducers (dexamethasone, phenytoin, carbamazepine, rifampin, rifabutin, rifapentine, phenobarbital): May significantly decrease lapatinib level. Avoid using together or gradually increase dose of lapatinib, as tolerated, to 4,500 mg/day. If the strong inducer is stopped, adjust lapatinib dose to recommended dose.

Strong CYP3A4 inhibitors (ketoconazole, itraconazole, clarithromycin, atazanavir indinavir, nefazodone, nelfinavir, ritonavir, saquinavir, telithromycin, voriconazole): May significantly increase lapatinib level. Avoid using together or reduce lapatinib dose to 500 mg/day. If the strong inhibitor is stopped, allow 1 week before increasing lapatinib dose.

Drug-food. *All food:* May increase exposure to drug. Advise patient to take at least 1 hour before or 1 hour after a meal.
Grapefruit: May increase drug level. Discourage use together.

Drug-herb. *St. John's wort:* May significantly decrease drug level. Discourage use together, or gradually increase lapatinib dose as tolerated to 4,500 mg/day.

EFFECTS ON LAB TEST RESULTS
• May increase total bilirubin, AST, and ALT levels. May decrease hemoglobin level.
• May decrease platelet and neutrophil counts.

CONTRAINDICATIONS & CAUTIONS
• Use cautiously in patients with left ventricular dysfunction; conditions that may decrease LVEF; severe hepatic impairment; hypokalemia; hypomagnesemia, or diarrhea.

NURSING CONSIDERATIONS
• Evaluate LVEF before starting treatment, and monitor during treatment.
• Correct hypokalemia and hypomagnesemia before start of treatment.
• Monitor for excessive diarrhea; give antidiarrheals and correct electrolyte abnormalities, as needed.
• Monitor blood counts for anemia and neutropenia.
• Interstitial lung disease and pneumonitis has occurred in patients during drug therapy. Monitor patient for pulmonary symptoms, including dyspnea, cough, hypoxia, and fever.

PATIENT TEACHING
• Tell patient to immediately report shortness of breath, palpitations, fatigue, diarrhea, and change in medications or OTC preparations to prescriber.

• Instruct patient not to divide doses but to take drug once daily, regardless of number of tablets per dose, 1 hour before or after a meal.
• Remind patient to take capecitabine only as prescribed.
• Advise patient that he will need routine blood tests to evaluate for adverse effects.

SAFETY ALERT!

mitoxantrone hydrochloride
mye-toe-ZAN-trone

Novantrone

Pharmacologic class: DNA-reactive agent; anthracenedione
Pregnancy risk category D

AVAILABLE FORMS
Injection: 2 mg/ml in 10-ml, 12.5-ml, 15-ml vials

INDICATIONS & DOSAGES
➤ **Combination initial therapy for acute nonlymphocytic leukemia**
Adults: Induction begins with 12 mg/m^2 I.V. daily on days 1 to 3, with 100 mg/m^2 daily of cytarabine on days 1 to 7. A second induction may be given if response isn't adequate. Maintenance therapy is 12 mg/m^2 on days 1 and 2, with cytarabine 100 mg/m^2 on days 1 to 5.
➤ **To reduce neurologic disability and frequency of relapse in chronic progressive, progressive relapsing, or worsening relapsing-remitting multiple sclerosis**
Adults: 12 mg/m^2 I.V. over 5 to 15 minutes every 3 months.
➤ **Advanced hormone-refractory prostate cancer**
Men: 12 to 14 mg/m^2 as a short I.V. infusion every 21 days. Drug is given as an adjunct to corticosteroid therapy.

ADMINISTRATION
I.V.
• Preparing and giving drug may be mutagenic, teratogenic, or carcinogenic. Follow facility policy to reduce risks.

Reactions may be *common*, uncommon, *life-threatening*, or COMMON AND LIFE-THREATENING.
Interaction may have a *rapid onset* or **delayed onset**.

• Dilute dose in at least 50 ml of normal saline solution for injection or D$_5$W injection. Don't mix with other drugs.
■ **Black Box Warning** Give slowly into a free-flowing I.V. infusion of normal saline solution or D$_5$W injection over at least 3 minutes. ■
■ **Black Box Warning** Never give subcutaneously, intra-arterially, or intramuscularly. ■
■ **Black Box Warning** Drug is not for intrathecal use. ■
■ **Black Box Warning** Severe local tissue damage may occur if there is extravasation. ■
• If extravasation occurs, stop infusion immediately and notify prescriber.
• Once vial is penetrated, undiluted solution may be stored for 7 days at room temperature or 14 days in refrigerator. Don't freeze.
• **Incompatibilities:** Amphotericin B, aztreonam, cefepime, doxorubicin liposomal, heparin sodium, hydrocortisone, other I.V. drugs, paclitaxel, piperacillin sodium and tazobactam sodium, propofol, sargramostim.

ACTION
Reacts with DNA, producing cytotoxic effect. Probably not specific to cell cycle.

Route	Onset	Peak	Duration
I.V.	Unknown	Unknown	Unknown

Half-life: Terminal half-life, 23 to 215 hours.

ADVERSE REACTIONS
CNS: *fever, headache,* **seizures.**
CV: **arrhythmias,** ECG abnormalities, **heart failure,** tachycardia.
EENT: conjunctivitis, sinusitis.
GI: *abdominal pain, bleeding, constipation, diarrhea, mucositis, nausea, stomatitis, vomiting.*
GU: *amenorrhea, menstrual disorder, UTI,* **renal failure.**
Hematologic: *myelosuppression,* anemia.
Hepatic: jaundice.
Metabolic: hyperuricemia.
Musculoskeletal: back pain.
Respiratory: *cough, dyspnea, upper respiratory tract infection,* pneumonia.
Skin: *alopecia, ecchymoses, local irritation or phlebitis, petechiae.*
Other: *fungal infections,* **sepsis.**

INTERACTIONS
None significant.

EFFECTS ON LAB TEST RESULTS
• May increase ALT, AST, bilirubin, GGT, and uric acid levels. May decrease hemoglobin level and hematocrit.
• May decrease leukocyte and granulocyte counts.

CONTRAINDICATIONS & CAUTIONS
• Contraindicated in patients hypersensitive to drug.
■ **Black Box Warning** Evaluate left ventricular ejection fraction (LVEF) before initiating treatment and prior to administering each dose of mitoxantrone to patients with multiple sclerosis. All patients with multiple sclerosis who have finished treatment should receive yearly, quantitative LVEF evaluation to detect late-occurring cardiac toxicity. ■
• Use cautiously in patients with previous exposure to anthracyclines or other cardiotoxic drugs, previous radiation therapy to mediastinal area, or heart disease. Significantly myelosuppressed patients shouldn't receive drug unless benefits outweigh risks.

NURSING CONSIDERATIONS
■ **Black Box Warning** Administer under the supervision of a physician experienced with cytotoxic chemotherapy. ■
• Give allopurinol. Hydrate patient before and during therapy to avoid uric acid nephropathy.
■ **Black Box Warning** Except when used to treat ANLL, mitoxantrone should generally not be given to patients with baseline neutrophil counts less than 1,500 cells/mm^3. Frequently monitor peripheral blood cell counts for all patients using drug. ■
• Closely monitor hematologic and laboratory chemistry parameters. Patient may require blood transfusion or RBC or WBC colony-stimulating factors.
• Avoid all I.M. injections if platelet count falls below 50,000/mm^3.
■ **Black Box Warning** Use of drug has been associated with cardiotoxicity. Monitor left ventricular ejection fraction before initiating therapy and prior to each

dose; risk of cardiotoxicity increases with cumulative dose of 140 mg/m^2, although toxicities may occur at any dose. Continue ongoing cardiac monitoring to detect late occurring cardiotoxicity. ■

• If severe nonhematologic toxicity occurs during first course, delay second course until patient recovers.

■ **Black Box Warning** Secondary AML has been reported with mitoxantrone therapy. ■

PATIENT TEACHING

• Advise patient to report any pain or burning at site of injection during or after administration.

• Tell patient that urine may appear blue-green within 24 hours after receiving drug and that the whites of his eyes may turn blue. These effects are not harmful but may persist during therapy.

• Advise patient to watch for signs and symptoms of bleeding and infection.

• Recommend that women consult prescriber before becoming pregnant.

SAFETY ALERT!

nelarabine
neh-LAR-uh-been

Arranon

Pharmacologic class: DNA demethylation agent; prodrug of cytotoxic deoxyguanosine
Pregnancy risk category D

AVAILABLE FORMS
Injection: 5 mg/ml in 50-ml vial

INDICATIONS & DOSAGES
➤ **T-cell acute lymphoblastic leukemia and T-cell lymphoblastic lymphoma in patients whose disease hasn't responded to or has relapsed after treatment with at least two chemotherapy regimens**
Adults: 1,500 mg/m^2 I.V. over 2 hours on days 1, 3, and 5. Repeat every 21 days.
Children: 650 mg/m^2 I.V. over 1 hour daily for 5 consecutive days. Repeat every 21 days.

ADMINISTRATION
I.V.
■ **Black Box Warning** Drug is for I.V. use only. ■

• Wear gloves and protective clothing when preparing drug, and avoid skin contact.

• Transfer undiluted dose to a polyvinylchloride infusion bag or glass container.

• Once prepared, drug may be stored for 8 hours at 86° F (30° C).

• For adults, infuse dose over 2 hours; for children, infuse over 1 hour.

• Dispose of drug according to facility's protocol for hazardous waste.

• **Incompatibilities:** None reported.

ACTION
Probably accumulates in leukemic cells, inhibiting DNA synthesis and causing cell death.

Route	Onset	Peak	Duration
I.V.	Immediate	2 hr	3–25 hr

Half-life: Parent drug, 30 minutes; active metabolite, 3 hours.

ADVERSE REACTIONS
CNS: *dizziness, fatigue, fever, headache, hypoesthesia, paresthesias, peripheral neuropathy, rigors, somnolence,* **demyelination peripheral neuropathies, seizures,** abnormal gait, asthenia, ataxia, confusion, decreased level of consciousness, depression, insomnia, pain.
CV: *edema, petechiae,* chest pain, hypotension, sinus tachycardia.
EENT: blurred vision, epistaxis, sinusitis.
GI: *constipation, diarrhea, nausea, vomiting,* abdominal distention, abdominal pain, anorexia, stomatitis.
Hematologic: FEBRILE NEUTROPENIA, LEUKOPENIA, NEUTROPENIA, THROMBOCYTOPENIA, anemia.
Metabolic: *hypoglycemia,* dehydration, hyperglycemia, hypocalcemia, hypokalemia, *hypomagnesemia.*
Musculoskeletal: *myalgia,* arthralgia, back pain, limb pain, muscle weakness.
Respiratory: *cough, dyspnea, pleural effusion,* wheezing.
Other: infection, weakness.

Reactions may be *common,* uncommon, *life-threatening,* or COMMON AND LIFE-THREATENING.
Interaction may have a *rapid onset* or *delayed onset.*

INTERACTIONS
Drug-drug. *Live vaccines:* Virus replication may occur; immunocompromised individuals may become ill. Don't give live vaccines to immunocompromised patients.

EFFECTS ON LAB TEST RESULTS
• May increase creatinine, transaminase, bilirubin, glucose, and AST levels. May decrease potassium, calcium, glucose, magnesium, albumin, and hemoglobin levels and hematocrit.
• May decrease WBC, platelet, and neutrophil counts.

CONTRAINDICATIONS & CAUTIONS
• Contraindicated in pregnant or breast-feeding women and in patients hypersensitive to drug or any of its components.
• Use cautiously if patient is receiving or has received intrathecal chemotherapy and in patients with severe renal or hepatic impairment.

NURSING CONSIDERATIONS
■ **Black Box Warning** Administer under the supervision of a physician experienced with chemotherapy. ■
• Monitor CBC at baseline and regularly throughout treatment.
■ **Black Box Warning** Monitor patient for signs of severe neurotoxicity, including ataxia, coma, confusion, excessive somnolence, Guillain-Barré–like symptoms, peripheral neuropathy, and seizures. For NCI Common Toxicity Criteria grade 2 or higher, stop treatment. Patient may not fully recover even after drug is stopped. ■
• Take steps to prevent hyperuricemia caused by tumor lysis syndrome. Appropriate care includes hydration, alkalinization of body fluids, and allopurinol.

PATIENT TEACHING
• *Alert:* Tell patient to immediately report tingling or numbness in hands or feet, problems with fine motor skills, unsteadiness when walking, weakness when getting out of a chair or climbing stairs, tripping while walking, or seizures. These may be signs of serious adverse effects.
• Explain the importance of regular blood tests to evaluate drug effectiveness and detect adverse effects.

• Tell patient to report being more tired or paler than usual, trouble breathing, unusual bruising or bleeding, or fever.
• Advise care when driving or operating hazardous machinery because drug may cause sleepiness or dizziness.
• Urge patient to avoid live-virus vaccines while taking this drug.

✳ NEW DRUG

nilotinib
nye-low-TIH-nibb

Tasigna

Pharmacologic class: kinase inhibitor
Pregnancy risk category D

AVAILABLE FORMS
Capsules: 200 mg

INDICATIONS & DOSAGES
➤ **Chronic and accelerated-phase Philadelphia chromosome–positive chronic myelogenous leukemia in patients resistant to or intolerant of imatinib**
Adults: 400 mg P.O. b.i.d. with water, at least 2 hours before or 1 hour after food.
Adjust-a-dose: If QTcF interval exceeds 480 msec, withhold drug; it if returns to less than 450 msec and within 20 msec of baseline within 2 weeks, resume therapy at previous dose. If QTcF interval is 450 to 480 msec after 4 weeks, reduce dose to 400 mg once daily; if QTcF interval returns to more than 480 msec, stop therapy. If neutrophil count is less than 1,000/mm³ or platelet count less than 50,000/mm³, stop therapy. If neutrophil count exceeds 1,000/mm³ and platelet count exceeds 50,000/mm³ within 2 weeks, resume therapy at previous dose. If blood counts stay low for more than 2 weeks, reduce dose to 400 mg P.O. once daily. If serum amylase, lipase, bilirubin, or hepatic transaminase levels are grade 3 or greater, withhold drug; when levels return to grade 1 or less, resume therapy. Withhold drug with other clinically significant moderate or severe toxicity. When toxicity resolves, resume at 400 mg P.O. once daily; increase to 400 mg P.O. b.i.d. when clinically appropriate.

PHARMACODYNAMICS
Chemotherapeutic action: Stops leukemic cell lines by inhibiting Bcr-Abl kinase.

PHARMACOKINETICS
Absorption: Increased with food.
Distribution: 98% protein-bound.
Metabolism: Mainly hepatic, inactive metabolites.
Excretion: Mainly in feces.

Route	Onset	Peak	Duration
P.O.	Unknown	3 hr	Unknown

Half-life: 17 hours.

ADVERSE REACTIONS
CNS: *asthenia, fatigue, fever, headache,* insomnia, dizziness, paresthesia.
CV: flushing, hypertension, palpitations, *peripheral edema,* **prolonged QT interval.**
EENT: *nasopharyngitis,* vertigo.
GI: abdominal discomfort, *abdominal pain,* anorexia, *constipation, diarrhea,* dyspepsia, flatulence, *nausea, vomiting.*
Hematologic: anemia, FEBRILE NEUTRO-PENIA, THROMBOCYTOPENIA, NEUTRO-PENIA, PANCYTOPENIA.
Hepatic: elevated lipase level.
Metabolic: *hyperglycemia,* hyperkalemia, hypocalcemia, hypokalemia, ***hypomagne-semia,*** hyponatremia, *hypophosphatemia,* weight gain or loss.
Musculoskeletal: *arthralgia, myalgia,* back pain, bone pain, limb pain, *muscle spasms,* musculoskeletal chest pain, pain in extremities.
Respiratory: *cough,* dysphonia, *dyspnea,* exertional dyspnea.
Skin: alopecia, dry skin, eczema, erythema, hyperhidrosis, night sweats, *pruritus, rash,* urticaria.

INTERACTIONS
Drug-drug. *Antiarrhythmics and other drugs that prolong QTc interval.* May further prolong QTc interval. Avoid using together.
CYP2C8, CYP2C9, CYP2D6, CYP3A4, UGT1A1 substrates, warfarin: May increase levels of these drugs. Avoid using together.
CYP3A4 inducers (carbamazepine, dexamethasone, phenobarbital, phenytoin, rifabutin, rifampin, rifapentin): May

decrease nilotinib level. Avoid using together, or consider increasing dosage.
CYP3A4 inhibitors (atazanavir, clarithro-mycin, indinavir, itraconazole, ketocona-zole, nefazodone, nelfinavir, ritonavir, saquinavir, telithromycin, voriconazole): May increase nilotinib level. Avoid using together, or consider reducing dose to 400 mg daily.
Midazolam: May increase midazolam level. Avoid using together.
P-glycoprotein substrates: May increase nilotinib levels. Avoid using together.
Drug-herb. *St. John's wort:* May decrease nilotinib level. Avoid using together.
Drug-food. *Food:* May increase drug level. Avoid eating 2 hours before and 1 hour after taking dose.
Grapefruit: May increase drug level. Avoid using together.

EFFECTS ON LAB TEST RESULTS
● May increase lipase, bilirubin, alkaline phosphatase, AST, ALT, potassium, and creatinine levels. May decrease albumin, sodium, potassium, calcium, phosphate, and hemoglobin levels.
● May decrease neutrophil and platelet counts.

CONTRAINDICATIONS & CAUTIONS
■ **Black Box Warning** Contraindicated in patients with prolonged QT-interval syndrome, hypokalemia, and hypo-magnesemia. Avoid use in patients with galactose intolerance, severe lactose deficiency, or glucose-galactose malabsorption. ■
■ **Black Box Warning** Obtain electro-cardiogram (ECG) to monitor the QTc at baseline, 7 days after initiation, and peri-odically thereafter, as well as following any dose adjustments. ■
● Use cautiously in patients with hepatic impairment, elevated lipase levels, or a history of pancreatitis.

NURSING CONSIDERATIONS
● Check patient's ECG before therapy, 7 days after starting therapy, when dosage is adjusted, and periodically thereafter.
● Monitor patient's phosphate, potassium, calcium, and sodium levels before and during therapy. Monitor the complete blood

count every 2 weeks for the first 2 months and then monthly thereafter.

• Assess patient for evidence of fluid retention, such as shortness of breath and swelling of hands, ankles, feet, or face.

• Check lipase, amylase, ALT, AST, and alkaline phosphatase levels periodically during therapy.

• If stopping a CYP3A4 inhibitor, allow an appropriate washout period before escalating the nilotinib dose.

• Caution women to avoid becoming pregnant during therapy because of the risk of fetal harm.

• It isn't known whether drug appears in breast milk. Advise women to avoid breast-feeding during therapy.

• Safety and efficacy haven't been established in children.

PATIENT TEACHING

• Instruct patient to immediately report an irregular heartbeat, shortness of breath, or swelling of the hands, ankles, feet, or face.

• Urge patient to immediately notify prescriber about a sudden onset of abdominal pain, nausea, and vomiting.

• Tell patient to avoid grapefruit during therapy.

• Instruct patient to take drug with water, and to restrict food intake for at least 2 hours before and 1 hour after taking the drug.

• Advise women of childbearing age to use an effective form of contraception while taking nilotinib and to notify prescriber immediately if pregnancy occurs.

• Advise women to stop breast-feeding during therapy because of the risk of toxicity to infant.

---

panitumumab
pan-eh-TOO-moo-mab

Vectibix

Pharmacologic class: monoclonal antibody
Pregnancy risk category C

AVAILABLE FORMS
Solution for infusion: 20 mg/ml in 5-ml, 10-ml, and 20-ml vials

INDICATIONS & DOSAGES

➤ **Human epidermal growth factor receptor-expressing metastatic colorectal cancer with disease progression during or following fluoropyrimidine-, oxaliplatin-, and irinotecan-containing regimens**
Adults: 6 mg/kg I.V. infusion over 60 minutes every 14 days. For doses greater than 1,000 mg, infuse over 90 minutes.

Adjust-a-dose: For patients with mild or moderate (grade 1 or 2) infusion reactions, reduce infusion rate by 50%. For patients with severe (grade 3 or 4) infusion reactions, stop drug permanently.

For skin toxicities grade 3 or greater, or if considered intolerable, stop drug. If toxicity doesn't improve to grade 2 or less within 1 month, permanently stop therapy. If toxicity improves to grade 2 or less, and patient is symptomatically improved after withholding 2 or fewer doses, restart treatment at 50% of original dose. If toxicity recurs, permanently stop drug. If toxicity doesn't recur, increase subsequent doses in increments of 25% of original dose until a 6-mg/kg dose is reached.

ADMINISTRATION
I.V.
• Dilute drug using aseptic technique. The solution should be colorless but may contain white or translucent particles that will be filtered out during infusion. Don't shake vials.

• Withdraw drug and dilute to a total volume of 100 ml with normal saline solution. For doses higher than 1,000 mg, dilute to 150 ml. Final concentration shouldn't exceed 10 mg/ml. Use within 6 hours if stored at room temperature or within 24 hours if refrigerated. Dispose of any unused drug.

• Give by I.V. infusion using a pump with a low–protein-binding 0.2- or 0.22-micrometer in-line filter. Don't give by I.V. push or bolus.

• Flush I.V. line with normal saline solution before and after giving drug.

• Refrigerate vials, don't freeze. Protect from sunlight.

• **Incompatibilities:** Other I.V. drugs and solutions.

ACTION

Inhibits actions between proteins and cell surface receptors that would normally allow proliferation of cells and new blood vessel growth.

Route	Onset	Peak	Duration
I.V.	Immediate	Unknown	Unknown

Half-life: 7½ days.

ADVERSE REACTIONS

CNS: *chills, fatigue, fever.*
CV: *peripheral edema,* hypotension.
EENT: *eyelash growth, ocular toxicities, oral mucositis.*
GI: *abdominal pain, constipation, diarrhea, nausea, vomiting,* mucosal inflammation, stomatitis.
Metabolic: HYPOMAGNESEMIA.
Respiratory: *cough, pulmonary toxicity*
Skin: *acne, acneiform dermatitis, dry skin, fissures, nail infection, pruritus, rash, redness,* **skin exfoliation, skin toxicity.**
Other: *anaphylaxis, severe infusion reaction,* general deterioration.

INTERACTIONS

None known.

EFFECTS ON LAB TEST RESULTS

• May decrease calcium and magnesium levels.

CONTRAINDICATIONS & CAUTIONS

• Use cautiously in patients with skin conditions, or preexisting lung or ocular disease.

NURSING CONSIDERATIONS

■ **Black Box Warning** Drug may cause severe infusion reactions, including anaphylaxis, bronchospasm, fever, chills, and hypotension. Monitor patient closely. Keep emergency treatment immediately available to treat severe infusion reactions. ■
■ **Black Box Warning** Monitor patient for severe dermatologic toxicities. Withhold or discontinue drug if severe dermatologic toxicities occur and monitor for inflammatory or infectious sequelae. ■
• Notify prescriber if patient develops severe eye or pulmonary toxicities. The

drug may need to be stopped or the dose lowered.
• Drug-induced diarrhea can be especially severe when combined with other chemotherapy drugs. Monitor patient for dehydration. Using with the irinotecan, bolus 5-fluorouracil, leucovorin regimen isn't recommended.
• Monitor patient's electrolytes, especially calcium and magnesium, periodically during and for 8 weeks after treatment. Supplementation may be needed.

PATIENT TEACHING

• Warn patient that drug can cause photosensitivity reactions and instruct him to wear a hat, sunscreen, and protective clothing, and to limit sun exposure.
• Warn patient about the risk of severe skin, eye, infusion-related, and pulmonary reactions. Advise him to report any skin changes, eye problems, or difficulty breathing to his prescriber.
• Diarrhea may be severe, especially if more than one chemotherapy drug is used. Remind patient to stay well hydrated.
• Tell women of childbearing age that contraception must be used during and for 6 months following treatment.
• Advise mothers to stop breast-feeding during and for 2 months after treatment ends.

SAFETY ALERT!

pegaspargase (PEG-L-asparaginase)

peg-AHS-per-jays

Oncaspar

Pharmacologic class: modified L-asparaginase
Pregnancy risk category C

AVAILABLE FORMS

Injection: 750 international units/ml

INDICATIONS & DOSAGES

➤ **As part of a multidrug chemotherapy regimen in the treatment of acute lymphoblastic leukemia, and acute lymphoblastic leukemia with hypersensitivity to asparaginase**

Reactions may be *common*, uncommon, *life-threatening*, or COMMON AND LIFE-THREATENING.
Interaction may have a *rapid onset* or **delayed onset**.

Adults and children older than 1 year:
2,500 international units/m^2 I.V. or I.M. every 14 days.

ADMINISTRATION
I.V.
● Drug may be a contact irritant, and solution must be handled and given with care. Wear gloves. Avoid inhalation of vapors and contact with skin or mucous membranes, especially in the eyes. If contact occurs, wash with generous amounts of water for at least 15 minutes.
● Don't use if cloudy or contains precipitate. Avoid excessive agitation of drug; don't shake.
● Don't freeze or use drug that has been frozen because freezing destroys drug's effectiveness.
● Give over 1 to 2 hours in 100 ml of normal saline solution or D$_5$W injection through an infusion that's already running.
● Discard unused portions. Use only one dose per vial; don't reenter vial.
● Don't use if stored at room temperature for longer than 48 hours. Keep refrigerated at 36° to 46° F (2° to 8° C).
● **Incompatibilities:** None reported, but don't mix with other I.V. drugs.
I.M.
● When giving I.M., limit volume given at a single injection site to 2 ml. If volume to be given exceeds 2 ml, use multiple injection sites.

ACTION
A modified version of the enzyme L-asparaginase that exerts cytotoxic effects by inactivating the amino acid asparagine, which tumor cells need to synthesize proteins.

Route	Onset	Peak	Duration
I.V., I.M.	Unknown	Unknown	Unknown

Half-life: Unknown.

ADVERSE REACTIONS
CNS: *coma, seizures, status epilepticus,* confusion, disorientation, dizziness, emotional lability, fatigue, headache, malaise, mental status changes, mood changes, paresthesia, parkinsonism, somnolence.

CV: chest pain, hypertension, hypotension, peripheral edema, subacute bacterial endocarditis, tachycardia.
EENT: epistaxis.
GI: *pancreatitis,* abdominal pain, anorexia, constipation, diarrhea, indigestion, flatulence, mouth tenderness, mucositis, nausea, severe colitis, vomiting.
GU: *renal failure,* hematuria, increased urinary frequency, proteinuria, renal dysfunction, severe hemorrhagic cystitis.
Hematologic: *agranulocytosis, disseminated intravascular coagulation, hemorrhage, leukopenia, pancytopenia, thrombocytopenia, thrombosis,* easy bruising, hemolytic anemia.
Hepatic: *liver failure,* ascites, fatty changes in liver, hypoalbuminemia, jaundice.
Metabolic: *hypoglycemia,* hyperglycemia, hyperuricemia, hyponatremia, hypoproteinemia, *metabolic acidosis,* uric acid nephropathy, weight loss.
Musculoskeletal: arthralgia, cramps, joint stiffness, myalgia, musculoskeletal pain, pain in limbs.
Respiratory: *bronchospasm,* cough, upper respiratory tract infection.
Skin: alopecia, ecchymoses, erythema, erythema simplex, fever blister, fungal changes, hand whiteness, injection pain or reaction, itching, localized edema, nail whiteness and ridging, petechial rash, purpura, rash, urticaria.
Other: *anaphylaxis, sepsis, septic shock,* hypersensitivity reactions, infection, night sweats.

INTERACTIONS
Drug-drug. *Aspirin, dipyridamole, heparin, NSAIDs, warfarin:* May cause imbalances in coagulation factors, predisposing patient to bleeding or thrombosis. Use together cautiously.
Methotrexate: May interfere with action of methotrexate. Check patient for decreased effectiveness.
Protein-bound drugs: May increase toxicity of other drugs that bind to proteins and may interfere with enzymatic detoxification of other drugs, especially in the liver. Check for toxicity, and use together cautiously.

EFFECTS ON LAB TEST RESULTS
- May increase BUN, creatinine, amylase, lipase, bilirubin, ALT, AST, uric acid, and ammonia levels. May decrease hemoglobin, sodium, and protein levels. May increase or decrease glucose level.
- May increase PT, INR, activated PTT, and thromboplastin. May decrease antithrombin III, WBC, RBC, platelet, and granulocyte counts.

CONTRAINDICATIONS & CAUTIONS
- Contraindicated in patients with pancreatitis or history of pancreatitis, in those who have had significant hemorrhagic events related to previous treatment with L-asparaginase, and in those with history of serious allergic reactions to drug, such as generalized urticaria, bronchospasm, laryngeal edema, hypotension, or other unacceptable adverse reactions.
- Use cautiously in patients with liver dysfunction; use only when clearly indicated in pregnant women.

NURSING CONSIDERATIONS
- Take preventive measures (including adequate hydration) before starting treatment. Hyperuricemia may result from rapid lysis of leukemic cells. Allopurinol may be ordered.
- I.M. use is preferred because it has the lowest risk of hepatotoxicity, coagulopathy, and GI and renal disorders.
- **Alert:** Monitor patient closely for hypersensitivity (including life-threatening anaphylaxis), especially those hypersensitive to other forms of L-asparaginase. Observe patient for 1 hour after giving drug and have emergency equipment and other drugs needed to treat anaphylaxis readily available. Moderate to life-threatening hypersensitivity requires stopping L-asparaginase.
- To assess effects of therapy, monitor patient's peripheral blood count and bone marrow. A drop in circulating lymphoblasts is often noted after therapy starts, sometimes accompanied by a marked rise in uric acid level.
- Obtain frequent amylase and lipase determinations to detect pancreatitis. Monitor patient's glucose level during therapy to detect hyperglycemia.

- Monitor patient for liver dysfunction when drug is used with hepatotoxic chemotherapeutic drugs.
- Drug may affect several plasma proteins; monitoring of fibrinogen, PT, INR, and PTT may be indicated.

PATIENT TEACHING
- Inform patient of risk of hypersensitivity reactions and importance of reporting them immediately.
- Tell patient not to take other drugs, including OTC preparations, until approved by prescriber because risk of bleeding is higher when pegaspargase is given with drugs such as aspirin. Drug may also increase toxicity of other drugs.
- Urge patient to report signs and symptoms of infection (fever, chills, and malaise); drug may suppress the immune system.
- Caution woman of childbearing age to avoid pregnancy and breast-feeding during therapy.

SAFETY ALERT!

procarbazine hydrochloride
proe-KAR-buh-zeen

Matulane, Natulan†

Pharmacologic class:
methylhydrazine derivative
Pregnancy risk category D

AVAILABLE FORMS
Capsules: 50 mg

INDICATIONS & DOSAGES
➤ **Adjunct treatment of Hodgkin lymphoma (stages III and IV), other cancers using nitrogen mustard, vincristine, procarbazine, prednisone (known as MOPP) regimen**
Adults: 2 to 4 mg/kg P.O. daily in single dose or divided doses for first week. Then, 4 to 6 mg/kg daily until WBC count falls below 4,000/mm^3, platelet count falls below 100,000/mm^3, or maximum response is obtained. Maintenance dose is 1 to 2 mg/kg daily after bone marrow recovery. For MOPP regimen, 100 mg/m^2 daily P.O. for 14 days of 28-day cycle.

Children: 50 mg/m^2 P.O. daily for first week; then 100 mg/m^2 until response or toxicity occurs. Maintenance dose is 50 mg/m^2 P.O. daily after bone marrow recovery.

ADMINISTRATION
P.O.
• Give drug at bedtime and in divided doses to decrease nausea and vomiting.

ACTION
Unknown. Thought to inhibit DNA, RNA, and protein synthesis.

Route	Onset	Peak	Duration
P.O.	Unknown	Unknown	Unknown

Half-life: 10 minutes.

ADVERSE REACTIONS
CNS: *hallucinations,* **coma,** confusion, depression, dizziness, headache, insomnia, nervousness, neuropathy, nightmares, paresthesia, syncope.
CV: flushing, hypotension, tachycardia.
EENT: nystagmus, photophobia, retinal hemorrhage.
GI: *nausea, vomiting,* abdominal pain, anorexia, constipation, diarrhea, dry mouth, dysphagia, **hematemesis, melena,** stomatitis.
GU: hematuria, nocturia, urinary frequency.
Hematologic: **anemia, bleeding tendency, leukopenia, thrombocytopenia,** eosinophilia, hemolytic anemia.
Hepatic: *hepatotoxicity,* jaundice.
Respiratory: *pleural effusion,* cough, pneumonitis.
Skin: dermatitis, hyperpigmentation, pruritus, rash, reversible alopecia.
Other: *secondary malignancies,* allergic reaction, gynecomastia, herpes outbreak.

INTERACTIONS
Drug-drug. *CNS depressants:* May cause additive depressant effects. Avoid using together.
Digoxin: May decrease digoxin level. Monitor digoxin level closely.
Drugs high in tyramine, local anesthetics, MAO inhibitors, sympathomimetics, tricyclic antidepressants: May cause tremor,

palpitations, and increased blood pressure. Monitor patient closely.
Levodopa: May cause sudden hypertensive crisis. Don't give within 2 to 4 weeks of procarbazine.
Methotrexate: The nephrotoxicity of methotrexate may be increased. Wait 72 hours or longer between giving the final dose of procarbazine and starting a high-dose methotrexate infusion.
Drug-food. *Caffeine:* May result in arrhythmias and severe hypertension. Discourage caffeine intake.
Foods high in tyramine (cheese, Chianti): May cause tremor, palpitations, and increased blood pressure. Monitor patient closely; advise him to avoid or limit intake.
Drug-lifestyle. *Alcohol use:* Mild disulfiram-like reaction may cause flushing, headache, nausea, and hypotension. Warn patient to avoid alcoholic beverages.

EFFECTS ON LAB TEST RESULTS
• May decrease hemoglobin level.
• May increase eosinophil count. May decrease platelet, RBC, and WBC counts.

CONTRAINDICATIONS & CAUTIONS
• Contraindicated in patients hypersensitive to drug and in those with inadequate bone marrow reserve as shown by bone marrow aspiration.
• Use cautiously in patients with impaired hepatic or renal function.

NURSING CONSIDERATIONS
■ **Black Box Warning** Give drug only under the supervision of a physician experienced with potent antineoplastic drugs. Adequate clinical and laboratory facilities should be available. ■
• Monitor CBC and platelet counts.
• Bone marrow depression begins 2 to 8 weeks after the start of treatment.
• Avoid all I.M. injections when platelet count is below 50,000/mm^3.
• RBC colony-stimulating factors may promote RBC production and decrease need for blood transfusions.
• Stop drug and notify prescriber if patient becomes confused or develops paresthesia or other neuropathy.
• The manufacturer recommends that if radiation or chemotherapeutic agents with

bone marrow depressant activity have been used, give patient a 1-month interval without such therapy before beginning procarbazine therapy.

PATIENT TEACHING
• To decrease nausea and vomiting, advise patient to take drug at bedtime and in divided doses.
• Tell patient to watch for fever, sore throat, fatigue, easy bruising, nosebleeds, bleeding gums, or tarry stools. Tell patient to take temperature daily.
• Warn patient to avoid alcohol during therapy. Urge him to stop drug and check with prescriber immediately if, after drinking alcohol, he experiences chest pain, rapid or irregular heartbeat, severe headache, or stiff neck.
• Instruct patient to avoid OTC medications that contain sympathomimetics and to avoid foods and drinks high in tyramine, such as wine, tea, coffee, cola, cheese, and bananas.
• Warn patient to avoid hazardous activities that require alertness and good motor coordination until CNS effects of drug are known.
• Caution woman of childbearing age to avoid becoming pregnant during therapy and to consult prescriber before becoming pregnant.

SAFETY ALERT!

rituximab
ri-TUX-i-mab

Rituxan

Pharmacologic class: monoclonal antibody
Pregnancy risk category C

AVAILABLE FORMS
Injection: 10 mg/ml in 10-ml and 50-ml single-use, sterile vials

INDICATIONS & DOSAGES
➤ **Previously untreated, follicular CD20-positive, B-cell non-Hodgkin lymphoma (NHL) with cyclo-phosphamide, vincristine, and**

prednisolone (CVP) chemotherapy regimen
Adults: 375 mg/m^2 I.V. given on day 1 of each CVP cycle, for up to eight doses.
➤ **Previously untreated low-grade, CD20-positive, B-cell NHL following first-line treatment with CVP chemotherapy**
Adults: For patients who fail to progress after six to eight cycles of CVP chemotherapy, give 375 mg/m^2 I.V. once weekly for four doses every 6 months for up to 16 doses.
➤ **Relapsed or refractory low-grade or follicular, CD20-positive, B-cell NIIL**
Adults: Initially, 375 mg/m^2 I.V. once weekly for four or eight doses. Retreatment for patients with progressive disease, 375 mg/m^2 I.V. infusion once weekly for four doses.
➤ **With methotrexate to reduce the signs and symptoms of moderate to severely active rheumatoid arthritis in patients who have had an inade-quate response to one or more tumor necrosis factor antagonists**
Adults: Two 1,000 mg I.V. infusions 2 weeks apart. To reduce the incidence and severity of infusion reactions, give methyl-prednisolone 100 mg I.V., or its equivalent, 30 minutes before each infusion.
➤ **Diffuse large B-cell, CD20-positive, non-Hodgkin lymphoma, given with cyclophosphamide-adriamycin-oncovin-prednisone, known as CHOP, or other anthracycline-based chemotherapy regimens**
Adults: 375 mg/m^2 I.V. given on day 1 of each chemotherapy cycle for up to eight infusions.

ADMINISTRATION
I.V.
• Give acetaminophen and diphenhy-dramine before each infusion.
• Protect vials from direct sunlight.
• Give as an infusion; don't give as I.V. push or bolus.
• Begin infusion at rate of 50 mg/hour. If no hypersensitivity or infusion-related events occur, increase rate by 50 mg/hour every 30 minutes, to maximum of 400 mg/hour. Start subsequent infusions at 100 mg/hour and increase by 100 mg/hour

---

Reactions may be *common*, uncommon, *life-threatening*, or COMMON AND LIFE-THREATENING.
Interaction may have a *rapid onset* or **delayed onset**.

every 30 minutes, to maximum of 400 mg/hour as tolerated.
• Dilute to yield 1 to 4 mg/ml in bag of D_5W or normal saline solution. Gently invert bag to mix solution.
• Discard unused portion left in vial.
• Diluted solutions are stable for 24 hours if refrigerated and for 12 hours at room temperature.
• **Incompatibilities.** Other I.V. drugs

ACTION
A murine and human monoclonal antibody directed against CD20 antigen found on the surface of normal and malignant B lymphocytes. Binding to this antigen mediates the lysis of the B cells.

Route	Onset	Peak	Duration
I.V.	Variable	Variable	6–12 mo

Half-life: Varies widely, possibly because of differences in tumor burden among patients and changes in CD-positive B-cell populations upon repeated therapy.

ADVERSE REACTIONS
CNS: *asthenia, fever, headache,* agitation, dizziness, fatigue, hypesthesia, hypertonia, insomnia, malaise, nervousness, pain, paresthesia, somnolence, vertigo.
CV: *hypotension,* **arrhythmias, bradycardia,** chest pain, edema, flushing, hypertension, peripheral edema, tachycardia.
EENT: conjunctivitis, lacrimation disorder, rhinitis, sinusitis, sore throat.
GI: *nausea,* abdominal pain or enlargement, anorexia, diarrhea, dyspepsia, taste perversion, vomiting.
GU: *acute renal failure.*
Hematologic: LEUKOPENIA, *neutropenia, thrombocytopenia,* anemia.
Metabolic: hyperglycemia, hypocalcemia, weight decrease.
Musculoskeletal: arthritis, back pain, myalgia.
Respiratory: *bronchospasm,* bronchitis, cough increase, dyspnea.
Skin: *pruritus, rash,* SEVERE MUCO-CUTANEOUS REACTIONS, pain at injection site, urticaria.
Other: *chills, rigors,* ANGIOEDEMA, *infusion reaction,* infection, *tumor lysis syndrome,* tumor pain.

INTERACTIONS
Drug-drug. *Cisplatin:* May cause renal toxicity. Monitor renal function tests.
Live virus vaccines: Virus replication may occur. Avoid vaccination with live virus vaccines.

EFFECTS ON LAB TEST RESULTS
• May increase glucose and LDH levels. May decrease calcium and hemoglobin levels.
• May decrease WBC, platelet, and neutrophil counts.

CONTRAINDICATIONS & CAUTIONS
• Contraindicated in patients with type I hypersensitivity or anaphylactic reactions to murine proteins or components of drug.

NURSING CONSIDERATIONS
■ **Black Box Warning** Deaths from infusion reactions have occurred. Monitor patient for infusion reaction complex, including hypoxia, pulmonary infiltrates, acute respiratory distress syndrome, MI, or cardiogenic shock. ■
• Monitor patient closely for signs and symptoms of hypersensitivity. Have drugs, such as epinephrine, antihistamines, and corticosteroids available to immediately treat such a reaction.
• Monitor patient's blood pressure closely during infusion. If hypotension, bronchospasm, or angioedema occurs, stop infusion and restart at half the rate when symptoms resolve.
• Withhold antihypertensives 12 hours before infusion because transient hypotension may occur.
• If serious or life-threatening arrhythmias occur, stop infusion. If patient develops significant arrhythmias, monitor cardiac function during and after subsequent infusions.
■ **Black Box Warning** Severe mucocutaneous reactions (including toxic epidermal necrolysis, Stevens-Johnson syndrome, paraneoplastic pemphigus, and lichenoid or vesiculobullous dermatitis) may occur 1 to 13 weeks after administration. Avoid further infusions and promptly start treatment of the skin reaction. ■
• Infusion-related reactions are most severe with the first infusion. Subsequent infusions are generally well tolerated.

■ **Black Box Warning** Acute renal failure requiring dialysis has been reported in the setting of tumor lysis syndrome following treatment of patients with NHL. ■

• *Alert:* JC virus infection resulting in progressive multifocal leukoencephalopathy has been reported in patients within 12 months of their last rituximab infusion. Monitor patient for new onset neurologic manifestations.

• Obtain CBC at regular intervals and more frequently in patients in whom cytopenias develop.

PATIENT TEACHING
• Tell patient to report symptoms of hypersensitivity, such as itching, rash, chills, or rigor, during and after infusion.
• Urge patient to watch for fever, sore throat, fatigue, easy bruising, nosebleeds, bleeding gums, or tarry stools. Tell him to take temperature daily.
• Advise breast-feeding women to stop breast-feeding until drug levels are undetectable.

---

sorafenib
sohr-uh-FEN-ib

Nexavar

Pharmacologic class: multi-kinase inhibitor
Pregnancy risk category D

AVAILABLE FORMS
Tablets: 200 mg

INDICATIONS & DOSAGES
➤ **Advanced renal cell carcinoma, hepatocellular carcinoma**
Adults: 400 mg P.O. b.i.d. at least 1 hour before or 2 hours after eating. Continue until disease progresses or unacceptable toxicity occurs.
Adjust-a-dose: If grade 2 skin toxicity (pain and swelling with normal activities) develops, continue treatment and use topical drugs to relieve symptoms. If symptoms don't improve in 1 week or if they occur a second or third time, stop treatment until toxicity resolves to grade 0 or 1 (able to perform daily activities). Resume treatment at 400 mg daily or

every other day. At fourth occurrence of grade 2 toxicity, stop treatment. If grade 3 skin toxicity (ulceration, blistering, severe, debilitating pain of hands and feet) or a second occurrence develops, stop treatment until toxicity resolves to grade 0 or 1. Resume treatment at 400 mg daily or every other day. At third occurrence of grade 3 toxicity, stop treatment.

ADMINISTRATION
P.O.
• Give drug with water, 1 hour before or 2 hours after a meal.

ACTION
Decreases tumor cell proliferation by interacting with multiple intracellular and cell-surface kinases that may influence growth of new blood vessels into a tumor.

Route	Onset	Peak	Duration
P.O.	Unknown	3 hr	Unknown

Half-life: 1 to 2 days.

ADVERSE REACTIONS
CNS: *asthenia, fatigue, headache, neuropathy,* depression, pyrexia.
CV: flushing, *hypertension.*
EENT: *hoarseness.*
GI: *abdominal pain, anorexia, constipation, diarrhea, nausea, vomiting,* dyspepsia, dysphagia, mucositis, stomatitis.
GU: erectile dysfunction.
Hematologic: *bleeding, hemorrhage, leukopenia, lymphopenia, neutropenia, thrombocytopenia,* anemia.
Metabolic: *weight loss,* hypothyroidism.
Musculoskeletal: *joint pain,* arthralgia, myalgia.
Respiratory: *cough, dyspnea.*
Skin: *alopecia, dry skin, erythema, hand-foot reaction, pruritus, rash,* acne, exfoliative dermatitis.
Other: flulike illness.

INTERACTIONS
Drug-drug. *CYP2B6 or CYP2C8 substrates:* May increase levels of these drugs. Use cautiously together.
CYP3A4 inducers (such as carbamazepine, dexamethasone, phenobarbital, phenytoin,

---

Reactions may be *common,* uncommon, *life-threatening,* or COMMON AND LIFE-THREATENING.
Interaction may have a *rapid onset* or *delayed onset.*

rifampin): May increase sorafenib metabolism and decrease its effects. Monitor patient.

Doxorubicin, drugs metabolized by the UGT1A1 pathway (such as irinotecan): May increase levels of these drugs. Use cautiously together.

Warfarin: May increase the risk of bleeding. Monitor PT, INR, and patient for bleeding.

Drug-herb. *St. John's wort:* May decrease drug effects. Discourage use together.

EFFECTS ON LAB TEST RESULTS

● May increase TSH, lipase, amylase, transaminase, and bilirubin levels. May decrease phosphate levels.

● May decrease RBC, WBC, and platelet counts.

CONTRAINDICATIONS & CAUTIONS

● Contraindicated in patients severely hypersensitive to drug or its components.

● Use cautiously in patients with bleeding disorders, healing wounds, current or previous hand-foot skin reactions, or liver, renal, or cardiac disease, such as hypertension, cardiac ischemia, or a history of MI.

NURSING CONSIDERATIONS

● To avoid serious drug interactions, take a careful drug history.

● Monitor patient closely for hand-foot skin reaction, especially during the first 6 weeks of treatment.

● Measure blood pressure weekly during the first 6 weeks of treatment to check for hypertension.

● If patient is scheduled for major surgery, inform the surgeon that patient is taking this drug; therapy should be stopped. Monitor incision for adequate healing before restarting.

● Monitor patient for symptoms of cardiac ischemia.

● Assess patient for unusual bruising or bleeding.

● Provide patient with contact information for cancer support groups and instructions for managing adverse effects.

● *Alert:* Warn women to avoid pregnancy during and for 2 weeks following treatment.

PATIENT TEACHING

● Tell patient to swallow tablet whole, with water, 1 hour before or 2 hours after a meal.

● Advise patient to keep appointments for blood tests and blood pressure checks.

● Explain that hair loss, nausea, vomiting, diarrhea, and fatigue are common.

● Inform patient that mild to moderate skin reactions are common. Tell him to notify prescriber if they occur. If they're severe, treatment may have to be stopped or dosage reduced. Urge patient to report pain, redness, blisters, or skin ulceration to prescriber immediately.

● Tell patient to report bleeding episodes right away.

● Tell patient to notify prescriber if chest pain or other serious heart problems develop.

● *Alert:* Drug may cause serious birth defects or fetal death. Advise women not to become pregnant during treatment and for at least 2 weeks after. Men should also avoid fathering children at this time.

---

sunitinib malate
soo-NIH-tih-nib

Sutent⌀

Pharmacologic class: protein-tyrosine kinase inhibitor
Pregnancy risk category D

AVAILABLE FORMS
Capsules: 12.5 mg, 25 mg, 50 mg

INDICATIONS & DOSAGES
➤ **GI stromal tumor that's progressing despite imatinib therapy or because patient is intolerant of imatinib; advanced renal cell carcinoma**
Adults: 50 mg P.O. once daily for 4 weeks, followed by 2 weeks off the drug. Repeat cycle.

Adjust-a-dose: Increase or decrease dosage in 12.5-mg increments based on individual safety and tolerability.

ADMINISTRATION
P.O.
● Give drug without regard for meals.

ACTION

A multi-kinase inhibitor targeting several receptor tyrosine kinases, which are involved in tumor growth, pathologic angiogenesis, and metastatic progression of cancer.

Route	Onset	Peak	Duration
P.O.	Rapid	6–12 hr	Unknown

Half-life: 40 to 60 hours; primary metabolite, 80 to 110 hours.

ADVERSE REACTIONS

CNS: *asthenia, dizziness, fatigue, fever, headache, peripheral neuropathy.*
CV: ***decreased left ventricular ejection fraction, thromboembolic events,*** *hypertension,* peripheral edema.
EENT: increased lacrimation, periorbital edema.
GI: ***GI perforation, pancreatitis,*** abdominal pain, *altered taste, anorexia,* appetite disturbance, burning sensation in mouth, *constipation, diarrhea,* dyspepsia, flatulence, *mucositis,* nausea, oral pain, *stomatitis,* vomiting.
Hematologic: BLEEDING, LEUKOPENIA, LYMPHOPENIA, NEUTROPENIA, THROMBOCYTOPENIA, anemia.
Metabolic: *dehydration, hypernatremia, hyperuricemia, hypokalemia,* **hyperkalemia,** hyponatremia, hypophosphatemia, hypothyroidism.
Musculoskeletal: *arthralgia, back pain, limb pain, myalgia.*
Respiratory: *cough, dyspnea.*
Skin: *alopecia, dry skin, hair color changes, hand-foot syndrome, rash, skin discoloration,* skin blistering.
Other: ***adrenal insufficiency,*** hypothyroidism.

INTERACTIONS

Drug-drug. *CYP3A4 inducers (such as carbamazepine, dexamethasone, phenobarbital, phenytoin, rifabutin, rifampin, rifapentine):* May decrease sunitinib level and effects. If use together can't be avoided, increase sunitinib dosage to 87.5 mg daily.
Strong CYP3A4 inhibitors (such as atazanavir, clarithromycin, indinavir, itraconazole, ketoconazole, nefazodone, nelfinavir, ritonavir, saquinavir, telithro- *mycin, voriconazole):* May increase sunitinib level and toxicity. If use together can't be avoided, decrease sunitinib dosage to 37.5 mg daily.
Drug-herb. *St. John's wort:* May cause an unpredictable decrease in drug level. Discourage use together.
Drug-food. *Grapefruit:* May increase drug level. Discourage use together.

EFFECTS ON LAB TEST RESULTS

● May increase AST, ALT, alkaline phosphatase, total and indirect bilirubin, amylase, lipase, creatinine, uric acid, and TSH levels. May decrease phosphorus and hemoglobin levels and hematocrit. May increase or decrease potassium and sodium levels.
● May decrease RBC, neutrophil, lymphocyte, leukocyte, and platelet counts.

CONTRAINDICATIONS & CAUTIONS

● Contraindicated in patients hypersensitive to drug or any of its components.
● Don't use in patients with non–small cell lung cancer.
● Use cautiously in patients with a history of hypertension, MI, angina, coronary artery bypass graft, symptomatic heart failure, stroke, transient ischemic attack, or pulmonary embolism.

NURSING CONSIDERATIONS

● Obtain CBC with platelet count and serum chemistries, including phosphate level, before each treatment cycle.
● Obtain baseline evaluation of ejection fraction in all patients before treatment. If patient had a cardiac event in the year before treatment, check ejection fraction periodically.
● Interrupt therapy or decrease dose in patients with an ejection fraction less than 50% and more than 20% below baseline.
● Monitor patient's blood pressure closely. If severe hypertension occurs, notify prescriber. Treatment may need to be held until blood pressure is controlled.
● Monitor patient for signs and symptoms of heart failure, especially if he has a history of heart disease.
● If patient has seizures, he may have reversible posterior leukoencephalopathy syndrome. Signs and symptoms include hypertension, headache, decreased alert-

---

Reactions may be *common,* uncommon, *life-threatening,* or COMMON AND LIFE-THREATENING.
Interaction may have a *rapid onset* or **delayed onset.**

ness, altered mental functioning, and vision loss. Stop treatment temporarily.
• If patient will be undergoing surgery or suffers trauma or severe infection, assess him for adrenal insufficiency (muscle weakness, weight loss, depression, salt craving, low blood pressure).
• Provide antiemetics or antidiarrheals as needed for adverse GI effects.

PATIENT TEACHING
• Advise patient to keep appointments for blood tests and periodic heart function evaluations.
• Tell patient about common adverse effects, such as diarrhea, nausea, vomiting, fatigue, mouth pain, and taste disturbance.
• Inform patient about changes that may occur in skin and hair, including color changes and dry, red, blistering skin of the hands and feet.
• Urge patient to tell prescriber about all prescribed and OTC drugs or herbal supplements.
• Warn patient not to consume grapefruit during therapy.
• Tell patient to notify his prescriber about unusual bleeding, trouble breathing, wheezing, severe or prolonged diarrhea or vomiting, or swelling of the hands or lower legs.

SAFETY ALERT!

temsirolimus
TEM-seer-OLE-ih-muss

Torisel

Pharmacologic class: kinase inhibitor
Pregnancy risk category D

AVAILABLE FORMS
I.V. solution: 25 mg/ml

INDICATIONS & DOSAGES
➤ **Advanced renal cell carcinoma**
Adults: 25 mg I.V. over 30 to 60 minutes once weekly until disease progresses or unacceptable toxicity occurs. Give diphenhydramine, 25 to 50 mg I.V. 30 minutes before each dose.

Adjust-a-dose: In patients with an absolute neutrophil count of less than 1,000/mm³, a platelet count of less than 75,000/mm³, or National Cancer Institute Common Terminology Criteria for Adverse Events grade 3 or greater adverse reactions, hold dose. Once toxicities have resolved to grade 2 or less, drug may be restarted, with dose reduced by 5 mg weekly to dose no lower than 15 mg/week.

ADMINISTRATION
I.V.
• Refrigerate drug and protect from light.
• Prepare solution only in glass, polypropylene, or polyolefin containers. Don't use polyvinyl chloride containers or administration sets.
• Inject 1.8 ml of provided diluent into vial of temsirolimus 25 mg/ml injection. The temsirolimus vial contains an overfill of 0.2 ml (30 mg per 1.2 ml). The drug concentration of the resulting solution is 10 mg/ml. A total volume of 3 ml will be obtained, including the overfill. Mix well.
• Further dilute in a 250-ml container (glass, polyolefin, or polyethylene) of normal saline solution. Mixture is stable for up to 24 hours at room temperature.
• Give drug using a polyethylene-lined administration set. Using an infusion pump, infuse drug over 30 to 60 minutes through an in-line filter of 5 microns or less.
• Complete infusion within 6 hours of second dilution.
• Always use diluent provided to prevent precipitation. Stability with solutions other than normal saline hasn't been evaluated.
• **Incompatibilities:** Other I.V. drugs.

ACTION
Binds to an intracellular protein, which halts the cell cycle, reducing tumor size.

Route	Onset	Peak	Duration
I.V.	Immediate	End of infusion	Unknown

Half-life: 17.3 hours.

ADVERSE REACTIONS
CNS: *asthenia,* depression, *dysgeusia, headache, insomnia,* depression, *pain, pyrexia.*

CV: *chest pain, edema,* hypertension, *hyperlipidemia, hypertriglyceridemia,* **venous thromboembolism,** thrombophlebitis.
EENT: conjunctivitis, *pharyngitis, rhinitis.*
GI: *abdominal pain, anorexia,* **bowel perforation,** *constipation, diarrhea, mucositis, nausea, vomiting.*
GU: *UTI,* **renal failure.**
Hematologic: *anemia,* THROMBO-CYTOPENIA, LEUKOPENIA.
Metabolic: HYPERGLYCEMIA, *hypophosphatemia, weight loss.*
Musculoskeletal: *arthralgia, back pain, myalgia.*
Respiratory: *cough, rhinitis, pharyngitis, dyspnea, epistaxis,* **interstitial lung disease,** pneumonia, **pulmonary embolism,** respiratory tract infection.
Skin: *acne, dry skin, nail disorder, pruritus, rash.*
Other: *chills,* hypersensitivity reaction, impaired wound healing, *infections.*

INTERACTIONS
Drug-drug. *ACE inhibitors:* Potential for angioedema. Monitor patient for difficulty swallowing, tongue swelling, and difficulty breathing.
Anticoagulants: May increase risk of bleeding. Use cautiously together and monitor bleeding times closely.
CYP3A4 inducers (such as carbamazepine, dexamethasone, phenobarbital, phenytoin, rifabutin, rifampin, rifampicin): May decrease temsirolimus level. Avoid using together, if possible. If not, increase temsirolimus dose up to 50 mg/week, as needed.
CYP3A4 inhibitors (such as atazanavir, clarithromycin, indinavir, itraconazole, ketoconazole, nefazodone, nelfinavir, ritonavir, saquinavir, telithromycin, voriconazole): May increase temsirolimus level. Avoid using together, if possible. If not, decrease dose to 12.5 mg/week as needed.
Live virus vaccines (such as bacillus Calmette Guérin; intranasal influenza; measles, mumps, rubella; oral polio; TY21a typhoid, varicella; yellow fever): May increase risk of infection. Avoid using together.
Sunitinib: May cause dose-limiting toxicity. Monitor patient carefully.

Drug-herb. *St. John's wort:* May decrease temsirolimus level. Discourage use together.
Drug-food. *Grapefruit juice:* May increase sirolimus levels, a metabolite of temsirolimus. Discourage use together.

EFFECTS ON LAB TEST RESULTS
● May increase alkaline phosphatase, AST, creatinine, glucose, total bilirubin, total cholesterol, and triglyceride levels. May decrease phosphorus, potassium, and hemoglobin levels.
● May decrease lymphocyte, neutrophil, platelet, and leukocyte counts.

CONTRAINDICATIONS & CAUTIONS
● Contraindicated in patients hypersensitive to drug or its metabolites (including sirolimus), polysorbate 80, or any other components.
● Contraindicated in pregnancy; may cause fetal harm.
● Use cautiously in men with partners of childbearing potential. Use of reliable birth control is recommended throughout treatment and for 3 months after.
● Use cautiously in patient with CNS tumors or anticoagulation therapy because of increased risk of intracerebral bleeding.
● Use cautiously in patients with hyperglycemia, hyperlipidemia, thrombocytopenia, immunosuppression, or infections, especially during postoperative period.
● It's unknown if drug or its metabolites appear in breast milk. Patient should either stop breast-feeding or stop drug.

NURSING CONSIDERATIONS
● Doses larger than 25 mg increase the risk of serious adverse effects. No specific treatment exists; monitor patient carefully.
● Because hypersensitivity reactions are common, give diphenhydramine 25 to 50 mg or a histamine 2 receptor antagonist (such as famotidine 20 mg or ranitidine 50 mg I.V.) 30 minutes before infusion.
● If reaction occurs, stop infusion and monitor patient for 30 to 60 minutes or more. As ordered, treatment may resume at a slower rate (up to 60 minutes).
● Monitor laboratory values regularly.

Reactions may be *common,* uncommon, *life-threatening,* or COMMON AND LIFE-THREATENING.
Interaction may have a *rapid onset* or **delayed onset.**

- Expect elevated triglyceride or cholesterol levels during treatment; start lipid-lowering medication as needed.
- Watch carefully for evidence of infection, especially after surgery.
- Monitor patient carefully for possible interstitial lung disease, bowel perforation, and renal failure.

PATIENT TEACHING

- Urge patient to give a complete list of all drugs he takes, to avoid potentially dangerous interactions.
- Inform patient that temsirolimus therapy increases the risk of renal failure.
- Explain that patient will need regular blood tests during therapy.
- Inform patient of the possibility of serious allergic reaction and tell him to report immediately any facial swelling or difficulty breathing.
- Tell patient that increased blood glucose is likely and may require the start or increase of insulin or other hypoglycemic agent. Tell him to report excessive thirst or increased volume or frequency of urination.
- Tell patient that increased triglycerides and cholesterol levels are likely and may require the start of or increase in lipid-lowering agents.
- Urge patient not to miss any infusion appointments to maintain effectiveness of treatment.
- Instruct patient to immediately report any infection, open wound, breathing problem, new abdominal pain, blood in stool, or other bleeding.
- Advise patient to avoid live vaccines and close contact with those who have received live vaccines.
- Tell women (and men with partners of childbearing age) to use reliable contraception during treatment and for 3 months after last dose.
- Tell patient and partners to notify prescriber right away about possible or confirmed pregnancy.
- Tell women to consult prescriber before breast-feeding.

SAFETY ALERT!

teniposide (VM-26)
teh-NIP-uh-side

Vumon

Pharmacologic class:
podophyllotoxin
Pregnancy risk category D

AVAILABLE FORMS
Injection: 10 mg/ml

INDICATIONS & DOSAGES
➤ **Refractory childhood acute lymphoblastic leukemia**
Children: Optimum dosage hasn't been established. Dosages ranging from 165 to 250 mg/m² I.V. once or twice weekly for 4 to 8 weeks have been used. Usually given with other chemotherapy.
Adjust-a-dose: Patients with both Down syndrome and leukemia are at higher risk for myelosuppression. Give first course of treatment at half the recommended dosage.

ADMINISTRATION
I.V.
- Drug contains benzyl alcohol. Avoid use in neonates.
- Preparation and administration of parenteral form of drug may be mutagenic, teratogenic, or carcinogenic. Follow institutional policy to reduce risks.
- Use containers and tubing that don't contain di(2-ethylhexyl)phthalate.
- Dilute drug in either D_5W or normal saline solution for injection to final concentration of 0.1, 0.2, 0.4, or 1 mg/ml. Don't agitate vigorously; precipitation may occur. Discard cloudy solutions. Prepare and store drug in glass containers.
- Flush administration apparatus and catheters with D_5W or normal saline solution before and after infusion of drug.
- Infuse over at least 30 to 60 minutes to prevent hypotension.
- Ensure correct placement of I.V. catheter. Extravasation can cause local tissue necrosis or sloughing.
- Occlusion of catheters can occur (including those centrally placed), particularly

during 24-hour infusions at 0.1 to
0.2 mg/ml. Monitor catheters carefully.
● Don't use a membrane-type in-line filter
because diluent may dissolve it.
● Monitor blood pressure every 30 minutes
during infusion. If systolic blood pressure
falls below 90 mm Hg, stop infusion and
notify prescriber.
● In normal saline solution or D_5W, concentrations of 0.1 to 0.4 mg/ml in glass
containers are chemically stable for up to
24 hours at room temperature. Give solutions with a concentration of 1 mg/ml
within 4 hours to reduce possible
precipitation. Refrigeration isn't
recommended.
● **Incompatibilities:** Idarubicin. Heparin
sodium may cause precipitation.

ACTION

A phase-specific cytotoxic drug that acts
in the late S or early G_2 phase of the cell
cycle, thus preventing cells from entering
mitosis.

Route	Onset	Peak	Duration
I.V.	Unknown	Unknown	Unknown

Half-life: 5 hours.

ADVERSE REACTIONS

CNS: fever.
CV: hypotension, *phlebitis.*
GI: *diarrhea, mucositis, nausea, vomiting.*
Hematologic: LEUKOPENIA, MYELO-
SUPPRESSION, NEUTROPENIA, THROMBO-
CYTOPENIA, *anemia.*
Skin: *extravasation at injection site,*
alopecia, rash.
Other: *infection,* **anaphylaxis, bleeding,**
hypersensitivity reactions.

INTERACTIONS

Drug-drug. *Methotrexate:* May increase
clearance and intracellular levels of
methotrexate. Avoid using together.
*Sodium salicylate, sulfamethizole, tolbu-
tamide:* May displace teniposide from
protein-binding sites and increase toxicity.
Avoid using together.

EFFECTS ON LAB TEST RESULTS

● May decrease hemoglobin level.
● May decrease WBC, platelet, and
neutrophil counts.

CONTRAINDICATIONS & CAUTIONS

● Contraindicated in patients hypersensitive
to drug or to polyoxyethylated castor oil, an
injection vehicle.

NURSING CONSIDERATIONS

■ **Black Box Warning** Administer under
the supervision of a physician experienced
with cancer chemotherapy. ■
● Severe myelosuppression with resulting
bleeding or infection may occur.
● Drug may be prescribed despite patient's
history of hypersensitivity. Treat such
patients with antihistamines and corticosteroids before infusion begins, and
observe continuously for first hour of
infusion and at frequent intervals
thereafter.
● Obtain baseline blood counts and renal
and hepatic function tests and monitor
regularly.
● Monitor blood pressure before and
during therapy. Hypotension can occur
from rapid infusion.
■ **Black Box Warning** Severe hypersensitivity reaction may occur. Have on hand
diphenhydramine, hydrocortisone, epinephrine, and emergency equipment to
establish an airway in case of anaphylaxis.
Signs of hypersensitivity include chills,
fever, urticaria, tachycardia, bronchospasm,
dyspnea, hypotension, and flushing. ■

PATIENT TEACHING

● Advise patient to report any pain or
burning at site of injection during or after
administration.
● Tell patient to report signs and symptoms
of infection (fever, sore throat, fatigue)
and bleeding (easy bruising, nosebleeds,
bleeding gums, tarry stools). Tell patient
to take temperature daily.
● Caution woman to avoid becoming
pregnant during therapy and to consult
prescriber before becoming pregnant.

Reactions may be *common,* uncommon, *life-threatening,* or COMMON AND LIFE-THREATENING.
Interaction may have a *rapid onset* or **delayed onset.**

SAFETY ALERT!

topotecan hydrochloride
toh-poh-TEE-ken

Hycamtin

Pharmacologic class: DNA
topoisomerase inhibitor
Pregnancy risk category D

AVAILABLE FORMS
Capsules: 0.25 mg, 1 mg
Injection: 4-mg single-dose vial
(preservative-free)

INDICATIONS & DOSAGES
➤ **Relapsed small cell lung cancer
(SCLC) in patients with a prior
complete or partial response who
are at least 45 days from the end of
first-line chemotherapy**
Adults: 2.3 mg/m²/day P.O. once daily for
5 consecutive days. Repeat every 21 days.
Round the calculated dose to the nearest
0.25 mg.
Adjust-a-dose: For patients with
moderate renal impairment (creatinine
clearance 30 to 49 ml/min) give
1.8 mg/m²/day. Hold subsequent
courses until neutrophils are greater
than 1,000 cells/mm³, platelets are
greater than 100,000 cells/mm³, and
hemoglobin is 9 g/dl or more. Reduce
the dose for subsequent courses to
0.4 mg/m²/day for patients who experience severe neutropenia (neutrophils
less than 500 cells/mm³ associated with
fever or infection or lasting 7 days or
more), neutropenia (neutrophils 500 to
1,000 cells/mm³ lasting beyond day 21
of the treatment course), platelet count
below 25,000 cells/mm³, or grade 3 or
4 diarrhea.
➤ **With cisplatin, stage-IVB, recurrent or persistent cervical cancer
unresponsive to surgery or radiation**
Adults: 0.75 mg/m² by I.V. infusion over
30 minutes on days 1, 2, and 3, followed
by 50 mg/m² cisplatin by I.V. infusion on
day 1. Repeat cycle every 21 days. Adjust
subsequent doses of each drug based on
hematologic toxicities.
➤ **Metastatic carcinoma of the ovary
after failure of first or subsequent**

**chemotherapy; small cell lung
cancer-sensitive disease after failure
of first-line chemotherapy**
Adults: 1.5 mg/m² I.V. infusion given over
30 minutes daily for 5 consecutive days,
starting on day 1 of a 21-day cycle. Give a
minimum of four cycles.
Adjust-a-dose: For patients with creatinine clearance of 20 to 39 ml/minute,
decrease dosage to 0.75 mg/m². If
severe neutropenia occurs, decrease
dosage by 0.25 mg/m² for subsequent
courses. Or, if severe neutropenia
occurs, give granulocyte colony-
stimulating factor after subsequent
course (before resorting to dosage
reduction) starting from day 6 of course
(24 hours after completion of topotecan
administration).

ADMINISTRATION
P.O.
● Avoid direct contact with capsule
contents.
● Give drug without regard to food.
● Do not crush or divide the capsule.
● If patient vomits after taking dose, do
not give a replacement dose.
I.V.
● Protect unopened vials from light.
● Reconstitute each 4-mg vial with 4 ml
sterile water for injection. Dilute appropriate volume of reconstituted solution in
either normal saline solution or D₅W
before giving.
● Lyophilized form contains no antibacterial preservative; use reconstituted
product immediately.
● Monitor insertion site during infusion.
Extravasation has been linked to mild
local reactions, such as erythema and
bruising.
● If stored at 68° to 77° F (20° to 25° C)
and exposed to normal lighting, reconstituted drug is stable for 24 hours.
● **Incompatibilities:** Dexamethasone,
fluorouracil, mitomycin, ticarcillin
disodium, and clavulanate potassium.

ACTION
Interacts with topoisomerase I, inducing
reversible single-strand DNA breaks.
Drug binds to the topoisomerase I–DNA
complex and prevents relegation of these
single-strand breaks.

Route	Onset	Peak	Duration
I.V.	Unknown	Unknown	Unknown

Half-life: 2 to 3 hours.

ADVERSE REACTIONS
CNS: *asthenia, fatigue, fever, headache.*
GI: *abdominal pain, anorexia, constipation, diarrhea, nausea, stomatitis, vomiting.*
Hematologic: *anemia,* LEUKOPENIA, NEUTROPENIA, THROMBOCYTOPENIA.
Hepatic: *hepatotoxicity.*
Musculoskeletal: *back and skeletal pain.*
Respiratory: *coughing, dyspnea.*
Skin: *alopecia,* rash.
Other: *sepsis.*

INTERACTIONS
Drug-drug. *Cisplatin:* May increase severity of myelosuppression. Use together with extreme caution.
Granulocyte colony-stimulating factor: May prolong duration of neutropenia. If granulocyte colony-stimulating factor is to be used, don't start it until day 6 of the course, 24 hours after completion of topotecan treatment.

EFFECTS ON LAB TEST RESULTS
● May increase ALT, AST, and bilirubin levels. May decrease hemoglobin level.
● May decrease WBC, platelet, and neutrophil counts.

CONTRAINDICATIONS & CAUTIONS
● Contraindicated in patients hypersensitive to drug or its components and in those with severe bone marrow depression.
● Contraindicated in pregnant or breast-feeding women.
● Safety and effectiveness of drug in children haven't been established.

NURSING CONSIDERATIONS
■ **Black Box Warning** Give drug only under the supervision of a physician experienced with cancer chemotherapeutic agents. ■
■ **Black Box Warning** Before first course of therapy is started, patient must have baseline neutrophil count more than 1,500/mm³ and platelet count more than 100,000/mm³. ■

● Monitor peripheral blood counts frequently. Don't give subsequent courses until neutrophil count recovers to more than 1,000 cells/mm³, platelet count recovers to more than 100,000/mm³, and hemoglobin level recovers to more than 9 mg/dl (with transfusion, if needed).
● Prepare drug under vertical laminar flow hood; wear gloves and protective clothing. If drug solution contacts skin, wash immediately and thoroughly with soap and water. If mucous membranes are affected, flush areas thoroughly with water.
● Bone marrow suppression indicates toxic levels of topotecan. The nadir occurs at about 11 days. Neutropenia isn't cumulative over time.
● Duration of thrombocytopenia is about 5 days, with nadir at 15 days. The nadir for anemia is 15 days. Blood or platelet transfusions may be needed.
● WBC colony-stimulating factors may promote cell growth and decrease risk for infection.

PATIENT TEACHING
● Urge patient to report promptly sore throat, fever, chills, or unusual bleeding or bruising.
● Caution women to avoid pregnancy or breast-feeding during therapy.
● Teach patient and family about drug's adverse reactions and need for frequent monitoring of blood counts.
● Advise patient that capsules can be taken without regard to food.
● Tell patient not to chew, crush, or divide capsules; they should be swallowed whole.

SAFETY ALERT!

trastuzumab
trass-too-ZOO-mab

Herceptin

Pharmacologic class: monoclonal antibody
Pregnancy risk category B

AVAILABLE FORMS
Lyophilized powder for injection:
440 mg/vial

Reactions may be *common*, uncommon, *life-threatening*, or COMMON AND LIFE-THREATENING.
Interaction may have a *rapid onset* or ***delayed onset.***

INDICATIONS & DOSAGES
➤ **Metastatic breast cancer in patients whose tumors overexpress the human epidermal growth factor receptor 2 (HER2) protein**

Adults: Loading dose of 4 mg/kg I.V. over 90 minutes. If tolerated, continue with 2 mg/kg I.V. weekly as 30-minute infusion. If patient hasn't previously received one or more chemotherapy regimens for their metastatic disease, drug is given with paclitaxel.

ADMINISTRATION
I.V.
● Reconstitute drug in each vial with 20 ml of bacteriostatic water for injection, 1.1% benzyl alcohol preserved, as supplied, to yield a multidose solution containing 21 mg/ml. Don't shake vial during reconstitution. Make sure reconstituted preparation is colorless to pale yellow and free of particulates. Immediately after reconstitution, label vial with expiration 28 days from date of reconstitution.
● If patient is hypersensitive to benzyl alcohol, reconstitute drug with sterile water for injection, use immediately, and discard unused portion. Avoid use of other reconstitution diluents.
● Determine dose based on loading dose of 4 mg/kg or maintenance dose of 2 mg/kg. Calculate volume of 21-mg/ml solution and withdraw this amount from vial and add it to an infusion bag containing 250 ml of normal saline solution. Don't use D$_5$W or dextrose-containing solutions. Gently invert bag to mix solution.
● Don't give as I.V. push or bolus.
● Infuse loading dose over 90 minutes. If well tolerated, infuse maintenance doses over 30 minutes.
● Vials are stable at 36° to 46° F (2° to 8° C). Discard reconstituted solution after 28 days. Don't freeze drug that has been reconstituted. Store solution of drug diluted in normal saline solution for injection at 36° to 46° F (2° to 8° C) before use; it's stable for up to 24 hours.
● **Incompatibilities:** Other I.V. drugs or dextrose solutions.

ACTION
A recombinant DNA-derived monoclonal antibody that selectively binds to HER2, inhibiting proliferation of tumor cells that overexpress HER2.

Route	Onset	Peak	Duration
I.V.	Unknown	Unknown	Unknown

Half-life: Range, 1 to 32 days; mean, 5¾ days.

ADVERSE REACTIONS
CNS: *asthenia, dizziness, fever, headache, insomnia, pain,* depression, neuropathy, paresthesia, peripheral neuritis.
CV: *peripheral edema,* **heart failure,** hypotension, tachycardia.
EENT: *pharyngitis, rhinitis,* sinusitis.
GI: *abdominal pain, anorexia, diarrhea, nausea, vomiting.*
GU: UTI.
Hematologic: *leukopenia,* anemia.
Musculoskeletal: *back pain,* arthralgia, bone pain.
Respiratory: *dyspnea, increased cough.*
Skin: *rash,* acne.
Other: ANAPHYLAXIS, *chills, flulike syndrome, infection,* allergic reaction, herpes simplex.

INTERACTIONS
Drug-drug. *Anthracyclines, cyclophosphamide:* May increase cardiotoxicity. Use together very cautiously.

EFFECTS ON LAB TEST RESULTS
● May decrease hemoglobin level.
● May decrease WBC count.

CONTRAINDICATIONS & CAUTIONS
● Contraindicated in patients hypersensitive to the drug.
● Use cautiously in elderly patients, in patients hypersensitive to drug or its components, and in those with cardiac dysfunction.
● Use with extreme caution in patients with pulmonary compromise, symptomatic intrinsic pulmonary disease (such as asthma, COPD), or extensive tumor involvement of the lungs.
● Safety and effectiveness of drug in children haven't been established.

NURSING CONSIDERATIONS
■ **Black Box Warning** Before beginning therapy, patient should undergo thorough

baseline cardiac assessment, including history and physical examination and methods to identify risk of cardiotoxicity. ■
■ **Black Box Warning** Assess patient for signs and symptoms of cardiac dysfunction, especially if he is receiving drug with anthracyclines and cyclophosphamide. ■
• Check for dyspnea, increased cough, paroxysmal nocturnal dyspnea, peripheral edema, or S_3 gallop. Treatment may be stopped in patients who develop a significant decrease in left ventricular function.
• Monitor patient receiving both drug and chemotherapy closely for cardiac dysfunction or failure, anemia, leukopenia, diarrhea, and infection.
• Drug is only for patients with metastatic breast cancer whose tumors have HER2 protein overexpression.
■ **Black Box Warning** Drug can cause serious infusion reactions and pulmonary toxicity. Interrupt infusion if patient experiences dyspnea or clinically significant hypotension. Strongly consider discontinuation for patients who develop anaphylaxis, angioedema, pneumonitis, or acute respiratory distress syndrome. ■
• Check for first-infusion symptom complex, commonly consisting of chills or fever. Give acetaminophen, diphenhydramine, and meperidine (with or without reducing rate of infusion). Other signs or symptoms include nausea, vomiting, pain, rigors, headache, dizziness, dyspnea, hypotension, rash, and asthenia and occur infrequently with subsequent infusions.

PATIENT TEACHING
• Tell patient about risk of first-dose infusion-related adverse reactions.
• Urge patient to notify prescriber immediately if signs or symptoms of heart problems occur, such as shortness of breath, increased cough, or swelling in arms or legs. Tell patient that these effects can occur after infusion is complete.
• Instruct patient to report adverse effects to prescriber.
• Advise woman to stop breast-feeding during drug therapy and for 6 months after last dose of drug.

hepatitis B immune globulin,
   human
immune globulin intramuscular
immune globulin intravenous
rabies immune globulin, human
respiratory syncytial virus
   immune globulin intravenous,
   human
Rh$_O$(D) immune globulin, human
Rh$_O$(D) immune globulin
   intravenous, human
tetanus immune globulin, human
varicella zoster immune globulin

---

hepatitis B immune globulin, human (HBIG)
hep-ah-TYE-tis

HepaGam B, HyperHEP B S/D,
Nabi-HB

Pharmacologic class: immune
serum
Pregnancy risk category C

AVAILABLE FORMS
Injection: 1-ml, 5-ml vials; 0.5-ml neonatal
single-dose syringe; 1-ml single-dose
syringe

INDICATIONS & DOSAGES
➤ **Hepatitis B exposure in high-risk
patients**
Adults and children: 0.06 ml/kg (usual
dose is 3 ml to 5 ml) I.M. as soon as
possible, but within 7 days after exposure
(within 14 days if sexual exposure). Repeat
dose 28 days after exposure if patient
doesn't elect to receive the hepatitis B
vaccine.
*Neonates born to hepatitis B surface
antigen (HBsAg)-positive patients:* 0.5 ml
I.M. within 12 hours of birth.
➤ **To prevent hepatitis B recurrence
following liver transplantation in
HBsAg-positive liver transplant
patients (HepaGam B only)**
Adults: 20,000 international units I.V. at
rate of 2 ml/minute. Give first dose given
simultaneously with the grafting of the
transplanted liver (anhepatic phase); then
daily on days 1 through 7, every 2 weeks
from day 14 through 12 weeks, monthly
from month 4 onward.
Adjust-a-dose: Adjust dosage in patients
who don't reach anti-HBs levels of
500 international units/L within the first
week after transplantation.

ADMINISTRATION
I.M.
• Inspect for discoloration or particulates.
Make sure drug is clear, slightly amber,
and moderately viscous.
• Inject into anterolateral thigh or deltoid
muscle in older children and adults; inject
into anterolateral thigh in neonates and
children younger than age 3.
I.V.
• Give HepaGam B through a separate I.V.
line using an I.V. administration set via
infusion pump.
• During preparation, don't shake vials;
avoid foaming.
• Set administration rate at 2 ml/minute.
Decrease rate of infusion to 1 ml/minute
or slower if the patient develops discomfort
or infusion-related adverse events, or
if there is concern about the speed of
infusion.

ACTION
Provides passive immunity to hepatitis B.

Route	Onset	Peak	Duration
I.M.	1–6 days	3–11 days	2 mo
I.V.	Unknown	Unknown	Unknown

Half-life: Antibodies to HBsAG, 21 days.

ADVERSE REACTIONS
CNS (I.V.): chills, fever, *headache.*
GI (I.V.): nausea, vomiting.
Musculoskeletal (I.V.): arthralgia, low
back pain, *myalgia.*
Skin: *pain and tenderness at injection
site,* urticaria.
Other: *anaphylaxis, angioedema, cold
symptoms or flu,* malaise.

INTERACTIONS
Drug-drug. *Live-virus vaccines:* May interfere with response to live-virus vaccines. Postpone routine immunization for 3 months.

EFFECTS ON LAB TEST RESULTS
None reported.

CONTRAINDICATIONS & CAUTIONS
• Contraindicated in patients with history of anaphylactic reactions to immune serum.
• Give to patients with coagulation disorders or thrombocytopenia only if benefit outweighs risk.
• Use cautiously in patients with specific IgA deficiency.

NURSING CONSIDERATIONS
• Obtain history of allergies and reactions to immunizations. Keep epinephrine 1:1,000 available.
• For postexposure prophylaxis (such as after needlestick or direct contact), give drug with hepatitis B vaccine.
• A vial of HBIG (human) that has been entered should be used promptly. Don't reuse or save for future use.
• The maltose contained in HepaGam B can interfere with some blood glucose monitoring systems, causing falsely elevated readings.
• Antibodies present in HepaGam B may interfere with some serological tests.
• **Look alike–sound alike:** This immune globulin provides passive immunity; don't confuse with hepatitis B vaccine. Both drugs may be given at same time. Don't mix in the same syringe.

PATIENT TEACHING
• Inform patient that pain and tenderness may occur at injection site.
• Tell patient to report signs and symptoms of hypersensitivity immediately.

immune globulin intramuscular (gamma globulin, IG, IGIM)
GamaSTAN S/D

immune globulin intravenous (IGIV)
Carimune NF, Flebogamma, Gammagard Liquid, Gamunex, Iveegam EN, Octagam, Privigen

Pharmacologic class: immune serum
Pregnancy risk category C

AVAILABLE FORMS
immune globulin intramuscular
Injection: 15% to 18% in 2-ml, 10-ml vials
immune globulin intravenous
Injection: 5% in 10-ml, 50-ml, 100-ml, and 200-ml vials (Flebogamma); 5% in 1-g, 2.5-g, 5-g, 10-g single-use bottles (Octagam)
Powder for injection: 1-g, 3-g, 6-g, 12-g vials (Carimune NF)
Solution for injection: 1-g, 2.5-g, 5-g, 10-g, 20-g vials (Gamunex); 10% in 5 g, 10 g, 20 g vials (Privigen)

INDICATIONS & DOSAGES
➤ **Primary immunodeficiency (IGIV)**
Carimune NF
Adults and children: 200 mg/kg I.V. monthly. Start with 0.5 to 1 ml/minute of 3% solution; gradually increase to 2.5 ml/minute after 15 to 30 minutes.
Flebogamma
Adults: 300 to 600 mg/kg I.V. every 3 to 4 weeks. Infuse at 0.5 mg/kg/minute and increase after 30 minutes to 5 mg/kg/minute.
Gammagard Liquid
Adults: 300 to 600 mg/kg I.V. every 3 to 4 weeks. Infuse at 0.8 mg/kg/minute and increase every 30 minutes to 8.9 mg/kg/minute.
GammaSTAN S/D
Adults and children: Initially, 1.3 ml/kg I.M. Maintenance 0.66 ml/kg (at least 100 mg/kg) every 3 to 4 weeks. Maximum single dose of IGIM is 30 to 50 ml in

---

Reactions may be *common*, uncommon, *life-threatening*, or COMMON AND LIFE-THREATENING.
Interaction may have a *rapid onset* or **delayed onset**.

adults and 20 to 30 ml in infants and small children.

Gamunex
Adults: 300 to 600 mg/kg I.V. every 3 to 40 weeks.

Iveegam EN
Adults and children: 200 mg/kg I.V. monthly, infused at 1 to 2 ml/minute for 5% solution. May increase to maximum of 800 mg/kg or give more often to produce desired effect.

Octagam
Adults and children: 300 to 600 mg/kg I.V. every 3 to 4 weeks. Start infusion at 30 mg/kg/hour for 30 minutes. If no discomfort is experienced, increase rate to 60 mg/kg/hour for 30 minutes. Rate can then be increased to maximum of 120 mg/kg/hour.

Privigen
Adults: 200 to 800 mg/kg every 3 to 4 weeks. Start infusion at 0.5 mg/kg/minute and increase slowly to 8 mg/kg/minute.

➤ **Chronic inflammatory demy-elinating polyneuropathy**
Adults: 2,000 mg/kg I.V. Gamunex in divided doses over 2 to 4 days every 3 weeks. Or, 1,000 mg/kg I.V. over 1 day every 3 weeks or 500 mg/kg I.V. on 2 consecutive days every 3 weeks.

➤ **Idiopathic thrombocytopenic purpura**
Carimune
Adults and children: 400 mg/kg I.V. for 2 to 5 consecutive days, depending on platelet count and immune response.

Gamunex
Adults: 2,000 mg/kg I.V. in divided doses over 2 days or 400 mg/kg I.V. in 5 doses over 5 days.

Privigen
Adults: 1,000 mg/kg I.V. for 2 days.

➤ **Pediatric HIV infection (IGIV)**
Children: 400 mg/kg I.V. once every 2 to 4 weeks.

➤ **Kawasaki syndrome**
Iveegam EN
Adults: 400 mg/kg I.V. daily over 2 hours for 4 consecutive days, or a single dose of 2,000 mg/kg over 10 hours. Start within 10 days of disease onset. Give with aspirin (100 mg/kg P.O. daily through day 14; then 3 to 5 mg/kg P.O. daily for 5 weeks).

➤ **Hepatitis A exposure (IGIM)**
Adults and children: 0.02 ml/kg I.M. as soon as possible after exposure. Up to 0.06 ml/kg may be given for prolonged or intense exposure.

➤ **Measles exposure (IGIM)**
Adults and children: 0.25 ml/kg I.M. within 6 days after exposure.

➤ **Measles postexposure prophylaxis (IGIM)**
Immunocompromised children: 0.5 ml/kg I.M. (maximum 15 ml) immediately after exposure.

➤ **Chickenpox exposure (IGIM)**
Adults and children: 0.6 to 1.2 ml/kg I.M. as soon as possible after exposure.

➤ **Rubella exposure in first trimester of pregnancy (IGIM)**
Women: 0.55 ml/kg I.M. as soon as possible after exposure (within 72 hours).

➤ **Guillain-Barré syndrome (IGIV)** ◆
Adults: 2,000 mg/kg I.V. over 2 to 5 days within 2 to 4 weeks of onset.
Children: 2,000 mg/kg I.V. over 2 days within 2 to 4 weeks of onset.

➤ **Severe exacerbation of myasthenia gravis (IGIV)** ◆
Adults: 1,000 to 2,000 mg/kg I.V. over 2 to 5 days.

ADMINISTRATION
I.M.
● Give in the anterolateral aspects of the upper thigh and the deltoid muscle of the upper arm. Divide doses larger than 10 ml and inject into several muscle sites to reduce pain and discomfort.
● Give drug soon after reconstitution.
● The gluteal region should not routinely be used. If necessary, only the upper outer quadrant should be used.
I.V.
● Before use, refrigerate Iveegam EN at 36° to 46°F (2° to 8°C).
● After reconstitution, Iveegam EN contains 50 mg of IgG/ml; Carimune NF contains at least 96% IgG; Octagam contains about 50 mg of protein/ml and at least 96% IgG.
● Most adverse reactions are related to a rapid infusion rate. If they occur, decrease infusion rate or stop infusion until reaction subsides. Resume infusion at a rate the patient can tolerate.

• Store Octagam at 36° to 46° F (2° to 8° C) for 24 months or at no higher than 77° F (25° C) for up to 18 months from the date of manufacture.

Carimune NF
• Use 15-micron in-line filter when giving. Reconstitute with normal saline solution, D_5W, or sterile water. Infusion rate is 0.5 to 1 ml/minute for 3% solution. After 15 to 30 minutes, increase rate to 1.5 to 2.5 ml/minute.

Gammagard Liquid
• Drug should be at room temperature during administration.
• Normal saline solution should not be used as a diluent. If dilution is preferred, D_5W may be used.
• The use of an in-line filter is optional.
• Begin infusion at 0.5 ml/kg/hour. If tolerated, gradually increase every 30 minutes to 5 ml/kg/hour.

Gamunex
• Incompatible with saline solutions. Compatible with D_5W, if needed.
• Infuse I.V. at a rate of 0.01 ml/kg/minute for first 30 minutes. If no problems, rate can be slowly increased to maximum of 0.08 ml/kg/minute.
• Store vials at 36° to 46° F (2° to 8° C). During first 18 months from the date of manufacture, store vials for up to 5 months at room temperature not exceeding 77° F (25° C); then vials must be used immediately or discarded. Don't freeze vials.

Iveegam EN
• Reconstitute Iveegam with sterile water for injection diluent provided. Use 15-micron in-line filter when giving drug. Infusion rate is 1 to 2 ml/minute for 5% solution.

Privigen
• If necessary dilute with D_5W
• Begin infusion at 0.5 mg/kg/min. If well tolerated, may increase gradually to 8 mg/kg/min.
• For chronic ITP, maximum infusion rate is 4 mg/kg/min.
• Infusion line may be flushed with D_5W or normal saline solution.

Octagam
• Octagam should be at room temperature during infusion. If using an infusion set (not mandatory), the filter size must be 0.2 to 200 microns. Initially, infuse at 30 mg/kg/hour for the first 30 minutes;

if tolerated, infuse at 60 mg/kg/hour for the second 30 minutes; if further tolerated, infuse at 120 mg/kg/hour for the third 30 minutes. If tolerated, infusion can be maintained at less than 200 mg/kg/hour. Adverse reactions usually disappear with slowing or stopping the infusion. For patients at risk for renal dysfunction, reduce infusion time to less than 200 mg/kg/hour.
• **Incompatibilities:** Other I.V. drugs.

ACTION
Provides passive immunity by increasing antibody titer. The primary component is IgG. It's unknown how it works for idiopathic thrombocytopenic purpura.

Route	Onset	Peak	Duration
I.V.	Immediate	Immediate	Unknown
I.M.	Unknown	2–5 hr	Unknown

Half-life: 21 to 24 days in immunocompromised patients.

ADVERSE REACTIONS
CNS: severe headache requiring hospitalization, faintness, fever, headache, malaise.
CV: chest pain, chest tightness, *heart failure, MI.*
GI: nausea, vomiting.
Musculoskeletal: hip pain, muscle stiffness at injection site.
Respiratory: *pulmonary embolism, transfusion related acute lung injury,* dyspnea.
Skin: erythema, urticaria, pain.
Other: *anaphylaxis, angioedema,* chills.

INTERACTIONS
Drug-drug. *Live-virus vaccines:* Length of time to wait before giving live-virus vaccinations varies with dose of immune globulin given. Check the recommendations of the American Academy of Pediatrics.

EFFECTS ON LAB TEST RESULTS
• May falsely elevate serum glucose level (for IGIV preparations containing maltose, such as Octagam).
• May cause positive Coombs test.

CONTRAINDICATIONS & CAUTIONS
• Contraindicated in patients hypersensitive to drug or its components.

Reactions may be *common*, uncommon, *life-threatening*, or COMMON AND LIFE-THREATENING.
Interaction may have a *rapid onset* or *delayed onset.*

• Use IGIV cautiously in patients with a history of CV disease or thrombotic episodes.
■ **Black Box Warning** Use IGIV cautiously in patients with renal dysfunction or a predisposition to renal failure, including patients with preexisting renal insufficiency, diabetes mellitus, volume depletion, sepsis, paraproteinemia, those older than age 65, and those receiving nephrotoxic drugs. ■

NURSING CONSIDERATIONS
• Obtain history of allergies and reactions to immunizations. Keep epinephrine 1:1,000 available to treat anaphylaxis.
• IGIV administration may be linked to thrombotic events.
• If patient is at risk for a thrombotic event, make sure infusion concentration is no more than 5% and start infusion rate no faster than 0.5 ml/kg/hour. Advance rate slowly only if well tolerated, to a maximum rate of 4 ml/kg/hour.
• Don't give as prophylaxis against hepatitis A if 6 weeks or more since exposure or onset of symptoms.

PATIENT TEACHING
• Explain to patient and family how drug will be given.
• Tell patient that local reactions may occur at injection site. Instruct him to notify prescriber promptly if adverse reactions persist or become severe.
• Inform patient of possible need for therapy more than once monthly to maintain adequate immunoglobulin G levels.

---

rabies immune globulin, human
RAY-beez

HyperRab S/D, Imogam Rabies-HT

Pharmacologic class: immune serum
Pregnancy risk category C

AVAILABLE FORMS
Injection: 150 international units/ml in 2-ml, 10-ml vials

INDICATIONS & DOSAGES
➤ **Rabies exposure**
Adults and children: 20 international units/kg I.M. at time of first dose of rabies vaccine. If anatomically feasible, up to the full dose is used to infiltrate wound area; remainder is given I.M. in a different site.

ADMINISTRATION
I.M.
• Give large volumes (5 ml) in adults only. The deltoid is the preferred area of injection.
• Don't give more than 5 ml I.M. at one injection site; divide doses over 5 ml and give at different sites.

ACTION
Provides passive immunity to rabies.

Route	Onset	Peak	Duration
I.M.	24 hr	Unknown	Unknown

Half-life: About 24 days.

ADVERSE REACTIONS
CNS: slight fever, headache, malaise.
Skin: pain, redness, and induration at injection site.

INTERACTIONS
Drug-drug. *Immunosuppressive agents (corticosteroids, chloroquine):* May interfere with the active antibody response to rabies vaccine. Avoid using together. If used together, do serologic testing for rabies antibody.
Live-virus vaccines (measles, mumps, or rubella): May interfere with response to vaccine. Postpone immunization, if possible.

EFFECTS ON LAB TEST RESULTS
None reported.

CONTRAINDICATIONS & CAUTIONS
• Repeated doses of rabies immune globulin are contraindicated in patients who have started to receive rabies vaccine immunization.
• Use with caution in patients hypersensitive to thimerosal or history of systemic allergic reactions to human immunoglobulin preparations; also use cautiously in those with immunoglobulin A deficiency.

NURSING CONSIDERATIONS
- Obtain history of animal bites, allergies, and reactions to immunizations. Have epinephrine 1:1,000 ready to treat anaphylaxis.
- Clean wound thoroughly with soap and water; this is best prophylaxis against rabies.
- Ask patient when last tetanus immunization was received; many prescribers order a booster at this time.
- Use only with rabies vaccine and immediate local treatment of wound. Don't give rabies vaccine and rabies immune globulin in same syringe or at same site. Give as soon as possible after exposure or through day 7. After day 8, antibody response to culture vaccine has occurred.
- Don't give live-virus vaccines within 3 months of rabies immune globulin.
- *Look alike–sound alike:* This immune serum provides passive immunity. Don't confuse with rabies vaccine, a suspension of killed microorganisms that confers active immunity. The two drugs are often used together prophylactically after exposure to rabid animals.

PATIENT TEACHING
- Inform patient that local reactions may occur at injection site. Instruct him to notify prescriber promptly if reactions persist or become severe.
- Tell patient that a tetanus shot also may be needed.
- Instruct patient in wound care.

---

respiratory syncytial virus (RSV) immune globulin intravenous, human (RSV-IGIV)
RespiGam

Pharmacologic class: immune globulin
Pregnancy risk category C

AVAILABLE FORMS
Injection: 50 mg ± 10 mg/ml in 20-ml, 50-ml single-use vial

INDICATIONS & DOSAGES
➤ **To prevent serious lower respiratory tract infections from RSV in children with broncho-pulmonary dysplasia (BPD) or who were born prematurely (35 weeks gestation or less)**
Premature infants and children younger than age 2: Single infusion monthly. Give 1.5 ml/kg/hour I.V. for 15 minutes; then, if condition allows higher rate, increase to 3.6 ml/kg/hour until infusion ends. Maximum recommended total dose per monthly infusion is 750 mg/kg.

ADMINISTRATION
I.V.
- Don't use turbid solution. Enter single-use vial only once. Don't shake; avoid foaming.
- Drug doesn't contain a preservative. Don't dilute before infusion.
- Use a constant infusion pump and an in-line filter with pore size larger than 15 microns.
- Give separately from other drugs.
- Begin infusion within 6 hours and end within 12 hours after vial is entered.
- **Incompatibilities:** Other I.V. drugs.

ACTION
Provides passive immunity to RSV.

Route	Onset	Peak	Duration
I.V.	Unknown	Unknown	> 1 mo

Half-life: 22 to 28 days.

ADVERSE REACTIONS
CNS: anxiety, dizziness, fever.
CV: chest tightness, flushing, hypertension, palpitations, tachycardia.
GI: abdominal cramps, diarrhea, gastroenteritis, vomiting.
Metabolic: fluid overload.
Musculoskeletal: arthralgia, myalgia.
Respiratory: crackles, dyspnea, *hypoxia, respiratory distress,* tachypnea, wheezing.
Skin: inflammation at injection site, rash, pruritus.
Other: *angioneurotic edema;* hypersensitivity reactions, including *anaphylaxis.*

INTERACTIONS
Drug-drug. *Live-virus vaccines (such as mumps, rubella, and especially measles):*

Reactions may be *common,* uncommon, *life-threatening,* or COMMON AND LIFE-THREATENING.
Interaction may have a *rapid onset* or *delayed onset.*

May interfere with response. If such vaccines are given during or within 10 months after RSV-IGIV, reimmunization is recommended, if appropriate.

EFFECTS ON LAB TEST RESULTS
None reported.

CONTRAINDICATIONS & CAUTIONS
• Contraindicated in patients severely hypersensitive to drug or other human immunoglobulin and selective immunoglobulin A deficiency.
• Children with fluid overload shouldn't receive drug.

NURSING CONSIDERATIONS
• Give first dose before RSV season (November to April) begins; give subsequent doses monthly throughout RSV season to maintain protection. Children with RSV should continue to receive monthly doses for duration of RSV season.
• Follow infusion rate guidelines; adverse reactions may be related to rate. Slower rates may be indicated especially in ill children with BPD.
• Assess cardiopulmonary status and vital signs before infusion, before each rate increase, and every 30 minutes thereafter until 30 minutes after infusion ends.
• Watch patient closely for signs and symptoms of fluid overload. Children with BPD may be more prone to this condition.
• *Alert:* If patient develops hypotension, anaphylaxis, or severe allergic reaction, stop infusion and give epinephrine 1:1,000. Patients with selective immunoglobulin A deficiency can develop antibodies to immunoglobulin A and have anaphylactic or allergic reactions to subsequent administration of blood products containing immunoglobulin A, including RSV-IGIV.

PATIENT TEACHING
• Explain to parents the importance of child receiving drug monthly throughout RSV season, even if he is already infected.
• Teach parents how drug is given and which adverse reactions are related to administration. Tell parents to report all adverse reactions promptly.

Rh$_o$(D) immune globulin, human (IGIM)
HyperRHO S/D Full Dose,
HyperRHO S/D Mini-Dose,
MICRhoGAM, RhoGAM

Rh$_o$(D) immune globulin intravenous, human (IGIV)
Rhophylac, WinRho SDF

Pharmacologic class: immune globulin
Pregnancy risk category C

AVAILABLE FORMS
IGIM
Injection: 300 mcg of Rh$_o$(D) immune globulin/vial (standard dose); 50 mcg of Rh$_o$(D) immune globulin/vial (microdose)
IGIV
Injection: 120 mcg, 300 mcg, 500 mcg, 1,000 mcg, 3,000 mcg

INDICATIONS & DOSAGES
➤ **Rh exposure after abortion, miscarriage, ectopic pregnancy, or childbirth**
Adults: Transfusion unit or blood bank determines fetal packed RBC volume entering patient's blood; one vial IGIM is given I.M. if fetal packed RBC volume is less than 15 ml. More than one vial I.M. may be needed if severe fetomaternal hemorrhage occurs; must be given within 72 hours after delivery or miscarriage.
➤ **To prevent Rh antibody formation after abortion or miscarriage**
Adults: Consult transfusion unit or blood bank. One IGIM microdose vial I.M. will suppress immune reaction to 2.5 ml Rh$_o$(D)-positive RBCs. Ideally, give within 3 hours, but may be given up to 72 hours after abortion or miscarriage.
➤ **Rh exposure after abortion, amniocentesis after 34 weeks' gestation, or other manipulations past 34 weeks' gestation with increased risk of Rh isoimmunization**
Adults: 120 mcg IGIV, given I.V. or I.M. within 72 hours of delivery, miscarriage, or manipulation.

➤ **To suppress Rh isoimmunization during pregnancy**
Adults: 300 mcg I.V. or I.M. at 28 weeks' gestation. If given early in pregnancy, give additional doses at 12-week intervals to maintain adequate levels of passively acquired anti-Rh antibodies. Then, within 72 hours of delivery, give 120 mcg I.M. or I.V. If 72 hours have elapsed, give drug as soon as possible, up to 28 days.

➤ **Incompatible blood transfusion**
Adults: 600 mcg I.V. every 8 hours or 1,200 mcg I.M. every 12 hours until total dose given. Total dose depends on volume of packed RBCs or whole blood infused. Consult blood bank or transfusion unit at once; must be given within 72 hours.

➤ **Idiopathic thrombocytopenic purpura in Rh$_o$(D) antigen-positive adults**
Adults: Initially, 50 mcg/kg I.V. as single dose or divided into two doses on separate days. If hemoglobin level is less than 10 g/dl, reduce first dose to 25 to 40 mcg/kg. Then, give 25 to 60 mcg/kg I.V. as needed to elevate platelet counts with specific individually determined dosage.

ADMINISTRATION

I.V.
• Reconstitute vials containing 600 or 1,500 units with 2.5 ml of 0.8% sodium chloride diluent provided by the manufacturer and vials containing 5,000 units with 8.5 ml of 0.8% sodium chloride diluent provided by the manufacturer. Slowly inject normal saline solution onto wall of vial and gently swirl until lyophilized pellet is dissolved. Don't shake.
• Give injection over 3 to 5 minutes.
• **Incompatibilities:** Other I.V. drugs.

I.M.
• IGIM preparations aren't for I.V. use.
• Give preferably in the anterolateral aspect of the upper thigh and the deltoid muscle of the upper arm.

ACTION
Mechanism of action not completely known. Suppresses active antibody response and formation of anti-Rh$_o$(D)

antibodies in Rh$_o$(D)-negative, D^u-negative persons exposed to Rh-positive blood. Rh$_o$(D) immune globulin I.V. may block platelet destruction in Rh$_o$(D) antigen–positive adults.

Route	Onset	Peak	Duration
I.V., I.M.	Unknown	Unknown	Unknown

Half-life: 24 to 30 days.

ADVERSE REACTIONS
CNS: *fever, headache, chills,* dizziness, weakness.
Skin: discomfort at injection site.
Other: *anaphylaxis.*

INTERACTIONS
Drug-drug. *Live-virus vaccines:* May interfere with response. Postpone immunization for 3 months, if possible.

EFFECTS ON LAB TEST RESULTS
• May affect the results of blood typing, the antibody screening test, and Coombs test.

CONTRAINDICATIONS & CAUTIONS
• Contraindicated in Rh$_o$(D)-positive or D^u-positive patients and in those previously immunized to Rh$_o$(D) blood factor. Contraindicated in patients with anaphylactic or severe systemic reaction to human globulin.
• Use extreme caution when giving drug to patients with immunoglobulin A deficiency.

NURSING CONSIDERATIONS
• Patients with immunoglobulin A deficiency may develop immunoglobulin A antibodies and have anaphylactic reaction; prescriber must weigh benefits of treatment against risk of hypersensitivity reactions before giving.
• Obtain history of allergies and reactions to immunizations. Keep epinephrine 1:1,000 ready to treat anaphylaxis.
• *Alert:* Immediately after delivery, send a sample of neonate's cord blood to laboratory for typing and cross-matching. Confirm if mother is Rh$_o$(D)-negative and D^u-negative. Give drug to mother only if infant is

$Rh_0(D)$- or D^u-positive. Administration must occur within 72 hours of delivery.
- This immune serum provides passive immunity to patient exposed to $Rh_0(D)$-positive fetal blood during pregnancy and prevents formation of maternal antibodies (active immunity), which would endanger future $Rh_0(D)$-positive pregnancies.
- Postpone vaccination with live virus vaccines for 3 months after administration of $Rh_0(D)$ immune globulin.
- Minidose preparations are recommended for patient undergoing abortion or miscarriage up to 12 weeks' gestation unless she is $Rh_0(D)$-positive or D^u-positive or has Rh antibodies, or unless the father or fetus is Rh-negative.

PATIENT TEACHING
- Explain how drug protects future $Rh_0(D)$-positive fetuses if used because of pregnancy, or explain other use, if indicated.
- Warn patient about adverse reactions related to drug.
- Reassure patient receiving this drug that there's no risk of HIV transmission.

tetanus immune globulin, human
BayTet

Pharmacologic class: immune globulin
Pregnancy risk category C

AVAILABLE FORMS
Injection: 250-unit vial or syringe

INDICATIONS & DOSAGES
➤ **Postexposure prevention of tetanus after injury, in patients whose immunization is incomplete or unknown**
Adults and children: 250 units deep I.M. injection.
➤ **Tetanus**
Adults and children: Single doses of 3,000 to 6,000 units I.M. have been used. Optimal dosage schedules haven't been established.

ADMINISTRATION
I.M.
- Don't give I.V. or I.D.
- Don't give in gluteal area.

ACTION
Provides passive immunity to tetanus.

Route	Onset	Peak	Duration
I.M.	Unknown	2–3 days	4 wk

Half-life: About 28 days.

ADVERSE REACTIONS
CNS: slight fever, pain.
GU: *nephrotic syndrome.*
Musculoskeletal: stiffness.
Skin: erythema at injection site.
Other: *anaphylaxis, angioedema,* hypersensitivity reactions.

INTERACTIONS
Drug-drug. *Live-virus vaccines:* May interfere with response. Postpone administration of live-virus vaccines for 3 months after giving tetanus immune globulin.

EFFECTS ON LAB TEST RESULTS
None reported.

CONTRAINDICATIONS & CAUTIONS
- Contraindicated in patients with thrombocytopenia or other coagulation disorders that would contraindicate I.M. injection unless benefits outweigh risks.
- Use cautiously in patients with history of previous systemic allergic reactions after giving human immunoglobulin preparations and in those allergic to thimerosal.

NURSING CONSIDERATIONS
- Obtain history of injury, tetanus immunizations, last tetanus toxoid injection, allergies, and reactions to immunizations. Keep epinephrine 1:1,000 available to treat hypersensitivity reaction.
- Tetanus immune globulin is used only if wound is more than 24 hours old or patient has had fewer than two tetanus toxoid injections.

- Thoroughly clean wound and remove all foreign matter.
- **Look alike–sound alike:** Don't confuse drug with tetanus toxoid. Tetanus immune globulin isn't a substitute for tetanus toxoid, which should be given at same time to produce active immunization. Don't give at same site as toxoid.
- Antibodies remain at effective levels for about 4 weeks, several times the duration of equine antitetanus antibodies, thereby protecting patients for incubation period of most tetanus cases.
- Don't give live-virus vaccines for 3 months after giving tetanus immune globulin.

PATIENT TEACHING
- Warn patient about local adverse reactions related to drug.
- Instruct patient to report serious adverse reactions promptly.
- Advise patient to complete full series of tetanus immunizations.
- Instruct patient to take acetaminophen to reduce fever and to apply cool compresses at injection site for comfort.

varicella zoster immune globulin (VZIG)

Pharmacologic class: immune serum
Pregnancy risk category C

AVAILABLE FORMS
Injection: 10% to 18% solution of the globulin fraction of human plasma containing 125 units of varicella zoster virus antibody (volume is about 2.5 ml or less)

INDICATIONS & DOSAGES
➤ **Passive immunization of susceptible immunodeficient patients after exposure to varicella (chickenpox or herpes zoster)**
Adults and children who weigh more than 40 kg (88 lb): 625 units I.M.
Children who weigh 30 to 40 kg (66 to 88 lb): 500 units I.M.
Children who weigh 20 to 30 kg (44 to 66 lb): 375 units I.M.

Children who weigh 10 to 20 kg (22 to 44 lb): 250 units I.M.
Children who weigh up to 10 kg (22 lb): 125 units I.M.

ADMINISTRATION
I.M.
- Give only by deep I.M. injection into a large muscle, such as gluteal muscle.
- Never give I.V.

ACTION
Provides passive immunity to varicella zoster virus in immunodeficient patients.

Route	Onset	Peak	Duration
I.M.	Unknown	Unknown	1 mo

Half-life: 21 days.

ADVERSE REACTIONS
CNS: headache, malaise.
GI: GI distress.
Respiratory: *respiratory distress.*
Skin: discomfort at injection site, rash.
Other: *anaphylaxis.*

INTERACTIONS
Drug-drug. *Live-virus vaccines:* May interfere with response. Postpone vaccination for 3 months after administration of VZIG.

EFFECTS ON LAB TEST RESULTS
None reported.

CONTRAINDICATIONS & CAUTIONS
- Contraindicated in patients with thrombocytopenia or history of severe reaction to human immune serum globulin or thimerosal; also contraindicated during pregnancy.

NURSING CONSIDERATIONS
- Obtain accurate patient history of allergies and reactions to immunizations. Keep epinephrine 1:1,000 ready to treat anaphylaxis.
- For maximum benefit, give as soon as possible after presumed exposure. Drug may be of benefit when given as late as 96 hours after exposure.
- Don't give in divided doses.

• Although usually restricted to children younger than age 15, VZIG may be given to adolescents and adults, if needed.

• VZIG isn't recommended for patients who are not immunosuppressed.

• *Look alike–sound alike:* VZIG provides passive immunity; don't confuse with varicella vaccine. Don't use these two drugs together.

PATIENT TEACHING

• Warn patient about local adverse reactions caused by the drug.

• Instruct patient to report serious adverse reactions to prescriber promptly.

• Suggest use of acetaminophen to reduce fever and cool compresses at injection site for comfort.

87

Immunomodulators

interferon alfa-2b, recombinant
interferon alfacon-1
interferon beta-1a
interferon beta-1b, recombinant
interferon gamma-1b
peginterferon alfa-2a
peginterferon alfa-2b

SAFETY ALERT!

interferon alfa-2b, recombinant (IFN-alpha 2)
in-ter-FEER-on

Intron A

Pharmacologic class: biologic
response modifier
Pregnancy risk category C

AVAILABLE FORMS
Solution for injection: 3, 5, 10 million
international units/dose in multidose
pens; 10 million international units/vial;
18 and 25 million international units
multidose vials
Powder for injection: 10, 18, 50 million
international units/vial with diluent

INDICATIONS & DOSAGES
➤ **Hairy cell leukemia**
Adults: 2 million international units/m^2
I.M. or subcutaneously, three times
weekly for 6 months or more.
➤ **Condylomata acuminata (genital
or venereal warts)**
Adults: 1 million international units for
each lesion intralesionally three times
weekly for 3 weeks.
➤ **AIDS-related Kaposi sarcoma**
Adults: 30 million international units/m^2
subcutaneously or I.M. three times weekly.
Maintain dose unless disease progresses
rapidly or intolerance occurs.
➤ **Chronic hepatitis B**
Adults: 30 to 35 million international units
weekly I.M. or subcutaneously, given as
5 million international units daily or
10 million international units three times
weekly for 16 weeks.

Children ages 1 to 17: 3 million international units/m^2 subcutaneously three
times weekly for first week; then increase
to 6 million international units/m^2 subcutaneously three times weekly (maximum is 10 million international units three
times weekly) for total of 16 to 24 weeks.
➤ **Chronic hepatitis C**
Adults: 3 million international units I.M.
or subcutaneously three times weekly. In
patients tolerating therapy with normaliza-
tion of ALT at 16 weeks of therapy, continue for 18 to 24 months. In patients who
haven't normalized the ALT, consider
stopping therapy.
➤ **Adjunct to surgical treatment in
patients with malignant melanoma
who are asymptomatic after surgery
but at high risk for systemic recurrence for up to 8 weeks after surgery**
Adults: Initially, 20 million international
units/m^2 by I.V. infusion 5 consecutive
days weekly for 4 weeks; then maintenance
dose of 10 million international units/m^2
subcutaneously three times weekly
for 48 weeks. If adverse effects
occur, stop therapy until they abate;
then resume therapy at 50% of the
previous dose. If intolerance persists,
stop therapy.
➤ **First treatment of clinically
aggressive follicular non-Hodgkin
lymphoma with chemotherapy
containing anthracycline**
Adults: 5 million international units
subcutaneously three times weekly for
up to 18 months.

ADMINISTRATION
I.V.
● Prepare infusion solution immediately
before use.
● Based on desired dose, reconstitute
appropriate vial strength of drug with
diluent provided. Withdraw dose and
inject into a 100-ml bag of normal saline
solution. Final yield of drug shouldn't
be less than 10 million international
units/100 ml.
● Infuse over 20 minutes.

Reactions may be *common,* uncommon, *life-threatening,* or COMMON AND LIFE-THREATENING.
Interaction may have a *rapid onset* or **delayed onset.**

• Store solution in refrigerator. Store powder before and after reconstitution in refrigerator. Use within 24 hours.
• **Incompatibilities:** Dextrose solutions.
I.M.
• Carefully monitor injection sites in patient with thrombocytopenia. Avoid I.M. injections if possible.
• In patients whose platelet count is below 50,000/mm³, give subcutaneously,
• Give drug at bedtime to minimize daytime drowsiness.
Subcutaneous
• For condylomata acuminata intralesional injection, use only 10 million-international unit vial because dilution of other strengths for intralesional use results in a hypertonic solution.
• Don't reconstitute drug in 10 million-international unit vial with more than 1 ml of diluent.
• Use tuberculin or similar syringe and 25G to 30G needle.
• Don't inject too deep beneath lesion or too superficially. As many as five lesions can be treated at one time.
• To ease discomfort, give in evening with acetaminophen.

ACTION
Unknown. May inhibit tumor or viral cell replication and modulate host immune response by enhancing macrophage activity and improving specific lymphocytes' cytotoxicity for target cells.

Route	Onset	Peak	Duration
I.V.	Unknown	15–60 min	4 hr
I.M., Subcut.	Unknown	3–12 hr	16 hr

Half-life: 3½ to 8½ hours.

ADVERSE REACTIONS
CNS: apathy, amnesia, *asthenia, depression,* difficulty in thinking or concentrating, *dizziness, fatigue, insomnia,* paresthesia, *somnolence,* anxiety, lethargy, nervousness, weakness, headache.
CV: *chest pain,* **cyanosis,** edema, hypotension.
EENT: conjunctivitis, earache, rhinorrhea, *sinusitis,* pharyngitis, rhinitis.
GI: *anorexia, diarrhea, dry mouth, dyspepsia, nausea, vomiting,* abdominal

pain, constipation, esophagitis, flatulence, stomatitis.
GU: decreased libido, impotence.
Hematologic: *leukopenia, thrombocytopenia,* anemia, *neutropenia.*
Hepatic: *hepatitis.*
Respiratory: *coughing, dyspnea.*
Skin: *alopecia, dryness, increased diaphoresis, pruritus, rash,* dermatitis.
Other: *flulike syndrome,* injection site reaction.

INTERACTIONS
Drug-drug. *Aminophylline, theophylline:* May reduce theophylline clearance. Monitor theophylline level.
CNS depressants: May increase CNS effects. Avoid using together.
Live-virus vaccines: May increase adverse reactions to vaccine or decrease antibody response. Postpone immunization.
Zidovudine: May cause synergistic adverse effects (higher risk of neutropenia). Carefully monitor WBC count.

EFFECTS ON LAB TEST RESULTS
• May increase calcium, phosphate, AST, ALT, LDH, alkaline phosphatase, and fasting glucose levels. May decrease hemoglobin level.
• May increase PT, INR, and PTT. May decrease WBC and platelet counts.

CONTRAINDICATIONS & CAUTIONS
• Contraindicated in patients hypersensitive to drug or its components.
• Use cautiously in patients with history of CV disease, pulmonary disease, diabetes mellitus, coagulation disorders, and severe myelosuppression.
• Depression and suicidal behavior have been linked to drug use; patients with psychotic disorders, especially depression, shouldn't continue drug treatment.
• *Alert:* Neurotoxicity and cardiotoxicity are more common in elderly patients, especially those with underlying CNS or cardiac impairment.

NURSING CONSIDERATIONS
■ **Black Box Warning** Alpha interferons cause or aggravate fatal or life-threatening neuropsychiatric, autoimmune, ischemic, and infectious disorders. Monitor patients closely with periodic clinical and labora-

tory evaluations. Withdraw patients with persistently severe or worsening signs or symptoms of these conditions from therapy. ■

• Ensure patient is well hydrated, especially at beginning of treatment.

• At start of treatment, monitor patient for flulike signs and symptoms, which tend to diminish with continued therapy. Premedicate patient with acetaminophen to minimize these symptoms.

• Periodically check for adverse CNS reactions, such as decreased mental status and dizziness, during therapy.

• Monitor CBC with differential, platelet count, blood chemistry and electrolyte studies, and liver function tests. Monitor ECG if patient has cardiac disorder or advanced stages of cancer.

• For patients who develop thrombocytopenia, exercise extreme care in performing invasive procedures; inspect injection site and skin frequently for signs and symptoms of bruising; limit frequency of I.M. injections; test urine, emesis fluid, stool, and secretions for occult blood.

• Severe adverse reactions may need dosage reduction to one-half or stoppage of drug until reactions subside.

• Use with blood dyscrasia–causing drugs, bone marrow suppressants, or radiation therapy may increase bone marrow suppression. Dosage reduction may be needed.

• For condylomata acuminata, maximum response usually occurs in 4 to 8 weeks. If results are not satisfactory after 12 to 16 weeks, a second course may be started. Patients with 6 to 10 condylomata may receive a second course of treatment; patients with more than 10 condylomata may receive additional courses.

PATIENT TEACHING

• Advise patient to avoid contact with persons with viral illness; patient is at increased risk for infection during therapy.

• Advise patient that laboratory tests will be performed before and periodically during therapy.

• Teach patient proper oral hygiene during treatment because bone marrow suppressant effects of interferon may lead to microbial infection, delayed healing, and bleeding gums. Drug also may decrease salivary flow.

• Advise patient to check with prescriber for instructions after missing a dose.

• Stress need to follow prescriber's instructions about taking and recording temperature and how and when to take acetaminophen.

• If patient will give drug to himself, teach him how to prepare injection and to use disposable syringe. Give him information on drug stability.

• Tell patient that drug may cause temporary partial hair loss; hair should return after drug is stopped.

• Advise patient to notify prescriber if signs or symptoms of depression occur.

SAFETY ALERT!

interferon alfacon-1
in-ter-FEER-on

Infergen

Pharmacologic class: biologic response modifier
Pregnancy risk category C

AVAILABLE FORMS
Injection: 9 mcg/0.3-ml, 15 mcg/0.5-ml vials

INDICATIONS & DOSAGES
➤ **Chronic hepatitis C viral infection in patients with compensated liver disease**
Adults: 9 mcg subcutaneously three times weekly for 24 weeks; for patients who don't respond or who relapse, 15 mcg subcutaneously three times weekly for up to 48 weeks.

Adjust-a-dose: For patients intolerant to higher doses, dose may be reduced to 7.5 mcg. Don't give doses below 7.5 mcg because decreased efficacy may result.

ADMINISTRATION
Subcutaneous
• Store drug in refrigerator at 36° to 46° F (2° to 8° C); don't freeze. Injection may be allowed to reach room temperature just before use.

• Avoid vigorous shaking.

• Discard unused portion.

Reactions may be *common*, uncommon, *life-threatening*, or COMMON AND LIFE-THREATENING.
Interaction may have a *rapid onset* or *delayed onset*.

ACTION
Induces gene-mediated biological responses that include antiviral, antiproliferative, and immunomodulatory effects and cytokine regulation.

Route	Onset	Peak	Duration
Subcut.	Unknown	24–36 hr	Unknown

Half-life. Unknown.

ADVERSE REACTIONS
CNS: *amnesia, anxiety, depression, dizziness, emotional lability, headache, insomnia, malaise, nervousness, paresthesia, suicidal ideation,* agitation, confusion.
CV: hypertension, palpitations, tachycardia, *chest pain.*
EENT: *pharyngitis, retinal hemorrhages, rhinitis, sinusitis,* conjunctivitis, ear pain, epistaxis, loss of visual acuity or visual field, tinnitus.
GI: *abdominal pain, anorexia, diarrhea, dyspepsia, nausea, vomiting,* constipation, decreased saliva, flatulence, hemorrhoids, taste perversion.
GU: dysmenorrhea, vaginitis.
Hematologic: *granulocytopenia, leukopenia, thrombocytopenia,* ecchymosis, lymphadenopathy, *lymphocytosis.*
Metabolic: hypothyroidism.
Respiratory: *congestion, cough, infection,* bronchitis, dyspnea.
Skin: *alopecia, erythema at injection site, pruritus, rash,* dry skin.
Other: *body pain, flulike symptoms,* hypersensitivity reactions, decreased libido, toothache.

INTERACTIONS
Drug-drug. *Drugs metabolized by cytochrome P-450:* May alter drug levels. Monitor changes in levels of these drugs.
Myelosuppressives: May cause added hematologic toxicities; use cautiously together. Monitor CBC and therapeutic or toxic level of myelosuppressive.

EFFECTS ON LAB TEST RESULTS
• May increase triglyceride and TSH levels. May decrease T_4 levels.
• May increase PT and INR. May decrease granulocyte, WBC, and platelet counts.

CONTRAINDICATIONS & CAUTIONS
• Contraindicated in patients hypersensitive to alpha interferons, to *Escherichia coli*–derived products, or to any component of product; and in patients with history of severe psychiatric disorders, autoimmune hepatitis, or decompensated hepatic disease.
• Use with caution in patients with history of cardiac disease and other autoimmune or endocrine disorders, in those with abnormally low peripheral blood cell counts, and in those receiving drugs that cause myelosuppression.

NURSING CONSIDERATIONS
■ **Black Box Warning** Alpha interferons may cause or aggravate fatal or lifethreatening neuropsychiatric, autoimmune, ischemic, and infectious disorders. Monitor patients closely with periodic clinical and laboratory evaluations. Withdraw patients with persistently severe or worsening signs or symptoms of these conditions from therapy. ■
• *Alert:* Depression and suicidal behavior have been linked to drug.
• Obtain the following laboratory tests before therapy, 2 weeks after it starts, and periodically during therapy: CBC with platelet count, and creatinine, albumin, bilirubin, TSH, and T_4 levels.
• *Alert:* If hypersensitivity reaction occurs, stop drug immediately and treat. Premedication with acetaminophen or ibuprofen may decrease adverse effects.
• Allow at least 48 hours to elapse between doses.
• Dosages and adverse reactions vary among different subtypes of drug. Don't use different subtypes in a single treatment regimen.

PATIENT TEACHING
• If drug is to be used at home, instruct patient on appropriate use, dosage, and administration. Give the patient information leaflet available from the manufacturer to the patient. Also teach patient proper disposal procedures for needles, syringes, drug containers, and unused drug.
• Instruct patient not to reuse needles or syringes or reenter vial.
• Urge patient not to use vial that's discolored or contains particulates.

• Tell patient that nonnarcotic analgesics and bedtime administration may be used to prevent or lessen flulike symptoms (headache, fever, malaise, muscle pain) related to therapy.
• Instruct patient to immediately report symptoms of depression.

SAFETY ALERT!

interferon beta-1a
in-ter-FEER-on

Avonex, Rebif

Pharmacologic class: biologic response modifier
Pregnancy risk category C

AVAILABLE FORMS
Avonex
Lyophilized powder for injection: 33 mcg (6.6 million international units)
Prefilled syringe: 30 mcg (6 million international units)/0.5 ml
Rebif
Parenteral: 22 mcg (6 million international units) and 44 mcg (12 million international units) per 0.5-ml prefilled syringe

INDICATIONS & DOSAGES
➤ **To slow accumulation of physical disability and decrease frequency of clinical worsening in patients with relapsing forms of multiple sclerosis (MS)**
Adults age 18 and older: 30 mcg Avonex I.M. once weekly. Or, initially, 8.8 mcg Rebif subcutaneously three times weekly for 2 weeks; then increase dose to 22 mcg three times weekly for another 2 weeks. Then increase to a maintenance dose of 44 mcg subcutaneously three times weekly.
Adjust-a-dose: For Rebif, in patients with leukopenia or elevated liver function test values (ALT greater than five times upper limit of normal), reduce dosage by 20% to 50% until toxicity is resolved. Stop treatment if jaundice or other signs of hepatic injury occur.
➤ **First MS attack if brain magnetic resonance imaging shows abnormalities consistent with MS**
Adults: 30 mcg Avonex I.M. once weekly.

ADMINISTRATION
Subcutaneous
• Visually inspect Rebif for particulate matter and discoloration before administration.
• Rotate sites of injection.
• Store Rebif in the refrigerator between 36° and 46° F (2° and 8° C). Don't freeze. Rebif may be stored at or below 77° F (25° C) for up to 30 days if away from heat and light.
I.M.
• To reconstitute lyophilized Avonex, inject 1.1 ml of supplied diluent (sterile water for injection) into vial and gently swirl to dissolve drug. Don't shake.
• Use drug as soon as possible; may be used up to 6 hours after being reconstituted if stored at 36° to 46° F (2° to 8° C).
• Rotate sites of injection.
• The Avonex and diluent vials are for single use only; discard unused portions.
• Store Avonex prefilled syringes in the refrigerator at 36° to 46° F (2° to 8° C). Once removed from refrigerator, warm to room temperature (about 30 minutes) and use within 12 hours. Don't use external heat sources, such as hot water, to warm syringe, or expose to high temperatures. Don't freeze. Protect from light.
• After giving each dose, discard any remaining product in the syringe.

ACTION
Unknown. Interacts with specific cell receptors found on the surface of cells. Binding of these receptors causes the expression of a number of interferon-induced gene products believed to mediate the biological actions of interferon beta-1a.

Route	Onset	Peak	Duration
Subcut.	Unknown	16 hr	Unknown
I.M.	Unknown	3–15 hr	Unknown

Half-life: I.M., 10 hours; subcutaneous, 69 hours.

ADVERSE REACTIONS
CNS: *asthenia, dizziness, fatigue, fever, headache, pain, sleep difficulty,* depression, **seizures, suicidal ideation or attempt, suicidal tendency,** abnormal coordination, ataxia, hypertonia, malaise, speech disorder, syncope.

Reactions may be *common,* uncommon, *life-threatening,* or COMMON AND LIFE-THREATENING.
Interaction may have a *rapid onset* or **delayed onset.**

CV: chest pain, vasodilation.
EENT: *abnormal vision, sinusitis,* decreased hearing, otitis media.
GI: *abdominal pain, diarrhea, dyspepsia, nausea,* anorexia, dry mouth.
GU: increased urinary frequency, ovarian cyst, urinary incontinence, vaginitis.
Hematologic: *lymphadenopathy, leukopenia, pancytopenia, thrombocytopenia,* anemia.
Hepatic: abnormal hepatic function, *autoimmune hepatitis,* bilirubinemia, hepatic injury, *hepatitis.*
Metabolic: hyperthyroidism, hypothyroidism.
Musculoskeletal: *back pain, muscle ache, skeletal pain,* arthralgia, muscle spasm.
Respiratory: *upper respiratory tract infection,* dyspnea.
Skin: *injection site reaction,* alopecia, ecchymosis at injection site, nevus, urticaria.
Other: *chills, flulike syndrome, infection,* hypersensitivity reactions, herpes simplex, herpes zoster, neutralizing antibodies.

INTERACTIONS
Drug-lifestyle. *Sun exposure:* May cause photosensitivity reactions. Advise patient to take precautions against sun exposure.

EFFECTS ON LAB TEST RESULTS
● May increase liver enzyme level. May decrease hemoglobin level and hematocrit. May increase or decrease thyroid function test levels.
● May increase eosinophil count. May decrease WBC and platelet counts.

CONTRAINDICATIONS & CAUTIONS
● Contraindicated in patients hypersensitive to natural or recombinant interferon beta, human albumin, or other components of drug.
● Use cautiously in patients with depression, seizure disorders, or severe cardiac conditions.
● It's unknown if drug appears in breast milk; a breast-feeding woman must either stop breast-feeding or stop drug.
● Safety and effectiveness of drug in chronic progressive MS or in children younger than age 18 haven't been established.

NURSING CONSIDERATIONS
● Monitor patient closely for depression and suicidal ideation. It isn't known if these symptoms are related to the underlying neurologic basis of MS or to the drug.
● Monitor WBC count, platelet count, and blood chemistries, including liver function tests. Rare but severe liver injury, including liver failure, may occur in patients taking Avonex.
● Give analgesics or antipyretics to decrease flulike symptoms.

PATIENT TEACHING
● Teach patient and family member how to reconstitute drug and give I.M.
● Caution patient not to change dosage or schedule of administration. If a dose is missed, tell him to take it as soon as he remembers. He may then resume his regular schedule. Tell patient not to take two injections within 2 days of each other.
● Show patient how to store drug.
● Inform patient that flulike signs and symptoms, such as fever, fatigue, muscle aches, headache, chills, and joint pain, are not uncommon at start of therapy. Acetaminophen 650 mg P.O. may be taken immediately before injection and for another 24 hours after each injection, to lessen severity of flulike signs and symptoms.
● Advise patient to report depression, suicidal thoughts, or other adverse reactions.
● Instruct patient to keep syringes and needles away from children. Also, instruct him not to reuse needles or syringes and to discard them in a syringe-disposal unit.
● Caution woman not to become pregnant during therapy because of the risk of spontaneous abortion. If pregnancy occurs, instruct patient to notify prescriber immediately and to stop drug.
● Advise patient to use sunscreen and avoid sun exposure while taking drug because photosensitivity may occur.
● Tell patient to store Rebif in the refrigerator between 36° to 46° F (2° to 8° C) and not to freeze. Rebif may also be stored at or below 77° F (25° C) for up to 30 days and away from heat and light.

SAFETY ALERT!

interferon beta-1b, recombinant
in-ter-FEER-on

Betaseron

Pharmacologic class: biologic response modifier
Pregnancy risk category C

AVAILABLE FORMS
Powder for injection: 9.6 million international units (0.3 mg)

INDICATIONS & DOSAGES
➤ **To reduce frequency of exacerbations in relapsing forms of multiple sclerosis**
Adults: 0.0625 mg subcutaneously every other day for weeks 1 and 2; then 0.125 mg subcutaneously every other day for weeks 3 and 4; then 0.1875 mg subcutaneously every other day for weeks 5 and 6; then 0.25 mg subcutaneously every other day thereafter.

ADMINISTRATION
Subcutaneous
• To reconstitute, inject 1.2 ml of supplied diluent (half-normal saline solution for injection) into vial and gently swirl to dissolve drug.
• Reconstituted solution contains 8 million international units (0.25 mg)/ml.
• Don't shake. Discard vial that contains particulates or discolored solution.
• Inject immediately after preparation.
• Rotate injection sites to minimize local reactions and observe site for necrosis.
• Store at room temperature. After reconstitution, if not used immediately, drug may be refrigerated for up to 3 hours.

ACTION
A naturally occurring antiviral and immunoregulatory drug derived from human fibroblasts. Drug attaches to membrane receptors and causes cellular changes, including increased protein synthesis.

Route	Onset	Peak	Duration
Subcut.	Unknown	1–8 hr	Unknown

Half-life: 8 minutes to 4¼ hours.

ADVERSE REACTIONS
CNS: depression, anxiety, emotional lability, depersonalization, *suicidal tendencies,* confusion, somnolence, *hypertonia, asthenia, migraine, seizures,* headache, pain, dizziness.
CV: palpitations, hypertension, tachycardia, peripheral vascular disorder.
EENT: laryngitis, *sinusitis, conjunctivitis,* abnormal vision.
GI: *diarrhea, constipation, abdominal pain, vomiting.*
GU: *menstrual bleeding or spotting, early or delayed menses, fewer days of menstrual flow, menorrhagia.*
Hematologic: LEUKOPENIA, *lymphadenopathy.*
Musculoskeletal: *myasthenia.*
Respiratory: dyspnea.
Skin: *inflammation, pain, necrosis at injection site, diaphoresis,* alopecia.
Other: breast pain, *flulike syndrome, pelvic pain,* generalized edema.

INTERACTIONS
None significant.

EFFECTS ON LAB TEST RESULTS
• May increase ALT and bilirubin levels.
• May decrease WBC and neutrophil counts.

CONTRAINDICATIONS & CAUTIONS
• Contraindicated in patients hypersensitive to interferon beta, human albumin, or components of drug.
• Use cautiously in women of childbearing age. Evidence is inconclusive about teratogenic effects, but drug may be an abortifacient.

NURSING CONSIDERATIONS
• *Alert:* Serious liver damage, including hepatic failure requiring transplant, can occur. Monitor liver function at 1, 3, and 6 months after therapy starts and periodically thereafter.
• Monitor patient for signs of depression.

Reactions may be *common,* uncommon, *life-threatening,* or COMMON AND LIFE-THREATENING.
Interaction may have a *rapid onset* or **delayed onset.**

PATIENT TEACHING
• Warn woman about dangers to fetus. If pregnancy occurs during therapy, tell her to notify prescriber and stop taking drug.
• Teach patient how to perform subcutaneous injections, including solution preparation, aseptic technique, injection site rotation, and equipment disposal. Periodically reevaluate patient's technique.
• Tell patient to take drug at bedtime to minimize mild flulike signs and symptoms that commonly occur.
• Advise patient to report suicidal thoughts or depression.
• Urge patient to immediately report signs or symptoms of tissue death at injection site.

interferon gamma-1b
in-ter-FEER-on

Actimmune

Pharmacologic class: biologic response modifier
Pregnancy risk category C

AVAILABLE FORMS
Injection: 100 mcg (2 million international units)/0.5-ml vial

INDICATIONS & DOSAGES
➤ **Chronic granulomatous disease, severe malignant osteopetrosis**
Adults with body surface area (BSA) greater than 0.5 m²: Give 50 mcg/m² (1 million international units/m²) subcutaneously three times weekly, preferably at bedtime.
Adults with a BSA 0.5 m² or less: 1.5 mcg/kg subcutaneously three times weekly.

ADMINISTRATION
Subcutaneous
• Discard unused drug. Each vial is for single use only and doesn't contain a preservative.
• Don't mix with other drugs in the same syringe.

ACTION
Interleukin-type lymphokine. Drug has potent phagocyte-activating properties and increases the oxidative metabolism of tissue macrophages.

Route	Onset	Peak	Duration
Subcut.	Unknown	7 hr	Unknown

Half-life: 6 hours.

ADVERSE REACTIONS
CNS: *fatigue,* chills, dizziness, *fever, headache.*
GI: *diarrhea, nausea, vomiting.*
Hematologic: *neutropenia, thrombocytopenia.*
Musculoskeletal: arthralgia, myalgia.
Skin: *erythema and tenderness at injection site,* rash.
Other: *flulike syndrome.*

INTERACTIONS
Drug-drug. *Myelosuppressives:* May increase myelosuppression. Monitor patient closely.
Zidovudine: May increase zidovudine level. Adjust dosage when used together.

EFFECTS ON LAB TEST RESULTS
• May increase liver enzyme levels.
• May decrease neutrophil and platelet counts.

CONTRAINDICATIONS & CAUTIONS
• Contraindicated in patients hypersensitive to drug or to genetically engineered products derived from *Escherichia coli.*
• Use cautiously in patients with cardiac disease, including arrhythmias, ischemia, or heart failure. The flulike syndrome commonly seen with high doses of drug can worsen these conditions.
• Use cautiously in patients with compromised CNS function or seizure disorders. CNS adverse reactions that may occur at high doses of drug can worsen these conditions.

NURSING CONSIDERATIONS
• Administer in the deltoid or anterior thigh muscle.

• *Alert:* The drug's activity is expressed in international units (1 million international units/50 mcg). This is equal to what was previously expressed as units (1.5 million units/50 mcg).

• Use myelosuppressives together with caution.

• Premedicate patient with acetaminophen to minimize signs and symptoms at start of therapy; these tend to diminish with continued therapy.

• Before beginning therapy and at 3-month intervals, monitor CBC, platelet count, renal and hepatic function tests, and urinalysis.

PATIENT TEACHING
• If patient will give drug to himself, teach him how to give it and how to dispose of used needles, syringes, containers, and unused drug.

• Instruct patient how to manage flulike signs and symptoms (fever, fatigue, muscle aches, headache, chills, joint pain) that commonly occur.

• Advise use of acetaminophen.

SAFETY ALERT!

peginterferon alfa-2a
peg-in-ter-FEER-on

Pegasys

Pharmacologic class: biologic response modifier
Pregnancy risk category C

AVAILABLE FORMS
Injection: 180 mcg/1 ml single-dose vials; 180 mcg/0.5 ml prefilled syringes

INDICATIONS & DOSAGES
➤ **Chronic hepatitis C with compensated hepatic disease in patients not previously treated with interferon alfa**
Adults: 180 mcg subcutaneously in abdomen or thigh, once weekly for 48 weeks. May be used with 800 to 1,200 mg ribavirin daily, divided b.i.d. depending on viral genotype.
➤ **Chronic hepatitis C (regardless of genotype) in HIV-infected patients**

who have not previously been treated with interferon
Adults: 180 mcg subcutaneously in abdomen or thigh, once weekly for 48 weeks. May be used with 800 mg ribavirin P.O. daily divided b.i.d.
➤ **Chronic hepatitis B who have compensated liver disease and evidence of viral replication and liver inflammation**
Adults: 180 mcg subcutaneously in abdomen or thigh, once weekly for 48 weeks.
Adjust-a-dose: For patients who experience moderate adverse reactions, decrease dose to 135 mcg subcutaneously once a week; for severe adverse reactions, decrease to 90 mcg subcutaneously once a week. For patients who experience hematologic reactions, if the absolute neutrophil count (ANC) is less than 750/mm^3, reduce dose to 135 mcg subcutaneously once a week; if the ANC is less than 500/mm^3, stop drug until ANC exceeds 1,000/mm^3 and restart at 90 mcg subcutaneously once a week. If platelet count is less than 50,000/mm^3, reduce dose to 90 mcg subcutaneously once a week; stop drug if platelet count drops below 25,000/mm^3. In patients with end-stage renal disease requiring hemodialysis, decrease dose to 135 mcg subcutaneously once a week. In chronic hepatitis C patients with ALT increases above baseline, decrease dose to 135 mcg subcutaneously once a week. For chronic hepatitis B patients with elevations in ALT more than five times the upper limit of normal (ULN), reduce dose to 135 mcg subcutaneously once a week or temporarily stop treatment; if less than 10 times the ULN, consider stopping treatment. For patients also taking ribavirin therapy, if hemoglobin level is less than 10 g/dl in patients with no cardiac disease, reduce ribavirin dose to 600 mg/day. If less than 8.5 g/dl in this population, stop ribavirin. If there is a greater than or equal to 2 g/dl decrease in hemoglobin level during any 4-week period in patients with history of stable cardiac disease, reduce ribavirin dose to 600 mg daily. If less than 12 g/dl despite 4 weeks at reduced dose, stop ribavirin. Don't use ribavirin in patients with a creatinine clearance less than 50 ml/minute.

Reactions may be *common,* uncommon, *life-threatening,* or COMMON AND LIFE-THREATENING.
Interaction may have a *rapid onset* or **delayed onset.**

ADMINISTRATION
Subcutaneous
• Vials and prefilled syringes are for single use only. Discard unused portion.
• Visually inspect drug for particulate matter and discoloration before administration; don't use if particulate matter is visible or product is discolored.

ACTION
Causes reversible decreases in leukocyte and platelet counts, partially through stimulation of production of effector proteins in vitro.

Route	Onset	Peak	Duration
Subcut.	Unknown	3–4 days	< 1 wk

Half-life: 80 hours.

ADVERSE REACTIONS
CNS: *depression, dizziness, fatigue, headache, insomnia, irritability, pain, pyrexia,* anxiety, asthenia, concentration impairment, memory impairment.
GI: *abdominal pain, anorexia, diarrhea, nausea,* dry mouth, *vomiting.*
Hematologic: NEUTROPENIA, *thrombocytopenia,* anemia, LYMPHOPENIA.
Musculoskeletal: *arthralgia, myalgia,* back pain.
Skin: *alopecia, pruritus,* dermatitis, increased sweating, rash.
Other: *injection site reaction, rigors.*

INTERACTIONS
Drug-drug. *Nucleoside reverse transcriptase inhibitors (NRTIs):* May cause severe and potentially fatal hepatic decompensation. If used together in patients coinfected with HIV who are taking NRTIs, monitor for toxicities.
Ribavirin: May cause additive hematologic toxicity. Monitor hematologic function.
Theophylline, other drugs metabolized by CYP1A2: May increase theophylline level and may interact with other drugs metabolized by this enzyme system. Monitor theophylline level and adjust dosage as needed.

EFFECTS ON LAB TEST RESULTS
• May increase ALT level. May decrease hemoglobin level and hematocrit.

• May decrease ANC, WBC, and platelet counts. May increase or decrease thyroid function test values.

CONTRAINDICATIONS & CAUTIONS
• Contraindicated in patients hypersensitive to interferon alfa-2a or any components of formulation.
• Contraindicated in patients with autoimmune hepatitis or decompensated liver disease (with moninfection or coinfection with HIV) before or during treatment with drug and in neonates and infants.
• Use cautiously in patients with a history of depression.
• Use cautiously in patients with baseline neutrophil counts less than 1,500/mm³, baseline platelet counts less than 90,000/mm³, or baseline hemoglobin level less than 10 g/dl.
• Use cautiously in patients with creatinine clearance less than 50 ml/minute.
• Use cautiously in patients with cardiac disease or hypertension, thyroid disease, autoimmune disorders, pulmonary disorders, colitis, pancreatitis, and ophthalmologic disorders.
• Use cautiously in elderly patients because they may be at increased risk for adverse reactions.
■ **Black Box Warning** Use cautiously in patients also taking ribavirin. Ribavirin may cause birth defects or fetal demise. Ribavirin is also known to cause hemolytic anemia which may worsen cardiac disease. ■
• Safety and effectiveness haven't been established in patients who have failed to respond to other alfa interferon treatments, in organ transplant recipients, and in patients who are also infected with hepatitis B.

NURSING CONSIDERATIONS
■ **Black Box Warning** Alpha interferons cause or aggravate fatal or life-threatening neuropsychiatric, autoimmune, ischemic, and infectious disorders. Monitor patients closely with periodic clinical and laboratory evaluations. Withdraw patients with persistently severe or worsening signs or symptoms of these conditions from therapy. ■
• Obtain CBC before treatment and monitor counts routinely during therapy. Stop

drug in patients who develop severe decrease in neutrophil or platelet counts.

• Stop drug if uncontrollable thyroid disease, hyperglycemia, hypoglycemia, or diabetes mellitus occurs during treatment.

• If persistent or unexplained pulmonary infiltrates or pulmonary dysfunction occur, stop drug.

• Stop drug if signs and symptoms of colitis occur, such as abdominal pain, bloody diarrhea, and fever. Symptoms should resolve within 1 to 3 weeks.

• Stop drug if signs and symptoms of pancreatitis occur, including fever, malaise, and abdominal pain.

• Obtain baseline eye examination and periodically monitor eye exams during treatment. Stop drug if new or worsening eye disorders occur.

• Monitor patient with impaired renal function for interferon toxicity.

• Use in women of childbearing age only when effective contraception is being used.

PATIENT TEACHING
• Teach patient proper way to give drug and dispose of needles and syringes.

• Tell patient to immediately report depression or suicidal ideation.

• Tell patient to report signs and symptoms of pancreatitis, colitis, eye disorders, or respiratory disorders.

• Advise patient to avoid driving or operating machinery if he feels dizzy, tired, confused, or sleepy.

■ **Black Box Warning** Tell patient to take extreme care to avoid pregnancy. ■

SAFETY ALERT!

peginterferon alfa-2b
peg-in-ter-FEER-on

PEG-Intron

Pharmacologic class: biological response modifier
Pregnancy risk category C

AVAILABLE FORMS
Injection: 50 mcg/0.5 ml, 80 mcg/0.5 ml, 120 mcg/0.5 ml, 150 mcg/0.5 ml

INDICATIONS & DOSAGES
➤ **Chronic hepatitis C in patients not previously treated with interferon alfa**
Adults: 1 mcg/kg subcutaneously once weekly for up to 1 year, on same day each week. The volume of PEG-Intron to be injected depends on the patient's weight and the vial strength used.
Adults who weigh 137 to 160 kg (302 to 353 lb): 150 mcg (0.5 ml) of 300-mcg/ml strength.
Adults who weigh 107 to 136 kg (236 to 300 lb): 120 mcg (0.5 ml) of 240-mcg/ml strength.
Adults who weigh 89 to 106 kg (196 to 234 lb): 96 mcg (0.4 ml) of 240-mcg/ml strength.
Adults who weigh 73 to 88 kg (161 to 194 lb): 80 mcg (0.5 ml) of 160-mcg/ml strength.
Adults who weigh 57 to 72 kg (126 to 159 lb): 64 mcg (0.4 ml) of 160-mcg/ml strength.
Adults who weigh 46 to 56 kg (101 to 123 lb): 50 mcg (0.5 ml) of 100-mcg/ml strength.
Adults who weigh 45 kg (99 lb) or less: 40 mcg (0.4 ml) of 100-mcg/ml strength.
➤ **Chronic hepatitis C in patients not previously treated with interferon alfa, combined with ribavirin**
Adults: 1.5 mcg/kg subcutaneously once weekly for 24 to 48 weeks on same day every week. The volume of PEG-Intron to be injected depends on the patient's weight and the vial strength used.
Adults who weigh more than 85 kg (more than 187 lb): 150 mcg (0.5 ml) of 300-mcg/ml strength.
Adults who weigh 76 to 85 kg (167 to 187 lb): 120 mcg (0.5 ml) of 240-mcg/ml strength.
Adults who weigh 61 to 75 kg (134 to 165 lb): 96 mcg (0.4 ml) of 240-mcg/ml strength.
Adults who weigh 51 to 60 kg (112 to 132 lb): 80 mcg (0.5 ml) of 160-mcg/ml strength.
Adults who weigh 40 to 50 kg (88 to 110 lb): 64 mcg (0.4 ml) of 160-mcg/ml strength.

Adults who weigh less than 40 kg (less than 88 lb): 50 mcg (0.5 ml) of 100-mcg/ml strength.

Adjust-a-dose: Decrease peginterferon alfa-2b dose by 50% in patients with WBC count less than 1,500/mm³, neutrophil count less than 750/mm³, or platelet count less than 80,000/mm³. Oral ribavirin dose can be continued. If hemoglobin level is less than 10 g/dl, reduce oral ribavirin dose by 200 mg. Stop both drugs if hemoglobin level is less than 8.5 g/dl, WBCs less than 1,000/mm³, neutrophil count less than 500/mm³, or platelet count less than 50,000/mm³. If symptoms improve and remain stable for 4 weeks, continue at present dose or resume previous dose.

If patient develops mild depression, continue peginterferon alfa-2b, but evaluate patient once weekly. In moderate depression, reduce peginterferon alfa-2b dose by 50% for 4 to 8 weeks and evaluate patient every week. In severe depression, stop peginterferon alfa-2b.

For patients with stable CV disease, decrease peginterferon alfa-2b dose by 50% and ribavirin dosage by 200 mg daily if hemoglobin level drops more than 2 g/dl in any 4-week period. Stop both drugs if hemoglobin level goes below 12 g/dl after 4 weeks of reduced dosages.

ADMINISTRATION
Subcutaneous
- To reconstitute the lyophilized peginterferon alfa-2b in the Redipen, hold the Redipen upright (dose button down) and press the two halves of the pen together until there is an audible click.
- Gently invert the pen to mix the solution. Don't shake.
- Keeping the pen upright, attach the supplied needle and select the appropriate peginterferon alfa-2b dose by pulling back on the dosing button until the dark bands are visible and turning the button until the dark band is aligned with the correct dose.
- The Redipen is for single use only.
- Reconstitute the peginterferon alfa-2b lyophilized product with only 0.7 ml of supplied diluent (sterile water for injection). Discard the remaining diluent.

- Swirl gently to dissolve completely.
- **Incompatibilities:** Don't add any other medication to solutions containing peg-interferon alfa-2b.

ACTION
Binds to specific membrane receptors on the cell surface, inducing certain enzymes, suppressing cell proliferation, immunomodulating activities, and inhibiting virus replication in virus-infected cells. Increases levels of effector proteins and body temperature, and decreases leukocyte and platelet counts.

Route	Onset	Peak	Duration
Subcut.	Unknown	15–44 hr	Unknown

Half-life: 40 hours.

ADVERSE REACTIONS
CNS: *anxiety, depression, dizziness, emotional lability, fatigue, fever, headache, insomnia, irritability,* **suicidal behavior,** hypertonia, malaise.
CV: flushing.
EENT: *pharyngitis,* sinusitis.
GI: *abdominal pain, anorexia, diarrhea, nausea,* dyspepsia, right upper quadrant pain, vomiting.
Hematologic: neutropenia, thrombo-cytopenia.
Hepatic: hepatomegaly.
Metabolic: *weight loss,* hyperthyroidism, hypothyroidism.
Musculoskeletal: *musculoskeletal pain, myalgia, arthralgia.*
Respiratory: cough.
Skin: *alopecia, dry skin, increased sweating, injection site inflammation or reaction, pruritus, rash,* injection site pain.
Other: *flulike symptoms, rigors, viral infection.*

INTERACTIONS
None reported.

EFFECTS ON LAB TEST RESULTS
- May increase serum bilirubin, uric acid, and ALT levels. May increase or decrease TSH level.
- May decrease hemoglobin.
- May decrease neutrophil and platelet counts.

CONTRAINDICATIONS & CAUTIONS
• Contraindicated in patients hypersensitive to drug or any of its components, in patients with autoimmune hepatitis or decompensated liver disease, in those with diabetes or thyroid disorders that can't be controlled with medication, in patients who have failed to respond to other alfa interferon treatment or have had an organ transplant, and in those with HIV or hepatitis B virus.
• Use cautiously in patients with psychiatric disorders, diabetes mellitus, CV disease, creatinine clearance less than 50 ml/minute, pulmonary infiltrates, pulmonary function impairment, or autoimmune, ischemic, or infectious disorders.

NURSING CONSIDERATIONS
• Obtain eye examination in patient with diabetes or hypertension before starting drug. Retinal hemorrhages, cotton-wool spots, and retinal artery or vein obstruction may occur.
■ **Black Box Warning** Drug may cause or aggravate fatal or life-threatening neuropsychiatric, autoimmune, ischemic, and infectious disorders. Monitor patients closely with periodic clinical and laboratory evaluations. In patient with persistently severe or worsening signs or symptoms of these conditions from therapy, withhold drug. In many but not all cases, these disorders resolve after stopping PEG-Intron therapy. ■
■ **Black Box Warning** If used in combination therapy with ribavirin, ensure extreme care to avoid pregnancy. Also, monitor patient for worsening cardiac disease secondary to anemia. ■
• Drug may cause or aggravate hypothyroidism, hyperthyroidism, or diabetes.
• Perform ECG on patient with history of MI or arrhythmias before starting drug.
• Start treatment in patient who is well hydrated.
• Monitor patient with history of MI or arrhythmias closely for hypotension, arrhythmias, tachycardia, cardiomyopathy, and signs and symptoms of MI.
• Monitor patient for depression and other mental health disorders. If symptoms are severe, stop drug and refer patient for psychiatric care.
• Monitor patient for signs and symptoms of colitis, such as abdominal pain, bloody diarrhea, and fever. Stop drug if colitis occurs. Symptoms should resolve 1 to 3 weeks after stopping drug.
• Monitor patient for signs and symptoms of pancreatitis or hypersensitivity reactions, and stop drug if these occur.
• Monitor patient with pulmonary disease for dyspnea, pulmonary infiltrates, pneumonitis, and pneumonia.
• Monitor patient with renal disease for signs and symptoms of toxicity.
• Monitor CBC count, platelets count, and AST, ALT, bilirubin, and TSH levels before starting drug and periodically during treatment.
• Notify prescriber if severe neutropenia or thrombocytopenia occurs.

PATIENT TEACHING
• Teach patient the appropriate use of the drug and the benefits and risks of treatment. Tell patient that adverse reactions may continue for several months after treatment is stopped.
• Tell patient to immediately report symptoms of depression or suicidal thoughts.
• Instruct patient on importance of proper disposal of needles and syringes and caution him against reuse of old needles and syringes.
• Tell patient that drug won't prevent transmission of hepatitis C virus (HCV) to others and may not cure hepatitis C or prevent cirrhosis, liver failure, or liver cancer that may result from HCV infection.
• Advise patient that laboratory tests are needed before starting therapy and periodically thereafter.
• Tell patient to take drug at bedtime and to use fever-reducing drugs to decrease risk of flulike signs and symptoms.
• Inform breast-feeding patient of the potential for adverse reactions in infants. Tell her to either stop using drug or stop breast-feeding.
■ **Black Box Warning** Tell patient to avoid pregnancy. ■

88

Immunosuppressants

alefacept
anakinra
azathioprine
basiliximab
certolizumab pegol
cyclosporine
cyclosporine, modified
daclizumab
efalizumab
etanercept
glatiramer acetate injection
infliximab
lymphocyte immune globulin
muromonab-CD3
mycophenolate mofetil
mycophenolate mofetil
  hydrochloride
mycophenolic acid
natalizumab
pimecrolimus
sirolimus
tacrolimus
tacrolimus (topical)

---

alefacept
ALE-fuh-sept

Amevive

Pharmacologic class:
immunosuppressant
Pregnancy risk category B

AVAILABLE FORMS
Powder for injection: 7.5-mg and 15-mg
single-dose vials

INDICATIONS & DOSAGES
➤ **Moderate to severe chronic
plaque psoriasis in candidates for
systemic therapy or phototherapy**
Adults: 7.5 mg I.V. bolus or 15 mg I.M.
once weekly for 12 weeks. Another
12-week course may be given if CD4+
T-lymphocyte count is normal and at least
12 weeks have passed since the previous
treatment.
Adjust-a-dose: Withhold dose if
CD4+ T-lymphocyte count is below
250 cells/mm³. Stop drug if CD4+ count
remains below 250 cells/mm³ for 1 month.

ADMINISTRATION
I.M.
● Reconstitute 15-mg vial of alefacept
with 0.6 ml of supplied diluent.
● Rotate I.M. injection sites so that the
new injection is given at least 1 inch away
from the old site, and not in an area that is
bruised, tender, or hard.
● After reconstitution, use product immediately or within 4 hours.
I.V.
● Reconstitute 7.5 mg vial with 0.6 ml of
the supplied diluent; 0.5 ml of the reconstituted solution contains 7.5 mg of alefacept.
● Swirl gently to avoid foaming.
● Inspect solution for particulate matter
and discoloration before administration.
● Prepare two syringes with 3.0 ml
normal saline for preadministration and
postadministration flush.
● Prime the winged infusion set with 3.0 ml
saline and insert the set into the vein.
● Attach the alefacept-filled syringe to the
infusion set and give the solution over no
more than 5 seconds.
● Flush the infusion set with 3.0 ml saline.
● Don't filter reconstituted solution during
preparation or administration.
● **Incompatibilities:** Don't reconstitute
with other diluents. Don't mix with other
drugs.

ACTION
An immunosuppressive protein that
interferes with lymphocyte activation and
reduces subsets of CD2+ T lymphocytes,
which reduces circulating total CD4+ and
CD8+ T-lymphocyte counts.

Route	Onset	Peak	Duration
I.M., I.V.	Unknown	Unknown	Unknown

Half-life: About 11 days.

ADVERSE REACTIONS
CNS: dizziness.
CV: coronary artery disorder.
EENT: pharyngitis.

GI: nausea.
Hematologic: LYMPHOPENIA.
Musculoskeletal: myalgia.
Respiratory: cough.
Skin: pruritus, *injection site pain, inflammation,* bleeding, edema or mass.
Other: *infection,* chills, *malignancy,* hypersensitivity reaction, accidental injury, antibody formation.

INTERACTIONS
Drug-drug. *Immunosuppressants, phototherapy:* May increase risk of excessive immunosuppression. Avoid using together.

EFFECTS ON LAB TEST RESULTS
• May decrease CD4+ and CD8+ T-lymphocyte counts.

CONTRAINDICATIONS & CAUTIONS
• Contraindicated in patients hypersensitive to drug or its components, in breast-feeding women, and in patients with HIV, a history of systemic malignancy, or important infection.
• Use cautiously in patients at high risk for malignancy, patients with chronic or recurrent infections, and pregnant women.
• Use cautiously in elderly patients because of their increased rate of infection and malignancies.
• Safety and effectiveness in children haven't been established.

NURSING CONSIDERATIONS
• Ensure that CD4+ T-lymphocyte count is normal before therapy. Monitor CD4+ T-lymphocyte count weekly for the 12-week course.
• Monitor patient carefully for evidence of infection or malignancy, and stop drug if it appears.
• Because effects on fetal development aren't known, give drug only if clearly needed. Enroll pregnant women receiving alefacept into the Biogen pregnancy registry at 1-800-811-0104.

PATIENT TEACHING
• Tell patient about potential adverse reactions.
• Urge patient to report evidence of infection immediately.

• Tell patient that blood tests will be done regularly to monitor WBC counts.
• Tell patient to notify prescriber if she is or could be pregnant within 8 weeks of receiving drug.
• Advise patient to either stop breast-feeding or stop using the drug because of the risk of serious adverse reactions in the infant.

---

anakinra
ann-ACK-in-rah

Kineret

Pharmacologic class: interleukin-1 receptor antagonist
Pregnancy risk category B

AVAILABLE FORMS
Injection: 100 mg/0.67 ml in a prefilled glass syringe

INDICATIONS & DOSAGES
➤ **To reduce signs and symptoms and slow progression of structural damage in moderately to severely active rheumatoid arthritis (RA) after one or more failures with disease-modifying antirheumatic drugs (DMARDs), alone or combined with DMARDs other than tumor necrosis factor (TNF)-blocking drugs**
Adults: 100 mg subcutaneously daily.
Adjust-a-dose: In patients with a creatinine clearance less than 30 ml/minute, give 100 mg subcutaneously every other day.

ADMINISTRATION
Subcutaneous
• Inject entire contents of prefilled syringe.
• Store drug in the refrigerator at 35° to 46° F (2° to 8° C). Don't freeze or shake.
• Protect drug from light.

ACTION
A recombinant, nonglycosylated form of the human interleukin-1 receptor antagonist (IL-1Ra). The level of naturally occurring IL-1Ra in synovium and synovial fluid from patients with RA isn't enough to compete with the elevated level of locally produced IL-1. Anakinra blocks the

---

biologic activity of IL-1 by competitively inhibiting IL-1 from binding to the interleukin-1 type receptor, which is expressed in various tissues and organs.

Route	Onset	Peak	Duration
Subcut.	Unknown	3–7 hr	Unknown

Half-life: 4 to 6 hours.

ADVERSE REACTIONS
CNS: *headache.*
EENT: *sinusitis.*
GI: abdominal pain, diarrhea, nausea.
Hematologic: *neutropenia.*
Respiratory: *upper respiratory tract infection.*
Skin: *ecchymosis, injection site reactions (erythema, inflammation, pain).*
Other: infection (cellulitis, pneumonia, bone and joint), flulike symptoms.

INTERACTIONS
Drug-drug. *Etanercept, other TNF-blocking drugs:* May increase risk of severe infection. Use together isn't recommended.
Vaccines: May decrease effectiveness of vaccines or may increase risk of secondary transmission of infection with live vaccines. Avoid using together.

EFFECTS ON LAB TEST RESULTS
• May increase eosinophil count. May decrease neutrophil, platelet, and WBC counts.

CONTRAINDICATIONS & CAUTIONS
• Contraindicated in patients hypersensitive to *Escherichia coli*–derived proteins or any components of the product, or in patients with active infections.
• Use drug cautiously in immuno-suppressed patients, those with a chronic infection, the elderly, and breast-feeding women.
• Safety and effectiveness in patients with juvenile RA haven't been established.

NURSING CONSIDERATIONS
• Don't start treatment if patient has active infection.
• Obtain neutrophil count before treatment, monthly for the first 3 months of treatment, and then quarterly for up to 1 year.

• Monitor patient for infections and injection site reactions.
• Stop drug if a serious infection develops.
• Monitor patient for possible anaphylactic reaction.
• ***Look alike–sound alike:*** Don't confuse anakinra with amikacin.

PATIENT TEACHING
• Tell patient to store drug in refrigerator and not to freeze or expose to excessive heat. Advise letting drug come to room temperature before giving dose.
• Teach patient proper dosage, administration, and needle and syringe disposal.
• Urge patient to rotate injection sites.
• Review signs and symptoms of allergic and other adverse reactions, especially signs of serious infections. Urge patient to contact prescriber if they arise.
• Inform patient that injection site reactions are common, usually mild, and typically last 14 to 28 days.
• Tell patient to avoid live-virus vaccines during therapy.

azathioprine
ay-za-THYE-oh-preen

Azasan, Imuran

Pharmacologic class: purine antagonist
Pregnancy risk category D

AVAILABLE FORMS
Powder for injection: 100 mg
Tablets: 25 mg, 50 mg, 75 mg, 100 mg

INDICATIONS & DOSAGES
➤ **Immunosuppression in kidney transplantation**
Adults: Initially, 3 to 5 mg/kg P.O. or I.V. daily, usually beginning on day of transplantation. Maintained at 1 to 3 mg/kg daily based on patient response and tolerance.
Adjust-a-dose: Give drug in lower doses to patients with oliguria in the posttransplant period and in those with impaired renal function. In patients receiving allopurinol, decrease azathioprine dose to one-fourth to one-third of the usual dose.

➤ **Severe, refractory rheumatoid arthritis**
Adults: Initially, 1 mg/kg P.O. as single dose or divided into two doses. Usual dose is 50 to 100 mg. If patient response isn't satisfactory after 6 to 8 weeks, dosage may be increased by 0.5 mg/kg daily to maximum of 2.5 mg/kg daily at 4-week intervals. Maintenance therapy should be at lowest effective dose. Attempt gradual dose reduction once the patient is stable. Reduce dosage by 0.5 mg/kg (about 25 mg daily) every 4 weeks.

ADMINISTRATION
P.O.
● Give drug after meals to minimize adverse GI effects.
I.V.
● Use only in patients who can't tolerate oral drugs.
● Reconstitute drug in 100-mg vial with 10 ml of sterile water for injection.
● Inspect for particles before use.
● Give by direct I.V. injection, or further dilute in normal saline solution for injection or D_5W solution and infuse over 30 to 60 minutes.
● **Incompatibilities:** None reported.

ACTION
May cause variable alterations in antibody production.

Route	Onset	Peak	Duration
P.O., I.V.	Unknown	Unknown	Unknown

Half-life: About 5 hours.

ADVERSE REACTIONS
CNS: fever.
GI: *nausea, vomiting,* anorexia, *pancreatitis,* steatorrhea, diarrhea, abdominal pain.
Hematologic: LEUKOPENIA, *myelosuppression,* macrocytic anemia, anemia, *pancytopenia,* THROMBOCYTOPENIA, *immunosuppression.*
Hepatic: *hepatotoxicity,* jaundice.
Musculoskeletal: arthralgia, myalgia.
Skin: rash, alopecia.
Other: *infections, increased risk of neoplasia.*

INTERACTIONS
Drug-drug. *ACE inhibitors:* May cause severe leukopenia. Monitor patient closely.

Allopurinol: May impair inactivation of azathioprine. Avoid using if possible; decrease azathioprine to one-third to one-fourth usual dose.
Co-trimoxazole and other drugs that interfere with myelopoiesis: May cause severe leukopenia, especially in renal transplant patients. Use cautiously together.
Cyclosporine: May decrease cyclosporine level. Monitor cyclosporine level closely.
Warfarin: May decrease action of warfarin. Monitor patient closely.

EFFECTS ON LAB TEST RESULTS
● May increase alkaline phosphatase, ALT, AST, and bilirubin levels. May decrease hemoglobin and uric acid levels.
● May decrease platelet, RBC, and WBC counts.

CONTRAINDICATIONS & CAUTIONS
● Contraindicated in patients hypersensitive to drug or its components.
● Use cautiously in patients with hepatic or renal dysfunction.
● Benefits must be weighed against risk when giving to patient with systemic viral infection, such as chickenpox or herpes zoster.
● Patients with rheumatoid arthritis previously treated with alkylating drugs, such as cyclophosphamide, chlorambucil, or melphalan, may be at risk for tumor development if treated with this drug.

NURSING CONSIDERATIONS
■ **Black Box Warning** Chronic immunosuppression with this drug increases the risk of neoplasia. Physicians using this drug should be very familiar with its risks. ■
● To prevent bleeding, avoid all I.M. injections when platelet count is below 100,000/mm³.
● Monitor CBC and platelet counts weekly for 1 month and then twice monthly. Notify prescriber if counts drop suddenly or become dangerously low. Drug may need to be temporarily withheld.
● Watch for early signs and symptoms of hepatotoxicity (such as clay-colored

---

Reactions may be *common,* uncommon, *life-threatening,* or COMMON AND LIFE-THREATENING.
Interaction may have a *rapid onset* or *delayed onset.*

stools, dark urine, pruritus, and yellow skin and sclera) and for increased alkaline phosphatase, bilirubin, AST, and ALT levels.

• Therapeutic response usually occurs within 8 weeks. Patients not improved after 12 weeks can be considered refractory to treatment.

• **Look alike–sound alike:** Don't confuse azathioprine with Azulfidine. Don't confuse Imuran with Inderal.

PATIENT TEACHING
• Warn patient to report even mild infections (colds, fever, sore throat, malaise), because drug is a potent immunosuppressant.
• Instruct patient to avoid conception during therapy and for 4 months after therapy stops.
• Warn patient that some hair thinning is possible.
• Tell patient taking drug for refractory rheumatoid arthritis that it may take up to 12 weeks to be effective.
• Advise patient to report unusual bleeding or bruising.
• Tell patient that drug may be taken with food to decrease nausea.
• Advise patient to use soft toothbrush and perform oral care cautiously.

basiliximab
ba-sil-IK-si-mab

Simulect

Pharmacologic class: monoclonal antibody
Pregnancy risk category B

AVAILABLE FORMS
Injection: 20-mg vials

INDICATIONS & DOSAGES
➤ **To prevent acute organ rejection in patients receiving renal transplantation when used as part of an immunosuppressive regimen that includes cyclosporine and corticosteroids**
Adults and children weighing 35 kg (77 lb) or more: 20 mg I.V. given within 2 hours before transplant surgery

and 20 mg I.V. given 4 days after transplantation.
Children weighing less than 35 kg: 10 mg I.V. given within 2 hours before transplant surgery and 10 mg I.V. given 4 days after transplantation.

ADMINISTRATION
I.V.
• Reconstitute with 5 ml sterile water for injection. Shake gently to dissolve powder.
• Use reconstituted solution immediately.
• Dilute reconstituted solution to 50 ml with normal saline solution or D_5W for infusion.
• When mixing solution, invert bag gently to avoid foaming. Don't shake.
• Infuse over 20 to 30 minutes.
• Drug may be given as a bolus injection, but doing so may cause nausea, vomiting, pain, and local reactions.
• Reconstituted solution may be refrigerated at 36° to 46° F (2° to 8° C) for up to 24 hours or kept at room temperature for 4 hours.
• **Incompatibilities:** Don't add or infuse other drugs simultaneously through same I.V. line.

ACTION
Binds specifically to and blocks the interleukin (IL)-2 receptor alpha chain on the surface of activated T lymphocytes, inhibiting IL-2–mediated activation of lymphocytes, a critical pathway in the cellular immune response involved in allograft rejection.

Route	Onset	Peak	Duration
I.V.	Unknown	Immediate	Unknown

Half-life: About 7¼ days in adults, 9½ days in children, 9 days in adolescents.

ADVERSE REACTIONS
CNS: *fever, headache, insomnia, tremor,* agitation, anxiety, asthenia, depression, dizziness, hypoesthesia, neuropathy, paresthesia, fatigue.
CV: *hypertension, leg or peripheral edema, arrhythmias, heart failure,* angina pectoris, atrial fibrillation, chest pain, abnormal heart sounds, aggravated hypertension, hypotension, tachycardia, generalized edema.

EENT: *pharyngitis, rhinitis,* abnormal vision, cataract, conjunctivitis, sinusitis.
GI: *abdominal pain, candidiasis, constipation, diarrhea, dyspepsia, nausea, vomiting, GI hemorrhage,* esophagitis, enlarged abdomen, flatulence, gastroenteritis, GI disorder, gum hyperplasia, melena, ulcerative stomatitis.
GU: *UTI,* abnormal renal function, albuminuria, bladder disorder, dysuria, frequent micturition, genital edema, hematuria, increased nonprotein nitrogen, oliguria, *renal tubular necrosis,* ureteral disorder, urine retention, impotence.
Hematologic: *anemia, hemorrhage, thrombocytopenia,* hematoma, polycythemia, purpura, thrombosis.
Metabolic: *hypercholesterolemia, hyperglycemia, hyperkalemia, hyperuricemia, hypokalemia, hypophosphatemia,* acidosis, dehydration, *diabetes mellitus,* fluid overload, hypercalcemia, hyperlipemia, hypertriglyceridemia, hypocalcemia, *hypomagnesemia,* hypoproteinemia, weight gain.
Musculoskeletal: arthralgia, arthropathy, back pain, bone fracture, cramps, hernia, leg pain, myalgia.
Respiratory: *dyspnea, upper respiratory tract infection, bronchospasm, pulmonary edema,* abnormal chest sounds, bronchitis, cough, pneumonia, pulmonary disorder.
Skin: *acne,* cyst, hypertrichosis, pruritus, rash, skin disorder or ulceration.
Other: *surgical wound complications, viral infection, hypersensitivity reactions, sepsis,* accidental trauma, infection, herpes zoster, herpes simplex.

INTERACTIONS
None significant.

EFFECTS ON LAB TEST RESULTS
• May increase calcium, cholesterol, glucose, lipid, and uric acid levels. May decrease hemoglobin, magnesium, phosphorus, and protein levels. May increase or decrease potassium level.
• May increase RBC count. May decrease platelet count.

CONTRAINDICATIONS & CAUTIONS
• Contraindicated in patients hypersensitive to drug or its components.

■ **Black Box Warning** Use cautiously and only under supervision of prescriber qualified and experienced in immunosuppressive therapy and organ transplantation. ■
• Use cautiously in elderly patients.

NURSING CONSIDERATIONS
• Severe acute hypersensitivity reactions can occur within 24 hours after administration. Make sure drugs for treating hypersensitivity reactions are readily available; withhold second dose if hypersensitivity reactions occur.
• Check for electrolyte imbalances and acidosis during drug therapy.
• Monitor patient's intake and output, vital signs, hemoglobin level, and hematocrit during therapy.
• Be alert for signs and symptoms of opportunistic infections during drug therapy.

PATIENT TEACHING
• Inform patient of potential benefits of and risks related to immunosuppressive therapy, including decreased risk of graft loss or acute rejection.
• Advise patient that immunosuppressive therapy increases risk of developing infection. Tell him to report signs and symptoms of infection promptly.
• Inform woman of childbearing age to use effective contraception before therapy starts and for 4 months after therapy ends.
• Instruct patient to report adverse effects immediately.
• Explain that drug is used with cyclosporine and corticosteroids.

✻ **NEW DRUG**

certolizumab pegol
SERT-oh-LIZ-u-mahb PEGH-ol

Cimzia

Pharmacologic class: tumor necrosis factor blocker
Pregnancy risk category B

AVAILABLE FORMS
Lyophilized powder for injection: 200 mg

Reactions may be *common,* uncommon, *life-threatening,* or COMMON AND LIFE-THREATENING.
Interaction may have a *rapid onset* or *delayed onset.*

INDICATIONS & DOSAGES

➤ **Crohn's disease when response to conventional therapy is inadequate**
Adults: Initially, 400 mg subcutaneously, then at 2 weeks and 4 weeks followed by a maintenance dose of 400 mg subcutaneously every 4 weeks, if adequate response.

ACTION

Selectively neutralizes TNFα, a pro-inflammatory cytokine responsible for stimulating the production of inflammatory mediators associated with Crohn's disease.
Absorption: 80% bioavailable after subcutaneous injection.
Distribution: Unknown.
Metabolism: Unknown.
Excretion: Unknown.

Route	Onset	Peak	Duration
Subcut.	Unknown	54–171 hr	Unknown

Half-life: 14 days.

ADVERSE REACTIONS

CNS: anxiety, bipolar disorder, suicide attempt.
CV: angina pectoris, arrhythmias, heart failure, hypertensive heart disease, myocardial infarction, pericardial effusion and pericarditis, vasculitis.
EENT: optic neuritis, retinal hemorrhage, uveitis.
GI: abdominal pain.
GU: urinary tract infection.
Hematologic: anemia, *leukopenia,* lymphadenopathy, *pancytopenia,* thrombophilia.
Hepatic: elevated liver enzymes, hepatitis.
Musculoskeletal: arthralgia, extremity pain.
Respiratory: *upper respiratory tract infection.*
Skin: alopecia, dermatitis, peripheral edema, erythema nodosum, urticaria, injection site pain and erythema.
Other: *tuberculosis and opportunistic infection, Stevens-Johnson syndrome, toxic epidermal necrolysis and erythema multiforme.*

INTERACTIONS

Drug-drug. *Anakinra:* May increase risk of serious infection and neutropenia. Avoid using together.

Live vaccines: May cause infection. Avoid using together.

EFFECTS ON LAB TEST RESULTS

● May falsely elevate PTT.

CONTRAINDICATIONS & CAUTIONS

● Use cautiously in patients with known hypersensitivity to other TNF blockers and those with underlying conditions that may increase the risk of infections
● Use cautiously in those with a history of recurrent infections or concomitant immunosuppressive therapy, or in those who have resided in regions where tuberculosis and histoplasmosis are endemic. Avoid use in patients with active infections.
● Use cautiously in patients with a history of central nervous system demyelinating disorder, hematologic disorders, or heart failure.

NURSING CONSIDERATIONS

● Each 400-mg dose requires two vials. Reconstitute each vial with 1 ml of sterile water for injection, using a 20-G needle. Gently swirl the vial without shaking. May take up to 30 minutes to fully reconstitute. Inspect vial for particulate matter and discoloration, and discard if present.
● Draw up each vial in its own syringe, switch each 20-G needle to a 23-G needle, and inject into separate sites in the abdomen or thigh.
● Reconstituted drug is stable for 2 hours at room temperature or for up to 24 hours if refrigerated.
■ **Black Box Warning** Monitor patient for signs and symptoms of tuberculosis, invasive fungal infection, and other opportunistic infections during and after treatment. Discontinue treatment if serious infection develops. Fatal infections have occurred. ■
● Before initiating therapy, evaluate patient for tuberculosis risk factors and test for latent tuberculosis infection.
● Before therapy, consider antituberculosis therapy in patients with past history of latent or active tuberculosis when adequate treatment can't be confirmed.
● Before therapy, evaluate patients at risk for hepatitis B virus (HBV) infection and test for previous HBV infection.

• Use during pregnancy only when benefits to mother outweigh the risks to fetus.

• It isn't known whether drug appears in breast milk. Advise stopping breast-feeding during therapy.

• Safety and efficacy haven't been established in children.

• Use cautiously in elderly patients because of increased risk for infection.

PATIENT TEACHING
■ **Black Box Warning** Teach patient to seek prompt medical attention if persistent fever, cough, shortness of breath, or fatigue develops. ■

• Advise patient to seek immediate medical attention for signs and symptoms of infection or for unusual bruising or bleeding.

• Instruct patient to seek immediate medical attention if any symptoms of severe allergic reaction develop.

• Tell patient to report signs and symptoms of heart failure.

---

cyclosporine
SYE-kloe-spor-een

Sandimmune

cyclosporine, modified
Gengraf, Neoral

Pharmacologic class:
immunosuppressive
Pregnancy risk category C

AVAILABLE FORMS
Capsules for microemulsion (modified):
25 mg, 50 mg, 100 mg
Capsules (nonmodified): 25 mg, 50 mg,
100 mg
Injection: 50 mg/ml
Oral solution (modified and nonmodified):
100 mg/ml

INDICATIONS & DOSAGES
➤ **To prevent organ rejection
in renal, hepatic, or cardiac
transplantation**
Adults and children: 15 mg/kg P.O. 4 to
12 hours before transplantation and
continue daily for 1 to 2 weeks postoperatively. Then reduce dosage by 5%

each week to maintenance level of 5 to
10 mg/kg daily. Or, 5 to 6 mg/kg I.V.
concentrate 4 to 12 hours before transplantation as a continuous infusion.
Postoperatively, repeat dose daily until
patient can tolerate P.O. forms.

For conversion from Sandimmune to
Gengraf or Neoral, use same daily dose
as previously used for Sandimmune.
Monitor blood levels every 4 to 7 days
after conversion, and monitor blood
pressure and creatinine level every
2 weeks during the first 2 months.
➤ **Severe, active rheumatoid arthritis (RA) that hasn't adequately
responded to methotrexate**
Adults: 2.5 mg/kg Gengraf or Neoral daily
P.O., taken b.i.d. as divided doses. Dosage
may be increased by 0.5 to 0.75 mg/kg
daily after 8 weeks and again after 12 weeks
to a maximum of 4 mg/kg daily. If no
response is seen after 16 weeks, stop
therapy.
➤ **Psoriasis**
Adults: 1.25 mg/kg Gengraf or Neoral
daily P.O. b.i.d. for at least 4 weeks.
Increase dosage by 0.5 mg/kg daily once
every 2 weeks as needed to a maximum
of 4 mg/kg daily.
Adjust-a-dose: For patients with adverse
effects such as hypertension, creatinine
level 30% above pretreatment level,
or abnormal CBC count or liver function
test results, decrease dosage by 25%
to 50%.

ADMINISTRATION
P.O.
• Give Neoral or Gengraf on an empty
stomach.
• Measure oral solution doses carefully in
an oral syringe. Don't rinse dosing syringe
with water. If syringe is cleaned, it must
be completely dry before reuse.
• To improve the taste of Sandimmune
oral solution, mix it with milk, chocolate
milk, or orange juice. Gengraf or Neoral
oral solution may be mixed with orange or
apple juice (not grapefruit juice); it's less
palatable when mixed with milk.
• Use a glass container to mix, and have
patient drink at once.
I.V.
• This form is usually reserved for patients
who can't tolerate oral drugs.

Reactions may be *common*, uncommon, *life-threatening*, or COMMON AND LIFE-THREATENING.
Interaction may have a *rapid onset* or **delayed onset**.

- Immediately before use, dilute each milliliter of concentrate in 20 to 100 ml of D_5W or normal saline solution for injection. Give at one-third the oral dose.
- Infuse over 2 to 6 hours.
- Protect diluted drug from light.
- **Incompatibilities:** Amphotericin B cholesteryl sulfate complex, magnesium sulfate.

ACTION
May inhibit proliferation and function of T lymphocytes and inhibit production and release of lymphokines.

Route	Onset	Peak	Duration
P.O.	Unknown	90 min–3 hr	Unknown
I.V.	Unknown	Unknown	Unknown

Half-life: Initial phase, about 1 hour; terminal phase, 8½ to 27 hours.

ADVERSE REACTIONS
CNS: *tremor, headache,* confusion, paresthesia, *seizures.*
CV: *hypertension,* flushing.
EENT: *gum hyperplasia,* sinusitis.
GI: *nausea, vomiting,* diarrhea, abdominal discomfort.
GU: NEPHROTOXICITY.
Hematologic: anemia, *leukopenia, thrombocytopenia.*
Hepatic: *hepatotoxicity.*
Metabolic: hyperglycemia.
Skin: *hirsutism,* acne.
Other: infections, *anaphylaxis.*

INTERACTIONS
Drug-drug. *Acyclovir, aminoglycosides, amphotericin B, cimetidine, co-trimoxazole, diclofenac, gentamicin, ketoconazole, melphalan, NSAIDs, ranitidine, sulfamethoxazole and trimethoprim, tacrolimus, tobramycin, vancomycin:* May increase risk of nephrotoxicity. Avoid using together.
Allopurinol, **azole antifungals,** *bromocriptine,* **caspofungin,** *cimetidine, clarithromycin, danazol, diltiazem, erythromycin, imipenem and cilastatin, methylprednisolone, metoclopramide,* **micafungin,** *nicardipine, prednisolone, verapamil:* May increase cyclosporine level. Monitor patient for increased toxicity.
Azathioprine, corticosteroids, cyclophosphamide, verapamil: May increase

immunosuppression. Monitor patient closely.
Carbamazepine, isoniazid, nafcillin, octreotide, **orlistat,** *phenobarbital,* **phenytoin, rifabutin, rifampin,** *ticlopidine:* May decrease immunosuppressant effect from low cyclosporine level. Cyclosporine dosage may need to be increased.
Digoxin, lovastatin, prednisolone: May decrease clearance of these drugs. Use together cautiously.
Mycophenolate mofetil: May decrease mycophenolate level. Monitor patient closely when cyclosporine is added to or removed from therapy.
Potassium-sparing diuretics: May induce hyperkalemia. Monitor patient closely.
Sirolimus: May increase sirolimus level. Take sirolimus at least 4 hours after cyclosporine dose. If separating doses isn't possible, monitor patient for increased adverse effects.
Vaccines: May decrease immune response. Delay routine immunization.
Drug-herb. *Astragalus, echinacea, licorice:* May interfere with drug's effect. Discourage use together.
St. John's wort: May reduce drug level, resulting in transplant failure. Discourage use together.
Drug-food. *Alfalfa sprouts:* May interfere with drug's effect. Discourage use together.
Grapefruit and grapefruit juices: May increase drug level and cause toxicity. Advise patient to avoid use together.
Drug-lifestyle. *Sunlight:* May increase risk of sensitivity to sunlight. Advise patient to avoid excessive sunlight exposure.

EFFECTS ON LAB TEST RESULTS
- May increase ALT, AST, bilirubin, BUN, creatinine, glucose, and LDL levels. May decrease hemoglobin and magnesium levels.
- May decrease platelet and WBC counts.

CONTRAINDICATIONS & CAUTIONS
- Contraindicated in patients hypersensitive to drug or polyoxyethylated castor oil (found in injectable form).
- Contraindicated in patients with RA or psoriasis with abnormal renal function, uncontrolled hypertension, or malignancies (Neoral or Gengraf).

NURSING CONSIDERATIONS

■ **Black Box Warning** Only experienced physicians should prescribe this drug. ■

■ **Black Box Warning** Psoriasis patients previously treated with psoralen and ultra-violet light A, methotrexate or other immunosuppressive agents, UVB, coal tar, or radiation therapy are at an increased risk for skin malignancies when taking Neoral or Gengraf. ■

● Drug can cause hepatotoxicity.

■ **Black Box Warning** Neoral and Gengraf may increase the susceptibility to infection and the development of neoplasia. ■

● Monitor elderly patient for renal impairment and hypertension.

■ **Black Box Warning** Monitor Sandimmune level at regular intervals. Absorption of oral solution can be erratic. ■

■ **Black Box Warning** Neoral and Gengraf have greater bioavailability than Sandimmune. A lower dose of Neoral or Gengraf may be needed to provide blood level similar to that achieved with Sandimmune. Monitor blood level when switching patients between these two brands. ■

● Gengraf is bioequivalent to and interchangeable with Neoral capsules.

■ **Black Box Warning** Always give with corticosteroids; however, don't give Sandimmune with other immuno-suppressants. ■

■ **Black Box Warning** Drug can cause systemic hypertension and nephrotoxicity. ■

● Use Neoral or Gengraf to treat RA or psoriasis.

● *Look alike–sound alike:* Don't confuse cyclosporine with cyclophosphamide or cycloserine. Don't confuse Sandimmune with Sandostatin.

RA

● Before starting treatment, measure blood pressure at least twice and obtain two creatinine levels to estimate baseline.

● Evaluate blood pressure and creatinine level every 2 weeks during first 3 months and then monthly if patient is stable.

● Monitor blood pressure and creatinine level after an increase in NSAID dosage or introduction of a new NSAID. Monitor CBC and liver function tests monthly if patient also receives methotrexate.

● If hypertension occurs, decrease dosage of Gengraf or Neoral by 25% to 50%.

If hypertension persists, decrease dosage further or control blood pressure with antihypertensives.

Psoriasis

● Measure blood pressure at least twice to determine a baseline.

● Evaluate patient for occult infection and tumors initially and throughout treatment.

● Obtain baseline creatinine level (on two occasions), CBC, and BUN, magnesium, uric acid, potassium, and lipid levels.

● Evaluate creatinine and BUN levels every 2 weeks during first 3 months and then monthly thereafter if patient is stable.

● If creatinine level is 25% above pre-treatment levels, repeat creatinine level measurement within 2 weeks. If creatinine level stays 25% to 50% above baseline, reduce dosage by 25% to 50%. If creatinine level is ever 50% above baseline, reduce dosage by 25% to 50%. Stop therapy if creatinine level isn't reversed after two dosage modifications.

● Monitor creatinine level after increasing NSAID dose or starting a new NSAID.

● Evaluate blood pressure, CBC, and uric acid, potassium, lipid, and magnesium levels every 2 weeks for the first 3 months and then monthly if patient is stable, or more frequently if a dosage is adjusted.

● If an adverse reaction occurs, reduce dosage by 25% to 50%.

● Improvement in psoriasis takes 12 to 16 weeks of therapy.

PATIENT TEACHING

● Encourage patient to take drug at same time each day and to be consistent with relation to meals.

● Teach patient how to measure dosage and mask taste of oral solution. Tell him not to take drug with grapefruit juice.

● Instruct patient to fill glass with water after dose and drink it to make sure he consumes all of drug.

● Advise patient to take drug with meals if nausea occurs.

● Advise patient to take Neoral or Gengraf on an empty stomach.

● Tell patient being treated for psoriasis that improvement may not occur until after 12 to 16 weeks of therapy.

● Stress that drug shouldn't be stopped without prescriber's approval.

Reactions may be *common*, uncommon, *life-threatening*, or COMMON AND LIFE-THREATENING.
Interaction may have a *rapid onset* or *delayed onset*.

• Explain to patient the importance of frequent laboratory monitoring while receiving therapy.
• Tell patient to avoid people with infections because drug lowers resistance to infection.
• Advise patient to perform careful oral care and to see a dentist regularly because drug can cause gum disease.
• Advise woman to use barrier contraception, not hormonal contraceptives, during therapy. Advise her of the potential risk during pregnancy and the increased risk of tumors, high blood pressure, and renal problems.
• Warn patient to wear protection in the sun and to avoid excessive sun exposure.

daclizumab
da-KLIZ-yoo-mab

Zenapax

Pharmacologic class: interleukin-2 receptor antagonist
Pregnancy risk category C

AVAILABLE FORMS
Injection: 25 mg/5 ml

INDICATIONS & DOSAGES
➤ **To prevent acute organ rejection in patients receiving renal transplants with an immunosuppressive regimen that includes cyclosporine and corticosteroids**
Adults: 1 mg/kg I.V. Standard course of therapy is five doses. Give first dose no more than 24 hours before transplantation; remaining four doses are given at 14-day intervals.

ADMINISTRATION
I.V.
• Protect undiluted solution from direct light.
• Dilute in 50 ml of sterile normal saline solution. To avoid foaming, don't shake.
• If drug contains particulates or is discolored, don't use.
• Give over 15 minutes via a central or peripheral line.

• Drug may be refrigerated at 36° to 46° F (2° to 8° C) for 24 hours and is stable at room temperature for 4 hours.
• Discard unused solution after 24 hours.
• **Incompatibilities:** Other drugs infused through same I.V. line.

ACTION
Inhibits interleukin-2 (IL-2) binding to prevent IL-2–mediated activation of lymphocytes, a critical pathway in the cellular immune response against allografts. Once in circulation, drug impairs response of immune system to antigenic challenges.

Route	Onset	Peak	Duration
I.V.	Unknown	Unknown	Unknown

Half-life: 20 days.

ADVERSE REACTIONS
CNS: anxiety, depression, dizziness, fatigue, fever, generalized weakness, headache, insomnia, pain, prickly sensation, tremor.
CV: aggravated hypertension, edema, chest pain, hypertension, hypotension, tachycardia, thrombosis.
EENT: blurred vision, pharyngitis, rhinitis.
GI: abdominal distention, abdominal pain, constipation, diarrhea, dyspepsia, epigastric pain, flatulence, gastritis, hemorrhoids, nausea, pyrosis, vomiting.
GU: *oliguria, renal tubular necrosis,* dysuria, hydronephrosis, renal damage, renal insufficiency, urinary tract bleeding, urinary tract disorder, urine retention.
Hematologic: *bleeding and clotting disorders,* lymphocele.
Metabolic: dehydration, *diabetes mellitus,* fluid overload.
Musculoskeletal: arthralgia, leg cramps, musculoskeletal or back pain, myalgia.
Respiratory: *hypoxia, pulmonary edema,* abnormal breath sounds, atelectasis, congestion, coughing, crackles, dyspnea, pleural effusion.
Skin: acne, hirsutism, impaired wound healing without infection, increased sweating, night sweats, pruritus, rash.
Other: *anaphylaxis, severe infection,* limb edema, shivering.

INTERACTIONS
Drug-drug. *Corticosteroids, cyclosporine, mycophenolate mofetil:* May increase

mortality, especially in patients taking antilymphocyte antibody therapy, and in those in whom severe infections develop. Monitor patient closely.

EFFECTS ON LAB TEST RESULTS
None reported.

CONTRAINDICATIONS & CAUTIONS
• Contraindicated in patients hypersensitive to drug or its components.
■ **Black Box Warning** Use cautiously and only under supervision of prescriber experienced in immunosuppressive therapy and management of organ transplantation. ■

NURSING CONSIDERATIONS
• *Alert:* Using cyclosporine, mycophenolate mofetil, and corticosteroids with this drug may be life-threatening. Monitor patients for increased risk of lympho-proliferative disorders and opportunistic infections.
• *Alert:* Monitor patient for severe, acute hypersensitivity reactions when giving each dose. Reactions may include anaphylaxis, hypotension, bronchospasm, loss of consciousness, injection site reactions, edema, and arrhythmias. If a severe reaction occurs, stop drug. Keep drugs for anaphylactic reactions immediately available.

PATIENT TEACHING
• Tell patient to consult prescriber before taking other drugs during therapy.
• Advise patient to practice infection prevention precautions.
• Inform patient that neither he nor any household member should receive vaccinations unless medically approved.
• Urge patient to immediately report wounds that fail to heal, unusual bruising or bleeding, fever, or any sign of allergic reaction.
• Advise patient to drink plenty of fluids during drug therapy and to report painful urination, bloody urine, or decreased urine volume.
• Instruct woman of childbearing age to use effective contraception before therapy starts and to continue for 4 months after therapy stops.

efalizumab
eh-fah-LEE-zoo-mab

Raptiva

Pharmacologic class:
immunosuppressant
Pregnancy risk category C

AVAILABLE FORMS
Injection: 125-mg single-use vial

INDICATIONS & DOSAGES
➤ **Chronic moderate to severe plaque psoriasis when systemic therapy or phototherapy is appropriate**
Adults: A single dose of 0.7 mg/kg subcutaneously followed by weekly doses of 1 mg/kg subcutaneously, beginning 1 week after first dose. Maximum single dose, 200 mg.

ADMINISTRATION
Subcutaneous
• Reconstitute the drug immediately before use.
• To reconstitute, inject 1.3 ml of sterile water for injection into the vial. Swirl gently for less than 5 minutes to dissolve powder. Don't shake.
• Use only sterile water as the diluent, and use a vial only once.
• Solution should be colorless to pale yellow and free of particulates. If not used immediately, store at room temperature for up to 8 hours.
• Don't add other drugs to solution.
• Rotate injection sites.
• Keep powder refrigerated, and protect vials from light.

ACTION
Binds to a leukocyte function antigen and decreases its expression, thus inhibiting the action of T lymphocytes at sites of inflammation, including psoriatic skin.

Route	Onset	Peak	Duration
Subcut.	1–2 days	Unknown	25 days

Half-life: Unknown.

ADVERSE REACTIONS
CNS: *stroke,* fever, *headache, pain.*
GI: *nausea.*

Reactions may be *common,* uncommon, *life-threatening,* or **COMMON AND LIFE-THREATENING.**
Interaction may have a *rapid onset* or **delayed onset.**

Musculoskeletal: back pain, myalgia.
Skin: acne.
Other: *chills,* flulike syndrome, hypersensitivity reaction, *infection.*

INTERACTIONS
Drug-drug. *Immunosuppressants:* May increase the risk of infection and malignancy if used together. Use with other immunosuppressants isn't recommended. *Vaccines:* May decrease or negate immune response to vaccine. Avoid using together.

EFFECTS ON LAB TEST RESULTS
• May increase alkaline phosphatase level.
• May increase leukocyte and lymphocyte counts. May decrease platelet count.

CONTRAINDICATIONS & CAUTIONS
• Contraindicated in patients hypersensitive to drug or its components and in patients with significant infection.
■ **Black Box Warning** Increased risk of infections including bacterial sepsis, invasive fungal disease and progressive leukoencephalopathy. Patient should be up to date with immunizations prior to beginning therapy. ■
• Use cautiously in patients with chronic infection or history of recurrent infection and in those with history of or high risk for malignancy.

NURSING CONSIDERATIONS
■ **Black Box Warning** Notify prescriber if patient develops signs of infection. ■
• Watch for evidence of thrombocytopenia. Check patient's platelet count monthly during initial treatment and then every 3 months.
• Monitor patient for worsening of psoriasis during or after therapy.

PATIENT TEACHING
• Tell patient to take the drug exactly as prescribed.
• Explain that platelet counts will be monitored during therapy.
• Urge patient to immediately report evidence of severe thrombocytopenia, such as bleeding gums, bruising, or petechiae.
• Tell patient to report weight changes because dose may need to be changed.
• Advise patient to report any infection or worsening psoriasis.

• Advise patient to hold off receiving vaccines during therapy because the immune response may be inadequate.
• Caution patient to immediately report pregnancy or suspected pregnancy.

etanercept
ee-tan-ER-sept

Enbrel

Pharmacologic class: tumor necrosis factor (TNF) blocker
Pregnancy risk category B

AVAILABLE FORMS
Injection: 25-mg multiuse vial
Prefilled syringe: 25 mg/0.5 ml, 50 mg/ml

INDICATIONS & DOSAGES
➤ **To reduce signs and symptoms of moderately to severely active polyarticular-course juvenile rheumatoid arthritis (RA) in patients whose response to one or more disease-modifying antirheumatic drugs has been inadequate**
Children ages 2 to 17: 0.8 mg/kg subcutaneously weekly (maximum 50 mg/week). For children weighing 63 kg (138 lb) or more, give weekly dose using the prefilled syringe. For children weighing 31 to 62 kg (68 to 136 lb), give total weekly dose as two subcutaneous injections, either on the same day or 3 or 4 days apart using the multiuse vial. For children weighing less than 31 kg (68 lb), give weekly dose as single subcutaneous injection using the correct volume from the multiuse vial. Glucocorticoids, NSAIDs, or analgesics may be continued during treatment. Use with methotrexate hasn't been studied in pediatric patients.
➤ **RA, psoriatic arthritis, ankylosing spondylitis**
Adults: 50 mg subcutaneously once weekly using the 50-mg/ml single-use prefilled syringe. Methotrexate, glucocorticoids, salicylates, NSAIDs, or analgesics may be continued during treatment.
➤ **Chronic moderate to severe plaque psoriasis in patients who are**

candidates for systemic therapy or phototherapy
Adults: 50 mg subcutaneously twice weekly, 3 to 4 days apart for 3 months. Then, reduce dose to 50 mg subcutaneously once weekly. Give dose using 50-mg/ml single-use prefilled syringes.

ADMINISTRATION
Subcutaneous
● Give 50-mg dose as one subcutaneous injection using a 50-mg/ml single-use prefilled syringe or as two 25-mg subcutaneous injections using multiuse vial. Give the two 25-mg injections on the same day or 3 to 4 days apart.
● Store prefilled syringe at 36° to 46° F (2° to 8° C), but let it reach room temperature (15 to 30 minutes) before use.
● Reconstitute multiple-use vial aseptically with 1 ml of supplied sterile bacteriostatic water for injection (0.9% benzyl alcohol). Use a 25G needle rather than the supplied vial adapter if the vial will be used for multiple doses. Don't filter reconstituted solution when preparing or giving drug. Inject diluent slowly into vial. Refrigerate in vial for up to 14 days at 36° to 46° F (2° to 8° C).
● Minimize foaming by gently swirling during dissolution rather than shaking. Dissolution takes less than 10 minutes.
● Don't use solution if it's discolored or cloudy, or if it contains particulate matter.
● Separate injection sites by at least 1 inch, rotate regularly, and never use areas where skin is tender, bruised, red, or hard. Use sites on the thigh, abdomen, and upper arm.
● *Alert:* Needle covers of diluent syringe and prefilled syringe contain latex and shouldn't be handled by persons sensitive to latex.
● **Incompatibilities:** Don't add other drugs or diluents to solution.

ACTION
Binds specifically to TNF and blocks its action with cell surface TNF receptors, reducing inflammatory and immune responses found in RA.

Route	Onset	Peak	Duration
Subcut.	Unknown	72 hr	Unknown

Half-life: About 5 days.

ADVERSE REACTIONS
CNS: *headache,* asthenia, dizziness.
EENT: *rhinitis,* pharyngitis, sinusitis.
GI: abdominal pain, dyspepsia.
Respiratory: *upper respiratory tract infections,* cough, respiratory disorder.
Skin: *injection site reaction,* rash.
Other: *infections,* **malignancies.**

INTERACTIONS
Drug-drug. *Anakinra:* Increased rate of serious infection when used together. Use together cautiously.
Cyclophosphamide: May increase risk of solid malignancies. Concurrent use not recommended.
Sulfasalazine: May cause decreased neutrophil count. Monitor patient carefully.
Vaccines: May affect normal immune response. Postpone live-virus vaccine until therapy stops.

EFFECTS ON LAB TEST RESULTS
None reported.

CONTRAINDICATIONS & CAUTIONS
● Contraindicated in patients hypersensitive to drug or its components, in those with sepsis, and in those receiving a live vaccine.
● Drug isn't indicated for use in children younger than age 2.
● Use cautiously in patients with underlying diseases that predispose them to infection, such as diabetes, heart failure, or history of active or chronic infections. Also use cautiously in RA patients with preexisting or recent onset of demyelinating disorders, including multiple sclerosis, myelitis, and optic neuritis.

NURSING CONSIDERATIONS
● Methotrexate, glucocorticoids, salicylates, NSAIDs, or analgesics may be continued during treatment in adults.
■ **Black Box Warning** Anti-TNF therapies that include drug may affect defenses against infection. If serious infection occurs, stop therapy and notify prescriber. ■
■ **Black Box Warning** Infections including bacterial sepsis and tuberculosis have

---

been reported. Evaluate patient's risk factors and test for latent tuberculosis. Begin treatment for latent tuberculosis prior to therapy with etanercept. ■

• *Alert:* Don't give live vaccines during therapy.

• If possible, bring patients with juvenile RA up-to-date with all immunizations before starting treatment.

• *Alert:* Histoplasmosis, coccidioido mycosis, blastomycosis, and other opportunistic infections may develop with use of this drug.

• Use of this drug may increase the risk of lymphoma.

PATIENT TEACHING

• If patient will be self-administering drug, advise him about mixing and injection techniques, including rotation of injection sites.

• Instruct patient to use puncture-resistant container for disposal of needles and syringes.

• Tell patient that injection site reactions generally occur within first month of therapy and decrease thereafter.

• Inform patient of importance of avoiding live vaccine administration during therapy.

• Stress importance of alerting other health care providers of etanercept use.

• Instruct patient to promptly report signs and symptoms of infection to prescriber, including persistent fever, cough, shortness of breath or fatigue.

• Advise woman to stop breast-feeding during therapy.

SAFETY ALERT!

glatiramer acetate injection
glah-TEER-ah-mer

Copaxone

Pharmacologic class: biologic response modifier
Pregnancy risk category B

AVAILABLE FORMS
Injection: 20 mg glatiramer acetate and 40 mg mannitol, USP, in a single-use prefilled syringe

INDICATIONS & DOSAGES
➤ **Reduce frequency of relapse in patients with relapsing-remitting multiple sclerosis**
Adults: 20 mg subcutaneously daily.

ADMINISTRATION
Subcutaneous
• Give drug only subcutaneously.
• Drug doesn't contain preservatives; discard if solution contains particulate matter.
• Don't try to expel the air bubble from the prefilled syringe. This may lead to loss of drug and an incorrect dose.
• Store drug in refrigerator (36° to 46° F [2° to 8° C]); allow drug to warm to room temperature for 20 minutes before use. If refrigeration is not available, may store at room temperature for up to 1 month.

ACTION
May modify immune processes responsible for the pathogenesis of multiple sclerosis.

Route	Onset	Peak	Duration
Subcut.	Unknown	Unknown	Unknown

Half-life: Unknown.

ADVERSE REACTIONS
CNS: *anxiety, asthenia,* abnormal dreams, agitation, confusion, emotional lability, *fever,* migraine, nervousness, *pain,* speech disorder, stupor, syncope, tremor, vertigo.
CV: *chest pain, palpitations, vasodilation,* hypertension, tachycardia.
EENT: *rhinitis,* ear pain, eye disorder, laryngismus, nystagmus.
GI: *diarrhea, nausea, anorexia,* bowel urgency, gastroenteritis, *GI disorder,* oral candidiasis, salivary gland enlargement, ulcerative stomatitis, *vomiting.*
GU: *urinary urgency,* **vaginal hemorrhage,** abnormal Papanicolaou smear, amenorrhea, *dysmenorrhea,* hematuria, impotence, menorrhagia, *vaginal candidiasis.*
Hematologic: *lymphadenopathy,* ecchymosis.
Metabolic: weight gain.
Musculoskeletal: *arthralgia, back pain, hypertonia,* footdrop, neck pain.
Respiratory: *dyspnea, bronchitis,* hyperventilation.
Skin: *diaphoresis, injection site reaction, pruritus, rash,* eczema, erythema or

hemorrhage, nodule, skin atrophy, urticaria, warts.

Other: *flulike syndrome, infection,* bacterial infection, chills, cyst, dental caries, herpes simplex and zoster, *peripheral and facial edema.*

INTERACTIONS
None significant.

EFFECTS ON LAB TEST RESULTS
None reported.

CONTRAINDICATIONS & CAUTIONS
• Contraindicated in patients hypersensitive to drug or mannitol.

NURSING CONSIDERATIONS
• Immediate postinjection reactions may occur; symptoms include flushing, chest pain, palpitations, anxiety, dyspnea, constriction of the throat, and urticaria. They typically are transient and self-limiting and don't need specific treatment. Onset of postinjection reaction may occur several months after treatment starts, and patients may have more than one episode.
• Patient may experience at least one episode of transient chest pain, which usually begins at least 1 month after treatment starts; it isn't accompanied by other signs or symptoms and doesn't appear to be clinically important.

PATIENT TEACHING
• Instruct patient how to self-inject drug. Supervise first injection.
• Explain need for aseptic self-injection techniques and warn patient against reuse of needles and syringes. Periodically review proper disposal of needles, syringes, drug containers, and unused drug.
• Tell patient to notify prescriber about planned, suspected, or known pregnancy.
• Tell woman to notify prescriber if she is breast-feeding.
• Advise patient not to change drug or dosage schedule or to stop drug without medical approval.
• Tell patient to notify prescriber immediately if dizziness, hives, profuse sweating, chest pain, difficulty breathing, or if severe pain occurs after drug injection.

infliximab
in-FLICKS-ih-mab

Remicade

Pharmacologic class: tumor necrosis factor (TNF) blocker
Pregnancy risk category B

AVAILABLE FORMS
Lyophilized powder for injection: 100-mg vial

INDICATIONS & DOSAGES
➤ **Moderately to severely active Crohn's disease; reduction in the number of draining enterocutaneous and rectovaginal fistulas and maintenance of fistula closure in patients with fistulizing Crohn's disease**
Adults: 5 mg/kg I.V. infusion over at least 2 hours. Repeat at 2 and 6 weeks, then every 8 weeks thereafter. For patients who respond and then lose their response, consider 10 mg/kg. Patients who don't respond by week 14 are unlikely to respond with continued therapy. In those patients, consider stopping drug.
Children age 6 to 17: For Crohn's disease, 5 mg/kg I.V. infusion over at least 2 hours. Repeat at 2 and 6 weeks, then every 8 weeks thereafter.
➤ **Moderately to severely active rheumatoid arthritis**
Adults: 3 mg/kg I.V. infusion over at least 2 hours. Repeat at 2 and 6 weeks after first infusion and every 8 weeks thereafter. Dose may be increased up to 10 mg/kg, or doses may be given every 4 weeks if response is inadequate. Use with methotrexate.
➤ **Moderate to severe ulcerative colitis**
Adults: Induction dose, 5 mg/kg I.V. over at least 2 hours. Repeat at 2 and 6 weeks, then every 8 weeks thereafter.
➤ **Ankylosing spondylitis**
Adults: 5 mg/kg I.V. infusion over at least 2 hours. Repeat at 2 and 6 weeks, then every 6 weeks thereafter.
➤ **Psoriatic arthritis, with or without methotrexate**
Adults: 5 mg/kg I.V. infusion over at least 2 hours. Repeat at 2 and 6 weeks after first infusion, then every 8 weeks thereafter.

➤ **Chronic severe plaque psoriasis**
Adults: 5 mg/kg I.V. infusion over at least 2 hours. Repeat dose in 2 and 6 weeks, then give 5 mg/kg every 8 weeks thereafter.

ADMINISTRATION
I.V.
● Reconstitute with 10 ml sterile water for injection, using syringe with 21G or smaller needle. Don't shake; gently swirl to dissolve powder. Solution should be colorless to light yellow and opalescent. It may also develop a few translucent particles; don't use if other types of particles develop or discoloration occurs.
● Dilute total volume of reconstituted drug to 250 ml with normal saline solution for injection. Infusion concentration range is 0.4 to 4 mg/ml.
● Use an in-line, sterile, nonpyrogenic, low–protein-binding filter with a pore size less than 1.2 micrometer.
● Begin infusion within 3 hours of preparation and give over at least 2 hours.
● **Incompatibilities:** Other I.V. drugs.

ACTION
Binds to human tumor necrosis factor (TNF)-alpha to neutralize its activity and inhibit its binding with receptors, thereby reducing the infiltration of inflammatory cells and TNF-alpha production in inflamed areas of the intestine.

Route	Onset	Peak	Duration
I.V.	Unknown	Unknown	Unknown

Half-life: 9½ days.

ADVERSE REACTIONS
CNS: *fatigue, fever, headache,* dizziness, depression, insomnia, malaise, pain, systemic and cutaneous vasculitis.
CV: *hypertension,* chest pain, flushing, hypotension, pericardial effusion, tachycardia.
EENT: *pharyngitis, rhinitis, sinusitis,* conjunctivitis.
GI: *abdominal pain, diarrhea, dyspepsia, nausea, intestinal obstruction,* constipation, flatulence, oral pain, ulcerative stomatitis, vomiting.
GU: *UTI,* dysuria, increased urinary frequency.

Hematologic: *leukopenia, neutropenia, pancytopenia, thrombocytopenia,* anemia, hematoma.
Musculoskeletal: *arthralgia, back pain,* arthritis, myalgia.
Respiratory: *coughing, upper respiratory tract infections,* bronchitis, dyspnea, respiratory tract allergic reaction.
Skin: *rash,* acne, alopecia, candidiasis, dry skin, eczema, erythema, erythematous rash, increased sweating, maculopapular rash, papular rash, urticaria.
Other: abscess, chills, ecchymosis, flulike syndrome, hot flashes, peripheral edema, toothache.

INTERACTIONS
Drug-drug. *Abatacept, anakinra:* May increase the risk of serious infections and neutropenia. Avoid using together.
Vaccines: May affect normal immune response. Postpone live-virus vaccine until therapy stops.

EFFECTS ON LAB TEST RESULTS
● May increase liver enzyme level. May decrease hemoglobin level and hematocrit.
● May decrease WBC and platelet counts.
● May cause false-positive antinuclear antibody test result.

CONTRAINDICATIONS & CAUTIONS
● Contraindicated in patients hypersensitive to murine proteins or other components of drug. Doses greater than 5 mg/kg are contraindicated in patients with moderate to severe heart failure.
● Use cautiously in elderly patients and in patients with active infection, history of chronic or recurrent infections, a history of hematologic abnormalities, or preexisting or recent onset of CNS demyelinating or seizure disorders; or in those who have lived in regions where histoplasmosis is endemic.

NURSING CONSIDERATIONS
● *Alert:* Watch for infusion-related reactions, including fever, chills, pruritus, urticaria, dyspnea, hypotension, hypertension, and chest pain during administration and for 2 hours afterward. If an

infusion-related reaction occurs, stop drug, notify prescriber, and give acetaminophen, antihistamines, corticosteroids, and epinephrine.
• Give for Crohn's disease and ulcerative colitis only after patient has an inadequate response to conventional therapy.
• Consider stopping treatment in patient who develops significant hematologic abnormalities or CNS adverse reactions.
• Notify prescriber for symptoms of new or worsening heart failure.
• **Alert:** Histoplasmosis, coccidioido-myocosis, blastomycosis, and other opportunistic infections may develop with use of this drug.
■ **Black Box Warning** Watch for development of lymphoma and infection. A patient with chronic Crohn's disease and long-term exposure to immunosuppressants is more likely to develop lymphoma and infection. ■
• Drug may affect normal immune responses. Patient may develop auto-immune antibodies and lupus-like syndrome; stop drug if this happens. Symptoms should resolve.
■ **Black Box Warning** Drug may cause disseminated or extrapulmonary tuberculosis and fatal opportunistic infections. ■
■ **Black Box Warning** Evaluate patient for latent tuberculosis infection with a tuberculin skin test. Treat latent tuberculosis infection before therapy. ■
• *Look alike–sound alike:* Don't confuse Remicade with Renacidin.

PATIENT TEACHING
• Tell patient about infusion-reaction symptoms and adverse effects and the need to report them promptly.
• Advise patient to seek immediate medical attention for signs and symptoms of infection, including persistent fever, cough, shortness of breath, or fatigue; or unusual bleeding or bruising.
• Tell woman to stop breast-feeding during therapy.
• Tell patient that before he receives vaccines, he should alert prescriber to therapy.
• Advise parent to get child up-to-date for all vaccines before therapy.

lymphocyte immune globulin (antithymocyte globulin [equine], ATG, LIG)
LIM-foh-site

Atgam

Pharmacologic class: immunoglobulin
Pregnancy risk category C

AVAILABLE FORMS
Injection: 50 mg of equine IgG/ml in 5-ml ampules

INDICATIONS & DOSAGES
➤ **To prevent acute renal allograft rejection**
Adults and children: 15 mg/kg I.V. daily for 14 days; then alternate-day therapy for 14 days. Give first dose within 24 hours of transplantation.
➤ **Acute renal allograft rejection**
Adults and children: 10 to 15 mg/kg I.V. daily for 14 days. Additional alternate-day therapy to total of 21 doses can be given. Start therapy when rejection is diagnosed.
➤ **Aplastic anemia**
Adults: 10 to 20 mg/kg I.V. daily for 8 to 14 days. Additional alternate-day therapy to total of 21 doses can be given.

ADMINISTRATION
I.V.
• Don't use solutions that are older than 12 hours, including actual infusion time.
• Dilute concentrated drug for injection before giving. Dilute required dose in 250 to 1,000 ml of half-normal or normal saline solution. Final concentration of drug shouldn't exceed 4 mg/ml.
• Allow diluted drug to reach room temperature before infusion.
• When adding drug to infusion solution, make sure container is inverted so drug doesn't contact air inside container. Gently rotate or swirl container to mix contents; don't shake because this may cause excessive foaming or denature the drug protein.
• Infuse with an in-line filter with a pore size of 0.2 to 1 micron over at least 4 hours (most institutions use 4 to 8 hours) into a vascular shunt, arterial venous fistula, or high-flow central vein.

Reactions may be *common*, uncommon, *life-threatening*, or COMMON AND LIFE-THREATENING.
Interaction may have a *rapid onset* or **delayed onset**.

• Refrigerate at 35° to 47° F (2° to 8° C). Concentrate is heat sensitive. Don't freeze.
• **Incompatibilities:** Don't dilute with dextrose solutions or those with a low salt concentration because a precipitate may form. Proteins in drug can be denatured by air. Drug is unstable in acidic solutions.

ACTION
Unknown. Inhibits cell-mediated immune responses either by altering T-cell function or eliminating antigen-reactive T cells.

Route	Onset	Peak	Duration
I.V.	Immediate	5 days	Unknown

Half-life: About 6 days.

ADVERSE REACTIONS
CNS: *seizures,* headache, malaise.
CV: *chest pain, hypotension,* edema, iliac vein obstruction, tachycardia, thrombophlebitis.
EENT: *laryngospasm.*
GI: *diarrhea, nausea, vomiting,* abdominal distention, epigastric pain, hiccups, stomatitis.
GU: renal artery stenosis.
Hematologic: LEUKOPENIA, THROMBO-CYTOPENIA, *aplastic anemia,* hemolysis, lymphadenopathy.
Metabolic: hyperglycemia.
Musculoskeletal: *arthralgia, myalgia.*
Respiratory: *dyspnea, pulmonary edema.*
Skin: *pruritus, rash, urticaria.*
Other: *anaphylaxis,* chills, febrile reactions, hypersensitivity reactions, infections, night sweats, serum sickness.

INTERACTIONS
None significant.

EFFECTS ON LAB TEST RESULTS
• May increase liver enzyme and glucose levels. May decrease hemoglobin level.
• May decrease WBC and platelet counts.

CONTRAINDICATIONS & CAUTIONS
• Contraindicated in patients hypersensitive to drug.
• Use cautiously in patients receiving additional immunosuppressive therapy (such as corticosteroids or azathioprine) because of increased risk of infection.

NURSING CONSIDERATIONS
• *Alert:* Do an I.D. skin test at least 1 hour before first dose. Give an I.D. dose of 0.1 ml of a 1:1,000 lymphocyte immune globulin along with a contralateral normal saline control. Marked local swelling or erythema larger than 10 mm indicates increased risk of severe systemic reaction such as anaphylaxis. Severe reactions to skin test, such as hypotension, tachycardia, dyspnea, generalized rash, or anaphylaxis, usually preclude further use of drug. Anaphylaxis may still occur in patients with negative skin tests.
■ **Black Box Warning** Drug should only be used by physicians experienced in immunosuppressive therapy in the treatment of renal transplant or aplastic anemia patients. ■
• Monitor patient for hypotension, respiratory distress, and chest, flank, or back pain, which may indicate anaphylaxis or hemolysis.
• Keep airway adjuncts and anaphylaxis drugs at bedside during administration.
• Watch for signs and symptoms of infection, such as fever, sore throat, malaise.

PATIENT TEACHING
• Instruct patient to report adverse drug reactions promptly, especially signs and symptoms of infection (fever, sore throat, fatigue).
• Tell patient to immediately report discomfort at I.V. insertion site because drug can cause a chemical phlebitis.
• Advise woman to avoid pregnancy during therapy.

muromonab-CD3
myoo-roh-MOH-nab

Orthoclone OKT3

Pharmacologic class: monoclonal antibody
Pregnancy risk category C

AVAILABLE FORMS
Injection: 1 mg/1 ml in 5-ml ampules

INDICATIONS & DOSAGES
➤ **Acute allograft rejection in renal transplant patients; steroid-resistant hepatic or cardiac allograft rejection**
Adults: 5 mg I.V. daily for 10 to 14 days.
Children: Initially, 2.5 mg/day (if 30 kg or less) or 5 mg/day (if more than 30 kg) I.V. as a single bolus over less than 1 minute for 10 to 14 days. Daily dosage may need 2.5-mg increment increases to decrease CD3+ cells.

ADMINISTRATION
I.V.
● Draw solution into syringe through low–protein-binding 0.2- or 0.22-micron filter. Discard filter and attach needle for I.V. bolus injection.
● Give bolus over less than 1 minute.
● Don't shake or freeze.
● **Incompatibilities:** Other I.V. drugs.

ACTION
A murine monoclonal antibody that reacts in the T-lymphocyte membrane with CD3, needed for antigen recognition. Depletes blood of CD3+ T cells, restoring allograft function and reversing rejection.

Route	Onset	Peak	Duration
I.V.	Immediate	Unknown	1 wk

Half-life: Unknown.

ADVERSE REACTIONS
CNS: *asthenia, fever, headache, tremor,* **meningitis, seizures,** confusion, depression, dizziness, fatigue, lethargy, malaise, nervousness, somnolence.
CV: *edema, hypertension, hypotension, tachycardia,* **arrhythmia, bradycardia, cardiac arrest, heart failure, shock,** chest pain, **vascular occlusion,** vasodilation.
EENT: photophobia, tinnitus.
GI: *diarrhea, nausea, vomiting,* abdominal pain, anorexia, GI pain.
GU: **anuria,** renal dysfunction.
Hematologic: anemia, leukocytosis, **leukopenia, thrombocytopenia.**
Musculoskeletal: arthralgia, myalgia.
Respiratory: *dyspnea,* **acute respiratory distress syndrome,** hyperventilation, **hypoxia,** pneumonia, **pulmonary edema,** respiratory congestion, wheezing.
Skin: diaphoresis, pruritus, *rash.*

Other: **anaphylaxis,** *chills,* **cytokine release syndrome,** hypersensitivity reactions, pain in trunk area.

INTERACTIONS
Drug-drug. *Immunosuppressants:* May increase risk of infection. Consider reducing immunosuppressant dosage. Use together cautiously.
Indomethacin: May increase muromonab-CD3 level, causing encephalopathy and other CNS effects. Monitor patient closely.
Live-virus vaccines: May increase replication and effects of vaccine. Use together cautiously.

EFFECTS ON LAB TEST RESULTS
● May increase BUN and creatinine levels.
● May cause abnormal urine cytologic study results.

CONTRAINDICATIONS & CAUTIONS
● Contraindicated in patients hypersensitive to drug or other products of murine (mouse) origin, in those who have history of seizures or are predisposed to seizures, in pregnant or breast-feeding women, and in patients with uncontrolled hypertension.
● Contraindicated in those with antimurine antibody titers of 1:1,000 or more or fluid overload, as evidenced by chest X-ray or weight gain greater than 3% the week before treatment.

NURSING CONSIDERATIONS
■ **Black Box Warning** Drug should be used only by physicians experienced in immunosuppressive therapy and management of solid organ transplant patients. ■
● Never give I.M.
● Obtain chest X-ray within 24 hours before starting drug treatment.
● Assess patient for signs and symptoms of fluid overload before treatment.
■ **Black Box Warning** Give therapy in facility equipped and staffed for cardio-pulmonary resuscitation, where patient can be monitored closely. ■
● Most adverse reactions develop within 30 minutes to 6 hours after first dose.
● Before giving drug, pretreat patient with an antipyretic to reduce risk of pyrexia and chills. Treat temperature over 100° F (38° C) with antipyretics before giving drug, and evaluate risk of infection.

Reactions may be *common,* uncommon, *life-threatening,* or COMMON AND LIFE-THREATENING.
Interaction may have a *rapid onset* or *delayed onset.*

• **Alert:** Methylprednisolone 8 mg/kg
1 to 4 hours before first dose to reduce
the severity of infusion reaction.
• Patients may develop antibodies to drug,
which can lead to loss of effectiveness and
more severe adverse reactions if a second
course is attempted.

PATIENT TEACHING
• Inform patient of expected adverse
reactions.
• Reassure patient that reactions will
diminish as treatment progresses.
• Tell patient to avoid people with infections because drug lowers resistance to
infection.
• Advise woman to avoid pregnancy
during therapy.

---

mycophenolate mofetil
my-koe-FIN-oh-late

CellCept

mycophenolate mofetil hydrochloride
CellCept Intravenous

mycophenolic acid
Myfortic

Pharmacologic class: mycophenolic
acid derivative
Pregnancy risk category D

AVAILABLE FORMS
mycophenolate mofetil
Capsules: 250 mg
Powder for oral suspension: 200 mg/ml
Tablets: 500 mg
mycophenolate mofetil hydrochloride
Injection: 500 mg/vial
mycophenolic acid
Tablets (extended-release): 180 mg,
360 mg

INDICATIONS & DOSAGES
➤ **To prevent organ rejection in
patients receiving allogenic renal
transplants**
Adults: 1 g I.V. or P.O. (regular-release)
b.i.d. with corticosteroids and cyclosporine. Or, 720 mg extended-release

tablets P.O. b.i.d. 1 hour before or 2 hours
after food.
*Children with a body surface area
(BSA) greater than 1.19 m²:* 400 mg/m²
extended-release tablets b.i.d. up to a
maximum of 720 mg b.i.d. Children with
a BSA of 1.19 to 1.58 m² may be dosed
with either three 180-mg tablets b.i.d. or
one 180-mg tablet plus one 360-mg tablet
b.i.d. for a total daily dosage of 1,080 mg.
Children with a BSA greater than 1.58 m²
can receive either four 180-mg tablets
b.i.d. or two 360-mg tablets b.i.d. for a
total daily dosage of 1,440 mg.
*Children 3 months to 18 years (mycophe-
nolate mofetil oral suspension only):*
600 mg/m² P.O. b.i.d., maximum dose
is 1 g b.i.d.
Adjust-a-dose: For patients with
severe chronic renal impairment
outside of immediate posttransplant
period, avoid doses above 1 g b.i.d.
If neutropenia develops, interrupt
or reduce dosage.
➤ **To prevent organ rejection in
patients receiving allogenic cardiac
transplant**
Adults: 1.5 g P.O. or I.V. b.i.d. with cyclosporine and corticosteroids.
➤ **To prevent organ rejection in
patients receiving allogenic hepatic
transplants**
Adults: 1 g I.V. b.i.d. over no less than
2 hours or 1.5 g P.O. b.i.d. with cyclosporine and corticosteroids.
Adjust-a-dose: If neutropenia develops,
stop or reduce dosage.

ADMINISTRATION
P.O.
• Don't crush tablets; don't open or crush
capsules.
• Avoid inhaling powder in capsule or
having it contact skin or mucous membranes. If contact occurs, wash skin thoroughly with soap and water, and rinse eyes
with water.
• The extended-release tablets are not
interchangeable with other forms.
I.V.
• Reconstitute and dilute to 6 mg/ml using
14 ml of D₅W.
• Never give by rapid or bolus I.V.
injection. Infuse drug over at least
2 hours.

- Use within 4 hours of reconstitution and dilution.
- **Incompatibilities:** Other I.V. drugs or solutions.

ACTION
Inhibits proliferative response of T and B lymphocytes, suppresses antibody formation by B lymphocytes, and may inhibit recruitment of leukocytes into sites of inflammation and graft rejection.

Route	Onset	Peak	Duration
P.O.	Unknown	30–75 min	7–18 hr
P.O. (extended-release)	Unknown	1½–2¾ hr	8–17 hr
I.V.	Unknown	Unknown	10–17 hr

Half-life: About 18 hours.

ADVERSE REACTIONS
CNS: *asthenia, fever, headache, pain, tremor, dizziness, insomnia, **progressive multifocal leukoencephalopathy.***
CV: *chest pain, edema, hypertension.*
EENT: *pharyngitis.*
GI: *abdominal pain, constipation, diarrhea, dyspepsia, nausea, oral candidiasis, vomiting, **hemorrhage.***
GU: *hematuria, UTI, **renal tubular necrosis.***
Hematologic: *anemia,* LEUKOPENIA, THROMBOCYTOPENIA, *hypochromic anemia, leukocytosis.*
Metabolic: *hypercholesterolemia, hyperglycemia, **hyperkalemia,** hypokalemia, hypophosphatemia.*
Musculoskeletal: *back pain.*
Respiratory: *cough, dyspnea, infection, bronchitis, pneumonia.*
Skin: *acne, rash.*
Other: *infection, sepsis.*

INTERACTIONS
Drug-drug. *Acyclovir, ganciclovir, other drugs that undergo renal tubular secretion:* May increase risk of toxicity for both drugs. Monitor patient closely.
Antacids with magnesium and aluminum hydroxides: May decrease mycophenolate absorption. Separate dosing times.
Azathioprine: Inhibits purine metabolism. Don't use together.
Cholestyramine: May interfere with enterohepatic recirculation, reducing

mycophenolate bioavailability. Avoid using together.
Phenytoin, theophylline: May increase both drug levels. Monitor drug levels closely.
Probenecid, salicylates: May increase mycophenolate level. Monitor patient closely.
Vaccines, live: May decrease vaccine's effectiveness. Avoid using together.
Drug-herb. *Cat's claw, echinacea:* May increase immunostimulation. Discourage use together.
Drug-food. *Food:* May delay absorption of extended-release form. Advise patient to take Myfortic on an empty stomach.

EFFECTS ON LAB TEST RESULTS
- May increase cholesterol and glucose levels. May decrease phosphorus and hemoglobin levels. May increase or decrease potassium level.
- May decrease platelet count. May increase or decrease WBC count.

CONTRAINDICATIONS & CAUTIONS
- Contraindicated in patients hypersensitive to drug, its ingredients, or mycophenolic acid and in patients sensitive to polysorbate 80.
- Use cautiously in patients with GI disorders.
- Oral suspension contains aspartame; use cautiously in patients with phenylketonuria or those who restrict intake of phenylalanine.

NURSING CONSIDERATIONS
- **Black Box Warning** Increased risk of infection and lymphoma may result from immunosuppression. ■
- **Black Box Warning** Drug should only be use by health care providers experienced in immunosuppressive therapy and management of renal, cardiac, or hepatic transplant patients. ■
- Start drug therapy within 24 hours after transplantation. Use I.V. form in patients unable to take oral forms.
- I.V. form can be given for up to 14 days; switch patient to capsules or tablets as soon as oral drugs can be tolerated.
- *Alert:* Drug may cause progressive multifocal leukoencephalopathy (PML). Consider PML in patients reporting neurologic symptoms.

PATIENT TEACHING
- Warn patient not to open or crush capsules nor to cut, crush, or chew extended-release tablets, but to swallow them whole on an empty stomach.
- Stress importance of following treatment as prescribed.
- Inform patient of the importance of follow-up visits and ongoing lab tests during therapy
- Tell woman to have a pregnancy test 1 week before therapy begins.
- ■ **Black Box Warning** Instruct woman to use two forms of contraception during therapy and for 6 weeks afterward, even if she has a history of infertility. Tell her to notify prescriber immediately if she suspects pregnancy. ■
- ■ **Black Box Warning** Warn patient of the increased risk of lymphoma and other malignancies. ■

---

natalizumab
nah-tah-LIZ-yoo-mab

Tysabri

Pharmacologic class: monoclonal antibody
Pregnancy risk category C

AVAILABLE FORMS
Injection: 300 mg/15 ml single-use vials

INDICATIONS & DOSAGES
➤ **To slow the accumulation of physical disabilities and reduce the frequency of clinical exacerbations in relapsing forms of multiple sclerosis (MS) for patients who failed to respond or were unable to tolerate other therapies. Or moderate to severe Crohn disease in patients with inadequate response or intolerance to conventional therapy.**
Adults: 300 mg I.V. over 1 hour every 4 weeks.

ADMINISTRATION
I.V.
- Dilute 300 mg in 100 ml normal saline solution.
- Invert I.V. bag gently to mix solution; don't shake.

- Infuse over 1 hour; don't give by I.V. push or bolus.
- Flush I.V. line with normal saline solution after infusion is complete.
- Refrigerate solution and use within 8 hours if not used immediately.
- **Incompatibilities:** Don't mix or infuse with other drugs. Don't use any diluent other than normal saline solution.

ACTION
May block interaction between adhesion molecules on inflammatory cells and receptors on endothelial cells of vessel walls.

Route	Onset	Peak	Duration
I.V.	Unknown	Unknown	Unknown

Half-life: 7 to 15 days.

ADVERSE REACTIONS
CNS: *progressive multifocal leuko-encephalopathy (PML),* depression, fatigue, headache, somnolence, vertigo.
CV: chest discomfort.
EENT: tonsillitis.
GI: *abdominal discomfort, diarrhea, gastroenteritis.*
GU: *UTI, vaginitis,* amenorrhea, dysmenorrhea, irregular menstruation, urinary frequency, urinary urgency, ovarian cyst.
Metabolic: weight increase or decrease.
Musculoskeletal: *arthralgia,* extremity pain, muscle cramps, swollen joints.
Respiratory: *lower respiratory tract infection.*
Skin: *rash,* dermatitis, pruritus, urticaria, night sweats.
Other: hypersensitivity reaction, infusion-related reaction, *tooth infections,* herpes, infection, rigors, seasonal allergy, cholelithiasis.

INTERACTIONS
Drug-drug. *Corticosteroids, other antineoplastics, immunosuppressants, and immunomodulating agents:* May increase risk of infection. Avoid using together.

EFFECTS ON LAB TEST RESULTS
- May increase liver function test values and lymphocyte, monocyte, eosinophil, basophil, and nucleated RBC counts.
- May cause transient decrease in hemoglobin.

CONTRAINDICATIONS & CAUTIONS
• Contraindicated in patients hypersensitive to drug or its components or in those with current or past history of PML. Use with other immunosuppressants isn't recommended.
• Safety and efficacy in patients with chronic progressive MS haven't been established.

NURSING CONSIDERATIONS
■ **Black Box Warning** Only prescribers registered in the TOUCH Prescribing Program may prescribe drug. Contact the TOUCH Prescribing Program at 1-800-456-2255. ■
• Report serious opportunistic and atypical infections to Biogen Idec at 1-800-456-2255 and to the FDA's MedWatch Program at 1-800-FDA-1088.
• The safety and efficacy of natalizumab treatment beyond 2 years are unknown.
■ **Black Box Warning** Drug may cause PML. Withhold drug immediately at the first signs or symptoms suggestive of PML. Symptoms include clumsiness; progressive weakness; and visual, speech, and sometimes personality changes. ■
• Obtain a brain MRI before starting therapy.
• *Alert:* Watch for evidence of hypersensitivity reaction during and for 1 hour after infusion, which may include dizziness, urticaria, fever, rash, rigors, pruritus, nausea, flushing, hypotension, dyspnea, and chest pain.
• If hypersensitivity reaction occurs, stop drug and notify prescriber.
• Patients who develop antibodies to drug have an increased risk of infusion-related reaction.
• Discontinue drug in patients with jaundice or other evidence of significant liver injury. Elevated serum hepatic enzymes and elevated total bilirubin levels may occur as early as 6 days after the first dose.

PATIENT TEACHING
• Tell patient to read the "Medication Guide for Tysabri" before each infusion.
• Urge patient to immediately report progressively worsening symptoms persisting over several days, including changes in thinking, eyesight, balance, or strength.

• Advise patient to inform all health care providers caring for him that he's receiving this drug.
• Tell patient to schedule follow-up appointments with prescriber at 3 and 6 months after the first infusion, then at least every 6 months thereafter.
• Urge patient to immediately report rash, hives, dizziness, fever, shaking chills, or itching while drug is infusing or up to 1 hour afterward.
• Tell patient about the potential for liver injury.

pimecrolimus
py-meck-roh-LY-mus

Elidel

Pharmacologic class: topical immunomodulator
Pregnancy risk category C

AVAILABLE FORMS
Cream: 1% 30-g, 60-g, and 100-g tubes. Base contains benzyl alcohol, cetyl alcohol, oleyl alcohol, and stearyl alcohol.

INDICATIONS & DOSAGES
➤ **Short- and intermittent long-term treatment of mild to moderate atopic dermatitis in nonimmuno-compromised patients in whom the use of other conventional therapies is deemed inadvisable, or in patients with inadequate response to or intolerance of conventional therapies**
Adults and children age 2 and older: Apply a thin layer to the affected skin b.i.d. and rub in gently and completely.

ADMINISTRATION
Topical
• Drug may be used on all skin surfaces, including the head, neck, and intertriginous areas.
• Clear infections at treatment sites before using.
• Don't use with occlusive dressing.

ACTION
Unknown. Inhibits T-cell activation and prevents the release of inflammatory cytokines and mediators from mast cells.

Reactions may be *common*, uncommon, *life-threatening*, or COMMON AND LIFE-THREATENING.
Interaction may have a *rapid onset* or **delayed onset**.

Route	Onset	Peak	Duration
Topical	Unknown	Unknown	Unknown

Half-life: Unknown.

ADVERSE REACTIONS

CNS: *headache, fever.*
EENT: *nasopharyngitis,* otitis media, sinusitis, pharyngitis, tonsillitis, eye infection, nasal congestion, rhinorrhea, sinus congestion, rhinitis, epistaxis, conjunctivitis, earache.
GI: gastroenteritis, abdominal pain, vomiting, diarrhea, nausea, constipation, loose stools.
GU: dysmenorrhea.
Musculoskeletal: back pain, arthralgias.
Respiratory: *upper respiratory tract infections, bronchitis, cough, asthma,* pneumonia, wheezing, dyspnea.
Skin: *application site reaction (burning, irritation, erythema, pruritus),* skin infections, impetigo, folliculitis, molluscum contagiosum, herpes simplex, varicella, papilloma, urticaria, acne.
Other: *influenza,* flulike illness, hypersensitivity, toothache, bacterial infection, staphylococcal infection, viral infection.

INTERACTIONS

Drug-drug. *Cytochrome P-450 inhibitors (such as erythromycin, itraconazole, ketoconazole, fluconazole, calcium channel blockers):* May affect metabolism of pimecrolimus. Use together cautiously.
Drug-lifestyle. *Natural or artificial sunlight exposure:* May worsen atopic dermatitis. Advise patient to avoid or minimize sunlight exposure.

EFFECTS ON LAB TEST RESULTS
None reported.

CONTRAINDICATIONS & CAUTIONS
• Contraindicated in patients hypersensitive to drug or its components, in patients with Netherton syndrome, and in immunocompromised patients.
• Contraindicated in patients with active cutaneous viral infections or infected atopic dermatitis.
■ **Black Box Warning** Contraindicated in children under age 2. ■

• Use cautiously in patients with varicella zoster virus infection, herpes simplex virus infection, or eczema herpeticum.
• Safety of use in pregnant women hasn't been established.

NURSING CONSIDERATIONS
• *Alert:* Use drug only after other therapies have failed because of the risk of cancer.
■ **Black Box Warning** Avoid continuous long-term use of drug and limit application to areas of involvement of atopic dermatitis. ■
• If symptoms persist longer than 6 weeks, reevaluate the patient.
• May cause local symptoms such as skin burning. Most local reactions start within 1 to 5 days after treatment, are mild to moderately severe, and last no longer than 5 days.
• Monitor patient for lymphadenopathy. If lymphadenopathy occurs and its cause is unknown, or if the patient develops acute infectious mononucleosis, consider stopping drug.
• Drug use may cause papillomas or warts. Consider stopping drug if papillomas worsen or don't respond to conventional treatment.
• It's unknown if drug appears in breast milk. Serious adverse reactions may occur in breast-feeding infants exposed to drug. Patient should either stop breast-feeding or stop treatment.

PATIENT TEACHING
• Inform patient that this drug is for external use only and that he should use it as directed.
• Tell patient to report adverse reactions.
• Tell patient not to use with an occlusive dressing.
• Instruct patient to wash hands after application if hands are not treated.
• Tell patient to stop therapy after signs and symptoms have resolved. If symptoms persist longer than 6 weeks, tell him to contact his prescriber.
• Tell patient to resume treatment at first signs of recurrence.
• Stress that patient should minimize or avoid exposure to natural or artificial sunlight (including tanning beds and UVA-UVB treatment) while using this drug.

• Tell patient to expect application site reactions but to notify his prescriber if reaction is severe or persists for longer than 1 week.

---

sirolimus
sir-AH-lih-mus

Rapamune

Pharmacologic class:
immunosuppressant
Pregnancy risk category C

AVAILABLE FORMS
Oral solution: 1 mg/ml
Tablet: 1 mg, 2 mg

INDICATIONS & DOSAGES
➤ **With cyclosporine and cortico-steroids, to prevent organ rejection in patients receiving renal transplants**
Adults and adolescents: Initially, 6 mg P.O. as one-time dose as soon as possible after transplantation; then maintenance dose of 2 mg P.O. once daily.
Children age 13 and older who weigh less than 40 kg (88 lb): First dose is 3 mg/m² P.O. as one-time dose after transplantation; then 1 mg/m² P.O. once daily.
Adjust-a-dose: For patients with mild to moderate hepatic impairment, reduce maintenance dose by about one-third. It isn't necessary to reduce loading dose. Two to 4 months after transplant in patients with low to moderate risk of graft rejection, taper off cyclosporine over 4 to 8 weeks. While tapering cyclosporine, adjust sirolimus dose every 1 to 2 weeks to obtain levels between 12 and 24 nanograms/ml. Base dosage adjustments on clinical status, tissue biopsies, and laboratory findings.
  Maximum daily dose shouldn't exceed 40 mg. If a daily dose exceeds 40 mg due to a loading dose, give the loading dose over 2 days. Monitor trough concentrations at least 3 to 4 days after a loading dose.

ADMINISTRATION
P.O.
• Give drug consistently either with or without food.

• Dilute oral solution before use. After dilution, use immediately and discard oral solution syringe.
• When diluting oral solution, empty correct amount into glass or plastic (not Styrofoam) container holding at least ¼ cup (60 ml) of either water or orange juice. Don't use grapefruit juice or any other liquid. Stir vigorously and have patient drink immediately. Refill container with at least ½ cup (120 ml) of water or orange juice, stir again, and have patient drink all contents.
• A slight haze may develop during refrigeration, which doesn't affect potency of drug. If haze develops, bring to room temperature and shake until haze disappears.
• Store away from light, and refrigerate at 36° to 46° F (2° to 8° C). After opening bottle, use contents within 1 month. If needed, store bottles and pouches at room temperature (up to 77° F [25° C]) for several days. Drug may be kept in oral syringe for 24 hours at room temperature.

ACTION
Inhibits T-cell activation and proliferation that occurs in response to antigenic and cytokine stimulation. Also inhibits antibody formation.

Route	Onset	Peak	Duration
P.O.	Unknown	1–3 hr	Unknown

Half-life: About 62 hours.

ADVERSE REACTIONS
CNS: *anxiety, asthenia, depression, fever, headache, insomnia, pain, tremor,* confusion, dizziness, emotional lability, hypertonia, hypesthesia, hypotonia, malaise, neuropathy, paresthesia, somnolence, syncope.
CV: *chest pain, edema, hypertension, peripheral edema,* **atrial fibrillation, heart failure, hemorrhage,** hypotension, palpitations, peripheral vascular disorder, tachycardia, thrombophlebitis, ***thrombosis,*** vasodilatation.
EENT: *pharyngitis,* abnormal vision, epistaxis, cataract, conjunctivitis, deafness, ear pain, otitis media, rhinitis, sinusitis, tinnitus.
GI: *abdominal pain, constipation, diarrhea, dyspepsia, nausea, vomiting,* anorexia, ascites, dysphagia, enlarged

---

Reactions may be *common,* uncommon, *life-threatening,* or COMMON AND LIFE-THREATENING.
Interaction may have a *rapid onset* or **delayed onset.**

abdomen, eructation, esophagitis, flatulence, gastritis, gastroenteritis, gingivitis, gum hyperplasia, hernia, ileus, peritonitis, mouth ulceration, oral candidiasis, stomatitis.

GU: *UTI, kidney tubular necrosis, toxic nephropathy,* albuminuria, bladder pain, dysuria, glycosuria, hematuria, hydronephrosis, impotence, kidney pain, nocturia, oliguria, pelvic pain, pyuria, scrotal edema, testis disorder, urinary frequency, urinary incontinence, urine retention.

Hematologic: *anemia,* THROMBOCYTOPENIA, *leukopenia, thrombotic thrombocytopenia purpura,* ecchymosis, leukocytosis, polycythemia.

Hepatic: *hepatic artery thrombosis, hepatotoxicity.*

Metabolic: *hypercholesteremia,* HYPERKALEMIA, *hyperlipidemia, hypokalemia, hypophosphatemia, weight gain, hypoglycemia, acidosis,* Cushing syndrome, *diabetes mellitus,* dehydration, hypercalcemia, hyperglycemia, hyperphosphatemia, hypervolemia, hypocalcemia, *hypomagnesemia,* hyponatremia, weight loss.

Musculoskeletal: *arthralgia, back pain,* arthrosis, bone necrosis, leg cramps, myalgia, osteoporosis, tetany.

Respiratory: *atelectasis, cough, dyspnea, upper respiratory tract infection, interstitial lung disease, asthma,* bronchitis, *hypoxia,* lung edema, pleural effusion, pneumonia.

Skin: *acne, rash,* fungal dermatitis, hirsutism, pruritus, skin hypertrophy, skin ulcer, sweating.

Other: *sepsis,* abnormal healing, including fascial dehiscence and anastomotic disruption (wound, vascular, airway, ureteral, biliary), abscess, cellulitis, chills, facial edema, flu syndrome, infection, lymphadenopathy, lymphocele.

INTERACTIONS
Drug-drug. *Aminoglycosides, amphotericin B, other nephrotoxic drugs:* May increase risk of nephrotoxicity. Use with caution.

Bromocriptine, cimetidine, clarithromycin, clotrimazole, danazol, erythromycin, fluconazole, indinavir, itraconazole, metoclopramide, nicardipine, ritonavir, verapamil, other drugs that inhibit CYP3A4:

May increase blood levels of sirolimus. Monitor sirolimus levels closely.

Carbamazepine, phenobarbital, phenytoin, rifabutin, rifapentine, other drugs that induce CYP3A4: May decrease blood levels of sirolimus. Monitor patient closely.

Cyclosporine: May increase sirolimus level and toxicity. Give sirolimus 4 hours after cyclosporine; monitor levels and adjust dose, as needed.

Diltiazem: May increase sirolimus levels. Monitor sirolimus level, as needed.

HMG-CoA reductase inhibitors or fibrates: May increase risk of rhabdomyolysis with the combination of sirolimus and cyclosporine. Monitor patient closely.

Ketoconazole: May increase rate and extent of sirolimus absorption. Avoid using together.

Live-virus vaccines: May reduce vaccine effectiveness. Avoid using together.

Rifampin: May decrease sirolimus level. Alternative therapy to rifampin may be prescribed.

Drug-food. *Grapefruit juice:* May decrease drug metabolism. Discourage use together.

Drug-lifestyle. *Sun exposure:* May increase risk of skin cancer. Advise patient to avoid sunlight exposure.

EFFECTS ON LAB TEST RESULTS
● May increase BUN, creatinine, liver enzyme, cholesterol, and lipid levels. May decrease sodium, magnesium, and hemoglobin levels. May increase or decrease phosphate, potassium, glucose, and calcium levels.
● May increase RBC count. May decrease platelet count. May increase or decrease WBC count.

CONTRAINDICATIONS & CAUTIONS
● Contraindicated in patients hypersensitive to active drug, its derivatives, or components of product.
● Use cautiously in patients with hyperlipidemia and impaired liver or renal function.
■ **Black Box Warning** Safety and effectiveness of sirolimus as immunosuppressive therapy haven't been established in liver or lung transplant patients. ■

NURSING CONSIDERATIONS

■ **Black Box Warning** Using this drug with tacrolimus or cyclosporine may cause hepatic artery thrombosis, leading to graft loss and death in liver transplant patients. ■

■ **Black Box Warning** Only those experienced in immunosuppressive therapy and management of renal transplant patients should prescribe drug. ■

● *Alert:* This drug has been associated with angioedema; using it with ACE inhibitors increases the risk. Monitor the patient closely.

● Use drug in regimen with cyclosporine and corticosteroids; have patient take drug 4 hours after cyclosporine dose.

● Cyclosporine withdrawal in patients with high risk of graft rejection isn't recommended. This includes patients with Banff grade III acute rejection or vascular rejection before cyclosporine withdrawal, those who are dialysis dependent, those with serum creatinine level greater than 4.5 mg/dl, black patients, patients with retransplants or multiorgan transplants, and patients with high panel of reactive antibodies.

● After transplantation, give antimicrobial prophylaxis for *Pneumocystis jiroveci (carinii)* for 1 year and for cytomegalovirus for 3 months.

■ **Black Box Warning** Patients taking drug are more susceptible to infection and lymphoma. ■

● Monitor renal function tests because use with cyclosporine may cause creatinine level to increase. Adjustment of immunosuppressive regimen may be needed.

● Monitor cholesterol and triglyceride levels. Treatment with lipid-lowering drugs during therapy isn't uncommon. If hyperlipidemia is detected, additional interventions, such as diet and exercise, should begin.

● Check for rhabdomyolysis.

● Monitor drug levels in patients age 13 and older who weigh less than 40 kg (88 lb), patients with hepatic impairment, those also receiving drugs that induce or inhibit CYP3A4, and patients in whom cyclosporine dosing is markedly reduced or stopped.

PATIENT TEACHING

● Teach patient how to properly store, dilute, and give drug.

● Advise woman about risks during pregnancy. Tell her to use effective contraception before and during therapy and for 12 weeks after stopping therapy.

● Tell patient to take drug consistently with or without food to minimize absorption variability.

● Tell patient to take drug 4 hours after cyclosporine to avoid drug interactions.

● Advise patient to wash area with soap and water if drug solution touches skin or mucous membranes.

---

tacrolimus
tack-ROW-lim-us

Prograf

Pharmacologic class: macrolide
Pregnancy risk category C

AVAILABLE FORMS
Capsules: 0.5 mg, 1 mg, 5 mg
Injection: 5 mg/ml

INDICATIONS & DOSAGES
➤ **To prevent organ rejection in allogenic liver, kidney, or heart transplant**

Adults: For patients who can't take drug orally, give 0.03 to 0.05 mg/kg/day (liver or kidney) or 0.01 mg/kg/day (heart) I.V. as continuous infusion at least 6 hours after transplant. Switch to oral therapy as soon as possible, with first dose 8 to 12 hours after stopping I.V. infusion. For renal transplant, give oral dose within 24 hours of transplantation after renal function has recovered. Initial P.O. dosages: For liver transplant, give 0.1 to 0.15 mg/kg daily in two divided doses every 12 hours; for kidney transplant, give 0.2 mg/kg daily in two divided doses every 12 hours; for heart transplant, give 0.075 mg/kg daily in two divided doses every 12 hours. Adjust dosages based on patient response.

Children (liver transplant only): Initially, 0.03 to 0.05 mg/kg daily I.V.; then 0.15 to 0.2 mg/kg daily P.O. on schedule similar to that of adults, adjusted as needed.

Reactions may be *common,* uncommon, *life-threatening,* or COMMON AND LIFE-THREATENING.
Interaction may have a *rapid onset* or **delayed onset.**

Adjust-a-dose: Give lowest recommended P.O. and I.V. dosages to patients with renal or hepatic impairment.

ADMINISTRATION
P.O.
● Give drug 1 hour before or 2 hours after a meal.
● Don't give with grapefruit juice.
I.V.
● Dilute drug with normal saline solution for injection or D₅W injection to 0.004 to 0.02 mg/ml before use.
● Monitor patient continuously during first 30 minutes and frequently thereafter for signs and symptoms of anaphylaxis.
● Store diluted infusion solution for up to 24 hours in glass or polyethylene containers. Don't store drug in a polyvinyl chloride container because of decreased stability and potential for extraction of phthalates.
● **Incompatibilities:** Solutions or I.V. drugs with a pH above 9, such as acyclovir and ganciclovir.

ACTION
Exact mechanism unknown. Inhibits T-cell activation, which results in immunosuppression.

Route	Onset	Peak	Duration
P.O., I.V.	Unknown	1½–3 hr	Unknown

Half-life: 33 to 56 hours.

ADVERSE REACTIONS
CNS: *asthenia, delirium, fever, headache, insomnia, pain, paresthesia, tremor,* **coma.**
CV: *peripheral edema,* hypertension.
GI: *abdominal pain, anorexia, ascites, constipation, diarrhea, nausea, vomiting.*
GU: *abnormal renal function, oliguria, UTI.*
Hematologic: THROMBOCYTOPENIA, *anemia, leukocytosis.*
Metabolic: *hyperglycemia,* HYPER-KALEMIA, *hypokalemia,* HYPO-MAGNESEMIA.
Musculoskeletal: *back pain.*
Respiratory: *atelectasis, dyspnea, pleural effusion.*
Skin: *burning, photosensitivity, pruritus, rash,* alopecia.

INTERACTIONS
Drug-drug. *Azole antifungals, bromo-criptine, cimetidine, clarithromycin, cyclo-sporine, danazol, diltiazem, erythromycin, methylprednisolone, metoclopramide, nicardipine, verapamil:* May increase tacrolimus level. Watch for adverse effects.
Carbamazepine, phenobarbital, pheny-toin, **rifamycins:** May decrease tacrolimus level. Monitor effectiveness of drug.
Cyclosporine: May increase risk of excess nephrotoxicity. Avoid using together.
Immunosuppressants (except adrenal corticosteroids): May oversuppress immune system. Monitor patient closely, especially during times of stress.
Inducers of cytochrome P-450 enzyme system: May increase tacrolimus metabo-lism and decrease blood levels. Dosage adjustment may be needed.
Inhibitors of cytochrome P-450 enzyme system (phenobarbital, phenytoin, rifampin): May decrease tacrolimus metabolism and increase blood level. Dosage adjustment may be needed.
Live-virus vaccines: May interfere with immune response to live-virus vaccines. Postpone routine immunizations.
Nephrotoxic drugs, such as aminoglyco-sides, amphotericin B, cisplatin, cyclo-sporine: May cause additive or synergistic effects. Monitor patient closely. Don't use tacrolimus simultaneously with cyclosporine. Stop cyclosporine at least 24 hours before starting tacrolimus.
Potassium-sparing diuretics: May cause severe hyperkalemia. Don't use together.
Sirolimus: May increase risk of wound healing complications, renal impairment, and insulin-dependent post-transplant dia-betes mellitus in heart transplant patients. Avoid using together.
Drug-herb. *St. John's wort:* May decrease drug level. Discourage use together.
Drug-food. *Any food:* May inhibit drug absorption. Urge patient to take drug on empty stomach.
Grapefruit juice: May increase drug level. Discourage patient from taking together.

EFFECTS ON LAB TEST RESULTS
● May increase BUN, creatinine, and glucose levels. May decrease magnesium and hemoglobin levels. May increase or

decrease potassium level and cause abnormal liver function test values.
●May decrease WBC and platelet counts.

CONTRAINDICATIONS & CAUTIONS
● Contraindicated in patients hypersensitive to drug.
● I.V. form is contraindicated in patients hypersensitive to castor oil derivatives.

NURSING CONSIDERATIONS
■ **Black Box Warning** Patient has increased risk for infections, lymphomas, and other malignant diseases. Only health care providers experienced in immunosuppressive therapy and management of organ transplant patients should use this drug. ■
● *Alert:* Because of risk of anaphylaxis, use injection only in patients who can't take oral form. Keep epinephrine 1:1,000 and oxygen available.
● Children with normal renal and hepatic function may need higher dosages than adults.
● Patients with hepatic or renal dysfunction should receive lowest dosage possible.
● Use with adrenal corticosteroids for all indications. For heart transplant patients, also use with azathioprine or mycophenolate mofetil.
● Don't use tacrolimus simultaneously with cyclosporine. Stop either drug at least 24 hours before initiating the other.
● Monitor patient for signs and symptoms of neurotoxicity and nephrotoxicity, especially if patient is receiving a high dose or has renal or hepatic dysfunction.
● Monitor patient for signs and symptoms of hyperkalemia, such as palpitations and muscle weakness or cramping. Obtain potassium levels regularly. Avoid potassium-sparing diuretics during drug therapy.
● Monitor patient's glucose level regularly. Also monitor patient for signs and symptoms of hyperglycemia, such as dizziness, confusion, and frequent urination. Treatment of hyperglycemia may be needed. Insulin-dependent posttransplant diabetes may occur; in some cases, it's reversible.

PATIENT TEACHING
● Advise patient to check with prescriber before taking other drugs during therapy.
● Urge patient to report adverse reactions promptly.
● Tell diabetic patient that glucose levels may increase.

tacrolimus (topical)
tack-ROW-lim-us

Protopic

Pharmacologic class: macrolide
Pregnancy risk category C

AVAILABLE FORMS
Ointment: 0.03%, 0.1%

INDICATIONS & DOSAGES
➤ **Moderate to severe atopic dermatitis in patients unresponsive to other therapies or unable to use other therapies because of potential risks**
Adults: Thin layer of 0.03% or 0.1% strength applied to affected areas b.i.d. and rubbed in completely.
Children age 2 and older: Thin layer of 0.03% strength applied to affected areas b.i.d. and rubbed in completely.

ADMINISTRATION
Topical
● In patients with infected atopic dermatitis, clear infections at treatment site before using drug.
● Don't use with occlusive dressings.
● Use only the 0.03% ointment in children ages 2 to 15.

ACTION
Unknown. Probably acts as an immune system modulator in the skin by inhibiting T-lymphocyte activation, which causes immunosuppression. Drug also inhibits the release of mediators from mast cells and basophils in skin.

Route	Onset	Peak	Duration
Topical	Unknown	Unknown	Unknown

Half-life: Unknown.

Reactions may be *common*, uncommon, *life-threatening*, or COMMON AND LIFE-THREATENING.
Interaction may have a *rapid onset* or *delayed onset*.

ADVERSE REACTIONS
CNS: *headache,* hyperesthesia, asthenia, insomnia, *fever,* pain.
CV: peripheral edema.
EENT: *otitis media, pharyngitis,* rhinitis, sinusitis, conjunctivitis.
GI: diarrhea, vomiting, nausea, abdominal pain, gastroenteritis, dyspepsia.
GU: dysmenorrhea.
Musculoskeletal: back pain, myalgia.
Respiratory: *increased cough,* **asthma,** pneumonia, bronchitis.
Skin: *burning, pruritus, erythema, infection, herpes simplex,* eczema herpeticum, pustular rash, *folliculitis,* urticaria, maculopapular rash, fungal dermatitis, acne, sunburn, tingling, benign skin neoplasm, vesiculobullous rash, dry skin, varicella zoster, herpes zoster, eczema, exfoliative dermatitis, contact dermatitis.
Other: *flulike symptoms, accidental injury, infection,* facial edema, alcohol intolerance, periodontal abscess, cyst, *allergic reaction.*

INTERACTIONS
Drug-drug. *Calcium channel blockers, cimetidine, CYP3A4 inhibitors (erythromycin, itraconazole, ketoconazole, fluconazole):* May interfere with effects of tacrolimus. Use together cautiously.
Drug-lifestyle. *Sun exposure:* May cause phototoxicity. Advise patient to avoid excessive sunlight or artificial ultraviolet light exposure.

EFFECTS ON LAB TEST RESULTS
None reported.

CONTRAINDICATIONS & CAUTIONS
• Contraindicated in patients hypersensitive to drug.
■ **Black Box Warning** Don't use in children less than 2 years of age. Only 0.03% ointment is indicated for children 2 to 15 years of age. ■
• Don't use in immunocompromised patients or in patients with Netherton syndrome or generalized erythroderma.
• *Alert:* Use only after other therapies have failed because of the risk of cancer.

NURSING CONSIDERATIONS
■ **Black Box Warning** Use drug only for short-term or intermittent long-term therapy. Rare cases of malignancy have been reported. ■
• If signs and symptoms of atopic dermatitis don't improve within 6 weeks, reevaluate patient to confirm the diagnosis.
• Use of this drug may increase the risk of varicella zoster, herpes simplex virus, and eczema herpeticum.
• Consider stopping drug in patients with lymphadenopathy if cause is unknown or acute mononucleosis is diagnosed.
• Monitor all cases of lymphadenopathy until resolution.
• Local adverse effects are most common during the first few days of treatment.

PATIENT TEACHING
• Tell patient to wash hands before and after applying drug and to avoid applying drug to wet skin.
• Urge patient not to use bandages or other occlusive dressings.
• Tell patient not to bathe, shower, or swim immediately after application because doing so could wash the ointment off.
• Tell patient to stop treatment when the signs and symptoms resolve.
• Advise patient to avoid or minimize exposure to natural or artificial sunlight.
• Caution patient not to use drug for any disorder other than that for which it was prescribed.
• Encourage patient to report adverse reactions.
• Tell patient to store the ointment at room temperature.

89

Antiglaucoma drugs

betaxolol hydrochloride
bimatoprost
brimonidine tartrate
carteolol hydrochloride
dorzolamide hydrochloride
latanoprost
levobunolol hydrochloride
timolol maleate
travoprost

---

betaxolol hydrochloride
beh-TAX-oh-lol

Betoptic, Betoptic S

Pharmacologic class: beta blocker
Pregnancy risk category C

AVAILABLE FORMS
Ophthalmic solution: 0.5%
Ophthalmic suspension: 0.25%

INDICATIONS & DOSAGES
➤ **Chronic open-angle glaucoma, ocular hypertension**
Adults: Instill 1 or 2 drops of 0.5% solution or 0.25% suspension b.i.d.

ADMINISTRATION
Ophthalmic
• Shake suspension well.
• Apply light finger pressure on lacrimal sac for 1 minute after instilling drug.
• Don't touch tip of dropper to eye or surrounding tissue.

ACTION
Unknown. Reduces aqueous formation and may increase outflow of aqueous humor.

Route	Onset	Peak	Duration
Ophthalmic	30–60 min	2 hr	> 12 hr

Half-life: Unknown.

ADVERSE REACTIONS
CNS: *stroke,* depressive neurosis, insomnia.

CV: *arrhythmias, heart block, heart failure,* palpitations.
EENT: *eye stinging on instillation causing brief discomfort,* erythema, itching, keratitis, occasional tearing, photophobia.
Respiratory: *bronchospasm, asthma.*

INTERACTIONS
Drug-drug. *Calcium channel blockers:* May cause AV conduction disturbances, ventricular failure, and hypotension if significant systemic absorption occurs. Monitor patient closely.
Cardiac glycosides: May cause excessive bradycardia if significant systemic absorption occurs. Patient may need ECG monitoring.
Dipivefrin, ophthalmic epinephrine: May produce mydriasis. Use together cautiously.
Inhaled hydrocarbon anesthetics: May prolong severe hypotension if significant systemic absorption occurs. Tell anesthesiologist that patient is receiving ophthalmic betaxolol.
Insulin, oral antidiabetics: May cause hypoglycemia or hyperglycemia if significant systemic absorption occurs. May need to adjust dosage of antidiabetics.
Phenothiazines: May have additive hypotensive effects; may increase risk of adverse effects if significant systemic absorption occurs. Monitor patient closely.
Prazosin: May increase risk of orthostatic hypotension in early phases of use together. Help patient stand slowly until effects are known.
Reserpine: May cause excessive beta blockade. Monitor patient closely.
Systemic beta blockers: May have additive effects. Monitor patient closely.
Verapamil: May increase effects of both drugs. Monitor cardiac function closely and decrease dosages as necessary.
Drug-lifestyle. *Cocaine use:* May inhibit betaxolol's effects. Tell patient about this interaction.
Sun exposure: May cause photophobia. Advise patient to wear sunglasses.

Reactions may be *common,* uncommon, *life-threatening,* or COMMON AND LIFE-THREATENING.
Interaction may have a *rapid onset* or **delayed onset.**

EFFECTS ON LAB TEST RESULTS
None reported.

CONTRAINDICATIONS & CAUTIONS
● Contraindicated in patients hypersensitive to drug and in those with sinus bradycardia, greater than first-degree AV block, cardiogenic shock, or overt heart failure.
● Use cautiously in patients with restricted pulmonary function, diabetes mellitus, hyperthyroidism, or history of heart failure.

NURSING CONSIDERATIONS
● Stabilization of intraocular pressure (IOP)–lowering response may take a few weeks. Determine IOP after 4 weeks of treatment.

PATIENT TEACHING
● Teach patient how to instill drug. Advise him to wash hands before and after instillation and to apply light finger pressure on lacrimal sac for 1 minute after instilling drug. Warn him not to touch tip of dropper to eye or surrounding tissue. Tell him to shake suspension well before instilling.
● Encourage patient to comply with twice-daily regimen.
● Tell patient to remove contact lenses before instilling drug. Lenses may be reinserted about 15 minutes after using drops.
● Advise patient to ease sun sensitivity by wearing sunglasses.

---

bimatoprost
by-MAT-oh-prost

Lumigan

Pharmacologic class: prostaglandin analogue
Pregnancy risk category C

AVAILABLE FORMS
Ophthalmic solution: 0.03%

INDICATIONS & DOSAGES
➤ **Increased intraocular pressure in patients with open-angle glaucoma or ocular hypertension**
Adults: Instill 1 drop in conjunctival sac of affected eye once daily in the evening.

ADMINISTRATION
Ophthalmic
● Don't touch tip of dropper to eye or surrounding tissue.
● If more than one ophthalmic drug is being used, give drugs at least 5 minutes apart.
● Store drug in original container between 59° and 77° F (15° and 25° C).

ACTION
Has ocular hypotensive activity, which selectively mimics the effects of naturally occurring prostaglandins. Drug may also increase outflow of aqueous humor.

Route	Onset	Peak	Duration
Ophthalmic	4 hr	8–12 hr	Unknown

Half-life: 45 minutes.

ADVERSE REACTIONS
CNS: headache, asthenia.
EENT: *conjunctival hyperemia, growth of eyelashes, ocular pruritus,* allergic conjunctivitis, asthenopia, blepharitis, cataract, conjunctival edema, eye discharge, tearing, and pain, eyelash darkening, eyelid erythema, foreign body sensation, increase in iris pigmentation, ocular burning, dryness, and irritation, photophobia, pigmentation of the periocular skin, superficial punctate keratitis, visual disturbance.
Respiratory: *upper respiratory tract infection.*
Skin: hirsutism.
Other: *infection.*

INTERACTIONS
None known.

EFFECTS ON LAB TEST RESULTS
● May cause abnormal liver function test values.

CONTRAINDICATIONS & CAUTIONS
● Contraindicated in patients hypersensitive to bimatoprost, benzalkonium chloride, or other ingredients in product.
● Contraindicated in patients with angle-closure glaucoma or inflammatory or neovascular glaucoma.
● Use cautiously in patients with renal or hepatic impairment.

• Use cautiously in patients with active intraocular inflammation (iritis, uveitis), aphakic patients, pseudophakic patients with torn posterior lens capsule, and patients at risk for macular edema.

NURSING CONSIDERATIONS

• Temporary or permanent increased pigmentation of iris and eyelid, as well as increased pigmentation and growth of eyelashes, may occur.
• Patient should remove contact lenses before using solution. Lenses may be reinserted 15 minutes after administration.

PATIENT TEACHING

• Tell patient receiving treatment in only one eye about potential for increased brown pigmentation of iris, eyelid skin darkening, and increased length, thickness, pigmentation, or number of lashes in treated eye.
• Teach patient how to instill drops, and advise him to wash hands before and after instilling solution. Warn him not to touch tip of dropper to eye or surrounding tissue.
• If eye trauma or infection occurs or if eye surgery is needed, tell patient to seek medical advice before continuing to use multidose container.
• Advise patient to immediately report eye inflammation or lid reactions.
• Advise patient to apply light pressure on lacrimal sac for 1 minute after instillation to minimize systemic absorption of drug.
• Tell patient to remove contact lenses before using solution and that lenses may be reinserted 15 minutes after administration.
• If patient is using more than one ophthalmic drug, tell him to apply them at least 5 minutes apart.
• Stress importance of compliance with recommended therapy.

brimonidine tartrate

bri-MOE-ni-deen

Alphagan P

Pharmacologic class: selective alpha₂ agonist
Pregnancy risk category B

AVAILABLE FORMS

Ophthalmic solution: 0.1%, 0.15%, 0.2%

INDICATIONS & DOSAGES

➤ **To reduce intraocular pressure in open-angle glaucoma or ocular hypertension**
Adults: 1 drop in affected eye t.i.d., about 8 hours apart.

ADMINISTRATION

Ophthalmic
• Don't touch tip of dropper to eye or surrounding tissue.

ACTION

Reduces aqueous humor production and increases uveoscleral outflow.

Route	Onset	Peak	Duration
Ophthalmic	Unknown	30 min–2½ hr	Unknown

Half-life: 2 hours.

ADVERSE REACTIONS

CNS: asthenia, dizziness, headache.
CV: hypertension, hypotension.
EENT: *allergic conjunctivitis, ocular hyperemia, pruritus,* abnormal vision, allergic reaction, blepharitis, burning, conjunctival edema, hemorrhage, or inflammation, dryness, eyelid edema or erythema, follicular conjunctivitis, foreign body sensation, increased tearing, pain, pharyngitis, photophobia, rhinitis, sinus infection or inflammation, stinging, superficial punctate keratopathy, visual disturbances, visual field defect, vitreous floaters, worsened visual acuity.
GI: dyspepsia, oral dryness.
Respiratory: bronchitis, cough, dyspnea.
Skin: rash.
Other: flulike syndrome.

INTERACTIONS

Drug-drug. *Apraclonidine, dorzolamide, pilocarpine, timolol:* May have additive IOP-lowering effects. Use cautiously together.
Antihypertensives, beta blockers, cardiac glycosides: May further decrease blood pressure or pulse. Monitor vital signs.
CNS depressants: May increase effects. Use cautiously together.
MAO inhibitors: May increase effects. Avoid using together.

Reactions may be *common*, uncommon, *life-threatening*, or COMMON AND LIFE-THREATENING.
Interaction may have a *rapid onset* or *delayed onset*.

Tricyclic antidepressants: May interfere with brimonidine's effect. Use cautiously together.
Drug-lifestyle. *Alcohol use:* May increase CNS-depressant effect. Urge patient to avoid alcohol.

EFFECTS ON LAB TEST RESULTS
None reported.

CONTRAINDICATIONS & CAUTIONS
● Contraindicated in patients hypersensitive to drug or benzalkonium chloride and in those taking MAO inhibitors.
● Use cautiously in patients with CV disease, cerebral or coronary insufficiency, hepatic or renal impairment, depression, Raynaud phenomenon, orthostatic hypotension, or thromboangiitis obliterans.

NURSING CONSIDERATIONS
● Monitor IOP because drug effect may reverse after first month of therapy.

PATIENT TEACHING
● Tell patient to wait at least 15 minutes after instilling drug before wearing soft contact lenses.
● Caution patient to avoid hazardous activities because of risk of decreased mental alertness, fatigue, or drowsiness.
● Advise patient to avoid alcohol.
● If patient is using more than one opthalmic drug, tell him to apply them at least 5 minutes apart.

---

carteolol hydrochloride
KAR-tee-oh-lol

Ocupress

Pharmacologic class: nonselective beta blocker
Pregnancy risk category C

AVAILABLE FORMS
Ophthalmic solution: 1%

INDICATIONS & DOSAGES
➤ **Chronic open-angle glaucoma, intraocular hypertension**
Adults: One drop into conjunctival sac of each affected eye b.i.d.

ADMINISTRATION
Ophthalmic
● Don't touch tip of dropper to eye or surrounding tissue.
● Apply light finger pressure on lacrimal sac for 1 minute after instilling to minimize systemic absorption.
● If more than one ophthalmic drug is being used, give at least 10 minutes apart.

ACTION
Exact mechanism unknown. Reduces intraocular pressure by decreasing aqueous humor production.

Route	Onset	Peak	Duration
Ophthalmic	Unknown	2 hr	12 hr

Half-life: Unknown.

ADVERSE REACTIONS
CNS: asthenia, dizziness, headache, insomnia.
CV: *arrhythmias, bradycardia,* hypotension, palpitations.
EENT: *burning, conjunctival hyperemia, edema, ocular tearing, transient eye irritation,* abnormal corneal staining, blepharoconjunctivitis, blurred and cloudy vision, corneal sensitivity, decreased night vision, photophobia, ptosis, sinusitis.
GI: constipation, diarrhea, nausea, taste perversion, vomiting.
Respiratory: *bronchospasm,* dyspnea.

INTERACTIONS
Drug-drug. *Aminophylline, theophylline:* May act antagonistically, reducing the effects of one or both drugs. May reduce elimination of theophylline. Monitor theophylline levels and patient closely.
Catecholamine-depleting drugs such as reserpine, oral beta blockers: May cause additive effects and development of hypotension or bradycardia. Monitor patient closely; monitor vital signs.
Clonidine: May cause significant increase in blood pressure when either drug is started or stopped. Monitor blood pressure if used together.
Epinephrine: May cause an initial hypertensive episode followed by bradycardia. Stop beta blocker 3 days before anticipated epinephrine use. Monitor patient closely.

Glucagon: May decrease the effect of glucagon. Monitor for therapeutic effect; consider oral glucose supplement if appropriate.

Insulin: May mask symptoms of hypoglycemia as a result of beta blockade (such as tachycardia). Use together cautiously in patients with diabetes.

Prazosin: May increase risk of orthostatic hypotension in early phases of use together. Assist patient to stand slowly until effects are known.

Verapamil: May increase effects of both drugs. Monitor cardiac function closely and decrease dosages as necessary.

Drug-lifestyle. *Sun exposure:* May cause photophobia. Advise patient to wear sunglasses.

EFFECTS ON LAB TEST RESULTS
None reported.

CONTRAINDICATIONS & CAUTIONS
• Contraindicated in patients hypersensitive to drug or its components and in those with bronchial asthma, severe COPD, sinus bradycardia, second- or third-degree AV block, overt cardiac failure, or cardiogenic shock.
• Use cautiously in patients hypersensitive to other beta blockers; in those with non-allergic bronchospastic disease, diabetes mellitus, hyperthyroidism, or decreased pulmonary function; and in breast-feeding women.

NURSING CONSIDERATIONS
• Monitor vital signs.
• *Alert:* Stop drug at first sign of cardiac failure, and notify prescriber.

PATIENT TEACHING
• If patient is using more than one topical ophthalmic drug, tell him to apply them at least 5 minutes apart.
• Teach patient how to instill drops. Advise him to wash hands before and after instillation, and warn him not to touch tip of dropper to eye or surrounding tissue.
• Advise patient to apply light finger pressure on lacrimal sac for 1 minute after drug instillation to minimize systemic absorption.

• Tell patient to remove contact lenses before instilling drug.
• Instruct patient to keep bottle tightly closed when not in use and to protect it from light.
• Tell patient that drug is a beta blocker and, although given topically, may be absorbed systemically, causing adverse effects. Advise patient to monitor heart rate and blood pressure closely, to report slow heart rate to prescriber, and, if signs or symptoms of serious adverse reactions or hypersensitivity occur, to stop drug and notify prescriber immediately.
• Stress importance of compliance with recommended therapy.
• Advise patient to ease sun sensitivity by wearing sunglasses.

dorzolamide hydrochloride
dor-ZOLE-ah-mide

Trusopt

Pharmacologic class: carbonic anhydrase inhibitor, sulfonamide
Pregnancy risk category C

AVAILABLE FORMS
Ophthalmic solution: 2%

INDICATIONS & DOSAGES
➤ **Increased intraocular pressure (IOP) in patients with ocular hyper-tension or open-angle glaucoma**
Adults and children: One drop into conjunctival sac of each affected eye t.i.d.

ADMINISTRATION
Ophthalmic
• Don't touch tip of dropper to eye or surrounding tissue.
• Apply light finger pressure on lacrimal sac for 1 minute after instilling to minimize systemic absorption.
• If more than one ophthalmic drug is being used, give at least 10 minutes apart.

ACTION
Decreases aqueous humor secretion, presumably by slowing the formation of bicarbonate ions. This reduces sodium and fluid transport, reducing IOP.

Reactions may be *common,* uncommon, *life-threatening,* or COMMON AND LIFE-THREATENING.
Interaction may have a *rapid onset* or **delayed onset.**

Route	Onset	Peak	Duration
Ophthalmic	1–2 hr	2–3 hr	8 hr

Half-life: 4 months.

ADVERSE REACTIONS
CNS: asthenia, fatigue, headache.
EENT: *blurred vision, dryness, lacrimation, ocular allergic reaction, ocular burning, stinging, and discomfort, photophobia, superficial punctate keratitis,* iridocyclitis.
GI: *bitter taste,* nausea.
GU: urolithiasis.
Skin: rash.

INTERACTIONS
Drug-drug. *Oral carbonic anhydrase inhibitors, salicylates:* May cause additive effects. Avoid using together.

EFFECTS ON LAB TEST RESULTS
None reported.

CONTRAINDICATIONS & CAUTIONS
• Contraindicated in patients hypersensitive to drug or its components.
• Use cautiously in patients with hepatic or renal impairment.

NURSING CONSIDERATIONS
• Normal IOP is 10 to 21 mm Hg.

PATIENT TEACHING
• Teach patient how to instill drops. Advise him to wash hands before and after instillation, and warn him not to touch tip of dropper to eye or surrounding tissue.
• Tell patient that drug is a sulfonamide and, although it's given topically, it can be absorbed systemically. Advise patient to apply light finger pressure on lacrimal sac for 1 minute after drug instillation to minimize systemic absorption.
• Tell patient to stop drug and notify prescriber immediately if signs or symptoms of serious adverse reactions or hypersensitivity occur, including eye inflammation and eyelid reactions.
• Tell patient not to wear soft contact lenses during therapy.
• Stress importance of compliance with recommended therapy.

latanoprost
lah-TAN-oh-prost

Xalatan

Pharmacologic class: prostaglandin analogue
Pregnancy risk category C

AVAILABLE FORMS
Ophthalmic solution: 0.005% (50 mcg/ml)

INDICATIONS & DOSAGES
➤ **Increased intraocular pressure (IOP) in patients with ocular hypertension or open-angle glaucoma who are intolerant or who had insufficient response to other IOP-lowering medications**
Adults: Instill 1 drop in conjunctival sac of each affected eye once daily at bedtime.

ADMINISTRATION
Ophthalmic
• Don't allow tip of dispenser to contact eye or surrounding tissue. Serious damage to eye and subsequent vision loss may be caused by contaminated solutions.
• Apply light finger pressure on lacrimal sac for 1 minute after instilling drug to minimize systemic absorption.
• If more than one ophthalmic drug is being used, give at least 5 minutes apart.

ACTION
Thought to increase outflow of aqueous humor, thereby lowering IOP.

Route	Onset	Peak	Duration
Ophthalmic	3–4 hr	8–12 hr	Unknown

Half-life: 3 hours (from aqueous humor).

ADVERSE REACTIONS
CV: angina pectoris.
EENT: *blurred vision, burning, foreign body sensation, increased brown pigmentation of the iris, itching, stinging,* conjunctival hyperemia, dry eye, excessive tearing, eye pain, eyelash changes, lid crusting or edema, lid discomfort, photophobia, punctate epithelial keratopathy.
Musculoskeletal: muscle, joint, or back pain.

Respiratory: upper respiratory tract infection.
Skin: allergic skin reaction, rash.
Other: cold, flulike syndrome.

INTERACTIONS
Drug-drug. *Eyedrops that contain thimerosal:* May cause precipitation of eyedrops. Give at least 5 minutes apart.

EFFECTS ON LAB TEST RESULTS
None reported.

CONTRAINDICATIONS & CAUTIONS
• Contraindicated in patients hypersensitive to drug, benzalkonium chloride, or other components of drug.
• Use cautiously in patients with impaired renal or hepatic function.
• Use cautiously in breast-feeding women; it's unknown if drug appears in breast milk.
• Safety and effectiveness of drug in children haven't been established.

NURSING CONSIDERATIONS
• Don't give drug while patient is wearing contact lenses.
• Giving drug more frequently than recommended may decrease its IOP-lowering effects; don't exceed once-daily dosing.
• Drug may gradually change eye color, increasing amount of brown pigment in iris. This change in iris color occurs slowly and may not be noticeable for months or years. Increased pigmentation may be permanent.

PATIENT TEACHING
• Inform patient of risk that iris color may change in treated eye.
• Teach patient how to instill drops, and advise him to wash hands before and after instilling solution. Warn him not to touch tip of dropper to eye or surrounding tissue.
• Advise patient to apply light finger pressure on lacrimal sac for 1 minute after instillation to minimize systemic absorption.
• Instruct patient to report reactions in the eye, especially eye inflammation and lid reactions.
• Tell patient who wears contact lenses to remove them before instilling solution and

not to reinsert the lenses until 15 minutes have elapsed.
• If patient is using more than one topical ophthalmic drug, tell him to apply them at least 5 minutes apart.
• If patient develops another eye condition (such as trauma or infection) or needs eye surgery, advise him to contact prescriber about continued use of multidose container.
• Stress importance of compliance with recommended therapy.

levobunolol hydrochloride
LEE-voe-BYOO-no-lahl

AKBeta, Betagan

Pharmacologic class: nonselective beta blocker
Pregnancy risk category C

AVAILABLE FORMS
Ophthalmic solution: 0.25%, 0.5%

INDICATIONS & DOSAGES
➤ **Chronic open-angle glaucoma, ocular hypertension**
Adults: One or two drops once daily (0.5%) or b.i.d. (0.25%).

ADMINISTRATION
Ophthalmic
• Don't let tip of dropper touch patient's eye or surrounding tissue.
• Apply light finger pressure on lacrimal sac for 1 minute after instilling drug to minimize systemic absorption.

ACTION
Thought to reduce formation, and possibly increase outflow, of aqueous humor.

Route	Onset	Peak	Duration
Ophthalmic	1 hr	2–6 hr	24 hr

Half-life: Unknown.

ADVERSE REACTIONS
CNS: *syncope,* depression, headache, insomnia.
CV: *hypotension,* **bradycardia, heart failure,** slight reduction in resting heart rate.

EENT: *transient eye stinging and burning,* blepharoconjunctivitis, corneal punctate staining, decreased corneal sensitivity, erythema, itching, keratitis, photophobia, tearing.
GI: nausea.
Respiratory: *bronchospasm.*
Skin: urticaria.

INTERACTIONS
Drug-drug. *Dipivefrin, epinephrine, systemically administered carbonic anhydrase inhibitors, topical miotics:* May further reduce intraocular pressure (IOP). Use together cautiously.
Metoprolol, propranolol, other oral beta blockers: May increase ocular and systemic effects. Use together cautiously.
Reserpine, other catecholamine-depleting drugs: May increase hypotensive and bradycardiac effects. Monitor blood pressure and heart rate closely.
Drug-lifestyle. *Sun exposure:* May cause photophobia. Advise patient to wear sunglasses.

EFFECTS ON LAB TEST RESULTS
None reported.

CONTRAINDICATIONS & CAUTIONS
● Contraindicated in patients hypersensitive to drug and in those with bronchial asthma, sinus bradycardia, second- or third-degree AV block, cardiac failure, cardiogenic shock, or history of bronchial asthma or severe COPD.
● Use cautiously in patients with chronic bronchitis, emphysema, diabetes mellitus, hyperthyroidism, or myasthenia gravis.
● Safe use in pregnant or breast-feeding women hasn't been established.

NURSING CONSIDERATIONS
● Normal IOP is 10 to 21 mm Hg.

PATIENT TEACHING
● Teach patient how to instill drug. Advise him to wash hands before and after instillation and to apply light finger pressure on lacrimal sac for 1 minute after drops are instilled.
● Warn patient not to touch tip of dropper to eye or surrounding tissue.
● Advise elderly patient to report shortness of breath, chest pain, or heart irregularities

to prescriber. Drug may be absorbed systemically and produce signs and symptoms of beta blockade.
● Advise patient to carry medical identification at all times during therapy.

---

timolol maleate
tye-MOE-lol

Betimol, Istalol, Timoptic, Timoptic-XE

Pharmacologic class: nonselective beta blocker
Pregnancy risk category C

AVAILABLE FORMS
Ophthalmic gel: 0.25%, 0.5%
Ophthalmic solution: 0.25%, 0.5%

INDICATIONS & DOSAGES
➤ **To reduce intraocular pressure (IOP) in ocular hypertension or open-angle glaucoma**
Adults: Initially, 1 drop of 0.25% solution in each affected eye b.i.d.; maintenance dosage is 1 drop once daily. If no response, instill 1 drop of 0.5% solution in each affected eye b.i.d. If IOP is controlled, reduce dosage to 1 drop daily. Or, 1 drop of gel in each affected eye once daily. Or, for Istalol, initially 1 drop 0.5% solution in each affected eye once daily in the morning. If response is unsatisfactory, concomitant therapy may be considered.

ADMINISTRATION
Ophthalmic
● Don't touch tip of dropper to eye or surrounding tissue.
● Apply light finger pressure on lacrimal sac for 1 minute after instilling drug to minimize systemic absorption.
● Give other ophthalmic drugs at least 10 minutes before giving gel form of drug.

ACTION
Thought to reduce formation, and possibly increase outflow, of aqueous humor.

Route	Onset	Peak	Duration
Ophthalmic	30 min	1–2 hr	12–24 hr

Half-life: Unknown.

ADVERSE REACTIONS

CNS: *syncope, **stroke,*** confusion, depression, dizziness, fatigue, hallucinations, lethargy.

CV: *hypotension, **arrhythmia, bradycardia, cardiac arrest, heart block, heart failure,*** palpitations, slight reduction in resting heart rate.

EENT: *burning and stinging* (Istalol), blepharitis, conjunctivitis, decreased corneal sensitivity with long-term use, diplopia, keratitis, minor eye irritation, ptosis, visual disturbances.

Metabolic: hyperglycemia, hyperuricemia.

Respiratory: ***bronchospasm in patients with history of asthma,*** dyspnea, respiratory infection.

INTERACTIONS

Drug-drug. *Aminophylline, theophylline:* May act antagonistically, reducing effects of one or both drugs; may also reduce elimination of theophylline. Monitor theophylline level and patient closely.

Calcium channel blockers, cardiac glycosides, quinidine: May increase risk of adverse cardiac effects if large amounts of timolol are systemically absorbed. Use together cautiously.

Cimetidine: May increase beta blocker effects. Consider another H_2 agonist or decrease dose of beta blocker.

Epinephrine: May cause a hypertensive episode, followed by bradycardia. Stop beta blocker 3 days before starting epinephrine. Monitor patient closely.

Insulin, oral antidiabetic agents: May mask symptoms of hypoglycemia (such as tachycardia) as a result of beta blockade. Use together cautiously in patients with diabetes.

Oral beta blockers: May increase ocular and systemic effects. Use together cautiously.

Prazosin: May increase risk of orthostatic hypotension in early phases of use together. Assist patient to stand slowly until effects are known.

Reserpine, other catecholamine-depleting drugs: May increase hypotensive and bradycardia-induced effects. Avoid using together.

Verapamil: May increase effects of both drugs. Monitor cardiac function closely and decrease dosages as necessary.

EFFECTS ON LAB TEST RESULTS

● May increase BUN, potassium, glucose, and uric acid levels.

CONTRAINDICATIONS & CAUTIONS

● Contraindicated in patients hypersensitive to drug and in those with bronchial asthma, sinus bradycardia, second- or third-degree AV block, cardiac failure, cardiogenic shock, or history of bronchial asthma or severe COPD.

● Use cautiously in patients with non-allergic bronchospasm, chronic bronchitis, emphysema, diabetes mellitus, hyperthyroidism, or cerebrovascular insufficiency.

NURSING CONSIDERATIONS

● Monitor diabetic patients carefully. Systemic beta-blocking effects can mask some signs and symptoms of hypoglycemia.

● Some patients may need a few weeks of treatment to stabilize pressure-lowering response. Determine IOP after 4 weeks of treatment.

● Drug can be used safely in patients with glaucoma who wear conventional polymethylmethacrylate (PMMA) hard contact lenses.

● ***Look alike–sound alike:*** Don't confuse timolol with atenolol, or Timoptic with Viroptic.

PATIENT TEACHING

● Teach patient how to instill drops. Advise him to wash hands before and after instillation and to apply light finger pressure on lacrimal sac for 1 minute after drops are instilled. Warn patient not to touch tip of dropper to eye or surrounding tissue.

● Instruct patient using gel to invert container and shake once before each use. Also tell him to use other ophthalmic drugs at least 10 minutes before applying gel.

● Tell patient to instill drug without contact lenses in place. Lenses may be reinserted about 15 minutes after drug use.

● Drug may be absorbed systemically and produce signs and symptoms of beta blockade. Advise patient to monitor pulse rate and report slow rate to prescriber.

● Tell patient to report difficulty breathing or chest pain to prescriber.

Reactions may be *common,* uncommon, *life-threatening,* or COMMON AND LIFE-THREATENING.
Interaction may have a *rapid onset* or ***delayed onset.***

travoprost
TRA-voe-prost

Travatan, Travatan Z

Pharmacologic class: prostaglandin
analogue
Pregnancy risk category C

AVAILABLE FORMS
Ophthalmic solution: 0.004%

INDICATIONS & DOSAGES
➤ **To reduce intraocular pressure
(IOP) in patients with open-angle
glaucoma or ocular hypertension
who can't tolerate or who respond
inadequately to other IOP-lowering
drugs**
Adults: One drop in conjunctival sac of
each affected eye once daily at bedtime.

ADMINISTRATION
Ophthalmic
• Don't touch tip of dropper to eye or
surrounding tissue.
• Apply light finger pressure on lacrimal
sac for 1 minute after instilling drug to
minimize systemic absorption.
• If using more than one ophthalmic drug,
give them at least 5 minutes apart.
• Store drug between 36° and 77° F
(2° and 25° C).

ACTION
Thought to reduce IOP by increasing
uveoscleral outflow.

Route	Onset	Peak	Duration
Ophthalmic	Unknown	30 min	Unknown

Half-life: 45 minutes.

ADVERSE REACTIONS
CNS: anxiety, depression, headache, pain.
CV: *bradycardia,* angina pectoris, chest
pain, hypertension, hypotension.
EENT: *eye discomfort, eye pain, eye
pruritus, decreased visual acuity, foreign
body sensation, ocular hyperemia,* abnormal vision, blepharitis, blurred vision,
cataract, conjunctival hyperemia, conjunctivitis, dry eye, eye disorder, iris discoloration, keratitis, lid margin crusting,
photophobia, sinusitis, subconjunctival
hemorrhage, tearing.
GI: dyspepsia, GI disorder.
GU: prostate disorder, urinary incontinence, UTI.
Metabolic: hypercholesterolemia.
Musculoskeletal: arthritis, back pain.
Respiratory: bronchitis.
Other: accidental injury, cold syndrome,
infection.

INTERACTIONS
Drug-herb. *Areca, jaborandi:* May
increase effects. Discourage use together.

EFFECTS ON LAB TEST RESULTS
• May increase cholesterol level.

CONTRAINDICATIONS & CAUTIONS
• Contraindicated in patients hypersensitive
to drug, benzalkonium chloride (Travatan),
or other drug components; in pregnant
women or women trying to become
pregnant; and in those with angle-closure,
inflammatory, or neovascular glaucoma.
• Use cautiously in patients with renal or
hepatic impairment, active intraocular
inflammation (iritis, uveitis), or risk
factors for macular edema.
• Use cautiously in aphakic patients
and pseudophakic patients with a torn
posterior lens capsule.

NURSING CONSIDERATIONS
• Temporary or permanent increased
pigmentation of the iris and eyelid may
occur as well as increased pigmentation
and growth of eyelashes.
• Patient should remove contact lenses
before instilling drug and reinsert them
15 minutes after administration.
• If a pregnant woman or a woman
attempting to become pregnant accidentally
comes in contact with drug, thoroughly
cleanse the exposed area with soap and
water immediately.
• Travatan contains benzalkonium chloride.
Travatan Z does not.

PATIENT TEACHING
• Teach patient how to instill drops, and
advise him to wash hands before and
after instilling solution. Warn him not to
touch tip of dropper to eye or surrounding
tissue.

- Advise patient to apply light finger pressure on lacrimal sac for 1 minute after instillation to minimize systemic absorption of drug.
- Tell patient to remove contact lenses before administration and explain that he can reinsert them 15 minutes afterward.
- Tell patient receiving treatment in only one eye about potential for increased iris pigmentation, eyelid darkening, and increased length, thickness, pigmentation, or number of lashes in the treated eye.
- If eye trauma or infection occurs or if eye surgery is needed, advise patient to seek medical advice before continuing to use the multidose container.
- Advise patient to immediately report eye inflammation or lid reactions.
- If patient is using more than one ophthalmic drug, tell him to apply them at least 5 minutes apart.
- Stress importance of compliance with recommended therapy.
- If a pregnant woman or a woman attempting to become pregnant accidentally comes in contact with drug, tell her to thoroughly cleanse the exposed area with soap and water immediately.

90

Miotics and mydriatics

atropine sulfate
carbachol (intraocular)
carbachol (topical)
phenylephrine hydrochloride
pilocarpine hydrochloride
pilocarpine nitrate
scopolamine hydrobromide

---

atropine sulfate
A-troe-peen

Atropine 1, Atropisol, Isopto
Atropine

Pharmacologic class:
antimuscarinic
Pregnancy risk category C

AVAILABLE FORMS
Ophthalmic ointment: 1%
Ophthalmic solution: 0.5%, 1%, 2%

INDICATIONS & DOSAGES
➤ **Acute iritis, uveitis**
Adults: Instill 1 to 2 drops up to q.i.d.
or apply small strip of ointment to
conjunctival sac up to t.i.d.
Children: Instill 1 to 2 drops of 0.5%
solution up to t.i.d. or apply small
strip of ointment to conjunctival sac
up to t.i.d.
➤ **Cycloplegic refraction**
Adults: One to two drops of 1% solution
1 hour before refraction. Or, apply 0.3 to
0.5 cm of ointment to the conjunctival sac
one to three times daily. Apply ointment
several hours before the procedure.
Children: One to two drops of 0.5% solution in each eye b.i.d. for 1 to 3 days
before eye examination and 1 hour before
refraction. Or, 0.3 cm of ointment in the
conjunctival sac t.i.d. daily for 1 to 3 days
before the procedure. Apply ointment
several hours before the procedure.

ADMINISTRATION
Ophthalmic
● Don't touch tip of dropper to eye or
surrounding tissue.

● Apply light finger pressure on
lacrimal sac for 2 to 3 minutes after
instilling drug to minimize systemic
absorption.

ACTION
Anticholinergic action leaves the pupil
under unopposed adrenergic influence,
causing it to dilate.

Route	Onset	Peak	Duration
Ophthalmic	Unknown	30 min– 3 hr	7–10 days

Half-life: Unknown.

ADVERSE REACTIONS
CNS: confusion, headache, somnolence.
CV: tachycardia.
EENT: *blurred vision,* conjunctivitis,
contact dermatitis of eye, eye dryness,
hyperemia, increased intraocular pressure
(IOP), irritation, ocular congestion with
long-term use, ocular edema, photophobia,
transient stinging and burning.
GI: abdominal distention in infants, dry
mouth.
Skin: dryness.

INTERACTIONS
Drug-lifestyle. *Sun exposure:* May cause
photophobia. Advise patient to wear
sunglasses.

EFFECTS ON LAB TEST RESULTS
None reported.

CONTRAINDICATIONS & CAUTIONS
● Contraindicated in patients hypersensitive to drug or belladonna
alkaloids and in those with glaucoma
or adhesions between the iris
and lens.
● Don't use atropine in infants age
3 months or younger because of possible
link between cycloplegia and development
of amblyopia.
● Use cautiously in elderly patients
and in others who may have increased
IOP.

NURSING CONSIDERATIONS
• *Alert:* Treat drops and ointment as poison (not for internal use); signs of poisoning are disorientation and confusion. Antidote of choice is physostigmine salicylate I.V. or I.M.
• Watch patient for signs and symptoms of glaucoma, including increased IOP, ocular pain, headache, and progressive blurring of vision; notify prescriber if they occur.
• Excessive use in children or in certain susceptible patients, including those with spastic paralysis, brain damage, or Down syndrome, may produce systemic symptoms of atropine poisoning.

PATIENT TEACHING
• Teach patient how to self-instill drug. Advise him to wash hands before and after instillation and to apply light finger pressure on lacrimal sac for 2 to 3 minutes after instillation. Warn patient not to touch tip of dropper or tube to eye or surrounding tissue.
• Warn patient to avoid hazardous activities, such as operating machinery or driving, until temporary blurring subsides.
• Advise patient to ease photophobia by wearing dark glasses or staying out of bright light.

---

carbachol (intraocular)
KAHR-buh-kawl

Carbastat, Miostat

carbachol (topical)
Carboptic, Isopto Carbachol

Pharmacologic class: direct-acting parasympathomimetic
Pregnancy risk category C

AVAILABLE FORMS
Intraocular injection: 0.01%
Topical ophthalmic solution: 0.75%, 1.5%, 2.25%, 3%

INDICATIONS & DOSAGES
➤ **To produce pupillary miosis in ocular surgery**
Adults: Before or after securing sutures, 0.5 ml (intraocular form) instilled gently into anterior chamber.
➤ **To reduce intraocular pressure in the treatment of glaucoma**
Adults: 1 or 2 drops (topical form) instilled every 4 to 8 hours.

ADMINISTRATION
Ophthalmic
• Don't touch tip of dropper to eye or surrounding tissue.
• Apply light finger pressure on lacrimal sac for 1 minute after instilling drug to minimize systemic absorption.

ACTION
A cholinergic that causes contraction of the sphincter muscles of the iris, resulting in miosis. Also produces ciliary spasm, deepening of the anterior chamber, and vasodilation of conjunctival vessels of the outflow tract.

Route	Onset	Peak	Duration
Intraocular	Seconds	2–5 min	24–48 hr
Ophthalmic (topical)	10–20 min	Unknown	4–8 hr

Half-life: Unknown.

ADVERSE REACTIONS
CV: *cardiac arrhythmia,* flushing, hypotension, syncope.
EENT: *transient stinging and burning,* bullous keratopathy, ciliary and conjunctival injection, conjunctival vasodilation, corneal clouding, eye and brow pain, iritis, retinal detachment, salivation, spasm of eye accommodation.
GI: diarrhea, epigastric distress, GI cramps, vomiting.
GU: frequent urge to urinate, tightness in bladder.
Respiratory: *asthma.*
Other: diaphoresis.

INTERACTIONS
Drug-drug. *Pilocarpine:* May cause additive effects. Use together cautiously.

Reactions may be *common,* uncommon, *life-threatening,* or COMMON AND LIFE-THREATENING.
Interaction may have a *rapid onset* or **delayed onset.**

Topical NSAIDs: May inactivate carbachol. Monitor patient for clinical effect.

EFFECTS ON LAB TEST RESULTS
None reported.

CONTRAINDICATIONS & CAUTIONS
• Contraindicated in patients hypersensitive to drug and in those with conditions in which cholinergic effects, such as constriction, are undesirable (acute iritis, some forms of secondary glaucoma, pupillary block glaucoma, or acute inflammatory disease of the anterior chamber).
• Use cautiously in patients with acute heart failure, bronchial asthma, peptic ulcer, hyperthyroidism, GI spasm, Parkinson disease, and urinary tract obstruction.

NURSING CONSIDERATIONS
• In case of toxicity, give atropine parenterally.
• Drug is used in open-angle glaucoma, especially when patients are resistant or allergic to pilocarpine hydrochloride or nitrate.
• **Alert:** Patients with hazel or brown irises may need stronger solutions or more frequent instillation because eye pigment may absorb drug.
• If tolerance to drug develops, prescriber may switch to another miotic for a short time.
• **Look alike–sound alike:** Don't confuse Isopto Carbachol with Isopto Carpine.

PATIENT TEACHING
• Teach patient how to instill drug. Advise him to wash hands before and after instillation and to apply light finger pressure on lacrimal sac for 1 minute after drops are instilled. Warn him not to exceed recommended dosage.
• Warn patient to avoid hazardous activities, such as operating machinery or driving, until temporary blurring subsides. Reassure patient that blurred vision usually diminishes with prolonged use.

• Tell glaucoma patient that long-term use may be needed. Stress compliance. Tell him to remain under medical supervision for periodic tests of intraocular pressure.
• Warn patient to use caution during night driving and while performing other hazardous activities in reduced light.

phenylephrine hydrochloride
fen-ill-EF-rin

AK-Dilate, Altafrin ◇ , Mydfrin, Neofrin, Prefrin Liquifilm ◇ , Relief ◇

Pharmacologic class:
sympathomimetic amine, adrenergic
Pregnancy risk category C

AVAILABLE FORMS
Ophthalmic solution: 0.12%, 2.5%, 10%

INDICATIONS & DOSAGES
➤ **Mydriasis without cycloplegia**
Adults and children: Instill 1 drop of 2.5% or 10% solution before examination. May repeat in 1 hour, as needed. May need to apply topical anesthetic before use to prevent stinging and dilution from lacrimation.
➤ **Mydriasis and vasoconstriction**
Adults and adolescents: Instill 1 drop of 2.5% or 10% solution.
Children: Instill 1 drop of 2.5% solution.
➤ **Chronic mydriasis**
Adults and adolescents: Instill 1 drop of 2.5% or 10% solution b.i.d. or t.i.d.
Children: Instill 1 drop of 2.5% solution b.i.d. or t.i.d.
➤ **Posterior synechiae
(adhesion of iris)**
Adults and children: To prevent or break posterior synechiae in patients with anterior uveitis, instill 1 drop of 10% solution three or more times daily in combination with atropine sulfate ophthalmic solution or ointment. To prevent posterior synechiae after iridectomy, instill 1 drop of 10% solution once or twice daily; give in combination with atropine sulfate ophthalmic solution or ointment if inflammation is

severe. Don't use 10% concentration in children younger than 1.

➤ **Minor eye irritations**
Adults and children: Instill 1 or 2 drops of the 0.12% solution in affected eye up to q.i.d., as needed.

ADMINISTRATION
Ophthalmic
● Don't touch tip of dropper to eye or surrounding tissue.
● Apply light finger pressure on lacrimal sac for 1 minute after instilling drug to minimize systemic absorption.
● Don't use brown solution or solution that contains precipitate.

ACTION
Dilates the pupil by contracting the dilator muscle.

Route	Onset	Peak	Duration
Ophthalmic	Rapid	10–90 min	3–7 hr

Half-life: Unknown.

ADVERSE REACTIONS
CNS: brow ache, headache.
CV: *hypertension with 10% solution, MI,* palpitations, PVCs, tachycardia.
EENT: allergic conjunctivitis, blurred vision, increased intraocular pressure (IOP), keratitis, lacrimation, reactive hyperemia of eye, rebound miosis, transient eye burning or stinging on instillation.
Skin: dermatitis, diaphoresis, pallor.
Other: trembling.

INTERACTIONS
Drug-drug. *Atropine (topical), cyclopentolate, homatropine, scopolamine:* May increase pupil dilation. Use together cautiously.
Beta blockers, MAO inhibitors: May cause arrhythmias because of increased pressor effect. Use together cautiously.
Levodopa: May reduce mydriatic effect of phenylephrine. Use together cautiously.
Tricyclic antidepressants: May increase cardiac effects of epinephrine. Use together cautiously.
Drug-lifestyle. *Sun exposure:* May cause photophobia. Advise patient to wear sunglasses.

EFFECTS ON LAB TEST RESULTS
● May lower IOP in normal eyes or in open-angle glaucoma; may cause false-normal tonometry readings.

CONTRAINDICATIONS & CAUTIONS
● Contraindicated in patients hypersensitive to drug, in those with angle-closure glaucoma, and in those who wear soft contact lenses.
● Use cautiously in patients with marked hypertension, cardiac disorders, advanced arteriosclerotic changes, type 1 diabetes, or hyperthyroidism; in children with low body weight; and in elderly patients.

NURSING CONSIDERATIONS
● Systemic adverse reactions are least likely with 0.12% and 2.5% solutions and most likely with 10% solution.
● *Look alike–sound alike:* Don't confuse Mydfrin with Midrin.

PATIENT TEACHING
● Teach patient how to instill drug. Advise him to wash hands before and after instillation and to apply light finger pressure on lacrimal sac for 1 minute after drops are instilled. Warn him not to touch tip of dropper to eye or surrounding tissue.
● Warn patient not to exceed recommended dosage because systemic effects can result. Monitor blood pressure and pulse rate.
● Tell patient not to use brown solution or solution that contains precipitate.
● Warn patient to avoid hazardous activities, such as operating machinery or driving, until temporary blurring subsides.
● Advise patient to contact prescriber if condition persists longer than 12 hours after stopping drug.
● Advise patient to ease photophobia by wearing dark glasses.

Reactions may be *common,* uncommon, *life-threatening,* or COMMON AND LIFE-THREATENING.
Interaction may have a *rapid onset* or *delayed onset.*

pilocarpine hydrochloride
pie-low-KAR-peen

Akarpine, Isopto Carpine, Pilocar, Pilopine HS

pilocarpine nitrate
Pharmacologic class: direct-acting parasympathomimetic
Pregnancy risk category C

AVAILABLE FORMS
pilocarpine hydrochloride
Ophthalmic gel: 4%
Ophthalmic solution: 0.25%, 0.5%, 1%, 2%, 3%, 4%, 5%, 6%, 8%, 10%
pilocarpine nitrate
Ophthalmic solution: 1%, 2%, 4%

INDICATIONS & DOSAGES
➤ **Primary open-angle glaucoma**
Adults and children: Instill 1 or 2 drops of 1% to 4% solution every 4 to 12 hours; adjust concentration and frequency to control intraocular pressure (IOP). Or apply 1.3-cm (½-inch) ribbon of 4% gel into the lower conjunctival sac once daily at bedtime.
➤ **Emergency treatment of acute angle-closure glaucoma**
Adults and children: Instill 1 drop of 2% solution every 5 to 10 minutes for three to six doses; then 1 drop every 1 to 3 hours until IOP is controlled.
➤ **Mydriasis caused by mydriatic or cycloplegic drugs**
Adults and children: Instill 1 drop of 1% solution.

ADMINISTRATION
Ophthalmic
• Don't touch tip of dropper to eye or surrounding tissue.
• Apply light finger pressure on lacrimal sac for 1 minute after instilling to minimize systemic absorption.
• If both solution and gel are used, the solution should be applied first; the gel is then applied at least 5 minutes later.

ACTION
A cholinergic that causes contraction of iris sphincter muscles, resulting in miosis, and that produces ciliary spasm, deepening of the anterior chamber, and vasodilation of conjunctival vessels of the outflow tract.

Route	Onset	Peak	Duration
Ophthalmic	10–30 min	30–85 min	4–8 hr

Half-life: Unknown.

ADVERSE REACTIONS
CV: hypertension, tachycardia.
EENT: *blurred vision, brow pain, myopia,* changes in visual field, ciliary spasm, conjunctival irritation, keratitis, lacrimation, lens opacity, periorbital or supraorbital headache, retinal detachment, salivation, transient stinging and burning.
GI: diarrhea, nausea, vomiting.
Respiratory: *pulmonary edema,* bronchiolar spasm.
Other: diaphoresis.

INTERACTIONS
Drug-drug. *Carbachol, echothiophate:* May cause additive effects. Avoid using together.
Cyclopentolate, ophthalmic belladonna alkaloids such as atropine, scopolamine: May decrease pilocarpine's antiglaucoma effect and block mydriatic effects of these drugs. Avoid using together.
Phenylephrine: May decrease dilation by phenylephrine. Avoid using together.

EFFECTS ON LAB TEST RESULTS
None reported.

CONTRAINDICATIONS & CAUTIONS
• Contraindicated in patients hypersensitive to drug and in conditions in which cholinergic effects, such as constriction, are undesirable (acute iritis, some forms of secondary glaucoma, pupillary block glaucoma, or acute inflammatory disease of the anterior chamber).
• Use cautiously in patients with acute cardiac failure, bronchial asthma, peptic ulcer, hyperthyroidism, GI spasm, urinary tract obstruction, and Parkinson disease.

NURSING CONSIDERATIONS
• Monitor vital signs.
• *Alert:* Patients with hazel or brown irises may need stronger solutions or more

frequent instillation because eye pigment may absorb drug.
- **Look alike–sound alike:** Don't confuse Isopto Carpine with Isopto Carbachol.

PATIENT TEACHING
- Instruct patient to apply gel at bedtime because it will blur vision. Warn him to avoid hazardous activities, such as operating machinery or driving, until temporary blurring subsides.
- Teach patient how to instill drug. Advise him to wash hands before and after instillation and to apply light finger pressure on lacrimal sac for 1 minute after drops are instilled. Warn patient not to touch applicator tip to eye or surrounding tissue.
- Tell patient that if other glaucoma medications and gel are used at bedtime, to apply the drops first; the gel is then applied at least 5 minutes later.
- Warn patient that transient brow pain and nearsightedness are common at first but usually disappear in 10 to 14 days.
- Advise patient to carry medical identification at all times during therapy.

---

scopolamine hydrobromide
skoe-POL-a-meen

Isopto Hyoscine

Pharmacologic class:
antimuscarinic, anticholinergic
Pregnancy risk category NR

AVAILABLE FORMS
Ophthalmic solution: 0.25%

INDICATIONS & DOSAGES
➤ **Cycloplegic refraction**
Adults: Instill 1 or 2 drops of 0.25% solution 1 hour before refraction.
Children: Instill 1 drop of 0.25% solution b.i.d. for 2 days before refraction.
➤ **Iritis, uveitis**
Adults: Instill 1 or 2 drops of 0.25% solution once daily to q.i.d.
Children: Instill 1 drop of 0.25% solution once daily to q.i.d.

ADMINISTRATION
Ophthalmic
- Don't touch tip of dropper to eye or surrounding tissue.
- Apply light finger pressure on lacrimal sac for 1 minute after instilling drug to minimize systemic absorption.

ACTION
Leaves the pupil under unopposed adrenergic influence, causing it to dilate.

Route	Onset	Peak	Duration
Ophthalmic	Rapid	15–45 min	< 1 wk

Half-life: Unknown.

ADVERSE REACTIONS
CNS: acute psychotic reactions, confusion, delirium, hallucinations, headache, somnolence.
CV: edema, tachycardia.
EENT: *blurred vision, photophobia,* conjunctivitis, eye dryness, increased intraocular pressure, ocular congestion with prolonged use, transient stinging and burning.
GI: dry mouth.
Skin: contact dermatitis, dryness.

INTERACTIONS
Drug-lifestyle. *Sun exposure:* May cause photophobia. Advise patient to wear sunglasses.

EFFECTS ON LAB TEST RESULTS
None reported.

CONTRAINDICATIONS & CAUTIONS
- Contraindicated in patients hypersensitive to drug and in those with shallow anterior chamber, angle-closure glaucoma, or adhesions between the iris and lens.
- Contraindicated in children with previous severe systemic reaction to atropine.
- Use cautiously in patients with cardiac disease and in infants, small children, and elderly patients.

NURSING CONSIDERATIONS
- Observe patients closely for adverse CNS effects, such as disorientation and delirium.
- Drug may be used in patients sensitive to atropine because it's faster acting and has

---

a shorter duration of action and fewer adverse reactions.

PATIENT TEACHING
● Teach patient how to instill drug. Advise him to wash hands before and after instillation and to apply light finger pressure on lacrimal sac for 1 minute after drops are instilled. Warn him to avoid touching tip of dropper to eye or surrounding tissue.
● Warn patient to avoid hazardous activities, such as operating machinery or driving, until temporary blurring subsides.
● Advise patient to ease sun sensitivity by wearing dark glasses.
● Instruct patient to carry medical identification at all times during therapy.
● Tell parents to avoid getting drug into child's mouth.
● Teach parents to wash their own hands and the child's hands after administration.

91

Nasal drugs

beclomethasone dipropionate
budesonide
ciclesonide
flunisolide
fluticasone propionate
(See Chapter 57, MISCELLANEOUS
RESPIRATORY DRUGS.)
olopatadine hydrochloride
oxymetazoline hydrochloride
phenylephrine hydrochloride
pseudoephedrine hydrochloride
pseudoephedrine sulfate
tetrahydrozoline hydrochloride
triamcinolone acetonide

---

beclomethasone dipropionate
be-kloe-METH-a-sone

Beconase AQ

Pharmacologic class:
corticosteroid
Pregnancy risk category C

AVAILABLE FORMS
Nasal spray: 42 mcg/metered spray

INDICATIONS & DOSAGES
➤ **To relieve symptoms of seasonal or perennial rhinitis, to prevent nasal polyp recurrence after surgical removal**
Adults and children 12 years and older:
1 or 2 sprays in each nostril b.i.d.
Children ages 6 to 12: 1 spray into each nostril b.i.d.

ADMINISTRATION
Intranasal
• Pump nasal spray three or four times before first use.
• Shake before use; pump once or twice before first use each day.

ACTION
May reduce nasal inflammation by inhibiting mediators of inflammation.

Route	Onset	Peak	Duration
Intranasal	5–7 days	3 wk	Unknown

Half-life: 15 hours.

ADVERSE REACTIONS
CNS: headache, light-headedness.
EENT: *mild, transient nasal burning and stinging,* dryness, epistaxis, nasal congestion, nasopharyngeal fungal infections, rhinorrhea, sneezing, watery eyes.
GI: nausea.
Metabolic: growth velocity reduction in children and adolescents.

INTERACTIONS
None significant.

EFFECTS ON LAB TEST RESULTS
None reported.

CONTRAINDICATIONS & CAUTIONS
• Contraindicated in patients hypersensitive to drug and in those with untreated localized infection involving the nasal mucosa.
• Not recommended for children less than 6 years.
• Use cautiously, if at all, in patients with active or quiescent respiratory tract tuberculous infections or untreated fungal, bacterial, or systemic viral or ocular herpes simplex infections.
• Use cautiously in patients who have recently had nasal septal ulcers, nasal surgery, or trauma until wound healing occurs.

NURSING CONSIDERATIONS
• Observe patient for fungal infections.
• Drug isn't effective for acute exacerbations of rhinitis. Decongestants or antihistamines may be needed.

PATIENT TEACHING
• Advise patient to pump nasal spray three or four times before first use.
• To instill, instruct patient to blow nose to clear nasal passages, shake container, tilt head slightly forward, and insert

---

Reactions may be *common,* uncommon, *life-threatening,* or COMMON AND LIFE-THREATENING.
Interaction may have a *rapid onset* or **delayed onset.**

nozzle into nostril, pointing away from septum. Tell him to hold other nostril closed and inhale gently while spraying, hold breath for a few seconds, and exhale through the mouth. Next, have him shake container and repeat in other nostril.
• Tell patient to pump nasal spray once or twice before first use each day. He should clean the cap and nosepiece of the activator in warm water every day, and then allow them to air-dry.
• Advise patient to use drug regularly, as prescribed, because its effectiveness depends on regular use.
• Explain that unlike decongestants, drug doesn't work right away. Most patients notice improvement within a few days, but some may need 2 to 3 weeks.
• Warn patient not to exceed recommended dosage because of risk of hypothalamic-pituitary-adrenal axis suppression.
• Tell patient to notify prescriber if signs and symptoms don't improve within 3 weeks or if nasal irritation persists.
• Teach patient good nasal and oral hygiene.

budesonide
byoo-DES-oh-nide

Rhinocort Aqua

Pharmacologic class: corticosteroid
Pregnancy risk category B

AVAILABLE FORMS
Nasal spray: 32 mcg/metered spray

INDICATIONS & DOSAGES
➤ **Symptoms of seasonal or perennial allergic rhinitis**
Adults and children age 6 and older:
1 spray in each nostril once daily. Maximum recommended dose for adults and children 12 and older is 4 sprays per nostril once daily (256 mcg daily). Maximum recommended dose for children ages 6 to 12 is 2 sprays per nostril once daily (128 mcg daily).

ADMINISTRATION
Intranasal
• Shake before each actuation.

ACTION
May reduce nasal inflammation by inhibiting mediators of inflammation.

Route	Onset	Peak	Duration
Intranasal	10 hr	2 wk	Unknown

Half-life: Unknown.

ADVERSE REACTIONS
EENT: epistaxis, nasal irritation, pharyngitis.
Respiratory: *bronchospasm,* cough.

INTERACTIONS
None significant.

EFFECTS ON LAB TEST RESULTS
None reported.

CONTRAINDICATIONS & CAUTIONS
• Contraindicated in patients hypersensitive to drug or its components and in those who have had recent septal ulcers, nasal surgery, or nasal trauma until total healing has occurred.
• Contraindicated in those with untreated localized nasal mucosa infections.
• Use cautiously in patients with tuberculous infections, ocular herpes simplex, or untreated fungal, bacterial, or systemic viral infections.

NURSING CONSIDERATIONS
• Systemic effects of corticosteroid therapy may occur if recommended daily dose is exceeded.

PATIENT TEACHING
• Tell patient to avoid exposure to chickenpox or measles.
• To instill drug, instruct patient to shake container before use, blow nose to clear nasal passages, and tilt head slightly forward and insert nozzle into nostril, pointing away from septum. Tell him to hold other nostril closed and inhale gently while spraying. Next, have him shake container and repeat in other nostril.
• Advise patient not to freeze, break, incinerate, or store canister in extreme heat; contents are under pressure.
• Advise patient to store canister with valve upward.

- Warn patient not to exceed prescribed dosage or use drug for long periods because of risk of hypothalamic-pituitary-adrenal axis suppression.
- Tell patient to notify prescriber if signs or symptoms don't improve or if they worsen in 3 weeks.
- Teach patient good nasal and oral hygiene.
- Tell patient to use drug within 6 months of opening the protective aluminum pouch.
- Instruct patient not to share drug because this could spread infection.

---

ciclesonide
si-CLEH-son-ide

Omnaris

Pharmacologic class:
nonhalogenated glucocorticoid
Pregnancy risk category C

AVAILABLE FORMS
Nasal spray: 50 mcg/metered spray

INDICATIONS & DOSAGES
➤ **Symptoms of perennial allergic rhinitis**
Adults and children age 12 and older:
2 sprays in each nostril once daily (200 mcg/day).
➤ **Symptoms of seasonal allergic rhinitis**
Adults and children age 6 and older:
2 sprays in each nostril once daily (200 mcg/day).

ADMINISTRATION
Intranasal
- Before first use, gently shake container, then prime by spraying eight times. If not used for 4 consecutive days, gently shake and reprime with 1 spray or until a fine mist appears.

ACTION
Hydrolyzed by the nasal mucosa to a biologically active metabolite with anti-inflammatory properties.

Route	Onset	Peak	Duration
Nasal	1–2 days	1–5 wk	Unknown

Half-life: Unknown.

ADVERSE REACTIONS
CNS: headache.
EENT: epistaxis, nasopharyngitis, ear pain, nasal discomfort.
Metabolic: growth retardation.

INTERACTIONS
None significant.

EFFECTS ON LAB TEST RESULTS
None reported.

CONTRAINDICATIONS & CAUTIONS
- Contraindicated in patients hypersensitive to the drug or its components.
- Contraindicated in patients who have had recent nasal septal ulcers, nasal surgery, or nasal trauma until healing has occurred.
- Use cautiously in patients who have changed from systemic to inhaled corticosteroids; renal insufficiency, steroid withdrawal (pain, lassitude, depression) or acute worsening of symptoms may occur.
- Use cautiously in immunosuppressed patients or in those with wounds; corticosteroids suppress the immune system.
- Use cautiously in children; may cause a decline in growth rate.
- Use cautiously in breast-feeding women.

NURSING CONSIDERATIONS
- Monitor infants born to mothers using drug during pregnancy for hypoadrenalism.
- Monitor patients who are switched from systemic to inhaled corticosteroids for worsening of symptoms and other side effects of withdrawal.
- Monitor children for decline in growth rate; potential to regain growth after drug is stopped hasn't been studied.
- Monitor patient for nasal side effects.

PATIENT TEACHING
- Teach patient how to use the spray properly. Refer patient to package insert.
- Instruct patient to contact his prescriber if he has no relief from symptoms after 1 week.
- Advise patient to use drug around the same time every day, as directed.
- Warn patient to avoid exposure to people with infections, such as chickenpox or measles; corticosteroids have immuno-suppressant effects.

Reactions may be *common*, uncommon, *life-threatening*, or COMMON AND LIFE-THREATENING.
Interaction may have a *rapid onset* or **delayed onset**.

• Tell patient to discard the bottle after 120 actuations following initial priming or 4 months after removal from foil pouch, whichever occurs first.

---

flunisolide
floo-NISS-oh-lide

Aerobid, Nasarel

Pharmacologic class: corticosteroid
Pregnancy risk category C

AVAILABLE FORMS
Nasal spray: 25 mcg/spray, 29 mcg/spray

INDICATIONS & DOSAGES
➤ **Symptoms of seasonal or perennial rhinitis**
Adults: Starting dose is 2 sprays in each nostril b.i.d. If needed, dosage may be increased to 2 sprays in each nostril t.i.d. Maximum total daily dose is 8 sprays in each nostril per day.
Children ages 6 to 14: Starting dose is 1 spray in each nostril t.i.d. or 2 sprays in each nostril b.i.d. Maximum total daily dose is 4 sprays in each nostril per day.

ADMINISTRATION
Intranasal
• Before use, prime the nasal spray by pushing down on the pump five or six times until a fine mist appears. If the pump hasn't been used for 5 days or more, the spray must be primed again.

ACTION
Exact mechanism unknown. Decreases nasal inflammation, mainly by stabilizing leukocyte lysosomal membranes.

Route	Onset	Peak	Duration
Intranasal	Unknown	Unknown	Unknown

Half-life: 1 to 2 hours.

ADVERSE REACTIONS
CNS: dizziness, headache.
EENT: *mild, transient nasal burning and stinging,* epistaxis, nasal dryness, nasal congestion, pharyngitis, sneezing, watery eyes.
GI: nausea, vomiting.

Respiratory: cough.
Other: *aftertaste,* hypersensitivity reaction, loss of taste and smell.

INTERACTIONS
None significant.

EFFECTS ON LAB TEST RESULTS
None reported.

CONTRAINDICATIONS & CAUTIONS
• Contraindicated in patients hypersensitive to drug and in those with untreated localized infection involving nasal mucosa.
• Use cautiously, if at all, in patients with active or quiescent respiratory tract tuberculous infections or untreated fungal, bacterial, or systemic viral or ocular herpes simplex infections.
• Use cautiously in patients who have recently had nasal septal ulcers, nasal surgery, or nasal trauma.

NURSING CONSIDERATIONS
• Drug isn't effective for acute exacerbations of rhinitis. Decongestants or antihistamines may be needed.
• *Look alike–sound alike:* Don't confuse flunisolide with fluocinonide, fluticasone, or Flumadine.

PATIENT TEACHING
• Tell patient to avoid exposure to chickenpox or measles.
• Instruct patient to shake container before use, blow nose to clear nasal passages, tilt head slightly forward, and insert nozzle into nostril, pointing away from septum. Tell him to hold other nostril closed and inhale gently while spraying. Have him repeat procedure in other nostril. Tell him to clean nosepiece with warm water daily.
• Explain that drug doesn't work right away. Most patients notice improvement within a few days, but some may need 2 to 3 weeks.
• Advise patient to use drug regularly, as prescribed.
• Warn patient not to exceed recommended dosage to avoid hypothalamic-pituitary-adrenal axis suppression.
• Tell patient to stop drug and notify prescriber if signs and symptoms don't diminish in 3 weeks or if nasal irritation persists.

✹ NEW DRUG

olopatadine hydrochloride
oh-loh-PAT-ah-dine

Patanase

Pharmacologic class: histamine$_1$-receptor antagonist
Pregnancy risk category C

AVAILABLE FORMS
Nasal spray: 665 mcg/100 ml

INDICATIONS & DOSAGES
➤ **Seasonal allergic rhinitis**
Adults and children age 12 years and older: 2 sprays into each nostril b.i.d.

ACTION
Selectively antagonizes H$_1$-receptor activity.
Absorption: Rapidly absorbed.
Distribution: 55% protein-bound, primarily to albumin.
Metabolism: Not extensively metabolized.
Excretion: 70% excreted in urine.

Route	Onset	Peak	Duration
Intranasal	Rapid	¼–2 hr	Unknown

Half-life: 8 to 12 hours.

ADVERSE REACTIONS
CNS: dizziness, fatigue, headache, malaise, somnolence.
EENT: nasal septum perforation, epistaxis, pharyngolaryngeal pain, postnasal drip, nasopharyngitis, throat irritation.
GI: *bitter taste,* dry mouth, thirst, abdominal pain, diarrhea, nausea.
GU: UTI, occult blood in urine.
Respiratory: cough, influenza.

INTERACTIONS
Drug-drug. *CNS depressants:* May cause additive sedative effects. Use together cautiously.
Drug-lifestyle. *Alcohol:* May increase CNS depression. Discourage using together.

EFFECTS ON LAB TEST RESULTS
● May increase CPK levels.

CONTRAINDICATIONS & CAUTIONS
● Contraindicated in patients hypersensitive to drug or its components.

NURSING CONSIDERATIONS
● Monitor nasal passages for ulceration before and during therapy.
● Monitor for somnolence.
● Give drug only if benefit to mother outweighs risk to fetus.
● Appearance of drug in breast milk isn't known. Use only if benefits to mother outweigh risk to child.
● Safety and efficacy haven't been established in children under age 12.
● Use cautiously in elderly patients because they may have impaired liver, renal, or cardiac function.

PATIENT TEACHING
● Tell patient to prime the spray before initial use, and again when spray hasn't been used for more than 7 days.
● Caution patient to avoid hazardous activities until drug effects are known.
● Tell patient to notify prescriber if epistaxis or nasal ulcerations occur.
● Warn patient to avoid spraying drug into eyes.
● Advise patient to avoid alcohol use while taking drug.

oxymetazoline hydrochloride
ox-i-met-AZ-oh-leen

Afrin ◇ , Dristan 12 Hour Nasal ◇ , Duramist Plus 12 Hour ◇ , Duration ◇ , Genasal ◇ , Neo-Synephrine 12 Hour Spray ◇ , Nostrilla ◇ , Vicks Sinex ◇

Pharmacologic class: sympathomimetic
Pregnancy risk category C

AVAILABLE FORMS
Nasal solution: 0.05% ◇

INDICATIONS & DOSAGES
➤ **Nasal congestion**
Adults and children age 6 and older: 2 to 3 sprays of 0.05% solution in each nostril b.i.d. Don't use for more than 3 days.

Reactions may be *common,* uncommon, *life-threatening,* or COMMON AND LIFE-THREATENING.
Interaction may have a *rapid onset* or **delayed onset.**

ADMINISTRATION
Intranasal
● Don't exceed two doses in a 24-hour period.
● Have patient sit upright and tilt head back slightly.
● Have patient occlude opposite nostril during administration.
● Wait 1 to 2 minutes between sprays.
● Rinse tip of container with hot water and dry with a clean tissue.

ACTION
Thought to cause local vasoconstriction of dilated arterioles, reducing blood flow and nasal congestion.

Route	Onset	Peak	Duration
Intranasal	5–10 min	6 hr	< 12 hr

Half-life: Unknown.

ADVERSE REACTIONS
CNS: anxiety, dizziness, headache, insomnia, restlessness.
CV: *CV collapse,* hypertension, palpitations.
EENT: dryness of nose and throat, increased nasal discharge, rebound nasal congestion or irritation, sneezing, stinging.
Other: systemic effects in children.

INTERACTIONS
None significant.

EFFECTS ON LAB TEST RESULTS
None reported.

CONTRAINDICATIONS & CAUTIONS
● Contraindicated in patients hypersensitive to drug and in children younger than age 6.
● Use cautiously in patients with hyperthyroidism, cardiac disease, hypertension, or diabetes mellitus.
● Use cautiously in those with difficulty urinating because of an enlarged prostate.

NURSING CONSIDERATIONS
● Monitor patient for rebound congestion or systemic effects.
● Don't give to children younger than age 6.

PATIENT TEACHING
● Teach patient how to use drug.
● Caution patient not to share drug because this could spread infection.
● Tell patient not to exceed recommended dosage and to use only when needed.
● Inform patient that prolonged use may result in rebound congestion.
● *Alert:* Warn patient that excessive use may cause slow or rapid heart rate, high blood pressure, dizziness, and weakness.

---

phenylephrine hydrochloride
fen-ill-EF-rin

Afrin Children's Pump Mist ◇,
Little Noses Gentle Formula ◇,
Neo-Synephrine ◇, Rhinall ◇,
Rhinall-10 Children's Flavored
Nose Drops ◇, Vicks Sinex Ultra
Fine Mist ◇

Pharmacologic class: adrenergic
Pregnancy risk category C

AVAILABLE FORMS
Nasal solution: 0.125%, 0.25%, 0.5%, 1%

INDICATIONS & DOSAGES
➤ **Nasal congestion**
Adults and children age 12 and older: 2 to 3 drops or 1 to 2 sprays in each nostril every 4 hours, p.r.n. Don't use for longer than 3 to 5 days.
Children ages 6 to 12: 2 to 3 drops or 1 to 2 sprays of 0.25% solution in each nostril every 4 hours, p.r.n.
Children ages 2 to 6: 2 to 3 drops of 0.125% solution every 4 hours, p.r.n.

ADMINISTRATION
Intranasal
● Give 1% solution no more often than every 4 hours. Don't give the 1% solution to children younger than age 12 unless directed by prescriber.
● To instill nose drops, have patient lie down and tilt his head back. Insert dropper no more than ⅓ inch into nostril. Don't touch side of nose. Patient should remain supine with head back for 2 minutes after dose.

• Tilt patient's head back slightly to give nasal spray. Gently occlude opposite nostril.
• When giving more than one spray, wait 1 to 2 minutes between sprays.
• Rinse tip of spray under hot water and dry with a clean tissue.

ACTION
Causes local vasoconstriction of dilated arterioles, reducing blood flow and nasal congestion.

Route	Onset	Peak	Duration
Intranasal	Rapid	Unknown	30 min–4 hr

Half-life: Unknown.

ADVERSE REACTIONS
CNS: dizziness, headache, nervousness, psychological disturbances, restlessness, tremor.
CV: *palpitations, tachycardia,* hypertension, pallor, PVCs.
EENT: dryness of nasal mucosa, rebound nasal congestion, transient burning or stinging.
GI: nausea.
Other: hypersensitivity reactions, sweating.

INTERACTIONS
Drug-drug. *Beta blockers:* May cause hypertension, then bradycardia. Avoid using together.
MAO inhibitors, methyldopa, tricyclic antidepressants: May potentiate the pressor response of phenylephrine. Avoid using within 14 days of an MAO inhibitor.

EFFECTS ON LAB TEST RESULTS
None reported.

CONTRAINDICATIONS & CAUTIONS
• Contraindicated in patients hypersensitive to drug.
• Use cautiously in patients with hyperthyroidism, marked hypertension, type 1 diabetes mellitus, cardiac disease, or advanced arteriosclerotic changes; in children with low body weight; and in elderly patients.

NURSING CONSIDERATIONS
• Monitor patient for systemic adverse effects.
• Don't use in children who are younger than age 2.

PATIENT TEACHING
• Teach patient how to use drug.
• Caution patient not to share drug because this could spread infection.
• Tell patient not to exceed recommended dosage and to use only when needed.
• Advise patient to contact prescriber if signs and symptoms persist longer than 3 days.
• Inform patient that prolonged use may result in rebound congestion.

pseudoephedrine hydrochloride
soo-dow-e-FED-rin

Cenafed◊, Decofed◊, Dimetapp Decongestant Pediatric◊, Dimetapp, Maximum Strength, Non-Drowsy◊, Genaphed◊, PediaCare Infants' Decongestant Drops◊, Sudafed◊, Triaminic◊

pseudoephedrine sulfate
Drixoral Non-Drowsy Formula◊

Pharmacologic class: adrenergic
Pregnancy risk category C

AVAILABLE FORMS
pseudoephedrine hydrochloride
Capsules: 30 mg◊, 60 mg◊
Drops: 7.5 mg/0.8 ml◊
Oral solution: 15 mg/5 ml◊, 30 mg/5 ml◊
Tablets: 30 mg◊, 60 mg◊
Tablets (chewable): 15 mg◊
Tablets (extended-release): 120 mg◊, 240 mg◊
pseudoephedrine sulfate
Tablets (extended-release): 120 mg (60 mg immediate-release, 60 mg delayed-release)◊

INDICATIONS & DOSAGES
➤ **To decongest nose and eustachian tube**
Adults and children older than age 12: 60 mg P.O. every 4 to 6 hours; or 120 mg P.O. extended-release tablet every 12 hours; or 240 mg P.O. extended-release tablet once daily. Maximum dosage is 240 mg daily.

Reactions may be *common,* uncommon, *life-threatening,* or COMMON AND LIFE-THREATENING.
Interaction may have a *rapid onset* or **delayed onset.**

Children ages 6 to 12: 30 mg P.O. every 4 to 6 hours. Maximum dosage is 120 mg daily.
Children ages 2 to 5: 15 mg P.O. every 4 to 6 hours. Maximum dosage is 60 mg daily.

ADMINISTRATION
P.O.
• Don't crush or break extended-release forms.

ACTION
Stimulates alpha receptors in the respiratory tract, constricting blood vessels, shrinking swollen nasal mucous membranes, increasing airway patency, and reducing tissue hyperemia, edema, and nasal congestion.

Route	Onset	Peak	Duration
P.O.	30 min	30–60 min	4–12 hr

Half-life: Unknown.

ADVERSE REACTIONS
CNS: *anxiety, nervousness,* dizziness, headache, insomnia, transient stimulation, tremor.
CV: *palpitations, arrhythmias, CV collapse,* tachycardia.
GI: anorexia, dry mouth, nausea, vomiting.
GU: difficulty urinating.
Respiratory: *respiratory difficulties.*
Skin: pallor.
Other: diaphoresis.

INTERACTIONS
Drug-drug. *Antihypertensives:* May inhibit hypotensive effect. Monitor blood pressure closely.
MAO inhibitors (phenelzine, tranylcypromine): May cause severe headache, hypertension, fever, and hypertensive crisis. Avoid using together.
Methyldopa, reserpine: May increase pressor response. Monitor patient closely.

EFFECTS ON LAB TEST RESULTS
None reported.

CONTRAINDICATIONS & CAUTIONS
• Contraindicated in patients with severe hypertension or severe coronary artery disease, in those receiving MAO inhibitors, and in breast-feeding women. Extended-release forms are contraindicated in children younger than age 12.
• Use cautiously in patients with hypertension, cardiac disease, diabetes, glaucoma, hyperthyroidism, and prostatic hyperplasia.

NURSING CONSIDERATIONS
• Elderly patients are more sensitive to drug's effects. Extended-release tablets shouldn't be given to elderly patients until safety with short-acting preparations has been established.

PATIENT TEACHING
• Tell patient not to crush or break extended-release forms.
• Warn against using OTC products containing other sympathomimetics.
• Instruct patient not to take drug within 2 hours of bedtime because it can cause insomnia.
• Tell patient to stop drug and notify prescriber if he becomes unusually restless.

---

tetrahydrozoline hydrochloride
tet-rah-hi-DRAZ-oh-leen

Tyzine

Pharmacologic class:
sympathomimetic
Pregnancy risk category C

AVAILABLE FORMS
Nasal solution: 0.05%, 0.1%

INDICATIONS & DOSAGES
➤ **Nasal congestion**
Adults and children older than age 6: 2 to 4 drops or 3 to 4 sprays of 0.1% solution in each nostril no more than every 3 hours, p.r.n.
Children ages 2 to 6: Give 2 to 3 drops of 0.05% solution in each nostril no more than every 3 hours, p.r.n.

ADMINISTRATION
Intranasal
• Instill nose drops with patient in lateral head-low position.

- Give spray with patient's head tilted back slightly. Wait 1 to 2 minutes between sprays.
- Rinse spray tip in hot water and dry with a clean tissue.

ACTION
Thought to cause local vasoconstriction of dilated arterioles, reducing blood flow and nasal congestion.

Route	Onset	Peak	Duration
Intranasal	Few min	Unknown	4–8 hr

Half-life: Unknown.

ADVERSE REACTIONS
EENT: rebound nasal congestion, sneezing, transient burning or stinging.

INTERACTIONS
Drug-drug. *Bromocriptine, catechol-O-methyltransferase inhibitors, such as tolcapone:* May increase the effects of these drugs. Monitor patient for increased clinical response and adverse effects.
MAO inhibitors: May cause headache, hypertension, and hyperpyrexia. Avoid using tetrahydrozoline within 14 days of stopping an MAO inhibitor.
Tricyclic antidepressants: May decrease the effects of tetrahydrozoline. Monitor patient for clinical effect.
Drug-herb. *St. John's wort:* May increase adverse effects of herb. Discourage use together.

EFFECTS ON LAB TEST RESULTS
None reported.

CONTRAINDICATIONS & CAUTIONS
- Contraindicated in patients hypersensitive to drug and in children younger than age 2. The 0.1% solution is contraindicated in children younger than age 6.
- Use cautiously in patients with hyperthyroidism, hypertension, or diabetes mellitus.

NURSING CONSIDERATIONS
- Drug should be used for only 3 to 5 days.
- Overdose in young children may cause oversedation.

PATIENT TEACHING
- Teach patient how to use drug.
- Caution patient not to share drug because this could spread infection.
- Tell patient not to exceed recommended dosage and to use only as needed for 3 to 5 days.

triamcinolone acetonide
trye-am-SIN-oh-lone

Nasacort AQ

Pharmacologic class: corticosteroid
Pregnancy risk category C

AVAILABLE FORMS
Nasal spray: 55 mcg/spray

INDICATIONS & DOSAGES
➤ **Treatment of nasal symptoms of seasonal and perennial allergic rhinitis**
Adults and children 12 years and older: 2 sprays in each nostril daily; may decrease to 1 spray in each nostril daily for allergic disorders. Adjust to minimum effective dosage.
Children ages 6 to 11: 1 spray in each nostril daily. Maximum dosage is 2 sprays in each nostril daily. Adjust to minimum effective dosage.

ADMINISTRATION
Intranasal
- Shake well before use.

ACTION
Unknown. A glucocorticoid with anti-inflammatory properties.

Route	Onset	Peak	Duration
Intranasal	Unknown	1½–4 hr	Unknown

Half-life: AQ form, about 3 hours.

ADVERSE REACTIONS
CNS: *headache,* fever.
EENT: *nasal irritation,* burning, dry mucous membranes, epistaxis, irritation, nasal and sinus congestion, otitis media, pharyngitis, rhinitis, sinusitis, sneezing, stinging, throat discomfort.
GI: dyspepsia, nausea, vomiting.
Respiratory: *asthma symptoms,* cough.

Reactions may be *common,* uncommon, *life-threatening,* or COMMON AND LIFE-THREATENING.
Interaction may have a *rapid onset* or *delayed onset.*

INTERACTIONS
None significant.

EFFECTS ON LAB TEST RESULTS
None reported.

CONTRAINDICATIONS & CAUTIONS
• Contraindicated in patients hypersensitive to drug or its components and in those with untreated mucosal infection.
• Use with caution, if at all, in patients with active or quiescent tuberculous infection of respiratory tract and in patients with untreated fungal, bacterial, or systemic viral infection or ocular herpes simplex.
• Use cautiously in patients already receiving systemic corticosteroids because of increased likelihood of hypothalamic-pituitary-adrenal axis suppression.
• Use cautiously in breast-feeding women and in those with recent nasal septal ulcers, nasal surgery, or trauma because drug may inhibit wound healing.

NURSING CONSIDERATIONS
• *Alert:* Excessive doses may cause signs and symptoms of hyperadrenocorticism and adrenal axis suppression; stop drug slowly.
• *Look alike–sound alike:* Don't confuse triamcinolone with Triaminicin.

PATIENT TEACHING
• Urge patient to read patient instruction sheet contained in each package before using drug for first time.
• To instill, instruct patient to shake container before use, blow nose to clear nasal passages, tilt head slightly forward, and insert nozzle into nostril, pointing away from septum. Tell him to hold other nostril closed and inhale gently while spraying. Next, have patient shake container and repeat procedure in other nostril.
• Instruct patient to avoid getting aerosol in eyes. If this occurs, tell him to rinse with copious amounts of cool tap water.
• Stress importance of using drug on a regular schedule because its effectiveness depends on regular use. Warn patient not to exceed prescribed dosage because serious adverse reactions can occur.

• Tell patient to notify prescriber if signs and symptoms don't diminish or if condition worsens in 2 to 3 weeks.
• Warn patient to avoid exposure to chickenpox or measles and, if exposed, to notify prescriber.
• Instruct patient to watch for and report signs and symptoms of nasal infection. Drug may need to be stopped and appropriate local therapy given.

92

Ophthalmic anti-infectives

ciprofloxacin hydrochloride
erythromycin
gatifloxacin
gentamicin sulfate
moxifloxacin hydrochloride
ofloxacin 0.3%
sulfacetamide sodium 1%, 10%,
  15%, 30%
tobramycin

---

ciprofloxacin hydrochloride
si-proe-FLOX-a-sin

Ciloxan

Pharmacologic class:
fluoroquinolone
Pregnancy risk category C

AVAILABLE FORMS
Ophthalmic ointment: 0.3% (base)
Ophthalmic solution: 0.3% (base)

INDICATIONS & DOSAGES
➤ **Corneal ulcers caused by *Pseudo-monas aeruginosa*, *Staphylococcus aureus*, *S. epidermidis*, *Streptococcus pneumoniae*, and possibly *Serratia marcescens* and *Streptococcus viridans***
Adults and children older than age 12:
Give 2 drops in affected eye every 15 minutes for first 6 hours; then 2 drops every 30 minutes for remainder of first day. On the second day, 2 drops hourly. On days 3 to 14, 2 drops every 4 hours.
➤ **Bacterial conjunctivitis caused by *Haemophilus influenzae*, *S. aureus*, *S. epidermidis*, and possibly *S. pneumoniae***
Adults and children older than age 12:
Give 1 or 2 drops into conjunctival sac of affected eye every 2 hours while awake for first 2 days. Then, 1 or 2 drops every 4 hours while awake for next 5 days. Or ½-inch ribbon into the conjunctival sac t.i.d. for the first 2 days, then ½-inch ribbon b.i.d. for the next 5 days.

ADMINISTRATION
Ophthalmic
● Apply light finger pressure on lacrimal sac for 1 minute after drops are instilled.

ACTION
Inhibits bacterial DNA gyrase, an enzyme needed for bacterial replication.

Route	Onset	Peak	Duration
Ophthalmic	Unknown	Unknown	Unknown

Half-life: 3 to 5 hours.

ADVERSE REACTIONS
EENT: *local burning or discomfort, white crystalline precipitate in superficial portion of corneal defect in patients with corneal ulcers,* allergic reactions, conjunctival hyperemia, foreign body sensation, itching.
GI: bad or bitter taste in mouth.

INTERACTIONS
None significant.

EFFECTS ON LAB TEST RESULTS
None reported.

CONTRAINDICATIONS & CAUTIONS
● Contraindicated in patients hypersensitive to drug or other fluoroquinolones.
● It's unknown if drug appears in breast milk after application to eye; however, drug given systemically appears in breast milk. Use cautiously in breast-feeding women.

NURSING CONSIDERATIONS
● *Alert:* Stop drug at first sign of hypersensitivity, such as rash, and notify prescriber. Serious hypersensitivity reactions, including anaphylaxis, may occur in patients receiving systemic drug.
● A topical overdose may be flushed from eyes with warm tap water.
● If corneal epithelium is still compromised after 14 days of treatment, continue therapy.
● Institute appropriate therapy if superinfection occurs. Prolonged use may result

---

Reactions may be *common*, uncommon, *life-threatening*, or COMMON AND LIFE-THREATENING.
Interaction may have a *rapid onset* or **delayed onset**.

in overgrowth of nonsusceptible organisms, including fungi.

• *Look alike–sound alike:* Don't confuse Ciloxan with Cytoxan.

PATIENT TEACHING

• Tell patient to clean eye area of excessive discharge before instilling.

• Teach patient how to instill drops or apply ointment. Advise him to wash hands before and after using drug and not to touch tip of dropper to eye or surrounding tissues.

• Instruct patient to apply light finger pressure on lacrimal sac for 1 minute after drops are instilled.

• Advise patient that drug may cause temporary blurring of vision or stinging after administration. If these symptoms become pronounced or worsen, contact prescriber.

• Tell patient to avoid wearing contacts while treating bacterial conjunctivitis. If approved by prescriber, tell patient to wait at least 15 minutes after instilling drops before inserting contact lenses.

• Tell patient not to share drug, washcloths, or towels with family members and to notify prescriber if anyone develops same signs or symptoms.

• Stress importance of compliance with recommended therapy.

---

erythromycin
er-ith-roe-MYE-sin

Ilotycin

Pharmacologic class: macrolide
Pregnancy risk category B

AVAILABLE FORMS
Ophthalmic ointment: 0.5%

INDICATIONS & DOSAGES
➤ **Acute and chronic conjunctivitis, other eye infections**
Adults and children: Apply a ribbon of ointment about 1 cm long directly to infected eye up to six times daily, depending on severity of infection.

➤ **Chlamydial ophthalmic infections (trachoma)**
Adults and children: Apply small amount to each eye b.i.d. for 2 months or b.i.d. on first 5 days of each month for 6 months.
➤ **To prevent ophthalmia neonatorum caused by** *Neisseria gonorrhoeae* **or** *Chlamydia trachomatis*
Neonates: Apply a ribbon of ointment about 1 cm long in lower conjunctival sac of each eye shortly after birth.

ADMINISTRATION
Ophthalmic
• Don't use for infection unless causative organism has been identified.
• To prevent ophthalmia neonatorum, apply ointment no later than 1 hour after birth. Use drug in neonates born either vaginally or by cesarean birth. Gently massage eyelids for 1 minute to spread ointment. Use new tube for each neonate.

ACTION
Inhibits protein synthesis; usually bacteriostatic, but may be bactericidal in high concentrations or against highly susceptible organisms.

Route	Onset	Peak	Duration
Ophthalmic	Unknown	Unknown	Unknown

Half-life: Unknown.

ADVERSE REACTIONS
EENT: blurred vision, itching and burning eyes, slowed corneal wound healing.
Skin: dermatitis, urticaria.
Other: overgrowth of nonsusceptible organisms with long-term use.

INTERACTIONS
None significant.

EFFECTS ON LAB TEST RESULTS
• May interfere with fluorometric determinations of urine catecholamines.

CONTRAINDICATIONS & CAUTIONS
• Contraindicated in patients hypersensitive to drug.
• Use cautiously in breast-feeding women.

NURSING CONSIDERATIONS
• Use drug only when sensitivity studies show it's effective against infecting

organisms; don't use in infections of unknown cause.
• Store drug at room temperature in tightly closed, light-resistant container.

PATIENT TEACHING
• Tell patient to clean eye area of excessive discharge before application.
• Teach patient how to apply drug. Advise him to wash hands before and after applying ointment, and warn him not to touch tip of applicator to eye or surrounding tissue.
• Tell patient that vision may be blurred for a few minutes after applying ointment. Instruct patient to keep eyes closed for 1 to 2 minutes after applying drug.
• Advise patient to watch for and report signs and symptoms of sensitivity (itching lids, redness, swelling, or constant burning).
• Tell patient not to share drug, washcloths, or towels with family members and to notify prescriber if anyone develops same signs or symptoms.
• Stress importance of compliance with recommended therapy.

---

gatifloxacin
ga-ti-FLOKS-a-sin

Zymar

Pharmacologic class:
fluoroquinolone
Pregnancy risk category C

AVAILABLE FORMS
Solution: 0.3%

INDICATIONS & DOSAGES
➤ **Bacterial conjunctivitis**
Adults and children age 1 and older:
Instill 1 drop into affected eye every 2 hours while patient is awake, up to eight times daily for 2 days. Then instill 1 drop up to q.i.d. for 5 more days.

ADMINISTRATION
Ophthalmic
• Apply gentle pressure to the inside corner of the eyelid for 1 to 2 minutes after instilling drop.

ACTION
Inhibits DNA gyrase and topoisomerase, preventing cell replication and division.

Route	Onset	Peak	Duration
Ophthalmic	Unknown	Unknown	Unknown

Half-life: Unknown.

ADVERSE REACTIONS
CNS: headache.
EENT: *conjunctival irritation, increased lacrimation, keratitis, papillary conjunctivitis,* chemosis, conjunctival hemorrhage, discharge, dry eyes, eye irritation, eyelid edema, pain, red eyes, reduced visual acuity.
GI: taste disturbance.

INTERACTIONS
None reported.

EFFECTS ON LAB TEST RESULTS
None reported.

CONTRAINDICATIONS & CAUTIONS
• Contraindicated in patients hypersensitive to drug or other quinolones.
• Safety and effectiveness in infants less than 1 year have not been established.
• Use cautiously in pregnant or breast-feeding women.

NURSING CONSIDERATIONS
• Solution isn't for injection sub-conjunctivally or into the anterior chamber of the eye.
• Systemic drug may cause serious hypersensitivity reactions. If allergic reaction occurs, stop drug and treat symptoms.
• Monitor patient for superinfection.

PATIENT TEACHING
• Urge patient to immediately stop drug and seek medical treatment if evidence of a serious allergic reaction develops, such as itching, rash, swelling of the face or throat, or difficulty breathing.
• Instruct patient to apply gentle pressure to inside corner of eyelid for 1 to 2 minutes after instilling drop.
• Tell patient not to wear contact lenses during treatment.
• Warn patient to avoid touching the applicator tip to anything, including eyes and fingers.

• Teach patient that prolonged use may encourage infections with nonsusceptible bacteria.

---

gentamicin sulfate
jen-ta-MYE-sin

Genoptic, Genoptic S.O.P., Gentak

Pharmacologic class:
aminoglycoside
Pregnancy risk category C

AVAILABLE FORMS
Ophthalmic ointment: 0.3% (base)
Ophthalmic solution: 0.3% (base)

INDICATIONS & DOSAGES
➤ **External ocular infections (conjunctivitis, keratoconjunctivitis, corneal ulcers, blepharitis, blepharoconjunctivitis, meibomianitis, and dacryocystitis) caused by susceptible organisms, especially** *Pseudomonas aeruginosa, Proteus, Klebsiella pneumoniae, Escherichia coli,* **and other gram-negative organisms**
Adults and children: 1 to 2 drops in affected eye every 4 hours. In severe infections, up to 2 drops every hour. Or, apply ointment to lower conjunctival sac b.i.d. or t.i.d.

ADMINISTRATION
Ophthalmic
• Store drug away from heat.
• Apply light finger pressure on lacrimal sac for 1 minute after drops are instilled.
• Wait at least 10 minutes before instilling other eyedrops.

ACTION
Thought to inhibit protein synthesis; usually bactericidal.

Route	Onset	Peak	Duration
Ophthalmic	Unknown	Unknown	Unknown

Half-life: Unknown.

ADVERSE REACTIONS
EENT: burning, stinging, or blurred vision with ointment, conjunctival hyperemia, transient irritation from solution.

Other: overgrowth of nonsusceptible organisms with long-term use.

INTERACTIONS
None significant.

EFFECTS ON LAB TEST RESULTS
None reported.

CONTRAINDICATIONS & CAUTIONS
• Contraindicated in patients hypersensitive to drug.
• Use cautiously in patients with history of sensitivity to aminoglycosides because cross-sensitivity may occur.

NURSING CONSIDERATIONS
• Obtain culture before giving drug. Therapy may begin before culture results are known.
• Solution isn't for injection into conjunctiva or anterior chamber of eye.
• If ophthalmic gentamicin is given together with systemic gentamicin, monitor gentamicin level.
• Systemic absorption from excessive use may cause toxicities.

PATIENT TEACHING
• Tell patient to clean eye area of excessive discharge before instilling drug.
• Teach patient how to instill drops or apply ointment. Advise him to wash hands before and after applying ointment or solution and not to touch tip of dropper or tube to eye or surrounding tissues.
• Instruct patient to apply light finger pressure on lacrimal sac for 1 minute after drops are instilled.
• Tell patient to wait at least 10 minutes before instilling other eyedrops.
• Instruct patient to stop drug and notify prescriber if signs and symptoms of sensitivity (itching lids, swelling, or constant burning) occur.
• Advise patient not to share drug, washcloths, or towels with family members and to notify prescriber if anyone develops same signs or symptoms.
• Tell patient that vision may be blurred for few minutes after application of ointment.
• **Alert:** Stress importance of following recommended therapy. *Pseudomonas* infections can cause complete vision loss within 24 hours if infection isn't controlled.

moxifloxacin hydrochloride
mocks-ah-FLOX-a-sin

Vigamox

Pharmacologic class:
fluoroquinolone
Pregnancy risk category C

AVAILABLE FORMS
Solution: 0.5%

INDICATIONS & DOSAGES
➤ **Bacterial conjunctivitis**
Adults and children age 1 and older:
1 drop into affected eye t.i.d. for 7 days.

ADMINISTRATION
Ophthalmic
• Place gentle pressure on lacrimal duct for 1 to 2 minutes after instilling drop.

ACTION
Inhibits DNA gyrase and topoisomerase, preventing cell replication and division.

Route	Onset	Peak	Duration
Ophthalmic	Unknown	Unknown	Unknown

Half-life: 13 hours.

ADVERSE REACTIONS
CNS: fever.
EENT: conjunctivitis, dry eyes, increased lacrimation, keratitis, ocular discomfort, pain, or pruritus, otitis media, pharyngitis, reduced visual acuity, rhinitis, subconjunctival hemorrhage.
Respiratory: increased cough.
Skin: rash.
Other: infection.

INTERACTIONS
None reported.

EFFECTS ON LAB TEST RESULTS
None reported.

CONTRAINDICATIONS & CAUTIONS
• Contraindicated in patients hypersensitive to drug or other fluoroquinolones.
• Use cautiously in pregnant or breast-feeding women.

NURSING CONSIDERATIONS
• Systemic drug may cause serious hypersensitivity reactions. If allergic reaction occurs, stop drug and treat symptoms.
• Monitor patient for superinfection.
• Solution isn't for injection subconjunctivally or into anterior chamber of the eye.
• *Look alike–sound alike:* Don't confuse Vigamox with Avonex.

PATIENT TEACHING
• Tell patient to stop drug and seek medical treatment immediately if evidence of hypersensitivity reaction develops, such as itching, rash, swelling of the face or throat, or difficulty breathing.
• Tell patient not to wear contact lenses during treatment.
• Instruct patient not to touch dropper tip to anything, including eyes and fingers.

---

ofloxacin 0.3%
oh-FLOX-a-sin

Ocuflox

Pharmacologic class:
fluoroquinolone
Pregnancy risk category C

AVAILABLE FORMS
Ophthalmic solution: 0.3%

INDICATIONS & DOSAGES
➤ **Conjunctivitis caused by** *Staphylococcus aureus, S. epidermidis, Streptococcus pneumoniae, Enterobacter cloacae, Haemophilus influenzae, Proteus mirabilis,* **and** *Pseudomonas aeruginosa*
Adults and children older than age 1:
Give 1 or 2 drops in conjunctival sac every 2 to 4 hours daily while patient is awake, for first 2 days; then q.i.d. for up to 5 additional days.
➤ **Bacterial corneal ulcer caused by** *S. aureus, S. epidermidis, S. pneumoniae, P. aeruginosa, Serratia marcescens,* **and** *Propionibacterium acnes*
Adults and children older than age 1:
Give 1 or 2 drops every 30 minutes while patient is awake and 1 or 2 drops 4 and 6 hours after patient goes to bed on days 1

Reactions may be *common,* uncommon, *life-threatening,* or COMMON AND LIFE-THREATENING.
Interaction may have a *rapid onset* or **delayed onset.**

and 2. On day 3, 1 or 2 drops hourly while patient is awake; continue for 4 to 6 days. Then, 1 or 2 drops q.i.d. for an additional 3 days or until cured.

ADMINISTRATION
Ophthalmic
• Apply light finger pressure on lacrimal sac for 1 minute after drug instillation.

ACTION
Inhibits bacterial DNA gyrase, an enzyme needed for bacterial replication.

Route	Onset	Peak	Duration
Ophthalmic	Unknown	Unknown	Unknown

Half-life: 4 to 8 hours.

ADVERSE REACTIONS
EENT: *transient ocular burning or discomfort,* chemical conjunctivitis or keratitis, eye dryness, eye pain, itching, lacrimation, periocular or facial edema, photophobia, redness, stinging.

INTERACTIONS
None significant.

EFFECTS ON LAB TEST RESULTS
None reported.

CONTRAINDICATIONS & CAUTIONS
• Contraindicated in patients hypersensitive to drug or other fluoroquinolones and in breast-feeding women.

NURSING CONSIDERATIONS
• Stop drug if improvement doesn't occur within 7 days. Prolonged use may result in overgrowth of nonsusceptible organisms, including fungi.
• Solution isn't for injection into conjunctiva or anterior chamber of the eye.
• *Look alike–sound alike:* Don't confuse Ocuflox with Ocufen.

PATIENT TEACHING
• If an allergic reaction occurs, tell patient to stop drug and notify prescriber. Serious acute hypersensitivity reactions may need emergency treatment.
• Tell patient to clean excessive discharge from eye area before application.
• Teach patient how to instill drops. Advise him to wash hands before and after instilling solution, and warn him not to touch tip of dropper to eye or surrounding tissue.
• Advise patient to apply light finger pressure on lacrimal sac for 1 minute after drug instillation.
• Tell patient not to share drug, washcloths, or towels with family members and to notify prescriber if anyone develops same signs or symptoms.
• Stress importance of compliance with recommended therapy.
• Warn patient not to use leftover drug for new eye infection.
• Remind patient to discard drug when it's no longer needed.

sulfacetamide sodium 1%
sul-fah-SEE-tah-mide

sulfacetamide sodium 10%
Bleph-10, Cetamide, OcuSulf-10, Sulf-10

sulfacetamide sodium 15%
Isopto Cetamide, Sulfacel-15

sulfacetamide sodium 30%
Bleph-15

Pharmacologic class: sulfonamide
Pregnancy risk category C

AVAILABLE FORMS
Ophthalmic ointment: 10%
Ophthalmic solution: 10%, 15%, 30%

INDICATIONS & DOSAGES
➤ **Inclusion conjunctivitis, corneal ulcers, chlamydial infection**
Adults and children: 1 or 2 drops into lower conjunctival sac every 2 to 3 hours. Increase interval as condition responds. The usual duration of treatment is 7 to 10 days. Apply 0.5 inch of 10% ointment into conjunctival sac t.i.d. to q.i.d. and at bedtime. Ointment may be used at night along with drops during the day.
➤ **Trachoma**
Adults and children: 2 drops into lower conjunctival sac every 2 hours with systemic sulfonamide or tetracycline.

ADMINISTRATION
Ophthalmic
- Store drug away from heat in tightly closed, light-resistant container.
- Apply light finger pressure on lacrimal sac for 1 minute after drops are instilled.
- Wait at least 5 to 10 minutes before instilling other eyedrops.

ACTION
Bacteriostatic; bactericidal in high concentrations. Prevents uptake of PABA, a metabolite of bacterial folic acid synthesis.

Route	Onset	Peak	Duration
Ophthalmic	Unknown	Unknown	Unknown

Half-life: Unknown.

ADVERSE REACTIONS
EENT: burning, eye itching, headache or brow pain, pain on instillation of drops, periorbital edema, photophobia, slowed corneal wound healing with ointment.
Other: overgrowth of nonsusceptible organisms.

INTERACTIONS
Drug-drug. *Gentamicin (ophthalmic):* May cause in vitro antagonism. Avoid using together.
Local anesthetics (procaine, tetracaine), PABA derivatives: May decrease sulfacetamide sodium action. Wait 30 minutes to 1 hour after instilling anesthetic or PABA derivative before instilling sulfacetamide.
Silver preparations: May cause precipitate formation. Avoid using together.
Drug-lifestyle. *Sun exposure:* May cause photophobia. Advise patient to avoid excessive sunlight exposure.

EFFECTS ON LAB TEST RESULTS
None reported.

CONTRAINDICATIONS & CAUTIONS
- Contraindicated in patients hypersensitive to sulfonamides and children younger than age 2 months.
- Contraindicated in epithelial herpes simplex keratitis, vaccinia, varicella, and many other viral diseases of the cornea and conjunctiva; in mycobacterial or fungal diseases of ocular structures; and after uncomplicated removal of a corneal foreign body (corticosteroid combinations).
- Use cautiously in patients with severe dry eye. Ointment may have a negative effect on corneal epithelial healing.

NURSING CONSIDERATIONS
- Drug is often used with oral tetracycline to treat trachoma and inclusion conjunctivitis.
- ***Look alike–sound alike:*** Don't confuse Bleph-10 (sulfacetamide sodium) with Blephamide (sulfacetamide sodium and prednisolone acetate).

PATIENT TEACHING
- Tell patient to clean excessive discharge from eye area before application.
- Teach patient how to instill drops or apply ointment. Advise him to wash hands before and after applying ointment or solution and not to touch tip of dropper to eye or surrounding tissue.
- Instruct patient to apply light finger pressure on lacrimal sac for 1 minute after drops are instilled.
- Warn patient that eyedrops burn slightly.
- Advise patient to watch for and report signs and symptoms of sensitivity (itching lids, swelling, or constant burning).
- Tell patient to wait at least 5 to 10 minutes before instilling other eyedrops.
- Warn patient that solution may stain clothing.
- Tell patient to minimize sensitivity to sunlight by wearing sunglasses and avoiding prolonged exposure to sunlight.
- Advise patient not to use discolored solution.
- Tell patient not to share drug, washcloths, or towels with family members and to notify prescriber if anyone develops same signs or symptoms.
- Stress importance of compliance with recommended therapy.
- Advise patient to alert prescriber if no improvement occurs.

Reactions may be *common*, uncommon, *life-threatening*, or COMMON AND LIFE-THREATENING.
Interaction may have a *rapid onset* or **delayed onset**.

tobramycin
toe-bra-MYE-sin

AKTob, Tobrex

Pharmacologic class:
aminoglycoside
Pregnancy risk category B

AVAILABLE FORMS
Ophthalmic ointment: 0.3%
Ophthalmic solution: 0.3%

INDICATIONS & DOSAGES
➤ **External ocular infections by susceptible bacteria**
Adults and children: In mild to moderate infections, instill 1 or 2 drops into affected eye every 4 hours, or apply 1-cm strip of ointment every 8 to 12 hours. In severe infections, instill 2 drops into infected eye every 30 to 60 minutes until condition improves; then reduce frequency. Or, apply 1-cm strip of ointment every 3 to 4 hours until condition improves; then reduce frequency to b.i.d. to t.i.d.

ADMINISTRATION
Ophthalmic
• When two different ophthalmic solutions are used, allow at least 10 minutes between instillations.
• Apply light finger pressure on lacrimal sac for 1 minute after drops are instilled.

ACTION
Thought to inhibit protein synthesis; usually bactericidal.

Route	Onset	Peak	Duration
Ophthalmic	Unknown	Unknown	Unknown

Half-life: 2 to 3 hours.

ADVERSE REACTIONS
EENT: blurred vision with ointment, burning or stinging on instillation, conjunctival erythema, increased lacrimation, lid itching or swelling.

INTERACTIONS
None significant.

EFFECTS ON LAB TEST RESULTS
None reported.

CONTRAINDICATIONS & CAUTIONS
• Contraindicated in patients hypersensitive to drug or other aminoglycosides.

NURSING CONSIDERATIONS
• **Alert:** Tobramycin ophthalmic solution isn't for injection.
• If topical ocular tobramycin is given with systemic tobramycin, carefully monitor levels.
• Prolonged use may result in overgrowth of nonsusceptible organisms, including fungi.
• **Look alike–sound alike:** Don't confuse tobramycin with Trobicin or Tobrex with TobraDex.

PATIENT TEACHING
• Tell patient to clean excessive discharge from eye area before application.
• Teach patient how to instill drops or apply ointment. Advise him to wash hands before and after applying and to avoid touching tip of dropper to eye or surrounding tissue.
• Instruct patient to apply light finger pressure on lacrimal sac for 1 minute after drops are instilled.
• Tell patient to wait at least 10 minutes before instilling other eyedrops.
• Advise patient to watch for itching lids, swelling, or constant burning. Tell him to stop drug and notify prescriber if these signs and symptoms develop.
• Tell patient not to share drug, washcloths, or towels with family members and to notify prescriber if anyone develops same signs or symptoms.
• Stress importance of compliance with recommended therapy.

93

Ophthalmic anti-inflammatories

bromfenac
dexamethasone
dexamethasone sodium
   phosphate
difluprednate
fluorometholone
fluorometholone acetate
ketorolac tromethamine
prednisolone acetate
prednisolone sodium phosphate

---

bromfenac
BROM-fen-ak

Xibrom

Pharmacologic class: NSAID
Pregnancy risk category C

AVAILABLE FORMS
Ophthalmic solution: 0.09%

INDICATIONS & DOSAGES
➤ **Inflammation and pain after cataract surgery**
Adults: 1 drop in each eye b.i.d., starting 24 hours after surgery and continuing for 2 weeks.

ADMINISTRATION
Ophthalmic
● Ask patient if he's sensitive to sulfites, aspirin, or other NSAIDs before treatment. Drug contains sulfite, which may cause allergic-type reactions, including anaphylaxis and life-threatening or less severe asthmatic episodes, in patients sensitive to sulfites.
● Begin treatment at least 24 hours after surgery and continue for 2 weeks. Starting treatment less than 24 hours after surgery or giving for longer than 14 days increases risk of ocular adverse effects.
● After giving drop, have patient close his eyes and apply gentle pressure to lacrimal sac for 1 to 2 minutes.

ACTION
Blocks prostaglandin synthesis by inhibiting cyclooxygenase 1 and 2.

Route	Onset	Peak	Duration
Ophthalmic	Unknown	Unknown	Unknown

Half-life: Unknown.

ADVERSE REACTIONS
CNS: headache.
EENT: abnormal sensation in the eye, burning, conjunctival hyperemia, eye irritation, eye pain, eye pruritus, eye redness, iritis, keratitis, stinging.

INTERACTIONS
Drug-drug. *Drugs that affect coagulation:* May further increase bleeding tendency or prolong bleeding time. Avoid using together, if possible, or monitor patient closely for bleeding.
Topical corticosteroids: May delay healing. Avoid using together, if possible, or monitor healing closely.

EFFECTS ON LAB TEST RESULTS
None reported.

CONTRAINDICATIONS & CAUTIONS
● Contraindicated in patients hypersensitive to drug or its ingredients. Drug contains sulfite, which may cause allergic-type reactions, including anaphylaxis and life-threatening or less severe asthmatic episodes in patients sensitive to sulfites.
● Use cautiously in patients with bleeding tendencies, those taking anticoagulants, and those sensitive to aspirin products, phenylacetic acid derivatives, and other NSAIDs.
● Use cautiously in patients who have had complicated or repeat ocular surgeries or those with corneal denervation, corneal epithelial defects, diabetes mellitus, ocular surface diseases (such as dry-eye syndrome), or rheumatoid arthritis because of the increased risk of corneal adverse effects, which may threaten sight.
● Use in pregnant women only if potential benefit justifies risk; avoid use late in pregnancy because NSAIDs may cause premature closure of the ductus

---

Reactions may be *common*, uncommon, *life-threatening*, or COMMON AND LIFE-THREATENING.
Interaction may have a *rapid onset* or **delayed onset**.

arteriosus, a necessary structure of fetal circulation.
• Use cautiously in breast-feeding women.

NURSING CONSIDERATIONS
• Sulfite sensitivity is more common in patients with asthma than in those without asthma. If patient has asthma, monitor closely.
• If patient takes an anticoagulant, watch closely for increased bleeding.

PATIENT TEACHING
• Teach patient how to instill the drops.
• Instruct patient to start therapy 24 hours after surgery and to continue for 14 days.
• Tell patient not to use for longer than 2 weeks after surgery or to save unused amount for other conditions.
• Tell patient the signs and symptoms of adverse effects. If bothersome or serious adverse effects occur, advise patient to stop therapy and contact prescriber.
• Tell patient to store drug at room temperature.
• Advise patient not to use while wearing contact lenses.

---

dexamethasone
dex-a-METH-a-sone

Maxidex

dexamethasone sodium phosphate

Pharmacologic class: corticosteroid
Pregnancy risk category C

AVAILABLE FORMS
Ophthalmic solution: 0.1%
Ophthalmic suspension: 0.1%

INDICATIONS & DOSAGES
➤ **Uveitis; iridocyclitis; inflammatory conditions of eyelids, conjunctiva, cornea, anterior segment of globe; corneal injury from chemical or thermal burns, or penetration of foreign bodies; allergic conjunctivitis; suppression of graft rejection after keratoplasty**
Adults and children: Initially, 1 or 2 drops of solution into conjunctival sac every 1 to

2 hours. Decrease to 1 drop every 4 hours when favorable response is noted. As condition improves, taper to 1 drop t.i.d. or q.i.d. to control symptoms, then, to b.i.d., then once daily. Treatment may extend from a few days to several weeks. Or, give 1 or 2 drops of suspension in the conjunctival sac. In severe disease, drops may be used hourly, being tapered to discontinuation as inflammation subsides. In mild disease, drops may be used up to four to six times daily.

ADMINISTRATION
Ophthalmic
• Shake suspension well before use.
• Apply light finger pressure on lacrimal sac for 1 minute after instillation.

ACTION
Suppresses edema, fibrin deposition, capillary dilation, leukocyte migration, capillary proliferation, and collagen deposition.

Route	Onset	Peak	Duration
Ophthalmic	Unknown	Unknown	Unknown

Half-life: Unknown.

ADVERSE REACTIONS
EENT: burning, stinging, or red eyes, cataracts, corneal ulceration, defects in visual acuity and visual field, discharge, discomfort, dry eyes, foreign body sensation, glaucoma worsening, increased intraocular pressure, increased susceptibility to viral or fungal corneal infection, interference with corneal wound healing, mild blurred vision, optic nerve damage with excessive or long-term use, ocular pain, photophobia, thinning of cornea.
Other: adrenal suppression with excessive or long-term use, systemic effects.

INTERACTIONS
None significant.

EFFECTS ON LAB TEST RESULTS
None reported.

CONTRAINDICATIONS & CAUTIONS
• Contraindicated in patients hypersensitive to any component of drug.

• Contraindicated in those with ocular tuberculosis or acute superficial herpes simplex (dendritic keratitis), vaccinia, varicella, or other fungal or viral diseases of cornea and conjunctiva; in patients with acute, purulent, untreated infections of eye; and in those who have had uncomplicated removal of superficial corneal foreign body.

• Use cautiously in patients with corneal abrasions that may be infected (especially with herpes).

• Use cautiously in patients with glaucoma (any form) because intraocular pressure may increase. Dosage of glaucoma drugs may need to be increased to compensate.

• Safe use in pregnant and breast-feeding women hasn't been established.

NURSING CONSIDERATIONS

• Drug isn't for long-term use.

• Watch for corneal ulceration, which may require stopping drug.

• Corneal viral and fungal infections may be worsened by corticosteroid application.

• **Look alike–sound alike:** Don't confuse dexamethasone with desoximetasone. Don't confuse Maxidex with Maxzide.

PATIENT TEACHING

• Tell patient to shake suspension well before use.

• Teach patient how to instill drops. Advise him to wash hands before and after applying solution, and warn him not to touch tip of dropper to eye or surrounding tissue.

• Tell patient to apply light finger pressure on lacrimal sac for 1 minute after instillation.

• Advise patient that he may use eye pad with ointment.

• Warn patient not to use leftover drug for new eye inflammation; doing so may cause serious problems.

• **Alert:** Warn patient to call prescriber immediately and to stop drug if visual acuity changes or visual field diminishes.

• Tell patient not to share drug, washcloths, or towels with family members and to notify prescriber if anyone develops same signs or symptoms.

• Stress importance of compliance with recommended therapy.

• Tell patient who wears contact lenses to check with prescriber before using lenses again.

✱ NEW DRUG

difluprednate

die-FLU-pred-nate

Durezol

Pharmacologic class: corticosteroid
Pregnancy risk category C

AVAILABLE FORMS

Ophthalmic emulsion: 0.05%

INDICATIONS & DOSAGES

➤ **Inflammation and pain associated with ocular surgery**

Adults: One drop into the conjunctival sac of the affected eye q.i.d. beginning 24 hours after surgery for 2 weeks, then decrease to b.i.d. for one week, and then taper according to response.

ACTION

May inhibit the release of arachidonic acid, a precursor of inflammatory mediators, such as prostaglandins and leukotrienes.
Absorption: Minimal systemic absorption.
Distribution: Unknown.
Metabolism: Undergoes deacetylation to an active metabolite.
Excretion: Unknown.

Route	Onset	Peak	Duration
Ophthalmic	Rapid	Unknown	Unknown

Half-life: Unknown.

ADVERSE REACTIONS

EENT: *anterior chamber cells, anterior chamber flare, blepharitis, ciliary and conjunctival hyperemia, conjunctival edema, corneal edema,* eye inflammation, *eye pain,* iritis, *photophobia, posterior capsule opacification,* punctate keratitis, reduced visual acuity.

INTERACTIONS

None reported.

EFFECTS ON LAB TEST RESULTS

None reported.

Reactions may be *common,* uncommon, *life-threatening,* or COMMON AND LIFE-THREATENING.
Interaction may have a *rapid onset* or **delayed onset.**

CONTRAINDICATIONS & CAUTIONS
- Contraindicated in patients with ocular tuberculosis, epithelial herpes simplex keratitis (dendritic keratitis), vaccinia, varicella, or other fungal or viral diseases of ocular structures.
- Use cautiously in patients with glaucoma (any form) because intraocular pressure may increase.
- Use cautiously in patients with a history of herpes simplex; drug may prolong or worsen the condition.

NURSING CONSIDERATIONS
- Drug isn't intended for long-term use; if used for 10 days or more, monitor intraocular pressure. Watch for ocular bacterial, fungal or viral infections.
- Drug may delay healing after cataract surgery; examine with slit lamp biomicroscopy and, if appropriate, fluorescein staining, if used for more than 28 days.
- Safe use in pregnant women hasn't been established.
- Appearance of drug in breast milk isn't known. Use cautiously in breast-feeding women.
- Safety and efficacy haven't been established in children.

PATIENT TEACHING
- Teach patient how to instill drops. Advise him to wash his hands before and after applying the drug, and warn him not to touch tip of dropper to eye or surrounding tissue.
- Advise patient to contact prescriber if pain develops or redness, itching, or inflammation worsens.
- Tell patient who wears contact lenses to check with prescriber before using lenses again.
- Advise patient to store drug at room temperature in protective carton away from light, and to keep unused vials in foil pouch.

fluorometholone
flur-oh-METH-oh-lone

FML, FML Forte

fluorometholone acetate
Flarex

Pharmacologic class: corticosteroid
Pregnancy risk category C

AVAILABLE FORMS
fluorometholone
Ophthalmic ointment: 0.1%
Ophthalmic suspension: 0.1%, 0.25%
fluorometholone acetate
Ophthalmic suspension: 0.1%

INDICATIONS & DOSAGES
➤ **Inflammatory and allergic conditions of cornea, conjunctiva, sclera, anterior uvea**
Adults and children older than age 2 (acetate form not for use in children of any age): 1 drop of 0.1% or 0.25% suspension every 1 to 2 hours or ½ inch ointment every 4 hours during the first 1 to 2 days in severe cases. For mild to moderate inflammation, or when severe cases respond to treatment, 1 drop b.i.d. to q.i.d. or ½ inch ointment one to three times daily. For fluorometholone acetate, 1 to 2 drops q.i.d.; may give 2 drops every 2 hours during the initial 24 to 48 hours of treatment.

ADMINISTRATION
Ophthalmic
- Shake suspension well before use.
- Apply light finger pressure on lacrimal sac for 1 minute after instillation.
- Wait at least 10 minutes before giving any other eye preparations.

ACTION
Suppresses edema, fibrin deposition, capillary dilation, leukocyte migration, capillary proliferation, and collagen deposition.

Route	Onset	Peak	Duration
Ophthalmic	Unknown	Unknown	Unknown

Half-life: Unknown.

ADVERSE REACTIONS

EENT: increased intraocular pressure (IOP), thinning of cornea, interference with corneal wound healing, corneal ulceration, increased susceptibility to viral or fungal corneal infections, glaucoma worsening, discharge, discomfort, ocular pain, foreign body sensation, cataracts, decreased visual acuity, diminished visual field, optic nerve damage with excessive or long-term use.

Other: systemic effects, adrenal suppression with excessive or long-term use.

INTERACTIONS

None significant.

EFFECTS ON LAB TEST RESULTS

None reported.

CONTRAINDICATIONS & CAUTIONS

• Contraindicated in patients with vaccinia, varicella, acute superficial herpes simplex (dendritic keratitis), other fungal or viral eye diseases, ocular tuberculosis, or acute, purulent, untreated eye infections.
• Use cautiously in patients with corneal abrasions that may be contaminated (especially with herpes).
• Safety and effectiveness of fluorometholone in children younger than age 2 haven't been established. Fluorometholone acetate not for use in children of any age.

NURSING CONSIDERATIONS

• Treatment may last from a few days to several weeks, but avoid long-term use. Monitor IOP.
• Drug is less likely to increase IOP with extended use than other ophthalmic anti-inflammatories (except medrysone).
• In chronic conditions, withdraw treatment by gradually decreasing frequency of applications.

PATIENT TEACHING

• Tell patient to shake container well before use.
• Teach patient how to instill drops or apply ointment. Advise him to wash hands before and after using either form, and warn him not to touch tip of dropper to eye or surrounding tissue.

• Advise patient to apply light finger pressure on lacrimal sac for 1 minute after instillation.
• Tell patient not to use any other eye preparation for at least 10 minutes.
• Urge patient to call prescriber immediately and to stop drug if visual acuity decreases or visual field diminishes.
• Tell patient not to share drug, washcloths, or towels with family members and to notify prescriber if anyone develops same signs or symptoms.
• Warn patient not to use leftover drug for new eye inflammation; it may cause serious problems.
• Advise patient to consult prescriber if condition doesn't improve after 2 days. Don't stop treatment prematurely.
• Tell patient to store drug in tightly covered, light-resistant container.

---

ketorolac tromethamine
KEE-toe-role-ak

Acular, Acular PF, Acular LS

Pharmacologic class: NSAID
Pregnancy risk category C

AVAILABLE FORMS

Acular
Ophthalmic solution: 0.5% in 3-ml, 5-ml, and 10-ml containers
Acular PF
Ophthalmic solution: 0.5% in 4-ml vials
Acular LS
Ophthalmic solution: 0.4% in 5-ml containers

INDICATIONS & DOSAGES

➤ **Relief from ocular itching caused by seasonal allergic conjunctivitis (Acular)**
Adults and children age 3 and older:
1 drop into conjunctival sac in each eye q.i.d.
➤ **Postoperative inflammation in patients who have had cataract extraction (Acular)**
Adults and children age 3 and older:
1 drop to affected eye q.i.d. beginning 24 hours after cataract surgery and continuing through first 2 weeks of postoperative period.

Reactions may be *common,* uncommon, *life-threatening,* or COMMON AND LIFE-THREATENING.
Interaction may have a *rapid onset* or **delayed onset.**

> **Reduce ocular pain, burning, and stinging after corneal refractive surgery (Acular LS)**

Adults and children age 3 and older: 1 drop q.i.d. to affected eye, as needed, for up to 4 days after surgery.

> **Reduce pain and photophobia after incisional refractive surgery (Acular PF)**

Adults and children age 3 and older: 1 drop q.i.d. to affected eye, as needed, for up to 3 days after surgery.

ADMINISTRATION
Ophthalmic

● Apply light finger pressure on lacrimal sac for 1 minute after instillation.
● Store drug away from heat in a dark, tightly closed container and protect from freezing.

ACTION
Thought to inhibit the action of cyclo-oxygenase, an enzyme responsible for prostaglandin synthesis. Prostaglandins mediate the inflammatory response and cause miosis.

Route	Onset	Peak	Duration
Ophthalmic	Unknown	Unknown	Unknown

Half-life: 4 hours.

ADVERSE REACTIONS
CNS: headache (Acular LS).
EENT: *transient stinging and burning on instillation,* conjunctival hyperemia, corneal edema, corneal infiltrates, iritis, ocular edema and ocular pain (Acular LS), ocular inflammation (Acular), ocular irritation, ocular pain, superficial keratitis, superficial ocular infections.
Other: hypersensitivity reactions.

INTERACTIONS
None significant.

EFFECTS ON LAB TEST RESULTS
None reported.

CONTRAINDICATIONS & CAUTIONS
● Contraindicated in patients hypersensitive to components of drug and in those wearing soft contact lenses.

● Use cautiously in patients with bleeding disorders or those hypersensitive to other NSAIDs or aspirin. Use cautiously in breast-feeding women.

NURSING CONSIDERATIONS
● *Look alike–sound alike:* Don't confuse Acular with Acthar.

PATIENT TEACHING
● Teach patient how to instill drops. Advise him to wash hands before and after instilling solution, and warn him not to touch tip of dropper to eye or surrounding tissue.
● Advise patient to apply light finger pressure on lacrimal sac for 1 minute after instillation.
● Stress importance of compliance with recommended therapy.
● Tell patient not to instill drops while wearing contact lenses.
● Advise patient to report excessive bleeding or bruising to prescriber.
● Remind patient to discard drug when it's no longer needed.

prednisolone acetate (suspension)
pred-NISS-oh-lone

Pred Forte, Pred Mild

prednisolone sodium phosphate (solution)

Pharmacologic class: corticosteroid
Pregnancy risk category C

AVAILABLE FORMS
prednisolone acetate
Ophthalmic suspension: 0.12%; 1%
prednisolone sodium phosphate
Ophthalmic solution: 0.9%, 0.11%

INDICATIONS & DOSAGES
> **Inflammation of palpebral and bulbar conjunctiva, cornea, and anterior segment of globe**

Adults and children: 1 or 2 drops into eye. In severe conditions, may be used hourly, tapering as inflammation subsides. In mild or moderate inflammation or when a favorable response is attained in severe conditions, dosage may be reduced to 1 or 2 drops every 3 to 12 hours.

ADMINISTRATION
Ophthalmic
• Shake suspension and check dosage before giving to ensure correct strength. Store in tightly covered container.
• Apply light finger pressure on lacrimal sac for 1 minute after instillation.

ACTION
Suppresses edema, fibrin deposition, capillary dilation, leukocyte migration, capillary proliferation, and collagen deposition.

Route	Onset	Peak	Duration
Ophthalmic	Unknown	Unknown	Unknown

Half-life: Unknown.

ADVERSE REACTIONS
EENT: cataracts, corneal ulceration, discharge, discomfort, foreign body sensation, glaucoma worsening, increased intraocular pressure (IOP), increased susceptibility to viral or fungal corneal infection, interference with corneal wound healing, optic nerve damage with excessive or long-term use, visual acuity and visual field defects.
Other: adrenal suppression with excessive or long-term use, systemic effects.

INTERACTIONS
None significant.

EFFECTS ON LAB TEST RESULTS
None reported.

CONTRAINDICATIONS & CAUTIONS
• Contraindicated in patients with acute, untreated, purulent ocular infections; acute superficial herpes simplex (dendritic keratitis); vaccinia, varicella, or other viral or fungal eye diseases; or ocular tuberculosis.
• Use cautiously in patients with corneal abrasions that may be contaminated (especially with herpes).

NURSING CONSIDERATIONS
• *Look alike–sound alike:* Don't confuse prednisolone with prednisone.

PATIENT TEACHING
• Teach patient how to instill drops. Advise him to wash hands before and after instillation, and warn him not to touch tip of dropper to eye or surrounding area.
• Advise patient to apply light finger pressure on lacrimal sac for 1 minute after instillation.
• Tell patient on long-term therapy to have IOP tested frequently.
• Tell patient not to share drug, washcloths, or towels with family members and to notify prescriber if anyone develops same signs or symptoms.
• Stress importance of compliance with recommended therapy.
• Tell patient to notify prescriber if improvement doesn't occur within several days or if pain, itching, or swelling of eye occurs.
• Warn patient not to use leftover drug for new eye inflammation because serious problems may occur.

Reactions may be *common,* uncommon, *life-threatening,* or COMMON AND LIFE-THREATENING.
Interaction may have a *rapid onset* or **delayed onset.**

94

Ophthalmic vasoconstrictors and antihistamines

azelastine hydrochloride
epinastine hydrochloride
ketotifen fumarate
naphazoline hydrochloride
oxymetazoline hydrochloride
tetrahydrozoline hydrochloride

---

azelastine hydrochloride
ah-ZELL-ass-teen

Optivar

Pharmacologic class: H_1 receptor antagonist
Pregnancy risk category C

AVAILABLE FORMS
Ophthalmic solution: 0.05%

INDICATIONS & DOSAGES
➤ **Pruritus from allergic conjunctivitis**
Adults and children age 3 and older:
Instill 1 drop into affected eye b.i.d.

ADMINISTRATION
Ophthalmic
● Keep bottle tightly closed when not in use.

ACTION
Inhibits the release of histamine and other mediators from cells involved in the allergic response.

Route	Onset	Peak	Duration
Ophthalmic	3 min	Unknown	8 hr

Half-life: 22 hours.

ADVERSE REACTIONS
CNS: *headache,* fatigue.
EENT: *bitter taste, transient eye burning or stinging,* conjunctivitis, eye pain, pharyngitis, rhinitis, temporary blurring.
Respiratory: *asthma,* dyspnea.
Skin: pruritus.
Other: flulike syndrome.

INTERACTIONS
None reported.

EFFECTS ON LAB TEST RESULTS
None reported.

CONTRAINDICATIONS & CAUTIONS
● Contraindicated in patients hypersensitive to any of drug's components.
● Contraindicated for irritation related to contact lenses.

NURSING CONSIDERATIONS
● Drug is for ophthalmic use only. Don't inject or give orally.

PATIENT TEACHING
● Instruct patient not to touch any surface, eyelid, or surrounding areas with tip of dropper.
● Tell patient to keep bottle tightly closed when not in use.
● Advise patient not to wear contact lens if eye is red.
● Warn patient that soft contact lenses may absorb the preservative benzalkonium.
● Instruct patient who wears soft contact lenses and whose eyes aren't red to wait at least 10 minutes after instilling drug before inserting contact lenses.

---

epinastine hydrochloride
ep-ih-NAS-teen

Elestat

Pharmacologic class: H_1 receptor antagonist and mast cell stabilizer
Pregnancy risk category C

AVAILABLE FORMS
Ophthalmic solution: 0.05%

INDICATIONS & DOSAGES
➤ **To prevent pruritus from allergic conjunctivitis**
Adults and children age 3 and older:
Instill 1 drop into each eye b.i.d. Continue

---

treatment as long as allergen is present, even if symptoms resolve.

ADMINISTRATION
Ophthalmic
• Drug is for ophthalmic use only. Don't inject or give orally.
• Keep bottle tightly closed when not in use.

ACTION
Inhibits release of mediators from cells involved in hypersensitivity reactions, temporarily preventing pruritus.

Route	Onset	Peak	Duration
Ophthalmic	Immediate	Unknown	8 hr

Half-life: About 12 hours.

ADVERSE REACTIONS
CNS: headache.
EENT: *cold symptoms,* burning eyes, hyperemia, increased lymph nodes near eyes, pharyngitis, pruritus, rhinitis, sinusitis.
Respiratory: increased cough, *upper respiratory tract infection.*

INTERACTIONS
None reported.

EFFECTS ON LAB TEST RESULTS
None reported.

CONTRAINDICATIONS & CAUTIONS
• Contraindicated in patients hypersensitive to drug or its components.
• Contraindicated for irritation related to contact lenses.
• Use cautiously in pregnant or breast-feeding women.
• Safety and effectiveness haven't been established in children younger than age 3.

NURSING CONSIDERATIONS
• Monitor patient for signs and symptoms of infection.
• Soft contact lenses may absorb the preservative benzalkonium.

PATIENT TEACHING
• Teach patient proper instillation technique. Instruct him not to touch any surface, eyelid, or surrounding areas with tip of dropper.

• Caution patient not to use drops to treat contact lens–related eye irritation and not to wear contact lenses if eyes are red.
• Warn patient that soft contact lenses may absorb the preservative benzalkonium.
• Advise patient to report adverse reactions to drug.
• Tell patient to keep bottle tightly closed when not in use.
• Instruct patient who wears soft contact lenses and whose eyes aren't red to wait at least 10 minutes after instilling drug before inserting contact lenses.

ketotifen fumarate
kee-toe-TYE-fen

Alaway◊ , Zaditor◊

Pharmacologic class: H₁ receptor antagonist and mast cell stabilizer
Pregnancy risk category C

AVAILABLE FORMS
Ophthalmic solution: 0.025%

INDICATIONS & DOSAGES
➤ **To temporarily prevent eye itching from allergic conjunctivitis; or the temporary relief of itchy eyes due to pollen, ragweed, grass, animal hair, and dander**
Adults and children age 4 and older: Instill 1 drop in each affected eye every 8 to 12 hours.

ADMINISTRATION
Ophthalmic
• Drug is for ophthalmic use only. Don't inject or give orally.
• Close bottle tightly when not in use.

ACTION
Stabilizes mast cells to inhibit release of mediators involved in hypersensitivity reactions and blocks action of histamine at the H₁ receptor, temporarily preventing itching of the eye.

Route	Onset	Peak	Duration
Ophthalmic	Within min	Unknown	Unknown

Half-life: Unknown.

Reactions may be *common,* uncommon, *life-threatening,* or COMMON AND LIFE-THREATENING.
Interaction may have a *rapid onset* or **delayed onset.**

ADVERSE REACTIONS
CNS: *headache.*
EENT: *conjunctival infection, rhinitis,*
burning or stinging of eyes, conjunctivitis,
dry eyes, eye discharge, eye pain, eyelid
disorder, itching of eyes, keratitis,
lacrimation disorder, mydriasis, ocular
allergic reactions, ocular rash, pharyngitis,
photophobia.
Other: flulike syndrome.

INTERACTIONS
None significant.

EFFECTS ON LAB TEST RESULTS
None reported.

CONTRAINDICATIONS & CAUTIONS
• Contraindicated in patients hypersensitive
to components of drug.
• Contraindicated for irritation related to
contact lenses.

NURSING CONSIDERATIONS
• Soft contact lenses may absorb the
preservative benzalkonium. Contact lenses
shouldn't be inserted until 10 minutes
after drug is instilled.
• To prevent contaminating dropper
tip and solution, don't touch eyelids
or surrounding areas with dropper tip
of bottle.

PATIENT TEACHING
• Teach patient the proper technique for
instilling drops.
• Advise patient not to wear contact
lens if eye is red. Warn him not to use
drug to treat contact lens–related
irritation.
• Instruct patient who wears soft contact
lenses and whose eyes aren't red to wait
at least 10 minutes after instilling drug
before inserting contact lenses.
• Advise patient to report adverse
reactions.
• Advise patient to keep bottle tightly
closed when not in use.

naphazoline hydrochloride
naf-AZ-oh-leen

AK-Con, Albalon, All Clear◊,
Clear Eyes◊, Naphcon◊, 20/20
Eye Drops◊

Pharmacologic class:
sympathomimetic
Pregnancy risk category C

AVAILABLE FORMS
Ophthalmic solution: 0.012%◊,
0.02%◊, 0.03%◊, 0.1%

INDICATIONS & DOSAGES
➤ **Ocular congestion, irritation,
itching**
Adults: Instill 1 or 2 drops into the conjunctival sac of affected eye(s) every 3 to
4 hours, up to q.i.d.

ADMINISTRATION
Ophthalmic
• Store drug in tightly closed container.

ACTION
Thought to cause vasoconstriction by local
adrenergic action on the blood vessels of
the conjunctiva.

Route	Onset	Peak	Duration
Ophthalmic	10 min	Unknown	2–6 hr

Half-life: Unknown.

ADVERSE REACTIONS
CNS: dizziness, headache, nervousness,
weakness.
EENT: blurred vision, eye irritation,
increased intraocular pressure, keratitis,
lacrimation, photophobia, pupillary
dilation, transient eye stinging.
GI: nausea.
Skin: diaphoresis.

INTERACTIONS
Drug-drug. *Anesthetics:* Cyclopropane
and halothane may sensitize the
myocardium to sympathomimetics;
local anesthetics may increase t
he absorption of topical drugs.
Monitor patient for increased adverse
effects.

Beta blockers: May cause more systemic adverse effects. Monitor patient for adverse systemic effects.
MAO inhibitors, maprotiline, tricyclic antidepressants: May cause hypertensive crisis if naphazoline is systemically absorbed. Use together cautiously.

EFFECTS ON LAB TEST RESULTS
None reported.

CONTRAINDICATIONS & CAUTIONS
• Contraindicated in patients hypersensitive to drug's ingredients and in those with acute angle-closure glaucoma.
• Use of 0.1% solution is contraindicated in infants and small children.
• Use cautiously in patients with hyperthyroidism, cardiac disease, hypertension, or diabetes mellitus.

NURSING CONSIDERATIONS
• Drug is most widely used ocular decongestant.
• Rebound congestion and conjunctivitis may occur with frequent or prolonged use.

PATIENT TEACHING
• Teach patient how to instill drug. Advise him to wash hands before and after instillation and to apply light finger pressure on lacrimal sac for 1 minute after drops are instilled. Warn him not to touch tip of dropper to eye or surrounding tissue.
• Warn patient not to exceed recommended dosage to avoid rebound congestion and conjunctivitis.
• Tell patient to notify prescriber if sun sensitivity, blurred vision, pain, or lid swelling develops.
• Instruct patient not to use OTC preparations longer than 72 hours without consulting prescriber.

oxymetazoline hydrochloride
ox-i-met-AZ-oh-leen

OcuClear ◇ , Visine L.R. ◇

Pharmacologic class: direct-acting sympathomimetic amine
Pregnancy risk category C

AVAILABLE FORMS
Ophthalmic solution: 0.025%

INDICATIONS & DOSAGES
➤ **Relief from eye redness caused by minor eye irritation**
Adults and children age 6 and older: Instill 1 to 2 drops in affected eye every 6 hours, as needed.

ADMINISTRATION
Ophthalmic
• Don't use if solution has become cloudy or changed color.
• Apply light finger pressure on lacrimal sac for 1 minute after drug instillation.

ACTION
Acts on alpha-adrenergic receptors in the arterioles of the conjunctiva to produce vasoconstriction, resulting in decreased conjunctival congestion.

Route	Onset	Peak	Duration
Ophthalmic	5 min	Unknown	6 hr

Half-life: Unknown.

ADVERSE REACTIONS
CNS: headache, insomnia, light-headedness, nervousness.
CV: irregular heartbeat, palpitations, tachycardia.
EENT: *transient stinging on first instillation,* blurred vision, increased intra-ocular pressure, keratitis, lacrimation, reactive hyperemia with excessive doses or prolonged use.
Other: trembling.

INTERACTIONS
Drug-drug. *Anesthetics:* Cyclopropane and halothane may sensitize the myocardium to sympathomimetics; local anesthetics may increase the absorption

of topical drugs. Monitor patient for increased adverse effects.

Beta blockers: May cause more systemic adverse effects. Monitor patient for adverse systemic effects.

MAO inhibitors, maprotiline, tricyclic antidepressants: If significant systemic absorption of oxymetazoline occurs, use together may increase pressor effect of oxymetazoline. Avoid using together.

EFFECTS ON LAB TEST RESULTS
None reported.

CONTRAINDICATIONS & CAUTIONS
• Contraindicated in patients hypersensitive to drug or its components and in those with angle-closure glaucoma.
• Use cautiously in patients with hyperthyroidism, cardiac disease, hypertension, eye disease, infection, or injury.

NURSING CONSIDERATIONS
• *Alert:* Don't confuse Visine with Visken.

PATIENT TEACHING
• Teach patient how to instill drops. Advise him to wash hands before and after instillation, and warn him not to touch tip of dropper to eye or surrounding tissue.
• Instruct patient to apply light finger pressure on lacrimal sac for 1 minute after drug instillation.
• Advise patient to stop drug and consult prescriber if eye pain occurs, if vision changes, or if redness or irritation continues, worsens, or lasts for longer than 72 hours.

---

tetrahydrozoline hydrochloride
tet-rah-hi-DRAZ-oh-leen

Atazine◇, Geneye◇, Murine Tears Plus◇, Opti-Clear◇, Optigene 3◇, Visine ◇

Pharmacologic class:
sympathomimetic
Pregnancy risk category C

AVAILABLE FORMS
Ophthalmic solution: 0.05% ◇

INDICATIONS & DOSAGES
➤ **Conjunctival congestion, irritation, and allergic conditions**
Adults and children older than age 2: Instill 1 to 2 drops of 0.05% solution up to q.i.d., or as directed by prescriber.

ADMINISTRATION
Ophthalmic
• Apply light finger pressure on lacrimal sac for 1 minute after drops are instilled.

ACTION
Thought to cause vasoconstriction by local adrenergic action on the blood vessels of the conjunctiva.

Route	Onset	Peak	Duration
Ophthalmic	Few min	Unknown	1–4 hr

Half-life: Unknown.

ADVERSE REACTIONS
CNS: dizziness, drowsiness, headache, insomnia, tremor.
CV: *arrhythmias.*
EENT: eye irritation, increased intraocular pressure, keratitis, lacrimation, pupillary dilation, transient eye stinging.

INTERACTIONS
Drug-drug. *Anesthetics:* Cyclopropane and halothane may sensitize the myocardium to sympathomimetics; local anesthetics may increase the absorption of topical drugs. Monitor patient for increased adverse effects.
Beta blockers: May cause more systemic adverse effects. Monitor patient for adverse systemic effects.
Guanethidine, MAO inhibitors, tricyclic antidepressants: May cause hypertensive crisis if tetrahydrozoline is systemically absorbed. Avoid using together.

EFFECTS ON LAB TEST RESULTS
None reported.

CONTRAINDICATIONS & CAUTIONS
• Contraindicated in patients hypersensitive to drug or its components and in those with angle-closure glaucoma or other serious eye disease.

• Use cautiously in patients with hyperthyroidism, heart disease, hypertension, or diabetes mellitus.

NURSING CONSIDERATIONS
• Rebound congestion may occur with frequent or prolonged use.
• *Alert:* Don't confuse Visine with Visken.

PATIENT TEACHING
• Teach patient how to instill drug. Advise him to wash hands before and after instillation and to apply light finger pressure on lacrimal sac for 1 minute after drops are instilled. Warn him not to touch tip of dropper to eye or surrounding tissue.
• Warn patient not to exceed recommended dosage to avoid rebound congestion.
• Tell patient to stop drug and notify prescriber if redness or irritation persists or increases or if no relief occurs within 2 days.
• Warn patient not to share eyedrops.

95

Antagonists and antidotes

acamprosate calcium
activated charcoal
charcoal
deferasirox
digoxin immune Fab
dimercaprol
disulfiram
edetate calcium disodium
flumazenil
hydroxocobalamin
  (See Appendix, VITAMINS AND MINERALS.)
lanthanum carbonate
methylnaltrexone bromide
naloxone hydrochloride
naltrexone
naltrexone hydrochloride
physostigmine salicylate
pralidoxime chloride
protamine sulfate
pyridostigmine bromide
sevelamer carbonate
sevelamer hydrochloride
sodium polystyrene sulfonate
succimer

SAFETY ALERT!

acamprosate calcium
a-kam-PRO-sate

Campral✐

Pharmacologic class: synthetic
amino acid neurotransmitter
analog
Pregnancy risk category C

AVAILABLE FORMS
Tablets (delayed-release): 333 mg

INDICATIONS & DOSAGES
➤ **Adjunct to management of
alcohol abstinence**
Adults: 666 mg P.O. t.i.d.
Adjust-a-dose: In patients with creatinine
clearance of 30 to 50 ml/minute, give
333 mg t.i.d. Do not use in patients with
severe renal impairment (creatinine
clearance 30 ml/min or less).

ADMINISTRATION
P.O.
• Don't crush or break tablets.
• Give drug without regard for food.

ACTION
Restores the balance of neuronal excitation
and inhibition, probably by interacting
with glutamate and gamma-aminobutyric
acid neurotransmitter systems, thus
reducing alcohol dependence.

Route	Onset	Peak	Duration
P.O.	Unknown	3–8 hr	Unknown

Half-life: 20 to 33 hours.

ADVERSE REACTIONS
CNS: abnormal thinking, amnesia,
anxiety, asthenia, depression, dizziness,
headache, insomnia, paresthesia,
somnolence, *suicidal thoughts,*
syncope, tremor, pain.
CV: hypertension, palpitations, peripheral
edema, vasodilation.
EENT: abnormal vision, pharyngitis,
rhinitis.
GI: abdominal pain, anorexia, constipation, *diarrhea,* dry mouth, dyspepsia,
flatulence, increased appetite, nausea,
taste disturbance, vomiting.
GU: impotence.
Metabolic: weight gain.
Musculoskeletal: arthralgia, back pain,
chest pain, myalgia.
Respiratory: bronchitis, dyspnea,
increased cough.
Skin: increased sweating, pruritus, rash.
Other: accidental injury, chills, decreased
libido, flulike symptoms, infection.

INTERACTIONS
None significant.

EFFECTS ON LAB TEST RESULTS
• May increase ALT, AST, bilirubin,
blood glucose, and uric acid levels.
May decrease hemoglobin level and
hematocrit.
• May decrease platelet count.

CONTRAINDICATIONS & CAUTIONS
• Contraindicated in patients allergic to drug or its components and in those whose creatinine clearance is 30 ml/minute or less.
• Use cautiously in pregnant or breast-feeding women, elderly patients, patients with moderate renal impairment, and patients with a history of depression and suicidal thoughts or attempts.

NURSING CONSIDERATIONS
• Use only after the patient successfully becomes abstinent from drinking.
• Drug doesn't eliminate or reduce withdrawal symptoms.
• Monitor patient for development of depression or suicidal thoughts.
• Drug doesn't cause alcohol aversion or a disulfiram-like reaction if used with alcohol.

PATIENT TEACHING
• Tell patient to continue the alcohol abstinence program, including counseling and support.
• Advise patient to notify his prescriber if he develops depression, anxiety, thoughts of suicide, or severe diarrhea.
• Caution patient's family or caregiver to watch for signs of depression or suicidal ideation.
• Tell patient that drug may be taken without regard to meals, but that taking it with meals may help him remember it.
• Tell patient not to crush, break, or chew the tablets but to swallow them whole.
• Advise women to use effective contraception while taking this drug. Tell patient to contact her prescriber if she becomes pregnant or plans to become pregnant.
• Explain that this drug may impair judgment, thinking, or motor skills. Urge patient to use caution when driving or performing hazardous activities until drug's effects are known.
• Tell patient to continue taking acamprosate and to contact his prescriber if he resumes drinking alcohol.

activated charcoal
Actidose◇, Actidose-Aqua◇, Actidose with Sorbitol◇, CharcoAid◇, CharcoAid 2000◇, Liqui-Char◇

charcoal
Charcoal Plus DS◇, CharcoCaps◇

Pharmacologic class: adsorbent
Pregnancy risk category C

AVAILABLE FORMS
activated charcoal
Granules: 15 g◇
Liquid: 12.5 g◇, 15 g*◇, 25 g*◇, 30 g*◇, 50 g*◇
Oral suspension: 15 g◇, 30 g◇
Powder: 15 g◇, 30 g◇, 40 g◇, 120 g◇, 240 g◇
charcoal
Capsules: 260 mg◇
Tablets: 250 mg◇

INDICATIONS & DOSAGES
➤ **Flatulence, dyspepsia, diarrhea**
Adults: 500 to 520 mg (charcoal) P.O. after meals or at first sign of discomfort. Repeat as needed, up to 5 g daily.
➤ **Poisoning**
Adults and children from 1 to 12 years weighing over 32 kg (71 lbs): 50 to 60 g P.O. of drug in sorbitol base.
Children aged 1 to 12 years weighing 16 to 32 kg (38 to 71 lbs): 25 to 30 g P.O. (sorbitol base).
Adults and children older than 1 year: 5 to 60 g P.O. (aqueous base). Dosage should be from 8 to 10 times the amount of poison ingested, if known. If amount of poison ingested is not known, a dosage of at least 20 to 30 g should be given.

ADMINISTRATION
P.O.
• Give after emesis is complete because activated charcoal absorbs and inactivates ipecac syrup.
• For best effect, give within 30 minutes after poison ingestion.
• Mix powder (most effective form) with tap water to consistency of thick syrup.

Add small amount of fruit juice or flavoring to make mix more palatable. Don't mix with ice cream, milk, or sherbet; these decrease adsorptive capacity of activated charcoal.
• Give by large-bore nasogastric tube after lavage, if needed.
• If patient vomits shortly after administration, repeat dose.
• Space doses at least 1 hour apart from other drugs if treatment is for indications other than poisoning.

ACTION
Adheres to many drugs and chemicals, inhibiting their absorption from the GI tract. Also reduces volume of intestinal gas and relieves related discomfort.

Route	Onset	Peak	Duration
P.O.	Immediate	Unknown	Unknown

Half-life: Unknown.

ADVERSE REACTIONS
GI: *black stools,* **intestinal obstruction,** nausea, constipation.

INTERACTIONS
Drug-drug. *Acetaminophen, barbiturates, carbamazepine, digitoxin, digoxin, furosemide, glutethimide, hydantoins, methotrexate, nizatidine, phenothiazines, phenylbutazone, propoxyphene, salicylates, sulfonamides, sulfonylureas, tetracyclines, theophyllines, tricyclic antidepressants, valproic acid:* May reduce absorption of these drugs. Give charcoal at least 2 hours before or 1 hour after other drugs.
Acetylcysteine, ipecac: May inactivate these drugs. Give charcoal after vomiting has been induced by ipecac; remove charcoal by nasogastric tube before giving acetylcysteine.
Drug-food. *Milk, ice cream, sherbet:* May decrease adsorptive capacity of drug. Discourage use together.

EFFECTS ON LAB TEST RESULTS
None reported.

CONTRAINDICATIONS & CAUTIONS
• None known

NURSING CONSIDERATIONS
• Although there are no known contraindications, drug isn't effective for treating all acute poisonings.
• **Alert:** Drug is commonly used for treating poisoning or overdose with acetaminophen, aspirin, atropine, barbiturates, dextropropoxyphene, digoxin, poisonous mushrooms, oxalic acid, parathion, phenol, phenytoin, propantheline, propoxyphene, strychnine, or tricyclic antidepressants. Check with poison control center for use in other types of poisonings or overdoses.
• **Alert:** Don't aspirate or allow patient to aspirate charcoal powder; this may result in death.
• Follow treatment with stool softener or laxative to prevent constipation unless sorbitol is part of product ingredients. Preparations made with sorbitol have a laxative effect that lessens risk of severe constipation or fecal impaction.
• If preparation with sorbitol is used, maintain patient's fluid and electrolyte needs.
• Don't use charcoal with sorbitol in fructose-intolerant patients or in children younger than age 1.
• **Alert:** Drug is ineffective for poisoning or overdose of cyanide, mineral acids, caustic alkalis, and organic solvents; it's not very effective for overdose of ethanol, lithium, methanol, and iron salts.
• **Look alike–sound alike:** Don't confuse Actidose with Actos.

PATIENT TEACHING
• Explain use and administration of drug to patient (if awake) and family.
• Warn patient that stools will be black until all the charcoal has passed through the body.
• Instruct patient to drink 6 to 8 glasses of liquid per day because drug can cause constipation.

deferasirox
deh-fah-RASS-ih-rocks

Exjade

Pharmacologic class: heavy metal antagonist
Pregnancy risk category B

AVAILABLE FORMS
Tablets for oral suspension: 125 mg, 250 mg, 500 mg

INDICATIONS & DOSAGES
➤ **Chronic iron overload caused by blood transfusions (transfusional hemosiderosis)**
Adults and children age 2 and older: Initially, 20 mg/kg P.O. daily on an empty stomach 30 minutes before eating. Monitor serum ferritin level monthly and adjust dose every 3 to 6 months by 5 or 10 mg/kg based on ferritin trends. Don't exceed 30 mg/kg daily. Consider stopping therapy if serum ferritin level drops below 500 mcg/L.

ADMINISTRATION
P.O.
• Give drug to patient at same time each day, about 30 minutes before he eats.
• Tablets may be dissolved in water, orange juice, or apple juice.

ACTION
Binds with high affinity to iron, allowing mainly fecal excretion.

Route	Onset	Peak	Duration
P.O.	Unknown	1½–4 hr	Unknown

Half-life: 8 to 16 hours.

ADVERSE REACTIONS
CNS: *fever, headache,* dizziness, fatigue.
CV: leukocytoclastic vasculitis.
EENT: *nasopharyngitis, pharyngolaryngeal pain,* acute tonsillitis, auditory disturbances, ear infection, pharyngitis, rhinitis, visual disturbances.
GI: *abdominal pain, diarrhea, nausea, vomiting.*
GU: *acute renal failure.*

Hematologic: *agranulocytosis, neutropenia, thrombocytopenia.*
Hepatic: *liver toxicity.*
Musculoskeletal: back pain, joint pain.
Respiratory: *cough,* bronchitis, respiratory tract infection.
Skin: rash, urticaria, leukocytoclastic vasculitis.
Other: influenza, hypersensitivity reactions, *(including anaphylaxis and angioedema).*

INTERACTIONS
Drug-drug. *Aluminum-containing antacids:* May decrease iron chelation. Avoid using together.
Other iron chelators: May increase risk of toxic effects. Avoid using together.
Drug-food. *Any food:* May decrease drug effects. Give to patient with an empty stomach at least 30 minutes before eating.

EFFECTS ON LAB TEST RESULTS
• May increase transaminase and creatinine levels.

CONTRAINDICATIONS & CAUTIONS
• Contraindicated in patients hypersensitive to deferasirox or any component of the drug.
• Use cautiously in breast-feeding women and patients with renal impairment, hepatic impairment, hearing loss, or vision disturbances.

NURSING CONSIDERATIONS
• *Alert:* Monitor liver function regularly. If unexplained, persistent or progressive increase in serum transaminase levels occur, interrupt or stop treatment.
• *Alert:* In patients who are at increased risk of complications, have renal conditions, the elderly, have comorbid conditions or who are receiving other drugs that depress renal function, monitor serum creatinine closely. If level increases, notify prescriber. Dose may need adjustment or interruption, or drug may need to be stopped.
• Periodically evaluate patient for proteinuria.
• Test patient's hearing and visual acuity before starting drug and yearly thereafter.
• Monitor patient for rash. If mild or moderate, treatment may continue. If

---

Reactions may be *common*, uncommon, *life-threatening*, or COMMON AND LIFE-THREATENING.
Interaction may have a *rapid onset* or *delayed onset.*

severe, drug may be stopped or dose reduced. Patient also may need corticosteroids.
• Maintain adequate hydration for patients experiencing nausea and vomiting.

PATIENT TEACHING
• Tell patient to take drug at about the same time each day, on an empty stomach, 30 minutes before eating.
• Caution patient not to chew or swallow tablets.
• Instruct patient to dissolve tablets in water, orange juice, or apple juice; drink the mixture; swirl a small amount of the same liquid in the glass to pick up any remaining drug; and swallow that as well.
• Tell patient not to take aluminum-containing antacids at the same time.
• Inform patient of the need for monthly blood tests to evaluate the effectiveness of therapy and detect possible side effects.
• Tell patient to report changes in hearing or vision, rash, abdominal pain, yellowing of skin or eyes, pale stools, or dark urine.
• Urge patient to avoid driving or operating hazardous equipment if he becomes dizzy.

---

digoxin immune Fab (ovine)
di-JOX-in

Digibind, DigiFab

Pharmacologic class: antibody fragment
Pregnancy risk category C

AVAILABLE FORMS
Injection: 38-mg vial (Digibind), 40-mg vial (DigiFab)

INDICATIONS & DOSAGES
➤ **Life-threatening digoxin toxicity**
Adults and children: Base dosage on ingested amount or level of digoxin. When calculating amount of antidote, round up to the nearest whole number.
    For digoxin tablets, calculate number of antidote vials as follows: multiply ingested amount by 0.8; then divide answer by 0.5. For example, if patient takes 25 tablets of 0.25 mg digoxin, the ingested amount is 6.25 mg. Multiply 6.25 mg by

0.8 and divide answer by 0.5 to obtain 10 vials of antidote.
    For digoxin capsules, divide the ingested dose in milligrams by 0.5. For example, if patient takes 50 capsules of 0.2 mg, the ingested amount is 10 mg. Divide 10 mg by 0.5 to obtain 20 vials of antidote.
    If digoxin level is known, determine the number of antidote vials as follows: multiply the digoxin level in nanograms per milliliter by patient's weight in kilograms; then divide by 100. For example, if digoxin level is 4 nanograms/ml, and patient weighs 60 kg, multiply together to obtain 240. Divide answer by 100 to obtain 2.4 vials; then round up to 3 vials.
➤ **Acute toxicity or if estimated ingested amount or digoxin level is unknown**
Adults and children: Consider giving 10 vials of digoxin immune Fab and observing patient's response. Follow with another 10 vials if indicated. Dosage should be effective in most life-threatening cases in adults and children but may cause volume overload in young children.

ADMINISTRATION
I.V.
• Reconstitute drug immediately before use with 4 ml sterile water for injection.
• For children or other patients who need small doses, reconstitute 38-mg vial Digibind with 38 ml of normal saline solution to yield 1 mg/ml; reconstitute 40-mg vial DigiFab with 40 ml of normal saline solution to yield 1 mg/ml.
• If cardiac arrest seems imminent, drug may be given by direct injection.
• For intermittent infusion, further dilute with normal saline solution for injection to an appropriate volume.
• Infuse drug over 30 minutes through a 0.22-micron membrane filter.
• Refrigerate powder for injection. Reconstituted solutions may be refrigerated 4 hours.
• **Incompatibilities:** None reported.

ACTION
Binds molecules of unbound digoxin and digitoxin, making them unavailable for binding at site of action on cells.

Route	Onset	Peak	Duration
I.V.	30 min	End of infusion	15–20 hr

Half-life: 15 to 20 hours.

ADVERSE REACTIONS
CV: *heart failure, rapid ventricular rate, worsening low cardiac output.*
Metabolic: *hypokalemia.*
Other: *anaphylaxis,* hypersensitivity reactions.

INTERACTIONS
None significant.

EFFECTS ON LAB TEST RESULTS
• May decrease potassium level.
• May interfere with digitalis immunoassay measurements until drug is cleared from the body (about 48 hours).

CONTRAINDICATIONS & CAUTIONS
• Use cautiously in patients allergic to sheep proteins and in those who have previously received antibodies.

NURSING CONSIDERATIONS
• In patients allergic to sheep proteins and in those who have previously received antibodies, skin testing is recommended because drug is derived from digoxin-specific antibody fragments obtained from immunized sheep.
• Drug is used for life-threatening overdose in patients with anaphylaxis, severe hypotension, or cardiac arrest and in those with ventricular arrhythmias (such as ventricular tachycardia or fibrillation), progressive bradycardia (such as severe sinus bradycardia), or second- or third-degree AV block not responsive to atropine.
• Heart failure and rapid ventricular rate may result by reversal of cardiac glycoside's therapeutic effects.
• Monitor potassium level closely.
• In most patients, signs of digitalis toxicity disappear within a few hours.

PATIENT TEACHING
• Explain use and administration of drug to patient and family.
• Instruct patient to report adverse reactions promptly.

dimercaprol
dye-mer-KAP-rawl

BAL in Oil

Pharmacologic class: heavy metal antagonist
Pregnancy risk category C

AVAILABLE FORMS
Injection: 100 mg/ml

INDICATIONS & DOSAGES
➤ **Severe arsenic or gold poisoning**
Adults and children: 3 mg/kg deep I.M. every 4 hours for 2 days; then q.i.d. on third day; then b.i.d. for 10 days.
➤ **Mild arsenic or gold poisoning**
Adults and children: 2.5 mg/kg deep I.M. q.i.d. for 2 days; then b.i.d. on third day; then once daily for 10 days.
➤ **Mercury poisoning**
Adults and children: Initially, 5 mg/kg deep I.M.; then 2.5 mg/kg daily or b.i.d. for 10 days.
➤ **Acute lead encephalopathy or lead level greater than 100 mcg/ml**
Adults and children: 4 mg/kg deep I.M.; then every 4 hours with edetate calcium disodium for 2 to 7 days. Use separate sites. For less-severe poisoning, reduce dose to 3 mg/kg after first dose.

ADMINISTRATION
I.M.
• **Alert:** Don't give drug I.V.; give by deep I.M. route only.
• Don't let drug contact skin because it may cause a skin reaction.
• Drug has an unpleasant, garlicky odor.
• Solution with slight sediment is usable.

ACTION
Forms complexes with heavy metals to create chelates that are renally excreted.

Route	Onset	Peak	Duration
I.M.	Unknown	30–60 min	4 hr

Half-life: Unknown.

ADVERSE REACTIONS
CNS: *fever;* headache, paresthesia, anxiety.

Reactions may be *common,* uncommon, *life-threatening,* or COMMON AND LIFE-THREATENING.
Interaction may have a *rapid onset* or **delayed onset.**

CV: *transient increase in blood pressure, tachycardia.*
EENT: blepharospasm, conjunctivitis, lacrimation, rhinorrhea.
GI: *nausea, vomiting,* excessive salivation, *abdominal pain, burning sensation in lips, mouth, and throat.*
Musculoskeletal: muscle pain or weakness.
Other: pain or tightness in throat, chest, or hands.

INTERACTIONS
Drug-drug. *Iron:* May cause toxic metal complex. Take iron 24 hours after last dimercaprol dose.

EFFECTS ON LAB TEST RESULTS
● May block thyroid uptake of ^{131}I, decreasing values.

CONTRAINDICATIONS & CAUTIONS
● Contraindicated in patients with hepatic dysfunction (except postarsenical jaundice) or iron, cadmium, or selenium poisoning; also contraindicated in those allergic to peanuts.
● Don't use in pregnant women except for life-threatening acute poisoning.
● Use cautiously in patients with hypertension, G6PD deficiency, or oliguria.

NURSING CONSIDERATIONS
● Use antihistamine to prevent or relieve mild adverse reactions.
● Keep urine alkaline to prevent renal damage.

PATIENT TEACHING
● Explain use and administration of drug to patient and family.
● Instruct patient to report adverse reactions promptly.

disulfiram
dye-SUL-fi-ram

Antabuse

Pharmacologic class: aldehyde dehydrogenase inhibitor
Pregnancy risk category C

AVAILABLE FORMS
Tablets: 250 mg, 500 mg

INDICATIONS & DOSAGES
➤ **Adjunct to management of alcohol abstinence**
Adults: 250 to 500 mg P.O. as single dose in morning for 1 to 2 weeks or in evening if drowsiness occurs. Maintenance dosage is 125 to 500 mg P.O. daily (average 250 mg) until permanent self-control is established. Treatment may continue for months or years.

ADMINISTRATION
P.O.
● **Alert:** Never give until patient has abstained from alcohol for at least 12 hours. He should clearly understand consequences of drug and give permission for its use. Use drug only in patients who are cooperative, well motivated, and receiving supportive psychiatric therapy.

ACTION
Blocks oxidation of alcohol at the acetaldehyde stage. Excess acetaldehyde produces a highly unpleasant reaction in the presence of even small amounts of alcohol.

Route	Onset	Peak	Duration
P.O.	1–2 hr	Unknown	14 days

Half-life: Unknown.

ADVERSE REACTIONS
CNS: drowsiness, headache, fatigue, delirium, depression, neuritis, peripheral neuritis, polyneuritis, restlessness, psychotic reactions.
EENT: optic neuritis.
GI: metallic or garlicky aftertaste.
GU: impotence.
Skin: acneiform or allergic dermatitis, occasional eruptions.

Other: *disulfiram reaction precipitated by alcohol use.*

INTERACTIONS

Drug-drug. *Barbiturates:* May prolong duration of barbiturate effect. Closely monitor patient.

CNS depressants: May increase CNS depression. Use together cautiously.

Coumarin anticoagulants: May increase anticoagulant effect. Adjust dosage of anticoagulant.

Isoniazid: May cause ataxia or marked change in behavior. Avoid using together.

Metronidazole: May cause psychotic reaction. Avoid using together.

Midazolam: May increase midazolam level. Use together cautiously.

Paraldehyde: May cause toxic level of acetaldehyde. Avoid using together.

Phenytoin: May increase toxic effect of phenytoin. Monitor phenytoin level closely, and adjust dose as necessary.

Tricyclic antidepressants, especially amitriptyline: May cause transient delirium. Closely monitor patient.

Drug-herb. *Herbal preparations containing alcohol:* May cause disulfiram reaction. Warn patient against using together. Alcohol reaction may occur as long as 2 weeks after single drug dose.

Drug-food. *Caffeine:* May increase elimination half-life of caffeine. Tell patient to watch for effects.

Drug-lifestyle. *Alcohol use:* May cause disulfiram reaction including flushing, tachycardia, bronchospasm, sweating, nausea and vomiting, or death. Warn patient not to use products containing alcohol, including back rub preparations, cough syrups, liniments, and shaving lotion, or to drink alcoholic beverages.

EFFECTS ON LAB TEST RESULTS

● May increase cholesterol level.

CONTRAINDICATIONS & CAUTIONS

● Contraindicated in patients hypersensitive to drug or other thiram derivatives used in pesticides and rubber vulcanization; in those with psychoses, myocardial disease, or coronary occlusion; in those receiving metronidazole, paraldehyde, alcohol, or alcohol-containing products; and in those experiencing alcohol intoxication or who have ingested alcohol in preceding 12 hours.

● Don't give drug during pregnancy.

● Use with caution in patients also receiving phenytoin therapy and in those with diabetes mellitus, hypothyroidism, seizure disorder, cerebral damage, nephritis, or hepatic cirrhosis or insufficiency.

NURSING CONSIDERATIONS

■ **Black Box Warning** Never give drug to a patient when in a state of alcohol intoxication, or without his full knowledge. ■

● Perform complete physical examination and laboratory studies, including CBC, SMA-12, and transaminase level, before therapy and repeat regularly.

● Disulfiram reaction may result from alcohol use, with flushing, throbbing headache, dyspnea, nausea, copious vomiting, diaphoresis, thirst, chest pain, palpitations, hyperventilation, hypotension, syncope, anxiety, weakness, blurred vision, confusion, and arthropathy.

● *Alert:* A severe disulfiram reaction can cause respiratory depression, CV collapse, arrhythmias, MI, acute heart failure, seizures, unconsciousness, and death.

● The longer the patient remains on the drug, the more sensitive he becomes to alcohol.

● *Look alike–sound alike:* Don't confuse Antabuse with Anturane.

PATIENT TEACHING

■ **Black Box Warning** Caution patient's family that drug should never be given to patient without his knowledge; severe reaction or death could result if patient drinks alcohol. ■

● Tell patient to carry medical identification that identifies him as a disulfiram user.

● Mild reactions may occur in sensitive patient with blood alcohol levels of 5 to 10 mg/dl; symptoms are fully developed at 50 mg/dl; unconsciousness typically occurs at 125 to 150 mg/dl level. Reaction may last from 30 minutes to several hours or as long as alcohol remains in blood.

● Reassure patient that drug-induced adverse reactions (unrelated to alcohol use), such as drowsiness, fatigue, impotence, headache, peripheral neuritis, and metallic or garlic taste, subside after about 2 weeks of therapy.

Reactions may be *common*, uncommon, *life-threatening*, or COMMON AND LIFE-THREATENING.
Interaction may have a *rapid onset* or **delayed onset**.

• Advise patient not to drink alcoholic beverages or use products containing alcohol, including topical preparations and mouthwash.
• Have patient verify content of OTC products with pharmacist before use.

---

edetate calcium disodium
ED-e-tate

Calcium Disodium Versenate, Calcium EDTA

Pharmacologic class: heavy metal antagonist
Pregnancy risk category B

AVAILABLE FORMS
Injection: 200 mg/ml

INDICATIONS & DOSAGES
➤ **Acute lead encephalopathy or lead levels greater than 70 mcg/dl**
Adults and children: Use in conjunction with dimercaprol. Consult published protocols and specialized references for dosage recommendations.
➤ **Lead poisoning without encephalopathy or asymptomatic with lead levels less than 70 mcg/dl**
Adults and children: 1 g/m² I.V. or I.M. daily in divided doses spaced 8 to 12 hours apart for 5 days.

ADMINISTRATION
I.V.
• Dilute 5-ml ampule with 500 ml or 250 ml of D₅W or normal saline solution for injection to yield 2 mg/ml to 4 mg/ml, respectively.
• Infuse half of daily dose over 1 hour and remaining infusion at least 12 hours later. Or, give by slow infusion over at least 8 hours.
• **Incompatibilities:** Amphotericin B, dextrose 10% in water, hydralazine hydrochloride, invert sugar 10% in normal saline solution, invert sugar 10% in water, lactated Ringer's solution, Ringer's injection, ⅙ M sodium lactate.
I.M.
• Add lidocaine or procaine hydrochloride to I.M. solution to minimize pain. Watch for local reactions.

ACTION
Forms stable, soluble complexes with metals, particularly lead.

Route	Onset	Peak	Duration
I.V., I.M.	1 hr	24–48 hr	Unknown

Half-life: 20 minutes to 1¼ hours.

ADVERSE REACTIONS
CNS: fever, tremors, headache, paresthesia, malaise, fatigue.
CV: hypotension, rhythm irregularities.
EENT: histamine-like reactions (including sneezing, congestion, and lacrimation).
GI: cheilosis, nausea, vomiting, anorexia, excessive thirst.
GU: *nephrotoxicity with renal tubular necrosis, leading to fatal nephrosis,* proteinuria, hematuria.
Hematologic: *transient bone marrow suppression,* anemia.
Metabolic: zinc deficiency, hypercalcemia.
Musculoskeletal: myalgia, arthralgia.
Skin: rash.
Other: pain at I.M. injection site, chills.

INTERACTIONS
Drug-drug. *Insulin:* May interfere with action of insulin by binding with zinc. Adjust insulin dosage as directed.

EFFECTS ON LAB TEST RESULTS
• May increase ALT, AST, and calcium levels. May decrease hemoglobin level and hematocrit.

CONTRAINDICATIONS & CAUTIONS
• Contraindicated in patients with anuria, hepatitis, or acute renal disease.
• Use with caution in patients with mild renal disease. Dosage may be reduced.

NURSING CONSIDERATIONS
■ **Black Box Warning** Because rapid I.V. use may increase intracranial pressure, I.M. route may be preferred for lead encephalopathy. I.V. infusion is still recommended whenever possible. ■
• Monitor fluid intake and output, urinalysis, BUN level, and ECG daily.
• To avoid toxicity, use with dimercaprol; don't mix in same syringe.
• *Look alike–sound alike:* Don't confuse edetate calcium disodium with edetate

---

disodium. Both drugs may be abbreviated EDTA; clarify drug order with prescriber.

PATIENT TEACHING
• Explain use of drug to patient and family.
• Tell patients with lead encephalopathy to avoid excess fluids.

---

flumazenil
floo-MAZ-eh-nill

Romazicon

Pharmacologic class:
benzodiazepine antagonist
Pregnancy risk category C

AVAILABLE FORMS
Injection: 0.1 mg/ml in 5-ml and 10-ml multiple-dose vials

INDICATIONS & DOSAGES
➤ **Complete or partial reversal of sedative effects of benzodiazepines after anesthesia or conscious sedation**
Adults: Initially, 0.2 mg I.V. over 15 seconds. If patient doesn't reach desired level of consciousness after 45 seconds, repeat dose. Repeat at 1-minute intervals, if needed, until cumulative dose of 1 mg has been given (first dose plus four more doses). Most patients respond after 0.6 to 1 mg of drug. In case of resedation, dosage may be repeated after 20 minutes, but never give more than 1 mg at any one time or exceed 3 mg in any 1 hour.
Children age 1 year and older: 0.01 mg/kg I.V. over 15 seconds. If patient doesn't reach desired level of consciousness after 45 seconds, repeat dose. Repeat at 1-minute intervals, if needed, until cumulative dose of 0.05 mg/kg or 1 mg, whichever is lower, has been given (first dose plus four more doses).
➤ **Suspected benzodiazepine overdose**
Adults: Initially, 0.2 mg I.V. over 30 seconds. If patient doesn't reach desired level of consciousness after 30 seconds, give 0.3 mg over 30 seconds. If patient still doesn't respond adequately, give 0.5 mg over 30 seconds. Repeat 0.5-mg doses, as needed, at 1-minute intervals until cumulative dose of 3 mg has been given. Most

patients with benzodiazepine overdose respond to cumulative doses between 1 and 3 mg; rarely, patients who respond partially after 3 mg may need additional doses, up to 5 mg total. If patient doesn't respond in 5 minutes after receiving 5 mg, sedation is unlikely to be caused by benzodiazepines. In case of resedation, dosage may be repeated after 20 minutes, but never give more than 1 mg at any one time or exceed 3 mg in any 1 hour.

ADMINISTRATION
I.V.
• Store drug in vial until use.
• Make sure airway is secure and patent.
• Compatible solutions include D_5W, lactated Ringer's injection, and normal saline solution.
• To minimize pain at injection site, inject drug over 15 to 30 seconds into large vein through free-flowing solution.
• Monitor patient for signs of extravasation.
• Drug is stable in a syringe for 24 hours.
• **Incompatibilities:** None reported.

ACTION
Competitively inhibits the actions of benzodiazepines on the GABA-benzodiazepine receptor complex.

Route	Onset	Peak	Duration
I.V.	1–2 min	6–10 min	Variable

Half-life: 54 minutes.

ADVERSE REACTIONS
CNS: *dizziness, abnormal or blurred vision, headache, **seizures**, agitation, emotional lability, tremor, insomnia.*
CV: ***arrhythmias**, cutaneous vasodilation, palpitations.*
GI: *nausea, vomiting.*
Respiratory: dyspnea, hyperventilation.
Skin: *diaphoresis.*
Other: *pain at injection site.*

INTERACTIONS
Drug-drug. *Antidepressants, drugs that may cause seizures or arrhythmias:* May increase risk of seizures or arrhythmias. Don't use flumazenil when overdose involves more than one drug, especially when seizures (from any cause) are likely.

Reactions may be *common*, uncommon, ***life-threatening***, or COMMON AND LIFE-THREATENING.
Interaction may have a *rapid onset* or ***delayed onset***.

EFFECTS ON LAB TEST RESULTS
None reported.

CONTRAINDICATIONS & CAUTIONS
• Contraindicated in patients hypersensitive to flumazenil or benzodiazepines, in those with evidence of serious tricyclic antidepressant overdose, and in those who have received benzodiazepines to treat a potentially life-threatening condition, such as status epilepticus.
• Use cautiously in patients with head injury, psychiatric disorders, or alcohol dependence.
• Use cautiously in patients at high risk for developing seizures and in those who have recently received multiple doses of a parenteral benzodiazepine, who display signs of seizure activity, or who may be at risk for benzodiazepine dependence, such as intensive care unit patients.

NURSING CONSIDERATIONS
• Monitor patient closely for resedation that may occur after reversal of benzodiazepine effects; drug's duration of action is the shortest of all benzodiazepines. Length of monitoring period depends on specific drug being reversed. Monitor patient closely after doses of long-acting benzodiazepines, such as diazepam, or after high doses of short-acting benzodiazepines, such as 10 mg of midazolam. In most cases, severe resedation is unlikely in patients who fail to show signs of resedation 2 hours after a 1-mg dose.
■ **Black Box Warning** Monitor patients for seizures, especially those who have been on benzodiazepines for long-term sedation or in overdose cases where patients are showing signs of serious cyclic antidepressant overdose. ■

PATIENT TEACHING
• Warn patient not to perform hazardous activities within 24 hours of procedure because of resedation risk.
• Tell patient to avoid alcohol, CNS depressants, and OTC drugs for 24 hours.
• Give family necessary instructions or provide patient with written instructions. Patient won't recall information given after the procedure; drug doesn't reverse amnesic effects of benzodiazepines.

lanthanum carbonate
LAN-thah-num

Fosrenol

Pharmacologic class: non-calcium, non–aluminum phosphate binder
Pregnancy risk category C

AVAILABLE FORMS
Tablets (chewable): 500 mg, 750 mg, 1 g

INDICATIONS & DOSAGES
➤ **To reduce phosphate level in patients with end-stage renal disease (ESRD)**
Adults: Initially, 250 to 500 mg P.O. t.i.d. with meals. Adjust every 2 to 3 weeks by 750 mg daily until reaching desired phosphate level. Reducing phosphate level to less than 6 mg/dl usually requires 1,500 to 3,000 mg daily.

ADMINISTRATION
P.O.
• Give drug with or just after a meal.
• Remind patient to chew tablets completely before swallowing them.

ACTION
Inhibits phosphate absorption by binding to phosphate released during digestion and forming highly insoluble lanthanum-phosphate complexes.

Route	Onset	Peak	Duration
P.O.	Unknown	Unknown	Unknown

Half-life: 53 hours.

ADVERSE REACTIONS
CNS: *headache.*
CV: *hypotension.*
EENT: *rhinitis.*
GI: *constipation, diarrhea, nausea, vomiting,* abdominal pain.
Metabolic: hypercalcemia.
Respiratory: bronchitis.
Other: *dialysis graft occlusion or complication.*

INTERACTIONS
None reported.

EFFECTS ON LAB TEST RESULTS
• May increase calcium level.

CONTRAINDICATIONS & CAUTIONS
• No known contraindications.
• Use cautiously in breast-feeding women and patients with acute peptic ulcer, ulcerative colitis, Crohn's disease, or bowel obstruction.

NURSING CONSIDERATIONS
• Monitor patient for bone pain and skeletal deformities.
• Check serum phosphate levels during dosage adjustment and regularly as needed throughout treatment.
• Drug isn't recommended for children because it's deposited in developing bone, including the growth plate.

PATIENT TEACHING
• Urge patient to follow a low-phosphorus diet. Assist with meal planning as needed.
• Tell patient to take drug with or immediately after meals.
• *Alert:* Remind patient to chew tablets completely before swallowing them.
• Instruct patient to avoid taking lanthanum within 2 hours of oral drugs known to interact with antacids.
• Explain that the most common side effects are nausea and vomiting and that they tend to subside over time.

✳ NEW DRUG

methylnaltrexone bromide
mehth-eel-NAHL-trek-zone

Relistor

Pharmacologic class: peripherally acting μ-opioid receptor antagonist
Pregnancy risk category B

AVAILABLE FORMS
Injection: 12 mg/0.6 ml single-use vial

INDICATIONS & DOSAGES
➤ **Opioid-induced constipation in those receiving palliative care for advanced illness when response to laxatives is insufficient**

Adults weighing less than 38 kg (84 lb): 0.15 mg/kg subcutaneously every other day, as needed.
Adults weighing 38 to 61 kg (84 to 134 lb): 8 mg subcutaneously every other day, as needed.
Adults weighing 62 to 114 kg (136 to 251 lb): 12 mg subcutaneously every other day, as needed.
Adults weighing more than 114 kg (251 lb): 0.15 mg/kg subcutaneously every other day, as needed.
Adjust-a-dose: If creatinine clearance is less than 30 ml/minute, reduce dose by one-half.

ACTION
Antagonizes GI μ-opioid receptors, preventing opioid-induced slowing of GI motility and transit time.
Absorption: Peaks about ½ hour after subcutaneous administration.
Distribution: 11% to 15.3% protein-bound.
Metabolism: Converts to methyl-6-naltrexol isomers (5% of total) and methyl-naltrexone sulfate (1.3% of total) in the liver.
Excretion: 50% excreted in urine, less in feces as unchanged drug.

Route	Onset	Peak	Duration
Subcut.	Unknown	30 min	Unknown

Half-life: About 8 hours.

ADVERSE REACTIONS
CNS: *dizziness.*
GI: *abdominal pain, flatulence, nausea, diarrhea.*

INTERACTIONS
None reported.

EFFECTS ON LAB TEST RESULTS
None reported.

CONTRAINDICATIONS & CAUTIONS
• Contraindicated in patients hyper-sensitive to the drug and in those with known or suspected mechanical GI obstruction.
• Use cautiously in patients with peritoneal catheters.

NURSING CONSIDERATIONS
• Administer no more than one dose within 24 hours.

Reactions may be *common*, uncommon, *life-threatening*, or COMMON AND LIFE-THREATENING.
Interaction may have a *rapid onset* or *delayed onset*.

• To determine injection volume for the 0.15 mg/kg dose, multiply patient's weight in pounds by 0.0034 and round up to the nearest 0.1 ml, or multiply patient's weight in kilograms by 0.0075 and round up to the nearest 0.1 ml.

• Store drug at room temperature, away from light.

• After drawn into a syringe as directed, drug is stable at room temperature for 24 hours.

• Give injections subcutaneously into the abdomen, thighs, or upper arms.

• Drug will relieve opioid-induced constipation without affecting opioid-mediated analgesic effects.

• Orthostatic hypotension may occur with overdose. Monitor patient's vital signs closely, and provide supportive care as needed.

• Don't use in pregnant women unless the benefits outweigh risk to fetus.

• It's unknown whether the drug is excreted in breast milk. Avoid use in breast-feeding women.

• Safety and efficacy in children haven't been established.

PATIENT TEACHING

• Inform patient that drug may be effective within a few minutes to a few hours after administration.

• Instruct patient to discontinue therapy, and notify prescriber if severe or persistent diarrhea occurs.

• Tell patient that vial is for single-use only; remaining drug should be discarded.

• Advise patient to avoid injecting the drug into areas where the skin is tender, bruised, red, or hard and to avoid areas with scars or stretch marks.

• Warn patient that no more than one dose should be taken within a 24-hour period.

• Advise women of childbearing age to notify prescriber if pregnancy is desired or if it occurs.

naloxone hydrochloride
nal-OX-one

Pharmacologic class: opioid antagonist
Pregnancy risk category B

AVAILABLE FORMS
Injection: 0.02 mg/ml, 0.4 mg/ml, 1 mg/ml

INDICATIONS & DOSAGES
➤ **Known or suspected opioid-induced respiratory depression, including that caused by pentazocine, propoxyphene methadone, nalbuphine and butorphanol**
Adults: 0.4 to 2 mg I.V., I.M., or subcutaneously. Repeat dose every 2 to 3 minutes, p.r.n. If patient doesn't respond after 10 mg have been given, question diagnosis of opioid-induced toxicity.
Children: 0.01 mg/kg I.V.; then, second dose of 0.1 mg/kg I.V., if needed. If I.V. route isn't available, drug may be given I.M. or subcutaneously in divided doses.
Neonates: 0.01 mg/kg I.V., I.M., or subcutaneously. Repeat dose every 2 to 3 minutes, p.r.n.
➤ **Postoperative opioid depression**
Adults: 0.1 to 0.2 mg I.V. every 2 to 3 minutes, p.r.n. Repeat dose within 1 to 2 hours, if needed.
Children: 0.005 to 0.01 mg I.V. repeated every 2 to 3 minutes, p.r.n.

ADMINISTRATION
I.V.
• Give continuous infusion to control adverse effects of epidural morphine.
• Dilute 2 mg of drug in 500 ml D_5W or normal saline solution to yield a concentration of 0.004 mg/ml.
• Titrate rate to patient's response.
• If 0.02 mg/ml isn't available, adult concentration (0.4 mg) may be diluted by mixing 0.5 ml with 9.5 ml of sterile water for injection to make neonatal concentration (0.02 mg/ml).
• **Incompatibilities:** Alkaline solutions, amphotericin B cholesteryl sulfate, preparations containing bisulfite, sulfite, long-chain or high-molecular-weight anions.

I.M.
● Use mixtures within 24 hours. After 24 hours, discard.
Subcutaneous
● Use mixtures within 24 hours. After 24 hours, discard.

ACTION
May displace opioid analgesics from their receptors (competitive antagonism); drug has no pharmacologic activity of its own.

Route	Onset	Peak	Duration
I.V.	1–2 min	5–15 min	Variable
I.M., Subcut.	2–5 min	5–15 min	Variable

Half-life: 30 to 81 minutes in adults; 3 hours in neonates.

ADVERSE REACTIONS
CNS: *seizures,* tremors.
CV: *ventricular fibrillation,* tachycardia, hypertension with higher than recommended doses, hypotension.
GI: nausea, vomiting.
Respiratory: *pulmonary edema.*
Skin: diaphoresis.
Other: withdrawal symptoms in opioid-dependent patients with higher than recommended doses.

INTERACTIONS
None significant.

EFFECTS ON LAB TEST RESULTS
None reported.

CONTRAINDICATIONS & CAUTIONS
● Contraindicated in patients hypersensitive to drug.
● Use cautiously in patients with cardiac irritability or opioid addiction. Abrupt reversal of opioid-induced CNS depression may result in nausea, vomiting, diaphoresis, tachycardia, CNS excitement, and increased blood pressure.

NURSING CONSIDERATIONS
● Duration of action of the opioid may exceed that of naloxone, and patients may relapse into respiratory depression.
● Respiratory rate increases within 1 to 2 minutes.

● *Alert:* Drug is only effective for reversing respiratory depression caused by opioids and not for other drug-induced respiratory depression, including that caused by benzodiazepines.
● Patients who receive drug to reverse opioid-induced respiratory depression may exhibit tachypnea.
● Monitor respiratory depth and rate. Provide oxygen, ventilation, and other resuscitation measures.
● *Look alike–sound alike:* Don't confuse naloxone with naltrexone.

PATIENT TEACHING
● Reassure family that patient will be monitored closely until effects of opioid resolve.

---

naltrexone
nal-TREX-one

Vivitrol

naltrexone hydrochloride
ReVia

Pharmacologic class: opioid antagonist
Pregnancy risk category C

AVAILABLE FORMS
naltrexone
Injection: 380 mg/vial dose kit
naltrexone hydrochloride
Tablets: 25 mg, 50 mg, 100 mg

INDICATIONS & DOSAGES
➤ **Adjunct for maintaining opioid-free state in detoxified patients**
Adults: Initially, 25 mg P.O. If no withdrawal signs occur within 1 hour the patient may be started on 50 mg every 24 hours the following day. From 50 to 150 mg may be given daily, depending on schedule prescribed.
➤ **Alcohol dependence**
Adults: 50 mg P.O. once daily or 380 mg I.M. in the gluteal muscle once monthly.

ADMINISTRATION
P.O.
● Keep container tightly closed and protect from light.

Reactions may be *common,* uncommon, *life-threatening,* or COMMON AND LIFE-THREATENING.
Interaction may have a *rapid onset* or *delayed onset.*

I.M.
- Use only the diluent, needles, and other components supplied with the dose kit. Don't substitute.
- Administer I.M. into gluteal muscle. Avoid giving I.V., subcutaneously, or inadvertently into fatty tissue. Monitor the injection site.

ACTION
Probably reversibly blocks the effects of I.V. opioids by competitively occupying opiate receptors in the brain.

Route	Onset	Peak	Duration
P.O.	15–30 min	1 hr	24 hr
I.M.	Unknown	2–3 days	> 30 days

Half-life: About 4 hours.

ADVERSE REACTIONS
CNS: *insomnia, anxiety, nervousness, headache, suicidal ideation,* depression, dizziness, fatigue, somnolence.
GI: *nausea, vomiting, abdominal pain,* anorexia, constipation, increased thirst.
GU: delayed ejaculation, decreased potency.
Hepatic: *hepatotoxicity.*
Musculoskeletal: *muscle and joint pain.*
Skin: *injection site reaction,* rash.
Other: chills.

INTERACTIONS
Drug-drug. *Products that contain opioids:* May decrease effect of opioid. Avoid using together.
Thioridazine: May increase somnolence and lethargy. Monitor patient closely.

EFFECTS ON LAB TEST RESULTS
- May increase AST, ALT, and LDH levels.
- May increase lymphocyte count.

CONTRAINDICATIONS & CAUTIONS
- Contraindicated in patients hypersensitive to drug or dependent on opioids, those receiving opioid analgesics, those who fail the naloxone challenge test or who have a positive urine screen for opioids, or those in acute opioid withdrawal.
- **Black Box Warning** Contraindicated in patients with acute hepatitis or liver failure. ■
- Use cautiously in patients with mild hepatic disease or history of recent hepatic disease.

NURSING CONSIDERATIONS
- **Black Box Warning** Discontinue drug if patient develops symptoms and/or signs of acute hepatitis. ■
- Don't begin treatment for opioid dependence until patient receives naloxone challenge, a test of opioid dependence. If signs and symptoms of opioid withdrawal persist after naloxone challenge, don't give drug.
- Patient must be completely free from opioids before taking naltrexone or severe withdrawal symptoms may occur. Patients who have been addicted to short-acting opioids, such as heroin and meperidine, must wait at least 7 days after last opioid dose before starting drug. Patients who have been addicted to longer-acting opioids such as methadone should wait at least 10 days.
- In an emergency, patient may be given an opioid analgesic, but dose must be higher than usual to overcome naltrexone's effect. Watch for respiratory depression from the opioid; it may be longer and deeper.
- For patients expected to be noncompliant because of history of opioid dependence, use a flexible maintenance-dose regimen of 100 mg on Monday and Wednesday and 150 mg on Friday.
- Use drug only as part of a comprehensive rehabilitation program.
- *Look alike–sound alike:* Don't confuse naltrexone with naloxone.

PATIENT TEACHING
- Advise patient to carry medical identification and to tell medical personnel that he takes naltrexone.
- Tell patient that drug can block the effects of opioids or opioid-like drugs, including heroin, pain medicine, antidiarrheals, or cough medicine.
- *Alert:* Warn patient if he uses large doses of heroin or any other opioid; serious injury, coma, or death can occur.
- Advise patient who previously used opioids that he may be more sensitive to lower doses of opioids once naltrexone therapy is stopped.

• ■ **Black Box Warning** Tell patient to report adverse effects, especially those related to liver injury, to prescriber immediately. ■

• Tell caregiver of alcohol-dependent patient to monitor him closely for signs of depression or suicide ideation and to report this immediately to prescriber.

• Give patient the names of nonopioid drugs that he can continue to take for pain, diarrhea, or cough.

• Tell patient to report pain, swelling, tenderness, induration, bruising, pruritis, or redness at the injection site.

---

physostigmine salicylate (eserine salicylate)
fis-oh-STIG-meen

Pharmacologic class:
cholinesterase inhibitor
Pregnancy risk category C

AVAILABLE FORMS
Injection: 1 mg/ml

INDICATIONS & DOSAGES
➤ **Reversal of drug-induced anti-cholinergic effects**
Adults: 0.5 to 2 mg slow I.V. or I.M. not to exceed 1 mg/minute I.V. repeated every 20 minutes as needed until patient responds or develops adverse cholinergic effects. Give additional 1 to 4 mg I.V. or I.M. every 30 to 60 minutes if life-threatening problems, such as coma, seizures, and arrhythmias, recur.
Children: Only for life-threatening situations. Give 0.02 mg/kg I.M. or slow I.V. at 0.5 mg/minute or slower, and repeat every 5 to 10 minutes until patient responds, adverse anticholinergic reactions develop, or a total dose of 2 mg has been given. Or, give 0.03 mg/kg or 0.9 mg/m² as needed.

ADMINISTRATION
I.V.
• Use only clear solution. Darkening may indicate loss of potency.
• Position patient to ease breathing. Keep atropine injection available.

• Give drug at controlled rate; use direct injection at no more than 1 mg/minute in adults or 0.5 mg/minute in children.
• Monitor vital signs frequently, especially respirations. Provide respiratory support, as needed.
• **Incompatibilities:** None reported.
I.M.
• Use only clear solution. Darkening may indicate loss of potency.

ACTION
Inhibits acetylcholinesterase, blocking destruction of acetylcholine from the parasympathetic and somatic efferent nerves. Acetylcholine accumulates, promoting increased stimulation of the receptors.

Route	Onset	Peak	Duration
I.V.	3–5 min	5 min	45 min–1 hr
I.M.	3–5 min	20–30 min	45 min–1 hr

Half-life: 1 to 2 hours.

ADVERSE REACTIONS
CNS: *restlessness, excitability, seizures,* muscle weakness.
CV: *bradycardia,* hypotension, palpitations, irregular pulse.
EENT: miosis, lacrimation.
GI: *diarrhea, excessive salivation,* nausea, vomiting, epigastric pain.
GU: urinary urgency.
Respiratory: *bronchospasm, bronchial constriction, respiratory paralysis,* dyspnea.
Skin: diaphoresis.

INTERACTIONS
Drug-drug. *Anticholinergics, atropine, local and general anesthetics, procainamide, quinidine:* May reverse cholinergic effects. Observe patient for lack of drug effect.
Ganglionic blockers: May decrease blood pressure. Avoid using together.
Neuromuscular blockers (succinylcholine): May increase neuromuscular blockade, respiratory depression. Use together cautiously.
Drug-herb. *Jaborandi tree, pill-bearing spurge:* May have additive effect. Ask patient about use of herbal remedies, and advise caution.

Reactions may be *common*, uncommon, *life-threatening*, or COMMON AND LIFE-THREATENING.
Interaction may have a *rapid onset* or **delayed onset.**

EFFECTS ON LAB TEST RESULTS
None reported.

CONTRAINDICATIONS & CAUTIONS
● Contraindicated in patients with mechanical obstruction of the intestine or urogenital tract; in patients with asthma, gangrene, diabetes, CV disease, or vagotonia; and in patients receiving choline esters or depolarizing neuromuscular blockers.
● Use cautiously in pregnant patients and those with epilepsy, parkinsonism, or bradycardia.

NURSING CONSIDERATIONS
● *Alert:* Watch closely for adverse reactions, particularly CNS disturbances. Raise side rails of bed if patient becomes restless or hallucinates. Adverse reactions may indicate drug toxicity.
● Effectiveness is typically immediate and dramatic but may be short-lived. Patient may need repeated dosages.
● Drug contains benzyl alcohol and has been associated with fatal "gasping syndrome" in premature infants.
● Drug contains sulfites, which may cause an allergic reaction in susceptible people.

PATIENT TEACHING
● Inform patient of need for drug, explain its use and adverse reactions, and answer any questions or concerns.
● Tell patient to report adverse reactions promptly.
● Instruct patient to report discomfort at I.V. site.

---

pralidoxime chloride (2-PAM chloride, 2-pyridine-aldoxime methochloride)
pra-li-DOX-eem

Protopam Chloride

Pharmacologic class: quaternary ammonium oxime
Pregnancy risk category C

AVAILABLE FORMS
Injection: 1 g/20 ml in 20-ml vial

INDICATIONS & DOSAGES
➤ **Antidote for organophosphate poisoning**
Adults: 1 to 2 g in 100 ml of normal saline solution by I.V. infusion over 15 to 30 minutes. Repeat in 1 hour if muscle weakness persists. Additional doses may be given cautiously. I.M. or subcutaneous injection may be used if I.V. isn't feasible.
➤ **Cholinergic crisis in myasthenia gravis**
Adults: 1 to 2 g I.V.; then 250 mg I.V. every 5 minutes, p.r.n.

ADMINISTRATION
I.V.
● Reconstitute by adding 20 ml of sterile water for injection to vial containing 1 g of drug.
● Dilute by adding 100 ml of normal saline solution.
● Infuse over 15 to 30 minutes. Too-rapid infusion may cause tachycardia, laryngospasm, and muscle rigidity.
● If patient has pulmonary edema, give drug by slow I.V. push over 5 minutes. Don't exceed 200 mg/minute.
● **Incompatibilities:** None reported.
I.M.
● Visually inspect parenteral drug products for particulate matter and discoloration before administration, whenever solution and container permit.
Subcutaneous
● Visually inspect parenteral drug products for particulate matter and discoloration before administration, whenever solution and container permit.

ACTION
Reactivates cholinesterase inactivated by organophosphorus pesticides and related compounds, permitting degradation of accumulated acetylcholine and facilitating normal functioning of neuromuscular junctions.

Route	Onset	Peak	Duration
I.V.	Unknown	5–15 min	Unknown
I.M.	Unknown	10–20 min	Unknown
Subcut.	Unknown	Unknown	Unknown

Half-life: 1½ hours.

ADVERSE REACTIONS
CNS: dizziness, headache, drowsiness.

CV: tachycardia.
EENT: blurred vision, diplopia, impaired accommodation.
GI: nausea.
Musculoskeletal: muscle weakness.
Respiratory: hyperventilation.
Other: mild to moderate pain at injection site.

INTERACTIONS
Drug-drug. *Barbiturates:* May increase anticholinesterase level. Use together cautiously to treat seizures.

EFFECTS ON LAB TEST RESULTS
● May increase liver enzyme levels.

CONTRAINDICATIONS & CAUTIONS
● Contraindicated in patients hypersensitive to drug.
● Use cautiously in patients with myasthenia gravis (overdose may trigger myasthenic crisis) and in those with impaired renal function.
● Safety and effectiveness in children have not been established.

NURSING CONSIDERATIONS
● Initially, remove secretions, maintain patent airway, and institute mechanical ventilation, if needed. After dermal exposure to organophosphate, remove patient's clothing and wash his skin and hair with sodium bicarbonate, soap, water, and alcohol as soon as possible. A second washing may be needed. When washing patient, wear protective gloves and clothes to avoid exposure.
● Draw blood for cholinesterase level before giving drug.
● Use drug only in hospitalized patients; have respiratory and other supportive measures available. If possible, obtain accurate medical history and chronology of poisoning. Give drug as soon as possible after poisoning; drug is most effective if started within 24 hours after exposure.
● To improve muscarinic effects and block accumulation of acetylcholine from organophosphate poisoning in adults, give atropine 2 to 4 mg I.V. with pralidoxime if cyanosis isn't present; if cyanosis is present, give atropine I.M. Give atropine every 5 to 10 minutes until signs of atropine toxicity (flushing, tachycardia,

dry mouth, blurred vision, excitement, delirium, and hallucinations) appear; maintain atropinization for at least 48 hours.
● Observe patient for 48 to 72 hours if he ingested poison. Delayed absorption may occur from lower bowel. It's difficult to distinguish between toxic effects produced by atropine or organophosphate compounds and those resulting from pralidoxime.
● In a patient with myasthenia gravis being treated for overdose of cholinergics, watch for signs of rapid weakening. He can pass quickly from cholinergic crisis to myasthenic crisis and need more cholinergics to treat myasthenia. Keep edrophonium available for differentiating diagnoses.
● Avoid use of aminophylline, morphine, phenothiazine-like tranquilizers, reserpine, succinylcholine, and theophylline in patients with organophosphate poisoning.
● Drug isn't effective against poisoning caused by phosphorus, inorganic phosphates, or organophosphates with no anticholinesterase activity.
● *Look alike–sound alike:* Don't confuse pralidoxime with pramoxine or pyridoxine.

PATIENT TEACHING
● Explain use and administration of drug to patient and family.
● Tell patient to report adverse effects.
● Caution patient treated for organophosphate poisoning to avoid contact with insecticides for several weeks.

---

protamine sulfate
PROE-ta-meen

Pharmacologic class: heparin antagonist
Pregnancy risk category C

AVAILABLE FORMS
Injection: 10 mg/ml

INDICATIONS & DOSAGES
➤ **Heparin overdose**
Adults: Base dosage on venous blood coagulation studies, usually 1 mg neutralizes not less than 100 units of heparin. Give

by slow I.V. injection over 10 minutes in doses not to exceed 50 mg.

ADMINISTRATION
I.V.
- Have emergency equipment available to treat anaphylaxis or severe hypotension.
- Give slowly by direct injection. Excessively rapid administration may cause acute hypotension, bradycardia, pulmonary hypertension, dyspnea, transient flushing, and a feeling of warmth.
- **Incompatibilities:** Cephalosporins, diatrizoate meglumine 52% and diatrizoate sodium 8%, diatrizoate sodium 60%, ioxaglate meglumine 39.3% and ioxaglate sodium 19.6%, penicillins.

ACTION
Forms a physiologically inert complex with heparin sodium.

Route	Onset	Peak	Duration
I.V.	30–60 sec	Unknown	2 hr

Half-life: Unknown.

ADVERSE REACTIONS
CNS: lassitude.
CV: *bradycardia, circulatory collapse,* hypotension, transient flushing.
GI: nausea, vomiting.
Respiratory: *acute pulmonary hypertension,* dyspnea, *pulmonary edema.*
Other: *anaphylaxis, anaphylactoid reactions,* feeling of warmth.

INTERACTIONS
None significant.

EFFECTS ON LAB TEST RESULTS
None reported.

CONTRAINDICATIONS & CAUTIONS
- Contraindicated in patients hypersensitive to drug.

NURSING CONSIDERATIONS
- Base postoperative dose on coagulation studies, and repeat activated PTT time 15 minutes after administration.
- Calculate dosage carefully. One milligram neutralizes 100 units of heparin, depending on salt (heparin calcium or

heparin sodium) and source of heparin (beef or pork).
- Risk of hypersensitivity reaction increases in patients hypersensitive to fish, in vasectomized or infertile men, and in patients taking protamine-insulin products.
- Monitor patient continually.
- Watch for spontaneous bleeding (heparin rebound), especially in dialysis patients and in those who have undergone cardiac surgery.
- Drug may act as an anticoagulant in very high doses.
- *Look alike–sound alike:* Don't confuse protamine with Protopam or Pro-Amatine.

PATIENT TEACHING
- Explain use and administration of drug to patient and family.
- Tell patient to report adverse effects.

---

pyridostigmine bromide
peer-id-oh-STIG-meen

Mestinon*, Mestinon-SR†, Mestinon Timespans, Regonol

Pharmacologic class:
cholinesterase inhibitor
Pregnancy risk category C

AVAILABLE FORMS
Injection: 5 mg/ml in 2-ml ampules or 5-ml vials
Syrup: 60 mg/5 ml
Tablets: 30 mg (for military use only), 60 mg
Tablets (extended-release): 180 mg

INDICATIONS & DOSAGES
➤ **Antidote for nondepolarizing neuromuscular blockers**
Adults: 10 to 20 mg I.V., preceded by atropine sulfate 0.6 to 1.2 mg I.V.
➤ **Myasthenia gravis**
Adults: 60 to 120 mg P.O. every 3 or 4 hours. Average dosage is 600 mg daily, but dosages up to 1,500 mg daily may be needed. For I.M. or I.V. use, give ⅓₀ of oral dose. Dosage must be adjusted for each patient, based on response and tolerance. Or, 180 to 540 mg extended-release

tablets P.O. daily or b.i.d., with at least 6 hours between doses.

Children ♦: 7 mg/kg P.O. daily in five or six divided doses.

Neonates: 5 mg P.O. every 4 to 6 hours or 0.05 to 0.15 mg/kg I.M. every 4 to 6 hours.

➤ **Preexposure prophylaxis against the deadly effects of nerve agent soman**

Adults in military combat: 30 mg P.O. every 8 hours, starting at least several hours before soman exposure.

Adjust-a-dose: Smaller doses may be required in patients with renal disease. Adjust dosage to achieve desired effect.

ADMINISTRATION
P.O.
• Don't crush extended-release tablets.
• If patient has trouble swallowing, give syrup form. If patient can't tolerate sweet flavor, give over ice chips.
I.V.
• Don't use solution if it contains particulate matter or is discolored.
• Position patient to ease breathing. Keep atropine injection available, and be prepared to give it immediately.
• Monitor vital signs frequently, especially respirations. Provide respiratory support as needed.
• Give injection no faster than 1 mg/minute. Rapid infusion may cause bradycardia and seizures.
• If patient's muscle weakness is severe, prescriber will determine if it results from drug toxicity or worsening myasthenia gravis. Test dose of edrophonium I.V. will aggravate drug-induced weakness but will temporarily relieve disease-induced weakness.
• **Incompatibilities:** Alkaline solutions.
I.M.
• Don't use solution if it contains particulate matter or is discolored.

ACTION
Inhibits acetylcholinesterase, blocking destruction of acetylcholine from the parasympathetic and somatic efferent nerves. Acetylcholine accumulates, promoting increased stimulation of the receptors.

Route	Onset	Peak	Duration
P.O.	20–30 min	2 hr	3–6 hr
P.O. (extended-release)	30–60 min	1–2 hr	6–12 hr
I.V.	2–5 min	Unknown	2–4 hr
I.M.	15 min	Unknown	2–4 hr

Half-life: 1 to 3 hours, depending on route.

ADVERSE REACTIONS
CNS: headache with high doses, weakness, syncope.
CV: *bradycardia, cardiac arrest,* hypotension, thrombophlebitis.
EENT: miosis, rhinorrhea.
GI: *nausea, vomiting,* abdominal cramps, diarrhea, excessive salivation, increased peristalsis.
GU: urinary frequency, urinary urgency.
Musculoskeletal: muscle cramps, muscle fasciculations, muscle weakness, tingling in extremities.
Respiratory: *bronchospasm, bronchoconstriction,* increased bronchial secretions.
Skin: rash, diaphoresis.

INTERACTIONS
Drug-drug. *Aminoglycosides:* May prolong or enhance muscle weakness. Use together cautiously.
Anticholinergics, atropine, corticosteroids, general or local anesthetics, magnesium, procainamide, quinidine: May antagonize cholinergic effects. Observe patient for lack of drug effect.
Ganglionic blockers: May increase risk of hypotension. Monitor patient closely.
Succinylcholine: May prolong the phase I block of the depolarizing muscle relaxant. Avoid using together.

EFFECTS ON LAB TEST RESULTS
None reported.

CONTRAINDICATIONS & CAUTIONS
• Contraindicated in patients hypersensitive to anticholinesterases or bromides and in those with mechanical obstruction of the intestinal or urinary tract.
• Use cautiously in patients with bronchial asthma, bradycardia, arrhythmias, epilepsy, recent coronary occlusion, vagotonia, renal impairment, hyperthyroidism, or peptic ulcer.

Reactions may be *common,* uncommon, *life-threatening,* or COMMON AND LIFE-THREATENING.
Interaction may have a *rapid onset* or **delayed onset.**

- Use cautiously in patients taking beta blockers for hypertension or glaucoma.
- Use cautiously in pregnant and breast-feeding women; drug appears in breast milk.

NURSING CONSIDERATIONS

- *Alert:* If taken immediately before or during soman exposure, drug may be ineffective and may worsen soman's effects. At the first sign of soman poisoning, stop drug and immediately start atropine and pralidoxime.
- Stop all other cholinergics before giving this drug.
- Monitor and document patient's response after each dose. Optimum dosage is difficult to judge.
- *Alert:* Regonol contains benzyl ethanol preservative, which may cause toxicity in neonates if given in high doses.
- *Look alike–sound alike:* Don't confuse pyridostigmine with physostigmine.

PATIENT TEACHING

- When giving drug for myasthenia gravis, stress importance of taking exactly as prescribed, on time, in evenly spaced doses. For extended-release tablets, tell patient to take at same time each day, at least 6 hours apart.
- Advise patient not to crush or chew extended-release tablets.
- Explain that patient may have to take drug for life.
- Advise patient to wear or carry medical identification that identifies his myasthenia gravis.
- Stress to military personnel importance of taking nerve agent antidotes, atropine and pralidoxime, rather than this drug at the first sign of nerve-agent poisoning.

sevelamer carbonate
seh-VELL-ah-meer

Renvela

sevelamer hydrochloride
Renagel

Pharmacologic class: polymeric phosphate binder
Pregnancy risk category C

AVAILABLE FORMS

sevelamer carbonate
Tablets (film-coated): 800 mg
sevelamer hydrochloride
Tablets (film-coated): 400 mg, 800 mg

INDICATIONS & DOSAGES

➤ **To control phosphorus level in chronic kidney disease patients on dialysis**
Adults not taking a phosphate binder: Initially, 800 to 1,600 mg (one to two 800-mg tablets or two to four 400-mg tablets) with each meal, based on phosphorus level. If phosphorus level is greater than 5.5 and less than 7.5 mg/dl, start with 800 mg t.i.d. with meals. If phosphorus level is greater than or equal to 7.5 and less than 9 mg/dl, start with two 800-mg tablets t.i.d., or three 400-mg tablets t.i.d. with meals. If phosphorus level is greater than or equal to 9 mg/dl, start with 1,600 mg t.i.d. (two 800-mg tablets or four 400-mg tablets) with meals.
Adults switching from calcium acetate: Initially, if taking one 667-mg calcium acetate tablet per meal, start with 800 mg per meal. If taking two 667-mg calcium acetate tablets per meal, start with two 800-mg tablets or three 400-mg tablets per meal. If taking three 667-mg calcium acetate tablets per meal, start with three 800-mg tablets or five 400-mg tablets per meal.
Adjust-a-dose: If phosphorus level is greater than 5.5 mg/dl, increase by one tablet per meal at 2-week intervals. If phosphorus level is 3.5 to 5.5 mg/dl, maintain current dose. If phosphorus level is less than 3.5 mg/dl, decrease dose by one tablet per meal.

ADMINISTRATION
P.O.
- Don't cut, crush, or allow patient to chew tablets.
- Give drug with meals.
- Drug may bind to other drugs and decrease their bioavailability. Give other drugs 1 hour before or 3 hours after this drug.
- Take special precautions when using antiarrhythmics or anticonvulsants with this drug.

ACTION
Inhibits intestinal phosphate absorption and decreases phosphorus levels.

Route	Onset	Peak	Duration
P.O.	Unknown	Unknown	Unknown

Half-life: Unknown.

ADVERSE REACTIONS
CNS: *headache, pain,* fever.
CV: *hypertension,* **thrombosis.**
GI: *diarrhea, dyspepsia, vomiting, nausea,* constipation, flatulence.
EENT: *nasopharyngitis.*
Musculoskeletal: *limb pain, arthralgia,* back pain.
Respiratory: *bronchitis, dyspnea,* increased cough, upper respiratory infection.
Skin: *pruritus.*

INTERACTIONS
Drug-drug. *Ciprofloxacin:* May decrease the effectiveness of ciprofloxacin. Give 1 hour before or 3 hours after sevelamer.

EFFECTS ON LAB TEST RESULTS
None reported.

CONTRAINDICATIONS & CAUTIONS
- Contraindicated in patients hypersensitive to drug or its components and in those with hypophosphatemia or bowel obstruction.
- Use cautiously in patient with dysphagia, swallowing disorders, severe GI motility disorders, or major GI tract surgery.

NURSING CONSIDERATIONS
- Monitor calcium, bicarbonate, and chloride levels.

- Watch for symptoms of thrombosis (numbness or tingling of limbs, chest pain, shortness of breath), and notify prescriber if they occur.

PATIENT TEACHING
- Instruct patient to take with meals and to adhere to prescribed diet.
- **Alert:** Inform patient that tablets must be taken whole because contents expand in water. Tell him not to cut, crush, or chew.
- Tell patient to take other drugs as directed, but they must be taken either 1 hour before or 3 hours after sevelamer.
- Inform patient about common adverse reactions. Teach patient signs and symptoms of thrombosis, such as numbness, tingling in arms or legs, or chest pain, and to report these immediately.

---

sodium polystyrene sulfonate
pol-ee-STYE-reen

Kayexalate, Kionex, SPS

Pharmacologic class: cation-exchange resin
Pregnancy risk category C

AVAILABLE FORMS
Powder: 1-lb jar (3.5 g/tsp)
Suspension: 15 g/60 ml*

INDICATIONS & DOSAGES
➤ **Hyperkalemia**
Adults: 15 g P.O. daily to q.i.d. in water or sorbitol (3 to 4 ml/g of resin). Or, mix powder with appropriate medium—aqueous suspension or diet appropriate for renal failure—and instill through a nasogastric tube. Or, 30 to 50 g/dl of sorbitol every 6 hours as warm emulsion deep into sigmoid colon (20 cm).
Children: 1 g/kg of body weight/dose P.O. every 6 hours, as needed.

ADMINISTRATION
P.O.
- Don't heat resin; this impairs drug's effect. Mix resin only with water or sorbitol for P.O. use. Never mix with orange juice (high potassium content) to disguise taste.
- Chill oral suspension for greater palatability.

• Oral administration is preferred because drug should remain in intestine for at least 30 minutes.
• If sorbitol is given, mix with resin suspension.
• Consider giving in solid form. Resin cookie and candy recipes are available; ask pharmacist or dietitian to supply.
Rectal
• Premixed forms (SPS and others) are available. If preparing manually, mix polystyrene resin only with water or sorbitol for rectal use. Don't use mineral oil for P.R. administration to prevent impaction; ion exchange needs aqueous medium. Sorbitol content prevents impaction.
• Prepare P.R. dose at room temperature. Stir emulsion gently during administration.
• Use #28 French rubber tube for rectal dose; insert 20 cm into sigmoid colon. Tape tube in place. Or, consider an indwelling urinary catheter with a 30-ml balloon inflated distal to anal sphincter to aid in retention. This is especially helpful for patients with poor sphincter control. Use gravity flow. Drain returns constantly through Y-tube connection. Place patient in knee-chest position or with hips on pillow for a while if back leakage occurs.
• After P.R. administration, flush tubing with 50 to 100 ml of nonsodium fluid to ensure delivery of all drug. Flush rectum to remove resin.
• Prevent fecal impaction in elderly patients by giving resin P.R. Give cleansing enema before P.R. administration. Have patient retain enema for 6 to 10 hours if possible, but 30 to 60 minutes is acceptable.

ACTION
Exchanges sodium ions for potassium ions in the intestine: 1 g of sodium polystyrene sulfonate is exchanged for 0.5 to 1 mEq of potassium; the resin is then eliminated. Much of the exchange capacity is used for calcium, magnesium, and possibly fats and proteins.

Route	Onset	Peak	Duration
P.O., P.R.	2–12 hr	Unknown	Unknown

Half-life: Unknown.

ADVERSE REACTIONS
GI: *constipation, diarrhea with sorbitol emulsions,* fecal impaction, anorexia, gastric irritation, nausea, vomiting.
Metabolic: hypokalemia, hypocalcemia, *hypomagnesemia,* sodium retention.

INTERACTIONS
Drug-drug. *Antacids and laxatives containing magnesium and calcium:* May cause systemic alkalosis and reduce potassium exchange capability. Avoid using together. If it can't be avoided, separate doses by several hours.

EFFECTS ON LAB TEST RESULTS
• May increase sodium level. May decrease potassium, calcium, and magnesium levels.

CONTRAINDICATIONS & CAUTIONS
• Contraindicated in patients hypersensitive to drug and in those with hypokalemia.
• Use cautiously in patients with severe heart failure, severe hypertension, or marked edema. Drug provides 100 mg sodium/g.

NURSING CONSIDERATIONS
• Watch for constipation with oral or nasogastric administration. Give 10 to 20 ml of 70% sorbitol syrup every 2 hours, p.r.n. to produce one or two watery stools daily.
• Monitor potassium level at least once daily. Treatment may result in potassium deficiency and is usually stopped when potassium is reduced to 4 or 5 mEq/L.
• Watch for signs of hypokalemia: irritability, confusion, arrhythmias, ECG changes, severe muscle weakness or even paralysis, and digitalis toxicity in digitalized patients.
• When hyperkalemia is severe, polystyrene resin alone isn't adequate for lowering potassium. Dextrose 50% with regular insulin I.V. push may also be given.
• Watch for symptoms of other electrolyte deficiencies (magnesium, calcium) because drug is nonselective. Monitor calcium level in patients receiving sodium polystyrene therapy for more than 3 days. Supplementary calcium may be needed.

• Watch for sodium overload. Drug contains about 100 mg sodium/g. About one-third of resin's sodium is retained.

PATIENT TEACHING
• Explain use and administration of drug to patient.
• Advise patient to report adverse reactions promptly.
• Teach patient about low-potassium diet.

---

succimer
SUX-i-mer

Chemet

Pharmacologic class: heavy metal
Pregnancy risk category C

AVAILABLE FORMS
Capsules: 100 mg

INDICATIONS & DOSAGES
➤ **Lead poisoning in children with lead levels greater than 45 mcg/dl**
Children: Initially, 10 mg/kg or 350 mg/m² every 8 hours for 5 days. Because capsules come only in 100 mg, round dose to nearest 100 mg, as appropriate (see table). Then reduce frequency of administration to every 12 hours for another 2 weeks.

Weight in kg (lb)	Dose (mg)
> 45 (> 100)	500
35–44 (76–100)	400
24–34 (56–75)	300
16–23 (36–55)	200
8–15 (18–35)	100

ADMINISTRATION
P.O.
• If necessary, open capsule and sprinkle contents on small amount of soft food. Or, pour beads from capsule onto a spoon, have patient swallow them, and follow that with flavored beverage.

ACTION
A chelating drug that forms water-soluble complexes with lead and increases its excretion in urine.

Route	Onset	Peak	Duration
P.O.	Unknown	1–2 hr	Unknown

Half-life: 48 hours.

ADVERSE REACTIONS
CNS: *drowsiness, dizziness, sensorimotor neuropathy, sleepiness, paresthesia, headache.*
CV: *arrhythmias.*
EENT: plugged ears, cloudy film in eyes, otitis media, watery eyes, sore throat, rhinorrhea, nasal congestion.
GI: *nausea, vomiting, diarrhea, anorexia, abdominal cramps, hemorrhoidal symptoms, metallic taste in mouth, loose stools.*
GU: decreased urination, difficult urination, proteinuria.
Hematologic: *neutropenia,* increased platelet count, intermittent eosinophilia.
Musculoskeletal: *leg, kneecap, back, stomach, rib, or flank pain.*
Respiratory: cough, head cold.
Skin: papular rash, herpetic rash, mucocutaneous eruptions, pruritus.
Other: *flulike syndrome,* candidiasis.

INTERACTIONS
Drug-drug. *Other chelating drugs (such as edetate calcium disodium):* May cause unknown adverse effects. Separate administration times by 4 weeks.

EFFECTS ON LAB TEST RESULTS
• May increase AST, ALT, alkaline phosphatase, and cholesterol levels.
• May increase eosinophil and platelet counts.
• May cause false-positive urine ketone results.

CONTRAINDICATIONS & CAUTIONS
• Contraindicated in patients hypersensitive to drug.
• Use cautiously in patients with compromised renal function.

NURSING CONSIDERATIONS
• Measure severity of poisoning by initial lead level and by rate and degree of rebound of lead level. Use severity as a guide for more frequent lead monitoring.
• Monitor patient at least once weekly for rebound lead levels. Elevated levels and associated symptoms may return

---

Reactions may be *common*, uncommon, *life-threatening*, or COMMON AND LIFE-THREATENING.
Interaction may have a *rapid onset* or **delayed onset**.

rapidly after drug is stopped because of redistribution of lead from bone to soft tissues and blood.

• Monitor transaminase levels before and at least weekly during therapy. Transient mild elevations may occur.

• Course of treatment lasts 19 days and may be repeated if indicated by weekly monitoring of lead levels.

• Minimum of 2 weeks between courses is recommended unless high lead levels indicate need for immediate therapy.

• Don't give with other chelating drugs. Patient who has received edetate calcium disodium with or without dimercaprol may use succimer after a 4-week interval.

PATIENT TEACHING

• Explain drug use and administration to parents and child. Stress importance of complying with frequent blood tests.

• Tell parents of young child who can't swallow capsules that capsule can be opened and its contents sprinkled on a small amount of soft food. Or, beads from capsule may be poured on a spoon and followed with flavored beverage.

• Tell parents to give child adequate fluids.

• Assist parents with identifying and removing sources of lead in child's environment. Chelation therapy isn't a substitute for preventing further exposure.

• Tell parents to notify prescriber if rash occurs. Tell them allergic or other muco-cutaneous reactions may occur each time drug is used.

96

Electrolyte balancing drugs

calcium acetate
calcium chloride
calcium citrate
calcium glubionate
calcium gluconate
calcium lactate
calcium phosphate, dibasic
calcium phosphate, tribasic
magnesium chloride
magnesium sulfate
potassium acetate
potassium bicarbonate
potassium chloride
potassium gluconate
sodium chloride

---

calcium acetate
PhosLo Gelcaps

calcium chloride

calcium citrate ◊
Citracal ◊, Citracal Liquitab ◊

calcium glubionate
Calciquid

calcium gluconate

calcium lactate ◊
Cal-Lac ◊

calcium phosphate, dibasic ◊

calcium phosphate, tribasic
Posture ◊

Pharmacologic class: calcium salts
Pregnancy risk category NR;
C (PhosLo)

AVAILABLE FORMS
calcium acetate
Contains 253 mg or 12.7 mEq of elemental calcium/g
Capsules: 333.5 mg, 667 mg
Gelcaps: 667 mg
Tablets: 667 mg

calcium chloride
Contains 270 mg or 13.5 mEq of elemental calcium/g
Injection: 10% solution in 10-ml ampules, vials, and syringes
calcium citrate
Contains 211 mg or 10.6 mEq of elemental calcium/g
Tablets: 250 mg, 950 mg ◊
Tablets (effervescent): 500 mg of elemental calcium ◊
calcium glubionate
Contains 64 mg or 3.2 mEq elemental calcium/g
Syrup: 1.8 g/5 ml
calcium gluconate
Contains 90 mg or 4.5 mEq of elemental calcium/g
Injection: 10% solution in 10-ml ampules and vials, 10-ml or 50-ml vials
Powder for oral suspension: 346.7 elemental calcium/15 ml
Tablets: 500 mg ◊, 650 mg ◊, 1 g ◊
calcium lactate
Contains 130 mg or 6.5 mEq of elemental calcium/g
Capsules: 500 mg (96 mg elemental calcium)
Tablets: 100 mg, 650 mg (84.5 mg elemental calcium)
calcium phosphate, dibasic
Contains 230 mg or 11.5 mEq of elemental calcium/g
Tablets: 500 mg ◊
calcium phosphate, tribasic
Contains 400 mg or 20 mEq of elemental calcium/g
Tablets: 600 mg ◊

INDICATIONS & DOSAGES
➤ **Hypocalcemic emergency**
Adults: 7 mEq to 14 mEq calcium I.V. May give as a 10% calcium gluconate solution, 2% to 10% calcium chloride solution.
Children: 1 mEq to 7 mEq calcium I.V.
Infants: Up to 1 mEq calcium I.V.
➤ **Hypocalcemic tetany**
Adults: 4.5 mEq to 16 mEq calcium I.V. Repeat until tetany is controlled.

Reactions may be *common*, uncommon, **life-threatening**, or COMMON AND LIFE-THREATENING.
Interaction may have a *rapid onset* or **delayed onset**.

Children: 0.5 to 0.7 mEq/kg calcium I.V. t.i.d. to q.i.d. until tetany is controlled.
Neonates: 2.4 mEq/kg calcium I.V. daily in divided doses.

➤ **Adjunctive treatment of magnesium intoxication**
Adults: Initially, 7 mEq I.V. Base subsequent doses on patient's response.

➤ **During exchange transfusions**
Adults: 1.35 mEq I.V. with each 100 ml citrated blood.
Neonates: 0.45 mEq I.V. after each 100 ml citrated blood.

➤ **Hyperphosphatemia**
Adults: 1,334 to 2,000 mg P.O. calcium acetate or 2 to 5.2 g calcium ion t.i.d. with meals. Most dialysis patients need 3 to 4 tablets with each meal.

➤ **Dietary supplement**
Adults: 500 mg to 2 g P.O. daily.

➤ **Hyperkalemia with secondary cardiac toxicity**
Adults: 2.25 mEq to 14 mEq I.V. Repeat dose after 1 to 2 minutes, if needed.

ADMINISTRATION
P.O.
- Give drug with a full glass of water.
- Give 1 to 1½ hours after meals if GI upset occurs.

I.V.
- Calcium salts are not interchangeable; verify preparation before use.
- Give calcium chloride only by I.V. route. When adding to parenteral solutions that contain other additives (especially phosphorus or phosphate), watch for precipitate. Use an in-line filter.
- When giving calcium gluconate as injection, give only by I.V. route.
- Monitor ECG when giving calcium I.V. Stop drug and notify prescriber if patient complains of discomfort.
- Extravasation may cause severe necrosis and tissue sloughing. Calcium gluconate is less irritating to veins and tissues than calcium chloride.

Direct injection
- Don't use scalp veins in children.
- Warm solution to body temperature before giving it.
- For calcium chloride, give at 1 ml/minute (1.5 mEq/minute); for calcium gluconate, 2 ml/minute.

- Give slowly through a small needle into a large vein or through an I.V. line containing a free-flowing, compatible solution.
- After injection, keep patient recumbent for 15 minutes.

Intermittent infusion
- Infuse diluted solution through an I.V. line containing a compatible solution.
- For calcium gluconate, don't exceed 200 mg/minute.
- **Incompatibilities:** Drug will precipitate if given with sodium bicarbonate or other alkaline drugs. Calcium chloride: amphotericin B, chlorpheniramine, dobutamine. Calcium gluconate: amphotericin B, dobutamine, fluconazole, indomethacin sodium trihydrate, methylprednisolone sodium succinate, prochlorperazine edisylate.

I.M.
- Use I.M. calcium gluconate only in emergencies when no I.V. route is available because of irritation of tissue by calcium salts.
- Give I.M. in gluteal muscle in adults and in side of the thigh in infants.

ACTION
Replaces calcium and maintains calcium level.

Route	Onset	Peak	Duration
P.O.	Unknown	Unknown	Unknown
I.V.	Immediate	Immediate	30 min–2 hr
I.M.			

Half-life: Unknown.

ADVERSE REACTIONS
CNS: tingling sensations, sense of oppression or heat waves with I.V. use, syncope with rapid I.V. use.
CV: *bradycardia, arrhythmias, cardiac arrest with rapid I.V. use,* mild drop in blood pressure, vasodilation.
GI: *constipation,* irritation, chalky taste, *hemorrhage,* nausea, vomiting, thirst, abdominal pain.
GU: polyuria, renal calculi.
Metabolic: hypercalcemia.
Skin: local reactions, including burning, necrosis, tissue sloughing, cellulitis, soft-tissue calcification with I.M. use.

INTERACTIONS
Drug-drug. *Atenolol, tetracyclines:* May decrease bioavailability of these drugs and calcium when oral preparations are taken together. Separate dosing times.
Cardiac glycosides: May increase digoxin toxicity. Give calcium cautiously, if at all, to digitalized patients.
Ciprofloxacin, levofloxacin, lomefloxacin, moxifloxacin, norfloxacin, ofloxacin:
May decrease effects of quinolone. Give calcium carbonate at least 6 hours before or 2 hours after quinolone.
Fosphenytoin, phenytoin: Use together may decrease absorption of both drugs. Avoid using together, or monitor levels carefully.
Sodium polystyrene sulfonate: May cause metabolic acidosis in patients with renal disease and a reduction of the resin's binding of potassium. Separate drugs by several hours.
Thiazide diuretics: May cause hypercalcemia. Avoid using together.
Verapamil: May reduce effects and toxicity of verapamil. Monitor patient closely.
Drug-food. *Foods containing oxalic acid (rhubarb, spinach), phytic acid (bran, whole-grain cereals), phosphorus (dairy products, milk):* May interfere with calcium absorption. Discourage use together.

EFFECTS ON LAB TEST RESULTS
• May increase calcium level.

CONTRAINDICATIONS & CAUTIONS
• Contraindicated in cancer patients with bone metastases and in those with ventricular fibrillation, hypercalcemia, hypophosphatemia, or renal calculi.

NURSING CONSIDERATIONS
• Use all calcium products with extreme caution in digitalized patients and patients with sarcoidosis and renal or cardiac disease. Use calcium chloride cautiously in patients with cor pulmonale, respiratory acidosis, or respiratory failure.
• *Alert:* Double-check that you are giving the correct form of calcium; resuscitation cart may contain both calcium gluconate and calcium chloride.
• Monitor calcium levels frequently. Maintain calcium level of 9 to 10.4 mg/dl. Don't allow level to exceed 12 mg/dl.

Hypercalcemia may result after large doses in chronic renal failure. Report abnormalities.
• Signs and symptoms of severe hypercalcemia may include stupor, confusion, delirium, and coma. Signs and symptoms of mild hypercalcemia may include anorexia, nausea, and vomiting.
• *Look alike–sound alike:* Don't confuse calcium with calcitriol, calcium gluconate with calcium glubionate, or calcium chloride with calcium gluconate.

PATIENT TEACHING
• Tell patient to take oral calcium 1 to 1½ hours after meals if GI upset occurs.
• Tell patient to take oral calcium with a full glass of water.
• Tell patient to report anorexia, nausea, vomiting, constipation, abdominal pain, dry mouth, thirst, or polyuria.
• Warn patient that, in the meal before he takes calcium, he shouldn't have rhubarb, spinach, bran and whole-grain cereals, or dairy products; these foods may interfere with calcium absorption.
• Inform patient that some products may contain phenylalanine or tartrazine.

magnesium chloride
Slow-Mag ◊

magnesium sulfate

Pharmacologic class: magnesium salt
Pregnancy risk category C (chloride injection); A (sulfate injection)

AVAILABLE FORMS
magnesium chloride
Injection: 20% in 50-ml vials
Tablets (delayed-release): 64 mg
magnesium sulfate
Injectable solutions: 10%, 12.5%, 50% in 2-, 5-, 10-, 20-, and 30-ml ampules, vials, and prefilled syringes

INDICATIONS & DOSAGES
➤ **Mild hypomagnesemia**
Adults: 1 g I.V. by piggyback or I.M. every 6 hours for four doses, depending on magnesium level. Or, 3 g P.O. every 6 hours for four doses.

Reactions may be *common*, uncommon, *life-threatening*, or COMMON AND LIFE-THREATENING.
Interaction may have a *rapid onset* or *delayed onset.*

➤ **Symptomatic severe hypo-magnesemia, with magnesium 0.8 mEq/L or less**
Adults: 5 g I.V. in 1 L of solution over 3 hours. Base subsequent doses on magnesium level.

➤ **Magnesium supplementation**
Adults: 64 mg (one tablet) P.O. t.i.d.

➤ **Magnesium supplementation in total parenteral nutrition (TPN)**
Adults and children: 8 to 24 mEq I.V. daily added to TPN solution.
Infants: 2 to 10 mEq I.V. daily added to TPN solution. Each 2 ml of 50% solution contains 1 g, or 8.12 mEq, magnesium sulfate.

➤ **Seizures associated with epilepsy, glomerulonephritis, or hypothyroidism**
Adults: 1 g I.M. or I.V.

➤ **Severe pre-eclampsia or eclampsia**
Adults: 4 to 5 g I.V. in 250 ml of solution. Simultaneously, give up to 10 g I.M. (5 g or 10 ml of the undiluted 50% solution in each buttock.) Base subsequent doses on magnesium level. Do not exceed 30 to 40 g in a 24 hour period.

➤ **Barium poisoning**
Adults: 1 to 2 g magnesium sulfate I.V.

➤ **Cerebral edema**
Adults: 2.5 g (25 ml of a 10% solution) I.V.

ADMINISTRATION
P.O.
- Give drug with food.
- Store between 20° and 25° C (68° and 77° F).

I.V.
- Concentration should be 200 mg/ml or less.
- Inject bolus dose slowly at a rate of 150 mg/minute or less, or use infusion pump for continuous infusion to avoid respiratory or cardiac arrest. Maximum infusion rate is 150 mg/minute. Rapid drip causes feeling of heat.
- For severe hypomagnesemia, watch for respiratory depression and evidence of heart block. Respirations should be better than 16 breaths/minute before giving dose.
- **Incompatibilities:** Alcohol (in large amounts), alkali carbonates and bicarbonates, amiodarone, amphotericin B, calcium chloride, calcium gluconate, cefepime,

ciprofloxacin, clindamycin, cyclosporine, dobutamine, drotrecogin alfa, heavy metals, hydralazine, hydrocortisone sodium succinate, I.V. fat emulsion 10%, phytonadione, polymyxin B, procaine, quinolones, salicylates, sodium bicarbonate, soluble phosphates, vitamin B complex.

I.M.
- Undiluted 50% solutions may be given by deep I.M. injection to adults. Dilute solutions to 20% or less for use in children.

ACTION
Replaces magnesium and maintains magnesium level; as an anticonvulsant, reduces muscle contractions by interfering with release of acetylcholine at myoneural junction.

Route	Onset	Peak	Duration
P.O.	Unknown	4 hr	4–6 hr
I.V.	Immediate	Unknown	30 min
I.M.	1 hr	Unknown	3–4 hr

Half-life: Unknown.

ADVERSE REACTIONS
CNS: toxicity, *weak or absent deep tendon reflexes,* flaccid paralysis, drowsiness, stupor.
CV: slow, weak pulse, ***arrhythmias,*** *hypotension,* **circulatory collapse,** flushing.
GI: diarrhea.
Metabolic: hypocalcemia.
Respiratory: *respiratory paralysis.*
Skin: diaphoresis.
Other: hypothermia.

INTERACTIONS
Drug-drug. *Alendronate, fluoroquinolones, nitrofurantoin, penicillamine, sodium polystyrene sulfonate, tetracyclines:* May decrease bioavailability with oral magnesium supplements. Separate doses by 2 to 3 hours.
Cardiac glycosides: May cause serious cardiac conduction changes. Use together with caution.
CNS depressants: May have additive effect. Use together cautiously.
Neuromuscular blockers: May cause increased neuromuscular blockage. Use together cautiously.

EFFECTS ON LAB TEST RESULTS
• May increase magnesium level. May decrease calcium level.

CONTRAINDICATIONS & CAUTIONS
• Contraindicated in patients with myocardial damage or heart block, coma, and in pregnant women in actively progressing labor.
• Use parenteral magnesium with caution in patients with impaired renal function.

NURSING CONSIDERATIONS
• Keep I.V. calcium available to reverse magnesium intoxication.
• Test knee-jerk and patellar reflexes before each additional dose. If absent, notify prescriber and give no more magnesium until reflexes return; otherwise, patient may develop temporary respiratory failure and need cardiopulmonary resuscitation or I.V. administration of calcium.
• Check magnesium level after repeated doses.
• Monitor fluid intake and output. Output should be 100 ml or more during 4-hour period before dose.
• Monitor renal function.
• After giving to toxemic pregnant woman within 24 hours before delivery, watch neonate for signs and symptoms of magnesium toxicity, including neuromuscular and respiratory depression.
• *Look alike–sound alike:* Don't confuse magnesium sulfate with manganese sulfate.

PATIENT TEACHING
• Explain use and administration of drug to patient and family.
• Tell patient to report adverse effects.

---

potassium acetate

Pharmacologic class: potassium salt
Pregnancy risk category C

AVAILABLE FORMS
Injection: 2 mEq/ml in 20-, 50-, and 100-ml vials, 4 mEq/ml in 50-ml vial

INDICATIONS & DOSAGES
➤ **Hypokalemia**
Adults: No more than 20 mEq/hour in concentration of 40 mEq/L or less. Total

24-hour dose shouldn't exceed 150 mEq (3 mEq/kg in children).
➤ **To prevent hypokalemia**
Adults: Dosage is individualized to patient's needs, not to exceed 150 mEq daily. Give as an additive to I.V. infusions. Usual dose is 20 mEq/L, infused at no more than 20 mEq/hour.
Children: Individualize dose; don't exceed 3 mEq/kg daily. Give as an additive to I.V. infusions.

ADMINISTRATION
I.V.
• Use only in life-threatening hypokalemia or when oral replacement isn't feasible.
• Don't give undiluted potassium. Maximum concentration is 80 mEq/L.
• Don't add potassium to a hanging bag. Mix well to avoid layering.
• To prevent pain, use largest peripheral vein and a well-placed small-bore needle.
• Give only by infusion, never I.V. push or I.M. Watch for pain and redness at infusion site.
• Give slowly as diluted solution; rapid infusion may cause fatal hyperkalemia.
• **Incompatibilities:** None reported.

ACTION
Replaces potassium and maintains potassium level.

Route	Onset	Peak	Duration
I.V.	Immediate	Immediate	Unknown

Half-life: Unknown.

ADVERSE REACTIONS
CNS: paresthesia of limbs, listlessness, mental confusion, weakness or heaviness of legs, flaccid paralysis, pain, fever.
CV: *arrhythmias, cardiac arrest, heart block,* ECG changes, hypotension.
GI: nausea, vomiting, abdominal pain, diarrhea.
Metabolic: *hyperkalemia.*
Respiratory: *respiratory paralysis.*
Skin: redness at infusion site.

INTERACTIONS
Drug-drug. *ACE inhibitors, digoxin, potassium-sparing diuretics:* May increase risk of hyperkalemia. Use together with caution.

Reactions may be *common,* uncommon, *life-threatening,* or COMMON AND LIFE-THREATENING.
Interaction may have a *rapid onset* or *delayed onset.*

Digoxin: May cause digoxin toxicity, from hypokalemia. Stop potassium cautiously if patient is taking digoxin.

EFFECTS ON LAB TEST RESULTS
• May increase potassium level.

CONTRAINDICATIONS & CAUTIONS
• Contraindicated in patients with severe renal impairment with oliguria, anuria, or azotemia.
• Contraindicated in those with untreated Addison's disease, acute dehydration, heat cramps, hyperkalemia, hyperkalemic form of familial periodic paralysis, or conditions linked to extensive tissue breakdown.
• Use cautiously in patients with cardiac disease or renal impairment.

NURSING CONSIDERATIONS
• During therapy, monitor ECG, renal function, fluid intake and output, and potassium, creatinine, and BUN levels. Never give potassium postoperatively until urine flow is established.
• Many adverse reactions may reflect hyperkalemia.
• *Look alike–sound alike:* Potassium preparations aren't interchangeable; verify preparation before use.

PATIENT TEACHING
• Explain use and administration to patient and family.
• Tell patient to report adverse effects, especially pain at insertion site.

---

potassium bicarbonate
K-Lyte, Klor-Con/EF

Pharmacologic class: potassium salt
Pregnancy risk category C

AVAILABLE FORMS
Tablets (effervescent): 25 mEq, 50 mEq

INDICATIONS & DOSAGES
➤ **To prevent hypokalemia**
Adults and children: Initially, 20 mEq P.O. daily, in divided doses. Adjust dosage, as needed.

➤ **Hypokalemia**
Adults and children: 40 to 100 mEq P.O. divided into two to four daily doses. Don't exceed 150 mEq P.O. daily in adults and 3 mEq/kg daily P.O. in children.

ADMINISTRATION
P.O.
• Dissolve tablets completely in 4 to 8 ounces of cold water.
• Available in lime, fruit punch, citrus, or orange.

ACTION
Replaces potassium and maintains potassium level.

Route	Onset	Peak	Duration
P.O.	Unknown	4 hr	Unknown

Half-life: Unknown.

ADVERSE REACTIONS
CNS: paresthesia of limbs, listlessness, confusion, weakness or heaviness of legs, flaccid paralysis.
CV: *arrhythmias,* ECG changes, hypotension, *heart block, cardiac arrest.*
GI: *nausea, vomiting, abdominal pain,* diarrhea.

INTERACTIONS
Drug-drug. *ACE inhibitors, digoxin, potassium-sparing diuretics:* May cause hyperkalemia. Use with extreme caution. Monitor potassium levels.

EFFECTS ON LAB TEST RESULTS
• May increase potassium level.

CONTRAINDICATIONS & CAUTIONS
• Contraindicated in patients with severe renal impairment with oliguria, anuria, or azotemia; untreated Addison's disease; or acute dehydration, heat cramps, hyperkalemia, hyperkalemic form of familial periodic paralysis, or other conditions linked to extensive tissue breakdown.
• Use cautiously in patients with cardiac disease or renal impairment.

NURSING CONSIDERATIONS
• Don't give potassium supplements postoperatively until urine flow has been established.

• *Alert:* Potassium preparations aren't interchangeable; verify preparation before use. Never switch potassium products without prescriber's order. Potassium chloride can't be given instead of potassium bicarbonate.
• Use I.V. potassium chloride when oral replacement isn't feasible.
• Monitor fluid intake and output and BUN, potassium, and creatinine levels.

PATIENT TEACHING
• Tell patient to take drug with meals and sip slowly over 5 to 10 minutes.
• Tell patient to report adverse effects.
• Warn patient not to use salt substitutes at the same time, except with prescriber's permission.

SAFETY ALERT!

potassium chloride
Apo-K*†, Cena-K, K 10†, Kaon-Cl, Kaon-Cl-10, Kay Ciel, K-Dur 20✐, K-Lor, Klor-Con, Klor-Con 8, Klor-Con 10, Klor-Con/25, Klor-Con M10, Klor-Con M15, Klor-Con M20, Klotrix, K-Lyte/Cl, K-Tab, Micro-K, Micro-K 10, Micro-K LS, Potasalan

Pharmacologic class: potassium salt
Pregnancy risk category C

AVAILABLE FORMS
Capsules (controlled-release): 8 mEq, 10 mEq
Injection concentrate: 1.5 mEq/ml, 2 mEq/ml
Injection for I.V. infusion: 0.1 mEq/ml, 0.2 mEq/ml, 0.3 mEq/ml, 0.4 mEq/ml
Oral liquid: 20 mEq/15 ml, 30 mEq/15 ml, 40 mEq/15 ml
Powder for oral administration: 15 mEq/packet, 20 mEq/packet, 25 mEq/packet
Tablets (controlled-release): 6.7 mEq, 8 mEq, 10 mEq, 20 mEq
Tablets (extended-release): 8 mEq, 10 mEq, 15 mEq, 20 mEq

INDICATIONS & DOSAGES
➤ **To prevent hypokalemia**
Adults and children: Initially, 20 mEq of potassium supplement P.O. daily, in

divided doses. Adjust dosage, as needed, based on potassium levels.
➤ **Hypokalemia**
Adults and children: 40 to 100 mEq P.O. in two to four divided doses daily. Maximum dose of diluted I.V. potassium chloride is 40 mEq/L at 10 mEq/hour. Don't exceed 200 mEq daily in adults and 3 mEq/kg daily in children. Further doses are based on potassium levels and blood pH. Give I.V. potassium replacement only with monitoring of ECG and potassium level.
➤ **Severe hypokalemia**
Adults and children: Dilute potassium chloride in a suitable I.V. solution of less than 80 mEq/L, and give at no more than 40 mEq/hour.
Further doses are based on potassium level. Don't exceed 400 mEq I.V. daily in adults and 3 mEq/kg I.V. daily in children. Give I.V. potassium replacement only with monitoring of ECG and potassium level.

ADMINISTRATION
P.O.
• Make sure powders are completely dissolved before giving.
• Enteric-coated tablets are not recommended because of increased risk of GI bleeding and small-bowel ulcerations.
• Tablets in wax matrix may lodge in the esophagus and cause ulceration in cardiac patients with esophageal compression from an enlarged left atrium. Use sugar-free liquid form in these patients and in those with esophageal stasis or obstruction. Have patient sip slowly to minimize GI irritation.
• Don't crush sustained-release forms.
I.V.
• Use only when oral replacement isn't feasible or when hypokalemia is life-threatening.
• Give by infusion only, never I.V. push or I.M. Give slowly as dilute solution; rapid infusion may cause fatal hyperkalemia.
• If burning occurs during infusion, decrease rate.
• **Incompatibilities:** Amikacin, amoxicillin, amphotericin B, azithromycin, diazepam, dobutamine, ergotamine, etoposide with cisplatin and mannitol, fat emulsion 10%, methylprednisolone, penicillin G, phenytoin, promethazine.

Reactions may be *common,* uncommon, *life-threatening,* or COMMON AND LIFE-THREATENING.
Interaction may have a *rapid onset* or *delayed onset.*

ACTION
Replaces potassium and maintains potassium level.

Route	Onset	Peak	Duration
P.O.	Unknown	Unknown	Unknown
I.V.	Immediate	Immediate	Unknown

Half-life: Unknown.

ADVERSE REACTIONS
CNS: paresthesia of limbs, listlessness, confusion, weakness or heaviness of limbs, flaccid paralysis.
CV: *postinfusion phlebitis, **arrhythmias, heart block, cardiac arrest,*** ECG changes, hypotension.
GI: nausea, vomiting, abdominal pain, diarrhea.
Metabolic: *hyperkalemia.*
Respiratory: *respiratory paralysis.*

INTERACTIONS
Drug-drug. *ACE inhibitors, digoxin, potassium-sparing diuretics:* May cause hyperkalemia. Use together with extreme caution. Monitor potassium level.

EFFECTS ON LAB TEST RESULTS
• May increase potassium level.

CONTRAINDICATIONS & CAUTIONS
• Contraindicated in patients with severe renal impairment with oliguria, anuria, or azotemia; with untreated Addison's disease; or with acute dehydration, heat cramps, hyperkalemia, hyperkalemic form of familial periodic paralysis, or other conditions linked to extensive tissue breakdown.
• Use cautiously in patients with cardiac disease or renal impairment.

NURSING CONSIDERATIONS
• Patients at an increased risk of GI lesions include those with scleroderma, diabetes, mitral valve replacement, cardiomegaly, or esophageal strictures, and in elderly or immobile patients.
• Drug is commonly used orally with potassium-wasting diuretics to maintain potassium levels.
• Monitor ECG and electrolyte levels during therapy.

• Monitor renal function. After surgery, don't give drug until urine flow is established.
• Many adverse reactions may reflect hyperkalemia.
• Patient may be sensitive to tartrazine in some of these products.
• ***Look alike–sound alike:*** Potassium preparations aren't interchangeable; verify preparation before use and don't switch products.

PATIENT TEACHING
• Teach patient how to prepare powders and how to take drug. Tell patient to take with or after meals with full glass of water or fruit juice to lessen GI distress.
• Teach patient signs and symptoms of hyperkalemia, and tell patient to notify prescriber if they occur.
• Tell patient to report discomfort at I.V. insertion site.
• Warn patient not to use salt substitutes concurrently, except with prescriber's permission.
• Tell patient not to be concerned if wax matrix appears in stool because the drug has already been absorbed.

potassium gluconate
Kaon*, Kaylixir*

Pharmacologic class: potassium salt
Pregnancy risk category C

AVAILABLE FORMS
Elixir: 20 mEq/15 ml*
Tablets: 500 mg (83 mg potassium) ◊, 595 mg (99 mg potassium) ◊

INDICATIONS & DOSAGES
➤ **To prevent hypokalemia**
Adults and children: Initially, 20 mEq of potassium supplement P.O. daily, in divided doses. Adjust dosage, as needed, based on potassium level.
➤ **Hypokalemia**
Adults and children: 40 to 100 mEq P.O. divided into two to four daily doses. Use I.V. potassium chloride when oral replacement isn't feasible. Don't exceed 150 mEq P.O. daily in adults and 3 mEq/kg daily P.O. in children.

ADMINISTRATION
P.O.
- Have patient sip liquid potassium slowly to minimize GI irritation.
- Give drug with meals, with a full glass of water or fruit juice.

ACTION
Replaces potassium and maintains intracellular and extracellular potassium levels.

Route	Onset	Peak	Duration
P.O.	Unknown	Unknown	4 hr

Half-life: Unknown.

ADVERSE REACTIONS
CNS: paresthesia of limbs, listlessness, confusion, weakness or heaviness of legs, flaccid paralysis.
CV: *arrhythmias,* ECG changes.
GI: *nausea, vomiting, abdominal pain,* diarrhea.

INTERACTIONS
Drug-drug. *ACE inhibitors, digoxin, potassium-sparing diuretics:* May cause hyperkalemia. Use with caution. Monitor potassium level.

EFFECTS ON LAB TEST RESULTS
- May increase potassium level.

CONTRAINDICATIONS & CAUTIONS
- Contraindicated in patients with severe renal impairment with oliguria, anuria, or azotemia; untreated Addison's disease; or acute dehydration, heat cramps, hyperkalemia, hyperkalemic form of familial periodic paralysis, or other conditions linked to extensive tissue breakdown.
- Use cautiously in patients with cardiac disease or renal impairment.

NURSING CONSIDERATIONS
- *Alert:* Give oral potassium supplements with caution because different forms deliver varying amounts of potassium. Never switch products without prescriber's order.
- Don't give potassium supplements postoperatively until urine flow has been established.
- Monitor ECG, fluid intake and output, and BUN, potassium, and creatinine levels.

PATIENT TEACHING
- Advise patient to sip liquid potassium slowly to minimize GI irritation. Also tell him to take drug with meals, with a full glass of water or fruit juice.
- Warn patient not to use potassium gluconate with a salt substitute, except with prescriber's permission.
- Teach patient signs and symptoms of hyperkalemia, and tell him to notify prescriber if they occur.

SAFETY ALERT!

sodium chloride
Slo-Salt, Slo-Salt-K, Sustain

Pharmacologic class: sodium salt
Pregnancy risk category C

AVAILABLE FORMS
Injection: Half-normal saline solution 25 ml, 50 ml, 150 ml, 250 ml, 500 ml, 1,000 ml; normal saline solution 2 ml, 3 ml, 5 ml, 10 ml, 20 ml, 25 ml, 30 ml, 50 ml, 100 ml, 150 ml, 250 ml, 500 ml, 1,000 ml; 3% sodium chloride solution 500 ml; 5% sodium chloride solution 500 ml; 14.6% sodium chloride solution 20 ml, 40 ml, 200 ml; 23.4% sodium chloride solution 30 ml, 50 ml, 100 ml, 200 ml
Tablets: 220 mg (with 18 mg calcium carbonate and 15 mg potassium chloride), 650 mg, 1 g, 2.25 g ◇
Tablets (slow-release): 410 mg (with 150 mg potassium chloride) ◇, 600 mg ◇

INDICATIONS & DOSAGES
➤ **Fluid and electrolyte replacement in hyponatremia caused by electrolyte loss or in severe salt depletion**
Adults: Dosage is individualized. Use 3% or 5% solution only with frequent electrolyte level determination and only slow I.V. Don't exceed 100 ml/hour or 400 ml/24 hour. For 0.45% solution, dose according to deficiencies, over 18 to 24 hours. For 0.9% solution, dose according to deficiencies, over 18 to 24 hours.
➤ **Prevention of heat prostration**
Adults: 1 g P.O. with each glass of water, or as directed by prescriber.

Reactions may be *common,* uncommon, *life-threatening,* or COMMON AND LIFE-THREATENING.
Interaction may have a *rapid onset* or ***delayed onset.***

ADMINISTRATION

P.O.
● For treatment of heat cramps, give dose with each glass of water.

I.V.
● Don't confuse 14.6% form with 23.4% form when adding to parenteral nutrient solutions with normal saline solution for injection, and never give without diluting. Read label carefully.
● Infuse 3% and 5% solutions slowly and cautiously to avoid pulmonary edema. Use only for critical situations, and observe patient continually. Infuse through central line, if possible.
● In neonates, never use the bacteriostatic injection.
● If infusing peripherally, infuse into the largest vein possible, using a well-placed small-bore needle to prevent pain. Infuse slowly.
● **Incompatibilities:** Amphotericin B, chlordiazepoxide, diazepam, fat emulsion, mannitol, methylprednisolone sodium succinate, phenytoin sodium.

ACTION

Replaces sodium and chloride and maintains levels.

Route	Onset	Peak	Duration
P.O.	Unknown	Unknown	Unknown
I.V.	Immediate	Immediate	Unknown

Half-life: Unknown.

ADVERSE REACTIONS

CV: *aggravation of heart failure,* thrombophlebitis, edema when given too rapidly or in excess.
Metabolic: hypernatremia, *aggravation of existing metabolic acidosis with excessive infusion.*
Respiratory: *pulmonary edema.*
Skin: local tenderness, tissue necrosis at injection site.
Other: abscess.

INTERACTIONS

None significant.

EFFECTS ON LAB TEST RESULTS

● May increase sodium level. May decrease potassium level.
● May cause electrolyte imbalance.

CONTRAINDICATIONS & CAUTIONS

● Contraindicated in patients with conditions in which sodium and chloride administration is detrimental.
● Sodium chloride 3% and 5% injections contraindicated in patients with increased, normal, or only slightly decreased electrolyte levels.
● Use cautiously in elderly or post-operative patients and in patients with heart failure, circulatory insufficiency, renal dysfunction, or hypoproteinemia.

NURSING CONSIDERATIONS

● Monitor electrolyte levels.

PATIENT TEACHING

● Explain use and administration of drug to patient and family.
● Tell patient to report adverse reactions promptly.
● *Alert:* Tell elderly patients and patients with heart failure, circulatory insufficiency, renal dysfunction, or malnutrition to consult prescriber before taking OTC tablets.
● Advise patient to follow prescriber or product label directions carefully.
● Tell patient that wax matrix of slow-release tablets may appear in stool.

97
Nutritional drugs

amino acid infusions,
  crystalline
amino acid infusions in
  dextrose
amino acid infusions with
  electrolytes
amino acid infusions with
  electrolytes in dextrose
amino acid infusions for hepatic
  failure
amino acid infusions for high
  metabolic stress
amino acid infusions for renal
  failure
dextrose
fat emulsions

SAFETY ALERT!

amino acid infusions, crystalline
a-MEE-noh

Aminosyn, Aminosyn II, Aminosyn-
PF, Aminosyn-RF, FreAmine III,
Novamine, Premasol, Travasol,
TrophAmine

amino acid infusions in dextrose
Aminosyn II with Dextrose,
Travasol in Dextrose

amino acid infusions with electrolytes
Aminosyn with Electrolytes,
Aminosyn II with Electrolytes,
FreAmine III with Electrolytes,
ProcalAmine with Electrolytes,
Travasol with Electrolytes

amino acid infusions with electrolytes in dextrose
Aminosyn II with Electrolytes in
Dextrose

amino acid infusions for hepatic failure
HepatAmine, Hepatasol

amino acid infusions for high metabolic stress
Aminosyn-HBC, BranchAmin,
FreAmine HBC

amino acid infusions for renal failure
Aminess, Aminosyn-RF,
NephrAmine, RenAmin

Pharmacologic class: protein
substrate
Pregnancy risk category C

AVAILABLE FORMS
Injection: 250 ml, 500 ml, 1,000 ml,
2,000 ml containing amino acids in
various concentrations
amino acid infusions, crystalline
Aminosyn: 3.5%, 5%, 7%, 8.5%, 10%
Aminosyn II: 3.5%, 5%, 7%, 8.5%,
10%, 15%
Aminosyn-PF: 7%, 10%
Aminosyn-RF: 5.2%
FreAmine III: 8.5%, 10%
Novamine: 11.4%, 15%
Premasol: 6%, 10%
Travasol: 5.5%, 8.5%, 10%
TrophAmine: 6%, 10%
amino acid infusions in dextrose
Aminosyn II: 3.5% in 5% dextrose, 3.5%
in 25% dextrose, 4.25% in 10% dextrose,
4.25% in 20% dextrose, 4.25% in 25%
dextrose, 5% in 25% dextrose
Travasol: 2.75% in 5% dextrose, 2.75%
in 10% dextrose, 2.75% in 25% dextrose,
4.25% in 5% dextrose, 4.25% in 10%
dextrose, 4.25% in 25% dextrose
amino acid infusions with electrolytes
Aminosyn: 3.5%, 7%, 8.5%
Aminosyn II: 3.5%, 7%, 8.5%, 10%
FreAmine III: 3%, 8.5%
ProcalAmine: 3%
Travasol: 3.5%, 5.5%, 8.5%
**amino acid infusions with electrolytes
in dextrose**
Aminosyn II: 3.5% with electrolytes in 5%
dextrose, 3.5% with electrolytes in 25%
dextrose, 4.25% with electrolytes in 10%

dextrose, 4.25% with electrolytes in 20% dextrose, 4.25% with electrolytes in 25% dextrose
amino acid infusions for hepatic failure
HepatAmine: 8%
Hepatasol: 8%
amino acid infusions for high metabolic stress
Aminosyn-HBC: 7%
BranchAmin: 4%
FreAmine HBC: 6.9%
amino acid infusions for renal failure
Aminess: 5.2%
Aminosyn-RF: 5.2%
NephrAmine: 5.4%
RenAmin: 6.5%

INDICATIONS & DOSAGES
➤ **Total parenteral nutrition (TPN) in patients who can't or won't eat**
Adults: 1 to 1.5 g/kg I.V. daily.
Children weighing more than 10 kg (22 lb): 20 to 25 g I.V. daily for first 10 kg; then 1 to 1.25 g/kg I.V. daily for each kilogram over 10 kg.
Children weighing less than 10 kg: 2 to 4 g/kg I.V. daily.
➤ **Nutritional support in patients with cirrhosis, hepatitis, or hepatic encephalopathy**
Adults: 80 to 120 g of amino acids (12 to 18 g of nitrogen) I.V. daily of formulation for hepatic failure.
➤ **Nutritional support in patients with high metabolic stress**
Adults: 1.5 g/kg I.V. daily of formulation for high metabolic stress.
➤ **Nutritional support in patients with renal failure**
Adults: Aminosyn-RF 300 to 600 ml added to 70% dextrose I.V. daily. NephrAmine 250 to 500 ml added to 70% dextrose I.V. daily. Aminess 400 ml added to 70% dextrose I.V. daily. RenAmin 250 to 500 ml I.V. daily.
Children: 0.5 to 1 g/kg/day. Individualize dosage. Maximum recommended dose is 1 g/kg/day.

ADMINISTRATION
I.V.
• Infuse amino acids only in I.V. fluids or TPN solution.
• Limit peripheral infusions to 2.5% amino acids and 10% dextrose.

• Control infusion rate carefully with infusion pump. If infusion rate falls behind, notify prescriber; don't increase rate to catch up.
• Check infusion site often for erythema, inflammation, irritation, tissue sloughing, necrosis, and phlebitis.
• **Incompatibilities:** Bleomycin, ganciclovir, and indomethacin. Because of high risk of incompatibility with other substances, add only needed nutritional products.

ACTION
Provides a substrate for protein synthesis or increases conservation of existing body protein.

Route	Onset	Peak	Duration
I.V.	Immediate	Immediate	Unknown

Half-life: Unknown.

ADVERSE REACTIONS
CNS: fever.
CV: thrombophlebitis, edema, *thrombosis*, flushing.
GI: nausea.
GU: glycosuria, osmotic diuresis.
Metabolic: REBOUND HYPOGLYCEMIA WHEN LONG-TERM INFUSIONS ARE ABRUPTLY STOPPED, *hyperosmolar hyperglycemic nonketotic syndrome,* hyperglycemia, *metabolic acidosis,* alkalosis, hypophosphatemia, hyperammonemia, electrolyte imbalances, weight gain.
Musculoskeletal: osteoporosis.
Skin: tissue sloughing at infusion site from extravasation.
Other: *catheter-related sepsis,* hypersensitivity reactions.

INTERACTIONS
Drug-drug. *Tetracycline:* May reduce protein-sparing effects of infused amino acids because of its antianabolic activity. Monitor patient.

EFFECTS ON LAB TEST RESULTS
• May increase ammonia and liver enzyme levels. May decrease magnesium, phosphate, and potassium levels. May increase or decrease glucose level.

CONTRAINDICATIONS & CAUTIONS

• Contraindicated in patients with anuria and in those with inborn errors of amino acid metabolism, such as maple syrup urine disease and isovaleric acidemia.
• Standard amino acid formulations are contraindicated in patients with severe renal failure or hepatic disease.
• Use cautiously in children and neonates.
• Use cautiously in patients with renal or hepatic impairment or failure or diabetes.
• Use cautiously in patients with cardiac disease or insufficiency; drug may cause circulatory overload.

NURSING CONSIDERATIONS

• Patients with fluid restriction may tolerate only 1 to 2 L.
• When diabetic patient receives drug, his insulin requirements may increase.
• Some products contain sulfites. Check contents before giving to patients with sulfite sensitivity.
• Safe and effective use of parenteral nutrition requires knowledge of nutrition and clinical expertise in recognizing and treating complications. Frequent evaluations of patient and laboratory studies are needed.
• Obtain baseline electrolyte, glucose, BUN, calcium, and phosphorus levels before therapy; monitor these levels periodically throughout therapy.
• Check fractional urine for glycosuria every 6 hours initially, and then every 12 to 24 hours in stable patients. Abrupt onset of glycosuria may be an early sign of impending sepsis.
• Assess body temperature every 4 hours; elevation may indicate sepsis or infection.
• Watch for extraordinary electrolyte losses that may occur during nasogastric suction, vomiting, diarrhea, or drainage from GI fistula.
• If patient has chills, fever, or other signs of sepsis, replace I.V. tubing and bottle and send tubing and bottle to the laboratory to be cultured.
• **Look alike–sound alike:** Don't confuse Aminosyn with amikacin.

PATIENT TEACHING

• Explain need for supplement to patient and family, and answer any questions.
• Tell patient to report adverse reactions promptly.

---

dextrose (d-glucose)
DEKS-trohse

Pharmacologic class: carbohydrate caloric agent
Pregnancy risk category C

AVAILABLE FORMS

Injection: 3-ml ampule (10%); 10 ml (25%); 25 ml (5%); 50 ml (5% and 50% available in vial, ampule, and Bristoject); 70-ml pin-top vial (70% for additive use only); 100 ml (5%); 150 ml (5%); 250 ml (5%, 10%); 500 ml (5%, 10%, 20%, 30%, 40%, 50%, 60%, 70%); 650 ml (38.5%); 1,000 ml (2.5%, 5%, 10%, 20%, 30%, 40%, 50%, 60%, 70%); 2,000 ml (50%, 70%)

INDICATIONS & DOSAGES

➤ **Fluid replacement and caloric supplementation in patients who can't maintain adequate oral intake or are restricted from doing so**
Adults and children: Dosage depends on fluid and caloric requirements. Use peripheral I.V. infusion of 2.5%, 5%, or 10% solution or central I.V. infusion of 20% solution for minimal fluid needs. Use a 10% to 25% solution to treat acute hypoglycemia in neonate or older infant (2 ml/kg). Use a 50% solution to treat insulin-induced hypoglycemia (20 to 50 ml). Solutions of 10%, 20%, 30%, 40%, 50%, 60%, and 70% are diluted in admixtures, usually amino acid solutions, for total parenteral nutrition (TPN) given through a central vein.

ADMINISTRATION

I.V.
• Use central vein to infuse dextrose solutions at concentrations above 10%.
• Use infusion pump when giving dextrose solution with amino acids for TPN.
• Never infuse concentrated solution rapidly. Rapid infusion may cause hyperglycemia and fluid shift. Maximum infusion rate is 0.8 g/kg/hour.
• Check injection site often for irritation, tissue sloughing, necrosis, and phlebitis.
• **Incompatibilities:** Ampicillin sodium, cisplatin, diazepam, erythromycin lacto-

---

bionate, 10% and 25% fat emulsion solutions, phenytoin, procainamide, solutions of 10% thiopental and above, whole blood.

ACTION
A simple water-soluble sugar that minimizes glyconeogenesis and promotes anabolism in patients whose oral caloric intake is limited.

Route	Onset	Peak	Duration
I.V.	Immediate	Immediate	Unknown

Half-life: Unknown.

ADVERSE REACTIONS
CNS: *unconsciousness in hyperosmolar hyperglycemic nonketotic syndrome,* fever, confusion.
CV: *worsened hypertension and heart failure with fluid overload in susceptible patients,* phlebitis, venous sclerosis, tissue necrosis with prolonged or concentrated infusions, especially when given peripherally.
GU: glycosuria, osmotic diuresis.
Metabolic: hypovolemia, hypervolemia, hyperglycemia, dehydration, and hyperosmolarity with rapid infusion of concentrated solution or prolonged infusion, *hypoglycemia from rebound hyperinsulinemia with rapid termination of long-term infusions.*
Respiratory: PULMONARY EDEMA.
Skin: sloughing and tissue necrosis if extravasation occurs with concentrated solutions.

INTERACTIONS
Drug-drug. *Corticosteroids:* May cause salt and water retention and increase potassium excretion. Monitor glucose, sodium, and potassium levels.

EFFECTS ON LAB TEST RESULTS
● May increase or decrease glucose level.

CONTRAINDICATIONS & CAUTIONS
● Contraindicated in patients with allergy to corn or corn products.
● Contraindicated in patients in diabetic coma while glucose level remains excessively high.
● Use of concentrated solutions is contraindicated in patients with intracranial or intraspinal hemorrhage; in dehydrated

patients with delirium tremens; and in patients with severe dehydration, anuria, diabetic coma, or glucose-galactose malabsorption syndrome.
● Use cautiously in patients with cardiac or pulmonary disease, hypertension, renal insufficiency, urinary obstruction, or hypovolemia.

NURSING CONSIDERATIONS
● *Alert:* Never stop hypertonic solutions abruptly. Have dextrose 10% in water available to treat hypoglycemia if rebound hyperinsulinemia occurs.
● Don't give concentrated solutions I.M. or subcutaneously.
● Monitor glucose level carefully. Prolonged therapy with D₅W can cause reduction of pancreatic insulin production and secretion.
● Check vital signs frequently. Report adverse reactions promptly.
● Monitor fluid intake and output and weight carefully. Watch closely for signs and symptoms of fluid overload.
● Monitor patient for signs of mental confusion.

PATIENT TEACHING
● Explain need for supplement to patient and family, and answer any questions.
● Tell patient to report adverse reactions promptly.

SAFETY ALERT!

fat emulsions
Intralipid 10%, Intralipid 20%, Intralipid 30%, Liposyn II 10%, Liposyn II 20%, Liposyn III 10%, Liposyn III 20%, Liposyn III 30%

Pharmacologic class: lipids
Pregnancy risk category C

AVAILABLE FORMS
Injection: 50 ml (20%), 100 ml (10%, 20%), 200 ml (10%, 20%), 250 ml (10%, 20%), 500 ml (10%, 20%, 30%)

INDICATIONS & DOSAGES
■ **Black Box Warning** Death in preterm infants after infusion of I.V. fat emulsions have occurred. Adhere strictly to the

recommended total daily dose. Hourly I.V. infusion rate should not exceed 1 g/kg in 4 hours. ■

➤ **Adjunct to total parenteral nutrition (TPN) to provide adequate source of calories**
Adults: 1 ml/minute I.V. for 15 to 30 minutes (10% emulsion) or 0.5 ml/minute I.V. for 15 to 30 minutes (20% emulsion). If no adverse reactions occur, increase rate to deliver 250 ml (20% Liposyn) or 500 ml (10% Liposyn; 10% or 20% Intralipid) over the first day; don't give more than 2.5 g/kg (10%) or 3 g/kg (20%) daily. For 30% Liposyn III, initial infusion rate is the equivalent of 0.1 g fat/minute for the first 15 to 30 minutes. If no adverse reactions occur, increase infusion rate to equivalent of 0.2 g fat/minute. The admixture shouldn't contain more than 330 ml of Liposyn III 30% on first day of therapy. If patient has no adverse reactions, increase dose the next day. Daily dosage shouldn't exceed 2.5 g of fat/kg of body weight.
Children: 0.1 ml/minute for 10 to 15 minutes (10% emulsion) or 0.05 ml/minute I.V. for 10 to 15 minutes (20% emulsion). If no adverse reactions occur, increase rate to deliver 1 g/kg over 4 hours; don't give more than 3 g/kg daily. For 30% Liposyn, initial infusion rate is no more than 0.01 g fat/minute for the first 10 to 15 minutes. If no adverse reactions occur, change rate to permit infusion of 0.1 g fat/kg/hour. Daily dosage shouldn't exceed 3 g of fat/kg of body weight. Fat emulsion supplies 60% of daily caloric intake; protein-carbohydrate TPN should supply remaining 40%.
Premature infants: Begin at 0.5 g fat/kg/24 hours (2.5 ml Intralipid 20%, 1.7 ml Liposyn III 30%) and may be increased in relation to the infant's ability to eliminate fat. Maximum recommended dosage is 3 g fat/kg/24 hours.
➤ **Fatty acid deficiency**
Adults and children: 8% to 10% of total caloric intake I.V.

ADMINISTRATION
I.V.
● Don't use if it separates or becomes oily.
● Drug may be mixed in same container with amino acids, dextrose, electrolytes, vitamins, and other nutrients.

● Because lipids support bacterial and fungal growth, change all tubing before each infusion, and check infusion site daily.
● Use an infusion pump to regulate rate. Rapid infusion may cause fluid or fat overload.
● Refrigeration isn't needed unless part of an admixture.
● **Incompatibilities:** Acyclovir, albumin, amikacin, aminophylline, amphotericin B, ampicillin sodium, ascorbic acid injection, calcium chloride, calcium gluconate, cyclosporine, dopamine, doxorubicin, doxycycline, droperidol, fluorouracil, ganciclovir, gentamicin, haloperidol, heparin sodium, hydromorphone hydrochloride (HCl), iron dextran, levorphanol tartrate, lorazepam, magnesium chloride, methyldopate HCl, midazolam HCl, minocycline HCl, morphine sulfate, nalbuphine HCl, ondansetron HCl, penicillin G, pentobarbital sodium, phenobarbital sodium, phenytoin sodium, potassium chloride, potassium phosphates, ranitidine HCl, sodium bicarbonate, sodium chloride solution, sodium phosphates, vitamin B complex.

ACTION
Provides neutral triglycerides, predominantly unsaturated fatty acids; acts as a source of calories and prevents fatty acid deficiency. When substituted for dextrose as a source of calories, fat emulsions decrease carbon dioxide production.

Route	Onset	Peak	Duration
I.V.	Immediate	Immediate	Unknown

Half-life: Unknown.

ADVERSE REACTIONS
Early reactions
CNS: headache, sleepiness, dizziness, fever.
CV: chest and back pains, flushing.
EENT: pressure over eyes.
GI: nausea, vomiting.
Hematologic: hypercoagulability.
Respiratory: dyspnea, cyanosis.
Skin: diaphoresis, irritation at infusion site.
Other: hypersensitivity reactions.

Reactions may be *common*, uncommon, *life-threatening*, or COMMON AND LIFE-THREATENING.
Interaction may have a *rapid onset* or **delayed onset**.

Delayed reactions
CNS: *focal seizures,* fever.
Hematologic: *thrombocytopenia,*
leukopenia, leukocytosis.
Hepatic: hepatomegaly.
Other: splenomegaly.

INTERACTIONS
None significant.

EFFECTS ON LAB TEST RESULTS
● May increase bilirubin, lipid, and liver enzyme levels.
● May decrease platelet count. May increase or decrease WBC count.

CONTRAINDICATIONS & CAUTIONS
● Contraindicated in patients with severe egg allergies, hyperlipidemia, lipid nephrosis, or acute pancreatitis with hyperlipidemia.
● Use cautiously in patients with severe hepatic or pulmonary disease, anemia, or blood coagulation disorders including thrombocytopenia, and in patients at risk for fat embolism.
● Use cautiously in jaundiced or prema-ture infants.

NURSING CONSIDERATIONS
● Watch for adverse reactions, especially during first half of infusion.
● Monitor lipid levels closely when patient is receiving fat emulsion therapy. Lipemia must clear between doses.
● Monitor hepatic function carefully in long-term therapy.
● Check platelet count frequently in neonates.
■ **Black Box Warning** Carefully monitor triglyceride levels and free fatty acids in infants, especially premature and jaundiced infants. ■
● Available products differ mainly by their fatty acid components.

PATIENT TEACHING
● Explain need for fat emulsion therapy, and answer any questions.
● Tell patient to report adverse reactions promptly.

conivaptan hydrochloride
imiquimod
isotretinoin
mecasermin
minoxidil
orlistat
pregabalin
raloxifene hydrochloride
riluzole
sapropterin dihydrochloride
tetrabenazine
tretinoin
varenicline tartrate

---

conivaptan hydrochloride
kah-nih-VAP-tan

Vaprisol

Pharmacologic class: arginine
vasopressin receptor antagonist
Pregnancy risk category C

AVAILABLE FORMS
Injection: 20 mg/4 ml

INDICATIONS & DOSAGES
➤ **Euvolemic hyponatremia (as from
SIADH, hypothyroidism, adrenal
insufficiency, pulmonary disorders)
and hypervolemic hyponatremia in
hospitalized patients**
Adults: Loading dose of 20 mg I.V. over
30 minutes; then 20 mg I.V. by continuous
infusion over 24 hours for 1 to 3 days. If
sodium level isn't rising at desired rate,
increase to 40 mg/day by continuous
infusion. Don't give for more than 4 days
after loading dose.
Adjust-a-dose: If sodium level rises more
than 12 mEq/L in 24 hours, stop infusion.
If hyponatremia persists or recurs and the
patient has had no adverse neurologic
effects from the rapid rise in sodium
level, restart infusion at a reduced dose.
If patient develops hypotension or hypovolemia, stop infusion. Monitor vital
signs and volume status often. If hyponatremia persists once the patient is no
longer hypotensive and volume returns
to normal, restart infusion at a reduced
dose.

ADMINISTRATION
I.V.
● Dilute only with D₅W. For the loading
dose, add 20 mg to 100 ml of D₅W. Gently
invert bag to ensure complete mixing.
Infuse over 30 minutes. For continuous
infusion, add 40 mg to 250 ml of D₅W.
Gently invert bag to ensure complete
mixing. Infuse over 24 hours.
● Give via a large vein, and change
infusion site every 24 hours.
● Solution is stable for 24 hours at room
temperature.
● **Incompatibilities:** Lactated Ringer's
solution, normal saline solution. Don't
mix or infuse with other I.V. drugs.

ACTION
Increases free water eliminated by
kidneys, inhibiting inappropriate or
excessive arginine vasopressin (antidiuretic hormone) secretion. Typically,
this causes increased net fluid loss,
increased urine output, and decreased
urine osmolality.

Route	Onset	Peak	Duration
I.V.	Unknown	2–4 hr	12 hr

Half-life: 5 hours.

ADVERSE REACTIONS
CNS: *headache,* confusion, fever,
insomnia.
CV: atrial fibrillation, hypertension,
hypotension, orthostatic hypotension.
GI: constipation, diarrhea, dry mouth,
nausea, oral candidiasis, *vomiting.*
GU: frequency, hematuria, polyuria, UTI.
Hematologic: anemia.
Metabolic: *hypoglycemia,* hypokalemia,
dehydration, hyperglycemia, ***hypomagne-
semia,*** hyponatremia.
Respiratory: pneumonia.
Skin: erythema.
Other: *infusion site reactions, thirst.*

Reactions may be *common,* uncommon, *life-threatening,* or COMMON AND LIFE-THREATENING.
Interaction may have a *rapid onset* or ***delayed onset.***

INTERACTIONS
Drug-drug. *Amlodipine:* May increase amlodipine level and half-life. Monitor blood pressure.

Digoxin: May increase digoxin level. Monitor patient, and adjust digoxin dose, as needed.

Midazolam: May increase midazolam level. Monitor patient for respiratory depression and hypotension.

Potent CYP3A4 inhibitors (clarithromycin, indinavir, itraconazole, ketoconazole, ritonavir): May seriously increase levels and toxic effects. Use together is contraindicated.

Simvastatin: May increase simvastatin level. Monitor patient for signs of rhabdomyolysis, including muscle pain, weakness, and tenderness.

EFFECTS ON LAB TEST RESULTS
● May decrease potassium, magnesium, sodium, and hemoglobin levels and hematocrit. May increase or decrease blood glucose level.

CONTRAINDICATIONS & CAUTIONS
● Contraindicated in patients with hypovolemic hyponatremia, patients hypersensitive to drug or its components, and those taking potent CYP3A4 inhibitors, such as clarithromycin, indinavir, itraconazole, ketoconazole, or ritonavir.
● Use cautiously in hyponatremic patients with underlying heart failure and patients with hepatic or renal impairment.

NURSING CONSIDERATIONS
● Monitor sodium level and neurologic status regularly during therapy.
● **Alert:** Rapid correction of sodium level may cause osmotic demyelination syndrome. Monitor patient's sodium level and volume status.
● Drug may cause significant infusion site reactions, even with proper dilution and administration. Rotate infusion site every 24 hours to reduce risk of reaction.

PATIENT TEACHING
● Inform patient that he may experience low blood pressure when standing. If he feels dizzy or faint, advise him to sit or lie down.

● Advise patient to promptly report signs and symptoms of hypoglycemia, such as feeling shaky, nervous, tired, sweaty, cold, hungry, confused, irritable, or impatient.
● Emphasize the importance of reporting an unusually fast heartbeat or weakness.
● Tell patient that analgesics and moist heating pads can be used to treat pain and inflammation at the infusion site.
● Inform patient that the infusion will be given for a maximum of 4 days after the loading dose.

imiquimod
ih-mih-KWI-mahd

Aldara

Pharmacologic class: immune response modifier
Pregnancy risk category C

AVAILABLE FORMS
Cream: 5% in single-use packets containing 250 mg

INDICATIONS & DOSAGES
➤ **External genital and perianal warts**
Adults and adolescents age 12 and older: Apply thin layer to affected area three times weekly before normal sleeping hours and leave on skin for 6 to 10 hours. Continue treatment until genital or perianal warts clear completely or maximum of 16 weeks.
➤ **Typical, nonhyperkeratotic, nonhypertrophic actinic keratoses on the face or scalp in immunocompetent adults**
Adults: Wash area with mild soap and water and dry at least 10 minutes. Apply cream to face or scalp, but not both concurrently, twice weekly at bedtime, and wash off after about 8 hours. Treat for 16 weeks.
➤ **Superficial basal cell carcinoma**
Adults: Wash area with mild soap and water and allow to dry thoroughly. Apply a thin layer of cream to a 1-cm margin around the biopsy-confirmed area five times a week at bedtime; wash off after about 8 hours. Treat for 6 weeks.

ADMINISTRATION
Topical
● Wash area with mild soap and water and dry completely before applying cream.
● Discard unused portion of single-use packet.

ACTION
Has no direct antiviral activity in cell culture. Drug induces mRNA-encoding cytokines including interferon alfa at the treatment site.

Route	Onset	Peak	Duration
Topical	Unknown	Unknown	Unknown

Half-life: About 20 hours.

ADVERSE REACTIONS
CNS: headache.
Musculoskeletal: myalgia.
Skin: local itching, burning, pain, soreness, erythema, ulceration, edema, erosion, induration, flaking, excoriation.
Other: *fungal infection,* flulike symptoms.

INTERACTIONS
None significant.

EFFECTS ON LAB TEST RESULTS
None reported.

CONTRAINDICATIONS & CAUTIONS
● Drug isn't recommended for treatment of urethral, intravaginal, cervical, rectal, or intra-anal human papillomavirus disease.
● Safety of drug in breast-feeding women is unknown.

NURSING CONSIDERATIONS
● Don't use until genital or perianal tissue is healed from previous drug or surgical treatment.
● Patient usually experiences local skin reactions at site of application or surround-ing areas. Use nonocclusive dressings, such as cotton gauze, or cotton under-garments in management of skin reactions. Patient's discomfort or severity of the local skin reaction may require a rest period of several days. Resume treatment once reaction subsides.
● Drug isn't a cure; new warts may develop during therapy.

● Maximum tumor diameter of superficial basal cell carcinoma should be 2 cm or smaller. Cream may be applied to neck, trunk, or arms and legs (excluding hands and feet).
● Assess treatment site for clearance 12 weeks posttreatment.

PATIENT TEACHING
● Advise patient that effect of cream on transmission of genital or perianal warts is unknown. New warts may develop during therapy; drug isn't a cure.
● Tell patient to use cream only as directed and to avoid contact with eyes, lips, or nostrils.
● Tell patient to wash hands before and after applying cream.
● Tell patient to wash the area with mild soap and water and dry completely before applying cream.
● Advise patient to apply cream in thin layer over affected area and rub in until cream isn't visible. Advise patient to avoid excessive use of cream. Tell him not to occlude area after applying cream and to wash with mild soap and water 6 to 10 hours after application of cream.
● Advise patient that mild local skin reactions, such as redness, erosion, excoriation, flaking, and swelling at site of application or surrounding areas, are common. Tell him that most skin reactions are mild to moderate. Advise him to report severe skin reactions promptly.
● Instruct uncircumcised man being treated for warts under the foreskin to retract foreskin and clean area daily.
● Advise patient that drug can weaken condoms and vaginal diaphragms and that use together isn't recommended.
● Advise patient to avoid sexual contact while cream is on the skin.
● Advise patient to minimize or avoid exposure to sunlight and other UV light; encourage sunscreen use.
● Tell patient to store drug at tempera-tures below 86° F (30° C) and to avoid freezing.
● Tell patient to discard partially used packets and not to reuse.

Reactions may be *common,* uncommon, *life-threatening,* or COMMON AND LIFE-THREATENING.
Interaction may have a *rapid onset* or **delayed onset.**

isotretinoin
eye-so-TRET-i-noyn

Accutane, Amnesteem, Claravis, Sotret

Pharmacologic class: retinoic acid derivative
Pregnancy risk category X

AVAILABLE FORMS
Capsules: 10 mg, 20 mg, 30 mg, 40 mg

INDICATIONS & DOSAGES
➤ **Severe nodular acne that's unresponsive to conventional therapy**
Adults and adolescents: 0.5 to 2 mg/kg P.O. daily in two divided doses with food for 15 to 20 weeks.

ADMINISTRATION
P.O.
● Before use, have patient read patient information and sign accompanying consent form.
● Give drug with or shortly after meals to facilitate absorption.

ACTION
May normalize keratinization, reversibly decrease size of sebaceous glands, and make sebum less viscous and less likely to plug follicles.

Route	Onset	Peak	Duration
P.O.	Unknown	3 hr	Unknown

Half-life: 30 minutes to 39 hours.

ADVERSE REACTIONS
CNS: *pseudotumor cerebri,* depression, **psychosis, suicidal ideation or attempts, suicide, aggressive and violent behavior,** emotional instability, headache, fatigue.
EENT: *conjunctivitis, epistaxis, drying of mucous membranes, dry nose,* corneal deposits, dry eyes, hearing impairment (sometimes irreversible), decreased night vision, visual disturbances.
GI: nonspecific GI symptoms, *nausea, vomiting, abdominal pain, dry mouth,* anorexia, gum bleeding and inflammation, *acute pancreatitis,* inflammatory bowel disease.

Hematologic: *increased erythrocyte sedimentation rate,* anemia, **thrombocytosis.**
Hepatic: *hepatitis.*
Metabolic: *hypertriglyceridemia,* hyperglycemia.
Musculoskeletal: *rhabdomyolysis,* skeletal hyperostosis, tendon and ligament calcification, premature epiphyseal closure, decreased bone mineral density and other bone abnormalities, back pain, arthralgia, arthritis, tendinitis.
Skin: *cheilitis, cheilosis, fragility, rash, dry skin, facial skin desquamation, petechiae, pruritus, nail brittleness,* thinning of hair, skin infection, peeling of palms and toes, photosensitivity reaction.

INTERACTIONS
Drug-drug. *Corticosteroids:* May increase risk of osteoporosis. Use together cautiously.
Medicated soaps, cleansers, and coverups, preparations containing alcohol, topical resorcinol peeling agents (benzoyl peroxide): May have cumulative drying effect. Use together cautiously.
Micro-dosed progesterone hormonal contraceptives ("minipills") that don't contain estrogen: May decrease effectiveness of contraceptive. Advise patient to use different contraceptive method.
Phenytoin: May increase risk of osteomalacia. Use together cautiously.
Tetracyclines: May increase risk of pseudotumor cerebri. Avoid using together.
Products containing vitamin A, vitamin A: May increase toxic effects of isotretinoin. Avoid using together.
Drug-food. *Any food:* May increase absorption of drug. Advise patient to take drug with milk, a meal, or shortly after a meal.
Drug-lifestyle. *Alcohol use:* May increase risk of hypertriglyceridemia. Discourage use together.
Sun exposure: May increase photosensitivity reaction. Advise patient to avoid excessive sunlight exposure.

EFFECTS ON LAB TEST RESULTS
● May increase AST, ALT, alkaline phosphatase, triglyceride, glucose, and uric acid levels.
● May increase platelet count and erythrocyte sedimentation rate.

CONTRAINDICATIONS & CAUTIONS
• Contraindicated in patients hypersensitive to parabens (used as preservatives), vitamin A, or other retinoids.
■ **Black Box Warning** Contraindicated in woman of childbearing potential, unless patient has had two negative pregnancy test results before beginning therapy, will begin drug therapy on second or third day of next menstrual period, and will comply with stringent contraceptive measures for 1 month before therapy, during therapy, and for at least 1 month after therapy. ■
• Use cautiously in patients with a history of mental illness or a family history of psychiatric disorders, asthma, liver disease, diabetes, heart disease, osteoporosis, genetic predisposition for age-related osteoporosis, history of childhood osteoporosis, weak bones, anorexia nervosa, osteomalacia, or other disorders of bone metabolism.

NURSING CONSIDERATIONS
• Patient must have negative results from two urine or serum pregnancy tests; one is performed in the office when the patient is qualified for therapy, the second during the first 5 days of the next normal menstrual period immediately preceding the beginning of therapy. For patients with amenorrhea, the second test should be done at least 11 days after the last unprotected act of sexual intercourse. A pregnancy test must be repeated every month before the patient receives the prescription.
■ **Black Box Warning** If pregnancy does occur during treatment, discontinue drug immediately and refer patient to an obstetrician-gynecologist experienced in reproductive toxicity. ■
• Monitor baseline lipid studies, liver function tests, and pregnancy tests before therapy and at monthly intervals.
• Regularly monitor glucose level and CK levels in patients who participate in vigorous physical activity.
• Most adverse reactions occur at doses exceeding 1 mg/kg daily. Reactions are generally reversible when therapy is stopped or dosage is reduced.
• *Alert:* If patient experiences headache, nausea and vomiting, or visual disturbances, screen for papilledema. Signs and symptoms of pseudotumor cerebri

require stopping the drug immediately and beginning neurologic interventions promptly.
■ **Black Box Warning** To minimize the risk of fetal exposure, the drug is only available through a restricted FDA-approved distribution program called iPLEDGE. ■
• A second course of therapy may begin 8 weeks after completion of the first course, if necessary. Improvements may continue after first course is complete.
• Patients may be at increased risk of bone fractures or injury when participating in sports with repetitive impact.
• Spontaneous reports of osteoporosis, osteopenia, bone fractures, and delayed healing of bone fractures have occurred in patients taking drug. To decrease this risk, don't exceed recommended doses and duration.
• *Look alike–sound alike:* Don't confuse Accutane with Accupril or Accolate.

PATIENT TEACHING
■ **Black Box Warning** Warn woman of childbearing age that, if this drug is used during pregnancy, severe fetal abnormalities may occur. Advise her to either abstain from sex or use two reliable forms of contraception simultaneously for 1 month before, during, and for 1 month after treatment. An isotretinoin medication guide must be given to the patient each time isotretinoin is dispensed, as required by law. ■
• Advise patient to take drug with or shortly after meals to facilitate absorption.
• Tell patient to immediately report visual disturbances and bone, muscle, or joint pain.
• Warn patient that contact lenses may feel uncomfortable during therapy.
• Warn patient against using abrasives, medicated soaps and cleansers, acne preparations containing peeling drugs, and topical products containing alcohol (including cosmetics, aftershave, cologne) because they may cause cumulative irritation or excessive drying of skin.
• Tell patient to avoid prolonged sun exposure and to use sunblock. Drug may have additive effect if used with other drugs that cause photosensitivity reaction.

Reactions may be *common,* uncommon, *life-threatening,* or COMMON AND LIFE-THREATENING.
Interaction may have a *rapid onset* or **delayed onset.**

• Tell women that manufacturer will supply urine pregnancy tests for monthly testing during therapy.

• Warn patient that transient exacerbations may occur during therapy.

• Warn patient not to donate blood during therapy and for 1 month after stopping drug because drug could harm fetus of a pregnant recipient.

• Tell patient to report adverse reactions immediately, especially depression, suicidal thoughts, persistent headaches, and persistent GI pain.

---

mecasermin
meh-KAH-sur-men

Increlex

Pharmacologic class: human insulin growth factor
Pregnancy risk category C

AVAILABLE FORMS
Injection: 10 mg/ml

INDICATIONS & DOSAGES
➤ **Growth failure in children with severe primary insulin growth factor-1 (IGF-1) deficiency or children with growth-hormone gene deletion who have developed neutralizing antibodies to growth hormone**
Children age 2 and older: Initially, 0.04 to 0.08 mg/kg twice daily subcutaneously. If well tolerated for at least one week, may increase by 0.04 mg/kg per dose, to the maximum dose of 0.12 mg/kg given twice daily.

ADMINISTRATION
Subcutaneous
• Reduce dose if hypoglycemia occurs despite adequate food intake.
• Give dose about 20 minutes before or after a meal or snack.
• Hold dose if patient is unable to eat.
• Do not increase dose to make up for 1 or more omitted doses.
• Rotate sites for injection (thigh, abdomen, buttocks, or upper arm). New injections should be given at least 1 inch from previ-

ous injection site(s) and never into areas where the skin is tender, bruised, red, or hard or lacks fatty tissue.

ACTION
Promotes growth because synthetic drug is identical to endogenous insulin-like growth factor-binding protein-3 (IGFBP-3) and IGF-1.

Route	Onset	Peak	Duration
Subcut.	1 hr	5–17½ hr	Unknown

Half-life: 10.7 to 16.1 hours.

ADVERSE REACTIONS
CNS: *headache,* dizziness, *intracranial hypertension, pain.*
EENT: *tonsillar hypertrophy,* otitis media, papilledema.
GI: vomiting.
GU: hematuria, ovarian cysts.
Hematologic: *iron deficiency anemia,* lymphadenopathy.
Metabolic: hyperglycemia, *hypoglycemia.*
Musculoskeletal: *muscle atrophy,* arthralgia, bone pain, scoliosis.
Skin: injection site reaction.
Other: *enlarged thyroid,* snoring.

INTERACTIONS
None known.

EFFECTS ON LAB TEST RESULTS
• May increase AST, LDH, and transaminase levels. May increase or decrease glucose level.

CONTRAINDICATIONS & CAUTIONS
• Contraindicated in patients with closed epiphyses, active or suspected cancer, or allergy to drug or its components. I.V. use is also contraindicated. Don't use in place of growth hormone or for other causes of growth failure.
• Use cautiously in pregnant or breast-feeding women.

NURSING CONSIDERATIONS
• Make sure patient has had a baseline ophthalmic examination before therapy.
• Monitor glucose level carefully, especially in small children, whose oral intake can be inconsistent.
• Check patient regularly for adenotonsillar enlargement. Ask parent or caregiver if the

child has developed snoring, sleep apnea, or reduced hearing.
• Monitor patient for changes typical of acromegaly.
• Monitor child experiencing rapid growth closely for development of a limp, hip or knee pain, or progression of scoliosis (if present).
• Safety and effectiveness in children younger than age 3 are not known.

PATIENT TEACHING
• Explain that drug must be kept refrigerated and protected from direct light and avoid freezing.
• Tell parent that vials are stable for 30 days after opening if kept refrigerated.
• Warn parent not to use cloudy drug.
• Tell parent to give drug 20 minutes before or after a meal or snack and to withhold dose if the child can't or won't eat.
• Teach parent how to inject drug and dispose of syringes properly.
• Tell parent to inject drug subcutaneously into child's upper arm, upper thigh, stomach area, or buttocks. Caution against injecting it into a muscle or vein.
• To decrease injection site reactions, advise parent to rotate the injection site for each dose.
• Tell parent to regularly monitor the child's glucose level. Review signs and symptoms of hypoglycemia, including dizziness, tiredness, hunger, irritability, sweating, nausea, and a fast or irregular heartbeat.
• Advise parent and child to keep a quick source of sugar (such as orange juice, glucose gel, or candy) readily available in case hypoglycemia occurs.
• Explain that child should avoid hazardous activities while the dose is being adjusted. Hypoglycemia can cause unconsciousness, seizures, or death.
• Advise parent to have the child's tonsils checked regularly and to monitor child for enlarged tonsils and snoring or sleep apnea.
• Tell parent to notify prescriber if child develops nausea and vomiting with headache, hypoglycemic episodes, limping, hip or knee pain, snoring, trouble swallowing, earaches, or breathing problems.

minoxidil (topical)
mi-NOX-i-dill

Men's Rogaine◊, Minoxidil Extra Strength for Men◊, Rogaine for Men◊, Rogaine Extra Strength for Men◊, Rogaine for Women◊, Theroxidil◊

Pharmacologic class: direct-acting vasodilator
Pregnancy risk category C

AVAILABLE FORMS
Topical Foam: 5%
Topical solution: 2%◊, 5%◊

INDICATIONS & DOSAGES
➤ **Androgenetic alopecia**
Adults: 1 ml of solution or half a capful of foam applied to affected area b.i.d. Maximum daily dose is 2 ml of solution.

ADMINISTRATION
Topical
• Don't use 5% solution in women.
• Dry hair and scalp thoroughly before application.

ACTION
Stimulates hair growth, possibly by dilating arterial microcapillaries around hair follicles.

Route	Onset	Peak	Duration
Topical	Unknown	Unknown	Unknown

Half-life: Unknown.

ADVERSE REACTIONS
CNS: headache, dizziness, faintness, light-headedness.
CV: edema, chest pain, hypertension, hypotension, palpitations, increased or decreased pulse rate.
EENT: sinusitis.
GI: diarrhea, nausea, vomiting.
GU: UTI, renal calculi, urethritis.
Metabolic: weight gain.
Musculoskeletal: back pain, tendinitis.
Respiratory: bronchitis, upper respiratory infection.
Skin: *irritant dermatitis, dry skin or scalp, flaking, local erythema, pruritus,*

Reactions may be *common*, uncommon, *life-threatening*, or COMMON AND LIFE-THREATENING.
Interaction may have a *rapid onset* or *delayed onset.*

allergic contact dermatitis, eczema, hypertrichosis, worsening of hair loss.

INTERACTIONS

Drug-drug. *Petroleum jelly, topical corticosteroids, topical retinoids, other drugs that may increase skin absorption:* May increase risk of systemic effects of minoxidil. Avoid using together.

EFFECTS ON LAB TEST RESULTS

None reported.

CONTRAINDICATIONS & CAUTIONS

● Contraindicated in patients hypersensitive to drug or components of solution.
● Use cautiously in patients older than age 50 and in those with cardiac, renal, or hepatic disease.

NURSING CONSIDERATIONS

● Patient needs to have normal, healthy scalp before beginning therapy because absorption of drug through irritated skin may cause adverse systemic effects.
● Treatment will most likely succeed in patients with balding area smaller than 4 inches (10 cm) that developed within past 10 years.

PATIENT TEACHING

● Teach patient how to apply drug. Tell him to dry hair and scalp thoroughly before application and not to apply drug to other body areas. Tell patient not to use drug on irritated or sunburned scalp or with other drugs on scalp. Tell him to thoroughly wash hands after application.
● Warn patient to avoid inhaling any spray or mist from drug and to avoid spraying around eyes because solution contains alcohol and may be irritating.
● Inform patient that more frequent applications or using more than 2 ml daily won't increase hair growth but instead may increase adverse reactions. Tell patient not to double the dose for missed applications.
● Teach patient to monitor pulse rate and body weight.
● Advise patient that therapy will be prolonged and will continue for at least 4 months before clinical effects appear. Tell him that drug must be used daily for optimal results. Almost half of patients

will experience moderate to dense hair growth.
● Tell patient that stopping drug may cause loss of new hair growth. New hair growth is usually fine and may be colorless but will resemble existing hair after continued treatment.

---

orlistat
ORE-lah-stat

Alli ◊ , Xenical

Pharmacologic class: lipase inhibitor
Pregnancy risk category B

AVAILABLE FORMS

Capsules: 60 mg ◊ , 120 mg

INDICATIONS & DOSAGES

➤ **To manage obesity, including weight loss and weight maintenance with a reduced-calorie diet; to reduce risk of weight gain after previous weight loss**
Adults and children ages 12 to 16: 120 mg P.O. t.i.d. with or up to 1 hour after each main meal containing fat.
➤ **Weight loss (OTC)**
Adults age 18 and older: One 60-mg capsule P.O. with each meal containing fat. Dosage shouldn't exceed 3 capsules a day.

ADMINISTRATION

P.O.
● Give drug with each main meal containing fat (during or up to 1 hour after the meal).

ACTION

Forms a bond with active site of gastric and pancreatic lipases, inactivating them. As a result, enzymes can't hydrolyze dietary triglycerides into absorbable free fatty acids and monoglycerides. The undigested triglycerides are not absorbed, resulting in caloric deficit.

Route	Onset	Peak	Duration
P.O.	Unknown	Unknown	Unknown

Half-life: 1 to 2 hours.

ADVERSE REACTIONS

CNS: *headache,* dizziness, fatigue, sleep disorder, anxiety, depression.
CV: pedal edema.
EENT: otitis.
GI: *flatus with discharge, fecal urgency, fatty or oily stool, oily spotting, increased defecation, abdominal pain,* fecal incontinence, nausea, infectious diarrhea, rectal pain, vomiting.
GU: menstrual irregularity, vaginitis, UTI.
Musculoskeletal: *back pain, leg pain,* arthritis, myalgia, joint disorder, tendinitis.
Respiratory: *influenza, upper respiratory tract infection,* lower respiratory tract infection.
Skin: rash, dry skin.
Other: tooth and gingival disorders.

INTERACTIONS

Drug-drug. *Cyclosporine:* May decrease cyclosporine levels, risking organ rejection in transplant patients. Avoid using together.
Fat-soluble vitamins (such as vitamins A and E and beta-carotene): May decrease absorption of vitamins. Separate doses by 2 hours.
Pravastatin: May slightly increase pravastatin levels and lipid-lowering effects of drug. Monitor patient.
Warfarin: May change coagulation values. Monitor INR.

EFFECTS ON LAB TEST RESULTS
None reported.

CONTRAINDICATIONS & CAUTIONS
● Contraindicated in patients hypersensitive to drug or its components and in those with chronic malabsorption syndrome or cholestasis.
● Use cautiously in patients with history of hyperoxaluria or calcium oxalate nephrolithiasis or those at risk for anorexia nervosa or bulimia.
● Use cautiously in patients receiving cyclosporine therapy because of potential changes in cyclosporine absorption related to variations in dietary intake.

NURSING CONSIDERATIONS
● Exclude organic causes of obesity, such as hypothyroidism, before starting drug therapy.

● Drug is recommended for use in patients with an initial body mass index (BMI) of 30 or more or those with a BMI of 27 or more and other risk factors (such as hypertension, diabetes, or dyslipidemia).
● ***Alert:*** Drug may cause pancreatitis. Monitor the patient closely.
● In diabetic patients, dosage of oral antidiabetic or insulin may need to be reduced because improved metabolic control may accompany weight loss.
● As with other weight-loss drugs, potential for misuse exists in certain patients (such as those with anorexia nervosa or bulimia).
● ***Look alike–sound alike:*** Don't confuse Xenical with Xeloda.

PATIENT TEACHING
● Advise patient to follow a nutritionally balanced, reduced-calorie diet that derives only 30% of its calories from fat. Tell him to distribute daily intake of fat, carbohydrate, and protein over three main meals. If a meal is occasionally missed or contains no fat, tell patient that dose of drug can be omitted.
● Advise patient to adhere to dietary guidelines. GI effects may increase when patient takes drug with high-fat foods, specifically when more than 30% of total daily calories come from fat.
● Drug reduces absorption of some fat-soluble vitamins and beta-carotene.
● Tell patient with diabetes that weight loss may improve his glycemic control, so dosage of his oral antidiabetic (such as a sulfonylurea or metformin) or insulin may need to be reduced during drug therapy.
● Tell woman of childbearing age to inform prescriber if pregnancy or breast-feeding is planned during therapy.

---

pregabalin
pray-GAB-ah-lin

Lyrica

Pharmacologic class: CNS drug
Pregnancy risk category C
Controlled substance schedule V

AVAILABLE FORMS
Capsules: 25 mg, 50 mg, 75 mg, 100 mg, 150 mg, 200 mg, 225 mg, 300 mg

INDICATIONS & DOSAGES
➤ **Fibromyalgia**
Adults: 75 mg P.O. b.i.d. (150 mg/day). May increase to 150 mg b.i.d. (300 mg/day) within 1 week, based on patient response. If pain relief insufficient with 300 mg/day increase to 225 mg b.i.d. (450 mg/day).
➤ **Diabetic peripheral neuropathy**
Adults: Initially, 50 mg P.O. t.i.d. May increase to 100 mg P.O. t.i.d. within 1 week.
➤ **Postherpetic neuralgia**
Adults: Initially, 75 mg P.O. b.i.d. or 50 mg P.O. t.i.d. May increase to 300 mg/day in two or three equally divided doses within 1 week. If pain relief insufficient after 2 to 4 weeks, may increase to 300 mg b.i.d. or 200 mg t.i.d.
➤ **Partial onset seizures**
Adults: Initially, 75 mg P.O. b.i.d. or 50 mg P.O. t.i.d. Range, 150 to 600 mg/day. Dosage may be increased to maximum 600 mg/day.
Adjust-a-dose: If creatinine clearance is 30 to 60 ml/minute, give 75 to 300 mg/day in two or three divided doses. If clearance is 15 to 30 ml/minute, give 25 to 150 mg/day in one dose or divided into two doses. If clearance is less than 15 ml/minute, give 25 to 75 mg/day in one dose. If patient undergoes hemodialysis, give one supplemental dose according to these guidelines. If patient takes 25 mg daily, give 25 or 50 mg. If patient takes 25 to 50 mg daily, give 50 or 75 mg. If patient takes 75 mg daily, give 100 or 150 mg.

ADMINISTRATION
P.O.
● Give drug without regard for food.

● Don't stop drug abruptly. Instead, taper gradually over at least 1 week.

ACTION
May contribute to analgesic and anti-convulsant effects by binding to sites in CNS.

Route	Onset	Peak	Duration
P.O.	Unknown	1½–3 hr	Unknown

Half-life: 6½ hours.

ADVERSE REACTIONS
CNS: *ataxia, dizziness, somnolence, tremor,* abnormal gait, abnormal thinking, amnesia, anxiety, asthenia, confusion, depersonalization, euphoria, headache, hypesthesia, hypertonia, incoordination, myoclonus, nervousness, nystagmus, pain, paresthesia, stupor, twitching, vertigo.
CV: *edema, PR interval prolongation.*
EENT: blurred or abnormal vision, conjunctivitis, diplopia, eye disorder, otitis media, tinnitus.
GI: *dry mouth,* abdominal pain, constipation, flatulence, gastroenteritis, vomiting.
GU: anorgasmia, impotence, urinary incontinence, urinary frequency.
Metabolic: HYPOGLYCEMIA, *weight gain,* increased or decreased appetite.
Musculoskeletal: arthralgia, back and chest pain, leg cramps, myalgia, myasthenia, neuropathy.
Respiratory: bronchitis, dyspnea.
Skin: ecchymosis, pruritus.
Other: *accidental injury, infection,* allergic reaction, decreased libido, flu syndrome.

INTERACTIONS
Drug-drug. *CNS depressants:* May have additive effects on cognitive and gross motor function. Monitor patient for increased dizziness and somnolence.
Pioglitazone, rosiglitazone: May cause additive fluid retention and weight gain. Monitor patient closely.
Drug-lifestyle. *Alcohol use:* May have additive depressant effects on cognitive and gross motor function. Discourage alcohol use.

EFFECTS ON LAB TEST RESULTS
● May increase CK level.
● May decrease platelet count.

CONTRAINDICATIONS & CAUTIONS
• Contraindicated in patients hypersensitive to drug or its components.
• Use cautiously in patients with New York Heart Association class III or class IV heart failure.

NURSING CONSIDERATIONS
• Monitor patient's weight and fluid status, especially if he has heart failure.
• Check for changes in vision.
• *Alert:* Watch for signs of rhabdomyolysis, such as dark, red, or cola-colored urine; muscle tenderness; generalized weakness; or muscle stiffness or aching.

PATIENT TEACHING
• Explain that drug may be taken without regard to food.
• Warn patient not to stop drug abruptly.
• Caution patient to avoid hazardous activities until drug's effects are known.
• Instruct patient to watch for weight changes and water retention.
• Advise patient to report vision changes and malaise or fever accompanied by muscle pain, tenderness, or weakness.
• Tell women to immediately report planned or suspected pregnancy.
• Tell a man who plans to father a child that he should consult prescriber about possible risks to fetus.
• If patient has diabetes, urge him to inspect his skin closely for ulcer formation.

---

raloxifene hydrochloride
rah-LOX-i-feen

Evista⬥

Pharmacologic class: selective estrogen receptor modulator
Pregnancy risk category X

AVAILABLE FORMS
Tablets: 60 mg

INDICATIONS & DOSAGES
➤ **To prevent or treat osteoporosis; to reduce the risk of invasive breast cancer in postmenopausal women with osteoporosis and postmeno-** **pausal women at high risk for invasive breast cancer**
Postmenopausal women: 60 mg P.O. once daily.

ADMINISTRATION
P.O.
• Give drug without regard for food.
• Stop drug at least 72 hours before prolonged immobilization and resume only after patient is fully mobilized.

ACTION
Reduces resorption of bone and decreases overall bone turnover. These effects on bone are manifested as reductions in serum and urine levels of bone turnover markers and increases in bone mineral density.

Route	Onset	Peak	Duration
P.O.	Unknown	Unknown	24 hr

Half-life: 27½ hours.

ADVERSE REACTIONS
CNS: depression, insomnia, fever, migraine.
CV: chest pain.
EENT: *sinusitis,* pharyngitis, laryngitis.
GI: nausea, dyspepsia, vomiting, flatulence, gastroenteritis, abdominal pain.
GU: vaginitis, UTI, cystitis, leukorrhea, endometrial disorder, vaginal bleeding.
Metabolic: weight gain.
Musculoskeletal: *arthralgia,* myalgia, arthritis, leg cramps.
Respiratory: increased cough, pneumonia.
Skin: rash, diaphoresis.
Other: *infection, flulike syndrome, hot flashes,* breast pain, peripheral edema.

INTERACTIONS
Drug-drug. *Cholestyramine:* May cause significant reduction in absorption of raloxifene. Avoid using together.
Highly protein-bound drugs (such as clofibrate, diazepam, diazoxide, ibuprofen, indomethacin, naproxen): May interfere with binding sites. Use together cautiously.
Warfarin: May cause a decrease in PT. Monitor PT and INR closely.

EFFECTS ON LAB TEST RESULTS
• May increase calcium, inorganic phosphate, total protein, albumin, hormone-binding globulin, and apolipoprotein A

Reactions may be *common,* uncommon, *life-threatening,* or COMMON AND LIFE-THREATENING.
Interaction may have a *rapid onset* or *delayed onset.*

levels. May decrease total and LDL cholesterol levels and apolipoprotein B levels.

CONTRAINDICATIONS & CAUTIONS
• Contraindicated in women hypersensitive to drug or its components; in women who are pregnant, planning to get pregnant, or breast-feeding; and in children.
■ **Black Box Warning** Increased risk of venous thromboembolism and death from stroke. Contraindicated in women with a history of, or active venous thromboembolism. Consider the risk-benefit balance in women at risk for stroke. ■
• Use cautiously in patients with severe hepatic impairment.
• Safety and efficacy of drug haven't been evaluated in men.

NURSING CONSIDERATIONS
• Watch for signs of blood clots. Greatest risk of thromboembolic events occurs during first 4 months of treatment.
• Report unexplained uterine bleeding; drug isn't known to cause endometrial proliferation.
• Watch for breast abnormalities; drug isn't known to cause an increased risk of breast cancer.
• Effect on bone mineral density beyond 2 years of drug treatment isn't known.
• Use with hormone replacement therapy or systemic estrogen hasn't been evaluated and isn't recommended.

PATIENT TEACHING
• Advise patient to avoid long periods of restricted movement (such as during traveling) because of increased risk of venous thromboembolic events.
• Inform patient that hot flashes or flushing may occur and that drug doesn't aid in reducing them.
• Instruct patient to practice other bone loss-prevention measures, including taking supplemental calcium and vitamin D if dietary intake is inadequate, performing weight-bearing exercises, and stopping alcohol consumption and smoking.
• Tell patient that drug may be taken without regard for food.
• Advise patient to report unexplained uterine bleeding or breast abnormalities during therapy.

• Explain adverse reactions and instruct patient to read patient package insert before starting therapy and each time prescription is renewed.

riluzole
RILL-you-zole

Rilutek

Pharmacologic class: benzothiazole
Pregnancy risk category C

AVAILABLE FORMS
Tablets: 50 mg

INDICATIONS & DOSAGES
➤ **Amyotrophic lateral sclerosis**
Adults: 50 mg P.O. every 12 hours, taken on empty stomach 1 hour before or 2 hours after a meal.

ADMINISTRATION
P.O.
• Give drug at least 1 hour before or 2 hours after meals to improve bioavailability.

ACTION
May protect motor neurons from excitotoxic effects of glutamate by inhibiting glutamate release, inactivating some sodium channels, and interfering with transmitter binding.

Route	Onset	Peak	Duration
P.O.	Unknown	Unknown	Unknown

Half-life: 12 hours with repeated doses.

ADVERSE REACTIONS
CNS: *asthenia,* headache, aggravation reaction, hypertonia, depression, dizziness, insomnia, malaise, somnolence, vertigo, circumoral paresthesia.
CV: hypertension, tachycardia, palpitations, orthostatic hypotension, phlebitis, peripheral edema.
EENT: rhinitis, sinusitis.
GI: *nausea,* abdominal pain, vomiting, dyspepsia, anorexia, diarrhea, flatulence, stomatitis, dry mouth, oral candidiasis.
GU: UTI, dysuria.
Metabolic: weight loss.
Musculoskeletal: back pain, arthralgia.

Respiratory: *decreased lung function,* increased cough.
Skin: pruritus, eczema, alopecia, exfoliative dermatitis.
Other: tooth disorder.

INTERACTIONS
Drug-drug. *Allopurinol, methyldopa, sulfasalazine:* May increase risk of hepatotoxicity. Monitor liver function closely.
Cytochrome P-450 inducers (omeprazole, rifampin): May increase riluzole elimination. Monitor for lack of effect.
Cytochrome P-450 inhibitors (amitriptyline, caffeine, phenacetin, quinolones, theophylline): May decrease riluzole elimination. Watch for adverse effects.
Drug-food. *Any food:* May decrease drug bioavailability. Advise patient to take drug 1 hour before or 2 hours after meals.
Charbroiled foods: May increase elimination of drug. Discourage use together.
Drug-lifestyle. *Alcohol use:* May increase risk of hepatotoxicity. Discourage excessive use.
Smoking: May increase drug elimination. Discourage patient from smoking.

EFFECTS ON LAB TEST RESULTS
• May increase AST, ALT, bilirubin, and GGT levels.

CONTRAINDICATIONS & CAUTIONS
• Contraindicated in patients with history of severe hypersensitivity to drug or its components.
• Use cautiously in patients with hepatic or renal dysfunction, in elderly patients, and in women and Japanese patients who may have lower metabolic capacity to eliminate drug than men and white patients, respectively.

NURSING CONSIDERATIONS
• Elevated baseline liver function studies (especially bilirubin) rule out therapy. Perform liver function studies periodically during therapy. In many patients, drug may increase aminotransferase level; if level exceeds five times upper limit of normal or if clinical jaundice develops, notify prescriber.

PATIENT TEACHING
• Tell patient to take drug at same time each day. If a dose is missed, tell him to take next tablet when planned.
• Instruct patient to take drug on an empty stomach to facilitate full dose absorption.
• Instruct patient to report fever to prescriber, who may order a WBC count.
• Warn patient to avoid hazardous activities until CNS effects of drug are known and to limit alcohol use during therapy.
• Tell patient to store drug at room temperature, protect from bright light, and keep out of children's reach.

✱ NEW DRUG

sapropterin dihydrochloride
SAP-roh-TEHR-in die-high-droh-KLOR-ighd

Kuvan

Pharmacologic class: enzyme cofactor
Pregnancy risk category C

AVAILABLE FORMS
Tablets: 100 mg

INDICATIONS & DOSAGES
➤ **Hyperphenylalaninemia caused by tetrahydrobiopterin-responsive phenylketonuria (PKU)**
Adults and children age 4 and older:
Initially, 10 mg/kg P.O. once daily with food. If phenylalanine level hasn't decreased from baseline after 4 weeks, increase dose to 20 mg/kg. Stop treatment if patient has no response after 4 weeks at 20 mg/kg.

ACTION
Activates residual phenylalanine hydroxylase to improve the oxidative metabolism of phenylalanine.

Route	Onset	Peak	Duration
P.O.	Varies	Unknown	24 hr

Half-life: About 7 hours.

ADVERSE REACTIONS
CNS: fever, *headache, seizures, spinal cord injury.*

CV: *MI,* peripheral edema.
EENT: nasal congestion, *pharyngo-laryngeal pain, rhinorrhea.*
GI: abdominal pain, diarrhea, gastritis, nausea, vomiting.
GU: polyuria, *testicular cancer.*
Hematologic: *neutropenia.*
Respiratory: cough, *upper respiratory tract infection.*
Skin: rash.
Other: contusion, infection.

INTERACTIONS
Drug-drug. *Drugs that alter folate metabolism (such as methotrexate):* May decrease sapropterin effects. Use together cautiously.
Levodopa: May worsen neurologic symptoms. Use together cautiously.
Phosphodiesterase-5 inhibitors (sildenafil, tadalafil, vardenafil): May cause hypotension. Avoid using together.

EFFECTS ON LAB TEST RESULTS
● May decrease neutrophil count.

CONTRAINDICATIONS & CAUTIONS
● Contraindicated in patients hypersensitive to drug or its components.
● Use cautiously in patients with hepatic impairment and in breast-feeding women.

NURSING CONSIDERATIONS
● Give drug only under supervision of practitioner experienced in treating PKU. Monitor phenylalanine level before and during treatment.
● Dissolve tablet in 4 to 8 oz (120 to 240 ml) of water or apple juice, and give within 15 minutes.
● Give with food to increase absorption, preferably at the same time each day.
● Symptoms of overdose include mild headache and dizziness. If they occur, withhold drug for 24 hours and then resume at previous dose.
● Monitor patient's neurologic status and renal and hepatic function test results.
● Watch patient for signs of infection.
● Protect tablets from moisture. Store at room temperature in a tightly closed container.
● Use only when potential benefits to the mother outweigh risk to the fetus.

● It isn't known whether drug appears in breast milk.
● Because of potential harm to the infant, patient should either stop breast-feeding or stop drug, taking into account the drug's importance to the mother.
● Safety and effectiveness haven't been established in children younger than age 4.
● These patients may have increased adverse effects.

PATIENT TEACHING
● Advise patient to follow a phenylalanine-restricted diet.
● Tell patient to take drug with food at about the same time each day.
● Instruct patient to dissolve tablet in 4 to 8 ounces of water or apple juice and to take within 15 minutes.
● Tell patient to report fever or other signs of infection.
● Caution women to avoid becoming pregnant and to notify prescriber if pregnancy is suspected.
● Advise women not to breast-feed during therapy because drug may appear in breast milk.
● Tell patient to store drug in a tightly sealed container at room temperature.

✱ NEW DRUG

tetrabenazine
teh-tra-BEN-ah-azine

Xenazine

Pharmacologic class: monoamine depleter
Pregnancy risk category C

AVAILABLE FORMS
Tablets: 12.5 mg, 25 mg

INDICATIONS & DOSAGES
➤ **Chorea associated with Huntington's disease**
Adults: Initially 12.5 mg P.O. daily in the morning. After 1 week, increase dose to 12.5 mg P.O. b.i.d. Titrate dose by 12.5 mg at weekly intervals, as needed. Maximum dose, 25 mg. If dose of 37.5 to 50 mg is needed, administer t.i.d. Patients requiring

---

more than 50 mg/day should be genotyped for CYP2D6 metabolism.

Adjust-a-dose: In patients who are extensive or intermediate CYP2D6 metabolizers, slowly titrate doses above 50 mg at weekly intervals by 12.5 mg as needed and tolerated. Maximum daily dose is 100 mg; maximum single dose, 37.5 mg. In patients who are poor CYP2D6 metabolizers, maximum daily dose is 50 mg; maximum single dose, 25 mg.

ACTION
Thought to reversibly deplete monoamines from nerve terminals.

Route	Onset	Peak	Duration
P.O.	Rapid	1–1½ hr	Unknown

Half-life: Metabolite α-HTBZ, 4 to 8 hours; β-HTBZ, 2 to 4 hours.

ADVERSE REACTIONS
CNS: *sedation, somnolence, insomnia, depression, anxiety, extrapyramidal symptoms, fatigue, falling,* balance difficulty, parkinsonism, bradykinesia, dizziness, irritability, obsessive reaction, dysarthria, unsteady gait, headache.
GI: *nausea,* vomiting.
GU: dysuria.
Metabolic: decreased appetite.
Respiratory: *upper respiratory infection,* dyspnea, bronchitis.
Skin: head laceration, ecchymosis.

INTERACTIONS
Drug-drug. *CYP2D6 inhibitors (fluoxetine, paroxetine, quinidine):* May increase metabolite exposure. Reduce tetrabenazine dose as directed.
Drugs that prolong QTc interval (amiodarone, chlorpromazine, moxifloxacin, procainamide, quinidine, sotalol, thioridazine, ziprasidone): May cause arrhythmias. Avoid use together.
Neuroleptic drugs (chlorpromazine, haloperidol, olanzapine, risperidone): May increase risk of neuroleptic malignant syndrome and extrapyramidal effects. Use together cautiously.
Reserpine: May increase effects of tetrabenazine. Wait 20 days after reserpine therapy before starting tetrabenazine.

Monoamine oxidase inhibitors: May increase risk of serious, sometimes fatal adverse reactions. Avoid using together.
Drug-lifestyle. *Alcohol:* May increase sedative effects. Discourage using together.

EFFECTS ON LAB TEST RESULTS
• May increase ALT, AST, and serum prolactin levels.

CONTRAINDICATIONS & CAUTIONS
• Contraindicated in patients who are actively suicidal and in those with depression who aren't receiving treatment or aren't being adequately treated. Contraindicated in those with hepatic impairment and in those receiving a monoamine oxidase inhibitor or reserpine. Use cautiously in patients at risk for aspiration pneumonia. Avoid use in patients with congenital long QT syndrome and in those with a history of arrhythmias.

NURSING CONSIDERATIONS
■ **Black Box Warning** Drug may increase the risk for depression and suicidal thinking. Monitor patient closely. Patient who requires more than 50 mg/day should be genotyped for CYP2D6 metabolism. ■
• *Alert:* Watch for signs of neuroleptic malignant syndrome (extrapyramidal effects, hyperthermia, autonomic disturbance), which is rare but commonly fatal. Drug may worsen mood, cognition, rigidity, and functional capacity. If these findings persist, reevaluate the need for the drug.
• Monitor for dysphagia; patient may be at increased risk for aspiration.
• Monitor electrocardiogram; drug may increase QTc interval.
• Monitor prolactin and estrogen levels. Elevated prolactin levels and low estrogen levels may increase the risk for osteoporosis.
• Patient should receive regular ophthalmologic exams during therapy.
• If drug is stopped without tapering, monitor patient for chorea, which may occur within 12 to 18 hours after last dose.
• If restarting drug within 5 days of last dose, restart at previous dosage; if more than 5 days, retitrate dose.
• Overdose may cause acute dystonia, oculogyric crisis, nausea and vomiting,

---

Reactions may be *common*, uncommon, *life-threatening*, or COMMON AND LIFE-THREATENING.
Interaction may have a *rapid onset* or *delayed onset*.

sweating, sedation, hypotension, confusion, diarrhea, hallucinations, inflammatory response, and tremor. Monitor vital signs and heart rhythm, and provide sympto-matic treatment.
• Safety and efficacy haven't been estab-lished. Use cautiously.
• It isn't known if drug appears in breast milk. Because of potential adverse effects to infant, patient should stop taking the drug or stop breast-feeding.
• Safety and efficacy haven't been established.
• Use cautiously in elderly patients.

PATIENT TEACHING
• Advise patient to avoid hazardous activities that require alertness and good psychomotor coordination until the effects of drug are known.
• Advise patient and his family to imme-diately report mood swings or suicidal thoughts.
• Warn patient to avoid alcohol during therapy.
• Tell women of childbearing age to notify practitioner immediately if pregnancy occurs or about any plans to become pregnant or to breast-feed.

tretinoin (retinoic acid, vitamin A acid)
TRET-i-noyn

Atralin, Avita, Rejuva-A†, Renova, Retin-A, Retin-A Micro, StieVA-A†

Pharmacologic class: retinoid
Pregnancy risk category C

AVAILABLE FORMS
Cream: 0.02%, 0.025%, 0.05%, 0.1%
Gel: 0.05%, 0.01%, 0.025%
Microsphere gel: 0.04%, 0.1%

INDICATIONS & DOSAGES
➤ **Acne vulgaris**
Adults and children: Clean affected area and lightly apply once daily at bedtime.
➤ **Adjunctive use in the mitigation of fine facial wrinkles in patients who use comprehensive skin care and sunlight avoidance programs (Renova)**

Adults: Apply a small, pea-sized amount (¼ inch or 5 mm in diameter) to cover the entire face lightly, once daily in the evening.

ADMINISTRATION
Topical
• Clean area thoroughly before application and avoid getting drug in eyes, mouth, or mucous membranes.

ACTION
Inhibits comedones by increasing epider-mal cell mitosis and turnover.

Route	Onset	Peak	Duration
Topical	Unknown	Unknown	Unknown

Half-life: Unknown.

ADVERSE REACTIONS
Skin: *feeling of warmth, slight stinging, local erythema, peeling,* chapping, swelling, blistering, crusting, temporary hyperpigmentation or hypopigmentation.

INTERACTIONS
Drug-drug. *Topical drugs containing benzoyl peroxide, resorcinol, salicylic acid, or sulfur:* May increase risk of skin irritation. Avoid using together.
Topical minoxidil or photosensitizing drugs (fluoroquinolones, phenothiazines, sulfonamides, tetracyclines, thiazides): May increase risk of skin irritation. Avoid using together.
Drug-lifestyle. *Abrasive cleansers, medicated cosmetics, skin preparations containing alcohol:* May increase risk of skin irritation. Discourage use together.
Sun exposure: May increase photosensi-tivity reaction. Advise patient to avoid excessive sunlight exposure.

EFFECTS ON LAB TEST RESULTS
None reported.

CONTRAINDICATIONS & CAUTIONS
• Contraindicated in patients hypersensitive to drug or its components and in those with sunburn.
• Use cautiously in patients with eczema.

NURSING CONSIDERATIONS
• Initially, drug may be applied every 2 to 3 days using a lower concentration to reduce irritation.

- Relapses typically occur within 3 to 6 weeks after therapy is stopped.
- *Look alike–sound alike:* Don't confuse tretinoin with trientine.

PATIENT TEACHING
- Instruct patient to clean area thoroughly before application and to avoid getting drug in eyes, mouth, or mucous membranes.
- Tell patient to wash hands after application.
- Tell patient to wash face with mild soap no more than b.i.d. or t.i.d. Warn patient against using strong or medicated cosmetics, soaps, or other skin cleansers. Also advise him to avoid topical products containing alcohol, astringents, spices, and lime because they may interfere with drug's actions.
- Tell patient using drug for treatment of fine wrinkles to wait 20 minutes after washing face to apply drug, and to avoid washing face or applying another skin product or cosmetic for 1 hour after application.
- Tell patient that normal use of cosmetics is allowed.
- Advise patient not to stop drug if temporary worsening of inflammatory lesions occurs. If severe local irritation develops, advise patient to stop drug temporarily and notify prescriber. Dosage will be readjusted when application is resumed. Some redness and scaling are normal reactions.
- Warn patient that he may experience increased sensitivity to wind or cold temperatures.
- Instruct patient to minimize exposure to sunlight or ultraviolet rays during treatment. If he becomes sunburned, he should delay therapy until sunburn subsides. Tell patient who can't avoid exposure to sunlight to use SPF-15 sunblock and to wear protective clothing.
- Warn patient that he may have a temporary increase in lesions, which will improve in 2 to 3 weeks.

varenicline tartrate
vah-RENN-ih-kleen

Chantix◆

Pharmacologic class: nicotinic acetylcholine receptor partial agonist
Pregnancy risk category C

AVAILABLE FORMS
Tablets: 0.5 mg, 1 mg

INDICATIONS & DOSAGES
➤ **Smoking cessation**
Adults: Starting 1 week before patient stops smoking, give 0.5 mg P.O. once daily on days 1 through 3. Days 4 through 7, give 0.5 mg P.O. b.i.d. Day 8 through the end of week 12, give 1 mg P.O. b.i.d. If patient successfully stops smoking, give an additional 12-week course to help with long-term success.
Adjust-a-dose: In patient with severe renal impairment, 0.5 mg P.O. once daily. Adjust as needed to maximum of 0.5 mg b.i.d. In patient with end-stage renal disease who is undergoing dialysis, 0.5 mg once daily.

ADMINISTRATION
P.O.
- Give drug with full glass of water after a meal.

ACTION
Blocks the effects of nicotine by binding at alpha$_4$ beta$_2$ neuronal nicotinic acetylcholine receptors. Drug also provides some of nicotine's effects to ease withdrawal.

Route	Onset	Peak	Duration
P.O.	4 days	3–4 hr	24 hr

Half-life: 24 hours.

ADVERSE REACTIONS
CNS: *abnormal dreams, headache, insomnia,* altered attention or emotions, anxiety, asthenia, depression, dizziness, fatigue, irritability, lethargy, malaise, nightmares, restlessness, sensory disturbance, sleep disorder, somnolence.

Reactions may be *common,* uncommon, *life-threatening,* or COMMON AND LIFE-THREATENING.
Interaction may have a *rapid onset* or **delayed onset.**

CV: chest pain, edema, hot flush, hypertension.
EENT: altered taste, epistaxis.
GI: *nausea,* abdominal pain, constipation, diarrhea, dry mouth, dyspepsia, flatulence, gingivitis, vomiting.
GU: menstrual disorder, polyuria.
Metabolic: decreased appetite, increased appetite, thirst.
Musculoskeletal: arthralgia, back pain, muscle cramps, myalgia.
Respiratory: dyspnea, upper respiratory tract disorder.
Skin: rash.
Other: flulike illness.

INTERACTIONS
Drug-drug. *Nicotine-replacement therapy:* May increase nausea, vomiting, dizziness, dyspepsia, and fatigue. Monitor patient closely.

EFFECTS ON LAB TEST RESULTS
• May increase liver function test values.

CONTRAINDICATIONS & CAUTIONS
• Use cautiously in pregnant or breast-feeding women, elderly patients, and patients with severe renal impairment or pre-existing psychiatric illness.

NURSING CONSIDERATIONS
• Assess patient's readiness and motivation to stop smoking.
• *Alert:* Monitor patient for changes in behavior, agitation, depressed mood, suicidal ideation, suicidal behavior and worsening of pre-existing psychiatric illness and report immediately.
• Notify prescriber if patient develops intolerable nausea; dosage reduction may be needed.
• Temporarily monitor levels of drugs—such as theophylline, warfarin, and insulin—after patient stops smoking to be sure levels are still within therapeutic range.

PATIENT TEACHING
• Provide patient with educational materials and needed counseling.
• Instruct patient to choose a date to stop smoking and to begin treatment 1 week before this date.

• Advise patient to take each dose with a full glass of water after eating.
• Teach patient to gradually increase the dose over the first week to a target of 1 mg in the morning and 1 mg in the evening.
• Explain that nausea and insomnia are common and usually temporary. Urge him to contact the prescriber if adverse effects are persistently troubling; a dosage reduction may help.
• Urge patient to continue trying to abstain from smoking if he has early lapses after successfully quitting.
• Tell patient that dosages of other drugs he takes may need adjustment when he stops smoking.
• Advise patient to use caution when driving or operating machinery until effects of the drug are known.
• Instruct family to observe patient for changes in behavior and mood including agitation, depression, suicidal ideation or behavior and worsening of pre-existing psychiatric illness; report changes to healthcare provider immediately.
• If woman plans to become pregnant or to breast-feed, explain the risks of smoking and the risks and benefits of taking drug to aid smoking cessation.

Appendices

Pregnancy risk categories

The FDA has assigned a pregnancy risk category to each drug based on available clinical and preclinical information. The five categories (A, B, C, D, and X) reflect a drug's potential to cause birth defects. Although drugs should ideally be avoided during pregnancy, sometimes they're needed; this rating system permits rapid assessment of the risk-benefit ratio. Drugs in category A are generally considered safe to use in pregnancy; drugs in category X are generally contraindicated.

- A: Adequate studies in pregnant women have failed to show a risk to the fetus.
- B: Animal studies haven't shown a risk to the fetus, but controlled studies haven't been conducted in pregnant women; or animal studies have shown an adverse effect on the fetus, but adequate studies in pregnant women haven't shown a risk to the fetus.
- C: Animal studies have shown an adverse effect on the fetus, but adequate studies haven't been conducted in humans. The benefits from use in pregnant women may be acceptable despite potential risks.
- D: The drug may cause risk to the fetus, but the potential benefits of use in pregnant women may be acceptable despite the risks (such as in a life-threatening situation or a serious disease for which safer drugs can't be used or are ineffective).
- X: Studies in animals or humans show fetal abnormalities, or adverse reaction reports indicate evidence of fetal risk. The risks involved clearly outweigh potential benefits.
- NR: Not rated.

Controlled substance schedules

Drugs regulated under the jurisdiction of the Controlled Substances Act of 1970 are divided into the following groups or schedules:

- Schedule I (C-I): High abuse potential and no accepted medical use. Examples include heroin, marijuana, and LSD.
- Schedule II (C-II): High abuse potential with severe dependence liability. Examples include opioids, amphetamines, and some barbiturates.
- Schedule III (C-III): Less abuse potential than schedule II drugs and moderate dependence liability. Examples include nonbarbiturate sedatives, nonamphetamine stimulants, anabolic steroids, and limited amounts of certain opioids.
- Schedule IV (C-IV): Less abuse potential than schedule III drugs and limited dependence liability. Examples include some sedatives, anxiolytics, and nonopioid analgesics.
- Schedule V (C-V): Limited abuse potential. This category includes mainly small amounts of opioids, such as codeine, used as antitussives or antidiarrheals. Under federal law, limited quantities of certain C-V drugs may be purchased without a prescription directly from a pharmacist if allowed under specific state statutes. The purchaser must be at least age 18 and must furnish suitable identification. All such transactions must be recorded by the dispensing pharmacist.

Quick guide to combination drugs

This guide lists trade names and generic ingredients of common combination drugs.

222†: aspirin, codeine phosphate, and caffeine citrate

282 MEP†: aspirin, codeine phosphate, caffeine citrate, and meprobamate

292†: aspirin, codeine phosphate, and caffeine citrate

Accuretic: quinapril and hydrochlorothiazide

Aceta with Codeine: acetaminophen and codeine phosphate

Activella: ethinyl estradiol and norethindrone acetate

ACTOPlus MET: pioglitazone hydrochloride and metformin hydrochloride

Adderall: dextroamphetamine sulfate, dextroamphetamine saccharate, amphetamine aspartate, and amphetamine sulfate

Advicor: niacin and lovastatin

Advil Cold and Sinus Caplets ◇: pseudoephedrine hydrochloride and ibuprofen

Aggrenox: aspirin and dipyridamole

AK-Poly-Bac ◇: polymyxin B sulfate and bacitracin zinc

Alavert Allergy & Sinus D-12 Hour ◇: loratadine and pseudoephedrine sulfate

Aldactazide: spironolactone and hydrochlorothiazide

Alka-Seltzer Gold ◇: sodium bicarbonate, citric acid, and potassium bicarbonate

Alka-Seltzer Original ◇: aspirin, citric acid, and phenylalanine

Allegra-D ◇: fexofenadine hydrochloride and pseudoephedrine sulfate

Allerest Maximum Strength Tablets ◇: pseudoephedrine hydrochloride and chlorpheniramine maleate

Alor: aspirin and hydrocodone bitartrate

Aludrox ◇: aluminum hydroxide and magnesium hydroxide

Anexsia: acetaminophen and hydrocodone bitartrate

Angeliq: drospirenone and estradiol

Apresazide: hydrochlorothiazide and hydralazine hydrochloride

Arthrotec: diclofenac sodium and misoprostol

Ascriptin ◇: aspirin, magnesium hydroxide, aluminum hydroxide, and calcium carbonate

Atacand HCT: candesartan cilexetil and hydrochlorothiazide

Atripla: efavirenz, emtricitabine, and tenofovir disoproxil fumarate

Avalide: irbesartan and hydrocholorothiazide

Avandamet: rosiglitazone hydrochloride and metformin hydrochloride

Avandaryl: glimepiride and rosiglitazone hydrochloride

AZOR: amlodipine and olmesartan medoxomil

Benicar HCT: olmesartan medoxomil and hydrochlorothiazide

BenzaClin: clindamycin and benzoyl peroxide

Benzamycin: erythromycin and benzoyl peroxide

Bicillin C-R: penicillin G benzathine and procaine

BiDil: isosorbide dinitrate and hydralazine

Blephamide Sterile Ophthalmic Ointment: sulfacetamide sodium and prednisolone acetate

Bronchial Capsules: theophylline and guaifenesin

Bronkaid Dual Action Tablets: ephedrine sulfate and guaifenesin

Caduet: amlodipine and atorvastatin

Cafergot: ergotamine tartrate and caffeine

Capital with Codeine: acetaminophen and codeine phosphate

Capozide: captopril and hydrochlorothiazide

Children's Advil Cold ◇: pseudoephedrine and ibuprofen

Chlor-Trimeton Allergy-D ◇: chlorpheniramine maleate and pseudoephedrine sulfate

Citracal + D ◇: calcium with cholecalciferol

Claritin-D: loratadine and pseudoephedrine

ClimaraPro: estradiol and levonorgestrel

Clorpres: chlorthalidone and clonidine hydrochloride

Co-Gesic: acetaminophen and hydrocodone bitartrate

Col-Probenecid: colchicine and probenecid

Combigan: brimonidine tartrate and timolol maleate

CombiPatch: estradiol and norethindrone

Combivent: ipratropium bromide and albuterol

Combivir: lamivudine and zidovudine

Comvax: *Haemophilus* b PRP, *Neisseria meningitidis* OMPC, and hepatitis B surface antigen

Contac Severe Cold & Flu Caplets ◊: acetaminophen, dextromethorphan hydrobromide, pseudoephedrine hydrochloride, and chlorpheniramine maleate

Coricidin 'D' Cold, Flu, & Sinus ◊: chlorpheniramine maleate, acetaminophen, and pseudoephedrine sulfate

Coricidin HBP Cold & Flu ◊: chlorpheniramine maleate and acetaminophen

Cortisporin Ophthalmic Suspension: polymyxin B sulfate, neomycin sulfate, and hydrocortisone

Corzide: nadolol and bendroflumethiazide

Cyclomydril Ophthalmic: cyclopentolate hydrochloride and phenylephrine hydrochloride

DAPTACEL: diphtheria toxoid, tetanus toxoid and acellular pertussis vaccine adsorbed

Darvocet: acetaminophen and propoxyphene napsylate

Decadron Phosphate with Xylocaine: dexamethasone phosphate and lidocaine hydrochloride

Deconamine ◊: pseudoephedrine hydrochloride and chlorpheniramine maleate

Dical-D ◊: calcium (as phosphate tribasic) with cholecalciferol

Di-Gel Advanced ◊: magnesium hydroxide and calcium carbonate, and simethicone

Diovan HCT: valsartan and hydrochlorothiazide

Donnatal: atropine sulfate, scopolamine hydrobromide, hyoscyamine sulfate, and phenobarbital

Donnatal Elixir: atropine sulfate, scopolamine hydrobromide, ethanol, hyoscyamine hydrobromide or sulfate, and phenobarbital

Dristan Sinus Caplets ◊: pseudoephedrine hydrochloride and ibuprofen

Duac: clindamycin and benzoyl peroxide

Duetact: pioglitazone and glimepiride

Dyazide: triamterene and hydrochlorothiazide

Dyflex-G Tablets: dyphylline and guaifenesin

Dyline-GG Tablets: dyphylline and guaifenesin

Empirin with Codeine: aspirin and codeine phosphate

Endocet: acetaminophen and oxycodone hydrochloride

Entex PSE: pseudoephedrine and guaifenesin

Epzicom: abacavir and lamivudine

Equagesic: meprobamate and aspirin

Eryzole: erythromycin ethylsuccinate and sulfisoxazole

Estratest: esterified estrogens and methyltestosterone

Excedrin ◊: aspirin, acetaminophen, and caffeine

Excedrin P.M. ◊: acetaminophen and diphenhydramine

Extra Strength Alka-Seltzer ◊: aspirin, citric acid, and sodium bicarbonate

femhrt: ethinyl estradiol and norethindrone acetate

Ferro-Sequels ◊: ferrous fumarate and docusate sodium

Fioricet: acetaminophen, butalbital, and caffeine

Fioricet with Codeine: acetaminophen, butalbital, caffeine, and codeine

Fiorinal: aspirin, butalbital, and caffeine

Fiorinal with Codeine: aspirin, butalbital, caffeine, and codeine

Gaviscon Tablets: aluminum hydroxide and magnesium trisilicate

Gelusil Tablets ◊: aluminum hydroxide, magnesium hydroxide, and simethicone

Glucovance: glyburide and metformin

Glyceryl-T Capsules: theophylline and guaifenesin

Haley's M-O ◊: mineral oil and magnesium hydroxide

Helidac: bismuth subsalicylate, metronidazole, tetracycline hydrochloride

Hyzaar: losartan and hydrochlorothiazide

Inderide LA: propranolol hydrochloride and hydrochlorothiazide

Janumet: sitagliptin and metformin hydrochloride

Kaodene Nonnarcotic ◊ **:** kaolin and pectin in bismuth subsalicylate liquid

Kapectolin ◊ **:** kaolin and pectin in suspension

Kolyum: potassium, chloride (from potassium gluconate and potassium chloride)

Lexxel: enalapril maleate and felodipine

Librax: chlordiazepoxide hydrochloride and methscopolamine nitrate

Limbitrol: chlordiazepoxide and amitriptyline

Lopressor HCT: metoprolol tartrate and hydrochlorothiazide

Lorcet: acetaminophen and hydrocodone bitartrate

Lortab: acetaminophen and hydrocodone bitartrate

Lortab ASA: aspirin and hydrocodone bitartrate

Lotensin HCT: benazepril and hydrochlorothiazide

Lotrel: amlodipine and benazepril hydrochloride

Lotrisone: clotrimazole and betamethasone dipropionate

Maalox Suspension ◊ **:** aluminum hydroxide, magnesium hydroxide, and simethicone

Maalox TC Suspension ◊ **:** aluminum hydroxide and magnesium hydroxide

Magnaprin ◊ **:** aspirin, magnesium hydroxide, aluminum hydroxide, and calcium carbonate

Marax: theophylline, ephedrine sulfate, and hydroxyzine hydrochloride

Maxitrol Ointment/Ophthalmic Suspension: dexamethasone, neomycin sulfate, and polymyxin B sulfate

Maxzide: triamterene and hydrochlorothiazide

Metaglip: glipizide and metformin

Metimyd Ophthalmic Ointment/ Suspension: sulfacetamide sodium and prednisolone acetate

Micardis HCT: telmisartan and hydrochlorothiazide

Midrin: isometheptene mucate, dichloralphenazone, and acetaminophen

Minizide: prazosin and polythiazide

Monopril HCT: fosinopril sodium and hydrochlorothiazide

Motrin Sinus Headache Tablets: pseudoephedrine hydrochloride and ibuprofen

Mudrane GG-2 Tablets: theophylline and guaifenesin

Murocoll 2: scopolamine hydrobromide and phenylephrine hydrochloride

Mycolog-II: triamcinolone acetonide and nystatin

Mylanta ◊ **:** aluminum hydroxide, magnesium hydroxide, and simethicone

Neosporin G.U. Irrigant: neomycin sulfate and polymyxin B sulfate

Neosporin Ophthalmic Ointment: polymyxin B sulfate, neomycin sulfate, and bacitracin zinc

Neosporin Ophthalmic Solution: polymyxin B sulfate, neomycin sulfate, and gramicidin

Neosporin Plus Pain Relief Ointment ◊ **:** polymyxin B sulfate, bacitracin zinc, and neomycin sulfate

Neutra-phos ◊ **:** phosphorus, sodium, potassium

Norco: acetaminophen and hydrocodone bitartrate

Norgesic: orphenadrine citrate, aspirin, and caffeine

Novo-gesic C8†: acetaminophen, codeine phosphate, and caffeine

Opcon-A Ophthalmic Solution ◊ **:** naphazoline hydrochloride and pheniramine maleate

Ornex No Drowsiness Caplets ◊ **:** acetaminophen and pseudoephedrine hydrochloride

Panacet: acetaminophen and hydrocodone bitartrate

Panasal: aspirin and hydrocodone bitartrate

Pediazole: erythromycin ethylsuccinate and sulfisoxazole

Pepcid Complete ◊ **:** calcium carbonate, magnesium hydroxide, and famotidine

Percocet: acetaminophen and oxycodone hydrochloride

Percodan: aspirin, oxycodone hydrochloride and oxycodone terephthalate

Perloxx: acetaminophen and oxycodone hydrochloride

Polysporin Ophthalmic Ointment: polymyxin B sulfate and bacitracin zinc

Polytrim Ophthalmic: trimethoprim sulfate and polymyxin B sulfate

Posture-D ◊ : calcium (as phosphate tribasic) with cholecalciferol

Pred-G S.O.P.: prednisolone acetate and gentamicin sulfate equivalent to gentamicin base

Prefest: estradiol and norgestimate

Premphase: conjugated estrogens and medroxyprogesterone

Prempro: conjugated estrogen and medroxyprogesterone

Preven: ethinyl estradiol and levonorgestrel

Prevpac: lansoprazole, amoxicillin, clarithromycin

Primatene Tablets: ephedrine hydrochloride and guaifenesin

Prinzide: lisinopril and hydrochlorothiazide

Prosed/DS Tablets: methenamine, phenyl salicylate, methylene blue, benzoic acid, atropine sulfate, and hyoscyamine sulfate

PYLERA: bismuth subcitrate potassium, metronidazole, and tetracycline hydrochloride

Pyridium Plus: phenazopyridine, butabarbital, and hyoscyamine

Quinaretic: quinapril hydrochloride and hydrochlorothiazide

Rauzide: bendroflumethiazide and powdered Rauwolfia serpentina

Rebetron: ribavirin and interferon alpha-2b

Renese-R: polythiazide and reserpine

Reprexain: hydrocodone bitartrate and ibuprofen

Rifamate: isoniazid and rifampin

Rifater: isoniazid, rifampin, and pyrazinamide

Riopan ◊ : magaldrate and simethicone

Roxicet: acetaminophen and oxycodone hydrochloride

Roxilox: acetaminophen and oxycodone hydrochloride

Semprex-D: acrivastine and pseudoephedrine hydrochloride

Senokot-S ◊ : docusate sodium and sennosides

Simcor: niacin and simvastatin

Sinus-Relief ◊ : acetaminophen and pseudoephedrine hydrochloride

Sinutab Maximum Strength Without Drowsiness ◊ : acetaminophen and pseudoephedrine hydrochloride

Soma Compound: carisoprodol and aspirin

Soma Compound with Codeine: carisoprodol, aspirin, and codeine phosphate

Suboxone: buprenorphine and naloxone

Symbicort: budesonide and formoterol fumarate dihydrate

Symbyax: olanzapine and fluoxetine

Synophylate-GG Syrup: guaifenesin and theophylline sodium glycinate

Talacen: acetaminophen and pentazocine hydrochloride

Talwin: aspirin and pentazocine hydrochloride

Talwin NX: naloxone and pentazocine hydrochloride

Tarka: trandolapril and verapamil

Tekturna HCT: aliskiren hemifumarate and hydrochlorthiazide.

Tenoretic: atenolol and chlorthalidone

Terak with Polymyxin B Sulfate Ophthalmic Ointment: polymyxin B sulfate and oxytetracycline hydrochloride

Teveten HCT: eprosartan and hydrochlorothiazide

Theomax DF Syrup: theophylline, ephedrine sulfate, hydroxyzine hydrochloride

Timolide: timolol maleate and hydrochlorothiazide

Titralac Plus ◊ : calcium carbonate and simethicone

TobraDex: dexamethasone and tobramycin

Triaminic Cold & Allergy ◊ : pseudoephedrine hydrochloride and chlorpheniramine maleate

TriHIBIT: *Haemophilus* b conjugated to inactivated tetanus toxoid diphtheria toxoid, tetanus toxoid, and acellular pertussis vaccine adsorbed

Trizivir: abacavir sulfate, zidovudine, and lamivudine

Truvada: emtricitabine and tenofovir

Tuinal Pulvules: amobarbital sodium and secobarbital sodium

Tussionex Pennkinetic: chlorpheniramine polistirex and hydrocodone polistirex.

Twinrix: inactivated hepatitis A and recombinant HBsAg protein

Tylenol PM Extra Strength ◊ : acetaminophen and diphenhydramine

Tylenol with codeine: acetaminophen and codeine phosphate

Tylox: acetaminophen and oxycodone hydrochloride

Ultracet: acetaminophen and tramadol hydrochloride

Uniretic: moexipril hydrochloride and hydrochlorothiazide

Urimax Tablets: methenamine, sodium biphosphate, phenyl salicylate, methylene blue, and hyoscyamine sulfate

Urised Tablets: methenamine, phenyl salicylate, methylene blue, benzoic acid, atropine sulfate, and hyoscyamine sulfate

Vanquish ◊ : aspirin, acetaminophen, caffeine, aluminum hydroxide, and magnesium hydroxide

Vaseretic: enalapril maleate and hydrochlorothiazide

Vasocidin Ophthalmic Solution: sulfacetamide sodium and prednisolone phosphate

Vicodin: acetaminophen and hydrocodone bitartrate

Vicoprofen: hydrocodone bitartrate and ibuprofen

Vytorin: ezetimibe and simvastatin

Zestoretic: lisinopril and hydrochlorothiazide

Ziac: bisoprolol fumarate and hydrochlorothiazide

Zincfrin ◊ : phenylephrine hydrochloride and zinc sulfate

Zydone: acetaminophen and hydrocodone bitartrate

Zyrtec-D 12-hour Extended-Release Tablets: cetirizine hydrochloride and pseudoephedrine hydrochloride

Common combination drugs: Indications and dosages

AMPHETAMINES

Adderall
Adderall XR
Controlled Substance Schedule (CSS) II

GENERIC COMPONENTS
Tablets
5 mg: 1.25 mg dextroamphetamine sulfate, 1.25 mg dextroamphetamine saccharate, and 1.25 mg amphetamine aspartate, and 1.25 mg amphetamine sulfate
7.5 mg: 1.875 mg dextroamphetamine sulfate, 1.875 mg dextroamphetamine saccharate, 1.875 mg amphetamine aspartate, and 1.875 mg amphetamine sulfate
10 mg: 2.5 mg dextroamphetamine sulfate, 2.5 mg dextroamphetamine saccharate, 2.5 mg amphetamine aspartate, and 2.5 mg amphetamine sulfate
12.5 mg: 3.125 mg dextroamphetamine sulfate, 3.125 mg dextroamphetamine saccharate, 3.125 mg amphetamine aspartate, and 3.125 mg amphetamine sulfate
15 mg: 3.75 mg dextroamphetamine sulfate, 3.75 mg dextroamphetamine saccharate, 3.75 mg amphetamine aspartate, and 3.75 mg amphetamine sulfate
20 mg: 5 mg dextroamphetamine sulfate, 5 mg dextroamphetamine saccharate, 5 mg amphetamine aspartate, and 5 mg amphetamine sulfate
30 mg: 7.5 mg dextroamphetamine sulfate, 7.5 mg dextroamphetamine saccharate, 7.5 mg amphetamine aspartate, and 7.5 mg amphetamine sulfate
Capsules (extended-release)
5 mg: 1.25 mg dextroamphetamine sulfate, 1.25 mg dextroamphetamine saccharate, 1.25 mg amphetamine aspartate, and 1.25 mg amphetamine sulfate
10 mg: 2.5 mg dextroamphetamine sulfate, 2.5 mg dextroamphetamine saccharate, 2.5 mg amphetamine aspartate, and 2.5 mg amphetamine sulfate
15 mg: 3.75 mg dextroamphetamine sulfate, 3.75 mg dextroamphetamine saccharate, 3.75 mg amphetamine aspartate, and 3.75 mg amphetamine sulfate
20 mg: 5 mg dextroamphetamine sulfate, 5 mg dextroamphetamine saccharate, 5 mg amphetamine aspartate, and 5 mg amphetamine sulfate
25 mg: 6.25 mg dextroamphetamine sulfate, 6.25 mg dextroamphetamine saccharate, 6.25 mg amphetamine aspartate, and 6.25 mg amphetamine sulfate
30 mg: 7.5 mg dextroamphetamine sulfate, 7.5 mg dextroamphetamine saccharate, 7.5 mg amphetamine aspartate, and 7.5 mg amphetamine sulfate

DOSAGES
Narcolepsy
Adults and children age 12 and older: Initially, 10 mg immediate-release tablet daily. Increase by 10 mg weekly to maximum dose of 60 mg in 2 or 3 divided doses every 4 to 6 hours.
Children ages 6 to 12: Initially, 5 mg immediate-release tablet P.O. daily. Increase by 5 mg at weekly intervals to maximum dose of 60 mg in divided doses.
Attention deficit hyperactivity disorder
Adults: 20 mg extended-release capsules P.O. daily.
Adolescents ages 13 to 17: Initially, 10 mg extended-release capsule P.O. daily. Increase after 1 week to 20 mg daily if needed.
Children age 6 and older: Initially, 5 mg immediate-release tablet P.O. daily or b.i.d. Increase by 5 mg at weekly intervals until optimal response. Dosage should rarely exceed 40 mg.
Children ages 6 to 12: Give 10 mg extended-release capsule P.O. daily in a.m. Increase by 5 to 10 mg in weekly intervals to a maximum dose of 30 mg.
Children ages 3 to 5: Initially, 2.5 mg immediate-release tablet P.O. daily. Increase by 2.5 mg at weekly intervals until optimal response. Divide total daily dose into 2 or 3 doses and give 4 to 6 hours apart.

ANALGESICS

Alor 5/500
Damason-P
Lortab ASA
CSS III

GENERIC COMPONENTS
500 mg aspirin and 5 mg hydrocodone
bitartrate

DOSAGES
Moderate to moderately severe pain
Adults: 1 or 2 tablets every 4 hours.
Maximum dosage, 8 tablets in 24 hours.

Anexsia 5/325
Norco 5/325
CSS III

GENERIC COMPONENTS
325 mg acetaminophen and 5 mg
hydrocodone bitartrate

DOSAGES
Moderate to moderately severe pain
Adults: 1 to 2 tablets every 4 to 6 hours.
Maximum dosage, 12 tablets in 24 hours.

Anexsia 5/500
Co-Gesic
Lorcet HD
Lortab 5/500
Panacet 5/500
Vicodin
CSS III

GENERIC COMPONENTS
500 mg acetaminophen and 5 mg
hydrocodone bitartrate

DOSAGES
Moderate to moderately severe pain
Adults: 1 to 2 tablets every 4 to 6 hours.
Maximum dosage, 8 tablets in 24 hours.

Anexsia 7.5/325
Norco 7.5/325
CSS III

GENERIC COMPONENTS
325 mg acetaminophen and 7.5 mg
hydrocodone bitartrate

DOSAGES
Moderate to moderately severe pain
Adults: 1 to 2 tablets every 4 to 6 hours.
Maximum dosage, 12 tablets in 24 hours.

Anexsia 7.5/650
Lorcet Plus
CSS III

GENERIC COMPONENTS
650 mg acetaminophen and 7.5 mg
hydrocodone bitartrate

DOSAGES
Arthralgia, bone pain, dental pain,
headache, migraine, moderate pain
Adults: 1 to 2 tablets every 4 hours.
Maximum dosage, 6 tablets in 24 hours.

Anexsia 10/660
Vicodin HP
CSS III

GENERIC COMPONENTS
660 mg acetaminophen and 10 mg
hydrocodone bitartrate

DOSAGES
Arthralgia, bone pain, dental pain,
headache, migraine, moderate pain
Adults: 1 tablet every 4 to 6 hours.
Maximum dosage, 6 tablets in 24 hours.

Capital with Codeine
Tylenol with Codeine Elixir
CSS V

GENERIC COMPONENTS
120 mg acetaminophen and 12 mg
codeine phosphate/5 ml

DOSAGES
Mild to moderate pain
Adults and children 12 years and older:
15 ml every 4 hours as needed.

Darvocet-A500
CSS IV

GENERIC COMPONENTS
500 mg acetaminophen and 100 mg
propoxyphene napsylate

DOSAGES
Mild to moderate pain
Adults: 1 tablet every 4 hours. Maximum dosage, 6 tablets in 24 hours.

Darvocet-N50
CSS IV

GENERIC COMPONENTS
325 mg acetaminophen and 50 mg propoxyphene napsylate

DOSAGES
Mild to moderate pain
Adults: 2 tablets every 4 hours. Maximum dosage, 12 tablets in 24 hours.

Darvocet-N100
CSS IV

GENERIC COMPONENTS
650 mg acetaminophen and 100 mg propoxyphene napsylate

DOSAGES
Mild to moderate pain
Adults: 1 tablet every 4 hours. Maximum dosage, 6 tablets in 24 hours.

Empirin with Codeine No. 3
CSS III

GENERIC COMPONENTS
325 mg aspirin and 30 mg codeine phosphate

DOSAGES
Fever and mild to moderate pain
Adults: 1 to 2 tablets every 4 hours. Maximum dosage, 12 tablets in 24 hours.

Empirin with Codeine No. 4
CSS III

GENERIC COMPONENTS
325 mg aspirin and 60 mg codeine phosphate

DOSAGES
Fever and mild to moderate pain
Adults: 1 tablet every 4 hours. Maximum dosage, 6 tablets in 24 hours.

Endocet 5/325
Percocet 5/325
Roxicet
CSS II

GENERIC COMPONENTS
325 mg acetaminophen and 5 mg oxycodone hydrochloride

DOSAGES
Moderate to moderately severe pain
Adults: 1 tablet every 6 hours. Maximum dosage, 12 tablets in 24 hours.

Endocet 7.5/325
Percocet 7.5/325
CSS II

GENERIC COMPONENTS
325 mg acetaminophen and 7.5 mg oxycodone hydrochloride

DOSAGES
Moderate to moderately severe pain
Adults: 1 tablet every 6 hours. Maximum dosage, 8 tablets in 24 hours.

Endocet 7.5/500
Percocet 7.5/500
CSS II

GENERIC COMPONENTS
500 mg acetaminophen and 7.5 mg oxycodone hydrochloride

DOSAGES
Moderate to moderately severe pain
Adults: 1 tablet every 6 hours. Maximum dosage, 8 tablets in 24 hours.

Endocet 10/325
Percocet 10/325
CSS II

GENERIC COMPONENTS
325 mg acetaminophen and 10 mg oxycodone hydrochloride

DOSAGES
Moderate to moderately severe pain
Adults: 1 tablet every 6 hours. Maximum dosage, 6 tablets in 24 hours.

Fioricet with Codeine
CSS III

GENERIC COMPONENTS
325 mg acetaminophen, 50 mg butalbital, 40 mg caffeine, and 30 mg codeine phosphate

DOSAGES
Headache, mild to moderate pain
Adults: 1 to 2 capsules every 4 hours. Maximum dosage, 6 capsules in 24 hours.

Fiorinal with Codeine
CSS III

GENERIC COMPONENTS
325 mg aspirin, 50 mg butalbital, 40 mg caffeine, and 30 mg codeine phosphate

DOSAGES
Headache, mild to moderate pain
Adults: 1 to 2 tablets or capsules every 4 hours. Maximum dosage, 6 tablets or capsules in 24 hours.

Lorcet 10/650
CSS III

GENERIC COMPONENTS
650 mg acetaminophen and 10 mg hydrocodone bitartrate

DOSAGES
Moderate to moderately severe pain
Adults: 1 tablet every 4 to 6 hours. Maximum dosage, 6 tablets in 24 hours.

Lortab 2.5/500
CSS III

GENERIC COMPONENTS
500 mg acetaminophen and 2.5 mg hydrocodone bitartrate

DOSAGES
Moderate to moderately severe pain
Adults: 1 to 2 tablets every 4 to 6 hours. Maximum dosage, 8 tablets in 24 hours.

Lortab 7.5/500
CSS III

GENERIC COMPONENTS
500 mg acetaminophen and 7.5 mg hydrocodone bitartrate

DOSAGES
Moderate to moderately severe pain
Adults: 1 tablet every 4 to 6 hours. Maximum dosage, 8 tablets in 24 hours.

Lortab 10/500
CSS III

GENERIC COMPONENTS
500 mg acetaminophen and 10 mg hydrocodone bitartrate

DOSAGES
Moderate to moderately severe pain
Adults: 1 tablet every 4 to 6 hours. Maximum dosage, 6 tablets in 24 hours.

Lortab Elixir
CSS III

GENERIC COMPONENTS
167 mg acetaminophen and 2.5 mg/5 ml hydrocodone bitartrate

DOSAGES
Moderately severe pain
Adults: 15 ml every 4 to 6 hours. Maximum dosage, 90 ml/day.

Norco 325/10
CSS III

GENERIC COMPONENTS
325 mg acetaminophen and 10 mg hydrocodone bitartrate

DOSAGES
Moderate to moderately severe pain
Adults: 1 tablet every 4 to 6 hours. Maximum dosage, 6 tablets in 24 hours.

Percocet 2.5/325
CSS II

GENERIC COMPONENTS
325 mg acetaminophen and 2.5 mg oxycodone hydrochloride

DOSAGES
Moderate to moderately severe pain
Adults: 1 to 2 tablets every 4 to 6 hours.
Maximum dosage, 12 tablets in 24 hours.

Percocet 10/650
CSS II

GENERIC COMPONENTS
650 mg acetaminophen and 10 mg
oxycodone hydrochloride

DOSAGES
Moderate to moderately severe pain
Adults: 1 tablet every 4 hours. Maximum
dosage, 6 tablets in 24 hours.

Percodan
CSS II

GENERIC COMPONENTS
325 mg aspirin, 4.5 mg oxycodone
hydrochloride, and 0.38 mg oxycodone
terephthalate

DOSAGES
Moderate to moderately severe pain
Adults: 1 tablet every 6 hours. Maximum
dosage, 12 tablets in 24 hours.

Roxicet 5/500
Roxilox
Tylox
CSS II

GENERIC COMPONENTS
500 mg acetaminophen and 5 mg
oxycodone hydrochloride

DOSAGES
Moderate to moderately severe pain
Adults: 1 tablet every 6 hours.

Roxicet Oral Solution
CSS II

GENERIC COMPONENTS
325 mg acetaminophen and 5 mg/5 ml
oxycodone hydrochloride

DOSAGES
Moderate to moderately severe pain
Adults: 5 ml every 6 hours. Maximum
dosage, 60 ml in 24 hours.

Talacen
CSS IV

GENERIC COMPONENTS
650 mg acetaminophen and 25 mg
pentazocine hydrochloride

DOSAGES
Mild to moderate pain
Adults: 1 tablet every 4 hours. Maximum
dosage, 6 tablets in 24 hours.

Talwin Compound
CSS IV

GENERIC COMPONENTS
325 mg aspirin and 12.5 mg pentazocine
hydrochloride

DOSAGES
Moderate pain
Adults: 2 tablets every 6 to 8 hours.
Maximum dosage, 8 tablets in 24 hours.

Talwin NX
CSS IV

GENERIC COMPONENTS
0.5 mg naloxone and 50 mg pentazocine
hydrochloride

DOSAGES
Moderate to severe pain
Adults: 1 to 2 tablets every 3 to 4 hours.
Maximum dosage, 12 tablets daily.

Tylenol with Codeine No. 2
CSS III

GENERIC COMPONENTS
300 mg acetaminophen and 15 mg
codeine phosphate

DOSAGES
Fever, mild to moderate pain
Adults: 1 to 2 tablets every 4 hours.
Maximum dosage, 12 tablets in 24 hours.

Tylenol with Codeine No. 3
CSS III

GENERIC COMPONENTS
300 mg acetaminophen and 30 mg
codeine phosphate

DOSAGES
Fever, mild to moderate pain
Adults: 1 to 2 tablets every 4 hours.
Maximum dosage, 12 tablets in 24 hours.

Tylenol with Codeine No. 4
CSS III

GENERIC COMPONENTS
300 mg acetaminophen and 60 mg
codeine phosphate

DOSAGES
Fever, mild to moderate pain
Adults: 1 tablet every 4 hours. Maximum
dosage, 6 tablets in 24 hours.

Tylox 5/500
CSS II

GENERIC COMPONENTS
500 mg acetaminophen and 5 mg
oxycodone hydrochloride

DOSAGES
Moderate to moderately severe pain
Adults: 1 capsule every 6 hours.
Maximum dosage, 8 capsules in 24 hours.

Vicodin ES
CSS III

GENERIC COMPONENTS
750 mg acetaminophen and 7.5 mg
hydrocodone bitartrate

DOSAGES
Moderate to moderately severe pain
Adults: 1 tablet every 4 to 6 hours.
Maximum dosage, 5 tablets in 24 hours.

Zydone 5/400
CSS III

GENERIC COMPONENTS
400 mg acetaminophen and 5 mg
hydrocodone bitartrate

DOSAGES
Moderate to moderately severe pain
Adults: 1 to 2 tablets every 4 to 6 hours.
Maximum dosage, 8 tablets in 24 hours.

Zydone 7.5/400
CSS III

GENERIC COMPONENTS
400 mg acetaminophen and 7.5 mg
hydrocodone bitartrate

DOSAGES
Moderate to moderately severe pain
Adults: 1 tablet every 4 to 6 hours.
Maximum dosage, 6 tablets in 24 hours.

Zydone 10/400
CSS III

GENERIC COMPONENTS
400 mg acetaminophen and 10 mg
hydrocodone bitartrate

DOSAGES
Moderate to moderately severe pain
Adults: 1 tablet every 4 to 6 hours.
Maximum dosage, 6 tablets in 24 hours.

ANTIACNE DRUGS

Estrostep 21
Estrostep Fe

GENERIC COMPONENTS
Tablets
1 mg norethindrone and 20 mcg ethinyl
estradiol, 1 mg norethindrone and 30 mcg
ethinyl estradiol, or 1 mg norethindrone
and 35 mcg ethinyl estradiol and 75 mg
ferrous fumarate

DOSAGES
Women older than age 15: 1 tablet P.O.
daily.

Ortho Tri-Cyclen

GENERIC COMPONENTS
Tablets
0.18 mg norgestimate and 35 mcg ethinyl
estradiol
0.215 mg norgestimate and 35 mcg
ethinyl estradiol
0.25 mg norgestimate and 35 mcg ethinyl
estradiol

DOSAGES
Women older than age 15: 1 tablet P.O. daily.

ANTIBACTERIALS

Pediazole

GENERIC COMPONENTS
Granules for oral suspension
Erythromycin ethylsuccinate (equivalent of 200 mg erythromycin activity) and 600 mg sulfisoxazole per 5 ml when reconstituted according to manufacturer's directions

DOSAGES
Acute otitis media
Children: 50 mg/kg/day erythromycin and 150 mg/kg/day sulfisoxazole in divided doses q.i.d. for 10 days. Give without regard to meals. Refrigerate after reconstitution; use within 14 days.

ANTIDIABETICS

Avandamet

GENERIC COMPONENTS
Tablets
2 mg rosiglitazone and 500 mg metformin
2 mg rosiglitazone and 1 g metformin
4 mg rosiglitazone and 500 mg metformin
4 mg rosiglitazone and 1 g metformin

DOSAGES
Adults: 4 mg rosiglitazone with 500 mg metformin, once per day or in divided doses. Not for initial therapy; adjust using individual drugs alone then switch to the appropriate dosage of the combination product. See package insert for details on adjusting dosage based on use of other drugs and previous dosage levels.

Glucovance

GENERIC COMPONENTS
Tablets
1.25 mg glyburide and 250 mg metformin
2.5 mg glyburide and 500 mg metformin
5 mg glyburide and 500 mg metformin

DOSAGES
Adults: 1 tablet daily P.O., usually in the morning. Not for initial therapy; adjust using the individual drugs alone, then switch to the appropriate dosage of the combination product.

Metaglip

GENERIC COMPONENTS
Tablets
2.5 mg glipizide and 250 mg metformin
2.5 mg glipizide and 500 mg metformin
5 mg glipizide and 500 mg metformin

DOSAGES
Adults: 1 tablet per day with a meal; adjust dose based on patient response. Maximum dose, 20 mg glipizide with 2,000 mg metformin daily.

ANTIGOUT DRUGS

Col-Probenecid

GENERIC COMPONENTS
Tablets
500 mg probenecid and 0.5 mg colchicine

DOSAGES
Adults: 1 tablet P.O. daily for 1 week, then 1 tablet P.O. b.i.d. Adjust dosage based on symptoms and uric acid levels. Maximum dosage, 4 tablets daily.

ANTIHYPERTENSIVES

Accuretic
Quinaretic

GENERIC COMPONENTS
Tablets
10 mg quinapril and 12.5 mg hydrochlorothiazide
20 mg quinapril and 12.5 mg hydrochlorothiazide
20 mg quinapril and 25 mg hydrochlorothiazide

DOSAGES
Adults: 1 tablet P.O. per day in the morning. Adjust drug using the individual

products, then switch to appropriate dosage of the combination product.

Atacand HCT

GENERIC COMPONENTS
Tablets
16 mg candesartan and 12.5 mg hydrochlorothiazide
32 mg candesartan and 12.5 mg hydrochlorothiazide

DOSAGES
Adults: 1 tablet P.O. daily in the morning. Adjust dosage using the individual products, then switch to appropriate dosage.

Avalide

GENERIC COMPONENTS
Tablets
150 mg irbesartan and 12.5 mg hydrochlorothiazide
300 mg irbesartan and 12.5 mg hydrochlorothiazide
300 mg irbesartan and 25 mg hydrochlorothiazide

DOSAGES
Adults: 1 tablet P.O. daily. Adjust dosage with individual products, then switch to combination product when patient's condition is stabilized. Maximum daily dose, 300 mg irbesartan and 25 mg hydrochlorothiazide.

Benicar HCT

GENERIC COMPONENTS
Tablets
20 mg olmesartan and 12.5 mg hydrochlorothiazide
40 mg olmesartan and 12.5 mg hydrochlorothiazide
40 mg olmesartan and 25 mg hydrochlorothiazide

DOSAGES
Adults: 1 tablet P.O. per day in the morning. Adjust dosage using the individual products, then switch to the combination product when patient's adjustment schedule is stable.

Capozide

GENERIC COMPONENTS
Tablets
25 mg captopril and 15 mg hydrochlorothiazide
50 mg captopril and 15 mg hydrochlorothiazide
25 mg captopril and 25 mg hydrochlorothiazide
50 mg captopril and 25 mg hydrochlorothiazide

DOSAGES
Adults: 1 to 2 tablets P.O. daily, in the morning. Adjust dosage using the individual products, then switch to the combination product when patient's adjustment schedule is stable.

Clorpres

GENERIC COMPONENTS
Tablets
15 mg chlorthalidone and 0.1 mg clonidine hydrochloride
15 mg chlorthalidone and 0.2 mg clonidine hydrochloride
15 mg chlorthalidone and 0.3 mg clonidine hydrochloride

DOSAGES
Adults: 1 to 2 tablets per day P.O. in the morning. Adjust dosage using the individual products, then switch to the combination product when patient's adjustment schedule is stable.

Corzide

GENERIC COMPONENTS
Tablets
40 mg nadolol and 5 mg bendroflumethiazide
80 mg nadolol and 5 mg bendroflumethiazide

DOSAGES
Adults: 1 tablet P.O. per day in the morning. Adjust dosage using the individual products, then switch to the combination product when patient's adjustment schedule is stable.

Diovan HCT

GENERIC COMPONENTS
Tablets
80 mg valsartan and 12.5 mg hydrochlorothiazide
160 mg valsartan and 12.5 mg hydrochlorothiazide
160 mg valsartan and 25 mg hydrochlorothiazide
320 mg valsartan and 12.5 mg hydrochlorothiazide
320 mg valsartan and 25 mg hydrochlorothiazide

DOSAGES
Adults: 1 tablet per day P.O. Not for initial therapy; start using each component first.

Hyzaar

GENERIC COMPONENTS
Tablets
50 mg losartan and 12.5 mg hydrochlorothiazide
100 mg losartan and 12.5 mg hydrochlorothiazide
100 mg losartan and 25 mg hydrochlorothiazide

DOSAGES
Adults: 1 tablet per day P.O. in the morning. Not for initial therapy; start using each component and if desired effects are obtained, Hyzaar may be used.

Inderide

GENERIC COMPONENTS
Tablets
40 mg propranolol hydrochloride and 25 mg hydrochlorothiazide

DOSAGES
Adults: 1 tablet P.O. b.i.d. Adjust dosage using the individual products, then switch to the combination product when patient's adjustment schedule is stable. Maximum total daily dose shouldn't exceed 160 mg propranolol and 50 mg hydrochlorothiazide

Lexxel

GENERIC COMPONENTS
Extended-release tablets
5 mg enalapril maleate and 2.5 mg felodipine
5 mg enalapril maleate and 5 mg felodipine

DOSAGES
Adults: 1 tablet per day P.O. Adjust dosage using the individual products, then switch to the combination product when patient's adjustment schedule is stable. Make sure that patient swallows tablet whole. Don't cut, crush, or allow him to chew.

Lopressor HCT

GENERIC COMPONENTS
Tablets
50 mg metoprolol and 25 mg hydrochlorothiazide
100 mg metoprolol and 25 mg hydrochlorothiazide
100 mg metoprolol and 50 mg hydrochlorothiazide

DOSAGES
Adults: 1 tablet P.O. per day. Adjust dosage using the individual products, then switch to the combination product when patient's adjustment schedule is stable.

Lotensin HCT

GENERIC COMPONENTS
Tablets
5 mg benazepril and 6.25 mg hydrochlorothiazide
10 mg benazepril and 12.5 mg hydrochlorothiazide
20 mg benazepril and 12.5 mg hydrochlorothiazide
20 mg benazepril and 25 mg hydrochlorothiazide

DOSAGES
Adults: 1 tablet per day P.O. in the morning. Adjust dosage using the individual products, then switch to the combination product when patient's adjustment schedule is stable.

Lotrel

GENERIC COMPONENTS
Capsules
2.5 mg amlodipine and 10 mg benazepril
5 mg amlodipine and 10 mg benazepril
5 mg amlodipine and 20 mg benazepril
5 mg amlodipine and 40 mg benazepril
10 mg amlodipine and 20 mg benazepril
10 mg amlodipine and 40 mg benazepril

DOSAGES
Adults: 1 tablet P.O. daily in the morning. Monitor patient for hypertension and adverse effects closely over first 2 weeks and regularly thereafter.

Methyldopa and hydrochlorthiazide

GENERIC COMPONENTS
Tablets
250 mg methyldopa and 15 mg hydrochlorothiazide
250 mg methyldopa and 25 mg hydrochlorothiazide
500 mg methyldopa and 30 mg hydrochlorothiazide
500 mg methyldopa and 50 mg hydrochlorothiazide

DOSAGES
Adults: 1 tablet P.O. daily, in the morning. Adjust dosage using the individual products, then switch to the combination product when patient's adjustment schedule is stable.

Micardis HCT

GENERIC COMPONENTS
Tablets
40 mg telmisartan and 12.5 mg hydrochlorothiazide
80 mg telmisartan and 12.5 mg hydrochlorothiazide
80 mg telmisartan and 25 mg hydrochlorothiazide

DOSAGES
Adults: 1 tablet P.O. per day; may be adjusted up to 160 mg telmisartan and 25 mg hydrochlorothiazide, based on patient's response.

Monopril-HCT

GENERIC COMPONENTS
Tablets
10 mg fosinopril and 12.5 mg hydrochlorothiazide
20 mg fosinopril and 12.5 mg hydrochlorothiazide

DOSAGES
Adults: 1 tablet P.O. per day in the morning. Adjust dosage using the individual products, then switch to appropriate dosage of the combination product.

Prinzide
Zestoretic

GENERIC COMPONENTS
Tablets
10 mg lisinopril and 12.5 mg hydrochlorothiazide
20 mg lisinopril and 12.5 mg hydrochlorothiazide
20 mg lisinopril and 25 mg hydrochlorothiazide

DOSAGES
Adults: 1 tablet per day P.O. taken in the morning. Adjust dosage using the individual products, then switch to the combination product when patient's adjustment schedule is stable.

Tarka

GENERIC COMPONENTS
Tablets
1 mg trandolapril and 240 mg verapamil
2 mg trandolapril and 180 mg verapamil
2 mg trandolapril and 240 mg verapamil
4 mg trandolapril and 240 mg verapamil

DOSAGES
Adults: 1 tablet P.O. per day, taken with food. Adjust dosage using the individual products, then switch to the combination product when patient's adjustment schedule is stable. Make sure that patient swallows tablet whole. Don't cut, crush, or allow him to chew.

Tenoretic

GENERIC COMPONENTS
Tablets
50 mg atenolol and 25 mg chlorthalidone
100 mg atenolol and 25 mg chlorthalidone

DOSAGES
Adults: 1 tablet P.O. daily in the morning. Adjust dosage using the individual products, then switch to appropriate dosage of the combination product.

Teveten HCT

GENERIC COMPONENTS
Tablets
600 mg eprosartan and 12.5 mg hydrochlorothiazide
600 mg eprosartan and 25 mg hydrochlorothiazide

DOSAGES
Adults: 1 tablet P.O. each day. Establish dosage with each component alone before using the combination product; if blood pressure isn't controlled on 600 mg/25 mg tablet, 300 mg eprosartan may be added each evening.

Uniretic

GENERIC COMPONENTS
Tablets
7.5 mg moexipril and 12.5 mg hydrochlorothiazide
15 mg moexipril and 12.5 mg hydrochlorothiazide
15 mg moexipril and 25 mg hydrochlorothiazide

DOSAGES
Adults: Give ½ to 2 tablets per day. Not for initial therapy. Adjust dose to maintain appropriate blood pressure.

Vaseretic

GENERIC COMPONENTS
Tablets
5 mg enalapril maleate and 12.5 mg hydrochlorothiazide
10 mg enalapril maleate and 25 mg hydrochlorothiazide

DOSAGES
Adults: 1 to 2 tablets per day P.O. in the morning. Adjust dosage using the individual products, then switch to the combination product when patient's adjustment schedule is stable.

Ziac

GENERIC COMPONENTS
Tablets
2.5 mg bisoprolol and 6.25 mg hydrochlorothiazide
5 mg bisoprolol and 6.25 mg hydrochlorothiazide
10 mg bisoprolol and 6.25 mg hydrochlorothiazide

DOSAGES
Adults: 1 tablet daily P.O. in morning. Initial dose is 2.5/6.25 mg tablet P.O. daily. Adjust dosage within 1 week; optimal antihypertensive effect may require 2 to 3 weeks.

ANTIMIGRAINE DRUGS

Cafergot, Migergot

GENERIC COMPONENTS
Tablets
1 mg ergotamine tartrate and 100 mg caffeine
Suppositories
2 mg ergotamine tartrate and 100 mg caffeine

DOSAGES
Adults: 2 tablets P.O. at the first sign of attack. Follow with 1 tablet every 30 minutes, if needed. Maximum dose is 6 tablets per attack. Don't exceed 10 tablets per week. Or, 1 suppository P.R. at first sign of attack; follow with second dose after 1 hour, if needed. Maximum dose is 2 suppositories per attack. Don't exceed 5 suppositories per week. Don't combine this drug with ritonavir, nelfinavir, indinavir, erythromycin, clarithromycin, or troleandomycin, as serious vasospasm could occur.

ANTIPLATELET DRUGS

Aggrenox

GENERIC COMPONENTS
Capsules
25 mg aspirin and 200 mg dipyridamole

DOSAGES
Adults: To decrease risk of stroke, 1 capsule P.O. b.i.d. in the morning and evening. Swallow capsule whole; may be taken with or without food.

ANTIRETROVIRALS

Combivir

GENERIC COMPONENTS
Tablets
150 mg lamivudine and 300 mg zidovudine

DOSAGES
Adults and children age 12 and older: 1 tablet P.O. b.i.d.

Epzicom

GENERIC COMPONENTS
Tablets
600 mg abacavir with 300 mg lamivudine

DOSAGES
Adults: 1 tablet daily, taken without regard to food and in combination with other antiretrovirals.

Trizivir

GENERIC COMPONENTS
Tablets
300 mg abacavir sulfate, 150 mg lamivudine, and 300 mg zidovudine

DOSAGES
Adults and adolescents who weigh 40 kg (88 lb) or more: 1 tablet P.O. b.i.d., alone or with other antiretrovirals.

Truvada

GENERIC COMPONENTS
Tablets
200 mg emtricitabine with 300 mg tenofovir

DOSAGES
Adults and adolescents weighing more than 40 kg (88 lb): 1 tablet daily, taken without regard to food and in combination with other antiretrovirals.

ANTIULCER DRUGS

Helidac

GENERIC COMPONENTS
Tablets
262.4 mg bismuth subsalicylate, 250 mg metronidazole, and 500 mg tetracycline hydrochloride

DOSAGES
Active duodenal ulcers associated with Helicobacter pylori infection
Adults: 2 chewable bismuth subsalicylate tablets, 1 metronidazole tablet, and 1 tetracycline capsule P.O. q.i.d. for 14 days along with a prescribed H_2 antagonist.

Prevpac

GENERIC COMPONENTS
Daily administration pack
Two 30-mg lansoprazole capsules, four 500-mg amoxicillin capsules, and two 500-mg clarithromycin tablets.

DOSAGES
Adults: Divide pack equally to take twice daily, morning and evening.

DIURETICS

Aldactazide

GENERIC COMPONENTS
Tablets
25 mg spironolactone and 25 mg hydrochlorothiazide
50 mg spironolactone and 50 mg hydrochlorothiazide

DOSAGES
Adults: One to eight 25-mg spironolactone and 25-mg hydrochlorothiazide tablets daily. Or, one to four 50-mg spironolactone and 50-mg hydrochlorothiazide tablets daily.

Dyazide

GENERIC COMPONENTS
Capsules
37.5 mg triamterene and 25 mg hydrochlorothiazide

DOSAGES
Adults: 1 to 2 tablets daily.

Maxzide

GENERIC COMPONENTS
Tablets
37.5 mg triamterene and 25 mg hydrochlorothiazide
75 mg triamterene and 50 mg hydrochlorothiazide

DOSAGES
Adults: 1 tablet daily.

Moduretic

GENERIC COMPONENTS
Tablets
5 mg amiloride and 50 mg hydrochlorothiazide

DOSAGES
Adults: 1 to 2 tablets per day with meals.

HEART FAILURE DRUGS

BiDil

GENERIC COMPONENTS
Tablets
20 mg isosorbide dinitrate and 37.5 mg hydralazine

DOSAGES
Adults: 1 to 2 tablets P.O. t.i.d.

LIPID-LOWERING DRUGS

Advicor

GENERIC COMPONENTS
Tablets
20 mg lovastatin and 500 mg niacin
20 mg lovastatin and 750 mg niacin
20 mg lovastatin and 1,000 mg niacin
40 mg lovastatin and 1,000 mg niacin

DOSAGES
Adults: 1 tablet daily P.O. at night.

Vytorin

GENERIC COMPONENTS
Tablets
10 mg ezetimibe with 10, 20, 40, or 80 mg simvastatin

DOSAGES
Adults: 1 tablet daily, taken in the evening in combination with a cholesterol-lowering diet and exercise. Dosage of simvastatin in the combination may be adjusted based on patient response. If given with a bile sequestrant, must be given at least 2 hours before or 4 hours after the bile sequestrant.

MENOPAUSE DRUGS

Activella
femhrt

GENERIC COMPONENTS
Tablets
2.5 mcg ethinyl estradiol and 0.5 mg norethindrone acetate (femhrt)
5 mcg ethinyl estradiol and 1 mg norethindrone acetate (femhrt)
0.5 mg ethinyl estradiol and 0.1 mg norethindrone acetate (Activella)
1 mg ethinyl estradiol and 0.5 mg norethindrone acetate (Activella)

DOSAGES
Signs and symptoms of menopause; to prevent osteoporosis
Women with intact uterus: 1 tablet P.O. daily.

Prefest

GENERIC COMPONENTS
Tablets
1 mg estradiol and 0.09 mg norgestimate

DOSAGES
Moderate to severe symptoms of menopause; to prevent osteoporosis
Women with intact uterus: 1 tablet per day P.O. (3 days of pink tablets: estradiol alone; followed by 3 days of white tablets: estradiol and norgestimate combination; continue cycle uninterrupted).

Premphase

GENERIC COMPONENTS
Tablets
0.625 mg conjugated estrogens; 0.625 mg conjugated estrogens with 5 mg medroxyprogesterone

DOSAGES
Moderate to severe symptoms of menopause; to prevent osteoporosis
Women with intact uterus: 1 tablet per day P.O. Use estrogen alone on days 1 to 14 and estrogen-medroxyprogesterone tablet on days 15 to 28.

Prempro

GENERIC COMPONENTS
Tablets
0.3 mg conjugated estrogen and 1.5 mg medroxyprogesterone
0.45 mg conjugated estrogen and 1.5 mg medroxyprogesterone
0.625 mg estrogen and 2.5 mg medroxyprogesterone
0.625 mg conjugated estrogen and 5 mg medroxyprogesterone

DOSAGES
Symptoms of menopause; to prevent osteoporosis
Women with intact uterus: 1 tablet per day P.O.

MISCELLANEOUS CARDIAC DRUGS

Caduet

GENERIC COMPONENTS
Tablets
2.5 mg amlodipine with 10 mg, 20 mg, or 40 mg atorvastatin
5 mg amlodipine with 10 mg, 20 mg, 40 mg, or 80 mg atorvastatin
10 mg amlodipine with 10 mg, 20 mg, 40 mg, or 80 mg atorvastatin

DOSAGES
Adults, boys, and postmenarchal girls age 10 and older: Determine the most effective dose for each component. Then select the most appropriate combination product.

OPIOID AGONIST

Suboxone
CSS III

GENERIC COMPONENTS
Sublingual tablets
2 mg buprenorphine and 0.5 mg naloxone
8 mg buprenorphine and 2 mg naloxone

DOSAGES
Opioid dependence
Adults: 12 to 16 mg S.L. once daily, after induction with S.L. buprenorphine.

PSYCHOTHERAPEUTICS

Limbitrol
Limbitrol DS

GENERIC COMPONENTS
Tablets
5 mg chlordiazepoxide and 12.5 mg amitriptyline
10 mg chlordiazepoxide and 25 mg amitriptyline

DOSAGES
Adults: 10 mg chlordiazepoxide with 25 mg amitriptyline 3 to 4 times per day up to 6 times daily. For patients who don't tolerate the higher doses, 5 mg

chlordiazepoxide with 12.5 mg amitriptyline 3 to 4 times per day. Reduce dosage after initial response.

---

perphenazine and amitriptyline

GENERIC COMPONENTS
Tablets
2 mg perphenazine and 10 mg amitriptyline
2 mg perphenazine and 25 mg amitriptyline
4 mg perphenazine and 10 mg amitriptyline
4 mg perphenazine and 25 mg amitriptyline
4 mg perphenazine and 50 mg amitriptyline

DOSAGES
Adults: 2 to 4 mg perphenazine with 10 to 50 mg amitriptyline 3 to 4 times daily. Reduce dosage after initial response.

Symbyax

GENERIC COMPONENTS
Capsules
3 mg olanzapine and 25 mg fluoxetine
6 mg olanzapine and 25 mg fluoxetine
6 mg olanzapine and 50 mg fluoxetine
12 mg olanzapine and 25 mg fluoxetine
12 mg olanzapine and 50 mg fluoxetine

DOSAGES
Adults: 1 capsule daily in the evening. Begin with 6 mg/25 mg capsule and adjust according to efficacy and tolerability.

RESPIRATORY TRACT DRUGS

Loratadine and pseudoephedrine ◇

GENERIC COMPONENTS
Extended-release tablets
5 mg loratadine and 120 mg pseudoephedrine

DOSAGES
Adults: 1 tablet every 12 hours.

Claritin-D 24 Hour

GENERIC COMPONENTS
Extended-release tablets
10 mg loratadine and 240 mg pseudoephedrine

DOSAGES
Adults: 1 tablet every day.

Combivent

GENERIC COMPONENTS
Metered dose inhaler
18 mcg ipratropium bromide and 90 mcg albuterol

DOSAGES
Bronchospasm with COPD in patients who require more than a single bronchodilator
Adults: Two inhalations q.i.d. Not for use during acute attack. Use caution with known sensitivity to atropine, soy, or peanuts.

Vaccines and toxoids: Indications and dosages

Haemophilus b conjugate
vaccines

Haemophilus b conjugate
vaccine, diphtheria CRM 197
protein conjugate (HbOC)
HibTITER

Haemophilus b conjugate
vaccine, diphtheria toxoid
conjugate (PRP-D)
Prohibit

Haemophilus b conjugate
vaccine, meningococcal
protein conjugate, hepatitis B
Comvax

Haemophilus b conjugate
vaccine, meningococcal
protein conjugate (PRP-OMP)
PedvaxHIB

Haemophilus b conjugate,
tetanus toxoid conjugate
(PRP-T)
ActHIB

Pharmacologic class: vaccine
Pregnancy risk category C

AVAILABLE FORMS
***Haemophilus influenzae type b* (HIB)
conjugate vaccine, diphtheria CRM
197 protein conjugate**
Injection: 10 mcg of purified HIB saccharide and about 25 mcg CRM 197 protein
per 0.5 ml
**HIB conjugate vaccine, diphtheria
toxoid conjugate**
Injection: 25 mcg of HIB capsular polysaccharide and 18 mcg of diphtheria
toxoid protein per 0.5 ml
HIB conjugate vaccine, hepatitis B
Injection: 7.5 mcg of HIB capsular polysaccharide and 5 mcg hepatitis B surface
antigen per 0.5 ml

**HIB conjugate vaccine, meningo-
coccal protein conjugate**
Injection: 7.5 mcg of HIB PRP and
125 mcg *N. meningitides* OMPC per
0.5 ml
**HIB conjugate vaccine, tetanus
toxoid conjugate**
Injection: 10 mcg HIB capsular polysaccharide, 24 mcg tetanus toxoid

INDICATIONS & DOSAGES
➤ **Immunization against HIB
infection**
*Conjugate vaccine, diphtheria CRM$_{197}$
protein conjugate*
Infants: 0.5 ml I.M. at age 2 months.
Repeat at 4 months and 6 months. Give
booster dose at age 15 months.
*Previously unvaccinated children ages
15 months to 6 years:* 0.5 ml I.M. Booster
dose isn't needed.
*Previously unvaccinated infants ages 12 to
14 months:* 0.5 ml I.M. Give booster dose
at age 15 months (but no sooner than
2 months after first vaccination).
*Previously unvaccinated infants ages 7 to
11 months:* 0.5 ml I.M. Repeat in
2 months, for a total of two doses. Give
booster dose at age 15 months (but no
sooner than 2 months after last vaccination).
*Previously unvaccinated infants ages 2 to
6 months:* 0.5 ml I.M. Repeat in 2 months
and again in 4 months for total of three
doses. Give booster at age 15 months.
*Conjugate vaccine, diphtheria toxoid
conjugate*
*Previously unvaccinated children ages
15 to 71 months:* 0.5 ml I.M. Booster dose
isn't needed.
Conjugate vaccine, hepatitis B
Infants born to HBsAg negative mothers:
0.5 ml I.M. at ages 2, 4, and 12 to
15 months for a total of three doses. Infants
who received a dose of hepatitis B vaccine
at or shortly after birth can still receive the
full three-dose series of Comvax.
*Conjugate vaccine, meningococcal
protein conjugate*
Infants: 0.5 ml I.M. at age 2 months;
repeat at age 4 months. Give booster
dose at age 12 months.

Previously unvaccinated children ages 15 months to 6 years: 0.5 ml I.M. Booster dose isn't needed.

Premature infants follow same schedule as full-term infants.

Previously unvaccinated infants ages 12 to 14 months: 0.5 ml I.M. Give booster dose at age 15 months (but no sooner than 2 months after first vaccination).

Previously unvaccinated infants ages 7 to 11 months: 0.5 ml I.M.; repeat in 2 months. Give booster dose at age 15 months (but no sooner than 2 months after last vaccination).

Previously unvaccinated infants ages 2 to 6 months: 0.5 ml I.M.; repeat in 2 months. Give booster dose at age 12 months.

Conjugate vaccine, tetanus toxoid conjugate

Infants: 0.5 ml I.M. at age 2 months. Repeat at ages 4 and 6 months. Give booster doses at ages 15 to 18 months.

Previously unvaccinated infants ages 7 to 11 months: 0.5 ml I.M. Repeat in 2 months, for a total of two doses. Give booster doses at ages 15 to 18 months.

Previously unvaccinated infants ages 12 to 14 months: 0.5 ml I.M. Repeat in 2 months, for a total of two doses.

Diphtheria and tetanus toxoids and acellular pertussis vaccine adsorbed (DTaP)
Daptacel, Infanrix, TRIPACEL†, Tripedia

Tetanus toxoid and reduced diphtheria toxoid and acellular pertussis vaccine adsorbed (Tdap)
ADACEL, Boostrix

Pharmacologic class: vaccine/toxoid
Pregnancy risk category C

AVAILABLE FORMS
DTaP
Daptacel
Injection: 15 limit flocculation (Lf) units diphtheria toxoid, 5 Lf units tetanus toxoid, 10 mcg pertussis toxoid adsorbed per 0.5 ml

Infanrix
Injection: 25 Lf units diphtheria toxoid, 10 Lf units tetanus toxoid, 25 mcg inactivated pertussis toxins adsorbed per 0.5 ml

Tripedia
Injection: 6.7 Lf units diphtheria toxoid, 5 Lf units tetanus toxoid, 46.8 mcg acellular pertussis vaccine adsorbed per 0.5 ml

TDAP
Adacel
Injection: 5 Lf units tetanus toxoid, 2 Lf units diphtheria toxoid, 2.5 mcg detoxified pertussis toxins adsorbed per 0.5 ml

Boostrix
Injection: 5 Lf units tetanus toxoid, 2.5 Lf units diphtheria toxoid, 8 mcg inactivated pertussis toxins adsorbed per 0.5 ml

INDICATIONS & DOSAGES
➤ **Primary immunization (Daptacel, Infanrix, Tripedia)**
Children ages 6 weeks to 7 years: Give 0.5 ml I.M. 4 to 8 weeks apart for three doses (6 to 8 weeks for Daptacel) and a fourth dose at least 6 months after the third dose.

➤ **Booster immunization**
Children ages 6 weeks to 7 years: Daptacel may be given to complete the immunization series in children who have received at least one dose of whole-cell DTP vaccine.

Infanrix is indicated as a fifth dose in children ages 4 to 6 before entering school in those who received at least one dose of whole-cell DTP vaccine, unless the fourth dose was given after the fourth birthday.

If Tripedia was used for the first four doses, a fifth dose is recommended at age 4 to 6 before entering school. If the fourth dose was given after age 4, a fifth dose isn't needed.

Adults and children age 11 to 64 (ADACEL): 0.5 ml I.M. as a single dose at least 5 years after the last DTaP vaccination.

Children and adolescents age 10 to 18 (Boostrix): 0.5 ml I.M. as a single dose at least 5 years after the last DTaP vaccination.

Diphtheria and tetanus toxoids, acellular pertussis adsorbed, hepatitis B (recombinant), and inactivated poliovirus vaccine combined
Pediarix

Pharmacologic class: vaccine/toxoid
Pregnancy risk category C

AVAILABLE FORMS
Injection: 0.5-ml single-dose vials and disposable, prefilled Tip-Lok syringes

INDICATIONS & DOSAGES
➤ **Active immunization**
Children ages 6 weeks to 7 years: Primary series is three 0.5-ml doses I.M. at 6- to 8-week intervals (preferably 8), usually starting at age 2 months; may start at age 6 weeks.

Hepatitis A vaccine, inactivated
Havrix, Vaqta

Pharmacologic class: vaccine
Pregnancy risk category C

AVAILABLE FORMS
Havrix
Injection: 720 enzyme-linked immunosorbent assay (ELISA) units (ELU)/0.5 ml; 1,440 ELU/ml
Vaqta
Injection: 25 units/0.5 ml, 50 units/ml

INDICATIONS & DOSAGES
➤ **Active immunization against hepatitis A virus; with immune globulin, to prevent hepatitis A in those exposed to virus or who travel to endemic areas**
Adults: 1,440 ELU Havrix or 50 units Vaqta I.M. as single dose. For booster dose, give 1,440 ELU Havrix 6 to 12 months after first dose or 50 units Vaqta I.M. 6 to 18 months after first dose. Booster is recommended for prolonged immunity.
Children ages 12 months to 18 years: 720 ELU Havrix or 25 units Vaqta I.M. as

single dose. Then, give booster dose of 720 ELU Havrix 6 to 12 months after first dose or 25 units Vaqta I.M. 6 to 18 months after first dose. Booster is recommended for prolonged immunity.

Hepatitis B vaccine, recombinant
Engerix-B, Recombivax HB, Recombivax HB Dialysis Formulation

Pharmacologic class: vaccine
Pregnancy risk category C

AVAILABLE FORMS
Injection: 5 mcg HBsAg/0.5 ml (Recombivax HB, pediatric and adolescent form with or without preservative); 10 mcg HBsAg/0.5 ml (Engerix-B, pediatric and adolescent form); 10 mcg HBsAg/ml (Recombivax HB, adult form); 20 mcg HBsAg/ml (Engerix-B, adult form); 40 mcg HBsAg/ml (Recombivax HB dialysis form)

INDICATIONS & DOSAGES
➤ **Immunization against infection from all known subtypes of hepatitis B virus (HBV), primary preexposure prophylaxis against HBV, postexposure prophylaxis when given with hepatitis B immune globulin (HBIG)**
Engerix-B
Adults age 20 and older: Initially, 20 mcg I.M.; then second dose of 20 mcg I.M. after 30 days. A third dose of 20 mcg I.M. is given 6 months after the first dose.
Adjust-a-dose: For adults undergoing dialysis or receiving immunosuppressants, initially, 40 mcg I.M. (divided into two 20-mcg doses and given at different sites). Then second dose of 40 mcg I.M. in 30 days, a third dose after 2 months, and final dose of 40 mcg I.M. 6 months after first dose.
Adolescents ages 11 to 19: Initially, 10 mcg (pediatric and adolescent form) I.M.; then second dose of 10 mcg I.M. 30 days later. Give third dose of 10 mcg I.M. 6 months after first dose. Or, 20 mcg (adult form) I.M.; then second dose of 20 mcg I.M. 30 days later. Give third dose of 20 mcg I.M. 6 months after first dose.

Neonates and children up to age 10:
Initially, 10 mcg I.M.; then second dose of 10 mcg I.M. 30 days later. Give third dose of 10 mcg I.M. 6 months after first dose.

Recombivax HB
Adults age 20 and older: Initially, 10 mcg I.M.; then second dose of 10 mcg I.M. after 30 days. Give third dose of 10 mcg I.M. 6 months after first dose.

For adults undergoing dialysis, initially, 40 mcg I.M. (use dialysis form, which contains 40 mcg/ml); then second dose of 40 mcg I.M. in 30 days, and final dose of 40 mcg I.M. 6 months after first dose. A booster or revaccination may be indicated if anti-HBs level is below 10 mIU/ml 1 to 2 months after third dose.

Infants, children, and adolescents age 19 or younger: Initially, 5 mcg I.M.; then second dose of 5 mcg I.M. after 30 days. Give third dose of 5 mcg I.M. 6 months after first dose. Or, in adolescents ages 11 to 15, give 10 mcg (1 ml adult form) I.M.; then second dose of 10 mcg 4 to 6 months later.

Infants born of HBsAg-positive mothers or mothers of unknown HbsAg status: Initially, 5 mcg I.M.; then second dose of 5 mcg I.M. after 30 days. Give third dose of 5 mcg I.M. 6 months after first dose.

Infants born of HBsAg-negative mothers: Initially, 5 mcg I.M.; then second dose of 5 mcg I.M. after 30 days. Give third dose of 5 mcg I.M. 6 months after first dose.

Note: If the mother is found to be HbsAg-positive within 7 days of delivery, also give the infant a dose of HBIG (0.5 ml) in the opposite anterolateral thigh.

➤ **Chronic hepatitis C infection**
Engerix-B
Adults: Initially, 20 mcg I.M.; then second dose of 20 mcg I.M. after 30 days. Give third dose of 20 mcg I.M. 6 months after first dose.

Human papillomavirus recombinant vaccine, quadrivalent
Gardasil

Pharmacologic class: virus antigen
Pregnancy risk category B

AVAILABLE FORMS
Injection: 0.5 ml single-dose vial

INDICATIONS & DOSAGES
➤ **To prevent cervical cancer, genital warts, cervical adenocarcinoma in situ, and cervical, vulval, and vaginal intraepithelial neoplasias caused by human papillomavirus (HPV) types 6, 11, 16, and 18**
Women and girls ages 9 to 26 years: Three separate I.M. injections of 0.5 ml each. Give second injection 2 months after first, then give third injection 6 months after the first.

Influenza virus vaccine live, intranasal
FluMist

Pharmacologic class: vaccine
Pregnancy risk category C

AVAILABLE FORMS
Intranasal spray: 0.2 ml

INDICATIONS & DOSAGES
➤ **Active immunization to prevent disease caused by influenza A and B viruses**
Adults younger than age 50 and children older than age 9: 0.2-ml intranasal dose (0.1 ml in each nostril) once each season.
Children ages 2 through 8 not previously vaccinated with FluMist: Two intranasal doses of 0.2 ml (0.1 ml in each nostril) 60 days apart for the first season.
Children ages 2 through 8 previously vaccinated with FluMist: 0.2-ml intranasal dose (0.1 ml in each nostril) once each season.

Measles, mumps, and rubella virus vaccine, live
M-M-R II

Pharmacologic class: vaccine
Pregnancy risk category C

AVAILABLE FORMS
Injection: Single-dose vial containing at least 1,000 tissue culture infective doses (TCID$_{50}$), 20,000 TCID$_{50}$ of mumps strain, and 1,000 TCID$_{50}$ rubella virus per 0.5-ml dose.

INDICATIONS & DOSAGES
➤ **Routine immunization**
Adults: 0.5 ml subcutaneously. Patients born after 1957 should receive two doses at least 1 month apart.
Children: 0.5 ml subcutaneously. A two-dose schedule is recommended, with first dose given between 12 to 15 months (6 to 12 months in high-risk areas) and second dose given either at ages 4 to 6 or 11 to 12.

Measles virus vaccine, live
Attenuvax

Pharmacologic class: vaccine
Pregnancy risk category C

AVAILABLE FORMS
Injection: Single-dose vial containing not less than 1,000 tissue culture infective doses ($TCID_{50}$) of measles virus derived from the more attenuated line of Enders attenuated Edmonston strain (grown in chick embryo culture); available in 10- and 50-dose vials

INDICATIONS & DOSAGES
➤ **Immunization**
Adults and children age 15 months and older: 0.5 ml (1,000 units) subcutaneously. A two-dose schedule is recommended, with first dose given at 15 months (12 months in high-risk areas) and second dose given at ages 4 to 6 or 11 to 12.
➤ **Measles outbreak control**
Adults: Revaccinate school personnel born in or after 1957 if they lack evidence of measles immunity. If outbreak is in a medical facility, revaccinate all workers born in or after 1957 if they lack evidence of immunity.
Children: If cases occur in children younger than age 1, vaccinate children as young as age 6 months. Revaccinate all students and siblings if they lack documentation of measles immunity.

Meningococcal (groups A, C, Y, and W-135) polysaccharide diphtheria toxoid conjugate vaccine (MCV4)
Menactra

Meningococcal polysaccharide vaccine, groups A, C, Y and W-135 combined (MPSV4)
Menomune A/C/Y/W-135

Pharmacologic class: vaccine
Pregnancy risk category C

AVAILABLE FORMS
Injection: 0.5 ml single-dose vials

INDICATIONS & DOSAGES
➤ **Active immunization for the prevention of invasive meningococcal disease caused by *Neisseria meningitidis* serogroups A, C, Y, W-135**
Adults and children ages 2 to 55: Give 0.5 ml I.M. MCV4 as a single dose, preferably in the deltoid muscle.
Adults and children over 2 years: Give 0.5 ml subcutaneously MPSV4 as a single dose, preferably in the upper-outer triceps area.

Mumps virus vaccine, live
Mumpsvax

Pharmacologic class: vaccine
Pregnancy risk category C

AVAILABLE FORMS
Injection: Single-dose vial containing at least 20,000 tissue culture infective doses ($TCID_{50}$) of attenuated mumps virus derived from Jeryl Lynn mumps strain (grown in chick embryo culture) per 0.5 ml and vial of diluent; single-dose vial containing at least 5,000 $TCID_{50}$ of the U.S. Reference Mumps Virus in each 0.5 ml

INDICATIONS & DOSAGES
➤ **Immunization**
Adults and children age 1 and older: Two doses recommended for both children and

adults, separated by at least 4 weeks.
0.5 ml (20,000 units) subcutaneously.

Not recommended in children younger than age 12 months; revaccinate children vaccinated before age 12 months. Routine childhood immunization at ages 12 to 15 months and a second dose at ages 4 to 6 years.

Pneumococcal vaccine, polyvalent
Pneumovax 23

7-valent conjugate vaccine
Prevnar

Pharmacologic class: vaccine
Pregnancy risk category C

AVAILABLE FORMS
Injection: 25 mcg each of 23 polysaccharide isolates/0.5 ml (Pneumovax), 2 mcg each of 6 polysaccharide isolates, and 4 mcg of polysaccharide isolate/0.5 ml (Prevnar)

INDICATIONS & DOSAGES
➤ **Pneumococcal immunization**
Adults and children age 2 and older:
0.5 ml, Pneumovax I.M. or subcutaneously.
➤ **Immunization against *Streptococcus pneumoniae* and otitis media (Prevnar)**
Infants ages 6 weeks to 6 months: 0.5 ml I.M. at 2 month intervals for three doses, then a fourth dose of 0.5 ml I.M. at 12 to 15 months.
Children ages 7 to 11 months, previously unvaccinated: 0.5 ml I.M.; three doses with at least 4 weeks between first and second doses, and 8 weeks between second and third doses.
Children age 12 to 23 months, previously unvaccinated: Two doses of 0.5 ml I.M. at least 2 months apart.
Children age 24 months to 9 years, previously unvaccinated: 0.5 ml I.M. as single dose.
Healthy children ages 24 to 59 months who have not completed any recommended schedule for pneumococcal vaccine:
0.5 ml I.M. (one dose).
Children with underlying medical conditions, ages 24 to 59 months who

have received three doses: 0.5 ml I.M. (one dose).
Children with underlying medical conditions, ages 24 to 59 months who have recieved less than 3 doses: 0.5 ml I.M.; two doses at least 8 weeks apart.

Poliovirus vaccine, inactivated (IPV)
IPOL

Pharmacologic class: vaccine
Pregnancy risk category C

AVAILABLE FORMS
0.5-ml prefilled syringe: Mixture of three types of poliovirus (types 1, 2, and 3) grown in tissue culture

INDICATIONS & DOSAGES
➤ **Poliovirus immunization**
Unvaccinated adults: 0.5 ml subcutaneously or I.M.; give second dose 4 to 8 weeks later. Give third dose 6 to 12 months later.
Children: 0.5 ml subcutaneously or I.M. at ages 2 months and 4 months. Give third dose at ages 6 to 18 months. Give a reinforcing dose of 0.5 ml subcutaneously before entry into school at ages 4 to 6.

Rabies vaccine, human diploid cell (HDCV)
Imovax Rabies, RabAvert

Pharmacologic class: vaccine
Pregnancy risk category C

AVAILABLE FORMS
I.M. injection: 2.5 international units rabies antigen/ml, in single-dose vial with diluent

INDICATIONS & DOSAGES
➤ **Postexposure antirabies immunization**
Adults and children: Five 1-ml doses of HDCV I.M. Give first dose as soon as possible after exposure; give additional doses on days 3, 7, 14, and 28 after first dose. If no antibody response occurs after this primary series, booster dose is recommended.

➤ **Postexposure antirabies immunization in previously immunized people**
Adults and children: 1 ml I.M. immediately and 1 ml I.M. 3 days later.
➤ **Preexposure preventive immunization for persons in high-risk groups**
Adults and children: Three 1-ml injections I.M. Give first dose on day 0 (first day of therapy), second dose on day 7, and third dose on day 21 or 28. Or, 0.1 ml I.D. on same dosage schedule.

Rotavirus, live
RotaTeq

Pharmacologic class: vaccine
Pregnancy risk category C

AVAILABLE FORMS
Oral suspension: rotavirus outer capsid protein (2.2×10^6 infectious units of G1, 2.8×10^6 infectious units of G2, 2.2×10^6 infectious units of G3, 2×10^6 infectious units of G4, and 2.3×10^6 infectious units of rotavirus attachment protein P1A[8]) per 2 ml

INDICATIONS & DOSAGES
➤ **Prevention of rotavirus gastroenteritis**
Children ages 6 to 12 weeks: 2 ml P.O. Give second dose 4 weeks later, followed by third dose at 10 weeks. Do not give third dose after the patient reaches 32 weeks of age.

Rubella and mumps virus vaccine, live
Biavax II

Pharmacologic class: vaccine
Pregnancy risk category C

AVAILABLE FORMS
Injection: Single-dose vial containing not less than 1,000 tissue culture infective doses ($TCID_{50}$) of Wistar RA 27/3 rubella virus (propagated in human diploid cell culture) and not less than 20,000 $TCID_{50}$ of Jeryl Lynn mumps strain (grown in chick embryo cell culture)

INDICATIONS & DOSAGES
➤ **Rubella and mumps immunization**
Adults and children age 1 and older: 0.5 ml subcutaneously.

Rubella virus vaccine, live attenuated (RA 27/3)
Meruvax II

Pharmacologic class: vaccine
Pregnancy risk category C

AVAILABLE FORMS
Injection: Single-dose vial containing not less than 1,000 tissue culture infective doses ($TCID_{50}$) of Wistar RA 27/3 strain of rubella virus (propagated in human diploid cell culture)

INDICATIONS & DOSAGES
➤ **Rubella immunization**
Adults and children age 1 and older: 0.5 ml or 1,000 units subcutaneously. Give second dose at least 1 month later. Follow routine childhood schedule of first dose at 12 to 15 months of age and second dose at 4 to 6 years of age.

Smallpox vaccine, dried
Dryvax

Smallpox vaccine, live
ACAM2000

Pharmacologic class: vaccine
Pregnancy risk category C (dried); D (live)

AVAILABLE FORMS
Injection: About 100 million pock-forming units (pfu) per ml (dried); about 2.5-12.5×10^5 plaque-forming units per 0.0025 ml (ACAM2000)

INDICATIONS & DOSAGES
➤ **Active immunization to prevent smallpox disease**
Adults and children: One drop of vaccine (dried) deposited over the deltoid or triceps muscle, followed by a multiple-puncture technique into the superficial layers of skin (two or

three needle punctures for primary vaccination and 15 for revaccination). One drop of ACAM2000 given by scarification using 15 jabs of bifurcated needle by trained provider. Don't give by intradermal, subcutaneous, I.M., or I.V. route.

tetanus toxoid, adsorbed

tetanus toxoid, fluid

Pharmacologic class: vaccine
Pregnancy risk category C

AVAILABLE FORMS
tetanus toxoid, adsorbed
Injection: 5 limit flocculation (Lf) units inactivated tetanus/0.5-ml dose, in 0.5-ml syringes and 5-ml vials
tetanus toxoid, fluid
Injection: 4 Lf units inactivated tetanus/7.5-ml vials

INDICATIONS & DOSAGES
➤ **Primary immunization to prevent tetanus**
Adults and children age 7 and older:
0.5 ml (adsorbed) I.M. 4 to 8 weeks apart for two doses; then give third dose 6 to 12 months after second.
Children ages 6 weeks to 6 years:
Although use isn't recommended in children younger than age 7, the following dosage schedule may be used: 0.5 ml (adsorbed) I.M. for two doses, each 4 to 8 weeks apart, followed by a third dose 6 to 12 months after the second dose. Diphtheria and tetanus toxoids and acellular pertussis vaccine adsorbed (DTaP) is recommended for active immunization in children younger than age 7.
➤ **Booster dose to prevent tetanus**
Adults and children age 7 and older:
0.5 ml I.M. at 10-year intervals.
➤ **Postexposure prevention of tetanus**
Adults: For a clean, minor wound, give emergency booster dose if more than 10 years have elapsed since last dose. For all other wounds, give booster dose if more than 5 years have elapsed since last dose.

varicella virus vaccine
Varivax

Pharmacologic class: vaccine
Pregnancy risk category C

AVAILABLE FORMS
Injection: Single-dose vial containing 1,350 plague-forming units of Oka/Merck varicella virus (live)

INDICATIONS & DOSAGES
➤ **To prevent varicella zoster (chickenpox) infections**
Adults and children age 13 and older:
0.5 ml subcutaneously; then, second 0.5-ml dose 4 to 8 weeks later.
Children ages 1 to 12: Give 0.5 ml subcutaneously.

zoster vaccine, live
Zostavax

Pharmacologic class: vaccine, live attenuated
Pregnancy risk category C

AVAILABLE FORMS
Injection: Lyophilized vaccine of 19,400 plaque-forming units in a single-dose vial with supplied diluent

INDICATIONS & DOSAGES
➤ **Prevention of herpes zoster (shingles)**
Adults age 60 and older: One reconstituted vial subcutaneously as a single dose preferably in the upper arm.

Recommended pediatric immunizations

Vaccine	Birth	1 mo	2 mo	4 mo	6 mo	12 mo	15 mo	18 mo	19–23 mo	2–3 yr	4–6 yr
Hepatitis B	HepB	HepB		HepB		HepB					
Rotavirus			Rota	Rota	Rota						
Diphtheria, tetanus, pertussis			DTaP	DTaP	DTaP		DTaP				DTaP
H. influenzae type b			Hib	Hib	Hib	Hib					
Pneumococcal			PCV	PCV	PCV	PCV					PPSV
Inactivated poliovirus			IPV	IPV		IPV					IPV
Influenza						Influenza (yearly)					
Measles, mumps, rubella						MMR					MMR
Varicella						Varicella					Varicella
Hepatitis A						HepA (2 doses)				HepA series	
Meningococcal										MCV	

Vaccine	7–10 yr	11–12 yr	13–18 yr
Diphtheria, tetanus, pertussis		Tdap	Tdap
Human papillomavirus		HPV (3 doses)	HPV series
Meningococcal	MCV4	MCV4	MCV
Pneumococcal	PPSV		
Influenza	Influenza (yearly)		
Hepatitis A	HepA series		
Hepatitis B	HepB series		
Inactivated Poliovirus	IPV series		
Measles, mumps, rubella	MMR series		
Varicella	Varicella series		

▨ Range of recommended ages
▨ Catch up immunization
▨ Certain high-risk groups

For details on the pediatric immunization schedule see:
http://www.cdc.gov/vaccines/recs/schedules/child-schedule.htm

Recommended adult immunizations

Vaccine	19–26 yr	27–49 yr	50-59 yr	60-64 yr	≥65 yr
Tetanus, diphtheria, pertussis (Td/Tdap)	Substitute 1-time dose of Tdap for Td booster; then boost with Td every 10 yr				Td booster every 10 yr
Human papillomavirus (HPV)	3 doses (females)				
Varicella	2 doses				
Zoster				1 dose	
Measles, mumps, rubella (MMR)	1 or 2 doses		1 dose		
Influenza			1 dose annually		
Pneumococcal (polysaccharide)	1 or 2 doses				1 dose
Hepatitis A	2 doses				
Hepatitis B	3 doses				
Meningococcal	1 or more doses				

Vaccine	Indication								
	1	2	3a	3b	4	5	6	7	8
Tetanus, diphtheria, pertussis (Td/Tdap)	1-dose Td booster every 10 yr substitute 1 dose of Tdap for Td								
Human papillomavirus	3 doses for females ≤ 26 yr (0, 2, 6 mo)								
Measles, mumps, rubella (MMR)	1 or 2 doses								
Varicella	2 doses (0, 4–8 wk)								
Influenza	1 dose TIV annually								1 dose TIV or LAIV annually
Pneumococcal (polysaccharide)	1–2 doses	1–2 doses							1–2 doses
Hepatitis A	2 doses (0, 6–12 mo, or 0, 6–18 mo)								
Hepatitis B	3 doses (0, 1–2, 4–6 mo)								
Meningococcal	1 or more doses								
Zoster	1 dose								

For all persons in this category who meet the age requirements and who lack evidence of immunity.

Recommended if some other risk factor is present.

Contraindicated.

Indication key:
1. Pregnancy
2. Immunocompromising conditions (excluding human immunodeficiency virus [HIV]), medications, radiation
3. HIV infection, CD4+ T lymphocyte count a. < 200 cells/μL b. ≥ 200 cells/μL
4. Diabetes, heart disease, chronic pulmonary disease, chronic alcoholism
5. Asplenia (including elective splenectomy and terminal complement component deficiencies)
6. Chronic liver disease
7. Kidney failure, end-stage renal disease, recipients of hemodialysis
8. Health care workers
For more details, see http://www.cdc.gov/vaccines/recs/schedules/adult-schedule.htm

Vitamins and minerals: Indications and dosages

vitamin A (retinol)
Aquasol A, Palmitate-A

Pregnancy risk category A if dose is under 800 mcg retinol equivalents; C if dose exceeds 800 mcg retinol equivalents; X for Aquasol

AVAILABLE FORMS
Capsules: 10,000 international units ◊, 15,000 international units ◊, 25,000 international units
Injection: 2-ml vials (50,000 international units/ml with 0.5% chlorobutanol, polysorbate 80, butylated hydroxyanisole, butylated hydroxytoluene)
Tablets: 5,000 international units ◊

INDICATIONS & DOSAGES
➤ **RDA**
Men and boys older than age 14: Give 900 mcg retinol equivalent (RE) or 3,000 international units.
Women and girls older than age 14: Give 700 mcg RE or 2,330 international units.
Children ages 9 to 13: Give 600 mcg RE or 2,000 international units.
Children ages 4 to 8: Give 400 mcg RE or 1,330 international units.
Children ages 1 to 3: Give 300 mcg RE or 1,000 international units.
Infants ages 7 to 12 months: 500 mcg or 1,665 international units.
Neonates and infants younger than age 6 months: 400 mcg RE or 1,330 international units.
Pregnant women ages 14 to 18: Give 750 mcg RE or 2,500 international units.
Pregnant women ages 19 to 50: Give 770 mcg RE or 2,564 international units.
Breast-feeding women ages 14 to 18: Give 1,200 mcg RE or 4,000 international units.
Breast-feeding women ages 19 to 50: Give 1,300 mcg RE or 4,330 international units.

➤ **Severe vitamin A deficiency**
Adults and children older than age 8: Give 100,000 international units I.M. or 100,000 to 500,000 international units P.O. for 3 days; then 50,000 international units P.O. or I.M. for 2 weeks, followed by 10,000 to 20,000 international units P.O. for 2 months. Follow with adequate dietary nutrition and RE vitamin A supplements.
Children age 8 and younger: 17,500 to 35,000 international units I.M. daily for 10 days.
➤ **Maintenance dose to prevent recurrence of vitamin A deficiency**
Children ages 1 to 8: Give 5,000 to 10,000 international units P.O. daily for 2 months; then adequate dietary nutrition and RE vitamin A supplements.

vitamin B complex

cyanocobalamin (vitamin B₁₂)
Big ShotB12, CaloMist, Crystamine, Crysti 1000, Cyanoject, Cyomin, Nascobal, Rubesol-1000, TwelvecResin-K.

hydroxocobalamin (vitamin B₁₂)
CYANOKIT, Hydro-Crysti-12, LA-12

Pregnancy risk category A ; C if dose exceeds RDA

AVAILABLE FORMS
cyanocobalamin
Injection: 100 mcg/ml, 1,000 mcg/ml
Intranasal spray: 25 mcg/spray, 500 mcg/spray
Tablets ◊ : 25 mcg ◊, 50 mcg ◊, 100 mcg ◊, 250 mcg ◊, 500 mcg ◊, 1,000 mcg ◊, 5,000 mcg ◊
Lozenges: 50 mcg ◊, 100 mcg ◊, 250 mcg ◊, 500 mcg ◊

hydroxocobalamin
Injection: 1,000 mcg/ml; 2.5 g/vial

INDICATIONS & DOSAGES
➤ **RDA for cyanocobalamin**
Adults and children age 14 and older:
2.4 mcg.
Children ages 9 to 13: Give 1.8 mcg.
Children ages 4 to 8: Give 1.2 mcg.
Children ages 1 to 3: Give 0.9 mcg.
Infants ages 6 months to 1 year: 0.5 mcg.
*Neonates and infants younger than age
6 months:* 0.4 mcg.
Pregnant women: 2.6 mcg.
Breast-feeding women: 2.8 mcg.
➤ **Vitamin B$_{12}$ deficiency from
inadequate diet, subtotal gastrectomy,
or other condition, disorder, or
disease, except malabsorption,
related to pernicious anemia or
other GI disease**
Adults: 30 mcg hydroxocobalamin I.M.
daily for 5 to 10 days, depending on
severity of deficiency. Maintenance dose
is 100 to 200 mcg I.M. once monthly or
500 mcg gel intranasally once weekly. For
subsequent prophylaxis, advise adequate
nutrition and daily RDA vitamin B12
supplements.
Children: 1 to 5 mg hydroxocobalamin
in single doses of 100 mcg I.M. over 2 or
more weeks, depending on severity of
deficiency. Maintenance dose is 60 mcg/
month I.M. For subsequent prophylaxis,
advise adequate nutrition and daily RDA
vitamin B12 supplements.
➤ **Pernicious anemia or vitamin B$_{12}$
malabsorption**
Adults: Initially, 100 mcg cyanocobalamin I.M. or subcutaneously daily
for 6 to 7 days. If response is observed,
100 mcg I.M. or subcutaneously every
other day for 7 doses, then 100 mcg
every 3 to 4 days for 2 to 3 weeks; then
100 mcg I.M. or subcutaneously once
monthly.
Children: 30 to 50 mcg I.M. or subcutaneously daily over 2 or more weeks; then
100 mcg I.M. or subcutaneously monthly
for life.

➤ **Maintenance therapy for remission of pernicious anemia after I.M.
vitamin B$_{12}$ therapy in patients
without nervous system involvement;
dietary deficiency, malabsorption
disorders, and inadequate secretion
of intrinsic factor**
Adults: Initially, one spray in one nostril
once weekly (Nascobal). Give at least 1
hour before or after hot foods or liquids.
Or one spray in each nostril daily (total
daily dose of 50 mcg CaloMist). May
increase to one spray in each nostril twice
daily (total daily dose of 100 mcg) as
needed.
➤ **Prevention of methylmalonic
aciduria**
Mothers and their neonates: 5,000 mcg
cyanocobalamin I.M. daily to the mother
prepartum, then 1,000 mcg I.M. daily to
the neonate for 11 days, with a protein-
restricted diet.
➤ **Methylmalonic aciduria**
Neonates: 1,000 mcg cyanocobalamin
I.M. daily.
➤ **Schilling test flushing dose**
Adults and children: 1,000 mcg
hydroxocobalamin I.M. as single dose.
➤ **Cyanide poisoning**
Adults: Initially, 5 g I.V. over 15 minutes.
Based on patient's condition may repeat
5 g dose I.V. over 15 minutes to 2 hours.

---

folic acid (vitamin B$_9$)
Folvite

Pregnancy risk category A

AVAILABLE FORMS
Injection: 10-ml vials (5 mg/ml with
1.5% benzyl alcohol, 5 mg/ml with 1.5%
benzyl alcohol and 0.2% ethylenediaminetetraacetic acid)
Tablets: 0.4 mg ◊ , 0.8 mg ◊ , 1 mg

INDICATIONS & DOSAGES
➤ **RDA**
Adults and children age 14 and older:
Give 400 mcg.
Children ages 9 to 13: Give 300 mcg.
Children ages 4 to 8: Give 200 mcg.
Children ages 1 to 3: Give 150 mcg.
Infants ages 7 months to 1 year: 80 mcg.

Neonates and infants younger than age 6 months: 65 mcg.
Pregnant women: 600 mcg.
Breast-feeding women: 500 mcg.
➤ **Megaloblastic or macrocytic anemia from folic acid or other nutritional deficiency, hepatic disease, alcoholism, intestinal obstruction, or excessive hemolysis**
Adults and children age 4 and older: 0.4 to 1 mg P.O., I.M., or subcutaneously daily. After anemia caused by folic acid deficiency is corrected, proper diet and RDA supplements are needed to prevent recurrence.
Children younger than age 4: Up to 0.3 mg P.O., I.M., or subcutaneously daily.
Pregnant and breast-feeding women: 0.8 mg P.O., I.M., or subcutaneously daily.
➤ **To prevent fetal neural tube defects during pregnancy**
Adults: 0.4 mg P.O. daily.
➤ **To prevent megaloblastic anemia during pregnancy to prevent fetal damage**
Adults: Up to 1 mg P.O., I.M., or subcutaneously daily throughout pregnancy.
➤ **Test for folic acid deficiency in patients with megaloblastic anemia without masking pernicious anemia**
Adults and children: 0.1 to 0.2 mg P.O. or I.M. for 10 days while maintaining a diet low in folate and vitamin B12.
➤ **Tropical sprue**
Adults: 3 to 15 mg P.O. daily.

leucovorin calcium (citrovorum factor, folinic acid)

Pregnancy risk category C

AVAILABLE FORMS
Injection: 1-ml ampule (3 mg/ml with 0.9% benzyl alcohol); 10 mg/ml in 5-ml vial; 50-mg, 100-mg, 350-mg, 500-mg vials for reconstitution (contains no preservatives)
Tablets: 5 mg, 10 mg, 15 mg, 25 mg

INDICATIONS & DOSAGES
➤ **Overdose of folic acid antagonist (methotrexate, trimethoprim, or pyrimethamine)**
Adults and children: I.M. or I.V. dose equivalent to weight of antagonist given. For methotrexate overdose, up to 75 mg I.V. infusion within 12 hours, followed by 12 mg I.M. every 6 hours for four doses. For adverse effects after average doses of methotrexate, 6 to 12 mg I.M. every 6 hours for four doses.
➤ **Leucovorin rescue after high methotrexate dose in treatment of malignant disease**
Adults and children: 10 mg/m² P.O., I.M., or I.V. every 6 hours until methotrexate level falls below 5 × 10⁻⁸ M.
➤ **Megaloblastic anemia from congenital enzyme deficiency**
Adults and children: 3 to 6 mg I.M. daily.
➤ **Folate-deficient megaloblastic anemia**
Adults and children: Up to 1 mg I.M. daily. Duration of treatment depends on hematologic response.
➤ **To prevent hematologic toxicity from pyrimethamine or trimethoprim therapy**
Adults and children: 400 mcg to 5 mg I.M. with each dose of folic acid antagonist. Oral dosages of 10 to 35 mg once daily or 25 mg once weekly may also be used.
➤ **Hematologic toxicity from pyrimethamine or trimethoprim therapy**
Adults and children: 5 to 15 mg I.M. daily.
➤ **Palliative treatment of advanced colorectal cancer**
Adults: 20 mg/m² I.V.; then fluorouracil 425 mg/m² I.V. or 200 mg/m² I.V. (over 3 minutes or longer) followed by fluorouracil 370 mg/m² daily for 5 consecutive days. Repeat at 4-week intervals for two additional courses; then at intervals of 4 to 5 weeks, if tolerated.

niacin (nicotinic acid, vitamin B₃)
Niacor◇, Niaspan◇, Slo-Niacin◇

niacinamide◇ (nicotinamide◇)

Pregnancy risk category A; C if dose exceeds RDA

AVAILABLE FORMS
niacin
Capsules (timed-release): 125 mg◇, 250 mg◇, 400 mg◇, 500 mg
Tablets: 50 mg◇, 100 mg◇, 250 mg◇, 500 mg
Tablets (extended-release): 250 mg◇, 500 mg◇, 750 mg◇, 1,000 mg◇
niacinamide
Tablets: 50 mg◇, 100 mg◇, 125 mg◇, 250 mg◇, 500 mg◇

INDICATIONS & DOSAGES
➤ **RDA**
Adult men and boys ages 14 to 18: Give 16 mg
Adult women and girls ages 14 to 18: Give 14 mg.
Children ages 9 to 13: Give 12 mg.
Children ages 4 to 8: Give 8 mg.
Children ages 1 to 3: Give 6 mg.
Infants ages 7 months to 1 year: 4 mg.
Neonates and infants younger than age 6 months: 2 mg.
Pregnant women: 18 mg.
Breast-feeding women: 17 mg.
➤ **Pellagra**
Adults: 300 to 500 mg P.O. daily in divided doses.
Children: 100 to 300 mg P.O. daily in divided doses.
➤ **Hartnup disease**
Adults: 50 to 200 mg P.O. daily.
➤ **Niacin deficiency**
Adults: Up to 100 mg P.O. daily.
➤ **Hyperlipidemias, especially with hypercholesterolemia**
Adults: 250 mg P.O. daily at bedtime. Increase at 4- to 7-day intervals up to 1.5 to 2 g P.O. daily divided b.i.d. to t.i.d. Maximum 6 g daily. Or, 1 to 2 g extended-release tablets P.O. daily at bedtime.

paricalcitol
Zemplar

Pregnancy risk category C

AVAILABLE FORMS
Capsules: 1 mcg, 2 mcg, 4 mcg
Injection: 2 mcg/ml, 5 mcg/ml

INDICATIONS & DOSAGES
➤ **To prevent or treat secondary hyperparathyroidism in patients with stage 3 or 4 chronic kidney disease**
Adults: Initial dose is based on baseline intact parathyroid hormone (iPTH) levels. If iPTH is less than or equal to 500 picograms (pg)/ml, give 1 mcg P.O. daily or 2 mcg P.O. three times weekly, no more often than every other day. If iPTH is greater than 500 pg/ml, give 2 mcg P.O. daily or 4 mcg P.O. three times weekly, no more often than every other day. Adjust dose at 2- to 4-week intervals, based on iPTH levels.
➤ **To prevent or treat secondary hyperparathyroidism in patients with chronic renal failure**
Adults: 0.04 to 0.1 mcg/kg (2.8 to 7 mcg) I.V. no more often than every other day during dialysis. Doses as high as 0.24 mcg/kg (16.8 mcg) may be safely given. If satisfactory response isn't observed, increase dosage by 2 to 4 mcg at 2- to 4-week intervals.

pyridoxine hydrochloride (vitamin B₆)
Aminoxin, Vitelle Nestrex

Pregnancy risk category A; C if dose exceeds RDA

AVAILABLE FORMS
Injection: 100 mg/ml
Tablets: 25 mg◇, 50 mg◇, 100 mg◇, 250 mg◇, 500 mg◇
Tablets (enteric-coated): 20 mg◇

INDICATIONS & DOSAGES
➤ **RDA**
Adults ages 19 to 50: Give 1.3 mg.
Men age 51 and older: 1.7 mg.

Women age 51 and older: 1.5 mg.
Boys ages 14 to 19: Give 1.3 mg.
Girls ages 14 to 19: Give 1.2 mg.
Children ages 9 to 13: Give 1 mg.
Children ages 4 to 8: Give 0.6 mg.
Children ages 1 to 3: Give 0.5 mg.
Infants ages 7 months to 1 year: 0.3 mg.
Neonates and infants younger than age 6 months: 0.1 mg.
Pregnant women: 1.9 mg.
Breast-feeding women: 2 mg.
➤ **Dietary vitamin B₆ deficiency**
Adults: 2.5 to 10 mg P.O., I.V., or I.M. daily for 3 weeks; then 2 to 5 mg daily as supplement to proper diet.
➤ **Seizures related to vitamin B₆ deficiency or dependency**
Adults and children: 100 mg I.V. or I.M. in single dose.
➤ **Vitamin B₆-responsive anemias or dependency syndrome (inborn errors of metabolism)**
Adults: Up to 500 mg P.O., I.V., or I.M. daily until symptoms subside; then same dosage daily for life.
➤ **To prevent vitamin B₆ deficiency during drug therapy with isoniazid or penicillamine**
Adults: 10 to 50 mg P.O. daily.
➤ **To prevent seizures during cycloserine therapy**
Adults: 100 to 300 mg P.O. daily.
➤ **Antidote for isoniazid poisoning**
Adults: 4 g I.V.; then 1 g I.M. every 30 minutes until amount of pyridoxine given equals amount of isoniazid ingested.

thiamine hydrochloride (vitamin B₁)
Betaxin†, Thiamiject†, Thiamilate

Pregnancy risk category A; C if dose exceeds RDA

AVAILABLE FORMS
Injection: 100 mg/ml
Tablets: 50 mg ◇, 100 mg ◇, 250 mg ◇, 500 mg
Tablets (enteric-coated): 20 mg ◇

INDICATIONS & DOSAGES
➤ **RDA**
Adult men: 1.2 mg.
Adult women: 1.1 mg.

Boys ages 14 to 18: Give 1.2 mg.
Girls ages 14 to 18: Give 1 mg.
Children ages 9 to 13: Give 0.9 mg.
Children ages 4 to 8: Give 0.6 mg.
Children ages 1 to 3: Give 0.5 mg.
Infants ages 7 months to 1 year: 0.3 mg.
Neonates and infants younger than age 6 months: 0.2 mg.
Pregnant women: 1.4 mg.
Breast-feeding women: 1.4 mg.
➤ **Beriberi**
Adults: Depending on severity, 5 to 30 mg I.M. t.i.d. for 2 weeks; then dietary correction and multivitamin supplement containing 5 to 30 mg thiamine daily for 1 month.
Children: Depending on severity, 10 to 25 mg I.V. or I.M. daily. For noncritically ill children, 10 to 50 mg P.O. daily in divided doses for several weeks with adequate diet.
➤ **Wet beriberi with myocardial failure**
Adults and children: 10 to 30 mg I.V. t.i.d.
➤ **Wernicke encephalopathy**
Adults: Initially, 100 mg I.V.; then 50 to 100 mg I.V. or I.M. daily until patient is consuming a regular balanced diet.

sodium fluoride
Fluor-A-Day†, Fluoritab, Fluorodex, Flura, Flura-Drops, Flura-Loz, Karidium, Luride, Luride, Lozi-Tabs, Luride-SF, Lozi-Tabs, Pediaflor, Pedi-Dent†, Pharmaflur, Pharmaflur df, Pharmaflur 1.1, Phos-Flur

sodium fluoride, topical
ACT◇, Fluorigard◇, Fluorinse, Gel-Kam, Gel-Tin◇, Karigel, Karigel-N, Luride, Minute-Gel, MouthKote F/R◇, Point-Two, Prevident, Stop Gel◇, Thera-Flur, Thera-Flur-N

Pregnancy risk category NR

AVAILABLE FORMS
Sodium fluoride
Drops: 0.125 mg/drop, 0.25 mg/drop, 0.2 mg/ml, 0.5 mg/ml
Lozenges: 1 mg
Tablets: 1 mg

Tablets (chewable): 0.25 mg, 0.5 mg, 1 mg
Sodium fluoride, topical
Gel: 0.1%, 0.5%, 1.2%, 1.23%
Gel Drops: 0.5%
Rinse: 0.02%◇, 0.04%◇

INDICATIONS & DOSAGES
➤ To prevent dental caries
Adults and children older than age 6: Give 5 to 10 ml of rinse or thin ribbon of gel applied to teeth with toothbrush or mouth trays for at least 1 minute at bedtime.
If fluoride ion level in drinking water is less than 0.3 parts/million (ppm)
Children ages 6 to 16: Give 1 mg P.O. daily.
Children ages 3 to 5: Give 0.5 mg P.O. daily.
Infants and children ages 6 months to 2 years: 0.25 mg P.O. daily.
If fluoride ion level in drinking water is 0.3 to 0.6 ppm
Children ages 6 to 16: Give 0.5 mg P.O. daily.
Children ages 3 to 5: Give 0.25 mg P.O. daily.
➤ Osteoporosis
Adults: Up to 60 mg P.O. daily with calcium, vitamin D, or estrogen.

---

trace elements

chromium (chromic chloride)
Chroma-Pak, Chromic Chloride

copper (cupric sulfate)
Cupric Sulfate

iodine (sodium iodide)
Iodopen

manganese (manganese chloride, manganese sulfate)

selenium (selenious acid)
Sele-Pak, Selepen

zinc (zinc sulfate)
Zinca-Pak

Pregnancy risk category C

AVAILABLE FORMS
Chromium
Injection: 4 mcg/ml, 20 mcg/ml

Copper
Injection: 0.4 mg/ml, 2 mg/ml
Iodine
Injection: 100 mcg/ml
Manganese
Injection: 0.1 mg/ml
Selenium
Injection: 40 mcg/ml
Zinc
Injection: 1 mg/ml,
5 mg/ml

INDICATIONS & DOSAGES
➤ To prevent individual trace element deficiencies in patients receiving long-term total parenteral nutrition (TPN)
Chromium
Adults: 10 to 15 mcg I.V. daily.
Metabolically stable adults with intestinal fluid loss: 20 mcg I.V. daily.
Children: 0.14 to 0.2 mcg/kg I.V. daily.
Copper
Adults: 0.5 to 1.5 mg I.V. daily.
Children: 20 mcg/kg I.V. daily.
Iodine
Adults: 1 to 2 mcg/kg I.V. daily.
Pregnant and lactating women, children: 2 to 3 mcg/kg I.V. daily.
Manganese
Adults: 0.15 to 0.8 mg I.V. daily.
Children: 2 to 10 mcg/kg I.V. daily.
Selenium
Adults: 20 to 40 mcg I.V. daily.
Children: 3 mcg/kg I.V. daily
Zinc
Adults: 2.5 to 4 mg I.V. daily. Add 2 mg daily for acute catabolic states.
Stable adults with fluid loss from the small bowel: Give an additional 12.2 mg zinc per liter of TPN solution, or an additional 17.1 mg per kg of stool or ileostomy output.
Full-term infants and children younger than age 5: Give 100 mcg/kg I.V. daily.
Premature infants weighing up to 3 kg (3.3 to 7 lb): 300 mcg/kg I.V. daily.

vitamin C (ascorbic acid)
Ascor L 500, Cecon ◇, Cenolate ◇,
Cevi-Bid ◇, Dull-C ◇, Flavorcee ◇,
Vicks Vitamin C Drops ◇, Vita-C ◇

*Pregnancy risk category A; C if
dose exceeds RDA*

AVAILABLE FORMS
Capsules: 500 mg ◇
Capsules (timed-release): 500 mg ◇,
1,000 mg ◇
Crystals: 1,000 mg/¼ tsp ◇
Injection: 500 mg/ml
Lozenges: 25 mg ◇
Oral solution: 100 mg/ml ◇
Powder: 60 mg/¼ tsp ◇, 1,060 mg/¼ tsp ◇
Tablets: 250 mg ◇, 500 mg ◇,
1,000 mg ◇, 1,500 mg ◇
Tablets (chewable): 100 mg ◇, 250 mg ◇,
500 mg ◇, 1,000 mg ◇
Tablets (timed-release): 500 mg ◇,
1,000 mg ◇

INDICATIONS & DOSAGES
➤ **RDA**
Men age 19 and older: 90 mg.
Women age 19 and older: 75 mg.
Boys ages 14 to 18: Give 75 mg.
Girls ages 14 to 18: Give 65 mg.
Children ages 9 to 13: Give 45 mg.
Children ages 4 to 8: Give 25 mg.
Children ages 1 to 3: Give 15 mg.
Infants ages 7 months to 1 year: 50 mg.
Neonates and infants up to age 6 months:
40 mg.
Pregnant women: 80 to 85 mg.
Breast-feeding women: 115 to 120 mg.
➤ **Frank and subclinical scurvy**
Adults: Depending on severity, 100 to
250 mg P.O., I.V., I.M., or subcutaneously
daily; then 70 to 150 mg daily for
maintenance.
Children: Depending on severity, 100 to
300 mg P.O., I.V., I.M., or subcutaneously
daily; then at least 30 mg daily for
maintenance.
➤ **Extensive burns, delayed fracture
or wound healing, postoperative
wound healing, severe febrile or
chronic disease states**
Adults: 300 to 500 mg I.V., I.M., or
subcutaneously daily for 7 to 10 days;
1 to 2 g daily for extensive burns.

Children: 100 to 200 mg P.O., I.V., I.M.,
or subcutaneously daily.
➤ **To prevent vitamin C deficiency
in patients with poor nutritional
habits or increased requirements**
Adults: 70 to 150 mg P.O., I.V., I.M., or
subcutaneously daily.
Children: At least 40 mg P.O., I.V., I.M.,
or subcutaneously daily.
Infants: At least 35 mg P.O., I.V., I.M.,
or subcutaneously daily.
Pregnant and breast-feeding women:
70 to 150 mg P.O., I.V., I.M., or subcutaneously daily.
➤ **To acidify urine**
Adults: 4 to 12 g P.O. daily in divided
doses.
➤ **Macular degeneration**
Adults: 500 mg daily in combination
with beta carotene, vitamin E, zinc, and
copper.

vitamin D

cholecalciferol (vitamin D₃)
Delta-D ◇, Maximum-D

ergocalciferol (vitamin D₂)
Calciferol, Drisdol

*Pregnancy risk category A;
C if dose exceeds RDA*

AVAILABLE FORMS
cholecalciferol
Capsules: 250 mcg (10,000 international
units)
Tablets: 10 mcg (400 international units),
25 mcg (1,000 international units)
ergocalciferol
Capsules: 1.25 mg (50,000 international
units)
Injection: 12.5 mg (500,000 international
units)/ml
Oral liquid: 200 mcg (8,000 international
units)/ml in 60-ml dropper bottle ◇

INDICATIONS & DOSAGES
➤ **RDA for cholecalciferol or
ergocalciferol**
Adults older than age 70: Give 15 mcg
(600 international units).
Adults ages 51 to 70: Give 10 mcg
(400 international units).

Infants, children, and adults up to age 50:
Give 5 mcg (200 international units).
Pregnant or breast-feeding women: 5 mcg
(200 international units).
➤ **Rickets and other vitamin D
deficiency diseases**
Adults: Initially, 10,000 international
units P.O. or I.M. daily; expect to increase, based on response, to maximum
of 500,000 international units daily.
Children: 1,500 to 5,000 international
units P.O. or I.M. daily for 2 to 4 weeks;
repeat after 2 weeks, if needed. Or, give
single dose of 600,000 international units.
After correction of deficiency, maintenance includes adequate diet and RDA
supplements.
➤ **Hypoparathyroidism**
Adults: 625 mcg to 5 mg ergocalciferol
P.O. daily with calcium supplement
Children: 1.25 mg to 5 mg of ergocalciferol P.O. daily with calcium
supplement.
➤ **Familial hypophosphatemia**
Adults: 250 mcg to 1.5 mg P.O. daily of
ergocalciferol with phosphate supplement.
Children: 1 to 2 mg P.O. daily of ergocalciferol with phosphate supplement,
increased in 250- to 500-mcg increments
at 3- to 4-month intervals based on
response.

vitamin D analogue

doxercalciferol
Hectorol

Pregnancy risk category B

AVAILABLE FORMS
Capsules: 0.5 mcg, 2.5 mcg
Injection: 2 mcg/ml

INDICATIONS & DOSAGES
➤ **Secondary hyperparathyroidism
in dialysis patients with chronic
kidney disease**
Adults: Initially, 10 mcg P.O. three times
weekly at dialysis. Adjust dosage as
needed to lower intact parathyroid
hormone (iPTH) levels to 150 to
300 picograms (pg)/ml. Increase dose
by 2.5 mcg at 8-week intervals if iPTH
level hasn't decreased by 50% and fails

to reach target range. Maximum dose is
20 mcg P.O. three times weekly. If iPTH
levels fall below 100 pg/ml, suspend
drug for 1 week; then give dose of at
least 2.5 mcg less than last dose Or, 4 mcg
I.V. bolus 3 times a week at the end of
dialysis about every other day. Adjust
dose as needed to lower iPTH levels to
150 to 300 pg/ml. Dosage may be
increased by 1 to 2 mcg at 8-week intervals if the iPTH level isn't decreased by
50% and fails to reach target range.
Maximum dose is 18 mcg weekly. If
iPTH levels go below 100 pg/ml, suspend
drug for 1 week, then resume at a dose
that's at least 1 mcg P.O. lower than the
last dose.
➤ **Secondary hyperparathyroidism
in predialysis patients with stage 3
or 4 chronic kidney disease**
Adults: 1 mcg P.O. daily. Adjust dosage
as needed to lower iPTH levels to 35 to
70 pg/ml for stage 3 or 70 to 110 pg/ml
for stage 4. Increase dosage at 2-week
intervals by 0.5 mcg if levels are above
70 pg/ml for stage 3 or above 110 pg/ml
for stage 4. If level falls below 35 pg/ml
for stage 3 or 70 pg/ml for stage 4, suspend treatment for 1 week, then give dose
at least 0.5 mcg lower than last dose.
Maximum dose, 3.5 mcg daily.

vitamin E (tocopherols)
Aquasol E ◇

Pregnancy risk category A

AVAILABLE FORMS
Capsules: 100 international units ◇ ,
200 international units ◇ , 400 international units ◇ , 600 international units ◇ ,
1,000 international units ◇
Drops: 50 international units/ml
Tablets: 100 international units ◇ ,
200 international units ◇ , 400 international units ◇ , 500 international
units ◇ , 600 international units ◇ ,
1,000 international units ◇

INDICATIONS & DOSAGES
Note: RDAs for vitamin E have been
converted to α-tocopherol equivalents
(α-TE). One α-TE equals 1 mg of D-α
tocopherol, or 1.49 international units.

➤ **RDA**
Adults and children ages 14 to 18: Give 15 mg.
Children ages 9 to 13: Give 11 mg.
Children ages 4 to 8: Give 7 mg.
Children ages 1 to 3: Give 6 mg.
Infants ages 7 months to 1 year: 5 mg.
Neonates and infants younger than age 6 months: 4 mg.
Pregnant women: 15 mg.
Breast-feeding women: 19 mg.
➤ **Vitamin E deficiency in premature neonates and in patients with impaired fat absorption**
Adults: Depending on severity, 60 to 75 international units P.O. daily.
Children: 1 international unit/kg daily.

---

vitamin K analogue

phytonadione (vitamin K₁)
AquaMEPHYTON, Mephyton

Pregnancy risk category C

AVAILABLE FORMS
Injection (emulsion): 2 mg/ml, 10 mg/ml
Tablets: 5 mg

INDICATIONS & DOSAGES
➤ **RDA**
Men age 19 and older: 120 mcg.
Women age 19 and older, including pregnant and breast-feeding women: 90 mcg.
Children ages 14 to 18: Give 75 mcg.
Children ages 9 to 13: Give 60 mcg.
Children ages 4 to 8: Give 55 mcg.
Children ages 1 to 3: Give 30 mcg.
Infants ages 7 months to 1 year: 2.5 mcg.
Neonates and infants younger than age 6 months: 2 mcg.
➤ **Hypoprothrombinemia caused by vitamin K malabsorption, drug therapy, or excessive vitamin A dosage**
Adults: Depending on severity, 2.5 to 25 mg P.O., I.M., or subcutaneously, repeated and increased up to 50 mg as needed.
➤ **Hypoprothrombinemia caused by effect of oral anticoagulants**
Adults: 2.5 to 10 mg P.O., I.M., or subcutaneously, based on PT and INR; repeat if

needed within 12 to 48 hours after oral dose or within 6 to 8 hours after parenteral dose. In emergency, 10 to 50 mg slow I.V. at rate not to exceed 1 mg/minute, repeated every 4 hours as needed.
➤ **To prevent hemorrhagic disease of newborn**
Neonates: 0.5 to 1 mg I.M. within 1 hour after birth.
➤ **Hemorrhagic disease of newborn**
Neonates: 1 mg subcutaneously or I.M. Higher doses may be needed if mother has been receiving oral anticoagulants.

Therapeutic drug monitoring guidelines

Drug	Laboratory test monitored	Therapeutic ranges of test
aminoglycoside antibiotics (amikacin, gentamicin, tobramycin)	Amikacin peak Amikacin trough Creatinine Gentamicin, tobramycin peak Gentamicin, tobramycin trough	20–30 mcg/ml 1–8 mcg/ml 0.6–1.3 mg/dl 4–12 mcg/ml < 2 mcg/ml
amphotericin B	BUN CBC with differential and platelets Creatinine Electrolytes (especially potassium and magnesium) Liver function	5–20 mg/dl ***** 0.6–1.3 mg/dl Potassium: 3.5–5 mEq/L Magnesium: 1.5–2.5 mEq/L Sodium: 135–145 mEq/l Chloride: 98–106 mEq/L *
ACE inhibitors (benazepril, captopril, enalapril, enalaprilat, fosinopril, lisinopril, moexipril, quinapril, ramipril, trandolapril)	Creatinine BUN Potassium WBC with differential	0.6–1.3 mg/dl 5–20 mg/dl 3.5–5 mEq/L *****
antibiotics	Cultures and sensitivities WBC with differential	 *****
biguanides (metformin)	CBC Creatinine Fasting glucose Glycosylated hemoglobin	***** 0.6–1.3 mg/dl 70–110 mg/dl 4%–7% of total hemoglobin
carbamazepine	BUN Carbamazepine CBC with differential Liver function Platelet count	5–20 mg/dl 4–12 mcg/ml ***** * 150–450 × 10³/mm³
clozapine	WBC with differential	*****
corticosteroids (cortisone, hydrocortisone, prednisone, prednisolone, triamcinolone, methylprednisolone, dexamethasone, betamethasone)	Electrolytes (especially potassium) Fasting glucose	Potassium: 3.5–5 mEq/L Magnesium 1.7–2.1 mEq/L Sodium 135–145 mEq/L Chloride 98–106 mEq/L Calcium 8.6–10 mg/dl 70–110 mg/dl

***** For those areas marked with asterisks, the following values can be used:

Hemoglobin: Women: 12–16 g/dl
   Men: 14–18 g/dl
Hematocrit: Women: 37%–48%
   Men: 42%–52%
RBCs: 4–5.5 × 10⁶/mm³
WBCs: 5–10 × 10³/mm³

Differential: Neutrophils: 45%–74%
   Bands: 0%–8%
   Lymphocytes: 16%–45%
   Monocytes: 4%–10%
   Eosinophils: 0%–7%
   Basophils: 0%–2%

Monitoring guidelines

Wait until after the third dose is given to check drug levels. Obtain blood for peak level 30 minutes after I.V. infusion ends or 60 minutes after I.M. administration. For trough levels, draw blood just before next dose. Dosage may need to be adjusted accordingly. Recheck after three doses. Monitor creatinine and BUN levels and urine output for signs of decreasing renal function. Monitor urine for increased proteins, cells, and casts.

Monitor creatinine, BUN, and electrolyte levels at least weekly during therapy. Regularly monitor blood counts and liver function test results during therapy.

Monitor WBC with differential before therapy, monthly during the first 3 to 6 months, then periodically for the first year. Monitor renal function and potassium level periodically.

Monitor WBC with differential weekly during therapy. Specimen cultures and sensitivities will determine the cause of the infection and the best treatment.

Check renal function and hematologic values before starting therapy and at least annually thereafter. If the patient has impaired renal function, don't use metformin because it may cause lactic acidosis. Monitor response to therapy by periodically evaluating fasting glucose and glycosylated hemoglobin levels. A patient's home monitoring of glucose levels helps monitor compliance and response.

Monitor blood counts and platelets before therapy, monthly during the first 2 months, then yearly. Liver function, BUN, and urinalysis should be checked before and periodically during therapy.

Before starting, patient must have a baseline WBC count of at least 3,500/mm³ and a baseline absolute neutrophil count (ANC) of at least 2,000/mm³. During the first 6 months of therapy, monitor patient weekly. If acceptable WBC and ANC values are maintained, reduce monitoring to every other week. After 6 months of monitoring without leukopenia, monitor every 4 weeks. WBC count and ANC must be monitored weekly for at least 4 weeks after stopping drug.

Monitor electrolyte and glucose levels regularly during long-term therapy.

(continued)

* For those areas marked with one asterisk, the following values can be used:

ALT: 7–56 units/L
AST: 5–40 units/L
Alkaline phosphatase: 17–142 units/L
LDH: 60–220 units/L
GGT: < 40 units/L

Total bilirubin: 0.2–1 mg/dl

Drug	Laboratory test monitored	Therapeutic ranges of test
digoxin	Creatinine	0.6–1.3 mg/dl
	Digoxin	0.8–2 nanograms/ml
	Electrolytes	Potassium: 3.5–5 mEq/L
		Magnesium: 1.7–2.1 mEq/L
		Sodium: 135–145 mEq/L
		Chloride: 98–106 mEq/L
		Calcium: 8.6–10 mg/dl
erythropoietin	CBC with differential	*****
	Hematocrit	Women: 36%–48%
		Men: 42%–52%
	Platelet count	150–450 × 10³/mm³
	Serum ferritin	10–383 mg/dl
	Transferrin saturation	220–400 mg/dl
ethosuximide	CBC with differential	*****
	Ethosuximide	40–100 mcg/ml
	Liver function	*
gemfibrozil	CBC	*****
	Lipids	Total cholesterol: < 200 mg/dl
		LDL: < 100 mg/dl
		HDL: Women: 40–75 mg/dl
		Men: 37–70 mg/dl
		Triglycerides: 10–150 mg/dl
	Liver function	*
	Serum glucose	70–100 mg/dl
heparin	Partial thromboplastin time (PTT)	1.5–2.5 times control
	Hematocrit	*****
	Platelet count	150–450 × 10³/mm³
HMG-CoA reductase inhibitors (atorvastatin, fluvastatin, lovastatin, pravastatin, rosuvastatin, simvastatin)	Lipids	Total cholesterol: < 200 mg/dl
		LDL: < 100 mg/dl
		HDL: Women: 40–75 mg/dl
		Men: 37–70 mg/dl
		Triglycerides: 10–150 mg/dl
	Liver function	*
insulin	Fasting glucose	70–110 mg/dl
	Glycosylated hemoglobin	4%–7% of total hemoglobin
isotretinoin	CBC with differential	*****
	Liver function	*
	Lipids	Total cholesterol: < 200 mg/dl
		LDL: < 130 mg/dl
		HDL: Women: 40–75 mg/dl
		Men: 37–70 mg/dl
		Triglycerides: 10–160 mg/dl
	Platelet count	150–450 × 10³/mm³
	Pregnancy test	Negative

***** For those areas marked with asterisks, the following values can be used:

Hemoglobin: Women: 12–16 g/dl
  Men: 14–18 g/dl
Hematocrit: Women: 37%–48%
  Men: 42%–52%
RBCs: 4–5.5 × 10⁶/mm³
WBCs: 5–10 × 10³/mm³

Differential: Neutrophils: 45%–74%
  Bands: 0%–8%
  Lymphocytes: 16%–45%
  Monocytes: 4%–10%
  Eosinophils: 0%–7%
  Basophils: 0%–2%

Monitoring guidelines

Check digoxin levels just before the next dose or at least 6 to 8 hours after the last dose. To monitor maintenance therapy, check drug levels at least 1 to 2 weeks after therapy is initiated or changed. Make any adjustments in therapy based on entire clinical picture, not solely on drug levels. Also, check electrolyte levels and renal function periodically during therapy.

After therapy is initiated or changed, monitor the hematocrit twice weekly for 2 to 6 weeks until stabilized in the target range and a maintenance dose determined. Monitor hematocrit regularly thereafter.

Check drug level 8 to 10 days after therapy is initiated or changed. Periodically monitor CBC with differential, liver function tests, and urinalysis.

Therapy is usually withdrawn after 3 months if response is inadequate. Patient must be fasting to measure triglyceride levels. Periodically obtain blood counts during the first 12 months.

When drug is given by continuous I.V. infusion, check PTT every 4 hours in the early stages of therapy, and daily thereafter. When drug is given by deep subcutaneous injection, check PTT 4 to 6 hours after injection, and daily thereafter. Periodically during therapy, check platelet counts and hematocrit and test for occult blood in stools.

Perform liver function tests at baseline, 6 to 12 weeks after therapy is initiated or changed, and about every 6 months thereafter. If adequate response isn't achieved within 6 weeks, consider changing the therapy.

A patient's home monitoring of glucose levels helps measure compliance and response. Glycosylated hemoglobin level is a good measure of long-term control.

Use a serum or urine pregnancy test with a sensitivity of at least 25 milli-international units/ml. Perform one test before therapy and a second test during the first 5 days of the menstrual cycle before therapy begins or at least 11 days after the last unprotected act of sexual intercourse, whichever is later. Repeat pregnancy tests monthly. Obtain baseline liver function tests and lipid levels; repeat every 1 to 2 weeks until a response is established (usually 4 weeks).

(continued)

* For those areas marked with one asterisk, the following values can be used:

ALT: 7–56 units/L
AST: 5–40 units/L
Alkaline phosphatase: 17–142 units/L
LDH: 60–220 units/L
GGT: < 40 units/L
Total bilirubin: 0.2–1 mg/dl

Drug	Laboratory test monitored	Therapeutic ranges of test
linezolid	Amylase	35–118 international units/L
	CBC with differential	*****
	Cultures and sensitivities	
	Liver function	*
	Lipase	10–150 units/L
	Platelet count	150–450 × 10³/mm³
lithium	Creatinine	0.6–1.3 mg/dl
	CBC	*****
	Electrolytes (especially potassium and sodium)	Potassium: 3.5–5 mEq/L Magnesium: 1.7–2.1 mEq/L Sodium: 135–145 mEq/L Chloride: 98–106 mEq/L
	Fasting glucose	70–110 mg/dl
	Lithium	0.6–1.2 mEq/L
	Thyroid function tests	TSH: 0.2–5.4 microunits/ml T₃: 80–200 nanogram/dl T₄: 5.4–11.5 mcg/dl
methotrexate	CBC with differential	*****
	Creatinine	0.6–1.3 mg/dl
	Liver function	*
	Methotrexate	Normal elimination: ~ 10 micromol 24 hours postdose ~ 1 micromol 48 hours postdose < 0.2 micromol 72 hours postdose
	Platelet count	150–450 × 10³/mm³
nonnucleoside reverse transcriptase inhibitors (nevirapine, delavirdine, efavirenz)	Amylase	35–118 international units/L
	CBC with differential and platelets	*****
	Liver function	*
	Lipids (efavirenz)	Total cholesterol: < 200 mg/dl LDL: < 100 mg/dl HDL: Women: 40–75 mg/dl Men: 37–70 mg/dl Triglycerides: 10–150 mg/dl
phenytoin	CBC	*****
	Phenytoin	10–20 mcg/ml
procainamide	ANA titer	Negative
	CBC	*****
	Liver function	*
	N-acetylprocainamide (NAPA)	10–30 mcg/ml
	Procainamide	3–10 mcg/ml

(continued)

***** For those areas marked with asterisks, the following values can be used:

Hemoglobin: Women: 12–16 g/dl
   Men: 14–18 g/dl
Hematocrit: Women: 37%–48%
   Men: 42%–52%
RBCs: 4–5.5 × 10⁶/mm³
WBCs: 5–10 × 10³/mm³
	Differential: Neutrophils: 45%–74%
	Bands: 0%–8%
	Lymphocytes: 16%–45%
	Monocytes: 4%–10%
	Eosinophils: 0%–7%
	Basophils: 0%–2%

Monitoring guidelines

Obtain baseline CBC with differential and platelet count. Repeat weekly, especially if more than 2 weeks of therapy are received. Monitor liver function tests and amylase and lipase levels during therapy.

Checking drug levels is crucial to the safe use of the drug. Obtain level immediately before next dose. Monitor level twice weekly until stable. Once at steady state, level should be checked weekly; when the patient is on the appropriate maintenance dose, levels should be checked every 2 or 3 months. Monitor CBC; creatinine, electrolyte, and fasting glucose levels; and thyroid function test results before therapy starts and periodically thereafter.

Monitor drug levels according to dosing protocol. Monitor CBC with differential, platelet count, and liver and renal function test results more frequently when therapy starts or changes and when methotrexate levels may be elevated, such as when the patient is dehydrated.

Obtain baseline liver function tests and monitor closely during the first 12 weeks of therapy. Continue to monitor regularly during therapy. Check CBC with differential and platelet count before therapy and periodically during therapy. Monitor lipid levels during efavirenz therapy. Monitor amylase level during efavirenz and delavirdine therapy.

Monitor drug level immediately before next dose and 7 to 10 days after therapy starts or changes. Obtain a CBC at baseline and monthly early in therapy. Watch for toxic effects at therapeutic levels. Adjust the measured level for hypoalbuminemia or renal impairment, which can increase free drug levels.

Measure drug levels 6 to 12 hours after a continuous infusion is started or immediately before the next oral dose. Combined procainamide and NAPA levels can be used as an index of toxicity when renal impairment exists. Obtain CBC, liver function tests, and ANA titer periodically during longer-term therapy.

(continued)

* For those areas marked with one asterisk, the following values can be used:

ALT: 7–56 units/L
AST: 5–40 units/L
Alkaline phosphatase: 17–142 units/L
LDH: 60–220 units/L
GGT: < 40 units/L
Total bilirubin: 0.2–1 mg/dl

Drug	Laboratory test monitored	Therapeutic ranges of test
quinidine	CBC	*****
	Creatinine	0.6–1.3 mg/dl
	Electrolytes (especially potassium)	Potassium: 3.5–5 mEq/L
		Magnesium: 1.7–2.1 mEq/L
		Sodium: 135–145 mEq/L
		Chloride: 98–106 mEq/L
	Liver function	*
	Quinidine	2–6 mcg/ml
sulfonylureas	Fasting glucose	70–110 mg/dl
	Glycosylated hemoglobin	4%–7% of total hemoglobin
theophylline	Theophylline	10–20 mcg/ml
thiazolidinediones (rosiglitazone, pioglitazone)	Fasting glucose	70–110 mg/dl
	Glycosylated hemoglobin	4%–7% of total hemoglobin
	Liver function	*
thyroid hormones	Thyroid function tests	TSH: 0.2–5.4 microunits/ml
		T_3: 80–200 nanogram/dl
		T_4: 5.4–11.5 mcg/dl
valproate sodium, valproic acid, divalproex sodium	Ammonia	15–45 mcg/dl
	BUN	5–20 mg/dl
	CBC with differential	*****
	Creatinine	0.6–1.3 mg/dl
	Liver function	*
	Platelet count	150–450 × 10³/mm³
	PTT	10–14 seconds
	Valproic acid	50–100 mcg/ml
vancomycin	Creatinine	0.6–1.3 mg/dl
	Vancomycin	20–40 mcg/ml (peak)
		5–15 mcg/ml (trough)
warfarin	INR	For an acute MI, atrial fibrillation, treatment of pulmonary embolism, prevention of systemic embolism, tissue heart valves, valvular heart disease, or prophylaxis or treatment of venous thrombosis: 2–3
		For mechanical prosthetic valves or recurrent systemic embolism: 2.5–3.5

***** For those areas marked with asterisks, the following values can be used:

Hemoglobin: Women: 12–16 g/dl
  Men: 14–18 g/dl
Hematocrit: Women: 37%–48%
  Men: 42%–52%
RBCs: 4–5.5 × 10⁶/mm³
WBCs: 5–10 × 10³/mm³

Differential: Neutrophils: 45%–74%
  Bands: 0%–8%
  Lymphocytes: 16%–45%
  Monocytes: 4%–10%
  Eosinophils: 0%–7%
  Basophils: 0%–2%

(continued)

Monitoring guidelines

Obtain levels immediately before next oral dose and 30 to 35 hours after therapy starts or changes. Periodically obtain blood counts, liver and kidney function test results, and electrolyte levels. With more specific assays, therapeutic levels are < 1 mcg/ml.

Monitor response to therapy by periodically evaluating fasting glucose and glycosylated hemoglobin levels. Patient should monitor glucose levels at home to help measure compliance and response.

Obtain drug levels right before next dose of sustained-release oral product and at least 2 days after therapy starts or changes.

Monitor response by evaluating fasting glucose and hemoglobin A$_{1c}$ levels. Obtain baseline liver function test results, and repeat tests periodically during therapy.

Monitor thyroid function test results every 2 to 3 weeks until appropriate maintenance dose is determined and annually thereafter.

Monitor liver function test results, ammonia level, coagulation test results, renal function test results, CBC, and platelet count at baseline and periodically during therapy. Liver function test results should be closely monitored during the first 6 months.

Drug levels may be checked with the third dose administered, at the earliest. Draw peak levels 1.5 to 2.5 hours after a 1-hour infusion or I.V. infusion is complete. Draw trough levels within 1 hour of the next dose administered. Renal function can be used to adjust dosing and intervals.

Check INR daily, beginning 3 days after therapy starts. Continue checking it until therapeutic goal is achieved, and monitor it periodically thereafter. Also, check level 7 days after change in dose or start of a potentially interacting therapy.

* For those areas marked with one asterisk, the following values can be used:

ALT: 7–56 units/L
AST: 5–40 units/L
Alkaline phosphatase: 17–142 units/L
LDH: 60–220 units/L
GGT: < 40 units/L
Total bilirubin: 0.2–1 mg/dl

Cytochrome P-450 enzymes and common drug interactions

Cytochrome P-450 enzymes, identified by "CYP" followed by numbers and letters identifying the enzyme families and subfamilies, are found throughout the body (primarily in the liver) and are important in the metabolism of many drugs. This table lists common drug-drug interactions based on substrates, inducers, and inhibitors that can influence drug metabolism.

CYP enzyme	Substrates
1A2	acetaminophen, aminophylline, amitriptyline, betaxolol, caffeine, chlordiazepoxide, clomipramine, clozapine, cyclobenzaprine, desipramine, diazepam, doxepin, flutamide, fluvoxamine, haloperidol, imipramine, mirtazapine, naproxen, olanzapine, pimozide, ropinirole, tacrine, theophylline, verapamil, warfarin, zileuton, zolmitriptan
2C9	alosetron, amiodarone, amitriptyline, bosentan, carvedilol, clomipramine, dapsone, diazepam, diclofenac, flurbiprofen, fluvastatin, glimepiride, glipizide, ibuprofen, imipramine, indomethacin, losartan, mirtazapine, montelukast, naproxen, omeprazole, phenytoin, pioglitazone, piroxicam, ritonavir, sildenafil, tolbutamide, torsemide, vardenafil, voriconazole, warfarin, zafirlukast, zileuton
2C19	amitriptyline, carisoprodol, celecoxib, citalopram, clomipramine, cyclophosphamide, desogestrel, diazepam, doxepin, escitalopram, esomeprazole, fenofibrate, fluoxetine, glyburide, imipramine, irbesartan, lansoprazole, mephenytoin, omeprazole, pantoprazole, pentamidine, phenytoin, phenobarbital, rabeprazole, voriconazole, warfarin
2D6	amitriptyline, amphetamine, aripiprazole, atomoxetine, betaxolol, captopril, carvedilol, chlorpheniramine, chlorpromazine, clomipramine, clozapine, codeine, cyclobenzaprine, delavirdine, desipramine, dextromethorphan, donepezil, doxepin, fentanyl, flecainide, fluoxetine, fluphenazine, fluvoxamine, haloperidol, hydrocodone, imipramine, labetalol, loratadine, maprotiline, meperidine, methadone, methamphetamine, metoprolol, mexiletine, mirtazapine, morphine, nefazodone, nortriptyline, oxycodone, paroxetine, perphenazine, procainamide, propafenone, propoxyphene, propranolol, risperidone, tamoxifen, thioridazine, timolol, tolterodine, tramadol, trazodone, venlafaxine
3A	albuterol, alfentanil, alprazolam, amiodarone, amitriptyline, amlodipine, amprenavir, aripiprazole, atazanavir, atorvastatin, bosentan, bromocriptine, buspirone, busulfan, carbamazepine, chlordiazepoxide, chlorpheniramine, citalopram, clarithromycin, clomipramine, clonazepam, clorazepate, cocaine, colchicine, corticosteroids, cyclophosphamide, cyclosporine (neural), dapsone, delavirdine, dexamethasone, diazepam, diltiazem, disopyramide, docetaxel, doxepin, doxorubicin, doxycycline, efavirenz, enalapril, eplerenone, ergotamine, erythromycin, escitalopram, esomeprazole, estrogens, ethosuximide, etoposide, felodipine, fentanyl, fexofenadine, finasteride, flurazepam, flutamide, fluvastatin, haloperidol, ifosfamide, imatinib, imipramine, indinavir, isosorbide, isradipine, itraconazole, ketamine, ketoconazole, lansoprazole, lidocaine, loratadine, losartan, lovastatin, methadone, methylprednisolone, miconazole, midazolam, mirtazapine, montelukast, nefazodone, nevirapine, nicardipine, nifedipine, nimodipine, nisoldipine, ondansetron, paclitaxel, pantoprazole, pioglitazone, pravastatin, prednisone, quinidine, quinine, rabeprazole, rifabutin, ritonavir, saquinavir, sertraline, sildenafil, simvastatin, tacrolimus, tamoxifen, teniposide, testosterone, tolterodine, trazodone, triazolam, troleandomycin, vardenafil, verapamil, vinca alkaloids, voriconazole, warfarin, zileuton, zolpidem

Inducers	Inhibitors
carbamazepine, cigarette smoking, insulin, omeprazole, phenobarbital, phenytoin, primidone, rifampin, ritonavir	atazanavir, caffeine, cimetidine, ciprofloxacin, clarithromycin, enoxacin, erythromycin, fluvoxamine, grapefruit juice, interferon, isoniazid, ketoconazole, levofloxacin, mexiletine, norethindrone, norfloxacin, omeprazole, paroxetine, tacrine, ticlopidine, zileuton
carbamazepine, phenobarbital, phenytoin, primidone, rifampin	amiodarone, atazanavir, chloramphenicol, cimetidine, co-trimoxazole, delavirdine, disulfiram, fluconazole, fluoxetine, fluvastatin, fluvoxamine, isoniazid, itraconazole, ketoconazole, lovastatin, metronidazole, omeprazole, ritonavir, sertraline, sulfinpyrazone, ticlopidine, trimethoprime, zafirlukast
carbamazepine, phenytoin, prednisone, rifampin	cimetidine, delavirdine, esomeprazole, felbamate, fluconazole, fluoxetine, fluvoxamine, ketoconazole, lansoprazole, omeprazole, sertraline, ticlopidine, topiramate
carbamazepine, dexamethasone, phenobarbital, phenytoin, primidone	amiodarone, bupropion, celecoxib, chloroquine, chlorpheniramine, cimetidine, citalopram, cocaine, delavirdine, fluoxetine, fluphenazine, fluvoxamine, haloperidol, methadone, nefazodone, paroxetine, perphenazine, propafenone, propoxyphene, quinidine, quinine, ritonavir, rosiglitazone, sertraline, terbinafine, thioridazine, venlafaxine
barbiturates, carbamazepine, glucocorticoids, griseofulvin, nafcillin, nevirapine, oxcarbazepine, phenytoin, primidone, rifabutin, rifampin	amprenavir, atazanavir, bromocriptine, clarithromycin, cimetidine, cyclosporine (neural), danazol, delavirdine, diltiazem, erythromycin, fluconazole, fluoxetine, fluvoxamine, fosamprenavir, grapefruit juice, imatinib, indinavir, isoniazid, itraconazole, ketoconazole, metronidazole, miconazole, nefazodone, nelfinavir, nicardipine, nifedipine, norfloxacin, omeprazole, prednisone, quinidine, quinine, rifabutin, ritonavir, saquinavir, sertraline, troleandomycin, verapamil, zafirlukast

Drugs that prolong the QTc interval

Changes in a patient's heart rate can affect the QT interval of his ECG. To account for such changes, you can use a formula such as the one below. Such formulas let you determine the corrected QT (QTc) interval.

$$\frac{QT\ interval}{\sqrt{R\text{-}R\ internal}} = QTc\ interval$$

For men younger than age 55, a normal QTc interval is 350 to 430 msec; for women younger than age 55, a normal QTc interval is 350 to 450 msec.

A prolonged QTc interval may cause fatal arrhythmias, including ventricular tachycardia and torsades de pointes. The causes of a prolonged QTc interval include disorders such as hypokalemia, hypomagnesemia, renal failure, and heart failure. These drugs may also cause an abnormal QTc interval.

albuterol
amantadine
amiodarone
arformoterol
aripiprazole
arsenic trioxide
azithromycin
celecoxib
chloral hydrate
chloroquine
chlorpromazine
cisapride
clarithromycin
clindamycin
clozapine
cyclobenzaprine
diphenhydramine
disopyramide
dofetilide
dolasetron
domperidone
doxorubicin
droperidol
efavirenz
erythromycin
famotidine

felbamate
fexofenadine
flecainide
fluconazole
fluphenazine
formoterol
foscarnet
fosphenytoin
furosemide
gemifloxacin
granisetron
halofantrine
haloperidol
halothane
hydroxyzine
ibutilide
indapamide
isoproterenol
isradipine
itraconazole
ketoconazole
levofloxacin
levomethadyl
lithium
maprotiline
mefloquine

mesoridazine
methadone
moexipril
moxifloxacin
naratriptan
nicardipine
nilotinib
octreotide
ofloxacin
ondansetron
oxytocin
palonosetron
papaverine
pentamidine
perphenazine
pimozide
prednisolone
prednisone
procainamide
propafenone
quetiapine
quinidine
quinine
ranolazine
risperidone
salmeterol

serotonin reuptake inhibitors
sotalol
sparfloxacin
sulfamethoxazole
sumatriptan
tacrolimus
tamoxifen
telithromycin
terbutaline
tetrabenazine
thioridazine
tizanidine
trazodone
tricyclic antidepressants
trimethoprim
trifluoperazine
vardenafil
vasopressin
voriconazole
vorinostat
ziprasidone
zolmitriptan

Dialyzable drugs

The amount of a drug removed by dialysis differs among patients and depends on several factors, including the patient's condition, the drug's properties, length of dialysis and dialysate used, rate of blood flow or dwell time, and purpose of dialysis. This table indicates the effect of conventional hemodialysis on selected drugs.

Drug	Level reduced by hemodialysis	Drug	Level reduced by hemodialysis
acebutolol	Yes	buspirone	No
acetaminophen	Yes (may not influence toxicity)	busulfan	Yes
		captopril	Yes
acetazolamide	No	carbamazepine	No
acetylcysteine	Yes	carbenicillin	Yes
acyclovir	Yes	carboplatin	Yes
albuterol	No	carisoprodol	Yes
allopurinol	Yes	carmustine	No
alprazolam	No	carvedilol	No
amantadine	No	cefaclor	Yes
amikacin	Yes	cefadroxil	Yes
amiodarone	No	cefazolin	Yes
amitriptyline	No	cefepime	Yes
amlodipine	No	cefotaxime	Yes
amoxicillin	Yes	cefotetan	Yes (only by 20%)
amoxicillin and clavulanate potassium	Yes	cefoxitin	Yes
		cefpodoxime	Yes
amphotericin B	No	ceftazidime	Yes
ampicillin	Yes	ceftibuten	Yes
ampicillin and sulbactam sodium	Yes	ceftizoxime	Yes
		ceftriaxone	No
aprepitant	No	cefuroxime	Yes
arsenic trioxide	No	cephalexin	Yes
ascorbic acid	Yes	cephradine	Yes
aspirin	Yes	chloral hydrate	Yes
atenolol	Yes	chlorambucil	No
atorvastatin	No	chloramphenicol	Yes (very small amount)
atropine	No		
auranofin	No	chlordiazepoxide	No
azathioprine	Yes	chlorpheniramine	Yes
aztreonam	Yes	chlorpromazine	No
bivalirudin	Yes	chlorthalidone	No
bretylium	No	cimetidine	Yes
bumetanide	No	ciprofloxacin	Yes (only by 10%)
bupropion	No	cisplatin	No

Drug	Level reduced by hemodialysis	Drug	Level reduced by hemodialysis
clavulanic acid	Yes	famciclovir	Yes
clindamycin	No	famotidine	No
clofibrate	No	fenoprofen	No
clonazepam	No	filgrastim	No
clonidine	No	flecainide	No
clorazepate	No	fluconazole	Yes
cloxacillin	No	flucytosine	Yes
codeine	No	fluorouracil	No
colchicine	No	fluoxetine	No
cortisone	No	flurazepam	No
co-trimoxazole	Yes	foscarnet	Yes
cyclophosphamide	Yes	fosinopril	No
deferoxamine	Yes	furosemide	No
desloratadine	No	gabapentin	Yes
dexamethsone	No	ganciclovir	Yes
diazepam	No	gemcitabine	Yes
diazoxide	Yes	gemfibrozil	No
diclofenac	No	gemifloxacin	Yes
dicloxacillin	No	gentamicin	Yes
didanosine	Yes	glipizide	No
digoxin	No	glyburide	No
digoxin immune Fab	No	guanfacine	No
diltiazem	No	haloperidol	No
diphenhydramine	No	heparin	No
dipyridamole	No	hydralazine	No
disopyramide	Yes	hydrochlorothiazide	No
dopamine	No	hydroxyzine	No
doripenem	Yes	ibuprofen	No
doxazosin	No	ifosfamide	Yes
doxepin	No	imipenem	Yes
doxorubicin	No	imipramine	No
doxycycline	No	indapamide	No
emtricitabine	Yes	indomethacin	No
enalapril	Yes	insulin	No
enoxaparin	No	irbesartan	No
epoetin alfa	No	iron dextran	No
ertapenem	Yes	isoniazid	No
erythromycin	Yes (only by 20%)	isosorbide	Yes
ethacrynic acid	No	isradipine	No
ethambutol	Yes (only by 20%)	kanamycin	Yes
ethosuximide	Yes	ketoconazole	No

Drug	Level reduced by hemodialysis	Drug	Level reduced by hemodialysis
labetalol	No	nabumetone	No
lamivudine	No	nadolol	Yes
lansoprazole	No	nafcillin	No
lapatinib	yes	nalmefene	No
levetiracetam	Yes	naltrexone	No
levocetirizine	No	naproxen	No
levofloxacin	No	nelfinavir	No
lidocaine	No	nicardipine	No
linezolid	Yes	nifedipine	No
lisinopril	Yes	nimodipine	No
lithium	Yes	nitazoxanide	No
lomefloxacin	No	nitrofurantoin	Yes
lomustine	No	nitroglycerin	No
loratadine	No	nitroprusside	Yes
lorazepam	No	nizatidine	No
mannitol	No	norfloxacin	No
maraviroc	Yes	nortriptyline	No
mechlorethamine	No	octreotide	yes
mefenamic acid	No	ofloxacin	Yes
meperidine	No	olanzapine	No
meprobamate	Yes	omeprazole	No
mercaptopurine	Yes	oxazepam	No
meropenem	Yes	paclitaxel	No
mesalamine	Yes	paroxetine	No
metformin	Yes	penicillin G	Yes
methadone	No	pentamidine	No
methotrexate	Yes	pentazocine	Yes
methyldopa	Yes	pentobarbital	No
methylprednisolone	Yes	perindopril	Yes
metoclopramide	No	phenobarbital	Yes
metolazone	No	phenylbutazone	No
metoprolol	Yes	phenytoin	No
metronidazole	Yes	piperacillin	Yes
mexiletine	Yes	piroxicam	No
miconazole	No	prazosin	No
midazolam	No	prednisone	No
minocycline	No	pregabalin	Yes
minoxidil	Yes	primidone	Yes
misoprostol	No	procainamide	Yes
morphine	No	promethazine	No
		propoxyphene	No

Drug	Level reduced by hemodialysis	Drug	Level reduced by hemodialysis
propranolol	No	triazolam	No
protriptyline	No	trimethoprim	Yes
pseudoephedrine	No	valacyclovir	Yes
pyrazinamide	Yes	valganciclovir	Yes
pyridoxine	Yes	valproic acid	No
quinapril	No	valsartan	No
quinidine	No	vancomycin	Yes
quinine	No	venlafaxine	No
ramipril	No	verapamil	No
ranitidine	Yes	vigabatrin	Yes
rifampin	No	wartarin	No
ritodrine	Yes	zolpidem	No
rituximab	No	zonisamide	Yes
rosiglitazone	No		
salsalate	Yes		
sertraline	No		
sotalol	Yes		
stavudine	Yes		
streptomycin	Yes		
sucralfate	No		
sulbactam	Yes		
sulfamethoxazole	Yes		
sulfisoxazole	No		
sulindac	No		
tazobactam	Yes		
telbivudine	Yes (by 23%)		
temazepam	No		
theophylline	Yes		
ticarcillin	Yes		
ticarcillin and clavulanate	Yes		
timolol	No		
tirofiban	Yes		
tobramycin	Yes		
tocainide	Yes		
tolbutamide	No		
topiramate	Yes		
topotecan	Yes		
torsemide	No		
tramadol	No		
trandolapril	Yes		
trazodone	No		

Abbreviations to avoid

The Joint Commission requires every health care facility to develop a list of approved abbreviations for staff use. Certain abbreviations should be avoided because they're easily misunderstood, especially when handwritten. The Joint Commission has identified a minimum list of dangerous abbreviations, acronyms, and symbols. This do-not-use list includes the following items.

Abbreviation	Intended meaning	Misinterpretation	Correction
U or *u*	unit	Frequently misinterpreted as a "0" or a "4," causing a tenfold or greater over-dose	Write "unit."
IU	international unit	Frequently misinterpreted as I.V. or 10	Write "international unit."
q.d., q.o.d. Q.D., QD, Q.O.D., QOD	every day, every other day	Mistaken for each other. The period after the "q" has sometimes been mis-interpreted as "i," the "o" can be mistaken for "i," and the drug has been given q.i.d. rather than daily.	Write them out.
Trailing zero (5.0 mg)	5 mg	Frequently misinterpreted dosage, such as: 50 mg	Never write a zero by itself after a decimal point and always use a zero before a decimal point if no other number is present.
Lack of leading zero (.5 mg)	0.5 mg	5 mg	
MS, MSO₄, MgSO₄	morphine sulfate magnesium sulfate	Confused with each other	Write "morphine sulfate" or "magnesium sulfate."

(continued)

In addition to the minimum required list, the following items should also be considered when expanding the do-not-use list.

Abbreviation	Intended meaning	Misinterpretation	Correction
MTX	methotrexate	Misinterpreted as Mustar-gen (mechlorethamine hydrochloride)	Use the complete spelling for drug names.
DIG	digoxin	Misinterpreted as digitoxin	Use the complete spelling for drug names.
HCTZ	hydrochlorothiazide	Misinterpreted as hydro-cortisone (HCT)	Use the complete spelling for drug names.
ara-A	vidarabine	Misinterpreted as cytara-bine (ara-C)	Use the complete spelling for drug names.
μg	microgram	Frequently misinterpreted as "mg"	Write "mcg."
cc	cubic centimeter	Frequently misinterpreted as U (units)	Write "ml" for milliliters.
A.S., A.D., and AU	Latin abbreviations for left ear, right ear, and both ears, respectively	Frequently misinterpreted as O.S., O.D., and OU	Write "left ear," "right ear," or "both ears."
OD	once daily	Frequently misinterpreted as "O.D." (*oculus dexter*—right eye)	Don't abbreviate "daily." Write it out.
OJ	orange juice	Frequently misinterpreted as "O.D." (*oculus dexter*—right eye) or "O.S." (*oculus sinister*—left eye) Drugs meant to be diluted in orange juice may be given in the eye.	Write it out.
qn.	nightly or at bedtime	Frequently misinterpreted as "q.h." (every hour)	Write out "nightly" or "at bedtime."
S.C. SQ	subcutaneous	Mistaken as SL for sub-lingual or "5 every"	Use "SubQ," "subQ," or write out "subcutaneous."
D/C	discharge or discon-tinue	Frequently misinterpreted	Write "discharge" or "dis-continue."
h.s.	half-strength or bed-time	Frequently misinterpreted as the other	Write out "half-strength" or "at bedtime."
T.I.W.	three times per week	Frequently misinterpreted as three times per day or twice weekly	Write it out.

©*The Joint Commission, 2008. Reprinted with permission.*

Herbal supplements

If your patient is taking an herbal supplement, ask him some general questions, such as why he's taking the herb and how long he has been taking it. Find out if the condition he's trying to treat has been diagnosed. If so, is he taking or has he taken prescription or OTC drugs for the condition?

If your patient is taking a prescription or OTC drug and an herbal supplement, explain that drug–herb interactions can occur, and advise him to report any unusual signs or symptoms.

For nursing considerations and patient-teaching information on specific herbal supplements, see the table below.

Herb and reported uses	Nursing considerations	Patient teaching
Aloe • Burns and skin irritation • Cathartic • To ease discomfort of defecation	• Herb's laxative effects are apparent within 10 hours of ingestion. • Monitor patient for signs of dehydration. Elderly patients are particularly at risk. • Monitor electrolyte levels, especially potassium, after long-term use. • If patient is using herb topically, monitor wound for healing.	• Caution patient that if he delays seeking medical diagnosis and treatment, his condition could worsen. • If patient is taking digoxin or another drug to control his heart rate, a diuretic, or a corticosteroid, warn him not to take herb without consulting his health care provider. • Advise patient not to take herb for longer than 1 to 2 weeks at a time without consulting his health care provider.
Chamomile • Antibacterial, antiviral • Diarrhea, flatulence, stomatitis, motion sickness • Hemorrhagic cystitis • Sedation, relaxation • Skin inflammation, wounds, burns	• **ALERT:** Patients sensitive to ragweed and chrysanthemums or other Compositae family members (arnica, yarrow, feverfew, tansy, artemisia) may be more susceptible to contact allergies and anaphylaxis. Patients with hay fever or bronchial asthma caused by pollens are more susceptible to anaphylactic reactions.	• Advise patient against use during pregnancy. • If patient is taking an anticoagulant, advise him not to use herb because of possible enhanced anticoagulant effects. • Advise patient that herb may enhance an allergic reaction or make existing symptoms worse in susceptible patients. • Instruct parent not to give herb to any child before checking with an experienced practitioner.
Cranberry • Asthma • Fever • Kidney stones • UTI	• Tinctures may contain up to 45% alcohol. • Herb's ability to prevent bacteria from adhering to the bladder wall seems important in preventing UTIs. • Herb is safe for pregnant and breast-feeding women. • When consumed regularly, herb may be effective in reducing the frequency of bacteriuria with pyuria in women with recurrent UTIs.	• Advise patient that an appropriate antibiotic is usually needed to treat an active UTI. • If patient is using herb to prevent a UTI, advise him to notify his health care provider if signs or symptoms of a UTI appear. • If patient has diabetes, inform him that the juice contains sugar but that sugar-free supplements and juices are available. • Only the unsweetened, unprocessed juice is effective in preventing bacteria from adhering to the bladder wall.

Herb and reported uses	Nursing considerations	Patient teaching
Echinacea • Abscesses, burns, eczema, skin ulcers • Immune system stimulant • Prevention of common cold, upper respiratory infections • Upper respiratory tract infection	• Daily dose depends on the preparation and potency but shouldn't exceed 8 weeks. Consult specific manufacturer's instructions for parenteral administration, if applicable. • Herb is considered supportive treatment for infection; it shouldn't be used in place of antibiotic therapy. • Herb is usually taken at the first sign of illness and continued for up to 14 days. Regular prophylactic use isn't recommended. • A liquid preparation is recommended because herb is thought to function in the mouth and should have direct contact with the lymph tissues at the back of the throat.	• Advise patient not to delay seeking appropriate medical evaluation for a prolonged illness. • Advise patient that prolonged use may result in overstimulation of the immune system and possible immune suppression. Herb shouldn't be used longer than 14 days for supportive treatment of infection. • The herb should be stored away from direct light. • Warn patients to keep all herbal products away from children and pets.
Ephedra • Appetite suppressant • Asthma • Chills, cough, cold, flu, fever, headache, edema, nasal congestion • CV stimulant • Respiratory tract diseases, mild bronchospasm	• Compounds containing herb may be linked to several deaths and more than 800 adverse effects, many of which appear to be dose related. • Patients with eating disorders may abuse this herb. • **ALERT:** Pills containing herb have been combined with other stimulants such as caffeine and sold as "natural" stimulants in weight loss products. Death from overstimulation may occur. • Signs and symptoms of toxic reaction include diaphoresis, dilated pupils, muscle spasms, fever, and cardiac and respiratory failure. • If overdose occurs, perform gastric lavage and give activated charcoal. Treat spasms with diazepam, replace electrolytes with I.V. fluids, and prevent acidosis with sodium bicarbonate infusions.	• Advise patient not to use this herb in place of getting the proper medical evaluation for a prolonged illness. • **ALERT:** The FDA has banned the sale of dietary supplements containing this herb because of unreasonable risk of injury or illness. • Advise patient with thyroid disease, hypertension, CV disease, or diabetes to avoid using herb. • Advise patient not to use herb. Dosages that are purported to produce psychoactive or hallucinogenic effects are toxic to the heart. • Advise patient to watch for adverse reactions, particularly chest pain, shortness of breath, palpitations, dizziness, and fainting. • Warn patient to keep all herbal products away from children and pets.
Feverfew • Abortifacient • Asthma • Menstrual cramps • Migraine headache • Mouthwash • Psoriasis • Rheumatoid arthritis • Tranquilizer	• If patient is taking an anticoagulant, monitor appropriate coagulation values, such as INR, PTT, and PT. Also, observe patient for abnormal bleeding. • Rash or contact dermatitis may indicate sensitivity to herb. Patient should stop use immediately. • Abruptly stopping the herb may cause "postfeverfew syndrome," involving tension headaches, insomnia, joint stiffness and pain, and lethargy.	• Use during pregnancy isn't recommended. • Educate patient about the risk of abnormal bleeding when combining herb with an anticoagulant, such as warfarin or heparin, or an antiplatelet, such as aspirin or another NSAID. • Caution patient that a rash or abnormal skin alteration may indicate an allergy to herb. Instruct patient to stop taking the herb if a rash appears.
Flax • Constipation • Diarrhea • Diverticulitis	• When herb is used internally, it should be taken with more than 5 oz of liquid per tablespoon of flaxseed.	• Warn patient not to treat chronic constipation or other GI disturbances or ophthalmic injury with herb before seeking appropriate medical evaluation because doing so may delay

Herb and reported uses	Nursing considerations	Patient teaching
Flax *(continued)* • Externally as poultice for skin inflammation • Irritable bowel syndrome	• Cyanogenic glycosides may release cyanide; however, the body only metabolizes these to a certain extent. At therapeutic doses, flax doesn't elevate cyanide ion level. • Although herb may decrease a patient's cholesterol level or increase bleeding time, it isn't necessary to monitor cholesterol level or platelet aggregation.	diagnosis of a potentially serious medical condition. • Discourage use during pregnancy. • Instruct patient to drink plenty of water when taking flaxseed. • Instruct patient not to take any drug for at least 2 hours after taking herb.
Garlic • Atherosclerosis prevention • Cholesterol and triglyceride levels reduction • Colds, coughs, fever, and sore throat • GI tract cancers prevention • HDL cholesterol level increase • MI and stroke prevention	• Herb isn't recommended for patients with diabetes, insomnia, pemphigus, organ transplants, or rheumatoid arthritis or for postsurgical patients. • Consuming excessive amounts of raw garlic increases the risk of adverse reactions. • Monitor patient for signs and symptoms of bleeding. • Herb may lower glucose level. If patient is taking an antidiabetic, watch for signs and symptoms of hypoglycemia, and monitor his glucose level. • **ALERT:** Advise parents not to use oil to treat inner ear infection in children.	• Advise patient not to delay seeking appropriate medical evaluation because doing so may delay diagnosis of a serious medical condition. • Advise patient to consume herb in moderation, to minimize the risk of adverse reactions. • Discourage heavy use of herb before surgery. • If patient is using herb to lower his cholesterol levels, advise him to notify his health care provider and to have his cholesterol levels monitored. • Advise patient that using herb with anticoagulants may increase the risk of bleeding. • If patient is using herb as a topical antiseptic, avoid prolonged exposure to the skin because burns can occur.
Ginger • Antiemetic • Anti-inflammatory, antiarthritic • Antispasmodic • Antitumorigenic • Colic, flatulence, indigestion • Hypercholesterolemia, burns, ulcers, depression, impotence, liver toxicity	• Adverse reactions are uncommon. • Monitor patient for signs and symptoms of bleeding. If patient is taking an anticoagulant, monitor PTT, PT, and INR carefully. • Use in pregnant patients is questionable, although small amounts used in cooking are safe. It's unknown if ginger appears in breast milk. • Herb may interfere with the intended therapeutic effect of conventional drugs. • If overdose occurs, monitor patient for arrhythmias and CNS depression.	• If woman is pregnant, advise her to consult an experienced practitioner before using herb medicinally. • Educate patients to look for signs of bleeding, such as nosebleeds or excessive bruising. • Warn patient to keep all herbal products away from children and pets.
Ginkgo • Cerebral insufficiency, dementia, and circulatory disorders • Headaches, asthma, colitis, impotence, depression, altitude sickness, tinnitus, cochlear deafness, vertigo, pre-	• Extracts are considered standardized if they contain 24% flavonoid glycosides and 6% terpene lactones. • Treatment should continue for at least 6 to 8 weeks, but therapy beyond 3 months isn't recommended. • **ALERT:** Seizures have been reported in children after ingestion of more than 50 seeds.	• If patient is taking the herb for motion sickness, advise him to begin taking it 1 to 2 days before taking the trip and to keep taking it for the duration of his trip. • Inform patient that the therapeutic and toxic components of ginkgo can vary significantly from product to product. Advise him to obtain herb from a reliable source.

Herb and reported uses	Nursing considerations	Patient teaching
Ginkgo *(continued)* menstrual syndrome, macular degeneration, diabetic retinopathy, and allergies • Pancreatic cancer and schizophrenia adjunct	• Patients must be monitored for possible adverse reactions, such as GI problems, headaches, dizziness, allergic reactions, and serious bleeding. • Toxicity may cause atonia and adynamia.	• Warn patient to keep all herbal products away from children and pets. • Advise patient to stop use at least 2 weeks before surgery.
Ginseng, Asian • Fatigue and lack of concentration, atherosclerosis, bleeding disorders, colitis, diabetes, depression, and cancer • Health and strength recovery after sickness or weakness	• The German Commission E doesn't recommend using herb for longer than 3 months. • Herb may strengthen the body and increase resistance to disease. • **ALERT:** Reports have circulated of a severe reaction known as the ginseng abuse syndrome in patients taking more than 3 g/day for up to 2 years: Increased motor and cognitive activity with diarrhea, nervousness, insomnia, hypertension, edema, and skin eruptions.	• Inform patient that the therapeutic and toxic components can vary significantly from product to product. Advise him to obtain herb from a reliable source.
Green tea • To prevent cancer, hyperlipidemia, atherosclerosis, dental caries, headaches • Wounds, skin disorders, stomach disorders, and infectious diarrhea • CNS stimulant, mild diuretic, antibacterial, topical astringent	• Daily consumption should be limited to fewer than 5 cups, or the equivalent of 300 mg of caffeine, to avoid the adverse effects of caffeine. • Prolonged high caffeine intake may cause restlessness, irritability, insomnia, palpitations, vertigo, headache, and adverse GI effects. • The adverse GI effects of chlorogenic acid and tannin can be avoided if milk is added to the tea mixture. • The tannin content in tea increases the longer it's left to brew; this increases the antidiarrheal properties of the tea. • The first signs of a toxic reaction are vomiting and abdominal spasm.	• Advise patient that heavy consumption may be associated with esophageal cancer secondary to the tannin content in the mixture. • Tell patient that the first signs of toxic reaction are vomiting and abdominal spasm. • Tell patient that herb interferes with iron absorption from supplements or multivitamins.
Hawthorn • Atherosclerosis • Blood pressure regulation • Cardiotonic and sedative • Mild heart conditions	• High doses may cause hypotension and sedation. Monitor patient for CNS adverse effects, and monitor blood pressure. • Herb may interfere with digoxin's effects or serum monitoring. • Observe patient closely for adverse reactions, especially adverse CNS reactions.	• Advise patient that when he fills a prescription, he should tell the pharmacist of any herb or dietary supplement he's taking. • Advise patient to avoid herb because of toxic adverse effects. • Warn patient to keep all herbal products away from children and pets.
Horse chestnut • Analgesic, anticoagulant, antipyretic, astringent, expectorant, and tonic	• **ALERT:** The nuts, seeds, twigs, sprouts, and leaves of horse chestnut are poisonous and can be lethal. • Standardized formulations remove most of the toxins and standardize the amount of aescin.	• Inform patient that the FDA considers herb unsafe and that death may occur. • Advise patient not to confuse horse chestnut with sweet chestnut, used as a food.

Herb and reported uses	Nursing considerations	Patient teaching
Horse chestnut *(continued)* • Chronic venous insufficiency, varicose veins, leg pain, tiredness, tension, and leg swelling and edema • Lymphedema, hemorrhoids, and enlarged prostate • Skin ulcers, phlebitis, leg cramps, cough, and diarrhea	• Signs and symptoms of toxicity include loss of coordination, salivation, hemolysis, headache, dilated pupils, muscle twitching, seizures, vomiting, diarrhea, depression, paralysis, respiratory and cardiac failure, and death. • Monitor patient for signs of toxicity. • Monitor glucose level in patients taking antidiabetics for hypoglycemia.	• Warn patient to keep the herb away from children. Consumption of amounts of leaves, twigs, and seeds equaling 1% of a child's weight may be lethal.
Kava • Nervous anxiety, stress, and restlessness • Skin diseases, including leprosy • Intestinal problems, otitis, and abscesses • Urogenital infections, including chronic cystitis, venereal disease, uterine inflammation, menstrual problems, and vaginal prolapse • Wound healing, headaches, seizure disorders, the common cold, respiratory tract infection, tuberculosis, and rheumatism	• Patient shouldn't use herb with conventional sedative-hypnotics, anxiolytics, MAO inhibitors, other psychopharmacologic drugs, levodopa, or antiplatelet drugs without first consulting a health care provider. • Use for longer than 3 months may be habit forming. • Herb can cause drowsiness and may impair motor reflexes. • Patients should avoid taking herb with alcohol because of increased risk of CNS depression and liver damage. • Periodic monitoring of liver function tests and CBC may be needed. • Toxic doses can cause progressive ataxia, muscle weakness, and ascending paralysis, all of which resolve when herb is stopped. Extreme use (more than 300 g per week) may increase GGT levels.	• Tell patient oral use is probably safe for 3 months or less, but use for longer than 3 months may be habit forming. • Warn patient to avoid taking herb with alcohol because of increased risk of CNS depression and liver damage. • **ALERT:** Tell patient that the FDA has linked herb to liver problems including cirrhosis, hepatitis, and liver failure. Herb users should immediately contact their health care provider if their skin or eyes begin to yellow, or they experience severe itching, easy bruising, dark urine, or bloody vomit.
Melatonin • Insomnia, jet lag, shift-work disorder, blind entrainment, immune system enhancement, tinnitus, depression, and benzodiazepine withdrawal • Cancer therapy adjunct, antiaging product, and pregnancy and cluster headaches preventative • Skin protection against ultraviolet light	• Monitor patient for excessive daytime drowsiness. • May increase human growth hormone levels.	• Warn patient to avoid hazardous activities until full extent of CNS depressant effect is known. • If patient wishes to conceive, tell her that herb may have a contraceptive effect. However, herb shouldn't be used as birth control. • Although no chemical interactions have been reported, tell patient that herb may interfere with therapeutic effects of conventional drugs. • Warn patient about possible additive effects if taken with alcohol. • Advise patient not to use herb for prolonged periods because safety data aren't available.

Herb and reported uses	Nursing considerations	Patient teaching
Milk thistle • Dyspepsia, liver damage from chemicals, Amanita mushroom poisoning, supportive therapy for inflammatory liver disease and cirrhosis, loss of appetite, and gall bladder and spleen disorders • Liver protectant	• Mild allergic reactions may occur, especially in people allergic to members of the Astertaceae family, including ragweed, chrysanthemums, marigolds, and daisies. • Don't confuse seeds or fruit with other parts of the plant or with blessed thistle.	• Warn woman not to take this herb while pregnant or breast-feeding. • Tell patient to stay alert for possible allergic reactions, especially if allergic to ragweed, chrysanthemums, marigolds, or daisies. • Warn patient not to take herb for liver inflammation or cirrhosis before seeking appropriate medical evaluation because doing so may delay diagnosis of a potentially serious medical condition.
Passion flower • Sedative, hypnotic, analgesic, antispasmodic, menstrual cramps, pain, migraines • Neuralgia, generalized seizures, hysteria, nervous agitation, and insomnia • Topically for cuts and bruises	• Monitor patient for possible adverse CNS effects. • A disulfiram-like reaction may produce nausea, vomiting, flushing, headache, hypotension, tachycardia, ventricular arrhythmias, and shock leading to death. • Patients with liver disease and alcoholics shouldn't use herbal products that contain alcohol.	• Because sedation is possible, caution patient to avoid hazardous activities. • Warn patient not to take herb for chronic pain or insomnia before seeking medical attention because doing so may delay diagnosis of a potentially serious medical condition. • Caution pregnant patient to avoid this herb.
Saw palmetto • BPH and coughs and congestion from colds, bronchitis, or asthma • Mild diuretic, urinary antiseptic, and astringent	• Herb should be used cautiously for conditions other than BPH because data about its effectiveness in other conditions are lacking. • Obtain a baseline prostate-specific antigen (PSA) value before patient starts taking herb because it may cause a false-negative PSA result. • Saw palmetto may not alter prostate size. • Laboratory values didn't change significantly in clinical trials using dosages of 160 mg to 320 mg daily.	• Warn patient not to take herb for bladder or prostate problems before seeking medical attention because doing so could delay diagnosis of a potentially serious medical condition. • Tell patient to take herb with food to minimize GI effects. • Caution patient to promptly notify health care provider about new or worsened adverse effects. • Warn woman to avoid herb if planning pregnancy, if pregnant, or if breast-feeding.
St. John's wort • Mild to moderate depression, anxiety, sciatica, and viral infections, including herpes simplex virus, hepatitis C, influenza virus, murine cytomegalovirus, and poliovirus • Bronchitis, asthma, gallbladder disease, nocturnal enuresis, gout, and rheumatism	• Recommended duration of therapy for depression is 4 to 6 weeks; if no improvement occurs, a different therapy should be considered. • Monitor patient for response to herbal therapy, as evidenced by improved mood and lessened depression. • By using standardized extracts, patient can better control the dosage. Studies have used forms of standardized 0.3% hypericin as well as hyperforin-stabilized version of the extract. • Serotonin syndrome may cause dizziness, nausea, vomiting, headache, epigastric pain, anxiety, confusion, restlessness, and irritability.	• Instruct patient to consult a health care provider for a thorough medical evaluation before using herb. • If patient takes herb for mild to moderate depression, explain that several weeks may pass before effects occur. Tell patient that a new therapy may be needed if no improvement occurs in 4 to 6 weeks. • Inform patient that herb interacts with many other prescription and OTC products and may reduce their effectiveness. • Tell patient that herb may cause increased sensitivity to direct sunlight. Recommend protective clothing, sunscreen, and limited sun exposure.

Herb and reported uses	Nursing considerations	Patient teaching
St. John's wort *(continued)*	• Because herb decreases the effect of certain prescription drugs, watch for signs of drug toxicity if patient stops using the herb. Drug dosage may need to be reduced. • Herb has mutagenic effects on sperm and egg cells. It shouldn't be used by pregnant patients, women planning pregnancy, or men wishing to father a child.	• Inform patient that a sufficient wash-out period is needed after stopping an antidepressant before switching to herb. • Tell patient to report adverse effects to a health care provider. • Warn patient to keep all herbal products away from children and pets.
Tea tree oil • Contusions, inflammation, myalgia, burns, hemorrhoids, and vitiligo • Tonsillitis and lotion for dermatoses	• Because of systemic toxicity, herb shouldn't be used internally. • Essential oil should be used externally only after being diluted. • Herb may cause burns or itching in tender areas and shouldn't be used around nose, eyes, and mouth. • 100% pure essential oil is rarely used and should be used only with close supervision by a health care provider.	• Explain that a few drops are sufficient in mouthwash, shampoo, or sitz bath. • Caution patient not to apply oil to wounds or to skin that's dry or cracked. • Warn patient to keep all herbal products away from children and pets.

Acknowledgments

We would like to thank the following companies for granting us permission to include their drugs in the full-color photoguide. We would also like to thank Facts & Comparisons for the use of their resources.

Abbott Laboratories
Biaxin®, Biaxin® XL, Depakote®, Depakote® Sprinkle, E-Mycin®, Ery-Tab®, Hytrin®, Kaletra™, Synthroid®, Vicodin®, Vicodin ES®

Akrimax Pharmaceuticals
Inderal®, Inderal LA®

AstraZeneca LP
Arimidex®, Crestor®, Prilosec®, Tenormin®, Toprol-XL®, Zestril®

Aventis Pharmaceuticals
Allegra®, Ambien®, DiaBeta®, Lasix®, Trental®

Axcan Pharma
Carafate®

Bayer Healthcare Pharmaceuticals
Nexavar®

Biovail Pharmaceuticals, Inc.
Cardizem®, Cardizem® CD, Cardizem® LA, Vasotec®

Bristol-Myers Squibb Company
BuSpar®, Cefzil®, Coumadin®, Monopril®, Pravachol®, Reyataz®, Sinemet®, Sinemet CR®

CV Therapeutics
Ranexa®

Elan Pharmaceuticals, Inc.
Frova™

Forest Pharmaceuticals, Inc.
Campral®, Celexa®, Lexapro™

Gilead Sciences
Viread®

GlaxoSmithKline
Copyright GlaxoSmithKline. Used with permission.
Avandia®, Combivir ®, Imitrex®, Retrovir®, Zantac®

Janssen Pharmaceutica, Inc.
Risperdal®, Risperdal M-Tab®

King Pharmaceuticals, Inc.
Levoxyl®

Eli Lilly and Company
Cymbalta®, Evista®, Prozac®, Strattera™
Copyright 2008 Eli Lilly and Company.
Used with permission.

Mallinckrodt, Inc.
Pamelor®, Restoril®

McNeil-PPC, Inc.
Concerta®

MedPointe Pharmaceuticals
Soma®

Merck & Co., Inc.
Used with permission of Merck & Co., Inc.
Cozaar®, Crixivan®, Fosamax®, Januvia®, Mevacor®, Pepcid®, Prinivil®, Singulair®, Zocor®

Merck Santé
An associate of Merck KGaA, Darmstadt, Germany.
Glucophage®, Glucophage® XR

Merck/Schering-Plough Pharmaceuticals
Used with permission of Merck/Schering-Plough Pharmaceuticals.
Zetia™

Novartis Pharmaceuticals
Diovan®, Enablex®, Lescol®, Lotensin®, Ritalin®, Ritalin SR®, Stalevo®,
Used by permission

Ortho-McNeil Pharmaceutical
Floxin®, Levaquin®, Tylenol® with
Codeine No. 3, Ultracet®

Otsuka Pharmaceutical Company, Ltd.
Abilify®

Pfizer
Used with permission of Pfizer, Inc.
Accupril®, Calan®, Cardura®, Celebrex®,
Chantix®, Detrol®, Diflucan®, Dilantin
Kapseals®, Glucotrol®, Glucotrol XL®,
Lipitor®, Lopid®, Medrol®, Micronase®,
Neurontin®, Nitrostat®, Norvasc®,
Procardia XL®, Provera®, Relpax®,
Sutent®, Viagra®, Xanax®, Zithromax®,
Zoloft®

**Procter and Gamble
Pharmaceuticals, Inc.**
Actonel©, Macrobid®

Purdue Pharma L.P.
OxyContin®

Ranbaxy, Inc.
Isoptin SR®

Roche Laboratories, Inc.
Bumex®, Klonopin®, Naprosyn®,
Ticlid®, Valium®
Reprinted with the permission of Roche
Laboratories Inc. All rights reserved.

Sanofi-Synthelabo, Inc.
Demerol®, Uroxatral®

Sankyo Pharma
Benicar™

**Schering Corporation and Key
Pharmaceuticals, Inc.**
Clarinex™, K-Dur®

Schwarz Pharma
Verelan®

Sepracor, Inc.
Lunesta®

Sucampo Pharmaceuticals, Inc.
Amitiza®

Tap Pharmaceuticals, Inc.
Prevacid®

Teva Pharmaceuticals
Azilect®

UCB Pharmaceuticals, Inc.
Lortab®

URL Pharma
Bactrim DS®

Warner Chilcott Laboratories, Inc.
Eryc®, Estrace®, Sarafem®

Wyeth Pharmaceuticals
Effexor®, Effexor XR®, Premarin®
The appearance of these tablets and
capsules is a registered trademark of
Wyeth Pharmaceuticals, Philadelphia,
Pennsylvania.

Index

t refers to a table; **boldface** refers to full-color photographs.

t refers to a table; **boldface** refers to full-color photographs.

t refers to a table; **boldface** refers to full-color photographs.

t refers to a table; **boldface** refers to full-color photographs.

t refers to a table; **boldface** refers to full-color photographs.

t refers to a table; **boldface** refers to full-color photographs.

t refers to a table; **boldface** refers to full-color photographs.

---

t refers to a table; **boldface** refers to full-color photographs.

New Directions in Cultural Policy Research

Series Editor
Eleonora Belfiore
Department of Social Sciences
Loughborough University
Loughborough, UK

New Directions in Cultural Policy Research encourages theoretical and empirical contributions which enrich and develop the field of cultural policy studies. Since its emergence in the 1990s in Australia and the United Kingdom and its eventual diffusion in Europe, the academic field of cultural policy studies has expanded globally as the arts and popular culture have been re-positioned by city, regional, and national governments, and international bodies, from the margins to the centre of social and economic development in both rhetoric and practice. The series invites contributions in all of the following: arts policies, the politics of culture, cultural industries policies (the 'traditional' arts such as performing and visual arts, crafts), creative industries policies (digital, social media, broadcasting and film, and advertising), urban regeneration and urban cultural policies, regional cultural policies, the politics of cultural and creative labour, the production and consumption of popular culture, arts education policies, cultural heritage and tourism policies, and the history and politics of media and communications policies. The series will reflect current and emerging concerns of the field such as, for example, cultural value, community cultural development, cultural diversity, cultural sustainability, lifestyle culture and eco-culture, planning for the intercultural city, cultural planning, and cultural citizenship.

More information about this series at
http://www.palgrave.com/gp/series/14748

Ben Walmsley

Audience Engagement in the Performing Arts

A Critical Analysis

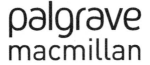

Ben Walmsley
School Performance Cultural
Industries
University of Leeds
Leeds, West Yorkshire, UK

New Directions in Cultural Policy Research
ISBN 978-3-030-26652-3   ISBN 978-3-030-26653-0   (eBook)
https://doi.org/10.1007/978-3-030-26653-0

Cover image: Miemo Penttinen - miemo.net/Getty images
Cover design by eStudioCalamar

This Palgrave Macmillan imprint is published by the registered company Springer Nature Switzerland AG
The registered company address is: Gewerbestrasse 11, 6330 Cham, Switzerland

Acknowledgements

I would like to dedicate this book to audiences. Audiences are the lifeblood of the performing arts and this book highlights the ways in which they have been marginalised for centuries. Audiences are extraordinary; they perform myriad roles in sustaining the arts, acting as critics, fans, champions, donors, and sense-makers. Since the first time I went to the theatre I have been fascinated by what happens to audiences in the course of a live performance. We can call this catharsis, or we can call it transformation, or even just entertainment; but something happens when audiences engage and are engaged with live performance that is special. So this book constitutes an extended plea for audiences to be taken more seriously and represents a tribute to their passion and commitment.

This book has been fuelled by, and is partly based on, a significant body of empirical research that I conducted with audiences between 2010 and 2015. I am constantly moved and humbled by the generosity and depth of insight provided by audience research participants, and without their openness of spirit this book would never have come to fruition. So a huge thanks must be extended to all those who participated in my audience research projects. Research of this type is also dependent on the generosity of arts organisations, so I also want to acknowledge the moral and logistical support of colleagues from Melbourne Theatre Company (especially Ann Tonks), Leeds Playhouse (then West Yorkshire Playhouse), Slung Low (particularly Alan Lane), Unlimited Theatre (Jon Spooner), Transform (Amy Letman), Yorkshire Dance (Wieke Eringa and Antony Dunn), and Love

Arts Leeds. Thanks are also due to Brooklyn Museum, National Theatre of Scotland and Watershed for permission to reproduce their images and capture their inspiring audience engagement activities via case studies.

Prolonged periods of research cannot take place without funding, so I'd like to acknowledge the support of Leeds Metropolitan University (now Leeds Beckett University), which offered me a research fellowship back in 2010 that enabled me to undertake research in Melbourne and kick-started my ensuing career as an audience researcher. I'd also like to thank the Arts and Humanities Research Council, Arts Council England and Nesta, who have funded several of my research projects over the past ten years and who continue to champion empirical audience research. In these times of apparent austerity and considering the increasing pressure to support STEM-based research, it feels more vital than ever to support arts and humanities research, and these organisations have consistently supported research into the arts. Publishers also play a key role in commissioning and disseminating research, of course, and so I would also like to thank the dedicated team at Palgrave Macmillan for their belief, support, and encouragement.

The School of Performance and Cultural Industries at the University of Leeds offers the perfect environment to undertake audience research and the School has generously funded two research sabbaticals over the past five years that have enabled me to develop this monograph. So I'd like to acknowledge my wonderful colleagues at the University the Leeds and my inspiring audience research peers, who have shaped and supported this publication in all sorts of ways. Some have read and fed back on early drafts—especially members of the School's Audience Experience and Engagement Group. Particular thanks are due to Anna Upchurch, Maria Barrett, Matthew Reason, Joslin McKinney, Kirsty Sedgman, and Ruth Rentschler, who have acted as formal or informal reviewers and as constant inspirations of how to conduct audience research with care, humour, humanity, and rigour. Tragically, Anna Upchurch left us far too soon, but as a founder editor of this book series (alongside Ele Belfiore) and the most generous of colleagues one could ever hope for, Anna persuaded me to write this book in the first place, so I will be forever in her debt and I hope that this book represents some small part of her wonderful academic legacy.

Finally, I'd like to formally thank my partner, Fabien, and my family and friends, who have patiently supported the development of this monograph and seen me through the inevitably challenging moments that arise in writing a sole-authored book.

CONTENTS

List of Figures

LIST OF TABLES

CHAPTER 1

Introduction

A PLEA FOR AUDIENCES

Back in the 1970s, the French philosopher and playwright Jean-Paul Sartre made a famous plea for intellectuals in his acclaimed essay *Plaidoyer pour les intellectuals* (Sartre 1976). In his essay, Sartre argued that society can't complain about its intellectuals without accusing itself, because we attract the intellectuals that we deserve and create. Despite the facile marketing soundbite that the contemporary customer is king, the same could certainly be said about today's performing arts audiences, who are often ignored, blamed and even derided by a sector that generally fails to listen to them or engage with them on equal terms.

Another French dramatist, Antonin Artaud, invoked the metaphor of the Fall to explain how audiences have been disempowered and disassociated from the public and are therefore irrevocably doomed in their illusory search for judgement and catharsis (cited in Blau 1990, p. 42). Indeed since the time of Plato, audiences have been variously, but consistently, feared, vilified, victimised, ignored, patronised, pacified, mollified, homogenised, ridiculed, abused, segmented, and even killed-off (both literally and metaphorically). This all points towards the reality that the audience (whatever that slippery construct might mean, and *to whom*) has fallen from grace.

© The Author(s) 2019
B. Walmsley, *Audience Engagement in the Performing Arts*,
New Directions in Cultural Policy Research,
https://doi.org/10.1007/978-3-030-26653-0_1

1

This unhappy state of affairs is aggravated by the apparent antipathy exhibited towards audiences by many arts professionals and even, somewhat extraordinarily, by audience scholars themselves. Herbert Blau (1990) rightly claims that there is a tradition of disdainful and disconcerted ambivalence towards the audience and that many people who work in the theatre perceive audiences as "a kind of usurper or intruder" (p. 40). This historical and prevalent disdain towards audiences shapes the academic and sociological context of this book, which embarks from the acknowledgement that audiences have been systematically, and sometimes cynically, sidelined, undermined and alienated by scholars, artists, managers, producers, arts organisations, policymakers, and society more broadly. So it is now time to plead on behalf of audiences; and via an in-depth critical analysis of audience research in the performing arts, this monograph makes the case for a more sustained, more authentic, more relational, and ultimately more effective engagement with audiences.

The underlying premise of this book is that we are currently living in a climate of quixotic thinking and theory regarding audience behaviour and engagement. Whilst on the one hand, some scholars, especially in media studies, are hailing the "end" or even the "death" of the audience (Livingstone and Das 2015) and conferences in the arts sector are devoted to "the people formerly known as the audience" (Rosen 2012), in actual fact, performing arts audiences are thriving, especially the commercial audiences in London's West End and on Broadway. What is interesting to observe, however, is how audience behaviour and expectations are changing, as the next generation of "prosumers" matures and as factors such as big data, co-creation, participation, digital engagement, and live streaming continue to impact on the sector. As traditional sources of arts funding start to dissipate and alternative income sources such as philanthropy and crowdfunding continue to rise, audiences are increasingly being targeted as donors, which further complicates and potentially compromises their relationships with artists and arts organisations. Mindful of this evolving context, this book will prioritise audiences and their *lived experiences* and explore the implications of changing audience expectations and evolving practices of engagement for artists, arts managers, marketers, cultural leaders, policymakers, and, of course, for audiences themselves.

The terminology surrounding audiences is particularly unhelpful in shedding light on the audience experience with core terms such as "theatre", "spectator", and "audience" all reflecting *one* particular sensory response to the performing arts. There is thus an urgent need to clarify the underlying terms that describe and denote the act of being an audience member and to critique the pernicious etymological associations that conspire to reduce this complex, multisensory pursuit. I will address this endeavour later in this introductory chapter.

Questions of audience engagement naturally beg the fundamental question of what an audience actually *is* and *does*. To what extent do audiences constitute a congregation, a collective, a community, or even a public? How do people transform into an audience and how might they best prepare for this transformation? Blau poses an important question in his deconstruction of the audience project: "To play the part of an audience is to play the part of *not playing* a part, and how *do* you rehearse for that?" (1990, p. 298, original italics). This question goes to the heart of audience engagement because it challenges both the ability and the preparedness of artists and performing arts organisations to develop their audiences aesthetically. As a theorist, Blau defines the audience as a constructed consciousness, an initiated body of thought and desire (1990, p. 25). But as the practitioner Stanislavsky points out, playing to no audience is "like listening for an echo in a place without resonance" (cited in Blau 1990, p. 255). As Stanislavsky intimates here, one of the primary roles of the audience is to provide resonance and meaning; and yet surprisingly little research is dedicated to this hermeneutic endeavour.

Helen Freshwater (2009) rightly contends that without the audience there *is* no real performance. Considering this indubitable primacy of the audience, it is quite simply astonishing that empirical research of and with performing arts audiences remains both contested as a scholarly endeavour and immature as an academic field. In fact, as Kirsty Sedgman (2016) notes, audience research is often dismissed as futile and even inimical.

> Audience research is frequently considered *nonproductive* as, through talking about the experience, audiences will only be able to explicate a pale approximate shadow of it; and at its worst, audience research is seen as potentially *destructive*, as what audiences remember afterwards will be not the ineffable experience itself but the shadow experience as it was described. (p. 24)

Sedgman goes on to heed Bourdieu's portentous warning about the "implacable hostility to those who try to advance the understanding of the work of art and of aesthetic experience" because this presents a "mortal threat to the pretension [...] of thinking of oneself as an ineffable individual" (p. 25). So audience research emerges as a sociological power game governed by the rules of cultural capital—a game in which some powerful cultural gatekeepers have a vested interest in silencing audiences and therefore in undermining audience research. To some extent, then, audience research is not only a policy tool but actually a political act, because it challenges established thinking regarding who actually has the right to express an opinion on questions of cultural engagement and aesthetic experience.

There can be no doubt that scholarship has systematically overlooked audience research in the past. As Susan Bennett observes, "what a theory of theatre audiences needs is not the neglect it has historically received, but a systematic, if cautious, approach that would make clearer the relationship between the art form [...] and the audience [...] that supports it" (1997, p. 17). However even revered audience scholars such as Bennett appear to be ambivalent towards empirical audience research, claiming that the performing arts sector itself is making such significant progress in understanding audiences that there is "little need or merit" in academics seeking to replicate its efforts (2006, pp. 226–228).

Fortunately, this beleaguered perspective on audience research is not shared by the vast majority of contemporary researchers, some of whom, like Janelle Reinelt, have abandoned their historic disregard for empirical research and come to value its ability to explicate audiences' experiences on their own terms.

> Most of the recent scholarship on reception in theatre and performance studies points to a lack of sustained attention to spectator research, or more specifically, to the kind of research that tells us what spectators experience, how they make meanings or feel feelings in relation to theatre, and how they come to value "assisting at performance." These features have been much less investigated and interpreted than the theoretical framing of the problems of the audience [...] or the description of the reception of particular performances. (Reinelt 2014, p. 337)

Reinelt's reflection here represents the high degree of consensus amongst audience researchers that the field has suffered from a significant over-reliance on theoretical approaches to explicating the audience experience. Even Blau, that most theoretical of audience scholars, acknowledges, albeit implicitly, the urgent need for an empirical approach.

> We simply do not know, in any reliable – no less ideal or accountable – sense, *who is there* nor, in the absence of the classical subject, *where to look*. We are despite this still likely to generalize – as I have said and maybe done –

about what the audience, with its disparate, cross-purposed, alienated, and incalculable perceptions, feels and felt. (1990, pp. 355–356, original italics)

Katya Johanson summarises the research context pithily, noting that "the audience has been all too absent from past scholarly performing arts studies" (2013, p. 168). This deficiency is not only a methodological and epistemological failure on the behalf of audience studies in the performing arts; it represents a perplexing and counter-intuitive conundrum, considering that the *actual* audience is "more complex and interesting" than the *ideal* audience that has long received the attention of scholars (Johanson 2013, p. 170). The net result of this deficient research context is that over the past few decades, and indeed centuries, theoretical scholars have conspired to: make general assumptions about audiences; speak on their behalf; assume a simplistic homogeneity of reception and response; and construct reductive notions of "bad" or "ideal" audiences (Sedgman 2016, p. 17). In short, audience research has not historically been very audience-friendly.

This general disregard for audiences is also apparent within the performing arts sector itself, where artists often either praise or vilify audiences both in the rehearsal room and in the auditorium, treating them with "a kind of benign paternalism" and creating a "phantom audience that we as makers, project, out of an admixture of experience, hearsay and blind anxiety" rather than "the real people who actually watch a performance" (Chris Goode, cited in Sedgman 2016, p. 161). As Conway and Leighton put it, the role of the audience member as "an active, skilled and discerning participant in the consumption process" has been sorely neglected (2012, p. 37). Caroline Heim (2010) echoes this damning verdict, observing that the active role of the audience has been significantly "undervalued" in contemporary practice and that audiences are often just treated as "a homogeneous mass incapable of creativity" (p. 1) or of holding a "unique personality" (p. 21). In light of the fact that audiences are "living, dynamic and heterogeneous" and contribute "crucial meanings" to performances (ibid.), Heim laments the current state of audience engagement in Western theatres, where walking out and clapping are often the only opportunities for audiences to actually express a critical response (2016, p. 35). Heim rightly concludes that the fact that audiences often cherish and sometimes "almost deify" their theatre programmes (p. 133) signifies their hunger for engagement beyond the short temporal sphere and space of a performance itself.

With the rise of digital media and producer disintermediation, global audiences are becoming increasingly powerful. Digital communications technologies are giving audiences more agency than ever before to signal and tailor their leisure and entertainment preferences. This rising power means that audiences are of growing interest to media and social media platforms and also to research councils and governments, who are starting to invest heavily in areas such as digital storytelling and immersive media. Even supra-governments like the European Union are allocating significant budgets to audience research, conscious no doubt of the historic connection between arts engagement and active citizenship (Walmsley 2018). Yet despite this shift in focus, policymakers, artists, producers, marketers, and even audience scholars often perpetuate narrow and reductive configurations of arts audiences. In her groundbreaking short book *Theatre & audience*, Helen Freshwater calls for a rejection of "the notion of 'the audience' as a singular or homogeneous entity" in favour of "a detailed interrogation of diverse and sometimes unexpected responses, and an ethnographic engagement with the range of cultural conditions which inform an individual's viewing position" (2009, p. 28). This current book responds to Freshwater's call by placing centre stage the diversity and complexity of audiences' projects and experiences; it takes a fiercely audience-centric stance and explores the implications of changing expectations and practices for the myriad stakeholders who are concerned with, and reliant on, audiences.

DEFINING AUDIENCES

As I suggested earlier, audience research is plagued by loose, woolly terminology that often perpetuates ambiguity and hinders attempts to cohere a scholarly community around it. To begin with the core term itself, the word "audience" is undoubtedly what Josephine Machon labels a "vexed term" (2013, p. 98). Its Latin roots (from *audire*, to hear) suggest a group of passive listeners, who simply engage their ears at one step removed from performance. Despite its Latin etymology, the term also lacks a gerund, which makes it difficult to articulate concisely the precise activity that audiences actually engage in. The term "spectator" at least has a gerund ("spectating") and even a related noun ("spectatorship") which of course denotes the act of spectating. But again the Latin origins (*spectare*) reduce what audiences do to the deployment of one of their senses, evoking this time a group of voyeurs who observe or gaze at a performance from a distance. Related terms such as "theatre" (from the Greek *theatron*, a place for *viewing*) similarly delimit the audience experience to an act of spectatorship.

The terminology surrounding the act of engaging with the performing arts is thus more than vexed; it is reductive and deceptive, and singularly fails to capture the rich multisensory and phenomenological complexity of the act.

Certain theatre practitioners hold the view that the role that audiences play in the performing arts, or at least the role that they *want* them to play, is so far removed from traditional notions of spectatorship that the word "audience" is no longer valid. Jerzy Grotowski, for example, claimed that the term "audience" was no longer relevant because he wanted to remove any kind of distance or separation between performers and audiences (cited in Ben Chaim 1984, pp. 47–48). In light of the rise of immersive and one-on-one performances and of co-created and participatory work, and even with the hindsight of Boal's Forum theatre, we might justifiably conclude that boundaries between performers and audiences are blurring almost to the point of oblivion. So we can see already that audiences are increasingly being perceived as an endangered species, not just because younger audiences are shunning traditional performance genres and venues, but also in the sense that their artistic and social functions are morphing into something fundamentally different: audiences are perhaps gradually transitioning into *co*-performers.

Despite this radical, if gradual, transformation of the audience project, traditional modes of performance still prevail, and it seems that we are stuck with our reductive terminology, at least for the time being. However, as audience studies has developed and grown in confidence, scholars have started to neologise. John Fiske (1992), for example, notably deployed the neologism of "audiencing", which he borrowed from cultural studies to describe the active pursuit of *being* an audience member. Reason and Londelof (2016) have since adopted the term into performance studies and elaborated an effective definition:

> 'Audiencing' describes the work of the spectator. It describes acts of attention, of affect, of meaning-making, of memory, of community. A focus on audiencing recognizes that attention is a constructive or performative act, that spectators bring performances into being through the nature of their variously active, distractive or contested attention. (p. 17)

This definition helpfully broadens the scope of the act of being an audience member and starts to encapsulate its aesthetic, interpretive, social and psychological qualities. However, welcome though this new term assuredly is, when I began to write this book I still felt poorly served by the audience lexicon and found myself often searching in vain for an abstract noun to convey the wider concept of what some scholars refer to as "spectatorship". This struggle reflected Bruce McConachie's observation that there is no adequate English word that encompasses all that an audience does in the context of the performing arts (2008, p. 3). "Spectatorship" simply doesn't work for me because of its negative connotations of sitting on the edge of something, of passively observing without really taking part. So I have coined the term "audiency" here to connote the general *state* of audiencing and the conceptual theorisation *of* it.

It is of course not just the core terms of audiency that remain slippery, problematic, and contested: many, if not most, of the terms used to describe audiences and their relationship to the performing arts are laden with value judgements (Freshwater 2009, pp. 2–3). "Audience development", "audience enrichment", "participation", "co-creation", and "engagement" are all either ambiguous, loaded, or both: whilst "audience development" and "enrichment" suggest some kind of cultural deficit amongst audiences, "participation", "co-creation", and "engagement" are vague to the point of being meaningless, at least when used in isolation. They are perhaps typical examples of what Clive Gray (2015) might refer to as deliberate policy ambiguity. In other words, the vague nature of these concepts can serve politicians' and policymakers' interests by remaining elusive or hard to pin down; it is therefore difficult to evaluate any policy-related progress (or rather lack of progress) against them. Caroline Heim translates this idea adroitly to the field of audience research, arguing that "approaching, writing about and conceptualising audiences and what they do is slippery, risky, complex and full of paradox" (2016, p. 5).

Even with our growing armoury of dedicated concepts and terms, audience researchers still struggle to pin down the act of audiency. This is probably a result of the significant role ambiguity that affects audiences. I mentioned earlier in the chapter that audiences are now often expected to fund or crowdfund their favourite artists and organisations, and in the transactional context of relationship marketing, this makes total sense. However, Heim (2016) characterises audiences variously as guests, fans, groupies, critics, communities, consumers, co-creators, co-performers, and co-conspirators. For Josephine Machon, audiences alternate between passive consumers, witnesses, associates, clients, guests, co-producers, protagonists, and "creative comrades" (2013, p. 73). For companies like Lone

Twin they are partners who share an equal role in a common artistic endeavour (Sedgman 2016, p. 14). This role complexity illustrates the significant dissonance surrounding audiency and audiencing, and highlights the tensions that infiltrate the relationships that different stakeholders try to develop with audiences. For example, to consider an audience member as a guest and as a donor appears inherently paradoxical; and how can co-creators also function as critics and consumers? Audience development theory tries to square these circles through its notion of *laddering*, taking audiences on a journey from outsider to co-performer, for example. Marketers and fundraisers might explain the dissonance via segmentation theory. But ultimately, audiences are active agents whose performance encounters are messy and individualised (Sedgman 2016, p. 16). What matters, and is of interest, therefore, is perhaps less what audiences *do* and more how we actually *engage* them.

Audience Engagement

Alongside "audience", "engagement" is the other core concept that drives the focus of this book. So for the purposes of this book it is important to define precisely how I understand "engagement" and to justify the privileged conceptual role that I have accorded it. Despite the fact that in the past two decades the arts marketing and cultural policy literature has witnessed an exponential rise in the deployment of the term "engagement" (Walmsley 2019), very few authors have actually attempted to define the concept, never mind differentiate it from similarly relational concepts such as "participation" and "involvement" (Brodie et al. 2011). As we have already seen, audience studies has adopted and been content with what Martin Barker refers to as "loose and vague concepts" for far too long (2006, p. 128); "engagement" is undoubtedly an exemplar of a loose and vague concept, and my first objective here is therefore to attempt to synthesise existing definitions of the term in order to produce a meaningful and workable definition.

There exists a significant gap in understanding about what actually constitutes *audience engagement*. I will argue in the course of this book that this epistemological lacuna is serving to hamper the progression of audience research as an emerging academic field and as an area of exponential growth in the arts and cultural sector, and in the wider creative industries. This book will therefore shine a light on engagement and on its constituent processes.

In the context of this book, engagement incorporates a much more complex and nuanced approach to developing relationships with audiences than crass attempts to market to them or simply allow them to participate or even co-produce. This is because active participation is not a given: it is made possible by the particularities of an event (Sedgman 2016, p. 13). However, I want to push Sedgman's analysis further by framing engagement as a *philosophy* underpinned by an audience-centric ethos that recognises audiences as *partners* in processes of artistic *exchange*. Indeed engagement has been aptly described as "a unifying philosophy" that combines marketing, education, artistic programming, and development to maximise impact on audiences (Brown and Ratzkin 2011, p. 8).

Many of the surprisingly few definitions that do exist perceive engagement primarily as a psychological process or state (Brodie et al. 2011, p. 253). Brodie et al. trace the theoretical roots of engagement to relationship marketing's focus on interactive experience and value co-creation, which, they maintain, offers "a transcending view of relationships, which contrasts with a more traditional, transactional view of marketing relationships" (ibid.). Vincs et al. (2009) certainly belong to this strand of research, defining engagement as being "compelled, drawn in, connected to what is happening, interested in what will happen next" (cited in Vincs 2013, p. 135). This definition successfully highlights two clear goals and manifestations of engagement: namely to captivate audiences concurrently, in the moment of appreciating a work of art; and to draw them into the future creative life of an artist or organisation. It also foregrounds the key concepts of immersion and flow that we shall explore in Chapter 3.

Susan Ashley (2014) provides a broader, sociological definition of engagement, characterising it as "a process for generating, improving or repairing relationships between institutions of culture and society at large" (p. 261). This is a particularly useful definition in the context of the cultural policy imperative for subsidised arts organisations to become more relevant to their diverse communities. Engagement is a necessarily broad term, which is used by organisations to describe their attempts to occupy audiences' attention, to involve them, to establish meaningful contact, and even to assure impact (Ashley 2014, p. 262). However, Ashley warns that engagement can also lead to "misrecognition, lack of parity and the subordination of some publics to management and regulation" and that it can be undermined by the "political agenda-setting, conflicting subjectivities and power relations inherent in intercultural communication" (p. 263).

Engagement activities can thus result in "problematic and unequal encounters" unless audiences are encouraged to "assert their own agency" and make their own choices in the way they use the arts as a "resource" (ibid.). Like audience research, engagement, then, is a political act that is open to manipulation and abuse. Like power, it is perhaps not something that is often relinquished but something that must be *seized*. This is where the politics of participation and co-creation come into play, and we will therefore scrutinise these proliferating phenomena very carefully in the course of this book.

In their erudite discussion of arts encounters and their apparent impacts, Belfiore and Bennett (2007) expound an interactive model of engagement based on factors pertaining to the individual, the artwork, and the environment, which we might interpret in terms of the subjective, the aesthetic, and the social. Lynne Conner (2013) provides a more prosaic, but nonetheless insightful, definition of engagement, associating the term with the deployment of gears that enable a mechanism to function (p. 37). Likewise, audiences, she suggests, engage in the process of art-making when they feel a vital part of its engine. In a similar vein, Steven Tepper defines engagement as "to interlock" or "involve" (2008, p. 363). Following Conner, Tepper's definition reflects a post-structural perspective of audiency, which perceives audiences as people who "actively connect to art – discovering new meanings, appropriating it for their own purposes, creatively combining different styles and genres, offering their own critique" (ibid.). Taking a similarly emancipated stance, Campanelli describes engagement in terms of "emotional connection and empowerment" (cited in Brodie et al. 2011, p. 266), whilst Sashi (2012) claims that effective engagement establishes intimate bonds, which culminate in enduring relational exchanges between producers and customers, and which can effect both loyalty and delight, transforming customers into fans.

Jennifer Radbourne (2013) approaches engagement from a marketing perspective and contends that engagement is all about "converging" with audiences. Radbourne observes an evolving context wherein audiences are increasingly seeking appropriation, connectivity and transformation through their arts experiences; she argues therefore that the role of modern arts and cultural organisations is to "converge" creators with consumers of art (p. 155). Supporting a number of existing studies into audience motivation, Radbourne concludes that performing arts audiences' primary goal is emotional engagement, which can most effectively be secured via immersion in the arts experience (p. 153). Brown and Ratzkin (2011) also explore engagement from the perspective of arts marketing, offering a helpful deconstruction of the concept by discerning six diverse audience typologies of engagement, ranging from reading and critical review to insight seeking and active learning (p. 2). The authors also delineate what they regard as different *stages* of engagement, which we will explore further in Chapter 2. This more plural understanding is also adopted by McConachie, who rightly claims that an adequate understanding of audiency must encompass many aspects of engagements with performances (2008, p. 7). The consensus between these researchers is that there is not a one-size-fits-all model of audience engagement.

In summary, then, theoretical definitions coalesce around the notion of engagement as a psychological process which aims to develop intimate, meaningful, converged, and enduring relationships with audiences by involving them in interactive, immersive, and hermeneutic experiences. This in turn emancipates and empowers audiences and generates deep connections by enabling audiences to become an invaluable part of the art-making process. Engagement emerges therefore as both a strategic management process (or a psychological manipulation) and a sociocultural benefit.

In order to appreciate the ultimate goal of the engagement process, it is important to consider what these meaningful and enduring relationships might look like from the demand side. The development of the wider economy from the services economy of the late Twentieth Century to the experience economy of the new millennium (Pine and Gilmore 1999) is perhaps one of the most familiar tropes of twenty-first century marketing. However, since the turn of the millennium, scholars such as Bill Sharpe (2010) have started to argue that experiences per se are no longer sufficient for the post-postmodern consumer, who is actually seeking a particular kind of experience—namely one which is shared, meaningful, valuable, and enduring. This focus on meaning reflects Silvia's (2005) finding that audiences' meaning-making is positively correlated to their aesthetic enjoyment. Sharpe's thesis is essentially that art acts as the currency in this new economy, "the currency of experience, putting our unique individual experiences into motion amongst us as shared meaning" (p. 2). This new economy of meaning is characterised by participatory modes of engagement, both within the arts and beyond them, and the ultimate goal of this engagement is aesthetic and spiritual enrichment.

Commentators on the creative economy are currently fixated on the so-called *attention economy*, a perspective that regards consumer attention as a scarce resource and therefore as a "cultural problem" (Crawford 2015). Within museum studies, Stephen Bitgood's (2010) research with museum audiences links attention closely with engagement and suggests that engagement encompasses a number of intellectual, perceptual, and affective processes, including learning, flow, inquiry, and immersion. Based on his extensive research in this area, Bitgood has developed an "attention-value model", which designates engagement as the third stage of audiences' attention process, following the prior states of focus and captivation. In other words, audience focus and captivation are prerequisites of engagement, which represents the most difficult level for audiences to reach as it requires "deep sensory-perceptual, mental and/or affective involvement" alongside "some type of exertion or concentration" (Bitgood 2010). This returns us neatly to the chapter's opening citation, which pondered how audiences can rehearse for being an audience member (Blau 1990, p. 298). Engagement has emerged here as an integral component of effective audiencing; as a state of mind and body that demands not only the deep immersion of audiences but also the careful mediation of producers. Suffice to say that engagement does not happen by itself.

The Case for Engagement

There are many rationales for dedicating an entire monograph to audience engagement, but perhaps the most compelling is the mounting evidence that the goal of being engaged is actually the primary motivation behind audiences' decision to attend the performing arts. McConachie regards this as a physiological transformation, claiming that as audience members, we seek "emotional engagement and the chemical changes it brings to our brains [...] the means for a direct jolt" (2008, pp. 95–96). There is also growing consensus that engaging audiences on a macro scale is imperative not only to the long-term health of the arts and cultural sector but more importantly to the cultural vitality of our communities (Brown and Ratzkin 2011, p. 35). This is a view increasingly shared within cultural policy and it is gradually starting to effect a more community-based and participatory approach to arts funding, which is incrementally shifting its focus from artistic quality to social relevance.

From the organisational perspective, the ultimate goal of engagement is "to enable arts organizations to develop empathy with their audiences and communities, communicate persuasively to them, engage meaningfully with them, and shape resonant and relevant arts experiences and programmes with them and for them" (Baxter et al. 2013, p. 117). This relational perspective on engagement supports our earlier synthesis of existing definitions of engagement, which framed it as both a strategic management process and a sociocultural benefit. As business-minded leaders might say, engagement is a win-win. Yet it remains under-theorised, under-researched, and under-utilised, especially in the context of the performing arts, where it is often tacked onto core promotional activity as an adjunct or afterthought.

As Maxine Greene notes, informed engagement with the arts does not happen automatically or naturally; it requires reflective time and dialogue (Greene 1995, cited in Reason 2013, p. 106). Reason goes on to add that "the unthinking, unblinking eye of passive consumption can only be countered by ensuring that spectators are actively processing and evaluating their experiences and as a result become cultural producers of meaning" (2013, p. 110). This point responds to Blau's rhetorical question regarding how audiences can prepare (or *be prepared*) for their audiencing activity. Just as the co-production of cultural products cannot happen without artists to co-produce them, so is the co-creation of meaning dependent on some form of mediation, which I am referring to here as "engagement". As Deleuze argued, effective engagement can enable a work of art to leave the domain of representation to become experience (cited in Machon 2013, p. 109). Based on our previous discussion, we can now develop the Deleuzian theory by adding that effective engagement can enable a work of art to leave the domain of experience to become meaning. This, again, is the process increasingly referred to by audience scholars as "enrichment".

This book takes a fresh approach to engagement by placing it at the heart of the enquiry into audiency. It offers fresh insights into the concept drawn from arts marketing and cultural policy, such as evolving theories of consumer behaviour, value creation and co-creation and changing perspectives on the politics and practices of participation and audience development. As such, the book has the ambitious aim of broadening and reconfiguring the paradigm of audience studies.

AUDIENCE STUDIES

Attempts to research performing arts audiences in any consistent and coherent way have been held back by the significant fragmentation that characterises the wider field of audience studies. At its best, audience studies is radically interdisciplinary, and in an academic context where interdisciplinarity is increasingly extolled, this rich potential for cross-pollination is undoubtedly the field's greatest strength. At its worst, however, audience studies is fractured and dispersed across such a diverse range of traditionally incompatible fields, disciplines, and sub-disciplines that attempts to collaborate become mired in methodological dispute. Consequently, findings and developments in one particular field often get lost in translation, or even worse, ignored. Audience researchers come in many different guises, and they emerge (often in a defensive minority) in conferences dedicated to arts marketing, arts management, cultural studies, cultural policy, theatre studies, performance studies, dance studies, opera studies, media studies, film studies, reception theory, critical theory, semiotics, and dramaturgy. The implications of this are that audience research is generally marginalised in and by the academy.

As we shall see in Chapter 5, audience research is plagued by myriad methodological challenges, ranging from the positive bias of audiences and memory recall issues to researchers' poor grasp of methods and their inherent confirmation bias. These issues combine to undermine and delegitimise audience scholarship, which is often disregarded by social scientists and civil servants, in particular, as being overly narrative or anecdotal. These methodological issues are compounded by tensions between theory and practice—notably by scholars' perceptions of a lack of rigour in arts evaluation and by practitioners' perceptions of academic idealism amongst scholars. Neither of these perceptions is fully misguided: sector research on audiences and their experiences is often indeed biased and advocatory, whereas academic research is often overly theoretical and/or impracticable. Audience research is also hampered by ambiguous and whimsical cultural policy imperatives (which very rarely value audiences' experiences per se), and by the utter complexity of capturing what are invariably ineffable, multisensory experiences.

So where does all this leave audience studies? In his aspirational essay on the future of audience research, Martin Barker calls for a "fully elaborate research paradigm [...] combining a theoretical framework, working concepts, methods of enquiry, research implements, and paradigmatic studies" (2006, p. 129). This is perhaps a natural response to the prevalent critique that audience research "never transcends clever description" (ibid.). Barker's call to develop one research paradigm with one theoretical framework certainly represents a lofty goal; but it is surely a problematic one in what is an inherently plural, disparate, and radically interdisciplinary field that draws on so many different research paradigms and traditions. However, Barker is right to allude that in order to achieve widespread recognition and legitimacy as an academic field, audience studies does need to become less fragmented and more coherent; and the search for suitable theoretical frameworks, methods, and paradigms is certainly an underlying objective of this book.

RESEARCHING AUDIENCES

In his comprehensive exploration of the dynamics of performance and perception Willmar Sauter adds his voice to the growing chorus of audience researchers who acknowledge the marginal existence traditionally accorded to audiences. Sauter maintains that in order to gain a deeper understanding of audiences' experiences, both during and after performances, we need to develop radically different research strategies (2000, pp. 26–27). This book responds to Sauter's call by advocating for an interdisciplinary and triangulated approach to audience research that places aspects of experience and engagement at its heart. It does this partly by showcasing research that shares these relational objectives.

A prime example of this relational approach to audience research is Radbourne et al.'s (2013) edited collection entitled *The audience experience: A critical analysis of audiences in the performing arts*, which offers a range of different perspectives on audience experience and engagement. One of these perspectives is offered by Lisa Baxter et al. (2013), who make a powerful case for change in audience research strategies, calling for more creative and innovative methods of enquiry into audience engagement, and contending, justifiably, that arts organisations need to shift their focus from financial to experiential value:

> For arts organizations operating in an experience economy, it is important to understand how they can deliver value through understanding the experiences they create and manage. It is not enough to count 'bums on seats'. They need to know and understand the ways in which the arts experiences they offer hold value for their audiences, and what kind of value that is, whether it be a good night out or a meaningful aesthetic experience. [...] arts organizations need to use insight to put the audience at the centre of their creative and professional practices. (p. 117)

Although explicitly challenging arts organisations to engage in questions of cultural and experiential value, this exhortation also represents an implicit challenge to the myriad arts funders who do indeed count "bums on seats"; and it directly contradicts Susan Bennett's curious contention that the sector is making such considerable progress in understanding audiences by itself that academic research in this area is becoming redundant.

Dwight Conquergood also advocates for a more creative and sophisticated approach to audience research, claiming, for example, that the method of participant-observation succeeds in privileging the body "as a site of knowing" (cited in Kattwinkel 2003, p. xi). Conquergood argues that the acts of speaking, listening and acting enable researchers to gather experiential knowledge as opposed to the purely exterior knowledge gleaned from detached observation. As we shall see in Chapter 5, this tension between anthropological and ethnographic engagement is indicative of the many mysteries and idiosyncrasies that characterise empirical audience research. Indeed, as became evident during the discussions that took place over the two-year *International Network for Audience Research in the Performing Arts*,[1] the tensions, complexities and paradoxes that are seemingly inherent to audience research are actually one of the drivers for many audience scholars. For instance, my own research with audiences has unearthed a deep sense of ambivalence amongst theatre-goers regarding the extent to which they perceive themselves as individuals or a collective. Many audience members, including myself, see themselves as simultaneously both, which often establishes an inner psychological and ontological tension as we oscillate between contradictory modes of being: we like to share in the communal buzz before a performance, the collective silences, the common gasps, the shared applause, and the atavistic sense of *communitas* delivered by a standing ovation; and yet we rail at the noise or cognitive dissonance that interrupts our flow or hinders our goal of escapism, and argue, sometimes fervently, with those who offer alternative interpretations of a performance from our own. In order to deal with this inner conflict, we are beginning as a research community to acknowledge the fact that audience members generate "elaborate viewing strategies" as they develop

---

[1] This was a research network funded by the Arts and Humanities Research Council (AHRC) led by the University of Leeds (UK) in conjunction with Deakin University, Melbourne, that ran initially from January 2017 to December 2018. See https://audience-research.leeds.ac.uk.

their engagement with the performing arts (Sedgman 2016, p. 16). Audiences' experiences are therefore increasingly being represented as multidirectional and multifarious; and like wider questions of cultural value, the precise nature of these experiences will inevitably always lie beyond scholars' grasp. This, at least for me, is what makes audience research particularly intriguing.

Scope and Aims

In light of this confession, the aim of this book is certainly not to completely demystify the audience experience. Audiency is intriguing and mystifying, and the job of audience studies must therefore be to communicate its rich complexity. So the core aim of this book is to explore and reveal audiences as they manifest themselves in situ, based on empirical studies and on critical insights derived from audience theories and histories. As I intimated at the start of this chapter, this book is intended as a plea for audiences, at least in the sense that it aspires to place audiences back in their rightful place at the heart of scholarship into their own experiences. The book approaches audiences and audience engagement from a range of what I consider to be complementary perspectives: cultural value, marketing, and co-creation. It considers the role that different methods and methodologies can play in elucidating audiences' experiences with the performing arts and investigates how existing and emerging technologies can inform our understanding of how to engage audiences.

I have chosen to explore audience engagement within the specific context of the performing arts, and I therefore draw predominantly on theories, empirical studies and case examples from theatre, dance, music, opera, and musical theatre. I decided to limit the focus of this book to the performing arts for several reasons. One personal and pragmatic reason is that most of my own audience research has been conducted with audiences of theatre and dance. A logical and academic reason is that the field of performance studies covers all of these art forms and sometimes theorises about them generically. A strategic reason for the performing arts focus is to apply insights from other fields and sectors in order to galvanise thinking about engagement within the performing arts and recommend enhancements, especially from the museums sector: as Lynne Conner notes, museums have led the field in acknowledging and facilitating audiences' cultural right to interpret art and the performing arts have much to learn from them in this endeavour (2013, p. 148). A more epistemological rationale is certainly that the different genres that comprise the performing arts share a number of underlying commonalities, including of course the existential requirement for a live audience. Monica Prendergast (2006) expresses the exceptionality of live performance beautifully, arguing that it offers "a crucial counterbalance to the prevailing forces of film, television and other mass media" (cited in Sedgman 2016, p. 12). She goes on to argue that performing arts audiences are "generally more challenged – aesthetically, affectively and cognitively – in their reception and interpretation of live performance" and that the shared presence in live performance offers potential for "authentic, meaningful interactions between performers and spectators in a way that is not possible in most media-based forms" (ibid.). These provocative ideas and claims will be scrutinised extensively in the course of this book.

Considering the core focus on the book, I have made extensive use of research from theatre studies, performance studies, musicology, arts marketing, and cultural policy studies. However, for the reasons outlined above, the book also draws heavily on scholarship from cognate fields such as museology, philosophy, psychology, and sociology. As we have seen, audience studies is an inherently *cross*-disciplinary field and I very much hope that this book will offer readers a unique perspective on audience engagement that breaks down established silos between different academic fields to offer something genuinely *inter*disciplinary. In homage to the many notable audience researchers who have undertaken pioneering work in the field, this book advocates for a rigorous and empirical approach to audience research. However, in lieu of presenting a body of fresh empirical findings, it provides an overview of an existing body of empirical audience research, including my own, and therefore makes a predominantly theoretical case for empirical research. As such, it aims to provide a robust defence against persisting accusations amongst theoretical researchers of audiences that empirical work is often anecdotal and overly subjective, and therefore of limited worth.

The personal perspective I bring to this book is that of a theatre producer and manager turned academic. As a practitioner, I worked most closely with marketing and production teams in the service of theatre audiences. As an academic, my career began with a Ph.D. in French theatre and philosophy that provided a critical comparison of the plays of Jean-Paul Sartre and Eugène Ionesco and their respective contributions to twentieth-century humanism. I now describe myself as an audience researcher, and ally myself most closely to the complementary fields of arts marketing, arts management and cultural policy studies. This diverse scholarly context has influenced me, I suspect, to explore audiences in a genuinely interdisciplinary way, and it has certainly shaped my perspective that at the heart of audience research lies a mutual exchange of value wherein audiences should play the role of strategic partners in the artistic mission fulfilment of performing arts organisations. This belief constitutes the underlying thesis of this book.

Ultimately, I hope that this book represents a call to action to both academics and practitioners to engage more authentically and rigorously with audiences. I hope that it contributes to the growing body of audience research that respects audiences and engages with them actively and on equal terms. I hope that it helps to further galvanise the currently fractured community of academics cohered loosely around audience research. I hope that it inspires performing arts organisations to invest time and money in dedicated audience research and engagement activity. I hope that it enhances thinking on cultural value and moves marketing of the arts away from a transactional, consumption-based approach towards the relational mode required by effective engagement and meaningful enrichment.

As we shall see in the following chapter, there is growing consensus amongst scholars that audience research needs a new theoretical framework. For too long, audience studies has been splintered across seemingly incompatible disciplines that generally dialogue in different languages, spaces, and modes. By taking a radically interdisciplinary approach that combines scholarship from art form specific fields such as performance studies and musicology with insights from museology, psychology, philosophy, sociology, arts marketing, arts management, and cultural policy studies, this book ultimately outlines a new empirical and theoretical framework for audience studies.

References

Ashley, S. L. T. 2014. 'Engage the world': Examining conflicts of engagement in public museums. *International Journal of Cultural Policy*, 20(3), pp. 261–280.
Barker, M. 2006. I have seen the future and it is not here yet …; or, on being ambitious for audience research. *The Communication Review*, 9(2), pp. 123–141.
Baxter, L., O'Reilly, D. and Carnegie, E. 2013. Innovative methods of inquiry into arts engagement. In: Radbourne, J., Glow, H. and Johanson, K. (eds.) *The audience experience: A critical analysis of audiences in the performing arts.* Bristol, Intellect, pp. 113–128.

Belfiore, E. and Bennett, O. 2007. Determinants of impact: Towards a better understanding of encounters with the arts. *Cultural Trends*, 16(3), pp. 225–275.

Ben Chaim, D. 1984. *Distance in the theatre: The aesthetics of audience response*. London, Ann Arbor.

Bennett, S. 1997. *Theatre audiences: A theory of production and reception*. 2nd ed. London, Routledge.

Bennett, S. 2006. Theatre audiences, redux. *Theatre Survey*, 47(2), pp. 225–230.

Bitgood, S. 2010. An attention-value model of museum visitors. Available from: https://airandspace.si.edu/rfp/exhibitions/files/j1-exhibition-guidelines/3/An%20Attention-Value%20Model%20of%20Museum%20Visitors.pdf [Accessed 5 April 2019].

Blau, H. 1990. *The audience*. Baltimore, The John Hopkins University Press.

Brodie, R. J., Hollebeek, L. D., Juric, B. and Ilic, A. 2011. Customer engagement: Conceptual domain, fundamental propositions, and implications for research. *Journal of Service Research*, 14(3), pp. 252–271.

Brown, A. S. and Ratzkin, R. 2011. *Making sense of audience engagement: A critical assessment of efforts by nonprofit arts organizations to engage audiences and visitors in deeper and more impactful arts experiences*. San Francisco, The San Francisco Foundation.

Conner, L. 2013. *Audience engagement and the role of arts talk in the digital era*. New York, Palgrave Macmillan.

Conway, T. and Leighton, D. 2012. "Staging the past, enacting the present": Experiential marketing in the performing arts and heritage sectors. *Arts Marketing: An International Journal*, 2(1), pp. 35–51.

Crawford, M. 2015. *The world beyond your head: How to flourish in an age of distraction*. London, Penguin.

Fiske, J. 1992. Audiencing: A cultural studies approach to watching television. *Poetics*, 21, pp. 345–359.

Freshwater, H. 2009. *Theatre & audience*. London, Palgrave Macmillan.

Gray, C. 2015. Ambiguity and cultural policy. *Nordic Journal of Cultural Policy*, 1(18), pp. 66–80.

Heim, C. L. 2010. *Theatre audience contribution: Facilitating a new text through the post-performance discussion*. Saarbrücken, Lambert.

Heim, C. 2016. *Audience as performer: The changing role of theatre audiences in the Twenty-First Century*. London and New York, Routledge.

Johanson, K. 2013. Listening to the audience: Methods for a new era of audience research. In: Radbourne, J., Glow, H. and Johanson, K. (eds.) *The audience experience: A critical analysis of audiences in the performing arts*. Bristol, Intellect, pp. 159–171.

Kattwinkel, S. 2003. Introduction. In: Kattwinkel, S. (ed.) *Audience participation: Essays on inclusion in performance*. Westport, CT, Praeger, pp. ix–xviii.

Livingstone, S. and Das, R. 2015. The end of audiences? Theoretical echoes of reception amid the uncertainties of use. In: Hartley, J., Burgess, J. and Bruns, A. (eds.) *A companion to new media dynamics*. Chichester, Wiley, pp. 104–121.

Machon, J. 2013. *Immersive theatres: Intimacy and immediacy in contemporary performance*. London, Palgrave Macmillan.

McConachie, B. 2008. *Engaging audiences: A cognitive approach to spectating in the theatre*. New York, Palgrave Macmillan.

Pine, B. J. and Gilmore, J. H. 1999. *The experience economy: Work is theatre and every business a stage*. Boston, Harvard Business School.

Radbourne, J. 2013. Converging with audiences. In: Radbourne, J., Glow, H. and Johanson, K. (eds.) *The audience experience: A critical analysis of audiences in the performing arts*. Bristol, Intellect, pp. 143–158.

Radbourne, J., Glow, H. and Johanson, K. (eds.). 2013. *The audience experience: A critical analysis of audiences in the performing arts*. Bristol, Intellect.

Reason, M. 2013. The longer experience: Theatre for young audiences and enhancing engagement. In: Radbourne, J., Glow, H. and Johanson, K. (eds.) *The audience experience: A critical analysis of audiences in the performing arts*. Bristol, Intellect, pp. 95–111.

Reason, M. and Londelof, A. M. (eds.). 2016. *Experiencing liveness in contemporary performance: Interdisciplinary perspectives*. London, Routledge.

Reinelt, J. G. 2014. What UK spectators know: Understanding how we come to value theatre. *Theatre Journal*, 66(3), pp. 337–361.

Rosen, J. 2012. The people formerly known as the audience. In: Mandiberg, M. (ed.) *The social media reader*. New York, New York University Press, pp. 13–16.

Sartre, J.-P. 1976. A plea for intellectuals. In: Sartre, J.-P. (ed.) *Between existentialism and Marxism*. New York, William Morrow, pp. 228–285.

Sashi, C. M. 2012. Customer engagement, buyer-seller relationships, and social media. *Management Decision*, 50(2), pp. 253–272.

Sauter, W. 2000. *The theatrical event: Dynamics of performance and perception*. Iowa City, University of Iowa Press.

Sedgman, K. 2016. *Locating the audience: How people found value in National Theatre Wales*. Bristol, Intellect.

Sharpe, B. 2010. *Economies of life: Patterns of health and wealth*. Axminster, Triarchy Press.

Silvia, P. J. 2005. Emotional responses to art: From collation and arousal to cognition and emotion. *Review of General Psychology*, 9(4), pp. 342–357.

Tepper, S. J. 2008. The next great transformation: Leveraging policy and research to advance cultural vitality. In: Tepper, S. J. and Ivy, B. (eds.) *Engaging art: The next great transformation of America's cultural life*. Oxon, Routledge, pp. 363–383.

Vincs, K. 2013. Structure and aesthetics in audience responses to dance. In: Radbourne, J., Glow, H. and Johanson, K. (eds.) *The audience experience: A critical analysis of audiences in the performing arts*. Bristol, Intellect, pp. 129–142.

Walmsley, B. 2018. A plea for audiences: From active spectatorship to enactive audiency. In: Bonet, L. and Négrier, E. (eds.) *Breaking the fourth wall: Proactive audiences in the performing arts.* Elverum, Kunnskapsverket, pp. 196–209.

Walmsley, B. 2019. The death of arts marketing: A paradigm shift from consumption to enrichment. *Arts and the Market*, 9(1), pp. 32–49.

CHAPTER 2

Understanding Audiences: A Critical Review of Audience Research

INTRODUCTION

The aim of this chapter is to provide a critical overview of the existing literature on audience research and audience engagement in order to ascertain what we already know about audiences in the performing arts and to identify any significant epistemological gaps. The chapter will survey the seminal contributions to this rapidly emerging field and identify the recurrent themes that characterise the scholarly contributions to it thus far, which I have identified and categorised as follows: the pacification of audiences; power, elitism, and class; cultural policy, participation, and co-creation; immersive performance; performance venues, spaces and places; performance as ritual; reception theory and semiotics; research methodologies; the audience experience; value and impact research; young audiences; arts marketing and management; audience engagement and enrichment. Whilst this is certainly not intended as an exhaustive categorisation of audience research, it is proposed here as an emerging taxonomy that will hopefully help to construct a paradigm for audience studies in the performing arts and, in so doing, offer a useful point of anchorage for scholars in the field. As Martin Barker insists, audience research remains a loose and fragmented field that lacks not only a scholarly home but also a coherent set of questions and principles around which scholars might cohere:

© The Author(s) 2019
B. Walmsley, *Audience Engagement in the Performing Arts,*
New Directions in Cultural Policy Research,
https://doi.org/10.1007/978-3-030-26653-0_2

The question I want us to ask – and I regard our ability to ask and answer it as a sign of the potential maturity of audience research as a field of work – is this: what are our ambitions for our field? What are the kinds of questions we want to be able to ask and answer? (2006, p. 127)

As we saw in the previous chapter, until relatively recently, audience research in the performing arts was hindered by a stubborn refusal amongst many scholars to conduct empirical work. The field has also been hampered by a dearth of academic research into audiences in the performing arts. As a broader field, audience studies has to date been overly dominated by cultural studies and media studies, and this is where it is still most likely to be located in the shadowy groves of academe. However, as cross-, inter-, and trans-disciplinary research continues its steep and steady climb up the research agenda, audience researchers are starting to emerge in other areas of academia, not least in departments of theatre, performance studies, and music. However, as audience research proliferates, there is a real danger that scholars will fail to work in a truly interdisciplinary way across established disciplinary divides; that audience studies gets "stuck at the level of *accumulation*" and loses sight of existing research in fields such as cultural studies (Barker 2006, pp. 126–127, original italics). With this in mind, this chapter will draw on insights from a diverse range of fields and structure itself in a transdisciplinary way that generally privileges recurrent ideas and themes over the fields that happened to generate them.

THE PACIFICATION OF AUDIENCES

One of the most dominant tropes in the existing scholarship is that performing arts audiences have been systematically quietened over the past two centuries. A number of scholars, including Lynne Conner, Richard Butsch, and Caroline Heim, have written extensively about this, arguing that as the arts became sacralised in the Nineteenth Century during the class wars, audiences were deliberately pacified by theatre managers—closed off from the human interaction that was now reserved for the stage itself and obscured in a darkened auditorium where social engagement became impracticable. As Butsch (2008) notes, this pacification of audiences was effected by a combination of factors, including changing trends in theatre architecture, the rise of realism, developments in stage lighting and set design that required a contrasting darkness in the auditorium, and management

imperatives to raise box office income by welcoming more women to matinee performances, which in turn required a softer etiquette. However, as
Judith Fisher (2003) observes, even before these influences emerged, most
eighteenth-century theatre performances were actually "relatively quiet"
once the opening music started, and most spectators "behaved themselves"
(p. 66). There thus remains debate and disagreement regarding the relative
bawdiness of pre-Enlightenment audiences, which suggests that claims of
constant noise and ubiquitous audience participation have been deliberately
exaggerated in order to serve the agenda of what some might call a roman-
tic revisionism of theatre history to support the case for re-democratising
audience engagement and reviewing established theatre etiquette.

Regardless of why and to what extent the dynamics in the auditorium
shifted, the net result was that the focal point, and therefore the power,
shifted away from audiences towards producers and performers. However,
much as these shifting power dynamics might well explain the subsequent
disempowerment of the audience voice, both literally and metaphorically,
the discourse surrounding the cynical quietening of audiences needs to be
problematised, because the growing number of calls for audiences to be
allowed to become more vocal (Sedgman 2018) lie in opposition to recent
findings regarding the drivers and impacts of arts attendance—particularly
the pursuit of flow experiences, which are reliant on individual concentration, immersion and peace (Walmsley 2011). There is also an underlying assumption that audiences are communities or collectives rather than
crowds or disparate groups of individuals engaged in diverse objectives and
pursuits, and this tension between homogeneity and heterogeneity still
pervades a good proportion of audience research.

Power, Elitism, and Class

As we saw in Chapter 1, audiency has always been, or at least always been
perceived to be, a political act. Whilst practitioners such as Brecht and
Boal consciously exploited the *explicitly* political act of theatre-going, the
implicitly political aspect of being part of a social collective has been noted
by many philosophers and commentators stemming back to Plato, who
warned how audiences could easily be activated by the dangerous persuasive
rhetoric and emotional manipulation that lie at the heart of performance
(Hall 2010). Audiences' perceived propensity for manipulation has long
effected a culture of mistrust towards audiences and fostered a prejudiced
view of them as "disorderly crowds and unruly subjects" (Butsch 2008,

p. 24). In his treatise on what he labels "the citizen audience", Butsch contends that institutions often cast audiences in the role of the "Other" (2008, p. 3). As we will see in the course of this book, this "othering" often serves to objectify audiences, diminishing their intellectual and interpretive capacities and alienating them from both the encoding and decoding phase of the creative endeavour.

In his eponymous theoretical study *The audience*, Herbert Blau (1990) suggests that the issue is not simply about who speaks and who listens, but rather "who constructs meanings and in what positions of language" (p. 8). Blau goes on to argue that variant social interests combine to "disarticulate the process of signification, the signifier itself, from [...] the dominant and oppressive systems of meaning" (ibid.). According to Blau, then, audiences are often deliberately excluded from processes of interpretation because meaning-making is in and of itself a highly political and politicised process and one which is therefore primarily concerned with retaining power. Caroline Heim expands on this idea, illustrating how audiences' voices have been systematically silenced:

> Due to changes in theatre architecture, the rise in power of arts professionals, changes in audience demographics, and the rise of a commodity culture, contemporary audience contribution has been largely relegated to laughter and applause. (2012, p. 189)

The disempowerment of audiences is a familiar trope in audience research and the cynical dislocation of the act of audiency from acts of interpretation represents a political and epistemological problem that has partly fuelled the rise of scholarship into audience engagement and enrichment. Indeed this problem is one of the core foci of this monograph and it will be explored in due course in relation to cultural value, research methodologies, arts marketing, co-creation, and digital engagement.

Considering the prevailing demographic of performing arts audiences, this disempowerment functions on a much wider scale than in the often unseen world of theatres and concert halls and it is to a large extent essentially an issue of class discrimination. Although this book is primarily concerned with actual (as opposed to potential) audience members, it is important to note that audience research has been greatly influenced over the past few decades by Pierre Bourdieu, whose work on cultural capital has served to highlight how entrenched processes of social elitism exclude many social groups from the act of audiency altogether, creating a culture where "a narrow band of voices militates against change and innovation" (Jancovich 2011, p. 279). This cultural elitism is illustrated on a national scale by Butsch (2008), who traces the development and dominance of upper-middle class audiences in the United States during the Eighteenth and Nineteenth Centuries. These audiences carved out for themselves a preciously guarded cultural haven between what they perceived as "uncultivated" working class audiences on one side and the "unappreciative rich" on the other (p. 69).

Class has been woefully under-explored by audience researchers. As Willmar Sauter argued almost two decades ago now, the encounters between performers and spectators need to be studied much more closely "in terms of psychology, gender relations, class formations, genre expectations, and other contextual conditions" (2000, p. 48). Given that questions of class are central to attempts to diversify audiences, and that this objective lies at the heart of cultural policy strategies across the globe, it is quite simply astonishing that more sector and academic research has not been dedicated to the particular issues (and notably barriers to engagement) encountered by working class audiences. The rare exceptions to this research lacuna are David Wright's (2015) extensive exploration of cultural taste and Maria Barrett's (2015) meticulous ethnographic study of working class audiences, effected through a case study of Liverpool's Royal Court Theatre. Barrett's research presents a Bourdieusian analysis of theatre-going in the city of Liverpool, highlighting, for example, the particular methodological challenges faced when working with working class audiences (who may be suspicious of "academics" and "interviews") alongside the significant roles that programming, casting, audience participation, architecture, seating, nostalgia and sociability can all play in establishing a welcoming aesthetic that speaks to a working class habitus. The barriers encountered by working class audiences are reflected of course in the significant challenges faced by working class artists, which merely compound the persistent under-representation of the working class voice in the performing arts sectors and serve to alienate working class audiences even further (O'Brien et al. 2018).

Cultural Policy, Participation and Co-creation

Largely influenced by sociology, and particularly once again by the work of Bourdieu, cultural policy research is increasingly dominated by the politics of cultural engagement. Put quite simply, many cultural policy scholars are now concerned essentially with who does and doesn't engage with the arts and why/why not. Accordingly, there is a rapidly growing body of work dedicated to aspects of what has historically been referred to as audience development, but which might more accurately and appropriately be referred to as audience diversification. Whilst this work is undeniably important, partly for the reasons outlined above, it is arguably serving to marginalise audience research within cultural policy studies and, rightly or wrongly, shift the professional policy focus away from the phenomenology of the audience experience. This imbalance was partly addressed in the significant body of work funded by the UK's Arts and Humanities Research Council (2013) under the auspices of its Cultural Value Project (see Chapter 4), which called for more research into the lived experiences of audiences.

Despite this hefty (and continuing) intervention, it is important to note the significant scholarly shift over the past two decades towards questions of participation and non-participation. Indeed according to a recent thematic analysis of peer-reviewed journal articles published between 2007 and 2016 in ten leading arts marketing journals, 16% of all articles relating to arts marketing or audience engagement were primarily focused on participation, which emerged overall as the 3rd most popular topic (Walmsley 2019). Typical examples of these publications are Keaney and Oskala's (2007) article, which explores the reasons for and barriers to older people engaging with the arts, and Jancovich's (2011) critical analysis of New Labour's policy drive to increase cultural participation amongst under-represented groups in the UK. Collectively, this significant body of work, which finds its natural home in *Cultural Trends*, provides an objective evaluation of who is participating in different manifestations of the arts and culture together with a predominantly subjective analysis of why this might be the case and what managers and policymakers might do about it. As such, although it is vital from a cultural policy studies perspective, the insights it offers into audiences' experiences per se are somewhat limited, and this particular genre of scholarship thus inevitably lies on the periphery of audience research.

Despite the recent renaissance in scholarship on cultural participation and democracy, audience researchers have always been interested in a different aspect of participation, namely *how* audiences participate in the arts. This is an important distinction because it demarcates audience studies as a discipline that explores the *how and why* of engagement, rather than the *who and why not*. So the *nature* of participation has always been a core question for audience researchers who, as we have already seen in this review, have long wrestled with debates about active versus passive engagement and traced the decline of vocal audience participation. A perfect illustration of audience research into participation is offered by Gareth White's (2013) study of what he refers to as the "aesthetics of the invitation". White's book offers a rare insight into how well conceived participation can foster a more embodied mode of interpretation amongst audiences and into the role that risk can play in determining whether audiences take up an invitation to participate.

As we shall see in the next section of this review, the rise in participatory arts practice has engendered a new subgenre of audience research that coheres specifically around immersive performance. But before we move on to explore this particular genre, we must pause to acknowledge the rising scholarly interest in co-production and co-creation, which indeed is now such a significant (although vastly under-explored) field of study that I will dedicate an entire chapter of this book to it.

The novelty of co-creation has been overemphasised in the literature. Although scholars are right to respond to the rise in co-created activity within the performing arts in recent years, co-creation, whether understood as the co-creation of art (product) or the co-creation of value and meaning (process), has actually been a feature of the performing arts since time immemorial, and it was certainly a core aspect of both Ancient Greek and Shakespearean performance. In more recent memory, the Russian actor, director, and producer Vsevolod Meyerhold was highly aware back in 1929 that plays remain unfinished until they reach an audience, acknowledging that "the crucial version" of a production is "made by the spectator" (Blau 1990, p. 279). Blau expresses a seemingly vain hope that co-created art might offer new insights into the audience experience:

> What happened over the last generation was that we sometimes thought we might see something else by not looking at all, while returning the theater to more or less nonverbal, elemental forms of play and alternative playing spaces in which the old narrative atrocities would be dispersed and the audience could perform. (1990, p. 94)

Blau appears to regard co-creation in a cynical light as a kind of phenomenological bad faith, a doomed attempt by producers and directors to break the fourth wall and conjoin performers with audiences: "We gaze, in separation, at what we cannot touch, though we fear to be touched by that at which we gaze" (ibid., p. 84). This separates him from more contemporary audience researchers, including myself, whose empirical work with audiences has highlighted the potential for co-creation to extend live engagement with art and develop empathy with artists (Walmsley 2013b, 2016). In a similar vein, and in direct contrast to Blau, Caroline Heim explores co-creation in terms of "gestural, verbal and paralingual performance" and characterises the special interrelationship between actors and audiences as a "co-presence" (2012, p. 146). So once again there are divergent views amongst audience researchers—on this occasion regarding the potential of co-creation to deepen engagement and deepen relationships between audiences and artists.

IMMERSIVE PERFORMANCE

As if in response to this challenge, the past decade has witnessed a flurry of research into audiences of immersive performance, which has rekindled interest in audience research and provided vital insights to audience studies. At the core of this body of work lies Josephine Machon's (2013) influential monograph *Immersive theatres: Intimacy and immediacy in contemporary performance*, which combines a critical commentary on immersive performance with interviews conducted with leading proponents of the genre. Machon defines immersive practice in relation to the relative degree of audience involvement, arguing essentially that what delineates immersive performance is "a prioritisation of the sensual world that is unique to each immersive event" alongside a heightened focus on the "significance of space and place" (p. 70). In immersive theatre, Machon contends, audiences are "integral to the experiential heart of the work and central to the form and aesthetic of the event" (p. 72). This is a useful description of certain types of immersive performance, but in an era where many companies and artists have latched onto the term as a catchy promotional hook, it fails to really distinguish immersive work from other participatory genres of performance. However, Machon goes on to explore audiences' motivations for engaging with immersive work, claiming convincingly that in an increasingly digital world, audiences are hungry for visceral experiences which remind them what it means to feel alive. As she puts it: "Immersive practice creates a space for reinvigorating human interaction and exchange" (p. 72).

It is this focus on viscerality and exchange that starts to demarcate immersive performance as a genre that might offer privileged phenomenological insights into audiences' experiences and qualify them as something fundamentally different from many other performance experiences. Indeed by drawing on Debord, Machon illustrates how audiences of immersive performance play the role of "*viveurs*" (p. 72) as opposed to the unemancipated *voyeurs* pitied by Rancière. This suggests that immersive performance can invoke a particular form of co-creation that empowers audiences to become a living component of live performance—at least fleetingly, because Machon goes on to clarify that the disparate roles played by audiences alternate between passive consumers, witnesses, associates, clients, guests, co-producers, protagonists, and even "creative comrades" (p. 73). Considering audience members' propensity to engage with artists on equal terms and to engage with art via multiple senses, Machon concludes that the term "audience" has become a "vexed term" (p. 98) which reduces the audience project to that of a passive audio witness, whereas in reality immersive performance can have an "affective potential for empowerment and communitas" and therefore act as "a democratising force" (p. 150). So there is a strong suggestion in Machon's work that immersive performance, at its most authentic, can act as a welcome antidote to the centuries of calculated disempowerment of audiences and serve as a positive emancipatory force. This positive assessment of immersive performance is echoed in the most recent addition to the field, *Staging spectators in immersive performance*, where the editors argue that immersive experiences can mobilise audiences through processes of "affective rationality" (Kolesch et al. 2019).

Jennifer Radbourne approaches immersive performance from an arts marketing perspective and appears to concur with Mahon that this contemporary genre can foster deeper relationships with audiences:

> Marketing in the arts is now driven by an audience quest for appropriation, connectivity and transformation through the arts experience. New immersive models of performance, presentation, production and distribution, are required in order to attract and retain audiences. (2013, p. 147)

Radbourne and her Deakin University colleagues have developed a significant body of work on performing arts audiences that is largely focused on investigating the dimensions of the audience experience (Radbourne et al. 2013) and how audiences perceive artistic quality and impact

(Radbourne et al. 2009, 2010). Radbourne's observation about arts marketing cited above illustrates how audiences' needs and desires are evolving as they seek deeper and more transformative connections with art and artists, and she distinguishes immersive performance as an ideal model to meet these changing consumer needs. However, as its title suggests, Adam Alston's (2016) book *Beyond immersive theatre: Aesthetics, politics and productive participation* takes a much more critical stance. Alston questions the extent to which the "productive audiences" often hailed by immersive practitioners might justifiably be judged to be empowered. Through a range of extended case studies, Alston explores how the putative empowerment of immersed audiences actually stands up to political scrutiny. Ultimately, Alston argues that immersive aesthetics are often influenced in practice by neoliberalism, which can sometimes manifest as a commercial experience machine, and he calls on immersive practitioners to challenge what he perceives to be a negative political interference on a potentially liberating genre.

Lynne Conner (2013) is equally critical of immersive performance. In the course of her exhortation for a genuine and dialogic engagement with audiences, Conner dismisses immersive performances such as Punchdrunk's *Sleep no more* as "a kind of meta-spectating" that "invites audience members to actively shape each other's experience, even if that shaping is limited to shoving other spectators out of the way" (p. 146). She also questions whether immersive performance pushes audience members "towards analysis and evaluation of the arts event itself" or "to render meaning once they pull off their masks" (pp. 146–147). In a thinly veiled critique of contemporary practice reminiscent of Alston's charge of neoliberalism, Conner concludes that arts organisations need to consider their audiences as "a collection of individual subjects who think and feel – as opposed to groupings of demographics who consume" (p. 160). So as with co-creation, the jury seems to be out on whether immersive performance ultimately offers any deeper type or mode of engagement than traditional performance.

PERFORMANCE VENUES, SPACES, AND PLACES

The previous section on immersive performance highlighted the significant role that place and space can play in influencing the nature of audiences' experiences. As Bourdieu (1991) noted, arts venues act as physical manifestations of cultural capital and habitus, and they can elicit profound feelings of unworthiness and incompetence amongst those who are new to them.

As we observed earlier in the chapter, a very small number of audience researchers are engaging with this theory under the wider theme of class. But the role of the arts venue, or perhaps the location of an arts event, is so important in the context of audience engagement that it warrants its own independent scrutiny, and various audience researchers have focused on aspects of place and space, either expressly or spontaneously, precisely because of its fundamental impact on audiences' overall experiences of art.

As Douglas Brown notes: "A fundamental ingredient of presenting quality arts and entertainment experiences to contemporary audiences is the imaginative design, management and use of the places in which they happen" (2011, p. 103). Brown's concise history of the design and architecture of arts venues highlights how they have evolved over the centuries from the open public fora of Classical Greece to the socially exclusive Victorian spaces that contained segregated entrances, exits, and seating, and back to more open, but now more intimate, contemporary social spaces. As Janelle Reinelt observes, audience members often invest "in the occasion of the performance rather than the performance itself" (2014, p. 358) and so these more social spaces are fit-for-purpose. However, considering the strong consensus in the literature regarding the vital role that arts venues play in audiences' artistic encounters, the charge that "arts facilities have not evolved or adapted to the changing expectations and needs of contemporary artists, audiences and communities" is of particular concern (Brown 2013, p. 52). Alan Brown's manifold empirical studies of performing arts audiences have led him to conclude that: "Inviting audiences to spaces they do not want to visit is a losing proposition, especially when they *do* show up and feel out of place" (p. 53, original italics). Brown's research illustrates how audiences often identify with and even personify arts spaces, promoting them in their minds to core determinants of their overall experience.

> Consumers have deep-seated feelings about arts spaces, describing them as 'friendly', 'welcoming', or 'cold', or 'intimidating' – attributes often ascribed to people. [...] Venues also take on symbolic meanings, either based on actual experience or transmitted through social networks. (2013, p. 53)

From an arts marketing perspective, then, venues are strongly correlated with consumer satisfaction and have a powerful impact on perceptions and word-of-mouth. But as Brown suggests here, their role is far more than simply an augmented product: arts spaces play an important sociological role in their communities, and audiences engage with them on a deeply personal level that may or may not be connected to the art that takes place within them. This perhaps, at least partly, explains the popularity of site-specific, site-responsive, and immersive performance, which, as we saw in the previous section, is characterised by its integral relationship with place.

Aspects of place and space are undeniably central to questions of audience development, audience engagement and audience enrichment: venues and artistic locations either enhance or detract; they appeal or repel. Although limited research has been conducted into young audiences' perceptions of arts venues, a comprehensive six-year study of Australian audiences aged 14–25 revealed that venues' social and communal spaces are often as much of an attraction for young people as the performances themselves (O'Toole et al. 2014, p. 9). The study highlighted the fact that younger audiences want to feel "comfortable", "special", and welcome in an arts venue; they seek "a sense of belonging" to a place that is "special, classy or cool" (pp. 50–51). They like the idea of "a place where certain behaviours and protocols were to be followed; a place tinged with excitement and expectation" (ibid.). Younger audiences often sense disappointment and anti-climax when venues lack any palpable "atmosphere" or close soon after a performance, because they appreciate the "buzz and excitement" of a busy public space (pp. 54–55). Studies dedicated to young audiences are vitally important (although also markedly rare) not simply because young audiences are of course *the* future audiences of the arts and thus their *sine qua non*, but also because they represent a microcosm of audiences more broadly and can therefore provide fresh insights into audience research: The fresh eyes and honesty often exhibited by young audiences can help to circumnavigate methodological challenges such as positive bias that we will explore in detail in Chapter 5.

When it comes to venues, the findings of studies of young audiences tend to reinforce the audience research undertaken with adult audiences—which again is sadly rare on the ground. A wonderful exception to this gap is Karen Burland and Stephanie Pitts' (2012) study of *The Spin*—a weekly jazz club in Oxford (UK). As the authors describe it, *The Spin* takes place in an intimate room above a pub with a bar at the back and a small stage at the front. Seats are arranged in café style with standing room at the back. The researchers selected the club because it had been recently nominated for Jazz Venue of the Year and so they felt it would provide an opportunity to explore what is special about venues and how they impact on audiences' overall experiences. Their findings highlighted the significance of the small, intimate and social nature of the space, which participants compared with being a football fan, sharing with others "feelings of intimacy, connectedness and despair and joy [...] surrounded by a like-minded crowd" (pp. 534–35). It transpired that jazz audiences want to feel part of the performance, which involves "being close enough to the music that it is totally immersing" (p. 537). When deciding where to go to see a live performance, participants seemed to be searching for the "ideal" jazz gig, which they articulated mainly in terms of the atmosphere and venue, the performers and fellow audience members (p. 537). Cognisant again of the sociological role played by the venue, the authors conclude that:

> *The Spin*'s success must, in part, be related to its choice to develop a community, or "club", of like-minded individuals who support its activities almost as a matter of routine, suggesting that the current focus on developing new audiences may be better dedicated to understanding how to sustain current audiences and increase their loyalty to events within particular venues. (Burland and Pitts 2012, p. 538)

The Spin is partly a case study in fandom, and as such it highlights the role that arts clubs might play in developing more loyal followers, from both new and existing audiences.

It cannot be a coincidence that several significant audience studies are based on jazz. Just as young audiences represent a microcosm of general arts audiences, jazz seems to offer up a particularly intense example of audiencing. This is probably a result of the factors elucidated in the previous case study, namely: intimacy, proximity to performers, and opportunities for fandom and socialisation. This working hypothesis is supported by another study of jazz, which similarly accentuates the particularly social and relational aspects of jazz attendance:

> For the audience members interviewed, a significant factor in their choice of jazz performance was whether the venue allowed for them to make direct connections, physical or emotional, with the musicians. [...] They wanted to be close to the musicians, see them interact with each other and see them play as clearly as they could hear them. (Brand et al. 2012, p. 642)

Alongside this further evidence of the arts providing an ideal opportunity for enhanced socialisation, there are insights into kinaesthetic and educational engagement here which will be developed later in the book. But for now, let's focus our attention on the concept of intimacy and on its antithetical concept of "distance".

Distance emerges as a niche but nonetheless important area of audience research—not least because of its phenomenological implications. As Blau observes, distance impacts upon audiences in both a literal and metaphorical sense: "Up too close you can't think, too far back you can't feel. If proximity blurs vision, there is a point beyond which there is an astigmatism in distance" (1990, p. 117). Blau is suggesting here that there is an optimal distance between audiences and performers. Bearing in mind Machon's research into immersive performance and our earlier discussion about jazz, Blau's theory appears to be contested by audiences themselves, who often appear keen to actually touch performers and even push fellow spectators out of the way to achieve this! However, the theoretical viewpoint propagated by Blau is supported by phenomenologists, who make a clear distinction between everyday and aesthetic distance: "Our engagement during the theatrical experience may be intense, but it is not the kind of engagement that occurs in life experience. The difference is a function of distance" (Ben Chaim 1984, p. ix). Although Daphna Ben Chaim's philosophical exploration of the aesthetics of audience response clarifies that there is no unified theory of distance amongst aestheticians, she draws heavily on Edward Bullough and Jean-Paul Sartre to argue that the performing arts function through the deliberate manipulation of distance by artists and that audiences need to be complicit in this in order to derive emotional engagement. So distance ultimately emerges as an enabler of audience engagement.

The natural conclusion to draw from phenomenologists and aestheticians is that distance functions differently in art from in real life because art is always a *conceit*. This reflects the broader consensus in this section of the review that performing arts venues can hold exceptional qualities that are integral to audiences' artistic experiences. Heim's research with audiences and performers drives this point home, highlighting succinctly the communitarian value of arts venues and reinforcing the inherently relational nature of the performing arts: "People nowadays have relatively few opportunities to physically commune with each other and feel part of a community, so arts venues have the potential to become community spaces" (2016, p. 123). We will explore this communitarian aspect of audiency further in the following section.

Performance as Ritual

As we saw earlier in the chapter, scholars remain divided on the extent to which audiencing can be considered a collaborative pursuit. Blau, for example, asserts that the notion of the theatre audience as a community can only ever be fictitious (1990, p. 11). For Blau, who was heavily influenced by Sartre, theatre-going represents a kind of futile wish-fulfilment, the ultimate goal of which (i.e. to possess the Other, in form of the performer and/or the fellow audience member) is always ultimately doomed. Blau is ultimately cynical about the audience project, claiming that the desired goals of permanence and collective experience remain de facto elusive:

> The dative of an audience is this alienated zone where a repeated impermanence is the thing itself and where there is an intersection, too, of being and *being more*, more than *one*, the proximity of separation in a space of desire that precedes or exceeds any sort of collectivity. (1990, p. 346, original italics)

In Blau's opinion, audiences can only ever exist as temporary postulates because: "An audience without a history is not an audience" (p. 16). What Blau neglects here is not simply the fact that some audience groups do indeed share a long history of collective arts experiences (as the case study of *The Spin* made clear) but also the potential for *communitas*, a shared state of liminality which delivers communal experience and meaning. He also disregards the value and impact of temporary communities and experiences. According to Victor Turner (1975), communitas "can only be evoked easily when there are many occasions outside the ritual on which communitas has been achieved" (p. 56). This is seemingly a positive sign for audiences, who, as Stanley Fish observed, often arrive at performances as part of "interpretive communities" and approach productions with a "similar language" (cited in Kattwinkel 2003, p. xii). This suggests that audiences are not always as heterogeneous, nor indeed as disconnected, as theorists might lead us to believe. Susan Kattwinkel interprets communitas as a desire amongst audience members to "feel like they are creating and expressing common sentiment along with the performers and each other; a goal of active spectatorship" (pp. x–xi). There are some interesting and significant implications here, which collectively highlight the need for arts organisations to engage their audiences collectively, to develop them as a congregation, or at least to encourage and facilitate this act of communal active spectatorship.

For Turner, communitas is enabled by the ritualistic nature of performance and by its ability to replace the routine of everyday life with special "dramatic time" (1982, p. 9). Dramatic time allows for what Turner refers to as "ergotropic behaviour" (p. 9), which is characterised by participants' arousal and heightened emotional activity. This behaviour leads participants into a numinous, hypertrophic state that encourages them to de-sacralise society and ultimately to be transformed (p. 10). Although Turner's highly influential theories of performance emerged well before the rise of empirical audience research, his notions of arousal and hypertrophy have since been supported by biometric, psychobiological and neurobiological enquiries into audiency. To that extent, Turner's work might be judged to be somewhat prescient, foreshadowing numerous recent studies that have highlighted the strong emotional impact of the performing arts on audiences as well as its spiritual and physiological impacts (Walmsley 2013a). However, despite the enduring legacy of Turner's work in performance studies, in her inspirational book *Dancing in the streets: A history of collective joy*, Barbara Ehrenreich (2007) criticises Turner's narrow focus on communitas as a manifestation of social structure. Ehrenreich develops the concept by focusing on the psychological drivers that underscore the state of communitas, drawing closely on Durkheim's concept of "collective effervescence", which she interprets as "ritually induced passion or ecstasy that cements social bonds" (pp. 2–3) and leads to "communal excitement" (p. 35). This Classical interpretation of communitas nods to the more prevalent theory of catharsis, which will be explored in the following chapter. For now, it is important to note Ehrenreich's depiction of the performing arts as a joyful communal ritual. It is also worth noting that Ehrenreich's observations are supported by insights from cognitive science, where experiments have revealed that rhythm can indeed enhance group solidarity (McConachie 2008, p. 73).

So once again, there is dissonance in the literature regarding the extent to which audiencing can ever be a genuinely collective experience. The theoretical dividing line appears to be between the spiritualists and anthropologists on the one side and the rationalists and phenomenologists on the other: although phenomenologists believe they have proved that the Self can never be at one with or possess the Other, many anthropologists have borne witness to ritual practice which presents itself as a communal rite. This brings into question the relationship between art and ritual, and in response to this it is important to acknowledge the high degree of consensus amongst audience researchers that art represents a quintessential human ritual. Indeed as Ehrenreich notes, art is one of the few remaining rituals we have left and we run the risk of losing it altogether. This brings us back to the insights offered by relational aesthetics, which pertinently suggests that art offers "spaces where we can elaborate alternative forms of sociability, critical models and moments of constructed conviviality" (Bourriaud 2002, p. 44).

RECEPTION THEORY AND SEMIOTICS

One of the main attempts to place audiences back at the heart of audience research came with the development of reception theory, and Susan Bennett's *Theatre audiences* remains a seminal text for audience researchers working in this tradition. Bennett's monograph originally dates back to 1990 and it was therefore one of the first books to apply both reader-response and spectatorship theories to the context of the performing arts (Freshwater 2009). Bennett was influenced by a number of cultural theorists including Roland Barthes, who famously argued in his *Death of the author* that critics should take a less biographical approach to literary analysis and focus more on the interpretation of readers in the acknowledgment that interpretation takes place within a complex network of intertextuality, at the heart of which lie "interpretive communities" (Fish, cited in Bennett 1997, p. 40). The notion of interpretive communities will be central to this book and as such this book owes much to the audience-centred thinking proffered by Barthes, Fish and Bennett.

Bennett's book champions what she calls the "productive and emancipated" role that audiences play in critical theory and in explicating what is undoubtedly a complex social phenomenon (1997, p. 1). Bennett laments the developments in production values and mores that engendered the damaging separation of audiences from the stage (p. 3) and the epistemological biases that led to much dramatic theory neglecting the role of audience interpretation (p. 4) and culminated in a situation characterised by the fact that discussions of audience reception remain "simple and cursory" (p. 7). In tracing the development of theatre practice over the course of the Twentieth Century, Bennett highlights the primary role that political (and notably Brechtian) theatre played in emancipating the audience project, shifting the culture of performance from a "hermetically sealed" to a "cooperative" venture where audiences were no longer conceived as passive receivers but as active participants and producers of meaning (p. 30). This shift was precipitated by the rebalancing of power away from texts and writers towards directors and dramaturgs that was notable in much European theatre in the latter half of the Twentieth Century. Bennett's study was instrumental in shifting thinking about audiences into a new empirical terrain, partly by insisting that the audience project needed to be explored through "social co-ordinates" (p. 86), including "proxemic relations" and the interplay between and amongst performers and audiences (pp. 131–32). As Kirsty Sedgman argues, Bennett's work succeeded in breaking theatre scholarship away from considering audiences' responses to performance as "natural outcomes of performance intention" (2016, p. 8). However, Sedgman justifiably goes on to critique Bennett's contribution for its overridingly theoretical focus on the "culturally specific paratheatrical determinants of audience reception" (ibid.).

Marco De Marinis (1987) distinguishes between two different levels of reception: the "extra-textual" level of "the real (empirical) receiver" and the "intra-textual" level of "the implied (the hypothetical, ideal, virtual) receiver" (p. 102). According to De Marinis, extra-textual reception involves the effective activation of reading strategies whereas intra-textual reception is concerned with "the manner of interpretation anticipated by the text and written into it" (ibid.). This is a useful distinction because it highlights both the need for empirical research to make fully informed judgements about reception and the fact that by concentrating only on the hypothetical or ideal audience member, theoretical scholars wilfully ignore the semiotic and dramaturgical impact on audiences, their individual viewing strategies and subjective responses, and thus engage primarily in what can only be called assumption. As De Marinis puts it, the ideal or "model" spectator "represents a hypothetical construct and is simply part of a theoretical metalanguage" (ibid.). This implicit call to prioritise the live performance over the text as the ultimate moment of reception was taken up by a number of audience scholars including Vasile Popovici, who rightly argued that "the dialogical nature of the dramatic genre is not to be found in the internal organisation of the play: it is revealed at the level of the performance" (1984, p. 111). Popovici and De Marinis thus also helped to move audience research closer to the audience.

In theory, semiotics represented a concerted attempt to analyse precisely how performance was revealed during performance. In his influential monograph *The theatrical event: Dynamics of performance and reception*, Willmar Sauter (2000) offers a useful summary of the development of audience research. Although in many ways this study argues strongly against a semiotic approach to performance studies, Sauter rightly credits semiotics with placing performance "right back in the centre of the debate" (2000, p. 24). This point is emphasised by Martin Barker (2006), who goes so far as to credit the very emergence of audience research, at least in Europe, to the rise of semiotics within its home of cultural studies:

> For good or bad, audience research in the UK, and consequentially in the rest of Europe, was born under the star of Stuart Hall's "encoding-decoding" model—a model that sought to offer a conceptualization of text-audience relations which could simultaneously treat texts properly as such (as culturally formed items) and also capture their ideological functions. (p. 128)

However, in Sauter's view, semiotics dehumanised and commodified performance; and Sauter's own lasting contribution to audience research was to characterise performance as a "communicative event" that can be "traced to hermeneutic theories, both as a philosophical approach and as an empirical system" (p. 12). This is the view shared by most contemporary audience researchers, who have adopted the intersubjective and co-created perspective of interpretation and meaning-making championed by hermeneutics.

Bruce McConachie (2008) places another nail in the coffin of semiotics by positioning it in opposition to cognitive science. McConachie argues that like certain other post-structuralist theories of audiences' experiences, semiotics merely condemns the audience project to the world of illusion:

> For some poststructuralist theorists such as Jean Baudrillard, who build on the assumptions of semiotics, spectators rarely get beyond illusory signifiers; they are mostly doomed to a world of simulations that can never touch the Real. But [...] the world on stage is not entirely fictional. (p. 48)

Like the phenomenologists whom we explored earlier in relation to distance and communality, the post-structuralists condemn the audience project to the realms of fiction and bad faith. To counter this, and by drawing on documentary theatre as an example, McConachie convincingly illustrates how via a process of "conceptual blending" audiences can in reality be exposed to "a high level of actuality" and happily accept "a minimally intrusive level of fictionality" (pp. 48–49). This culminates, McConachie argues, in a situation whereby audiences "do not believe they are participating in an unreal illusion when they 'live in the blend' of a performance". Unlike semiotic theory, cognitive studies can provide scientific *evidence* for audiences' ability to blend fiction with reality and run "multiple conceptions simultaneously" (p. 50).

A final critique that can justifiably be levelled at reception and semiotic studies is that they fail to explore what Schoenmakers (1990) refers to as "reception results" (i.e. the impact of performance on audiences post hoc). Through their exclusive focus on the decoding of the performance itself, these approaches neglect the vitally important hermeneutic aspects of audiency and as such remain epistemologically flawed. In summary, history has not been kind to reception theory and semiotics, at least in the field of audience studies, where scholars have now moved on to adopt a wide array of empirical methods that enable more sensitive and longitudinal enquiries into audiences' arts experiences and that finally identify audiences themselves as the rightful subjects of audience research.

RESEARCH METHODOLOGIES

Chapter 5 is dedicated to a thorough critical review of the different methods and methodologies deployed by audience researchers. The aim of this section is rather to review recent studies that themselves provide valuable insights into different methodological approaches to audience research.

Martin Barker (2006) certainly provides such an insight in a state-of-the-field article which sets out his ambitions for audience research. Barker's greatest expressed ambition for audience research is to be able to state "with sufficient precision to be checkable the conditions that have to be met for an audience member to be said to have attained an unconditionally positive experience from a cultural encounter" (p. 130). Barker is a stoic champion of rigorous mixed-methods audience research and he rightly bemoans the fact that tried and tested methods in one field (such as media studies) often fail to be replicated in others (such as performance studies). As the above citation suggests, replicability is vital to Barker, because he is keen to harbour audience research from persistent charges of description and anecdotalism. To this end, Barker has been part of a research team that has conducted two of the largest scale audiences studies ever undertaken, with almost 25,000 participants responding to a survey on *The Lord of the Rings* in 2004 and over 36,000 responding to a subsequent study of New Line Cinema and Peter Jackson's adaptation of *The Hobbit* (Barker and Mathijs 2016). Barker is right to rail that audience studies has thus far "been content with loose and vague concepts", and he is equally justified in his call for the field to establish its own working concepts and methods of enquiry (2006, p. 128).

However, audience studies has always been an inherently cross-disciplinary and heterogeneous field, and it is certainly unlikely, and probably undesirable, than any one theoretical framework will ever emerge. If a paradigm is ever to be determined for audience studies then it will need to be a catholic one which leaves room for diverse traditions and methods. Like Barker, Kirsty Sedgman is a strong advocate for both diversity and rigour in audience research and both scholars call for a "defragmentation" of the field. Sedgman also urges the discipline towards greater self-reflexivity, arguing that "rigorous audience projects must embed in their analysis an examination of the political and interpersonal implications of the process of research itself" (forthcoming). In other words, the methodologies and methods selected by audience researchers always colour the ensuing "findings", which are therefore always contingent and contextual. Accordingly, qualitative audience research can only ever be interpretative, and possibly even doubly so, since it generally constitutes "an act of interpreting an act of interpretation" (Sedgman 2017, p. 315).

Lisa Baxter, Daragh O'Reilly and Liz Carnegie have also made a significant contribution to developing research methodologies with audiences. Much of their work champions, applies and evaluates innovative and participatory methods of inquiry into arts engagement, including creative and interactive techniques such as guided visualisation. These researchers operate under the guiding principle that: "Audience research participants should be treated as active partners rather than simply sources of data" in order to elicit "richer, deeper insights" (Baxter et al. 2013, p. 127). Their work, and that of Lisa Baxter in particular, offers alternative approaches that not only open up audience research to participants who might struggle to communicate their arts engagement in verbal terms but that also align with the creative questions under scrutiny. Moreover, these creative approaches can also facilitate the emergence of non-conscious responses to arts engagement.

Creative methods can be particularly effective with non-traditional audience groups, such as children and participants suffering from dementia, for example. Like Baxter, Matthew Reason deploys a range of creative methods, including drawing and movement, to "deepen and extend the kinds of responses" collected from audience participants (2010, p. 15). As Reason points out, audiences' responses to performances can act as "a kind of countersignature" to them, morphing and modifying them along the way; and although these responses can be intellectual or rational, they can equally be embodied, kinaesthetic and/or intuitive (p. 28). These disparate types of response clearly require divergent research methods, and Reason emphasises the need for synergy between different philosophies and methodologies of audience research:

> The key concern here is the nature of spectatorship and the relationship between what we might term 'the experience' of performance and any one individual's conscious, reflective ability to externalise that experience. These concerns are at once methodological, asking what is knowable about our own and other people's experiences; and also philosophical, directly interrogating the fundamental question of what it means to experience art. (2010, p. 15)

As Sedgman (forthcoming) concludes, there are many different ways to research audiences but it is never a neutral act.

As we observed earlier in the chapter, Bruce McConachie (2008) takes a very particular approach to audience engagement and strives to make developments through cognitive science. Cognisant of the entrenched prejudices and methodological divides that have hampered audience research over the past few decades, McConachie rightly insists that "cognitive and cultural approaches to audiences need not be antithetical" (p. 5). Nevertheless, he argues that in order to make progress, audience scholars need to "move beyond postshow interviews, audience surveys, and similar methods" and deploy the more scientific tools offered by disciplines such as experimental linguists and neuroscience (pp. 15–16). Like Barker, he is minded to support methodological approaches that have the potential to generate irrefutable evidence about audiences, claiming that "an approach to spectatorship grounded in falsifiable theories and empirical knowledge has a better chance of discovering some critical and historical truths than do theories that cannot be validated scientifically" (p. 14). However, there exists an inner tension within McConachie's work, which on the one hand claims that divergent methods should coexist whilst on the other establishes an implicit hierarchy between interpretivist and positivist research. This is indicative of the wider tension that persists in the field and that often prevents the mixed-methods or triangulated approach that the field desperately needs. We will explore these challenges further in Chapter 5.

The Audience Experience

It has become apparent in the course of this review that scholars are increasingly moving away from theoretical approaches to audience research and investing their efforts in explicating audiences' diverse and complex experiences of the performing arts through empirical methods. Helen Freshwater, for example, advocates for a cultural studies approach to audience research, noting that a more embedded approach makes manifest the individual positionality inherent to the audience experience:

> Ultimately, cultural studies has come to be characterised by a rejection of the notion of 'the audience' as a singular or homogeneous entity, a detailed interrogation of diverse and sometimes unexpected responses, and an ethnographic engagement with the range of cultural conditions which inform an individual's viewing position. (2009, p. 28)

The following chapter will be dedicated to deconstructing the nature of audiences' diverse experiences of the performing arts. The aim of this section is to review how the key authors who focus explicitly on audiences' experiences explicate those experiences and to outline the implications of this for audience research more broadly.

As Freshwater intimates, one of the main reasons to prioritise audiences' experiences is to guard against the general objectification and homogenisation which audiences have faced for centuries.

> The common tendency to refer to an audience as 'it' and, by extension, to think of this 'it' as a single entity or a collective, risks obscuring the multiple contingencies of subjective response, context, and environment which condition an individual's interpretation of a particular performance event. (2009, p. 5)

Focussing research on audiences' lived experiences implies exploring the complexities inherent to these experiences and accepting the nature of audience engagement as plural and contingent. However, in an attempt to simplify this plurality, some scholars have strived to narrow the scope of audience research and delimit the inevitable contingencies. For example, Radbourne et al. (2009) attempt to "measure" the audience experience. Based on a qualitative study of audience engagement in three Australian performing arts organisations, the authors discern four core dimensions of the audience experience: knowledge, risk, authenticity, and collective engagement. They argue that if audiences' expectations in relation to these dimensions are satisfied, then audiences will be highly likely to return to an arts organisation, which, they maintain, represents a valid proxy for experiential "quality" (p. 28). The problem with this reduction is not simply the small sample size that the authors themselves concede; it is also that it diminishes the subjective nature of audiences' desires and fails to account for the artistic and emotional quality of their experiences, factors which have been demonstrated time and again to be primary determinants of positive engagement.

Once again there exists a tension in audience research between positivism and interpretivism, and in the context of the audience experience, this generally occurs across disciplinary divides such as arts management versus cultural or performance studies. We will explore the foci and contributions offered by arts management and marketing in due course, but at this stage it is important to note that many audience researchers working in this domain are keen to offer *solutions* to arts organisations and policymakers, and so their research is inevitably more utilitarian and applied. By contrast the research produced by cultural studies and performance scholars tends to be more conceptual and abstract. It covers, for example, aspects of liveness, play, and manipulation (Auslander 2008; De Marinis 1987; McConachie 2008); collective engagement and intersubjectivity (Blau 1990; Popovici 1984); suspending disbelief (Schechner 2003); immersion and flow (Csikszentmihalyi 1988; Machon 2013); embodied and enactive spectatorship (Bleeker and Germano 2014; Reynolds and Reason 2011); arousal and reward (Berlyne 1971; Silvia 2005); and catharsis and transformation (Golden 1973). These are the main topics that will shape the structure of the following chapter. They encapsulate and illustrate the myriad psychological, phenomenological, psychobiological, and spiritual elements that comprise audiences' experiences of the performing arts.

Value and Impact Research

One area of audience research that attracts scholars from many different disciplines is what I will refer to here as value and impact research. Studies in this area explore fundamental questions of why audiences engage with the performing arts, what they are seeking, what kind of value and benefits they incur, and how this value might impact both on audiences themselves and on society more broadly. These questions are naturally of interest to many different fields—for example, to cultural policy scholars who are investigating cultural value, to management scholars interested in aspects of strategic purpose and evaluation, to arts marketing scholars exploring consumer demands, to performance scholars investigating the role of dramaturgy, etc. This all makes for a rich body of cross-disciplinary research on the value and impact of the performing arts as perceived by audiences.

One small but significant strand of this work is research on audience motivation, which explores the artistic/aesthetic, social, and psychological aspirations of audiences. Konijn (1999) refers to these drivers as "the affective benefits of attending performances" and observes that these are underprivileged in performance studies (pp. 170–171). This is an understatement: as many scholars have noted, the vast majority of audience research still focuses on what we could call the *micro* context—i.e. immediate responses to a particular performance. What is lacking is sufficient research into the *meta* context—the accumulated longitudinal value incurred by audiences over many years of audiencing. A notable exception here is Janelle Reinelt's study of theatre spectatorship and value attribution, which demonstrated the longitudinal impact of different types of theatre on audiences, reporting, for example, how theatre encourages audiences to "think or feel deeply about aspects of human life, the current world situation, politics, or social issues" (2014, p. 354). Reinelt's study revealed how audiences attribute both intrinsic and instrumental value to their theatre-going activity, which they describe in terms ranging from an appreciation of language and acting to developing their world view (p. 354). In a policy and management context where arts organisations have to increasingly justify their very existence, longitudinal value and impact evaluation is of paramount importance, and so Chapter 4 will offer a detailed exploration of this theme.

There is also insufficient research into what we know to be significant differences in audiences' motivations for engaging with different art forms. For example, as we saw in the discussion of jazz, one recurrent theme in the literature on value and impact is audiences' desire to be in close proximity to performers. However, a tiny minority of audience researchers contend that this desire is inherently futile, in that the dynamic of performance is actually predicated on the distinction, distance and separation, rather than the unity and communion, between performers and spectators (Auslander 2008, pp. 55–56). Or, as Blau puts it: "A discourse on the audience must inevitably move across a spectrum of apprehension between the old fantasy of communion and the divisionary impasse" (1990, p. 25). Empirical research generally contests this pessimistic reading of the audience project. My own research with theatre audiences highlights a strong desire amongst certain audience typologies to join the inner circle of actors (Walmsley, forthcoming), and, of course, many audience members are actually performers themselves. Audience members often report feeling part of a communion with performers; they empathise, perceive the chemical buzz of the performance, and are conjoined in moments of collective flow. As Caroline Heim's work illustrates, there is a necessary reciprocity between performers and audiences that takes the form of an "unlimited symbiosis" wherein both parties "intuitively and consensually collaborate as co-performers and sometimes co-conspirators to create a performance" (2016, p. 53). So in many empirical studies undertaken with both audiences and performers, the communal and collaborative nature of performance emerges as a core component of impact, providing both groups with an empathic human experience that seems to supersede their physical distance.

The other significant studies into the value and impact of performance on audiences have been produced by McCarthy et al., Alan Brown, Jennifer Novak, Radbourne et al., Stephanie Pitts, Anne-Marie Hede and Tabitha White. McCarthy et al.'s (2004) *Gifts of the Muse* aimed to reframe the debate on the benefits of the arts by reviewing the totality of arts-related benefits; illustrating the relationship between private and public benefits; and dichotomising them into intrinsic benefits, including captivation and pleasure, and instrumental benefits, such as social capital and economic growth. A few years later, Brown (2006) provided an extended version of the framework, aimed at providing a kaleidoscopic "architecture of value" (p. 19) to visually articulate the arts experience. Brown's model maps a range of arts benefits by value cluster, which he delineates as follows: imprint of the arts experience; personal development; human interaction; communal meaning; and economic and social benefits. Brown and Novak's (2007) research into the intrinsic impacts of live performances moved these findings forwards by focusing on the *process* of value transfer. Based on extensive primary research of performing arts audiences in the United States, this mixed-methods study indicates that the single best predictor of audience satisfaction is captivation, which itself is generated most effectively by stoking audiences' sense of anticipation and getting them in the mood, which the authors construct as "readiness-to-receive". Captivation emerges therefore as the "lynchpin of impact" (pp. 10–11). This research is supported by Radbourne et al.'s (2009) findings, which link prior knowledge to a "richer experience" (p. 20), and by Pitts' (2005) qualitative research of a chamber music festival, which demonstrates how audiences' anticipation can be enhanced by pre-show activities such as introductory talks, which set the scene, provide a context, and create a sense of empathy between the performers and the spectators, drawing them into the action and opening up the "communication loop" (p. 260). White and Hede (2008) draw on a narrative methodology to explore the various dimensions of the impact of art on individuals. Their model portrays impact as a ripple effect, emanating outwards from the core artistic experience. Unlike the previous models, it combines individual and collective impact, depicting the blurred lines between the personal and social benefits of the arts, and it focuses on the important role that "enablers" such as context, access, and venues can play in maximising impact. The core manifestations of impact again reflect the now familiar themes from the literature—wellbeing, social bonding, aesthetic growth, vision, and empathy.

Young Audiences

A significant but sadly still niche subgenre of audience research is dedicated to studying young audiences. As well as constituting a vital audience segment in their own right, young audiences are also of course the future lifeblood of the performing arts; and in a context where they seem to be dying away, at least in some of the more traditional art forms such as classical music and opera, they are ripe subjects for audience development and engagement activity and the focus of much cultural policy. As audience research develops and evolves, scholars are increasingly investigating special subgroups such as prison audiences (e.g. Reason 2019) and intercultural audiences (e.g. Knowles 2010). One of the main achievements of these specialist foci is to shine a spotlight on a microcosm of "the audience", to provide insights into what we might term *hyper-audiencing*—highly tailored or specialised experiences of the performing arts designed for niche audience segments. Although there is not an abundant body of literature on young audiences per se, the studies that do exist succeed in providing fresh understanding of how a particular group of people, from a particular generation that shares particular traits and concerns, engages with the performing arts.

For example, O'Toole et al.'s (2014) extensive empirical study of young Australian audiences illustrates that for many young people, theatre-going is more of a social experience than a purely cultural experience. It also provides further evidence that theatre-going can strengthen family bonds and create shared memories. Young audiences seek "intense" experiences that are "transporting, relevant and connected to their own lives and concerns" (p. 9). Based on the findings of the study, O'Toole concludes that what happens before, during and after a performing arts experience impacts significantly on young audiences' overall experience (p. 11). Focusing on the significant need for arts education, the research team develops the concepts of "theatre confidence" and "theatre literacy" to describe what enables younger audiences to maximise their enjoyment of their theatre-going (ibid.). It could be argued, of course, that some of these findings are not specific to younger audiences. Many audience members seek social rather than cultural experiences and want to be transported by work that resonates with their lives. Similarly, all audience members are heavily influenced by what happens before, during, and after a performing arts encounter, as we saw in Brown and Novak's study. Most audience members could also benefit from further contextualisation of and education around a work of art.

However, what this study highlights is that younger audiences are particularly receptive to certain types of art and particular kinds of intervention. Many audience development studies emphasise the strong correlation between a positive formative experience of the arts and future arts participation, and so it is particularly important for artists and arts organisations to be mindful of what generally constitutes a positive experience for their younger audiences; and in a context where the creative arts are under pressure in school curricula, educational activity within arts venues themselves is more vital than ever before. Similar findings were derived from a large qualitative study of 40 young audiences of a chamber music concert in the UK (Dearn and Pitts 2017), which concluded that "the emotional, responsive listening of popular music conflicted with the etiquette of the concert hall and the structures of classical music" (p. 43). The study called for a renewed focus on music education to prepare and equip young people for all kinds of live music experiences. Like O'Toole et al.'s study, Dearn and Pitts' project highlighted the particular significance of the arts venue for younger audiences, who can easily feel conspicuous and alienated when presented with unfamiliar rites and rituals such as hidden dress codes, interval behaviour, and etiquette surrounding applause.

Matthew Reason has also conducted a significant body of research into child audiences. As discussed earlier in the chapter, Reason deploys a range of creative methods in his audience research and some of these (such as drawing) work particularly well with children when trying to elicit responses to performance. Reason (2008) is careful to point out that his role as an audience researcher is not to try to interpret children's drawings of performance but rather to use them to stimulate further discussion from the children themselves about their performance experiences. Reason's research with children has indicated that young audiences are particularly willing to accept illusion as reality and he highlights the extent to which stage characters can stimulate children's imaginations (pp. 346–347). However, his core conclusion is that children can be highly sophisticated audience members who possess "the ability to juggle contradictory interpretations and to see simultaneously on two levels [and] perform dual readings" (p. 353). This ability, he maintains, enables children "to pursue and preserve the magic of the illusion if they desire, but to do so in an empowered and enfranchised manner" (ibid.). Reason's work reminds us that the relationship between audience researchers and participants implies an inevitable imbalance of power, a theme we will return to in Chapter 5. It also reminds us to treat audiences with care and respect and to tailor our methods to their specific needs.

Arts Marketing and Management

I noted earlier in the chapter that arts management scholars tend to produce more utilitarian research that often seeks to inform management practice regarding audiences. Much of this work is located in the *International Journal of Arts Management, The Journal of Arts Management, Law and Society* and *Poetics*—journals that explicitly favour empirical research and often specifically request a dedicated focus on management implications. The tone, structure, and purport of this research tend to differ markedly from the audience scholarship produced in arts and humanities journals. This is partly because of the overt influence of business and management scholarship on the field, which tends to favour empirical and deductive research. Arts management is a relatively new academic field, and arts marketing is an even newer branch of it. Both fields suffer from a legitimacy problem as they are often viewed with suspicion from artists and management scholars alike (Colbert 2011); and both face issues of acceptance related to their language and methodologies (Piber and Chiaravalloti 2011, p. 241). This is particularly the case in audience research, where quantitative analyses of audiences tend to dominate and where qualitative research is often dismissed as narrative and anecdotal.

Arts marketing has probably evolved more notably than arts management over the past few decades, largely because it has managed to attract and embrace a more diverse range of scholars. It has been argued that since the 1980s there has been a shift in focus in arts marketing from product development to audience development but that despite this development scant attention has been paid to "building enduring relationships with existing audiences" to assist the long-term viability of performing arts organisations (Rentschler et al. 2001, p. 118). This criticism of arts marketing gets to the heart of debates about audience engagement and again highlights the urgent need to pour more resources into understanding what fundamentally motivates and moves audiences. Unfortunately, many arts marketers still spend the majority of their time designing publicity materials and segmenting their databases in order to tailor and push their promotional materials in ever more sophisticated ways. As I will argue Chapter 6, arts marketing needs to move beyond this transactional approach and catch up with not only the growing body of scholarship on audience engagement and enrichment but with audiences' desires themselves. As Hilary Glow (2013) maintains, the "new arts marketing discourse" focuses on audience engagement because arts organisations are "the orchestrators of social interaction with communities who are seeking opportunities for interactivity, participation, access and engagement" (pp. 38–39). Arts marketing scholars have nonetheless enriched the debates about audiences' experiences. As we shall see in the following chapter, they have dissected and qualified the nature of these experiences and some scholars continue to advocate strongly for the exceptional nature of arts and cultural experiences, which moves them well beyond the traditional foci of marketing.

AUDIENCE ENGAGEMENT AND ENRICHMENT

One of the core reasons for writing this book was to fill a gap in the literature on audience engagement and enrichment. Although we are witnessing a palpable shift from a culture of marketing to a culture of engagement, with scholars who research on areas related to arts marketing increasingly drawing on the language and tools of audience engagement (Walmsley 2019), as we saw in Chapter 1, engagement remains poorly defined and explicated in the scholarly literature and poorly understood and resourced in the performing arts sector. Considering that this book is dedicated to an exhaustive study of audience engagement, it would be redundant to produce a summary overview of the relevant literature at this stage. But it is important to highlight here the seminal studies that have influenced this emerging field and catalysed fresh thinking about audiences and their complex relationships with the performing arts.

Lynne Conner and Alan Brown are the two foremost figures in the development of thinking about audience engagement and enrichment. As a theatre and dance historian and cultural policy theorist, Conner has produced a significant body of work dedicated to audience research, including her highly influential monograph, *Audience engagement and the role of arts talk in the digital era* (Conner 2013). In the course of this groundbreaking book, Conner advocates for a de-sacralisation of the performing arts in favour of a renewed and more democratic engagement with audiences. As a solution to the current state of audience disengagement, where audiences are generally controlled, quietened and pacified, Conner promulgates a new culture of "arts talk", which she defines as "a spirit of vibrancy and engagement among and between people who share an interest in the arts" (p. 137) and describes as "a metaphor, an ethos, a call to arms and a way of doing business" (p. 167). Drawing on Heidegger, Gadamer, and Habermas, Conner argues that a deeply pleasurable audience experience is reliant on the hermeneutic opportunity to discuss and interpret meaning which, she argues, is in turn dependent on successful facilitation based on principles of social learning. Conner's call to arms is underpinned by her (2004) essay on audience enrichment, which offered a compelling definition of this new concept:

> The radical notion here is that a viable philosophy and practice of audience enrichment is centered on the assumption that what an audience really wants is the opportunity to co-author the arts experience. They don't want to be told what the art means. They want the opportunity to participate — in an intelligent and responsible way — in *telling* its meaning. They want to have a real forum (or several forums) for the interplay of ideas, experience, data, and feeling that makes up the arts experience.

Conner's work has undoubtedly shaped the development of audience studies in the context of the performing arts and already left a lasting legacy. Not least, it has helped to position audience engagement at the heart of audience research and explicated its ultimate goal of enrichment.

Alan Brown is a leading American arts consultant, speaker, and writer, and I have already cited his work liberally in this literature review because, like Conner, his impact on both scholarship and practice has been hugely influential. Alongside his work on value and impact, one of Brown's most significant contributions to thinking on audiences has been his co-authored study with Rebecca Ratzkin entitled *Making sense of audience engagement* (Brown and Ratzkin 2011). The authors' stated aim here was to provide a critical assessment of arts organisations' efforts to "engage audiences and visitors in deeper and more impactful arts experiences" (p. 1). In the course of this endeavour, Brown and Ratzkin outline a typology of audience members dependent on their propensity for engagement and develop a useful Arc of Engagement model, which depicts five chronological stages through which audience members ideally progress (build-up, intense preparation, artistic exchange, post-processing, and impact echo) to construct "unique experiences around a shared work of art" (pp. 2 and 7).

The combined impact of this body of work has been to increase awareness around different modes of audience engagement and to shift the focus slightly away from the quality of art towards the quality of audiences' engagement with it. This in itself has served to move audiences up the stakeholder management ladder and rebalance the power dynamic with artists and producers. It has also promoted awareness of a "total" audience experience and raised questions about the role and remit of arts marketing, programming, and education.

Conclusion

Until relatively recently audience research has been dominated by theoretical studies which have been based largely on assumptions about an ideal and homogenised audience. Audience scholars have traditionally manifested a pernicious fear and suspicion of real audience members and have shied away from empirical enquiries of or with them. In this sense, audience research has lagged behind other social sciences. However, this review has illustrated the diverse interests of audience researchers that are increasingly combining to make the field richer and more coherent. I have argued in this chapter that audience studies is predominantly interested in the *how and why* of engagement and that it should leave questions of *who and who not* to sociology and cultural policy studies.

In this review, I have attempted to draw out a taxonomy of audience research, and I have developed this typology by highlighting what I perceive to be the complementary subgenres that comprise the emerging field of audience studies. As I intimated in the introduction, academic fields require an underlying paradigm, a coherent set of questions and principles around which scholars can cohere. So it is important to delineate what audience studies is, what it does, and how it goes about doing it; such was the underlying aim of this chapter. Based on my analysis of the literature, we can conclude that in the context of the performing arts, audience studies increasingly concerns itself with understanding different kinds of audiences' diverse experiences with the arts and with artists. This involves exploring the impact of performance genres, places and spaces, as well as underlying traditions and power dynamics. Scholars working in the field increasingly derive from a broad range of disciplines, which in turn is diversifying the range of methods deployed to investigate audiencing, and this cross-disciplinary approach is starting to yield rich results.

The extensive review of the extant literature on performing arts audiences was structured thematically rather than chronologically. It is thus easy to appreciate the core themes that emerge in such a review, and I have classified these as outlined in the introduction into thirteen major topics, some of which certainly remain much more established than others. However, the lack of chronology makes it harder to identify the trends that characterise audience research and thus the likely future direction of travel for audience research. Some of these are easier to discern than others. There is obviously a strong correlation between developments in the performing arts themselves and the research that circumnavigates them. So there is clearly a trend towards researching audiences of co-created and immersive performance, for example. As the field of audience studies develops, supported by the rise in interdisciplinary research, there is also a convergence between scholarship from traditionally disparate fields, such as arts management, cultural policy studies, performance studies, psychology, and sociology. Less apparent from a review of the literature is perhaps the steady growth in creative and psychobiological research methods, which we will explore in Chapter 5. Another less visible trend is probably the emergent growth in research of diverse audiences, such as working class and cross-cultural audiences, and in studies of audiences in locations such as prisons and hospitals. As the arts and health agenda gains in prominence and spreads throughout the globe, we are likely to see scholars moving into this new research space to accompany their colleagues in arts therapy and applied performance. What is certain is that although audience studies is gaining traction and momentum as a field, scholars of performing arts audiences still face a complex set of challenges, not least the methodological disparities and gaps which will be explored in greater depth in Chapters 4 and 5.

As we have seen in the course of this chapter, many audience researchers have highlighted the cynical disempowerment of audiences which has effected a dislocation of the act of audiency from acts of interpretation over the past few centuries. Audiences may have been "enlightened" in terms of their ability to access art, but this enlightenment has not yet culminated in the stable interpretive communities imagined by Stanley Fish. This is certainly a result of calculated alienation and disempowerment; but it has also come about through indifference and because of a lack of understanding about the complex role that audiences actually play in the performing arts process. In the following chapter, we will therefore deconstruct the experiences that audiences have whilst engaging with the performing arts.

References

Alston, A. 2016. *Beyond immersive theatre: Aesthetics, politics and productive participation*. London, Palgrave Macmillan.

Arts and Humanities Research Council. 2013. *Cultural Value Project* [Internet]. London, Arts and Humanities Research Council. Available from: http://www.ahrc.ac.uk/Funded-Research/Funded-themes-and-programmes/Cultural-Value-Project/Pages/default.aspx [Accessed 25 June].

Auslander, P. 2008. *Liveness: Performance in a mediatized culture*. 2nd ed. Oxon, Routledge.

Barker, M. 2006. I have seen the future and it is not here yet ...; or, on being ambitious for audience research. *The Communication Review*, 9(2), pp. 123–141.

Barker, M. and Mathijs, E. 2016. Introduction: The World Hobbit Project. *Participations* [Online], 13(2), pp. 158–174.

Barrett, M. 2015. Diversity and social engagement: Cultivating a working class theatre audience. In: ENCACT (ed.) *The ecology of culture: Community engagement, co-creation, cross-fertilization*. Lecce, ENCACT, pp. 47–61.

Baxter, L., O'Reilly, D. and Carnegie, E. 2013. Innovative methods of inquiry into arts engagement. In: Radbourne, J., Glow, H. and Johanson, K. (eds.) *The audience experience: A critical analysis of audiences in the performing arts*. Bristol, Intellect, pp. 113–128.

Ben Chaim, D. 1984. *Distance in the theatre: The aesthetics of audience response*. London, Ann Arbor.

Bennett, S. 1997. *Theatre audiences: A theory of production and reception*. 2nd ed. London, Routledge.

Berlyne, D. E. 1971. *Aesthetics and psychobiology*. New York, Appleton.

Blau, H. 1990. *The audience*. Baltimore, The John Hopkins University Press.

Bleeker, M. and Germano, I. 2014. Perceiving and believing: An enactive approach to spectatorship. *Theatre Journal*, 66, pp. 363–383.

Bourdieu, P. 1991. *The love of art: European art museums and their public.* Stanford, CA, Stanford University Press.

Bourriaud, N. 2002. *Relational aesthetics.* Dijon, Les Presses du Réel.

Brand, G., Sloboda, J., Saul, B. and Hathaway, M. 2012. The reciprocal relationship between jazz musicians and audiences in live performances: A pilot qualitative study. *Psychology of Music*, 40(5), pp. 634–651.

Brown, A. 2013. All the world's a stage: Venues and settings, and their role in shaping patterns of arts participation. In: Radbourne, J., Glow, H. and Johanson, K. (eds.) *The audience experience: A critical analysis of audiences in the performing arts.* Bristol, Intellect, pp. 49–66.

Brown, A. S. 2006. An architecture of value. *Grantmakers in the Arts Reader*, 17(1), pp. 18–25.

Brown, A. S. and Novak, J. L. 2007. *Assessing the intrinsic impacts of a live performance.* San Francisco, WolfBrown.

Brown, A. S. and Ratzkin, R. 2011. *Making sense of audience engagement: A critical assessment of efforts by nonprofit arts organizations to engage audiences and visitors in deeper and more impactful arts experiences.* San Francisco, The San Francisco Foundation.

Brown, D. 2011. The 21st century venue. In: Walmsley, B. (ed.) *Key issues in the arts and entertainment industry.* Oxford, Goodfellow, pp. 103–121.

Burland, K. and Pitts, S. 2012. Rules and expectations of jazz gigs. *Social Semiotics*, 22(5), pp. 523–543.

Butsch, R. 2008. *The citizen audience: Crowds, publics, and individuals.* New York, Routledge.

Colbert, F. 2011. Management of the arts. In: Towse, R. (ed.) *A handbook of cultural economics.* 2nd ed. Cheltenham, Edward Elgar, pp. 261–265.

Conner, L. 2004. Who gets to tell the meaning? Building audience enrichment. *GIA Reader* [Online], 15(1).

Conner, L. 2013. *Audience engagement and the role of arts talk in the digital era.* New York, Palgrave Macmillan.

Csikszentmihalyi, M. 1988. The flow experience and its significance for human psychology. In: Csikszentmihalyi, M. and Csikszentmihalyi, I. S. (eds.) *Optimal experience: Psychological studies of flow in consciousness.* Cambridge, Cambridge University Press, pp. 15–35.

Dearn, L. K. and Pitts, S. E. 2017. (Un)popular music and young audiences: Exploring the classical chamber music concert from the perspective of young adult listeners. *Journal of Popular Music Education*, 1(1), pp. 43–62.

De Marinis, M. 1987. Dramaturgy of the spectator. *The Drama Review*, 31(2), pp. 100–114.

Ehrenreich, B. 2007. *Dancing in the streets: A history of collective joy.* London, Granta.

Fisher, J. W. 2003. Audience participation in the eighteenth-century London theatre In: Kattwinkel, S. (ed.) *Audience participation: Essays on inclusion in performance.* Westport, CT, Praeger, pp. 55–69.

Freshwater, H. 2009. *Theatre & audience.* London, Palgrave Macmillan.

Glow, H. 2013. Challenging cultural authority: A case study in participative audience engagement. In: Radbourne, J., Glow, H. and Johanson, K. (eds.) *The audience experience: A critical analysis of audiences in the performing arts.* Bristol, Intellect, pp. 35–48.

Golden, L. 1973. The purgation theory of catharsis. *Journal of Aesthetics and Art Criticism,* 31(4), pp. 473–491.

Hall, E. 2010. *Greek tragedy: Suffering under the sun.* Oxford, Oxford University Press.

Heim, C. L. 2012. 'Argue with us!': Audience co-creation through post-performance discussions. *New Theatre Quarterly,* 28(2), pp. 189–197.

Heim, C. 2016. *Audience as performer: The changing role of theatre audiences in the Twenty-First Century.* London and New York, Routledge.

Jancovich, L. 2011. Great art for everyone? Engagement and participation policy in the arts. *Cultural Trends,* 20(3–4), pp. 271–279.

Kattwinkel, S. 2003. Introduction. In: Kattwinkel, S. (ed.) *Audience participation: Essays on inclusion in performance.* Westport, CT, Praeger, pp. ix–xviii.

Keaney, E. and Oskala, A. 2007. The golden age of the arts? Taking Part survey findings on older people and the arts. *Cultural Trends,* 16(4), pp. 323–355.

Knowles, R. 2010. *Theatre and interculturalism.* London, Macmillan.

Kolesch, D., Schütz, T. and Nikoleit, S. (eds.) 2019. *Staging spectators in immersive performance.* Oxon and New York, Routledge.

Konijn, E. A. 1999. Spotlight on spectators: Emotions in the theatre. *Discourse Processes,* 28(2), pp. 169–194.

Machon, J. 2013. *Immersive theatres: Intimacy and immediacy in contemporary performance.* London, Palgrave Macmillan.

McCarthy, K. F., Ondaatje, E. H., Zakaras, L. and Brooks, A. 2004. *Gifts of the muse: Reframing the debate about the benefits of the arts.* Santa Monica, CA, RAND.

McConachie, B. 2008. *Engaging audiences: A cognitive approach to spectating in the theatre.* New York, Palgrave Macmillan.

O'Brien, D., Brook, O. and Taylor, M. 2018. *Panic! Social class, taste and inequalities in the creative industries.* London, Arts and Humanities Research Council.

O'Toole, J., Adams, R.-J., Anderson, M., Burton, B. and Ewing, R. (eds.) 2014. *Young audiences, theatre and the cultural conversation.* Dordrecht, Springer.

Piber, M. and Chiaravalloti, F. 2011. Ethical implications of methodological settings in arts management research: The case of performance evaluation. *The Journal of Arts Management, Law, and Society,* 41, pp. 240–266.

Pitts, S. E. 2005. What makes an audience? Investigating the roles and experiences of listeners at a chamber music festival. *Music and Letters*, 86(2), pp. 257–269.

Popovici, V. 1984. Is the stage-audience relationship a form of dialogue? *Poetics*, 13(1–2), pp. 111–118.

Radbourne, J. 2013. Converging with audiences. In: Radbourne, J., Glow, H. and Johanson, K. (eds.) *The audience experience: A critical analysis of audiences in the performing arts*. Bristol, Intellect, pp. 143–158.

Radbourne, J., Glow, H. and Johanson, K. 2010. Measuring the intrinsic benefits of arts attendance. *Cultural Trends*, 19(4), pp. 307–324.

Radbourne, J., Glow, H. and Johanson, K. (eds.) 2013. *The audience experience: A critical analysis of audiences in the performing arts*. Bristol, Intellect.

Radbourne, J., Johanson, K., Glow, H. and White, T. 2009. The audience experience: measuring quality in the performing arts. *International Journal of Arts Management*, 11(3), pp. 16–29.

Reason, M. 2008. Did you watch the man or did you watch the goose? Children's responses to puppets in live theatre. *New Theatre Quarterly*, 24(4), pp. 337–354.

Reason, M. 2010. Asking the audience: Audience research and the experience of theatre. *About Performance* 10, pp. 15–34.

Reason, M. 2019. A prison audience: Women prisoners, Shakespeare and spectatorship. *Cultural Trends*, 28(2–3), pp. 86–102.

Reinelt, J. G. 2014. What UK spectators know: Understanding how we come to value theatre. *Theatre Journal*, 66(3), pp. 337–361.

Rentschler, R., Radbourne, J., Carr, R. and Rickard, J. 2001. Relationship marketing, audience retention and performing arts organisation viability. *International Journal of Nonprofit and Voluntary Sector Marketing*, 7(2), pp. 118–130.

Reynolds, D. and Reason, M. (eds.) 2011. *Kinesthetic empathy in creative and cultural practices*. Bristol, Intellect.

Sauter, W. 2000. *The theatrical event: Dynamics of performance and perception*. Iowa City, University of Iowa Press.

Schechner, R. 2003. *Performance theory*. 2nd ed. London, Routledge.

Schoenmakers, H. 1990. The spectator in the leading role: Developments in reception and audience research within theatre studies. In: Sauter, W. (ed.) *New directions in theatre research*. Stockholm and Copenhagen, Munksgaard, Nordic Theatre Studies, pp. 93–106.

Sedgman, K. 2016. *Locating the audience: How people found value in National Theatre Wales*. Bristol, Intellect.

Sedgman, K. 2017. Audience experience in an anti-expert age: A survey of theatre audience research. *Theatre Research International*, 42(3), pp. 307–322.

Sedgman, K. 2018. *The reasonable audience: Theatre etiquette, behaviour policing, and the live performance experience*. London, Palgrave Macmillan.

Sedgman, K. Forthcoming. On rigour in theatre audience research. *Contemporary Theatre Review*.

Silvia, P. J. 2005. Emotional responses to art: From collation and arousal to cognition and emotion. *Review of General Psychology*, 9(4), pp. 342–357.

Turner, V. 1975. *Dramas, fields, and metaphors: Symbolic action in human society.* Ithaca and London, Cornell University Press.

Turner, V. 1982. *From ritual to theatre: The human seriousness of play.* New York, PAJ.

Walmsley, B. 2011. Why people go to the theatre: A qualitative study of audience motivation. *Journal of Customer Behaviour*, 10(4), pp. 335–351.

Walmsley, B. 2013a. 'A big part of my life': A qualitative study of the impact of theatre. *Arts Marketing: An International Journal*, 3(1), pp. 73–87.

Walmsley, B. 2013b. Co-creating theatre: Authentic engagement or inter-legitimation? *Cultural Trends*, 22(2), pp. 108–118.

Walmsley, B. 2016. From arts marketing to audience enrichment: How digital engagement can deepen and democratize artistic exchange with audiences. *Poetics*, 58, pp. 66–78.

Walmsley, B. 2019. The death of arts marketing: A paradigm shift from consumption to enrichment. *Arts and the Market*, 9(1), pp. 32–49.

Walmsley, B. Forthcoming. Theatre fans: A typology of serious leisure seekers. In: Sedgman, K. (ed.) *Theatre fandom.* Iowa City, University of Iowa Press.

White, G. 2013. *Audience participation in theatre: Aesthetics of the invitation.* Basingstoke, Palgrave Macmillan.

White, T. R. and Hede, A.-M. 2008. Using narrative inquiry to explore the impact of art on individuals. *Journal of Arts Management, Law and Society*, 38(1), pp. 19–35.

Wright, D. 2015. *Understanding cultural taste: Sensation, skill and sensibility.* London, Palgrave Macmillan.

CHAPTER 3

Deconstructing Audiences' Experiences

INTRODUCTION

We have already seen that audiences' experiences of the performing arts are complex, contested, undervalued, and under-researched. This is possibly because performance takes place in multiple contexts that are simultaneously real and imagined, and "there remains an uncertainty around how best to capture that which happens in the hinterlands of performance" (Whalley and Miller 2017, p. 78). As Whalley and Miller note, the act of audiencing does not have "clean edges", and so audience researchers need to "open up the debate around the terminology available to capture experiences of exchange in performance, and consider terms that might help to communicate the complexity of the relationship between audience and the performance, especially in those instances where roles are flexible and open to negotiation" (2017, p. 77). The core aim of this chapter is therefore to push at the edges of audience research and to open up the field to different terms and concepts that might help to elucidate audiences' experiences of the performing arts. The chapter is therefore concerned with some of the most fundamental questions of audiency: What is going on when audiences engage or are engaged with performance? How important is the live element of audiences' experiences? What kinds of experiences do audiences have when they engage with the performing arts? Which elements and phenomena characterise and differentiate these experiences from

© The Author(s) 2019
B. Walmsley, *Audience Engagement in the Performing Arts*,
New Directions in Cultural Policy Research,
https://doi.org/10.1007/978-3-030-26653-0_3

other kinds of experiences? Can audiences' experiences be truly restorative or even transformative?

The chapter will begin with a theoretical discussion of the nature of performing arts experiences. It will then investigate the role that liveness plays within these experiences before moving on to explore the relative agency that audiences have in engaging with performance. This will segue into a discussion on the phenomenology of audiency, including the roles of empathy, intersubjectivity, and immersion. Towards the end of the chapter we will explore the concepts of embodied and enactive spectatorship and discuss how the psychological principles of arousal and reward contribute towards audience engagement. The chapter will conclude with a critical appraisal of the age-old concept of catharsis and assessment of the extent to which audiences' experiences might be deemed to be transformative.

Qualifying Audiences' Experiences

The conceptual development of arts marketing, and of experiential marketing in particular, has engendered a wide-ranging debate about the nature of audiences' arts experiences. One of the earliest and most significant interventions in this debate was offered by Hirschman and Holbrook (1982)who famously classified arts experiences as *hedonic*. Their argument was essentially that audiences engage with the arts primarily to fulfil their personal wishes and fantasies. In their 1982 article, Hirschman and Holbrook described aesthetic experiences as *autotelic*, which they interpreted as intrinsically motivated and consumed as ends in themselves. This hedonic perspective is now shared by many arts marketers who regard cultural products as *symbolic* because they believe that "consumers" use them "to construct, sustain, and enact identity projects" (Colbert and St-James 2014, p. 569). This conceptual understanding of cultural products as symbolic reflects the value and impact research which suggests that audiences use the arts to self-actualise (Brown 2006). It also echoes the perspective of relational aestheticians that the arts exist as a means to a greater social end.

However, Carù and Cova (2003)claim that the hedonic or experiential approach lacks a solid theoretical foundation and call for a clearer definition of the conceptual domain of experience. Following Abrahams, the authors make an important distinction between memorable or "extraordinary" experiences and more mundane or "ordinary" experiences, describing extraordinary experiences as framed, intense, and stylised (p. 275). In a marketing context (often referred to as the experience economy) where consumers are encouraged to expect all of their experiences to be extraordinary, Carù and Cova urge scholars and marketers to take a more critical stance on what actually constitutes the extraordinary.

In contrast to arts marketing scholars, many performance theorists focus on the ludic aspects of the audience experience. A classic example of this strand of research is the work of Bruce McConachie, who argues that audiencing is fundamentally a play experience.

> As the background emotion underlying all theatrical engagement, playing frames and qualifies the sometimes negative feelings that a performance can arouse in audiences, assuring them from the start that any psychological pain they might experience will be temporary and perhaps even purgative. [...] While playing, humans and other mammals get an infusion of energy, which they usually attempt to maintain at an optimal level. (2008, p. 51)

In this interpretation of audiencing, play emerges as an ideal state of mind, a necessary mode of engagement for a positive and cathartic experience. In a play state, audience members "frame" their experiences and therefore accept the particular traditions and conventions related to performance (Goffman, cited in McConachie 2008, p. 53). Play therefore emerges in the literature as an enabler of audiency, a mindset required of audiences if they are to engage in and benefit from the quasi-fictional stage-world. This apparent requirement of audiences to enter into a playful state or to willingly suspend their disbelief (as Samuel Taylor Coleridge famously wrote about readers) functions as a form of *cognitive estrangement* (Buchanan 2010) that enables audiences to sacrifice their sense of realism in order to achieve aesthetic pleasure. As Penny Bundy puts it: "In live theatre the spectator is able to move backwards and forwards between a focus on the fictional world of the play and a focus on the acting and other aspects of stagecraft that have produced it" (2014, p. 119).

Influenced no doubt by Coleridge, Richard Schechner (2003) makes a distinction between belief (ritual) and suspension of disbelief (aesthetic drama). However, McConachie rejects both Coleridge's and Schechner's theories by developing the notion of conceptual blending, a process whereby, he claims, audiences are able to blend the fluid constructs of actor, character, and identity and also blend reality with fiction to run multiple conceptions of the world simultaneously during their performance experiences (2008, p. 42) and perform dual readings of performance (Reason 2008).

As we saw in the previous chapter, the extent to which presentational art inculcates 'passive' engagement amongst audiences remains contested. McConachie argues that the audiencing can never be passive because "human vision is always selective and discriminating" (2008, p. 56). Indeed McConachie's advocacy for an empirical approach to audience research—in his case underpinned by cognitive science—serves to capture the breadth and complexity of audiences' experiences of the performing arts and, in so doing, highlights the historic inability of performance studies to explicate these experiences in scientific terms. Matthew Reason (2010) concurs that audiencing requires a complex combination of different modes of active engagement:

> The possibility that the theatre audience is engaged in a kind of doing is an interesting one. It might be considered a kind of imaginative doing, as audiences suspend disbelief; or an emotional doing, as spectators invest sympathy with the characters or performance. The audience experience might also be considered an intersubjective doing, through kinaesthetic empathy with the movement and presence of people in space. (p. 19)

Reason's insistence on the active nature of audiencing is shared by the majority of audience researchers, who accept that sitting quietly in a darkened auditorium does not equate to a passive experience. As is the case with McConachie, Reason's creative methods enable him to demonstrate and illustrate the embodied nature of audiencing and to move the debate far beyond the tired terminology of spectatorship. Indeed it could be argued that empirical audience research has itself played a role in emancipating the spectator, not merely by giving audiences a voice but by proving beyond all doubt that their cognitive and bodily faculties represent the *sine qua non* of performance. In that sense, empirical research has proven what certain practitioners knew to be true several decades ago, namely that when audiences "abandon their position as spectators" they can be "drawn into the circle of action that restores collective energy" (Artaud, cited in Machon 2013, p. 117). This collective endeavour of course functions as much as a social and sociological experience as an aesthetic one, and Reason's emphasis on the intersubjective nature of audiencing reminds us of the very simple fact that many audiences engage with the performing arts primarily to socialise with others.

LIVENESS

Perhaps the most enticing and differentiating aspect of the performing arts, and, of course, the overriding element that unites them all, is *liveness*. Indeed liveness represents the main rationale for dedicating this extended study of audience engagement to the performing arts as opposed to the arts in general. Engaging with an exhibit in a museum or a painting in a gallery, for instance, is phenomenologically different from being part of a live audience immersed in a dedicated space alongside artists and fellow audience members for a sustained period of time. We know from existing studies that audiences seek different personal, social and aesthetic goals, and report fundamentally different experiences, when walking into a museum or gallery from those who venture into performing arts venues. Slater (2007), for example, highlights the peace and solace sought by gallery visitors, whilst a large scale study of museum-going by Morris Hargreaves McIntryre (2007) reveals contemplation as a core driver of attendance. It goes without saying that audiences of theatre, opera, music and dance are not primarily motivated by peace and solace (although classical music can of course offer a contemplative experience). Indeed as Iain Mackintosh observes, performing arts audiences often find themselves in a situation which is "essentially anarchic" and where "anything might happen" (1992, p. 2). Mackintosh continues to argue that it is the sense of danger, community and shared experience that demarcates live theatrical occasions from cinematic performances.

Many of these differentiators are picked up also by Martin Barker (2013, p. 20), who identifies seven core aspects of liveness:

1. Physical co-presence with performers and performance
2. Simultaneity with performance
3. Direct engagement and absence of intervening (technological) mediation
4. Sense of the local within the experience
5. Sense of interaction with performers
6. Sense of interaction with others in the audience
7. Intensified experiences/participation through sensing any of the above.

We might easily add to this list the following elements of live performance: audiences' sense of precarity and risk; their freedom to set their own gaze and curate their own personal viewing experience; the multisensory impact of production elements; the sense of chemistry and buzz; the venue or location and its wider opportunities for (enhanced) socialisation, etc. This again highlights the fact that the audience experience is fundamentally different in a performing arts setting from that of many other mediated arts and leisure activities. However, it is noteworthy that in Barker's study, even audiences for live-streamed events appreciated the sense of simultaneity with performers and enjoyed the "sense of danger" generated by this awareness, seemingly inured to the fact that live editing is regardless an act of mediation (p. 26). Along with the other scant research into live streaming (e.g. Bakhshi and Whitby 2014; Nesta 2010), this suggests quite strongly that the live element of simulcasts is more important that the filmed or streamed element, and that the various advantages proffered by this relatively new format can actually enhance the audience experience of live performance. As Barker concludes, "liveness is a complex phenomenon, with many separable components" (p. 31).

Liveness emerges as both a driver for and benefit of performing arts attendance in a wide range of empirical studies. Caroline Heim (2016), for example, reports that in over half of the 106 audience interviews she conducted for her *Audience as performer* book, participants spontaneously used the word "live" to explain either their experience of theatre, their motivations for attending or to distinguish their theatre attendance from their cinema-going (p. 146). Similarly, Reinelt et al.'s study revealed liveness to be one of the core values that audiences ascribe to theatre-going (Reinelt 2014, pp. 353–354). The huge significance of the live experience was reflected also in O'Toole et al.'s (2014) study, which found that younger audiences are particularly attracted to the "liveness and immediacy" of theatre (p. 9), principally because of the physical co-presence it offered them with performers:

> Young people enjoyed anything that occurred on stage which heightened their awareness of the actors being 'real people'. For instance, they delighted in commenting on actor sweat and spit. [...] Being physically present in the same space as the performers either increased emotional response to the work or heightened spectator awareness of their own emotional response. (p. 122)

Likewise, Burland and Pitts' (2012) study of jazz club members characterised the live performance of jazz as a fundamentally different experience from recorded jazz, largely as a result of its risky and co-creative potential:

"Spontaneity and uncertainty offer a sense of excitement as does the immediacy of the event: the sense that the music is being formed 'in the moment' and that the audience is part of that process resonates with research on jazz musicians and audiences" (p. 527). So live performance is often described by audiences as delivering an almost intoxicating sense of liveness. This liveness can manifestly heighten audiences' emotions and offer them a sense of ownership of their chosen art form.

However, certain theorists refute this differentiating condition of live performance. Auslander is the chief detractor here, claiming essentially that the inevitable distance, both literal and metaphorical, between performers and audience members inherently thwarts the latter's apparent desire for communion:

> Live performance places us in the living presence of the performers, other human beings with whom we desire unity and can imagine achieving it, because they are there, in front of us. Yet live performance also inevitably frustrates that desire since its very occurrence presupposes a gap between performer and spectator. [...] By reasserting the unbridgeable distinction between audience and performance, live performance foregrounds its own fractious nature and the unlikelihood of community in a way that mediatized representations, which never hold out the promise of unity, do not. (2008, p. 66)

Auslander's assumptions regarding audiences desiring a "unity" with performers is very rarely reflected in empirical studies. However, audience research *is* replete with testimonies of the visceral pleasure audiences derive from the liveness and proximity of performers performing in front of them as a synchronous and unmediated presence. The audience participants in Burland and Pitts' (2012) study, for example, make a distinction between the "intimacy" of their jazz club and the "sterility" of larger venues, where they can't see artists "up close and personal" (p. 528). Meanwhile, other studies (e.g. Konijn 1999) highlight the importance that audience members ascribe to watching artists and stagecraft first-hand and appreciating technical skill in-the-moment and before their own eyes.

As an antithesis to Auslander's thesis that live performance offers scarcely more "spontaneity, community, presence, and feedback between performers and audience" than mediatised performance (2008, p. 63), I would cite the extraordinary rise of immersive and one-on-one performance, which suggests to me that both performers and audiences are becoming increasingly aware of and hungry for the unique communal and dialogic opportunities afforded by these emerging genres. The phenomenal success of companies such as Punchdrunk also attests to the rise of a type of spontaneous, intimate, social and self-curated performance that lies well beyond the reach of even gaming and virtual reality; and the year-on-year rise in live audiences witnessed on Broadway, in London's West End, at the Edinburgh Festivals and across China appears to challenge Auslander's ultimate conclusion that "any change in the near future is likely to be toward a further diminution of the symbolic capital associated with traditional live events" (ibid., p. 187). Despite audiences' abounding thick descriptions of what we might regard as an almost animalistic engagement with performers, Blau continues to assert that the tangible benefits of live proximity to performers are actually null.

> The audience can be made to see, as Grotowski once insisted they see, the actors sweat. Even so, the ontological distinctions between, say, theater and film are often superficially made, and made superficial by much of what we see on stage, where the actor may very well be sweating, though for all its affective and ideational substance, it could just as well be on film. (p. 142)

As often, Blau's theoretical cynicism is not borne out in audience testimony, where the affect (and effect) of live creative labour appears to be especial.

Daphna Ben Chaim (1984) also explores live performance from the ontological perspective of "distance", the manipulation of which she lists as one of the distinctive features of twentieth-century theatre (p. 78). In her rigorous overview of different theoretical perspectives of distance provided by leading philosophers, dramatists, and performance and film scholars from the past century, Ben Chaim argues that dramatists' manipulation of distance requires heightened awareness amongst audiences. She concludes that although a unified theory of distance remains ultimately elusive, the most basic principle of distance lies in audiences' tacit awareness of the *fictitious* nature of their experiences, which enables them to "experience emotions without danger" (p. 74). This is a significant point that sheds fresh light on the concept of catharsis by suggesting that the arts offer a safe haven for audiences to play out and expunge their emotions. As Norman Holland has argued:

Our emotions in the literary situation seem stronger than in everyday life... Within the literary 'as if', because consciously we know we need only fantasy in response, we sink down to deeper levels of our mind. The aesthetic stance inhibits our motor activity; it therefore engages our moral and intellectual selves, not in suppressing or judging our deeper feelings, but in accepting and transforming them. Our 'rind' of higher ego-functions, our 'core' of deeply repressed ego – these make up a richer, longer kind of self than our ordinary one. (1968, p. 102)

We will revisit the concept of catharsis later in the chapter; what is intriguing in Holland's thesis here is the connection of audiencing with a super ego or "extraordinary self". Although it might appear somewhat counter-intuitive to suggest that the fictional worlds created by the performing arts can enable audiences to experience emotions in deeper and more powerful ways than in real life, this hypothesis could well explain the growing consensus that emotional engagement is actually audience members' biggest driver of attendance (Heim 2016; Walmsley 2011). So whatever theorists make of the ontological properties of liveness in live performance, it is incontrovertibly something that is tangible and that matters, and matters deeply, to audiences.

RECEPTION AND MANIPULATION

The debates around liveness expose deeper underlying tensions about how audience research is conceived and conducted. For example, in his musings on dramaturgy and semiotics, Marco De Marinis (1987) argues that we should consider the audience as an active subject of dramaturgy rather than as an object of the writer, director, or dramaturg. De Marinis highlights the various "receptive operations" that audiences carry out, including perception, interpretation, aesthetic appreciation, memorisation, emotive, and intellectual response, and considers that it is only through these activities that the performance text or score "achieves its fullness, becoming realized in all its semantic and communicative potential" (p. 101). This is an interesting theoretical development, which casts audience members in the role of dramaturgs who can exert at least some element of control over the otherwise manipulative processes of performance which, according to De Marinis, "seeks to induce in each spectator a range of definite transformations, both intellectual (cognitive) and affective (ideas, beliefs, emotions, fantasies, values, etc.)" (ibid.). The potential of performance to manipulate audiences, both emotionally and morally or politically, is relatively uncontested by theoreticians; indeed entire movements and genres such as Brecht's Epic Theatre have been built upon the critique of "bourgeois' theatre captivating audiences emotionally rather than transforming them politically (Sartre 1961). As Helen Freshwater observes, audiences have even been subjected to direct abuse in the theatre, with companies such as Forced Entertainment castigating them as "voyeurs" (2009, p. 52). This kind of assault constitutes the kind of shock that Artaud envisaged in his Theatre of Cruelty, designed to engender an intense emotional response amongst the audience (Ben Chaim 1984, p. 46).

As we saw in the previous chapter, Willmar Sauter's work is particularly useful in distinguishing reception theory from semiotics. In focussing on the primary role of performance (and indeed culture more broadly) as a "communicative event" (2000, p. 20), Sauter manages to shift the focus of audience research away from the hackneyed communication science of encoding and decoding towards a phenomenological understanding of meaning-making and engagement:

> The field of semiotics, which was in vogue at the time, was not very useful in empirical reception studies: spectators do not perceive 'signs' which they describe and interpret for a scholar; they perceive 'meaning' – and they have fun! Semiotics had no way of accounting for the pleasure and the enjoyment which spectators experience in the theatre.

For Sauter, then, audiencing represents an interpretive interaction that ultimately constitutes "a joint act of understanding" between audiences and performers (p. 2). This focus on the interpretive mode of audiency aligns Sauter with De Marinis and also with Susan Bennett (1997), who observes that the traditional reader-response approach to audience studies was severely compromised by the development of post-structuralist theory (p. 34). Sauter identifies four main categories of audience response: describing, interpreting, evaluating, and expressing emotions (p. 180). However, he goes on to assert that the only "crucial" factor that determines whether audiences evaluate performance in a positive light is the quality of the acting, regardless of the nature of the performance or the genesis of the spectator. This is a curious and spurious conclusion, which once again reduces the audience experience and completely negates the semioticians' perspective of audiences as interpreters of texts and signs. It therefore counters De Marinis's useful categorisation of audiences as active dramaturgs in their own right and ignores the significant roles played by lighting, sound and scenography. This appears particularly odd in light of Sauter's earlier argument that the communicative field between presentation and perception constitutes three aspects: "the sensory, artistic, and symbolic modes of communication" (p. 6).

A Phenomenological Project

Despite his debatable views on acting, Sauter's prioritisation of perception over reception has made a significant impact on audience research, partly because perception "carries connotations that tie it to phenomenology" (Sauter 2000, p. 5). Sauter has undoubtedly influenced a whole new generation of audience scholars, including Kirsty Sedgman, who maintains that "phenomenology has the capacity to reveal how audiences' responses are creative acts in themselves [because] emotional and embodied responses have a significant and legitimate role in the analysis of performance" (2016, p. 9). As we shall see in the following chapter, phenomenological approaches are starting to dominate the discourse on cultural value and it is both appropriate and necessary, therefore, that audience research develops in a way such that it enables further explication of audiences' actual experiences of performance.

Phenomenologists' long-held fascination with performance is perhaps explained by performance's "addiction to otherness" (Blau 1990, p. 52). A perfect example of this synergy is Jean-Paul Sartre, who as an accomplished playwright went so far as to actually explore phenomenology *through* performance, and vice versa. Sartre dedicated almost a third of his major tome *Being and nothingness*, which he described as a "phenomenological ontology", to an exploration of "being-for-others", the sometimes hellish battles of the self to (co-)exist in a world with others whose "self" it can never fully understand or capture. For example, Sartre argues that: "In the phenomenon of the look, the Other is in principle that which cannot be an object" (cited in Blau 1990, p. 275). Blau applies Sartre's theory to the field of performance and interprets this particular theorem as the audience's doomed attempt to objectify the performer through its gaze. For Blau, the Other presents as "an absent cause" and the performer's presence is "always in jeopardy" (p. 52). Following this logic, audiences' hunger for a meaningful communion with performers is what Sartre might have labelled an ontological act of bad faith, because audiences can never fully get what they desire from performers and their ultimate project (namely to *capture*

74   B. WALMSLEY

or *possess* the performer) is thus doomed to fail with the audience cast as Tantalus endlessly trying to reach his unattainable fruit. This cynical reading of the audience project might sound negative enough, but Blau goes on to argue that audiences actually act in a *dual* manifestation of bad faith:

> If the audience is moved, it is moved by a curious twist of empathy that involves a double loss. For in identifying with the actor who 'becomes' the character, the members of the audience neither complete the self nor identify with each other. (p. 256)

This somewhat nihilistic reading of audiences' phenomenological drivers for engaging with performance challenges the increasingly prevalent trope in audience studies regarding the transformative nature of the performance experience. Indeed a few recent studies (e.g. Radbourne 2013; Radbourne et al. 2010) have heralded self-actualisation as primary to the audience project. This dissonance represents another instance of theoretical scholars disregarding or even disparaging the lived experiences of audiences. It is perhaps no surprise therefore that Bennett (1997) concurs with Blau on this point, drawing on Ubersfeld to argue that the audience experience can only ever be dissatisfying.

> The spectator cannot arrest or touch the object of desire. Indeed desire moves from object to object and should it stop and fix on a particular object, then the role of the spectator is relinquished, the theatrical experience denied. Pleasure is thus limited by the essential situation of spectatorial dissatisfaction; not only because the spectator is not able to possess the object of desire but because, if he or she did, it would be something other than that which was desired. The spectator cannot experience pleasure without experiencing its limits. (p. 73)

Bennett is intimating here that the only role played by the audience is that of spurned lover, perhaps because she is using the visual terminology accorded to the spectator, who gazes at the stage like an impotent *voyeur*.

A possible route out of the apparent impasses established by theories of reception and perception is offered by Sartre himself, who argues that aesthetic experiences can only occur when audiences shift from the perceptual to the *imaginative* mode of consciousness (cited in Ben Chaim 1984, p. 15). Ben Chaim maintains that audiences' engagement during a performance experience may well be intense, but that they differ from the kind of engagement that occurs in life experiences because of the function of *distance* (1984, p. ix). This is because the gaze that the Self fixes on the Other is exacerbated in the performance arena because of the distance (or fourth wall) that is imposed between audiences and performers by traditional performance spaces. This distance is both literal and ontological, and it creates a very specific relationship between spectators and performers. So there appears to be something fundamentally different about the distance and otherness that exists between audiences and performers from that which exists in real life or even between audiences and other audience members. Ben Chaim suggests that the difference is established by the heightened emotional state of audiences, which effects what Sartre calls "a magical potency" (1984, p. 16). As we shall observe in the following section, many scholars explicate this magic in terms of empathy.

EMPATHY

As noted earlier, the potential for emotional engagement offered by "bourgeois" performance presented Brecht with a dramaturgical problem because it developed empathy between audience members and stage characters that apparently inhibited the former from thinking objectively. Empathy has always been a significant and contested phenomenon for performance theorists, some of whom go so far as to categorise it as audiences' strongest aesthetic experience (Konijn 1999, p. 187). The concept of empathy arises in both intrinsic and instrumental approaches to audience research, because it emerges as both an integral part of a performing arts experience and a knock-on benefit that audiences apparently develop as they learn to identify with stage characters. Empathy is therefore a regular feature in value and impact research and in related models and frameworks of cultural value.

The focus in audience research on audiences' motivations for attending the performing arts and for the ensuing benefits that they derive from this engagement was introduced in the previous chapter. A synthesis of this body of literature indicates strongly that the overriding driver of attendance, and by far the most significant impact that the performing arts have on audiences, is emotional engagement. In the context of deconstructing audiences' experiences, it is important to note the primary sources of this impact, and several studies (e.g. Burland and Pitts 2012; Konijn 1999; Walmsley 2011) conclude that one of these is the technical or performance skills of the artists, which generally dictate audiences' levels of involvement, identification, engagement and empathy, and influence the longitudinal impact of a given performance. As Konijn expresses it, "the audience does not only come to witness events full of suspense, emotion, and interesting trials and tribulations that appear as real as possible but also to enjoy the skill with which the illusion is produced" (1999, p. 188).

As I noted earlier in the chapter, Matthew Reason characterises audiencing as a kind of "intersubjective doing" which involves an element of what he calls "kinaesthetic empathy with the movement and presence of people in space" (Reason 2010, p. 19). Kinaesthetic empathy is an interesting and complex concept, which we will return to in due course when we explore the notion of embodied spectatorship. What is significant here is the relationship between intersubjectivity and empathy—with performers, with stage characters, and with other audience members. Audiencing emerges therefore as a deeply empathic activity because it involves three levels (as well as different modes) of empathy. Vasile Popovici supports Reason's perspective on intersubjectivity, highlighting the dialogic nature of the stage–audience relationship (1984, p. 114). Similarly, Whalley and Miller interpret what they refer to as the "affective transmission" from performers to audiences as an "intersubjective exchange" (2017, p. 78). But as these somewhat narrow foci reveal, the intersubjectivity between audience members themselves often gets lost in the literature as scholars focus almost obsessively on the dyadic audience–performer relationship—and this despite the profound influence of relational aesthetics, which effectively foregrounded human relations and the social context of arts experiences.

Audiences appear to have an ambivalent attitude towards other audience members, and based on my own research with audiences, this seems to be because they can either hinder or enhance engagement. Noise produced from fellow audience members is of course a classic disrupter of engagement. But when audience members empathise and engage with the people around them, they can actually develop close social bonds. This is illustrated beautifully in Burland and Pitts' (2012) study of a jazz club, where a participant reported sharing "feelings of intimacy, connectedness and despair and joy" with fellow audience members and experiencing sensations of "connectedness and belonging" because they "knew the players", were "with friends" and "surrounded by a like-minded crowd" (pp. 534–535). These empirical insights support the triadic model of empathy explored above and promote this as a core source of audience satisfaction and impact. Bruce McConachie explains how this process happens in action:

> Put us together in an auditorium and our bodies and minds are like the inside of a good violin; we resonate and amplify emotions with each other.

> Emotional contagion in a theatre is automatic and usually very quick. Audiences will tend to laugh, cry, and even gasp simultaneously. The more spectators join together in one emotion, the more empathy shapes the emotional response of the rest. (2008, p. 97)

Or, as Hatfield et al. explain it, as a consequence of mimicry, people tend to "catch" each other's emotions (cited in Heim 2016, p. 21). Heim's own studies also reveal how audience members "catch or are infected by the contagion of laughter, crying and even applause" (p. 22) and illustrate how this positive type of contagion can actually merge them into a community (p. 112).

This evidence of the potential for audiency to develop a sense of communion and communitas is borne out by biometric research, which provides a psychobiological illustration of how the brainwaves and heartbeats of live audiences start to sync as they become collectively immersed in live performance. So empathy and intersubjectivity emerge as physiological and biological as well as psychological and sociological phenomena—phenomena whose true cultural significance remain seriously undervalued. McConachie (2008) also draws on cognitive science to investigate empathy via processes of neurological mirroring, and determines that:

> spectators paying attention to performers will automatically mirror their rhythms, whether the performers express them in movement or sound [...]. Both visual and aural mirroring operations link neurological response directly to the motor system, which, in turn, is mostly hardwired to our emotions. Spectatorial empathy appears to be strongest when combinations of sound and movement entrain our bodies. (p. 71)

McConachie insists that empathy is not an emotion in its own right, but that it "readily leads viewers to emotional engagements" (p. 75). His argument that the generation of empathy is heightened when sound and movement are combined suggests that the performing arts are ideally placed to invoke empathetic engagement amongst audiences. This of course reflects our earlier discussion of performance as ritual and again highlights its potential to invoke a state of liminality and/or communitas.

IMMERSION AND FLOW

Earlier in the chapter, we qualified arts experiences as hedonic. Santoro and Troilo describe hedonic experiences as "a combined response from the emotions, senses, imagination, and intellect" and claim that consumers engage in hedonic activity to create an "absorbing experience" (Radbourne et al. 2009, p. 18). Indeed postmodern consumption more broadly has been described as "an immersion into experiential moments of enchanted, multifaceted and spectacular encounters" (Firat and Dholakia 1998, p. 101). If this holds for consumption in general, then it is certainly a powerful driver for engagement in the performing arts, where research has demonstrated an overriding audience motivation for meaningful emotional encounters (Walmsley 2011). Boehner et al. (2008) note that aesthetic experiences are "bound by the ineffable: indescribable and irreducible aspects of being". The authors contend that aesthetic experiences are "tied to the particular, invoke the senses, command an immersion of the whole self, and result in a heightened form of engagement" (n.p.). The aim of this section is to shed some fresh light on these ineffable experiences by focussing in depth on the aspect of immersion.

Immersion in a piece or work of art is variably referred to as captivation or 'flow'. Flow is a psychological concept that was discovered and coined by the Hungarian-American psychologist Mihaly Csikszentmihalyi and it essentially refers to a state of total captivation and absorption in the task at hand. Although it has never actually been applied to the act of audiency by Csikszentmihalyi himself, flow has been drawn on effectively by commentators such as Alan Brown (2006) to encapsulate audiences' recurrent accounts of being "lost in the moment" or "losing track of time". Csikszentmihalyi describes flow as an autotelic, optimal experience, which is "rewarding in and of itself" (1988b, p. 8). He provides a range of phenomenological explanations to qualify this claim, including the links between flow and self-improvement, self-congruence, self-harmony, happiness, escapism, and timelessness. Because self-congruence is heightened during moments of optimal experience, Csikszentmihalyi maintains that the pursuit of flow becomes "one of the central goals of the self" (1988a, p. 24), the apotheosis of its strivings and pursuit of wellbeing.

The concept of flow is reflected and referenced in a wide body of literature exploring the value and purpose of arts and leisure experiences. For example, John Dewey credits the arts with providing exemplary, "clarified and intensified" experiences, free from the distractions of everyday life (1980, p. 46). Belfiore and Bennett go even further, framing flow as the very pinnacle of value: "the value of the arts resides in our complete commitment and absorption when creating or enjoying a work of art" (2008, p. 97). This hypothesis was seemingly confirmed in Brown and Novak's (2007) deductive analysis of the intrinsic impacts of live performance, where captivation correlated most highly with satisfaction, representing therefore what the researchers referred to as "the lynchpin of impact" (p. 11). Immersion and flow thus emerge as relatively reliable proxies for impact in the performing arts, at least for concurrent or immediate impact; and to the delight of producers, programmers, ethnographers and sometimes even audiences themselves, flow is often visibly manifest in the audience:

> Through their facial expressions, body language and audible reactions, audiences communicate impact as it is happening. There is no mistaking the silence of rapture during a concert, the moments of shared emotion in a theater when the plot takes a dramatic twist or the post-performance buzz in the lobby. All are reliable evidence of intrinsic impact. (Brown and Novak 2007, p. 5)

De Marinis too notes that audiences' engagement can be physically manifest in various ways, including sweating, changes in heartbeat, muscular tension, and pupil dilation, and claims that this state of heightened interest is itself aroused by the more basic psychophysiological states of amazement or surprise (1987, p. 109), which Artaud might well have articulated as "shock".

One of the problems with the theoretical explorations of flow is that it tends to focus on the individual audience member. In light of our recent discussion regarding the empathy and intersubjectivity that can emerge *between* audience members, it is interesting to speculate whether flow might be understood as a *collective* phenomenon, reflecting, for example, moments that audiences often describe as those where they could "hear a pin drop". In his educational study of the Montessori classroom, Keith Sawyer (2007) offers some useful insights in this context by defining the spontaneous collaboration of group creativity as *group flow*. Sawyer establishes a range of ideal conditions for this phenomenon of group flow, including close listening, complete concentration, good communication, and equal participation. It is easy to appreciate from this analysis how performance might offer the optimal conditions for group flow, and how these might also facilitate the emotional contagion that we explored earlier.

We can't really conclude a discussion of immersion without making at least scant reference to immersive performance itself. Machon (2013) argues that immersive practice earns its name because its multisensory form facilitates audiences' immersion and generates an embodied and lasting memory of the event (p. 43). Indeed in describing immersive performance as "an embodied event" (p. 83), Machon expresses the need for audience researchers to acknowledge "the combination of sensation and sentience that impacts on cognition, proprioception and kinaesthesia" and to focus on audiences' "somatic modes of attention" (p. 112). In the following section, we will therefore hone in on theories of embodiment and enaction in order to highlight uncognitive responses to performance.

EMBODIED AND ENACTIVE SPECTATORSHIP

Performance studies research is increasingly challenging the conception of audiencing as a passive form of engagement as part of what has been labelled a "corporeal turn" (Reynolds and Reason 2011). For example, Reason (2010) argues that the audience experience is embodied because audiences do not just watch and listen to a performance but experience it with their whole bodies (p. 19). In her exegesis of immersive performance, Machon provides a helpful contextualisation of Reason's notion of intersubjectivity by highlighting what she refers to as "the shared milieu of subjectivities of sensory engagement within and between our own individual body and the bodies of others directly around us" (2013, p. 112). So there is a strong connection between embodiment and empathy, which demarcates embodiment as another aspect of live performance that conjoins audience members with performers and with one another. Embodied responses to the performing arts remain woefully under-researched, partly because of the cognitive bias in Western thinking and scholarship but largely because of methodological skills gaps. However, there are increasing indications that this particular avenue of research will prove fruitful in deconstructing audiences' experiences in a robust and scientific way.[1]

This notion of the performing arts audience as active and bodily engaged is an important one, and it adds further weight to the re-categorisation of performance as a process or experience rather than a product. As McConachie notes, embodied emotions shape cognitive processing and generate meanings (2008, p. 68). Embodied engagement signifies that

---

[1] See Chapter 5 for a discussion of the neuroscientific and biometric techniques that led to these particular findings.

audiencing is far removed from a simple act of consumption, which is fleeting and primarily cognitive. Audiencing, on the other hand, can function on an instinctive, irrational, and even atavistic level.

> Rational reflection becomes part of, or is secondary to, the visceral experience. Often, this results in a comprehension of the work that does not engage logical sense, but instead *understands* the work on a deeper level without necessarily being able to describe or explain this. (Machon 2013, p. 106, original italics)

Many researchers have described audiences' experiences as ineffable. Whilst this hyperbolic assessment of audiencing does seem to run contrary to the many rich and nuanced articulations of the audience experience that we have already explored, it does convey the limitations of language for encapsulating the entirety of the audience experience that I have identified elsewhere (see Walmsley 2018). One of the reasons behind the limitations of linguistic and rational or cognitive responses to performance is of course the multisensory nature of the genre. The domination of the role of performers (i.e. speech, movement, and/or song) in the literature obscures the other audio-visual, olfactory, and tactile elements of performance, which are therefore neglected in audience research. Fortunately, the growing body of work on immersive performance, lighting and scenography is starting to address this gap, partly under the influence of Joslin McKinney (2013), who rightly acknowledges that scenographic spectacle can make a direct appeal to audience members' bodies, and communicate images and ideas that they hold in common (p. 74).

Evidence of the embodied nature of the performing arts experience is also presented in numerous empirical studies. For example, surveys conducted as part of Reinelt et al.'s *Theatre spectatorship and value attribution* project found "ample evidence of an embodied act of receiving and processing the experience" (Reinelt 2014, p. 349). Reason and Reynold's (2010) study of dance audiences probed these embodied acts further, discovering that many audience members imagined themselves dancing whilst watching dance and even tried to 'invest' themselves into the dancers' bodies. The study captured audiences' "sensual", "escapist", and "multisensory" responses to dance, which in turn affected their breathing, posture, and energy (p. 71). The authors concluded that this variety of audience response establishes kinaesthetic engagement as "a key source of pleasure and motivation for many dance spectators" (ibid.). In their subsequent book, however, Reynolds and Reason (2011) rightly acknowledge the potentially harmful nature of kinaesthetic empathy when it is manipulated by adverse power networks. As we saw in the previous chapter, Adam Alston's (2016) research into audiences of immersive performance provides some telling examples of the negative aspects of this particular type of engagement.

Theories of embodiment (or embodied cognition) are closely related to those of enaction since both traditions accept the role of the unconscious and focus on how experiences are felt by the human body. It is worth, therefore, pausing to reflect on the insights that audience research can glean from theories of enaction. Enaction can be interpreted as a response to the "explanatory gap" of cognitivism, which perpetuated the mind–body dualism established by Descartes and resurfaced the "phenomenological mind-body problem" of how the brain can have experiences (Thompson 2007, p. 3). Thompson argues convincingly that cognitive science is incomplete: by focussing on cognition, he claims, it has neglected emotion, affect, and motivation. In its insistence that humans construct and co-construct knowledge and meaning through their "sensorimotor interactions" with their environments (ibid.) enaction offers an alternative perspective from theories of cognition that is more closely aligned with the empathic, embodied and intersubjective nature of performance and audiency. It is perhaps no surprise, then, that Bleeker and Germano (2014) have led the call for an "enactive approach to spectatorship" that could help us to understand performance as a process "that is both profoundly embodied and deeply cultural" (p. 383).

Enaction implies audience immersion; it situates audiences at the heart of artistic experiences and acknowledges that they are engaged in performance in a deeply phenomenological way. An enactive approach to audiency is holistic in that it embraces the cognitive, the embodied and the social.

> From an Enaction perspective, perception, like the rest of cognition, is not only embodied and embedded, it is also ecologically extended. Spectators use their material and social surroundings as well as their bodies and brains to take action and make meaning during a performance. (McConachie 2013, p. 186)

Embodied and enactive perspectives thus establish a useful theoretical framework for audience research. They not only speak to developing trends in performance such as immersive practice but also underpin the hermeneutic and co-creative processes that lie at the heart of the audience project itself.

AROUSAL AND REWARD

Philosophers and psychologists have always been interested in questions of artistic production and appreciation. But as Berlyne (1971) claims in his monograph *Aesthetics and microbiology*, epistemological progress in this area has been hampered by weak theorisation and by the reduction of complex phenomenological questions to simplistic lines of enquiry such as what motivates artists to produce art; what might constitute an "artistic personality"; and how we might measure creative or aesthetic potential. This suggests that like arts marketing, the field of psychology has historically neglected to focus on complex notions of cultural engagement. As Paul Silvia (2005) contends, the study of art and emotions "languished during much of the last century", and as a result "the study of emotional responses to art has remained curiously detached from the psychology of emotions" (p. 342). This disciplinary divide remains a significant problem for audience research and it is therefore important to devote some space here to investigating emotion psychology.

One of Berlyne's major contributions to this field was to foreground the hedonic qualities of art by highlighting what he called its 'arousal modifying collative properties', namely: complexity, novelty, uncertainty, and conflict. Berlyne's theory was essentially that these four apparently divergent properties had two core similarities: firstly, their dependence on comparing (or collating) incoming information with expected information (e.g. the potential gap between audiences' expectations and the live event); and secondly, their common ability to affect the intensity of arousal. In summary, Berlyne claimed that stimuli that were either low or high (but not moderate) in complexity, novelty, uncertainty and conflict were likely to increase arousal, and that people's preferences for art could be framed in terms of "how collative properties of art affect the arousal systems of reward" (Silvia 2005, p. 344). Berlyne's work notably influenced the theories of hedonic consumption that we explored at the beginning of the chapter and that have been defined as the "multisensory, fantasy and emotive aspects" of audience experience (Hirschman and Holbrook 1982, p. 92).

Despite these theoretical advances, it is important to note that Berlyne's work has been critiqued for overemphasising the role of arousal as a mechanism of reward and preference as well as for advocating a single system of arousal and reward (Silvia 2005). New approaches to the experimental aesthetics movement of the 1970s have demonstrated that emotional responses to art are much more differentiated than simply arousing or rewarding, and emotion psychologists have discovered that emotions are much more complex than simply states of high arousal. However, although the psychobiological assumptions behind Berlyne's arousal model have now been widely discredited, three of his four original core properties (novelty, complexity, and uncertainty) have been positively correlated by psychologists with feelings of aesthetic interest and enjoyment (Silvia 2005, p. 345). Silvia's own research has indicated that audiences have a more enjoyable experience of art when they feel that they have grasped its meaning; but Silvia cautions against a simplistic view of positive affective responses to art, which are likely to champion global, undifferentiated emotional concepts (p. 351). Instead he calls for aestheticians to adopt the "appraisal theories" developed by emotional psychologists—theories which, he argues, offer "an expansive set of new ideas, hypotheses, and research directions" (p. 354). These appraisal theories find consensus in their acceptance of audiences' subjective evaluations of their aesthetic experiences and in their acknowledgement of the complexity of emotions involved.

CATHARSIS AND TRANSFORMATION

Let us now return to the notion of catharsis, which we mentioned briefly earlier in the chapter in relation to play and distance in order to ascertain how these qualities might effect a safe space for audiences to experience heightened emotions. Catharsis is a complex concept, the precise interpretation of which has of course triggered centuries of critical debate, not least amongst philosophers and performance theorists. The dominant view of catharsis remains the so-called "purgation theory", which holds that tragic drama can arouse emotions of pity and fear in an audience, which it then quells or purges in the resolution. Butcher (cited in Bennett 1981, p. 207) elucidates the concept further, describing the "emotional cure" wrought by the alleviation of pity and fear, which are "artificially stirred" in the audience and then "universalized" to lift spectators out of themselves into a state of "sympathetic ecstasy". There is a strong resonance here with the notion of *enthousiasmos*, the ritualistic possession trance (Ehrenreich 2007, p. 35) that we explored in the previous chapter. The purgation theory of catharsis also reflects Falassi's typologies of ritual, which identify the "rite of purification" as "a cleansing, or chasing away of evil" (1987, pp. 4–6). It is clear to see here how notions of arousal, embodiment and enaction are also implicated in this particular interpretation of catharsis, which again illustrates their centrality to the theoretical framework of audiency.

But there remains strong opposition to the purgation theory. According to Golden (1973, p. 473), there are three main schools of thought in this category: those who see catharsis as a "moral purification"; those who perceive it as a "structural purification in which the development of the plot purifies the tragic deed of its moral pollution"; and a third group who recognise the concept as "a form of intellectual clarification in which the concepts of pity and fear are clarified by the artistic representation of them". Nussbaum (1986) promulgates this third interpretation, although she rejects Golden's focus on the intellect, arguing that clarification derives from emotions. With the possible exception of Nussbaum, these critiques of the purgation theory all neglect the increasing evidence of audiences *embodying* their responses to performance; so whether or not there is a "purging", it appears that the purgation theory remains the closest to the enactive perspective explored earlier. McConachie (2008) appears to concur with this analysis, claiming that audiences want to be moved to emotional extremes that "provide a kind of catharsis that is good for our bodies" (p. 65). He goes on to assert that emotional purging in the form of laughing and crying helps to regulate audiences' "homeostasis" or "physiological thermostats" and that this "may be the closest that cognitive science can come to the Aristotelian notion of catharsis" (p. 111).

The notion of "regulation", or perhaps "resetting", is an interesting development in the theorisation of catharsis, and it challenges the dominant interpretation of catharsis as effecting some kind of transformation. This tension between the restorative versus the transformative properties of the arts has marked debates about audiences and performance since Aristotelian times. As we have seen, it notably preoccupied Brecht and fellow proponents of his Epic Theatre, and it continues to divide audience researchers to this day. Whalley and Miller (2017) articulate the contemporary terms of the debate perfectly in their synopsis of Rancière's theory of emancipation:

What remains in question is whether the spectator is transformed through this moment of emancipation or whether the specific exchanges are contingent, tied to the room or the location in which they are enacted. (p. 25)

Arts and cultural organisations pepper their mission statements with claims of transforming audiences and communities. But although there is growing narrative evidence of this transformation, the ability of the performing arts to effect any tangible or durable transformation on its audiences remains uncertain.

CONCLUSION

We have seen in the course of this chapter that audiences' experiences of the performing arts have been classified as framed, intense, hedonic, autotelic, stylised, and playful. This is essentially because they are based on cultural "products" that are aesthetic, symbolic, and live. This complexity can often make audiences' experiences appear noumenal and ineffable, and many audience researchers have indeed described them as such. However, we have seen in this chapter that it is possible to deconstruct audiences' experiences into their constituent parts; and although the sum of these experiences will always be greater than their parts, if we are ever to make real progress in audience studies then it is vital to understand the properties of the experiences that motivate audiences to engage with the performing arts and that generate the impacts they incur from them. Artistic experiences can certainly be "extraordinary" but we must heed the critique offered by Carù and Cova (2003) that any claims to the extraordinary must be carefully qualified.

Audiences' experiences of the performing arts combine cognitive, sensual, aesthetic, kinaesthetic, emotional, social, intellectual, imaginative, enactive, and spiritual responses to performance. Many of these responses appear to be linked to the proviso that performance is experienced live by audiences who can feel close to artists and witness art-making and stagecraft up-close and personally. Despite what the theorists might say, the empiricists have revealed the exceptional qualities of live performance in myriad studies of different art forms; and there seems to be growing consensus that live performance can create fictional worlds that enable audience members to locate their super egos, or their extraordinary selves, and undergo an emotional or spiritual restoration or even transformation. However, there is another notable dichotomy between theoretical and empirical researchers regarding the transformative nature of audiency and the role that performers play therein. Whilst the theoreticians perceive the audience project to be ultimately disappointing and irretrievably doomed, the empiricists, informed by audiences themselves, bear witness to the sometimes cathartic and transformative potential of performance that can enable audiences to self-actualise. Theories of distance and catharsis suggest that this transformation might be a result of the magical quality of emotion.

Empathy emerges as a prerequisite of audiencing, and as a condition of intersubjectivity, it must be acknowledged as a core aspect of relational art. Empathy appears to lead to mirroring and emotional contagion, which can restore collective energy, effect a state of communitas, and ultimately develop a sense of community amongst a regular audience. Processes of amazement, shock, arousal, group flow, embodiment, enaction, and catharsis seem to feed into and enable this process and demarcate performance as a multisensory cultural experience rather than a creative product. Audience research thus needs to move beyond cognitive theory and embrace perspectives offered by these emerging theories. However, even then, the potential of these processes to effect any durable kind of emancipation or transformation amongst audiences remains decidedly uncertain.

References

Alston, A. 2016. *Beyond immersive theatre: Aesthetics, politics and productive participation.* London, Palgrave Macmillan.

Auslander, P. 2008. *Liveness: Performance in a mediatized culture.* 2nd ed. Oxon, Routledge.

Bakhshi, H. and Whitby, A. 2014. *Estimating the impact of live simulcast on theatre attendance: An application to London's National Theatre.* London, Nesta.

Barker, M. 2013. 'Live at a cinema near you': How audiences respond to digital streaming of the arts. In: Radbourne, J., Glow, H. and Johanson, K. (eds.) *The audience experience: A critical analysis of audiences in the performing arts.* Bristol, Intellect, pp. 15–34.

Belfiore, E. and Bennett, O. 2008. *The social impact of the arts: An intellectual history.* Basingstoke, Palgrave Macmillan.

Ben Chaim, D. 1984. *Distance in the theatre: The aesthetics of audience response.* London, Ann Arbor.

Bennett, K. C. 1981. The purging of catharsis. *British Journal of Aesthetics,* 21(3), pp. 204–213.

Bennett, S. 1997. *Theatre audiences: A theory of production and reception.* 2nd ed. London, Routledge.

Berlyne, D. E. 1971. *Aesthetics and psychobiology.* New York, Appleton.

Blau, H. 1990. *The audience.* Baltimore, The John Hopkins University Press.

Bleeker, M. and Germano, I. 2014. Perceiving and believing: An enactive approach to spectatorship. *Theatre Journal,* 66, pp. 363–383.

Boehner, K., Sengers, P. and Warner, S. 2008. Interfaces with the ineffable: meeting aesthetic experience on its own terms. *ACM Transactions on Computer-Human Interaction* [Online], 15(3), pp. 1–39.

Brown, A. S. 2006. An architecture of value. *Grantmakers in the Arts Reader,* 17(1), pp. 18–25.

Brown, A. S. and Novak, J. L. 2007. *Assessing the intrinsic impacts of a live performance.* San Francisco, WolfBrown.

Buchanan, I. 2010. *A dictionary of critical theory.* Oxford, Oxford University Press.

Bundy, P. 2014. Engagement and liveness. In: O'Toole, J., Adams, R.-J., Anderson, M., Burton, B. and Ewing, R. (eds.) *Young audiences, theatre and the cultural conversation.* Dordrecht, Springer, pp. 115–127.

Burland, K. and Pitts, S. 2012. Rules and expectations of jazz gigs. *Social Semiotics,* 22(5), pp. 523–543.

Carù, A. and Cova, B. 2003. Revisiting consumption experience: A more humble but complete view of the concept. *Marketing Theory,* 3, pp. 267–286.

Colbert, F. and St-James, Y. 2014. Research in arts marketing: Evolution and future directions. *Psychology and Marketing,* 31(8), pp. 566–575.

Csikszentmihalyi, M. 1988a. The flow experience and its significance for human psychology. In: Csikszentmihalyi, M. and Csikszentmihalyi, I. S. (eds.) *Optimal experience: Psychological studies of flow in consciousness.* Cambridge, Cambridge University Press, pp. 15–35.

Csikszentmihalyi, M. 1988b. Introduction. In: Csikszentmihalyi, M. and Csikszentmihalyi, I. S. (eds.) *Optimal experience: Psychological studies of flow in consciousness.* Cambridge, Cambridge University Press, pp. 3–14.

De Marinis, M. 1987. Dramaturgy of the spectator. *The Drama Review,* 31(2), pp. 100–114.

Dewey, J. 1980. *Art as experience.* New York, Perigee Books.

Ehrenreich, B. 2007. *Dancing in the streets: a history of collective joy.* London, Granta.

Falassi, A. 1987. *Time out of time: Essays on the festival.* Albuquerque, NM, University of New Mexico Press.

Fırat, A. F. and Dholakia, N. 1998. *Consuming people: From political economy to theaters of consumption.* London, Routledge.

Freshwater, H. 2009. *Theatre & audience.* London, Palgrave Macmillan.

Golden, L. 1973. The purgation theory of catharsis. *Journal of Aesthetics and Art Criticism,* 31(4), pp. 473–491.

Heim, C. 2016. *Audience as performer: The changing role of theatre audiences in the Twenty-First Century.* London and New York, Routledge.

Hirschman, E. C. and Holbrook, M. B. 1982. Hedonic consumption: emerging concepts, methods and propositions. *Journal of Marketing*, 46(3), pp. 92–101.

Holland, N. 1968. *The dynamics of literary response*. New York, Oxford University Press.

Konijn, E. A. 1999. Spotlight on spectators: Emotions in the theatre. *Discourse Processes*, 28(2), pp. 169–194.

Machon, J. 2013. *Immersive theatres: Intimacy and immediacy in contemporary performance*. London, Palgrave Macmillan.

Mackintosh, I. 1992. *Architecture, actor and audience*. London, Routledge.

McConachie, B. 2008. *Engaging audiences: A cognitive approach to spectating in the theatre*. New York, Palgrave Macmillan.

McConachie, B. 2013. Introduction: Spectating as sandbox play. In: Shaughnessy, N. (ed.) *Affective performance and cognitive science: Body, brain and being*. London, Bloomsbury, pp. 183–198.

McKinney, J. 2013. Scenography, spectacle and the body of the spectator. *Performance Research*, 18(3), pp. 63–74.

Morris Hargreaves McIntyre 2007. *Audience knowledge digest: why people visit museums and galleries, and what can be done to attract them*. Manchester, Morris Hargreaves McIntyre.

Nesta 2010. *Beyond live: Digital innovation in the performing arts*. London, Nesta.

Nussbaum, M. C. 1986. *The fragility of goodness: Luck and ethics in Greek tragedy and philosophy*. Cambridge, Cambridge University Press.

O'Toole, J., Adams, R.-J., Anderson, M., Burton, B. and Ewing, R. (eds.). 2014. *Young audiences, theatre and the cultural conversation*. Dordrecht, Springer.

Popovici, V. 1984. Is the stage-audience relationship a form of dialogue? *Poetics*, 13(1–2), pp. 111–118.

Radbourne, J. 2013. Converging with audiences. In: Radbourne, J., Glow, H. and Johanson, K. (eds.) *The audience experience: A critical analysis of audiences in the performing arts*. Bristol, Intellect, pp. 143–158.

Radbourne, J., Glow, H. and Johanson, K. 2010. Measuring the intrinsic benefits of arts attendance. *Cultural Trends*, 19(4), pp. 307–324.

Radbourne, J., Johanson, K., Glow, H. and White, T. 2009. The audience experience: Measuring quality in the performing arts. *International Journal of Arts Management*, 11(3), pp. 16–29.

Reason, M. 2008. Did you watch the man or did you watch the goose? Children's responses to puppets in live theatre. *New Theatre Quarterly*, 24(4), pp. 337–354.

Reason, M. 2010. Asking the audience: Audience research and the experience of theatre. *About Performance*, 10, pp. 15–34.

Reason, M. and Reynolds, D. 2010. Kinesthesia, empathy, and related pleasures: An inquiry into audience experiences of watching dance. *Dance Research Journal*, 42(2), pp. 49–75.

Reinelt, J. G. 2014. What UK spectators know: Understanding how we come to value theatre. *Theatre Journal*, 66(3), pp. 337–361.

Reynolds, D. and Reason, M. (eds.). 2011. *Kinesthetic empathy in creative and cultural practices*. Bristol, Intellect.

Sartre, J.-P. 1961. Beyond bourgeois theatre. *The Tulane Drama Review*, 5(3), pp. 3–11.

Sauter, W. 2000. *The theatrical event: Dynamics of performance and perception*. Iowa City, University of Iowa Press.

Sawyer, K. 2007. *Group genius: The creative power of collaboration*. New York, Basic Books.

Schechner, R. 2003. *Performance theory*. 2nd ed. London, Routledge.

Sedgman, K. 2016. *Locating the audience: How people found value in National Theatre Wales*. Bristol, Intellect.

Silvia, P. J. 2005. Emotional responses to art: From collation and arousal to cognition and emotion. *Review of General Psychology*, 9(4), pp. 342–357.

Slater, A. 2007. 'Escaping to the gallery': Understanding the motivations of visitors to galleries. *International Journal of Nonprofit and Voluntary Sector Marketing*, 12, pp. 149–162.

Thompson, E. 2007. *Mind in life: Biology, phenomenology, and the sciences of mind*. Cambridge, MA, Harvard University Press.

Walmsley, B. 2011. Why people go to the theatre: A qualitative study of audience motivation. *Journal of Customer Behaviour*, 10(4), pp. 335–351.

Walmsley, B. 2018. Deep hanging out in the arts: An anthropological approach to capturing cultural value. *International Journal of Cultural Policy*, 24(2), pp. 227–291.

Whalley, J. and Miller, L. 2017. *Between us: Audiences, affect and the in-between*. London, Palgrave.

CHAPTER 4

Capturing, Interpreting, and Evaluating Cultural Value

INTRODUCTION

Questions pertaining to cultural value are notoriously complex, and the aim of this chapter is certainly not to provide any reductive resolutions to what is not only a live and endless debate but one which might justifiably be labelled a "wicked problem" (Rittel and Webber 1973). By this I imply, following Rittel and Webber's characterisation, that questions of cultural value lack a definitive formulation; exist as symptoms of other problems; evade testable solutions; and have no "stopping rule". In other words, many questions of and about cultural value are more than intractable; they are ultimately irresolvable. Once that this uncomfortable truth has been established, discussions around and about cultural value counter-intuitively become more interesting and fruitful.

The main reason that questions pertaining to cultural value are irresolvable is probably that the concept itself comprises two of the most slippery and subjective terms in the human lexicon: "culture" and "value". It lies well beyond the project of this chapter to attempt to explicate the concept of culture, and in any case, this monograph is predominantly concerned with how culture is experienced by audiences within the performing arts. "Value", however, *is* of primary concern to this book, because it is a highly contested notion that lies at the heart of questions of audience engagement and enrichment. So the core aim of this chapter is to critically explore the contested notions of value that are relevant to the performing arts and to

© The Author(s) 2019
B. Walmsley, *Audience Engagement in the Performing Arts*,
New Directions in Cultural Policy Research,
https://doi.org/10.1007/978-3-030-26653-0_4

ascertain what insights these might provide into capturing and interpreting the impact of the performing arts on audiences.

The reason this chapter focuses on cultural value rather than on the value or impact of the performing arts for audiences more narrowly is because there are age-old debates about cultural value which establish a clear philosophical and epistemological context for an informed discussion about the role that the arts play in audiences' lives. Most recently, these debates have been influenced by the rise of the so-called cultural economy, which, amongst a wider raft of arguments about the positive role that culture can play in the economy, has encouraged polity to occasionally locate meaning beyond consumerism (Taylor 2015). It has been argued, for example, that "art is the currency of experience" that drives the new "economy of meaning" and that this economy is governed by "inalienable value" (Sharpe 2010, p. 2). In other words, human beings have a sacrosanct right to artistic experiences that cannot be denied even by utilitarian approaches to polity. This right is of course enshrined by the United Nations as a basic human right under Article 27 of the Universal Declaration of Human Rights, which declares that "everyone has the right freely to participate in the cultural life of the community" and "enjoy the arts" (United Nations 1948, p. 77). This is clearly a vague aspiration, which fails to qualify "participation" and to provide any evaluative framework for what "enjoying the arts" might entail.

Based on these historical, philosophical, theoretical, and political contexts, the research agenda for this chapter can be summarised around a series of core questions:

1. What do we know about cultural value and what is the purpose of asking questions about it?
2. *Who* wants to know *what* about cultural value? *Why* and *how* do they want to know?
3. In what sense are experiences of the performing arts significant to audiences?
4. What are the most effective ways to evaluate these experiences?
5. What are the implications of this for arts organisations and for cultural policy more broadly?

These questions will shape the structure of the chapter, which will begin with a critical summary of the existing debates about cultural value.

THE CULTURAL VALUE DEBATES

At the heart of the philosophical debates into cultural value lies over two centuries of "abstraction" evident in the dualistic separation between economics and aesthetics which was influenced by utilitarianism (Taylor 2015). At the heart of the policy debates lies the age-old tension between intrinsic and instrumental value (Belfiore and Bennett 2008). And at the heart of the political debates lies a seemingly intractable hierarchy of knowledge, where qualitative insights are generally subordinated to quantitative data, which are widely deemed to constitute the only suitable and sufficient "evidence" to measure the policy impact (or cost-benefit) of arts and cultural activity (EPPI Centre 2010). In many Western societies, this is perhaps the natural culmination of several decades of neoliberal attempts to co-opt economic logics into the public policy case for the arts (Taylor 2015). So although debates about cultural value are certainly not new, what *is* relatively new is the attempts of politicians, civil servants, policymakers, and academics to *measure* cultural value for the purposes of calculating return on public investment and informing future funding decisions.

Despite this political pressure to measure cultural value, myriad academic studies have challenged the premise of trying to *quantify* the impact of the arts (e.g. Matarasso 1996; Vuyk 2010; Walmsley 2012), whilst others have noted the dominant rationalist and successionist models of causation on which many cultural policy analyses are predicated (e.g. Galloway 2009; Sanderson 2000). Even cultural economists such as David Throsby (2006) concede that certain expressions of cultural value transcend valuation as they are rooted in shared social experiences. A broad conclusion of the growing number of critical qualitative studies on this topic is that attempts to quantify the effects of the arts at the level of social impact (e.g. through Subjective Wellbeing or Social Return on Investment methods) are flawed and deeply problematic, essentially because they are not sophisticated or reflexive enough to account for notions of context and praxis (Oliver and Walmsley 2011) nor for the immensurable realms of emotion and spirituality (Holden 2012). As Calvin Taylor argues, in its attempts to avoid a descent into self-reflexivity, the aesthetic runs the risk of sacrificing its "specificity to utilitarianism by finding an external logic – social value and economic value being two conspicuous contemporary examples" (2015, p. 17). The benefits of a more reflexive approach to exploring the value and impact of the arts are further elucidated by Carol Scott, who warns that when public funding decisions rely on measurable results rather than valuable outcomes, cultural policy risks falling back into "the bind of instrumentality" (2010, p. 2). I will return to these arguments later in the chapter when I explore the relative strengths and weaknesses of the diverse methodological approaches to explicating cultural value.

Qualitative research into the impact of the arts has certainly succeeded in elucidating the multiple dimensions of the audience experience outlined in Chapter 3, but it still struggles to close the epistemological gap between *perceived* and *actual* cultural experiences. One reason for this is that "the *how* of the cognitive processes that occur while audiences are watching a performance is largely out of reach to audience research that by definition takes place after the event. In some sense, therefore, the primary experience is available only through the refraction of conscious reflection" (Reason and Reynolds 2010, p. 71). So the more fruitful avenue for cultural value scholars and audience researchers is perhaps not to investigate what value *is*, but rather how it might be reliably *expressed*, reflexively and intersubjectively. What else is lacking, it seems, is a deeper understanding of the *processes* (rather than the *outcomes*) of arts engagement (cf. Hewison 2014).

Mindful of the fact that none of the recent attempts to capture cultural value "commanded widespread confidence", the UK's Arts and Humanities Research Council (AHRC) put out a call in 2013 to fund "ambitious research projects" that might cumulatively "establish a framework that will advance the way in which we talk about the value of cultural engagement and the methods by which we evaluate that value" (Arts and Humanities Research Council 2013). The call particularly targeted projects that aimed to explicate the phenomenology of cultural experiences and encounters. In foregrounding the subjective and intersubjective experiences of cultural audiences and participants, the project represented an open challenge to the Green and Magenta Book approaches[1] that had been championed and/or adopted in recent UK studies on cultural value (e.g. EPPI Centre 2010; O'Brien 2010). Indeed by calling for proposals that would consider the "actual experience" of culture and the arts rather than their "ancillary effects", the Cultural Value Project seemed to cast aspersions on Government-backed research such as the Culture and Sport Evidence

---

[1] The Green Book is produced for the UK Government by HM Treasury to provide guidance for public sector bodies on how to appraise proposals before committing funds to a policy, programme, or project. The Magenta Book provides complementary guidance on the evaluation of ensuing policies, programmes, and projects.

(CASE) programme and question its reliance on instrumental public policy methods such as cost-benefit analysis and subjective wellbeing, which are apparently used to great effect in transport and even health (O'Brien 2010). This highlights one of the core underlying tensions in cultural policy and management—namely the often implicit calls for exceptionalism that are well established on a supra-governmental level in France's successful negotiation of the *exception culturelle*, which considers cultural goods and services as exceptions to commercial entities in international treaties and agreements. So the precedent exists on a policy level to treat (and therefore value) the arts and culture in a different way from other, more tangible, areas of government.

Cognisant of the epistemological vacuum in credible research on audiences' lived experience of the arts and culture, the Cultural Value Project aimed to "articulate a set of evaluative approaches and methodologies suitable to assessing the different ways in which cultural value is manifested" (Arts and Humanities Research Council 2013). The diverse and comprehensive responses that this call produced comprised a rich, polyvocal and critical account of the impacts of the arts on individuals and communities. In their reflections on the 70 original studies that comprised the project, the authors of the summative report noted that: "Academic research on the effects and impacts of the arts is fragmented and fractured, something reflected in the dichotomies that underpin the debate and often distort it" (Crossick and Kaszynska 2016, p. 15). The key findings from this national multi-methods study were that arts and cultural engagement can help to develop reflective individuals and more highly engaged citizens; promote healing, health, and wellbeing; and underpin learning, creative thinking and cognitive development. However, the report called for further research into claims regarding the ability of the arts and culture to build peace and resolve conflict; regenerate communities and cities in a sustainable way; and generate economic impact. Ultimately, the report advocated for more mixed-methods and longitudinal studies of value and impact to support or challenge existing claims of cultural value.

One of the Cultural Value Project's studies that is of particular relevance here is the British Theatre Consortium's *Theatre Spectatorship and Value Attribution* research, which aimed to "reopen the question of what cultural engagement does for people" (Reinelt 2014, p. 340). The following statement of aims captures the tensions between different approaches to exploring cultural value in a clear and illuminating way:

We advocate a multivalenced approach to cultural value which, while not dismissing economic and instrumental approaches, rests on a comprehensive understanding of the processes of value attribution based on individual appropriation of the phenomenal experience of 'being there'. We seek to understand how these experiences coalesce and intermingle with the experiences of others to produce additional values, thus going beyond the 'aggregate of individuals' to highlight how cultural activity might contribute to public value. By emphasizing the processual aspects of value attribution, we hope to bypass the problems associated with the agon of 'intrinsic' and 'instrumental' values. Value emerges in the relationship between the performance, the spectator, and the network of associations which the experience triggers. (pp. 346–347)

What is significant here is the foregrounding of a "multivalenced" approach to cultural value that combines an instrumental focus on outcomes with an intrinsic focus on subjective experience and an acknowledgment of the processual and emergent nature of aesthetic value.

A Third Way: Embracing Complexity

These kinds of study demonstrate that there exists a third way between the dichotomous poles of self-reflexivity and utilitarianism that have divided scholars of cultural value for centuries: namely to accept that art and culture has its own internal logic (or value) and try to capture both the particular and the universal nature of this through reflexive (as opposed to self-reflexive) phenomenological or anthropological enquiries into both intrinsic and instrumental value and their related impact. Taylor (2015) links the particular with a naïve pursuit of *authenticity* and the universal with *reification*, and, following the Japanese philosopher Kojin Karatani, argues that what is actually required is "the ability to read both simultaneously as dynamic polar but mutually conditioning opposites. This is *abstraction* and moreover it is real" (p. 18). This suggests that a possibly fruitful avenue of research lies in a simultaneous investigation of the particular (or individual) and general (or universal) value of the arts, and ideally of the crossover between the two. Taylor intimates that Aristotle's call for people to strive to "live well" in their communities might also provide not only an escape from the predominance of utilitarian conceptions of value but also a possible third way between the individual and the universal.

With this in mind, scholars might benefit from exploring which narratives or manifestations of value might "cut through" the morass of personal and anecdotal stories about the impact of the arts and gain the traction and longevity that quantitative data often attracts, especially amongst managers, civil servants, politicians, and policymakers. Like Aristotle, they might also do well to focus more on how the arts might help people to live sustainably and live well. This third way would require a nuanced and assuredly postmodern approach to cultural value that embraces rather than eschews the complex and often paradoxical nature of its constituent parts.

Theories of complexity are becoming ever more popular as ways of conceptualising the impacts of policy initiatives (Burns 2007). This shift has been gradually effected as growing numbers of researchers have accepted the severe limitations of identifying any simple, linear causality within complex systems and contexts. As we have seen already in this chapter, the arts have been regarded by philosophers as a particularly complex and ambiguous pursuit for centuries—perhaps, as White and Hede argue, because "the impact of art is a complex and multilayered concept that is experienced and understood in a variety of ways contingent on each individual's experience and perspective" (2008, p. 32). This focus on the contingent nature of cultural experience reinforces the epistemological challenges described earlier and serves to strengthen the case for a more reflexive and phenomenological approach.

Further evidence of the complexity involved in exploring the value of the arts can be found in the increasingly prevalent reference to the arts sector as an "ecology" (e.g. Giannachi and Stewart 2005; Holden 2015; Knell 2007; Sharpe 2010). There is something primal and inherently relational about this metaphor, which reflects not only the key social role that the arts have always played in human lives, whether for mimetic or liminal purposes (Schechner 2003; Turner 1969), but also their inherent fragility and inter-dependence. John Holden's description of culture as "temporary phenomena with deep roots and complex enabling factors" (2015, p. 3) encapsulates not only the ephemeral nature of culture and cultural experiences (which of course pose their own methodological problems for audience researchers) but also the diverse and convoluted ecosystem required to produce and facilitate them. Bill Sharpe (2010) also draws on the ecology metaphor to illustrate his claim that the "economy of experience [...] is properly understood within an ecological context" (pp. 32–33). Sharpe's thesis is highly significant in this context, not only because it contributes to the cultural value debates by reasserting the primacy of artistic over economic impact, but more importantly because it once again shifts the very terms of the debate away from the utilitarian concern with the relative value of commensurable objects and towards an enactive focus on interpersonal experience:

> since our cultural systems are inherently social and historical, individual experience always arises in the extended interaction of the members of a community amongst themselves and within their wider context. (Sharpe 2010, p. 31)

Although this assertion is helpful in once again highlighting the all-important role of context, it nevertheless exposes one of the most problematic aspects of the cultural value debates in its reliance on assumptions about the audience experience. Indeed the voice of the audience is all too often missing not only from discussion on cultural value but, perhaps even more worryingly, from audience research itself. The remainder of this chapter and the whole of the following chapter will therefore focus on how to capture and interpret cultural value from the perspective of audiences themselves, placing them at the heart of the cultural value debates in line with the book's overall philosophy of audience-centricity.

THE AUDIENCE VOICE

As we saw in the introduction to this book, audiences are often deliberately or mistakenly underprivileged in audience research. There are many political, philosophical, and methodological reasons for this somewhat counterintuitive state of affairs, but one of the net results is that all sorts of problematic assumptions and extrapolations are made by researchers, who often frame themselves as a proxy for the audience voice. One such example is Herbert Blau (1990), who towards the end of his seminal monograph *The Audience* highlights the complexities inherent to interpreting the audience experience, which he characterises as "disparate, cross-purposed, alienated, and incalculable" (p. 355). Although audience research agencies, and even many marketing departments in performing arts organisations, often bemoan the challenges of locating their audiences beyond those who actually buy tickets, from the perspective of qualitative researchers, the notion that audiences are hard to find and alienated is nonsensical. The additional charge that audiences' arts experiences are "incalculable" is clearly anathema to anyone who spends their time trying to capture and interpret them.

A primary focus for empirical audience researchers is of course to understand what makes audiences engage with the performing arts in the first place. One of the most comprehensive qualitative studies into audience motivation is presented in Bergadaà and Nyeck's (1995) comparative review of the underlying motivations of theatre-goers and -makers. This groundbreaking research identified four motivational typologies behind theatre-going: escapism and entertainment; edutainment; personal enrichment; and social hedonism. The researchers then matched these motivations against the underlying personal values of hedonism, social conformism, personal development, and communal pleasure, respectively. These findings were broadly confirmed by my own extensive qualitative study of theatre-going, which concluded that the key driver for attendance was the pursuit of emotional experiences and impact, followed by edutainment, escapism, and spending quality time with partners, friends, and family (Walmsley 2011). There is increasing evidence that audiences are seeking meaningful, and even spiritual, experiences when engaging with the performing arts. In my study, for example, an audience participant talked about going on "pilgrimages" to see certain actors (Walmsley 2013, p. 83) whilst others also described their experiences in religious terms: "I love undergoing the communion thing – it's more of a religious experience, it's sacred to me". This trend may partly explain the current popularity of site-specific, site-sensitive and immersive forms of theatre, which all bring audiences into closer proximity and intimacy with performers (and, indeed, with each other). These empirical findings serve to contest Blau's theoretical claim that audiences' perceptions are alienated and incalculable.

THE IMPACT OF THE ARTS ON AUDIENCES

As we shall see in Chapter 6, the ultimate goal of marketing has been described as creating value for customers and capturing value from them in return (Kotler and Armstrong 2010, p. 26). Unlike many definitions of marketing, this particular definition is useful for arts marketers as it places value and audiences at the heart of marketing activity and therefore broadens traditional perceptions of what marketing entails to include aspects of audience engagement. But like the cultural value debates, it inevitably raises questions about how audiences perceive the value they derive from the arts and what reciprocal value performing arts organisations can capture from their audiences in return. Derrick Chong (2010) also raises the issue of value, questioning whether arts marketers are perceived as image promoters or value creators. This is a contentious issue for both arts professionals and scholars, as it exposes tensions between traditional marketers, who champion a product-led and/or transactional approach, and progressive marketers, who favour an audience-led or relational approach.

Despite these philosophical and professional tensions, more innovative forms of audience research and arts evaluation are starting to provide fresh insights into audiences' own perceptions of value. For example, various recent empirical studies into the audience experience (e.g. Brown and Novak 2007; Foreman-Wernet and Dervin 2013; Heim 2016; New Economics Foundation 2008; O'Toole et al. 2014; Radbourne et al. 2010; Walmsley 2013; White and Hede 2008) have articulated value in the following terms: emotional impact, stimulation, and flight; engagement and captivation; knowledge and risk; authenticity, beauty, and truth; aesthetic growth, learning, and challenge; energy and tension; happiness and improved wellbeing; shared experience, co-creation, and atmosphere; community immersion; personal resonance and inspiration; empowerment and renewal; self-expression, self-awareness, and self-actualisation; improved social skills, better relationships, and family cohesion. As we have seen, some studies (see, for example, Burland and Pitts 2012; Pitts 2005; White and Hede 2008) also highlight the significant role played by performance spaces, places and venues in "enabling" impact to occur and enhancing or diminishing its effect on audiences. These and similar qualitative studies of the audience experience have revealed how the arts are perceived to function as a vehicle towards self-identification and self-actualisation, especially for young audiences; they are believed by many audience participants to facilitate acculturation, socialising, relationship-building, and meaning-making. It is interesting to note here that audiences tend to discuss their arts experiences in holistic terms, transcending the reductive dichotomy between intrinsic and instrumental value that has long characterised debates into cultural value. So there is a significant (and ever-growing) body of qualitative and quantitative "evidence" regarding the value (both intrinsic and instrumental) that audiences place on their arts experiences, which reveals the terms in which audiences conceive of and articulate this value.

These qualitative insights into the value and impact of the arts provide much fertile ground for cultural policymakers, artists, producers, and arts marketers. On a strategic level, they indicate perhaps what kinds of epithets might yield the best results in marketing copy—for example, "emotional", "stimulating", "captivating", "authentic", "tense", "atmospheric", "inspiring", etc. might all persuade audiences that their conscious and unconscious artistic goals will be realised. On a higher plane, these insights suggest that artists, producers, and marketers could enhance and enrich the impact of the performing arts by facilitating captivation (through a tailored use of venue atmospherics, for example); by providing richer background context (e.g. via a pre-show talk); and by maximising audiences' collective experience (e.g. by facilitating a post-show discussion). But above all, these findings highlight the need for a fresh conceptualisation of the value exchange at the heart of the marketing concept and for a new form of relationship marketing that is "interactive, longitudinal, individual and contextual" (Payne et al. 2008, p. 93). We will return to this contention at length in Chapter 6. For now, it is just worth noting two things:

1. We already know the benefits and impacts that audiences claim to derive from the arts, as the summary of the impact research above demonstrates beyond any reasonable doubt;
2. What we lack are robust and uncontested ways of evaluating them.

Over and above the methodological issues that plague audience research that have already been discussed in this chapter, the problems that beset arts evaluation are partly caused by funders' obsession with instrumental value and partly caused by arts organisations' mistaken obsession with hitting marketing targets and maximising financial value. These utilitarian biases are compounded by the inherent complexities of evaluating artistic value, which encourages organisations to take paths of lesser resistance and evaluate *proxies* for artistic value. Some scholars (e.g. Boorsma and Chiaravalloti 2010; Walmsley 2012) are now therefore calling on arts organisations to evaluate their activities according to artistic, rather than predominantly financial, objectives and to give audiences an active voice in this artistic evaluation. This culture shift will require a fundamental reconceptualisation of value, from the traditional dominance of quantifiable metrics such as ticket price and yield towards a broader focus on aesthetic and social (i.e. cultural) value.

Arts Evaluation

As intimated throughout the course of this chapter, there are a number of significant challenges faced by researchers who try to evaluate the value and impact of the performing arts. Arguably the main challenge is to develop and deploy nuanced, multidimensional evaluation frameworks that are sensitive enough to capture the subtle complexities of the multisensory audience experience and interpret them in a meaningful and appropriate way for multiple stakeholders. Although this can appear at first sight to constitute an impossible endeavour, as O'Toole et al.'s discussion of theatre indicates, this really means in essence that we need to deploy audience research methods that can capture and account for diverse manifestations of value such as cognitive development, sensual engagement, embodied experience, mimesis, and hyper-emotion.

> Theatre [...] engages the intellect, the emotions and the senses. It invites its audience to peer into the private worlds of others where emotions, ideas, relationships are laid bare. In response, engaged spectators claim that they experience more intense emotion than is available to them in their everyday lives. (O'Toole et al. 2014, p. 115)

This depiction of the multifarious nature of the performing arts encapsulates the significant methodological challenges faced by evaluators and once again highlights the inability of econometric or utilitarian approaches to shed any meaningful light on questions of cultural value, particularly from the audience perspective. In an attempt to circumnavigate this issue and develop more sensitive quantitative measures of audiences' cultural experiences, in recent years, several countries (including Australia, Scotland, England, Singapore, and China) have experimented with a new artistic evaluation tool referred to variously as Culture Counts, Quality Metrics, Consumer Insight Toolkit, and Impact and Insight Toolkit. The core aim of this tool(kit) is apparently "to establish a deeper conversation between an organisation and its audiences" (Nicholas Serota, cited in Hemley 2018)[2] via a nuanced metrics framework involving the triangulation of assessments of self, peer and public.

The current version of the framework (see Arts Council England 2018) comprises the following nine core metrics:

- Presentation: it was well produced and presented
- Distinctiveness: it was different from things I've experienced before
- Rigour: it was well thought through and put together
- Relevance: it had something to say about the world in which we live
- Challenge: it was thought-provoking
- Captivation: it was absorbing and held my attention
- Meaning: it meant something to me personally

[2] Sir Nicholas Serota is currently the Chair of Arts Council England.

- Enthusiasm: I would come to something like this again
- Local impact: it is important that it's happening here.

A further three metrics are available for self and peer assessment only (i.e. not for audiences):

- Originality: it was groundbreaking
- Risk: the artists/curators really challenged themselves
- Excellence: it is one of the best examples of its type that I have seen.

Although this evaluation framework has been championed by a small number of academics and indeed by the national arts funder Arts Council England and regional funding body Western Australia, it has equally been subjected to fierce criticism and rejected by the Canada Council as well as the Australian state funding body Creative Victoria. The main critique levelled at the framework is that it represents a time-consuming and reductive proxy for artistic value that is open to political abuse:

> Metrics-based approaches to understanding the value of culture imply homogeneity of artistic purpose, invite political manipulation and demand time, money and attention from cultural organisations without proven benefit. (Phiddian et al. 2017, p. 174)

The framework was developed over time from significant empirical research with both arts organisations and audiences, and it therefore offers a relatively complex and multidimensional evaluation system that triangulates the perspectives of three core stakeholder groups. However, over and above the significant academic critique, the framework has been criticised by audiences for its unemotional and cognitive bias. For example, one participant in the Manchester Metrics pilot project fed back that: "The questions/measures were all very dry and didn't give an opportunity to rate things within the arts that are important to me – excitement, wonder, joy" (Bunting and Knell 2014, p. 59). Another participant reflected that: "I was invited to explore how the piece made me think, but not how it made me feel" (ibid.). This, and the obvious reality that as a survey it circumnavigates any direct dialogue between artists, arts organisations, and audiences, challenges Serota's claim that it can establish deeper conversations with audiences.

It is perhaps understandable that some performing arts organisations and funding bodies are keen to find the "holy grail" of artistic evaluation, and at first sight, multidimensional frameworks like this one do seem to offer a sensible step forward and some kind of compromise between qualitative and quantitative enquiry. But to reduce the complexity of performing arts experiences to a small number of metrics can only ever be self-defeating in that it reduces these experiences to the quantifiable level of products, which denies the potential for emotional and spiritual escapism that most audiences report seeking primarily from the performing arts in the first place. By focussing exclusively on the *outcomes* of the creative process, the tool fails to address questions of artistic *process* or *engagement* and is therefore particularly inadequate in evaluating co-created or participatory work. Moreover, the framework as it stands denies audiences the opportunity to reflect on a performance's originality, excellence or risk, presumably because audiences are deemed to be insufficiently qualified to comment on questions of overall quality and innovation. So despite its stated attempt to include audiences in artistic evaluation and deepen conversations with them, the framework actually perpetuates a hierarchy of cultural value by excluding them from what might be deemed to be the higher echelons of arts evaluation. Worse, perhaps, it opens the door for nepotism by enabling organisations to select their own peers, thus compromising any notion of objectivity; and if strategic decisions such as programming, commissioning or funding are ever to be informed by such a framework then transparency and objectivity are key.

As might be gleaned from the discussion thus far in this chapter, the main problem with any given arts evaluation tool is that it denies any space for praxis or context (qualities that were earlier demonstrated to be vital to cultural valuation) and inevitably reduces the act of evaluation to a crude, one-size-fits-all approach that fosters artistic homogeneity. On a simple and pragmatic level, the existence of such a tool raises the question of whether performing arts organisations should judge their Christmas shows, musicals and comedies in the same way that they judge their new work, existential dramas, and tragedies: can a pantomime ever be as challenging or meaningful as a Shakespearean history play? In the final analysis, even complex evaluation tools like the one explored here fall victim to one of the most common errors of research methods.

> Most approaches [...] fail to make sense of the contextual complexity of artistic activities, overestimating the general validity of methods and underestimating the richness and diversity of the contexts in which they might be applied. (Piber and Chiaravalloti 2011, p. 242)

Like the wider field of arts management, audience research faces the "twofold legitimacy problem" of being viewed with suspicion by the arts world whilst being derided by management scholars (Colbert 2011, p. 261). This often leads scholars, practitioners, and consultants working in the field to deploy quantitative and econometric methods that they don't fully understand in the hope of appearing scientific (Oman and Taylor 2018). This growing trend, often encouraged and even endorsed by policymakers in desperate search of advocacy data, represents a huge disservice to the arts and cultural sector and risks challenging its very credibility. Arts evaluation must be values-driven and as François Matarasso reminds us, the art of evaluation therefore lies in ensuring that the measurable never drives out the immeasurable (1996, p. 15).

CONCLUSION

This chapter has traced the history of the debates surrounding cultural value and explored how cultural value has been and can be captured, interpreted, and evaluated. We have seen that approaches to and conversations about both cultural value and arts evaluation are fraught, imbued with disciplinary bias, and influenced by political perspectives. Cultural value is an intractable concept and I have labelled it a "wicked problem"—both because it is a symptom of many other intractable problems (such as how to interpret and fund "culture" and how to capture intangible value) and because it is never very far away from discussions about the impact of the arts on audiences.

Despite the significant challenges posed by the ever-present spectre of cultural value, I have argued here that questions about and around cultural value are fruitful in and of themselves, as long as they don't culminate in yet another failed attempt to "solve" or resolve the Cultural Value debate itself. For artists, creative teams, producers, marketers, outreach workers, and audiences, questions about the value and impact of the arts are primary and these stakeholders are rarely interested or even included in academic debates about cultural value. There is a thirst in the arts and cultural sector globally for standardised evaluation methods and frameworks, and it is arguably the responsibility of audience researchers to work with all of these stakeholders to strive towards developing evaluation methodologies that are tailored towards their needs and fit-for-purpose. This is ostensibly the aim of toolkits such as Quality Metrics etc.; but as we have seen, these kinds of metrics-based tools fail from the outset because they restrict (and some might say prevent) a deeper engagement with audiences and thus fail to capture the primary goals of audiency.

What is needed, then, is a genuinely nuanced, multidimensional, and reflexive evaluation methodology. A reflexive approach to evaluation would reject the utilitarian conception of value as quantifiable, fixed, and given, and regard it instead as emergent, "constantly under negotiation and in-the-making" (Oliver and Walmsley 2011, p. 88). It would also reflect and articulate cultural value in the authentic language of artists, practitioners, and audiences (Walmsley 2012). An evaluation framework based on reflexivity would leave room for both Raymond Williams' (1958) conception of culture as ordinary and "everyday" and Matthew Arnold's (1869) perception of culture as the pursuit of perfection, thus embracing what we might describe as the three pillars of cultural policy: artistic excellence, audience participation, and public accessibility. It would also foster discussion about how the arts might promote Aristotle's "good life" and call to "live well". In a context where the role of the arts in enhancing health and wellbeing is rapidly moving up the political and social agenda, largely due to ageing and fractured populations, the therapeutic potential of the arts is perhaps more urgent than ever before. Whatever the policy goal, what has become clear in the course of this chapter is the imperative for effective and appropriate artistic impact assessment to embrace the complexity of the creative process and the audience experience; to put the value back into evaluation; and to ensure that the measurable never drives out the immeasurable.

Large national studies such as McCarthy et al.'s (2004) Gifts of the Muse study in the United States and the Arts and Humanities Research Council's Cultural Value Project in the UK have advocated for more mixed-methods and longitudinal studies of value and impact to support or challenge existing claims of cultural value. These calls reinforce the conclusion noted above that the most fruitful explorations into the value and impact of the arts will be those that foster open enquiry amongst the core potential beneficiaries of the arts. Although there is certainly no holy grail to find when seeking to capture and interpret cultural value or assess the impacts of the performing arts, it seems that ultimately only radically interdisciplinary and multi-perspectival approaches will ever be robust and nuanced enough to capture the contingency and contextual complexity of the creative process and the multidimensional complexity of the ensuing audience experience. We have seen in this chapter that the empirical imperative for audience researchers is to investigate how the value and impact of the arts might be reliably *expressed* by audiences, rather than to engage in the more abstract debate about what this value actually *is*. Ultimately, this might offer a much needed third way between the dichotomous poles of self-reflexivity and utilitarianism that have hampered debates on cultural value for centuries. Existing studies in the field indicate that reflexive, intersubjective, and polyvocal accounts of value are more grounded and enactive than quantitative measures, which reduce what is indisputably a complex and multidimensional phenomenon to an inappropriate set of metrics. Having said this, audience researchers also need to effect a methodological shift from anecdotes or "casual stories" to meaningful, potent and universal stories that will gain more traction than the widely discredited and often meaningless econometric data that they will supplant. In the following chapter, I will therefore hone in on the diverse array of methods deployed by audience researchers to elucidate the audience experience.

REFERENCES

Arnold, M. 1869. *Culture and anarchy: An essay in political and social criticism.* Oxford, Project Gutenberg.

Arts and Humanities Research Council. 2013. *Cultural Value Project* [Internet]. London, Arts and Humanities Research Council. Available from: http://www.ahrc.ac.uk/Funded-Research/Funded-themes-and-programmes/Cultural-Value-Project/Pages/default.aspx [Accessed 25 June].

Arts Council England. 2018. *Quality Metrics* [Internet]. London, Arts Council England. Available from: https://www.artscouncil.org.uk/quality-metrics/quality-metrics [Accessed 22 May].

Belfiore, E. and Bennett, O. 2008. *The social impact of the arts: An intellectual history.* Basingstoke, Palgrave Macmillan.

Bergadaà, M. and Nyeck, S. 1995. Quel marketing pour les activités artistiques: une analyse qualitative comparée des motivations des consommateurs et producteurs de théâtre. *Recherche et Applications en Marketing,* 10(4), pp. 27–46.

Blau, H. 1990. *The audience.* Baltimore, The John Hopkins University Press.

Boorsma, M. and Chiaravalloti, F. 2010. Arts marketing performance: An artistic-mission-led approach to evaluation. *The Journal of Arts Management, Law and Society,* 40(4), pp. 297–317.

Brown, A. S. and Novak, J. L. 2007. *Assessing the intrinsic impacts of a live performance.* San Francisco, WolfBrown.

Bunting, C. and Knell, J. 2014. *Measuring quality in the cultural sector: The Manchester Metrics pilot: Findings and lessons learned.* London, Arts Council England.

Burland, K. and Pitts, S. 2012. Rules and expectations of jazz gigs. *Social Semiotics,* 22(5), pp. 523–543.

Burns, D. 2007. *Systemic action research.* Bristol, Polity Press.

Chong, D. 2010. *Arts management.* 2nd ed. London, Routledge.

Colbert, F. 2011. Management of the arts. In: Towse, R. (ed.) *A handbook of cultural economics.* 2nd ed. Cheltenham, Edward Elgar, pp. 261–265.

Crossick, G. and Kaszynska, P. 2016. *Understanding the value of arts & culture. The AHRC Cultural Value Project.* Swindon, Arts and Humanities Research Council.

EPPI Centre 2010. *Understanding the drivers, impact and value of engagement in culture and sport: An overarching summary of the research.* London, DCMS.

Foreman-Wernet, L. and Dervin, B. 2013. In the context of their lives: How audience members make sense of performing arts experiences. In: Radbourne, J., Glow, H. and Johanson, K. (eds.) *The audience experience: A critical analysis of audiences in the performing arts.* Bristol, Intellect, pp. 67–82.

Galloway, S. 2009. Theory-based evaluation and the social impact of the arts. *Cultural Trends,* 18(2), pp. 125–148.

Giannachi, G. and Stewart, N. (eds.) 2005. *Performing nature: Explorations in ecology and the arts.* Bern, Lang.

Heim, C. 2016. *Audience as performer: The changing role of theatre audiences in the Twenty-First Century.* London and New York, Routledge.

Hemley, M. 2018. Arts Council to roll out toolkit to help theatre companies understand their audiences. *The Stage,* 5 July. Available from: https://www.thestage.co.uk/news/2018/arts-council-toolkit-theatre-companies-audiences/ [Accessed 5 July].

Hewison, R. 2014. *Cultural capital: The rise and fall of creative Britain.* London, Verso.

Holden, J. 2012. *New Year, new approach to wellbeing?* Available from: http://www.guardian.co.uk/culture-professionals-network/culture-professionals-blog/2012/jan/03/arts-heritage-wellbeing-cultural-policy [Accessed 5 January].

Holden, J. 2015. *The ecology of culture.* Swindon, Arts and Humanities Research Council.

Knell, J. 2007. *The art of living: A provocation paper.* London, Mission Models Money.

Kotler, P. and Armstrong, G. 2010. *Principles of marketing.* 13th ed. Upper Saddle River, NJ., Prentice Hall.

Matarasso, F. 1996. *Defining values: Evaluating arts programmes.* Stroud, Comedia.

McCarthy, K. F., Ondaatje, E. H., Zakaras, L. and Brooks, A. 2004. *Gifts of the muse: Reframing the debate about the benefits of the arts.* Santa Monica, CA, RAND.

New Economics Foundation 2008. *Capturing the audience experience: A handbook for the theatre.* London, New Economics Foundation.

O'Brien, D. 2010. *Measuring the value of culture: A report to the Department for Culture Media and Sport.* London, Department for Culture Media and Sport.

O'Toole, J., Adams, R.-J., Anderson, M., Burton, B. and Ewing, R. (eds.) 2014. *Young audiences, theatre and the cultural conversation.* Dordrecht, Springer.

Oliver, J. and Walmsley, B. 2011. Assessing the value of the arts. In: Walmsley, B. (ed.) *Key issues in the arts and entertainment industry.* Oxford, Goodfellow, pp. 83–101.

Oman, S. and Taylor, M. 2018. Subjective well-being in cultural advocacy: A politics of research between the market and the academy. *Journal of Cultural Economy,* 11(3), pp. 225–243.

Payne, A. F., Storbacka, K. and Frow, P. 2008. Managing the co-creation of value. *Journal of the Academy of Marketing Science,* 36, pp. 83–96.

Phiddian, R., Meyrick, J., Barnett, T. and Maltby, R. 2017. Counting culture to death: An Australian perspective on Culture Counts and Quality Metrics. *Cultural Trends,* 26(2), pp. 174–180.

Piber, M. and Chiaravalloti, F. 2011. Ethical implications of methodological settings in arts management research: The case of performance evaluation. *The Journal of Arts Management, Law, and Society,* 41, pp. 240–266.

Pitts, S. E. 2005. What makes an audience? Investigating the roles and experiences of listeners at a chamber music festival. *Music and Letters,* 86(2), pp. 257–269.

Radbourne, J., Glow, H. and Johanson, K. 2010. Measuring the intrinsic benefits of arts attendance. *Cultural Trends,* 19(4), pp. 307–324.

Reason, M. and Reynolds, D. 2010. Kinesthesia, empathy, and related pleasures: An inquiry into audience experiences of watching dance. *Dance Research Journal,* 42(2), pp. 49–75.

Reinelt, J. G. 2014. What UK spectators know: Understanding how we come to value theatre. *Theatre Journal,* 66(3), pp. 337–361.

Rittel, H. W. J. and Webber, M. M. 1973. Dilemmas in a general theory of planning. *Policy Sciences,* 4, pp. 155–169.

Sanderson, I. 2000. Evaluation in complex policy systems. *Evaluation,* 6, pp. 433–454.

Schechner, R. 2003. *Performance theory.* 2nd ed. London, Routledge.

Scott, C. A. 2010. Searching for the "public" in public value: Arts and cultural heritage in Australia. *Cultural Trends,* 19(4), pp. 273–289.

Sharpe, B. 2010. *Economies of life: Patterns of health and wealth.* Axminster, Triarchy Press.

Taylor, C. 2015. *Cultural value: A perspective from cultural economy.* Swindon, Arts and Humanities Research Council.

Throsby, D. 2006. The value of cultural heritage: What can economics tell us? In: Clark, K., ed. *Capturing the public value of heritage: The proceedings of the London Conference 25–26 January 2006.* London, English Heritage, pp. 40–44.

Turner, V. W. 1969. *The ritual process: Structure and anti-structure.* London, Routledge & K. Paul.

United Nations 1948. *Universal Declaration of Human Rights.* Paris, United Nations.

Vuyk, K. 2010. The arts as an instrument? Notes on the controversy surrounding the value of art. *International Journal of Cultural Policy,* 16(2), pp. 173–183.

Walmsley, B. 2011. Why people go to the theatre: A qualitative study of audience motivation. *Journal of Customer Behaviour,* 10(4), pp. 335–351.

Walmsley, B. 2012. Towards a balanced scorecard: A critical analysis of the Culture and Sport Evidence (CASE) programme. *Cultural Trends,* 21(4), pp. 325–334.

Walmsley, B. 2013. 'A big part of my life': A qualitative study of the impact of theatre. *Arts Marketing: An International Journal,* 3(1), pp. 73–87.

White, T. R. and Hede, A.-M. 2008. Using narrative inquiry to explore the impact of art on individuals. *Journal of Arts Management, Law and Society,* 38(1), pp. 19–35.

Williams, R. 1958. *Culture and society.* London, Chatto & Windus.

CHAPTER 5

Researching (with) Audiences

INTRODUCTION

Audience research is inherently and inevitably cross-disciplinary. This is because any deep and rigorous understanding of audiences' experiences of the performing arts needs to draw on a range of complementary methods drawn from different theoretical and empirical traditions and perspectives. As we saw in the previous chapter, one of the core objectives of any organisational or policy-level approach to audience research must be to strike a balance between measurable impact and immeasurable value. This implies that audience research must strive to capture, illustrate, and interpret the value and impact of audiences' experiences of the arts from a diverse range of disciplines, including positivist techniques that are primarily geared towards the statistical analysis of audiences' behaviours and experiences as well as those whose objectives are more anthropological and interpretivist. The core aim of this chapter is therefore to provide a critical overview of the most common quantitative, qualitative and bioscientific audience research methods, before exploring and illustrating how these different methods can be fruitfully combined and even systematically triangulated to provide a multiperspectival approach to audience research.

We have seen in the earlier chapters of this book that audiences are slippery and heterogeneous, and that their experiences are often described as ineffable. These structural and methodological challenges impact on

© The Author(s) 2019
B. Walmsley, *Audience Engagement in the Performing Arts*,
New Directions in Cultural Policy Research,
https://doi.org/10.1007/978-3-030-26653-0_5

anyone who tries to engage in audience research and they can some-times leave the field of audience studies feeling compromised and illegiti-mated. As an emerging academic field, audience studies is still struggling to cohere around a set of agreed methods and approaches that might lend it greater credibility not only amongst researchers from cogent fields, but also amongst arts workers and policymakers and, most importantly, with audiences themselves. As Katya Johanson (2013) acknowledges, audience research has been consistently criticised for its "lack of attention to issues of methodology", and its corresponding "lack of rigour", which suggests that "more comprehensive attention to appropriate data collection meth-ods is at least one of the requirements for improving the rigour, quality and extent of research on audience engagement" (p. 162). One of the core objectives of this chapter is therefore to draw together a set of methods that have been tried and tested by audience researchers and to place them into dialogue with newer, emerging methods that are starting to be adopted in the field in order to harness a comprehensive and complementary toolkit of rigorous audience research methods.

In the previous chapter, I provided a critical summary of the Cultural Value debates, which culminated in a call for audience researchers to inves-tigate how audiences *express* the value and impact of the arts rather than to continue to engage in more abstract and interminable debates about what this value actually *is*. Correspondingly, this chapter will focus on the empir-ical aspects of audience research. It will begin with a critical summary of quantitative audience research methods, including surveys, questionnaires, big data, stated and revealed preference techniques, and subjective wellbe-ing. It will then move on to explore qualitative approaches and methods, ranging from interviews and focus groups to narrative enquiry, ethnogra-phy and anthropology, deep hanging out, and participatory methods such as drawing, creative writing, cognitive mapping and guided visualisation. The chapter will conclude with a brief discussion of the rise of neurosci-entific methods and biometrics, which will lead to a broader discussion of mixed-methods and triangulated approaches to audience research.

The chapter is not intended to capture all of the methods deployed in audience research; nor does it aim to replicate the many excellent research methods sources available to empirical researchers working across the arts and social sciences. Instead the chapter seeks to understand the relative pros and cons of deploying different methods in the quest of elucidating the audience experience and to highlight the potential of fruitfully combining these to overcome the pernicious limitations of individual methods and approaches.

QUANTITATIVE METHODS

Despite the fact that statistical data analysis is often the favoured form of impact evaluation amongst key stakeholder groups such as politicians, civil servants, policymakers and arts funders, it is important to acknowledge that quantitative research often receives short shrift amongst artists, arts practitioners, and audience researchers. There are many valid and invalid reasons for this, and many of these were elucidated in the previous chapter. A valid source of distrust in quantitative research lies in the age-old adage that one can prove anything with statistics, and much of the advocacy-driven evaluation in the arts provides testimony to this fear. As Blau argues: "Statistical approaches to the sentiments and attitudes of an audience [...] – which mostly ascertain what they are looking for – make a mockery of it" (1990, p. 356). Some of the critiques levelled at Quality Metrics reflect this disdain for reducing audiences' emotional responses to relatively meaningless graphs.

Research methodologists have established that attitudinal data is best served by qualitative research, whilst quantitative research is best deployed to identify patterns and trends in significant data sets and analyse potential relationships between variables (Creswell 2014). So an *invalid* reason for dismissing quantitative research is the false belief that it can't shed any useful light on audience engagement. For example, significant headway has been made in recent years in understanding evolving patterns of arts attendance, which can now be segmented by a number of key geo-demographic and psychographic variables. These insights can in turn inform marketing and audience development activity, although skills gaps in interpreting box office data, sometimes brought about by an artistic fear or suspicion of numbers, often compounds the poor standing of quantitative research in the arts and cultural sector.

By far the most common audience research methods deployed by arts organisations are surveys and questionnaires. Although these tools are often poorly conceived and articulated and often suffer from poor response rates as a result of audiences' "survey fatigue", as core primary research methods, surveys, and questionnaires can provide organisations with timely, relevant data that is specific to their own audience groups. Although they too have been widely critiqued (see for example Taylor 2016), national cultural engagement surveys such as the UK's annual Taking Part survey, can nonetheless provide useful macro and baseline data that help to identify changing patterns and trends. So rather than be seen in oppositional terms, quantitative and qualitative research should actually be seen as a "continuum" (Alasuutari 1995, p. 7)—often one where the former can provide the "what" and the latter can explain the "why".

BIG DATA

Big data, in particular, has proven invaluable in helping audience researchers and marketers understand arts attendance on national scales. Big data is a generic term used to denote data sets that are too large or complex to be dealt with by traditional data-processing software. When gathered and analysed effectively, big data has the potential to deliver significant strategic benefits to performing arts organisations, not only in obvious areas of activity such as marketing and audience development but also potentially in producing and programming, and even in generating new business models (Lilley and Moore 2013). This strategic deployment of big data is referred to as "data-driven decision-making" or "DDD"; but, as Lilley and Moore point out, the arts and cultural sector is not yet reaping the benefits of DDD:

> The sector currently largely addresses data from too limited a perspective. Too often, the gathering and reporting of data is seen as a burden and a requirement of funding or governance rather than as an asset to be used to the benefit of the artistic or cultural institution and its work. This point of view is in danger of holding the sector back. It arises partly from the philosophy of dependence, subsidy and market failure which underpins much of the cultural sector including the arts and public service broadcasting. (2013, p. 3)

A good example of big data being used on a national scale is provided by the Audience Finder platform, which its developers and managers describe as follows:

> Audience Finder is the free national audience data and development tool, enabling cultural organisations to understand, compare and apply audience insight. Audience Finder brings together data on all UK households with data from over 800 cultural organisations: over 170 million tickets, 59 million transactions, approximately 280,000 surveys and web analytics from all the UK's major arts and cultural organisations. (The Audience Agency 2018)

Audience Finder relies on box office systems running on compatible technology to enable analysts to aggregate cultural consumption data on a national scale. It is now in operation across England, Scotland, and Wales and thus constitutes one of the largest cultural data sets in the world. Thanks to the increasingly sophisticated analysis and segmentation conducted by The Audience Agency and by its affiliate researchers, Audience Finder is starting to effect a step change in the way that arts and cultural organisations across the UK draw on their data in a strategic and comparative way to use it as an asset rather than a reporting tool. When cross-referenced against other large data sets, the platform can also provide nuanced comparative insights into audience behaviour in different genres across the sector. A perfect example of this nuance emerges in a recent study by Hanquinet et al. (2019), which found that ballet audiences were much more socially stratified than those for contemporary dance. It is easy to see how this kind of evidence-based sector-level insight might in future influence cultural policymaking in aspects of audience development and funding.

However, as sophisticated as Audience Finder undoubtedly is (and it is certainly the envy of many other national arts marketing and audience development agencies), it only really provides a snapshot in real time (a now-cast) of *what* arts audiences are doing and *how* they are behaving as consumers; as a blunt quantitative tool, it can't provide answers as to *why* audiences are buying or behaving in a certain way. For example, the platform has highlighted the fact that UK arts audiences aren't as loyal to specific venues as previously thought (i.e. they are more mobile, omnivorous and production-led) and that members of the public who identify their religious beliefs as atheistic or Jewish are significantly more likely to attend the arts than those who identify in other categories. Only qualitative research can provide meaningful explanations for these findings. So whilst big data platforms like Audience Finder can help arts organisations and policymakers to fund, plan, programme, market, and even operate in a more strategic way, the insights that they provide into audience behaviour and into questions of value and impact are inevitably blunt: big data can only ever produce *meaning* in tandem with other audience research methods.

Stated Preference Techniques

A more controversial and contested application of quantitative research comes in the form of stated preference techniques, which are increasingly used by government departments to provide cost-benefit analyses of public policies and spending. The main methods of stated preference techniques are contingent valuation and choice modelling. Contingent valuation is the most common stated preference technique, although it is used mainly for valuing environmental goods and services rather than the arts and culture. Contingent valuation (or willingness to pay) is based on asking people what they would be willing to pay for non-market goods or services. It relies on constructing a hypothetical market and then attaching hypothetical prices to these goods or services by asking people directly about their willingness to pay or to accept compensation for them (O'Brien 2010, p. 24). For example, a contingent valuation survey might ask participants how much they value the services provided by their local theatre and then aggregate this monetary value to calculate the overall cost-benefit to the taxpayer.

Another common stated preference technique is choice modelling (or conjoint analysis), which asks research participants to choose between prospective policy options by describing their relative characteristics and attributes. Instead of being asked directly about their willingness to pay for a good or service, as they would be under the contingent valuation method, participants' relative valuations are derived from their responses to a choice of options—for example whether a local arts venue should present more matinee performances or include a pre-theatre menu.

Both of these methods have been proposed at some point as reliable methods for assessing the value of the arts and culture, particularly by cultural economists. However, as Dave O'Brien points out, although stated preference techniques can capture option and "non-use" values, these techniques are costly; require significant expertise to implement correctly; and, if executed poorly, can produce misleading results (2010, pp. 26–27). They also assume that people are honest and reliable judges of their own wants and needs, and able to compare fundamentally different goods, services, and experiences. Another problem with these methods is that they aim to measure cultural value from the perspective of the general public rather than from audiences (or "users") themselves. Like much of the current scholarship in cultural policy, they therefore cast their gaze predominantly on people who choose *not* to engage with the subsidised arts as opposed to those who *do*. They are based, therefore, largely on hypotheticals and so fail to capture and interpret value and impact in any meaningful way from the perspective of engaged audiences.

Revealed Preference Techniques

Another accepted approach to providing a quantitative value for the arts and culture comes in the form of revealed preference techniques. Unlike contingent valuation methods, which are hypothesis based, revealed preference techniques assess how people *actually* behave in markets—for example whether the opening of a new arts centre makes a neighbourhood more or less attractive for house buyers to live in. There are two main methods used to reveal consumers' actual preferences: hedonic pricing and travel costs. Hedonic pricing captures the relationship between a good or a service and related market prices. So to refer back to the earlier example, the researcher would calculate the impact of the arts centre on house prices in the area. The travel costs method assesses the extent to which people value something based on the amount of time they are willing to spend travelling to consume or engage with it, and infers monetary values from standard travel costs. At first sight, this is a useful method for the arts sector to adopt, as we know from existing audience research that drive time is a significant determinant of attendance at a given venue and is used therefore for the purposes of geographic segmentation (Hill et al. 2003). However, the method lacks sophistication and can significantly undervalue audiences who benefit randomly from a naturally short travel time to a given venue.

The main advantage of revealed preference methods is that they are based on real, rather than hypothetical, markets and thus on what people actually do rather than what they claim they might do. The main drawbacks, however, are that they require a significant amount of complex primary research and rely on a highly questionable relationship between cause and effect.

Subjective Wellbeing

A more prevalent, if equally controversial and contested, approach to capturing cultural value is the method of subjective wellbeing. Subjective wellbeing (SWB) aims to calculate people's own internal judgements of what enhances their own wellbeing. Valuations of SWB are generally derived by evaluating the impact of an event or activity on wellbeing and then calculating the level of additional income that would be required for an individual to achieve the same change in wellbeing (O'Brien 2010). This technique of calculating SWB is referred to as income compensation. It is a highly contested method that has been deployed (some might argue manipulated) by academics, civil servants, and policymakers to make the financial case for arts funding, as demonstrated in the following citation:

> Headlines such as 'Dancing makes people as happy as a £1,600 pay rise' in the Telegraph emerge from the commissioning of language to tell a simple and selective story of cultural value. (Swinford 2014, cited in Oman and Taylor 2018, p. 230)

As illustrated here, the income compensation methodology is manifestly trite and it is based on two false premises: firstly, that the public is capable of isolating the value and benefits of complex, multidimensional cultural experiences; and secondly, that this value can (or indeed should) be expressed in monetary terms (Walmsley 2012).

The main advantage of SWB is that it reflects wider topical debates about the relationships between the arts and health and about how to evaluate the general state of a nation in uneconomic terms. However, the problem with attempts to measure wellbeing as a proxy for cultural value is that there remains "no definite set of indicators which can measure the contribution of culture and sport to quality of life and wellbeing, regardless of how these terms are defined" (Hamilton and Scullion, as cited in Galloway et al. 2005, p. 155). Perhaps precisely because they cannot be easily measured, the UK's Office of National Statistics recently decided to omit the arts, culture, and heritage from the headline measures of national wellbeing (Holden 2012). Evidence from other sectors too indicates that SWB is a highly affective construct that is strongly influenced by individual personality traits (Moum 2007). This might well have validity implications for adopting the methodology in the arts sector: for example, when interviewing generally positive people immediately after an emotional opera (Walmsley 2012). In this sense, then, SWB is subject to some of the same limitations as qualitative methods, in particular regarding questions of reliability and generalisability. The other main methodological problem is that there are literally hundreds of scales that claim to measure SWB despite the absence of a widely accepted definition of the term (Davern et al. 2007). The ultimate death knell for the method, though, is surely the now public indications that senior civil servants consider wellbeing econometrics a "dud technique" that is decades away from being robust enough for policymaking (Oman and Taylor 2018, p. 238).

Subjective wellbeing is perhaps an exemplar of the impossible environment that plagues arts and cultural evaluation. Oman and Taylor (2018) argue that the arts and cultural sector currently finds itself in "a double-bind: increasingly expected to look to new models and complicated quantitative techniques to prove its value and impact, while under-resourced to knowledgeably commission and evaluate these forms of research" (p. 230). They are half right in this assumption: most artists and arts organisations do not have the requisite expertise to commission econometric research—and why should they? But the rhetoric around the need to prove value and impact in econometric terms is overblown. Whilst in certain Western polities governmental culture departments do seem to want more parity with other departments in how they make evidence-based funding decisions, arts councils and regional governments seem to be increasingly interested in qualitative methodologies that might generate stories that are potent and universal, rather than figures that often become little more than a stick to beat the sector with. Even in the UK, the arts and culture have actually not been cut on the frontline as severely as they might have been since the financial crisis of 2008–2009, which suggests that the ongoing threats of "if you treasure it, measure it" remain somewhat hollow.

Quantitative methods certainly have their place in audience research but as Katya Johanson points out, quantitative studies "have lent themselves to measuring levels of impact or engagement, but have not necessarily been able to establish the factors that contribute to that engagement" (Johanson 2013, p. 169). In order to explore the potential of different qualitative methods to offer fresh insights into audience engagement, we will now turn our attention therefore to qualitative research.

QUALITATIVE METHODS

Qualitative approaches to research are widely credited with the potential to provide rich, nuanced and context-dependent analysis of phenomena that preclude a standardised or uniform approach (Rubin and Rubin 2005, p. 242). Unlike quantitative researchers, qualitative researchers are interested in *depth* rather than breadth; they seek to probe their interlocutors in order to unearth often hidden or unconscious values and beliefs; they aim to observe, engage with and get under the skin of their participants to better understand what makes people behave in the way they do, whilst striving to maintain a critical distance. Sometimes, qualitative researchers even cast their participants in the role of co-researchers, and explore research questions *with* them.

One of the core aims of qualitative research is to elicit what is generally now referred to as "thick description". According to Geertz (1973), thick description is microscopic and interpretive; it should interpret "the flow of social discourse"; and the goal of interpretation "consists in trying to rescue the 'said' of such discourse from its perishing occasions and fix it in pursuable terms" (pp. 20–21). So one of the strengths of good qualitative research is that it can interpret cultural activity in fine, granular detail and make the interpretation transferrable from one individual example to another. In other words, it can combine the particular with the universal, perhaps in the way that great literature or drama can.

Despite all of these potential strengths, it is important to note that qualitative audience research is plagued by a whole host of ethical and methodological challenges, including: vested interests of evaluators and commissioners of evaluation; a defensive tendency towards advocacy rather than objective evaluation; the lack of sufficiently affective language to describe artistic experiences; audiences' sense of responsibility for their own cultural experiences; their tendency to empathise with audience researchers; and their conflation of cultural value with other sociopolitical values (Johanson and Glow 2015). Qualitative research also struggles to address pernicious problems related to bias, contagion, memory, social class, and reliability.

There are two main forms of bias that impact on audience research: confirmation bias and positive bias. Confirmation bias is a form of cognitive bias whereby researchers search for, interpret or remember information in a way that confirms their preconceptions or working hypotheses (Miller et al. 2009). In audience research, this can manifest in a lack of scientific objectivity regarding the value and impact of the arts and culminate in an overly positive analysis of findings. As noted by White and Hede (2008), this is a problem that plagues entire fields such as cultural policy studies, which are "predisposed to homogeneity" and therefore shape a research culture that attempts "to prove that positive impacts exist rather than trying to reach a deeper understanding of what they may be" (p. 22). This issue is merely compounded by what Bourdieu (1984, p. 53) might well label an "interminable circuit of inter-legitimation"—namely, in this case, a research context where "researchers rich in cultural capital study audience members who are equally rich in cultural capital" (Johanson 2013, p. 165). This highlights the need for audience researchers to be open and reflexive about their own positionality and to sample audience participants in a scrupulously rigorous way, to include seemingly "incompetent" and "reluctant" audience members (ibid., p. 166).

Positive bias occurs as a result of audiences' tendency to overstate their positive aesthetic experiences.[1] This positive bias is compounded by the so-called "peak-end effect", whereby audiences' post-performance accounts of their experiences are overly influenced by their peak emotion during performances and the heightened emotion they may experience at the end, which may be impacted even further by the "contagion" of applause (Latulipe et al. 2011, p. 1836). Audience participants are therefore not always the most reliable of research participants, especially because those who self-select to partake in audience research tend to show too willing and often fulfil the role of fans. Moreover, audiences sometimes struggle to remember accurately how they felt or responded to moments in a performance that may have happened only an hour previously, never mind several years or decades ago.

Interviews and Focus Groups

Following the post-performance questionnaire and audience surveys, interviews and focus groups are by far the most common form of audience research. Although subject to all of the limitations described above, interviews provide manifold opportunities for "guided introspection", where audience participants are encouraged to "introspect or think aloud about themselves and their actions" (Wallendorf and Brucks 1993, p. 341). Whilst structured interviews are rare in audience research, they are useful for email interviews, for example, and have the advantage of producing more directly comparative data. In semi-structured, unstructured or open-ended interviews, questions can be nuanced, tailored and enhanced by probes and follow-ups to obtain the required detail, depth and thick description. Rubin and Rubin have characterised depth interviews as "a window on a time and on a social world that is experienced one person at a time" (2005, p. 14). As such, individual interviews offer ideal opportunities to capture and interpret cultural value and they therefore represent the backbone of qualitative audience research.

The inevitable challenge, however, is deciding on what terms to code (or decode and recode) the often abundant (and sometimes redundant)

---

[1] Indeed during a scoping event for the AHRC-funded International Network for Audience Research in the Performing Arts in April 2017, a recurrent issue raised by scholars and practitioners was the need to capture neutral and negative audience responses such as boredom.

qualitative data produced via interviews in order to analyse it and deci-
pher recurring themes. Alongside qualitative software analysis tools such
as NVivo, established analytical techniques such as discourse, thematic and
conversation analysis can prove helpful to audience researchers. Despite
these methodological crutches, it is at the analysis stage that limitations
such as confirmation bias are often most prevalent, as researchers make
sometimes arbitrary (or subconsciously biased) decisions about which participants, ideas, stories and quotations to privilege.

Audience researchers are starting to develop ever more creative
approaches to the standard participant interview. For example, the past
two decades have witnessed a flurry of interest in walking interviews, particularly amongst cultural geographers. Mobile conversations or walking
interviews have proven particularly adept not only at deconstructing participants' relationships with spaces, places, and cities, but also at encouraging them to respond in a significantly different way (Jones et al. 2008).
Moreover, conducting interviews outdoors or in a neutral space can shift
the power dynamic often skewed by researchers being on their home turf,
especially when this is in an 'ivory academic tower' or a potentially intimi-
dating sparkling new arts centre.

Focus groups also have an important role to play in audience research,
and particularly in organisational life, where busy marketing and audience
development staff may not always have the time to conduct a series of individual interviews. Although compromised on occasion by manifestations
of social dominance, shyness, and groupthink, focus groups can empower
engaged audience groups by giving them an active voice in an arts organisation. They can also be useful in generating collective interpretations in situations where a rapid consensus is required—for example to "test the pulse"
of small audience segment groups or to sound out audiences' views on
a proposed artistic or operational change. Like interviews, focus groups
require researchers to have strong listening, communication, and interpersonal skills; but in addition to the skills required to conduct an interview,
focus groups also demand excellent facilitation and moderation skills to
ensure that the discussion flows in a structured way and is not dominated
by a small number of individuals. Post-show discussions or talk-backs could
arguably be considered as a certain type of focus group, but in reality, these
events are often poorly facilitated (see Conner 2013) and used more as
a marketing incentive than to generate any research findings or co-create
value with audiences. The role of post-show discussions as a form of audience engagement will be elaborated upon in Chapter 7.

Narrative Enquiry

Despite the fact that narrative accounts provide an important framework for understanding cultural value and "remind us of the need to make the case for culture in a variety of ways" (O'Brien 2010, p. 8), narrative enquiry is under-utilised in audience research. According to Susan Chase (2005), narrative provides a structured method to organise events into a meaningful whole and to see the consequences of events and actions over time (p. 656). This can clearly pay rich dividends in the context of cultural value, particularly when we consider the insight from cognitive psychology that stories can be up to 22 times more powerful than facts alone (Bruner 2009). This is an adage well known to PR practitioners and scholars, and one that is deployed to great effect of course in activities such as advertising and propaganda. But in the context of the arts and culture, scholars and practitioners often shy away from stories in the belief that they are purely anecdotal, and therefore lack rigour or transferability. This takes us back to the discussion in the previous chapter regarding the need to capture stories that "cut through" the noise and approach the universal. Considering that this is one of the ultimate goals of playwrights, composers, directors, and choreographers, it is clearly an activity that the performing arts sector should excel at.

Narrative accounts generally take the form of stories, journal entries, diaries, and even life stories, autobiographies, photographs and performances (Seale 2012, p. 442). They therefore tend to present subjective accounts generated by individuals, usually in a less immediately mediated way that via other forms of qualitative research, where the researcher is more in control of the narrative. As McCormack maintains, narrative enquiry can prevent the nuances and complexity of the participant's experience from being simplified and fractured into smaller components or themes (cited in White and Hede 2008, p. 26). In their own narrative study of the impact of art on individuals, White and Hede (2008) respond to McCormack's theory by calling for a paradigm shift in modes of enquiry, highlighting the uncomfortable truth that impact is complex, subjective and contingent. By fostering deeply personal insights into impact, narrative accounts can capture effectively the subjective and contingent nature of impact and they thus offer rich possibilities for thick, microscopic description as well as more creative and reflexive manifestations of impact. In other words, they can capture impact on its own terms.

ETHNOGRAPHY AND ANTHROPOLOGY

There is much debate as to what actually distinguishes anthropology from ethnography and it is therefore sensible to regard them concurrently and in a holistic way. In his heralded lecture on the topic, Tim Ingold argues that the aim of anthropology is "to seek a generous, comparative but nevertheless critical understanding of human being and knowing in the world we all inhabit" (2007, p. 69). Unlike ethnography, which Ingold characterises as describing the lives of people with "an accuracy and sensitivity honed by detailed observation and prolonged first-hand experience" (ibid.), the main objective of anthropology is to engage in "participatory dialogue" (p. 87). A good example of the former approach is Penelope Woods' (2015) study of audience members at Shakespeare's Globe Theatre in London, which provides a number of meticulous insights into audiences' "skilful" viewing strategies. At their best, ethnographic and indeed auto-ethnographic accounts of audiency can provide rich and thick descriptions of audience engagement, replete with observational detail that is often lost in surveys, focus groups and interviews. At their worst, however, they can descend into banal description and assumption and certainly in the past have given audience research a reputation for being superficial and overly speculative.

Ingold clarifies the difference between ethnography and anthropology further by highlighting the immersive role of anthropologists, who function most effectively when they work and study *with* people:

> Immersed with them in an environment of joint activity, they learn to see things (or hear them, or touch them) in the ways their teachers and companions do. [...] anthropology, therefore, does more than furnish us with knowledge about the *world* [...]. It rather educates our perception of the world, and opens our eyes and minds to other possibilities of being. The questions we address are philosophical ones; of what it means to be a human being [...] and the balance of freedom or constraint in people's relations with others [...], of the connections between language and thought, between words and things [...]. (Ingold 2007, pp. 82–83, original italics)

So anthropological methods generally involve engaging actively with participants rather than observing from a distance how they behave. Ingold contends that anthropology thrives on what he calls "the sideways glance" (2007, p. 83); front-of-house staff in performing arts venues might well benefit from acting more like anthropologists by observing and discussing with audiences rather than providing touchpoints of effective customer service.

Netnography

A significant variant of ethnography is "netnography"—an emerging method which involves studying people's online interactions. Robert Kozinets defines netnography as "participant-observational research based in online fieldwork [which] uses computer-mediated communications as a source of data to arrive at the ethnographic understanding and representation of a cultural or communal phenomenon" (2010, p. 60). Netnography generally involves the detailed content analysis of participants' digital communications to provide a comparative and systematic textual analysis (Seale 2012). Kozinets maintains that netnography can help to generate new theories about emerging ideas and practices. This is particularly the case for digital engagement projects, where audiences may be engaged in and feeding back on innovative platforms and tools. A case study of digital engagement that involved an element of netnography is provided in Chapter 8, and it provides some insights into how the method can effectively respond to Martin Barker's call to investigate how audiences belong to interpretive communities, how researchers might begin to "draw boundaries" around such communities and how we might measure audience members' "degrees of commitment" to a community (2006, p. 130).

Deep Hanging Out

An anthropological audience research method that is gradually starting to gain traction in the field is "deep hanging out" (Geertz 1998; Walmsley 2018). There is very little literature available on deep hanging out, despite the fact it has been described as "the future of localized, long-term, close-in, vernacular field research" (Wogan 2004, p. 130). The term was coined (albeit disparagingly) by James Clifford in 1997 and rehabilitated by Geertz (1998) in the title of a book review he authored for *The New York Review of Books* to describe the fieldwork method of immersing oneself in a cultural, group or social experience on an informal level.

Deep hanging out is best understood as a research approach or umbrella method rather than a singular method in its own right. Like action research, it adopts and relies on more established qualitative methods such as mobile conversations, walking interviews, guided introspection and "interactive introspection" (Ellis 1991). In interactive introspection, although the researcher still encourages the participant to introspect, the ultimate focus becomes "the emergent experiences of both parties" (Ellis 1991, p. 30). In this sense, deep hanging out can be understood as a form of participatory action research (Burns 2007) because it can account for multiple realities and sometimes even liberate subjugated knowledge (Yu 2004). The aim of deep hanging out is to make the experiences and ideas of participants the primary material through which knowledge is generated in situ. To this end, participants are often treated as "co-researchers" in deep hanging out, following Moustakas's (1990) model of "heuristic research". Hartley and Benington argue that co-research "establishes a dialectical process of enquiry by drawing on the complementary perspectives, interests, skills, and knowledge bases of academics and practitioners" (2000, p. 463). This sometimes implies that a grounded theory approach provides the most suitable methodological framework for deep hanging out, because research questions can be co-designed according to the backgrounds and interests of all parties. Regardless, collaborative research approaches such as deep hanging out can bring a more democratic perspective to politically loaded topics like cultural value and help to circumnavigate confirmation bias.

In order to illustrate how deep hanging out works in practice and the kind of personal accounts of cultural value that it can solicit, I will now share a very short case study from a published article on cultural value (Walmsley 2018). This case study focuses on Gillian, one of ten co-researchers in a project which took place in Leeds (UK) in 2013–2014. Gillian has a longstanding interest in the arts, especially in creative writing. She regularly attends creative workshops, has sung in a choir, and regularly participates in and/or volunteers at arts festivals. Gillian's participation in the arts connects many aspects of her life, and having worked in several unfulfilling jobs in the past, she is now keen to focus her future employment prospects on the arts. Being involved in a research project on cultural value encouraged Gillian to reflect on the value that the arts bring to her life:

> I'd never really thought about why the arts are important to me until I was involved in this research. Being asked the question made me realise how much of my life has an arts or cultural link [...] and I've been inspired by people and institutions [...]. I've realised that this is where I'm happiest – being creative, being inspired by the arts and culture of the city and region.

It is plain to see even from this short excerpt that the simple act of participating in audience research can enhance the perceived value that participants derive from the arts. Indeed it is only through conscious reflection that individuals make sense of and invest meaning in their experiences (Reason

2010, p. 21). This is perhaps the core rationale behind audience engagement itself, and it illustrates how important methodological considerations are to both the academic field and the professional practice of audience engagement.

One of the advantages of deep hanging out over shorter-term qualitative methods such as depth interviews and focus groups is that it allows for a multiplicity of modes and moments of communication, and encourages the development of a longer-term, more honest and equal relationship between co-researchers. However, this type of co-research is intensive and time-consuming; it inevitably generates some significant ethical considerations; and it is certainly not without its limitations. The overriding consideration is perhaps to what extent deep hanging out constitutes a genuinely democratic or bidirectional process. This in turn raises questions of power and control between academic researchers and so-called co-researchers. My personal reflection on this is that deep hanging out generated the most equal power dynamic of any research process I have ever taken part in, as it genuinely realised Ingold's call for anthropologists to "immerse" themselves with participants "in an environment of joint activity" (2007, p. 82) following a process perhaps akin to what Margaret Ledwith (2007) has labelled "emancipatory action research" and "critical praxis".

Participatory Methods

With praxis in mind, one of the downsides of all of the qualitative methods explored thus far is that they rely on language as the predominant mode of communicating value and impact. Nobody can fully capture their aesthetic experiences in language and as any audience researcher will concede, some participants find it particularly challenging to articulate their responses to the performing arts in words. In the course of the project described above, several of our participants expressed frustration about the limitations of verbal communication and stressed the importance of artistic or aesthetic expressions of value. This means that audience researchers need to sometimes draw on methods that circumnavigate the limitations of the semantic.

Participatory methods such as sketching, painting, and singing provide opportunities to express cultural value and impact in its own terms, in nonverbal formats that are in keeping with the object of research. As Matthew Reason (2010) argues, the creative responses to a performance can create a dialogue between an audience member and his or her own artistic experience: for example, drawing can be disruptive, creative and intuitive.

Cognitive mapping is another creative method (used predominantly by cognitive psychologists) that has been used by impact evaluators to provide non-verbal insights into questions of belonging and empowerment. For example, Tomke Lask, one of the researchers on Liverpool's Impacts '08 project, was interested in how citizens perceived and lived in their cities before and after the city's year as European Capital of Culture. Lask (2011) was interested in exploring to what extent people's cognitive images of the city might change because of an artistic intervention, so she asked her participants to draw personal maps of Liverpool before the Capital of Culture year began and then about six months after the event. This creative method produced some visually arresting insights into the impact of culture and tapped into participants' subconsciousness in a way that language rarely does.

Guided visualisation is another participatory approach to audience research that has been used to positive effect. Guided visualisation is a form of creative facilitation that has been described as "an evocative technique that guides participants to a different state of mind" (Baxter et al. 2013, p. 118). In a guided visualisation process, research participants are taken on a short guided journey during which the researcher uses specific word prompts to "attune participants to the sensory, emotional, and other intangible elements of experience" in order to help them to re-experience a specific arts event in an immersive way (ibid.). Following the guided visualisation, participants are encouraged to note down, draw or discuss whatever immediately comes into their minds, which can evoke forgotten feelings, sensations and memories, and unlock hidden meanings. By re-immersing participants in a given context or environment, this experiential process can counteract some of the limitations and imperfections of conscious memory. Guided visualisation has been used in various arts settings, perhaps most notably as a form of arts therapy with dementia patients.

The visual matrix offers a similarly creative attempt to facilitate the post-experience sense-making of audiences. Visual matrix methodology is an image-led, group-based method that enables researchers to study "the aesthetic and affective aspects of audience experience" that "arise in the interaction *between*" artistic events and the cultural imaginaries of different audience groups (Froggett et al. 2019, p. 162). In a visual matrix, between 6 and 30 participants are assembled in a snowflake formation to enhance democratic group discussion as free from power imbalances as possible. Participants are encouraged by facilitators to offer images, thoughts and feelings aroused by the artistic event and/or by each other's associations (ibid., p. 166). The advantage of this method is that it is "group sensitive": because it is "attuned to affective and aesthetic impacts" (ibid., p. 162), the method enables groups to articulate lived experiences in a collective social setting, which to date remains relatively rare in audience research. Participatory methods such as guided visualisation and visual matrices can not only circumnavigate the limitations of language to capture the collective, multisensory and spiritual dimensions of the audience experience; they can also "take the research inquiry beyond 'harvesting' conscious information to 'mining' for beyond conscious insights" (Baxter 2010, p. 132). Moreover, they can also help arts organisations to develop fundamentally different kinds of relationships with their audiences: if audience research participants are treated as active partners rather than simply sources of data, organisations can reimagine the role of their audiences and create "people-focused enrichment strategies" that achieve the dual objective of fulfilling their artistic missions and delivering lasting value to their audiences (Baxter et al. 2013, p. 127). This provides further support for the recurrent theme in this book that audience research can engage audiences and be enriching in and of itself.

Neuroscience and Biometric Methods

The aim of biometric research is to investigate physiological signals, or what we might call embodied experiences, in order to reveal otherwise hidden human reactions and responses related to emotion, attention, cognition, and arousal. Like the participatory and creative research methods explored above, a key advantage of biometric methods is that they circumnavigate the traditional reliance on language and are in effect "semantically blind" (Vincs 2013, p. 138). Despite this clear benefit, it is therefore surprising to note that to date, very little biometric research has been carried out with arts audiences. However, thanks largely to the rapid development of cheaper technology such as smartwatches, biometric enquiries are gradually starting to supplant researchers' traditional reliance on hand-held devices, which required audiences to report their own perceptions of their neural activity and response and therefore seriously limited their reliability.

The few biometric studies that do exist suggest that the collective experience of being in a live audience can cause audiences' hearts to beat in synchrony and their brainwaves to sync. There is thus emerging evidence that a collective live arts experience can produce "common physiological reactions" in audience members which synchronise them as a group (University College London 2017). However, other neuroscientific studies (e.g. Gaser and Schlaug 2003; Seung et al. 2005) have indicated structural differences in how professional artists react as audiences, indicating, for example, that performers who listen to music exhibit different brain responses and auditory processes from those without musical training (Pitts 2013).

As a result of generally small sample sizes and the fact that biometric equipment is not yet sophisticated enough to produce holistic neuroscientific data, the most reliable results are achieved when biometric data from a variety of measures are combined. However, one of the few existing performance studies incorporating biometric data demonstrated that it is impossible to treat live performances as controlled laboratory experiments and highlighted the myriad challenges to contend with, including the risk of technology providing a distraction from the performance itself (Latulipe et al. 2011). This study also outlined the methodological benefits of evaluating audience *engagement* rather than the much more subjective and contentious variable of *enjoyment*.

Although audience researchers who engage with neuroscientific methods are few and far between, those who do so testify to their far-reaching implications, which, as Kim Vincs maintains, extend far beyond the arts themselves:

> Knowledge generated by contemporary neuroscience about how the brain perceives and understands patterns in sensory input through art is [...] simply another way of understanding the cultural forces that shape us, because brain function and cultural influence exist in a mutual relationship in which each shapes the other. (2013, p. 134)

Neuroscientific approaches to audience research can thus offer privileged insights into how our brains have evolved per se, and this is why teams of cognitive psychologists and neuroscientists (such as colleagues at UCL) are starting to become interested in audience research. Ultimately, however, although neuroscientific approaches to audience research such as biometric methods can help to circumnavigate the limitations of qualitative research such as bias, contagion, memory loss, peak-end effect, and reliability, they can only ever really prove *how* audiences' minds and bodies are responding to an external influence; they can't capture *why* given physiological responses are provoked. Like quantitative methods, therefore, they need to be used in tandem with qualitative methods in order to produce meaningful insights into audience behaviour.

MIXED-METHODS RESEARCH

Quantitative and qualitative methods can be effectively deployed in combination to analyse the same data (Alasuutari 1995, p. 6). Mixed-methods research (MMR) provides a robust alternative to the false dichotomy between qualitative vs. quantitative and constructivist vs. positivist research that culminated in the so-called paradigm wars of the 1900s (Flick 2016). MMR can be understood as:

> research in which more than one paradigmatic or methodological approach, method of data collection, and/or type of analysis strategy is integrated during the course of undertaking the research, regardless of how those approaches or methods might individually be classified, and with a common purpose that goes beyond that which could be achieved with either method alone. (Bazeley and Kemp 2012, p. 55)

Considering the overwhelming theoretical evidence that mixed-methods approaches to value and impact evaluation produce the most robust, nuanced and holistic results, it is astonishing how scarce mixed-methods studies actually are in the arts. As Kirsty Sedgman points out, there exists "a methodological lacuna within the discipline, which has not traditionally offered training in those analytical methods that study the interplay between qualitative and quantitative data" (2017, p. 310). However, certain high profile studies have successfully combined quantitative and qualitative methods to provide rich insights into the drivers, impact, and value of cultural engagement. For example, the diverse and innovative methods deployed by the evaluation team explored the impact of Liverpool's year as European Capital of Culture in 2008 in a holistic, longitudinal way before, during and after the event. The mixed-methods approach provided a genuine voice to the lived experiences of Liverpool residents; succeeded in exploring processes as well as outcomes; and contextualised impact data by assessing the surrounding narratives (Garcia et al. 2010, p. 5). The Impacts '08 evaluation comprised over 30 qualitative and quantitative research projects and incorporated a range of longitudinal evaluation methodologies, including stakeholder analysis, economic impact analysis, media impact analysis, business impact analysis, demographic analysis, and social anthropology. Specific research methods deployed by the team included depth interviews, focus groups, participant observation, cognitive mapping, surveys, questionnaires, and community workshops.

Mixed methods approaches currently appear to be more common in the visual arts and museums sector, perhaps because audiences in these kinds of spaces are more fluid and benefit from higher "dwell times" than their counterparts in the performing arts, who tend to be herded en masse into darkened performance spaces and then herded out again to the bar or the car park, with remarkably limited opportunities for meaning-making. So to a large extent, the growing field of visitor studies has succeeded where audience studies has thus far failed—namely in applying a range of empirical methods to deconstruct the audience experience. An excellent example of mixed-methods enquiry in museums are Dirk vom Lehn's studies of museum visitors' embodied and interactive responses to exhibitions (vom Lehn 2010; vom Lehn and Heath 2016). These innovative studies draw on a combination of video ethnography, sociological workplace studies, and conversation analysis to investigate the social role of museums in the situated context of the museum floor. Vom Lehn highlights the relative scarcity of audiences' individual and collective engagement with art and describes the process and benefits of his analytical approach as follows:

> The analysis of audiovisual data elaborates on the ways in which participants produce and make sense of particular actions. The analytical work focuses on the practices and reasoning that inform the practical accomplishment of every day, emergent, context embedded activities. (2010, p. 36)

This explanation of a complex methodological approach highlights the potential of mixed methods approaches to capture the complexity of situated engagement and the processes, rather than the outcomes, of audiences' meaning-making activities. It also confirms Johanson's affirmation that "[t]he challenge for the researcher of the audience experience is perhaps not to select the most appropriate technique, but to identify an appropriate combination of techniques" (2013, p. 170).

TRIANGULATION

Triangulation has been proposed by many scholars as a robust framework for a critical and reflexive approach to MMR. For example, Flick (2016) argues that we need to integrate mixed methods and triangulation into "a more comprehensive and more adequate concept of using multiple approaches in social research" (p. 46). Even within the narrow field of audience research itself, scholars such as Willmar Sauter have advocated for "systematic inquiries into the concepts we apply", arguing that a plural approach to the application of audience research methods "is part of the epistemological foundations of our discipline as well as the basis of the empirical work we accomplish" (2000, pp. 48–49).

Although triangulation was originally conceived as a means of validation (e.g. between individual methods, data sets, and researchers) it has now broadened out into a quest for "broader, deeper, more comprehensive understandings of what is studied", including the isolation of discrepancies and contradictions in the findings (ibid., p. 53). The aim of triangulation is not to pragmatically combine different methods, but rather to take into account their theoretical perspectives (ibid., p. 54). A triangulation approach must therefore be holistic and embedded in the research design; it must accept (and indeed celebrate) cross-disciplinary tensions and embark from a position of empirical transparency and openness.

There are different forms and schools of triangulation, however, and Flick (2016) advocates for "systematic triangulation". He outlines the core principles of this systematic approach as follows:

1. Investigator triangulation: collaboration between several researchers from different theoretical, epistemological, and methodological backgrounds;
2. Theory triangulation: explicitly using differing theoretical perspectives to generate research methods that approach an issue from several angles;
3. Methodological triangulation: not just the combination of methods but the triangulations of methodologies including appropriate methods and their theoretical, epistemological, and conceptual backgrounds;
4. Data triangulation: integrating the various theoretical and methodological perspectives into the research design so that the data generated offer a rich, meaningful and complex understanding of the research issue;
5. Systematic triangulation of perspectives: the integration of the diverse perspectives of all of the study's key stakeholder groups. (Flick 2016, pp. 54–55)

We can see here how systematic triangulation is fiercely *inter-* (rather than *cross-*) disciplinary, relying on interventions from a diverse range of investigators embarking on shared research questions from diverse theoretical perspectives. One key advantage of interdisciplinary research is that it can cope with the complexity of wicked problems such as cultural value, and it therefore represents an appropriate methodological approach to explore questions of audiences' multisensory experiences of the performing arts. In the case of audience research, systematic triangulation might also embrace the positions and perspectives of artists, composers, directors, choreographers, producers, programmers and audiences to produce a complex polyvocal account of the act of audiency.

Considering the complexity of the research questions involved in audience research and the significant limitations of any single method, it is hardly surprising that many empirical studies into the audience experience culminate in familiar findings and fail to attract the attention and legitimisation of key stakeholder groups such as policymakers. The advantage of mixed-method approaches, especially when they are embedded systematically into the research design, is that they can circumnavigate the biases and limitations of single methods and triangulate data in a way that offers a meaningful and complex response to the underlying problems and questions.

Conclusion

In the course of this chapter, I have provided a critical overview of the main research methods deployed by researchers to explicate the audience experience and endeavour to capture fresh insights into questions of cultural value and impact. This is an exciting time for audience research, partly because the drive towards interdisciplinary collaboration in the academy is encouraging audience scholars to pool their respective methodological traditions and methods, and this is starting to pay dividends in terms of triangulating what have traditionally been perceived to be competing and incompatible approaches to research. What is starting to emerge is a complementary toolkit of rigorous audience research methods that will support the emerging field of audience studies and hopefully increase its perceived legitimacy.

There remains a tension between theoretical and empirical approaches to audience research, both within the academy and between academics and arts practitioners. But with the rise of participatory culture, co-creation and co-research, audiences' voices are finally getting stronger and more potent, and this is effecting a step change in the role that audiences play in the research that is conducted about them. As we have seen in the course of this chapter, econometric methods such as preference techniques and Subjective Wellbeing are on the wane, whilst audience-centred, participatory and biometric research is in the ascendance. It seems, then, that the traditional fear and suspicion of audiences as active participants in their own phenomenon that characterised a significant amount of audience research in the last century is finally starting to dissipate.

However, audience researchers often find themselves embedded in disciplinary or departmental silos and demarcated as either qualitative or quantitative researchers. As with scholars of cultural value, they often struggle to find a third way between a quest for the particular and findings that are statistically valid and therefore scalable and generalisable. If audience researchers synthesised the ethnographic and anthropological philosophies of Geerz and Ingold, they might conclude that the ultimate role of the audience researcher is to generate a microscopic, generous and critical understanding of the value and impact of the arts from audiences' own perspective and then to interpret this in a comparative and transferrable way, which might succeed in combining the particular with the universal, in capturing both measurable impact and immeasurable value. To achieve this effectively, they may well need to draw in researchers from other disciplines and embrace established and emerging methods such as big data and biometrics.

This chapter has demonstrated how researching with audiences can in and of itself provide a powerful means of engagement, and in the following chapter, I will develop this idea by exploring the rise of audience engagement at the expense of arts marketing and by investigating the correlation between audience engagement and enrichment.

References

Alasuutari, P. 1995. *Researching culture: Qualitative method and cultural studies.* London, Sage.

Barker, M. 2006. I have seen the future and it is not here yet ...; or, on being ambitious for audience research. *The Communication Review*, 9(2), pp. 123–141.

Baxter, L. 2010. From luxury to necessity: The changing role of qualitative research in the arts. In: O'Reilly, D. and Kerrigan, F. (eds.) *Marketing the arts: A fresh approach.* London, Routledge, pp. 121–140.

Baxter, L., O'Reilly, D. and Carnegie, E. 2013. Innovative methods of inquiry into arts engagement. In: Radbourne, J., Glow, H. and Johanson, K. (eds.) *The audience experience: A critical analysis of audiences in the performing arts*. Bristol, Intellect, pp. 113–128.

Bazeley, P. and Kemp, L. 2012. Mosaics, triangles, and DNA: Metaphors for integrated analysis in mixed methods research. *Journal of Mixed Methods Research*, 6, pp. 55–72.

Blau, H. 1990. *The audience*. Baltimore, The John Hopkins University Press.

Bourdieu, P. 1984. *Distinction: A social critique of the judgement of taste*. Harvard, Harvard University Press.

Bruner, J. S. 2009. *Actual minds, possible worlds*. Cambridge, MA, Harvard University Press.

Burns, D. 2007. *Systemic action research*. Bristol, Polity Press.

Chase, S. E. 2005. Narrative inquiry: Multiple lenses, approaches, voices. In: Denzin, N. K. and Lincoln, Y. S. (eds.) *The Sage handbook of qualitative research*. 4th ed. Thousand Oaks, CA, Sage, pp. 651–679.

Conner, L. 2013. *Audience engagement and the role of arts talk in the digital era*. New York, Palgrave Macmillan.

Creswell, J. W. 2014. *Research design: Qualitative, quantitative, and mixed methods approaches*. 4th ed. London, Sage.

Davern, M. T., Cummins, R. A. and Stokes, M. A. 2007. Subjective wellbeing as an affective-cognitive construct. *Journal of Happiness Studies*, 8, pp. 429–449.

Ellis, C. 1991. Sociological introspection and emotional experience. *Symbolic Interaction*, 14(1), pp. 23–50.

Flick, U. 2016. Mantras and myths: The disenchantment of mixed-methods research and revisiting triangulation as a perspective. *Qualitative Inquiry*, 23(1), pp. 46–57.

Froggett, L., Muller, L. and Bennett, J. 2019. The work of the audience: Visual matrix methodology in museums. *Cultural Trends*, 28(2–3), pp. 162–176.

Galloway, S., Hamilton, C., Scullion, A. and Bell, D. 2005. *Quality of life and well-being: Measuring the benefits of culture and sport—Literature review and thinkpiece*. Edinburgh, Scottish Executive Social Research.

Garcia, B., Melville, R. and Cox, T. 2010. *Creating an impact: Liverpool's experience as European Capital of Culture*. Liverpool, University of Liverpool and Liverpool John Moores University.

Gaser, C. and Schlaug, G. 2003. Brains structures differ between musicians and non-musicians. *Journal of Neuroscience*, 23(27), pp. 9240–9245.

Geertz, C. 1973. *The interpretation of cultures: Selected essays*. New York, Basic Books.

Geertz, C. 1998. Deep hanging out. *The New York Review of Books*, 45(16), p. 69.

Hanquinet, L., O'Brien, D. and Taylor, M. 2019. The coming crisis of cultural engagement? Measurement, methods, and the nuances of niche activities. *Cultural Trends*, 28(2–3), pp. 198–219.

Hartley, J. and Benington, J. 2000. Co-research: A new methodology for new times. *European Journal of Work and Organizational Psychology*, 9(4), pp. 463–476.

Hill, L., O'Sullivan, C. and O'Sullivan, T. 2003. *Creative arts marketing*. 2nd ed. Oxford, Butterworth Heinemann.

Holden, J. 2012. *New Year, new approach to wellbeing?* Available from: http://www.guardian.co.uk/culture-professionals-network/culture-professionals-blog/2012/jan/03/arts-heritage-wellbeing-cultural-policy   [Accessed   5   January].

Ingold, T. 2007. Anthropology is not ethnography. In: *Proceedings of The British Academy 2008*. London, The British Academy, pp. 62–92.

Johanson, K. 2013. Listening to the audience: Methods for a new era of audience research. In: Radbourne, J., Glow, H. and Johanson, K. (eds.) *The audience experience: A critical analysis of audiences in the performing arts*. Bristol, Intellect, pp. 159–171.

Johanson, K. and Glow, H. 2015. A virtuous circle: The positive evaluation phenomenon in arts audience research. *Participations*, 12(1), pp. 254–270.

Jones, P., Bunce, G., Evans, J., Gibbs, H. and Hein, J. R. 2008. Exploring space and place with walking interviews. *Journal of Research Practice* [Online], 4(2).

Kozinets, R. 2010. *Netnography: Doing ethnographic research online*. London, Sage.

Lask, T. 2011. Cognitive maps: A sustainable tool for impact evaluation. *Journal of Policy Research in Tourism, Leisure and Events*, 3(1), pp. 44–62.

Latulipe, C., Carroll, E. A. and Lottridge, D. 2011. Evaluating longitudinal projects combining technology with temporal arts. In: *International Conference on Human Factors in Computing Systems*. Vancouver, BC.

Ledwith, M. 2007. On being critical: Uniting theory and practice through emancipatory action research. *Educational Action Research*, 15(4), pp. 597–611.

Lilley, A. and Moore, P. 2013. *Counting what counts: What Big Data can do for the cultural sector*. London, NESTA.

Miller, F. P., Vandome, A. F. and McBrewster, J. 2009. *Confirmation bias*. Saarbrücken, VDM Publishing.

Moum, T. 2007. A critique of "Subjective Wellbeing as an affective cognitive construct" by Davern, Cummins and Stokes. *Journal of Happiness Studies*, 8, pp. 451–453.

Moustakas, C. 1990. *Heuristic research: Design, methodology, and applications*. London, Sage.

O'Brien, D. 2010. *Measuring the value of culture: A report to the Department for Culture Media and Sport*. London, Department for Culture Media and Sport.

Oman, S. and Taylor, M. 2018. Subjective well-being in cultural advocacy: A politics of research between the market and the academy. *Journal of Cultural Economy*, 11(3), pp. 225–243.

Pitts, S. E. 2013. Amateurs as audiences: Reciprocal relationships between playing and listening to music. In: Radbourne, J., Glow, H. and Johanson, K. (eds.) *The audience experience: A critical analysis of audiences in the performing arts*. Bristol, Intellect, pp. 83–93.

Reason, M. 2010. Asking the audience: Audience research and the experience of theatre. *About Performance*, 10, pp. 15–34.

Rubin, H. J. and Rubin, I. 2005. *Qualitative interviewing: The art of hearing data*. 2nd ed. Thousand Oaks, CA; London, Sage.

Sauter, W. 2000. *The theatrical event: Dynamics of performance and perception*. Iowa City, University of Iowa Press.

Scale, C. 2012. *Researching society and culture*. London, Sage.

Sedgman, K. 2017. Audience experience in an anti-expert age: A survey of theatre audience research. *Theatre Research International*, 42(3), pp. 307–322.

Seung, Y., Kyong, J., Woo, S., Lee, B. and Lee, K. 2005. Brain activation during music listening in individuals with or without prior music training. *Neuroscience Research*, 52(4), pp. 323–329.

Taylor, M. 2016. Nonparticipation or different styles of participation? Alternative interpretations from Taking Part. *Cultural Trends*, 25(3), pp. 169–181.

The Audience Agency. 2018. *Audience Finder* [Internet]. The Audience Agency. Available from: https://www.theaudienceagency.org/audience-finder [Accessed 24 May].

University College London. 2017. *Audience members' hearts beat together at the theatre* [Internet]. London, University College London. Available from: https://www.ucl.ac.uk/news/slms/slms-news/slms/audience-members-hearts-beat-together?utm_content=buffer14d3c&utm_medium=social&utm_source=twitter.com&utm_campaign=buffer [Accessed 23 April].

Vincs, K. 2013. Structure and aesthetics in audience responses to dance. In: Radbourne, J., Glow, H. and Johanson, K. (eds.) *The audience experience: A critical analysis of audiences in the performing arts*. Bristol, Intellect, pp. 129–142.

vom Lehn, D. 2010. Examining "response": Video-based studies in museums and galleries. *International Journal of Culture, Tourism and Hospitality Research*, 4(1), pp. 33–43.

vom Lehn, D. and Heath, C. 2016. Action at the exhibit face: Video and the analysis of social interaction in museums and galleries. *Journal of Marketing Management*, 32(15–16), pp. 1441–1457.

Wallendorf, M. and Brucks, M. 1993. Introspection in consumer research: Implementation and implications. *Journal of Consumer Research*, 20(3), pp. 339–359.

Walmsley, B. 2012. Towards a balanced scorecard: A critical analysis of the Culture and Sport Evidence (CASE) programme. *Cultural Trends*, 21(4), pp. 325–334.

Walmsley, B. 2018. Deep hanging out in the arts: An anthropological approach to capturing cultural value. *International Journal of Cultural Policy*, 24(2), pp. 227–291.

White, T. R. and Hede, A.-M. 2008. Using narrative inquiry to explore the impact of art on individuals. *Journal of Arts Management, Law and Society*, 38(1), pp. 19–35.

Wogan, P. 2004. Deep hanging out: Reflections on fieldwork and multisited Andean ethnography. *Identities*, 11(1), pp. 129–139.

Woods, P. 2015. Skilful spectatorship? Doing (or being) audience at Shakespeare's Globe Theatre. *Shakespeare Studies*, 43, pp. 99–113.

Yu, J. E. 2004. Reconsidering participatory action research for organizational transformation and social change. *Journal of Organisational Transformation and Social Change*, 1(2–3), pp. 111–141.

CHAPTER 6

From Consumption to Enrichment: The Long Slow Death of Arts Marketing

INTRODUCTION

The aim of this chapter is to present a critical analysis of the main questions and issues pertaining to the marketing of the performing arts to audiences. Building on the conclusions of the previous chapters, and particularly on the insights into the audience experience explicated thus far in the book, this chapter will serve as a provocation to fundamentally reconfigure the arts marketing concept in order to reflect the conceptual evolution of the field towards notions and processes of audience engagement and enrichment. The chapter will expose the limitations of the traditional marketing mix for contemporary philosophies, modes and techniques of audience engagement and suggest an alternative, audience-centred paradigm fit for contemporary arts marketing scholarship and for twenty-first-century performing arts organisations. I will argue in the course of the chapter that we are currently witnessing a paradigm shift, as performing arts organisations and scholars continue to reject the outmoded principles of marketing and adopt a more engagement-based approach.

As an emerging academic field, arts marketing owes much to complementary, if exceptionally cross-disciplinary, academic disciplines such as arts management, business studies, cultural policy studies, cultural economics, museology, musicology, performance studies, psychology, sociology, semiotics, strategic management, and consumer behaviour (Dennis et al. 2011; O'Reilly 2011). The problem that will be elucidated in the course of this

© The Author(s) 2019
141
B. Walmsley, *Audience Engagement in the Performing Arts*,
New Directions in Cultural Policy Research,
https://doi.org/10.1007/978-3-030-26653-0_6

chapter is that traditionally, the focus has tended to fall on the marketing rather than the arts; that seemingly entrenched cross-disciplinary tensions have prevented the fully interdisciplinary approach required by this inherently hybrid discipline. So the underlying thesis behind this chapter is that it is time to redress the balance and reassert the primal role that arts and humanities research can play in tailoring the discipline back to its creative and not-for-profit origins. Ultimately, I will argue that as a term and as a concept, arts marketing has passed its sell-by date: having alienated artistic and audiences for decades, it is now finally being supplanted by the advent of socio-cultural phenomena such as co-creation and by the technological advancements that facilitate these developments. As processes of audience engagement start to eclipse the tired tactics of promotion, there is compelling evidence that we are finally witnessing a paradigm shift in arts marketing.

The History of Arts Marketing

The idea of extending the marketing concept to the not-for-profit sector was first advocated in the late 1960s by Levy and Kotler, who argued that marketing activities can no longer be "confined to the traditional economic units that have held them as their function" (1969, p. 67) because they are "everyone's business" (p. 68). This broadening of the concept was supported by other scholars such as Shapiro (1973), who confirmed just a few years later that marketing was recognised as an intrinsic element of not-for-profit organisations. By the end of the 1970s, what Hirschman (1983) refers to as "the intellectual battle for the acceptance of the broadened perspective of marketing" seemed to have been decisively won (p. 45), perhaps reflecting Debord's foreboding about the "autocratic reign of the market economy" (1992, n.p.).

In the arts, this somewhat pyrrhic victory of the market economy manifested in organisations adopting generic marketing tactics, while remaining highly sceptical about the supposed benefits of either an arts-led or holistic approach:

> There was no evidence of arts organisations embracing a marketing philosophy due to a fear of perceived complex administrative requirements, anti-management sentiment, not wishing to upset the status quo and the desire to keep a small but satisfied audience. There was also no indication of the need for a form of marketing which acknowledged the specific requirements

of the industry. Instead, the implementation of aspects of mainstream marketing was prevalent. (Fillis 2011, p. 12)

Supported both socially and philosophically by high profile movements such as the Frankfurt School and Debord's Situationists, the not-for-profit sector has long resisted the encroachment of neo-liberal terms and concepts. Steven Hadley's (forthcoming) comprehensive analysis of the advancement of audience development in Arts Council England testifies to the deep-seated resistance to marketing at a senior national policy level, bearing out Levy and Kotler's acknowledgement that "nonbusiness groups, institutions and organizations resist the term 'marketing' applied to their activities, feeling that it stigmatizes them by implying they value and seek money or success instead of less meretricious goals of social and professional kinds. This means there is a semantic and conceptual problem" (1969, p. 70). If there was a semantic and conceptual problem back in 1969, there is a conceptual crisis in the second decade of the Twenty-First Century where consumers are demanding an increasingly participatory and co-creative role in both production and meaning-making processes.

Kotler and Armstrong tried to circumnavigate this problem by redefining marketing in broader, less profit-focused terms, as an activity that involves "determining the needs and wants of target markets and delivering the desired satisfactions more effectively and efficiently than competitors do" (2010, p. 55). Kotler and Armstrong go on to describe the aim of marketing as creating value for customers and capturing value from them in return (p. 26). This definition of marketing is useful for arts marketers as it places value and audiences at the heart of marketing activity. But it inevitably raises questions about how audiences perceive the value they derive from the arts and what reciprocal value arts organisations can obtain from their audiences. Chong (2010) also raises the issue of value, questioning whether arts marketers are perceived as image promoters or value creators. This is a fundamental question, which goes to the heart of the debate that frames this chapter. But Chong's rhetorical question doesn't go far enough: perceptions are important, but what underlies these perceptions is how arts marketers perceive of themselves and, more fundamentally, which activities they actually prioritise.

Hill et al. (2003) define arts marketing as "an integrated management process which sees mutually satisfying exchange relationships with customers as the route to achieving organizational and artistic objectives" (p. 1). This definition succeeds in avoiding the supposition of profit and incorporates the realisation of artistic objectives; but although it incorporates the vital aspect of developing mutually beneficial relationships with audiences, it lacks the helpful focus on *value* evident in Kotler and Armstrong's and Chong's definitions. However, Hill et al. go on to develop their vision of arts marketing by articulating it as a process that seeks an interactive relationship with audiences via an integration of artistic objectives and management strategies. We can appreciate in this definition how scholars are now starting to critically apply marketing and management theory to the context of the arts, and how they are increasingly conceptualising arts marketing as an integrated process based on interactive relationships with audiences.

The conceptual development of arts marketing is the core focus of this chapter and it has been traced most effectively by Ruth Rentschler (1998) who provided a useful historical framework at the turn of the millennium. Based on a content analysis of journals covering topics related to arts marketing over the past few decades, Rentschler demarcated the field's conceptual development into three distinct eras: the Foundation Period (1975–1984); the Professionalization Period (1985–1994); and the Rediscovery Period (from 1995). Rentschler demonstrates how during the Foundation Period the arts sector (led by North America) started to diversify its offer; engage in audience analysis; and think more strategically about the potential benefits of marketing. The Professionalization Period witnessed arts organisations recruiting dedicated marketing staff and even establishing whole marketing departments as they strove to operate in a more tactical, strategic, and financially viable way and respond to their funders' increasing demands for stronger management and greater accountability. Over this period, they began to invest in strategic audience research in order to segment their audiences and differentiate between different stakeholder groups. It was also during the Professionalization Period that arts marketing began to come of age as an academic field: Rentschler recounts how from 1985 to 1994 five journals ran a combined total of six special issues on arts marketing and how towards the end of this phase, a wider interest in behavioural and social sciences began to manifest (1998, p. 92).

As Rentschler somewhat presciently anticipated back in 1998, the trend for a more strategic approach to arts marketing practice has continued into the new millennium, with audience analysis and segmentation gradually becoming standard practice in certain parts of the world. However, at the end of her analysis Rentschler also mused whether we might be on the cusp of a new era of arts marketing characterised by a wholesale adoption of relationship marketing based on a more collaborative approach. She called this potential new phase the Rediscovery Period, and in hindsight, it certainly does appear that the period from 1995 to around 2010 was marked by a rediscovery of what arts marketing actually entails, a time when performing artists and organisations started to play, collaborate, co-produce and co-create with audiences and wider communities. This is perhaps demonstrated most explicitly by the rise of live streaming and by the phenomenal popularity of immersive and site-specific or site-responsive work mastered in the UK by "new wave" companies such as Grid Iron, Punchdrunk, National Theatre of Scotland, and National Theatre Wales.

I would contend that these kinds of approaches have now in their turn also become mainstream. Marketing has become more about *people* than data; it is increasingly *relational* in that it takes place through various forms of *dialogue* with audiences; and in the context of the performing arts, it involves more than "anticipating customers' needs": it requires the inspiration to delight audiences by communicating the potential for lasting and meaningful experiences, pulling emotions and intelligence from people rather than pushing products into an increasingly saturated market. As Jennifer Radbourne (2013) argues, arts marketing has reached a state of "convergence" between creators and consumers, artists and audiences. This development is so marked, Radbourne suggests, that it demands a reconceptualisation of the entire arts marketing paradigm:

> Relationship marketing theory has been challenged by the new arts consumer who is on a quest for self-actualization where the creative or cultural experience is expected to fulfil a spiritual need that has very little to do with the traditional marketing plan of an arts company or organization [...] and who is changing the marketing paradigm. (2013, p. 146)

My argument here is therefore that arts marketing has now entered a fourth era, once which I will label the "Enrichment Period" (2007 to date). Semantically, this new era has once again been led by the United States, where Lynne Conner (2004) first introduced the phrase "audience enrichment"; but although audience enrichment programmes are now commonplace in the USA, the UK, and Australia are also at the forefront of this new approach to arts marketing in terms of both theory and practice.

Beginning with the fundamental principles of marketing, I will now trace the development of this new phase, demonstrating how arts marketing has transformed from the tactical application of strategic tools to a new conceptual paradigm characterised by the sociological processes of engagement discussed in Chapters 1 and 2.

The Marketing Concept

As a discreet discipline, arts marketing has struggled thus far to establish consensus around a coherent and compelling definition of its primary aims and objectives. It therefore suffers from charges of incoherence and illegitimacy (Colbert and St-James 2014). To date, its conceptual paradigm constitutes little more than a palimpsest of McKitterick's first definition of the marketing concept in 1957, which basically championed the production of products in response to the expressed or latent needs and desires of consumers to maximise profitability (Hirschman 1983, p. 46). The most persistent attempt to differentiate arts marketing conceptually has come from François Colbert (2007), who has repeatedly rejected a consumer-centric model in favour of a product-led approach. However, in recent years Colbert and other arts marketing scholars have acknowledged a shift away from "supply-side marketing" in the arts (Colbert and St-James 2014, p. 569) based predominantly on the still emerging cultures of co-creation and audience-centricity.

Marketing theory and practice are still essentially based around what is generally referred to as the "marketing mix". Marketing scholars and practitioners traditionally reference the 4Ps of marketing: the elements of product, place, price, and promotion (McCarthy 1964). "Product" refers to an organisation's market offering, which it tailors to meet the needs and desires of its customers. Products are affected by their features, quality, variety, design, branding, and related services. In the arts sector, this focus on products is highly problematic, as much of the sector exists to produce memorable experiences rather than tangible products. The second element of the marketing mix is "place", which defines where the product or experience is available to buy and/or be presented to the audience. As the performing arts are characterised predominantly by live performances, this element is hugely important, as it covers the significant experiential role played by venues: stadia, theatres, museums, art galleries, cinemas, concert halls, etc. In the performing arts sector, "place" is also markedly impacted by strategies and logistics of touring. The third element of the marketing mix is "price". Pricing strategies are developing apace in the performing arts, with strategies such as dynamic pricing becoming increasing popular; but it is worth noting here that in the predominantly non-profit and creative sector of the performing arts, profit and price are often secondary to artistic impact, audience development and accessibility. The fourth and final element of the mix is "promotion"—the mechanisms and activities which promote or advertise the product or experience to audiences and persuade them to buy or engage with it.

An updated version of the marketing mix is provided in the 7P model (Booms and Bitner 1981), also referred to as the Services Marketing Mix. This extended version of the mix includes the extra three elements of people, process and physical evidence. The "people" element covers customer service and any personal interaction between the product or experience and the customer or audience member. Its inclusion in the marketing mix represents an acknowledgement of the significant role that people play in selling and promoting products and augmenting experiences. In the performing arts, this could refer to a whole host of workers, from front-of-house staff to actors, producers and musicians, although arguably these are an essential part of the product or experience itself. The inclusion of the "process" element highlights the importance of the marketing process described above—the integrated range of marketing activities that comprise the ongoing dialogue between an organisation and its audiences. The final element is "physical evidence" (sometimes called the "physical environment"). This refers to buildings, packaging, flyers, uniforms, tickets programmes, and logos. Although these elements are important in positioning, promoting and enhancing a product or event, it could be argued that they are covered in the product, place, and promotion elements of the mix and therefore do not require their own separate element.

It is important to note here that both of these models have been widely critiqued by many marketing scholars. Constantinides (2006), for example, argues that the marketing mix fosters a normative, unstrategic approach, an internal orientation and a lack of interaction and personalisation that ignores the opportunities offered by digital marketing. He outlines the main areas of controversy surrounding the marketing mix as follows:

> Despite the background and status of the Mix as a major theoretical and practical parameter of contemporary marketing, several academics have at times expressed doubts and objections as to the value and the future of the Mix, proposing alternatives that range from minor modifications to total rejection. It is often evident in both the academic literature and marketing

> textbooks that the mix is deemed by many researchers and writers as inadequate to address specific marketing situations like the marketing of services, the management of relationships or the marketing of industrial products. (Constantinides 2006, p. 409)

With the advent of services marketing in the 1970s and its rapid development into a major sub-discipline of marketing in the 1980s and 1990s, focus started to shift away from production and the traditional predominance of the "product" towards aspects of consumption. This in turn effected a renewed appreciation of consumers and their different needs. Services, it was claimed, differed fundamentally from goods as a result of four key features: intangibility, heterogeneity, inseparability, and perishability—the so-called IHIP paradigm (Fisk et al. 1993). It was further argued that services offered no transfer of ownership (Lovelock and Gummesson 2004). There are self-evident synergies here with performing arts experiences, which are generally intangible, heterogeneous and perishable, if not inseparable, and whose ownership (at least legally) remains with the provider. The services marketing paradigm is therefore particularly apposite to the performing arts: as Rentschler puts it, "performing arts organisations are in a service industry in which the focus has shifted to meeting the needs of people [...] rather than a static relationship between the market and what can be taken out of it" (1998, p. 86).

Within this new context of service, Bernstein (2006) argues that modern consumers are principally concerned with satisfying their own requirements. The 4Ps focus on the seller's position, she claims, whereas a customer-focussed approach should reflect the buyer's mindset. Bernstein thus advocates replacing the 4Ps with 4Cs: customer value, customer costs, convenience, and communication. As discussed earlier, the focus on value is highly fitting from the arts marketing perspective; and although the inclusion of communication is potentially valuable, the persistent dominance of cost remains problematic and there is no mention here of the object or nature of any potential customer value. It is also important to distinguish service experiences from aesthetic experiences (Colbert and St-James 2014), because although aspects of service can impact significantly on arts experiences (Maher et al. 2011), they essentially define the surround or augmented product rather than the core aesthetic experience itself.

In an attempt to explicate the true nature of the arts exchange, other arts marketing scholars and audience researchers have recently incorporated aspects of hosting and hospitality. For example, Lynne Conner claims that we are now living in "the age of the hospitality economy" which requires arts spaces to "desacralize the normative etiquette" in an attempt to feel welcoming and inclusive (2004, pp. 156–157). As apposite as this provocation may appear, particularly in the domain of new audience development, the hospitality metaphor ultimately poses the same conceptual challenges as the service paradigm in that it fails to capture the specific nature of the core product or experience afforded by the arts. I would like to argue here, therefore, that the theoretical assumptions and traditions supporting arts marketing need to be rooted in the arts. This supports Fillis's view that "a contemporary interpretation of arts marketing should acknowledge its foundations in the application of the marketing mix but it needs to move forward on its own terms" (2011, p. 13). Let's now move on to consider on what bases we might make the case for what is commonly (and often disparagingly) termed "exceptionalism".

The Case for Exceptionalism

Like marketing, the performing arts are fundamentally based on a three-way process of interactive communication (B2C, C2B, and C2C, or artist/organisation to audience, audience to artist/organisation, and audience to audience). At face value, these commonalities make the performing arts an ideal "product" to market. However, the live and inherently interactive nature of the performing arts, the mystique surrounding their creative processes, the sociological complexities of cultural capital and taste, the diversity of the rapidly developing subgenres, and the complex psychology behind the audience experience actually make the performing arts one of the hardest "products" to market of all. Indeed many audiences and artists feel alienated by the application of generic marketing terminology such as "product" and "consumption" to something they perceive as profoundly experiential and even deeply spiritual.

So if the performing arts offer an atypical product for an atypical market, how can we define them in marketing terms and what implications might this have for arts marketers? We could borrow the cultural studies term "symbolic product" (Williams 1958), used to denote "prestige, pride and identity goods" (Khalil 2000). We could employ the more traditional marketing nomenclature of "intangible product", employed to describe products which can't be inspected or tried out in advance (Levitt 1981). We could argue that art is a "merit good", which civilised societies should provide in quantities greater than consumers actually demand

(Musgrave and Musgrave 1989). Or we could acknowledge the experiential nature of the arts and the autotelic, multisensory experiences that they offer, and opt for "hedonic products" (Hirschman and Holbrook 1982). In the creative industries, consumption is increasingly regarded as a non-utilitarian endeavour to fulfil personal wishes, feelings, and fantasies. This hedonic or experiential perspective on consumption takes account of the symbolic meanings of creative products alongside more subjective consumption goals such as fun, cheerfulness, sociability, and elegance (ibid.).

Pertinently for this chapter, Hirschman (1983) goes on to argue in a subsequent article that as a normative framework, the marketing concept is not applicable to art because of art's intrinsically motivated production values related to aspects of beauty, emotion, and aesthetics. For example, Hirschman maintains that artists prioritise audience groups (e.g. self, peers, experts, and the general public) whose desires they themselves seek to fulfil and that the arts sector often actually disfavours commercial creativity (p. 50). Such propositions would appear to be utterly reasonable in what is essentially a not-for-profit sector (but of course completely unreasonable in the commercial arts). Synthesising the earlier literature on the topic, Hirschman identifies five characteristics that differentiate artistic products: abstraction, subjectivity, non-utilitarianism, uniqueness and their holistic nature; she concludes that these distinctions demand a re-examination of the core theoretical premises of marketing and acknowledgement of its inherent scientific limitations.

In a similar vein, O'Sullivan (2013) argues for an egalitarian and emancipatory approach to arts marketing, calling for the adoption of an ethical framework which would champion audiences' "freedom to respond and participate fully and critically, untrammelled by manipulation or illusion" (p. 30). O'Sullivan ponders at length what the matter is with marketing and speculates what a more critical, co-operative and philosophical approach might render. He concludes, quite justifiably, that arts marketing "may have to find a new way of understanding what marketing means in order to be ethically consistent with its own aims" (ibid., p. 39). An example of what this new approach might look like, O'Sullivan suggests, is the potential for arts marketing to counteract marketing's inherent "distributive injustice" (Hansen 1981)—the strategic targeting of only the most attractive market segments—a practice that can only be judged as both unethical and antithetical for a public (and publicly funded) good.

Like Hirschman and O'Sullivan, Belfiore and Bennett (2008) also highlight the gap between the creative drivers of artists and the consumer demand that fuels the traditional marketing concept. This rejection of the utilitarian marketing ethos reflects the Marxist argument that consumption both implies and effects commodification (Blau 1990, p. 323). Following this line of argument, if arts marketing fell into the "broadening" trap and became too consumer-driven, it would defeat its own *raison d'être* and destroy the very uniqueness that makes the arts marketable in the first place. This paradox is what Debord (1992) might have referred to as "commodity logic". Many other scholars have highlighted the dangers of conflating cultural and market values, a phenomenon of course which Adorno (1991) blamed for cultural commodification and marketing's deliberate attempt to cynically manipulate the masses. Unlike commodities, the performing arts are holistic and often unknown before they are performed in front of a live audience, dealing in novelty and symbolic value (O'Connor 2008, p. 65).

This symbolic value is one of the core distinguishing features of the performing arts and it places them well beyond the neo-liberal realm of market values, which are driven by mass consumption. The underlying rationale for the assignment of symbolic value to the performing arts is their provenance in primal and tribal behaviour. Walter Benjamin (1970), for example, reminds us that artistic objects find their origins in rites, rituals, and cults, and he laments the lack of "aura" that they are granted in contemporary society—not least, perhaps, as a direct result of marketing, which conspires to reduce them to the level of any other sellable product. In tracing the "homology" between ritual and performance, Victor Turner (1982) also makes an implicit case for the exceptionalism of the performing arts, characterising the phenomenon of what he designates "dramatic time" as aroused, heightened, emotional, playful and liminal. From Benjamin and Turner's perspective, the performing arts are therefore deeply *sociological*; they exist as manifestations of human expression and understanding, rather than as marketable products.

Similarly nostalgic for the era of social ritual, Barbara Ehrenreich (2007) laments how in much of the Western world human beings have forgotten how to perform and listen together and instead chosen to wall themselves up in "a fortress of ego and rationality" (p. 9). In her extended call for collective artistic expression, Ehrenreich illustrates the supreme ability of the arts to generate "the ritually induced passion or ecstasy that cements social bonds" (pp. 2–3) and urges humankind to renew the bonds that hold its communities together (p. 10) and relocate its "ecstatic possibility" (p. 258). These calls to re-acknowledge and reassert that symbolic and ritual value of the arts reflect the Situationist tenet that art should reposition itself away from representation and "having" and instead move back towards "being" through dialogue and community relations (Debord 1992). Considering the reinvigorated calls in cultural policy circles for more diversity and participation in the arts alongside a more everyday approach to creative practice, this Situationism seems to mark the general direction of travel.

In this section alone, we have seen how artistic events have been characterised over recent years by theorists as symbolic, intangible, meritorious, prestigious, experiential, aesthetic, autotelic, multisensory, hedonic, abstract, subjective, non-utilitarian, unknown, unique, holistic, emotional, playful, liminal, ritualistic, dialogic, and communitarian. Bearing this complex range of epithets in mind, it seems fitting to adopt a more sociological approach to arts marketing by rejecting the reification of the arts altogether and reconceiving artistic events as extraordinary sociological experiences (Carù and Cova 2003) rather than reducible products. This rejection of product-based marketing implies a significant reconceptualisation of the entire marketing mix—an implication which is being championed in the course of this chapter.

The performing arts have been an itinerant art form ever since the days of the troubadours. Whilst touring has always been a mainstay of the performing arts, in recent years there has been a migration away from traditional performance spaces; and the rising trend of site-specific and site-responsive performance has seen performances emerge in a vast array of weird and wonderful spaces, from hotel rooms and tower blocks to swimming pools and ferries. In the UK, this trend has even led to new business models such as the national touring company model adopted by National Theatre of Scotland and National Theatre Wales and the commercial, site-responsive model adopted by Punchdrunk. This development has gradually refocused the attention of theatre-makers from places to spaces, which again challenges the relevance and suitability of the marketing mix in the context of the performing arts.

FROM MARKETING TO ENGAGEMENT

Very few scholars have ever assessed the state of arts marketing itself (Fillis 2011, p. 11). However, back in 1969 Levy and Kotler "took stock" of their field and pondered what might lie beyond marketing, which itself, they claimed, had supplanted sales and bartering (see Fig. 6.1). They suggested that "furthering" might be a more acceptable term for the marketing activities of non-profit organisations. Since then, we have of course

Fig. 6.1 Beyond marketing (Adapted from Levy and Kotler [1969, p. 68])

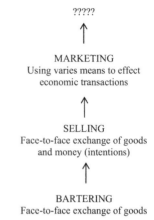

?????

↑

MARKETING
Using varies means to effect
economic transactions

↑

SELLING
Face-to-face exchange of goods
and money (intentions)

↑

BARTERING
Face-to-face exchange of goods

witnessed the so-called "participatory turn" (Ito 2007), which suggests, if not demands, a more collective and collaborative approach to "furthering" from inside and outside of a given organisation. In the context of the performing arts, the past few decades have also witnessed a strong focus on audience development, partly driven by the new public sector management demand for quantifiable evidence of social impact (O'Brien 2010). So there are significant sociological and political drivers that have encouraged (some might say forced) arts organisations to connect more closely and instrumentally with their audiences. But there are also strong artistic and technological drivers, such as co-creation (see Chapter 7) and digital marketing (Chapter 8), which have enabled the performing arts sector to engage on a creative level with audiences, both individually and collectively and both within and beyond the confines of a core artistic programme and venue.

Given the semantic and philosophical shift evident both in theory and in practice away from the language of product consumption towards a more relational engagement with an artistic experience, I would like to propose in this chapter that the concept of "marketing" is no longer the overarching activity that connects audiences to performing artists and their respective organisations. This thesis is based not only on the theories and insights explored thus far in the chapter; it is grounded in a comprehensive content analysis of peer-reviewed journal articles over the decade from 2007–2016, which revealed that over this ten-year period 3689 articles were published which contained the words "arts" and "engagement" in their abstracts, compared with only 1287 containing both "arts" and "marketing" (Walmsley 2019). This suggests that almost three times as many articles over this era focussed on notions of arts engagement as opposed to arts marketing.

This finding appears even more significant when compared with the analysis of the two previous decades: whereas in the era 1987–1996 (which roughly covers Rentschler's Professionalization Period) there were significantly more articles dedicated to arts marketing than to arts engagement, by the following decade this situation had been reversed, with almost 200 more articles mentioning "engagement" in their abstracts than "marketing" (see Table 6.1). The exponential growth in articles on "audience engagement" between 1997 and 2016 is also striking in the analysis, as is the sharp (if nascent) spike in articles published post-2006 mentioning "audience enrichment" in their abstracts. The overall growth in publications in the field is also worthy of note.

This does not mean, of course, that marketing activities no longer play a vital role in performing arts organisations: just as arts marketing should inform and support sales activity, engagement must support and complement marketing activity. But what I'm arguing here is that the ultimate strategic and artistic goal should be engagement rather than marketing. Indeed this content analysis appears to confirm Rentschler's hypothesis that towards the end of the last century we were on the cusp of a new era which "rediscovered" arts marketing as relational and collaborative. This "Rediscovery Period" (Rentschler 1998) witnessed a significant tipping point in arts management scholarship, as scholars for the first time gave priority to questions of engagement over notions of marketing. Figure 6.2 visually illustrates this tipping point and again highlights the growing dominance of the semantics of engagement over marketing.

Although the marketing literature has demonstrably witnessed an exponential rise in the deployment of the term "engagement" since 2006, as we saw in Chapter 1, very few authors have ever attempted to define or nuance

Table 6.1 Key abstract terms (1987–2016)

Decade	Arts + marketing	Arts + engagement	Arts + audience engagement	Arts + audience enrichment
1987–1996	193	111	9	1
1997–2006	595	790	38	1
2007–2016	1287	3689	309	7

No. of articles

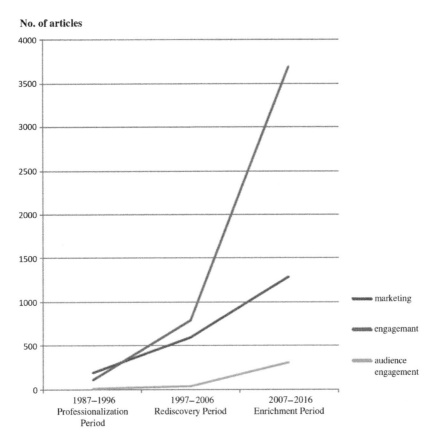

Fig. 6.2 Development of key abstract terms from 1987–2016 (Walmsley 2019)

the concept. Unlike marketing, then, the concept remains problematically under-theorised and under-developed. As noted in Chapter 1, Brodie et al. (2011) trace the theoretical development of engagement back to relationship marketing's focus on interactive experience and value co-creation in contrast to the more transactional relationships fostered by traditional marketing encounters. This supports Rentschler's thesis that in the Twenty-First Century, marketing has been "rediscovered" as more relational, as well as Radbourne's (2013) call for a more "converged" marketing paradigm. It also echoes the definitional discussion of engagement at the start of the book, where we saw how theoretical definitions cohere around perceptions

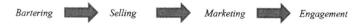

Bartering ➡ *Selling* ➡ *Marketing* ➡ *Engagement*

Fig. 6.3   The Consumer Exchange Model

of engagement as a psychological process that pursues intimate, meaningful and enduring relationships. In the performing arts, this is often achieved by involving audiences in interactive and co-creative experiences. So, to complete Levy and Kotler's conceptual model, the development of consumer exchange might look something like this (Fig. 6.3).

This shift perhaps mirrors the development of the wider economy from the services economy of the late Twentieth Century to the experience economy of the new millennium (Pine and Gilmore 1999). Since the turn of the millennium, scholars such as Bill Sharpe (2010) have started to argue that experiences per se are no longer sufficient for the post-postmodern consumer who is actually seeking a particular kind of experience (or engagement)—namely one which is shared, meaningful, valuable and lasting. In the context of the arts, Sharpe's thesis is essentially that art acts as the currency in this new economy of meaning, "the currency of experience, putting our unique individual experiences into motion amongst us as shared meaning" (p. 2). Table 6.2 illustrates the implications of an economy of meaning for traditional modes of production and consumption.

Table 6.2   Economic distinctions

Economy	Agrarian	Industrial	Service	Experience	Meaning
Economic offering	Commodities	Goods	Services	Experiences	Engagement opportunities
Economic function	Extract	Make	Deliver	Stage	(Co-)produce
Nature of offering	Fungible	Tangible	Intangible	Memorable	Meaningful
Key attribute	Natural	Standardised	Customised	Personal	Interpersonal
Seller	Trader	Manufacturer	Provider	Stager	(Co-)creator
Buyer	Market	User	Client	Guest	Co-creator
Factors of demand	Characteristics	Features	Benefits	Sensations	Value

Adapted from Pine and Gilmore (1999, p. 6)

The terms that populate this table illustrate the different expectations demanded of organisations by consumers in the experience economy. Notable developments from services to experiences include a focus on the personal, an expansion of distribution from short-term to long-term and a shift in demand from benefits to sensations. The implications of this semantic shift are far-reaching, and they highlight the need for today's organisations to create long-term, personal relationships with their "guests" by appealing to their senses and creating a sense of occasion. In turn, the shift from an experience economy to an economy of meaning implies an organisational responsibility to *engage* audiences on an interpersonal level to produce, or sometimes co-produce, memorable, meaningful, and "extraordinary" experiences (Carù and Cova 2003) and to co-create value from these experiences (see Chapter 7). This interpretation of the relational responsibilities and capabilities of arts organisations chimes closely with Dave Hesmondhalgh's definition of the wider cultural industries as those which "are most directly involved in the production of meaning" (2013, p. 16). This definition is based on Raymond Williams's (1981) understanding of culture as "a signifying system through which [...] a social order is communicated, reproduced, experienced and explored" (p. 13). So we can appreciate here that the notion of arts and cultural organisations as meaning-makers and producers of experience is actually nothing particularly new.

Pine and Gilmore highlight the need to enrich the consumer experience, evoking the concept of what they label the "sweet spot" to denote the holy grail of the experiential product, the "distinctive place" where the realms of aesthetics, escapism, education and entertainment overlap (1999, p. 43). In this ideal experience, the consumer is fully immersed and becomes an active participant. Significantly for this book, Pine and Gilmore use theatre as an exemplar for the staged experiences demanded by consumers (and therefore required of businesses) in the new economy. It follows, then, that the performing arts are ideally placed to excel in the experience economy. According to some commentators, this is essentially because the industry has always functioned in a constant state of creative flux: "Having thrived as a permanent 'industry' with inherently temporary arrangements, in a dynamic, multicultural and project-oriented environment, the arts context is the epitome of organisation for the 'new economy'" (Butler 2000, p. 343). The performing arts have always been in the business of producing experiences. The challenge for the sector now is to flourish in the economy of meaning, and it can only achieve this by developing meaningful modes of engagement with its audiences which in turn will engender intimate, enduring relationships of mutual value. Such is the ultimate goal of engagement.

Towards the beginning of the chapter, we saw how arts marketing has traditionally been conceptualised around a profit-centred marketing mix focussing on elements of product, price, place, and promotion. In the course of the chapter, we have seen how scholarship has shifted, in line with artistic practice and consumer demand, away from a transactional approach towards a relational philosophy, influenced by services marketing and then relationship marketing. The extent of this shift, evidenced in theory and in professional practice, and demonstrated empirically through the content analysis of peer-reviewed journal articles, constitutes nothing short of a paradigm shift in arts marketing, and arguably in marketing more generally.

If we agree that it is more appropriate to refer to the performing arts as an "experience" rather than a "product"; that "environment" is a more appropriate term than "place" to describe the aesthetic, physical, and ethical context of this experience; that "exchange" conveys the intimate, collaborative, and mutually valuable relationships inherent to the performing arts more effectively than "price"; and that "engagement" captures the more holistic and relational approach to relationship building more accurately than the reductive and transactional notion of "promotion", then we must accept the need to fundamentally reconfigure and reconceptualise the marketing mix. So I'd like to argue here that a reconceptualised marketing mix fit for the mid Twenty-First century would instead be based around 4E's: experience, exchange, environment, and engagement.

A Paradigm Shift from Consumption to Enrichment

Kuhn defines a paradigm as a fundamental set of assumptions shared by members of a scientific community (1970, cited in Lovelock and Gummesson 2004, p. 21). As Lovelock and Gummerson remind us, paradigms exist merely as "temporary postulates" whose conceptual validity "must always be open to challenge" (ibid.). This chapter has challenged the conceptual validity of the marketing paradigm. It has traced the development of production and consumption from goods and services through to experiences and engagement opportunities. In order to justify my claim that the underlying assumptions of arts marketing are no longer conceptually valid, I now want to go one step further and attempt to outline a fundamental set of assumptions surrounding audience enrichment, around which I hope the arts marketing community will cohere.

As discussed earlier in the chapter, the impact of macro factors such as increasing social participation and the development of interactive digital communications technologies has been so significant over the past few decades that the set of assumptions that led to the advent of arts marketing now lies in tatters. Younger generations are increasingly alienated by traditional approaches to marketing and twenty-first-century arts audiences are yearning for more meaningful modes of engagement; and we have seen already in this chapter that the service economy and even the experience economy have now had their day in the limelight. The new economy of meaning is characterised by participatory modes of engagement, both within the arts and beyond them. And the ultimate goal of this engagement is enrichment.

Enrichment is a complex concept, but it implies some kind of personal transformation, some aspiration to become a better person. In the context of the arts, this might imply some kind of creative or aesthetic development. If we recall the existing audience research into motivations for attending the performing arts (e.g. Bergadaà and Nyeck 1995; Walmsley 2011), it might equally imply an emotional, interpersonal, social or even spiritual development. And if we believe in a mission-based approach to strategic management, then the fact that many arts organisations claim to transform their audiences' lives suggests that their ultimate goal too should be one of enrichment.

The concept of "audience enrichment" is now prevalent in American arts organisations, where it is not uncommon to see "audience enrichment programs". We saw earlier in the chapter how the concept is rapidly gaining traction in the academic literature too (see Table 6.1). I would infer from this that we are going to witness a cross-pollination of enrichment into the vocabulary and everyday practice of arts engagement across the Western world, just as we have seen the exponential rise of engagement itself. Enrichment is then perhaps the next destination of arts marketing.

According to Lynne Conner (2004, n.p.), audience enrichment suggests a shift in power dynamics from the traditional producers of art to audiences.

> A viable philosophy and practice of audience enrichment is centered on the assumption that what an audience really wants is the opportunity to co-author the arts experience. They don't want to be told what the art means. They want the opportunity to participate — in an intelligent and responsible way — in telling its meaning. They want to have a real forum (or several forums) for the interplay of ideas, experience, data, and feeling that makes up the arts experience.

As Conner points out, the underlying power struggle here is about ownership of the meaning of the arts. This is interesting in light of my earlier contestation that services offer no transfer of ownership whatsoever. So enrichment involves empowerment and co-ownership. It gives audiences a voice, a say in what happens and a voice in the decoding process. In recent decades, much of the marketing focus in the performing arts has fallen on audience development and on maximising ticket sales. There are of course sound ethical, policy and business reasons to support this focus, despite the uncomfortable reality that audiences have remained stubbornly un-diverse. But it makes little strategic sense not to invest in the experiences of core audiences, because this is ultimately the key to long-term organisational sustainability.

CONCLUSION

The performing arts raise many challenges for arts professionals and scholars working in and around the field of arts marketing. I have argued in this chapter that the performing arts are so exceptional, so fundamentally different from the tangible products and ephemeral services of profit-based industries, that ultimately they challenge the very concept of marketing itself. This demands a reconceptualisation of the field and there is increasing evidence that arts organisations and scholars are responding to the new audience context and abandoning marketing in favour of engagement. This constitutes nothing less than a paradigm shift.

I have suggested here that a "4E" model might provide a more fitting conceptualization for this new paradigm, because it encapsulates the co-constructed, experiential, intimate value-based relationships that arts organisations are increasingly developing with their audiences. An engagement-based concept responds to this paradigm much more accurately and appropriately than the traditional marketing approach. We have seen in the course of this chapter that the ultimate goal of this engagement-based strategy in this new economy of meaning is *enrichment*. In the following chapter, we will see how the rising phenomenon of co-creation is enriching all parties in the triadic relationship that exists in the performing arts between artists, organisations, and audiences.

REFERENCES

Adorno, T. 1991. *The culture industry: Selected essays on mass culture.* London, Routledge.

Belfiore, E. and Bennett, O. 2008. *The social impact of the arts: An intellectual history.* Basingstoke, Palgrave Macmillan.

Benjamin, W. 1970. *Illuminations: Essays and reflections.* London, Fontana.

Bergadaà, M. and Nyeck, S. 1995. Quel marketing pour les activités artistiques: une analyse qualitative comparée des motivations des consommateurs et producteurs de théâtre. *Recherche et Applications en Marketing,* 10(4), pp. 27–46.

Bernstein, J. S. 2006. *Arts marketing insights: The dynamics of building and retaining performing arts audience.* San Francisco, Wiley.

Blau, H. 1990. *The audience.* Baltimore, The John Hopkins University Press.

Booms, B. H. and Bitner, M. J. 1981. Marketing strategies and organization structures for service firms. In: Donnelly, J. H. and George, W. R. (eds.) *Marketing of services.* Chicago, IL, American Marketing Association, pp. 47–51.

Brodie, R. J., Hollebeek, L. D., Juric, B. and Ilic, A. 2011. Customer engagement: Conceptual domain, fundamental propositions, and implications for research. *Journal of Service Research,* 14(3), pp. 252–271.

Butler, P. D. 2000. By popular demand: Marketing the arts. *Journal of Marketing Management,* 16(4), pp. 343–364.

Carù, A. and Cova, B. 2003. Revisiting consumption experience: A more humble but complete view of the concept. *Marketing Theory,* 3, pp. 267–286.

Chong, D. 2010. *Arts management.* 2nd ed. London, Routledge.

Colbert, F. 2007. *Marketing culture and the arts.* 3rd ed. Montreal, HEC Montreal.

Colbert, F. and St-James, Y. 2014. Research in arts marketing: Evolution and future directions. *Psychology and Marketing,* 31(8), pp. 566–575.

Conner, L. 2004. Who gets to tell the meaning? Building audience enrichment. *GIA Reader* [Online], 15(1).

Constantinides, E. 2006. The marketing mix revisited: Towards the 21st century marketing. *Journal of Marketing Management,* 22(3–4), pp. 407–438.

Debord, G. 1992. *Society of the spectacle.* London, Rebel Press.

Dennis, N., Larsen, G. and Macaulay, M. 2011. Terraforming arts marketing. *Arts Marketing: An International Journal* 1(1), pp. 5–10.

Ehrenreich, B. 2007. *Dancing in the streets: A history of collective joy.* London, Granta.

Fillis, I. 2011. The evolution and development of arts marketing research. *Arts Marketing: An International Journal*, 1(1), pp. 11–25.

Fisk, R. P., Brown, S. W. and Bitner, M. J. 1993. Tracking the evolution of the services marketing literature. *Journal of Retailing*, 69(1), pp. 61–103.

Hadley, S. Forthcoming. *Audience development and cultural policy*. London, Palgrave Macmillan.

Hansen, F. 1981. Contemporary research in marketing in Denmark. *Journal of Marketing*, 45(3), pp. 214–218.

Hesmondhalgh, D. 2013. *The cultural industries*. 3rd ed. London, Sage.

Hill, L., O'Sullivan, C. and O'Sullivan, T. 2003. *Creative arts marketing*. 2nd ed. Oxford, Butterworth Heinemann.

Hirschman, E. C. 1983. Aesthetics, ideologies and the limits of the marketing concept. *Journal of Marketing*, 47(3), pp. 45–55.

Hirschman, E. C. and Holbrook, M. B. 1982. Hedonic consumption: Emerging concepts, methods and propositions. *Journal of Marketing*, 46(3), pp. 92–101.

Ito, M. 2007. Introduction. In: Varnelis, K. (ed.) *Networked publics*. London, MIT Press, pp. 1–14.

Khalil, E. L. 2000. Symbolic products: Prestige, pride and identity goods. *Theory and Decision*, 49(1), pp. 53–77.

Kotler, P. and Armstrong, G. 2010. *Principles of marketing*. 13th ed. Upper Saddle River, NJ, Prentice Hall.

Levitt, T. 1981. Marketing intangible products and product intangibles. *Harvard Business Review*, 59, pp. 94–102.

Levy, S. J. and Kotler, P. 1969. Beyond marketing: The furthering concept. *California Management Review*, 12(2), pp. 67–73.

Lovelock, C. and Gummesson, E. 2004. Whither services marketing? In search of a new paradigm and fresh perspectives. *Journal of Service Research*, 7(1), pp. 20–41.

Maher, J. K., Clark, J. and Motley, D. G. 2011. Measuring museum service quality in relationship to visitor membership: The case of a children's museum. *International Journal of Arts Management*, 13(2), pp. 29–42.

McCarthy, E. J. 1964. *Basic marketing: A managerial approach*. Homewood, IL, Richard D. Irwin.

Musgrave, R. A. and Musgrave, P. B. 1989. *Public finance in theory and practice*. 5th ed. New York, McGraw-Hill.

O'Brien, D. 2010. *Measuring the value of culture: A report to the Department for Culture Media and Sport*. London, Department for Culture Media and Sport.

O'Connor, J. 2008. *The cultural and creative industries: A literature review*. 2nd ed. Newcastle-upon-Tyne, Creativity, Culture and Education.

O'Reilly, D. 2011. Mapping the arts marketing literature. *Arts Marketing: An International Journal*, 1(1), pp. 26–38.

O'Sullivan, T. 2013. Arts marketing and ethics: What you can and Kant do. In: O'Reilly, D., Rentschler, R. and Kirchner, T. A. (eds.) *The Routledge companion to arts marketing*. Abingdon, Routledge, pp. 29–47.

Pine, B. J. and Gilmore, J. H. 1999. *The experience economy: Work is theatre and every business a stage*. Boston, Harvard Business School.

Radbourne, J. 2013. Converging with audiences. In: Radbourne, J., Glow, H. and Johanson, K. (eds.) *The audience experience: A critical analysis of audiences in the performing arts*. Bristol, Intellect, pp. 143–158.

Rentschler, R. 1998. Museum and performing arts marketing: A climate of change. *Journal of Arts Management, Law, and Society*, 28(1), pp. 83–96.

Shapiro, B. P. 1973. Marketing for nonprofit organizations. *Harvard Business Review*, 51(5), pp. 123–132.

Sharpe, B. 2010. *Economies of life: Patterns of health and wealth*. Axminster, Triarchy Press.

Turner, V. 1982. *From ritual to theatre: The human seriousness of play*. New York, PAJ.

Walmsley, B. 2011. Why people go to the theatre: A qualitative study of audience motivation. *Journal of Customer Behaviour*, 10(4), pp. 335–351.

Walmsley, B. 2019. The death of arts marketing: A paradigm shift from consumption to enrichment. *Arts and the Market*, 9(1), pp. 32–49.

Williams, R. 1958. *Culture and society*. London, Chatto and Windus.

CHAPTER 7

Co-creating Art, Meaning, and Value

INTRODUCTION

In the previous chapter, we saw how arts professionals and scholars are turning away from traditional, transactional approaches to arts marketing and instead striving to understand how audiences can be engaged on a more relational level in their artistic encounters. Co-creative activities have now become an integral part of artistic experiences, as audiences engage and are engaged in cognitive, emotional, and imaginal practices to appropriate and make sense of cultural products and experiences (Caldwell 2001). Indeed marketing scholars have credited the co-creation of value between companies and consumers as the key process in what some of them refer to as "the new marketing logic"—a phenomenon they associate with "collaborative marketing" and "creative consumption" (Cova and Cova 2009, p. 88; Prahalad and Ramaswamy 2004b). However, as I argued in the last chapter, this new marketing logic is so profoundly different from the underlying paradigm of marketing that it is no longer really recognisable as marketing at all. The new paradigm governing the multidirectional relationships between art, artists, producers, arts organisations and audiences is based on a 4E model, which reflects the complementary aspects of enrichment: experience, exchange, environment, and engagement.

The aim of this chapter is to investigate why and how audiences' expectations and behaviours are changing and explore emerging theories, concepts and practices of co-creation, including active spectatorship, co-production,

© The Author(s) 2019

B. Walmsley, *Audience Engagement in the Performing Arts*,
New Directions in Cultural Policy Research,
https://doi.org/10.1007/978-3-030-26653-0_7

participation, play, interpretation and facilitation. The chapter will begin with a critical overview of co-creation and account for its definitional ambiguity. I will then review the drivers behind the emerging concepts of co-creation, situating them within wider sociological and technological contexts. Following a discussion of the political and related policy concerns that are shaping these phenomena, I will deconstruct the different components of co-creation and go on to argue that artists and arts organisations have a strategic, artistic and social responsibility to develop their audiences' co-creative skills, providing illustrations of how this can be achieved and discussing the potential impact. Finally, I will investigate how co-creation can be deployed to generate and extract meaning in a *collaborative* way, and how this, in turn, can effect a positive impact on audience engagement, providing a lifetime of value to audiences, artists and arts organisations, and establishing relationships and communities of interest based on a shared culture of artistic exchange.

What Is Co-creation?

It would be an understatement to contend that definitions of co-creation are divergent, ambiguous, shifting and contested. We have seen over the past few chapters of this book that many concepts pertaining to audience engagement lack any definitional coherence, and it has been acknowledged that the terminology surrounding arts participation in particular is in a problematic state of flux (Brown et al. 2011, p. 4). Thus far, scholars and practitioners have failed to cohere around a standard definition of what co-creation actually means or entails. Considering the rising popularity of co-creative practice, the lack of research into why audiences choose to engage with the arts in a more participatory way, and the value that they and others obtain from it, is both striking and inhibiting. However, it is perhaps of some comfort to learn that this lack of insight is not limited to the arts and culture: relatively little is known about how customers contribute to the co-creation of value in general (Payne et al. 2008). So one aim of this chapter is to close this epistemological gap through an extensive critical analysis of the various processes that comprise co-creation.

Grönroos (2011) forges a clear distinction between co-creation and co-production, arguing that the latter implies consumers participating in the production phases of the creative process whereas co-creation is linked to the creation of consumer value. There is some consensus about this demarcation in the literature, and personally, I find the separation between active involvement in the creative process and decoding or meaning-making activities a useful one: these are clearly two different modes of audience engagement that are likely to appeal to different kinds of participant at different phases of the production cycle. However, most scholars take a broader view of co-creation, perhaps because "co-production" has connotations of professional (B2B) collaborations, especially in the performing arts. For example, based on research with over 100 organisations actively engaged in participatory arts, Brown et al. (2011) define co-creation as an activity where audience members "contribute something to an artistic experience curated by a professional artist" (p. 15). This definition echoes Govier's description of co-creation as a "collaborative journey" that producers embark on with audiences in an attempt to create something new together (2009, p. 3). Govier's focus on novelty is replicated by Ind et al. (2012), for whom co-creation "suggests the interaction of individuals within a framework to evolve, re-define or invent something that is new" (p. 7). So for many scholars, co-creation implies a form of pro-am (B2C) collaboration deployed for the purpose of creative innovation.

However, it is important to acknowledge that co-creation does not always culminate in something *new*, and Charles Leadbeater's more generic depiction of co-creation as "the art of with" (2009, p. 5) provides a welcome alternative to what we might disparagingly refer to as the "novelty fetishism" prioritised in many accounts of co-creation and in the creative process (or even the creative industries) more broadly (Tanggaard 2014). Leadbeater goes on to elaborate his vision of this culture of *with*, highlighting the surprising irony evident in the lack of genuine engagement opportunities on offer even in a sector that has traditionally resisted the neo-liberal politics of consumption and commodification.

> The arts, and the modern avant garde in particular, has stood in opposition to this commodified, regimented world of *to* and *for*. The arts offer a space for contemplation and reflection, challenge and controversy, higher meanings and deeper purpose. Yet in its way the modern art world and modern arts institutions embody the principles of *to* and *for* just as powerfully as the modern factory or school. (Leadbeater 2009, p. 3)

Leadbeater's charge reflects the transactional and product-led approach to marketing the arts that I critiqued in the previous chapter, and it again highlights the urgent need to delineate new, more authentic modes of audience engagement. This broader, more democratic and open conception is also espoused by Hannah Rudman, who champions co-creation as "a new form of 'organizational porosity' – a mindset that allows for a free exchange of creative energy between an arts organization and its public" (as cited in Brown et al. 2011, p. 18). Rudman's definition is significant here, as it emphasises the need for a holistic organisational approach to co-creation; this is not a discreet area of activity that can happen "under the radar" or be "siloed off" into the bell jar of a particular department or project.

It is often assumed within both the academy and the professional arts sector that co-creation is a relatively new trend, but Claire Bishop reminds us that there is nothing fundamentally novel about it. Indeed Bishop argues that the arts enjoy a long tradition of participation and what she refers to as "activated spectatorship" (2004, p. 78). Citing the participatory qualities of 1920s German theatre, social sculpture, and performance art, Bishop rightly notes that a relational approach to art requires above all a critical assessment of its democratic or emancipatory outcomes.

> The tasks facing us today are to analyze *how* contemporary art addresses the viewer and to assess the *quality* of the audience relations it produces: the subject position that any work presupposes and the democratic notions it upholds, and how these are manifested in our experience of the work. (ibid., p. 78, original italics)

In other words, the true value of art resides in the responses that it triggers; and what matters, therefore, is the *quality* rather than the facticity of audience engagement. This focus on the quality of audience engagement is particularly important in light of John Knell's charge that "issues such as the *quality* of public engagement in cultural activities, and how innovation might recast public engagement, have been left unexamined" (2004, p. 4, original italics). These are important considerations that address the sociocultural functions of art explored in Chapter 4.

Another notable trend in the literature on co-creation is the argument that markets in general are shifting away from a company-centric model to a "forum-based" dynamic, where value is co-created "at multiple points of interaction" as consumers subject processes of value creation to scrutiny, analysis, and evaluation (Prahalad and Ramaswamy 2004a, pp. 6, 13). The metaphor of the market as a forum is an apt and productive one in the context of the performing arts, as it echoes Augusto Boal's Forum Theatre where as many "spect-actors" as possible were encouraged to "intervene directly on stage as part of the investigation of an oppressive social situation" (Dwyer 2004, p. 199). Like Bishop, Bourriaud, Debord and Leadbeater, Boal was interested in the political and emancipatory potential of collective artistic endeavour, in his case by producing theatre *with* audiences to liberate them from oppression. The very fact that we are striving here to consider the performing arts as a forum highlights how far we have travelled away from the social rituals of Ancient Greece, and even Shakespeare's Globe, where the performing arts really did function as a social forum, towards the consumption-based business of today's competitive leisure and entertainment markets.

Seemingly influenced by this consumption-based approach, Miranda Boorsma offers a fundamentally different perspective on co-creation, arguing that co-creation should be limited to the consumption phase of the artistic experience, where audiences strive to make sense of a work of art.

> A certain level of artistic freedom on the part of the artist is a necessary condition. The art consumer should not be actively involved before the artistic idea has developed its form. After that, however, the art consumer's role becomes crucial. Arts consumers play a central role as co-producers in the final stage of the art process by giving meaning to the artefact by means of their imaginative powers. (Boorsma 2006, p. 85)

This is a controversial standpoint, which presupposes the existence of an artistic elite that is uniquely capable of producing artistic works of original value. Boorsma justifies her rejection of co-production (to deploy Grönroos's binary distinction) by claiming that including audiences in product design and development will not only compromise artistic freedom but "lead to the production of safe, consumer-oriented arts products which, in the end, may not be what the audience either wants or needs" (Caust 2003, p. 58, cited in Boorsma 2006, p. 74). Boorsma warns that this "businesslike approach" constitutes the "arts marketing pitfall" (ibid.)—in other words, that when the traditional product-led approach to arts marketing is abandoned, artistic freedom, quality, and value is compromised. This represents an interestingly conservative view for a scholar who generally champions a relational perspective of art, and it is reminiscent of Andrew Keen's (2008) fulmination against the so-called "cult of the amateur", which, he argues, is blurring the distinction between trained experts and uninformed amateurs to the detriment of quality and truth.

These elitist arguments are challenged by many cultural producers, policymakers and scholars, who either question the objectivity of artistic quality or define it in much broader terms. A good example of the latter camp is Brian McMaster, the former Director of the Edinburgh International Festival, who contends that "excellence in culture occurs when an experience affects and changes an individual" (2008, p. 9). Another important challenge to Caust, Boorsma and Keen's position is provided by Leila Jancovich (2017), whose empirical study of audience participation contests the assumption that non-professional participants make safe, poor quality work. So let's proceed here on the basis that artistic quality and "excellence" are subjective, contested and experiential; art is not based (and therefore should not be judged) on technical merit alone but also on its transformational impact; and this impact can occur in myriad ways, modes and forms that are not always product- or producer-led.

Ultimately, we must accept that co-creation is likely to remain an ambiguous umbrella term for any number of participatory processes and practices that open up any part of the creative process to audiences and the wider public. The main problem with this is that the discussion and planning of co-creative practice tends to be dominated by attempts to engage audiences in the production phases of a project (despite Boorsma's appeal) at the expense of the decoding phases, where meaning is elaborated collectively. Co-creation is therefore adopted or rejected as a concept by many scholars and practitioners on narrow, partial or unclear terms. However, despite the ambiguities and tensions in the academic literature, the sparse definitions provided by scholars working in this small field do coalesce around a number of key ideas: collaboration, interaction, participation, invention, value, meaning, and exchange. These notions will be explored further in the following sections of the chapter, once we have explored their provenance.

Drivers of Co-creation

As discussed in the previous chapter and earlier in this chapter, the performing arts have traditionally functioned on a product-led model (Colbert 2007) designed to promote productions to predisposed audiences in order to entertain, challenge and/or educate them. However, we have also seen how audiences are starting to take back control and find or forge their way into artistic processes, particularly thanks to processes of co-creation. There are a number of factors and traditions that have driven this quiet revolution.

The renaissance of community and amateur arts is certainly one factor that is starting to impinge on the professional performing arts sector. In many Western countries, including the UK, the USA, and the Netherlands, this growth was spurred not only by the community arts movement of the 1970s and 1980s but also by the proliferation of outreach and education activity spearheaded by pioneering arts and cultural organisations and supported by sporadic policy initiatives. A prime example of this is Arts Council England's recent *Creative People and Places* programme. It could justifiably be argued that these movements and initiatives find their origins in cultural democracy—a tradition which encompasses three interrelated ideas:

1. Many cultural traditions co-exist in society and none of them should be allowed to dominate and become an 'official culture';
2. Everyone should be free to participate in cultural life;
3. Cultural life should be subject to democratic decision-making and control. (Goldbard and Adams 1990)

As well as influencing arts education and participation, cultural democracy has also influenced theories of creativity and cultural production. In essence, there has been a growing consensus that creativity is now a collective phenomenon rather than a special gift embodied in lone artists. As Csikszentmihalyi articulates it: "What we call creativity is a phenomenon that is constructed through an interaction between producers and audiences. Creativity is not the product of single individuals, but of social systems" (Csikszentmihalyi, cited in Pope 2005, p. 67). This collective perception of creativity has been embraced by a growing number of marketing scholars, including Terry O'Sullivan (2009), who describes audiences as "communities of consumption" or "consumities", and Chris Bilton, who notes that "cultural products are increasingly 'social' products, whose meaning and value is rewritten by audiences" (2017, p. 15). Whilst we might challenge the neo-liberal reduction of audience to the "consumption" of a "product" in these two citations, this relational perspective implies that art, which is perhaps the quintessential "cultural product", has no meaning in and of itself; it only derives meaning when it is experienced by an audience. This explains why Rancière (2011) is right to argue that audiences must be emancipated and that spectatorship can function as an aesthetic and political act. As we saw in Chapter 3, engaged audience members are active agents in an embodied, enactive and multisensory experience, and collectively, this act of audiency culminates in a powerful social phenomenon.

This focus on the active and collective experience of audiences is also a key characteristic of relational aesthetics. In his formative work in this emerging field Nicolas Bourriaud (2002) proposed that artistic practice and criticism should shift its focus away from the primacy of the artistic artefact or performance and embrace instead the discursive characteristics that engagement with art can produce. Influenced by Guy Debord (1992), who perceived the primary role of art as to stimulate dialogue and develop community relations, Bourriaud is interested in how art can *transform* the aesthetic project from an *object* into an *encounter* and, in so doing, unite artists and audiences in a common aesthetic endeavour. Relational art, he maintains, offers "spaces where we can elaborate alternative forms of sociability, critical models and moments of constructed conviviality" (Bourriaud 2006, p. 166). Bourriaud's ideas on relational art are regularly echoed in audience members' accounts of their performing arts experiences, as typified by one of Caroline Heim's (2016) participants who maintained: "You use the play as another avenue of communication". Grant Kester (2005) also notes the shift in contemporary art towards a more dialogical and socially engaged approach.

As we saw in the previous chapter, the insights offered by relational aesthetics are significant in that they attempt to move beyond the artistic product and beyond the traditional producer–consumer divide: they reflect the concerns of audience engagement and help to circumnavigate the passive and transactional relationships with audiences that are usually generated by marketing. Accordingly, Boorsma and Chiaravalotti (2010) maintain that arts marketing has evolved away from a functional approach towards a more relational view, which recognises artistic consumption as *experiential*. This, they contend, is serving to highlight the role of audiences in the creation and reception of art.

Perhaps in response to these and other calls for emancipation, over the past few decades artists and producers have gradually begun to open up their creative processes. This evolution has been fuelled by changing audience behaviours and expectations and by the dialogic opportunities offered by Web 2.0, social media and digital communications technologies (see Chapter 8). Arvidsson (2008) goes so far as to claim that the progressive inclusion of consumers in the creation of value represents one of the most significant trends in contemporary society. This kind of assessment of active consumer engagement has now become a trope, if not indeed a truism, which acknowledges the defining features of a postmodern audience that engages in "active and expressive ways" to form a culture of "making-and-doing" (Brown et al. 2011, p. 4). Arvidsson links this trend with an oversupply of knowledge workers who have learnt to seek out self-expression and self-realisation through social production, whilst Payne et al. (2008) identify three concrete factors behind this shift: technological breakthroughs; changes in industry logics; and changes in customer preferences and lifestyles. In the performing arts, these factors are manifest in developments like live streaming or simulcasting, which has spurred initiatives such as *NT Live* and National Theatre of Scotland's *5-Minute Theatre* (see Chapter 8).

Despite these sociological drivers of change, involving audiences in creative processes remains a highly controversial proposition. Many artists, writers, composers, directors, choreographers, and producers still fervently believe in the product-led model (albeit tacitly) and actively protect the freedom and independence of the artist. However, an increasing number of arts professionals advocate an "audience-focussed" approach, which appears to represent a hybrid model between the product-led and audience-led models. An audience-focussed approach to artistic development might involve marketing, engagement and education/outreach staff being involved in programming discussions and decisions, so that artistic decision-making contains an inherent audience focus. In other words, in an audience-focussed model, art is commissioned, produced, curated, presented and marketed with audiences very much in mind, albeit as passive stakeholder in the process. In an "audience-led" approach, audiences would have an active role in artistic decision-making and indeed in the strategic development of the organisation. Audiences might be represented on the board of directors and even have a say in the appraisal and recruitment of the leadership team. This book advocates for an "audience-centred" approach, wherein audiences are the primary stakeholders of the organisation, constituting its core focus and representing its very *raison d'être*. Audience-centred organisations are artistically led but empower audiences with a genuine artistic and strategic voice. Such organisations actively seek out opportunities for authentic co-creation but they retain the ultimate artistic vision and decision-making capabilities; they know when to stop engaging and *act*.

Another core driver of co-creation, particularly in the UK, the USA, Canada, and Australia, has been the concept of audience development. Audience development is yet another ambiguous and contested term, which was heavily influenced amongst cultural policymakers by notions of cultural democracy and which now covers a multitude of strategic activities ranging from audience recruitment and diversification to audience engagement and enrichment. The term has been helpfully and broadly defined as an ethos that "places the audience at the heart of everything the organisation does" (Arts Council England 2010). This aspirational definition reflects the audience-centred approach discussed earlier, and it is therefore the definition that reflects most closely the aims of audience engagement and thus the underlying philosophy of this book. A fuller definition of audience development, which highlights aspects of engagement and education, is offered by the international cultural strategy and research agency, Morris Hargreaves McIntyre:

> Audience development is a continual, actively managed process in which an organisation encourages each attender and potential attender to develop confidence, knowledge, experience and engagement across the full breadth of the art form to meet his or her full potential, whilst meeting the organisation's own artistic, social and financial objectives. (cited in European Commission 2015)

This is the quintessential depiction of the audience-centred organisation.

We can see from this analysis that co-creation is the product of a number of interrelated concepts, movements, and developments from both within the arts and cultural sector and from society at large. These include the community arts movement, cultural democracy, collective consumption, the emancipation of audiences, relational aesthetics, the rapid evolution of digital communications technologies, and audience development. In essence, co-creation represents a broadening perspective of creative production from the individual to the collective and a socially led reconceptualisation of creative consumption, alongside a democratisation of the ownership of their related processes. Co-creation remains contested and controversial and it is still in a state of flux and evolution, both within the academy and within the arts and cultural sector itself.

WHO IS CO-CREATION *FOR?*

Remarkably little research has been conducted into the marketing of co-creation or co-created work, so there remains a significant gap in knowledge regarding the potential target markets for and beneficiaries of this kind of activity. However, there is evidence that audience members with a professional or academic background in a given art form are not just more likely to attend artistic performances, but also to prepare in advance and report higher levels of anticipation and ultimate impact (Brown et al. 2011). There is also emerging evidence that although new audiences are potentially the biggest beneficiaries of co-creation, benefitting from the contextual insights and empathy with artists that co-creative activity can confer (Walmsley 2016), these participants can often feel anxious, insecure, alienated, conspicuous, incongruent or out of place (Walmsley 2013). Indeed my previous empirical research into co-creation revealed a tendency from some artists and producers to design co-creative activity specifically for highly engaged audience members, in effect "handpicking" participants for essentially "private" events (ibid., p. 113). This trend of course risks developing a solipsistic culture of "inter-legitimation" (Bourdieu 1984), which could merely alienate new audience members and reinforce existing perceptions of elitism. The issue of the openness of co-creative activity has significant repercussions on both policy and practice, because "finding better ways to engage with the public is necessary, not only to increase the legitimacy of decision-making but also to ensure that artistic practice is less self-referential" (Jancovich 2011, p. 279).

Questions of openness and empowerment are central to co-creative practice. As Whaley and Miller note, "the move to position audiences as partners seems to be informed by the anxiety around arts organisations losing cultural relevance. Implicit within this is the sense that it is within the gift of arts organisations to invite the audience in. It presupposes a them/us binary in which the power is held on one side" (Whalley and Miller 2017, p. 26). Decisions to co-create can, therefore, be cynical and self-interested, which can make them feel both tokenistic and inauthentic. Co-creation tends to be conceived by artists and producers and is often therefore framed by them to meet their own needs:

> Interactivity and immersion allow for more active involvement, leading to the language of co-creation, but always within a predetermined set of appropriate responses. In all these instances, and more besides, we seem to be surfacing

> the recognition that to be an audience continues to be a political act, one
> freighted with significant social and ideological implications. (Whalley and
> Miller 2017, p. 33)

So there is a live and urgent question about the extent to which co-creation
can offer opportunities for audience empowerment, autonomy and diversification. An obvious response to this question is that the potential impact of
a co-creative activity depends on its artistic intention and on the intended
beneficiary. This may sound obvious, but many (if not most) co-creative
projects are curated by professional artists and designed to enhance the
process or end product itself rather than offer a transformative audience
experience. If artists want to receive "expert" feedback, they may well pre-
fer to open up their creative process exclusively to peer artists and other
"desirable" customer groups (Payne and Frow 2005). Even if the process
is opened up, this is often to the artist's or producer's benefit, with audiences essentially crowdsourcing, imagineering or trialling artistic research
and development. A good example of this is The Royal Shakespeare Company's "R&D work in progress sharings", where audiences are invited into
The Other Place, the company's "creative engine room", to provide feedback on early iterations of productions such as *Matilda* (Royal Shakespeare
Company 2017).

As an audience researcher, I have observed and been actively involved in
a number of co-creative projects that have been designed by and for artists.
Whilst I am not arguing here that there is anything wrong with this per se,
there is a certain irony about a co-creative activity being designed primarily
with the artist in mind: as the RSC tacitly acknowledge, this approach is
more akin to traditional R&D. What I *would* argue is that the dominant
power dynamic noted by Whalley and Miller is indicative of and provides
further evidence for the underlying fear, suspicion, derision, and subjuga-
tion of audiences that was elaborated in Chapter 1. It is readily apparent
that artists and producers often underestimate the value and insight that
audiences can bring to both artistic development and sense-making. As we
have seen, it could and has been argued that a work of art has no significance
until an audience has enshrined it in meaning; and in the performing arts,
there is of course no performance at all without an audience (Freshwater
2009).

A telling example of a co-created activity geared exclusively towards
artists is the American choreographer Liz Lerman's Critical Response Process (CRP). CRP is a widely recognised and globally applied method that

nurtures the development of artistic works-in-progress through a four-step, facilitated dialogue between artists, peers, and audiences. CRP essentially helps artists to make the kind of work they want to make (Walmsley 2016). The role of the audience is to support the artist's creative process and artistic development by providing permission-based and highly structured constructive feedback. Again, and as with the RSC example above, there is nothing fundamentally wrong with this as a philosophy and creative approach; but CRP is limited in its audience appeal and engagement precisely because it is artist-led and artist-focussed. What is interesting is when the process is reconfigured into an audience-focussed process, designed to open up and contextualise artistic practices and develop empathy between audiences and artists. In the case study outlined in Chapter 8 (Respond), the positive impact of this shift in focus on non-attenders of a particularly alienating art form is profound. The simple lesson here is that genuine co-creation must be designed for both artists and audiences. Processes and activities that are both artist-led and artist-focussed are likely to alienate and intimidate all but a tiny minority of niche and culturally empowered audiences.

Brown and Ratzkin isolate six typologies of artistic engagement, the smallest and most deeply engaged of which, "active learners", are said to seek out "making and doing engagement opportunities that offer a way into the art" (2011, p. 24). Figure 7.1 displays Brown and Ratzkin's typologies according to participants' preferred style and mode of engagement. The framework provides a useful and workable psychographic segmentation model, and it highlights some of the most common forms and processes of co-creation, including critical review, talking, digital engagement and insight seeking.

Brown and Ratzkin rank these typologies on an engagement spectrum ranging from low appetite (= 1) to high appetite (= 6), as follows:

1. Readers
2. Critical reviewers
3. Casual talkers
4. Technology-based processors
5. Insights seekers
6. Active learners

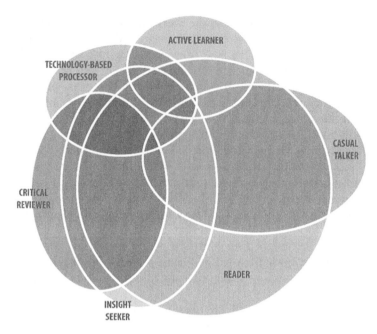

Fig. 7.1 Audience typologies with respect to engagement styles (*Source* Brown and Ratzkin [2011, p. 23])

A typology approach is helpful in informing discussions about co-creation, because the qualities, outcomes and potential beneficiaries of co-creation are always contingent on the underlying philosophy and rationale. However, I would contest the assumption that readers and critical reviewers all share a low appetite for arts engagement. All of these typologies are potential candidates for co-creation because they share a desire for active engagement with art. The problem, perhaps, is that artists, producers, and marketers are currently failing to engage typologies other than the active learner. This is very probably because the emphasis in co-creation is almost always on co-production rather than co-interpretation, which might appeal more to the more individual and reflective typologies outlined here. So the problem and area for development is perhaps not so much the audience but rather artists and arts organisations, who generally fail to provide a range of appealing opportunities for co-creation.

Now that we have considered the underlying theories and more common applications of co-creation, let's move on to explore some of its underlying processes in more depth.

PROCESSES OF CO-CREATION

Although co-creation might sometimes appear to be a relatively new concept in the performing arts, the participatory processes and practices that inform and inspire it are arguably as old as the arts themselves. Indeed Boorsma (2006) contends that the notion of art as autonomous only appeared with the modernists and claims that postmodernism has regenerated a vision of the arts as "a product of social interaction" (p. 75). This relational view of art, she argues, accepts the evolution of arts consumers from passive recipients into active participants. At the start of Chapter 3, I acknowledged the necessity to consider, critique and deconstruct terms that are deployed to describe and qualify the complex processes and relationships that connect audiences to performance. So I will now hone in on some of the most significant concepts that underpin this umbrella term of co-creation. The aim here is not to produce a detailed theoretical elaboration of all of these concepts (which lies well beyond the scope of this chapter) but rather to summarise the key ideas, aspects, and processes that mark them out as distinct and, in so doing, to highlight their potential complementarity in shaping co-creative practice.

PARTICIPATION

As noted earlier, the terminology surrounding arts participation is in a state of flux (Brown et al. 2011, p. 4). "Participation" itself is a particularly woolly term and to complicate matters, it is often used interchangeably with "audience development" and "co-creation". Like its sister terms, it is deployed and appropriated to cover a multitude of heterogeneous activities ranging from applause to blogging to community engagement. It is perhaps more useful, therefore, to talk about "participatory practice" rather than "participation" per se, because the former term implies an established philosophical approach to audience engagement that is distinct from audience development and narrower than co-creation. Jenkins and Bertozzi provide a useful description of what participatory practice might lead to and highlight its civic roots:

> A participatory culture might be defined as one where there are relatively low barriers to artistic expression and civic engagement, where there is strong support for creating and sharing what one creates with others, and where there is some kind of informal mentorship whereby what is known by the most experienced is passed along to novices. It is also a culture where members feel that their contributions matter and where they feel some degree of social connection with each other at least to the degree to which they care what other people think about what they have created. (Jenkins and Bertozzi 2008, p. 174)

I argued earlier that co-creation tends to be hierarchical and framed by the needs and interests of artists and producers. Participatory practice and culture, on the other hand, has its roots in the community arts movement. It is therefore, at least in theory, an audience-centred activity; more than that, it is often audience-led (representing what Brown et al. [2011] refer to as "audience-as-artist") and can even manifest as public engagement. So to return to Whalley and Miller's argument about empowerment, it is not about "letting the audience in" but more about co-designing, co-curating, co-programming, and co-performing.

Participatory practice is finally starting to take hold in mainstream arts organisations and venues, and the academic literature on participation is starting to burgeon, especially within cultural policy studies. Although there are different factions and tensions within the scholarly community of participatory arts, there is some consensus that participatory approaches can democratise the arts and culminate in the kind of "forum culture" referred to earlier in the chapter:

> By placing the users of art and culture and their different personal tastes and preferences in the center of cultural policy, arts advocacy and audience development consequently means that the classic cultural arenas – theatres, concert halls, cinemas, museums, and libraries – are regarded as democratic participatory platforms for exchanging and negotiating meanings and values. (Juncker and Balling 2016, p. 233)

Arts and cultural participation sits somewhere between the competing traditions of cultural democracy and the democratisation of culture. The challenge for scholars is essentially where to locate this kind of practice within the parameters of these two traditions, on a spectrum from participatory budgeting and decision-making at the cultural democracy end of the spectrum to the promotion of professional activity at the democratisation of culture end. So participation comes in many guises and is often philosophically and politically driven. Since this book is primarily focussing on the engagement of core or existing audiences, we will concentrate on how participatory practice impacts on this particular cohort, rather than communities or the general public more broadly. In other words, we will explore how participatory practice impacts on the democratisation of culture.

The American museum director Nina Simon has produced a significant body of work which explores how cultural institutions can use participatory techniques not simply to give visitors and audiences a genuine voice, but to develop experiences that are more valuable and compelling for everyone. Simon (2010) argues that participation is "a question of design and not just one of intention or desire". This is a useful (and indeed radical) proposition, because it again shifts the focus from *whether* arts and cultural organisations are engaging audiences through participatory practice to *how well* they are doing it. Simon highlights the importance of "scaffolding" participatory activities, demonstrating how participants "thrive on constraints, not open-ended opportunities for self-expression". She maintains that participatory organisations support "multidirectional content experiences".

> Participatory projects make relationships among staff members, visitors, community participants, and stakeholders more fluid and equitable. They open up new ways for diverse people to express themselves and engage with institutional practice. (Simon 2010)

As Matthew Reason might articulate it, they facilitate "intersubjective doing" (2010, p. 19). So we can see how participatory practice lies at the core of successful co-creation. It provides a guiding philosophy for engagement strategies and is starting to offer tried-and-tested techniques for deeper, richer engagement that can open up and democratise arts and cultural institutions.

PLAY

In my own empirical study of co-creation, one of the theatre directors involved said that he wanted his participants to "play wholeheartedly" and "come along for the ride" (Walmsley 2013, p. 114). This comment encouraged me to reflect on the role of play within the broader context of co-creation and led me to investigate some of its seminal theories. Play is generally understood by performance scholars as both positive and productive. Based on evidence from cognitive science, Bruce McConachie, for example, claims that "play has a positive impact on our wellbeing and on our homeostasis" (2008, p. 106). A perfect example of this is provided by Josephine Machon, who illustrates the interrelationship between play and interpretation:

> When an audience is encouraged to experience the layers of 'meaning' in the work by becoming part of the ludic play at the heart of the form itself, a dynamic curiosity is ignited; a curiosity that may seek to unearth narratives, themes or to just *be* within the work. (Machon 2013, p. 105)

Contrary to this unstructured ontological vision of play, other performance-based theories of play characterise it as a carefully managed process, a "framed activity where the frame both defines a space of freedom and provides a productive constraint" (Bayliss et al. 2009, p. 9). It is worth noting the focus on "constraints" here, which echoes the theories on participation detailed above. This suggests that playful co-creation incorporates constructive limitations which (perhaps counter-intuitively) facilitate participants' creativity.

Play is a process often deployed in rehearsals, of course, and particularly in devised or improvised work, where it enables directors and performers to experiment and innovate, to try out fresh ideas within a safe environment and within a given artistic vision or style. However, like co-creation, play is "risk-laden": for example, Bayliss et al.'s action research on play revealed that it can "unsettle, disturb and pressurise" participants (2009, p. 10). Play theorists present a paradoxical conceptualisation of play as both free and constrained, as creative and destructive, personal and collective, political and nihilistic:

> Play is a dance between creation and destruction, between creativity and nihilism. Playing is a fragile, tense activity, prone to breakdowns. Individual play is a challenge to oneself, to keep on playing. Collective play is a balancing act of egos and interests, of purposes and intentions. Play is always on the verge of destruction, of itself and of its players, and that is precisely why it matters. Play is a movement between order and chaos. (Sicart 2014, p. 3)

Sicart dedicates an entire book to exploring notions and processes of play. As revealed in the quotation above, he accepts the oxymorons inherent to play and seems to perceive it as profoundly *entrepreneurial*, at least if we accept Schumpeter's (1942) definition of economic innovation as "creative destruction". This is a productive connection, because in the context of co-creation, processes of play are often invoked to shape and develop something new, something risky, something that might push and challenge all sorts of artistic and organisational boundaries. Sicart acknowledges this implicitly in his reference to egos, interests, purposes, and intentions: play, like co-creation, is power-based and political in the sense that someone needs to frame and demarcate its boundaries and determine its ultimate purpose. Play, then, can be experienced as both pleasurable and painful, and its impact can be both positive and negative.

It is noteworthy here that Sicart characterises play as an almost liminal space that exists somewhere between order and chaos. Chaos theory informs us that behavioural patterns that might appear to be random can actually be integral to the effective development of natural ecosystems. Various scholars (e.g. Bilton 2007; Grobman 2005) have applied chaos theory to the context of arts management, particularly to illuminate the process of change management. For example, Grobman argues that organisational change should culminate in the adoption of "a quasi-equilibrium state, just short of the point where a system would collapse into chaos, at which the system maximizes its complexity and adaptability" (2005, p. 370). For Grobman, this entails a willingness by leaders to seek out contradictory attributes, engender a healthy level of anxiety and actually bring organisations to the "edge of chaos" (p. 351). The associations with play theory are self-evident here: like chaos, play is natural and creative; it fosters innovation and agility, and flourishes within the tension of a predetermined framework or equilibrium. As Sicart goes on to argue, the nature of this equilibrium is always contingent and open to negotiation.

> Play is autotelic – an activity with its own goals and purposes, with its own marked duration and spaces and its own conditions for ending. [...] Play is autotelic in its context, but it is also negotiated. Its autotelic nature is always being discussed and negotiated. We play by negotiating the purposes of play, how far we want to extend the influences of the play activity, and how much we play for the purpose of playing or for the purpose of personal expression. (Sicart 2014, p. 16)

The questions inherent to this theorisation of play shed fresh light on the purposes and impact of co-creation and provide a useful typological framework for it. For example, we might now ask of a co-creative activity whether its value is intrinsic or instrumental. What are its intended outcomes and who decides? Who are likely to be the main beneficiaries and why? Is a co-creative project valuable in and of itself or does it need to serve a higher (artistic) purpose?

Play and co-creation are thus indelibly linked: play theory can help us to explicate co-creation and processes of play are integral to co-creation because they provide a context for collective creativity. By incorporating aspects of experimentation, innovation and chaos, play can establish a safe space and a negotiable framework for productive and enjoyable co-creation. But as ever, the extent to which this potential is realised is dependent on the power dynamics (quite literally) at play.

INTERPRETATION

Many of the definitions of co-creation explored towards the beginning of this chapter coalesced around the notion of the collective elaboration of value, which is variously referred to in the literature as co-creating value, or collective meaning-making or sense-making. This suggests that artists and arts organisations should invest time in meaning-making activities in order to maximise their audiences' perceptions of the value of their artistic experiences. It also suggests that artists, producers, marketers and audiences need to possess (and ideally continuously develop) strong decoding and interpretive skills in order to derive as much value or meaning as possible. This is because in their "consumption" of art, audiences "integrate the resources offered by companies and combine them with their own resources to co-create and co-extract value from a consumption experience" (Cova and Cova 2009, p. 89). So in order to close the circle, or complete the artistic cycle, those who produce and "market" artistic experiences should also be in the business of building the requisite resources to decode and interpret them.

Like Miranda Boorsma, Chris Bilton (2017) is of the view that audiences should take an active role in the meaning-making process. This is essentially because audiences are inherently part of a triadic relationship with artists and fellow audience members:

> [...] the consumer is actively involved in creating meaning and value by associating the product with their own experiences, with the artist and with each other. Such extended meanings and interpretations can go well beyond

the producer's intentions, drawing on the collective imaginations and actions of audiences – but they remain umbilically connected to the product. (p. 82)

So there is a strong artistic case to be made for involving audiences actively in meaning-making processes, because this can uncover previously hidden meanings and interpretations and enhance the original value of a production or performance. Bilton argues persuasively that consumers of "cultural products" retain the right to reimagine them and add meanings of their own to them: "unlike other forms of product cultural products are not 'used up' by consumption, rather the uses of consumption change the product's meaning, making it more valuable not less" (pp. 99–100). In this sense, Bilton maintains, cultural products become paratexts which can be reimagined by successive audiences. Referring back to the previous chapter, we might add that this is essentially because in the performing arts, cultural products take the form of collective experiences, whose meaning can only ever be fully elaborated in a collaborative way.

The primary role of the audience in the meaning-making endeavour might at face value appear to be incontrovertible; but following the influence of Foucault and Derrida, some scholars insist on perceiving interpretation as illusory. Citing Artaud and Brecht as inspirations, Blau, for example, claims that theatre audiences are "beguiled into thinking" that plays are performed for them and "that by some consensus of perception they determine what the play means" (1990, p. 49). This suggests that plays have some kind of objective (or, as Derrida would say, "originary") meaning, the articulation of which lies beyond the capacity of mere audiences. Blau's studied disdain for audiences is revealed in his derisory slur that they "mostly miss the point" (p. 126). In our post-structuralist world, there are certainly divergent opinions about who owns the meaning-making process and who is empowered to (co-)create the meaning of artistic experiences. Blau quite rightly notes that meaning-making is "disarticulated" through "dominant and oppressive systems of meaning" (ibid., p. 8). The examples he provides here are the media and the self-referential theatre machine itself. The underlying philosophical question is the extent to which meaning-making is ever free and unfettered, and Blau reminds us of Heidegger's notion of "*Vorhabe*": "the forestructure of understanding in which interpretation is grounded" (p. 41). By this, Blau means that interpretation is partially preordained in that it is restricted by pre-existing linguistic and semiotic parameters, by social systems, by the "hermeneutic circle" (Gadamer 1989).[1]

In light of the rise of social media and the rise of immersive and co-created art, it is interesting to reflect on the extent to which audiences might have freed themselves from this dominance and oppression since the publication of Blau's monograph in 1990: although meaning-making is still very rarely facilitated by the professional arts sector, it is assuredly harder to contain and control. So although, as a core element of co-creation, meaning-making remains protected, prejudicial and political, in the past few decades it has certainly become more subjective and democratic. It was perhaps with this development in mind that Boorsma counselled arts organisations to actively develop their audiences' co-creative skills:

> If arts organizations want to survive in the competitive global world of tourism and leisure, they will have to develop their audiences' capacity to co-create and deepen their engagement through increasingly 'entire' experiences including recreational, social and learning experiences. (p. 77)

It is significant that Boorsma connects the co-creation of meaning with deep engagement here, and she is right to advocate for arts organisations performing a broader role that merely producing and/or presenting artistic content. As Hodgson (2002) reflects, in order to become "creative consumers", individuals need to be "shaped, guided and moulded" (p. 326). Interpretative skills are not innate and as the primary receivers of artistic work, audiences benefit from social and educational experiences that develop their capacity to sense-make. When audiences engage with a performance, they may or not decode or derive meaning from it depending on how they deploy their interpretative faculties:

> In a gaze we have at our disposal a natural instrument analogous to the blind man's stick. The gaze gets more or less from things according to the way in which it questions them, ranges over them or dwells on them. (Blau 1990, p. 377)

---

[1] Gadamer's interpretation of Heidegger's notion of the hermeneutic circle is that all interpretation is inherently *prejudicial* in the sense that it is always based on people's existing knowledge, concerns and interests (Malpas 2016).

In this sense, then, audience development, or education, is key, and it is fitting, therefore, that certain scholars insist on the need to develop audiences' critical response faculties. A natural context for this is of course within the school classroom, and O'Toole et al.'s (2014) study provides a revealing analysis of the potentially positive impact of developing younger audiences' capacities for meaning-making. For instance, there is consensus amongst almost all of the teachers and creative artists interviewed in the book that what the authors refer to as "theatre literacy" enabled young people to "master a complex theatre discourse that allowed them to describe, analyse and understand the experience of theatre" (p. 147). The authors go on to illustrate how providing young people with the appropriate critical tools to deconstruct a piece of theatre can develop their decoding and analytical skills.

> Theatre literate young people demonstrate the use of technical and meta-language, and the language of experience and pleasure. They are able to respond critically to a play, deconstructing both the text and the performance in depth, using learned conceptual frameworks. (p. 155)

However, some participants felt that their formal learning at school had encouraged them to be too analytical and critical in their responses, which "distanced" them from a live performance "because they were busy evaluating and deconstructing it" (p. 149). It is worth noting therefore that overanalysis can sometimes hamper engagement.

Developing audiences' interpretative skills is clearly a strategic goal that can bear rich dividends in the collective endeavour to elaborate the meaning(s) embedded in the performing arts. There is also evidence that it provides audiences with "eudaimonic pleasure"—the "deeply enjoyable critical attitude" extolled by Brecht (Heim 2016, p. 98). Despite these clear benefits, interpretation remains under-deployed, perhaps because of the entrenched habits and power structures delineated above. Some artists aren't interested in the meanings that audiences ascribe to their work; some producers never strive to listen to audiences' interpretations; and some scholars don't credit audiences with the ability (either cognitive or ontological) to interpret a work of art. This particular aspect of co-creation is therefore fraught with structural challenges ranging from apathy to disdain, which means that it is woefully neglected as a core component of the audience experience and an essential part of audience engagement.

> An audience member's pleasure is deeply tied with the opportunity to inter-
> pret the meaning and value of an arts event. [...] Without public oppor-
> tunities to articulate our individual decoding processes, the pleasure of the
> interpretive function is cut short and thus engagement is limited. (Conner
> 2004, pp. 1, 4)

As opportunities for collective meaning-making continue to be missed,
more and more audience members leave performances unsatiated and more
and more productions remain poorly explicated and under-critiqued.

FACILITATION

A potential remedy to this deficiency is provided by Lynne Conner (2013)
and her concept of "arts talk". Conner describes her concept as "a
metaphor, an ethos and [...] a call to arms" (p. 137) and she outlines
its underlying rationale as follows:

> Our goal should be to empower audiences to engage in constructive and
> pleasurable dialogue about the arts and to celebrate those audiences who,
> by virtue of their vital and engaged presence, can turn any arts space into a
> site of public assembly ripe for intellectual and emotional connection. (2013,
> p. 13)

Conner reminds us of Gadamer's contention that "meaningful conversation" can offer a resolution to the hermeneutic circle (ibid., p. 18).
In other words, bringing audiences into a structured dialogue can help
to generate fresh interpretations and produce original meaning that circumnavigates many of the linguistic and semiotic constraints inherent to
individual decoding. Citing Stanley Fish, Bennett rightly contends that
"texts are accorded value not by any intrinsic properties but by interpretive
communities" who develop strategies to provide opposing, and sometimes
even resistant, positions (1997, pp. 40–41; p. 56). This latter observation
is particularly evident in the interpretive approaches advocated by queer
and feminist theorists, for example, which further underline the Barthesian
resistance to the primary role of the author.

However, generating meaningful conversation requires excellent facilitation skills, and these are often sadly lacking in our arts and cultural institutions, which tend, perhaps as a result of this skills gap, to present "talk-
backs" or post-show Q&As which persist in their goal of casting audience
members as attentive listeners and which thus reduce, rather than facilitate,

opportunities for democratic dialogue and exchange. As Caroline Heim asserts:

> Most Western theatre companies that hold post-performance discussions follow either a question-and-answer or expert-driven model, both of which perpetuate an 'expert agenda' that can be seen as didactic and to devalue any audience contributions. [...] The expert-driven model fosters an intellectual environment in which audience contributions, if encouraged at all, are expected to conform to the cerebral thoughts of the expert in both expression and content. A large percentage of the audience, daunted and intimidated by the expert environment, are hesitant to contribute to the discussion or even ask questions. [...] Post-performance discussions have been relegated to educational or entertaining events that perpetuate a hegemonic hierarchy. (2012, pp. 189–190)

Heim's action research project on two theatre productions in Queensland, Australia culminated in the realisation that a carefully facilitated, nondirective and unstructured approach to post-show discussions helped to give audiences "a voice of authority" and generated "opinionated, expressive, articulate, and discerning" feedback that was "evaluative and interpretative, as well as fault-finding" (ibid., p. 194). It is important to note here the method's ability to unearth negative responses from the audience, as positive bias has been acknowledged as a particularly pernicious limitation of much audience research (Johanson and Glow 2015). Another significant finding of Heim's research was that a more empowering approach to post-show discussion served to maximise opportunities for audiences to co-create meaning and develop a community of interpretation:

> The audience critics were preoccupied with making meaning, negotiating meaning, and contributing meaning in an attempt to broaden and enrich their experience of the theatrical event. The audience regained their status as an interpretative community of critical contributors. (ibid., pp. 194–195)

The impact of this ad hoc community was palpable, as it apparently influenced the director's interpretation of one of the characters and led to subsequent changes in the way the actor portrayed the character. This provides a wonderful example of how engaging and emancipating audiences in a meaningful way after performances can develop a culture of co-creation in all senses of the term.

Heim's reflections on the benefits of adopting a more democratic model of audience feedback are shared by Lynne Conner, who equally advocates for independent facilitation. As Conner argues, when "invited properly, audiences will push beyond the discomfort of 'thinking' to get to the interpretive sphere" (2013, p. 109). Conner therefore advocates building what she calls "audience learning communities" (p. 101ff.) based on what she perceives to be the "fundamentals of productive talk" (p. 117ff.). Facilitation is the method she invokes to achieve these goals because she argues that "the best audience-centred interpretive experiences are rooted in good facilitation" (p. 117). Conner deconstructs productive talk into three operations: open talk, powerful questioning, and effective listening (p. 120). So these, she maintains, are the objectives of effective facilitators, who should "listen for meaning rather than for validation" (p. 164). There is surely an implicit criticism here of the solipsism and self-congratulation that characterise many post-performance events.

Although there is no scope here for a more thorough exploration of facilitation, it is worth noting that it is a process that is highlighted by other studies and scholars and one which has been demonstrated to deepen and broaden engagement.

> The richness of this [the theatre-going] experience, and therefore its potential to influence future theatre-going behaviours, can be enhanced and supported by well-crafted post-show discussions wherein meaning-making is scaffolded by thoughtful and strategic inputs from creative and educational facilitators [...] and by opportunities for open-ended discourse with friends, peers and mentors. Our research suggests that these opportunities for discussion and meaning-making beyond the time spent in the auditorium are critical. (O'Toole et al. 2014, p. 196)

We can appreciate here the repeated call for the "scaffolding" of co-creative interventions and also the significant potential of effective facilitation to perform the primary function of relational art in bringing people together to forge deeper social links, occasionally referred to as "enhanced socialization" (Nicholson and Pearce 2001, p. 460).

IMPACT

We have seen how co-creation is informed by theories related to collaboration, interaction, participation, invention, value, meaning and exchange, and also how it is underpinned by a number of underlying activities, including participation, play, interpretation and facilitation. In this final section of the chapter, we are going to reflect on the impact that co-creation can have on audiences, artists, arts organisations, and on the wider arts and cultural sector.

I have discussed several examples of how effective co-creation can deepen and broaden audiences' engagement and develop social communities of interpretation which can co-generate value and derive original meaning, providing a resolution to the hermeneutic circle. From a marketing perspective, co-creation has also been credited with providing "experiential interactions and encounters which customers perceive as helping them utilize their resources" (Payne et al. 2008, p. 87). In the context of the arts, this might imply aesthetic development (e.g. developing audiences' creative practice) or cognitive growth (e.g. developing school children's appreciation and knowledge of Shakespeare). This kind of intrinsic and instrumental impact can generate strategic opportunities for creating value, as long as producers align their creative processes with their audiences' interests and needs. So from a strategic marketing perspective, "planning for co-creation is outside-in as it starts from an understanding of the customer's value-creating processes, and aims at providing support for better co-creation of value" (Payne et al. 2008, p. 89). This suggests that co-creation should be embedded into the vision and strategic management of arts organisations in order to maximise mutual value.

However, this understanding of audiences' value-creating processes is essentially what is missing from both the research and practice of co-creation in the arts. As Brown et al. put it, whilst "an international debate rages about the value of the arts [...] missing in this debate is a dispassionate, critical assessment of the relative benefits and value of participatory arts practice versus receptive participation" (2011, p. 10). Whilst there is no space here for a thorough investigation of cultural value and impact (see Chapter 4), some of the key benefits of co-creation have been presented in the literature. From the audience perspective, such benefits have been described in terms of self-expression, self-realisation, aesthetic insight, as well as building confidence, creative thinking, communication and problem-solving skills (Arvidsson 2008; Brown et al. 2011).

From the perspective of artists, producers, and organisations, co-creation has been credited with maximising the lifetime value of desirable customer groups (Payne and Frow 2005); fulfilling the artistic mission (Boorsma 2006); and developing "artistic exchange relationships" (ibid., p. 77).

Indeed it has even been argued that value is compromised without some element of co-creation:

> The assumption that artistic value can be realized autonomously, independently of the patronage of arts consumers, is no longer valid. Artistic value goes beyond the product in terms of its form [and] emerges in the confrontation with an audience. (Boorsma 2006, pp. 75–76)

So again we can appreciate both the business and artistic case for investing in co-creation. But there is a wider impact at stake here, which takes us into the realm of audience development and education. Audience research has demonstrated how developing the interpretive skills of young people can empower them to generate their own meaning from the performing arts and encourage them to engage with a more diverse body of work.

> Once equipped with a conscious awareness of the skills and entitlement to construct their own meanings from their theatre experience, many young theatre-goers we interviewed articulated a desire to see work which challenged conventions (and therefore audience expectations) rather than affirmed them. They had transcended the fear of 'not liking' or 'not understanding' a theatre event, and embraced, equally, the prospect of being provoked and educated, or entertained. (O'Toole et al. 2014, p. 135)

Developing audiences' co-creative skills, then, can not only broaden their aesthetic tastes but also shift their perceptions of an art form and increase their likelihood to engage with it. This is particularly the case when co-creation occurs within a social or community setting:

> For most participants in customer co-production, similarly to other forms of social production, motivation is directly related to the pleasures that can be derived from community participation and contribution. (Arvidsson 2008, p. 335)

As Conner maintains, we desperately need a renaissance of "social interpretation" in the arts, and we can only achieve this by developing an "authorised audience" (2013, p. 40).

Despite the overwhelming evidence of the potentially positive impacts of co-creative activities, the overriding challenge in understanding and articulating the value of co-creation remains the lack of meaningful evaluation.

This is a problem that plagues many sectors and it often stems from reductive applications of marketing: "Improved ways of measuring the delivery of customer value are required. Marketing metrics and measures should meaningfully assess the value co-creation potential of customer relationships" (Payne et al. 2008, p. 89). In other words, if evaluators don't ask the right questions, they won't obtain meaningful answers. This again highlights the need for organisations to deploy the nuanced and tailored audience research methods explored in Chapter 5 and to adopt an engagement-based approach to developing relationships with audiences (strategies which are clearly interconnected).

CONCLUSION

Co-creation is an umbrella term which encompasses aspects of collaboration, interaction, invention, value, meaning, and exchange. In the course of this chapter, I have demonstrated that it is a slippery and ambiguous concept that resists a simple definition, and which, therefore, is both open to interpretation and vulnerable to misinterpretation and misappropriation. I have argued that co-creation might fruitfully be understood as a generic term, which has evolved theoretically via studies of processes of participation, play, interpretation, and facilitation.

We have seen in the course of this chapter how co-creation thrives on constraints, on skilful facilitation, and on careful planning, scaffolding, and evaluation. We have also seen that arts organisations would be wrong to believe that all audience members possess "the competencies enabling them to dialogue, play a particular role and integrate the products or services" that they offer (Cova and Cova 2009, p. 94). So it is beholden on arts organisations to develop the co-creative skills of their audiences: to enable them to participate; to encourage them to play; to educate and empower them to interpret; and to facilitate the full impact of arts engagement. This, in turn, can break down often pernicious barriers to engagement and develop audience members' aesthetic taste and their propensity for artistic risk.

Co-creation is undoubtedly in vogue, and this trend has been attributed to enduring communitarian values, which have engendered a more social approach to production and consumption (Arvidsson 2008). Co-creation is a natural heir of cultural democracy, although it is often deployed as an attempt (cynical or genuine) to democratise existing culture. It is also part of a wider "participatory turn" in society (Crawford et al. 2014), a phenomenon which we will explore more fully in the following chapter. Like questions of cultural value, practices and processes of co-creation are always political, because they are dependent on preordained power dynamics, and the power generally resides in the hands of artists and producers. I have therefore advocated here for an audience-centred approach to arts management and cultural policy, wherein audiences become the primary focus and *raison d'être* of artistically led organisations.

Audience-centred organisations actively seek out opportunities to co-create, and we have seen in the course of this chapter that co-creation can genuinely engage and empower audiences and culminate in democratic exchanges that can decode complex artistic messages and translate them into shared (albeit contested) meanings and values. So although there is undoubtedly a strong business case to be made for co-creation, perhaps the ultimate goals and benefits of co-creation are social and artistic: to derive collective meaning; to bring artists, producers and audiences together to co-create mutual long-term value by developing an interpretive community of artistic practice and exchange. Following Prahalad and Ramaswamy (2004a) and Boal, we might well conceive of this community as a *forum*; and if Csikszentmihalyi is correct in his assertion that creativity is the product of social systems, then arts and cultural organisations are uniquely placed to facilitate and even shape and lead these social forums.

If consumers in general are increasingly seeking experiences rather than products or services (Pine and Gilmore 1999), then arts audiences are hungry for *meaningful aesthetic* experiences. As Charles Leadbeater (2009) notes, the arts provide a space for higher meanings and deeper purpose; and as Lynne Conner argues, "deep pleasure resides in those opportunities to prepare, process, and analyse in order to be ready to interpret in a social setting" (2013, p. 67). To exclude audiences from active involvement in the creation or interpretation of a work of art is therefore to deny them the opportunity to find the deepest sense of purpose and pleasure, and to derive optimal meaning from their artistic engagement. When expressed in these stark terms, it is difficult to comprehend that this is what the majority of arts and cultural organisations continue to do, for this failure ultimately undermines most of their social and artistic missions.

Co-creation is on the rise, and as attention turns to high quality engagement opportunities, arts organisations have been cautioned that if they wish to survive in the increasingly competitive global world of tourism and leisure, they will have to develop their audiences' capacity to co-create and deepen their engagement (Boorsma 2006, p. 77). One proven way to achieve this is via digital communications technologies, and in the following chapter, I will explore how existing and emerging technologies can be harnessed to open up opportunities for co-creation and to elongate and ultimately enrich the audience experience.

REFERENCES

Arts Council England. 2010. *Audience development and marketing* [Internet]. London, Arts Council England. Available from: http://www.artscouncil.org. uk/information-sheet/audience-development-and-marketing-grants-for-the-arts [Accessed 2 June].

Arvidsson, A. 2008. The ethical economy of customer coproduction. *Journal of Macromarketing*, 28(4), pp. 326–338.

Bayliss, A., Hayles, D., Palmer, S. and Sheridan, J. G. 2009. (Re)searching through play: Play as a framework and methodology for collaborative design processes. *International Journal of Arts and Technology*, 2(1–2), pp. 5–21.

Bennett, S. 1997. *Theatre audiences: A theory of production and reception.* 2nd ed. London, Routledge.

Bilton, C. 2007. *Management and creativity: From creative industries to creative management.* Oxford, Blackwell.

Bilton, C. 2017. *The disappearing product: Marketing and markets in the creative industries.* Cheltenham, Edward Elgar.

Bishop, C. 2004. Antagonism and relational aesthetics. *October*, 110, pp. 51–79.

Blau, H. 1990. *The audience.* Baltimore, The John Hopkins University Press.

Boorsma, M. 2006. A strategic logic for arts marketing: Integrating customer value and artistic objectives. *The International Journal of Cultural Policy*, 12(1), pp. 73–92.

Boorsma, M. and Chiaravalloti, F. 2010. Arts marketing performance: An artistic-mission-led approach to evaluation. *The Journal of Arts Management, Law and Society*, 40(4), pp. 297–317.

Bourdieu, P. 1984. *Distinction: A social critique of the judgement of taste.* Harvard, Harvard University Press.

Bourriaud, N. 2002. *Relational aesthetics.* Dijon, Les Presses du Réel.

Bourriaud, N. 2006/1998. Relational aesthetics. In: Bishop, C. (ed.) *Participation.* London, Whitechapel Gallery, pp. 160–171.

Brown, A. S., Novak-Leonard, J. L. and Gilbride, S. 2011. *Getting in on the act: How arts groups are creating opportunities for active participation.* San Francisco, CA, The James Irvine Foundation.

Brown, A. S. and Ratzkin, R. 2011. *Making sense of audience engagement: A critical assessment of efforts by nonprofit arts organizations to engage audiences and visitors in deeper and more impactful arts experiences.* San Francisco, The San Francisco Foundation.

Caldwell, M. 2001. Applying General Living Systems Theory to learn consumers' sense making in attending performing arts. *Psychology & Marketing*, 18(5), pp. 497–511.

Colbert, F. 2007. *Marketing culture and the arts.* 3rd ed. Montreal, HEC Montreal.

Conner, L. 2004. Who gets to tell the meaning? Building audience enrichment. *GIA Reader* [Online], 15(1).

Conner, L. 2013. *Audience engagement and the role of arts talk in the digital era.* New York, Palgrave Macmillan.

Cova, B. and Cova, V. 2009. Faces of the new consumer: A genesis of consumer governmentality. *Recherche et Applications en Marketing*, 24(3), pp. 81–99.

Crawford, G., Gosling, V., Bagnall, G. and Light, B. 2014. Is there an app for that? A case study of the potentials and limitations of the participatory turn and networked publics for classical music audience engagement. *Information, Communication & Society*, 17(9), pp. 1072–1085.

Debord, G. 1992. *Society of the spectacle.* London, Rebel Press.

Dwyer, P. 2004. Making bodies talk in Forum Theatre. *Research in Drama Education: The Journal of Applied Theatre and Perfomance*, 9(2), pp. 199–210.

European Commission. 2015. *Study on audience development: How to place audiences at the centre of cultural organisations.* Brussels, European Commission.

Freshwater, H. 2009. *Theatre & audience.* London, Palgrave Macmillan.

Gadamer, H.-G. 1989. *Truth and method.* 2nd revised ed. New York, Crossroad.

Goldbard, A. and Adams, D. 1990. Cultural policy and cultural democracy. In: Goldbard, A. and Adams, D. (eds.) *Crossroads: Reflections on the politics of culture.* Talmage, CA, DNA Press, pp. 107–109.

Govier, L. 2009. *Leaders in co-creation: Why and how museums could develop their co-creative practice with the public, building on ideas from the performing arts and other non-museum organisations.* Leicester, University of Leicester.

Grobman, G. M. 2005. Complexity theory: A new way to look at organizational change. *Public Administration Quarterly*, 29(3–4), pp. 351–384.

Grönroos, C. 2011. Value co-creation in service logic: A critical analysis. *Marketing Theory*, 11(3), pp. 279–301.

Heim, C. 2016. *Audience as performer: The changing role of theatre audiences in the Twenty-First Century.* London and New York, Routledge.

Heim, C. L. 2012. 'Argue with us!': Audience co-creation through post-performance discussions. *New Theatre Quarterly*, 28(2), pp. 189–197.

Hodgson, D. 2002. "Know your customer": Marketing, governmentality and the "new consumer" of financial services. *Management Decision*, 40(4), pp. 318–328.

Ind, N., Fuller, C. and Trevail, C. 2012. *Brand together: How co-creation generates innovation and re-energizes brands.* London, Kogan Page.

Jancovich, L. 2011. Great art for everyone? Engagement and participation policy in the arts. *Cultural Trends*, 20(3–4), pp. 271–279.

Jancovich, L. 2017. The participation myth. *International Journal of Cultural Policy*, 23(1), pp. 107–121.

Jenkins, H. and Bertozzi, V. 2008. Artistic expression in the age of participatory culture. In: Tepper, S. J. and Ivey, B. (eds.) *Engaging art: The next great transformation of American cultural life*. New York, Routledge, pp. 171–195.

Johanson, K. and Glow, H. 2015. A virtuous circle: The positive evaluation phenomenon in arts audience research. *Participations*, 12(1), pp. 254–270.

Juncker, B. and Balling, G. 2016. The value of art and culture in everyday life: Towards an expressive cultural democracy. *The Journal of Arts Management, Law, and Society*, 46(5), pp. 231–242.

Keen, A. 2008. *The cult of the amateur: How blogs, MySpace, YouTube, and the rest of today's user-generated media are destroying our economy, our culture, and our values*. New York, Doubleday.

Kester, G. 2005. Conversation pieces: The role of dialogue in socially engaged art. In: Kocur, Z. and Leung, S. (eds.) *Theory in contemporary art since 1985*. Oxford, Blackwell, pp. 76–100.

Knell, J. 2004. *Whose art is it anyway?* London, The Intelligence Agency.

Leadbeater, C. 2009. *The art of with*. Manchester, Cornerhouse.

Machon, J. 2013. *Immersive theatres: Intimacy and immediacy in contemporary performance*. London, Palgrave Macmillan.

Malpas, J. 2016. Hans-Georg Gadamer. In: Zalta, E. N. (ed.) *The Stanford encyclopedia of philosophy* [Online]. Available from: https://plato.stanford.edu/archives/win2016/entries/gadamer [Accessed 19 April].

McConachie, B. 2008. *Engaging audiences: A cognitive approach to spectating in the theatre*. New York, Palgrave Macmillan.

McMaster, B. 2008. *Supporting excellence in the arts: From measurement to judgement*. London, Department for Culture Media and Sport.

Nicholson, R. E. and Pearce, D. G. 2001. Why do people attend events? A comparative analysis of visitor motivations at four south island events. *Journal of Travel Research*, 39(4), pp. 449–460.

O'Sullivan, T. 2009. All together now: A symphony orchestra audience as a consuming community. *Consumption, Markets and Culture*, 12(3), pp. 209–223.

O'Toole, J., Adams, R.-J., Anderson, M., Burton, B. and Ewing, R. (eds.). 2014. *Young audiences, theatre and the cultural conversation*. Dordrecht, Springer.

Payne, A. F. and Frow, P. 2005. A strategic framework for customer relationship management. *Journal of Marketing*, 69, pp. 167–176.

Payne, A. F., Storbacka, K. and Frow, P. 2008. Managing the co-creation of value. *Journal of the Academy of Marketing Science*, 36, pp. 83–96.

Pine, B. J. and Gilmore, J. H. 1999. *The experience economy: Work is theatre and every business a stage*. Boston, Harvard Business School.

Pope, R. 2005. *Creativity: Theory, history, practice*. London and New York, Routledge.

Prahalad, C. K. and Ramaswamy, V. 2004a. Co-creation experiences: The next practice in value creation. *Journal of Interactive Marketing*, 18(3), pp. 5–14.

Prahalad, C. K. and Ramaswamy, V. 2004b. *The future of competition: Co-creating unique value with customers*. Harvard, HBS Press.

Rancière, J. 2011. *The emancipated spectator*. London, Verso.

Reason, M. 2010. Asking the audience: Audience research and the experience of theatre. *About Performance* 10, pp. 15–34.

Royal Shakespeare Company. 2017. *Press release* [Internet]. Stratford-on-Avon, Royal Shakespeare Company. Available from: https://www.rsc.org.uk/press/releases/spring-mischief-festival-the-other-place-stratford-upon-avon-24-may-17-june [Accessed 10 November].

Schumpeter, J. 1942. *Capitalism, socialism and democracy*. New York, Harper.

Sicart, M. 2014. *Play matters*. Boston, MA, MIT Press.

Simon, N. 2010. *The participatory museum*. Santa Cruz, Museum 2.0.

Tanggaard, L. (ed.). 2014. *Fooling around: Creative learning pathways*. Charlotte, NC, Information Age Publishing.

Walmsley, B. 2013. Co-creating theatre: Authentic engagement or inter-legitimation? *Cultural Trends*, 22(2), pp. 108–118.

Walmsley, B. 2016. From arts marketing to audience enrichment: How digital engagement can deepen and democratize artistic exchange with audiences. *Poetics*, 58, pp. 66–78.

Whalley, J. and Miller, L. 2017. *Between us: Audiences, affect and the in-between*. London, Palgrave.

CHAPTER 8

Engaging Audiences Through Digital Technologies

INTRODUCTION

The previous chapter traced the rise of co-creative approaches to audience engagement and reviewed how these initiatives have the potential to enhance value and create artistic exchange relationships between audiences, artists and arts organisations. This chapter will move on to investigate how digital communications technologies are starting to transform philosophies and processes of audience engagement, occasionally by facilitating and enhancing co-creative projects themselves. The chapter will situate practices of digital engagement within the wider phenomena of participatory culture and social production, and acknowledge the implications of mass online migration for artists, producers, arts marketers and policymakers. This will entail a critical discussion of the relative utility of digital platforms in: supporting audience development initiatives; elongating the audience experience; and realising the core marketing objective of fostering two-way communication with audiences.

The literature on digital engagement in the arts is sparse, and although the arts sector has witnessed a sharp global rise in digital projects, not least through the proliferation of live streaming, surprisingly little empirical work has been undertaken to document or evaluate the impact of this trend. However, there are a small number of scholarly studies into digital engagement and these will be reviewed in the course of this chapter alongside Nesta's studies of NT Live—the Royal National Theatre's international programme of live streaming productions into cinemas.

© The Author(s) 2019
B. Walmsley, *Audience Engagement in the Performing Arts*,
New Directions in Cultural Policy Research,
https://doi.org/10.1007/978-3-030-26653-0_8

199

One aim of this chapter is to review the aims, objectives and outcomes of digital arts engagement projects; what *won't* be reviewed here are digital arts projects per se, as what we are focussed on in terms of *engagement* is essentially how digital communications technologies are impacting on the traditional marketing mix explored in Chapter 6: namely, artistic products and experiences; sales and distribution; pricing strategies; and promotional activity.

In order to illustrate how theories pertaining to digital engagement play out in practice, and to compensate in some way for the lack of academic literature on digital engagement in the arts, the chapter will conclude with four case studies. The first three case studies will present and review the activities of arts organisations that are acknowledged globally to be leading the way in the digital engagement of audiences: National Theatre of Scotland, Bristol's Watershed and New York's Brooklyn Museum. The final, extended, case study will provide a critical evaluation of a project funded by Nesta's Digital R&D Fund: Yorkshire Dance's *Respond*. The aim of this final case study is to illustrate and evidence the potential of digital communications technologies to create responsive, reflective and artist-led but audience-centred platforms, whilst critically reviewing the inherent challenges in maintaining active audience engagement remotely over a sustained period of time.

THE RISE OF DIGITAL ENGAGEMENT

As noted over a decade ago by Hannah Rudman (2006), interactive online communication is becoming an increasingly common feature of cultural consumption. The use of digital technology to engage audiences is a tangible manifestation of the wider cultural economy, which is characterised in part by a growing culture of participation. Crawford et al. (2014) characterise this "participatory turn" as a culture where everyday users engage more actively with online technologies than through the standard "read mode" (p. 1073). However, they also point out that the transformative potential of online engagement stems back several decades, citing Rheingold's (1993) argument regarding "the potential of the Internet to revitalize the public sphere and construct new forms of community, even before the advent of Web 2.0" (p. 1072). So it is important to avoid falling into the common trap of assuming that participation is something new: indeed as we saw in the previous chapter, the arts have enjoyed a long and proud tradition of "viewer participation" and "activated spectatorship" (Bishop, 2006, p. 78).

Ito (2007) relates this participatory turn to his concept of "networked publics", which he invokes to explain how online audiences engage actively with media to the point where they co-create or even reinvent it. This focus on collective participation provides an excellent example of what Cova (1999) calls "the linking value of consumption"; and a primary aim of this chapter is to explore how artists and arts organisations can harness digital technologies to engage their audiences collectively—or, in other words, to use the performing arts as a vehicle to create social bonds between them. Another practical example of this "linking value" is provided by Terry O'Sullivan's (2010) study of online engagement by a UK symphony orchestra, which found that respondents' motivations for participating in web forums included socially enhancing their cultural experiences and "obtaining privileged information" (p. 666). This reinforces Kozinets' (1999) argument that "information needs" drive people online; and it provides further evidence of audiences' desire to connect with other audience members, in this case through digital technology. This finding links back to the discussions of cultural value in Chapter 4, which highlighted the potential of the arts to facilitate social cohesion and strengthen human relationships.

O'Sullivan's study also highlights the importance of creating "a clear context for activity" in order to "manage relevant dialogue" through a "substantial online presence" (2010, p. 667). This indicates the need for digital engagement activities to be well designed, managed and resourced, just like any other type of co-creative activity. O'Sullivan concludes that "hosted online interactivity provides a distinctive opportunity for arts organisations to position themselves as an essential resource for [...] sustaining and enhancing arts experience" (p. 668). This is perhaps because, as Crawford et al. (2014) point out, online marketing enables "bidirectional communication"; and the "dynamic process of online attention" can lead to a form of "networked engagement – a necessary corollary to having a 'voice'" (p. 1081).

These studies suggest that the participatory turn has created a new generation of vocal, networked, and empowered audiences. However, there are some important caveats here that need to be acknowledged. The first caveat regards the "social risk" that audiences sometimes attach to participation and the "uncertainty" they attribute to their online identity (O'Sullivan 2010, p. 665). O'Sullivan notes that this insecurity can lead online audiences to feel alienated, which in turn can translate into a shyness or reluctance to post online for fear of appearing less complex or expert than their peers. Another caveat is that this new generation of empowered audience members is not always easy to reach and maintain. Sita Popat's (2006) work with online dance communities underscored the challenges of maintaining sustained digital engagement with a transient audience community. But in her discussion of the artist/participant relationship, Popat notes that interactive digital situations allow participants to "understand in detail how the artwork is created" (p. 33). Popat stresses the importance of participatory artists developing social interaction and hosting skills, and drawing on techniques of asynchronous communication in order to develop an effective partnership with audiences. This asynchronous interaction, she argues, "can support play, reflection and development in a journey through the creative cycle" (p. 35). So it seems that there are clear and tangible benefits to be reaped from persevering in coaxing unfamiliar participants and in drawing out their online identities.

In her powerful exhortation of taking a social learning and digital approach to audience engagement, Lynne Conner (2013) argues that a pleasurable audience experience is deeply connected to the hermeneutic opportunity to discuss and interpret meaning. Echoing Boorsma's theory on co-creation, Conner maintains that effective audience engagement is about process rather than outcome. Conner illustrates and elaborates the many benefits of digital engagement, including its ability to empower and embolden users by safeguarding their anonymity. Conner also stresses the importance of "honouring silence" in effective listening and notes that this is far easier online than face-to-face because of the different social mores attached to these different modes of dialogue. She adds that "periods of silence slow the pace and allow for a redistribution of power among the speakers". Conner demonstrates how effective online engagement can democratise discussion and increase audiences' access to paratextual insights, thus profoundly enhancing the "meaning-making operation" (p. 79). On the other hand, she acknowledges Keen's (2007) disdain for the rising cult of the amateur with a withering attack on the facile nature of the Facebook "Like", which she derides as "a gesture that eschews substantive feedback for quick, almost guerrilla-style intervention" (p. 89). Thus whilst effective digital engagement has been repeatedly demonstrated to facilitate creative dialogue, and therefore support the co-creation of meaning and value, it has also been revealed as a potential cause of facile reductionism, of what Daniel Kahneman (2011) might call "fast thinking".

Although it is important to remain critical of poorly planned and designed online projects, examples of effective digital engagement are now manifold. In the UK, high profile national digital initiatives such as The Space are transforming the way in which audiences engage with the performing arts and thus once again challenging the very premise of the marketing mix. The Space (www.thespace.org) is a relatively new digital collaboration between Arts Council England and the BBC. It describes itself as "a commissioner of art that employs technology to push the boundaries of creative expression" (The Space 2015). The Space provides an online platform to showcase artists who "nurture and develop projects on the cutting edge of the digital arts". It aims to "develop new models of participation that allow everybody to contribute".

The past few years have witnessed a significant increase in digital audience engagement tools, not least in the form of apps. Artory (www.artory.co.uk) is a digital engagement app that was launched as a pilot in 2015 to offer a "what's on" service for culture. The app gathered audience feedback and facilitated the collective promotion of arts and cultural events. In exchange for providing feedback and engaging in promotional activity, users earned so-called Art Miles, which they could redeem to receive exclusive offers at arts and cultural venues across Plymouth (UK). Ultimately, Artory aimed to measure the quality of cultural experiences and thus help organisations to better understand their audiences (Artory 2015). Along similar lines, Culture Counts (http://culturecounts.cc) is a new intrinsic measurement platform that captures artist, peer, and public feedback on the quality and reach of arts and cultural events (Culture Counts 2015). The aim of Culture Counts is essentially to enable cultural organisations to co-produce value metrics with their audiences and other key stakeholders on their terms. The platform combines survey insights with box office data and Google analytics to produce reports in real time, so that organisations can access feedback as it is produced; compare their feedback over time and against benchmark organisations; and quickly export it into graphs to send to their funders. Reliant on effective digital engagement of audiences and other key stakeholders, Culture Counts now forms a formal part of the artistic assessment process in Western Australia and has recently been introduced, to significant controversy (as we saw in Chapter 4), in England.

SOCIAL PRODUCTION

In the twenty-first-century networked culture of participation, the interrelationship between digital engagement and co-production is one of increasing significance. In Chapter 6, I discussed Debord's (1992) claim that art needs to reposition itself from its traditional mode of representation towards one of dialogue and community, and the academic studies of digital audience engagement reviewed above exemplify how some arts organisations are starting to embrace the digital to develop communities of artistic exchange based around a more relational and aesthetic approach to marketing. This shift in approach reflects not just the participatory turn explored earlier in the chapter but also the move towards what Benkler (2006) refers to as "social production". Adam Arvidsson (2008) credits the digitally networked environment with establishing the framework for this social production and with related phenomena such as fan culture. This framework, he argues, is built on the diffusion of networked information and communications technologies, "which have both lowered the price of access to the means of cultural and informational production and radically facilitated the autonomous organization of productive processes" (p. 328). Arvidsson claims that this social mode of production heralds "an ethical economy where value is related to social impact" (2008, p. 326). Arvidsson's focus on the ethical nature of social production complements Bill Sharpe's (2010) broader argument that human society comprises multiple "economies of life" that should function in a complex equilibrium to establish a balanced and effective ecosystem. Sharp, however, focusses more explicitly on artistic production, claiming that art is "the currency of the economy of experience" (p. 32).

EMPATHY

A possible justification behind Sharpe's claim lies in the role that art can play in facilitating empathy between one human being and another. This point marks a development of the argument proposed in Chapter 4 that the arts can function as an effective vehicle for relationship building and socialisation. Based as they are on live interactions between audiences and performers, the performing arts have been shown to be particularly powerful facilitators of human empathy, as discussed earlier in this book. What is relevant in the context of digital engagement is the role that technology can play in enhancing this core extrinsic benefit.

Clay Shirky (2009) claims that "technological changes and the rise of social networking mean that the age-old problem of synchronizing the performer and audience in space and time now has new solutions that no longer depend on traditional presenting organisations, venues, programming or marketing". This is an important argument, which highlights the potential of communications technologies to elongate the performer–audience relationship and transpose it offline and away from the constraints of synchronicity. This notion underlines Popat's earlier point about the benefits of asynchronous communication. A related benefit of the online interaction between performers and audiences is the disintermediation that it implies: audiences are increasingly engaging directly with performing artists online without needing to pass through organisational channels and mediation.

LIVE STREAMING

The rising trend of live streaming or "simulcasting" stems back to New York's Metropolitan Opera's live streaming of a production of Mozart's *The Magic Flute* on December 30, 2006. The international success of the Met's venture soon inspired others to follow suit, and an increasing number of large-scale arts organisations in the USA and Europe are now simulcasting their live productions, making live streaming the sector's fastest growing technology development (Nesta 2013; Towse 2013). Despite the ongoing, and sometimes heated, debate about whether live streaming is cannibalising live audiences (the Met claims that it is, whilst Nesta's latest research finds that it isn't), what is clear is that the phenomenon is impacting significantly both on the marketing mix and on the global arts ecology.

This impact is manifesting itself in a number of ways. There is emerging evidence that live streaming is starting to hamper cultural production, as venue producers and programmers increasingly offer valuable weekend slots to safe, live-streamed productions by global mega-brands like NT Live. This is likely to have a particularly negative impact on small regional producing organisations, which find themselves increasingly relegated to the more challenging mid-week slots. Another impact is on audience behaviour: whilst one study of London opera audiences seemed to indicate that attending a live broadcast increased audiences' motivation to see future simulcasts but not to see more live performance (Wise 2014), a recent study conducted for Nesta by Bakhshi and Whitby (2014), based on a big data set of 54 performing arts venues across England broadcasting the National Theatre's NT Live productions between 2009 and

2013, concluded that live streaming can actually boost live attendance in neighbourhoods where simulcasts are easily accessible. However, there is an important caveat to this study in that it was based on a meta-analysis of post-code based ticket transactions (rather than individual audience members) and failed to incorporate any qualitative audience research to explore possible explanations for this apparent behavioural shift.

Finally, simulcasting is almost irrevocably altering the audience experience of the performing arts. Exploratory research by Nesta (2010) on the 2009 NT Live season confirmed the significance of the live element of performance even for remote audiences, and concluded that live streaming can succeed in attracting new audiences into theatres. More surprisingly, it also indicated that remote audiences can actually enjoy a more emotionally engaging experience and are more likely to achieve a flow experience and feel "transported to another world" than if they watched the same performance live. Possible explanations for these findings proposed by survey participants included the ability to see actors "up close" and from a spacious, comfy seat. This supports White and Hede's (2008) thesis about the importance of *enablers* of artistic impact. Nesta's study concluded that whilst digital innovation can represent "a source of new and valuable theatrical experiences [...] better knowledge about what works with audiences, and what does not, in digital innovation is crucial for the competitive success of the UK's creative industries" (2010, p. 7). Such is the purpose of the following case study analysis.

Case Studies

Case Study 1: National Theatre of Scotland's Five Minute Theatre

On Monday 23rd June 2014, working in collaboration with The Space, National Theatre of Scotland (NTS) presented *The Great Yes, No, Don't Know, Five Minute Theatre Show*. The show comprised 24 hours of live theatre from Scotland and beyond on the topical theme of independence. This theatrical event was the latest edition of the company's much celebrated *Five-Minute Theatre* project, whose strapline reads: "created by anyone for an audience of everyone" (see Fig. 8.1).

To take part in *Five Minute Theatre*, successful applicants must create a five-minute-long piece of theatre, which must be performed in front of a live audience. It can be pre-recorded and sent to NTS; filmed live by one

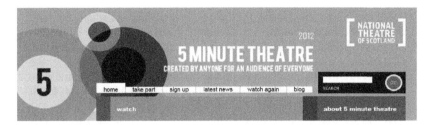

Fig. 8.1   Five Minute Theatre 2012 (Image courtesy of National Theatre of Scotland)

of NTS's roving crews; or filmed live at one of the company's performance hubs. There are very few restrictions on how participants can interpret "theatre" and anyone and everyone is actively encouraged to take part. The event's Producer, Marianne Maxwell, explained the rationale behind the project as follows:

> In our five year history, everything had changed, both in the potential ways we could communicate with audiences, artists and participants, but more importantly how they could communicate with us. We wanted to unite both these moments in time and the idea to open our doors and let whoever wanted to create theatre with us emerged. (Maxwell 2013)

Around 1000 people from all over the world participated in the first edition of *Five Minute Theatre* in 2011. The event gathered 6,300 unique viewers from 51 countries who visited the site 22,000 times. Since June 2011, the 207 individual shows, all performed in front of their own live audience, have been watched a further 28,000 times, creating a total *Five Minute Theatre* virtual audience of 50,000. However, in July 2012, the online audience for *Five Minute Theatre* was low compared with previous editions, rarely rising above 60. This led *The Scotsman*'s Theatre Critic, Joyce McMillan (2012) to comment that "NTS, having established this ground-breaking format, now needs to think hard about how to increase its impact and reach".

This temporary setback once again highlighted the challenges of maintaining online engagement with audiences over a sustained period of time and the disappointing figures led NTS to rethink its relationship with its audiences. Maxwell (2013) described the vital role that social media played in this process of re-engagement as follows:

Social media has been crucial in allowing us to talk about the audience and their connection with our work as anything other than passive. By embracing the power of our audiences' voices we have begun to refine the definition of audience members. This has led to hugely creative outcomes. [...] We are a theatre without walls ... *Five Minute Theatre* and the other audience engagement activity we plan absolutely reflect our core values. We are playful and provocative and we want to share that with as many people across the world as we can, building meaningful relationships in ways that suit our audience, in whatever way they choose to connect with us – physically or virtually.

Maxwell highlights here how successful digital engagement can help an arts organisation fulfil its mission and strategic objectives and develop more participatory and democratic relationships with its audiences on a global scale. This case study example provides a useful vindication of Lynne Conner's (2013) call for programming that "begins and ends with the audience's interests" (p. 99) and of her contention that when audiences are granted the authority to make meaning and feel that they are listened to, the potential to strengthen "a national dialogue around the arts" is significant. As Maxwell (2013) argues, the impact of this digital empowerment can be nothing short of game-changing.

As an idea it caught the imagination and was embraced. Technically we broke new ground and audience numbers and viewing figures were very high. However the most astonishing impact is how exciting it is to blur the lines between artists, audiences and participants, completely challenging what that means to a theatre company. The global impact of that seems to hold limitless potential: a connection with the National Theatre of Scotland is not restricted to a physical experience; now you can create, produce, watch, comment and chat with us no matter where you live. When you really think about that, it's revolutionary.

Case Study 2: Watershed (Bristol, UK)

In 1998, Watershed was a traditional arts centre in the south-west of England comprising two cinema screens, a photography gallery, an education department, and a café/bar. In 1999, Watershed entered into a collaborative agreement with the University of Bristol and invested heavily in high speed broadband. This strategic decision pushed the venue into spaces it wouldn't normally have entered and encouraged it to constantly innovate.

By getting rid of its old gallery content and co-producing new content with its audiences, Watershed realised that it was continually establishing new relationships and its staff became aware that they had to invest in these new relationships and get to know the people behind them. These developments quickly forced the management team to rethink radically what the venue now stood for and what art might mean for its new audiences, which in turn led to a wholesale rebrand that repositioned the venue as a co-creative space and recast its staff as cultural facilitators. As Managing Director Dick Penny puts it: "We understood that we were not just making and selling products, but offering an *experience*. As part of the capital project the public space in the building was flooded with free wireless, which transformed the spaces. Suddenly the social space became an active space where people did business, where people were not consuming, but getting active" (Penny 2009, p. 51). Through a creative use of technology, Watershed has handed over ownership of its building (at least physically and symbolically) to its audiences in what represents a genuine manifestation of social production (see Fig. 8.2).

This shift in production culture exemplifies the "bidirectional communication" and "networked engagement" promulgated by Crawford et al. as a precondition for audiences having a "voice" (p. 1081). Indeed, as Bill Sharpe notes, Watershed has become "a space that people and organisations naturally gravitate towards to stimulate creativity and to 'make something happen'". He goes on to claim that "Watershed operates in the economy of exchange" (Sharpe 2010, pp. 4–5). Sharpe's language is significant here, and it highlights the role that technology can play in opening up both arts spaces and their business models, and facilitating mutual exchange relationships between artists, producers, and audiences. Indeed the case of Watershed (like that of NTS) demonstrates how these traditionally separate functions are starting to blur and merge as digital communication technologies continue to break down traditional barriers to production, creation and engagement. As Sharpe puts it, Watershed has become a "perfect breeding ground" for producers; an "effective producer of producers" (pp. 79–80). What started out as a simple experiment to see what would happen if an arts centre flooded its spaces with high speed broadband has now become a *sine qua non*: Watershed's innovative use of technology has led it on a journey that has radically reshaped its mission and core purpose and enabled it to become one of the best networked arts venues in the UK, a champion of social engagement and production. However, as with NTS, the physical and rhetorical transference of ownership to audiences has not yet radically

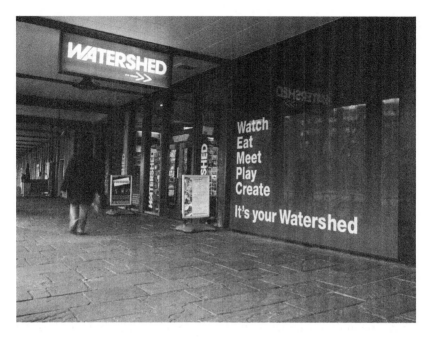

Fig. 8.2   Social production at Bristol's Watershed in 2010 (Image by Toby Farrow, courtesy of Watershed)

transformed the venue's business model into one where audiences could be fully described as partners.

Case Study 3: New York's Brooklyn Museum

Brooklyn Museum is one of the oldest and largest cultural organisations in the United States. Located in the New York borough of Brooklyn, its mission is "to act as a bridge between the rich artistic heritage of world cultures, as embodied in its collections and the unique experience of each visitor". The museum describes itself as "dedicated to the primacy of the visitor experience" and it draws on "both new and traditional tools of communication, interpretation, and presentation [...] to serve its diverse public as a dynamic, innovative, and welcoming center for learning through the visual arts" (Brooklyn Museum 2015).

From 1999 to 2016, the digital engagement strategy at Brooklyn Museum was overseen by its Vice Director of Digital Engagement and Technology, Shelley Bernstein. Shelley's role was to enhance the museum's visitor experience and community engagement through the innovative use of technology. This activity culminated in a series of digital initiatives including free public wifi, video competitions, user-generated content, projects designed specifically for mobile devices, and digitising the museum's vast collection of artwork. According to Bernstein (2013), one of the museum's most successful technology projects was its "comment kiosk". These iPad-based kiosks now sit in every exhibition (see Fig. 8.3), where they gather visitors' comments and email them automatically to the museum's curatorial and visitor services staff. Visitors' comments are moderated, but a selection (containing both positive and negative feedback) are posted on the kiosks in the gallery, on the website, and on the exhibition pages for other visitors to respond to. Bernstein argues that the kiosks offer the

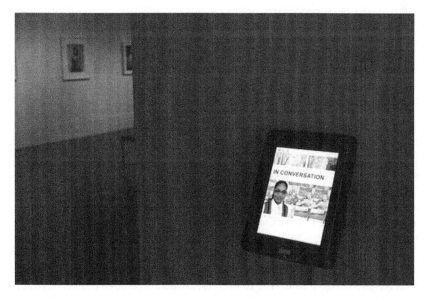

Fig. 8.3 An interactive comment kiosk at Brooklyn Museum (© 2004–2019 the Brooklyn Museum. Image courtesy of Brooklyn Museum, under Creative Commons License 3.0)

museum a novel way to learn from its visitors, as well as facilitating visitor to visitor communication.

Over time, the kiosks have become more interactive and the technology has enabled artists, curators, conservers, and educators to both pose and answer questions, which are then threaded into themes, ranked by popularity and posted on exhibition websites. This has facilitated a deeper, two-way engagement between visitors and the museum staff, and effected what staff estimate as a 40% rise in inspiring and insightful comments.

These three case studies illustrate how arts and cultural organisations are starting to harness digital technology to realise the fundamental goal of arts marketing: to develop and manage mutually satisfying value-based relationships with audiences. Through the innovative and appropriate use of digital communications technologies, National Theatre of Scotland, Watershed and Brooklyn Museum are engaging in open, creative dialogues with their audiences, which are enhancing the value of their audiences' cultural experiences and helping them to extract social and aesthetic meaning from them. Most performing arts organisations are still behind the technology curve; but these illustrative examples indicate how they in turn might draw on technology to maximise their cultural offering.

Case Study 4: Yorkshire Dance's Respond Project[1]

Introduction

The final case study of this chapter constitutes a critical evaluation of Respond (www.respondto.org)—a project funded by Nesta, the Arts and Humanities Research Council and Arts Council England through the Digital R&D Fund for the Arts. The core aim of this fund was to support ideas that use digital technology to develop new business models and enhance audience reach. The aim of Respond was to design and develop a digital adaptation of Liz Lerman's renowned Critical Response Process (CRP) that would enable participants to interact directly with artists and share their interpretations of artistic ideas and works-in-progress.

In March 2014 two dance artists, Hagit Yakira and Robbie Synge, were selected through a public vote to each create a new piece of dance. Between September and November 2014, the artists developed their respective

---

[1] I have published a full account of this project in *Poetics*. Please see Walmsley, B. 2016. From arts marketing to audience enrichment: How digital engagement can deepen and democratise artistic exchange with audiences. *Poetics*, 58, pp. 66–78.

pieces using the new Respond platform (see Fig. 8.4) to engage in a creative and extended dialogue with audiences, following the established four steps of Lerman's CRP: statements of meaning; artist's questions; neutral questions; and sharing opinions.

The core research purpose of the project was to investigate whether a new responsive online platform could successfully deepen and broaden audiences' engagement with contemporary dance and foster a culture of constructive critical enquiry between arts organisations, artists, and audiences. A related aim was to explore whether the platform could expand the audience reach of new dance works and benefit the creation and development process of new works of art. Particular research objectives included investigating whether the platform could enhance and demystify the creative process of contemporary dance and facilitate audiences' decoding processes, and evaluating to what extent it might increase empathy between

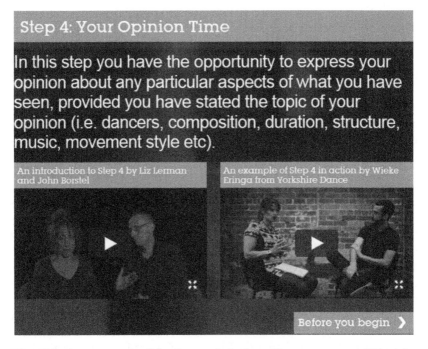

Fig. 8.4 A screen-grab of the Respond platform (Image courtesy of Breakfast Creatives)

artists and audiences. The project ultimately aspired to provide new insights into the benefits of artists engaging with a range of audiences via digital communications technologies throughout the creative process.

The research design followed a mixed-methods approach based on a combination of audience and participant surveys, discussion groups, depth interviews, content analysis of online discussion, and netnography. Primary research was undertaken with 32 participants sampled behaviourally across three distinct populations:

   I. Artists, producers, and frequent dance attenders;
   II. Infrequent dance attenders;
   III. Non-attenders (sampled from a range of ages, professions, and social groups).

Findings

The primary research produced a number of insightful findings that have significant implications for practices and processes of audience development and engagement. The research team observed that a high number of participants using the Respond platform during the first live week of the Critical Response Process (CRP1) were completing the four-step process in one sitting, as opposed to waiting for the artist's response and interacting with other participants. This was significant because the initial aim of the site was to foster a communal and interactive experience. The team thus became aware that participants were experiencing the platform independently and were sometimes acting in isolation, which made it question whether the online format and the language it was using on the platform were conducive to a communal online experience. The sense of an online community and the ability to view the experience of others seemed to be lacking from the site and so the experience was not reflective of how CRP usually functions amongst a group in dialogue, together in a physical space. Conversely, there was clear evidence that users were engaging deeply, emotively and reflexively with the dance clips and with the questions posed by the artists. Content analysis of online interactions also revealed that frequent attenders were focussing more on process, whereas infrequent and non-attenders appeared to be more focussed on emotions.

Both artists reported after CRP1 that they were impressed at the level and depth of user engagement. Compared with live CRP, Robbie Synge found the online process to be "more reflective, more expansive, a different mode of expression [...] the act of doing it is more generative". Robbie appreciated the fact that the platform gave him the opportunity to "re-read and reflect back on" his and other people's comments, but felt that it was missing what he called a "moment of dialogue". This point was reinforced by several survey participants, who called for "more interaction with others" and greater "collaboration and feedback". This finding led the project team to alter the functionality, look and feel of the platform before the next phase of the project (CRP2), in order to allow users to take part in live web chats and respond via subject threads to each other's online comments.

Despite the inevitable technical hitches at the start of the project, initial feedback from participants was predominantly positive, with 62% of respondents to the post-CRP1 survey reporting a positive experience of using this type of platform and 67% stating that they managed to convey their thoughts successfully. One of the infrequent attenders in the closed group fed back on her experience as follows:

> I had always loved dance but felt a lot of it was inaccessible to me because I didn't have 'the knowledge' and vocabulary to appreciate it fully. [...] Having not heard of Liz Lerman's work previously, I realized that it was possible to engage in dialogue with an artist/artistic work without opinionated, and often received, judgment playing a huge part in the process. [...] Creating, especially initial creation, is scary and I, therefore, also felt great respect and admiration for [the artists] – that they were actually prepared to offer up their creative works in progress and share/question that work in a dialogue with us.

There was consensus from the artists and participants that the platform encouraged a more "considered", "deep", "honest", "structured", "succinct", and "mindful" approach to critical response than a verbal, face-to-face exchange. Participants also fed back that the platform helped them to develop a "close relationship" with the artists and fellow participants, and to express their thoughts expansively and "in different ways". One infrequent attender confided that it made him feel "like an insider". However, a minority of participants missed the "layers of dialogue" that can emanate from a live discussion and felt that the physical absence of artists prevented non-verbal empathy and made the process feel a little "cold" and "impersonal". Others noted the inherent tension between the "snappy and superficial" habits encouraged by digital communications and the "thoughtful and analytical" process encouraged by CRP.

When asked if the process had affected their feelings about seeing the final performance, 86% of participants replied that it had had a positive impact. Positive responses here included participants feeling "intrigued", "involved", "important", "connected", and enjoying "a sense of ownership". This suggested that the platform had succeeded in generating a positive sense of anticipation, reminiscent of Brown and Novak's (2007) concept of "readiness-to-receive", which the study found to be a key predictor of captivation and ultimately of positive impact. Providing further insights into the role and power of anticipation, one non-attender responded as follows:

> I feel as if I'm now attached to the work and that I'm a part of the development, even if it's just as a viewer. I am looking forward to the performance more because I will be able to understand it in its entirety and read it with prior knowledge instead of just reading a quick blurb in a programme and attending like any other audience member. I feel somewhat privileged! It's quite lovely.

Another non-attender experienced an even greater transformation, communicating that the process had actually changed her outlook on contemporary dance: "I am looking forward to it more as my initial preconceptions of contemporary dance as an esoteric art form have been (mostly) dispelled". This evidence of the potential of the platform to serve as an effective audience development tool was also communicated by an infrequent attender, who fed back: "I feel more 'open' to dance now and more stimulated to read more about dance and [...] go and see more dance". These findings confirmed the conclusions of earlier studies regarding the particular needs and concerns of new audiences, as well as the positive role that context and paratextual insights can play in enhancing audience experience.

On the other hand, two participants (one non-attender, one infrequent attender) reported feeling "confused" following CRP1, and one frequent attender felt that the process had actually jeopardised his potential enjoyment of the ensuing performance: "I am looking forward to seeing the work; however I feel that I won't be able to enjoy it as much as I will be looking at it with informed analytical eyes". When asked whether the process had affected their ability to provide constructive feedback and whether it might encourage them to attend dance more frequently, almost all of the participants (89%) affirmed that the platform had challenged them to be more open, empathetic, questioning, and confident in providing feedback, in many different contexts. This again confirmed the findings of previous studies into the impact of effective digital engagement. But participants' predictions of the process's potential impact on their attendance patterns were mixed, with 55% reporting that it was unlikely to encourage them to attend dance performances more frequently. However, this figure was skewed negatively by the frequent attenders, with 62% of the infrequent non-attenders stating that it might indeed make them attend more often, offering yet further indication of the platform's potential capabilities to develop new audiences.

Three findings were particularly striking. Firstly, the contention from two of the participants that the digital engagement process had helped them to "do the hard work" before seeing the final performance indicates the ability of digital engagement during the creative process to remove a common barrier to artistic impact and enjoyment. One infrequent attender reported feeling that she had "done a lot of the thinking" during the two CRP weeks, so she imagined that seeing the performance would give her "a really rich experience" as opposed to "seeing it cold". She felt she would enjoy a "more embodied experience" and that it would be "less hard work". This confirmed Lynne Conner's argument that context can make cultural interpretation "cognitively easier" and enable deeper interpretations (2013, p. 113). It also reflected Matthew Reason's (2010) assertion that audiency is an embodied kinaesthetic experience, and provided tangible evidence of John Dewey's "rhythm of surrender and reflection" theory, which holds that reflection cannot occur during an absorbing experience (2005, p. 144). As Kahneman (2011) might put it, the platform facilitated the separation, whilst encouraging the complementarity, of two distinct modes of thinking: System 1 (fast, emotional and instinctive); and System 2 (slow, logical and deliberate).

Secondly, one participant commented that the experience had been transformative on a personal level. When asked how the process might affect the way she gave feedback in future, this participant replied:

> It's almost like a rebirth ... it has been incredibly profound [...]. I actually felt, during the process, what I had to say was taken seriously and perhaps valued and whatever thoughts I had were actually being recorded. And so, in a way, it forced me to think more about what I did think. But I think the whole CRP thing does that anyway; [...] you've got this kneejerk reaction,

which we all have nowadays. It makes you stand back and […] think, be
mindful about your first reactions.

This infrequent attender valued the "analytical and reflective" nature of
Respond and perceived it as an antidote to what she labelled "pundit culture". She felt that CRP's rejection of the "fix-it" (attempts to provide
any quick artistic "solutions") helped to avoid this trend towards punditry
by encouraging a more mindful, democratic and constructive approach to
delivering a critical response.[2] As such, this participant's views entwined
with the renowned film critic Mark Kermode (2013), who makes a strong
case for "slow reviewing". They were also akin to both Andrew Keen and
Lynne Conner's respective attacks on the rising cult of the amateur and
guerrilla-style online engagement.

Finally, the research findings indicated that digital platforms of this
nature might work more effectively with non- and infrequent attenders as
opposed to frequent attenders. This challenges the findings of some existing studies into co-creation (e.g. Walmsley 2013) that co-creative projects
generally attract a niche, highly engaged audience segment. It seems that
the key difference here is technology: non- and infrequent attenders communicated that they felt less intimidated to engage online, where they could
reflect in peace and enjoy some degree of anonymity. This supports existing
research findings regarding the benefits of digital anonymity, e.g. Conner's
assertion that the "face-to-facelessness" of digital platforms can generate
"a new kind of liquid courage when it comes to stating an opinion" (2013,
p. 80). Frequent attenders, on the other hand, felt that they learnt less and
found the film clips a little reductive.

When asked what changes participants would make to the platform,
the most common call was for more interaction with other participants.
Respondents also called for greater clarity and simplicity and for automated
email reminders, both to prompt them to engage with the platform more
frequently and to notify them when the artist had responded to their comments. Underlining the insights regarding empathy, it transpired to be very
important to almost all of the participants that artists did engage with their
responses. Mobile compatibility was another common request for future
versions of the platform. An interesting dilemma for the development team
emerged as several participants requested a mechanism that would allow

[2] On the online platform, participants received an automatic pop-up warning if the start of
their sentence seemed to be leading to a potential "fix-it".

them to revisit and amend their feedback. The danger here is that this might encourage groupthink and inhibit more immediate, spontaneous, original and visceral commentary. But participants seemed to want to be more in control of their online presence and be able to change and develop their comments as their views and ideas progressed along the process. They particularly praised the online journal for enabling them to do this in private.

Implications and Conclusions

The findings of this project have potentially significant implications for audiences, artists, arts organisations and policymakers. Respond has generated fresh insights into the benefits of sustained digital engagement between artists and audiences, including: encouraging greater reflexivity; encouraging a more generative creative process; empowering less frequent attenders to engage in artistic dialogue; facilitating a more kinaesthetic and absorbing engagement with live performance; and changing non-attenders' perceptions of unfamiliar artforms. The platform has therefore demonstrated its potential to serve as an effective audience development tool (for both new and existing audiences) and move audience relations well beyond the standard transactional processes into a more artistic and relational realm much more in tune with twenty-first-century marketing. This is precisely the kind of engagement that exemplifies Miranda Boorsma's (2006) conception of co-creation, whereby audiences give "meaning to the artefact by means of their imaginative powers" (p. 85). It also reflects the Situationist tenet that "art must move away from representation towards community and dialogue" (Debord 1992; Overend 2010, p. 2) and Bourriaud's definition of "relational art" as "intersubjective encounters [...] in which meaning is elaborated *collectively*" (cited in Bishop 2004, p. 54, original italics).

Furthermore, this kind of two-way interaction is indicative of an effective Integrated Marketing Communications (IMC) model, whereby "senders" and "receivers" are connected via a communications feedback loop which can facilitate the decoding process and increase customer loyalty and brand equity (Pickton and Broderick 2005). This research thus has profound implications for arts marketers and managers and has the potential to revolutionise the way in which arts organisations engage with their artists and audiences, bringing a whole new meaning and possible approach to Customer Relationship Management.

The biggest challenge during the lifecycle of the project was maintaining momentum amongst participants, especially amongst new audiences. The findings suggested that any future development of any such tool would need to focus on making the platform as sticky and interactive as possible: online users are accustomed to what one participant termed "a dopamine hit", and the platform could address this by providing automatic notifications when an artist or fellow participant has read and/or responded to a post. Another challenge is to maximise participants' dwell time on the platform and to encourage them to engage with the platform more reflectively. Challenges for organisations include the apparent need to provide professional development for artists to enhance their digital presence; to record their creative development in an interesting and high quality way; and to pose enticing and productive questions. Another obvious organisational challenge is the need to resource the facilitation of the online process during periods of intensive engagement. This confirms the findings of O'Sullivan's (2010) study discussed at the beginning of the chapter.

Ultimately, this type of digital engagement platform could provide the performing arts sector with a highly structured, tried-and-tested model for maximising audience development and engagement via digital communications technologies, which could potentially revolutionise arts organisations' digital engagement strategies and speed up the adoption of the more open, porous, dialogic, informally networked and digitised business models advocated by recent research in the arts (e.g. Bolton et al. 2011; Hewison and Holden 2011; Knell 2007). This kind of tool can demonstrably facilitate Steven Tepper's (2008) concept of engagement, whereby audiences actively connect to art; discover new meanings; and offer their own critique. It seems to encourage slow, structured critique and encourages participants to separate Kahneman's two distinct systems of thinking. There are therefore indications that it could even herald a new age of digital engagement that might provide an antidote to the punditry and kneejerk ephemerality that many popular social media platforms feed on by encouraging both artists and audiences to review artistic work more deliberately and dwell together more often online.

CONCLUSION

This chapter has investigated recent theories and practices of digital audience engagement and placed them within the wider context of an emerging culture of participation and within a wider ecology of an economy of experience and meaning. Digital platforms are undeniably changing the ways in which artists and arts organisations engage with their audiences. But as ever, whilst the early adopters are capitalising on the benefits of digital engagement, there is a long tail of laggards and luddites who are steadily falling behind the curve and not responding to the modern needs of their audiences. A good example of this is the Edinburgh Festivals, which were warned recently that unless they became leaders in the digital sphere and embraced the potential for digital platforms to improve social engagement and access, they risked being overtaken by their peers (BOP Consulting and Festivals and Events International 2015).

The case studies outlined in this chapter have illustrated and evidenced the potential of digital communications technologies to create responsive, reflective and artist-led but audience-centred platforms. Moreover, they have validated Rheingold's prediction back in 1993 that the Internet had the potential to "revitalize the public sphere and construct new forms of community". For whether digital platforms are facilitating cultural co-production at NTS; developing cultural networks at Watershed; adding meaning to audiences' visits to Brooklyn Museum; or encouraging slow reflexivity at Yorkshire Dance, what is clear is that they are empowering audiences all over the world and giving them an artistic voice.

At the same time, the case studies have highlighted the inherent challenges involved in maintaining digital audience engagement over a sustained period of time, confirming the findings of existing studies. There is a consensus in the academic literature that aspects of social risk and online insecurity can cause audiences to feel inferior and alienated, but also that effective design, social interaction and hosting skills can help to overcome these barriers to engagement. There is clearly a long way to go before the performing arts can claim to be delighting their audiences digitally or even responding to their basic online needs. But there is movement in the right direction, and a small number of trailblazers, some of whom have been showcased in this chapter, are starting to revolutionise their engagement with their audiences through the digital and reap rich dividends from these new value-based exchange relationships. It is to be hoped that the long tail will quickly follow suit so that a critical mass of audiences will soon have access to the kind of meaningful, reflexive digital engagement that the performing arts can assuredly excel at.

References

Artory. 2015. *Artory* [Internet]. Artory. Available from: http://www.artory.co.uk [Accessed 18 May].

Arvidsson, A. 2008. The ethical economy of customer coproduction. *Journal of Macromarketing*, 28(4), pp. 326–338.

Bakhshi, H. and Whitby, A. 2014. *Estimating the impact of live simulcast on theatre attendance: An application to London's National Theatre*. London, Nesta.

Benkler, Y. 2006. *The wealth of networks*. Princeton, NJ, Princeton University Press.

Bernstein, S. 2013. Moving toward a conversation. Available from: http://www. brooklynmuseum.org/community/blogosphere/2013/06/11/moving-toward-a-conversation [Accessed 5 August].

Bishop, C. 2004. Antagonism and relational aesthetics. *October*, 110, pp. 51–79.

Bishop, C. 2006. *Participation*. London, Whitechapel.

Bolton, M., Cooper, C., Antrobus, C., Ludlow, J. and Tebbutt, H. 2011. *Capital matters: How to build financial resilience in the UK's arts and cultural sector*. London, Mission Models Money.

Boorsma, M. 2006. A strategic logic for arts marketing: Integrating customer value and artistic objectives. *The International Journal of Cultural Policy*, 12(1), pp. 73–92.

BOP Consulting and Festivals and Events International. 2015. *Edinburgh Festivals: Thundering Hooves 2.0. A ten year strategy to sustain the success of Edinburgh's festivals*.

Brooklyn Museum. 2015. *About: Mission statement* [Internet]. New York, Brooklyn Museum. Available from: http://www.brooklynmuseum.org/about/mission. php [Accessed 18 May].

Brown, A. S. and Novak, J. L. 2007. *Assessing the intrinsic impacts of a live performance*. San Francisco, WolfBrown.

Conner, L. 2013. *Audience engagement and the role of arts talk in the digital era*. New York, Palgrave Macmillan.

Cova, B. 1999. From marketing to societing: When the link is more important than the thing. In: Brownlie, D., Saren, M., Wensley, R. and Whittington, R. (eds.) *Rethinking marketing: Towards critical marketing accountings*. London, Sage, pp. 64–83.

Crawford, G., Gosling, V., Bagnall, G. and Light, B. 2014. Is there an app for that? A case study of the potentials and limitations of the participatory turn and networked publics for classical music audience engagement. *Information, Communication & Society*, 17(9), pp. 1072–1085.

Culture Counts. 2015. *About* [Internet]. Available from: http://culturecounts. cc/about [Accessed 19 May].

Debord, G. 1992. *Society of the spectacle*. London, Rebel Press.

Dewey, J. 2005. *Art as experience*. New York, Perigee Books.

Hewison, R. and Holden, J. 2011. *The cultural leadership handbook: How to run a creative organization*. Farnham, Gower.

Ito, M. 2007. Introduction. In: Varnelis, K. (ed.) *Networked publics*. London, MIT Press, pp. 1–14.

Kahneman, D. 2011. *Thinking, fast and slow*. London; New York, Penguin.

Keen, A. 2007. *The cult of the amateur: How today's internet is killing our culture and assaulting our economy*. London, Nicholas Brealey.

Kermode, M. 2013. *Hatchet job: Love movies, hate critics*. London, Picador.

Knell, J. 2007. *The art of living: A provocation paper*. London, Mission Models Money.

Kozinets, R. 1999. E-tribalized marketing? The strategic implications of virtual communities of consumption. *European Management Journal*, 17(3), pp. 252–264.

Maxwell, M. 2013. *Five-Minute Theatre*. E-mail interview with Ben Walmsley. 25 March, Glasgow.

McMillan, J. 2012. Theatre reviews. *The Herald*, 19 July [Accessed 19 July].

Nesta. 2010. *Beyond live: Digital innovation in the performing arts*. London, Nesta.

Nesta. 2013. *Digital culture: How arts and cultural organisations in England use technology*. London, Nesta.

O'Sullivan, T. 2010. Dangling conversations: Web-forum use by a symphony orchestra's audience members. *Journal of Marketing Management*, 26(7–8), pp. 656–670.

Overend, D. 2010. *Underneath The Arches: Developing a relational theatre practice in response to a specific cultural site*. PhD, University of Glasgow.

Penny, D. 2009. Imagine an arts sector which works collaboratively to deliver excellence and engage the public. In: *Proceedings of the Arts Marketing Association Conference 21–23 July*. London, Arts Marketing Association, pp. 48–53.

Pickton, D. and Broderick, A. 2005. *Integrated marketing communications*. 2nd ed. Harlow, Pearson.

Popat, S. 2006. *Invisible connections: Dance, choreography and internet communities*. Oxon, Routledge.

Reason, M. 2010. Asking the audience: Audience research and the experience of theatre. *About Performance*, 10, pp. 15–34.

Rheingold, H. 1993. *The virtual community: Homesteading on the electronic frontier*. Reading, MA, Addison Wesley.

Rudman, H. 2006. New horizons. *Arts Professional*, 11 September, p. 20.

Sharpe, B. 2010. *Economies of life: Patterns of health and wealth*. Axminster, Triarchy Press.

Shirkey, C. 2009. *Here comes everybody: The power of organizing without organizations*. London; New York, Penguin.

Tepper, S. J. 2008. The next great transformation: Leveraging policy and research to advance cultural vitality. In: Tepper, S. J. and Ivy, B. (eds.) *Engaging art: The next great transformation of America's cultural life*. Oxon, Routledge, pp. 363–383.

The Space. 2015. *About* [Internet]. London, Available from: http://www.thespace.org/about [Accessed 18 May].

Towse, R. 2013. Performing arts. In: Towse, R. and Handke, C. (eds.) *Handbook on the digital creative economy*. London, Edward Elgar, pp. 311–321.

Walmsley, B. 2013. Co-creating theatre: Authentic engagement or inter-legitimation? *Cultural Trends*, 22(2), pp. 108–118.

White, T. R. and Hede, A.-M. 2008. Using narrative inquiry to explore the impact of art on individuals. *Journal of Arts Management, Law and Society*, 38(1), pp. 19–35.

Wise, K. 2014. *English touring opera: Opera in cinemas*. London, Creativeworks.

CHAPTER 9

Conclusions and Implications

Introduction

This book began with a plea for audiences—a plea to leave behind the fear, ridicule, homogenisation, vilification and victimisation which have traditionally characterised society's relationship with audiences, and to engage them as valid and informed subjects of their own research, as co-researchers, even. The book embarked from the thesis that at the heart of audience research lies a mutual exchange of value, wherein audiences can and should become strategic partners in the mission fulfilment of performing arts organisations—that is to say, in their own internal processes of enrichment and transformation. In the preceding chapters, we have seen how and why audiences are more than capable of playing this role. We have seen that they are increasingly demanding to play this role. But we have also seen that for many audiences, the doors to engagement and enrichment remain closed.

The past decade has witnessed a flurry of audience research, most of which appears to confirm the often hailed shift towards empiricism. By engaging directly and deeply with audiences, this shift is finally offering audiences a genuine voice in telling their own stories. As I stated at the beginning of the book, questions of audience engagement pose a number of fundamental questions regarding what an audience actually *is* and *does*. In advocating for an interdisciplinary approach to audience research that places questions of engagement at its heart, this book has responded to

© The Author(s) 2019
B. Walmsley, *Audience Engagement in the Performing Arts*,
New Directions in Cultural Policy Research,
https://doi.org/10.1007/978-3-030-26653-0_9

Willmar Sauter's (2000) call at the turn of the millennium to develop radically different research strategies. This is the only way to get beneath the surface of the audience project, to de-marginalise audiences and capture the rich complexity of their experiences of the performing arts.

This concluding chapter is structured into four sections. The first section draws out the key findings and conclusions from the preceding chapters and explores their implications for the evolving field of audience studies, and, most significantly, for the future of audience research in the performing arts. The second section hones in on the phenomenon of engagement and outlines how this core concept might be fruitfully reconceptualised to move the field and the performing arts sector forwards. Section three takes a more macro view and considers the implications of the findings for external stakeholders, including arts and cultural organisations, artists and arts professionals, and policymakers. It makes the case for audience-centric organisations fuelled by mutually beneficial relationships of artistic exchange. The final section draws out some overall conclusions and speculates about the likely direction of future research in the field.

THE EVOLUTION OF AUDIENCE STUDIES: TOWARDS A NEW PARADIGM

One of the most ambitious aims of this book was to reconfigure the paradigm of audience studies in the context of the performing arts. The core rationale for this was that audiences have traditionally been overly absent from audience research and treated with an odd admixture of disdain and paternalism, which of course represents a significant methodological and epistemological failure on behalf of the field. Through an extended critical exploration of different aspects of audience engagement, covering the audience experience, cultural value, research methods and methodologies, arts marketing, co-creation, and digital engagement, I have built the argument that audience studies should adopt an engagement-based paradigm. Engagement has been placed centre stage in my analysis of audience research because it encapsulates the embodied, relational and hermeneutic aspects of audiency required of twenty-first-century art. Researching audiences, audiencing, and audiency without a deep understanding of how audiences engage and *are* engaged with the performing arts will always be somewhat vacuous. However, the comprehensive review of existing audience research presented in Chapter 2 highlighted the welcome fact that audience scholars have now moved beyond the hypothetical "model" spectator towards a rich, multimodal exploration of the total audience experience. The assumptions that have been made for centuries about the "ideal" and homogenised audience have been supplanted by revelations about real audience members who deploy highly individualised and deeply personal strategies to engage with their chosen art forms.

I argued in Chapter 2 that audience studies is predominantly interested in the *how and why* of engagement and that it should leave questions of *who and who not* to sociology and cultural policy studies. In the course of the literature review which comprised that chapter I outlined an emerging taxonomy of extant audience research, which I deconstructed into the following core themes: the pacification of audiences; power, elitism and class; cultural policy, participation and co-creation; immersive performance; performance venues, spaces and places; performance as ritual; reception theory and semiotics; research methodologies; the audience experience; value and impact research; young audiences; arts marketing and management; and audience engagement and enrichment. The aim of this classification was not to reduce or restrict what is thankfully now a burgeoning field, but rather to anchor it, in another attempt to shore up its evolving paradigm. My proposed taxonomy can only be subjective, indicative and emergent; but it represents a critical summary of the core themes and traditions of research into performing arts audiences over the preceding decades and hopefully establishes a solid platform for future research in the field.

Audience studies ostensibly has much to learn from phenomenology, psychology, aesthetics, and anthropology, where mature theorisation on questions of distance, flow, arousal, empathy, and catharsis indicates that audiences' emotions are ultimately what transform ordinary everyday experiences into extraordinary aesthetic experiences. This suggests that audience scholars should follow Paul Silvia's (2005) advice and apply appraisal theories on emotional engagement, which would offer the field new ideas and research directions. They should also heed Miranda Boorsma's (2006) call to follow up insights from philosophical aesthetics, which perceive the arts as culturally and socially embedded. As the field of audience studies continues to evolve, supported by the serendipitous rise of interdisciplinary research, we are likely to see further convergence between scholars from traditionally disparate fields. Considering the complex social and managerial structures that contextualise the performing arts and the multifarious impacts that they have on individuals and communities, this can only be a positive development for audience research. But interdisciplinarity requires its own structures to support it, and so it is incumbent on audience scholars, and on their institutions and funders, to break free from twentieth-century silos and invest time and money in collaborative research; and if academic research is to impact on performing arts organisations and audiences, then the arts and higher education sectors will need to develop more embedded long-term collaborations that reflect the research requirements of both parties.

As we saw in Chapter 3, organic performance takes place within an aesthetic, symbolic and live context. Empirical research has revealed that this context can engender experiences for audiences that can be characterised as framed, intense, hedonic, autotelic, stylised, and playful. Audiences' experiences are complex and multisensory and they can therefore often appear noumenal and ineffable, but it is possible and indeed insightful to deconstruct audiences' experiences into their constituent parts in order to understand them more deeply without demystifying them completely. Audiences' experiences of the performing arts combine cognitive, sensual, aesthetic, kinaesthetic, emotional, social, intellectual, imaginative, enactive and spiritual responses to performance. Most researchers concur that many of these response modes are contingent on a live, relational experience of the performing arts, which offers intimate proximity to artists and privileged access to stagecraft. These are thus the inherent and differentiating qualities that demarcate the performing arts and make them so appealing to audiences. In order to facilitate an engagement-based culture, they are qualities that should therefore be borne in mind by artists, producers, and marketers when creating, programming, and promoting performances.

Questions of cultural value are never very far away from discussions about the impact of the arts on audiences; so these questions must also be imperative for audience studies. Scholars of cultural value and of audiences share a desire to capture the impact of the arts and culture, and both communities are continually exercised by seemingly intractable questions of methodology. The discussion in Chapter 4 revealed that investigations into cultural value and audience engagement also share a *political* element, because both fields are characterised by the vested interests of gatekeepers. As Whalley and Miller note, "to be an audience continues to be a political act, one freighted with significant social and ideological implications" (2017, p. 33). So there are many synergies between these two small loci of research, not least their combined impact on cultural policy and on society more broadly. What is needed, therefore, is a more coordinated research approach that might enable more rapid mechanisms for knowledge exchange, particularly in the area of evaluation methodologies, where both fields are separately advocating for nuanced, longitudinal, multidimensional and reflexive approaches to impact assessment that combine complementary methods in a tailored and systematic way. The conclusions offered in Chapter 4 suggest that a fruitful way forwards might be to focus on how the value and impact of the arts might be reliably *expressed* by audiences, rather than to engage in the more abstract debate about what this value actually *is*. This conclusion again supports the contention that empirical audience research offers a valuable impact in and of itself rather than a means to a constantly elusive end.

In Chapter 5, I explored the range of methods that are deployed by researchers to explicate audiences' engagement with the performing arts. This highlighted the issue that, like cultural value scholars, audience researchers often struggle to find a third way between the particular and the universal. This apparent tension between individual versus collective experience and impact is omnipresent in audience studies, and it still appears to compromise a good number of studies that choose not to take a mixed-methods approach. An ongoing challenge for the discipline is therefore to continue to develop a paradigm that captures the personal and the microscopic, whilst retaining the "generous" and critical eye necessary to interpret these personal findings in a comparative and transferrable way. A more scientific approach to narration and storytelling might support this endeavour and enable researchers to achieve the dual policy objective of communicating immeasurable value whilst demonstrating measurable impact.

In this first section of the concluding chapter we are principally concerned with the evolving paradigm of audience studies, and in Chapter 6, I called for a reconceptualisation of the tired old arts marketing paradigm towards an engagement-based model that would reflect the co-constructed, experiential and intimate value-based relationships that arts organisations are increasingly developing with their audiences. The performing arts offer audiences exceptional and extraordinary experiences that distance the sector from the product-centred paradigm offered by marketing, and there is increasing evidence that arts organisations and scholars are responding to the new audience context and prioritising engagement over marketing (Walmsley 2019). This conceptual shift has significant implications for audience studies as it strives to evolve as a field that is both interdisciplinary and audience-centred. Rather than engagement supplementing marketing, I have argued that marketing needs to augment engagement.

Engagement cannot be an afterthought; it must be embedded in professional arts practice and therefore embedded in the underlying paradigm of audience research and audience studies.

One particular aspect of audience engagement that is rapidly becoming a major sociocultural force is co-creation. In Chapter 7, we saw how co-creation functions as an ambiguous umbrella term that encompasses aspects of collaboration, interaction, invention, value, meaning, and exchange. In order to maximise the potential benefits of co-creation, we have seen how arts organisations need to develop the participatory skills of their audiences by encouraging them to play and empowering them to make meaning. Theories and practices of co-creation thus support the engagement model because they share a common focus on relational aesthetic experiences and intersubjective encounters. Like co-creation, effective engagement can develop audience members' aesthetic tastes and interpretive skills, and enhance their propensity for artistic risk. If we heed the advice of Caroline Heim (2016) and Josephine Machon (2013) and consider audience members as co-conspirators or creative comrades, then audience studies has much to learn from co-creation, which at its most effective acts as a powerful democratic force in arts and cultural organisations. In Chapter 8 we saw how digital communications technologies can also act as a democratising force, whilst simultaneously elongating and deepening audience engagement. Digital engagement can also enhance impact by providing a pre-performance context and offering diverse opportunities for post-performance sharing and interpretation, which in turn can generate a genuine culture of learning.

At the start of the book I cited Martin Barker's call for audience studies to develop an elaborate research paradigm that would combine a theoretical framework, working concepts, methods of enquiry, and paradigmatic studies (2006, p. 129). At this final stage of writing, it is now time to reflect on the extent to which this book has responded to this call. As I clarified in the introduction, it was never going to be feasible, nor indeed desirable, to develop *one* theoretical framework, nor even one, one-size-fits-all model of engagement. What has become clear is that audience studies is far too broad, even in the context of the performing arts, to ever be encapsulated within any one framework, and nor should any profoundly interdisciplinary field. However, as the core process of audiency, which itself subsumes other subsidiary processes, engagement does offer a plural and open framework that might inform a more suitable and sustainable paradigm for the field. This book does, therefore, represent a paradigmatic study of audience research. It also offers a critical exploration of working concepts and research methods that will hopefully inform the future development of the field and influence future research.

RECONCEPTUALISING ENGAGEMENT

As we saw in Chapter 1, audiences' attention is a dwindling resource and this makes the need for effective engagement all the more urgent. In the course of the opening chapter, I offered a summary overview of existing definitions of engagement, which I synthesised to conclude that engagement is essentially a psychological process which aims to develop intimate, meaningful, converged, and enduring relationships with audiences by involving them in interactive, immersive and hermeneutic experiences. Chapters 2 and 3 highlighted also the embodied and enactive aspects of engagement, so we should now modify our initial definition to qualify engagement also as a series of psychological and psychobiological processes that emancipate and empower audiences and generate deep connections by enabling audiences to become an invaluable part of the art-making process. So the ultimate goal of an engagement-based strategy in our new economy of meaning emerges as a form of *enrichment*; and based on the theorisation of engagement, captivation, immersion, and value undertaken in the previous chapters, we can discern a relatively simple model of enrichment as depicted in Fig. 9.1.

As illustrated in The Audience Enrichment Model, enrichment is dependent on the effective engagement of audiences and on their ensuing flow and immersion in art and artistic processes, including meaning-making processes, which generate growth and ultimately co-create personal, interpersonal and community-level value and impact. This is essentially why engagement is so significant. Engagement, flow/immersion, and learning/development are co-dependent processes which exist in a symbiotic relationship because effective engagement captivates and immerses audiences in art, which in turn facilitates aesthetic growth and personal development, which fuels future engagement. Stephen Bitgood's (2010) research with museum audiences helpfully deconstructed engagement into a number of intellectual, perceptual, and affective processes, including learning, inquiry, flow, and immersion. These processes are all reflected in the model but presented in a more circular way that frames engagement as a process to enrichment rather than an end goal in itself. Aesthetic growth and personal development are key aspects of engagement and various scholars have

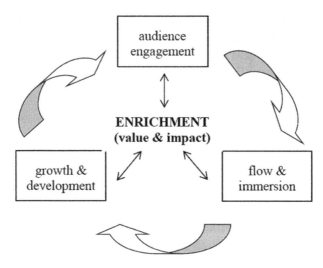

Fig. 9.1   The Audience Enrichment Model

highlighted the need for the sector to invest in the education and aesthetic growth of its audiences to help audiences "acclimatise" to artistic work (Machon 2013, p. 84).

As we saw in Chapter 6, audiences are increasingly seeking out more relational ways to engage with artists, and performing arts organisations are starting to offer innovative ways to facilitate this. The live element of the performing arts offers exceptional opportunities for audience engagement because, *pace* Philip Auslander, live performance *does* possess its own ontological integrity. As Auslander himself acknowledges, the ontology of live performance is based on the temporal and physical co-presence of performers and audience members (2008, p. 60). Auslander is partly right to assert that this co-presence rarely translates into a tangible benefit to audience members (because they are physically too far away from the performers, for example); but what he fails to acknowledge is that the ontology of live performance is based on the real and *potential* engagement of audiences and performers, as well as on the engagement of audiences with other audience members and, of course, with art itself. This triadic potential for engagement is another quality that demarcates live performance and sets it apart from mediated and mediatised arts and entertainment. The problem, as I have highlighted throughout this book, is that opportunities for audiences to engage with performers, each other, and art are almost always curtailed or completely missed. The implications of this for producers, performing arts organisations, funders and policymakers are clear: more time and money must be spent on conceiving, developing and delivering engagement opportunities; and alongside artistic quality, funding decisions should be dependent on the range and quality of engagement activities offered to audiences. Otherwise, Auslander will be proven right and live performance will continue to lose sway over easier and more accessible forms of leisure and entertainment.

This book has revealed how and why audiences should be treated as the active agents of their own aesthetic enrichment and highlighted how audiences' performance encounters are messy and individualised. There can never be, therefore, a one-size-fits-all approach to audience engagement. Engagement strategies and philosophies must embrace the diversity of audiences' unique experiences and therefore offer different touchpoints for engagement. I hope I have developed a convincing argument over the course of this book that engagement is above all a philosophy and a culture—one that must be underpinned by an audience-centric ethos which recognises audiences as equal partners in processes of artistic exchange.

A PLEA FOR AUDIENCE-CENTRIC ORGANISATIONS

The systematic disempowerment of audiences over the past two centuries is a familiar trope in audience research, and the cynical dislocation of audiencing and interpretation represents a political and aesthetic problem that has partly fuelled the rise of scholarship into co-creation, audience engagement and enrichment. In the course of this book, I have advocated the acceptance and adoption of an audience-centred model for the performing arts. By this I mean that audiences must finally be acknowledged, by both scholars and practitioners, as the primary stakeholders of performing arts organisations and placed at the heart of everything these organisations do. This is (sadly) a radical thesis, which rejects the traditional product- (and power-)led model that produced and still governs the field of arts marketing. However, it offers a compromise by moving beyond the fudge of an audience-focussed model whilst stopping short of the audience-led approach favoured by iconoclasts and by certain elements of the participatory arts sector. The reason for this audience-*centric* position is certainly not to stick to the middle ground, but rather to acknowledge that whilst audiences need to continue to be empowered and emancipated, they also need and desire to be challenged and delighted by artists and art, and from my own perspectives as an audience member, theatre producer and audience researcher, this can best be achieved via a vision that is artistically led.

Audience-centricity, then, implies placing audiences at the heart of artistically led and artistically vibrant organisations, and engaging them actively in all aspects of organisational activity. In other words, artists and arts organisations need to build and foster an open culture of engagement by developing "artistic exchange relationships" with audiences and treating them as creative partners. They need to consider their organisations, and their artistic spaces in particular, as social forums where audiences can interpret collectively, and collaboratively generate intrinsic cultural value. They need to facilitate these processes of meaning-making by developing their audiences' interpretive and imaginative powers (Boorsma 2006) and their ability to co-create both artistic experiences and value. Only then will audiences ever have the opportunity and requisite empowerment to become the "creative comrades" imagined by Machon (2013, p. 73).

Caroline Heim's case study of Chicago's Steppenwolf theatre depicts what this creative comradeship might look like in practice and illustrates how audience-centric organisations can reinvent traditionally closed artistic spaces as open civic spaces:

> Audience research indicated that Steppenwolf's audiences were predominantly lifelong learners who wanted plays 'to stimulate both introspection and debate'. The theatre now programmes post-show discussions for every performance they stage, inviting audiences to join them in a 'public square', which Artistic Director Martha Lavey describes as 'a civic cultural space activated by the work on stage where we can negotiate meaning in an interpretive community'. (Heim 2016, p. 104)

This example highlights the core functions that learning and engagement can play in developing communities of practice amongst audience groups and indicates how artists and performing arts organisations can themselves benefit by engaging their core audiences *collectively* to develop them as an artistic congregation. It thus supports the findings of Chapter 2, where we saw how the desirable goal of *communitas*, a shared liminal state which delivers communal experience and meaning, is facilitated when audiences share a common goal and attend performances with a shared vocabulary and history.

Regardless of the strong theoretical and philosophical case for an audience-centric model, there is also a strong business or strategic case to be made for embracing audiences as partners, not least that it can maximise their "lifetime value" (Payne and Frow 2005) and significantly increase organisations' earned income (Simon 2010). There is a moral and policy case to be made in that audiences invest and *are invested in* the arts and arts organisations, and so they have an inherent stake in and ownership of them. There is a social and economic case to be made for audience-centricity in that countless studies across the globe have now demonstrated the potentially positive impact that the arts can have on audiences' health and general wellbeing. There is an educational and sociological case to be made because the arts facilitate cognitive growth and fulfil the mimetic role of holding up a critical mirror to society. And, perhaps most importantly, there is a strong *artistic* case to be made for audience-centricity: many commentators agree that relinquishing control of a cultural project to participants can actually increase its relevance and impact (e.g. Arvidsson 2008; Department for Culture Media and Sport 2007).

This so-called "participation agenda" is of course opposed by detractors such as Brian McMaster (2008), who contend that a political focus on instrumental benefits can erode artistic excellence, and by others, such as Miranda Boorsma (2006), who claim that it endangers creative risk-taking and compromises artistic freedom. However, this protracted debate, which is at the heart of many of the policy tensions within national funding agencies, is far from Manichaean, as activities such as co-creation continue to blur and challenge the very terms of reference: "As artists collaborate, sample, remix and repurpose, they obscure the line between creator and observer and toy with fundamental presumptions of originality and authenticity that traditionally define artistic excellence" (Brown et al. 2011, p. 7). The focus on quality in this debate remains contested and is demonstrably beyond resolution. It might therefore make sense to alter the terms of the debate and shift the focus from the quality of the art to the quality of audience engagement. This is of course the underlying premise of relational aesthetics, and there are growing signs that the need to prioritise the quality of audience engagement might actually represent the next frontier. Practitioners like Nina Simon are trailblazing this approach and advocating for a reinvigorated focus on how engagement activities are actually *designed*, rather than whether they take place at all. So concepts and skills such as design thinking, facilitation, mediation and scaffolding are going to be of increasing importance to the sector, and they will need to be nurtured by arts leaders and policymakers alike.

The reason why these skills need to be prioritised is essentially that they facilitate meaning-making and confer value onto art and artistic experiences. To return to Stanely Fish's key term, they help to establish and solidify *interpretive communities,* these elusive forums where value is co-created by audiences who subject art to scrutiny, analysis and evaluation (Prahalad and Ramaswamy 2004). As a champion of audience enrichment, Lynne Conner (2013) is another strong advocate for facilitation and mediation skills; she urges arts workers to develop these skills in order to support the much needed renaissance of "social interpretation" in the arts, which, she maintains, can only be achieved by developing an "authorised audience" and by re-enfranchising "audience sovereignty" (p. 40).

The endeavour to develop an authorised audience implies a strong element of education, and another recurrent theme in this book has been the need for arts workers to promote arts education and guide their audiences so that they understand the "rules" of performance (Burland and Pitts 2012) and develop the appropriate skills to decode, interpret, deconstruct and make meaning of it (O'Toole et al. 2014). There is abundant evidence from extant empirical studies of performing arts audiences that the more *au fait* audiences become with the modes and codes of performance, the more critical they become and the more they start to feel part of a connected community of interest. This is all part and parcel of good hosting: designing engagement activities that will help audiences to feel included and at home. It is not education in a patronising, didactic or normative sense; it is about developing and enabling, about opening up possibilities for multiple and divergent interpretations rather than leading audiences to any predetermined decoding of intended meaning.

FINAL CONCLUSIONS

To describe the concept of "the audience" as a "vexed term" (Machon 2013, p. 98) is clearly an understatement. As a term, we have seen that "audience" is deceptive, reductive, elusive, problematic, and indicative of the cynical disempowerment and objectification of audiences that has been sustained for centuries. However, it seems that the battle to place audiences at the heart of research into their own experiences of the performing arts has almost been won. Nevertheless, audience research remains difficult. It is compromised by myriad methodological challenges and undermined by

rapidly evolving and often disingenuous policy and management imperatives that rarely value its legitimacy or integrity. I have argued in this book
that audience studies can only ever thrive as a field in its own right if it moves
beyond its disparate cross-disciplinarity to become fiercely *inter*disciplinary.
Fortunately, the rise of a culture of interdisciplinarity within the academy
is gradually encouraging audience scholars to collaborate in ever more creative and innovative ways and to learn how to compromise and even triangulate their respective positions, traditions and methods. This interdisciplinarity is already leading to some pioneering research—particularly, as
we have seen, in the areas of neuroscience and psychobiology, which are
starting to offer fresh insights (and, dare I say, *proof*) into how audiences
engage with the performing arts and the impacts that these art forms have
on them. This evidence of impact is vital from both a management and a
policy perspective, and it is, of course, of growing relevance to academics
too.

However, despite these advances, we urgently need *more* interdisciplinary research into audiences and into different *types* of audience. If the
ultimate goal of engagement is to enrich the lives of audiences and, in so
doing, enrich the work of artists and arts organisations, then we need an
even deeper understanding of how the various processes of engagement
co-function and of which amongst them might be the strongest predictor
variables of impact. If we are to shift our focus from assessing the quality of artistic products to evaluating the quality of audiences' experiences
and engagement—which would tangentially offer artists and policymakers
a possible solution to the quality assessment of community and participatory work—then we need to fund research into refined evaluation frameworks. As the rhetoric of cultural policy continues to shift towards questions
of cultural democracy and relevance, audience engagement offers a fresh
paradigm for audience studies that positions it ideally to exert a positive
influence in the policy and management sphere. From a policy perspective,
the impacts of engagement and co-creation need to be properly evaluated
in order to better understand the impact that they have on audiences, on
artists and organisations, on the wider sector, and on society at large. This
is one of the challenges inherent to the Cultural Value debate and any positive resolution to this challenge is likely to depend on finding and applying
appropriate anthropological methods. We need to move on methodolog-
ically from "casual stories" to meaningful, potent, and universal stories
that will gain more traction than the contested and meaningless econometric data that they will supplant. We need to evidence more rigorously

our repeated claims that the performing arts, audiencing, and audience engagement are transformative. There remains much work to do.

Audience engagement still has a lot to learn from aesthetics, both in its theoretical underpinnings and in its empirical endeavours. We have seen in this book how insights from biometric analysis, for example, are changing the way we understand audiences' intersubjective experiences and creating an evidence bank of the sociological benefits of artistic engagement. If artistic experiences can increase audiences' empathy and sync their brain waves and heart beats with fellow audience members, then the arts could find a renewed role in applied contexts of conflict resolution. Empathy has emerged in this book as a prerequisite condition of audiencing, essentially because it develops interpersonal engagement and supports emotional contagion, which in turn can restore collective energy and help to develop a sense of community amongst a regular audience. This is no small thing in light of the global rise in populism. In our postmodern world, people have relatively few opportunities to physically engage with one other and feel part of a community, and arts venues clearly have the potential, and some would argue the responsibility, to act as community spaces that bring diverse groups together in acts of enhanced socialisation (Heim 2016). With the demise of the community arts and arts centre movements, many arts venues have lost sight of this social aspect of their missions and sold their souls to the devil of marketing. Whilst marketing undoubtedly still has a vital role to play in supporting financial resilience, it is fundamentally different from engagement, and often continues to squeeze engagement out of the picture altogether. This constitutes an artistic, social and strategic error, because the misconstrued shift towards a culture of artistic consumption has undermined loyalty and artistic exchange, and wilfully ignored perhaps the ultimate virtue of aesthetic engagement—namely that it "implies no desire to possess or use the object" (Lord Shaftesbury cited in Ben Chaim 1984, p. 1). We have lost sight of the profound ability of the arts to offer an antidote to consumerism and materialism and to the wider neoliberal agenda. We have therefore neglected the inherently political role of the audience and of audience studies.

Machon argues that immersive artworks can function as "interstices" and "otherworldly-worlds" (2013, pp. 122 and 153). I would argue that *all* art has a public responsibility to offer an interstice, a small opening or aperture that can offer audiences a chink of light into an artist's practice or worldview. In reflecting on the term "interstice" I am reminded of the burgeoning literature on third and liminal spaces—in-between or "found" spaces that are politically neutral and therefore offer up ideal places to play and co-create. There is a wicked irony in the fact that just as we are really starting to appreciate the manifold creative benefits of these places and spaces, they are becoming scarcer and more remote as our cities proliferate and gentrify, pushing real estate prices up so high that artists and arts organisations are squeezed ever further outside them. There are significant implications here for policymakers, and specifically for local governments: creative spaces need to be preserved for the public and protected from the acquisitive development encouraged by the free market economy. Arts organisations, too, must look to their laurels and (co-)create neutral creative spaces where their local artists and communities can come together. As partners, their audiences can assist in this political endeavour.

Performing arts audiences are brimming with untapped potential: as the very people who make performance manifest, they are the only people who can make sense of and confer meaning on art. So as well as segmenting their databases into suitable target markets, performing arts organisations should be developing interpretive communities and forums which could become their lifeblood by co-creating artistic and organisational value and meaning. They should be converging audiences with performers. As Conner argues, audience engagement is concerned with offering audiences opportunities to prepare, process, and analyse so that they can interpret art in a social setting (2013, p. 67). We have seen that this concept is neither radical nor new and yet it has not yet become mainstream practice. To exclude audiences from active involvement in the creation or interpretation of a work of art is to deny them the opportunity to derive optimal meaning from their artistic engagement. Yet many performing arts organisations continue to treat their audiences as customers in defiance of their own artistic missions. As Ruth Rentschler (2007) notes, this constitutes a significant failure of governance and leadership. Many organisations still miss simple opportunities to deepen and elongate the engagement that they currently enjoy with audiences, which has led certain commentators to the depressing conclusion that in the contemporary performance culture, audiences' consumer power has become far more significant than their verbal power (Heim 2016, p. 130). This is strategic suicide in a sector, and indeed in a society, that is swiftly moving away from transactional modes of engagement. It represents nothing less than a significant policy, management, and artistic failure.

Considering that this book has devoted so much space to emerging theories, methods and practices, it seems fitting to conclude it with a little bit of futuregazing. What lies in store for audience studies and research? My analysis of the latest blogs, conferences and publications in the field suggests a steady growth in creative and psychobiological research methods alongside a greater focus on arts and health/wellbeing and marginalised audience groups. As governments and funders invest heavily in technology, video gaming, and digital art, we are likely to witness an exponential rise in digital engagement and in audience enquiries related to artificial intelligence, virtual reality and augmented reality. At the same time, as the attention economy makes its mark, commercial producers and streamers of creative content such as Netflix and Amazon are starting to realise that audience research in the live performing arts can offer rich and lucrative insights into cultural production and consumption. So we will probably see some convergence across the creative industries as researchers collaborate across disciplines to explore how work lands with audiences, how different narrative arcs and production elements affect them, and how creative content impacts on them, both concurrently and over their lifetimes. Artificial intelligence will probably play an increasing role in these investigations, for example by calculating "ideal" peaks and flows of plot lines in relation to audiences' attention spans.

As policy agendas shift away from the democratisation of culture and towards cultural democracy, we will certainly see renewed focus around questions of place-making, participation, and co-creation and an according rise in methods like Social Return on Investment. As arts organisations come under increasing pressure to welcome more diverse and representative audiences, I hope that we will also see a rise in design thinking and hospitality, with organisations acknowledging the enabling role of place and space, creating discursive social spaces, and ultimately becoming better hosts. These are significant sociocultural trends, and only a radically interdisciplinary approach to audience studies, based on the relational insights offered by the engagement paradigm, will be able to respond to them effectively to secure the privileged role of the performing arts well into the latter half of the century.

REFERENCES

Arvidsson, A. 2008. The ethical economy of customer coproduction. *Journal of Macromarketing*, 28(4), pp. 326–338.

Auslander, P. 2008. *Liveness: Performance in a mediatized culture*. 2nd ed. Oxon, Routledge.

Barker, M. 2006. I have seen the future and it is not here yet …; or, on being ambitious for audience research. *The Communication Review*, 9(2), pp. 123–141.

Ben Chaim, D. 1984. *Distance in the theatre: The aesthetics of audience response.* London; Ann Arbor, UMI Research Press.

Bitgood, S. 2010. An attention-value model of museum visitors. Available from: https://airandspace.si.edu/rfp/exhibitions/files/j1-exhibition-guidelines/3/An%20Attention-Value%20Model%20of%20Museum%20Visitors.pdf [Accessed 5 April 2019].

Boorsma, M. 2006. A strategic logic for arts marketing: Integrating customer value and artistic objectives. *The International Journal of Cultural Policy*, 12(1), pp. 73–92.

Brown, A. S., Novak-Leonard, J. L. and Gilbride, S. 2011. *Getting in on the act: How arts groups are creating opportunities for active participation.* San Francisco, CA, The James Irvine Foundation.

Burland, K. and Pitts, S. 2012. Rules and expectations of jazz gigs. *Social Semiotics*, 22(5), pp. 523–543.

Conner, L. 2013. *Audience engagement and the role of arts talk in the digital era.* New York, Palgrave Macmillan.

Department for Culture Media and Sport. 2007. *Culture on demand: Ways to engage a broader audience.* London, Department for Culture Media and Sport.

Heim, C. 2016. *Audience as performer: The changing role of theatre audiences in the Twenty-First Century.* London and New York, Routledge.

Machon, J. 2013. *Immersive theatres: Intimacy and immediacy in contemporary performance.* London, Palgrave Macmillan.

McMaster, B. 2008. *Supporting excellence in the arts: From measurement to judgement.* London, Department for Culture Media and Sport.

O'Toole, J., Adams, R.-J., Anderson, M., Burton, B. and Ewing, R. (eds.). 2014. *Young audiences, theatre and the cultural conversation.* Dordrecht, Springer.

Payne, A. F. and Frow, P. 2005. A strategic framework for customer relationship management. *Journal of Marketing*, 69, pp. 167–176.

Prahalad, C. K. and Ramaswamy, V. 2004. Co-creation experiences: The next practice in value creation. *Journal of Interactive Marketing*, 18(3), pp. 5–14.

Rentschler, R. 2007. Museum marketing: Understanding different types of audiences. In: Sandell, R. and Janes, R. R. (eds.) *Museum management and marketing.* London; New York, Routledge, pp. 345–365.

Sauter, W. 2000. *The theatrical event: Dynamics of performance and perception.* Iowa city, University of Iowa Press.

Silvia, P. J. 2005. Emotional responses to art: From collation and arousal to cognition and emotion. *Review of General Psychology*, 9(4), pp. 342–357.

Simon, N. 2010. *The participatory museum.* Santa Cruz, Museum 2.0.

Walmsley, B. 2019. The death of arts marketing: A paradigm shift from consumption to enrichment. *Arts and the Market*, 9(1), pp. 32–49.

Whalley, J. and Miller, L. 2017. *Between us: Audiences, affect and the in-between.* London, Palgrave.

INDEX